RAJ'S PRACTICAL MANAGEMENT OF PAIN

RAJ'S PRACTICAL MANAGEMENT OF PAIN

FOURTH EDITION

Honorio T. Benzon, M.D.

Professor of Anesthesiology
Senior Associate Chair for Academic Affairs
Northwestern University Feinberg School
  of Medicine
Chief, Division of Pain Medicine
Northwestern Memorial Hospital
Chicago, Illinois

James P. Rathmell, M.D.

Associate Professor of Anesthesia
Harvard Medical School
Director, Massachusetts General Hospital
  Pain Center
Department of Anesthesia and Critical Care
Massachusetts General Hospital
Boston, Massachusetts

Christopher L. Wu, M.D.

Associate Professor of Anesthesiology and
  Critical Care Medicine
Johns Hopkins University School of Medicine
Baltimore, Maryland

Dennis C. Turk, Ph.D.

John and Emma Bonica Professor of Anesthesiology
  and Pain Research
Department of Anesthesiology
University of Washington School of Medicine
Seattle, Washington

Charles E. Argoff, M.D.

Professor of Neurology
Albany Medical College
Director, Comprehensive Pain Program
Albany Medical Center
Albany, New York

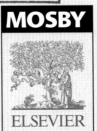

MOSBY

ELSEVIER

1600 John F. Kennedy Blvd.
Ste 1800
Philadelphia, PA 19103-2899

RAJ'S PRACTICAL MANAGEMENT OF PAIN   ISBN: 978-0-323-04184-3

Notice

Knowledge and best practice in this field are constantly changing. As new research and experience broaden our knowledge, changes in practice, treatment, and drug therapy may become necessary or appropriate. Readers are advised to check the most current information provided (i) on procedures featured or (ii) by the manufacturer of each product to be administered, to verify the recommended dose or formula, the method and duration of administration, and contraindications. It is the responsibility of the practitioner, relying on his or her experience and knowledge of the patient, to make diagnoses, to determine dosages and the best treatment for each individual patient, and to take all appropriate safety precautions. To the fullest extent of the law, neither the Publisher nor the Authors assume any liability for any injury and/or damage to persons or property arising out of or related to any use of the material contained in this book.

The Publisher

Library of Congress Cataloging-in-Publication Data

Raj's practical management of pain / editors, Honorio T. Benzon . . . [et al.].—4th ed.
    p. ; cm.
  Rev. ed. of: Practical management of pain. 2002.
  Includes bibliographical references and index.
  ISBN 978-0-323-04184-3
  1. Pain—Treatment.   2. Intractable pain—Treatment.   3. Analgesia.   I. Benzon, Honorio T.   II. Practical management of pain.   III. Title: Practical management of pain.
  [DNLM: 1. Pain—therapy.   2. Chronic Disease—therapy. WL 704 R161 2008]
RB127.P73 2008
616'.0472—dc22

2007044355

Executive Publisher: Natasha Andjelkovic
Developmental Editor: Janice Gaillard
Publishing Services Manager: Frank Polizzano
Project Manager: Rachel Miller
Design Direction: Steve Stave
Illustrations Manager: Ceil Nuyianes

Printed in China

Last digit is the print number: 9 8 7 6 5 4 3 2 1

To my family—Julieta, Hubert, Hazel, Paul, and Annalisa.

To my Chairs at Northwestern—Edward A. Brunner, M.D., Ph.D., Barry A. Shapiro, M.D., and M. Christine Stock, M.D.

To Prithvi Raj, M.D., for trusting us to continue his scholarly work.

Honorio T. Benzon, M.D.

To Nori Benzon, who had the patience and persistence to lead this project to completion.

To Dave Brown, Howard Schapiro, Rick Rosenquist, and Rick Rauck: trustworthy guides and much-needed friends.

To my wife and children—Bobbi, Lauren, James, and Cara—who have remained ever supportive through the minor interruptions of another book and the major interruptions of a move to Boston.

James P. Rathmell, M.D.

To Frederick W. Cheney, M.D., Professor Emeritus and former Chair of the Department of Anesthesiology at the University of Washington, for his efforts in attracting me to Seattle and for his support throughout my tenure;

and

to Lorraine M. Turk, more than a wife, a partner and my best friend, for her consistent and unyielding patience and understanding throughout our marriage.

Dennis C. Turk, Ph.D.

To my wife and best friend, Patty. Your continued love, support, and unending patience are immeasurable and are so cherished by me.

To our wonderful children, David, Melanie, and Emily. Watching your growth continues to astound me.

To Robert Y. Moore, M.D., Ph.D., Roscoe Brady, M.D., and John Halperin, M.D., for your guidance and your encouragement for me to fully develop my interest in pain medicine.

Charles E. Argoff, M.D.

Contributors

Bernard M. Abrams, M.D.
Clinical Professor of Neurology, University of Missouri—Kansas City School of Medicine, Kansas City, Missouri; Honorary Vice President (Neurology), Menorah Medical Center, Overland Park, Kansas; Dannemiller Memorial Education Foundation, San Antonio, Texas
Electromyography and Evoked Potentials

A. V. Apkarian, Ph.D.
Professor, Northwestern University Feinberg School of Medicine, Chicago, Illinois
Pain and Brain Changes

Charles E. Argoff, M.D.
Professor of Neurology, Albany Medical College; Director, Comprehensive Pain Program, Albany Medical Center, Albany, New York
History and Physical Examination of the Pain Patient; Skeletal Muscle Relaxants

Kjell Axelsson, M.D., Ph.D.
Professor, Department of Anesthesiology and Intensive Care, University Hospital, Örebro, Sweden
Intra-articular Analgesia

Mani Batra, M.D.
Staff Anesthesiologist, Virginia Mason Medical Center, Seattle, Washington
Nerve Blocks of the Head and Neck

Benoy Benny, M.D.
Assistant Professor, Physical Medicine and Rehabilitation, Baylor College of Medicine, Houston, Texas
Physical Medicine Techniques in Pain Management

Honorio T. Benzon, M.D.
Professor of Anesthesiology, Senior Associate Chair for Academic Affairs, Northwestern University Feinberg School of Medicine; Chief, Division of Pain Medicine, Northwestern Memorial Hospital, Chicago, Illinois
Low Back Pain; Pharmacology for the Interventional Pain Physician; Local Anesthetics for Regional Anesthesia and Pain Management; Neurolytic Blocking Agents: Use and Complications; Hip, Sacroiliac Joint, and Piriformis Injections; Outcomes, Efficacy, and Complications of the Treatment of Back Pain

Klaus Bielefeldt, M.D., Ph.D.
Associate Professor, University of Pittsburgh School of Medicine; Clinician and Director, Neurogastroenterology, Presbyterian University Hospital, Pittsburgh, Pennsylvania
Visceral Pain

David M. Biondi, D.O.
Director, Clinical Development—Neurology, Ortho-McNeil Janssen Scientific Affairs, Titusville, New Jersey
Headache Disorders

Hemmo Bosscher, M.D.
Clinical Assistant Professor, Department of Anesthesiology, Texas Tech University Health Sciences Center, Lubbock, Texas
Lumbosacral Epiduroscopy

Randall P. Brewer, M.D.
Clinical Assistant Professor of Neurology, Louisiana State University, Shreveport, Louisiana; Assistant Consulting Professor of Anesthesiology, Duke University, Durham, North Carolina; Director, Pain Institute, Willis Knighton Health System, Shreveport, Louisiana
Pain in Selected Neurologic Disorders

David L. Brown, M.D.
Edward Rotan Distinguished Professor, Department of Anesthesiology and Pain Medicine; Chairman, Department of Anesthesiology and Pain Medicine, University of Texas M.D. Anderson Cancer Center, Houston, Texas
Education, Training, and Certification in Pain Medicine

Chad M. Brummett, M.D.
Lecturer, University of Michigan Department of Anesthesiology, University of Michigan, Ann Arbor, Michigan
Facet Joint Pain

Allen W. Burton, M.D.
Professor of Anesthesiology and Pain Medicine; Chief of Pain Service, Clinical Medical Director Pain Center, University of Texas M.D. Anderson Cancer Center, Houston, Texas
Spinal Cord and Peripheral Nerve Stimulation

Asokumar Buvanendran, M.D.
Director of Orthopedic Anesthesia and Associate
Professor of Anesthesiology, Rush Medical College,
Chicago, Illinois
*Nonsteroidal Anti-inflammatory Drugs, Acetaminophen, and
COX-2 Inhibitors*

Alex Cahana, M.D.
Médecin Adjoint, Responsible, Postoperative and
Interventional Pain Unit, Department of
Anesthesiology, Pharmacology, and Intensive Care,
Geneva University Hospital, Geneva, Switzerland
*Organizing an Inpatient Acute Pain Management
Service*

Kenneth D. Candido, M.D.
Professor of Anesthesiology; Chief, Division of Pain
Management, Loyola University Medical School,
Maywood, Illinois
Nerve Blocks of the Head and Neck

David Casarett, M.D.
Associate Professor; Staff Physician, University of
Pennsylvania, Philadelphia VA Medical Center,
Philadelphia, Pennsylvania
Pain Management at the End of Life

Kwai-Tung Chan, M.D.
Assistant Professor, Physical Medicine and
Rehabilitation, Baylor College of Medicine, Houston,
Texas
Physical Medicine Techniques in Pain Management

Susan L. Charette, M.D.
Assistant Clinical Professor, Division of Geriatrics,
Department of Medicine, David Geffen School of
Medicine at UCLA, Los Angeles, California
Assessment of Pain in Older Patients

Steven P. Cohen, M.D.
Associate Professor, Johns Hopkins Medical Institutions,
Baltimore, Maryland; Colonel, Walter Reed Army
Medical Center, Anesthesiology Division, Washington,
D.C.
Neuraxial Agents; Facet Joint Pain; Lumbar Discography

Megan H. Cortazzo, M.D.
Assistant Professor, Department of Physical Medicine
and Rehabilitation, University of Pittsburgh School of
Medicine; Spine and Pain Center, Institute for
Rehabilitation and Research, Pittsburgh,
Pennsylvania
Major Opioids and Chronic Opioid Therapy

Edward C. Covington, M.D.
Assistant Professor of Psychiatry, Ohio University
College of Osteopathic Medicine, Athens, Ohio; Head,
Section of Pain Medicine, Neurological Institute,
Cleveland Clinic Foundation, Cleveland, Ohio
*Pain and Addictive Disorders: Challenge and
Opportunity*

Nessa Coyle, N.P., Ph.D.
Nurse Practitioner, Pain and Palliative Care Service,
Memorial Sloan-Kettering Cancer Center, New York,
New York
*Pain Management in the Home: Using Cancer Patients as a
Model*

Timothy R. Deer, M.D.
Clinical Professor, Department of Anesthesiology, West
Virginia University School of Medicine, Morgantown;
President and CEO, The Center for Pain Relief,
Charleston, West Virginia
*Intrathecal Drug Delivery: Overview of the Proper Use of
Infusion Agents*

Oscar de Leon-Casasola, M.D.
Professor of Anesthesiology and Oncology; University at
Buffalo School of Medicine; Chief, Pain Medicine,
Roswell Park Cancer Institute, Buffalo, New York
*Cancer Pain; Neurolysis of the Sympathetic Axis for Cancer
Pain Management*

Bonnie Deschner, M.D.
Assistant Professor of Anesthesiology, Virginia
Commonwealth University, Richmond, Virginia
Lower Extremity Peripheral Nerve Blocks

Robert H. Dworkin, Ph.D.
Professor of Anesthesiology, Neurology, Oncology, and
Psychiatry; Director, Anesthesiology Clinical Research
Center, University of Rochester School of Medicine and
Dentistry, Rochester, New York
Chronic Pain Clinical Trials: IMMPACT Recommendations

Michael Erdek, M.D.
Assistant Professor of Anesthesiology, Critical Care
Medicine, and Oncology, Johns Hopkins University
School of Medicine, Baltimore, Maryland
Pain in the Critically Ill Patient

Bruce A. Ferrell, M.D.
Professor, Division of Geriatrics, Department of
Medicine, David Geffen School of Medicine at UCLA,
Los Angeles, California
Assessment of Pain in Older Patients

Perry G. Fine, M.D.
Professor, University of Utah School of Medicine, Pain
Management Center, Department of Anesthesiology,
Salt Lake City, Utah
Pain Management at the End of Life

Scott M. Fishman, M.D.
Chief, Division of Pain Medicine; Professor of
Anesthesiology, Department of Anesthesiology and Pain
Medicine, University of California, Davis, Sacramento,
California
*Major Opioids and Chronic Opioid Therapy; Radiation
Safety and Use of Radiographic Contrast Agents in Pain
Medicine*

Kenneth A. Follett, M.D., Ph.D.
Professor and Chief, Section of Neurosurgery, University
of Nebraska Medical Center, Omaha, Nebraska
Neurosurgical Management of Pain

G. F. Gebhart, Ph.D.
Director, Center for Pain Research, Department of
Anesthesiology and Neurology, University of Pittsburgh
School of Medicine, Pittsburgh, Pennsylvania
Visceral Pain

Shiv K. Goel, M.B.
Clinical Assistant Professor of Anesthesiology,
University of Pittsburgh School of Medicine, Shadyside
Hospital, Pittsburgh, Pennsylvania
Postoperative Pain and Other Acute Pain Syndromes

Martin Grabois, M.D.
Professor and Chairman, Department of Physical Medicine and Rehabilitation, Baylor College of Medicine, Houston, Texas
Physical Medicine Techniques in Pain Management

Brock Gretter, M.D.
Associate Staff, Cleveland Clinic Foundation, Cleveland, Ohio
Intradiskal Procedures for the Management of Low Back Pain

Anil Gupta, M.B.B.S., Ph.D.
Senior Lecturer, University of Linköping, Linköping, Sweden; Associate Professor and Senior Consultant, Department of Anesthesiology and Intensive Care, University Hospital, Örebro, Sweden
Intra-articular Analgesia

Admir Hadzic, M.D., Ph.D.
Professor of Clinical Anesthesiology, Columbia University, College of Physicians and Surgeons; Attending Anesthesiologist, St. Luke's–Roosevelt Hospital Center, New York, New York
Lower Extremity Peripheral Nerve Blocks

Naeem Haider, M.D., M.B.B.S.
Assistant Professor of Anesthesiology, University of Michigan Medical School, Ann Arbor, Michigan
Phantom Limb Pain

Alicia Heapy, Ph.D.
Associate Research Scientist, Department of Psychiatry, Yale University School of Medicine, New Haven; Research Psychologist, VA Connecticut Healthcare System, West Haven, Connecticut
Psychological and Behavioral Assessment

James E. Heavner, D.V.M., Ph.D.
Professor, Anesthesiology and Physiology; Director, Pain and Anesthesia Research, Texas Tech University Health Sciences Center, Lubbock, Texas
Lumbosacral Epiduroscopy

Matthew D. Hepler, M.D.
Assistant Professor, Northwestern University Feinberg School of Medicine, Chicago, Illinois
Surgical Treatment of Lumbar Spinal Disorders

Marc A. Huntoon, M.D.
Associate Professor of Anesthesiology, Mayo Clinic College of Medicine, Mayo Clinic, Rochester, Minnesota
Interlaminar and Transforaminal Epidural Steroid Injections

Robert W. Hurley, M.D., Ph.D.
Assistant Professor in Anesthesiology, Johns Hopkins Medical Institutions, Baltimore, Maryland
Neuropathic Pain Syndromes; Neuraxial Agents

Kenneth C. Jackson II, Pharm.D.
Associate Professor, School of Pharmacy, Pacific University, Hillsboro, Oregon
Skeletal Muscle Relaxauts

Benjamin Johnson, M.D., M.B.A.
Associate Professor of Anesthesiology, Vanderbilt University School of Medicine; Pain Consultant, Howell Allen Clinic, Nashville, Tennessee
The History of Pain Medicine

Robert D. Kerns, Ph.D.
Professor, Departments of Psychology, Neurology, and Psychiatry, Yale University School of Medicine; Chief, Psychology Service, National Program Director, VA Connecticut Healthcare System, West Haven, Connecticut
Psychological and Behavioral Assessment

Timothy L. Lacy, M.D.
Staff Anesthesiologist and Pain Management Specialist, Holyoke Medical Center, Holyoke, Massachusetts
Anticonvulsants

Irfan Lalani, M.D.
Assistant Professor, Department of Anesthesiology and Pain Medicine, University of Texas M.D. Anderson Cancer Center, Houston, Texas
History and Physical Examination of the Pain Patient

Thomas M. Larkin, M.D.
Assistant Professor, Uniformed Services University of Health Sciences, F. Edward Hébert School of Medicine, Bethesda, Maryland; Attending Anesthesiologist, Walter Reed Army Medical Center, Washington, D.C.
Lumbar Discography

Elaina E. Lin, M.D.
Resident in Anesthesiology, Johns Hopkins Hospital, Baltimore, Maryland
Neuropathic Pain Syndromes; Outcomes, Efficacy, and Complications of Neuropathic Pain

Yuan-Chi Lin, M.D., M.P.H.
Associated Professor of Anaesthesia and Pediatrics, Harvard Medical School, Department of Anesthesiology, Perioperative and Pain Medicine, Children's Hospital Boston, Boston, Massachusetts
Acupuncture

Spencer S. Liu, M.D.
Clinical Professor of Anesthesiology, Weill Cornell Medical College; Director of Acute Pain Service, Hospital for Special Surgery, Department of Anesthesiology, New York, New York
Neuraxial Anesthesia; Outcomes, Efficacy, and Complications from Acute Postoperative Pain Management

Raymond Maciewicz, M.D., Ph.D.
Director, PBS Medical Consulting, Boston, Massachusetts
Dental and Facial Pain

David N. Maine, M.D.
Fellow in Pain Management, Johns Hopkins Hospital, Baltimore, Maryland
Outcomes, Efficacy, and Complications of Neuropathic Pain

Khalid Malik, M.B.B.S.
Assistant Professor of Anesthesiology, Northwestern University Feinberg School of Medicine; Northwestern Memorial Hospital, Chicago, Illinois
Low Back Pain; Local Anesthetics for Regional Anesthesia and Pain Management

Timothy P. Maus, M.D.
Assistant Professor of Radiology, Mayo Clinic College of Medicine, Rochester, Minnesota
Radiologic Assessment of the Patient with Spine Pain

Brenda C. McClain, M.D.
Associate Professor of Anesthesiology and (Adj)
Pediatrics, Yale University School of Medicine; Director
of Pediatric Pain Management Services, Yale–New
Haven Children's Hospital, New Haven, Connecticut
Chronic Pain Management in Children

Gary McCleane, M.D.
Consultant in Pain Management, Rampark Pain Centre,
Dollingstown, Northern Ireland, United Kingdom
Antidepressants as Analgesics

Brian McGeeney, M.D., M.P.H.
Assistant Professor of Neurology, Boston University
School of Medicine, Boston, Massachusetts
Anticonvulsants

Nashir R. Mehta, D.M.D., M.D.S.
Director, Craniofacial Pain Center; Professor and
Chairman, Department of General Dentistry; Assistant
Dean of International Relations, Tufts University School
of Dental Medicine, Boston, Massachusetts
Dental and Facial Pain

Nagy Mekhail, M.D., Ph.D.
Professor of Anesthesiology, Cleveland Clinic Lerner
College of Medicine of Case Western University;
Chairman, Department of Pain Management, Cleveland
Clinic, Cleveland, Ohio
*Intradiskal Procedures for the Management of Low Back
Pain; Minimally Invasive Procedures for Vertebral
Compression Fractures*

Douglas G. Merrill, M.D.
Professor, Department of Anesthesia, University of Iowa
Carver College of Medicine; Associate Hospital Director,
Medical Director, Ambulatory Surgery Center,
University of Iowa Hospitals and Clinics, Iowa City,
Iowa
*Health Care Policy, Quality Improvement, and Patient Safety
in Pain Medicine; Appendix of Useful CPT and ICD-9
Codes, Evaluation and Management Coding Template, and
Useful Internet Resources*

Harold Merskey, D.M.
Professor Emeritus, University of Western Ontario,
London, Ontario, Canada
Taxonomy and Classification of Chronic Pain Syndromes

Marjorie Meyer, M.D.
Associate Professor, University of Vermont College of
Medicine; Attending Physician, Obstetrics and
Gynecology, Fletcher Allen Health Care, Burlington,
Vermont
Managing Pain during Pregnancy and Lactation

James R. Miner, M.D.
Associate Professor of Emergency Medicine, University
of Minnesota Medical School; Research Director,
Department of Emergency Medicine, Hennepin County
Medical Center, Minneapolis, Minnesota
Pain Management in the Emergency Department

Beth H. Minzter, M.D., M.S.
Staff Director of Cancer Pain, Pain Management Center,
Cleveland Clinic Foundation, Department of Pain
Management, Division of Anesthesiology, Critical Care
Medicine and Comprehensive Pain Management,
Cleveland, Ohio
Organizing an Inpatient Acute Pain Management Service

Robert E. Molloy, M.D.
Residency Program Director, Department of
Anesthesiology, Northwestern University Feinberg
School of Medicine, Chicago, Illinois
Neurolytic Blocking Agents: Use and Complications

Antoun Nader, M.D.
Associate Professor of Anesthesiology, Northwesten
University Feinberg School of Medicine; Director, Acute
Pain Regional Anesthesiology, Northwestern Memorial
Hospital, Chicago, Illinois
Hip, Sacroiliac Joint, and Piriformis Injections

Patrick Narchi, M.D.
Physician, Anesthesia Department, Centre Clinical,
Soyaux, France
Truncal Blocks

Joseph M. Neal, M.D.
Anesthesiology Faculty, Virginia Mason Medical Center;
Clinical Professor of Anesthesiology, University of
Washington, Seattle, Washington
Upper Extremity Blocks

Krystof J. Neumann, M.D.
Visiting Instructor, University of Rochester School of
Medicine and Dentistry, Rochester, New York
Postoperative Pain and Other Acute Pain Syndromes

Jon B. Obray, M.D.
Instructor of Anesthesiology, Mayo Clinic College of
Medicine, Mayo Clinic, Rochester, Minnesota
Interlaminar and Transforaminal Epidural Steroid Injections

Marco Pappagallo, M.D.
Professor of Anesthesiology and Pain Management,
Mount Sinai School of Medicine, New York, New York
Anticonvulsants

Xavier Paqueron, M.D., Ph.D.
Physician, Anesthesia Department, Centre Clinical,
Soyaux, France
Truncal Blocks

Winston C. V. Parris, M.D.
Professor of Anesthesiology and Director, Pain
Programs, Duke University School of Medicine; Medical
Director, Pain and Palliative Clinic, Duke University
Medical Center, Durham, North Carolina
The History of Pain Medicine

Fred Perkins, M.D.
Associate Professor of Anesthesiology, Dartmouth
Medical School, Hanover, New Hampshire
*Preemptive Analgesia and Prevention of Chronic Pain
Syndromes after Surgery*

Sudhir Rao, M.D.
Assistant Professor of Pain Management, Baylor College of Medicine, Houston, Texas
Anticonvulsants

James P. Rathmell, M.D.
Associate Professor of Anesthesia, Harvard Medical School; Director, Massachusetts General Hospital Pain Center, Department of Anesthesia and Critical Care, Massachusetts General Hospital, Boston, Massachusetts
Education, Training, and Certification in Pain Medicine; Managing Pain during Pregnancy and Lactation; Radiation Safety and Use of Radiographic Contrast Agents in Pain Medicine

Scott S. Reuben, M.D.
Professor of Anesthesiology and Pain Medicine, Tufts University School of Medicine, Boston; Director, Acute Pain Services, Baystate Medical Center, Springfield, Massachusetts
Nonsteroidal Anti-inflammatory Drugs, Acetaminophen, and COX-2 Inhibitors

Christopher Robards, M.D.
Instructor of Anesthesiology, Mayo Clinic College of Medicine, Attending Anesthesiologist, Mayo Clinic, Jacksonville, Florida
Lower Extremity Peripheral Nerve Blocks

Richard W. Rosenquist, M.D.
Professor of Anesthesia, University of Iowa Carver College of Medicine; Medical Director, Center for Pain Medicine and Regional Anesthesia, University of Iowa Hospital and Clinics, Iowa City, Iowa
Phantom Limb Pain

I. Jon Russell, M.D., Ph.D.
Associate Professor of Medicine and Rheumatology; Director, University Clinical Research Center, University of Texas Health Service Center at San Antonio; Consultant Medicine Rheumatology, University Hospital, Audie Murphy Veterans Administration Hospital, San Antonio, Texas
Myofascial Pain Syndrome and Fibromyalgia Syndrome

Francis V. Salinas, M.D.
Clinical Assistant Professor of Anesthesiology, University of Washington School of Medicine; Staff Anesthesiologist, Virginia Mason Medical Center, Department of Anesthesiology, Seattle, Washington
Local Anesthetics for Regional Anesthesia and Pain Management

Michael D. Sather, M.D.
Chief Resident of Neurosurgery, University of Nebraska Medical Center, Department of Surgery, Section of Neurosurgery, Omaha, Nebraska
Neurosurgical Management of Pain

Michael F. Schafer, M.D.
Ryerson Professor and Chairman, Department of Orthopaedic Surgery, Northwestern University Feinberg School of Medicine, Chicago, Illinois
Surgical Treatment of Lumbar Spinal Disorders

Steven J. Scrivani, D.D.S., D.M.Sc.
Associate Professor, Craniofacial Pain and Headache Center, Tufts University School of Dental Medicine, Boston, Massachusetts
Dental and Facial Pain

Stelian Serban, M.D.
Assistant Professor of Anesthesiology and Pain Management; Director of Acute and Chronic Inpatient Pain Services, Mount Sinai School of Medicine, New York, New York
Anticonvulsants

Stephen D. Silberstein, M.D.
Professor of Neurology, Jefferson Medical College of Thomas Jefferson University; Director, Jefferson Headache Center, Philadelphia, Pennsylvania
Outcomes, Efficacy, and Complications of Headache Management

François Singelyn M.D., Ph.D.
Physician, Anesthesia Department, Centre Clinical, Soyaux, France
Truncal Blocks

Menno Sluijter, M.D., Ph.D.
Consultant, Institute for Anesthesiology and Pain, Swiss Paraplegic Center, Nottwil, Switzerland
Radiofrequency Treatment

Amol Soin, M.D.
Chairman, Ohio Pain Clinic, Beavercreek, Ohio; Pain Management Staff, Greene Memorial Hospital, Xenia, Ohio
Minimally Invasive Procedures for Vertebral Compression Fractures

Steven P. Stanos, D.O.
Assistant Professor, Department of Physical Medicine and Rehabilitation, Northwestern University Feinberg School of Medicine; Medical Director, Chronic Pain Care Center, Rehabilitation Institute of Chicago, Chicago, Illinois
Minor and Short-Acting Analgesics, Including Opioid Combination Products

Santhanam Suresh, M.D.
Director of Research, Children's Memorial Hospital; Associate Professor of Anesthesiology and Pediatrics, Northwestern University Feinberg School of Medicine, Chicago, Illinois
Chronic Pain Management in Children; Acute Pain Management in Children

Kimberly S. Swanson, Ph.D.
Senior Fellow, Department of Anesthesiology, University of Washington School of Medicine, Seattle, Washington
Psychological Interventions

Sally Tarbell, Ph.D.
Associate Professor of Pediatrics, Gastroenterology, and Nutrition, Medical College of Wisconsin, Milwaukee, Wisconsin
Chronic Pain Management in Children; Acute Pain Management in Children

Knox H. Todd, M.D., M.P.H.
Professor, Department of Emergency Medicine, Albert Einstein College of Medicine; Director, Pain and Emergency Medicine Institute, Beth Israel Medical Center, New York, New York
Pain Management in the Emergency Department

Dennis C. Turk, Ph.D.
John and Emma Bonica Professor of Anesthesiology and Pain Research, Department of Anesthesiology, University of Washington School of Medicine, Seattle, Washington
Psychological Interventions; Chronic Pain Clinical Trials: IMMPACT Recommendations

Mark D. Tyburski, M.D.
Assistant Chief, Department of Physical Medicine and Rehabilitation, Spine Clinic, The Permanente Medical Group, Sacramento/Roseville, California
Minor and Short-Acting Analgesics, Including Opioid Combination Products

M. van Kleef, M.D., Ph.D.
Professor, Head of the Department of Anesthesiology, University Hospital of Maastricht, The Netherlands
Radiofrequency Treatment

J. Van Zundert, M.D., Ph.D.
Head of Multidisciplinary Pain Center, University Hospital of Maastricht, The Netherlands
Radiofrequency Treatment

Renata Variakojis, M.D.
Assistant Professor, University of Chicago Pritzker School of Medicine, Chicago, Illinois
Pharmacology for the Interventional Pain Physician

Jeanine A. Verbunt, M.D., Ph.D.
Consultant in Rehabilitation Medicine/Research, Rehabilitation Foundation, Limburg, The Netherlands
Physical Rehabilitation for Patients with Chronic Pain

Christopher M. Viscomi, M.D.
Associate Professor of Anesthesiology, University of Vermont College of Medicine; Director, Acute Pain Service, Fletcher Allen Health Care, Burlington, Vermont
Managing Pain during Pregnancy and Lactation

Mitchell Wachtel, M.D.
Associate Professor, Department of Pathology, Texas Tech University Health Sciences Center, Lubbock, Texas
Lumbosacral Epiduroscopy

Howard J. Waldman, M.D., D.O.
Director, Rehabilitation Medicine, Director, Neurodiagnostic Laboratory, Headache and Pain Center, Leawood, Kansas
Electromyography and Evoked Potentials

David Walega, M.D.
Assistant Professor, Northwestern University Feinberg School of Medicine; Medical Director, Anesthesiology Pain Medicine Center, Northwestern Memorial Faculty Foundation, Chicago, Illinois
Pain Medicine Practice: Development of Outpatient Services for Chronic Pain; Appendix of Useful CPT and ICD-9 Codes, Evaluation and Management Coding Template, and Useful Internet Resources

Daniel T. Warren, M.D.
Academic Anesthesiologist, Pain Medicine Specialist, Virginia Mason Medical Center, Seattle, Washington
Neuraxial Anesthesia

Tabitha Washington, M.D.
Assistant Professor, Department of Anesthesiology, Dartmouth Medical School; Anesthesiologist, Dartmouth Hitchcock Clinic, Section of Pain Medicine, Lebanon, New Hampshire
Preemptive Analgesia and Prevention of Chronic Pain Syndromes after Surgery

Karin N. Westlund High, Ph.D.
Professor, Department of Physiology, University of Kentucky College of Medicine; Chandler Medical Center, Lexington, Kentucky
Pain Pathways: Peripheral Spinal, Ascending, and Descending Pathways

Brian A. Willams, M.D., M.B.A.
Associate Professor of Anesthesiology, University of Pittsburgh School of Medicine; Director, Outpatient Regional Anesthesia Service, University of Pittsburgh Medical Center—South Side Hospital, Pittsburgh, Pennsylvania
Postoperative Pain and Other Acute Pain Syndromes

Kayode A. Williams, M.D.
Assistant Professor in Anesthesiology, Johns Hopkins University School of Medicine, Baltimore, Maryland
Neuropathic Pain Syndromes

Harriët Wittink, Ph.D.
Professor of Lifestyle and Health, University of Applied Sciences Utrecht, Utrecht, The Netherlands
Physical Rehabilitation for Patients with Chronic Pain

Christopher L. Wu, M.D.
Associate Professor of Anesthesiology and Critical Care Medicine, Johns Hopkins University School of Medicine, Baltimore, Maryland
Postoperative Pain and Other Acute Pain Syndromes; Neuropathic Pain Syndromes; Outcomes, Efficacy, and Complications from Acute Postoperative Pain Management; Outcomes, Efficacy, and Complications of Neuropathic Pain

Daquan Xu, M.B., M.Sc., M.P.H.
Clinical Research Fellow of Anesthesiology, Columbia University College of Physicians and Surgeons/St. Luke's–Roosevelt Hospital Center, New York, New York
Lower Extremity Peripheral Nerve Blocks

Tony L. Yaksh, Ph.D.
Professor and Vice Chairman for Research, Department of Anesthesiology; Professor of Pharmacology, University of California, San Diego, School of Medicine, San Diego, California
A Review of Pain-Processing Pharmacology

Anthony Yarussi, M.D.
Clinical Assistant Professor of Anesthesia, University at Buffalo School of Medicine, Buffalo, New York
Cancer Pain

Foreword

The editors of the fourth edition of *Practical Management of Pain* have asked me to write a foreword for this edition, as I served as the lead editor for the first three editions of this text. This gives me a unique opportunity to reflect on the progress made in the field of pain medicine since the first edition published in 1980.

In 1978, as I arrived at the University of Cincinnati, I was asked by the Chairman, Philip Bridenbaugh, to organize a multidisciplinary pain clinic and to train anesthesia residents rotating through the department. I had successfully done that on two previous occasions at the UT Southwestern Medical School in Dallas and at Wadsworth Hospital, a UCLA-affiliated hospital in California. Organizing a multidisciplinary pain clinic wasn't easy in those times because pain management crossed several medical specialties, including anesthesiology, neurology, neurosurgery, psychiatry, and physical medicine and rehabilitation. At around the same time, I was asked by Year Book Medical Publishers to write a book on pain management. Other than Bonica's classic book *Management of Pain*, first published in 1953, there were no other comprehensive resources on pain management at the time, and, rather than write it myself, I decided to ask pain management experts to contribute chapters to the book. My goal was to create a resource for a pain trainee who had one year to learn everything about pain management, including organization and administration of a pain clinic, basic science relevant to clinical practice, equipment used in pain management, and all the clinically useful information I could think of. The book took some time to complete and be published, but it was successful and well received by all those who wanted to develop a career in pain medicine.

The second and third editions of the book published in 1992 and 2000, respectively. By that time pain management had become a strong field that was keenly monitored by the reimbursement and government regulatory agencies. Although it was accepted as a specialized area of medicine, its value was challenged by other specialties and insurance agencies. For the second and third editions the book was divided into sections and several noted leaders in the field were invited to edit individual sections.

Today, many physicians choose to have a career in pain management. They come from many different medical specialties and the book now has to reflect the advances in all those specialties, not just anesthesiology. The debate is still raging whether a single dedicated pain specialist can achieve better results in pain management than a group of specialists. The cost of such multidisciplinary clinics has been questioned, especially by the reimbursement agencies. The goal of pain clinics shouldn't be just short-term pain relief, but also the long-term improvement of the patient's function and quality of life. There is also a discrepancy in pain practices between developed, developing, and underdeveloped countries. Global epidemiology of pain is not precisely known, and neither is the number of pain physicians available per capita in many communities. We certainly have made advances in understanding the mechanisms of pain and the longitudinal natural course in some pain syndromes, but we are far from having a reliable treatment algorithm for an array of pain disorders. Today's challenge is to train pain physicians using a standardized curriculum during their residency and pain fellowship programs, followed by skilled practical training. Upon completion of training, periodic testing of competency is necessary. This will raise the standard of pain practice not only in the United States but all over the world.

I congratulate the editors of the fourth edition of *Practical Management of Pain* for embarking on and completing this challenging endeavor. Dr. Honorio Benzon deserves a particular mention for his dedication and scholarly direction of the new edition, to which I wish every success.

P. Prithvi Raj, M.D.

Preface

Raj's Practical Management of Pain has assumed an eminent position among the standard textbooks of pain medicine. I was truly honored when Dr. Raj recommended that I assume the responsibilities of the lead editor of the next edition of his classic book. I recruited Drs. James Rathmell, Christopher Wu, Dennis Turk, and Charles Argoff to serve as my coeditors. Each of them is well respected in their disciplines. They represent the specialties of anesthesiology, psychology, and neurology that, together with physical medicine and rehabilitation, provide the core of pain medicine.

This edition retains the successful format of the previous edition. It includes sections on general considerations; basic aspects; evaluation and assessment; clinical conditions; pharmacologic, psychological, and physical medicine treatments; nerve block techniques; interventional techniques; pain management as applied to special situations; and outcomes. Appendices on selected diagnoses and selected pain management billing codes are also included to expand the practical utility of the volume. The topics represent the multidisciplinary nature of pain medicine, and the authors are eminent authorities in their areas of expertise. Similar to the previous edition, the book includes an international group of authors, recognizing the scientific contributions of experts from around the world.

This book is intended for the pain clinicians looking for applications in their daily practice, pain researchers seeking adequate background on relevant topics, fellows reviewing for the pain medicine boards, and for residents who want a complete discussion of the breadth of the field. The book covers distillations of research on all relevant aspects of pain medicine, including current knowledge of mechanisms involved and strategies for assessing and treating people with chronic pain. It also covers practical applications of the various and diverse acute and chronic pain syndromes.

A project of this magnitude could not come to fruition without the efforts and assistance of a number of people. The contributors took time out of their busy academic, clinical, and administrative responsibilities to prepare their chapters. My coeditors spent an enormous amount of time finalizing the book. Our publishing team at Elsevier led by Executive Publisher Natasha Andjelkovic, Senior Developmental Editor Janice Gaillard, Design Manager Steven Stave, and Project Manager Rachel Miller did an excellent job of developing the book and keeping it on track. Everyone's hard work resulted in the distinguished quality of this book. To all the readers, we hope that we have prepared a comprehensive and attractive volume worthy of your reading.

Honorio T. Benzon, M.D.
Department of Anesthesiology
Northwestern University Feinberg School of
Medicine
Chicago, Illinois

Contents

PART

I

General Considerations

H. T. Benzon and J. Rathmell

1 The History of Pain Medicine

Winston C. V. Parris and Benjamin Johnson

History is a distillation of rumor.
THOMAS CARLYLE (1795-1881)

The management of pain, like the management of disease, is as old as mankind. In the view of Christians, the fall of Adam and Eve in the Garden of Eden produced for man (and woman) a long life of suffering disease and pain. This one act allegedly set the stage for several disease concepts, including the experience of pain in labor and delivery; the concept that hard work is painful; the notion that blood, sweat, and tears are needed to produce fruit; the introduction of pain and disease to human existence; the establishment of the fact that hell and its fires are painful; and the expectation that heaven is pure, delightful, spiritually pleasing, and, of course, pain-free. In these concepts, pain is viewed as a negative experience and one that is associated with disease, morbidity, and the dying process. Most diseases, including infections, plagues, metabolic disorders (e.g., diabetes mellitus), endocrine disorders, hypertension, and cancer, of course, afflict mankind spontaneously and usually cause significant pain, without any wrongdoing, negligence, or irresponsibility on the part of the afflicted person.

As we consider the historical perspective, humans have deliberately and knowingly inflicted on one another many experiences associated with pain—from the earliest wars to the more recent irrational shooting incidents in the Arkansas and Oregon public school systems, from the scourging of Jesus to the contemporary strife in the Middle East, the Rwandan genocide, the Irish "religious" fratricide, and the conflicts in Bosnia and the Balkans. All wars, including the great wars, World War I and World War II, the American Civil War, the Korean War, and the Vietnam War, have all been associated with untold pain, suffering, and death.

Although we as human beings have not learned from these painful episodes and continue to inflict pain on others, the advances and increasing sophistication of the 21st century have brought about new concepts of disease and the painful states that diseases produce. The social illnesses—veneral diseases, the pulmonary, cardiovascular, and neoplastic con-sequences of smoking, the trauma associated with automobile accidents, the pathology caused by drug abuse and drug misuse, and the proliferation of viral illnesses (e.g., acquired immunodeficiency syndrome) have all contributed further pain and suffering to our lot. Therefore any review of history and politics, economics, and social interrelationships of the world is inevitably a review of the history of pain. This chapter focuses on some of the major historical events that have influenced pain, its development, and its management and highlights the important phases that led to the current conceptualization of pain and its treatment as an independent specialty in modern medicine.

PAIN AND RELIGION

The early concept of pain as a form of punishment from supreme spiritual beings for sin and evil activity is as old as mankind.[1] In the book of *Genesis,* God told Eve that following her fall from grace, she would endure pain during childbirth: "I will greatly multiply your pain in childbearing; in pain you shall bring forth children, yet your desire shall be for your husband and he shall rule over you" (Genesis 3:16). This condemnation led early Christians to accept pain as a normal consequence of Eve's action and to view this consequence as being directly transferred to them. Thus any attempt to decrease the pain associated with labor and delivery was treated by early Christians with disdain and disapproval. It was not until 1847, when Queen Victoria was administered chloroform by James Simpson[2] for the delivery of her eighth child, Prince Leopold, that contemporary Christians, and in particular Protestants, accepted the notion that it was not heretical to promote pain-less childbirth as part of the obstetric process.

From the Old Testament, Job has been praised for his endurance of pain and suffering. Yet, Job's friends wondered whether these tribulations were an indication that he had committed some great sin for which God was punishing him. Their justification for this assumption was based in the book of *Proverbs,* which suggested that "no harm befalls the righteous" (Proverbs 12:21). Notwithstanding, Job was considered a faithful servant by God and was not guilty of any wrongdoing. In fact, he was described as a man who was "blameless and upright" and one who feared God and turned away from evil.[3]

In the 5th century, St. Augustine wrote that "all diseases of Christians are to be ascribed to demons; chiefly do they torment the fresh baptized, yea, even the guiltless newborn infant," implying that not even innocent infants escaped the work of demons. Today, major typhoons, hurricanes, fires, earthquakes, volcanoes, tsunamis, floods, droughts, and fires destroy hundreds, and at times thousands, of innocent, defenseless people. One ponders the rationale of such pain and suffering endured by otherwise good people while seemingly ruthless and evil persons apparently triumph and prosper in an atmosphere of luxury and comfort.

This paradox can be discouraging at times but is usually upheld by firm Christian belief. In the 1st century, many people who belonged to the Catholic Church were rebuked and suffered ruthless persecution, including death, because of their belief in Jesus as the Messiah. Some who were subsequently described as martyrs endured their suffering with the belief that they did it for the love of Christ, and they felt that their suffering identified them with Christ's suffering on the cross during his crucifixion.[4] This may be the earliest example of the value of psychotherapy as an important modality in managing pain. Thus many present-day cancer patients with strong Christian beliefs view their pain and suffering as part of their journey toward eternal salvation. This concept has led to several scientifically conducted and government-sponsored studies evaluating intercessory prayer as an effective modality for controlling cancer pain.

To fully appreciate the historical significance of pain, it is important to reflect on the origins of the "pain patient." The word *pain* comes from the Latin word *poena*, which means "punishment." The word *patient* is derived from the Latin word *patior*, meaning "to endure suffering or pain." Thus it is not too outrageous to appreciate that, in ancient days, persons who experienced pain were interpreted to have received punishment in the form of suffering that was either dispensed by the gods or offered up to appease the gods for transgressions.[5]

As epidural anesthesia has developed and the techniques have been refined so that mortality and morbidity are negligible, childbirth and delivery are increasingly considered relatively painless in most developed societies. Unfortunately, in many countries neither the personnel nor the technology is available and resources to provide such personnel and technology are inadequate, making childbirth a primitively painful and at times disastrous event. The history of anesthesia is full of instances wherein attempts to relieve pain were initially met with resistance and at times violence. In the mid-19th century, Crawford Long of Georgia attempted to develop and provide anesthesia, but contemporary Christians of that state considered him a heretic for his scholarly activity. As a result, he literally had to flee for his life from Georgia into Texas. Although surgical anesthesia was well developed by the late 19th century, religious controversy over its use required Pope Pius XII to give his approval before anesthesia could be extensively used for surgical procedures.[6] Pope Pius XII wrote, "The patient, desirous of avoiding or relieving pain, may without any disquietude of conscience, use the means discovered by science which in themselves are not immoral."

PAIN AND THE ANCIENT CULTURES

Disease, pain, and death have always been considered undesirable. The principles on which medicine was founded were based on measures to overcome human suffering from disease. Thus pain was usually thought of as either emanating from an injury or originating from the dysfunction of an internal organ or system. Traditionally, pain after physical injury (e.g., a gunshot wound or spear injury) was not considered problematic, since as soon as the offending injurious agent was removed or once the consequences of the offending injury were corrected, the patient either recovered rapidly or, on occasion, died.[7] On the other hand, pain from disease (e.g., the pain of an inflamed gallbladder or ruptured appendix) was regarded with more mystique, and treatment was usually tinged with superstitious tradition. The tribal concept of pain came from the belief that it resulted from an "intrusion" from outside the body. These "intruders" were thought to be evil spirits sent by the gods as a form of punishment. It was in this setting that the role of medicine men and shamans flourished, because these were the persons assigned to treat the pain syndromes associated with internal disease. Because it was thought that spirits entered the body by different avenues, the rational approach to therapy was aimed at blocking the particular pathway chosen by the spirit.

In Egypt, the left nostril was considered the specific site where disease entered. This belief was confirmed by the Papyri of Ebers and Berlin,[8] which stated that the treatment of headache involved expulsion of the offending spirit by sneezing, sweating, vomiting, urination, and even trephination. In New Guinea, it was believed that evil spirits entered via a spear or an arrow that then produced spontaneous pain.[7] Thus it was common for the shaman to occasionally purge the evil spirit from a painful offending wound and neutralize it with his special powers or his special medicines. Egyptians treated some forms of pain by placing an electric fish from the Nile over the wounds in order to control the pain.[9] The resulting electrical stimulation that produced pain relief actually works by a mechanism similar to transcutaneous electrical nerve stimulation, which is frequently used today to treat pain.

The Papyrus of Ebers, an ancient Egyptian manuscript, contains a wide variety of pharmacologic information and describes many techniques and recipes, some of which still have validity.[8] The Papyri describe the use of opium for the treatment of pain in children. Other concoctions for treating pediatric pain have included wearing amulets filled with a dead man's tooth (Omnibonus Ferraruis, 1577) as a treatment for teething pain. Although early documents specifically address the management of pain in children, it is unfortunate that even today the treatment of pediatric pain is far from optimal. This glaring deficiency was highlighted in 1977 by Eland, who demonstrated that in a population of children 4 to 8 years of age, only 50% received analgesics for postoperative pain.[3] The results are even more unsatisfactory for the treatment of chronic pain and cancer pain in children. It is unfortunate that the observations of earlier scholars have been ignored. Two erroneous assumptions—that (1) children are less sensitive to pain and (2) the central nervous system is relatively undeveloped in neonates—are partially responsible for this deficiency.

Early Native Americans believed that pain was experienced in the heart, whereas the Chinese identified multiple points in the body where pain might originate or might be self-perpetuating.[10] Consequently, attempts were made to drain the body of these "pain points" by inserting needles, a concept that may have given birth to the principles of acupuncture therapy, which is well over 2000 years old.[11]

The ancient Greeks were the first to consider pain to be a sensory function that might be derived from peripheral stimulation.[12] In particular, Aristotle believed that pain was a central sensation arriving from some form of stimulation of the flesh, while Plato hypothesized that the brain was the destination of all peripheral stimulation.[1] Aristotle advanced the notion that the heart was the originating source or processing center for pain. He based his hypothesis on the concept that an excess of vital heat was conducted by the blood to the heart where pain was modulated and perceived. Because of his great reputation, many Greek philosophers followed Aristotle and embraced the notion that the heart was the center for pain processing.[13] Another Greek philosopher, Stratton, and other distinguished Egyptians, including Herophilus and Eistratus, disagreed with Aristotle and proposed the concept that the brain was the site of pain perception as suggested by Plato. Their theories were reinforced by actual anatomic studies showing the connections of the peripheral and central nervous systems.[14]

Notwithstanding, controversies between the opposing theories of the brain and the heart as the center for pain continued, and it was not until 400 years later that the Roman philosopher Galen rejuvenated the works of the Egyptians Herophilus and Eistratus, and greatly reemphasized the model of the central nervous system. Although Galen's work was compelling, he received little recognition for it until the 20th century.

Toward the period of the Roman Empire, steady progress was made in understanding pain as a sensation similar to other sensations in the body. Developments made in anatomy, and to a lesser extent physiology, helped establish that the brain, not the heart, was the center for the processing of pain.[15]

While these advances were taking place, there were simultaneous advances in the development of therapeutic modalities, including the use of drugs (e.g., opium) as well as heat, cold, massage, trephining, and exercise to treat painful illnesses. These developments brought about the establishment of the principles of surgery for treating disease. Electricity was first used by the Greeks of that era as they exploited the power of the electrogenic torpedo fish (*Scribonius longus*) to treat the pain of arthritis and headache. Electrostatic generators were used in the late Middle Ages, as was the Leyden jar; these developments resulted in the reemergence of electrotherapy as a modality for managing medical problems, including pain. There was a relative standstill in the development of electrotherapy as a medical modality until the invention of the electric battery in the 19th century. Then several attempts were made to revive its use as an effective medical modality, but these concepts did not catch on and were largely used only by charlatans and obscure scientists and practitioners. Throughout the Middle Ages and the Renaissance, debate raged regarding the origin and processing center of pain. Fortunes fluctuated between proponents of the brain theory and proponents of the heart theory, depending on which theory was favored.

Heart theory proponents appeared to prosper when William Harvey, recognized for his discovery of the circulation, supported the heart as the focus for pain sensation. Descartes disagreed vehemently with the Harvey hypothesis, and his description of pain conduction from peripheral damage through nerves to the brain led to the first plausible pain theory, that is, the *specificity theory*.[16] It is interesting to note that the specificity theory followed Descartes' description by some 2 centuries. Several other theories followed the specificity theory and contributed to the foundation for understanding pain and pain mechanisms.

PAIN AND PAIN THEORIES

The specificity theory, originally proposed by Descartes, was formally revised by Schiff based on animal research. The fundamental tenet of the theory was that each sensory modality, including pain, was transmitted along an independent pathway. By examining the effect of incisions in the spinal cord, Schiff[16] demonstrated that touch and pain were independent sensations. Furthermore, he demonstrated that sectioning of the spinal cord deferentially resulted in the loss of one modality without affecting the other. Further work along the same lines by Bliz,[17] Goldscheider,[18] and von Frey[19] contributed to the concept that separate and distinct receptors existed for the modalities of pain, touch, warmth, and cold.

During the 18th and 19th centuries, new inventions, new theories, and new thinking emerged. This period was known as the Scientific Revolution, and several important inventions took place, including the discovery of the analgesic properties of nitrous oxide, followed by the discovery of the local anesthetic agents (e.g., cocaine). The study of anatomy was also developing rapidly as an important branch of science and medicine; most notable was the discovery of the anatomic division of the spinal cord into sensory (dorsal) and motor (ventral) divisions. In 1840, Mueller proposed that, based on anatomic studies, there was a straight-through system of specific nerve energies in which specific energy from a given sensation was transmitted along sensory nerves to the brain.[20] Mueller's theories led Darwin to propose the intensive theory of pain,[21] which maintained that the sensation of pain was not a separate modality but instead resulted from a sensory overload of sufficient intensity for any modality. This theory was modified by Erb[22] and then expanded by Goldscheider[18] to encompass the roles of both stimulus intensity and central summation of stimuli. Although the intensive theory was persuasive, the controversy continued, with the result that by the mid-20th century, the specificity theory was universally accepted as the more plausible theory of pain.

With this official blessing (although it was not unanimous) of the contemporary scientific community, strategies for pain therapy began to focus on identifying and interrupting pain pathways. This tendency was both a blessing and a curse. It was a blessing in that it led many researchers to explore surgical techniques that might interrupt pain pathways and consequently relieve pain, but it was a curse in that it blind-sided the medical community for more that half a century into believing that pain pathways and their interruption were the total answer to the pain puzzle. This trend was begun in the late 19th century by Letievant, who first described specific neurectomy techniques for treating neuralgic pain.[23] Afterward, various surgical interventions for chronic pain were developed and used, including rhizotomy, cordotomy, leucotomy, tractotomy, myelotomy, and several other operative procedures designed to interrupt the central nervous system and consequently reduce pain.[24] Most of these techniques were abysmal failures that not only did not relieve pain but also on occasion produced much more pain than was previously present. A major consequence lingers today—the notion that pain can be "fixed" by a surgical procedure or other modality.

PAIN AND DISEASE

The cardinal features of disease as recognized by early philosophers included calor, rubor, tumor, and dolor; the English translation is heat, redness, swelling, and pain. One of the important highlights in the history of pain medicine was the realization that even though heat, redness, and swelling may disappear, pain can continue long after and be unresponsive on occasion to different therapeutic modalities. When pain continues long after the natural pathogenetic course of disease has ended, a chronic pain syndrome develops with characteristic clinical features, including depression, dependency, disability, disuse, drug misuse, drug abuse, and, of course, "doctor shopping." John

Dryden once wrote, "For all the happiness mankind can gain is not in pleasure, but in rest from pain." Thus many fatal nonpainful diseases are not as feared as relatively trivial painful ones.

Throughout the ages, physicians and healers have focused their attention on managing pain. Thus in managing cancer, an important measure of successful treatment is the success with which any associated pain is managed. Although many technologic advances have been made in medicine, it is only within the past 10 to 20 years that significant strides have been made to deal with chronic pain as a disease entity per se—one requiring specialized study, specialized evaluation, and specialized therapeutic interventions. As better techniques and more effective methods for evaluation and treatment of pain, especially chronic pain, are developed, the management of this disease will be considered more complete and an important supplement to the great strides made in other areas of chronic disease management.

PAIN IN THE 20TH CENTURY

General anesthesia was formally discovered by William Morton in 1846; in 1847, Simpson used chloroform to provide anesthesia for labor and delivery.[9] Around the same time, the needle and the syringe were invented. Many local anesthetic agents were also discovered in that era. In 1888, Corning described the use of a local anesthetic, cocaine, for the treatment of nerve pain. Techniques for local and regional anesthesia for both surgery and pain disorders proliferated rapidly.

In 1907, Schlosser reported significant relief of neuralgic pain for long periods with alcohol injection of damaged and painful nerves. Reports of similar treatment came from the management of pain resulting from tuberculous and neoplastic invasion.[25] In 1926 and 1928, Swetlow and White, respectively, reported on the use of alcohol injections into thoracic sympathetic ganglia to treat chronic angina. In 1931, Dogliotti described the use of alcohol injected into the cervical subarachnoid space to treat pain associated with cancer.[26]

One consequence of war has been the development of new techniques and procedures to manage injuries. In World War I (1914-1918), numerous injuries were associated with trauma (e.g., dismemberment, peripheral vascular insufficiency, and frostbite). In World War II (1939-1946), not only peripheral vascular injuries but also phantom limb phenomena, causalgias, and many sympathetically mediated pain syndromes occurred. Leriche developed the technique of sympathetic neural blockade with procaine to treat the causalgic injuries of war.[27] John Bonica, himself an army surgeon during World War II, recognized the gross inadequacy of managing war injuries and other painful states of veterans with the existing unidisciplinary approaches.[28] This led him to propose the concept of a multidisciplinary, multimodal management for chronic pain. Bonica also highlighted the fact that pain of all kinds was being undertreated; his work has borne fruit, in that he is universally considered the "father of pain," and he was the catalyst for the formation of many established national and international pain organizations. The clinic he developed at the University of Washington in Seattle remains a model for the multidisciplinary management of chronic pain. As a result of his work, the American Pain Society and the International Association for the Study of Pain (IASP) have been formed, are still active, and continue to lead in pain research and pain management. Bonica's lasting legacy is the historic volume *The Management of Pain,* published in 1953.

Anesthesia as a specialty developed but was still associated with significant mortality and morbidity. Anesthesia departments were considered divisions of surgery, not reaching full autonomy until after World War II. Because of morbidity associated with general anesthesia and because several new local anesthetics were being discovered, regional anesthesia and its associated techniques began to flourish in the United States. Bonica also played a major role in advancing the use of epidural anesthesia to manage the pain associated with labor and delivery. Regional anesthesia suffered a significant setback in the United Kingdom with the negative publicity surrounding the 1954 cases of Wooley and Roe, who suffered serious and irreversible neurologic damage after spinal anesthesia. It took 3 more decades to fully overcome that setback and to see regional anesthesia widely accepted as safe and effective in the United Kingdom. Several persons contributing significantly to the development of regional anesthesia are Corning, Quincke-August Bier, Pitkin, Etherington-Wilson, Barker, and Adriani.

As recent society has developed and as science has prospered, the general public has come to consider pain to be unsatisfactory and unacceptable. As a result, demands have been made that resulted in the development of labor and delivery anesthesia services, acute pain services, and, more recently, chronic pain clinics. Bonica's vision was not only the development of those clinics but also the founding and maintenance of national and international pain organizations to promote research and scientific understanding of pain medicine. As a result, a tremendous amount of research continues, almost quadrupling each year.

An outstanding contribution in the field of research was the development and publication of the *gate control theory* by Melzack and Wall in 1965.[29] This theory, built on the preexisting and prevalent specificity and intensive theories, provided a sound scientific basis for understanding pain mechanisms and for developing other concepts on which sound hypotheses could be developed. The gate control theory emphasizes the importance of both of ascending and descending modulation systems and laid down a solid framework for the management of different pain syndromes. The gate control theory almost single-handedly legitimized pain as a scientific discipline, leading not only to many other research endeavors building on the theory but also to the maturity of pain medicine as a science.[30] As a consequence, the American Pain Society, the American Academy of Pain Medicine, the IASP, and the World Institute of Pain (WIP) flourish today as serious and responsible organizations dealing with various aspects of pain medicine, including education, science, certification, and credentialing of members of the specialty of pain medicine.

PAIN AND THE IMPACT OF PSYCHOLOGY

The history of pain medicine would be incomplete without acknowledging the noteworthy contributions of psychologists. Their influential research and clinical activities have been an integral part of a revolution in the conceptualization of the pain experience.[31] For example, in the early 20th century, the role of the cerebral cortex in the perception of pain was controversial, due to a lack of understanding of neuroanatomic pathways and the neurophysiologic mechanisms involved in pain perception.[32,33] This controversy largely ended with the introduction of the gate control theory by Wall and Melzack in 1965.[29] The gate control theory has stood the test of time, in that subsequent research using modern brain imaging techniques such as PET, fMRI, and SPECT has also described the activation of multiple cortical and subcortical sites of activity in the brain during pain perception. Further elaboration of the psychological aspects of the pain experience includes the three psychological dimensions of pain: sensory-discriminative, motivational-affective, and cognitive-evaluative.[34]

Psychological researchers have greatly advanced the field of pain medicine by reconceptualizing both the etiology of the pain experience and the treatment strategy. Early pain researchers conceptualized the pain experience as a product of either somatic pathology or psychological factors. However, psychological researchers have convincingly challenged this misconception by presenting research that illustrates the complex interaction between biomedical and psychosocial factors.[35-37]

This biopsychosiocial approach to the pain experience encourages the realization that pain is a complex perceptual experience modulated by a wide range of biopsychosocial factors, including emotions, social and environmental contexts, and cultural background, as well as beliefs, attitudes, and expectations. As the acutely painful experience transitions into a chronic phenomenon, these biopsychosocial abnormalities develop permanency. Thus, chronic pain affects all facets of a person's functional universe, at great expense to the individual and society. Consequently, logic dictates that this multimodal etiology of pain requires a multimodal therapeutic strategy for opti-mal cost-effective treatment outcomes.[38,39]

Additional contributions from the field of psychology include therapeutic behavioral modification techniques for the management of pain. Such techniques as cognitive behavioral intervention, guided imagery, biofeedback, and autogenic training are the direct results of using the concepts presented in the gate control theory. In addition, neuromodulatory therapeutic modalities such as transcutaneous electrical nerve stimulation (TENS), peripheral nerve stimulation, spinal cord stimulation, and deep brain stimulation are also logical offspring of the concepts presented in the gate control theory.

The evaluation of candidates for interventional medical procedures is another valuable historical contribution from the field of psychology. Not only is the psychologist's expertise in the identification of appropriate patients valuable for the success of therapeutic procedural interventions in the management of pain, but his or her expertise is helpful in identifying patients who are not appropriate candidates for procedural interventions. Thus, psychologists have contributed positively toward the cost-effectiveness and usefulness of diagnostic and therapeutic pain medicine.

PAIN AND PAIN INSTITUTIONS

The International Association for the Study of Pain

The IASP is the largest multidisciplinary international association in the field of pain. Founded in 1973 by John J. Bonica, MD, the IASP is a nonprofit professional organization dedicated to furthering research on pain and improving the care of patients experiencing pain. Membership is open to scientists, physicians, dentists, psychologists, nurses, physical therapists, and other health professionals actively engaged in pain, and to those who have special interest in the diagnosis and treatment of pain. The IASP has members in more than 100 national chapters.

The goals and objectives of IASP are to foster and encourage research of pain mechanisms and pain syndromes, and to help improve the management of patients with acute and chronic pain by bringing together scientists, physicians, and other health professionals of various disciplines and backgrounds who have interest in pain research and management. The goals of the IASP also include mandates to promote education and training in the field of pain, as well as to promote and facilitate the dissemination of new information in the field of pain. One of the instruments of dissemination is sponsorship of the journal *Pain*. In addition, the IASP promotes and sponsors a highly successful triennial World Congress as well as other meetings. IASP encourages the development of national chapters for the national implementation of the international mission of the IASP. The IASP also encourages the adoption of a uniform classification, nomenclature, and definition regarding pain and pain syndromes. The development of a uniform records system in regard to information relating to pain mechanisms, syndromes, and management is also a stated goal of the IASP, and education of the general public to the results and implications of current pain research is another mission of the IASP.

The IASP has partnered with the World Health Organization (WHO) in providing guidelines for chronic pain assessment and management especially in developing countries. Cancer pain awareness and its management have been noteworthy contributions of the IASP.

Special interest groups (SIGs) within the IASP have successfully promoted research, understanding, education, and enhanced pain management of the particular special interest. Areas of interest include pain in children, neuropathic pain, herbal medicine, and neuropathic pain, among others. The IASP also promotes and administers Chronic Pain Fellowship programs for deserving candidates all over the world.

The American Pain Society

Spurred by a burgeoning public interest in pain management and research as well as the formation of the Eastern and Western USA Chapters of the IASP, the American Pain Society (APS) was formed in 1977 as a result of a meeting of the Ad Hoc Advisory Committee on the Formation of a National Pain Organization. The need for a national organization of pain professionals was realized as growth of the IASP continued. The APS became the first national chapter of the IASP, and has constituent regional and state chapters. The APS has its own journal, *The Journal of Pain,* and holds national meetings. Its main function is to carry out the mission of the IASP on a national level.

Commission on the Accreditation of Rehabilitation Facilities

As pain clinics developed, it became clear that there was a need for credentialing, not only of pain centers and pain clinics, but also of pain clinicians. In 1983, the Commission on Accreditation of Rehabilitation Facilities (CARF) was the first to offer a system of accreditation for pain clinics and pain treatment centers. The CARF model was based on the rehabilitation system, and it quickly became clear that the orientation of CARF would be physical and psychosocial rehabilitation of patients suffering pain in contrast to modality treatment to reduce pain sensation. CARF standards mandated that multidisciplinary pain management programs offer medical, psychologic, and physical therapy modalities for pain management. Pain clinicians were not accredited by CARF, and it quickly became apparent that one could have an accredited pain center without having accredited pain clinicians. The CARF model gained modest acceptance among insurance carriers and third-party payers, primarily because of its emphasis on accountability and program evaluation. Its major goals included such objective measures as increased physical function, reduced medication intake, and return-to-work issues.

The American Academy of Pain Medicine

As CARF gained prominence, many pain clinicians realized that neither CARF nor the APS completely met their practice and professional needs. Furthermore, it became obvious that there was a major deficiency in evaluating the competence of pain physicians, in that there were no uniform standards for training and credentialing of these pain clinicians. Thus in 1983, at a meeting of the APS in Washington, DC, a group of physicians (of whom chapter author Winston Parris was privileged to be a member) formed the American Academy of Algology (the term *algology* is derived from the word *algos* [Greek for "pain"], and *logos* [Greek for "study"]). The name was changed 2 years later to the American Academy of Pain Medicine (AAPM), a name that is more acceptable in mainstream medicine.

This academy was formed to meet the needs and aspirations of pain physicians in the United States. Its major focus was to address the specific concerns of pain physicians and to enhance, authenticate, develop, and lead to the credentialing of pain medicine specialists. As a medical specialty society, the academy is involved in education, training, advocacy, and research in the specialty of pain medicine. The practice of pain medicine is multidisciplinary in approach, incorporating modalities from various specialties to ensure the comprehensive evaluation and treatment of the pain patient. AAPM represents the diverse scope of the field through membership from a variety of origins, including such specialties as anesthesiology, internal medicine, neurology, neurologic surgery, orthopedic surgery, physiatry, and psychiatry. The goals of the AAPM include the promotion of quality care of both patients experiencing pain as a symptom of a disease and patients with the primary disease of pain through research, education, and advocacy, and the advancement of the specialty of pain medicine.

As we enter the managed care era, it is clear that issues such as reimbursement, contract negotiations, fee scheduling, practice management, mergers, acquisitions, and other business-related matters are becoming increasingly important to pain practitioners. The political and business arms of the American Academy of Pain Medicine are becoming instrumental in helping guide physicians through the murky waters of managed care and pain medicine.

In an attempt to provide creditable credentialing in pain medicine, the AAPM sponsored the American College of Pain Medicine (ACPM), which organized, developed, and administered the first credentialing examination in 1992. Successful candidates received the Fellowship of the American College of Pain Medicine. In the process of attempting to receive recognition of the American Board of Medical Specialties (ABMS), the name was changed on the recommendation of the ABMS to the American Board of Pain Medicine (ABPM).

Since the development of AAPM, most of the organization's goals have been met:

1. The successful lobbying for a seat for pain medicine in the House of Delegates of the American Medical Association (AMA).
2. The successful establishment of a credentialing body, the American Board of Pain Medicine (formerly the American College of Pain Medicine), which offers annual credentialing examinations for eligible physicians. Among the many criteria, the minimum criterion is that candidates be ABMS board-certified in their primary specialty.
3. The establishment of *The Clinical Journal of Pain,* which initially served as the official journal of AAPM and has now been replaced with the journal *Pain Medicine.*

Additional goals include an attempt to establish uniform practice parameters and outcome measures for different pain modalities.

The American Board of Pain Medicine

The ABPM is the examination division of the AAPM, which serves the public by improving the quality of pain medicine through certification of pain specialists. It evaluates candidates who voluntarily appear for examination after a credentialing process and certifies them as *diplomates in pain medicine* if they successfully pass the examination process. This mission serves the public by helping ensure that the physicians passing the examination have an approved level of expertise and currency of knowledge in pain medicine. More than 2000 physicians have become diplomates of the ABPM.

The American Society of Regional Anesthesia and Pain Medicine

The American Society of Regional Anesthesia (ASRA) is the preeminent society on regional anesthesia. The society is based in the United States; other societies on regional anesthesia are based in Europe, Asia, and Latin America. Cognizant of the fact that anesthesiologists comprise the majority of pain medicine practitioners and interventional pain physicians and perform translational and clinical research, the ASRA started another annual meeting dealing exclusively with pain medicine. The annual meeting of the ASRA that deals with regional anesthesia is held in the spring, whereas their annual meeting on pain medicine is held in the fall. To better fulfill its mission, the ASRA has changed its name to the American Society of Regional Anesthesia and Pain Medicine and the name of their highly cited journal, *Regional Anesthesia*, to *Regional Anesthesia and Pain Medicine.* The journal is the official publication of the American, European, Asian and Oceanic, and Latin American Societies of Regional Anesthesia.

The American Society of Interventional Pain Physicians

The American Society of Interventional Pain Physicians (ASIPP) is a national organization representing the interests of interventional pain physicians in the United States. The society was founded in 1998 by Dr. Laxmaiah Manchikanti and associates for the purpose of improving the delivery of interventional pain management services to patients across the United States, whether in hospitals, ambulatory surgical centers, or medical offices. The ASIPP has an active political action committee, which has been instrumental in achieving numerous legislative victories benefiting its constituents and their patients. The goals of the ASIPP include the preservation of insurance coverage, coverage for interventional pain procedures, the advancement of patient safety, advancement of cost-effectiveness, and establishment of accountability in the performance of interventional procedures. Also included in the goals of the ASIPP are the pursuit of excellence in education in interventional pain management, the improvement of practice management, the enhancement of regulatory compliance, and the elimination of fraud and abuse. The ASIPP journal is indexed and called *Pain Physician.*

The American Academy of Hospice and Palliative Medicine

The American Academy of Hospice and Palliative Medicine (AAHPM) was founded in 1988 to advance the specialty of hospice medicine in the United States. The academy's goals include providing education and clinical practice standards, fostering research, facilitating personal and professional development, and sponsoring public policy advocacy for the terminally ill and their families. The academy's philosophy includes the belief that the proper role of the physician is to help the sick, even when cure is not possible. In addition, the academy aims to help patients achieve an appropriate and easy passage to death as one of the most important and rewarding services that a physician can provide. The academy endorses the philosophy that the medical profession should attend to all the needs of the dying patient and family, and should encourage and promote patient autonomy.

The American Academy of Orofacial Pain

The American Academy of Orofacial Pain (AAOP) is an organization of health care professionals dedicated to the alleviation of pain and suffering through education, research, and patient care in the field of orofacial pain and associated disorders. Goals of the AAOP include the establishment of acceptable criteria for the diagnosis and treatment of orofacial pain and temporomandibular disorders, sponsorship of annual meetings and a medical journal, and encouragement for the study of orofacial pain and tempo-romandibular disorders at undergraduate and postgraduate levels of dental education.

The American Academy of Pain Management

The American Academy of Pain Management (AAP Management), founded in 1988, is an inclusive interdisciplinary organization serving clinicians who treat people with pain through advocacy and education, and by setting standards of care. The AAP Management is open to a diverse group of pain clinicians, and emphasizes inclusivity of all health care specialties. The organization boasts a large, diverse membership and an online University of Integrated Studies that offers graduate-level online courses for health practitioners. In addition, there are various levels of pain credentialing available depending on the level of education of the student/practitioner.

American Society for Pain Management Nursing

Founded in 1990, the American Society for Pain Management Nursing (ASPMN) is an organization of professional nurses dedicated to promoting and providing optimal care of individuals with pain through education, standards, advocacy, and research. Their goals include providing access to specialized care for patients experiencing pain, providing education of the public regarding self-advocacy for their pain needs, and providing a network for nurses working in the pain management field. This society also sponsors educational conferences and is formulating a means of adding compensational value to the specialty of pain management nursing.

The National Headache Foundation

Founded in 1970, the National Headache Foundation (NHF) works to create an environment in which headaches are viewed as a legitimate health problem. The foundation's goals include the promotion of research into the causes and treatment of headache, and the education of the public regarding the legitimacy of headaches as a biologic disease.

The World Institute of Pain

The World Institute of Pain (WIP) is an international organization that aims to promote the best practice of pain medicine throughout the world. Its goals are to educate and train personnel of member pain centers by the utilization of local hands-on training international seminars and exchange of clinicians. Updating member pain centers with state-of-the-art pain information via newsletters, scientific seminars, and journal and book publications are additional goals. One of the most important goals of WIP is to develop an international examination process for testing and certifying qualified interventional pain physicians. Showing proficiency in both general pain knowledge and the safe performance of interventional procedures, the successful candidates are awarded the designation of *fellow of interventional pain practice* (FIPP). The journal of the WIP, *Pain Practice,* is indexed.

The World Society of Pain Clinicians

The World Society of Pain Clinicians (WSPC) is an international organization whose goals are to bring together clinicians with a common interest in the treatment of pain. Also, the goals are to stimulate education and learning in the field of pain, and to encourage the dissemination of information on pain throughout the world. The WSPC also endorses and encourages the audit and scientific research on all aspects of pain, especially treatment. The WSPC sponsors a biannual international congress of clinical aspects of pain and has its own journal, *Pain Clinic*.

The International Spine Interventional Society

The International Spine Interventional Society (ISIS) is a society of physicians interested in the development, implementation, and standardization of percutaneous techniques for precision diagnosis of spinal pain. The organization sponsors forums for exchange of ideas, encourages research undertaking, and holds public lectures. The mission of ISIS includes the consolidation of developments in diagnostic needle procedures, the identification and resolution of controversies, the public dissemination of developments, and the recommendation of standards of practice based on scientific data.

The International Neuromodulation Society

Founded in 1989, the International Neuromodulation Society (INS) is a multidisciplinary international society promoting therapeutic neuromodulation at a clinical and scientific level. The primary means of exchanging knowledge consist of regular scientific meetings and the journal *Neuromodulation*. The first national chapter of the INS was the American Neuromodulation Society.

American Pain Foundation

Founded in 1997 by three past presidents of the APS, the American Pain Foundation (APF) is an independent, nonprofit, grassroots organization serving people with pain through information, advocacy, and support. Its goals include serving as an information clearinghouse for people with pain, promoting recognition of pain as a critical health issue, and advocating for changes in professional training regulatory policies and health care delivery systems to ensure that people with pain have access to proper medical care. The APF was the first pain organization specifically formed to serve the interests of people experiencing pain associated with diverse disorders associated with the presence of significant pain.

The National Pain Foundation

Founded in 1998, the National Pain Foundation (NPF) seeks to advance the recovery of persons in pain through education, information, and support. The NPF empowers patients by helping them become actively involved in the design of their treatment plan. The organization's website has interactive features that encourage patients to identify the information that they need to manage their pain in the most understandable way. The NPF strives to fill the gap in the understanding, awareness, and accessibility of pain treatment options.

PAIN AND THE HOSPICE MOVEMENT

Hospice is a medieval term representing a welcome place of rest for pilgrims to the Holy Land. The concept of hospice dates back to the reign of Emperor Julian the Apostate when Fabiola, a Roman matron, created a place for sick and healthy travelers and cared for the dying.[40] Hospitals in general were regarded as Christian institutions, and in medieval times, most hospitals were used as hospices and vice versa.[41]

During the 11th century, several hospices were based in and operated by monasteries. The 17th century Catholic priest St. Vincent DePaul founded the Sisters of Charity in Paris as a home for the poor, the sick, and the dying. St. Vincent DePaul's work for the poor and the sick created a significant impact not only on the Catholic Church but also on other contemporary religions. The Protestant pastor Fliedner was so influenced that he founded Kaiserwerth 100 years later. Nuns from the Sisters of Charity and Kaiserwerth accompanied Florence Nightingale to Crimea to care for wounded soldiers and other citizens who were either sick or dying.[42]

In 1902, the Irish Sisters of Charity founded St. Joseph's Hospice, staffed by Cecily Saunders 50 years later. Dr. Saunders was the first full-time hospice medical officer, and she was regarded as the founder and medical director of St. Christopher's Hospice in England. She was initially trained as a nurse and served in the Second World War. After she became injured, she received training as a medical social worker. She subsequently developed a keen interest in terminal cancer patients and underwent training in medical school to become a physician. She emphasized the importance of taking the patient at his or her word during pain assessment and scheduling the dosing of opioids on a time-contingent basis as compared to an as-needed dosing schedule. She also advocated the need for frequent pain assessments so as to effectively manage cancer patients' pain. In addition, she sought to convince the medical community that it was totally unnecessary and inhumane for cancer patients to die in pain.[43] For all her efforts and leadership, she is regarded as the "mother of palliative care" and was knighted for her contributions to the hospice movement and the care of the dying cancer patient. Dame Saunders' views and works are widely taught in medical and nursing schools today and form the basis of palliative care.

PAIN AND THE FUTURE

Pain medicine has come a long way. A review of the history of pain demonstrates that until the time of Bonica, pain management was considered to be unimodal, unidisciplinary, and largely managed haphazardly and without any clear structural organization. Today, new drugs, innovative techniques, and creative procedures have expanded the scope of pain medicine. In addition, new research is contributing daily to modern concepts of pain and its management; these concepts are having positive effects on the development of pain medicine.

The contributions of the IASP, the WSPC, the AAPMed, the APS, and the many other international, national, regional, state, and local organizations devoted to pain and pain management are all having a significant impact on the dissemination of knowledge, promotion of research, and realization of networking on local, national, and international levels. Pain practitioners and investigators are no longer isolated, and a flurry of published manuscripts and textbooks now cover a wide array of pain medicine topics. Credentialing is well on its way, and two credible organizations are responsible for credentialing pain physicians in the United States. They include the diploma offered by the ABPM and the Certificate of Added Qualification by the American Board of Anesthesiology. Diplomas are offered by examination.

With the change in medical dynamics and the realities created by managed care and the different health maintenance organizations, pain medicine has had to redirect its strategies for effective delivery and fair reimbursement for services rendered. Many groups are dealing with these issues, and it is clear that the scientific community concerned with pain must develop reliable and reproducible outcome measures to maintain high quality and competence in the management of chronic pain.

The training of pain specialists is being given serious consideration, and it is likely that in addition to the current 1-year pain medicine fellowships, attempts will be made to establish residencies in pain medicine. It is clear that, in addition to offering these postgraduate measures, the administrators of medical schools must reevaluate their educational programs and must make their curricula more inclusive of pain medicine. With such changes taking place, the future of pain medicine looks bright as a result of the major contributions at all levels by dedicated and committed pain clinicians and researchers.

References

1. Procacci P, Maresca M: Evolution of the concept of pain. In Sicuteri F (ed): Advances in Pain Research and Therapy, vol. 20. New York, Raven Press, 1984, p 1.
2. Raj PP: Pain relief: Fact or fancy? Reg Anesth 1990;15:157.
3. Unruh AM: Voices from the past: Ancient views of pain in childhood. Clin J Pain 1992;8:247.
4. Caton D: The secularization of pain. Anesthesiology 1985; 62:93.
5. Warfield C: A history of pain relief. Hosp Pract 1988;7:121.
6. Jaros JA: The concept of pain. Crit Care Nurs Clin North Am 1991;1:1.
7. Procacci P, Maresca M: Pain concepts in Western civilization: A historical review. In Benedetti C (ed): Advances in Pain Research and Therapy, vol. 7. Recent Advances in the Management of Pain. New York, Raven Press, 1984, p 1.
8. Todd EM: Pain: Historical perspectives. In Aronoff GM (ed): Evaluation and Treatment of Chronic Pain. Baltimore, Urban and Schwarzenberg, 1985, p 1.
9. Castiglioni A: A History of Medicine. New York, Alfred A Knopf, 1947.
10. Lin Y: The Wisdom of India. London, Joseph, 1949.
11. Veith I: Huang Ti Ne Ching Su Wen. Baltimore, William & Wilkins, 1949.
12. Bonica JJ: Evolution of pain concepts and pain clinics. In Brena SF, Chapman SL (eds): Clinics in Anesthesiology: Chronic Pain: Management Principles 1985;3:1.
13. Bonica JJ: The Management of Pain. Philadelphia, Lea & Febiger, 1953.
14. Rey R: Antiquity. In History of Pain. XIII. Paris, Editions la Decouverte, 1993, p 19.
15. Keele KD: Anatomies of Pain. Oxford, Blackwell Science, 1957.
16. Schiff M: Lerbuch der Phusiologie der Muskel, und Nerven-physiologie, Schavenburg, Lahr, 1848.
17. Bliz M: Experimentelle Beitrag zur Lösung der Frage uber die spezifische Energie der Hautnerven. Z Biol 1884;20:141.
18. Goldscheider A: Die spezifische Energie der Gefuhlsnerven der Haut. Monatsschrift Prakt Germatol 1884;3:282.
19. von Frey M: Ber Verhandl Konig Sachs Ges Wiss. Beitr Zur Physiol des Schmerzsinnes 1894;45:185.
20. Mueller J: In Baly W (transl) Handbuch der Physiologie des Menschen. London, Taylor and Walton, 1840.
21. Darwin E: Zoonomia, or the Laws of Organic Life. London, J Johnson, 1794.
22. Erb WH: Krankheitender periperischen cerebrosphinalen Nerven. In Luckey G: Some recent studies of pain. Am J Psychol 1895;7:109.
23. Letievant E: Traites des Sections Nerveuses. Paris, JB Bailliere, 1873.
24. White JC, Sweet WH: Pain and the Neurosurgeon: A Forty-Year Experience. Springfield, Ill, Charles C Thomas, 1969.
25. Raj PP (ed): History of pain management. In Practical Management of Pain. Chicago, Year Book Medical Publishers, 1986, p 3.
26. Dogliotti AM: Traitement des syndromes douloureqx de la peripherie par alcoholisation sub-arachnoidienne. Presse Med 1931;39:1249.
27. Leriche R: Surgery of Pain. Baltimore, William & Wilkins, 1939.
28. Bonica JJ (ed): Cancer pain. In The Management of Pain (3rd ed.). Philadelphia, Lea & Febiger, 1990, p 400.
29. Melzack R, Wall PD: Pain mechanisms: A new theory. Science 1965;150:971.
30. Abram SE: Advances in chronic pain management since gate control. Reg Anesth 1993;18:66.
31. Turk DC, Okifuji A: Psychological factors in chronic pain: Evolution and revolution. J Consult Clin Psychol 2002;70:678.
32. Head H, Holmes G: Sensory disturbances from cerebral lesions. Brain 1911;34:102.
33. Marshall J: Sensory disturbances in cortical wounds with special reference to pain. J Neurol Neurosurg Psychiatry 1951;14:187.
34. Melzack R, Casey KL: Sensory, motivational and central control determinants of pain: A new conceptual model. In Kenshalo D (ed): The Skin Senses. Springfield, Ill, Charles C. Thomas, 1968, pp 423-443.
35. Fordyce WE: Psychological factors in the failed back. Int Disabil Stud 1988;10:29.
36. Fordyce WE: Behavioural science and chronic pain. Postgraduate Med J 1984;60:865.
37. Fordyce WE: Behavioral factors in pain. Neurosurg Clin N Am 1991;2:749.
38. Turk DC: Clinical effectiveness and cost-effectiveness of treatments for patients with chronic pain. Clin J Pain 2002;18:355.
39. Turk DC: Chronic non-malignant pain patients and health economic consequences. Eur J Pain 2002;6:353.
40. Craven J, Wald FS: Hospice case for dying patients. Am J Nurs 1993;75:1816.
41. Allan N: Hospice to hospital in the near east: An instance of continuity and change in late antiquity. Bull Hist Med 1990;64:446.
42. Campbell L: History of the hospice movement. Cancer Nurs 1986;9:333.
43. Saunders C: The last stages of life. Am J Nurs 1965;65:70.

2 Taxonomy and Classification of Chronic Pain Syndromes

Harold Merskey

DEFINING PAIN

The first task of the authors of any taxonomy is to know what they are talking about. Sometimes knowledge is taken for granted. A taxonomy of pain needs some understanding of the term itself. We all assume that we know the meaning of the word pain—and indeed we do. Nevertheless, for a long time, there was no unanimity about how to define pain. There still is no absolute unanimity but a consensus appears to have formed in favor of the definition of pain offered by the International Association for the Study of Pain in 1979[1] and subsequently published in the *Classification of Chronic Pain* produced by the International Association for the Study of Pain (IASP).[2] The definition of pain—"an unpleasant sensory and emotional experience associated with actual or potential tissue damage or described in terms of such damage"—was based upon an earlier one[3] that had achieved some recognition, which was intended to deal with the situation that whereas pain normally was understood to be the consequence of physically damaging stimulation or disorder in the body, many patients appeared to have pain but did not have overt tissue damage.

Morris[4] observed the key to the IASP definition is to dissolve any necessary connection between pain and tissue damage. It depends upon the usage of the word *pain* whether or not physical change is apparent. It is important to recognize that pain is always a subjective psychological state. At the same time, the note on this definition emphasized that pain "most often has a proximate physical cause."[3] The IASP definition has been adopted fairly broadly and helps minimize the idea that there is some sort of pain that patients imagine and that is not the same as the pain of "real injury or disease." In the personal opinion of this writer, much pain that is primarily organic in origin has an organic basis that is incompletely explained. Sometimes that happens for reasons of mere convenience, that is, every-day transient pain is usually not investigated nor does it need to be. At other times, it may happen because of difficulties in diagnosis even with chronic severe disorders. The lack of physical proof should never be taken on its own as a sufficient indicator of a psychological cause of pain.

THE NATURE OF CLASSIFICATION

Taxonomy means the arrangement of rules. *Taxonomy* as a term is derived from two Greek words—*tasso* and *nomia*—meaning "arrangement" and "rules." In other words, it deals with the principles of classification and not with the content of classifications. It is about how to set up a classification and not about the detail of what goes into it. It ordinarily applies to the science of the classification of living organisms. Classifications are also produced for nonliving organisms and material that was never alive.

There are two types of classification, natural and artificial. A *natural* classification deals with the material of physics and biology, and anything else in the natural world, such as types of stars or forms of animals, in other words, the material world. An *artificial* classification deals with the arrangement of the products of human activity, for example, the telephone directory.

In an artificial classification, there is no necessary connection between the basis on which the classification is produced and the inherent nature of the subject matter. Thus, the list of names in a telephone directory by alphabetical order is arbitrary but works extremely well.[5]

An ideal classification should not only be comprehensive it should also locate each item within it in a place of its own without overlap. The periodic table in chemistry is a wonderful example of scientific beauty and perfect or almost perfect classification wherein every element belongs in its own place relative to the other elements. In biology, a superior form of classification is phylogenetic by evolutionary relationships.

Medical classifications are established on a very different basis. In the International Classification of

Diseases (ICD-10),[6] the classification is arranged by causal agents such as infectious diseases or neoplasms; by systems of the body, such as cardiovascular or musculoskeletal; by symptom pattern and type of symptom as in psychiatric illnesses, and even by whether or not the condition or event is related to the artificial intervention of an operation. Illnesses or categories may be grouped by time of occurrence, such as congenital or perinatal disorders, and at the basic level are grouped as symptoms, signs, and abnormal clinical and laboratory findings.

In ICD-10, there is a code 080 for delivery in an uneventful case, including spontaneous breech delivery. Major groups are subdivided by system (e.g., neurology) and by symptom pattern (e.g., epilepsy or migraine); by the presence of hereditary or degenerative disease (e.g., Huntington's disease and hereditary ataxia); by location of disorder (e.g., extrapyramidal disorders); by anatomic and physiologic characteristics (e.g., extrapyramidal and movement disorders, such as Parkinson's disease and dystonia); by location (e.g., polyneuropathies), and by infectious and chemical causes. In those approaches, categories overlap repeatedly. Pain is found in the group of symptoms, signs, and clinical and laboratory findings as "R52–pain not elsewhere classified." This particular code excludes some 19 others that reflect pain in different parts of the body and excludes "psychogenic" pain (code F45.4) and renal colic (N33). Thus pain occurs at various levels of diagnosis and categorization in the ICD-10.

The overlap found in medicine is inevitable. There must always be some provision for conditions that are not well described and that will overlap with others that are well described. The purposes of medicine require attention to many different aspects of disease that enter into the classifications. That should be apparent from the examples cited.

WHICH PAINS NEED CLASSIFICATION

From the point of view of a pain practitioner, only some pains need classification and indeed it would be inappropriate to classify all pains in a chronic pain classification. A large proportion of the pain that human beings and other creatures experience in the world is brief and transitory. As a rule, it results in overt damage that needs its own appropriate treatment or passes off quickly. Pain is the most common symptom in the whole of medicine. Therefore any attempt to classify all pain would inevitably lead to an overall classification of medicine that would have a particular focus that is unnecessary for most medical cases. Those illnesses with pain that have needed a special classification are those where pain is a significant persistent problem. This conclusion still leaves a large field for a classification of pain but saves the pain specialist from having to write the classification for all the rest of medicine as well.

Among specific systems of classification, the ICD-10 is used worldwide for the purpose of documenting mortality and morbidity.[6] In the United States, a slightly modified version of the previous international system of classification, namely ICD-9CM, is used. (CM stands for Clinical Modification.) This modification is promoted by the US government to provide the additional data required by clinicians, researchers, epidemiologists, medical record librarians, and administrators of inpatient and outpatient community programs. In the United States, ICD-9CM is published by the Department of Health and Human Services, Public Health Services, Health Care Financing Administration.

The international system ICD-10 comprises a table of names and numerical codes for them. ICD-10 consists of three volumes. Volume I is a tabular list that contains the report of the International Conference for the 10th revision, the classification itself at the three- and four-character levels, a classification of the morphology of neoplasms, a special tabulation list for mortality and morbidity, definitions, and the nomenclature regulations. Volume II includes an instruction manual, and Volume III is an alphabetical index. The latter also includes expanded instructions on the use of the index.

In the United States, ICD-9CM coding has particular importance because of the 1988 Medical Catastrophic Coverage Act, which although later repealed, required the use of ICD-9 codes on "Medicare Part B" claims. This requirement continued with ICD-9CM and to date (March 2006) ICD-9CM has not been replaced within the United States. Pain specialists within the United States may feel that the ICD-9CM classification does not cover their requirements for appropriate billing of work done and may prefer a pain-based classification.

Of course, classifications have a number of purposes besides billing. The primary one is to exchange standardized information so that "stroke" or "cholecystitis" or "depressive disorder" has the same meaning to different colleagues. Meanings should be the same both within the same country and throughout the world. This should facilitate statistical comparisons of the occurrence and management of disease and serve as a basic tool for scientific progress by establishing standards of diagnosis and description that can be compared between workers within countries and internationally.

Such classification can help provide understanding of disorders but it does so only by giving shape to the advances of investigators, whether alone or in working groups, or in national and international organizations. Classifications also serve as a means of recognizing work done and providing standards for payment. This is one of the reasons for their relative popularity with both medical professionals and administrators.

Classifications, of necessity, cannot provide "absolute truth." Thus even when a classification recognizes a disorder as a "condition," a "disorder," or a "disease," it is not the classification that provides the knowledge that justifies these various titles but rather it is the existing level of scientific knowledge. To the extent that a classification identifies current scientific knowledge and claims it to be acceptable, it may establish unity, but classification as a rule only follows scientific knowledge.

This also means that just as classifications take material as they find them, they are not expected to provide perfect decisions or standards by which we state that something is "a disease," a "disorder," a "syndrome," or merely a "symptom." The one word out of these four for which the meaning is not in dispute is *symptom,* the patient's statement of a complaint. All four words involve or have involved some dispute as to whether they reflect the true nature of the phenomena with which physicians deal. Physicians become concerned about whether they recognize something as a disease or "only a syndrome" or "just a symptom." It is not the function of a classification to determine the answers to such questions. In fact, it can be extraordinarily hard to determine what constitutes a syndrome and whether diseases should have a fixed standard.[7]

THE INTERNATIONAL ASSOCIATION FOR THE STUDY OF PAIN CLASSIFICATION

The IASP classification focuses on chronic pain. A small number of pain syndromes that are not necessarily chronic were included for comparative purposes because they might be relevant to pain specialists (e.g., acute herpes zoster, burns with spasm, pancreatitis, prolapsed intervertebral disk) or because the acute version frequently becomes chronic. The classification is based on five axes. The first axis is anatomic localization, which was chosen for both historical and practical reasons. The historical reasons are that there was previous difficulty in establishing a chronic pain classification based upon etiology and that there was too much argument or potential argument about causes. It was also recognized that in essence pain is referred to parts of the body, and it is always a somatic symptom, whatever its cause. As well, location provides a useful means of distinction between different conditions. Accordingly, the IASP classification presents a list of relatively generalized syndromes followed by regional ones. The relatively generalized syndromes include peripheral neuropathy, stump pain, phantom pain, complex regional pain syndrome, central pain, syringomyelia, polymyalgia rheumatica, fibromyalgia, rheumatoid arthritis, and so forth. Pain of psychological origin is included. The relatively localized syndromes are subdivided according to whether they are in the head and neck, limbs, thorax, or abdomen, or whether they have a spinal or radicular distribution or origin.

The IASP classification set out to provide categories and codes for all the relevant conditions. Not all pain is continuously chronic. Some pain that is severe *and* chronic remits between episodes, for example, migraine and cluster headache, but these types of pain are also included under the rubric of chronic pain. Some chronic pain is pain that persists past what has usually been considered to be the normal time of healing. But that is not always the case and the decision as to what constitutes the normal time of healing is much argued. Indeed, it is now understood—as it was not so well understood in 1986 with the first edition of the classification—that pathophysiologic processes may well maintain pain long after the normal expectation of pain from injury has ended. I personally question whether we should even mention the normal time of healing in discussing chronic pain.

Be that as it may, the IASP Taxonomy Committee recognized that some pain persists despite apparent explanation, other pain persists with an explanation (e.g., the pain of osteoarthritis), and still other pain, which is not always continuous, can recur. These pains, by virtue of their intractability, were considered proper subjects for a classification of chronic pain.

MULTIPLE AXES

An anatomic classification alone is not sufficient. Some effort has to be made, even if it is tentative, to describe the nature of the pain and different types of pain, to note the system in which it occurs, and to set up a system that indicates which disturbance seems to be most responsible for the pain, to describe the features of the pain even though the features might vary within diagnoses, and to attribute cause when possible. Accordingly, the classification of chronic pain specifies five axes for describing pain.

The first axis is the anatomic axis, and the second axis is the system most related to the cause of the pain (besides the nervous system, which is always involved in pain). The systems identified were (1) central, peripheral, and autonomic nervous system and special senses; (2) psychological and social function of the nervous system (which was given a separate coding); (3) respiratory and vascular systems; (4) the musculoskeletal system and connective tissue; (5) cutaneous, subcutaneous tissue, and associated glands (e.g., breast, apocrine), the gastrointestinal system, the genitourinary system, other organs or viscera (e.g., thyroid, lymphatic); (6) unknown systems. A code was also allowed wherein more than one system was found to contribute to the pain.

The third axis describes the temporal characteristics of pain and the pattern of occurrence. A code was allowed for places where temporal patterns were not recorded but distinctions were made as follows: single episode, continuous or nearly continuous, nonfluctuating or fluctuating, recurring irregularly, paroxysmal (e.g., tic douloureux), occurring regularly (e.g., premenstrual pain), sustained with superimposed paroxysms and other combinations, and none of the above.

The fourth axis accepts statements of intensity and the fifth axis identifies etiology. Causes can include genetic or congenital disorders; operations; burns; infection; inflammation; neoplasm; toxic, metabolic, degenerative, mechanical, or functional (including psychophysiologic) causes; or those resulting from ideas (e.g., conversion hysteria or depressive hallucination—both of which are either hard to show or particularly rare).

The actual system has served well as a guide to making a diagnosis and in establishing priorities in making a diagnosis. It has served poorly as a means of exchanging information on certain cases of different sorts. Thus I do not think I have seen any example of a study in which pain was selected solely on the basis that it had a particular pattern on the third axis, such as *continuous* or *nearly continuous*. These features have of course been found and reported frequently in studies in which the patients were selected on other criteria (e.g., the anatomic location or the etiologic diagnosis, to take the first and the fifth axes). The system however does provide fairly well for individual codes to be given if they are required for a specific study of a group, mainly relying on the anatomic systemic and diagnostic axes (e.g., I, II, and V). The third axis, namely the temporal characteristics, only serves well to identify continuous or discontinuous pain and that is often merely a feature of the diagnosis and not a feature of the selection of cases or the exchange of information. The fourth axis also has contributed relatively little in its present shape, with intensity often being recorded separately from the diagnosis.

The codes can serve as a means to identify unique patterns. Each of the five axes provides a place in the code for a condition. However, Vervest and Schimmer[8] showed that not all the codes are unique and allowance is made for that by adding letters a, b, c, and so forth to the five-number code where necessary.

Chronic pain was defined as pain that had been present for more than 6 months. It was thought that although many pains became persistent and chronic at 3 months, a 6-month division did not present difficulties in practice and was fairly characteristic, serving as a good entry to the population treated by pain specialists. The term *chronic pain* was not intended, and still is not intended, to mean a particular syndrome or pattern, and the notion of "chronic pain syndrome" that tends to mix physical and psychological consequences of pain was not accepted by the Taxonomy Committee of the IASP. In its deliberations, the committee proceeded to adopt an anatomic classification as the starting point for its classification of chronic pain on a model originally developed by John Bonica.[9]

PARTICULAR DIAGNOSES

The provision of categories is particularly useful where existing knowledge of painful syndromes is weak. For example, the understanding of reflex sympathetic dystrophy, whose name was changed on the advice of a special subcommittee to *complex regional pain syndrome* (CRPS) type I, has served as a means for identifying criteria that would provide either a clinical means for agreement between different investigators or a special sample for research purposes. In this case, the first step taken in conjunction with the classification system was to define CRPS type I merely by its clinical phenomena and not by its theoretic

relationship to the sympathetic nervous system. The second step, taken more recently,[10] proposed changes to diagnostic criteria that provided both clinical diagnostic criteria for general use and more stringent research diagnostic criteria for specific research investigations. This seems to be a satisfactory solution to the problem of how many people may claim the label and what sort of cases concomitantly should be studied for research to establish convincing evidence in the findings of research. Other examples where the classification has been useful include pioneering the spread of understanding about relatively new syndromes (e.g., the syndrome of painful legs and moving toes [see reference 3] or the syndrome of paroxysmal hemicrania). In these cases, the classification has given an appropriate place to syndromes that have not yet entered the general lexicon although they are described in the literature.

PSYCHIATRIC ASPECTS OF CHRONIC PAIN

Psychiatric aspects of chronic pain may be coded in two ways. The first recognizes that patients seen in clinical practice often have some degree of emotional difficulty in association with chronic pain. In such cases, the psychological changes are most often anxiety or depression and may be attributed to the persistence of pain causing distress, loss of employment, altered marital relationships, decline in self-image, and so forth, as well as independent events that cause depression or anxiety (e.g., bereavement or illness in a close relative). In these circumstances, it is important to describe the psychological status of patients, to understand why they are troubled, and to provide appropriate treatments, which first of all may be better analgesia but in addition may include antidepressant medication and social support. Whenever psychological help is requested, it should include assistance with the emotional difficulties, whether it be supportive or cognitive therapy. Behavioral therapy, as such, usually has only a very limited role to play in management of the secondary effects of pain but assistance in adjustment to pain can be of great importance and can involve rehabilitation experts.

The second option in regard to psychiatry and pain would be to see the psychological illness as a cause of pain. This is thought to be much less common as a sustained cause of pain than was originally suggested. Headache from emotional problems and precordial pain from anxiety are fairly typical examples of situations in which some pain, but less often chronic pain, may be due to depression or anxiety disorders. In such cases, after physical examination, psychiatric methods of care are appropriate. But these hardly ever account for the great majority of patients with chronic pain and emotional disturbance. One explanation that was formerly favored suggests that the pain solves a problem, but that explanation seems less and less realistic as time goes by and psychiatry has failed to prove by systematic methods that sustained pain results from chronic emotional disorder. We provided psychological categories notwithstanding; thus the IASP system laid down the following categories: pain of psychological origin: muscle tension; delusional hallucinatory; hysterical conversion or hypochondriacal; and associated with depression. Factitious illness and malingering were not included as disorders that were thought appropriate to describe as part of the psychiatric condition. It appears that these categories are not used much.

INTERNATIONAL PSYCHIATRIC CLASSIFICATIONS

The classification of mental and behavioral disorders recommended by the World Health Organization[11] is a part of the overall international classification. Categories have been established with an eye to agreement with the layout of the *Diagnostic and Statistical Manual, Fourth Edition (DSM-IV)* of the American Psychiatric Association (APA),[12] which is well known in many countries. The ICD-10 classification of mental and behavioral disorders preserves parallel categories to those used in DSM-IV, although the descriptions are often different. However the ICD-10 classification does not use the "checklist approach" but rather gives a general description and major criteria required. The APA DSM-IV and DSM-IV TR (in which the explanatory text changed but not the codes) retain the same criteria as each other.

With respect to pain, the options in both systems are as follows. First, any particular diagnosis such as schizophrenia or depression of some sort may be made and indicated as a cause of the patient's pain, where it is understood that the diagnosis applies and pain may be accepted as resulting from such conditions. Then, the ICD-10 classification provides a category of Pain Disorder, Somatoform Persistent (F45.44). This category in essence corresponds to what DSM-IV now calls Persistent Somatoform Pain Disorder as well. In the ICD-10, the predominant complaint is of persistent, severe, and distressing pain that cannot be explained fully by a physiologic process or a physical disorder. It is presumed to be of psychological origin but pain occurring during the course of depressive disorder or schizophrenia is not included. Pain due to known or inferred psychophysiologic mechanisms such as muscle tension pain or migraine, but which is still believed to have a psychogenic cause, is coded under Psychological or Behavioral Factors Associated with Disorders or Diseases Classified Elsewhere (e.g., muscle tension pain or migraine). In ICD-10, the most common problem is to differentiate this disorder from the histrionic elaboration of organically caused pain. Thus this category essentially is meant to deal with pain that serves an unconscious motive. For a number of practical reasons, that is an extremely difficult proposition to prove clinically.

Under DSM-IV the criteria are similarly stringent but the diagnosis is made much more frequently, both in the United States and Canada. According to the description of chronic pain disorder in the DSM-IV, the word *somatoform* was dropped from the title.

Pain disorder is the predominant focus of the clinical presentation, and it must cause significant stress or impairment in social, occupational, or other important areas of functioning. Psychological factors must be judged to have an important role in the onset, severity, exacerbation, or maintenance of the pain, and the symptom or deficit is not intentionally produced. This condition is not to be diagnosed if the pain is better accounted for by a mood, anxiety, or psychotic disorder or if it meets criteria for dyspareunia.

These criteria have the effect of limiting the condition to one that is not associated with significant depression or anxiety or that results from a physical illness. Within DSM-IV, two versions of pain disorder were allowed. One is "pain disorder associated with psychological factors" wherein the necessary criteria are met as above without psychologic illness being present. The other is "pain disorder associated with both psychological factors and a general medical condition." In this case the same rules apply as for pain disorder on its own, but it is thought that a physical condition may be present but not sufficient to account for a large part of the syndrome. It is stated as follows: "Both psychological factors and a general medical condition are judged to have important roles in the onset, severity, exacerbation, or maintenance of the pain." The associated general medical condition or anatomic site of the pain is coded separately.

In my observation, many diagnosticians who are sincerely interested in the patient's welfare welcome this category as a means for diagnosing a distressing psychological state to which they do not see an adequate physiologic or general medical explanation. In my view, that is not the way it should be used. It would only logically be justifiable having regard to the criteria for the cognate diagnoses, if it could be demonstrated that there was some psychological cause that was unconsciously producing the symptom at the same time as producing anxiety or depression; in other words, what used to be called *hysteria*. For reasons discussed elsewhere,[13] the diagnosis of pain as "a conversion disorder" can rarely be adequately made. Persons with doubts should try to imagine whether they could produce, by thinking about it, a physical symptom such as paralysis that they would maintain consciously and whether they could produce a state of feeling of chronic pain in themselves by reflecting on it, and then ask how is it possible that pain could be produced unconsciously if it cannot even be done consciously? Overall then, psychological diagnoses as causes of pain are not favored by this writer except in very limited situations. Occasional patients with classic depressive illness develop severe headache that goes away when the depression is better. Occasional patients with postherpetic neuralgia have much worse pain when they become depressed and much less pain when the depression is treated, but these are relatively rare and do not reflect the bulk either of general medical, neurologic, or psychiatric practice.

CONCLUSION

In conclusion, classification is required in medical practice in order to identify like phenomena observed by practitioners. There is no absolute rule as to what is a syndrome or classification. The basis for the use of different classification systems is outlined in this chapter.

References

1. Lindblom U, Merskey H, Mumford JM, et al: Pain terms: A current list with definitions and notes on usage. Pain 1979;Suppl 3:S215-S221.
2. Merskey H, Bogduk N (eds): Classification of Chronic Pain: Descriptions of Chronic Pain Syndromes and Definitions of Pain Terms, 2nd ed. Seattle, Wash, International Association for the Study of Pain, 1994.
3. Merskey H, Spear FG: Pain: Psychological and Psychiatric Aspects. London, Bailliere, Tindall & Cassell, 1967.
4. Morris D: The challenges of pain and suffering. In Jensen TS, Wilson PR, Rice SC (eds): Chronic Pain. London, Arnold, 2003, pp. 1-13.
5. Galbraith DI, Wilson DG: Biological Science: Principles and Patterns of Life. Toronto, Holt, Reinhart & Winston, 1966.
6. World Health Organization: International Statistical Classification of Diseases and Related Problems, 10th Revision (ICD-10). Geneva, World Heath Organization, 1992.
7. Merskey H: Variable meanings for the definition of disease. J Med Philos 1986;11:215-232.
8. Vervest A, Schimmer G: Taxonomy of pain of the IASP (Letter). Pain 1988;34:318-321.
9. Bonica JJ. The Management of Pain. Philadelphia, Lea & Febiger, 1953.
10. Harden RN, Bruehl SP: Diagnostic criteria: The statistical derivation of the four criterion factors. In Stanton-Hicks M, Harden RN (eds): CRPS Current Diagnosis and Therapy. Seattle, Wash, IASP Press, 2005, pp 45-58.
11. World Health Organization: The ICD-10 Classification of Mental and Behavioural Disorders: Clinical Descriptions and Diagnostic Guidelines. Geneva, World Health Organization, 1992.
12. American Psychiatric Association: Diagnostic and Statistical Manual of Mental Disorders, 4th ed (DSM-IV). Washington, DC, American Psychiatric Association, 1994.
13. Merskey H: Pain disorder, hysteria, or somatization? (Commentary). Pain Res Manage 2004;9:67-71.

3 Organizing an Inpatient Acute Pain Management Service

Beth H. Minzter and Alex Cahana

The only pain that is easy to treat, is the pain of others.

SIR WILLIAM OSLER

THE RATIONALE

The magnitude of the problems of undertreatment of acute pain has been described and reviewed extensively,[1-5] and the adverse impact of untreated pain on the recovery profile of surgical patients has been elucidated. Consequently, adequate pain control is regarded as a vital component of acute rehabilitation.[6-9] Kehlet has elegantly described the benefits of postoperative analgesia, epidural analgesia, and ablation of the surgical stress response as well as their impact on overall improved rehabilitation and patient outcome.[10,11]

The sequelae associated with surgical procedures result from various components of the stress response and include cardiopulmonary, infectious, and thromboembolic complications, cerebral dysfunction, nausea and gastrointestinal paralysis, fatigue, and prolonged convalescence. Throughout the process of organizing an acute pain program, it is helpful to keep the following statements in mind:

- The relief of postoperative pain provides subjective comfort as well as the inhibition of nociceptive impulses triggered by surgical trauma and allows for full return of movement and activity.
- Surgical stress responses are mostly inhibited by the neuraxial administration of local anesthetics; the administration of other agents, systemically or neuraxially, as well as infiltration of a local anesthetic agent, appears to contribute little toward the reduction of the classic endocrine metabolic and catabolic response to operative procedures, particularly in procedures performed below the umbilicus.[11]
- Parenteral opioids exaggerate the perioperative immunodepression already triggered by the neuroendocrine response to surgery; in contrast, epidural anesthesia and analgesia preserve perioperative immune function.[12]
- Optimal analgesia alone does not reduce postoperative morbidity for several reasons. The pain relief provided is often too brief, the post-operative care program is not formulated to take advantage of the physiologic effects afforded by epidural analgesia, and active rehabilitation is neither provided nor supported. To optimize post-operative outcome and provide a time-, energy-, and cost-effective acute pain program, one ideally should consider a program with multimodal interventions, including stress reduction with appropriate techniques and effective dynamic pain relief enhanced by early mobilization and oral nutrition.[13]

Detailed practice guidelines for acute pain management of patients in the operative, postoperative, and trauma phases as well as of patients with cancer pain have been published and are readily available.[14-16] The organization of an acute pain service, however, requires much more than just convincing departmental and hospital administrators that there is a need for adequate pain management of these patients. This chapter discusses the administrative process of translating this medical need into an efficiently functioning, patient-oriented service.

The provision of postoperative analgesia by anesthesiologists is common practice. The proficiency of anesthesiologists in systemic and regional analgesia is obvious, and their skills in peripheral and neuraxial blockade have led to the creation of primarily anesthesiology-based pain services, such as at Geneva University Hospital (HUG). An anesthesiology-based service, however, is only one option. Implementation of an interdisciplinary or multidisciplinary approach to acute pain management may involve surgical and/or nursing colleagues. One such model either partly or wholly employs nurse practitioners to provide 24-hour coverage and continuity of care, with various degrees of physician supervision depending on physician availability and affordability. The limited out-of-the-operating room resources of an anesthesiology department may hamper the role of anesthesiologists in postoperative pain management, and this may lead to the consideration of alternative models. At Vanderbilt University Medical Center (VUMC), surgeons have historically managed postsurgical intravenous (IV) patient-controlled analgesia (PCA) opioid administration and anesthesiologists manage all other forms of acute postoperative pain therapy. We also manage IV PCA opioid administration in patients with more complex problems about whom we are consulted.[17,18]

The following types of problems illustrate the consultations for IV PCA opioid management:
- History of drug abuse
- Coexisting medical conditions and associated multiple drug administration
- Postoperative pain superimposed on chronic pain
- Pain refractory to conventional IV PCA therapy
- Pain of multiple origin and site (e.g., trauma)

PERSONAL INVENTORY

Before beginning to organize an acute pain program, one might ask: *Am I sure I want to do this?* This question may seem unnecessary, but the successful formation of a responsive pain service requires a great deal of forethought and a major investment in time, energy, and money.

To establish and maintain a pain service requires a serious commitment from the medical director and his or her team, which may clash with operating room anesthesia practice and other obligations an anesthesiologist may have. These responsibilities must be discussed with the department chairman in advance because they often present as the first and the most formidable obstacle to consistent care. Until this question is seriously contemplated and answered in the affirmative, it is likely that all future efforts in organizing a pain service will be in vain.

The second question to be addressed is: *Am I qualified to run this service?* Just feeling comfortable with the placement of epidural catheters or the management of postoperative pain is not all that is needed to direct an acute pain service; competent leadership and administrative abilities are also required to develop a responsive, efficient pain service.

The corollaries to be addressed honestly are: *Am I qualified by education and temperament to start and then manage an acute pain service? Do I understand the financial aspects of such an endeavor?* Organizing and operating a pain service require expertise in developing guidelines and marketing plans in addition to a multitude of administrative skills.

ASSESSMENT OF THE NEED

Once the challenge of organizing an acute pain management service is accepted, assessment of the need is mandatory. *Is there a market for the service? What is the mission statement of the service* (Box 3–1)? There are two models from which to choose concerning the

---

BOX 3–1. VANDERBILT UNIVERSITY MEDICAL CENTER INPATIENT PAIN CONSULTANTS MISSION STATEMENT

The impetus for erecting the Inpatient Pain Consultants (IPC) stems from a group of practitioners extremely distressed over the undertreatment of the inpatient population. This, along with research interest, initiated an 18-month process of designing an acute pain consultant service. Once our model was finalized, the concept of IPC was presented to the executive body of our institute, chairpersons of various departments, deans of the medical and nursing schools, and the chief administrator. The four domains of practice include the:

1. Formation of a fluent *clinical* practice, treating all inpatients whose chief complaint is acute pain.
2. Use of the director's academic background to perform active *research* in interventional pain management.
3. Dissemination of pain management *education* to students, residents, and attendings, as well as to nurses and other staff.
4. Formation of an *administrative* and medical policy for inpatient pain care to ensure safe, efficacious, and cost-effective management.

---

question of the organization of acute pain service: (1) acute versus chronic or (2) malignant versus benign. One of the authors (A.C.) believes that the distinction between these definitions of pain symptoms is inappropriate for organizational matters and feels it is akin to establishing one clinic for patients with severe congestive heart failure and another for patients with "less severe" congestive heart failure. For organizational purposes, the other author (B.H.M.) tends to distinguish between acute postoperative and intractable pain syndromes, whether acute or chronic in nature, and then, within the latter category, to differentiate between benign and malignant processes. She finds that such categorization is particularly useful when developing a consultation service as an extension of the more traditional postoperative pain service. Hence, there are two services: *inpatient* and *outpatient*. This distinction recognizes and allows for the different resources required for these patient populations.

An acute postoperative pain management service often requires 24-hour, 7-day-a-week medical coverage, with an appropriate call response time. Concerns regarding postoperative patients often need to be evaluated more urgently than consultations for other hospitalized patients who have pain issues, and expectations from both patients and referring physicians need to be recognized and addressed.

The consultation service must be comprehensive in its ability to provide an initial evaluation within 24 hours of a request and to provide daily follow-up visits and recommendations until everyone involved in the care of the patient agrees that the problem for which the consultation was requested has been handled. This often requires multiple phone calls, additional studies, and communication with several residents and attending physicians on various services. Familiarity with hospital facilities and ancillary services is crucial to provide comprehensive and professional consultation. Follow-up care may be necessary, and this demands collaboration with the outpatient pain center staff.

We have found that a resourceful nurse practitioner who is educated in pain management can be extremely helpful with initial evaluations, continuity of patient care and follow-up, coordination of clinical studies, operating room procedures, and billing issues and overall functioning of the service. In our experience, the input and networking provided by our nurse practitioner have been invaluable to the development and maintenance of both the acute and consultation arms of the inpatient service and have greatly enhanced patient and referring physician satisfaction.

When assessing the need, one must determine the size of the population to be served, the willingness of physicians from adjacent communities to refer their patients to one's institution, and the availability of ancillary facilities within the institution. While one must recognize the existence of competitors in a tight managed care environment, it is also crucial to identify other health care providers who are committed to inpatient pain control and to develop good working relationships with them. Collaborative efforts on a continuing basis often enable everyone involved to coordinate the services offered, and they expand one's market base in the long term, with overall improved outcome, referral satisfaction, and reimbursement. It is an error to assume that one is working in a vacuum—such shortsightedness eventually impedes the success of the pain service one is directing.

DEFINITION OF THE SERVICE

Once institutional and community needs have been identified and the mission statement has been formulated, it is necessary to define resources in accordance with one's therapeutic approach. The modalities necessary to treat acute pain effectively are diverse and demand varied resources. Although it is always better to obtain the necessary resources after a therapeutic approach has been chosen, in this imperfect world the process must often be reversed. It is common to tailor the service according to the availability of personnel, skills, medications, and equipment rather than to meet the requirements of the ideal therapeutic goals.

The feasibility of various treatment plans based on the availability of resources has been defined by the International Association for the Study of Pain (IASP) task force on the management of acute pain (Box 3–2 and Table 3–1).[19] We believe that, when possible, the

BOX 3–2. RESOURCE CHECKLIST

Oral/rectal non-opioid analgesics	_____
Oral/rectal opioid analgesics	_____
Parenteral opioids	_____
Subcutaneous, intramuscular	_____
Intravenous bolus, infusion	_____
Local anesthetic infiltration	_____
Patient-controlled analgesia	_____
Ketamine	_____
Nitrous oxide	_____
Transcutaneous electrical nerve stimulation (TENS)	_____
Plexus/neuraxial local anesthetics	_____
Interpleural local anesthetics	_____
Intraspinal opioids	_____
Expert treatment of psychological problems	_____
Comprehensive care using any combination of the options above	_____

organization of the service should allow for individualized care so that maximum improvement in outcome and optimal cost-effectiveness can be achieved. This necessitates anticipating the various therapeutic options that may be considered and requesting the necessary support and resources from the institution's administrative, business, and clinical departments when one is negotiating the development of the service.

After resources are defined in concert with the mission statement of the service, it is imperative to assess the safety of the proposed plan. Additional treatment options must meet the minimum requirements, as outlined previously. The principles of therapy to be implemented in the practice of pain medicine should allow one to:

1. Evaluate the source and severity of pain.
2. Understand the relationship between pain and other components of suffering and provide palliative measures.
3. Achieve and maintain adequate analgesia and incorporate it into the acute rehabilitation scheme.
4. Refine therapy based on individual needs.

After available resources are identified, the type of service that can be organized must be determined.[20] A *single-modality service* allows for the provision of analgesia with IV opioid systems to all inpatients and of regional analgesia in selected instances. This model can be nurse-based with physician supervision, and it offers a limited yet cost-effective method to treat postoperative patients.[21] A *multimodal service* includes diverse health care professionals from a variety of domains. They bring varied essential and valuable expertise that is important in optimizing the care of inpatients with pain problems. These practitioners may include psychologists, pharmacists, physical therapists, and a nutritionist (like we have in HUG). This multimodal service may function in a consul-

Table 3–1. Options for Acute Pain Treatment Based on Available Resources

ANALGESIC TECHNIQUE	PERSONNEL*	KNOWLEDGE	SKILLS†	EQUIPMENT‡	COMMENT§
Basic anxiety reduction	Any	Human nature			1, 8, 9
PO/PR non-opioids	A, B	Dose, range, side effects	M, N		1, 8, 9
PO/PR opioids	A, B	Dose, range, side effects	M, N		1, 8, 9
SC/IM opioids	A, B, G	Dose, range, side effects	M, N, O, R	T	1, 8, 9
IV opioids	A, B, G	Dose, range, side effects, loading, titration	M, N, O, P, R	T, U, W, X, Y	1, 8, 9
Local anesthetic infiltration	B	Anatomy, dose, range, side effects	M, R, S T		4, 7
Opioid PCA	A, C or E, G	Dose, range, side effects, PCA principles	M, N, P	U, V, X, Y	8, 9
Ketamine	C	Dose, range, side effects	M, N, P, R	U, W, X, Y	4
Nitrous oxide	B	Dose, range, side effects, administration	M, N, R	Delivery system	4, 8
TENS	A, B	Anatomy	M	Units, accessories	Adjunct therapy
Intraspinal opioids	A, C, E	Dose, range, side effects	M, N, P, Q, R	T, U, W, X, Z	1, 2, 8, 9
Plexus blocks	A, C	Dose, range, side effects, anatomy	M, N, P, Q, R, S	T, W, X, Y	2
Neuraxial block	A, C	Dose, range, side effects, anatomy	M, N, P, Q, R, S	T, U, W, X, Y, Z	1, 2, 3, 5, 6, 7, 8
Interpleural	A, C, D, E	Dose, range, side effects, anatomy	M, N, P, Q, R, S	T, U, W, X, Y, Z	1, 3, 7
Cryoanalgesia	E, D	Anatomy		Delivery system	1, 3, 7
Psychological support	A, B, C, D, E, F	Coping strategies	Relaxation, breathing exercises		Time-consuming, adjunct
Acute pain service	A, C, D, E, F, G	All of the above	M, N, O, P, Q, R, S leadership	All of the above	Policies, procedures, education, quality assurance

Personnel: A: Nurse; B: Physician; C: Anesthesiologist; D: Surgeon; E: Pain specialist; F: Psychologist; G: Pharmacist.
†*Skills*: M: Evaluate effects; N: Monitor; O: Injection technique; P: Start IV; Q: Block technique; R: Support ventilation; S: Treat convulsion.
‡*Equipment*: T: Needles, syringes; U: IV equipment; V: PCA equipment; W: PPV equipment; X: Oxygen; Y: Suction; Z: Epidural catheters.
§*Comments*: 1: Dose regularly; 2: Continuous infusion; 3: Tachyphylaxis; 4: Aspiration; 5: Possible hypotension; 6: Possible high block; 7: Possible convulsion; 8: Hypoventilation; 9: Antagonist available.
IM, intramuscular; IV, intravenous; PCA, patient-controlled analgesia; PO, by mouth; PR, by rectum; SC, subcutaneous; TENS, transcutaneous electrical nerve stimulation.

tant capacity for inpatients with complicated pain issues, such as patients with chronic pain suffering from acute exacerbations and postsurgical patients who are long-term opioid users.[22]

Depending on the geographic area (state) and the level of physician involvement, reimbursement for care rendered by an acute pain service ranges from 85% to 100% of the total fee. At HUG and VUMC, acute pain consultants (APCs) can recover 100% of charges billed by the nurse practitioner supervised by a physician. Additionally, under Swiss law the nurse practitioner has full consulting privileges, affording the service optimal staffing flexibility. These billing and prescriptive regulations differ according to state and geographic availability of health care personnel.

The most complex and expensive yet versatile service is a *multidisciplinary* or *interdisciplinary* type in which all practitioners meet regularly to evaluate inpatients and design individualized care plans. The goal is to implement the concept of balanced analgesia, a multifaceted regimen involving pharmacological treatment, physical medicine and rehabilitation, physical therapy, psychological support, alternative and behavioral medicine, neurology, anesthesiology, and invasive techniques. The rehabilitative approach prevails in this system, and palliative measures are employed in an effort to return the patient to functionality as soon as possible. Ideally, this service would provide 24-hour medical coverage and would be engaged actively in medical research, education, and continuous quality improvement.[23-25] Few hospitals have this type of fully integrated pain service that also provides advanced training in newer techniques of acute and interventional pain management. Practical limitations cause many institutions not to endorse this approach despite the favorable cost-benefit ratio when it is applied optimally to a carefully selected patient population.[26,27]

THE BUSINESS PLAN

Once it is determined that the client base comfortably matches the *assessment of need* so that the proposed acute pain service is both affordable and profitable, it is time to construct a business plan. Often this can be the most difficult phase, since the financial and business skills may be lacking. The purpose of the business plan is to describe the component arms of the service and to outline its organizational strategy, marketing plan, tentative schedule for implementation, and overall cost. This must occur before the first cent is spent on the project.

The business plan has two components. The first is a narrative that includes the mission statement (see Box 3–1), the structure, and the responsibilities of the service. This document must include job descriptions of the personnel involved as well as facility requirements and a marketing plan. Vital to this section are manuals for attending physicians and house staff and nursing personnel outlining guidelines and expectations (Appendices 3–1, 3–2, and 3–3). The second component is prepared as a spreadsheet. It includes estimates for fixed and variable incomes, the start-up capital necessary until revenues produce profits, and a month-by-month expenditure estimate for at least the first year (Fig. 3–1). These estimates need to be as detailed as possible and include an analysis of reimbursement issues.

The payer mix, or the percentage of the population that is served by health maintenance (HMO), preferred provider (PPO), and medical care (MCO) organizations, must be determined. It may be necessary to meet with local health plan administrators to assess whether preauthorization is necessary for reimbursement. To prepare for this section, the monthly patient load should be estimated and the number of patients needed to support service expenses calculated. If patient referral appears to be insufficient, explore other sources such as nonsurgical patients hospitalized with acute exacerbations of pain and cancer patients with pain. When assessing these sources, be sure that reimbursement will adequately cover the expense of additional time, energy, and personnel required to follow up and document inpatient daily care.

It is crucial to be aware of current Centers for Medicare and Medicaid Services (CMS) guidelines for documentation and billing and to remain informed about modifications as they occur (in Switzerland we call this TarMed). Not only can this have an impact on reimbursement, but also today's climate includes the possibility of severe fines and even criminal charges for fraud if there are discrepancies between CMS and physician interpretation of components of documentation. Examples of institutional suggestions regarding chart notation and consult documentation are found in Appendix 3–4A, B, and C.

FINANCE AND MARKETING

At the inception of the acute/inpatient pain service it is best to shift fixed costs (e.g., permanent employees) to variable costs (e.g., temporary) as much as possible. This provides financial flexibility as the patient load increases and the service needs change. Determining a revenue estimate requires assessing an approximate charge per patient. It is essential to develop several patient charge averages if different therapeutic modalities are to be employed. In the construction of the business plan, total revenue minus total cost will produce a *predicted* financial position. It is important to hope for the best and to plan for the worst-case scenario.

Billing and Collection

Even the well-organized service cannot succeed if efficient billing and collection services are not instituted initially. Employing an outside billing and collection service with a percentage-based contract is usually more reliable than using an internal group. However, if an internal billing and collection group is selected or mandated by the institution, then knowledgeable personnel, appropriate computer hardware, and software for data collection are prerequisites.

At HUG we use an internal billing service and designate specific personnel to handle our paperwork. The nurse practitioner, the director, and one of the physicians designed several billing sheets to simplify the system for the billing office personnel. We have worked closely with them to eliminate errors proactively and to educate and promote interest in our efforts (Appendix 3–5A, B, C). Residents, fellows, and attending physicians are continually reminded so that appropriate billing material is collected and documented in a timely and organized fashion; this is outlined carefully in the HUG acute/inpatient pain manual (see Appendix 3–2).

A computer-generated commercial spreadsheet with predesignated CPT (Current Procedural Terminology) codes was purchased to document and trend patient and procedure census as well as to stratify billing. The APC nurse practitioner keeps track of reimbursement, collections, changes in referral patterns, consultations, patient satisfaction, and predicted needs for the future with a variety of data entry systems modified to fit our needs. With this system, we can document growth as well as generate data to support future requests to the hospital administration to fund increasing equipment, space, and staffing demands (see Appendix 3–5D).

Payment for pain services may change from a fee-for-service model to a managed care model. Thus, the following points must be addressed:
- The price structure must be profitable and may or may not be reflected in reimbursement and collections.
- Analysis must include a review of CPT codes used over the previous 12 months to define case mix.

VUMC Inpatient Pain Consultants (IPC)

	Total annual	Jan	Feb	March	Apr	May	June	July	Aug	Sep	Oct	Nov	Dec
Patient census													
Epidural													
Nerve block													
Consults													
Total patient census													
Revenue													
Epidural													
Nerve block													
Consults													
Total revenue													
Deductions													
80% coverage													
Billing expenses													
Total deductions													
Net Revenue													
Program personnel													
Medical director													
Nurse practitioner													
Pain fellow													
Physical therapy													
Psychologist													
Social worker													
Total program personnel													
Office personnel													
Secretary/receptionist													
Office manager													
Total office personnel													

Figure 3–1. Sample spreadsheet used by Vanderbilt University Medical Center (VUMC) Inpatient Pain Consultants. (Courtesy of Vanderbilt University Medical Center, Nashville, Tenn.)

Administrative costs
Accounting fee
Quality assurance
Total administrative cost

Marketing costs
Advertising
Brochures
Announcements
Lectures/slides
Total marketing costs

Office operation
Books
Insurance program
Laundry/linen
Magazines
Medical supplies
Phone line
Postal/Fed Ex
Printing
Maintenance
Stationery
Office supply
Transcription
Miscellaneous
Total office operation

Property, equipment
Rental
Hardware/software
Startup equipment
Total property, equipment

Total Expenses

Net Operating Income

Figure 3–1, cont'd. Sample spreadsheet used by Vanderbilt University Medical Center (VUMC) Inpatient Pain Consultants. (Courtesy of Vanderbilt University Medical Center, Nashville, Tenn.)

- The actual CPT reimbursement must be calculated to define a negotiating basis with insurers.
- Capitation rates of similar contracts for other services in the region should be learned.
- A reasonable safeguard when negotiating capitation contracts is to determine renegotiation conditions if actual costs exceed the projected ones.[28,29] At HUG, we are not able to negotiate our own contracts, so we must rely on the administration. Each individual situation must be evaluated carefully to assess accurately the profit structure of the services offered to the institution.

Financing

Financing an inpatient service should be straightforward, based on hospital and departmental commitment. The tertiary care, academic institution should demand an efficient and highly capable acute pain consultant group to attend to its postoperative and oncology patient populations. If this is not the case, however, other options must be considered, similar to those pursued in the non-academic environment. Once capitalization requirements have been determined, a joint venture with physician or nonphysician investors may provide the necessary financing. There is a limited partnership between those who provide the capital and those who generate it. The relationship within the partnership is legally binding, and losses are limited to the extent of investment.

Another source of financing is a practice loan, wherein the practitioners borrow money using conventional loan sources. It is wise to obtain a credit line for unforeseen emergencies or faulty planning.

Finally, use of personal capital may generate funds, but we do not recommend this option unless there is assurance of a comprehensive consultation service with a committed referral base and a supportive community of physicians.

Marketing Plan

The last step in establishing an acute/inpatient consultation service is to have an overall marketing plan. Conventional medical education has not equipped most physician clinicians to understand and deal effectively with the dynamics of marketing and media. Help can be garnered from the hospital public relations office or from a private marketing firm. The marketing plan should reflect the budget allocated to the entire service. Marketing strategy must present a consistent message emphasizing the added value of the service to patient care. Ethical standards and medical practice may vary regionally, making marketing a delicate job. The components to be addressed include announcements and brochures, professionally prepared stationery, logo, newsletters, and websites. This advertisement does not replace concerned, compassionate, and effective care but rather explains the nature of the service to the general population.

Internal marketing is also important. Education is a vital part of marketing an acute pain service. Frequent interactions with other departments and their personnel (e.g., in the form of interdepartmental case conferences) is crucial to increasing the visibility of the service and expanding the referral base. In a teaching hospital, involvement of residents from other departments as well as from anesthesiology is helpful. The nurse practitioner or coordinator of the service can be instrumental in educating nurses, setting and changing institutional policies, and empowering the nursing staff in pain management issues.

It is also necessary to continuously assess patient satisfaction and to respond to changes in patient care needs. Quality assurance can be handled on a departmental or institutional level or internally by pain service personnel themselves. At HUG we ask patients a series of simple questions designed to measure overall patient satisfaction and the effectiveness of the service (Appendix 3–6C). The data are maintained and distributed to APC staff on a regular basis for review. We have modified all the policies and forms that pertain to epidural analgesia and opioids (see Appendix 3–6A and B) and have instituted accredited nursing programs regarding the importance of pain management, epidural analgesia, and monitoring parameters. Nurses from several patient units are involved in evaluating pain tools and equipment. Feedback is encouraged when these tools and equipment are implemented to optimize communication and patient care, comfort, and satisfaction.

Anesthesia residents rotate through the acute pain service separate from their outpatient responsibilities and are encouraged to follow the guidelines outlined in our APC manual. The pain fellows also rotate through the APC and are exposed to a variety of consultations. They are encouraged to follow these patients on an outpatient basis in the chronic clinic facility. Every effort is made to educate the residents and staff of other services, particularly our surgical colleagues, about acute pain management techniques and rehabilitation-oriented treatment modalities in an effort to improve patient outcome.

Marketing and funding of an acute and inpatient pain consultation service should be facilitated by the efforts of The Joint Commission (TJC) to make pain assessment and management a priority in the nation's health care system.

TJC's standard of pain care has created a new working framework that gives pain management much greater attention. The new standards expand the patient's right to adequate pain assessment and treatment, explicitly acknowledging that pain is a coexisting condition with a number of diseases and injuries and that it requires explicit attention. The new standards require staff education and competency determination and address education of patients and their families. Implementation and compliance with these standards should serve to make pain a top priority.

CONCLUSION

The need to treat pain adequately is well established, and the practice guidelines have been in existence for some time. This is due to the efforts of our predecessors, who coined terms such as multidisciplinary approach, programmed convalescence, balanced analgesia, and preemptive analgesia.[30-32] The distance between this medical need and its translation into a practical and attainable model is great. In these days of medico-legal liability and cost containment, barriers to the establishment of such a service may seem insurmountable. It is important to recognize the problems and pitfalls likely to be encountered during the creation and subsequent management of an acute inpatient pain service. By doing so, some problems can be avoided and appropriate responses to others can be formulated. An efficient and dynamic organizational framework can make acute pain practice feasible and successful. For practical tips please refer to items 1 through 9 of Appendix 3–7.

Acknowledgments

We remain indebted to Ramiah Ramasubramanian, MD, and Barbara Grimm, MSN, for their invaluable contributions to the original manuscript, and to John W. Downing, MD, for helping us make the Acute Pain Management Service at VUMC a reality. We are indebted to the teams of Post-operative and Interventional Pain Management Services for their Sisyphean work with very difficult patients and to Mr. Henrik Weibel for help in obtaining and maintaining the ISO 9001 certification of quality.

References

1. Macintyre PE, Ready LB: Acute Pain Management: A Practical Guide. Philadelphia, WB Saunders, 1996.
2. Ward SE, Gordon D: Application of the APS quality assurance standards. Pain 1994;56:199-306.
3. Miaskowski C, Nicholas R, Brody R, et al: Assessment of patient satisfaction utilizing the APS quality assurance guidelines on acute and cancer pain. J Pain Symptom Manage 1994;9:5-11.
4. Apfelbaum JL, Chen C, Mehta SS, et al: Postoperative pain experience: Results from a national survey suggest postoperative pain continues to be undermanaged. Anesth Analg 2003;97:534-540.
5. Schoenwald A, Clark CR: Acute pain in surgical patients. Contemp Nurse 2006;22:97-108.
6. Kehlet H: Multimodal approach to control postoperative pathophysiology and rehabilitation. Br J Anaesth 1997;78: 606-617.
7. Kehlet H: Organizing postoperative accelerated recovery programs. Reg Anesth 1996;21:149-151.
8. Kehlet H: Postoperative pain relief. Br J Anaesth 1994;72: 375-377.
9. Labat lecture: Surgical stress and postoperative outcome—From here to where? Reg Anesth Pain Med 2006;31:47-52.
10. Kehlet H: Effect of pain relief on the surgical stress response. Reg Anesth 1996;21:35-37.
11. Kehlet H: General outcome improvement overview. Reg Anesth 1996;21:5-8.
12. de Leon-Casasola OA: Immunomodulation and epidural anesthesia and analgesia. Reg Anesth 1996;21:24-25.
13. Kehlet H, Jensen TJ, Woolf CJ: Persistent post surgical pain: risks factors and prevention. Lancet 2006;367(9522): 1618-1625.
14. Ready LB: ASA Task Force on Pain Management: Practice guidelines for acute pain management in the perioperative setting. Anesthesiology 1995;82:1071-1081.
15. Carr DB, Jacox AK, Chapman CR, et al: Acute Pain Management: Operative or Medical Procedures and Trauma (Publ. No. 92-0032). Rockville, Md, Agency for Health Care Policy and Research, 1992.
16. Jacox AK, Carr DB, Payne R, et al: Management of Cancer Pain (Publ. No. 94-0592). Rockville, Md, Agency for Health Care Policy and Research, 1994.
17. Engelman E, Salengros JC, Paquot MC, et al: The acute pain service (APS): How we should have done it. Acta Anaesthesiol Belg 2006;57:233-238.
18. Stalder M, Schlander M, Braeckman M, et al: A cost-utility and cost-effectiveness analysis of an acute pain service. J Clin Anesth 2004;16:159-167.
19. Ready LB, Edwards WT: Management of Acute Pain: Task Force on Acute Pain. Seattle, IASP Publications, 1992.
20. Rowlingson JC: Developing a comprehensive pain evaluation and management center. ASA Refresher Courses 1997;265: 1-6.
21. Ghia JN: Development and organization of pain center. In Raj PP (ed): Practical Management of Pain, ed 2. St. Louis, Mosby-Year Book, 1992, pp 16-39.
22. Chrubasik S, Chrubasik J, Grote U, et al: Practicability of the multimodal postoperative approach. Reg Anesth 1996; 21(Suppl):43.
23. Kritchevsky SB, Simmons BP: CQI: Concepts and applications for physicians. JAMA 1991;266:1817-1823.
24. APS Quality of Care Committee: QI guidelines for the treatment of acute and cancer pain. JAMA 1995;274:1874-1880.
25. Deming WE: Out of Crisis. Cambridge, Mass, MIT Center for Advanced Engineering Study, 1986.
26. Hubbard L: An acute pain management service in a large hospital. Am J Pain Manage 1994;4:167-171.
27. Ferrell BR, Griffith H: Cost-related issues related to pain management. J Pain Symptom Manage 1994;9:221-234.
28. Abram SE, Gillespie BM: Standards of care and reimbursement issues in pain management. In Raj PP (ed): Practical Management of Pain, ed 2. St. Louis, Mosby-Year Book, 1992, pp 40-55.
29. Cohen MJM, Campbell JN (eds): Pain Treatment Centers at Crossroads: Progress in Pain Research and Management. Vol 7. Seattle, IASP Press, 1991.
30. Liu S, Carpenter RL, Neal JM: Epidural anesthesia and analgesia: Their role in postoperative outcome. Anesthesiology 82:1474-1506, 1995.
31. Wolf C, Chong M: Preemptive analgesia. Anesth Analg 77:362-379, 1993.
32. Katz J: Perioperative predictors of long-term pain after surgery. In Progress in Pain Research and Management, vol 8. Seattle, IASP Press, 1997.

Additional Readings

Postoperative and Intervention Quality Manual: ISO9001 norms, 2005, Geneva University Hospitals.
JCAHO and NPC monograph: Improving quality of pain management through measurement and action, 2003.

Vanderbilt University Medical Center

A-B-Cs
in
PAIN MANAGEMENT

The Pain Management Manual for House Staff

First Edition

1997

---

*Please contact Beth H. Minzter if interested in contents.
Courtesy of Vanderbilt University Medical Center, Nashville, Tenn.

	Manuel Qualité groupe antalgie interventionnelle	ANI.MAQ.01-V4.0 06-02-27 Page 1/20
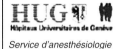 *Service d'anesthésiologie* *Département APS!*		

0.1 Objet

Ce document décrit le système de management et la manière de promouvoir la qualité au sein du Groupe Antalgie interventionnelle.

0.2 Liste des modifications apportées à la version antérieure

Nᵒ de version	Changements
ANI.MAQ.01-V1.0	sans objet
ANI.MAQ.01-V2.0	modifications selon interne I-2005 mis en oeuvre par les bulletin d'amélioration Nᵒ38 à 47
ANI.MAQ.01-V3.0	modification selon audit de certification, 1ᵉ partie, mis en oeuvre par les bulletin d'amélioration Nᵒ59, 61
ANI.MAQ.01-V4.0	modifications diverses en relation avec la diminution du volume d'activité de 50% suite au décisions de la RD du 23-11-2005 (cf points 1.2/6.4/8.4)

NB: seule la version présente en ligne sur le réseau intranet des HUG a valeur de référence.

0.3 Domaine d'application - responsabilités

Cf.: point 4

0.4 Documents applicables du système de management de la qualité

Cf.: point 1.2

0.5 Table des matières

---

*Courtesy of Geneva University Hospital.

3–3 Patient Care Resource Manual Clinical Guidelines

Review Responsibilities: Nursing Practice Committee
Last Revision: May 1998

EPIDURAL ANALGESIA ADMINISTRATION AND MANAGEMENT*

I. Outcome Goal

To ensure safe medication administration and pump function to all patients receiving epidural analgesia.

II. Policy

Epidural analgesia will be administered according to the following guidelines for the purpose of pain management. The guidelines do not apply to epidural catheters used for the purpose of anesthesia or to epidurals used in labor and delivery areas.

III. Specific Information

A. Does implementation require MD order?
_X_YES __NO

B. Guidelines applicable to:
__All patient care areas
_X_Adult areas only
__Pediatric areas only
__Critical Care/Stepdown areas only
__Selected areas (specify): __

C. Team members participating:
_X_RN
_X_LPN
__Care Partner/Patient Care Technician
__Other licensed staff (specify): __
__Other non-licensed staff (specify): __

D. Specific education required? _X_YES __NO
Completion of the Epidural Self Study Packet

IV. Protocol

A. An anesthesiologist or CRNA/CRNP will set up and administer the initial epidural infusion.

B. Only Acute Pain Consultants (APCs) may give additional medication through the epidural catheter.

C. RNs may change pump settings or modes per physician's order.

D. Epidural lines are not to be used for infusion of any other medications.

E. Post-operative Care:

1. When the patient enters PACU, the admitting nurse is responsible for requesting a full report of medication administered epidurally.

2. The PACU nurse will observe the patient for one hour before the patient is sent to a general care unit.

3. When the patient is transferred from the PACU, the receiving nurse must verify patient name, recent vital signs, medications, dose, and rate with the physician's order.

F. No parenteral/oral narcotics/sedatives given without consultation with APC.

G. Saline lock maintained during epidural infusion and for 8 hrs. after discontinuation

H. The infusion bag, tubing, and patient door should be labeled with a yellow "Epidural Narcotic Infusion" label.

I. Dressing changes will be performed by APC; nurses may stabilize dressings as necessary; if catheter comes out, it should be removed and saved for inspection by APC; infusion may be stopped.

J. Patient may ambulate only if sedation and motor function are within normal limits; ambulation must be assisted. (see K.4)

K. Monitoring:

1. Pain scale (0 = no pain to 10 = worst pain ever) and pain relief acceptable (yes/no) monitored q 4 hrs.

2. Respiratory rate and quality monitored q 2 hrs. × 12 hrs. then q 4 hrs.; respiratory rate/quality monitored q 2 hrs. × 8 hrs. with each bolus.

3. Sedation monitored q 4 hrs. per sedation scale:

0—None   Alert;
1—Mild   Occasionally drowsy, easy to arouse;

---

*Courtesy of Vanderbilt University Medical Center, Nashville, Tenn.

2—Moderate   Frequently drowsy, easy to arouse;

3—Severe   Somnolent, difficult to arouse; and

S—Sleeping   Normal sleep, easy to arouse.

4. Motor function monitored q 4 hrs. per Bromage scale:[†]

0 = no block (0%)   Full flexion of knees and feet possible;

1 = Partial (33%)   Just able to flex knees, full flexion of feet;

2 = Almost Complete (66%)   Unable to flex knees, still flexion in feet; and

3 = Complete (100%)   Unable to move legs or feet.

5. Site checked q shift and prn (for erythema, edema, site pain, or unusual drainage).

V.   Procedure(s)
   A. Operation of epidural infusion pump with optional PCA feature: refer to instruction manual maintained by floors and by SICU pharmacy.
   B. Changing medication bags: may be performed by RNs/LPNs. Infusion solutions must be changed every 72 hours unless the medication expires prior to 72 hours.
   C. Changing filters and tubing: May be performed by RNs/LPNs. Filters and tubing of continuous infusions should be changed every 72 hours.

VI. Nursing Implications:
   A. Code STAT for unresponsive patient. (STOP infusion.)
   B. Notify APC for
      1. Inadequate analgesia (pain scale ≥3 or worsening; unacceptable pain relief).
      2. RR < 8/min. (STOP infusion.); SBP < 80; T > 101.5 × 2 within 8 hrs.
      3. Increasing sedation (sedation 2–3). (STOP infusion.)
      4. Increasing motor block (Bromage >2).
      5. Concerns with catheter site or catheter connections dislodgment of catheter.
      6. Any other problems or concerns.

VII. Patient/Family Education
   A. Procedural expectations.
   B. Post-procedure vital sign and monitoring expectations.
   C. Activity expectations.
   D. Signs/symptoms to report to nurse.

VIII. Documentation
   A. Medication, concentration, prescribed dose/administration rate, volumes infused and left to count, boluses administered, and sedation/analgesia levels are to be documented as ordered while epidural analgesia is in use.
   B. Vital signs and other monitoring and assessment data are to be documented as ordered while epidural analgesia is in use.

IX.   Cross References:
   A. Patient Care Resource Manual
   B. Doctor's Order Set, Acute Pain Consultants
   C. Epidural infusion pump instruction manual
   D. Controlled Drug Record (MC No. 2334)

X.   References
   Ferrante, F.M., & VadeBoncouer, T.R. (Eds.) (1993). Postoperative Pain Management. New York: Churchill Livingstone.

XI.   Distribution
   A, B, C, D, F

XII. Contributors
   John W. Downing, MD, Director, OB/Regional Anesthesia
   Beth Minzter, MD, Director, Acute Pain Consultants
   Elizabeth Ryder, MSN, Brigham and Women's Hospital
   Barbara Grimm, MSN, Acute Pain Consultants

XIII. Endorsement
   Vanderbilt Nurse Practice Committee
   Acute Pain Consultants

_____   ____
Director, Acute Pain Consultants   Date

_____   ____
Director, Patient Care Services   Date
and Chief Nursing Officer

_____

[†]A modified Bromage scale will be used on the Controlled Drug Record (MC No. 2334).

3–4

A. Documentation Guidelines for Evaluation and Management Services

American Medical Association
Centers for Medicare and Medicaid*

CONTENT AND DOCUMENTATION REQUIREMENTS

LEVEL OF EXAM	PERFORM AND DOCUMENT
Problem focused	One to five elements identified by a bullet
Expanded problem focused	At least six elements identified by a bullet
Detailed	At least two elements identified by a bullet from each of six areas/systems *or* at least 12 elements identified by a bullet in two or more areas/systems
Comprehensive	At least two elements identified by a bullet from each of nine areas/systems

General Multisystem Examination

SYSTEM/BODY AREA	ELEMENTS OF EXAMINATION
Constitutional	• Measurement of any three of the following seven vital signs: (1) sitting or standing blood pressure, (2) supine blood pressure, (3) pulse rate and regularity, (4) respiration, (5) temperature, (6) height, (7) weight (May be measured and recorded by ancillary staff) • General appearance of patient (e.g., development, nutrition, body habitus, deformities, attention to grooming)
Eyes	• Inspection of conjunctivae and lids • Examination of pupils and irises (e.g., reaction to light and accommodation, size and symmetry) • Ophthalmoscopic examination of optic discs (e.g., size, C/D ratio, appearance) and posterior segments (e.g., vessel changes, exudates, hemorrhages)
Ears, nose, mouth, and throat	• External inspection of ears and nose (e.g., overall appearance, scars, lesions, masses) • Otoscopic examination of external auditory canals and tympanic membranes • Assessment of hearing (e.g., whispered voice, finger rub, tuning fork) • Inspection of nasal mucosa, septum, and turbinates • Inspection of lips, teeth, and gums • Examination of oropharynx: oral mucosa, salivary glands, hard and soft palates, tongue, tonsils, and posterior pharynx
Neck	• Examination of neck (e.g., masses, overall appearance, symmetry, tracheal position, crepitus) • Examination of thyroid (e.g., enlargement, tenderness, mass)
Respiratory	• Assessment of respiratory effort (e.g., intercostal retractions, use of accessory muscles, diaphragmatic movement) • Percussion of chest (e.g., dullness, flatness, hyperresonance) • Palpation of chest (e.g., tactile fremitus) • Auscultation of lungs (e.g., breath sounds, adventitious sounds, rubs)
Cardiovascular	• Palpation of heart (e.g., location, size, thrills) • Auscultation of heart with notation of abnormal sounds and murmurs Examination of: • Carotid arteries (e.g., pulse amplitude, bruits) • Abdominal aorta (e.g., size, bruits) • Femoral arteries (e.g., pulse amplitude, bruits) • Pedal pulses (e.g., pulse amplitude) • Extremities for edema and/or varicosities

*Centers for Medicare and Medicaid Services (CMS) website address: http://www.cms.hhs.gov.

General Multisystem Examination—cont'd

SYSTEM/BODY AREA	ELEMENTS OF EXAMINATION
Chest (breasts)	• Inspection of breasts (e.g., symmetry, nipple discharge) • Palpation of breasts and axillae (e.g., masses or lumps, tenderness)
Gastrointestinal (abdomen)	• Examination of abdomen with notation of presence of masses or tenderness • Examination of liver and spleen • Examination of presence or absence of hernia • Examination of anus, perineum and rectum, including sphincter tone, presence of hemorrhoids, rectal masses • Obtain stool sample for occult blood test when indicated
Genitourinary	Male • Examination of the scrotal contents (e.g., hydrocele, spermatocele, tenderness of cord, testicular mass) • Examination of the penis • Digital rectal examination of prostate gland (e.g., size, symmetry, nodularity, tenderness) Female Pelvic examination (with or without specimen collection for smears and cultures), including • Examination of external genitalia (e.g., general appearance, hair distribution, lesions) and vagina (e.g., general appearance, estrogen effect, discharge, lesions, pelvic support, cystocele, rectocele) • Examination of urethra (e.g., masses, tenderness, scarring) • Examination of bladder (e.g., fullness, masses, tenderness) • Cervix (e.g., general appearance, lesions, discharge) • Uterus (e.g., size, contour, position, mobility, tenderness, consistency, descent, or support) • Adnexa/parametria (e.g., masses, tenderness, organomegaly, nodularity)
Lymphatic	Palpation of lymph nodes in two or more areas • Neck • Axillae • Groin • Other
Musculoskeletal	• Examination of gait and station • Inspection and/or palpation of digits and nails (e.g., clubbing, cyanosis, inflammatory conditions, petechiae, ischemia, infections, nodes) Examination of joints, bones, and muscles of one or more of the following six areas: (1) head and neck; (2) spine, ribs, and pelvis; (3) right upper extremity; (4) left upper extremity; (5) right lower extremity; (6) left lower extremity. The examination of a given area includes: • Inspection and/or palpation with notation of presence of any misalignment, asymmetry, crepitation, defects, tenderness, masses, effusions • Assessment of range of motion with notation of any pain, crepitation, or contracture • Assessment of stability with notation of any dislocation (luxation), subluxation, or laxity • Assessment of muscle strength and tone (e.g., flaccid, cog wheel, spastic) with notation of any atrophy or abnormal movements
Skin	• Inspection of skin and subcutaneous tissue (e.g., rashes, lesions, ulcers) • Palpation of skin and subcutaneous tissue (e.g., induration, subcutaneous nodules, tightening)
Neurologic	• Test cranial nerves with notation of any deficits • Examination of deep tendon reflexes with notation of pathologic reflexes (e.g., Babinski) • Examination of sensation (e.g., by touch, pin, vibration, proprioception)
Psychiatric	• Description of patient's judgment and insight Brief assessment of mental status including: • Orientation to time, place, and person • Recent and remote memory • Mood and affect (e.g., depression, anxiety, agitation)

B. Acute Pain Consultant Admission Note

1. Preliminary:
   a. Date and time
   b. Place of examination
   c. Chart review
   d. Highlights of medical history
2. Current Medications:
3. Allergy:
4. Surgical Procedure Performed:
5. Intraoperative Course: (note significant points—hemodynamics, pain management, etc.)
6. Epidural Catheter:
   a. Approach: midline or lateral
   b. Site:
   c. Loss of resistance to injection of air or saline at:
   d. Length of catheter left in the epidural space
   e. Catheter marking at the skin:
   f. Complications/difficulties encountered
7. Clinical Status at the Time of Admission to APC:
   a. Level of consciousness
   b. Hemodynamics
   c. Pain—assessment on VAS/VNS
   d. Sensory level—four levels (RUL, LUL, RLL, LLL)
   e. Motor function—lower extremities
   f. Note on current epidural infusion (agents and rate of infusion)
8. Plan:

LLL, left lower level; LUL, left upper level; RLL, right lower level; RUL, right upper level; VAS, Visual Analogue Scale; VNS, Verbal Numeric Scale.

C. Epidural Placement Note

1. Preliminary note:
   a. Date and time
   b. Patient's ID
   c. Consent
   d. Chart review
   e. Vital signs: BP, HR, SpO_2
   f. Preloading
2. Aseptic technique
3. Position:
   a. Sitting
   b. Lateral
4. Infiltration—drug concentration and volume used
5. Interspace used and approach (midline or lateral)
6. Loss of resistance:
   a. Air or fluid
   b. Depth at which LOR was obtained
   c. Heme or CSF encountered (yes or no)
7. Length of the catheter left in the epidural space
   a. Ease of catheter placement
   b. Presence or absence of paresthesia
      If yes,
      (1) Where
      (2) How resolved
      (3) Negative administration on paresthesia
8. Catheter marking seen at the skin
9. Paraesthesia/blood in the catheter/aspiration for CSF: Yes or No
10. Test dose: LA used (concentration, epinephrine, volume used)
    Positive or negative for intravascular or subarachnoid injection
11. LA + opioid mixture: Note bolus injection and infusion (mL/hr and start time)
12. Sensory level obtained
13. Side effects (e.g., hypotension)—treatment
14. Complications (e.g., intravascular placement, accidental dural puncture)—management

CSF, cerebrospinal fluid; LA, local anesthetic; LOR, loss of resistance.

From American Medical Association Centers for Medicare and Medicaid Services.

A. Computer-Generated Sign-Out Sheet*

Vanderbilt University Medical Center sign-out sheet requested by GRIMULI on Jul 16 13:52

90   74 years M, MR#   , admitted on Jul 14

ATTD: DX: right lung cancer; right thoracoscopy, r pl thoracotomy, ru + rm lobectomies, mind, loa 7/14; CONDITION: stable; CODE STATUS:_____
ALLERGIES:
MEDS: ns; dopamine infusion; docusate sodium 100 bid; bisacodyl 10 bid; dilaudid/marcaine epidural; ipratropium 0.02% in 2.5 ml ns 0.5 q4h; albuterol 0.5% soln in 3ml ns 0.5 q4h; heparin inj 5000 q12h; pharmacy misc;

basal 7cc/h demand 3cc q 15 min T6-T7 CATHETER TORADOL 30MG IV Q6H X 4 DOSES

---

90   54 years F, MR#   , admitted on Jul 14

ATTD: DX: s/p III lung volume reduction; CONDITION: stable; CODE STATUS:_____
ALLERGIES: valium, levaquin;
MEDS: dilaudid/marcaine epidural; estrogen conjugated 1.25 qd; theophylline sr tab 100 q12h; famotidine 20 bid; ipratropium 0.02% in 2.5 ml ns 0.5 q4h; albuterol 0.5% soln in 3ml ns 0.5 q4h; heparin inj 5000 q12h; d5 1/4 ns + kcl 20 meq/l; pharmacy misc;

T5-T6 catheter basal 5cc/h demand 3cc q 15 min

---

90   70 years F, MR#   , admitted on Jul 12

ATTD: DX: right lung mass; CONDITION: good; CODE STATUS:_____
ALLERGIES:;
ABx: cefazolin inj 1000 q8h;
MEDS: bisacodyl 10 bid; pharmacy misc; dilaudid/marcaine epidural; furosemide 20 q12h; potassium chloride sr 10 q12h; docusate sodium 100 bid; vitamin e 400 qd; indomethacin 50 qd; omeprazole 20 qd; d5 1/2 ns + kcl 20 meq/l;

T7-T8 epidural, 9 cm. skin. Bupi 1/6% and Dilaudid 15 mcg. at 8 cc.

---

62   20 years F, MR#   , admitted on Jul 12

ATTD: DX: metastatic osteosarcoma; CONDITION: guarded; CODE STATUS:_____
ALLERGIES: tape; penicillin (rash); WEIGHT: 63.000 kgs;
MEDS: allopurinol 300 qd; nacl enteral (dosed in mg) 1000 tid; d5ns; morphine pca 1mg/ml; famotidine inj 20 q12h;

pt is DNR. may increase pca every hour by 5mg on basal as needed

---

4S4   72 years F, MR#   , admitted on Jul 16

ATTD: DX: pelvic support defect; CONDITION:_____ ; CODE STATUS:_____
ALLERGIES: demerol and contrast dye;
ABx: gentamicin inj 180 q24h; metronidazole inj 500 q6h; vancomycin inj 1000 q12h;
MEDS: famotidine inj 20 q12h; heparin inj 5000 q12h; d5 1/2 ns + kcl 20 meq/l; pharmacy misc; dilaudid/marcaine epidural;

lumber catheter basal rate 6cc/h demand 3cc q 15 min dilaudid 15mcg/cc bupi 1/5%

4S4   54 years F, MR#   , admitted on Jul 16

ATTD: DX: endometrial carcinoma for tah-bso; CONDITION: stable; CODE STATUS:_____
ALLERGIES:; WEIGHT: 113.398 kgs;
ABx: cefotetan inj 2000 q8h;
MEDS: d5 1/2 ns + kcl 20 meq/l; heparin inj 5000 q12h; pharmacy misc; dilaudid/marcaine epidural;

DOS s/p TAH-BSO for endometrial ca
PMH-HTN (on Hygroton 50mg po qd at home), depression (Prozac 20mg po qd)
Epidural
Foley in until epidural out
NPO

*Courtesy of Vanderbilt University Medical Center, Nashville, Tenn.

B. Acute Pain Consultant Special Report with Special Billing Information*

Vanderbilt University Medical Center	**APC report**	as of *7/16 14:26*

| | **90** | MR# | case# | 74y/o male |

21 **operative procedure:** right thoracoscopy, r pl thoracotomy, ru+rm lobectomies, mlnd, loa 7/14 ▸ Jul 14 16:00...
23 **attending:** ▸Jul 14 16:00...
24 **diagnosis:** right lung cancer ▸ Jul 14 16:00...

| | **90** | MR# | case# | 54y/o female |

21 **operative procedure:** s/p lll lung volume reduction ▸Jul 14 12:00...
24 **attending:** ▸Jul 14 12:00...

| | **90** | MR# | case# | 70y/o female |

31 **attending:** ▸Jul 12 14:00...
36 **diagnosis:** right lung mass ▸Jul 12 14:00...

| | **41** | MR# | case# | 17y/o female |

3 **diagnosis:** iup at 39 2/7 ega with pih ▸Jul 12 23:59...
61 **diagnosis:** failure to dilate ▸Jul 14 04:30...
62 **diagnosis:** s/p primary ltcs ▸Jul 14 04:30...

| | **4S4** | MR# | case# | 72y/o female |

1 **attending:** ▸Jul 16 06:30...
3 **diagnosis:** pelvic support defect ▸Jul 16 06:30...

| | **4S4** | MR# | case# | 54y/o female |

2 **attending:** ▸Jul 16 06:30...
5 **diagnosis:** endometrial carcinoma for tah-bso ▸Jul 16 06:30...

*Courtesy of Vanderbilt University Medical Center, Nashville, Tenn.

C. Placement/Procedure Billing Sheet*

APC REPORT				
				Date _____
STICKER NAME MED REC#: CASE#: ATTENDING AGE/SEX	SITE OF PAIN SURGICAL/MEDICAL DIAGNOSIS	REGIONAL ANESTHETIC PROCEDURE/DAILY CARE	RES Y/N	ATTENDING SIGNATURE
STICKER NAME MED REC#: CASE#: ATTENDING AGE/SEX	SITE OF PAIN SURGICAL/MEDICAL DIAGNOSIS	REGIONAL ANESTHETIC PROCEDURE/DAILY CARE	RES Y/N	ATTENDING SIGNATURE
STICKER NAME MED REC#: CASE#: ATTENDING AGE/SEX	SITE OF PAIN SURGICAL/MEDICAL DIAGNOSIS	REGIONAL ANESTHETIC PROCEDURE/DAILY CARE	RES Y/N	ATTENDING SIGNATURE
STICKER NAME MED REC#: CASE#: ATTENDING AGE/SEX	SITE OF PAIN SURGICAL/MEDICAL DIAGNOSIS	REGIONAL ANESTHETIC PROCEDURE/DAILY CARE	RES Y/N	ATTENDING SIGNATURE
STICKER NAME MED REC#: CASE#: ATTENDING AGE/SEX	SITE OF PAIN SURGICAL/MEDICAL DIAGNOSIS	REGIONAL ANESTHETIC PROCEDURE/DAILY CARE	RES Y/N	ATTENDING SIGNATURE

This report is to be used for femoral nerve blocks, OB post-op epidural narcotics, epidural catheters placed by APC team, and any other Acute Pain patients not on the computer APC Report.

Responsibilities:
SRNA/Resident: 1) Write progress note in chart, 2) Place sticker above.
Attending: 1) Complete/sign progress note, 2) Complete above information and sign.

Procedure column is to note femoral nerve block, continuous epidural placement, daily care follow-up, etc.

**ATTENTION BILLING DEPARTMENT: OB PATIENTS ARE TO BE BILLED DAILY CARE FOLLOW-UP FOR THE FOLLOWING DAY UNLESS OTHERWISE INDICATED.

2/10/1998

_____
*Courtesy of Vanderbilt University Medical Center, Nashville, Tenn.

D. Acute Pain Consultant Clinical Activity Report*

MONTH	Pts	CPT CODE	PROCEDURE	VUH FEE	PROCEDURE	CHARGED	WRITE OFF
Apr		01996	Daily Management				
Total Pts		62319	Epidural Placement/L				
OB Pts		62318	Epidural Placement/T				
		64417	Axillary Block				
		64450	Peripheral Block				
		99231	Hospital Care/1				
		99251	Inpatient Consult/1				
		99253	Inpatient Consult/3				
TOTAL							
May		01996	Daily Management				
Total Pts		62319	Epidural Placement/L				
OB Pts		62318	Epidural Placement/T				
		62350	Intrathecal Implant				
		64450	Peripheral Block				
		76005	Fluoroscopy				
		99251	Inpatient Consult/1				
		99255	Inpatient Consult/5				
		NC	Inpatient Consult				
TOTAL							
Jun		01996	Daily Management				
Total Pts		62319	Epidural Placement/L				
OB Pts		62318	Epidural Placement/T				
		62368	Pump Reprogramming				
		64450	Peripheral Block				
		95991	Pump Refill				
		99251	Inpatient Consult/1				
Jul		01996	Daily Management				
Total Pts		01996	Daily Management/IPC				
OB Pts		62319	Epidural Placement/L				
		62318	Epidural Placement/T				
		62350	Pump Implantation				
		62368	Pump Reprogram				
		64418	Suprascapular Block				
		64450	Peripheral Block				
		64510	Stellate Ganglion Bl				
		95991	Pump Refill				
		85396	Thromboelastogram				
		99241	Office Consult/1				
		99251	Inpatient Consult/1				
		99252	Inpatient Consult/2				
		99253	Inpatient Consult/3				
		99254	Inpatient Consult/4				
		99255	Inpatient Consult/5				
		NC	Inpatient Consult				

*Courtesy of Vanderbilt University Medical Center, Nashville, Tenn.

A. Computer-Generated Acute Pain Consultant Order Set*

Vanderbilt University Medical Center   **Wiz☺rder printout, Jul 16 13:56 for GRIMULI**

```
Epidural Analgesia Orders

 For post C-section patients:
1. Dilaudid (Hydromorphone) Preservative Free 0.25 mg per Epidural NOW
2. Morphine PF 1mg/ml: (Duramorph) 4 mg Epidural NOW

▾ APC Epidural Infusion Medications (w or w/o PCA)

 Always fill in basal (infusion) rate

 Fill in loading dose only if bolus is to be given in future

 Includes boluses: 3 cc every 15 min.

 Includes total lockout: 4 X rate + 12 (4 boluses)
3. Dilaudid (20 mcg/cc) & Bupivacaine 1/8% per 250 ml NS
4. Dilaudid (20 mcg/cc) & Bupivacaine 1/10% per 250 ml NS
5. Dilaudid (15 mcg/cc) & Bupivacaine 1/5% per 250 ml NS
6. other epidural medication orders ▸

 ▾
7. Click here for Meds & other Nursing orders - (APC) Benadryl 25-50 mg PO/IV q4-6h
prn pruritus
 ∟ (APC) compazine 10 mg PO/IV q6h prn nausea
 ∟ (APC) narcan 20-40 mcg IV q1h prn pruritus or nausea
 ∟ (APC) NO parenteral/oral narcotics/sedatives given without consultation with APC
 ∟ (APC) If pt. is unresponsive, call CODE STAT,notify APC & stop infusion;If RR
<8/min or sedation >2-3, stop infusion & call APC
 ∟ (APC) Lidocaine 2% w/epi, Plain Lido. 2%(10mlx2), Ephedrine x2 amp, Fentanyl
100mcg, Dilaudid PF(1mg/ml) x1ml & Narcan 0.4mg x2
 ∟ (APC) Bupivacaine PF .25% (30ml) at bedside
 ∟ (APC) while pt on epidural have Phenylephrine 10mg x 2 amps on unit
 ∟ (APC) In & out cath q6h prn for bladder distention & notify primary service
 ∟ (APC) monitor & document q4h: (1) pain using pain scale 0-10; (2) whether relief
acceptable or not
 ∟ (APC) monitor/document motor fxn q4h X48h after removal of epi cath; notify APC for
any motor/sensory deficits s/p cath removal
 ∟ (APC) respiratory rate & quality q2h X 12 hrs; then, q4h (q2h X 8 hrs. after each
bolus)
 ∟ (APC) temperature, pulse & blood pressure q4h
 ∟ (APC) sedation scale and motor function q4h & before ambulating. Pt. may ambulate
only if sedation & motor function WNL
 ∟ (APC) monitor/document site qshift for erythema, edema, site pain or unusual
drainage
 ∟ (APC)notify APC for (3)inadequate analgesia,unacceptable pain relief;
(4)RR<8,SBP<80,T>101.5 X2 within 8hr;(5)increas. sedation
 ∟ (APC) (6) motor block;(7) concerns about catheter site or connections;(8) any other
problems or concerns
 ∟ (APC) for ob pt. (post c-sect), call 1)ob anes junior resid.#0439,2) ob senior
resid. #1603, ob anes attending #1997
 ∟ (APC) for Acute Pain Consultants (non-OB), call 1) APC resident/fellow beeper
#1762; 2) APC attending beeper #3161
8. ◂ Return to previous list
```

*Courtesy of Vanderbilt University Medical Center, Nashville, Tenn.

B. Vanderbilt University Medical Center Controlled Drug Report*

Rx#_____ / _____ Pharmacy PCA _____

◎ Vanderbilt University Medical Center
CONTROLLED DRUG RECORD

Patient: _____ Room: _____

Drug: _____ Amount/total volume: _____

Date/Time: _____ / _____ By: _____ / _____

PCA   EPIDURAL   IV DRIP   TAB/CAPSULE   LIQUID   *(Circle One)*   addressograph

INITIAL ORDER: BASAL RATE: _____   DEMAND RATE: _____

INFUSION STARTED BY: _____ MD/RN/CRNA

TIME / DATE	VOLUME INF/ML	LEFT TO COUNT	BOLUS / GIVEN BY	RESP. RATE / QUALITY	SEDATION SCALE	PAIN SCALE	BROMAGE SCALE	SIGNATURE
		_____ ml	_____ DPH	Volume actually read on syringe				
			/					
			/					
			/					
			/					
			/					
			/					
			/					
			/					
			/					
			/					
			/					
			/					
			/					
			/					
			/					
			/					
			/					
			/					
		24 hour volume given						
			/					
			/					

Sedation Scale
0 = alert (none)
1 = occasionally drowsy; easy to arouse (mild)
2 = frequently drowsy; easy to arouse (moderate)
3 = somnolent; difficult to arouse (severe)
S = normal sleep; easy to arouse (sleeping)

Pain Scale
Use scale of 0 to 10 where:
0 = no pain, and
10 = worst pain imaginable

Motor Function
(modified Bromage Scale)
0 = no motor block
1 = inability to raise extended leg
2 = inability to flex knee
3 = inability to flex ankle

ORDER CHANGES
_____
_____

TOTAL VOLUME WASTED: _____   **NURSE/MD RECEIVING:** _____
WASTED BY: _____   **PHARMACIST VERIFYING**
WITNESSED BY: _____   **DOCUMENTATION:** _____

1. For oral solids and liquids, subtract each dose given from the beginning amount in the <u>left to count</u> column.
2. Record infusion volume/patient assessment at least every 4 hours or per protocols.
3. Replace infusion every 72 hours unless the medication expires prior to 72 hours. Notify pharmacy 2 hours in advance.
4. Document boluses as ML/HR & given by MD/RN/CRNA/patient.
5. Document additional medications on MAR, (Narcan, Reglan, ETC.) for epidurals only.
6. Two nurses must verify & record the amount left to count during the narcotic count or when patient transfers to another unit. Both nurses should sign on the appropriate line on signature column.
7. When infusion is completed, complete disposition record and return pink pharmacy copy. Original copy remains in medical record.

MC 2334 (1/98)   WHITE - Chart / CANARY - Pharmacy Disposition / PINK - Floor Copy / GOLD - Pharmacy Receipt

*Courtesy of Vanderbilt University Medical Center, Nashville, Tenn.

C. Quality Assurance Questions*

Quality Assurance Questionnaire:

MR # _____ Anesthesia case # _____ Surgery Date: __/__/__

Last Name: _____ First Name _____ Survey Date: __/__/__

Phone # (___) _____ Location: _____

1. Did staff explain your pain management in a way you could understand ?

yes ☐ no ☐

2. Were your preferences or requests concerning your pain management followed to

    your satisfaction ?   yes ☐ no ☐

3. Was your pain controlled to your satisfaction with your epidural ?   yes ☐ no ☐

4. Was your pain controlled to your satisfaction after your epidural was removed ?

yes ☐ no ☐

5. How would you rate your overall care by the pain service?

    Poor   ☐   Fair   ☐   Good   ☐   Very Good   ☐   Excellent   ☐

6. How could your pain management have been improved ?

_____

_____

_____

_____   *Thank You*

(Inpatient Pain Consultants)

_____
*Courtesy of Vanderbilt University Medical Center, Nashville, Tenn.

3–7 Organizational Framework for Acute Pain Management Service

1. Definitions before starting the plan:

Politics	**Strategy**	**Tactics**
Motor behind the strategy:		Mode of action:
Neutralizing		Persuasion
Associating		Negotiation
Symbiosis		Seduction

2. Checklist:

☐ Security ☐ Productivity ☐ Scientific reputation

☐ Efficacy ☐ Quality ☐ Market potential

☐ Efficiency ☐ Recognition ☐ etc.

☐ etc. ☐ etc.

3. Different general strategies:

ACTIONS	Direct	Indirect
Offensive	**Strategy of a challenger** (attack the leader)	**Strategy of a specialist** (attack the lay)
Defensive	**Strategy of a leader** (defend against a challenger)	**Strategy of a researcher** (development)

4. Analyzing reimbursement strategies:

	Reimbursement Medicaid	Reimbursement Private
Ambulatory intervention	yes	yes
Hospitalization	no	yes
Nonconventional therapy	no > yes	yes > no

5. Quality management strategy of any process:

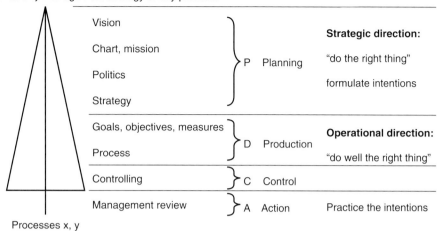

Processes x, y

Vision is the future position of the enterprise. It is the idea that will generate the profit. It is the ultimate goal. It should be analyzed according to SWOT (see below).
Mission is the answer to the question "how can we execute the vision?"
Politics defines the adversary. It is the detailed mission in regard to reality.
Chart vision, mission, and politics are grouped in a chart or an executive summary.
Strategy represents the execution of our political intentions. It depends on vision and politics and may change in time.

6. Priority (SWOT) analysis:

	Strength Internal resources can help to develop a competitive edge	**Weakness** Lack of internal resources
Opportunity To seize the occasion to advance where no one else did	**St-Op strategy** Ideal strategy to win (or stop) the opponent	**W-Op strategy** Ideal strategy to overcome (whop) the problems ahead
Threat Any change or situation that can menace the environment	**St-T strategy** Strategy to diminish damages	**W-T strategy** Defensive strategy to play it sure (not to get wet)

7. Why be certified?

The advantages of certification using industrial standards (like ISO 9001 norms) include:
- Increase of patient satisfaction due to longitudinal measurement (before and after treatment)
- Securitizing treatment procedures due to exact definition and taxonomy and clear responsibility attribution
- Enhanced traceability due to continuous recording of quality indicators and security data
- Clear direction due to ongoing internal auditing in face of nonconformities
- Continuous quality assurance as an enterprise culture due to corrective and preventive actions
- Heighten sense of awareness to quality among patients, other caregivers, and out of the institute partners

8. Definition of a process:

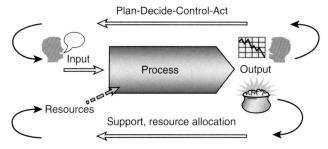

9. Architecture of a process:

We define 3 levels of process:
1. Process network
2. The process
3. Process elements

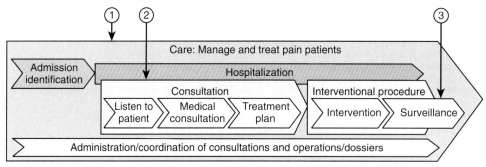

4 Pain Medicine Practice: Development of Outpatient Services for Chronic Pain

David Walega

HISTORY

The development of the multidisciplinary pain clinic is attributed to John Bonica, whose experiences while practicing medicine during World War II in a military hospital led him to develop a "pain center" concept in which patients with chronic pain disorders would have their special needs assessed and their pain symptoms evaluated and treated with a variety of modalities. This concept development was catalyzed by his frustration with managing complex pain patients as a lone practitioner and led him to include his colleagues in neurology, neurosurgery, orthopedics, and psychiatry in the evaluation and treatment plans. He later developed a multidisciplinary pain clinic at the University of Washington, a model from which many other pain centers were later developed.[1]

At present, pain centers in the United States number well over 3000, a number that continues to rise as life expectancies increase, populations age, the interest in pain treatment and treatment options grow, and the number of practicing pain specialists increase.

THE MODERN PAIN PRACTICE

There is no single blueprint or model for a successful pain practice. Within each individual pain practice there are variations of patient populations, disciplines involved, treatment philosophy, and modalities utilized. The International Association for the Study of Pain detailed four different types of pain programs: multidisciplinary pain centers, multidisciplinary pain clinics, pain clinics, and modality-oriented clinics.[2] The multidisciplinary pain centers and multidisciplinary pain clinics are the most com-

prehensive and are quite similar in focus, although the "centers" may focus on research and education in addition to clinical care, while "multidisciplinary clinics" may focus purely on clinical care. Pain clinics typically focus on a particular syndrome or disease (back pain, headache, complex regional pain syndrome, cancer pain), and modality-specific centers focus on specific treatments for a particular syndrome or disease (injection therapies; medication management; alternative, manual, or holistic therapies).[2]

MODELS FOR PAIN MEDICINE PRACTICE

There are multiple models for the practice of pain medicine. These include the academic or university-based pain center, institutional pain centers seen in military hospitals or the Veteran's Administration system, and the traditional private practice clinic, which may be hospital-based or freestanding in the community. These practices can be interdisciplinary, multidisciplinary, single-specialty, or a variant. Kirkady-Willis describes a team approach to management of back pain,[3] and states that in uncomplicated cases, a single team member can manage the problem (e.g., a therapist, internist, or injectionist), but in more complicated scenarios of chronic pain with functional impairment, coexisting psychological problems, or vocational issues, a more integrated team approach best serves the patient's interests. Cancer pain management, particularly in the context of palliative care, is a prime example of a complex, multidimensional pain dilemma, best solved when physical, psychological, and spiritual pain and suffering are addressed by a group with shared principles but differing areas of expertise.[4] Multidisciplinary care has been shown to be more effective in the treatment of spinal disorders than single specialty-care

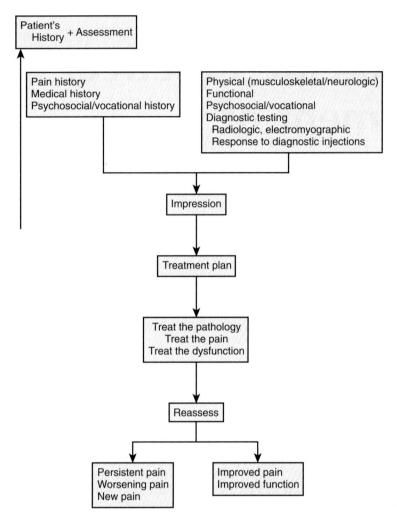

Figure 4–1. Algorithm for evaluation and treatment of chronic pain and cancer pain patients.

alone.[5-7] The team "captain" is the main treating practitioner, and in the context of a pain treatment center, this captain coordinates and facilitates care with other team members and retains control and focus over the treatment program for the patient.

In cases of chronic pain or cancer pain, thorough and multidimensional evaluation of the patient should take place, and a treatment plan should focus on each dimension of the patient's symptoms. Reassessment is necessary in order to propose and evaluate further treatment (Fig. 4–1).

A more recent trend in pain medicine is the integration of surgical and non-surgical specialties into a small interdependent group focused on one specialty area such as spinal disorders or pelvic pain.[8,9] The potential benefits of this model are numerous. The consumer-patient benefits from the concept of convenience and "one-stop shopping," obtaining multiple services, consultations, or treatments in one single location, perhaps on the same day. The feedback loop between patient and practitioners is tightened, giving the patient a greater confidence in follow-up and reassessment. Medical records are centralized and more accessible. Rapport and trust established between the patient and individual team members becomes transferable within the practice,

creating a group reputation, and subsequently a "brand" in the community. This model avoids the hassles and frustrations encountered by the pain patient being treated at multiple clinics with different physicians and therapists.[8] This "branding" is an important marketing concept and can lead to greater market share within the community and attract new or steady referrals to the group, sustaining the viability and financial heath of the practice.

Another advantage in this model is more facile communication between team members, as team members work in close proximity to one another. The opportunity to discuss management and broaden treatment options is significantly improved. Knowledge of the treatment options offered by each team member becomes obvious and inherent, and may lead to creation of treatment algorithms for particular patient types and a broad-focused treatment philosophy, which in turn can create a collegial atmosphere. Regular and frequent group interaction can also lead to innovation and improved efficiency.

Economic advantages of the multispecialty practice include lowered practice overhead costs and expenses through cost-sharing, reduced redundancy of services, and increased patient volume. An increased number of patients in such a broad-based practice may fuel the growth or expansion of other ancillary services within the practice, such as physical therapy, imaging (radiography, bone density testing, magnetic resonance imaging), or an ambulatory surgery center.

Challenges in such a model include differing philosophies in evaluation and treatment of patients, competition for financial resources, call coverage, allocation of space, equipment and ancillary personnel, as well as partnership parameters. Optimal financial, organizational, and personnel management become key issues in such a multispecialty setting, with interplay between all team members.

PRACTICE DEVELOPMENT

Deciding to create a new pain practice or pain center is dependent on many factors. A market analysis and feasibility study should be done to assess market saturation of similar specialty practices, financial and operating resources, space availability/cost, personnel needs for nursing, technical support, and administrative support, as well as payor mix, reimbursement history, and income potential.[10] A business plan should then be developed and used to integrate clinical, administrative, and economic needs and goals. The plan should identify patient volume and income requirements and include a plan for practice growth. The business plan should include space development as well as selection and implementation of medical information systems, with a specific focus on patient care, billing, collections, and accounts receivable tracking and payroll. The plan should also include the selection and purchase of equipment and supplies, recruitment of physicians, nurses, technicians, and administrative staff, and implementation of a marketing plan as well as contracting and negotiation with third party payors.[10]

Even the most comprehensive and detailed business plan can be thwarted by trends of decreasing reimbursements, increasing costs of operation, and increasing competition within the practice of pain medicine in a particular community. It is essential that compliance with evaluation and management documentation, coding, and practice billing policies be maintained. Furthermore, familiarity with state and federal regulations with regard to opiate prescription will remain a challenge to pain medicine practitioners throughout their careers.[11]

Often, a health care consultant is engaged to help physicians develop a practice model, feasibility study and market analysis, an implementation strategy, and a marketing plan. It is also helpful to use a consultant to continually assess problem areas within a practice that is already established. Potential areas for process improvement within a pain practice include coding, billing and reimbursement, compliance issues, insurance contract negotiation/renegotiation, patient satisfaction, expansion plans, and implementing new technologies like electronic medical records or new state-of-the-art equipment.

THE MULTIDISCIPLINARY OR MULTISPECIALTY PRACTICE MODEL

Building a multidisciplinary team and integrating it into a viable practice model is a complex task. Team building is dependent on communication, coordination, and consensus-building amongst several practitioner types (Box 4–1) all with varied inherent treatment philosophies. Large multidisciplinary practices and smaller multispecialty groups can develop treatment algorithms to address the individual needs of different patients. In the context of back pain, for example, patients can be triaged through a tiered treatment algorithm: conservative care (physical therapy, chiropractic care, anti-inflammatory medications, analgesics) for minor problems, interventional care (epidural steroid injections, medial branch blocks, diskography, percutaneous disk decompression), surgery (laminectomy, diskectomy, fusion) in cases of failed conservative care, neuromodulation (spinal cord or peripheral nerve stimulation, intrathecal drug delivery), or functional restoration when all other treatments have failed. How the patient is triaged depends on the individual history of pain and the severity of symptoms and clinical findings. Teams that communicate well can actively problem solve, weigh benefits and potential risks of different treatments, discuss interdisciplinary insights about the patient, and improve patient outcomes in more complex or chronic cases.

A recent study by Thunberg and Hallberg reviewed the organizational needs of pain clinics that treat patients with chronic nonmalignant pain and found that principles of "core knowledge of chronic pain"

BOX 4–1. POTENTIAL TEAM MEMBERS IN A MULTIDISCIPLINARY OR INTERDISCIPLINARY PAIN PRACTICE

- Family practitioner or internist
- Orthopedic surgeon
- Neurosurgeon
- Anesthesiologist
- Physiatrist
- Radiologist
- Occupational medicine specialist
- Vocational rehabilitation specialist
- Psychologist
- Social worker
- Chiropractor
- Physical therapist
- Nurse
- Administrative staff
- Case coordinator
- Case manager
- Attorney
- Patient
- Patient family/friends
- Employer

by team members, "mission clarity" within an interdisciplinary practice, and "integrational leadership" within the practice were paramount to success.[12]

EVALUATION OF CHRONIC PAIN AND CANCER PAIN PATIENTS WITHIN A PRACTICE

Pain is the most complex human health dilemma, integrating many aspects of the life experience, an experience that has a deleterious effect on almost every dimension of the human experience: the physiologic, sensory, affective, cognitive, behavioral, and sociocultural.[13-15] Thus in cases of chronic pain, every aspect or dimension of the human pain experience should be investigated and evaluated.

The *physiologic* dimension is the pain generator, or source of pain. The *sensory* dimension is the subjective experience of the patient, describing the quality, location, duration, and intensity of the pain experience. The *affective* dimension is the emotional component of anxiety or depression, which occurs as a response to pain. The *cognitive* dimension is the impact on thought processes and self-concept, on how the patient views life and the world he is living in. The *behavioral* aspect is the impact of the patient's pain on function, medication use, and use of medical resources. Finally, the *sociocultural* dimension is the impact of pain on society and culture as a whole.[15] Clearly, no single practitioner can address all of these complex issues in the context of a single medical specialty. Thus the more complex the pain problem, the more the multidisciplinary approach is needed to optimally care for a pain patient.

In the context of cancer pain management, multiple factors will guide the physician–patient relationship. With improvements in cancer detection, surgical technique, and chemotherapy options, cancer pain management does not necessarily equate with palliative care. Cancer patients can present with pain syndromes unrelated to their cancer (cervical or lumbar facet syndrome, spinal stenosis, myofascial pain), or with pain syndromes related to the cancer treatment (postsurgical nerve entrapment, chemotherapy-induced peripheral neuropathy, radiation neuritis). Another group of cancer pain patients may require pain treatment in the context of an incurable disease process, and may require more invasive treatment such as neuroablative techniques or neuraxial opiate delivery. Again, each case will vary with regard to intensity of interdisciplinary needs, and the pain practice should be structured to accommodate these varying clinical scenarios and differing patient needs.

PATIENT EDUCATION AND ADVOCACY

Patient education is incredibly important to the chronic pain patient, and it begins at the first evaluation. The pain clinic evaluation is a unique opportunity to help a patient and his or her family to understand a disease process, learn about anatomy, diagnosis, treatment options, expectations for im-

provement, and expectations for the future. As previously discussed, the clinical experience of pain can encompass nociception, psychological and social disorganization, sleep impairment, financial problems, frustration, and fear. All of these aspects should be addressed by the practitioner not only to improve patient outcome but also to improve patient satisfaction and reduce treatment dropout.[16]

A recent study investigated what patients expect from their first pain clinic visit.[16] The results are enlightening; an improved understanding of their pain was the most frequently stated expectation of patients attending a pain clinic. The severity of disability and emotional distress were strong influences shaping the expectations of the pain patient, but the need for understanding was strong amongst all patient types.

The Internet is another excellent accessible and practical resource for pain patients and their families or caregivers to find information on diagnoses, treatment options, and potential risks and benefits of treatment. This resource releases some of the burdens of one-on-one discussions from the pain physician. Furthermore, practices may benefit from developing an informational website for their patients or "virtual libraries" that can be accessed in a pain clinic waiting area. An "information prescription" with specific websites, contact information, or resources can provide patients with added depth of information that is not always amenable to an office visit or consultation scenario and can encourage patients to be actively involved in their own care and in the medical decision-making process encompassing a pain treatment plan.

Telemedicine in chronic pain practice is a new, developing trend. This modality has been used in a variety of medical settings, including monitoring response to therapy and counseling. A recent pilot study found that the use of telemedicine in the context of chronic pain management was feasible, user friendly, and cost effective.[17] For patients in rural areas, those with limited transportation resources or mobility issues, telemedicine may be a safe and effective alternative to regular office visits.

CREATING THE OPTIMAL PATIENT EXPERIENCE

In an increasingly competitive market in which pain practitioners practice and in which patient-consumers have many treatment options, it is important to retain and grow market share for a practice to survive. One way to reach this goal is through the creation of "optimal patient experience" in a pain medicine practice.

Access is one of the most important aspects of "optimal patient experience." Referrals for acute and subacute pain problems like acute herpes zoster, post–meningeal puncture headache, vertebral compression fracture, or severe radiculitis should be evaluated with moderate urgency within 24 to 48 hours of request. More chronic pain problems like generalized arthritis pain, myofascial pain syndromes, indolent back pain, and failed back surgery syndrome can typically be treated on a less urgent basis. Optimally, a screening system within the practice assesses the level of urgency in each individual case. Clearly, this requires education and training of scheduling and triage staff.

After the physician–patient relationship has been established, an environment of *continued access* should be maintained for patients. Chronic pain patients often have questions or problems regarding side effects of medications or treatments that have been initiated, and they may have changes in their clinical status or need further information about treatment options for the future. They may need to report progress on a regular basis, or report responses to diagnostic injections. Pain practices may benefit from using a *physician extender* such as a nurse practitioner or physician assistant to meet the special needs of the chronic pain patient population without compromising access, care, or treatment philosophy. E-mail may be an excellent method of providing access for patients, allowing the busy pain physician to answer patient queries easily and with greater flexibility and efficiency as compared to conventional telephone calls during busy clinic hours.[8]

Complementary or alternative therapies such as chiropractic care, massage therapy, acupuncture, hypnosis, and dietary/herbal therapy can play an important role in chronic pain treatment plans and optimizing the patient experience. Such therapies have shown benefit in certain chronic pain populations[18] and may foster increased autonomy and assumption of responsibility for the chronic pain patient. Cost of treatment and lack of insurance coverage for such services is an impediment to the use of these methods.

"Optimal patient experience" will encompass many of the pain patient's needs. A recent review discussed the special needs of the chronic pain patient that need to be addressed by the individual practitioner or team, summarized in Box 4–2.[8] Periodic reassessments and patient surveys address areas for process improvement or alterations in patient advocacy within a particular pain practice.

Understanding the impact of age on the chronic pain patient and how it affects the individual needs of the patient is also important in creating the "optimal patient experience." Recent literature confirms that younger chronic pain patients have greater psychosocial impairments than older populations, while physical impairments are higher in the older chronic pain population.[19] Thus ancillary services like cognitive and behavioral therapy may be more crucial in the younger patient, while physical therapy and reconditioning may be more important to promote to the older patient in an interdisciplinary practice.

THE DIFFICULT PAIN PATIENT

One of the unique challenges seen in pain practices is the management of the "difficult" patient. This

---

BOX 4–2. GOALS IN CHRONIC PAIN TREATMENT PLANS: PATIENT PERSPECTIVE

- Patient feels that his needs are taken seriously.
- Patient feels educated about his pain syndrome.
- Patient feels educated about the available treatment options.
- Patient understands the diagnosis.
- Patient understands the treatment or action plan.
- Patient feels that treatment is minimizing pain symptoms.
- Patient feels able to live with residual pain symptoms.
- Patient feels the impact of pain on functioning is improving.

From Messelink EJ: The pelvic pain centre. World J Urol 2001;19:
208-212.

---

unique patient type may be more liable to misuse or abuse prescription medications, cancel or "no-show" multiple appointments, engage in activities or behaviors that are counterproductive to their own pain care and functional restoration, or otherwise be noncompliant, threatening, disruptive, or abusive. The high prevalence of personality disorders and substance abuse/misuse in chronic pain populations can complicate the practice of pain medicine.[20] Dealing with such a patient once the doctor–patient relationship is established is an ethical issue. Even though a patient is not similarly obligated to a particular physician, once a physician–patient relationship has been initiated, the physician is ethically and legally obligated to provide services as long as the patient may require such service. Under special circumstances, however, a physician may terminate the physician–patient relationship while avoiding "patient abandonment." The American Medical Association provides guidance in such cases of patient termination outlined in Box 4–3.

CONCLUSION

Modern pain medicine practice has a great future, fueled by new therapies and techniques for diagnosis and treatment of multiple disorders as well as an increased number of well-trained specialists in the field. There are multiple ways in which a pain practice can be developed and implemented, depending on the community and resources available. A successful practice model is based on the principles of comprehensive, high-quality care, patient advocacy, customer service, and a team approach built in the context of a detailed business plan and ongoing process improvement. Earlier treatment, minimally

BOX 4–3. STEPS TO TERMINATE THE PHYSICIAN-PATIENT RELATIONSHIP

1. Give the patient written notice, preferably by certified mail, return receipt requested.
2. Provide the patient with a brief explanation for termination of the relationship. This should be a valid reason, such as noncompliance or failure to keep appointments.
3. Agree to continue to provide treatment and access to medical services for a reasonable period of time, such as 30 days, to allow the patient to secure care from another physician.
4. Provide resources and/or recommendations to help the patient locate another physician of like specialty.
5. Offer transfer of records to a newly designated physician upon signed patient authorization to do so.

From American Medical Association, Office of the General Counsel, Division of Health Law, American Medical Association, 1998, accessed via *www.ama-assn.org/ama/pub/category/4609.html* 10/26/06.

invasive techniques, and the Internet will continue to positively affect the practice of pain medicine and the development of pain medicine practices.

Challenges for the future include increased competition in the pain medicine marketplace, rising costs for delivery of care, and decreased reimbursement for services. These challenges can be met through increased physician activism, stronger research that supports evidence-based medicine in pain treatment, and pay-for-performance initiatives.

SUMMARY

- There are multiple viable pain practice models, all dependent on the individual community needs and resources.
- Multidisciplinary and interdisciplinary care is important in the treatment of complex pain patients and can exhibit fiduciary strength and financial viability when appropriately developed and implemented.
- Patient advocacy and education are essential in any pain medicine practice. As in many other aspects of modern culture, the Internet will have an increasing role in the practice of pain medicine in the future.
- Ongoing reevaluation and process improvement are important principles for the health and success of any modern pain medicine practice.

References

1. Bonica JJ: Multidisciplinary/interdisciplinary pain programs. In Bonica JJ, Loesser JD, Chapman CR, et al (eds): The Management of Pain, 2nd ed. Philadelphia, Lea & Febiger, 1990, pp 197-208.
2. Turk DC, Gatchel RJ: Multidisciplinary programs for rehabilitation of chronic low back pain patients. In Kirkaldy-Willis WH, Burton CV (eds): Managing Low Back Pain, 3rd ed. New York, Churchill Livingstone, 1999, pp 299-311.
3. Kirkaldy-Willis WH, Burton CV: A comprehensive outline of treatment. In Kirkaldy-Willis WH, Burton CV (eds): Managing Low Back Pain, 3rd ed. New York, Churchill Livingstone, 1999, pp 265-283.
4. Chapman E, Hughes D, Landy A, et al: Challenging the representations of cancer pain: Experiences of a multidisciplinary pain management group in a palliative care unit. Palliative and Supportive Care 2005;3:43-49.
5. Hazard RG: The multidisciplinary approach to occupational low back pain and disability. J Am Acad Orthop Surg 1994;2:157-163.
6. Hazard RG, Fenwick JW, Kalisch SM, et al: Functional restoration with behavioral support: A one year prospective study of patients with chronic low back pain. Spine 1989;14:157-161.
7. Lofland KR, Burns JW, Tsoutsouris J, et al: Predictors of outcome following multidisciplinary treatment of chronic pain: Effects of changes in perceived disability and depression. Int J Rehab Health 1997;3:221-232.
8. Messelink EJ: The pelvic pain centre. World J Urol 2001;19: 208-212.
9. Curcin A, Brokaw JP, Pylman ML, et al: The pros and cons of incorporating different spine specialties into one practice. Spineline 2006;8:26-28.
10. Rogers MT: Development of interdisciplinary spinal intervention centers. Pain Physician 2003;6:527-535.
11. Bloodworth D: Opioids in the treatment of chronic pain: Legal framework and therapeutic indications and limitations. Phys Med Rehabil Clin N Am 2006;17:355-379.
12. Thunberg KA, Hallberg LR: The need for organizational development of pain clinics: A case study. Disabil Rehabil 2002; 24:755-762.
13. Miaskowski C: Principles of pain assessment. In Pappagallo M (ed): The neurological basis of pain. New York, McGraw-Hill, 2005, pp 195-207.
14. Ahles TA, Blanchard EB, Rickdoschel JC: The multidimensional nature of cancer related pain. Pain 1983;17:277-288.
15. McGuire DB: The multidimensional phenomenon of cancer pain. In McGuire DB, Yarbro CH (eds): Cancer pain management. Philadelphia, Saunders, 1987, pp 1-4.
16. Petrie KJ, Framptom T, Large RG, et al: What do patients expect from their first visit to a pain clinic? Clin J Pain 2005;21:297-301.
17. Peng PW, Stafford MA, Wong DT, et al: Use of telemedicine in chronic pain consultation: A pilot study. Clin J Pain 2006;4:350-352.
18. Rossi P, DiLorenzi G, Faroni J, et al: Use of complementary and alternative medicine by patients with chronic tension-type headache: Results of a headache clinic survey. Headache 2006;46:662-631.
19. Wittink HM, Rogers WH, Lipman AG, et al: Older and younger adults in pain management programs in the United States: Differences and similarities. Pain Medicine 2006;7:151-163.
20. Dersh J, Polatin PB, Gatchel RJ: Chronic pain and psychopathology: Research findings and theoretical considerations. Psychosom Med 2002;64;773-786.

5 Health Care Policy, Quality Improvement, and Patient Safety in Pain Medicine Practice

Douglas G. Merrill

This chapter covers three distinct yet interrelated subjects. Health care policy, quality assessment and improvement systems, and patient safety are issues debated on national and international levels, and are elements of the daily practice of pain medicine. In each of three sections there is a discussion of the ways in which society and the specialty of pain medicine are affected by and respond to policy, and the manner in which the policies encroach upon the practice of each pain specialist.

The first section gives an overview of the issues confronting U.S. health care, including a history of health care policy and legislation—particularly the political background to the debate about health care coverage, a review of how health care policy currently interacts with the practice of pain medicine, and then a discussion of likely future trends in health care. The second section considers quality assessment and improvement programs, and some practical steps to take to create a "QA/QI" program in a pain practice. The final section discusses the patient safety movement both on a national scale and in terms of how each pain practitioner can expect to be involved.

Section I
Health Care Policy and the Practice of Pain Medicine

Health care policy is any regulation or activity that affects the delivery of health care. Health care policy is created by Federal, State, and local governments, by bureaucrats with no medical training, by legislators, and by appointed officials at all levels of regulatory and reimbursement agencies. It is created also by private payers and their medical directors; by judges, attorneys, and juries; by state workers' compensation medical directors and their administrators, and sometimes by their clerical staff. It is originated by hospital, ambulatory surgery center, and long-term care center administrators, practice managers, auditing and certifying organizations, physician specialty societies, state nursing and medical boards, and individual physicians and their staffs. These entities all create policy often as a by-product of the assumptions and decisions made in the course of the regular workday concerning individual patients or procedures, which then result in farther-reaching precedents and decisions about the way that medical care will be practiced and reimbursed.

The modern practice of pain medicine is subject to guidelines and regulation promulgated by these various entities, including practice and payment guidelines, requirements for equipment, electronic records, personnel training, medication management, coding compliance, HIPAA, and a host of other initiatives that all are a response in one way or another to societal concerns about health care quality and cost in general, and often about pain medicine quality and cost in particular.

Unmanaged painful conditions are recognized as a significant burden on the remainder of society and the country's economic health.[1] However, pain medicine has been largely overlooked by health policy researchers despite its significant cost to society and to patients and their families.[2,3] It is concerning that health care policy regarding pain management is created in such a vacuum of knowledge, but that concern deepens when it is appreciated that such policy has a proven and profound effect on the outcomes of patients' treatment, perhaps more so for pain patients than any other. One obvious example is society's reliance upon the tort system's link between the liability and the compensation—and thus the care—for injury and disability. This "system" is overly expansive and uneven at best in its response to real care needs.[4,5]

The importance of health to the success of any society ensures that its delivery will always be a centerpiece of government and private policy decisions. Health care policy is characterized by relatively constant flux primarily because its direction is controlled by the perennial interplay of partisan politics, moral outrage, religion, altruism, fear, blame, self-interest, misinformation, ignorance, and large amounts of money.[6-8] The result is a repetitive pastiche of legislative and regulatory short-term repairs rather than full programmatic reform. One misconception consequent to such tinkering is the belief that new issues confront today's health care policy makers, when in fact the same barriers to good care have been present for many years.

U.S. HEALTH CARE AND HEALTH CARE POLICY: THE SCOPE OF THE PROBLEM AND SOCIETY'S ROLE

The Cost of Health Care

The delivery of health services in this country is a giant enterprise. It is actually the largest industry in the nation with an economy of more than $1.6 trillion. The United States expends more annually on health care per capita than any other nation in the world, by a margin of almost 50% over its nearest "competitor," Switzerland. Even more striking is that the bill for the nation's health care is not just growing, it is *engulfing* the ability of the nation's workers to pay the tab. The growth rate in real per capita national health care spending averaged 4.1% over the last 55 years of the 20th century, while U.S. gross domestic product (GDP) rose at an annual rate of only 1.5%.[9] In fact, health care's "share" of GDP has risen from only 5.1% in 1960 to 13.1% in 1999, and is projected to be 16.5% by the end of 2006, 20% by 2015, and as high as 38% by the second half of this century (Fig. 5–1).[10]

All of these numbers outstrip those seen in the other developed countries, as represented by members of the Organization for Economic Cooperation and Development (OECD). Our nearest neighbors in per capita spending on health care are Switzerland and Norway, who in 2001 spent only 68% and 60% of what the United States does per citizen, respectively (Fig. 5–2). While 2001 expenditures on health care represented 13.9% of GDP in the United States, Switzerland's rate was 11.1%, Norway's was only 8.0% and the average expenditure of the 30 OECD countries was 8.1%. The growth rate of health care expenditures was also faster in this country, at 3.1%, whereas only 2.3% for Sweden and 2.8% for Norway, using the data for 2001.[11] By 2003, overall U.S. health care spending had risen to 15% of GDP while the average for the other 29 countries was only 8.4%.[12]

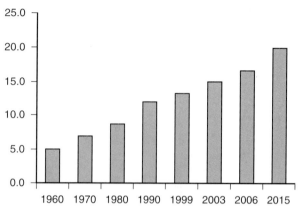

Figure 5–1. U.S. health care spending as a percentage of gross domestic product (GDP), 1960-2015. This graph shows the remarkable escalation in spending on health care in the United States with expected increases by 2015. Both the absolute value and the rate of increase greatly outstrip that of any other nation in the Organization for Economic Cooperation and Development (OECD). (From Chernew ME, Hirth RA, Culter DM: Increased spending on health care: How much can the United States afford? Health Aff 2003;22:15-25.)

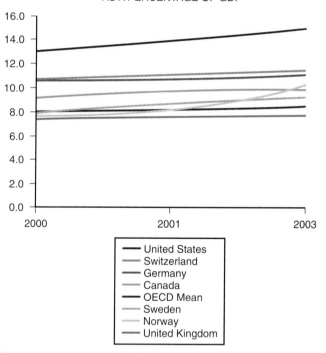

Figure 5–2. International health care spending as a percentage of gross domestic product (GDP). The notable findings are twofold: (1) The United States expends significantly more per capita on health care in relation to the GDP than any other country. (2) The gap is widening. This chart was assembled using data from the sources noted (see endnotes for specific citations).

Of note, the reason for this spending in the United States is not government coverage. The United States lags well behind other countries in the percentage of its citizens who are beneficiaries of public insurance programs and is much more dependent upon private insurance than are other countries (Fig. 5–3).[13]

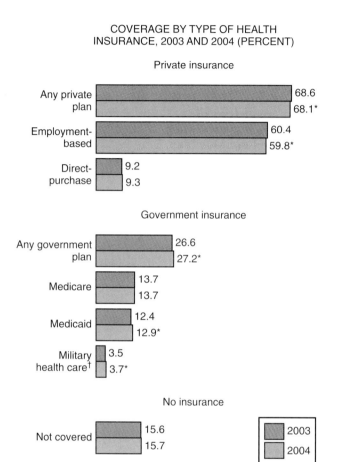

COVERAGE BY TYPE OF HEALTH INSURANCE, 2003 AND 2004 (PERCENT)

Private insurance

Any private plan — 68.6 / 68.1*
Employment-based — 60.4 / 59.8*
Direct-purchase — 9.2 / 9.3

Government insurance

Any government plan — 26.6 / 27.2*
Medicare — 13.7 / 13.7
Medicaid — 12.4 / 12.9*
Military health care[†] — 3.5 / 3.7*

No insurance

Not covered — 15.6 / 15.7

■ 2003
□ 2004

* Statistically different at the 90% confidence level.

[†] Military health care includes: CHAMPUS (Comprehensive Health and Medical Plan for Uniformed Services)/Tricare and CHAMPVA (Civilian Health and Medical Program of the Department of Veterans Affairs), as well as care provided by the Department of Veterans Affairs and the military.

Note: The estimates by type of coverage are not mutually exclusive; people can be covered by more than one type of health insurance during the year.

Figure 5–3. Health insurance coverage by type of plan, 2003-2004. This graph shows distribution of health care insurance coverage types in the United States for 2 years—2003 and 2004. The types are not mutually exclusive, such that many (most) private plans are also employment-based. The rate of private coverage and of the uninsured exceeds that found in other countries, and the rate of government-sponsored health care plans lags behind the international norms (see text). (From Health Insurance Coverage in America—2004 Data Update, #7415. The Henry J. Kaiser Family Foundation, November, 2005. This information was reprinted with permission from the Henry J. Kaiser Family Foundation. The Kaiser Family Foundation, based in Menlo Park, Calif, is a nonprofit, private operating foundation focusing on the major health care issues facing the nation and is not associated with Kaiser Permanente or Kaiser Industries.)

Why is health care more expensive in the United States and why is that cost escalating faster here than elsewhere? These questions are the subject of much debate and there is no shortage of answers. Our system is very inefficient, as measured by the high cost of administrative overhead compared to that of care systems in other countries.[14,15] One study found that 31% of health care expenditures were for administrative costs in the United States, while only 16.7% were so used in Canada. This "unnecessary" difference in administrative cost exceeds $752 per U.S. citizen per year.[16] Substantial costs also occur because public programs and the uninsured so severely underpay health care providers that they then charge the private carriers more in order to cover their own costs. This "cost shifting" is a massively inefficient means of paying for health care, and is responsible for approximately 13% of all private insurance costs. It is passed on to the employers as an approximately 9% additional cost for group health benefits, or a $900 "hidden tax" on each benefit package an employer buys.[17]

Two other reasons for higher costs of care in the United States are high labor costs for health care workers and poor bargaining power by the purchasers of health care.[18] Labor costs make up most of health care expenditure, and labor is more expensive in the United States because there is a relative shortage of workers here, primarily because talented and motivated U.S. citizens have so many good jobs to choose from other than health care. This is not true in many countries, where working as a physician or nurse is by far the best paying job available.

The many entities that purchase health care here are unable to bargain effectively for price breaks because of the labor shortages, because of the fragmented nature of their purchasing power, and because of the regulatory restraints such as those in the Bush administration's Medicare Part D program. This ineffectual bargaining position of the health care purchaser is also different from all other countries, where either the state is a single payer and effectively controls price (Canada), or the several private payers are able to collectively bargain with health care providers and are benefited by a mandated national health care budget, in addition to statutorily mandated employer-based insurance (as in Germany).[11,19]

Quality and Value

For all its cost, the value of the care being delivered in the United States has come into question in the past two decades.[20] Health care is *underused*, *overused*, and *misused*.[21] It is claimed that surgery is overused as much as 86% of the time and incurs significant risk,[22] yet the average citizen only gets 55% of the care he or she is supposed to receive.[23,24] However, another indicator of quality, accurate documentation of care, is often poorly performed and that might explain some portion of the apparent underuse of appropriate care.[25]

Misuse may cause as "few" as 44,000 and as many as 98,000 hospital deaths annually, according to the National Academy of Sciences' Institute of Medicine (IOM), but the number has been placed as high as 180,000 by others.[26] Others cite widespread evidence of poor quality, including a dire list compiled by Feazell and Marren[27]:

1. Medical error may cause 400,000 deaths in the United States every year.
2. Ninety-eight thousand of those deaths occur in hospitals.
3. Twenty-five percent of all hospital deaths are avoidable.
4. Thirty-three percent of hospital procedures incur risk without benefit.
5. Thirty-three percent of laboratory tests are never followed up by the ordering physician.
6. Thirty percent of acute care and 20% of chronic care rendered annually is not indicated.

A recent study showed that 3.4% of hospitalizations were marred by injury.[28] Injury during hospitalization may cost as much as 9.3 billion dollars per annum.[29] For all the money spent by the United States, it ranks only 29th in life expectancy and is dismally low in the sad statistic of infant mortality, resembling an undeveloped nation.[30] The United States suffers an infant mortality rate of 6.8 per 1000 live births or 26th among the 30 countries that make up the OECD, just ahead of Poland, the Slovak Republic, Mexico, and Turkey (Fig. 5–4).

More than 45 million of our citizens are uninsured, a condition that leaves them shut out of the health care system to the extent that as many as 18,000 deaths would be averted each year if there were no uninsured in this country.[31] While it comes as no surprise that better quality health is associated with health care coverage, not all health insurance is equal and data shows that those who are indigent and on Medicaid are not as healthy as those who can afford private insurance (Fig. 5–5).

Even with these quality deficits, health care financially devastates a growing portion of the U.S. public. Seventy-seven million, or nearly 40% of all adult Americans either have difficulty with medical bills, are in medical debt, or both. Two thirds of those people, or 30% of adult Americans, do not seek the health care they need as a result of this indebtedness.[32] Among the urban poor, more than two thirds of adults are victims of predatory medical billing and are currently in debt because of medical bills, or they have been referred to collections for medical debt, or both, to the extent that they have avoided seeking necessary health care.[33] Health care is taking over the American household budget (Fig. 5–6). Health costs are harder on the very poor, where such payments make up more than 15% of the household budget, as opposed to the wealthiest 20% of Americans, who spend only 3% of their incomes on health care (Fig. 5–7). Health debt is so significant that it now accounts for at least 25% of all personal bankruptcies in the United States.[34] This situation is the equivalent of the debtor's prisons of the 19th century, as the costs of basic needs are destroying the lives of those who cannot pay.

Health care delivery is also inequitable in its application in the United States across cultural, racial, economic, and geographic boundaries (Fig. 5–8).[35-38] This variability in access is important: simply

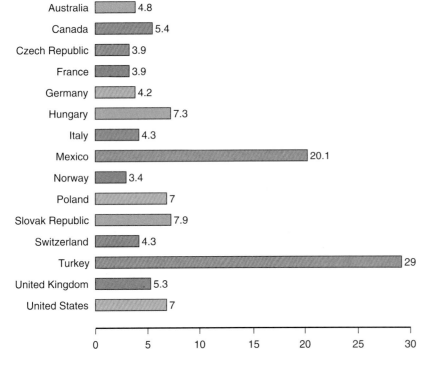

INFANT MORTALITY PER 1000 LIVE BIRTHS, 2002

Australia	4.8
Canada	5.4
Czech Republic	3.9
France	3.9
Germany	4.2
Hungary	7.3
Italy	4.3
Mexico	20.1
Norway	3.4
Poland	7
Slovak Republic	7.9
Switzerland	4.3
Turkey	29
United Kingdom	5.3
United States	7

Figure 5–4. Infant mortality by 1000 live births by Organization for Economic Cooperation and Development (OECD) nation, 2002. This graph shows the variation in infant mortality among countries represented by the OECD. Note the position of the United States at 7 per 1000 as opposed to the other "western" countries. (From OECD Health Data, 2006. Available at http://www.oecd.org/dataoecd/7/41/35530083.xls.)

HEALTH STATUS WITHIN HEALTH
INSURANCE COVERAGE TYPES, 2004

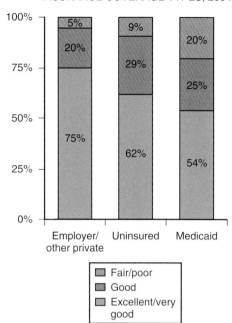

Medicaid also includes S-CHIP, other state programs,
Medicare, and military-related coverage. Data may not
total 100% due to rounding.

Figure 5–5. Effect of no insurance on health. This chart shows that patients with private health insurance rate their own health status higher than either those with no insurance or with Medicaid and other government-sponsored programs. (From Health Insurance Coverage in America—2004 Data Update, #7415. The Henry J. Kaiser Family Foundation, November, 2005. This information was reprinted with permission from the Henry J. Kaiser Family Foundation. The Kaiser Family Foundation, based in Menlo Park, Calif, is a nonprofit, private operating foundation focusing on the major health care issues facing the nation and is not associated with Kaiser Permanente or Kaiser Industries.)

PERSONAL SPENDING AS A PERCENTAGE
OF HOUSEHOLD SPENDING, 1970–2000

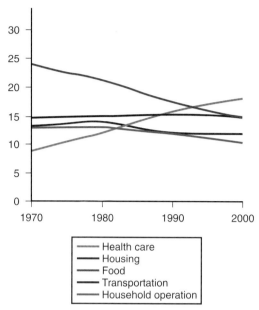

Figure 5–6. Personal spending as a percentage of household spending 1970-2000. This graph illustrates the rapid acceleration of health care as the primary cost to the average U.S. home, outstripping all others and now reaching more than 18% of the household budget. (Data from Reinhardt, UE, Hussey PS, Anderson GF: U.S. health care spending in an international context. Health Aff 2004;23:10-25.)

Figure 5–7. Health care expenditure by wealth quintile. This chart shows the disparity in the cost of health care to those in the lowest 20% income in the United States (who pay more than 15% of their income for health care) versus those in the middle and upper brackets, who pay 6% or less. Taken together with the known decreased access to care for those in the lower income levels, the fact that they have to pay more to get less is clear. (From www.bls.gov/cex/2004/Standard/quintile.pdf.)

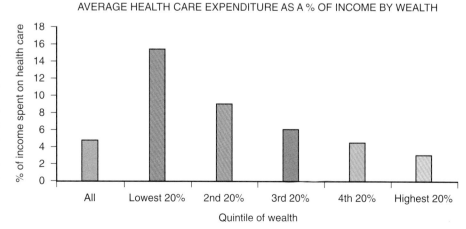

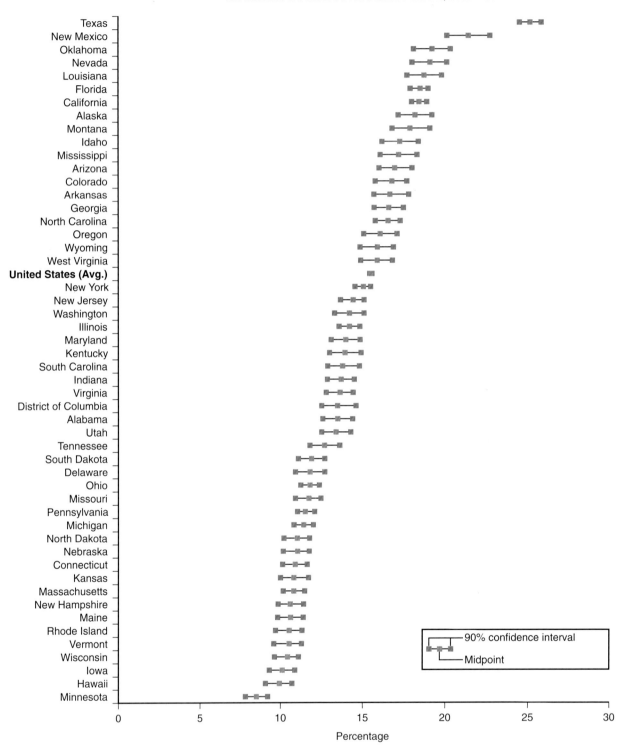

THREE-YEAR-AVERAGE PERCENTAGE OF PEOPLE WITHOUT
HEALTH INSURANCE COVERAGE BY STATE, 2002–2004

Figure 5–8. Variability of uninsured by state: average from 2002 to 2004. Variability would be expected in this system, where states administer non-Medicare programs. However, marked variability in the incidence of uninsured from state to state should be viewed the same as wide geographic variability in the use of medical procedures: It indicates poor quality of care. Three-hundred percent variation (e.g., Texas vs. Minnesota) indicates a significant negative impact on health care access, and therefore health. Those who would improve U.S. health care quality will need to address this issue. (From U.S. Census Bureau, Current Population Survey, 2003 to 2005 Annual Social and Economic Supplements. Available at http://www.census.gov/prod/2005pubs/p60-229.pdf.)

achieving equity in access to health care between Caucasian and African-American patients could save more than 80,000 lives per year, a target similar to that espoused by the IOM and the 100,000 Lives Campaign.[39]

Health care in almost any form is expensive, yet a link between money expended on services and the health of the recipients does not exist, suggesting that there is overuse of health care in the United States.[40] Examples of overuse specific to pain medicine are the routine use of magnetic resonance imaging scans for acute axial back pain and frequent use of invasive injection or implantation therapies applied in the absence of progressive improvement in pain or function. This latter example is displayed in the wide geographic variation in the application of these procedures around the country (Figs. 5–9 and 5–10).[41] Variation in care often (but not always) indicates poor quality and it is significant in the United States, where the use of surgery to treat lumbar disk herniation and to treat spinal stenosis each varies geographically by 8-fold and 12-fold, respectively.[42]

Some believe variability is caused by physicians who increased their procedural volumes to gain higher reimbursement, but that is disproved by the significant variation also extant in the care provided by salaried Veterans Administration physicians.[43] Rather, it is a symptom of the poor link between evidence and practice that is present in the United States (and elsewhere).[44]

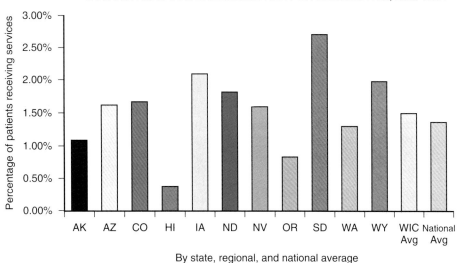

Figure 5–9. Variation in rate of application of spinal canal injections for chronic pain, 2003-2004. This chart shows the remarkable variation in spinal canal injections recorded by the Medicare carrier Noridian in the 11 states it served in 2003 and part of 2004. (From documents provided by the Noridian Administrative Service States' Carrier Advisory Committee during local contractor policy development process (LCD); prepared by the Centers for Medicare and Medicaid Services (CMS), Program Safety Contractor (PSC), August 2004.)

Figure 5–10. Inverse probability of receiving an injection anywhere but Texas. This graph shows the CMS data for six states with regard to three injections: cervical transforaminal epidural steroids; lumbar facet injection, single level; and epidural lysis of adhesions. The variation of care is most notable in that all bars to the right portray a diminished incidence of the use of these procedures with Texas serving as the baseline. Epidural neurolysis shows the most variation, with more than 80 times less use in Colorado per capita than in Texas. Such variation in care has been shown to be associated with a deficit in the quality of evidence for appropriate indications and is noted by health care policy experts as an indication of overuse. (From Merrill DG: Hoffman's glasses: Evidence-based medicine and the search for quality in the literature of interventional pain medicine. RAPM 2003;28: 547-560.)

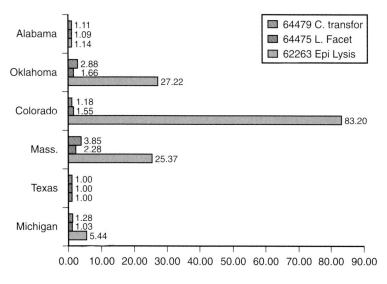

Care variation can be a pathway to discover best practice, so not all variation is a priori "bad."[45] Rather, variation is simply a signal indicating that something may be learned, that a best practice may be uncovered, and so measurement to detect variation is key to quality improvement.

Is the product worth the cost? High cost is not a guarantee of good health care; we know that higher costs are associated with increased delivery of care but no improvement in health outcomes or satisfaction.[46] In truth, geographic variation in resource use is greater than it is for quality.[47] Even as health care providers and policy makers decry the lack of quality and call for investment of large amounts of money to pay for new initiatives to increase safety and other beneficial programs, many modern policy makers are much more concerned about containing the costs of health care than in improving its quality. Their approach is not new. To varying degrees, each of these problems—access, inequity, inefficiency, and lack of value (high cost for poor quality)—has been the focus of government policy makers, health care professionals, social reformers, business and labor interests, economists, and the insurance industry for more than a century. Bodenheimer correctly notes, however, that in comparison to the push for lower costs, the quality movement is younger and the powerful advocates of decreasing cost may diminish the investment in and efficacy of widespread quality and safety programs now being touted.[48]

IS POOR QUALITY HEALTH DUE TO POOR QUALITY HEALTH CARE?

It is not the nature of this country's health care, but it is the nature of this country's social hierarchy and its inherent inequities that lead to poor quality health among its citizens.[49] There is a problem of poor application of medical science, but a bigger problem with the health of Americans is the lack of autonomy—a function of education—and the diminished social interaction that characterizes life for those in the lower socioeconomic strata of U.S. society. Great Britain, a country similar to the United States in many respects, is a much healthier nation, which appears to be related to a smaller difference between the quality of life among the highest and the lowest echelons of society in the United Kingdom.[50] There is a correlation between disease severity and lower economic and educational accomplishment in both societies. However, the United States has a purportedly "steeper gradient" in its socioeconomic status, and thus a greater incidence of poor health among the lowest levels of society compared to the highest. For instance, the U.S. infant mortality rate is 7 per 1000 live births, with a range of 5.8 for whites to 14.3 for blacks. By contrast, the U.K. numbers are 5.6 overall with "only" a doubling of the rate between the highest and lowest classes.[51]

A striking disparity also exists between the United States and Canada, where a recent study showed that, despite the much larger amount of money spent by the United States on health care, the health data of the populations are equivalent.[52] More alarming was the finding that the lowest income Americans are much more likely to be in poor health and to be disabled than the poorest Canadians. This is attributed to there being health care coverage in Canada for the indigent, who have complete access to preventive and emergency care, and there being no such coverage in the United States.

In essence, the severe flaws of the health care system in the United States mirror the flaws of the U.S. society as a whole. As Oliver Wendell Holmes noted in the 19th century:

Medicine, professedly founded on observation, is as sensitive to outside influences, political, religious, philosophical, imaginative, as is the barometer to the changes of atmospheric density. Theoretically it ought to go on its own straightforward inductive path, without regard to changes of government or to fluctuations of public opinion. But [there is] a closer relation between the Medical Sciences and the conditions of Society and the general thought of the time, than would at first be suspected.[53]

This close association between health care and the nature of society must be kept in mind as policy makers analyze the barriers to safe and efficient access to health care and consider policy to correct them. It is unlikely that the effect of any particular health care policy on the health of the citizenry will be apparent for years after it is created, due to the multiple factors that impact upon the health of any one individual, including genetics, education, income, and social networks.

HISTORY OF HEALTH CARE POLICY IN THE UNITED STATES

The observer of the realm of history cannot be disinterested . . . first, he must look at history from some locus in history; secondly, he is to a certain degree engaged in its ideological conflicts.

REINHOLD NIEBUHR[54]

Although the debate on quality is relatively new, a major determinant of quality is access to care, and that issue has driven national debate (and policy) for well over a century. The two factors that determine access to health care are the ability to pay and also the available supply of providers. The larger share of controversy in health care policy has surrounded the decisions as to who should pay how much for which care. However, in the wake of consolidation of hospital beds and the decreasing sizes of medical and nursing school classes relative to the growing population, the supply problem has become more significant. Both are wrapped up in the debate about how much is the right amount for a nation to pay for health care and who "deserves" to obtain it. Understanding the historical background of these issues

100 YEARS OF HEALTH CARE REFORM

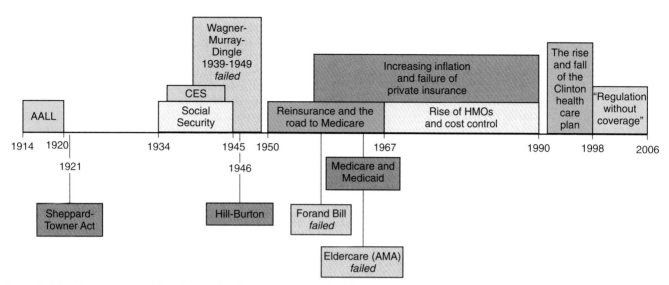

Figure 5–11. A health care political history timeline: 100 years of health care reform. AALL, American Association for Labor Legislation; AMA, American Medical Association; CES, Committee on Economic Security; HMO, Health Maintenance Organizations.

may illuminate the future direction the debates (and policy decisions) will take.

The Early 20th Century: Economy and Health Care

A careful study of health care over the past 100 years reveals a close intertwining of policy and the values of the society that created it (Fig. 5–11). Beginning in the late 19th and early 20th centuries, the United States became a more metropolitan and industrialized nation. The health of its people became complicated by their increased proximity to one another, the disruption of familial ties, an increasing number of new immigrants, with the social, cultural, and economic impact attendant to that influx, and the rise in relative personal anonymity that attached to these changes. Larger companies with often arcane bureaucratic organizations replaced family-run businesses. These changes resulted in polarization between employers and workers with an enlarging gap between the very poor and the very rich, and a marked increase in the population of each.[55] The new industrial-based economy placed many workers in situations in which they had fewer resources, either social or financial, upon which they could draw if they suffered significant disease and were unable to work.

These changes in the life of the nation were simultaneous with the rapid growth of the economy and the advances in medical and the biologic sciences that induced public and private funding of hospitals and recognition of the potential role of government and business in providing health care.[56] "Welfare capitalism" began to arise, as industries developed

benefits for unemployment, retirement, and illness primarily for white-collar employees.[57]

In response to these improved benefits for management and in an attempt to preserve wages for ill workers, the American Association for Labor Legislation (AALL) promulgated a plan to insure the poorest workers' wages (rather than pay for health care costs directly) in the event of illness. This was the beginning of a long history of basing insurance upon employment, which some historians believe instilled the modern prejudice against those citizens who do not work and so are not "worthy" of society's help regarding health care.

The early linkage between employment and health care insurance blossomed into the often fractious and ineffective century-long attempt to create a matrix of private insurance plans that would avoid a global, government-based public health care system. As such, health care became an oft-manipulated pawn in the disputes between labor and management, mixed with the support or lack thereof by the hospital and medical communities. The latter were concerned about the impact of any type of third-party insurer upon the nature of the patient-physician relationship. Through the first third of the 20th century, labor and industry traded places supporting or renouncing employer-funded health care insurance. In the 1920s, such a benefit was actually viewed by labor as potentially undermining the unionization movement, but by the 1930s the AFL and CIO were in favor of either national health insurance or an employer-based system, the latter seen as potentially valuable as a benefit that could be manipulated in collective bargaining.

The AALL's efforts failed, but the movement paved the way for passage of the Sheppard/Towner Act of 1921, which was a federal program to aid maternal health. However, it was poorly funded and devolved to primarily health education rather than actual care. Its opponents were successful in gradually eroding its funding even further as the decade wore on, despite recognition that public health programs, and those designed to aid maternal and child care in particular, were effective.

The Rise of Public Welfare: 1930-1950

The Great Depression spurred the recognition that public programs were needed to provide both stimulus to the economy and basic services to the citizens, many of whom were destitute and nonparticipants in any portion of the truncated private economy. Although many European countries conveyed most of their social insurance plans via work sites, the United States did not have this infrastructure in place. However, as payment for health care became more difficult in the growing Depression, hospitals created the Blue Cross plans and state medical societies created Blue Shield plans, exclusively for sale to those who had jobs. Remarkably, unlike the European nations, the first plans were only for the workers and excluded their families.[58] During and after the war, these new third-party payer programs were encouraged by the federal government by allowing these added benefits to be provided by employers without regard to the wage freezes during World War II and because the Internal Revenue Service ruled that employer costs for the premiums were tax-deductible in 1951.[56]

The rise of Social Security in 1935 as an income guarantee program designed to benefit the elderly was unaccompanied by benefits for health care. This separation was unlike programs that were starting in Great Britain, Canada, and Europe, where public benefits for retirement, disability, and health were integrated. This uniquely American omission has been blamed for years upon physicians, primarily the executives of the American Medical Association (AMA), who feared a loss of control of the physician-patient relationship, in case the federal government takes over as the primary payer for health care.[7,59,60] However, there was legitimate concern on the part of President Roosevelt and his administration that, while the future cost of old age pensions could be somewhat anticipated, the challenge of determining the price tag of health insurance for all citizens was unfathomable. Thus the actuarial hurdle made it just as unpalatable to the administration as it was to the AMA.[61]

World War II

The onset of World War II brought a dramatic increase in governmental health care coverage as a natural outgrowth of the military mobilization of so many citizens. The widespread acceptance of the social support programs provided to service members generated increased acceptance of governmental involvement in the health of the individual. In the years before WWII, the Wagner-Murray-Dingel (the original "WMD") health care bill was first introduced in the aftermath of the New Deal, when public health programs seemed more likely to succeed. WMD sought to widen the government's involvement in public health and maternal health care and to provide grants to bolster indigent care, disability insurance, and hospital construction. However, the war quieted progress on the bill in the ensuing congressional sessions for reasons that ranged from anticipation of 100% employment (and thus no need to provide benefits to the indigent) to concerns that national health care was exactly the kind of "fascism" against which the war effort was directed.[57]

This lack of concerted interest in public support of health care was abetted in the postwar era by the increase in employer-provided health care, an outgrowth of attempts to increase employment and inhibit unionization. This growth of employee benefits was directly fostered by government incentives for such benefits during the war, including the aforementioned tax exemptions for employer-provided health benefits. In only 15 years, from 1935 to 1950, the number of citizens with private hospital, surgical, and medical insurance rose from only 2 million people each to 55 million, 39 million, and 17 million, respectively.[57] Enrollment in the Blue Cross/Blue Shield plans alone rose from 1.4 million people before WWII to 60 million in 1951.[62] This expansion of private health insurance greatly inhibited the mandate for Congress to push for national health care coverage.

The Three-Layer Cake

By the late 1950s, however, it was apparent that private insurance held no room for the elderly or the indigent, and the movement toward what would eventually be Medicare and Medicaid began with the introduction of the Forand bill, a measure that would create health care insurance for old age pensioners via an increase in the Old Age Security Income (OASI) taxes. OASI was the Social Security pension program and it was only those participants, not the indigent, who were targeted by this legislation. However, the bill foundered upon debate over the need for "means-testing," the concerns of the American Medical Association (AMA) about socialized medicine disrupting the patient-physician relationship, and those within and outside government who worried that this would be the beginning of the end of private insurance.[57,63]

How best to care for the indigent and infirm was a question strongly debated throughout the 1950s and early 1960s. The Kerr-Mills bill designed a method whereby the federal government would defer to and subsidize individual state efforts to provide welfare, including health care for the poor and aged.[64] It passed, despite reformers concerns that means-testing to weed out those who could afford health care and the default of the administrative details to the states would be inefficient and unfair. It was also extremely limited in scope as it aimed government support only at the "hopelessly unproductive," such as the severely mentally ill or quadriplegic. This mealy progenitor of Medicaid did fail, as the majority of states were indeed ineffective at obtaining matching funds, with the result that almost all of the federal grant money was absorbed by the five most populous states.[57]

Repeated efforts to add health care to OASI were obstructed by opponents who claimed that the health care proposals would bankrupt the pension plan and by the vagaries of reelection politics. However, in 1964, bolstered by Lyndon Johnson's overwhelming reelection margin (2-to-1), a public who favored federal funding for health care for the elderly and a Democratic Congress, the various attempts to reform the system of health care delivery for the elderly and the indigent were successfully coalesced by the Chairman of the House Ways and Means Committee, Wilbur Mills.[65] The result was what has been called the "three layer cake"[66]:
1. Hospitalization for the elderly (Medicare Part A)
2. Voluntary supplementary insurance for physicians' fees (Medicare Part B)
3. Redesign of the Kerr-Mills bill for indigent care (Medicaid)

The bill was acceptable to private insurers (who welcomed the elimination of the poor and elderly from the risk pool), physicians (who did not have to share their pie with hospitals and were reimbursed for work done, rather than by a capitation system), and reformers, who at last saw progress on coverage for the elderly and indigent. Medicare and Medicaid were thus born in 1965 but, ironically, they stripped away the remaining sentiment for unitary national health coverage, despite experts' recognition that these three programs would not provide coverage for the working poor and would be inherently inflationary.[57]

Lost in America: The Indigent and the Working Poor

In the years that followed, private insurance did spread in terms of population covered, but still excluded the indigent, including the "working poor." The costs of health care delivery, including Medicare and Medicaid, rose dramatically as more Americans became covered for more and costlier medical care. Simultaneously, the economy was stagnant and the stock market was in decline. Combined with marked inflation this economic miasma was described as "stagflation." It led to price control imposition by President Nixon, a temporary move that did not stem the rising tide of health care costs. These economic woes, combined with polarization in Congress and among the public by the Vietnam War, and a Republican administration interested in expansion only of private medical care made difficult any further expansion of public coverage of health care.

Although by the early 1970s the public had supported national health insurance, it was an employer-based mandate and less a federal program that was envisioned by most voters. Thus Congress had the heart only for incremental change, but not federally funded and managed universal coverage.[67] The Nixon administration only offered changes aimed at restraint of consumers in private health care plans as a means of containing costs.

In Congress, more than 14 bills were introduced in an attempt to create coverage expansion and none had success in gaining clear popularity. The 1974 Kennedy-Mills bill melded public and private coverage, but was insufficiently supported by big labor, which anticipated an increase in Democratic control of the next Congress and hoped for a purely governmental solution. The intransigence of the unions effectively destroyed the compromise that was necessary and had seemed reachable.[68] Although the Democrats did win seats that autumn, the increasing cacophony of Watergate (Nixon resigned just days before the Ways and Means Committee vote on the compromise bill for national health insurance), the unfolding debacle in Vietnam, the failure of the bill to win support the preceding August, and most importantly, a painful economic recession all doomed the passage of sweeping public health care legislation.[69]

The Failure of Managed Care: Cost and Barriers to Access

In 1973, President Nixon had signed the Health Maintenance Organization and Resources Development bill, which stimulated the rise of Health Maintenance Organizations (HMOs) over the next several years. This was the watered-down, compromised Republican response to the original Kennedy Health Security Act of 1971. It even underfunded its own limited aims of stimulating the development of HMOs, dropping funding originally pegged at $5 billion down to just $375 million.[56]

Recognition of the need for health care cost control and the problem of economy-wide inflation prevented reformers from advancing the cause of universal health care coverage during President Ford's tenure. The situation did not alter much with President Carter's election. Although he had espoused universal health care during his campaign, his primary target in domestic affairs shifted to improving the economy once he was elected.[67]

With the onset of the Reagan administration, the emphasis in health care reform moved to "market solutions" rather than federal or state programs. Physicians, hospitals, and insurance companies distrusted government-run systems and everyone was disturbed by the escalating costs of the Medicare system. As a result, President Reagan's administration initially capped hospital payments and then introduced the Prospective Payment System (PPS). This took the form of the now well-known Diagnosis Related Groups (DRGs), created as the means of determining appropriate reimbursement for hospitals.[70]

Although PPS did slow the rise of hospital costs to Medicare, it did not suffice completely. National health care expenditures rose from $700 per capita in 1966 to $2500 in 1990. Of note, while all countries were facing health care cost escalation, the United States' experience was unique. In 1965 both the United States and Canada spent approximately 6% of GDP on health care. By 1990, the United States outspent every other developed nation by almost double and was spending 13% of its GDP on health care. Some historians attribute this unique inflation to the piecemeal administration of the health system in this country, characterizing it as a "fragmentary system that deferred health policy to private interests and squandered a quarter of its resources on the administrative task of sorting the insured from the uninsured."[57]

Simultaneously, private coverage became more expensive and elusive for the lower middle class, such that those who were employed formed 85% of the 38 million U.S. citizens without health insurance by 1990. The loss of coverage was relatively rapid: in 1977 only 13.8% of the population younger than age 65 years was uninsured, but by 1996 19.2% of that cohort was without health care coverage. This coverage loss was not equal across racial boundaries. While 6% of white Americans lost their health care coverage during this period, fully 11% of African Americans and 16% of Hispanic Americans lost theirs.[62] Unlike any other country in the world, the government did not step in to take up the cause of the uninsured. By the late 1990s, fewer than 25% of Americans were covered by public medical insurance, whereas no other developed country covered less than 87% of its citizens.[57]

In addition to loss of coverage, the type of coverage was changing during this era. Indemnity coverage, which allowed a patient to choose the provider and allowed the provider to determine which care options would be offered, decreased in availability precipitously and was open to only 33% of workers in 1998, down from 90% in 1988.[62] In 1978, Enthoven's concept of "managed competition"[71] spurred the move to managed care, such that enrollment in workplace-mandated managed care plans rose from only 4% of workers with health care coverage in 1977 to 86% in 1998. Cost for employment-associated health care coverage also rose significantly during that time, despite the hoped-for cost-savings of managed care. In 1977, employers and employees paid a combined $132 per month on average. By 1998 this number had risen to $341. Of even more import, the portion of this cost borne by the employee rose on average from $26 to $91 while real wages dropped 11% during this period. These figures make it apparent why the rising costs of health care became so very important to all Americans in the last quarter of the 20th century. This continued upward spiral of costs portrayed the failure of managed competition models to act like traditional market models for three reasons: health care is not a traditional service market (i.e., it is publicly subsidized and viewed as a public utility), the plans were placed with often involuntary enrollment (via employers), and the plans actively mediate access to "appropriate" services (the supplier determining demand).[72]

Managed care organizations (MCOs) conceived of "utilization management" techniques as the means to control the spiraling costs. Using primary care physicians as "gatekeepers" and preadmission hospital review techniques designed to prevent wasteful application of health care resources, these policies were touchstones for physician and nurse ire, as they were seen as inappropriate interference with medical judgment. These techniques also proved to be expensive in their own right, raising the already significant costs of administration of the health care system.[62]

In the end, these programs failed to stem the increased costs of care and by 1998 the cost of employment-based health care coverage had increased by 2.6 times, adjusting for inflation. The employee's share of this cost rose 3.5 times. This contributed to the decline in the number of workers with access to health care coverage due to a drop in real wages for low-skill workers, even as low-skill positions became a larger percentage of the available jobs in the shift to a service-based economy.[73,74] During this time, there was also a divergence between the losses of real wages by non–college-educated workers, while college-educated workers did not see such a decrement. This disparity has further contributed to the inequality of access to health care, as it mirrors the widening gap in the quality of life between those who can afford to go to college and those who cannot[75] (Fig. 5–12).

The Failure of the Clinton Plan

As President Clinton began his administration, he had made health care reform a cornerstone of his plans and was anticipating that MCOs would form the best way to accomplish universal coverage at the lowest possible prices. His attempt to use such private means failed, in large part because it was a too-complex system built not for efficiency but primarily crafted to earn support from both private and public funding advocates. The Clinton plan failed despite an apparent public mandate for radical reform, a Democratically controlled Congress, and its initial overwhelming support for the bill.

Two significant events simultaneously killed the Clinton plan (and universal health coverage) and bolstered the private market approach. First, the Office of Management and Budget, charged with evaluating the fiscal impact of all newly recommended legislation, determined that rather than saving money, the Clinton plan would actually increase the budget deficit by $74 billion over the first 6 years. Second, the business community began to report that the managed care organizations were containing costs so well that health care insurance premiums had dropped to their lowest level in two decades.[76] In reality, this "savings" was simply due to a drop in the originally inflated HMO premiums, caused by increased competition as more plans became available.

The impetus for radical reform evanesced due to this putative cost-containment.

NUMBER UNINSURED AND UNINSURED RATE, 1987–2004

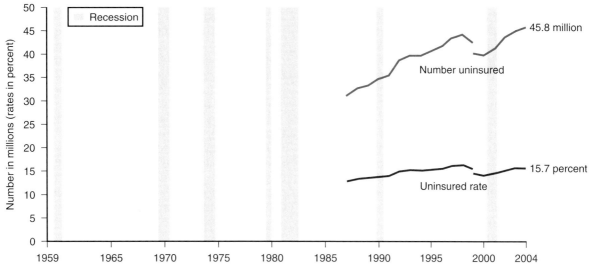

Notes: Respondents were not asked detailed health insurance questions before the 1988 Current Population Survey (CPS). Implementation of Census 2000-based population controls occurred for the 2000 ASEC, which collected data for 1999. These estimates also reflect the results of follow-up verification questions which were asked of people who responded "no" to all questions about specific types of health insurance coverage in order to verify whether they were actually uninsured. This change increased the number and percentage of people covered by health insurance, bringing the CPS more in line with estimates from other national surveys.

The data points are placed at the midpoints of the respective years.

A

NUMBER IN POVERTY AND POVERTY RATE, 1959–2004

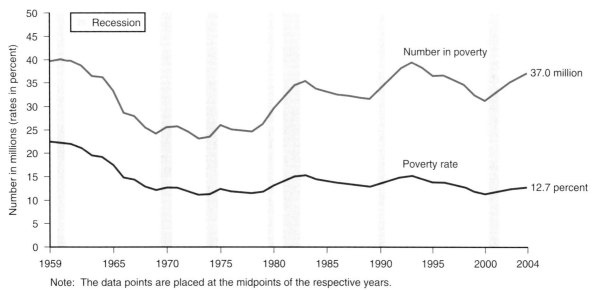

Note: The data points are placed at the midpoints of the respective years.

B

Figure 5–12. A, Number (in millions) and rate of uninsured in the United States, 1987-2004. Although the rate has only modestly increased, the total number of uninsured has crested at 45 million, with more than 5 million people added to that category in the most recent 4-year period. Methodologic changes explained in the graph's original caption are the reason for the break in the lines prior to 2000. ASEC, Annual Social and Economic Supplement. **B,** Number (in millions) in poverty and the rate of poverty, 1959-2004. This graph portrays a relatively flat rate of poverty but a sharp increase in absolute numbers, echoing the trend in the numbers and rate of the uninsured in the United States. (**A** from U.S. Census Bureau, Current Population Survey. 1988 Annual Social and Economic Supplements. Available at www.census.gov/prod/2005pubs/p60-229.pdf. **B** from U.S. Census Bureau, Current Population Survey, 1960 to 2005 Annual Social and Economic Supplements. Available at www.census.gov/prod/2005pubs/p60-229.pdf.)

The "one-two punch" of private success and the frightening potential costs of implementation fatally wounded the attempt to create a federal single-payer plan. More importantly, its failure set the stage for the conservative advocates of the private-payer system who would hold sway over the next two decades. By 1993 the conservatives had managed to raise doubt as to any real need for health care cost reform.[57] The reaction to the failed Clinton effort resulted in a flight to "market forces" and, for the remainder of his tenure, the "managed care back-lash" took primacy. The Congress even made efforts to roll back the federal government's involvement in Medicaid and to make Medicare a means-tested program like the debates of the early 1960s.[77]

This increasing dependence on MCOs led to the not unexpected exposure of their flaws as coverage providers, peaking with the public relations catastrophe of forced early discharge of new mothers.[72] The result was a series of legislative efforts to more tightly regulate MCOs. Nonetheless, the belief in "market forces" persisted and there was little improvement in coverage for the indigent, working or not, the unemployed, or those workers employed by small businesses.

The Flaw of Market-Driven Health Care: It's Not a Real Market

The ensuing Bush administration dedicated itself to the belief that employment-based private sources of health care are better able to manage the issues of quality and safety that face this country. However, "market-driven health care delivery" does not logically follow from the market experiences of our economy because, as Chen has noted, "None of us behaves as a wise cost-conscious consumer when we, or a loved one, are sick."[35]

Because the medical care consumer is not a "real" consumer, U.S. health care does not exist in a "real market."

For instance, despite the public espousal by a Republican congress for market driven health care, there is little evidence that innovative and lower cost solutions are welcome.

The case of specialty hospitals is but one example. The growth of that industry has been stopped by legislative moratoria passed repeatedly by Congress, which is concerned about the sustainability of the general hospital industry and charity care, should the proliferation of specialty hospitals continue in line with the inducements of market forces only.[78,79] Yet specialty hospitals provide safer and higher quality care than other hospitals.[80] Also, the health care system gains more in taxes from the work of these for-profit facilities than it "saves" in charity care performed by nonprofit hospitals.[81] Again, powerful political lobbies have thwarted data-driven health care policy.

The several states that have Certificate of Need regulation in force have also prevented the growth of health care supply.[82] These attempts by governments to slow demand by controlling supply of health care are not associated with higher quality.[83] As Bodenheimer noted, cost control and reduction in competitive forces in the medical marketplace does not aid quality, just as higher quality care may not aid cost control.[48] In fact, such controls are counterproductive, as stated by MedPAC[47]: "Encouraging efficiency through competition or price setting is difficult when markets have few suppliers."

The long-term result of such artificial restraint is that the United States is now in short supply of inpatient beds and will need to increase its hospital capacity by 40% over the next 10 years, at a phenomenal cost.[84] This is just one negative result of special interest driven policy restricting the potential of market driven reform and made despite clear data indicating a better path.

HEALTH CARE POLICY TODAY: QUALITY, COST, ACCESS, AND SUPPLY

Today, the financing and delivery of health care coverage in the United States remains grossly inefficient. The multiple sources of insurance, private and public, fail to cover almost 50 million Americans, including more than 20 million children, who therefore do not receive the medical care that they need.[85] It is estimated that a national health service that treated all patients without consideration of means would not only eliminate cost as a hurdle to access, but would save over $200 billion a year in the overhead costs that are now created by private health insurers, much of which is now spent in creating methodologies to decrease access to care.[86]

With increasing frequency, the employed are unable to afford insurance premiums, even when their employer offers help. The percentage of employees who are enrolled in such plans has dropped from 85.3% in 1998 to 80.3% in 2003 and it is little wonder why: during that same time, the annual cost of such coverage increased more than 40%, from about $2400 to $3400.[87] This affects more harshly the younger and lower income workers, as well as minorities (Fig. 5–13).

Medical Education and Physician Supply

The results of this inefficiency of coverage for health care include inadequate access to preventive health care, expensive and unnecessary use of emergency services, and a tremendous variation in health care access and outcomes among the different races and socioeconomic strata of the nation.[88,89] The rate of gain made in extending life expectancy in the United States that can be attributed to scientific discovery is diminishing and this is attributed to actual lack of access to care by Americans.[90] While the U.S. medical education is widely emulated, there is an imbalance between the high demand for care in the most rapidly growing areas of the country and the size of medical school classes.[91] This looming deficit of physician

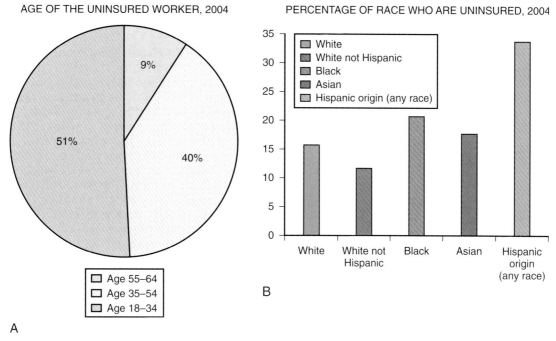

AGE OF THE UNINSURED WORKER, 2004

9%

51%

40%

☐ Age 55–64
☐ Age 35–54
☑ Age 18–34

A

PERCENTAGE OF RACE WHO ARE UNINSURED, 2004

☐ White
☑ White not Hispanic
☑ Black
☑ Asian
☐ Hispanic origin (any race)

White   White not   Black   Asian   Hispanic
         Hispanic   origin
                                        (any race)

B

Figure 5–13. A, Age of the uninsured worker. This chart illustrates the predilection for the burden of no health care insurance (and therefore poor access to health care) to fall upon younger workers, who tend to earn lower wages. **B,** Racial makeup of the uninsured, with each group shown as a percentage of the overall race's population. Thus, this graph shows that those uninsured who listed themselves as being of Hispanic origin (any race) form one third of all people who described themselves as of that racial origin in 2004. The uninsured population totals are 15% for whites, 11% for whites not Hispanic, 20% for blacks, and 17% for Asian. Thus, larger percentages of the black and Hispanic populations are uninsured, representing the racial inequity of health care access. (**A** from Health Insurance Coverage in America, 2004 Data Update, #7415. The Henry J. Kaiser Family Foundation, November, 2005, Table 16 "Characteristics of Uninsured Workers, 2004," pp. 42-43. This information was reprinted with permission from the Henry J. Kaiser Family Foundation. The Kaiser Family Foundation, based in Menlo Park, Calif, is a nonprofit, private operating foundation focusing on the major health care issues facing the nation and is not associated with Kaiser Permanente or Kaiser Industries. **B** from DeNavas-Walt C, Proctor BD, Lee CH: U.S. Census Bureau, Current Population Reports, P60-229, Income, Poverty, and Health Insurance Coverage in the United States: 2004. Washington, DC, U.S. Government Printing Office, 2005. Available at www.census.gov/prod/2005pubs/p60-229.pdf.)

supply can be expected to further diminish access to, and quality of care.

Financing for academic medical centers is decreasing while tuition for medical students already impoverishes them by graduation. In the wake of concerns about the safety of research, oversight regulation has been increased while funding for basic and clinical research wanes. Taken together, these trends will further erode the superb capabilities of medical training and innovation that have long characterized the U.S. medical education system. Of course, some would prefer a "leaner" medical system, and see physicians as an inefficient means of health care delivery. They may be satisfied to see interest in becoming a physician decline and health care delivery devolve to lower paid practitioners.[91]

HEALTH CARE POLICY AND PAIN PRACTICE: COST VERSUS EFFICACY

Pain medicine attracts attention in governmental and business sectors in keeping with the universality of the pain experience and the economic burden of pain and its relief. Pain's cost to society is high:

1. The cost to an employer for health care benefits for a worker with a chronic pain condition is $16,874 on average, whereas costs for an employee without pain are only $4849.[1]
2. The cost of interventional pain therapy was approximately $1.8 billion in 2001.[41]
3. Sixty percent of citizens on Social Security disability qualified because of chronic pain.[92]
4. Musculoskeletal diseases induce annual medical care expenditures of almost 3% of the gross domestic product.[93]
5. Chronic pain is the most costly generator of health care expenditures for adults of working age.[94]
6. The presence of either osteoarthritis or low back pain makes hospitalization three to four times more likely, and more than doubles the prescription drug expenditures of each afflicted patient.[95]
7. Suboptimal pain treatment induces as much as a sevenfold increase in the cost of health care.[96]

Despite this cost, most health care policy regarding pain is based on insufficient research, with the result that much of the policy created to date has been deleterious to patient care. Payment policies attributed to "managed care" have largely eviscerated access to multidisciplinary care for chronic pain patients, the one therapeutic approach that has proven to be of unquestioned value.[97-105] Policies truncating multidisciplinary benefits have been chosen despite research that has shown that those managed care plans that provided such benefits saw either no increase or an actual decrease in costs associated with pain care.[106] On the other hand, treating pain primarily with medication has been a significant cost to MCOs, as low back pain patients consume almost half of all the opioids paid for by such plans.[107]

SPECIFIC HEALTH CARE POLICY AND THE PAIN PRACTITIONER

With knowledge of the history of health care policy, the practitioner can more easily anticipate the impact of current programs on the management of a pain practice.

Current Procedural Terminology (CPT)

The use of the Current Procedural Terminology (CPT) can be challenging due to its extremely complex nature. The CPT was originally developed in 1966 by the Health Care Finance Administration (HCFA), which has become the Centers for Medicare and Medicaid Services (CMS). It is a coding system that allows the reporting of services, supplies, and equipment. In 2000, as part of HIPAA, CPT became the required coding system for use in all health care transaction reporting.

The codes are now maintained by and the process for their editing, creation, or deletion is managed by the American Medical Association. The process allows anyone to bring new codes or challenge the definitions or need for existing codes. The service codes, Level 1, are five-digit codes and two-digit modifiers. CMS has developed the Health Care Common Procedure Coding System (HCPCS) Level II codes for reporting product, supply, and other non-CPT services that are provided to patients. These are codes made up of a letter (A-S and V) followed by 4 digits, with two character modifiers.[108] HCPCS Level II codes can be modified by CMS via a process that is outlined on their website www.cms.hhs.gov/MedHCPCSGenInfo/Downloads/2007_alpha.pdf.

The CMS rules for use of CPT in billing are explicit in their requirement that as many codes be used (with various modifiers) as are needed to accurately describe a service, without *unbundling*. Usually any one service needs only one code while additional codes may be used to describe services that might have been provided concomitant to the first service, unless those codes are not allowed to be reported simultaneously (i.e., are bundled). *Unbundling* refers to the process of breaking down a service into its component parts and charging for them separately in an attempt to boost reimbursement. Such activity is considered abuse of the Medicare Trust and could lead to prosecution.

Resource Based Relative Value Scale

Once a service is properly coded, how much reimbursement it will generate must be determined. This is decided in part by the assigning of a relative value to each code. This process considers three components of the service: the work required of the provider, the practice expense, and the malpractice cost. The codification of this approach was accomplished when CMS introduced the Resource Based Relative Value Scale (RBRVS), effective January 1992. Relative value units (RVUs) derive from the RBRVS system and are the means of calculating how each CPT code is evaluated in terms of appropriate level of reimbursement, *relative* to all other CPT codes. These reimbursement levels are determined by CMS, based in part upon recommendations of the AMA Specialty Society RVS Update Committee, or RUC. The RUC makes recommendations to CMS regarding the practice expense (PE). The Practice Expense Review Committee (PERC), a subcommittee of RUC, reviews and recommends to the RUC the values to be used for direct practice expense, including clinical labor time, equipment, and supplies. RUC then applies these data in concert with the other two components of service value in making its recommendation to the CMS. In the final determination of reimbursement there is the additional factor of the geographic practice cost index that varies by region.

Specialty societies, such as the American Society of Anesthesiologists, play a major role in advising CMS by providing advisors to the CPT, RUC, and PERC committees. AMA appoints the physician members of the CPT Editorial Panel and these CPT panel members are subject to term limits. Specialties that have large Medicare case volumes have permanent membership on the RUC, with smaller specialties having the opportunity to be elected to one of three rotating 2-year RUC seats. Specialties recommend candidates for the PERC committee and the RUC chair appoints the PERC membership from among this group. Every specialty that has a seat in the AMA House of Delegates has an advisor at CPT and the RUC, who serves as an advocate for their specialty. This advocacy includes presenting codes to CPT, recommending values to the RUC for work and practice expense, and commenting on the presentations of other specialties. Each member of the CPT Editorial Panel and the RUC serves in the role of expert in coding (CPT) or in valuation (RUC). Procedural rules prevent the panel and committee members from advocating on behalf of their specialties, unlike the role of the advisers.

While the workings of the committees may seem arcane, they are a scrupulous methodology that strives to be fair to all, while requiring a scientific approach to the valuation of services. The CPT committee will entertain testimony from any entity that might wish to see a change in the CPT coding (adding, altering, or deleting a code). The RUC hears testimony only from physician specialty society representatives in determining valuation. The overriding principle is that CMS reimbursement valuations must be "budget neutral" so that the upward reevaluation of any CPT code's reimbursement—usually thereby favoring one or a few specialties—means a potential commensurate downgrading of other code valuations. CMS actually mandates that any alterations in valuation may not cause physician fee schedule payments to vary overall by more than $20 million from that which would have ensued had the changes not been made.[109]

Thus, the process is driven by evidence, and the demand for proof of efficacy or work valuation requires that members of the specialty participate in the surveys that determine what practice expense and work valuations actually are. Pain medicine has suffered over the years from two deficits: evidence in randomized controlled trials that interventional procedures are effective and a distinct lack of willingness of pain practitioners to fill out the surveys that then are taken before the RUC to help determine the amount of work and expense involved in the provision of the services in question. Inadequate survey responses have led directly to failed improvement in the valuation of pain codes.

As mentioned, new CPT codes can be requested by anyone. However, it costs an estimated $1,000,000 to create and value a new code.[110] Consequently, it should be reserved for those situations in which a service cannot be aptly described through the use of any existing code and should be for a service that is used with fair frequency, with 10,000 times a year having been suggested as a minimum requirement. The entity that recommends its acceptance must develop a code descriptor and the valuation process also requires the writing of clinical scenarios that describe patients and situations that would typify the use of the service and the new code. These are brought before the 20-member CPT Editorial Panel, composed of representatives of physician specialties and other health care provider organizations. There, the code is judged on the merits of the presentation and its apparent need, with particular attention paid to the volume of supportive high-level evidence published in the peer-reviewed literature.

If a code is accepted by CPT, it may be designated a category III code (experimental) and that is used for those services that the panel does not believe have yet amassed adequate evidence of appropriate indications or benefit. These type III codes will automatically "sunset" in 5 years if they are not brought before the panel with any interval data that portray a better understanding of their utility and indications. Alternatively, a code may be designated a category I code and go forward to the RUC and PERC for valuation. At this juncture, it is imperative that any providers who wish to see adequate reimbursement for a new code participate in the surveys. These are usually distributed via the appropriate specialty societies and are rigorous in comparing the work between the provision of the "new" service and the typical work of other, comparable services and codes.

If the survey participation is paltry, then the RUC may downgrade the value of the code.

All previously valued "old" codes are also eligible for a 5-year update. A similar process of surveying and calibration of the relative value of the work, practice expense, and malpractice component can be done at that time. Not surprisingly, specialties typically only bring codes forward in the 5-year review that are thought to be undervalued, whereas CMS typically brings forward codes thought to be overvalued. Because of its history of scrupulous attention to evidence and the high level of integrity in its processes and rules, RUC has an excellent record of having its recommendations accepted by CMS. Nonetheless, it is the responsibility of CMS to maintain values in the RBRVS. In the end, RUC is only an advisory body, albeit a very influential one.

The National Correct Coding Initiative

The National Correct Coding Initiative (NCCI) was developed before 1995 as a means to improve the likelihood that CPT coding for Medicare Part B work was done correctly. The edit policies are intended to minimize the chances that mutually exclusive codes are billed together, that component codes are unbundled from one another, and that codes for unassociated procedures that are performed at the same visit are adjusted in payment rate downward from the amounts that would be generated if the codes were done as stand-alone services.

Error in coding is a significant problem because accurate coding and modification is considered by CMS to be an important safeguard against fraud and abuse of the fee for service system.[111] Most providers are concerned about potential negative outcomes (fines and prosecution are at the top of the list) of overcoding, also known as "upcoding," so the errors that are usually made tend toward the cautious and result in "undercoding." These are, of course, deleterious to the income of the provider. Less experienced practitioners tend to miscode more often, although all physicians err in the choice of codes, particularly in the setting of a patient interaction that included multiple services.[112]

The evaluation and management (E and M) codes, the NCCI, and rules of medical necessity are the means by which CMS tries to prevent abuse and error in the billing of the Medicare Trust. It is absolutely imperative for practitioners to understand that CMS and the Office of the Inspector General (OIG) deem repeated error in coding as abusive. For instance, in March 2006, the OIG announced that it would pay particular attention to the coding of "consultations," because it has determined that fully one third of these were billed inappropriately, resulting in providers overcharging Medicare $1.1 billion in 2001.[113]

Some codes may not be billed simultaneously, because they are considered to be "bundled" as part of the same service, and documentation requirements to justify the use of modifiers to override the bundled "edits" are explicit. CMS maintains a website with updates to the CCI quarterly (www.cms.hhs.gov/

NationalCorrectCodInitEd/) and the reader is encouraged to routinely monitor the site. There, CMS posts information about concerns uncovered in audits of coding, such as the use of modifier-59, the "Distinct Procedure Service" code. This modifier is to be used only to describe distinctly *unassociated* services, such as procedures perpetrated at separate anatomic sites for different diagnoses, yet performed on the same day. CMS has determined that it will scrutinize the use of this modifier closely, because OIG found that in 2003 there were $59 million dollars in improper payments due to this modifier's misuse.[114] An excellent source of FAQs regarding the use of modifier-59 is located at www.cms.hhs.gov/National CorrectCodInitEd/downloads/modifier59.pdf.

Another target for audits will be the use of modifier-25, which is intended to unbundle E and M coding from other services. This code should be used if the E and M service is warranted as a separately billable service from whatever procedure or other service is being provided. However, the OIG found that 35% of the claims that used modifier-25 in 2003 were incorrect and that these billings resulted in overpayments by CMS of fully $538 million.[115] This amount of money will obviously keep this modifier's use in the spotlight for some time to come. Practitioners should be careful to charge only for an E and M service that they can justify *and document* as necessary in addition to the evaluation and management work that is already bundled into the valuation of the procedure that they are performing.

For example, a practitioner diagnoses a patient with lumbar facet arthropathy and performs lumbar facet injections. He or she is entitled to bill for the E & M service appropriate for the evaluation and diagnostic work attendant to the patient's facet problem, and to bill the codes that describe the injections. One week later, the patient returns for a scheduled second set of injections of the lumbar facets. Normally, a second evaluation and management code is unlikely to be necessary at that point and just the injection codes should be used. However, if the physician at this same visit also evaluated the patient's new complaint of neck pain and perhaps requests imaging studies of the cervical spine, communicates with physical therapists, and contacts the patient's primary care provider in regard to the new problem, then it would be reasonable to charge for an E & M code for the time and work performed regarding the cervical problem, identified with the -25 modifier and documented in the chart as a separate service from the facet injection.

Every practice should hold regular (monthly) meetings with a coding expert to be sure that its claims are being correctly managed with appropriate coding and that there is not an overuse of modifiers. If an outside billing agency is used, this should form a portion of their service. In addition to this work with the billing agency, however, practice managers and physicians should be willing to contract with another outside auditor to make certain on a quarterly or other regular basis that the bills going out match the work and the documentation of the work that occurred in the clinic.

Those physicians who practice ethical medicine and are fastidious in their adherence to appropriate coding practices, including the use of outside coding audits to make certain their coding is correct, are unlikely to fall afoul of the OIG or CMS for "fraud." Rather, CMS appears to be most concerned with those physicians who consistently inflate the services they provide, bill for services they do not provide, and those who perform procedures or examinations that are not only unwarranted, but "unbelievable." CMS has begun to identify what it considers to be "medically unlikely edits" and, when published, will identify what CMS considers these practices to be in pain medicine. There will be some controversy about how many levels of facet injections or other procedures may be accomplished in a day, for instance, but it will be up to the practitioner to comply regardless of his or her agreement. The best way to fight any such policies that the pain physician feels are inappropriate is to enlist the help of the professional societies and to use evidence-based medicine. However, evidence-based medicine is inadequate in pain medicine at this time, and the specialty will often find it difficult to argue with CMS policies for this reason.

Beware also that Medicare beneficiaries are being asked to act as members of "Senior Medicare Patrols" to aid in uncovering fraudulent billing practices.[116] The specter of "secret shoppers" is certainly disconcerting. Again, most practitioners will have no problem in this area, but the potential for the usual errors of vigilantism is high and even the most ethical of physicians should be prepared for yet another incursion into their practice by the well-meaning if not well-informed public.

International Classification of Diseases, 9th Revision, Clinical Modification (ICD-9-CM)

The ICD system was a product of the World Health Organization and was first considered for use as a classification of diseases for coding of hospital records in the 1940s. The Columbia Presbyterian Hospital of New York City first used it for its medical records system in 1951. Thereafter, adoption by other American hospitals progressed rapidly. By 1968, the ICD-8 was revised and adapted by the American Hospital Association (AHA) and the U.S. Public Health Service (PHS) for widespread use in American hospitals under the rubric ICDA-8. The current ICD-9-CM was developed between 1977 and 1979 and in 1988 the Congress mandated its use for any billing to Medicare after April 1, 1989.[117]

The ICD-9-CM classification is a product of the cooperation of the AHA, the Centers for Medicare and Medicaid Services (CMS), the National Center for Health Statistics (NCHS), and the American Health Information Management Association. Each year an open meeting of the Coordination and Maintenance Committee is held at CMS headquarters in Baltimore to consider revisions to the system. Any additions or deletions are published in the *Federal Register*. The next iteration is the ICD-10, which the WHO developed in 1993 as a revision that is markedly larger (5500 more codes than in the current version). It is slated to be the standard in the United States sometime in 2009, although physicians, hospitals, and payers have pressed significant resistance, as they foresee great costs in adapting the new system to their coding, billing, and payment software. It will also vastly increase the work for clerical staff and practitioners alike, because new, more technically complex codes will be required for many clinical situations.

Centers for Medicare and Medicaid Services and Local Carrier Reimbursement Policy

CMS maintains a website that directs the user to a search engine that can be used to glean information about which procedures are being reimbursed by the Medicare carriers in each region. This site is found at www.cms.hhs.gov/center/coverage.asp.

It also maintains information on National Coverage Decisions and official Technology Assessments. These are documents used by Medicare carriers and by some private payers to determine coverage for procedures and techniques for their beneficiaries. It is important for each practitioner to keep informed about these decisions, which potentially can have profound impact on local reimbursement patterns. The variation in carrier policy is sometimes profound and it is important for practitioners to remain vigilant concerning the denials that result from their billings. Only by systematically and repeatedly reviewing these reports can the practitioner be certain the carrier has not made an error. These reports will also uncover errors by the practice's coders who may not be aware of arcane rules specific to the carrier (Fig. 5–14).

Another website of value is www.cms.hhs.gov/center/provider.asp, where CMS displays information significant to all providers. Within this site it is possible to further narrow the focus by provider specialty, with pain information found primarily under the "Anesthesiologist" tab. Finally, a telephone list with hyperlinked Internet addresses to each of the Medicare carriers is located at www.cms.hhs.gov/MLNProducts/downloads/CallCenterTollNumDirectory.pdf. This is a good "bookmark" for every pain practice coder and manager's web browser.

Carrier Advisory Committees

Carrier advisory committees (CACs) are groups of physicians and other interested parties who advise the local and national carrier medical directors and officials about reimbursement policies. The value of participation on these committees cannot be overstated and pain practitioners should contact their state component and national specialty societies to offer their expertise to serve on a CAC or as an unofficial advisor.

The National Practitioner Databank

The **National Practitioner Databank (NPDB)** was created in 1989 as a result of the Health Care Quality Improvement Act originally signed by President Reagan in 1986. It is designed to amass information about all physicians with regard to any malpractice findings or licensure actions, as well as any clinical privilege restrictions or professional society sanctions. The stated intent is to ensure that no practitioner who has experienced any of these events will be able to move across state lines while suppressing the information. Beginning in 1992, anyone could query the database electronically. Various accreditation agencies and insurers for hospitals, other facilities, health maintenance organizations, and state licensure boards have made it a requirement that those entities query the NPDB in the course of accrediting practitioners. By 2005, more than 36 million queries to the NPDB had been processed since 1991 and 375,000 reports were being maintained.[118] In view of this amount of data, all practitioners should invest in a self-query annually to determine that their profile is accurate. The fee for a self-query is $8 and must be paid by credit card in advance.

The Health Insurance Portability and Accountability Act

The **Health Insurance Portability and Accountability Act (HIPAA)** was passed in 1996 and has been deemed the most significant and wide-reaching legislation since the introduction of Medicare and Medicaid.[119,120] Physicians, nurses, and administrators in facilities varying from private practice to endowed research laboratories have felt its affects. The primary intent of the Congress was twofold:

1. To improve the ability of the U.S. health care system to effectively communicate electronically with regard to patient information by establishing standard terminologies and protocols of transmission.
2. To ensure the privacy of that information.

In part, the hope was to decrease the high cost of health care administration, now pegged at 26 cents of every health care dollar spent in the United States.[121] The law has been slowly and gradually implemented, but by now all practitioners must have restructured their billing systems to comply with the regulations for HIPAA-compliant electronic transactions. The Privacy Rule and the Security Rule implementation dates came later but have all now passed. The final date for compliance is in regard to the National Provider Identifier (NPI), which will be in effect for all practitioners and health care entities except small health care plans by May 23, 2007. Small health care plans are also to be in compliance by May 23, 2008. The NPI is intended to decrease the array of identification methods used for health care plans, providers, and patients in order to decrease costs of administration. It may also have salutary effects on improving the validity of epidemiologic data.

Paravertebral facet joint nerve destruction – CPT ® Codes 64622-64627		AdminiStar	Cahaba	First Coast	Noridian	Trailblazer
721.0	Cervical spondylosis without myelopathy	X	X	X	X	X
721.1	Cervical spondylosis with myelopathy	X		X		X
721.2	Thoracic spondylosis without myelopathy	X	X	X	X	X
721.3	Lumbosacral spondylosis without myelopathy	X	X	X	X	X
721.41	Spondylosis with myelopathy thoracic region	X		X		X
721.42	Spondylosis with myelopathy lumbar region	X		X		X
721.90	Spondylosis of unspecified site without myelopathy		X			X
721.91	Spondylosis of unspecified site with myelopathy					X
722.4	Degeneration of cervical intervertebral disk	X			X	X
722.51	Degeneration of thoracic or thoracolumbar intervertebral disk	X			X	X
722.52	Degeneration of lumbar or lumbosacral intervterebral disk	X			X	X
722.6	Degeneration of intervertebral disk site unspecified					X
722.70	Intervertebral disk disorder with myelopathy unspecified region					X
722.71	Intervertebral disk disorder with myelopathy cervical region					X
722.72	Intervertebral disk disorder with myelopathy thoracic region					X
722.73	Intervertebral disk disorder with myelopathy lumbar region					X
722.81	Postlaminectomy syndrome of cervical region			X	X	X
722.82	Postlaminectomy syndrome of thoracic region			X	X	X
722.83	Postlaminectomy syndrome of lumbar region			X	X	X
723.0	Spinal stenosis in cervical region		X			
723.1	Cervicalgia			X		
724.01	Spinal stenosis of thoracic region		X			
724.02	Spinal stenosis of lumbar region		X			
724.1	Pain in thoracic spine			X		
724.2	Lumbago			X		
724.3	Sciatica			X		
733.13	Pathologic fracture of vertebrae				X	
733.82	Nonunion of fracture	X				
738.4	Acquired spondylolisthesis	X			X	
756.11	Congenital spondylolysis of lumbosacral region	X				
756.12	Spondylolisthesis congenital	X				
847.0	Neck sprain	X				
847.1	Thoracic sprain	X				
847.2	Lumbar sprain	X				

Figure 5–14. Variation in ICD-9 codes accepted as justification for billing of facet denervation by Medicare Carriers. This table, compiled by the American Society of Anesthesiologists, is a tabulated compilation of the varied policies of five different Medicare carriers with regard to which diagnoses would be accepted as justification for facet denervation procedures. Each practitioner should create a similar tabulation for the various private and public carriers to whom he or she bills, to be certain that their policies are kept in mind at the time of bill construction. This should diminish the incidence of rejections. (Table printed with permission of American Society of Anesthesiologists © 2006. Note also *Current Procedural Terminology* (CPT) is copyright 2005 American Medical Association. All Rights Reserved. No fee schedules, basic units, relative values, or related listings are included in CPT. The AMA assumes no liability for the data contained herein. Applicable FARS/DFARS restrictions apply to government use.)

The Security Rule was probably the most innocuous aspect of the new regulations, in that most practitioners are already cognizant of the obvious ethical need to keep electronic records safe from corruption by computer problems. The information specific to this rule is available at www.wedi.org, which is the website maintained by the Workgroup on Electronic Data Interchange (WEDI), the association of health care organizations, vendors, and government organizations that have created the standards for electronic health care media privacy and functionality. The practitioner who might be considering a new practice or new health information software product should ensure its compliance with HIPAA and with WEDI specifications. The best place to start such an evaluation is at the WEDI website.

The Privacy Rule has been the most obvious and onerous portion of HIPAA for clinicians. It requires health care providers and others who manage protected health information (PHI) to be in compliance with a strict methodology intended to safeguard the privacy of each patient's information. A summarized version of the regulations is available at www.hhs.gov/ocr/AdminSimpRegText.pdf. In short, without the patient's explicit permission, his or her health care information cannot be shared with any non-treating entity.

The legislation guarantees patients the right to view all their own health records. The practitioner has to have patient permission to share the health information in what HIPAA terms any "non-routine use or disclosure" but these permissions may be obtained at a single time on one form, an improvement in the final version of the rules.[122] This aspect of HIPAA has been the source of most misunderstandings by health care workers, and there have been significant lapses in quality health care as a result of reluctance to share critical information due to fear of HIPAA violations.[123] Ironically, it is doubtful that the medical care industry was ever as likely a source of patient privacy incursion as the finance industry or employers still remain. These sectors are unaffected by HIPAA.[124]

In addition, all practices must have a compliance plan that includes information about the rules, educational techniques used to inform staff of the practice about the rules, and identification of a person who will serve as the HIPAA compliance officer. Practices must monitor the activities of the employees to insure compliance with the privacy rules. An important aspect of the compliance plan is that there are to be regularly scheduled educational sessions with staff in which any potential privacy breeches are reviewed and employees are instructed in ways to avoid them. It is important that all medical practices document these educational events, who attended them, and that they all understood the rules and agreed to be compliant with them.

Another important aspect of HIPAA compliance is that there can be no punitive action taken against an employee who reports to the practice any potential or real rule violation. The intent is to encourage employees to help practices comply, and so the response to such notifications should be positive, include feedback to those who have erred, and prescribe follow-up audits to be sure that the errors are not recurring. All of the information on such activities should be kept in an HIPAA compliance binder that is maintained by the compliance officer.

The information surrounding HIPAA interpretation is fluid in nature. Current information is available at www.hipaa.org. This website is private but directs the user to multiple sites for information, including CMS sites and those of private consultants who can help a practice or practitioners create an HIPAA compliance plan. All practitioners should strongly consider the use of such consultants, because the penalties for noncompliance not only include fines, but also allow for criminal prosecution and imprisonment.

Health Insurance Portability and Accountability Act and Research

HIPAA compliance has required significant changes in many research organizations in view of much more restrictive approaches to patient recruitment. In part, this is because the regulations have been open to extremely variable interpretation by different Investigational Review Boards (IRBs). The end result has been slower accrual of research subjects and consequent delays and higher costs for studies. At least one group has successfully overcome these hurdles by employing more research assistants and paying more to subjects.[125] Of course, this means that all research becomes more expensive, driving up the cost of health care, a result at least partially antithetical to the original intent of the legislation.

Medicare Patient Advisory Commission

Medicare Patient Advisory Commission (MedPAC) is a commission that was created by Congress in 1997 to assess and analyze the Medicare program and to report their findings to Congress and the public twice a year. Seventeen commissioners are appointed by the Comptroller General of the General Accounting Office (GAO) and are physicians, nurses, health care policy analysts, academicians, executives in payer and managed care organizations, and board members of public nonprofit organizations, such as AARP. Their reports, supported by research done by a large staff of economic and health experts, are published in March and June of each year and are the source of much of what will occur in Medicare policy that follows. In the past, MedPAC has supported *"pay for performance"* *(P4P)*, improved care coordination among practitioners, and advocated that CMS create better technology assessment tools, ensuring that new technologies in health care are in future more carefully evaluated for best practice and cost effectiveness.[126]

Pay for Performance

The P4P programs propose to link rates of reimbursement to evidence of achievement of specific indicators of quality care. This initiative grew out of the IOM report and the resultant paradigms of care improvement embraced by the Leapfrog group and others. Its proponents believe that this will improve quality of care.[127] As well, this approach is seen as a means of saving money, in that it rewards efficiency and substitutes payment-for-quality in place of payment purely for volume of services provided.[128] This type of program has been extant in some private payer arrangements and primary care has now seen the institution of these policies by federal and state payers as well. The Integrated Health Care Association (IHA) began its P4P program in 2001.[129] Other payers have initiated "pay for participation" programs, in which practitioners and facilities can gain reimbursement by simply sharing outcome data, rather than by hitting a particular quality "mark."[130]

The incentive sizes that have been discussed usually range from 1% to 5% of a physician's total revenue.[131] Providing more money has increased quality in specific markets, but P4P is early in its evaluation.[132] One of the lessons learned at IHA is that larger amounts of payment will induce more rapid and widespread compliance with the program objectives and as a result IHA has instituted an increase in its bonus program that will reach as high as 10% by the end of the decade, up from an initial 1.5%. Some postulate that incentives as high as 20% will be necessary to effect quality improvement. It must be remembered that these are "holdbacks" and that the rewards of these programs will be extracted from the reimbursement of those who do not meet the P4P targets.[133]

Specialty societies have been invited to provide recommendations for appropriate measures of quality to be used in the production of P4P programs by CMS. The AMA has invested more than $5,000,000 on development of 140 measures that were expected to be ready for use by the end of 2006.[134] Measures for P4P can be outcome, process, or structural measures. The types of measures advocated for use in P4P programs should generally meet the following ten criteria[135]:

1. High volume—the diagnoses involved must be relatively common.
2. Gravity—the conditions that are to be affected must be significant.
3. Empirical evidence—process and structural measures may rest upon empirical evidence, but outcome measures require the more rigorous test of randomized controlled trials in the peer-reviewed literature.
4. Gap—there must be evidence that a significant difference exists between the current practice and the best practice.
5. Probability—there must be likelihood that the intervention being promulgated will improve the outcomes as desired.
6. Reliability—the measure (or "metric") is consistent when measured by various observers, at various points in time, and in various settings.
7. Validity—the metric is proven to actually measure its intended end point, and it is clearly defined so as not to be left open to interpretation by various stakeholders.
8. Feasibility—there must be a way to efficiently obtain the measurement.
9. Acceptance/approval—the metric should have been identified by such quality measurement organizations such as the National Quality Forum, the AMA's Physician Consortium for Performance Improvement, the National Committee on Quality Assurance, or by CMS itself.
10. Applicability in several settings—there must be utility of the metric in many practice settings, ideally ranging from the single-practitioner office to major medical centers.

P4P in Pain Medicine

As of this writing, P4P programs specific to pain medicine have not been created. However, at the request of CMS in 2005, the American Society of Anesthesiologists, the American Pain Society, the American Society of Regional Anesthesia and Pain Medicine, the North American Spine Society, the American Academy of Pain Medicine, and the International Spine Intervention Society collaborated on a recommendation to CMS for measures to be used for P4P in chronic pain medicine. Measures to be considered would have to conform to the above-noted characteristics.

Several potential measures were assayed for validity in terms of evidence in the scientific literature and expert consensus. In this review, it became clear that the most valid metric in the treatment of chronic pain patients would be the consideration of a comprehensive pain treatment plan, including patient- and practitioner-generated goals and therapeutic recommendations, and including coordination with the patient's other caregivers.

Pain practitioners recognize that, in those patients at risk to transition from acute to chronic pain, the role of fear and anxiety is of prime importance and that behavioral therapy can cause rapid and significant improvements in function by diminishing fear, anxiety, and associated catastrophizing.[136,137] A multidisciplinary approach to pain therapy that includes behavioral, vocational, and economic rehabilitation strategies is the most economic and effective approach to controlling and improving the pain and function of patients with chronic pain.[104,105,138,139] Indeed, detection of certain psychosocial risk factors early in the course of nonspecific low back pain may identify those patients who are at risk for development of chronic low back pain.[140]

Engaging patients in the process of setting their own goals for improvement and making the treatment plan "patient-centric" is an important factor in successful chronic pain care.[141] Finally, communication and coordination with other caregivers is a necessary aspect of appropriate pain care. CMS may make documentation of care coordination a part of most P4P programs, because, as the MedPAC notes, "Care is inefficient if providers do not coordinate across settings or assist beneficiaries in managing their conditions between visits."[47]

Six metrics were chosen as appropriate measures congruent with this evidence. The anticipated structure would be of reimbursement predicated upon documentation that the six tenets were *considered* in the care of each patient. Reimbursement would not be predicated upon the active performance of each item in all patients, as they would not always be applicable in all chronic pain patients. The six metrics chosen were as follows[142]:

1. Patient education about and inclusion in pain management planning when appropriate
2. Existence of a contingency plan for treatment of any future poorly controlled pain
3. Documentation of any potential or actual indications for behavioral-cognitive therapy and actions taken, if any, to provide such therapy
4. Indications and intent regarding consultation of other health care professionals, including physical or occupational therapists
5. The plans for follow-up assessments and a description of resources available to the patient for obtaining unplanned (emergent/urgent) follow-up care
6. Timely reporting of the patient's condition and the pain management plan to other health professionals attending the patient, to include at minimum the patient's primary care physician (if available)

Figure 5–15 shows one possible manner in which a health care form could be amended to allow these six steps to be efficiently documented on every patient.

P4P is another intuitively obvious quality and cost-cutting effort that has not yet been proven of value. Of note, early evidence suggests that it may not increase quality.[143] However, we are reminded that quality is only one target of this effort. Savings will become more likely as P4P "holdbacks" approach 10% or even higher in the years to come. The final nature and extent of the application of P4P will depend upon not only practitioner acceptance, but also upon how it is perceived by patients, who have been wary of such programs in the past.[144]

The Sustainable Growth Rate Formula and Physician Reimbursement

The Congress created the Sustainable Growth Rate (SGR) formula in 1997 as an effort to artificially cap

Behavioral Health: ________
Substance abuse: ________ Other: ________

EXAM: Mental Status: Awake and oriented Other: ________
Extremities: ________ Neurologic Exam: ________

Other pertinent positives: ________

IMPRESSION: ________
Recommendation(s): ________
Procedure(s): CESI # ___ LESI # ___ Other: ________ Fluoro used? Y N
Notes on procedure: ________

PLAN: ___ RTC p.r.n. or: ________
___ A. Did patient participate in pain management plan? Yes No N/A
___ B. Contingency plan for Rx of any future poorly controlled pain? Detail: ________
___ C. Behavioral Health Intervention indicated? Yes No If yes, action: ________
___ D. PMR, PT, or OT indicated? Yes No If yes, action: ________
___ E. What is plan for follow-up?: PCP or ________
___ F. Reporting to other health professionals attending the patient: PCP and/or ________

PHYSICIAN NAME (please print): ________
PHYSICIAN SIGNATURE: ________ Date___/___/___

INSERT PATIENT LABEL HERE

Virginia Mason Federal Way
ASC PAIN CLINIC

Figure 5–15. An example of an addendum to a pain clinic record using the pay for performance measures regarding a comprehensive care plan for chronic pain. This shows an example of a template that could be added to a pain clinic record that would allow for ease of documentation of either consideration or execution of the elements of a comprehensive pain management plan, such as might be included in a pay for performance program. Any pay for performance program should be designed to minimize the burden on the patient and the practitioner with regard to required documentation. "Virginia Mason Federal Way ASC Pain Clinic" is a trademark of the Virginia Mason Medical Center and Clinics.

the reimbursement of physicians. It was designed to use the country's overall economic condition (via the gross domestic product, or GDP) to determine annually the quantity of funds to be set aside for physician reimbursement. The four factors involved in the formula are annual assessments of the estimated percentage change in volume of service to Medicare beneficiaries, the number of Medicare fee-for-service enrollees, the 10-year estimated growth rate in the GDP, and any changes in expenditures engendered by law or regulations.

In the 1990s, when overall economic growth modestly outpaced Medicare volume increases, the SGR generated positive updates to physician reimbursement rates. Since 2001, there have been volume growth rates in Medicare that have outstripped those of the general economy. As a result, the updates have been negative over the past 5 years. The formula repeatedly has yielded annual decreases as much as 5% or more in physician reimbursement rates, despite annual increases in both the GDP and inflation. Indeed, if left uncorrected, this system would decrease physician reimbursement by fully 31% between 2006 and 2013, despite anticipated increases in practice overhead expenses by as much as 19% during that same time period.[145] The GDP is an inappropriate measuring stick for medical services. The more specific Medical Economic Index (MEI), which tracks inflation in the medical sector, would be a more appropriate index to use. However, MedPAC has also noted significant flaws in the CMS calculation of MEI that tend to overstate the productivity gains in services provided by health care workers.[146]

Each year (except for 2002 when the SGR 4.8% negative update was allowed to stand sending the anesthesia conversion factor down by 6.9%, in part due to the 5-year review but mostly due to the SGR),[147] Congress has—due to the avid lobbying of physician professional societies—overridden the results of the formula to insure that physician incomes were not crippled by the SGR.[148] Thus the SGR system has proven to be of no value as a means of "automating" or fairly capping CMS physician expenditures.

Why doesn't the SGR work? A significant flaw in the formula is that its design includes nonphysician costs—specifically medication costs—in calculating physicians' fees. This was not a part of the formula as enacted by Congress, but was inserted later by CMS administrators. It is inappropriate because most physicians neither control nor benefit from the cost of medications, inexpensive or expensive. As well, the formula includes laboratory and radiology technical costs. The system is also flawed because, although it uses a 10-year trailing method to calculate both physician fees and targets for physician expenditures, there is no provision to adjust incorrect evaluations of those historical amounts caused by errant calculations by the CMS staff. Thus the effects of documented errors, freely admitted by CMS, are perpetuated eternally.

At the time of this writing, it is not known how this formula will be amended, or if it will persist unchanged or in any form at all. Organized medicine is working hard to tie any implementation of a pay for performance policy by CMS to replacement of the SGR formula with an update system reflecting changes in the cost of providing care, such as is used in all other areas of the Medicare program.[149]

Physician and Nurse Supply

Although it may seem an obvious problem to those readers who have attempted to recruit qualified nurses and physicians to their practice, economists and health care policy makers dispute the very existence of a practitioner supply shortfall.[150,151] Indeed, some have deemed an oversupply of practitioners as the real problem with health care and attribute much of the upward pressure on costs to oversupply.[152] This attitude persists despite scholarly papers that show that the shortfall may reach 20% by 2020.[153-155] In part, a most likely cause of this dichotomy of fact and policy exists because of a paucity of objective research on the role of provider supply in the skewed market economics of health care.[156] None of this is academic, because the impact of the shortage on quality is well known: a lower ratio of physicians per capita is associated with lower quality care and higher death rates.[157]

The provider shortage exists because of inadequate numbers of training positions due in part to the policies generated by the belief that too many practitioners were the cause of increased health care costs. Undersupply also exists because practitioner dissatisfaction with the quality of life in a practice that is increasingly regulated and decreasingly reimbursed has led to early departure from full-time practice.[158,159] Recent legislation limiting hours for physicians in training and other patient safety measures have increased the costs of medical education sufficiently that academic centers' ability to increase training positions so as to improve physician and nursing supply is significantly impaired.[160] Diminished supply of physicians has a negative impact on quality of both specialty and primary care.[161,162] This shortfall has already diminished access to pain treatment.[163]

What is the future regarding practitioner supply? As with hospital beds, physician and nursing shortages will worsen. The next two decades will see an increasingly part-time and aging workforce provide the majority of health care. Continued use of foreign medical graduates will be the primary tool to fill the gap.[164] However, that trend will surely slow and may eventually stop as other countries improve their own health care reimbursement levels. In all likelihood, nonphysician provision will form an increasing percentage of providers.

National All Schedules Prescription Electronic Reporting Act and Opioid Regulation

Opioids are a cornerstone of analgesic treatment and play a significant role in the successful management of many acute and chronic organic pain problems.[165] Undertreatment with opioids is a common problem due to patient fear of addiction, physician fear of inducing addiction, and real concerns about potentially severe morbidities induced by their use. However, an increasingly common reason for underuse of opioids is fear of prosecution or loss of licensure. On average, one physician is arrested every day for "wrongful" opioid prescription practices.[166] The resulting fear of prosecution has created barriers to adequate pain care even for cancer patients.[167]

All pain practitioners must develop a practice policy regarding the provision of controlled substances. Recent legislation and regulation changes have whipsawed practitioners, making them liable for prosecution for either administering too little or too much opioid in their practice.[168,169] For the most part, state boards target only those physicians who dispense opioids without examining the patients and evaluating their ongoing need for the medications. In addition to the obvious need to examine regularly all patients in a practice who are on opioids, there must be regular documentation of their improvement or lack thereof regarding the medication's use, and a simple tallying of the volume of medication they actually do take.[170] Use of an opioid contract and strict adherence to its tenets are also recommended. Outcome monitoring systems are of value in even the most difficult patient populations and will help ensure patient compliance and document that the practice is in compliance with its own policies and procedures.[171] Finally, the use of postdated prescriptions to avoid the burden of monthly visits to obtain prescriptions for stable doses should be avoided. Although this practice is of obvious benefit to that vast majority of patients who are legitimate users of opioids for appropriate chronic pain control, the potential for abuse is significant enough that the Drug Enforcement Agency and other regulators have not uniformly viewed the practice as acceptable.[172]

Opioid prescription diversion has long been a problem in pain medicine practice.[173] Also, physicians do not have the resources available to monitor for medication abuse with certainty.[174] NASPER, The National All Schedules Prescription Electronic Reporting Act, was passed in 2005 as legislation intended to create a national program of electronic surveillance of controlled substance use. It is hoped that this law will provide practitioners with the missing link, as it will alert them to patient attempts to obtain opioids from multiple practitioners. The potential drawback to the legislation is that each state will engineer its own version of the tracking system and that the variability in design may thwart the intercommunication that is necessary for success.

Compensation for Injury and Disability and the Role of Litigation

The current system of compensation for injury based upon the assigned liability for that injury is driving the rate of putative injury higher and extends the individual patient's period of disability, slowing patients' recovery to function.[5] When one province in Canada instituted a no-fault system for management of automobile insurance, the number of claims for whiplash injuries dropped by 15% for women and 43% for men, while the number of days on average needed for resolution of claims and symptoms dropped by more than 50% for each gender group. One large meta-analysis of 129 studies and encompassing more than 20,000 patients found that the compensation status of the patient, including workers' compensation and litigation, was significantly and repeatedly associated with poor outcome after surgery.[175] Similarly, workers' compensation is associated with a more negative quality of life and poor symptom relief, even when function and work status is the same as for those injured workers who were not in a disability compensation program.[176]

Tying reimbursement to liability for injury leads to greater disability, even after solving for other factors, as has been validated in many studies, including those of patients outside North America.[177,178] The elimination of tort from the management of pain and disability is associated with improvement in health outcomes for the patient. Current disability programs, which focus entirely upon worker-reported pain and function for determination of monetary benefit, diminish the outcomes of treatment in part because they ignore the import of psychological stress in these injuries.[179] Because of their negative drag on the quality of clinical outcomes, it would be best if the adversarial and tort aspects of injury compensation were entirely eliminated.[180]

Malingering and Disability

Although malingering is a possible outcome of the current disability reimbursement system, research shows that outright falsification of injury by workers is rare.[181] Testing can be useful in determining the likely presence of malingering, or one of its less conscious manifestations.[182-184] However, even in the presence of some form of malingering, the significance of mental stress in the process of returning to work cannot be ignored if "pain treatment" is to be successful, and practitioners and policy makers must pay much more attention to the identification and treatment of such problems.[185]

Tort Reform

The U.S. malpractice tort system is a de facto health care policy. The incidence of lawsuit brought against physicians has risen even faster than the cost of medical care. In 1960 only one in every seven physicians was sued during their entire careers; now one in every seven is sued *every year*.[186] Although there is insufficient space here to fully cover the full issue of tort reform and health care policy, it is important to note its significance in the context of health care policy and patient safety. Perceived liability to malpractice claims impels physicians to deviate from "sound medical practice" and paradoxically increases the likelihood of such claims due to the practice of "defensive medicine."[187] The increases in invasive testing and procedures that are engendered by the concern for lawsuits imperil the safety of patients. This is exactly the opposite of the safer practice that the legal lobby often claims to be the merit of lawsuits. In fact, error occurs with equal frequency in tort and no-fault systems.[188] The other putative value of tort, patient compensation for injury due to medical errors, does not effectively or regularly occur in our tort-based system.[189]

Access to quality care has been improved in those states where tort reform has been accomplished and imperiled in those where such reform has been blocked.[190-192] Young physicians tend to locate in those areas where malpractice premiums are lower, meaning that higher premiums and lack of tort reform diminish access to care.[193] Thus two cornerstones of health care quality, access and safety, are impaired by the perpetuation of the current tort system.

The trial lawyer industry often derails consideration of malpractice reform by claiming that either a crisis does not actually exist or that the current higher premiums paid by physicians and hospitals are simply the result of either nefarious gouging or just poor management of assets by the insurance companies.[194] Failing this, some apologists for the trial lawyers claim that the costs of malpractice insurance to physicians are not a significant enough portion of their income to warrant change.[195] All of these arguments miss the point that patient safety is risked and that health care costs are inflated by the adversarial tort system. A recent study by the Agency for Health Care Research and Quality (AHRQ) has determined that those states in which malpractice award capitations have been enacted have seen on average a 3% to 4% reduction in overall health care expenditures.[196] Reform should proceed for both safety and savings, regardless of whether or not physicians are being sufficiently financially punished for negative medical outcomes.

Several options have been presented to alleviate the crisis, including the use of caps on monetary awards for noneconomic damages, enforced mediation, and no-fault systems.[197] Many policy makers recognize that tort reform would improve the quality of care, but believe any that reform measures should be coupled with mandated physicians' active involvement with safety system improvement activities.[198] In reality, physicians tend to provide better care when the threat of malpractice suits is eliminated and if they create systems within their practices to improve the "patient-centric" aspect of care, including more attention to the nonorganic aspects of patient maladies.[199]

Despite all this evidence, the institution of wider reforms or the logical adoption of "no fault" compensation for injuries sustained by patients seems unlikely.[200] Too much money is infused annually into the lobbying that supports the current system. Also, elected judges believe that their chances for reelection are enhanced if they support wealth re-

distribution through tort proceedings.[201] Thus the systems that are being advocated to improve health care quality have a ceiling effect or a maximum potential benefit imposed upon them, because they cannot undo the increased risk that patients will continue to face as a result of the tort system's hegemony in the state legislatures. As for the economic and psychological hardships that this system imposes on health care providers, only physician-initiated programs that focus on safety, quality assessment, and quality improvement programs, with rigorous attention to evidence-based guidelines provide any potential for decrease in malpractice liability.

Modern Health Care Reform

High Cost and High Dissatisfaction

Although there is controversy about the appropriate means, there is little disagreement that without significant change in the health system in the United States, the escalation in cost of health care will rapidly outstrip the rise in our nation's ability to pay it.[202]

The United States is unique in its quantity of spending on health care when compared to the 30-member OECD (Organization for Economic Cooperation and Development). As noted, Switzerland most closely approximates the cost per capita that the United States spends on health care and yet in 2002 it spent only 68 cents for every dollar of U.S. spending (Fig. 5–16).[11] For all the spending, we still are not

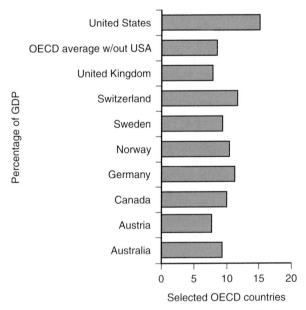

Figure 5–16. Percentage of gross domestic product (GDP) spent on health care: United States versus other "western" countries. This graph portrays the wide gap between the United States and other countries with regard to spending on health care. OECD, Organization for Economic Cooperation and Development. (From OECD Health Data, 2006. Available at www.oecd.org/dataoecd/60/28/35529791.xls.)

SATISFACTION WITH HEALTH CARE SYSTEM BY COUNTRY, 1999–2000

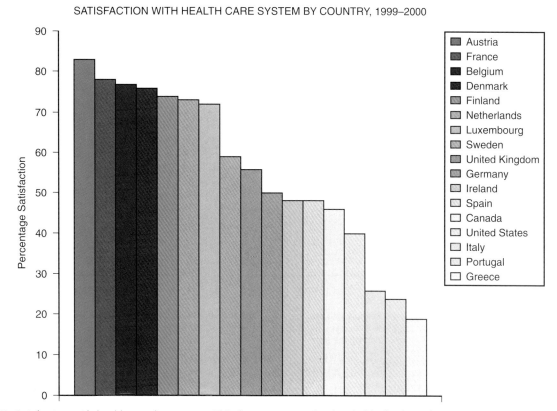

Figure 5–17. Satisfaction with health care by country. This figure portrays the decided lack of satisfaction by Americans with their health care system as contrasted to other countries. This sentiment is even more notable when the costs of the U.S. system are contrasted with other countries (see Figure 5–16). (From OECD www.oecd.org/dataoecd/5/53/22364122.pdf Table 8, p. 62.)

meeting the needs of our patients. The United States ranks 13th out of 17 countries in citizenry satisfaction with the health care system (Fig. 5–17).

They may have good reason for dissatisfaction. For instance, with an incidence that has doubled in the past 20 years, diabetes type 2 now affects more than 20 million Americans, has a death rate that has risen 22% in the 12 years to 225,000 per annum, is already the leading cause of renal failure, blindness, and non-traumatic induced amputation, and is expected to afflict one third of all children born in the year 2000. Yet funding for research on this fastest growing public health problem in the United States is being *cut*, with the result that even laboratories that have been contributing significant breakthroughs in genetic research to combat the disease are being forced to close.[203]

The problems of health care access persist. The United States leads all countries in coupling basic health care to wealth (Fig. 5–18), with minority patients still lagging behind white patients in access to care (see Fig. 5–13B) and in reaping the value of medical advance (Fig. 5–19).

**Health Care Access and Reform:
A Private or Public Solution?**

Access inequality is a problem that transcends the domain of health care and is rooted in the inequali-ties of our society, based upon bias in race, culture, and wealth.[36] Recent studies have confirmed that race, educational level achieved, socioeconomic status, and health care access barriers are the significant determinants of both healthy life expectancy and total life expectancy.[204-207] The cost of health care is so high that it provides a barrier to access and can by itself induce poverty.[34]

Those who would reform health care may generally be divided between those who believe that private or "market force" answers will work and those who believe that no solution can be delivered without the federal government taking the lead and establishing some version of universal health care coverage. The market force group sees health care as a utility that individuals may or may not purchase in relation to their own personal priorities and that such purchase should be made possible by improved economic status via employment-based coverage and full employment. The ethicist R.M. Hare summarized this approach as "Get the overall distribution of wealth right, and then treat health care much like groceries."[208]

However, the problem with this philosophy is twofold. First, higher income alone does not guarantee access because good quality care still is not uniformly distributed, because educational inequity and the biases surrounding race and culture persist.[209,210] Second, the cost of health care is now so high as to

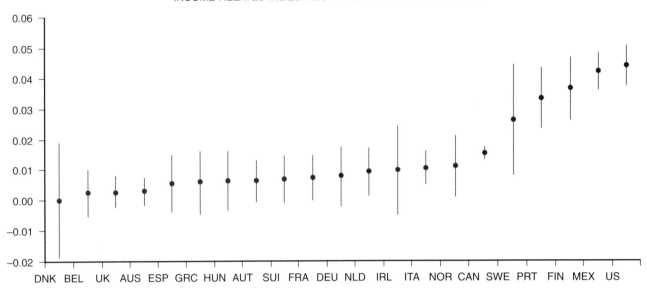

INCOME-RELATED INEQUITIES IN ACCESS TO CARE PERSIST

Note: The plotted points are horizontal inequity (HI) indices that summarize the inequality in the probability of at least one doctor visit (per annum) across income quintiles after need differences (variations in self-reported health) have been standardized. Positive values of HI indicate inequity favoring the rich.

Figure 5–18. Access inequity due to income, by country. This graph from the Organization for Economic Cooperation and Development (OECD) shows that the United States surpasses all other countries in the dismal statistic of inequity in access to care due to the barrier of income. The higher the index number, the more likely that lack of access is due to income. (From OECD www.oecd.org/dataoecd/53/10/32026026.pdf.)

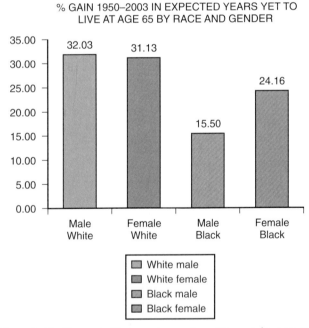

% GAIN 1950–2003 IN EXPECTED YEARS YET TO LIVE AT AGE 65 BY RACE AND GENDER

Figure 5–19. Change in life expectancy at age 65 years, by race and gender: 1950-2003. This graph illustrates the inequity between races of the beneficial improvement in health, as portrayed by life expectancy in the United States over the past five decades. The improved life expectancy of the older white male is double that of his black counterpart. Inequality of access to health care, diminished personal autonomy, and the wider impact of social inequities all play a role in creating these gaps. (From Health, United States, 2004; Table 27, p. 163. Available at www.cdc.gov/nchs/data/hus/hus04.pdf.)

preclude many of those who work even more than one job the ability to purchase coverage. Notably, even as employment has increased as the *potential* means for citizens to obtain their insurance (available to 77% of adult Americans in 1987 and 79% today) the percentage of American workers who can afford that coverage has fallen, primarily because the cost of health care has risen so greatly when compared to income (Fig. 5–20).[58] In part, this is due to a refusal by Congress to raise the minimum wage over the past decade.

Thus employment alone is not the means by which to ensure access to health care.

Even those who have espoused the power of market forces to achieve significant change cite four reasons that they no longer are optimistic about this likelihood:

1. Providers wield significant market power due to consolidation and lack of excess capacity.
2. The provider and payer systems are fragmented, causing markets to be inefficient.
3. Employers are ineffective in mandating increased efficiency and cost-containment: they are unwilling to offer competing health plans to their employees, and respond to higher costs and larger labor pools by increasing the employee share of premiums rather than working on decreasing costs.
4. Managed care plans have been less numerous and less competitive due to high market entry costs and high costs of administration, leading to few locally created MCOs that could conceivably compete with larger plans to drive down costs. As

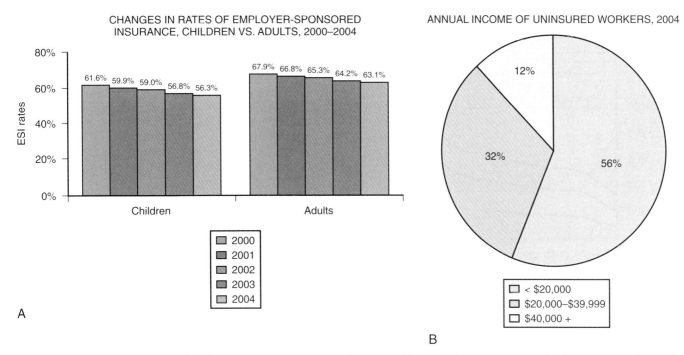

A

B

Figure 5–20. A, Changes in rates of employer insurance in the United States, child versus adults: 2000-2004. This figure portrays the steady decline in both adults and children covered by employer-sponsored insurance in the 5 years 2000-2004. ESI, employer-sponsored insurance. **B,** Annual income of uninsured workers in the United States. This pie chart emphasizes the undue burden of a lack of health care coverage on the poorest of the workers in the United States. (**A** from Health Insurance Coverage in America–2004 Data Update, #7415. The Henry J. Kaiser Family Foundation, November, 2005. **B** from Health Insurance Coverage in America, 2004 Data Update, #7415. The Henry J. Kaiser Family Foundation, November, 2005, Table 16 "Characteristics of Uninsured Workers, 2004," pp 42-43. This information was reprinted with permission from the Henry J. Kaiser Family Foundation. The Kaiser Family Foundation, based in Menlo Park, Calif, is a nonprofit, private operating foundation focusing on the major health care issues facing the nation and is not associated with Kaiser Permanente or Kaiser Industries.)

well, MCOs have been unsuccessful in limiting cost by restricting networks, in part due to consumer backlash as well the aforementioned lack of supply of medical providers.[202]

It appears that private market cost-control efforts also simply target the wrong people. Tactics like higher copayments or lower-cost managed care systems primarily affect only the people who are *not* spending the nation's health care resources. In reality, just 1% of the population accounts for fully 27% of health care expenditures each year, and 46% of those top spenders are older adults. Fully 69% of those costs are engendered by only the highest 10% of health care spenders.[211] As well, 74% of Medicare spending is for the care of citizens who earn less than $25,000 per year.[212] Thus those who are experiencing the majority of high-cost health care are indigent or elderly, or both, and are not affected by employment-linked health care initiatives nor are they capable of any response to initiatives that induce "cost-conscious choices" about their care.[213] Market forces and managed competition will not decrease the expenditures of those who are spending the most.

One more interesting note about the distribution of spending on care is that among those patients who are covered by private insurance (managed care or traditional models), the top 5% of spenders have annual expenses of $17,871. By contrast, the top 5% of *uninsured* spenders only spend $6651.[211] Certainly, the average uninsured patient is getting a far different brand of care than are insured patients, by almost threefold, yet cannot possibly spend (or save) his or her way into better quality care.[214]

FUTURE TRENDS

The exact programs in health care policy that will be enacted in the coming years are impossible to predict with assurance, yet some clues exist. The important factors to consider over the next 5 to 10 years will be as follows:

1. The state of the economy, and most particularly unemployment rates and inflation
2. Health care provider supply
3. The speed of health care providers in adoption of technologies to increase their patient capacity and decrease access problems[215]
4. Fiscal policy of the federal government regarding budgetary needs for defense, and the cost of servicing the national debt and other social support programs
5. Tort reform or lack thereof
6. Any legislation or policy further limiting research via regulation and decreased funding

EXPENDITURES IN BILLIONS OF DOLLARS
FOR SELECTED HEALTH CARE SECTORS

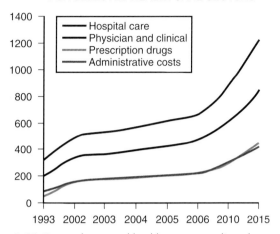

Figure 5–21. Past and expected health care expenditure by sectors, 1993-2015. This graph shows the past and expected increase in rate of rise of health care expenditures by sector. (From Borger C, Smith S, Truffer C, et al: Health spending projections through 2015: Changes on the horizon. Health Aff 2006;25:w61-w73.)

7. Continued ascendancy of conservatives who favor "market reforms" and hope to decrease taxation, as opposed to those who will promulgate public funded universal coverage[216]
8. Any increase in public desire for universal health care in response to a significant increase in the percentage of the American workforce being unable to afford health care coverage
9. The potential unknowns of pandemics or other widespread health events (leading to a heightened public awareness of the plight of the uninsured)
10. The rate of escalation in health care costs, expected now to be rampant in the first half of this century (Fig. 5–21)

Centralization will continue, with a decreasing number of payers and provider groups persisting. Technology costs and reimbursement strategies will continue to drive providers toward "centers of excellence" as larger payer organizations enjoy less competition. Technologic advance will inexorably provide more impressive care capability, but also higher cost, and it will become more obvious that a definite two-tiered system of care exists.[217]

Patients with pain will increase in number. This is because, as recent census data suggest, more patients will live longer but also will be active later in life, extending the period in which they will encounter injury and chronic breakdown of musculoskeletal systems.[218] Increased numbers of older adults will live in poverty. In view of the geographic mobility of our society, the traditional extended family networks will become ever less available to older patients. Even now, more of our nation's older population live alone than ever before, and living in isolation is associated with increased disability and worse health care outcomes.[219-222]

Greater Restrictions Will Be Placed upon Pain Care

With increasing costs and fewer payers, more restrictive managed care will again become the salient model, with spread of mandatory adherence to practice guidelines and reinstitution of gatekeeper strategies. The current lack of reliable literature justifying the use of various pain medicine techniques will become increasingly unacceptable to those who create payer guidelines. The emphasis on disease management paradigms combined with a dearth of evidentiary grounding in the literature will likely lead to the demise of many interventional techniques, because of their exclusion from guidelines and nonpayment.[41]

Some factors will continue to oppose the centralization of health care. These include the direct marketing of medications and therapies to patients via the media and use of the Internet by patients to gain advice and direction in therapeutic choices. However, this decentralization will not be significant regarding most pain therapies, because of the high cost of most techniques (interventional and noninterventional alike), the very small number of patients who can afford out-of-pocket purchases of those interventions, and the fact that few techniques can be obtained without the involvement of an (expensive) expert. As a result, patient access to pain care will be in large part controlled by increasingly restrictive payer guidelines. One exception to this will be the increased use of complementary and alternative medicine (CAM) techniques, because they are often directly available to the individual and do not necessitate expert involvement.

Controlling Cost at the Expense of Quality

For the same reasons that market forces have not made our health care system more efficient and less costly, they will not be the answer to the problem in the future. There may be some changes stimulated by the "consumer choice" movement, which may draw power from the increased use of medical savings accounts (MSAs) or health savings accounts (HSAs) and other programs aimed at moving the consumer closer to the cost. However, these programs are unlikely to be a significant solution, because costs are rising so quickly that consumers' savings are unlikely to be dependably powerful (or cohesive) forces. After all, the current national savings rate is zero.[223] In addition, these plans are extremely variable in terms of their cost-sharing provisions and may not induce any savings at all.[224]

One recent fad has been an increased interest in obtaining surgery overseas to decrease cost, or what has been dubbed "medical tourism." Hospitals and clinics in India, Mexico, and some Asian countries boast "U.S. trained doctors" and very low prices for surgical and dental interventions, sometimes for less than one-tenth the cost of the same procedures done in the United States.[225] Interest in such care has increased both on the part of uninsured patients and among insurance companies and some businesses. It is the opinion of some health care policy pundits that this is a direct result of "sloppiness" and inefficiency on the part of U.S. health care providers and might be a real alternative in the future as, in the words of Uwe Reinhardt, the overseas providers do "to the U.S. health care system what the Japanese auto industry did to American carmakers." However, this option will not be open to the indigent or the older population who are not able to travel.

Some experts consider the most likely future will see an increase in federally regulated price controls and decreases in provider market power due to more active enforcement of antitrust legislation.[202] Ironically, in the absence of government-backed strategies to increase the supply of providers, use of antitrust legislation and local limits on provider "power," such as certificate of need programs, will actually further decrease access, leading to decreased quality, and consequently higher rather than lower cost.

Current shortages of health care providers, coupled with the lack of excess capacity in the inpatient hospital system are secondary to the attempt to control costs over the past several decades. This resultant constricted supply of health care providers and beds already negatively affects the quality of care and will limit the success of efforts to improve it in the future.[89] Efforts continue to diminish incentives to potential new providers and to stunt the size of teaching centers through insufficient funding of medical education.[18] The likely outcome will be a continued decrease in the supply of available providers, leading to decreasing access and diminished quality of care.[226] Again, limiting access to care is being chosen as a means to diminish cost, without recognition that it hurts primarily those who already are unable to use the system, the indigent and the uninsured. This shortsighted policy will also deepen the divide between the two tiers of health care in the United States.

While this is happening, the insurance industry is moving to wall off the higher risk, chronically ill patient population, "covering" only the healthy sector of the population, and at that only with significant disincentives for health care use.[227] The increasingly obvious failure of the private sector to provide coverage for millions of Americans and the decreased access impelled by cost-cutting will make it likely that some form of larger governmental single payer program will be created to provide basic coverage for the growing number who cannot afford health insurance through private markets.[228] Such a new program might provide the basics of care to all citizens while private insurance will persist in a similar form to the current market to care for the upper economic tier of consumers.[11] It is likely that this "universal health care coverage" would require higher taxes and so will not occur until either the political hegemony in Washington changes back to the Democrats or if a more moderate Republican leadership is in power when the next health care crisis occurs.[229]

Alternatively, a widespread health crisis such as a pandemic that overstressed the limited provider supply could potentially make such universal coverage politically necessary even for the conservatives.

The cost for such a program is of course unknown, but the IOM study of 2003 stated that $6.61 per capita per annum would pay for such coverage for all citizens.[230] Another economic analysis shows that full coverage for all these citizens would increase the total of annual health care spending by between only 3% and 6% and take less than 1% of the GDP.[231] As the authors of that study point out, health care access leads to improvements in health, work status, earnings, and education.

As an alternative (or as a stopgap) to universal coverage, some have called for more rapid acceptance of the indigent with preventable disabling diseases into Medicaid and Medicare programs, hoping to forestall their descent into permanent complete disability and to save money overall by keeping such patients in the workforce.[232] Altruism aside, the relatively low cost of providing "free" health insurance to the uninsured would be paid for by these collateral benefits. One other more politically palatable option includes national health care via a single payer plan only for children, a platform that would be more difficult to denounce than insuring all adults.[233]

HEALTH CARE QUALITY AND SOCIETY'S HEALTH

It is understandable that the high cost of care here and its low quality when compared to other nations continue to be the focus of policy makers. Unfortunately, they too often ignore the underlying causes of poor health: the inequities of American societal structure. Inequity of health care access is not only driven by individual patient characteristics (gender, ethnicity, education, marital status, and employment), but also by the nature of their local environment: the economic standards, level of educational achievement, and the local practitioner specialty mix in the neighborhood.[234-236] Any policy attempting to improve health care quality and access will be limited in its success in direct proportion to the extent to which it ignores the wider environmental forces acting upon patients' lives.

As Marmot notes, however, the marked impact of non–health factors on patient health care quality does not absolve physicians and other members of the health care services of responsibility.[49] Rather, it places physicians in a peculiarly powerful position to help. Practitioners can effect change in the steep "social gradient," improving their patients' access to social services to improve literacy, prenatal care, early child development, job training, education, and improved living conditions for the poor and illiterate.

The Pain Medicine Practitioner as an Agent of Change

As pain practitioners, we are primary care providers who care for patients and their families at critical junctures in their lives, times when change is often imminent and when their resources are reduced. Pain care cannot be an isolated, needle-oriented discipline. A patient cannot be successfully treated for a physical complaint if the physician does not search for and treat the cultural, economic, employment-based, psychological, and social factors that abet the pain.[165,237-239] To provide excellent quality care, every therapeutic plan must be integrated with consideration of the patient's specific social situation and include access to those services and the personnel who can provide the support for the nonmedical hurdles. Pain care plans must provide aid for patients' lives outside the pain clinic and beyond the limits of prescription medication and deftly performed injections. Only such an integrated approach to the "whole patient" will ensure that we are providing the highest quality and the most effective care.[240,241]

By attending to the social support of the patients, the pain practitioner will see the efficacy of each intervention increase, which will in turn diminish the probability that the interventions will need to be repeated or the therapy plan intensified with "next steps," like implants or surgical procedures. Without such quality and the ability to prove that it exists, much of the therapy that pain practitioners now offer is at risk of elimination by payer and governmental guidelines. The remainder of this chapter discusses the medical aspects of providing safe care, in a manner consistent with regulatory requirements, and proving that it is of high quality. What we have learned to this point is that if pain medicine physicians attend to their patients' social ills and their somatic pain, the first steps will have been taken in raising the quality of the care in the clinic and in the nation's health care delivery system.

the financially and educationally impoverished, the isolated, those who live in economically and service-deprived neighborhoods, and those who live without hope of improved prospects.

- Over the past century, the political will to create cohesive reforms in health care policy has only occasionally crested above the restraint of special interests that benefit from the monopolies and market restrictions inherent in the current pastiche that is the U.S. health care system. It is unlikely that sufficient reform to provide health care to the 15% of Americans who are uninsured will occur before a catastrophic pandemic or another health crisis intervenes to make their plight apparent to every American.
- Health care policies that attempt to decrease costs by restricting access via gatekeepers, certificate of need programs, diminished support for medical education, and zealous cutbacks of provider income will lead to both higher costs and a starker demarcation of a two-tiered system of health care as greater percentages of the middle-class and impoverished will be unable to afford coverage.
- The pain practitioner must consequently be prepared to face two forces:
  a. Recurrent political targeting of physician reimbursement will remain the easiest (albeit ineffective) way to decrease costs of health care and will substitute for any politically more painful cohesive reform.
  b. The lack of sufficient scientific evidence for many of the expensive procedures in pain medicine will lead to their increasing circumscription.
- The pain practitioner's best defense against such restriction of care will be to consistently craft care plans with attention to the social and behavioral needs of the individual patient. In this way the highest quality and most effective care will be provided.

SUMMARY

- U.S. health care costs are inordinately high in comparison to the rest of the world and to the rest of the U.S. economy. The cost of health care is now and will be increasing at a higher rate than that seen previously.
- The high costs are due in part to the diminishing supply of providers, the poor position of service purchasers to negotiate for lower prices, and bloated administrative costs caused by the splintered systems dispersed among the many private and public payers, including those very high administrative costs engendered as they try to prohibit access by the "unqualified."
- The quality of U.S. health care is under increasing scrutiny by governmental and private payers, due in part to this upward spiral of cost and consequent questions of value.
- These high costs combined with inadequate minimum wages are preventing access to insurance and health care for increasing numbers of the working population. These barriers primarily affect the poor, who pay more than 15% of their incomes for health care.
- Health quality is partially determined by health care quality, but is also significantly affected by the other ills of U.S. society, including increasing numbers of

Section **II**

Quality Assessment and Improvement in the Pain Clinic

From the foregoing discussion of health care policy, it is a reasonable conclusion that a significant factor in the deficits of our nation's health is the broader social dysfunction of the nation: the inequities of education, income, employment, social support, and opportunity that still exist in this country. Nonetheless, we are cognizant that our health care system is also severely troubled. In the ensuing two sections, we discuss the topics of quality and patient safety separately. These sections review the practical efforts each pain physician can make to address those issues at the level he or she can control: in the pain clinic.

WHAT IS "QUALITY" IN HEALTH CARE: DO WE HAVE IT?

Quality as an issue in health care is a relatively recent phenomenon. Starr's massive and Pulitzer Prize winning 1982 review of health care policy and its relationship to society has no entry in its index for the word "quality" (or "value," or "outcome," for that matter).[242] Health care quality has been defined in many ways over the past several years, and it is important to recognize that the definition varies depending upon the profession of the one who answers.[243]

Lohr created a definition that the National Academy of Sciences' Institute of Medicine (IOM) has included in its discussion of quality[244]: "Quality is the degree to which health services for individuals and populations increase the likelihood of desired health outcomes and are consistent with current professional knowledge."

This definition, with its emphasis on targeting known "desired" goals of health and its link to evidence-based medicine is attractive to most physicians. As Donabedian wrote in his landmark paper on quality assessment in medicine in 1966[245]: "As such, the definition of quality may be almost anything anyone wishes it to be, although it is, ordinarily, a reflection of values and goals current in the medical care system and in the larger society of which it is a part.

Thus providers are not the only interested parties in defining and determining quality and so there are many available opinions as to what health care quality constitutes.[246] Here are six groups that might provide different definitions:

1. *The health care policy makers* represented by the National Academy of Sciences Institute of Medicine endorse Lohr's definition and have published three book-size reports on the deficits in quality of health care. They emphasize attention to evidence-based guidelines as a means to decrease unwarranted variation in care and errors in practice.
2. *Nursing staff* might agree in large part with Lohr's definition, but would add to it the nature of interpersonal relationships of the health care team. Patient satisfaction is also more frequently a part of nursing definitions of quality.[247,248]
3. *Administrators* desire efficiency of care and high patient satisfaction, in addition to evidence of quality as proven by accreditation by outside bodies such as Accreditation Association for Ambulatory Health Care (AAAHC), The Joint Commission (TJC), Commission on Accreditation of Rehabilitation Facilities (CARF), American Association for Accreditation of Ambulatory Surgery Facilities (AAAASF), and others.[243]
4. *Payers* are concerned about efficiency, cost of care, and fraud, such that they might define quality as the certainty that the care delivered was of benefit, was delivered for the least cost, and incurred the least waste possible.
5. *Patients* are naïve about the science of care and understandably assume that they are receiving the best technical quality at all times. Thus they often default to those aspects that they can assess: cordiality, efficiency, cleanliness, and other amenities such as timeliness, comfort of chairs, ease of parking, and climate control.
6. *Society.* Wyszewianski recognizes that a definition of quality is also held by "society." He notes that society is uniquely positioned to safeguard equality of access, and also has a stake in technical quality and cost effectiveness.[249]

A recommended addition to the "medical" definition that was offered by Lohr is one that recognizes the importance of process (the delivery of an intervention) as well as the structures that support that care in determining the actual outcome of the care.[245] This three-legged stool provides then opportunity for measurement (and improvement) of more than just report cards and leads to a more comprehensive definition of health care quality, if we add that which is suggested by Bowers and Kiefe[243]: "quality being the extent to which structure and process maximize the likelihood of good outcomes."

Again, the emphasis is on the "likelihood" of good outcomes, because high-quality care and good outcomes are not necessarily directly linked. As Chassin has described, the vagaries of the human condition mean that good quality medical care can be followed by poor outcome and excellent outcomes can occur despite poor care.[21]

QUALITY VERSUS VARIATION IN HEALTH CARE: MISUSE, OVERUSE, UNDERUSE, OR NONE OF THE ABOVE?

Another important definition of quality in health care is the absence of misuse, underuse, or overuse of therapy. These three embodiments of poor quality were originally cited by Donabedian in the 1960s and again by the IOM in 1990.[244,245] The process of avoiding or eliminating these three problems is inherent in the standards of evidence-based medicine and in the effort to assess for and to eliminate unwarranted variation in care patterns. It is important to recognize that variation may be good or bad, or neither. It may indicate significant overuse or underuse of a therapy and thereby signal that either the science of the therapy is poor or that it is being applied haphazardly.

However, before practice data can truly be defined as "variation," it must be assayed for any underlying reasons for diverse practices (including dissimilarities in supply and demand due to geographic economics and climate, for instance). Only if these factors are similar can any variation detected be linked to quality rather than just *associated* with confounding factors unrelated to quality.[250] For instance, an increased number of obstetricians in an area is often associated with a higher birthrate in that area, but physician supply does not cause pregnancy (or birth).[251]

An important example of misinterpretation of variation is found in the potentially influential monograph "The Care of Patients with Severe Chronic Illness: A Report on the Medicare Program by the Dartmouth Atlas."[252] Here the authors have counted the number of physician visits used by Medicare beneficiaries with various chronic medical conditions—filtered by hospital and by geographic region—and they have determined that the geographic regions where there are fewer physician visits are the same locations where the Medicare beneficiaries have higher levels of patient satisfaction and quality of care. From this they extrapolate to the conclusion that we have a surplus of physicians. One example cited is the contrast between the Mayo Clinic, where there are fewer physician visits, and nonintegrated health care systems in New York City and Los Angeles.

In reality, variation in health care practitioner visits may be associated with a diversity of genetic, cultural, and social situations. These three geographic areas are markedly different in their genetic, social, and cultural homogeneity, and in the percentage of older adults who live below the poverty level. They vary with regard to availability of nonphysician providers, and thus access to preventive care. As seen in Figure 5–8, these three areas are also quite different in their rate of uninsured, so we would be remiss to imagine that the health care quality would be the same in New York City or Los Angeles as it is in Minnesota.*

This study's conclusion is a reminder of the critical importance of risk adjustment for dissimilitude in population types when analyzing variation in clinical processes or outcomes. The value in finding variation in care is to provide a signal that there may be "best practices" that can be emulated, but best practices can only be determined if patient and disease characteristics are similar.[45] Not all variations are misuse, overuse, or underuse.

THE SEVEN PILLARS OF QUALITY

In 1990, Donabedian enumerated seven attributes, or "pillars," of health care quality[253]:
1. Efficacy—the ability of care to actually improve health
2. Effectiveness—how well care achieves improvement in health in the circumstances of "everyday practice"
3. Efficiency—the cost of any given improvement in health
4. Optimality—the point at which incremental increases in care begin to diminish in their return on investment, such that health may be improved, but in a less efficient manner
5. Acceptability of care to patients—accessibility, the practitioner-patient relationship, amenities of

care, patient valuations of care outcomes, patient estimation of care's economic worth
6. Legitimacy—considerations of the value of care by others than the patient receiving that care, the aspect of societal valuation as mentioned above
7. Equity—the balance between what individuals and what society considers to be appropriate distribution of care and resources

Donabedian continued, "quality cannot be judged by technical terms, by health care practitioners alone; that the preferences of individual patients and society at large have to be taken into account as well."

This last lesson should be kept in mind in choosing any single definition of "quality" as most appropriate.

WHAT FORCES PROPEL THE MODERN QUALITY MOVEMENT?

The concern about quality in health care became more intense in the latter 1980s as the systems of quality research and management that grew out of the business and manufacturing world were first applied to health care.[254] Despite the improved outcomes with some increased economy achieved by the application of these methods in some health care organizations, there was no wide penetration of the national health care delivery system by quality science.

In 1998, the IOM published its first large report detailing the problems in the quality of U.S. health care: "The urgent need to improve health care quality."[21] This was followed by "To Err is Human" in 1999, which focused on patient safety and claimed that between 40,000 and 98,000 patients die annually in hospitals due to quality defects in their care.[255] In addition, that report stated that 5.4% of patients suffered perioperative complications of which almost 50% were caused by caregiver error.

In addition to concerns about safety, five forces are driving the resurgence of concern about quality[256]:
1. Cost—health care expenditures have grown past the trillion-dollar mark and it is now the perception of many in business, government, and among the public that more than one third of that, or almost $400 billion dollars annually, is a waste of money.[23,257] Correct or not, this impression is a huge motivator for the modern concern about quality—and value—among those who are paying the bills for health care. This concern extends to pain medicine, because it is a high dollar item: in 1998, $26.3 billion was expended on the care of back pain alone.[2]
2. Variation in the application of care—geographic variation exists in cost and care, often without linkage between more care and better quality. This situation is a red flag for those who evaluate quality and who believe it reveals a lack of evidence for the value of that care (see Figs. 5–9 and Fig. 5–10).[258]

* The Dartmouth Atlas studied only the Medicare populations. However, a lack of health care access (insurance) before patients become eligible for Medicare would likely diminish their quality of health even after Medicare coverage begins.

3. The increase in for-profit health care delivery systems, specialty ("boutique") hospitals, and increased office-based surgery is a concern for some health care policy makers, who view these as potential drivers of increased cost. As well, there is a fear that such practice modes "skim" the most profitable segment of income from the traditional hospitals, leaving the larger nonprofit and public entities at risk for financial ruin. This same argument was a concern when ambulatory surgery centers were first introduced in the 1970s and is the impetus behind the Certificate of Need requirements that the American Hospital Association was able to lobby for in many states.[259]

4. The increase in medical malpractice litigation is seen by some as an indicator of poor quality.

5. The increased role of government and industry in scrutinizing health care and regulating its practice is due in part to the importance of these groups as the largest real purchasers/consumers of health care coupled with the business sector's internal history of quality innovation.

PATIENT SAFETY AND THE "CULTURE OF SAFETY"

There is reasonable debate as to whether or not a patient is safe and whether or not a specific error contributes to real morbidity.[260,261] However, the public, legislators, and payers are convinced that both patient safety and human error are significant problems in today's health care delivery system.[262,263] The health care industry is being urged to create a "culture of safety" at all levels of practice that will put in place processes that will eliminate or decrease the impact of human error.[264] The majority of error committed in health care is due to system defects, rather than just individual mishaps, as was pointed out in the IOM's *Crossing the Quality Chasm*. This book also presented a framework for improving health care quality with six specific targets for improvement[20]:

1. Safety
2. Effectiveness
3. Efficiency
4. Timeliness of care
5. Patient-centered care
6. Equitable care

This anxiety about safety has led to Medicare (CMS) contracts with Quality Improvement Organizations (QIOs) that spend in excess of $200 million dollars per year on them, despite evidence that QIOs do not make a difference in quality of care.[265] Congress appropriated more than $300 million dollars to the Agency for Health Care Research and Quality (AHRQ) in the 5 years that followed the publication of *To Err is Human*, yet there is still much on the IOM list that has not been addressed.[263]

Among these larger forces of business, government, and society, a lesson sometimes lost is that the individual practitioner can improve health care quality. If practitioners identify those outcomes that are desired, employ the tenets of evidence-based medi-cine to find "best practices," and measure both their delivery of those therapies (process) and the results of those therapies (outcomes), then it is more likely that quality will improve.[266] Adherence to evidence-based "best practice" begins with the individual practitioner, and is associated with significant improvement in patient outcomes, including mortality.[267]

CONTINUOUS QUALITY IMPROVEMENT OR TOTAL QUALITY MANAGEMENT DEFINED

Continuous quality improvement (or CQI) or total quality management (TQM) is a seven-step process that consists of the identification of desired knowledge, design of appropriate measures to obtain the necessary assessments, measurement, investigation of the measurements to find trends and best practices, return of that information to those who can effect change, implementation of change in practice to increase the incidence of best practice, and then remeasurement to assess the program of change. It is an outgrowth of the "total quality control" movement that spread from the business sector to health care in the 1980s.[268] Its origins may be traced to Walter Shewart's work in the 1920s, including the "Plan-Do-Study-Act" cycle that was further amplified by Deming in the 1970s.[254] In medicine, CQI has been valuable in creating significant improvement in practice patterns even among multiple practitioners in multiple sites across geographically large distances.[269]

HEALTH CARE QUALITY AND BUSINESS

The health care quality movement has attracted significant attention from the business community, the group that often pays the bill. Indeed, there is widespread belief that business management tools can provide the solutions to the health care quality problem.[246,270] Recognition of this potential industry crossover is the reason that the business community, so oddly placed as our nation's primary provider of health care insurance, has created powerful organizations such as the Leapfrog Group (www.leapfroggroup.org/home), the Bridges to Excellence program (www.bridgestoexcellence.org) and, in league with insurers, the Integrated Health Care Association (www.iha.org). Each of these organizations aims to push health care providers to embrace specific goals and behaviors that are likely to improve patient safety and outcome.[271] These organizations have recommended financial incentives (Pay for Performance, or P4P), public disclosure of hospital safety rankings ("report cards"), and institutional changes in quality methodologies and behaviors, including the use of electronic health records (EHRs) and computerized physician order entry (CPOE). They have spawned interest in these programs within CMS and pushed along the initiation of the CMS P4P programs that are growing in parallel to those being created by private payers.[272]

QUALITY ASSESSMENT AND QUALITY IMPROVEMENT: RISK ADJUSTMENT AND REPORT CARDS

Success in quality improvement by the employer-based initiatives has been mixed. This is in part due to the choice of quality initiatives with insufficient evidence of validity, as occurred when Leapfrog pushed for high-risk surgical procedures to be limited to only in those hospitals where their volume had already reached a chosen minimum level.[273] As well, participation has been voluntary and the financial incentives have been either paltry, easily gained, or both. Some revision of the Leapfrog criteria has occurred with recognition now of the importance of risk adjustment.[271]

One challenge is that the correlation between process measures (those most easily measured) and outcome measures (more difficult to measure) remains controversial in the most basic and oft-studied clinical circumstances (e.g., outcome of myocardial infarction treatment by hospital).[274] This critical aspect of the application of quality science must be certain before any real value can be attached to public reporting of hospital (or physician) performance. In addition, evidence is growing that, even when accurate, report cards alone do not induce improved performance.[270,275,276]

THE APPLICATION OF CONTINUOUS QUALITY IMPROVEMENT AND TOTAL QUALITY MANAGEMENT: NATIONAL SURGICAL QUALITY IMPROVEMENT PROGRAM

There is a known means to improve quality of care: the simple act of measuring clinical outcomes in a way in which they can be systematically analyzed and the information provided to the caregivers.[277-281] Using specific measures to guide improvement initiatives is the key to the success of the application of quality science. By contrast, monitoring broadly defined outcome measures (like mortality in hospital report cards) fail to effectively improve care because their causative factors are so many and are often independent of the practice of the caregivers under observation. The failures of a "shotgun" approach to measurement are exacerbated by a lack of risk adjustment.[282]

The Department of Veterans Affairs (VA) National Surgical Quality Improvement Program (NSQIP) was created by surgeons in the VA system and began in 1991 to collect data to allow assessment of surgical outcomes and quality among the many hospitals in the system.[277] Nurses hired specifically to work on the study collected the data. It included variables (e.g., preoperative serum albumin levels) to allow risk stratification of patients. Three important principles have been elucidated:

1. It is an absolute requirement that all evaluations of health care quality be amended by stratification of patient risk factors (risk adjustment). Not doing so introduces an error rate as high as 60% when comparing the unadjusted quality of programs.

2. Provider volume does *not* necessarily correlate with outcome. This finding disputes the Leapfrog tenet that outcomes are improved by directing surgical procedures to only those hospitals with "sufficient" volumes. Instead, there is no clearly safer "volume," but what is important is the quality of the program.[273] This is an example of the potentially very negative impact of identification of "obvious" quality goals before gathering adequate data.

3. Regular provision to surgeons of the results of their institution's outcomes allows identification of "best practice" and is an effective means of improving quality of care. This approach improved patient outcome measures such as mortality and length of stay by as much as 45%.

The VA system experience has further shown that there are aspects of the Leapfrog and 100,000 Life initiatives that are of value: the use of EHRs, CPOE, financial incentives for provider compliance with designated performance goals, and routine comprehensive quality measurement have led to improved quality and delivery of warranted care.[283]

However, there are still barriers to comprehensive CQI programs: physician-specific outcome monitoring is unlikely to be accurate because any single doctor treats too few patients for accurate statistical evaluation; in most settings, there is still a lack of extant evidence-based benchmarks; technical barriers still prevent accurate data collection.[284] Also, the lack of good data on the appropriate management of patients with multisystem disease means that the physician who holds back from treating one disease with guideline-specific treatments due to concern about disease–disease or disease–drug interactions would be "punished" if scrutinized under the current quality assessment and improvement paradigm.[285] This illustrates the difficulty of attributing specific patient outcomes to "causative" individual provider actions.

Iezzoni, a pioneer in risk adjustment science, notes that outcomes in health care cannot be simplistically linked directly to care, but are actually part of an equation she terms an "algebra of effectiveness." This "algebra" is determined by three factors: the patient's condition and inherent risk, the effectiveness of the treatment provided, and an unaccountable or uncontrollable set of random variables.[286] NSQIP has proven that collection of risk-adjusted data regarding surgery site outcomes, rather than physician-specific outcomes measurement, is a successful strategy for improving outcomes. Notably, the NSQIP data collection and analysis that was facility-specific was accurate enough that it prevented the planned closure of several "poorly" performing sites, once risk adjustment for patient comorbidity was invoked.[277] At this point in time, concentration on facility evaluation rather than upon individual physician is the only appropriate CQI approach in view of current technologic and evidence-based medicine's limitations.

QUALITY IMPROVEMENT IN PAIN MEDICINE

Community pain practice quality is improved if a cohesive program of measurement, identification of best practice, education, and reassessment are applied.[287,288] CQI programs may improve therapy quality by simply inducing a more extensive review of a patient's history. For instance, inquiry about patient risk adjustors may lead to the recognition of mental health issues that could significantly affect the outcomes of any pain treatment plan.[289] The use of baseline measures can both direct care and provide an understanding of the likely potential for meaningful improvement in function and pain scores by identifying risk factors for long-term treatment failure.[290,291] Verhoef and colleagues make the point that the best set of outcome measures for a pain practice will include some open-ended questions and also let patients take on part of the role of setting goals for their own therapy.[141] In this way, patients can be expected to be additionally motivated to reach those goals.

An active CQI program also will allow practitioners to evaluate the effects of the introduction of new therapies or treatment algorithms into their practices, and either prove or disprove their value.[292] CQI provides a means to achieve accreditation for facilities, and may even influence which quality measurements are adopted by regulatory agencies as sources of "grading" quality of care.[293] Finally, the use of a clinical database for monitoring patient outcomes also provides a sense of participation in the process for the staff whose work is being assessed, a key factor in their acceptance and enthusiasm for the benefits of CQI.[294]

The most significant hurdle in CQI for pain medicine is a lack of apparent benchmarks or national "best practices" that providers emulate. Using the literature to establish benchmarks is prone to error due to the significant positive bias in the reporting of success of techniques there.[295] Overall, the evidence is not clear as to which, if any, interventions improve many chronic pain states.[3]

The analysis of practice patterns among either partners or an unassociated local group of pain physicians is potentially an excellent source of evidence in those situations where there is a lack of randomized controlled trials in the peer-reviewed literature. Assessment programs that are under the mantel of "peer-review" statutes will allow participating physicians rapid and open means of sharing their own best practices with one another to attempt to increase the quality of the community's pain care. Such evaluation may be accomplished with very short questionnaires. Patient interest in and compliance with such assessments is usually avid.[296]

Pain medicine practitioners can find a useful template for CQI programs that can be used in their own practices in Patel and colleagues' description of such programs in mental health[297]:

Quality improvement programs are practice and system strategies that support efficiency, appropriate care, and acceptable outcome. Comprehensive approaches that support client and provider education; encourage consumers to take a more active role in their recovery; and make use of support structures, such as case management to coordinate care have *been shown to improve quality, in terms of both processes and outcomes of care.*

CONSTRUCTING A CQI PROGRAM FOR A PAIN PRACTICE

There are several steps that must be taken to create a CQI program for pain:

1. Identify the practitioners (physicians, nurses, therapists) who will be involved.
2. Gather those caregivers together to align their information goals and to craft a set of measures toward which all can agree that the program should be directed. A good starting point is the list put forth by the IOM[20]:
   a. Care should be *safe.*
   b. Care should be *effective* and based on proven *evidence and science.*
   c. Care should be *efficient* and *cost effective with no waste.*
   d. Care should be *timely*, with no waits or delays.
   e. Care should be *patient centered*: respect patient preference and give the patient control.
   f. Care should be *equitable* with no unequal treatment.
3. The most effective CQI program will start with the participants deciding what they personally feel are the most interesting (initial) questions to be answered. For instance, four or five separate practices in a delivery area might decide to evaluate the outcomes of referrals to physical and behavioral therapists in the area, or the value of a particular invasive pain technique.
4. Pick outcome measures that will allow accurate assessment of the problem. Weinstein and Deyo recommend separation of assessment into four domains: patient health status, cost, patient expectation, and clinical status.[298] Within these areas, indicators are chosen that answer the questions most important to the practitioners. Indicators are of three types[299]:
   a. *Structure measures* assess the characteristics of the practice or a facility, such as staff-to-patient ratios or patterns of diagnosis. These may alert the practitioner to unforeseen aspects of practice that are causing quality issues. For instance, a growth in the number of return visits of CRPS patients with increased dysfunction after an initial period of improvement could alert the care teams to an unrealized issue of reimbursement denials for the prolonged physical and behavioral therapy required in the care of this syndrome.
   b. *Process measures* assess how care is provided in the practice. For instance, the compliance audits regarding documentation by the practitioners and therapists that support evaluation and management coding fit into this category. The disadvantage to process measures is primarily in determining a link with outcome, as these must be considered surrogates for outcome in the many situations in which direct measurement of the outcomes is impeded by difficulty

with risk adjustment or other barriers. Another problem is that a process measure may seem of importance to health care workers (e.g., length of time spent in the recovery room after interventional procedures), but may not be valued by patients or payers. Finally, quality assessment is best if it considers a continuum of care, while process measures tend only to evaluate small pieces of care.[300]

c. *Clinical outcome measures* are those that most practitioners focus on, although an effective CQI program will monitor all three types. Examples of clinical outcome measures include use of repeated patient health status testing to determine health status longitudinally after interventions. In most practices it would be expected that some sort of evaluation of patients in this regard would be collated and sorted by diagnosis, demographics, and intervention. This is a critical step to monitor for overuse or underuse of medical therapies.

5. The chosen measures should have the following characteristics[301,302]:

a. *Relevance.* They should directly relate to the goals of the group and it should be true that the interventions of the group have an effect upon them.

b. *Timeliness.* The measures should be collected in a timely manner so as to relate them as closely as possible to the interventions that the practitioners wish to assess.

c. *Reliability.* The measures should be accurate and consistent no matter when or who is assessing and recording them.

d. *Validity.* The valid measure is sensitive to changes that the practitioner can effect.

e. *Precision.* The measures should be clearly defined and leave little potential for individual or erroneous interpretation.

f. *Cost effectiveness.* A CQI program costs money and the measures should be significant enough to your patients and your practice that they are worth the time and money expended on the process of collection and analysis.

g. *Provider control.* The variable measured must be one that the provider or organization can actually control or it is not worth measuring. For instance, measuring patient self-reported pain levels one year after intervention for a chronic pain condition is unlikely to reflect a process that the provider can control, due to the impact of the intervening health care and patient activity over the course of 1 year.

h. *Clear meaning.* The measure must be one that is easily understood by all concerned.

6. Terminology—once the practitioners have chosen the outcome measures that they determine are appropriate for use in the program, these terms must be adjusted to be in congruence with standard nomenclature. The accepted standard is a somewhat moving target, but SNOMED-CT (Systemized Nomenclature of Medicine—Clinical Terms) is produced by the College of American Pathologists (CAP) and has been designated for use by the NIH and National Library of Medicine (NLM) for use in electronic transfer of medical information in the United States. Thus all practitioners should make sure their own terms are "crosswalked" to SNOMED terms, so that they report data that is considered standardized by accreditation and certification bodies, and by payers in the years to come. This crosswalk process is done in one of four ways:

a. One can download all of SNOMED at the NLM site, which has licensed SNOMED for use by any entity within the United States. This site is www.nlm.nih.gov/research/umls but the data sets are raw and most practitioners would need help manipulating them.

b. The CAP has a complete version for sale at www.snomed.com, although the price may vary depending upon the nature of the entity requesting.

c. Apelon (www.apelon.com) has two products that will take care of the translation process. One is Mycroft, which is a translator that is free via web browser and allows the user to find the crossmatch in SNOMED for any other term. This requires a fair amount of time and may not be useful if there are a lot of terms to look up. The other option is Termworks, a translator that will automatically translate a body of terms (in a spreadsheet format). However, this product is obtained by subscription that, as of this writing, costs $800 per month. In the case of a large volume of terms, however, this may be a good tool to rapidly translate them, cutting down the hunting time that would otherwise be necessary.

7. *Risk adjustment* must be included in the design of the monitoring system in order for the measurements to have any utility for identifying high quality and best practice.[303] In the past, newly minted measures of quality have been introduced without attention to risk or scientific investigation to ascertain that they were valid estimators of outcome.[304] As NSQIP proved, without accounting for the severity of patient morbidity, "significant correlation" between care processes and clinical outcomes may prove spurious when such comorbidities are later considered.[277] Risk adjust-ment is a young and still potentially confounding science, and many of its controversies are yet unsolved.[305,306]

The vagaries of risk adjustment suggest that practitioners use tools of measurement that are already validated. For instance, it is true to say that age and diabetes are significant comorbidities that should be considered when determining likely outcome after surgery, but their relative import can vary depending upon which surgical procedure is under consideration, who is determining the severity of the comorbid condition, whether administrative or clinical determinants are used to determine presence of disease and its severity, or which administrative coding tool is used to identify the condition.[307,308] If a pain practitioner or group decides to create a completely new measure, careful attention to risk adjustment theory and its evaluation in the literature or appropriate texts is recommended.[309] Nonetheless, it is possible for small groups of clinical experts to choose risk adjustment indices with validity, if the process is done with bias controls and if there is involvement of biostatisticians and epidemiologic consultants.[310]

Risk adjustment in chronic pain practice poses very significant challenges, in view of the wide diversity in the types of adjustors that can be seen to be operant in the widely diverse population known as "chronic pain patients." The variegated nature of patients with multiple comorbid conditions ranging among physical disabilities, economic and social burdens, and mental health disorders makes construction of risk "cohorts" very difficult.[311] Risk adjustment in pain treatment outcome *research* is also a new science and more rigorous studies than yet exist in the literature are needed before clarity and certainty exist in this area.

SPECIFIC OUTCOME TOOLS AND MEASURES FOR YOUR PRACTICE

Box 5–1 lists some measures and tools that might be considered for a pain CQI program. These have been used in scientific studies to measure some of the variables that would be valuable to a pain program. The reader is cautioned however that a great deal of variation exists in the versions of some of these instruments published in the literature.[312]

Many organizations are attempting still to codify and make uniform the "dictionary" of terms that are used in quality databases. An excellent source of guidance in this endeavor is the document from the American Society of Anesthesiologists (ASA) titled "Guiding Principles for Management of Performance Measures by the American Society of Anesthesiologists," available on the ASA website www.asahq.org. Several organizations are involved in the effort to codify terminology in addition to the ASA, including the Anesthesia Patient Safety Foundation (APSF) and its Data Dictionary Taskforce, and international

---

BOX 5–1. EXAMPLES OF DATA MEASURES AND QUALITY ASSESSMENT TOOLS ADAPTABLE FOR QA AND QI IN PAIN PRACTICES

Basic Patient Information
Some of this information will be gleaned from the patient chart and some will require further questioning by the staff.

Demographics
Gender
Age
Ethnicity
Residential Zip Code
Referred: Y/N
Live alone Y/N
Care for self without help Y/N
Other caregivers/providers (list)

Disability and Litigation
Litigation active? Y/N
Legally Disabled? Y/N
—percentage?
Working? Y/N

Mental Health
DSM-IV codes assigned
Psychiatric hospitalization DRGs
Annual psychiatric hospitalization days

Patient Expectations
Expected degree of function return
Expected job status post treatment
Expected medication changes post treatment
Expected decrease in pain level post treatment

Costs[321,394]

Direct Health Care Costs
Physician visits

Emergency room and hospitalization costs
Physical therapist fees
Physical therapy modalities
Occupational therapy
Vocational rehabilitation therapy
Behavioral health therapy
Laboratory studies
Imaging costs
Professional home care
Stimulator or pump and implantation fees
Analgesic and behavioral medications
Alternative therapy costs

Indirect Health Care Costs
Litigation fees
Lost wages
Cost of housekeeping
Cost of other home care
Travel costs for care
Time expended by family, others in care

Tools
Be aware that multiple versions may exist in the literature for some of these. When available, the most definitive source is listed below.

Overall Quality of Life Status
SF-12 or 36 measures www.qualitymetric.com
U.S. National Health Interview Survey (US NHIS)
Spitzer's Quality of Life Uniscale—a one question set that records patient self-assessment of the past week in terms of their quality of life[395]
Spitzer's QOL Index—five items[395]

Continued

BOX 5–1. EXAMPLES OF DATA MEASURES AND QUALITY ASSESSMENT TOOLS ADAPTABLE FOR QA AND QI IN PAIN PRACTICES—cont'd

Pain- and Function-specific Questionnaires
TOPS (Treatment Outcomes in Pain Survey)[319]
PIQ-6 (Pain Impact Questionnaire) www.quality metric.com
DYNHA Acute Pain Impact (in development) www. qualitymetric.com
DYNHA Chronic Pain Impact (in development) www.qualitymetric.com
ASA 9 www.asahq.org/Newsletters/1998/06_98/ Choosing_0698.htm
The Fibromyalgia Impact Questionnaire[396]
Roland-Morris Back Pain[397]
Patient Specific Functional Scale[398]
Quebec Back Pain Questionnaire
Waddell Disability Index
West-Haven-Yale Multidimensional Pain Inventory (MPI)

Condition-specific Measures
These are somewhat more specialized tools that may work in pain assessment programs
Pain Disability Questionnaire[318]
Patient Specific Index/Patient Specific Functional Scale
Problem Elicitation Technique
Patient Generated Index
Canadian Occupational Performance Measure
Schedule for the Evaluation of Individual Quality of Life
Measure Yourself Medical Outcome Profile
Juvenile Arthritis Quality of Life Questionnaire

Risk Adjustment
Functional Comorbidity Index[320]

Patient Satisfaction
The Picker Patient Experience Questionnaire[399]— this is a superb assessment of how your practice measures up to the patient's expectations. It would be worth assessing at intermittent, fixed intervals to watch for trends and administrative areas that could be improved.

Measures Used in Health Quality and Function Studies
Utility measures—patient assessment of value of overall health state
Euroqol (EQ-5D)[400]—highly recommended as a short and insightful look at your patient's attitudes
Health Utility Index[321]
Generic measures—These measures quantify the patient's self assessment of overall health
Sickness Impact Profile[401]—progenitor of the Roland Morris questionnaire
Nottingham Health Profile[402]
SF-12, SF-36 www.qualitymetric.com

Work and Function
Work Limitations Questionnaire
Oswestry Disability Index
Simple Shoulder Test
Neck Disability Index
Short Musculoskeletal Functional Assessment

Pain
Visual Analog Scale (VAS) or Pain Intensity Difference (PID)—there are many confounding factors in the measurement of pain intensity; also there are validity concerns regarding the import of change over time (studies indicate that 2 points may be a valid cutoff for clinically significant improvement).[315]
Von Korff's Pain Scale[403]
Graded Chronic Pain Scale[323]
Neuropathic Pain Specific tools[404]
Neuropathic Pain Scale
Neuropathic Pain Symptom Inventory
Leeds Assessment of Neuropathic Symptoms and Signs (LANSS)
Neuropathic Pain Questionnaire (NPQ)[405]
Neuropathic Pain Screening Tool (NPST)
Neuropathic Pain Diagnostic Questionnaire (DN4)
Neuropathic Pain Screening Tool (NPST)

Palliative Care
Patient Needs Assessment Tool (PNAT)[406]

Data from references 314, 321, 391-393.

groups such as the World Health Organization (WHO). The number of societies, the importance of the task, and the lack of certainty in the area means that it should be expected that any database will need to be amenable to editing over the next decade. The benefit of such malleability of design, which will always cost money, is that the practitioners who use it will be better assured that they will be in compliance with the requirements of the accreditation agencies (e.g., TJC, AAAHC, and others), which will also be set and amended in the years to come.

The entire issue of *Spine* of December 15, 2000, is highly recommended reading, as it contains in-depth reviews of several of the back pain measurement tools.[313] Another excellent review is one concerning outcome measurement in low back pain by Resnik and Dobrykowski.[314] Obviously not all the listed measures will be applicable to every pain practice and the practitioner is urged to review the references in Box 5–1 for information as to how best to employ the various measures.

One important issue is the significance of any change observed in the various measures over time in each patient. Some of the recommended tools were developed primarily to look at patient cohorts, rather than an individual patient. This area of research is still emerging and the reader is encouraged to monitor the literature closely to help be sure that his or her use of the tools is valid.[315]

The Tools

The Brief Pain Inventory is adaptable to computer use, although it has not been validated for all pain conditions.[316] Another valuable tool is the modification of the SF-36, the Low-Back SF-36PF$_{18}$.[317] This instrument is also amenable to computer use and includes aspects of the SF-36, Oswestry, and Quebec back pain questionnaires. A newer instrument that may lend itself to prediction of outcomes is the Pain Disability Questionnaire (PDQ), which is a short list of 15 questions and uses a continuum line for responses similar to the visual analogue scales for pain rating that most chronic pain patients have seen.[318] It also may be used on a computer. TOPS (Treatment Outcomes of Pain Survey) is a valuable tool that includes the SF-36 and additional questions that are specific to pain medicine.[319] It has the added value of having been validated in clinical practice and as a research tool.

Over the next several years there will be advancement in the nomenclature of clinical outcomes monitoring, leading to more specific definitions of the vocabulary of pain quality databases. This will improve the comparability of data across databases and tools, further refinement of the science of pain management, and will increase the probability that we will be able to fix national benchmarks of quality and best practices.

A Risk Adjustment Tool for Pain Practice Continuous Quality Improvement

As mentioned, it is important within a pain practice to calibrate expectations of improvement in a given patient by factoring in comorbidities, any evident functional disabilities, and including other confounding conditions, such as ongoing litigation. One new index that allows for this is the Functional Comorbidity Index.[320]

Which Tool to Use and How?

Gathering data is probably best managed by using patient surveys before and after provision of services, with timing appropriate to the nature of the patient's condition and the expected effective duration of the intervention. Several very good reviews of the relative merits of these measurement tools advocate well for certain tools in certain patients or for certain conditions.[321-323]

Brevity and speed of both information entry (either by the patient or staff) and data analysis are salutatory aspects of an outcome measurement system and these should all be considered in determining which instruments will be used. The use of both a short general health assessment and a specific pain evaluation tool is probably the most basic approach. Using computerized surveys (e.g., in the waiting room)

improves data integrity by decreasing omitted responses and improving internal consistency.[324] They should be used instead of written surveys whenever possible.

WHAT IS THE VALUE OF CONTINUOUS QUALITY IMPROVEMENT TO A PAIN PRACTICE?

There are several ways that a QA/QI program can help a pain practice:

1. *Accreditation* of a pain practice facility is discussed in the section on safety. However, accreditation bodies are very interested in the nature of any CQI programs. Thus an added benefit of such a program, in addition to improved care for patients, is the approbation of accreditors.
2. *Payment for quality* is the newest impetus for providers and facilities to participate in quality improvement programs. Pay for performance (P4P) is the general term used to describe reimbursement programs that tie some portion of provider income to either process or outcome achievements. P4P will also effect changes in patient referral patterns as the gathered information on provider performance is made available to payers, employers, and patients.[130] Therefore, investment in a CQI program will have potential benefits in terms of patient census and reimbursement rates in the coming years.
3. *Benchmarking providers* in an objective and appropriate manner is another value of a well-crafted CQI program. By evaluating practice patterns among providers at a single site or among many sites, benchmarks can be identified which allow all physicians and staff to assess their own performances against other practitioners and thus elucidate "best practices." Allowing practitioners to see their own process outcome data and compare it to others working in the same facility has improved efficiency with no alteration in patient satisfaction.[325]

WHAT WILL A QA/QI PROGRAM COST?

Personnel

A busy practice will require between 0.5 and 1.0 full-time employees to manage data input. This staff person, if not completely occupied by this work, might also serve as the HIPAA compliance officer and oversee all the policies regarding the quality initiatives of the practice. Although relatively expensive, a registered nurse (RN) is of great value in this role.

Technology

It would be convenient if each practice location were to have access to an electronic health record (EHR) to allow automated capture of accurate data to provide evidence of quality. We may be some years away from an EHR in every procedure room and are even further away from an accurate EHR in every procedure room. Sadly, investment in those changes in infrastructure that might bolster improved quality is often squelched by the nature of reimbursement in our current medical system.[326]

In the meantime, therefore, it is appropriate to concentrate on inexpensive and already available means of capturing such data and transmitting it to practitioners.[25] Probably the most efficacious single site approach is to use a computer relational database (e.g., MS Access) to capture information gathered by more traditional methods, such as chart assessment by clerks and patient interviews by nurses. Such databases have been valuable in determining areas of potential cost savings, improvement in efficiency, and potential error and quality shortfalls.[325]

If the practitioner is not a skilled programmer, it is reasonable to hire one and build his or her own database with modes of risk adjustment, and automated capture of demographic and laboratory data. They can be built with a graphic user interface (GUI) that is intuitive for even the most non–technology-savvy staff member and that will allow patients to directly interface with waiting room kiosks. This can all be done with about 60 hours of programming (Fig. 5–22).

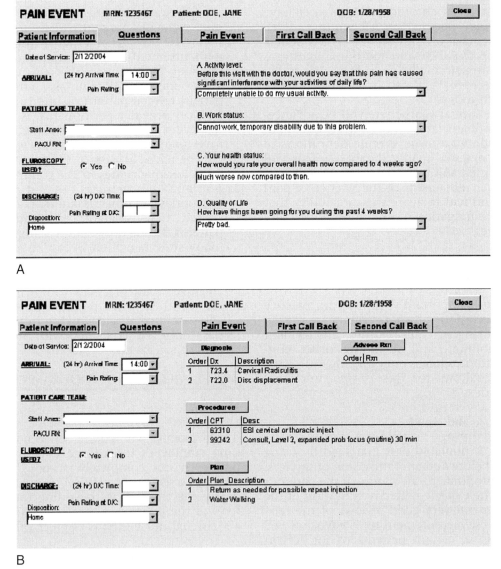

Figure 5–22. A, Pain clinic database: initial questions screen. This image shows a typical interface for recording the answers to an initial set of screening questions regarding the pain problem and quality of health as described by a patient upon his or her first visit to a pain clinic. Using the Microsoft Access Relational Database or similar technology, this user-friendly graphic interface allows clerical personnel to record the events and answers in a relational database that can then be used to monitor individual and collective patient outcomes for quality management in a pain practice. **B,** Pain clinic database: procedures screen. This image shows a typical interface for prompting and recording the events that typically occur on the day of a pain service, allowing the information to be placed into a relational database for quality management purposes.

Figure 5–22, cont'd. C, Pain clinic database: first callback screen. This image shows a typical interface for prompting and recording the questions and answers for phone calls to a pain patient, allowing the responses to be placed into a relational database for quality management purposes. (Microsoft Access is a registered trademark of Microsoft Corporation.)

Physicians and staff will spend somewhat less time helping with design and testing.[327] Licensing for the software and for the use of the AMA CPT codes will be needed and the purchase of additional computer monitors or kiosks may also be necessary, depending on the current configuration of technology at the clinic. In all, an investment of $10,000 to $15,000 would create a superb single-office product with automated reporting and measures very specific to the goals and practice patterns of the pain clinic whose practitioners created it.

CONCLUSIONS ABOUT QUALITY IMPROVEMENT IN PAIN PRACTICE

This chapter separates health care policy (and issues of cost), patient safety, and quality improvement as independent sections. However, all three must be considered when reviewing strategies to improve any one of them.[328] The following are necessary to improve pain CQI programs:

1. CQI programs should be used at each individual clinic to discover which processes and structures beget the best clinical outcomes.
2. The data for each clinic should be linked to all the others to create national quality benchmarks that will provide a means of identifying and duplicating best practices.
3. Innovations in care systems should be welcomed, but only in settings that allow their study in comparison to the best practices that already exist.
4. Evidence-based approaches to pain medicine must be improved. Practitioners must be scrupulous in evaluating procedures and therapies with rigorous doubt, eliminating those that do not prove

valuable in comparison to alternatives that may be more banal and less lucrative.
5. Access to high quality multidisciplinary care, including mental health care that may often be expensive and long-term, must be a priority of our specialty so that we can advocate for it to the payers, health care policy makers, and legislators who too frequently ignore the benefits of such care.[297]

Finally, pain medicine—and health care in general—needs more robust federal support for cheap methods to engender clinical measurement of outcomes, risk adjustment, and clinician feedback if quality improvement is to occur rapidly. Computerized systems should be made available to primary and ambulatory care facilities to allow for the identification of national benchmarks of care. Only in this way can we rapidly discover best practices and decrease the waste inherent in the current care model, where individual clinicians often practice in the dark with regard to evidence and to the effects of their own interventions.

SUMMARY

- The quality movement in health care is less than three decades old and is still evolving. However it is being rapidly driven by alarm among the public, payers, regulators, and the business community spurred by widespread evidence of unsafe care.
- The various stakeholders in health care define quality in different ways and physicians must consider these alternative attitudes as they work to improve and prove the value of their practices.

- At each clinic, a "culture of safety" must be established by creating new systems that will decrease the impact of human error on patient outcomes.
- Many of the current reforms aimed at improved safety and higher quality are based on as yet unproven theories and may well fall out of favor in the coming years.
- One certain way in which to improve quality is the measurement of practice to determine "best practice." This should be done by all practitioners and all facilities, monitoring measures of structure, process, and clinical outcomes.
- Use continuous quality improvement (CQI), also known as total quality management (TQM), techniques to increase the number of the practitioners who can replicate the best practices.
- Combining a practice that includes a comprehensive care approach that includes behavioral and vocational therapies with computer-based CQI strategies will improve the quality of care in pain medicine.

Section III
Patient Safety

TO ERR IS HUMAN

The publication of *To Err is Human* in 1999 was the Institute of Medicine's public alarm about patient safety and error in the health care delivery system.[255] The authors estimated that between 44,000 and 98,000 hospital deaths occur annually in the United States due to errors in medical care. In part, this conclusion was based on the Harvard Medical Practice Study of 1991, which found that the iatrogenic injury rate was 3.7% among U.S. hospitalized patients and that two thirds of these injuries could be prevented.[329] This numerical conclusion and the overall methodology of the IOM report have been thoughtfully contested regarding potentially flawed data interpretation and uneven evidence as to whether or not the cited errors are causal of adverse outcomes.[260,261,330] Despite the controversy, these reports focused the attention of practitioners, payers, patients, and the government on the need to improve the safety of patients within the health care system. Work remains to determine exactly how to most effectively and efficiently make those improvements.

THE RESPONSE

The speedy and wide acceptance of the IOM report's conclusions surprised even its most avid supporters.[331] Surprisingly, the groundswell of public and payer support for safety initiatives has moved so quickly that the need for further scientific examination of the underpinnings of the issue seems moot. The IOM report led to the launch of the "100,000 Lives" campaign, which was designed to save lives and improve patient care quality by identifying and eliminating six safety problems in health care (Box 5–2).[332] Concern that the move to fix the problem has been so rapid as to ignore the potential overstatement of the rate of error and the validity of the recommended solutions is resonant in HL Mencken's comment, as quoted by Forster and colleagues[260]: "For every complex problem, there is a solution that is simple, neat, and wrong."

BOX 5–2. SIX GOALS OF THE 100,000 LIVES CAMPAIGN

1. *Deploy rapid response teams or medical emergency teams.* Small interdisciplinary medical teams are dispatched to the bedside in anticipation of significant medical deterioration that could lead to cardiopulmonary arrest.
2. *Deliver reliable evidence-based care for acute myocardial infarctions.* Use the guidelines of the American College of Cardiology and American Heart Association to lessen the impact of or prevent myocardial infarction.
3. *Prevent adverse drug events through medication reconciliation.* Medication reconciliation is the process of reviewing the patient's medication orders before and after any change in caregiver or in site of care to monitor for any discrepancies in ordered versus administered medication.
4. *Prevent central-line infections.* Five components of care were identified by the Centers for Disease Control and Prevention (CDC) that if used will diminish the risk of infection: hand hygiene, maximal barrier protection (including gowns and gloves), chlorhexidine skin antisepsis, optimal site selection (subclavian vein in adults), and daily review of the indications for the catheter and removal as quickly as possible.
5. *Prevent surgical site infections.* The CDC recommended four practices to decrease surgical site infections: EBM-guided use of prophylactic antibiotics, as little hair removal via shaving the site as possible, perioperative glucose control (in the ICU after major cardiac surgery), and maintenance of perioperative normothermia after colorectal surgery.
6. *Prevent ventilator-assisted pneumonia.* Four practices were recommended: elevation of the head of the bed to between 30 and 45 degrees, daily "sedation vacation" with daily assessment for possible extubation, prophylaxis for peptic ulcer disease, and prophylaxis for deep vein thromboses.

From Berwick DM, Calkins DR, McCannon CJ, et al: The 100,000 lives campaign: Setting a goal and a deadline for improving health care quality. JAMA 2006;295:324-327.

A significant hurdle to the effort to improve safety is that there is insufficient data to assess health care safety or even definite identification of uniformly valid indicators of safety in health care.[333] Therefore which solutions, which information, and which technology will be of value in improving patient safety are as yet unknown.[44]

Large businesses, seeing the issue as one of poor quality in the face of high prices, organized themselves via the Leapfrog group and have created programs for change, while also pushing for new regulation and legislation to improve safety.[272] Three main goals were put forth: (1) public release of health care provider performance measurement, (2) wider use of information systems in clinical care, and (3) tying reimbursement to outcome quality achievement. These are variable in their evidentiary support for improving quality and they are all potentially very expensive.[266] Nonetheless, Leapfrog and its proponents quickly declared that the most important next step was and is the urging of the public to push for health care professionals to adopt these goals.[334] The Leapfrog group and its tenets have also imbued the discussion of patient safety in our health care system with an economic and political imperative that makes further objective evaluation of the true nature of health care's safety more difficult, even as new solutions are recommended.

Calls have come for widespread change in medical school curricula and the requirements for board certification to improve safety, well before any pilot studies have shown any of the changes valuable.[335,336] Also, the widespread and influential pay for performance programs (P4P) are being touted as a means of improving compliance with the safety imperatives that have been chosen, even while evidence for their efficacy is as yet insubstantial. New legislation has also created new patient safety organizations (PSOs) that will be charged with analyzing all newly (anonymously) reported errors,[337] even though error reporting is a complex and poorly understood behavior pattern,[338,339] and even though such programs are costly and have been uneven in achieving quality and safety improvement.[266,340] Nonetheless, the federal government at all levels has also weighed in substantially in favor of these programs.[341]

SUCCESS!

The Institute of Healthcare Improvement declared victory on June 14, 2006, stating that the 100,000 Lives Campaign had saved over 122,000 lives.[342] However, the support for this contention is a retrospective calculation of a statistical probability of how many lives "would have been lost" had the statistical analysis of 2004 been applied, versus the number of lives that were actually lost between January 2005 and June 2006.[343] Those who were skeptical of the mathematics that calculated the original numbers of lives at risk should be just as skeptical of the methodology used to verify this success.

NEXT STEPS FOR THE PAIN PRACTITIONER

Practitioners should work to discern practical ways to improve patient safety and the most efficient and economic means of practicing in congruence with the regulations and legislation now growing out of the public safety campaign. Whatever safety improvement programs are chosen, they should be repeatedly evaluated for efficacy as they go forward and abandoned if they are not efficient and effective.

TARGETING ERROR: HIGHLY RELIABLE ORGANIZATIONS AND KEEPING IT SIMPLE

In creating safer processes, it is best to focus on system change rather than on scrutiny of individual practitioner error, as system error is most causative of adverse events.[344] "Mistake-proofing" care will require minimizing variation in its delivery, monitoring the care of every patient's course of care for error, and adverse outcomes, and making care delivery systems within the clinic as simple as possible to avoid the complexities that lead to variation and error.[345] Such efforts have been effective in other industries such as aviation, nuclear power, and the military. Clinicians may feel that medical care is not amenable to the safety monitoring systems of other industries, yet emulation of highly reliable organizations (HROs) within these other industries do lead to improvements in safety in health care.[346,347] HROs succeed by making their systems as simple as possible, amenable to as little disruption as possible, and easy to understand.[348] They combine these three characteristics with a high priority placed on safety at the highest levels of the organization—including a willingness to spend money and person-power.[349]

Box 5–3 lists specific targets that the pain practitioner can emphasize in improving patient safety. It is critical to document these efforts and their results to be sure that resources are not wasted working on nonexistent issues and also to portray the diligence of the practice at the times when payers and regulators inquire as to safety efforts.

TREATMENT OUTCOME DATABASES: RECORDING ADVERSE EVENTS

Practitioners will best ensure their patients' safety by recording all adverse events in a database, the same database wherein they monitor all aspects of their patients' outcomes. Such an outcomes database or registry is vital for practitioners to discover their own best practices and to monitor for any trends that would reveal a lack of efficacy of therapeutic interventions. This topic is more completely covered in the section on Quality Assurance and Quality Improvement, but it is important to note that simple recording of adverse events, without affixing blame, can provide opportunities for solo physicians and large groups to spot trends in which certain care

BOX 5–3. INTERVENTIONS THAT MAY IMPROVE PATIENT SAFETY IN THE PAIN CLINIC

Facility Procedures and Structure

- Routinely and repetitively conduct drills for emergency situations, assigning specific roles to personnel in the case of patient medical emergencies, facility emergencies (e.g., power outage, fire, earthquake, severe weather), and selected adverse events in patient care.
- If locating/creating a new facility, site it as near to a hospital as is possible. Arrange to create a legal transfer agreement with that hospital.
- Furnish the facility with in-wall piped oxygen and suction, as well as adequate lighting and space to allow full access to patients by sufficient personnel in the case of an emergency.
- Consider accreditation by AAAHC, TJC, CARF, or other agency. If accreditation is not possible, consider annual inspection by one of these agencies for evaluation of your facility and practice regarding safety.
- Daily cleaning should include bactericidal cleansing of all surfaces contacted by staff, patients, or patient family members in all parts of the facility.
- Place hand cleanser dispensers in multiple locations readily available to all clinical and non-clinical staff.
- Drawers and supply cabinets should be clearly organized and standard in their organization between rooms.

Medication Management

- Use and enforce opioid/controlled substance contracts.
- Monitor and document patient response and frequency of renewals for opioids and sedatives.
- All medications used at the facility should be labeled (including an outdate, once opened) and carefully read aloud before being drawn up and before administration.
- All syringes should be labeled in a standard manner regarding label color, font, size, and information regarding outdate.
- The facility should be regularly inventoried (weekly or monthly) for outdating medication and other supplies.
- Use medication reconciliation techniques, confirming doses and frequency of all medications when there is a transition in caregiver, location, or date.
- Use computer technology to monitor for potential adverse drug events.
- Contract with a clinical pharmacist for consultation services as needed.
- Use protocols for monitoring the prescription of any medication that may lead to significant morbidity with continued use, such as NSAIDs, opioids, tricyclic antidepressants, and so on. These protocols should include timely and repetitive monitoring for known risks via either laboratory or electrocardiogram studies, or mandated office visits.
- Communicate prescriptions of all medications to all practitioners providing care to your patient.
- Any adverse drug events should be immediately reported and recorded in a database that is regularly reviewed for trend analysis. The patient should be notified about the adverse event. The patient's other caregivers outside the practice should be notified about the adverse drug event.
- Prompt attention by the staff should be focused on an open discussion and adjustment of protocols and policies by the end of the day to avoid any repetition of errors that occurred either with or without an adverse drug event.

Technology

- Track the outcomes of all care. Use relational database technology to allow evaluation of outcomes for trends, both positive and negative. Do not make this a punitive system, but provide information on outcomes to staff regularly to invite input on system changes that may avert negative events.
- Consider use of an electronic medical record.
- Use technology to allow integration of clinical and laboratory systems to insure all critical information is available at the point of care.
- Use a computerized physician order entry (CPOE) system that will also include outpatient prescription transmittal direct to pharmacy.
- Use a computer system to track patients' medications with automated alerts regarding potential drug interactions and anticoagulation use.
- Use technology to provide practitioners with all necessary reference material for decision support (e.g., medication dose, cross-reaction, and toxicity information).
- Use technology to insure accurate matching of patient identity, medication history, and current medications at each point of care. Consider use of a bar code system.
- Create or obtain audio-visual (e.g., VHS, DVD) materials about procedures and medications to allow patients to review them prior to obtaining informed consent for procedures or before beginning a new medication.

Staff

- Establish a pattern of regular use of hand cleansing by all personnel.
- Create and enforce protocols for hand-offs of patients between practitioners.
- Create and enforce protocols for two-person patient identification interaction.
- Use standard teams with assigned roles for medical and invasive procedures.

BOX 5–3. INTERVENTIONS THAT MAY IMPROVE PATIENT SAFETY IN THE PAIN CLINIC—cont'd

- Involve all staff in discussion of quality and safety issues and invite open and nonpunitive review of adverse events and trends with freedom of each staff member to contribute ideas for system improvement.
- Create a plan in advance to respond to adverse events, including honest discussions with patients and family as well as support for staff involved.
- Do not allow employees to work beyond the limits of their education and training.
- Monitor, track and report all practitioner work hours and do not allow them to extend beyond 80 hours in a week or more than 16 consecutive hours.
- Maintain sufficient staffing to ensure adequate care for sedated or recovering patients. These staff levels should be equivalent to or more intensive than the local standard of care as employed in the hospitals in the area.

Procedures
- Use full barrier protection during invasive procedures.
- Use appropriate prophylactic antibiosis.
- Use imaging technology when appropriate during invasive procedures.
- Use the minimum necessary contrast material.
- Develop and enforce the use of standard protocols for medical and invasive procedures, including sterile preparation and critical medication checks, such as anti-coagulants.
- Develop and enforce protocols to insure correct site invasive procedures, including marking the patient's body area prior to preparation and a pause for verbal confirmation among all staff present of patient identification and procedural intent.
- Follow State and other applicable regulations regarding radiation safety.

- Avoid patient sedation beyond loss of ability to discern and communicate paresthesia or other sensation change during neuraxial or perineural procedures.
- Refer procedures out that you rarely or never perform to higher volume practitioners or facilities. Monitor the outcomes of those patients.
- Provide both written and audio-visual informed consent materials and give patients time to review them, as well as to ask questions, prior to obtaining informed consent for procedures.
- Use supplemental oxygen and monitor oximetry whenever sedation is used.
- Use supplemental oxygen and monitor oximetry whenever the prone position is used.
- Mandate and enforce that all patients have a driver prior to beginning either sedation or any procedure.
- Obtain written agreement from the patient that they will not drive for 8 hours following a neuraxial procedure, sedation, or any procedure that could impair their motor skills.

Extra-facility
- Maintain close interaction with any provider also involved in your patient's care.
- Provide information about all controlled substance prescriptions you have begun as well as any other medication or treatment interventions you have made.
- Make direct phone contact with written confirmation regarding significant changes in condition or treatment plan.
- Create a transfer agreement with a hospital to prepare for a patient emergency.
- Participate in exchange of regular peer review of procedures and standards with other practitioners who have no economic stake in your practice or facility.

patterns are associated with significant rates of error or even injury.[350] Whether or not such adverse events are ever reported outside the practice, their scrutiny by the practitioners "in house" can improve care.[351,352] Box 5–4 lists some of the adverse events that might be included in a monitoring system.

TARGETING ERROR: MEDICATION ADVERSE EVENTS

Medication prescription is widely recognized as a source of patient injury in hospitals and in ambulatory care settings.[28,353,354] Recommended safety measures include adherence to evidence-based guidelines regarding medication prescription and use of CPOE.[355] However, compliance with guidelines in pain treatment has increased the use of opioids and other sedatives, sometimes leading to actual increases in adverse reactions in even the most careful and experienced institutions.[356] Institution of CPOE systems has even been associated with increases in mortality in even the most sophisticated environments.[357] The use of EHRs has not uniformly decreased cost or improved error rates, and has potentially increased medical liability in situations where they have not been reviewed and technical errors have been left unedited.[358,359] The important lesson is that all new programs and innovations in practice must be concurrently monitored for a prolonged period beyond initial implementation to be sure that the threat of error and adverse events truly has been lessened.[360-362] Such efforts by individual physicians and practices can also be a valuable part of larger drug surveillance efforts.[363]

**BOX 5–4. A LIST OF POTENTIAL ADVERSE EVENTS TO BE MONITORED
IN A PAIN PRACTICE SAFETY PROGRAM**

Procedural Events
Procedure on the wrong body part or location
Procedure performed on the wrong patient
Infection following a procedure
Unexpected death following a procedure
Unexpected hospitalization within 24 hours of a procedure
Unintentionally compromised nerve function following any procedure
Lack of consent or incongruous consent
Allergic reaction
Anaphylaxis
Abortion of procedure—anxiety
Abortion of procedure—other
Increased pain
Burn
CV—angina
CV—arrest
CV—CHF
CV—dysrythmia
CV—ECG changes
CV—hypertension
CV—hypotension
CV—infarction
Death
Dehiscence of wound
Dizziness
Electrolyte abnormality
Fainting
Fall
Fever—not MH
Headache
Hemorrhage
Itching
IV site pain
IV site infection
Malignant hyperthermia
Neurologic change
No home care
No instructions given
No ride available
Physician delay

Patient delay
Respiratory arrest/apnea
Respiratory asthma
Respiratory pneumothorax
Respiratory pulmonary edema
Return to OR
Sepsis
Signed out Against Medical Advice
Somnolence
Transient Neurologic Syndrome (TNS)
Urinary retention
Viscus perforation

Nonprocedural Care-related Adverse Events
Serious adverse event secondary to a medication prescription
Any medication prescription error requiring follow-up by pharmacist or physician
Serious injury to patient or other person secondary to misuse of a device or medication
Nerve injury, fall, or skin breakdown due to anesthetic body part following treatment
Allergic reaction to medication or other treatment
Patient fall while on site at facility for treatment
Patient fall while on medication that may impair balance or mentation
Patient involvement in motor vehicle accident subsequent/consequent to treatment
Any staff injury or patient injury while on site at facility for treatment
Patient misidentification
Release of any patient to an inappropriate or incorrect caregiver
HIPAA privacy or security rule violation
Incomplete medication list documentation
Incomplete allergy list documentation
Incomplete problem list documentation
Incomplete or incorrect "other provider" list
Inability to access health records at point of care
Omission of communication of any new prescription to all other medical providers of care to the patient

---

TARGETING ERROR: INFECTION CONTROL

Nosocomial infections can be devastating in the pain management environment. Those practices that include interventional therapy must be scrupulous in sterile technique. Surgical wound infection constitutes the second most common category of adverse events in health care.[329] In this setting, monitoring for patient wound infections or inappropriate use of antibiotics can have a positive effect on the rate of such events both inside the practice and in the community.[364] The outcomes of even minor procedures may be improved with routine use of sterile gowns and gloves. Also, attention should be paid to the very important although basic, step of adequate personal hygiene and hand washing repetitively throughout the day by both clinical and nonclinical staff.[365]

TARGETING ERROR: PROVIDER FATIGUE

Although operator fatigue has been recognized as a potential source of error in many industries, in health care it has received attention only recently, and little has been accomplished outside of creating new requirements for trainees.[366] Practitioners who have completed their training tend to work longer hours with less rest than is considered appropriate in almost any other work setting. This should be particularly concerning for those pain practices that employ interventional therapies. All aspects of cognition are adversely affected by fatigue, although there is insufficient evidence to pinpoint a specific amount of rest as "enough" in medicine. In general practitioners tend to ignore or discount the potential impact of fatigue on their own error rate.[367] Each practitioner is encouraged to create and follow personal and practicewide policies regarding continuous time spent in clinical activity.[368]

INFORMATION TECHNOLOGY AS A MEANS TO IMPROVE SAFETY

Technology can reduce error and the negative impact of error by three means:
1. Prevention, by provision of critical information at the point of care
2. Improved speed of response once an error has occurred
3. Tracking the occurrence of errors to allow monitoring for trends and to allow feedback to providers[369]

An example of the promise of safety improvement through innovative technology is in patient identification. Correct patient identification and elimination of wrong-site surgery has been identified by the IOM and TJC as a significant opportunity for improved safety.[370] The use of a bar coding system can virtually eliminate the potential for patient misidentification and also diminishes medication error. Unfortunately, high cost and slow speed of the systems have led to adoption by only 5% of U.S. hospitals.[371,372]

Bates and Gawande[369] note that other areas in which technology can help are
1. The calculation of medication doses
2. Communication of patient data between sometimes geographically or temporally separated practitioners
3. Providing references such as guidelines for care
4. Monitoring of patient outcomes, adverse events, and practice patterns

Systems that support clinicians with access to guidelines and medication error monitoring have improved quality of care and decreased error.[373]

BARRIERS TO TECHNOLOGY ADOPTION: COST AND STANDARDIZATION

Will the investment in database technology, EHR programs, hardware, and other technology be worth the costs? At this point it is not certain, because most studies of technology's impact on patient care and safety do not attend to the financial impact of such investment.[374] Cost is a large portion of the reason

that health care providers have not quickly adopted technology as a means of improving care.[375] In a measure of federal and state governments' belief in the IOM report on patient safety and the potential role of technology, several bills have been introduced and passed that subsidize the cost of introduction of technology at hospitals and offices.[369]

Other concerns that are holding back the widespread adoption of technology in practice include variations in standards in software design that would allow different systems in different practices to directly transfer data, particularly among older "legacy" databases. Considering the cost of implementation of new systems, including education of staff and acquisition costs for software and hardware, the inability of a new system to "read" the data already on hand in the practice is a significant disincentive.

SOME PRACTICAL TIPS TO IMPROVE PATIENT SAFETY

In the environment of national safety initiatives that emphasize significant investment in information technology, some of the simpler steps in improving patient safety may be overlooked. For an office that engages in interventional therapy, there are parallels to the safety features needed in offices that perform any kind of surgery. Recently Bridenbaugh[376] offered recommendations regarding safer office care, which include improved office emergency equipment, routinely updated and maintained by biotechnical personnel; training and certification of personnel in delivery of medication and resuscitative techniques; use of written practice policies and procedures that are routinely reviewed with the staff, including emergency procedures; use of monitoring that conforms to the same levels as would be expected in an accredited ambulatory surgical center or hospital; guidelines for sedation and anesthesia that conform to those of the American Society of Anesthesiologists; and compliance with any local or state standards of office safety and quality standards. One cheap but creative use of technology to improve patient safety at home is the simple handheld camera phone. This may serve as a means to monitor patient wound status, a technique that could be of value to a pain practice in which patients with invasive catheters are cared for at home.[377]

PATIENT SAFETY AND THE IMPAIRED DRIVER: CHRONIC PAIN AND ANALGESICS

A controversial topic is the role a physician plays in the determination of the automobile driving ability of his or her patients. Most state regulations require health care practitioners to report any patients who have a medical or surgical impairment that would make them unsafe, if they had not voluntarily given up driving. This is a significant concern for practitioners whose practice has a large percentage of older patients, many of whom may have vision or hearing impairments that warrant concern about safety while driving a car.[378]

However, additional concerns for the pain practitioner are those patients who are using opioid medication or who undergo procedures that may impair their motor skills or mentation. The real risk of driving in the setting of long-term use of opioids is uncertain, but there is likely impairment present for some patients.[379,380] It is also significant to consider that both opioid use and peripheral neuropathy are risk factors for impaired driving.[381] Some evidence exists that middle-aged drivers with chronic pain, with or without treatment, are involved more often in serious accidents than are drivers who do not report pain.[382] Recently, a study raised the possibility that just the presence of chronic pain of any severity is a risk for impaired driving skills when tested on a controlled course.[383]

PATIENTS UNDERGOING INJECTION THERAPY: SHOULD THEY HAVE A DRIVER?

Literature searches do not reveal a controlled study that provides the answer to this question. This author requires all patients undergoing interventional therapy to have a driver for the following reasons:

1. Most often the patient's original diagnosis entails some degree of neural dysfunction and therefore driving capability is probably already impaired.
2. Pain, which may actually increase during the initial treatment period, can cause mental distraction and muscle spasm that could impair driver focus and function.
3. The activity of driving very frequently will serve to exacerbate muscle spasm and is often among the activities that patients complain worsens their pain, so that driving is on the list of activities that we ask our patients not to practice any more than is absolutely necessary during the days that treatment is in progress.
4. Theoretically, even those procedures that do not intentionally block neural transmission (e.g., an epidural steroid injection with only steroid and normal saline) may cause a diminished motor response due to either volumetric compression on nerve tissue or increased pain after the injection.
5. We ask our patients to engage in therapeutic activities the day of their procedure, including use of massage, bath, and relaxation therapy. The efficacy of these measures is opposed by the stress associated with the activity of driving.
6. In our practice, we have found that patients who are required to organize a driver for their return home are less likely to immediately return to work after the procedure or to ignore postprocedure instructions.
7. Finally, with no definitive study in the literature showing that driving postinjection therapy is safe, and with plausible theoretic reasons to consider that such patients might be more prone to accidents, it is a reasonable and prudent precaution.

ACCREDITATION

It is strongly recommended that every practitioner invite an independent agency to inspect his or her practice annually to provide advice about improving the quality and safety of care delivered there, even if formal accreditation does not ensue. Options include state health departments, as well as either TJC (www.jointcommission.org/AccreditationPrograms/AmbulatoryCare/ed_amb.htm) or the AAAHC (www.aaahc.org/eweb/dynamicpage.aspx?webcode=home). Both of the latter will certify multiple- and single-specialty ambulatory surgical centers as well as physician practices and offices that practice pain medicine. If the program in question is a multidisciplinary program, another accrediting organization to consider is the CARF (www.carf.org/Providersaspx?content=content/Accreditation/Opportunities/MED/What.htm), which is willing to accredit what it terms "interdisciplinary pain rehabilitation programs."

Certainly full accreditation or even just a letter from an inspector describing a practice's positives and negative attributes—assuming the former outweigh the latter—can be valuable in contracting with third party payers as a means of proving a salutatory commitment to patient safety and practice quality. Such accreditation has been used successfully to decrease liability insurance for a facility and malpractice insurance for both a facility and the physicians who are part of its practice or ownership group. It is also probably true that such documentation would be of value in the event of any later tort action concerning a patient's safety.

WHAT TO DO WHEN AN ADVERSE EVENT DOES OCCUR

The intent of this section is to promote use of methods to diminish the likelihood of error and avoid adverse events. Nonetheless, adverse events will happen. How should the practitioner respond? Most often the initial impulse will be to deny the event, to "cover up" any role that error played in the outcome and to—at all costs—not implicate any practitioner as culpable when communicating with the affected patient.

However, recent work by the Anesthesia Patient Safety Foundation emphasizes the importance of open and frank communication with the patient and family involved, with open answers to even difficult questions.[384] An attitude of learning and correcting error rather than blaming the practitioners involved, combined with complete honesty about the events that occurred is recommended.[385,386] Above all, a strategy for dealing with patient injury should be worked out in advance among all the practice participants. The APSF has placed an "Adverse Event Protocol" on its website at www.apsf.org that is oriented toward an anesthetic adverse event (see drop down list under "resource center" and click on "clinical safety tools"). It would provide guidance in the pain clinic as well.

The practice's Adverse Event Plan should also include discussions with malpractice carriers and practice attorneys in advance of any events. Having a plan—and confidence in it—is the best approach to management of any breaches of patient safety. Always, such events should be examined closely to find the system flaws that led to any errors.

SAFETY CONCLUSIONS

Although the issue of patient safety programs may seem like a policy concern more fit for a hospital or even work on a national level, it is truly quite applicable to a single specialty clinic or practice, such as the pain practitioner's clinic. A "clinical microsystem" is a group of dedicated clinician teams with specific roles in the treatment of specific patient types or disease groups.[387] Such teams of clinicians, using the methods discussed here of measurement, monitoring, system revision and repeat evaluation, can be effective in creating safer care for their own patients and perhaps improving the care of the community as a whole. As noted above, the focus must be on the system, looking for areas in the stream of care provision that can be simplified and mistake-proofed, rather than on waiting for error to occur and then assigning blame or punishing the individual caregiver.[388]

The reader is encouraged to start small with a database to monitor a very few aspects of every patient's care and outcome, and to trial some of the methods listed here to evaluate whether or not there are improvements that can be made quickly and then monitored for efficacy. Attention to outside guidelines and recommendations for safe practice will also be necessary, both to ensure that the practice is safer and to maintain or improve income that will be increasingly tied to participation in safety programs dictated by others.

SUMMARY

- Patient safety may be improved by careful monitoring of adverse events and trends in care.
- A simple system of monitoring just a few aspects of *all* patients' care will improve chances of avoiding adverse events.
- Technology can be of value in decreasing the incidence of some errors in medication and patient identification.
- Use of protocols and adherence to practice policies are low-tech and relatively cheap ways to decrease error.
- Adverse events will occur, but caregivers and patients will benefit if a practice follows simple guidelines in their management of these events, including honest and forthright explication of any errors.

CONCLUSION

National health care policy will always fail in some measure to fix the poor health of the nation because the national malady is sustained by much more basic and widespread problems than can be repaired by improvements in health care policy. As well, it is unlikely that the effect of any particular health care policy on the health of the citizenry will be apparent for years after it is created, if then, due to the multiple factors that impact upon the health of any one individual, including genetics, education, income and social networks. Although we rightfully rue the high cost of health care and the unacceptably incongruous low quality of health that many of our citizens experience, a large portion of this conundrum exists because it is easier to spend money on (or to take it away from) the apparent ills of the health care delivery system than on those negative aspects of the societal structure that underpin our citizenry's ill health.

Continuing barriers to equitable access, increasing cost, and problems with quality will continue to push health care reform in the future. Experts believe that it is also likely that at some point there will be a governmental program that provides a guaranteed minimal level of care and coverage for "ordinary emergencies" but not for more expensive care, which will be left to those who can pay.[389] Unfortunately, even this minimal improvement will likely await a further deterioration in the system, because such significant reform will require that the majority of Americans feel that the crisis in health care delivery is "personal."[35] Some have suggested that if a pandemic or other actual health catastrophe does not intervene, it may require that fully 100 million Americans are without health care access before the public will support real reform of the delivery and financing of care.[281]

Thus it seems that even a more fundamental level of reform, perhaps as yet years distant, will only more strongly solidify the two-tiered system of health care that already exists, although it may successfully decrease the expensive use of emergency services and may increase the overall efficiency of the system by eliminating at least some of the confusion about who is eligible for what. However, it should be recognized that this will be but one more institutionalization of inequity in the society, and as such will hardly be considered a "final solution." Tinkering will continue at both national and state levels.

In the pain clinic, however, attention to an integrated system of care will provide both excellent quality care and superb outcomes, often with lowered costs and higher satisfaction. There are concrete means of improving quality of care at the level of the individual provider or practice. By using these techniques, each physician may become the most effective purveyor of change in our nation's health care system.[390] Seven practical disciplines in our individual practice of pain medicine will insure that we provide high value care, improve the state of health care in our community, and sustain our ability to maintain a significant and positive role in our patients' health care. We must each do the following:

1. Plan every patient's pain therapy as an integral part of the continuum of his or her access to complete health care.

2. Pay close attention to individual patient responses and needs in guiding therapy and avoid unexamined, reflexive therapeutic responses to diagnoses.
3. Integrate aggressive and creative CQI efforts into daily practice. Monitor every patient's outcome and include assessment of the overall value of each type of therapy that is purveyed.
4. Commit to patient safety via the integration of appropriate technology into medication management, CQI, and in communication with patients and other providers.
5. Restrict therapeutic interventions to medication and technology validated by evidence-based medicine, with the recognition that true EBM begins at the level of the individual practice and that it does not inhibit creativity but does demand that those who advocate the use of any treatment strategy carry the burden of proving its value.
6. Advocate for each patient, regardless of socioeconomic status, to have access to appropriate pain relief, including the application of all those mental health and social support benefits, opioids, and technologies that have been proven in the court of evidence-based medicine.
7. Measure and prove that pain therapies are of value, and anticipate that we will not be allowed to continue what we consider "best practice" for our patients if we cannot prove that value.[47]

If pain practitioners use quality science on a daily basis, measuring every patient's progress using the specific clinical structural, process and outcome measures agreed upon by their partners, and monitor the trends of those outcomes for best and lesser practices, then the quality of their patient care will rise steadily. The rewards will be those for which we have always strived: the improved health of our patients and our own satisfaction that we have been able to accomplish the best care of which we are capable.

References

1. White AG, Birnbaum HG, Mareva MN, et al: Economic burden of illness for employees with painful conditions. J Occup Environ Med 2005;47:884-892.
2. Luo X, Pietrobon R, Sun SX, et al: Estimates and patterns of direct health care expenditures among individuals with back pain in the United States. Spine 2003;29:79-86.
3. Wyatt M, Underwood MR, Scheel IB, et al: Back pain and health policy research. Spine 2004;29:E468-E475.
4. Deyo RA: Pain and public policy. N Engl J Med 2000;342:1211-1213.
5. Cassidy JD, Carroll LJ, Côté P, et al: Effect of eliminating compensation for pain and suffering on the outcome of insurance claims for whiplash injury. N Engl J Med 2000;342:1179-1186.
6. Morone JA: Morality, politics and health policy. In Mechanic D, Rogut LB, Colby DC, et al: (eds): Policy Challenges in Modern Health Care. New Brunswick, NJ, Rutgers University Press, 2005, pp 13-25.
7. Patel K. Rushefsky ME: Health Care Politics and Policy in America. Armonk, NY, ME Sharpe, 1999, pp 1-24.
8. Blendon RJ, Young JT, DesRoches CM: The uninsured, the working uninsured, and the public. Health Aff 1999;18:203-211.
9. Chernew ME, Hirth RA, Cutler DM: Increased spending on health care: How much can the United States afford? Health Aff 2003;22:15-25.
10. Borger C, Smith S, Truffer C, et al: Health spending projections through 2015: Changes on the horizon. Health Aff 2006;25:w61-w73 (published on line 02/22/2006; 10.1377/Healthaff.25.w61). Downloaded 05/28/2006.
11. Reinhardt UE, Hussey PS, Anderson GF: U.S. health care spending in an international context. Health Aff 2004;23:10-25.
12. Anderson GF, Frogner BK, Johns RA, et al: Health care spending and use of information technology in OECD countries. Health Aff 2006;25:819-831.
13. Colombo F, Tapay N. Private health insurance in OECD countries: The benefits and costs for individuals and health systems. OECD Health Working Papers No. 15, 2004. Available at www.oecd.org/dataoecd/34/56/33698043.pdf.
14. Mechanic D, Rogut LB, Colby DC, et al (eds): Policy Challenges in Modern Health Care. New Brunswick, NJ, Rutgers University Press, 2005, pp 1-12.
15. Available at http://www.oecd.org/document/16/0,2340,en_2825_495642_2085200_1_1_1_1,00.html
16. Woolhandler S, Campbell T, Himmelstein DU: Costs of health care administration in the United States and Canada. N Engl J Med. 2003;349:768-775.
17. Fox W, Pickering J: Payment level comparison between public programs and commercial health plans for Washington State hospitals and physicians. Milliman, Inc for Premera; May, 2006. Available at www.premera.com/stellent/groups/public/documents/pdfs/dynwat%385724_332932250_1636.pdf.
18. Anderson GF, Reinhardt UE, Hussey PS: It's the prices, stupid: Why the United States is so different from other countries. Health Aff 2003;23:89-105.
19. Giaimo S: Cost containment vs. solidarity in the welfare state: The case of German and American health care reform. AICGS, 1998; Policy papers #6. From www.jhu.edu/~aicgsdoc/ (202-332-9312).
20. Institute of Medicine: Crossing the Quality Chasm: A New Health System for the 21st Century. Washington, DC: National Academies Press, 2001.
21. Chassin MR, Galvin RW: The urgent need to improve health care quality. JAMA 1998;280:1000-1005.
22. Leape LL: Unnecessary surgery. Ann Rev Public Health 1992;13:363-383.
23. McGlynn EA, Asch SM, Adams J, et al: The quality of health care delivered to adults in the United States. N Engl J Med 2003;348:2635-2645.
24. Asch SM, Kerr EA, Keesey J, et al: Who is at greatest risk for receiving poor-quality care? N Engl J Med. 2006;354:1147-1155.
25. Steinberg EP: Improving the quality of care—Can we practice what we preach? (editorial). N Engl J Med 2003;348:2681-2683.
26. Leape LL: Error in medicine. JAMA 1994;272:1851-1857.
27. Feazell GL, Marren JP: The quality-value proposition in health care. J Health Care Fin 2003;30:1-29.
28. Meurer JR, Yang H, Guse CE, et al: Medical injuries among hospitalized children. Qual Safety Health Care 2006;202-207.
29. Zhan C, Miller MR: Excess length of stay, charge and mortality attributable to medical injuries during hospitalization. JAMA. 2003;290L:1868-1874.
30. OECD Factbook 2005—ISBN 92-64-01869-7—(c) OECD 2005. Downloaded 05/30/2006 at http://www.oecd.org/document/16/0,2340,en_2825_499502_2085200_1_1_1_1,00.html.
31. Derickson A: Health Security for All: Dreams of Universal Health care in America. Baltimore, Johns Hopkins University Press, 2005, p 160.
32. Doty MM, Edwards JN, Holmgren AL: Seeing red: Americans driven into debt by medical bills. Results from a national survey. Issue Brief (Commonwealth Fund). 2005;837:1-12.
33. O'Toole TP, Arbelaez JJ, Lawrence RS: Medical debt and aggressive debt restitution practices: Predatory billing among the urban poor. J Gen Int Med 2004;19:772-778.

34. Levitt JC: Transfer of financial risk and alternative financing solutions. J Health Care Fin 2004;30:21-32.
35. Chen JJ: A modernized medicine for our times: Reforming the American health care system. MURJ 2000;3:77-85.
36. Smedley BD, Stith AY, Nelson AR (eds): Unequal treatment confronting racial and ethnic disparities in health care. Wash, DC, National Academy Press, 2003.
37. National Health Care Disparities Report, 2005. Rockville, Md., Agency for Health Care Research and Quality, January 2006. Available at www.ahrq.gov/qual/nhdr05/nhdr05.htm.
38. Ross JS, Bradley EH, Busch SH: Use of health care services by lower-income and higher-income uninsured adults. JAMA 2006;295:2027-2036.
39. Woolf SH, Johnson RE, Fryer GE, et al: The health impact of resolving racial disparities: An analysis of U.S. mortality data. Am J Public Health 2004;94:2078-2081.
40. Wennberg JE, Fisher ES, Skinner JS: Geography and the debate over Medicare reform. Health Aff 2002; W96-W114. From http://content.healthaffairs.org/cgi/reprint/Healthaff.w2.96v1.
41. Merrill DG: Hoffman's glasses. RAPM 2003;28:547-560.
42. Birkmeyer NJ, Weinstein JN: Medical versus surgical treatment for low back pain: Evidence and clinical practice. Eff Clin Prac 1999. Available at http://wwws.acponline.org/journals/ecp/sepoct99/birkmeyer.htm.
43. Ashton CM, Petersen NJ, Souchek J, et al: Geographic variations in utilization rates in veterans affairs hospitals and clinics. N Engl J Med 1999;340:32-39.
44. Davis D: Quality, patient safety and implementation of best evidence. Health Q 2005;8:128-131.
45. Ballard DJ, Hopkins RS, Nicewander D: Variation in medical practice and implications for quality. In Ransom SB, Joshi MS, Nash DB (eds): The Health Care Quality Handbook. Chicago, Health Administration Press, 2005, pp 43-61.
46. Fisher ES, Wennberg DE, Sukel TA, et al: The implications of regional variations in Medicare spending. Part 2: Health outcomes and satisfaction. Ann Intern Med 2003;138:288-298.
47. MedPAC: Report to the Congress: Increasing the value of Medicare. June 2006. Available at www.MedPAC.gov.
48. Bodenheimer T: The movement for improved quality in health care. N Engl J Med 1999;340:488-492.
49. Marmot MG: Status syndrome: A challenge to medicine. JAMA 2006;295:1304-1307.
50. Banks J, Marmot M, Oldfield Z, et al: Disease and disadvantage in the United States and England. JAMA 2006;295:2037-2045.
51. Exworthy M, Bindman A, Davies J, et al: Evidence into policy and practice? Measuring the progress of U.S. and U.K. policies to tackle disparities and inequalities in the U.S. and U.K. health and health care. Mil Q 2006;84:75-109.
52. Sanmartin C, Berthelot JM, Ng E, et al: Comparing health and health care use in Canada and the United States. Health Aff 2006;25:1133-1142.
53. Weissmann G: Dr Holmes returns from Paris. In Weissmann G (ed):. Democracy and DNA. New York, Hill and Wang, 1995, pp 14-29.
54. Niebuhr R: Ideology and the scientific method. In Brown RM (ed): The Essential Reinhold Niebuhr. Binghamton, NY, Vail-Ballou Press, 1986, pp 205-217.
55. Henretta JA, Brody D, Dumenil L, et al: A maturing industrial society, 1877-1914. In America's History. Boston, Bedford-St. Martins, 2004, pp 573-601.
56. Patel K, Rushefsky ME: Health Care Politics and Policy in America. Armonk, NY, ME Sharpe, 1999, pp 25-54.
57. Gordon C: Dead on Arrival: The Politics of Health Care in Twentieth-Century America. Princeton, Princeton University Press, 2003, pp 12-45.
58. Glied SA: The employer-based health insurance system: Mistake or cornerstone? In Mechanic D, Rogut LB, Colby DC, et al (eds): Policy challenges in modern health care. New Brunswick, Rutgers University Press, 2005, pp 37-52.
59. Derickson A: Health Security for All: Dreams of Universal Health Care in America. Baltimore, Johns Hopkins University Press, 2005, pp 32-38.
60. Gordon C: Dead on Arrival: The Politics of Health Care in Twentieth-Century America. Princeton, Princeton University Press, 2003, pp 215-246.
61. Mayes R: Critical juncture: Health insurance subordinated to social security. In Universal Coverage: The elusive quest for national health insurance. Ann Arbor, Mich, University of Michigan Press, 2005, pp 17-29.
62. Gabel R: Job-based health insurance 1977-1998: The accidental system under scrutiny. Health Aff 1999;18:62-74.
63. Richmond JB, Fein R: The Health Care Mess: How We Got into It and What It Will Take to Get Out. Cambridge, Mass, Harvard University Press, 2005, pp 30-51.
64. Derickson A: Health Security for All: Dreams of Universal Health Care in America. Baltimore, Johns Hopkins University Press, 2005, pp 126-127.
65. Mayes R: Symbiotic attachment. In Universal Coverage: The Elusive Quest for National Health Insurance. Ann Arbor, Mich, University of Michigan Press, 2005, pp 61-80.
66. Starr P: The Social Transformation of American Medicine. New York, Basic Books, 1982, p 369.
67. Derickson A: Health Security for All: Dreams of Universal Health Care in America. Baltimore, Johns Hopkins University Press, 2005, pp 131-156.
68. Mayes R: Incrementalism's consequences. In Universal Coverage: The Elusive Quest for National Health Insurance. Ann Arbor, Mich, University of Michigan Press, 2005, pp 81-108.
69. Richmond JB, Fein R: The Health Care Mess: How We Got into It and What It Will Take to Get Out. Cambridge, Mass, Harvard University Press, 2005, pp 63-80.
70. Patel K, Rushefsky ME: Health Care Politics and Policy in America. Armonk, NY, ME Sharpe, 1999, pp 162-195.
71. Enthoven AC: Why managed care has failed to contain health costs. Health Aff 1993;12:27-43.
72. Rodwin MA: Promoting accountable managed health care: The potential role for consumer voice. From www.healthlaw.org/pubs/2000rodwin.html.
73. Grant DS, Wallace M: The political economy of manufacturing: Growth and decline across the American states, 1970-1985. Soc Forces 1994;73:33-63.
74. Beyers WB, Lindahl DP: Services and the new economic landscape. Eur Reg Sci Mtg paper. Aug-Sept, 1998.
75. Williams DR: Patterns and causes of disparities in health. In Mechanic D, Rogut LB, Colby DC, et al (eds): Policy Challenges in Modern Health Care. New Brunswick, Rutgers University Press, 2005, pp 115-134.
76. Mayes R: Locked in and crowded out. In Universal Coverage: The Elusive Quest for National Health Insurance. Ann Arbor, Mich, University of Michigan Press, 2005, pp 109-138.
77. Patel K, Rushefsky ME: Health Care Politics and Policy in America. Armonk, NY, ME Sharpe, 1999, pp 314-315.
78. Robinson JC: Entrepreneurial challenges to integrated health care. In Mechanic D, Rogut LB, Colby DC, et al (eds): Policy Challenges in Modern Health Care. New Brunswick, Rutgers University Press, 2005, pp 53-67.
79. Hackbarth GM: Physician owned specialty hospitals. From http://www.MedPAC.gov/search.
80. National Nosocomial Infection Surveillance (NNIS) System Report. Am J Infect Control 2003;31:481-498.
81. Kane NM: Medical bad debt: A growing public health crisis. Washington DC testimony before the House Ways and Means Committee June 22, 2004. http://waysandmeans.house.gov.
82. Schmidt K, Meagher TF: Specialty hospitals: positive contributors to health care delivery. J Nurs Adm 2005;35:323-325.
83. Popescu I, Vaughan-Sarrazin MS, Rosenthal GE: Certificate of need regulations and use of coronary revascularization after acute myocardial infarction. JAMA 2006;295:2141-2147.
84. Altman SH, Tompkins CP, Eilat E, et al: Escalating health care spending: Is it desirable or inevitable? Health Aff Jan-Jun 2003; W3_1.
85. Olson LM, Tang SS, Newacheck PW: Children in the United States with discontinuous health insurance coverage. N Engl J Med 353:382-391.

86. Woolhandler S, Himmelstein DU, Angell M, et al: Proposal of the physicians' working group for single-payer national health insurance. JAMA 2003;290:798-805.

87. USA Today: Briefly. May 5, 2006; B1.

88. Heslin KC, Andersen RM, Ettner SL, et al: Racial and ethnic disparities in access to physicians with HIV-related expertise: Findings from a nationally representative study. J Gen Int Med 2005;20:283-289.

89. Institute of Medicine: The health care delivery system. In IOM: The future of the public's health. Washington, DC, The National Academies Press, 2003, pp 212-267.

90. Leonhardt D: A health fix that is not a fantasy. New York Times April 12, 2006; C1.

91. Blumenthal D: New steam from an old cauldron—the physician supply debate. N Engl J Med 2004;350:1780-1787.

92. Turk DC, Rudy TE, Stieg RL: The disability determination dilemma: Toward a multiaxial solution. Pain 1988;34:217-229.

93. Yelin E: Cost of musculoskeletal diseases: Impact of work disability and functional decline. J Rheumatol 2003;30(S68):8-11.

94. Loeser JD: Economic implications of pain management. Acta Anaesthesiol Scand 1999;43:957-959.

95. Mapel DW, Shainline M, Paez K, et al: Hospital, pharmacy and outpatient costs for osteoarthritis and chronic back pain. J Rheumatol 2004;31:573-583.

96. Goldberg GA, Kim SS, Seifeldin R, et al: Health care costs associated with suboptimal management of persistent pain. Man Care 2003;12(8S):14-17.

97. Jensen IB, Bergstrom G, Ljungquist T, et al: A 3-year follow-up of a multidisciplinary rehabilitation program for back and neck pain. Pain 2005;115:273-283.

98. Turk DC, Burwinkle TM: Clinical outcomes, cost-effectiveness, and the role of psychology in treatments for chronic pain sufferers. Prof Psych Res Prac 2005;36:602-610.

99. Brose W: Interdisciplinary pain rehabilitation programs: The peer-reviewed, nationally-recognized evidence: Help for chronic pain sufferers. Presented at American Academy of Pain Medicine, Orlando, Fla, 2004. Available at www.helppain.net/transcriptFL.pdf.

100. Glied S, Cuellar A: Better behavioral health care coverage for everyone. N Engl J Med 2006;354:1415-1417.

101. Stieg RL: Financing the treatment of chronic pain: Models for risk-sharing among pain medicine physician, health care payers and consumers. Pain Med 2000;1:78-88.

102. Worrel LM, Krahn LE, Sletten CD, et al: Treating fibromyalgia with a brief interdisciplinary program: Initial outcomes and predictors of response. Mayo Clin Proc 2001;76:384-390.

103. Stadler M, Schlannder M, Braeckman M: A cost-utility and cost-effectiveness analysis of an acute pain service. J Clin Anesth 2004;16:159-167.

104. Turk DC: Clinical effectiveness and cost-effectiveness of treatments for patient with chronic pain. Clin J Pain 2002;18:355-365.

105. Flor H, Fydrich T, Turk DC: Efficacy of multidisciplinary pain centers: A meta-analytic review. Pain 1992;49:221-230.

106. Goldman JJ, Frank RF, Burnam MA: Behavioral health insurance parity for federal employees. N Engl J Med 2006;354:1378-1386.

107. Vogt MT, Kwoh K, Cope DK: Analgesic usage for low back pain: Impact on health care costs and service use. Spine 2005;30:1075-1081.

108. American Medical Association: Physicians' Current Procedural Terminology. Chicago, American Medical Association, 2005, pp 10-15.

109. CMS Final Rule. *Federal Register*, November 21, 2005, p. 70119. From www.acro.org/pdf/Final%20Rule%Physicians%20Nov2005.pdf.

110. Avitzur O: How members can make changes in coding that impact practice. Neurol Today 2004;4:70-73.

111. Carter D: Medicare cost controls and program compliance: The rationale of physician claims edits. J Med Prac Management 2002;18:115-119.

112. Duszak R, Sacks D, Manowczak J: CPT coding by interventional radiologists: Accuracy and implications. J Vasc Interv Radiol 2001:12:447-454.

113. http://oig.hhs.gov/oei/reports/oei-09-02-00030.pdf.

114. Levinson DR: Use of modifier 59 to bypass Medicare's National Correct Coding Initiative edits. OEI-03-02-00771. November, 2005. Available at www.oig.hhs.gov.

115. Levinson DR: Use of modifier 25. OEI-03-02-00771. November, 2005. Available at www.oig.hhs.gov.

116. Grey M, Yehieli M: Preventing Medicare fraud among health providers and organizations (part I): An overview for senior Medicare patrols of schemes, scams, and interventions with health organizations and providers. Available at http://www.smpresource.org/eSeries/Content/ahqaNavigationMenu/SMPResources/Webinars/ProviderFraud/ProviderFraudTrainingPartII.ppt.

117. Hart AC, Hopkins CA (eds): Ingenix ICD-9-CM. Available at www.ingenixonline.com.

118. Available at www.npdb-hipdb.hrsa.gov

119. Available at www.hhs.gov/ocr/hipaa/

120. Feld AD: The Health Insurance Portability and Accountability Act (HIPAA): Its broad effect on practice. Am J Gastroenterol 2005;100:1440-14443.

121. Jones ED: WEDI, HIPAA, and U. ASA Newsletter 2002, p 66. From www.asahq.org/Newletters/2002/jones.html.

122. Available at www.hhs.gov/news/press/2002pres/20020809.html

123. Wielawski IM: HIPAA, TB, and me. Health Aff 2006;25:1127-1132.

124. Rothstein MA, Talbott MK: Compelled disclosure of health information: Protecting against the greatest potential threat to privacy. JAMA 2006;295:2882-2885.

125. Wolf MS, Bennett CL: Local perspective of the impact of the HIPAA privacy rule on research. Cancer 2006;106:474-479.

126. Available at www.medpac.gov

127. Epstein AM, Lee TH, Hamel MB: Paying physicians for high-quality care. N Engl J Med. 2004;350:406-410.

128. Hackbarth GM: Medicare payment to physicians. Statement before the Subcommittee on Health, Common Energy and Commerce, U.S. House of Representatives; Nov 17, 2005. From http://www.MedPAC.gov/search/searchframes.cfm

129. Available at www.iha.org.

130. Birkmeyer NJO, Birkmeyer JD: Strategies for improving surgical quality—Should payers reward excellence or effort? N Engl J Med 2006;354:864-870.

131. Strunk B, Hurley R: Paying for quality: Health plans try carrots instead of sticks. Issue Brief Cent Stud Health Syst Change 2004;82:1-4.

132. Grabowski DC, Angelelli JL: The relationship of Medicaid payment rates, bed constraint policies, and risk-adjusted pressure ulcers. Health Serv Res 2004;39:793-812.

133. Milgate K, Cheng SB: Pay-for-performance: The MedPAC perspective. Health Aff 2006;25:413-419.

134. Available at www.asa-assn.org/ama/pub/category/2946.html.

135. Bierstein K: Pay for performance in ambulatory anesthesia. SAMBA annual meeting, May, 2006.

136. den Boer JJ, Oostendorp RAB, Beems T, et al: Continued disability and pain after lumbar disc surgery: The role of cognitive-behavioral factors. Pain 2006;123:45-52.

137. Vlaeyen JW, De Jong J, Geilen M, et al: The treatment of fear of movement/(re)injury in chronic low back pain: Further evidence on the effectiveness of exposure in vivo. Clin J Pain 2002;18:251-261.

138. Kroenke K: Patients presenting with somatic complaints: Epidemiology, psychiatric co-morbidity and management. Int J Methods Psych Res 2003;12:34-43.

139. Lin EHB, Katon W, Von Korff M, et al: Effect of improving depression care on pain and function outcomes among older adults with arthritis: A randomized controlled trial. JAMA 2003;290:2428-2434.

140. Pincus T, Vlaeyen JWS, Kendal NAS: Cognitive-behavioral therapy and psychosocial factors in low back pain: Directions for the future. Spine 2002;27:E133-E138.

141. Verhoef MJ, Mulkins A, Boon H: Integrative health care: How can we determine whether patients benefit? J Alt Comp Med 2005;11:S57-S65.
142. Data from www.asahq.org/Washington/ASA5ProposedMeasures.pdf.
143. Rosenthal MB, Frank RG, Li Z, et al: Early experience with pay-for-performance from concept to practice. JAMA 2005;294:1788-1793.
144. Pereira AG, Pearson SD: Patient attitudes toward physician financial incentives. Arch Intern Med 2001;161:1313-1317.
145. Dorman T: Unsustainable growth rate: Physician perspective. Crit Care Med 2006;34:S78-S81.
146. Moore J: Statement of Justin Moore before the House Ways and Means Committee. http://waysandmeans.house.gov/hearings.asp?fomrmode=view&id=3075
147. Federal Register 66(212):55320.
148. Eng WK: SVR, SGR and you: Why you need the ASAPAC. ASA Newsletter 2006;70:38.
149. Iglehart JK: Linking compensation to quality—Medicare payments to physicians. N Engl J Med 2005;353:870-872.
150. Reinhardt U: Does the Aging of the population really drive the demand for health care? Health Aff 2003;22:27-39.
151. Garber AM, Sox HC: The U.S. physician workforce: Serious questions raised, answers needed. Ann Int Med 2004;141:732-734.
152. Reinhardt UE: Analyzing cause and effect in the U.S. physician workforce. Health Aff (Millwood) 2002;21:165-166.
153. Cooper R: Weighing the evidence for expanding physician supply. Ann Intern Med 2004;141:705-714.
154. Cooper RA, Getzen TE, Mckee HJ, et al: Economic and demographic trends signal in impending physician shortage. Health Aff (Millwood) 2002;21:140-154.
155. Schubert A, Eckhout G, Cooperider T, et al: Evidence of a current and lasting national anesthesia personnel shortfall: Scope and implications. Mayo Clin Proc 2001;76:995-1010.
156. Gold M, Kuo S, Taylor EF: Translating research to action: Improving physician access in public insurance. J Amb Care Manage 2006;29:36-50.
157. Jarman B, Gault S, Alves B, et al: Explaining differences in English hospital death rates using routinely collected data. BMJ 1999;318:1515-1520.
158. Landon BE, Reschovsky JC, Pham HH, et al: Leaving medicine: The consequences of physician dissatisfaction. Med Care 2006;44:234-242.
159. Pedre VM: Letter. Ann Int Med 2005;142:473.
160. Nuckols TK, Escarce JJ: Residency work-hours reform: A cost analysis including preventable adverse events. J Gen Int Med 2005;20:873-878.
161. Ho V, Wirthlin D, Yun H, et al: Physician supply, treatment, and amputation rates for peripheral arterial disease. J Vasc Surg 2005;42:81-87.
162. Laditka JN, Laditka SB, Probst JC: More may be better: Evidence of a negative relationship between physician supply and hospitalization for ambulatory care sensitive conditions. Health Serv Res 2005;40:1148-1166.
163. Mishra R: A shortage slows down surgeries: HMOs, image cited in lack of anesthesiologists. Boston Globe, January 11, 2001;A-1.
164. Wilson JF: U.S. needs more physicians soon but how many more is debatable. Ann Int Med 2005;143:469-472.
165. Gordon DB, Dahl JL, Miaskowski C, et al: American Pain Society recommendations for improving the quality of acute and cancer pain management. Arch Intern Med 2005;165:1574-1580.
166. Ziegler D, Lovrich NP: Pain relief, prescription drugs, and prosecution: A four-state survey of chief prosecutors. J Law Med Ethics 2003;31:75-100.
167. Imbalance and inconsistency continue in DEA policy on medical use of opioids. Topics Pain Management 2006;May:6-7.
168. Foxhall K: DEA enforcement versus pain practice. Prac Pain Man 2005;Sept/Oct:42-49.
169. Gilson AM, Joranson DE: U.S. policies relevant to the prescribing of opioid analgesics for the treatment of pain in patients with addictive disease. Clin J Pain 2002;18:S91-S98.
170. Mehendale AW, Patrick D, Goldman M: Managing chronic pain patients in the new millennium: Clinical basis and regulatory viewpoint from Texas, USA. Pain Prac 2004;4:105-129.
171. Brown TG, Topp J, Ross D: Rationales, obstacles and strategies for local outcome monitoring systems in substance abuse treatment settings. J Subs Abuse Treat 2003;24:31-42.
172. Heit HA, Covington E, Good PA: Dear DEA. Pain Med 2004;5:303-308.
173. Hurwitz W: The challenge of prescription drug misuse: a review and commentary. Pain Med 2005;6:152-161.
174. Katz NP, Sherburne S, Beach M, et al: Behavioral monitoring an urine toxicology testing in patients receiving long-term opioid therapy. Anesth Analg 2003;97:1097-1102.
175. Harris I, Mulford J, Solomon M, et al: Association between compensation status and outcome after surgery. JAMA 2005;293:1644-1652.
176. Atlas SJ, Yuchiao C, Kammann E, et al: Long-term disability and return to work among patients who have a herniated lumbar disc: The effect of disability compensation. J Bone Joint Surg Am 2000;82:4-15.
177. Blyth F, March LM, Nicholas MK, et al: Chronic pain, work performance, and litigation. Pain 2003;103:41-47.
178. Suter PB: Employment and litigation: Improved by work, assisted by verdict. Pain 2003;100:249-257.
179. Tisza SM, Mottl JR, Matthews DB: Current trends in workers' compensation stress claims. Curr Op Psych 2003;16:571-574.
180. Bellamy R: Compensation neurosis: Financial reward for illness as nocebo. Clin Orthop 1997;336:94-106.
181. Eliashof BA, Streltzer J: Psychological impairment. In Demeter SL, Andersson GBJ (eds): Disability Evaluation, 2nd ed. St. Louis, Mosby, 2003, pp 583-595.
182. Fishbain DA, Cutler R, Rosomoff HL, et al: Chronic pain disability exaggeration/malingering and submaximal effort research. Clin J Pain 1999;15:244-274.
183. Arbisi PA, Butcher JN: Psychometric perspectives on detection of malingering of pain: Use of the Minnesota mulitphasic personality inventory-2. Clin J Pain 2004;20:383-391.
184. Rogers R. Introduction. In Rogers R (ed): Clinical Assessment of Malingering and Deception, 2nd ed. New York, Guilford, 1997, pp 1-22.
185. Franche RL, Krause N: Readiness for return to work following injury or illness: Conceptualizing the interpersonal impact of health care, workplace, and insurance factors. J Occup Rehabil 2002;12:233-256.
186. Kereiakes DJ, Willerson JT: Health care on trial: America's medical malpractice crisis. Circ 2004;109:2939-2941.
187. Budetti PP: Tort reform and the patient safety movement. JAMA 2005;293:2660-2662.
188. Davis P, Lay-Yee L, Briant R, et al: Preventable in-hospital medical injury under the "no fault" system in New Zealand. Qual Saf Health Care 2003;12:251-256.
189. Studdert DM, Mello MM, Brennan TA: Medical malpractice. N Engl J Med 2004;350:283-292.
190. Menachemi N, Brooks RG, Clawson A, et al: Continuing decline in service delivery for family physicians: Is the malpractice crisis playing a role? Q Manage Health Care 2006;15:39-45.
191. Kessler DP, Sage WM, Becker DJ: Impact of malpractice reforms on the supply of physician services. JAMA 2005;293:2618-2625.
192. Mello MM, Studdert DM, DesRoches CM, et al: Effects of a malpractice crisis on specialist supply and patient access to care. Ann Surg 2005;242:621-628.
193. Robinson P, Xu X, Keeton K, et al: The impact of medical legal risk on obstetrician-gynecologist supply. Ob Gyn 2005;105:1296-1302.
194. Baker T: The Medical Malpractice Myth. Chicago, University of Chicago Press, 2005.
195. Rodwin MA, Chang HJ, Clausen J: Malpractice premiums and physicians' income: Perceptions of a crisis conflict with empirical evidence. Health Aff 2006;25:750-758.

196. Hellinger FJ, Encinosa WE: The impact of State laws limiting malpractice damage awards on health care expenditures. Am J Public Health 2006;Jun 29; PMID 16809580. From www.ncbi.nlm.nih.giv/entrez/query. fcgi?db=pubme&cmd=Retrieve&dopt=Abstract&list_uids=16809580&query_hl=1&itool=pubmed_docsum.

197. Dauer EA, Marcus LJ: Adapting mediation to link resolution of medical malpractice disputes with health care quality improvement. Law Cont Prob 1997;60:186-218.

198. Schoenbaum SC, Bovbjerg RR: Malpractice reform must include steps to prevent medical injury. Ann intern Med 2004;140:51-53.

199. Forster HP, Schwartz J, DeRenzo E: Reducing legal risk by practicing patient-centered medicine. Arch Intern Med 2002; 162:12178-1219.

200. Dauer EA: A therapeutic jurisprudence perspective on legal responses to medical error. J Leg Med 2003;24:37-50.

201. Helland E, Tabarrok A: Exporting tort awards. Regulation 2000; 23:21-26. From http://catoinstitute.org/pubs/regulation/regv 23n2/helland.pdf.

202. Nichols LM, Ginsburg PB, Berenson RA, et al: Are market forces strong enough to deliver efficient health care systems? Confidence is waning. Health Aff 2004;23:8-21.

203. Urbina I: Rising diabetes threat meets a falling budget. New York Times, May 16, 2006;155:A-1.

204. Winkleby MA, Jatulis DE, Frank E, et al: Socioeconomic status and health: How education, income, and occupation contribute to risk factors for cardiovascular disease. Am J Pub Health 1992;82:816-820.

205. Chen E, Martin AD, Matthews KA: Understanding health disparities: The role of race and socioeconomic status in children's health. Am J Pub Health 2006;96:702-708.

206. Guralnik JM, Land KC, Blazer D, et al: Educational status and active life expectancy among older blacks and whites. N Engl J Med 1993;329:110-116.

207. Chang CF, Nocetti D, Rubin RM: Healthy life expectancy for selected race and gender subgroups: The case of Tennessee. South Med J 2005;98:977-984.

208. Hare RM: Essays on bioethics. Oxford, Oxford Press, 2002, p 212.

209. Regidor E, Ronda E, Pascual C, et al: Decreasing socioeconomic inequalities and increasing health inequalities in Spain: A case study. Am J Pub Health 2006;96:102-109.

210. Fisher ES, Wennberg DE, Stukel TA, et al: The implications of regional variations in Medicare spending. Part 1: The content, quality and accessibility of care. Ann Int Med 2003; 138:273-287.

211. Berk ML, Monheit AC: The concentration of health care expenditures, revisited. Health Aff 2001;20:9-18.

212. Centers for Medicare and Medicaid Services, Medicare 2000: Thirty-five years of improving American's health and security. Baltimore, CMS, 2000.

213. Enthoven AC: Choice in health care (letter). Health Aff 2006;25:566-567.

214. Appel SJ, Giger JN, Davidhizar RE: Opportunity cost: The impact of contextual risk factors on the cardiovascular health of low-income rural southern African American women. J Cardio Nurs 2005;20:315-324.

215. Freudenheim M: Pressures put more flex in family doctors' schedules. New York Times, June 24, 2006;B1.

216. Toner R, Kornblut AE: Wounds salved, Clinton returns to health care. New York Times, June 9, 2006;A1.

217. Vandenburgh H: Emerging trends in the provision and consumption of health services. Soc Spec 2001;21:279-291.

218. Lyman R: Census report foresees no crisis over aging generation's health. New York Times, Mar 10, 2006;A1, A17.

219. Fountain H: The lonely American just got a bit lonelier. New York Times July 2, 2006;Sect 4:12 (Week).

220. Waite LJ, Hugfies ME: At risk on the cusp of old age: Living arrangements and functional status among black, white and Hispanic adults. J Gerontol B Psychol Sci Soc Sci 1999;54: S136-S144.

221. Davis MA, Murphy SP, Neuhaus JM, et al: Living arrangements affect dietary quality for U.S. adults aged 50 years and older: NHANES III 1988-1994. J Nutr 2000;130:2256-2264.

222. Saluter AF. Marital status and living arrangements. From www.census.gov/prod/1/pop/profile/95/10_ps.pdf downloaded 06/30/2006.

223. Available at http://articles.moneycentral.msn.com/Investing/Extra/USSavingsRateFallsToZero.aspx.

224. Remler DK, Glied SA: How much more cost sharing will health savings accounts bring? Health Aff 2006;25:1070-1078.

225. Kher U: Outsourcing your heart. Time Magazine May, 29, 2006. From www.time.com/time/archive/preview/0,1196429,00.html.

226. Konetzka RT, Zhu J, Volpp KG: Did recent changes in Medicare reimbursement hit teaching hospitals harder? Acad Med 2005;80:1069-1074.

227. Robinson JC: Reinvention of health insurance in the consumer era. JAMA 2004;291:1880-1886.

228. Mullan F: A founder of quality assessment encounters a troubled system firsthand. Health Aff 2001;20:137-141.

229. Kronek R: Financing health care—finding the money is hard and spending it well is even harder. N Engl J Med 2005; 352:1252-1254.

230. Institute of Medicine: The Future of the Public's Health. Washington, DC, National Academies Press, 2003, p 148.

231. Hadley J, Holahan J: Covering the uninsured: How much would it cost? Health Aff 2003;10:1377.

232. Martin T: Going blind on our watch. Health Aff 2006;25: 1121-1126.

233. Oberlander J: The U.S. health care system: On a road to nowhere? CMAJ 2002;167:163-168.

234. Cagney KA, Browning CR, Wen M: Racial disparities in self-rated health at older ages: What difference does the neighborhood make? The J Gerontol Ser B: Psychol Sci Soc Sci 2005;60:S181-S190.

235. Zhong-Cheng L, Wilkins R, Kramer MS: Effect of neighbourhood income and maternal education on birth outcomes: A population-based study. CMAJ 2006;174:1415-1421.

236. Litaker D, Koroukian SM, Love TE: Context and health care access: Looking beyond the individual. Med Care 2005;43: 531-540.

237. Long D: Conquering pain. Neurosurgery 2000;46:257.

238. Mounce K: Back pain. Rheumatology 2002;41:1-5.

239. Macfarlane GJ, Thomas E, Papageorgiou AC, et al: Employment and physical work activities as predictors of future low back pain. Spine 1997;22:1143-1149.

240. Vlaeyen JWS, Morley S: Cognitive-behavioral treatments for chronic pain: What works for whom? Clin J Pain 2005; 21:1-8.

241. Jacobson SA, Folstein MF: Psychiatric perspectives on headache and facial pain. Otolaryngol Clin N Am 2003;36: 1187-1200.

242. Starr P: The Social Transformation of American Medicine. New York, Basic Books, 1982.

243. Bowers MR, Kiefe CI: Measuring health care quality: Comparing and contrasting the medical and the marketing approaches. Am J Med Qual 2002;17:136-144.

244. Lohr KN (ed): Medicare: A strategy for quality assistance, vol. I. Washington, DC, National Academy Press, 1990.

245. Donabedian A: Evaluating the quality of medical care. Milbank Q 1966;44:166-203.

246. Blumenthal D: Quality of care—What is it? N Engl J Med 1996;335:891-894.

247. Tovey EJ, Adams AE: The changing nature of nurses' job satisfaction: An exploration of sources of satisfaction in the 1990. J Adv Nursing 1999;30:150-158.

248. Hinshaw AS: Nursing knowledge for the 21st century: Opportunities and challenges. J Nurs Schol 2000;32:117-123.

249. Wyszewianski L: Basic concepts of health care quality. In Ransom SB, Joshi MS, Nash DB (eds): The Health Care Quality Handbook. Chicago, Health Administration Press, 2005, pp 25-42.

250. Cooper RA: Evidence for expanding physician supply (letter). Ann Int Med 2005;142:474.

251. Dranove D, Wehner P: Physician-induced demand for childbirths. J Health Econ. 1994;13:61-73.

252. Available at www.dartmouthatlas.org/atlases/2006_Atlas_Exec_Summary.pdf.
253. Donabedian A: The seven pillars of quality. Arch Path Lab Med. 1990;114:1115-1118.
254. Stoecklein M: Quality improvement systems, theories and tools. In Ransom SB, Joshi MS, Nash DB (eds): The Health Care Quality Handbook. Chicago, Health Administration Press, 2005, pp 63-86.
255. Kohn LT, Corrigan JM, Donaldson (eds): To Err Is Human. Washington, DC, National Academy Press, 1999.
256. Berwick DM, Godfrey AB, Roessner J: Curing health care, 1st ed. San Francisco, Jossey-Bass, 1990, pp 1-17.
257. Braden BR, Cowan CA, Lazenby HC, et al: National health expenditures, 1997. Health Care Fin Rev 1998;20:83-126.
258. Gandjour A, Telzerow A, Lauterback KW, et al: European comparison of costs and quality in the treatment of acute back pain. Spine 2003;30:969-975.
259. Casalino LP, Devers KJ, Brewster LR: Focused factories? Physician-owned specialty facilities. Health Aff 2003;22:56-67.
260. Forster AJ, Shojania KG, van Walraven C: Improving patient safety: Moving beyond the "hype" of medical errors. CMAJ 2005;173:893-894.
261. Hayward RA, Hofer TP: Estimating hospital deaths due to medical errors: Preventability is in the eye of the reviewer. JAMA 2001;286:415-420.
262. Blendon RJ, DesRoches CM, Bordie M, et al: Views of practicing physicians and the public on medical errors. N Engl J Med 2002;347:1933-1940.
263. Bleich S: Medical errors: Five years after the IOM report. The Commonwealth Fund publ #830. Available at www.cmwf.org.
264. Milstead JA: The culture of safety. Policy Polit Nurs Pract 2005;6:51-54.
265. Snyder C, Anderson G: Do quality improvement organizations improve the quality of hospital care for Medicare beneficiaries? JAMA 2005;293:2900-2907.
266. Brennan TA, Gawande A, Thomas E, et al: Accidental deaths, saved lives and improved quality. N Engl J Med 2005;353:1404-1409.
267. Peterson ED, Roe MT, Mulgund J, et al: Association between hospital process performance and outcomes among patients with acute coronary syndromes. JAMA 2006;295:1912-1920.
268. Gann MJ, Restuccia JD: Total quality management in health care: a view of current and potential research. Med Care Rev 1994;51:467-500.
269. Ferguson TB, Peterson ED, Coombs LP: Use of continuous quality improvement to increase use of process measures in patients undergoing coronary artery bypass graft surgery. JAMA 2003;290:49-56.
270. Blumenthal D, Epstein AM: The role of physicians in the future of quality management. N Engl J Med 1996;335:1328-1331.
271. Birkmeyer JD, Dimick JB: Potential benefits of the new leapfrog standards: Effect of process and outcome measures. Surgery 2004;135:569-575.
272. Galvin RS, Delbanco S, Milstein A: Has the Leapfrog group had an impact on the health care market? Health Aff 2005;24:228-233.
273. Khuri SF, Henderson WG: The case against volume as a measure of quality of surgical care. World J Surg 2005;29:1222-1229.
274. Bradley EH, Herrin J, Elbel B: Hospital quality for acute myocardial infarction: Correlation among process measures and relationship with short-term mortality. JAMA 2006;296:72-78.
275. Baker DW, Einstadter D, Thomas C, et al: The effect of publicly reporting hospital performance on market share and risk-adjusted mortality at high-mortality hospitals. Med Care 2003;41:729-740.
276. Dranove D, Kessler D, McClellan M, et al: Is more information better? The effects of "report cards" on health care providers. J Polit Econ 2003;111:555-588.
277. Khuri SF: Quality, advocacy, health care policy, and the surgeon. Ann Thorac Surg 2002;74:641-649.
278. Lambert MJ, Whipple JL, Hawkins EJ, et al: Is it time for clinicians to routinely track patient outcome? A meta-analysis. Clin Psychol Sci Pract 2003;10:288-301.
279. Lambert JM, Hansen NB, Finch AE: Patient-focused research; using patient outcome data to enhance treatment effects. J Consult Clin Psychol 2001;159-172.
280. Evans E, Yih-Ing H. Pilot-testing a statewide outcome monitoring system: Overview of the California treatment outcome project (CALTOP). J Psych Drugs 2004;SARC S2:109-114.
281. Fuchs VR, Emanuel EJ: Health care reform: Why? What? When? Health Aff 2005;24:1399-1414.
282. Chassin MR: Is health care ready for six sigma quality? Milbank Q 1998;76:565-591.
283. Asch SM, McGlynn EA, Hogan MM, et al: Comparison of quality of care for patients in the Veterans Health Administration and patients in a national sample. Ann Int Med 2004;141:938-945.
284. Landon BE, Normand ST, Blumenthal D: Physician clinical performance assessment. JAMA 2003;290:1183-1189.
285. Wachter RM: Expected and unanticipated consequences of the quality and information technology revolutions. JAMA 2006;295:2780-2783.
286. Iezzoni L: Risk adjustment for measuring health care outcomes, 3rd ed. Ann Arbor, MI, Health Administration Press, 2004.
287. Miller EH, Belgrade JM, Cook M, et al: Institutionwide pain management improvement through the use of evidence-based content, strategies, resources, and outcomes. Qual Manag Health Care 1999;7:28-40.
288. Bell A, Wheeler R: Improving the pain management standard of care in a community hospital. Cancer Pract 2002;10(S1):S45-S51.
289. Frankenburg FR, Zanarini MC: The association between borderline personality disorder and chronic medical illnesses, poor health-related lifestyle choices, and costly forms of health care utilization. Clin Psychiatry 2004;65:1660-1665.
290. Enthoven P, Skargren E, Oberg B: Clinical course in patients seeking primary care for back or neck pain: A prospective 5-year follow-up of outcome and health care consumption with subgroup analysis. Spine 2004;29:2458-2465.
291. Skargren EI, Oberg BE. Predictive factors for 1-year outcome of low-back and neck pain in patients treated in primary care: comparison between the treatment strategies chiropractic and physiotherapy. Pain 1998;77:201-207.
292. Turk DC, Burwinkle TM: Assessment of chronic pain in rehabilitation: Outcome measures in clinical trials and clinical practice. Rehab Psychol 2005;50:56-64.
293. Heinemann AW: Putting outcome measurement in context: A rehabilitation psychology perspective. Rehab Psychol 2005;50:6-14.
294. Fortuna D, Vizioli M, Contini A, et al: Assessing clinical performance in cardiac surgery: Does a specialized clinical database make a difference? Interact Cardiovasc Thorac Surg 2006;5:123-127.
295. Jones AF, Kent S: Small clinical cost studies can improve physician practice patterns. J Ambul Care Manage 1999;22:28-35.
296. Chen PP, Chen J, Gin T, et al: Out-patient chronic pain service in Hong Kong: Prospective study. Hong Kong Med J 2004;10:150-155.
297. Patel KK, Butler B, Wells KB: What is necessary to transform the quality of mental health care. Health Aff 2006;25:681-693.
298. Weinstein JN, Deyo RA: Clinical research; issues in data collection. Spine 2000;25:3104-3109.
299. Donabedian A. An Introduction to Quality Assurance in Health Care. Oxford, Oxford University Press, 2002, pp 45-58.
300. Rubin HR, Pronovost P, Diette GB: The advantages and disadvantages of process-based measures of health care quality. Intern J Qual Health Care 2001;13:469-474.
301. Lee KY, Hanold LS, Koss RG, et al: Statistical tools for quality improvement. In Ransom SB, Joshi MS, Nash DB (eds): The Health Care Quality Handbook. Chicago, Health Administration Press, 2005, pp 145-166.

302. Hummel PJ, Spellman Gamble TA: Reporting and analysis. In Norris TE, Fuller SS, Goldberg HI, et al. (eds): Informatics in Primary Care. New York, Springer-Verlag, 2002, pp 187-213.

303. Greenfield S, Apolone G, McNeil BJ, et al: The importance of co-existent disease in the occurrence of postoperative complications and one-year recovery in patients undergoing total hip replacement. Med Care 1993;31:141-154.

304. Silber JH, Rosenbaum PR: A spurious correlation between hospital mortality and complication rates: The importance of severity adjustment. Med Care 1997;35:OS77-OS92.

305. Iezzoni LI: The risks of risk adjustment. JAMA 1997;278: 1600-1607.

306. Iezzoni LI: Assessing quality using administrative data. Ann Int Med 1997;127:666-674.

307. Iezzoni LI: Ash AS, Shwartz M, et al: Predicting in-hospital deaths from coronary artery bypass graft surgery: Do different severity measures give different predictions? Med Care 1998;36:28-39.

308. Aronsky D, Haug PJ, Lagor C, et al: Accuracy of administrative data for identifying patients with pneumonia. Am J Med Qual 2005;20:319-328.

309. Daley J, Ash A, Iezzoni LI: Validity and reliability of risk adjusters. In Iezzoni LI (ed): Risk Adjustment for Measuring Health Care Outcomes, 3rd ed. Chicago, Health Administration Press, 2003, pp 207-230.

310. Jenkins KJ, Gauvreau K, Newburger JW, et al: Consensus-based method for risk-adjustment for surgery for congenital heart disease. J Thorac Cardio Surg 2002;123:110-118.

311. Iezzoni LI: Risk adjusting rehabilitation outcomes: An overview of methodologic issues. Am J Phys Med Rehabil 2004; 83:316-326.

312. Grotle M, Brox JI, Vollestad NK: Functional status and disability questionnaires: What do they assess? A systematic review of back-specific outcome questionnaires. Spine 2004;30:130-140.

313. Bombardier C: Spine focus issue introduction: Outcome assessments in the evaluation of treatment of spinal disorders. Spine 2000;24:3097-3099.

314. Resnik L, Dobrykowski E: Outcome measurement for patients with low back pain. Ortho Nurs 2005;24:14-24.

315. Farrar JT, Portenoy RK, Berlin JA, et al: Defining the clinically important difference in pain outcome measures. Pain 2000;88:287-294.

316. Keller S, Bann CM, Dodd SL, et al: Validity of the Brief Pain Inventory for use in documenting the outcomes of patients with noncancer pain. Clin J Pain 2004;20:309-318.

317. Davidson M, Keating JL, Eyres S: A low back-specific version of the SF-36 physical functioning scale. Spine 2004;29: 586-594.

318. Anagnostis C, Gatchel RJ, Mayer TG: The pain disability questionnaire. Spine 2004;29:2290-2302.

319. Ho MJ, LaFleur J: The treatment outcomes of pain survey (TOPS): A clinical monitoring and outcomes instrument for chronic pain practice and research. J Pain Palliat Care Pharmacother 2004;18:49-59.

320. Groll DL, To T, Bombardier C, et al: The development of a comorbidity index with physical function as the outcome. J Clin Epidemiol 2005;58:595-602.

321. Beaton DE, Schemitsch E: Measures of health-related quality of life and physical function. Clin Ortho Rel Res 2003;413: 90-105.

322. Deyo RA, Battie M, Beurskens AJHM, et al: Outcome measures for low back pain research: A proposal for standardized use. Spine 1998;23:2003-2013.

323. Von Korff M, Jensen MP, Karoly P: Assessing global pain severity by self-report in clinical and health services research. Spine 2000;24:3140-3151.

324. Hanscom B, Lurie JD, Homa K, et al: Computerized questionnaires and the quality of survey data. Spine 2002;27: 1797-1801.

325. Merrill DG: Benchmarking in the ambulatory surgery center. SAMBA annual meeting, May 2003.

326. Leatherman S, Berwick D, Iles D, et al: The business case for quality: Case studies and an analysis. Health Aff 2003;22: 17-30.

327. Merrill DG: Use of an outcomes database in a community pain clinic (abstract). Presented at the ASRAPM autumn meeting, 2005. Abstract ID A27. Available at www.asra.com.

328. Lee TH: A broader concept of medical errors. N Engl J Med 2002;347:1965-1967.

329. Leape LL, Brennan TA, Laird NM, et al: The nature of adverse events in hospitalized patients: Results from the Harvard Medical Practice Study II. N Engl J Med 1991;324:377-384.

330. Brennan TA: The Institute of Medicine report on medical errors—Could it do harm? N Engl J Med 2000;342: 1123-1125.

331. Leape LL, Epstein AM: A series on patient safety. N Engl J Med 2002;347:1272-1274.

332. Berwick DM, Calkins DR, McCannon CJ, et al: The 100 000 lives campaign: Setting a goal and a deadline for improving health care quality. JAMA 2006;295:324-327.

333. Zhan C, Kelley E, Yang HP: Assessing patient safety in the United States: Challenges and opportunities. Med Care 2005;43(3S):I42—I47.

334. Milstein A, Galvin RS, Delbanco SF, et al: Improving the safety of health care: The Leapfrog initiative. Eff Clin Pract 2000;6:313-316.

335. Halbach JL, Sullivan L: To err is human 5 years later (letter). JAMA 2005;294:1758-1759.

336. Kachalia A, Johnson JK, Miller S, et al: The incorporation of patient safety into board certification examinations. Acad Med 2006;81:317-325.

337. Klein CA: The patient safety and quality improvement act of 2005. Nurse Pract 2005;30:14.

338. Naveh E, Katz-Navon T, Stern Z: Readiness to report medical treatment errors: The effects of safety procedures, safety information, and priority of safety. Med Care 2006;44: 117-123.

339. Espin S, Levinson W, Regehr G, et al: Error or "act of God?" A study of patients' and operating room team members' perceptions of error definition, reporting and disclosure. Surgery 2006;139:6-14.

340. Leape LL: Reporting of adverse events. N Engl J Med 2002; 347:1633-1638.

341. Couig MP: Patient safety: A priority in the U.S. Department of Health and Human Services. Nurs Admin Q 2005;29:88-96.

342. Available at www.ihi.org.

343. Hackbarth AD, McCannon CJ, Martin L: The hard count: Calculating lives saved in the 100,000 lives campaign. ACP Guide for Hospitals, April 2006. Available at www.ihi.org/NR/rdonlyres/AA1B05AD-5DFF-45D6-8A2F-05C69C9C2860/0/ihiarticle.pdf.

344. Leape LL, Berwick DM, Bates DW: What practices will most improve safety? JAMA 2002;288:501-507.

345. Hinckley CM: Make no mistake—Errors can be controlled. Qual Saf Health Care 2003;12:359-365.

346. Webster CS: The nuclear power industry as an alternative analogy for safety in anaesthesia and a novel approach for the conceptualization of safety goals. Anaesthesia 2005;60: 1115-1122.

347. Gaba DM, Singer SJ, Sinaiko AD, et al: Differences in safety climate between hospital personnel and naval aviators. Human Factors 2003;45:173-185.

348. Gaba DM: Improving patient safety by implementing strategies of high reliability organization theory. Euroanesthesia 2005;17RC3:243-246. Available at www.euroanesthesia.org/education/rc2005vienna/17RC3.pdf.

349. Johnstone PAS: Sailorproofing quality (editorial). Q Manage Health Care 2004;13:96-98.

350. Keyes GR, Singer R, Iverson RE, et al: Analysis of outpatient surgery center safety using an Internet-based quality improvement and peer review program. Plast Reconstr Surg 2004;113:1760-1770.

351. Altman DE, Clancy C, Blendon RJ: Improving patient safety five years after the IOM report. N Engl J Med 2004;351: 2041-2043.

352. Plews-Ogan ML, Nadkarni MM, Forren S, et al: Patient safety in the ambulatory setting: A clinician-based approach. J Gen Int Med 2004;19:719-725.

353. Gandhi TK, Weingart SN, Borus J, et al: Adverse drug events in ambulatory care. N Engl J Med 2003;348:1556-1564.

354. McPhillips HA, Stille CJ, Smith D, et al: Potential medication dosing errors in outpatient pediatrics. J Pediatr 2005;147: 761-767.

355. Taylor LK, Kawasumi Y, Bartlett G, et al: Inappropriate prescribing practices: The challenge and opportunity for patient safety. Health Care Q 2005;8:81-85.

356. Villa H, Smith RA, Augustyniak MJ: The efficacy and safety of pain management before and after implementation of hospital-wide pain management standards: Is patient safety compromised by treatment based solely on numerical pain ratings? Anesth Analg 2005;101:474-480.

357. Han YY, Carcillo JA, Shekhar TV, et al: Unexpected increased mortality after implementation of a commercially sold computerized physician order entry system. Pediatrics 2005;116: 1506-1512.

358. Vigoda MM, Lubarsky DA: Failure to recognize loss of incoming data in an anesthesia record-keeping system may have increased medical liability. Anesth Analg 2006;102:1798-1802.

359. Sidorov J: It ain't necessarily so: The electronic health record and the unlikely prospect of reducing health care costs. Health Aff 2006;25:1079-1085.

360. Weir VL: Preventing adverse drug events. Nurs Manage 2005;36:24-30.

361. Jensen LS, Merry AF, Webster CS, et al: Evidence-based strategies for preventing drug administration errors during anaesthesia. Anaesthesia 2004;59:493-504.

362. Institute for Health Care Improvement: Getting started kit: Prevent adverse drug events (medication reconciliation) how-to guide. Available at www.ihi.org.

363. Trontell A: Expecting the unexpected—Drug safety, pharmacovigilance, and the prepared mind. N Engl J Med 2004;351: 1385-1387.

364. Burke JP: Infection control—A problem for patient safety. N Engl J Med 2003;348:651-655.

365. Coffin SE, Zaoutis TE: Infection control, hospital epidemiology, and patient safety. Infect Dis Clin N Am 2005;19: 647-665.

366. Gaba DM, Howard SK: Fatigue among clinicians and the safety of patients. N Engl J Med 2002;347:1249-1255.

367. Patel VL, Currie LM: Clinical cognition and biomedical informatics: Issues of patient safety. Int J Med Inform 2005; 74:869-885.

368. Oklahoma Nurses Association 2005 House of Delegates: Implications of fatigue on patient safety. Oklahoma Nurse 2005;50:7-8.

369. Bates DW, Gawande AA: Improving safety with information technology. N Engl J Med 2003;348:2526-2534.

370. Available at www.jointcommission.org/PatientSafety/ NationalPatientSafetyGoals/.

371. Wright AA, Katz IT: Bar coding and patient safety. N Engl J Med. 2005;353:329-331.

372. Rao AC, Burke DA, Dighe AS: Implementation of bar coded wristbands in a large academic medical center: Impact on point of care error rates. Point of Care 2005;4:119-122.

373. Quinn MM, Mannion J: Improving patient safety using interactive, evidence-based decision support tools. J Qual Patient Safety 2005;31:678-683.

374. Schmidek JM, Weeks WB: What do we know about financial returns on investments in patient safety? J Qual Patient Safety 2005;31:690-699.

375. McNeil B: Shattuck lecture—Hidden barriers to improvement in the quality of care. N Engl J Med 2001;345:1612-1620.

376. Bridenbaugh PO: Office-based anesthesia: Requirements for patient safety. Anesth Prog 2005;52:86-90.

377. Wertenberger S: The development of a patient safety program across the continuum of care. Nurs Admin Q 2005;29: 303-307.

378. Brown LH: Senior drivers: risks, interventions, and safety. Nurs Pract 2006;31:38-49.

379. Vainio A, Ollila J, Matikainen E: Driving ability in cancer patients receiving long-term morphine analgesia. Lancet 1995;346:667-670.

380. Galski T, Williams JB, Ehle HT, et al: Effects of opioids on driving ability. J Pain Symptom Manage 2000;19:200-208.

381. Lotfipour S, Conley B, Vaca F: Consequences of older adult motor vehicle collisions. Top Emerg Med 2006;28:39-47.

382. Lagarde E, Chastang JF, Lafont S, et al: Pain and pain treatment were associated with traffic accident involvement in a cohort of middle-aged workers. J Clin Epidemiol 2005;58: 524-531.

383. Veldhuijzen DS, van Wijck AJM, Wille F, et al: Effect of chronic nonmalignant pain on highway driving performance. Pain 2006;122:28-35.

384. Gaba DM: What to do after an adverse event. APSF Newsletter 2006;21:4.

385. Eichhorn EH: Patient perspectives personalize patient safety. APSF Newsletter 2005;20:61-66.

386. Available at www.ihi.org/IHI/Topics/PatientSafety/Safety General/Literature/WhenThingsGoWrongRespondingTo AdverseEvents.htm.

387. Mohr JJ, Batalden PB: Improving safety on the front lines: The role of clinical microsystems. Qual Saf Health Care 2002;11:45-50.

388. Vincent C: Understanding and responding to adverse events. N Engl J Med 2003;348:1051-1056.

389. Hare RM: Essays on bioethics. Oxford, Oxford Press, 2002, p 218.

390. Kennedy P, Pronovost P: Shepherding change: How the market, health care providers, and public policy can deliver quality care for the 21st century. Crit Care Med 2006;34: S1-S6.

391. Korthals-de Bos I, van Tulder M, van Dieten H, et al: Economic evaluations and randomized trials in spinal disorders: Principles and methods. Spine 2004;29:442-448.

392. Iezzoni LI: Data from surveys or asking patients. In Iezzoni LI (ed): Risk Adjustment for Measuring Health Care Outcomes, 3rd ed. Chicago, Health Administration Press, 2003, pp 163-177.

393. Pengel LHM, Refshauge KM, Maher CG: Responsiveness of pain, disability, and physical impairment outcomes in patients with low back pain. Spine 2004;29:879-883.

394. Wade DT: Outcome measures for clinical trials. Am J Phys Med Rehabil 2003;82(Suppl):S26-S31.

395. Sloan JA, Loprinzi CL, Kuross SA, et al: Randomized comparison of four tools measuring overall quality of life in patients with advanced cancer. J Clin Oncol 1998;16:3662-3673.

396. Burckhardt CS, Clark CR, Bennett RM: The Fibromyalgia Impact Questionnaire: Development and validation. J Rheumatol 1991;18:728-733.

397. Roland M, Morris R: A study of the natural history of back pain. Part I: Development of a reliable and sensitive measure of disability in low-back pain. Spine 1983;8:141-144.

398. Westaway MD, Stratford PW, Binkley JM: The patient-specific functional scale: Validation of its use in persons with neck dysfunction. J Orthop Sports Phys Ther 1998;27:331-338.

399. The Picker patient experience questionnaire: Development and validation using data from in-patient surveys in five countries. Int J Qual Health Care 2002;14:353-358.

400. Brooks R: EuroQol: The current state of play. Health Pol 1996;37:53-72.

401. Bergner M: Health status measures: An overview and guide for selection. Ann Rev Public Health 1987;8:191-210.

402. Jenkinson C, Fitzpatrick R, Argyle M: The Nottingham health profile: An analysis of its sensitivity in differing illness groups. Soc Sci Med 1988;27:1411-1414.

403. Von Korff M, Ormel J, Keefe FJ: Grading the severity of chronic pain. Pain 1992;50:133-149.

404. Benzon HT: The neuropathic pain scales. Reg Anesth Pain Med 2005;30:417-421.

405. Krause SJ, Backonja MM: Development of a neuropathic pain questionnaire. Clin J Pain 2003;19:306-314.

406. Coyle N, Goldstein ML, Passik S, et al: Development and validation of a patient needs assessment tool (PNAT) for oncology clinicians. Cancer Nursing 1996;19:81-92.

6 Education, Training, and Certification in Pain Medicine

James P. Rathmell and David L. Brown

THE EVOLUTION OF PAIN MEDICINE AS A SUBSPECIALTY

As knowledge expands and the need for detailed skills arises, specialization ensues. This is a natural progression. It has become impossible for any physician to become an expert in every field. There has long been a discomfort with specialization despite an unflagging progression in that direction. The urge to both specialize and remain unspecialized dates back to the earliest recorded history in medicine. The first specializations were between the barber-surgeons and the internists, and a rivalry of sorts remains to this day. Writing about Ambrose Paré, the 16th century physician who elevated the role of the barber-surgeons to that of other physicians, the present-day surgeon and historian Sherwin Nuland reflects on the ongoing distinction between internist and surgeon[1]:

> Surgery is an exercise in the use of the intellect. Heckling internists, with tongues barely in check, would prefer that surgical specialists be viewed merely as dexterous craftsman who carry out the routing errands assigned to them by their more cerebrally endowed medical overseers. I attribute this teasing raillery to a kind of good-natured fraternal envy, not so much of our celebrity status, but rather of the visibility of the cures we surgeons achieve and the particular personal gratification we have while doing it.

In the United States, anesthesiology has progressed toward further specialization, first with the establishment of critical care, then pain management (now pain medicine), and more recently pediatric anesthesiology and cardiothoracic anesthesiology. The addition of pain medicine as a subspecialty of anesthesiology is just one recent example of the growth of medical specialties. With specialization comes a conscious effort to focus practice to become intricately familiar with a more limited realm. The obvious result is a loss of the skills and knowledge needed to practice in the broader parent specialty. In pain medicine, many now view this as a full time vocation. The scientific meetings and journals that keep pain medicine specialists up-to-date have little overlap with those that are designed to serve anesthesiologists practicing in the operating room. The only common thread between the technical skills needed in the pain clinic and those required for anesthesiology in the operating rooms is expertise with neural blockade. The pain medicine practitioner must acquire a vastly different skill set than those practicing anesthesiology, including expanding their skills as diagnosticians.

Much has been written about the origins of pain medicine as a distinct discipline and anesthesiologists have played a primary role since the start.[2] It really started with the introduction of effective general anesthetics in the mid-19th century, when surgical pain could be separated from operation. Almost 100 years later, the late John Bonica, an anesthesiologist and recognized father of the specialty we now call pain medicine, developed his career promoting multidisciplinary pain care and formal training of specialists. From his life's work we now have extensive ongoing efforts to recognize and treat pain effectively, to train subspecialists, and to conduct basic and clinical research to further our understanding of pain and its treatment. The International Association for the Study of Pain (IASP) founded in 1974, its U.S. chapter, the American Pain Society (APS), and the journal *Pain* are legacies left by Dr. Bonica for our patients.

Accredited fellowship training in pain medicine is a relatively recent development. Before 1992, training was frequently obtained in academic anesthesiology departments, including those of Bonica, Bridenbaugh, Carron, Haugen, Moore, Raj, Winnie, and others, and subsequently in programs run by their trainees. These unaccredited programs advanced the specialty, widened interest in pain medicine as a career, and propagated pain care in smaller and smaller communities across the country. Outside of the United States, this type of informal training remains the rule for those seeking expertise in pain medicine. In the United States, the American Board of Anesthesiology (ABA) developed interest in certifying pain medicine training. Through the leadership of Dr. William Owens in his roles on both the ABA and the Residency Review Committee (RRC), and through his representations of the subspecialty to the American Board of Medical Specialties (ABMS), formal training programs were accredited and physicians were certified. Drs. Stephen Abram and John Rowlingson were both key members of the group that assisted Dr. Owens in moving the new subspecialty forward.

The first programs recognized by the Accreditation Council for Graduate Medical Education (ACGME) were accredited in 1992. The number of ACGME-accredited programs and the number of trainees in accredited programs has grown steadily over the past decade, reaching just over 100 training programs that turn out about 300 new pain specialists each year. The ABA working in parallel with the ACGME developed a subspecialty certification examination in pain medicine, first named the "Certificate of Added Qualifications in Pain Management" and now titled "Subspecialty Certification in Pain Medicine." The first

examination was given in 1993. The number of candidates sitting for the examination has steadily grown since the first examination was given.

Dr. Bonica's original push to develop multidisciplinary pain care recently evolved into collaboration between four specialties agreeing to a single and unified set of program requirements for all ACGME-accredited pain fellowships, regardless of sponsoring specialty. The RRCs for anesthesiology, neurology, physical medicine, and rehabilitation and psychiatry agreed on these requirements in late 2005 and the ACGME Board approved their implementation for 2007 (Box 6–1).[3] These requirements will standardize pain fellowship training and hopefully produce a more comprehensive and multidisciplinary focused physician. There are other groups that are also encouraging a more comprehensive approach to pain care, with the linked American Academy of Pain Medicine and the American Board of Pain Medicine devoting energy to a multidisciplinary approach. There remain a number of experienced pain specialists who believe that eventually the ACGME-accredited fellowships will be extended to 2 years in order to cover an expanding knowledge base. Equally important in the evolution of the discipline is the creation of academic physicians within the fellowships who undertake research programs to add

---

BOX 6–1. ACGME-RECOMMENDED CURRICULUM FOR PAIN MEDICINE

I. Didactic Curriculum
 A. Assessment of pain
  1. Anatomy, physiology, and pharmacology of pain transmission and modulation
  2. General principles of pain evaluation and management including neurologic examination, musculoskeletal examination, psychological assessment
  3. Diagnostic studies: x-ray study, magnetic resonance imaging (MRI), computed tomography (CT), and clinical nerve function studies
  4. Pain measurement in humans: experimental and clinical
  5. Psychosocial aspects of pain, including cultural and cross-cultural considerations
  6. Taxonomy of pain syndromes
  7. Pain of spinal origin including radicular pain, zygapophysial joint disease, discogenic pain
  8. Myofascial pain
  9. Neuropathic pain
  10. Headache and orofacial pain
  11. Rheumatologic aspects of pain
  12. Complex regional pain syndromes
  13. Visceral pain
  14. Urogenital pain
  15. Cancer pain, including palliative and hospice care
  16. Acute pain
  17. Assessment of pain in special populations: patients with ongoing substance abuse, older adults, pediatric patients, pregnant women, the physically disabled, and the cognitively impaired
  18. Functional and disability assessment
 B. Treatment of pain
  1. Drug treatment I: opioids
  2. Drug treatment II: antipyretic analgesics
  3. Drug treatment III: antidepressants, anticonvulsants, and miscellaneous drugs
  4. Psychological and psychiatric approaches to treatment, including cognitive-behavioral therapy and treatment of psychiatric illness
  5. Prescription drug detoxification concepts
  6. Functional and vocational rehabilitation
  7. Surgical approaches
  8. Complementary and alternative treatments in pain management
  9. Hospice and palliative care
  10. Treatment of pain in pediatric patients
 C. General topics
  1. Epidemiology of pain
  2. Gender issues in pain
  3. Placebo response
  4. Multidisciplinary pain medicine

BOX 6–1. ACGME-RECOMMENDED CURRICULUM FOR PAIN MEDICINE—cont'd

5. Organization and management of a pain center
6. Continuing quality improvement, utilization review, and program evaluation
7. Patient and provider safety
8. Designing, reporting, and interpreting clinical trials of treatment for pain
9. Ethical standards in pain management and research
10. Animal mode of pain, ethics of animal expectation

D. Interventional pain treatment
1. Airway management skills
2. Sedation/analgesia
3. Fluoroscopic imaging and radiation safety
4. Pharmacology of local anesthetics and other injectable medications, including radiographic contrast agents and steroid preparations (This must include treatment of local anesthetic systemic toxicity.)
5. Trigger point injections
6. Peripheral and cranial nerve blocks and ablation
7. Spinal injections including epidural injections: interlaminar, transforaminal, nerve root sheath injections, and zygapophysial joint injections
8. Discography and intradiskal/percutaneous disk treatments
9. Joint and bursal injections, including sacroiliac, hip, knee, and shoulder joint injections
10. Sympathetic ganglion blocks
11. Epidural and intrathecal medication management
12. Spinal cord stimulation
13. Intrathecal drug administration systems

II. Clinical Curriculum
A. The elements of pain medicine training from disciplines relevant to pain medicine:
1. Anesthesiology: the fellow will demonstrate competency in:
   a. Obtaining intravenous access in a minimum of 15 patients
   b. Basic airway management, including a minimum of mask ventilation in 15 patients and endotracheal intubation in 15 patients
   c. Provider course in basic life support and advanced cardiac life support
   d. Management of sedation, including direct administration of sedation to a minimum of 15 patients
   e. Administration of neuraxial analgesia, including placement of a minimum of 15 thoracic or lumbar epidural injections using an interlaminar technique
2. Neurology: minimum of 5 observed patient examinations, 15 CT and/or MRI studies
3. Physical medicine and rehabilitation: hands-on experience in the musculoskeletal and neuromuscular assessment of 15 patients and demonstrated proficiency in the clinical examination and rehabilitation plan development of a minimum of 5 patients
4. Psychiatry: conduct a complete mental status examination on a minimum of 15 patients and demonstrate this ability in 5 patients to a faculty observer

B. Core Clinical Curriculum
1. Outpatient (continuity clinic) pain experience: primary responsibility for 50 different patients followed up over at least 2 months
2. Inpatient chronic pain experience: minimum of 15 new patients
3. Acute pain inpatient experience: management of patients with acute pain, minimum of 50 new patients
4. Interventional experience: minimum of 25 patients who undergo interventional procedures
5. Cancer pain: longitudinal involvement with a minimum of 20 patients
6. Palliative care experience: longitudinal involvement with a minimum of 10 patients
7. Pediatric experience: strongly encouraged
8. Advanced education in interventional pain medicine:
   a. Image-guided spinal injection techniques, cervical spine: 15 procedures
   b. Image-guided spinal injection techniques, lumbar spine: 25 procedures
   c. Injection of motor joint or bursa: 10 procedures
   d. Trigger point injection: 20 procedures
   e. Sympathetic blockade: 10 procedures
   f. Neurolytic techniques including chemical and radiofrequency treatment for pain: 5 procedures
   g. Intradiskal procedures, including discography: 10 procedures
   h. Placement of permanent spinal drug delivery system: 3 procedures

From ACGME Recommended Curriculum for Pain Medicine Accreditation Council for Graduate Medical Education. Available at www.acgme.org.

new knowledge to this very needed practice of medicine.

As outlined, pain and its consequences draw on resources from all medical disciplines. Dr. Bonica's experiences during World War II suggested that each medical specialist had unique expertise to bring to patients suffering in pain; hence his consistent and effective promotion of a multidisciplinary process for pain care. Also thanks largely to Dr. Bonica, anesthesiology has led the development of formal training programs. Indeed the majority of currently accredited programs reside within academic anesthesiology departments and most program directors are anesthesiologists. Specialists from other disciplines have also focused their clinical and research efforts on pain. The most obvious example is neurology where the majority of clinical treatment and research about headache has arisen. Physical medicine and rehabilitation (PM&R) has also had a focus and expertise in functional restoration, and physiatrists lead many chronic pain rehabilitation programs. And, of course, psychiatrists have been closely involved where pain, depression, and substance abuse overlap. During the last decade, specialists from these other disciplines have been seeking subspecialty training in pain medicine with increasing regularity.

The range of practitioners declaring themselves as pain medicine specialists is extraordinary, from clinics that provide largely or solely cognitive-behavioral approaches to chronic pain through functional restoration programs all the way to the type of clinic that offers nothing more than injections of various sorts. "Interventional pain medicine" is a phrase that has been coined for those techniques that involve minimally invasive treatments and minor surgery as part of their application, including neural blockade and implantable analgesic devices. Despite the paucity of scientific evidence to guide pain practitioners, particularly evidence to support the use of many interventional modalities, many techniques appear to have efficacy based on limited observational data and have been adopted into widespread use. As practitioners, we are left to choose among available treatment modalities, often with only anecdotal and personal experience to guide us in treating a group of desperate patients with intractable pain who are willing to accept almost any treatment, even that which remains unproven. There is no single practice pattern that any pain specialist can point to as the correct way to treat patients with chronic pain. Training programs vary widely in the scope of what they train practitioners to do. The best pain medicine practitioners strike a reasonable balance between interventional and noninterventional management. This practice pattern is sustainable and those adopting a balanced style of practice will be able to adapt to evolving scientific evidence that appears in support of pain treatment, regardless of the type of treatment. A balance between treatment modalities also allows practitioners to switch from one mode to another or incorporate multiple treatment approaches simultaneously. Use

of these interventional modalities is just a small part of the armamentarium of the skilled pain practitioner.

TRAINING AND CREDENTIALING IN INTERVENTIONAL PAIN MEDICINE

In our rapidly changing world of modern health care, new technologies are appearing at a dizzying rate. Many of these new treatments require physicians to acquire detailed new knowledge and technical skills. The introduction of new techniques typically extends from centers in the public or private sector, where the ideas are conceived and tested in a limited realm among innovators. From there, anecdote can often take over, and many techniques in pain medicine have blossomed into widespread use with nothing more than word-of-mouth to propagate their use. The use of pulsed radiofrequency treatment for pain is one such example where clinical application has preceded detailed clinical testing.[4]

In the United States and Europe, industry often leads innovation by testing and leading the introduction of new devices. When the innovation appears to have merit in limited trials, many devices have been introduced to the market with approval through the Food and Drug Administration's 510K "substantially similar device" process with little or no data regarding efficacy. Once on the market, the means by which practitioners decide to adopt new technologies, the speed of progression of these new techniques, and—of great importance—the means by which practitioners gain enough expertise to introduce new techniques into their own practices, are all highly variable and seemingly without any rational or consistent approach.

Interventional pain medicine is evolving as a distinct discipline that requires detailed new knowledge and expertise. Familiarity with radiographic anatomy for the conduct of image-guided injection and the minor surgical skills needed to place implanted devices such as spinal cord stimulators and implanted drug delivery systems are just a few of the techniques that practitioners must master. As we set out to introduce new interventional techniques to our own pain practices, we must be sure that we have been properly trained to conduct these techniques to assure safety and success.

Adequate exposure to these newer treatment alternatives during the fellowship training period is necessary to assure appropriate application and optimize patient outcomes. Although we do not have scientific data that define the average minimum level of experience that will be necessary to achieve competence, especially for complex procedures that are associated with significant risks, logic dictates that there is a minimum number of these procedures that trainees should be exposed to during a fellowship. The ACGME has established requirements for average minimal numbers of epidural, spinal, and peripheral nerve blocks necessary for accreditation of anesthesiology residency programs. Other medical subspecialties also require a minimum number of specified procedures to achieve and maintain competence: subspecialty training in gastroenterology has a requirement of performing a minimum of 100 esophagogastroduodenoscopies and 100 colonoscopies with polyp removal[5] during formal training and subspecialty training in cardiovascular disease requires 100 cardiac catheterizations to demonstrate minimum proficiency.[6] Indeed the ACGME's RRC for anesthesiology has accepted revised Program Requirements for Pain Medicine Training Programs that specify minimum exposure of trainees for various techniques, including image-guided spinal injection techniques, cervical and lumbar spine; sympathetic blockade; neurolytic block, including radiofrequency treatment for pain; intradiskal procedures, including discography; spinal cord stimulation; and placement of permanent spinal drug delivery system (see Box 6–1). For those techniques that are now widely accepted as a core part of pain practice, we must assure that our trainees gain enough experience to conduct these procedures independently. One key element of the ACGME deliberations about unified pain training is to acknowledge that not all pain fellows will have experience in the wide variety of interventional techniques. Rather, it is hoped that these fellows will gain an understanding of all available options for patients with pain, and yet demonstrate and have competence documented in only those techniques for which formal training is made available during fellowship training.

It is difficult to define the techniques that are core for a pain practitioner, but it does seem that detailed knowledge of radiographic anatomy of the spine and the minor surgical skills required to implant spinal cord stimulators and place permanent spinal drug delivery systems are among those skills most practicing pain physicians would expect a new graduate from a pain fellowship to have. New techniques are appearing at a staggering rate, and we cannot rely on pain fellowship programs to provide all of the technical training that is needed. Stronger standards for minimal training following fellowship are also urgently needed. Some pain practitioners believe that all too many of their colleagues find it perfectly acceptable to attend a brief weekend course and then introduce a highly technical new treatment into practice without additional study, training, or oversight.[7] Intradiskal electrothermal therapy (IDET), nucleoplasty, and radiofrequency treatment are among the many techniques that are showing promise and each requires a set of unique knowledge and skills to be used safely and effectively. Practitioners themselves must take the lead in obtaining adequate training *before* proceeding with any new and unfamiliar technique. The weekend workshop is just a start, often a good start—the best workshops will give practitioners a detailed understanding of anatomy, pathophysiology of disease related to the use of the new technique, patient selection, conduct of the procedure, outcomes, and avoidance, management, and recognition of complications. Box 6–2 is

---

BOX 6–2. SUGGESTED TRAINING AND EXPERIENCE WHEN INTRODUCING A NEW TECHNIQUE INTO CLINICAL PRACTICE

1. *Study the new technique*, the published literature, and gain a detailed knowledge of all aspects of the technique.
2. *Attend a workshop*, preferably a hands-on cadaver-based workshop that allows introduction to the technique in as realistic a setting that can be assembled.
3. *Plan* adequate time for your initial procedures.
4. *Get help* at the bedside during initial conduct of new procedures—perhaps another experienced practitioner at your institution, an invited expert to assist, or team up with a colleague in a related discipline.
5. *Inform your patients* that you are introducing a new technique and include this discussion as part of the informed consent process.
6. *Examine your outcomes* carefully in the initial stages of using any new technique and compare them with those of your colleagues and the published literature.

From Lubenow TR, Rathmell JP: Let's take a rational approach to technical training in pain medicine. Am Soc Anesth Newsl 2005;69:6-8, with permission.

---

a suggested method for practitioners introducing a new technique into clinical practice.[8]

FUTURE DIRECTIONS

The field of evidence-based medicine has emerged as a new paradigm to guide practicing physicians. This field endeavors to educate practitioners about how to frame specific questions based on the clinical problems they are faced with every day. They then venture to the published scientific literature with focused questions about prevention, treatment, and diagnosis of a specific clinical condition. Many evidence-based medicine centers offer concise and periodically updated summaries about specific clinical conditions. The idea is to get the best information available to the practicing clinician. It describes the best available evidence and if there is no good evidence it says so. In pain medicine, we are faced with an expanding array of treatment options that strike us as logical developments that *should* provide pain relief for our patients. However, there is a dearth of clinical evidence to guide rational choice and application of the majority of these emerging treatments. So how are we to decide when to apply them?

Merrill[9] recently presented a detailed analysis of the current state of evidence guiding the use of interventional treatments in the field of pain medicine. He points out the frequent flaws in existing studies (largely the lack of valid comparators, such as no treatment) and concludes that "the practice of invasive pain medicine teeters at a particularly critical juncture . . . crippled by a lack of vigorous self-evaluation of its role in the treatment of chronic pain." Merrill goes on to detail the means by which we, as scientists and clinicians, can proceed to build a better body of evidence for the treatments we are using. But the field of pain medicine is young and early in development, and it is perhaps unreasonable to expect an accumulation of randomized clinical trials just yet.

New treatments evolve slowly in clinical medicine. Applying the scientific method in clinical medicine begins with an observation. Perhaps a chance observation that a certain drug typically used for another purpose provides analgesia to a given patient. If the drug is readily available, a clinician may choose to try treatment on other patients with similar presentations. If an academic sort, the clinician may choose to report the limited success in a case series. Case series are a valuable beginning, the very beginning of emerging new ideas. If the problem is uniform and prevalent enough, the new treatment may gain the attention of investigators willing to assemble a randomized clinical trial. All too often, sound treatments are never tested for lack of interest or funding. Those that are tested tend to be those under patent where a manufacturer proceeds with these large endeavors understandably in hope of financial return in the event the treatment proves useful. Patients who are suffering from severe and intractable pain are desperate and they can easily be convinced that desperate measures, however new or unproven, are warranted.

How then are we to proceed? Our patients are begging for us to try anything that offers a glimmer of hope in reducing their pain, and we as scientists embrace the rigor of the scientific method and want desperately to do what is best for our patients. We have treatment after treatment that makes logical sense and shows early promise in case series and observational studies, but little data that support an evidence-based approach to practice. Using acute low back pain with sciatica as an example, a number of evidence-based reports have emerged to guide clinicians.[10] The only modalities that are rated as "beneficial" or "likely to be beneficial" are advice for the patient to stay active, nonsteroidal anti-inflammatories, behavioral therapy, and multidisciplinary treatment programs. Use of opioid analgesics, acupuncture, back schools, epidural steroid injections, and spinal manipulation were all judged to be of "unknown effectiveness." Yet, in actual clinical practice in the United States, a short course of opioid analgesic and early intervention with epidural steroid injections is common. To complicate matters, the use of fluoroscopic guidance and directing injections to the affected level using an interlaminar or transforaminal approach is gaining widespread acceptance, with only uncontrolled case series to guide us as clinicians. To complicate treatment options, those with persistent pain and contained disk herniations now have a dizzying array of treatment options including laser diskectomy, thermal disk decompression, and vacuum disk extraction, all using Food and Drug Administration–approved devices with only uncontrolled observational studies that suggest effectiveness.[11] The new devices are intellectually appealing as they are minimally invasive, yet only open surgical diskectomy has proven superior to conservative management in patients with persistent sciatica due to intervertebral disk prolapse.[12]

The evidence-based medicine movement gives little guidance to practitioners whose tools are still under development. They simply remind us that no evidence regarding many of our techniques exists. Without declaring a moratorium on all interventional pain techniques, Merrill[9] offers the individual practitioner advice: monitor your own outcomes using valid measures, be more reflective and systematic in studying your own outcomes and patterns of care, and provide this information to your patients as part of the decision-making process. As pain practitioners we have an expanding range of treatment options available to us, few with convincing evidence of efficacy superior to alternate treatments. We must evaluate each patient and use the limited evidence available to us today to guide compassionate and rational, if not evidence-based, use of therapy for our desperate patients.

References

1. Nuland SB: The gentle surgeon: Ambrose Paré. In Nuland SB (ed): Doctors: The Biography of Medicine. New York, Knopf, 1988, p 94.
2. Rathmell JP, Brown DL: The evolution of training in pain medicine in the United States. American Society of Anesthesiologists Newsletter, November 2002.
3. Program Requirements for Fellowship Education in Pain Medicine. Available at http//www.acgme.org/acWebsite/downloads/RRC_progReq/sh_multiPainPR707_TCC.pdf.
4. Richebe P, Rathmell JP, Brennan TJ: Immediate early genes after pulsed radiofrequency treatment: Neurobiology in need of clinical trials. Anesthesiology 2005;102:1-3.
5. Program Requirements for Residency Education in Gastroenterology. Available at http://www.acgme.org/acWebsite/downloads/RRC_progReq/144pr799.pdf.
6. Program Requirements for Residency Education in Cardiovascular Disease. Available at http://www.acgme.org/acWebsite/downloads/RRC_progReq/141pr799.pdf.
7. Rathmell JP: The injectionists. Reg Anesth Pain Med 2004;29:305-306.
8. Lubenow TR, Rathmell JP: Let's take a rational approach to technical training in pain medicine. Am Soc Anesth Newsl 2005;69:6-8.
9. Merrill DG: Hoffman's glasses: Evidence-based medicine and the search for quality in the literature of interventional pain medicine. Reg Anesth Pain Med 2003;28:547-560.
10. van Tulder M, Koes B: Low back pain and sciatica: Acute. In Clinical Evidence: Concise 8. London, BMJ Publishing Group, 2002, pp 226-228.
11. Maroon JC: Current concepts in minimally invasive discectomy. Neurosurgery 2002;51(Suppl 2):137-145.
12. Gibson JNA, Grant IC, Wadell G: The Cochrane review of surgery for disc prolapse and degenerative lumbar spondylosis. Spine 1999;24:1820-1832.

PART

II

Basic Considerations

D. Turk and C. Argoff

7 Pain Pathways: Peripheral, Spinal, Ascending, and Descending Pathways

Karin N. Westlund High

The neural circuits that are responsible for pain and the reactions to pain[1] can be termed the *pain system*[2-4] or perhaps more appropriately, the *pain systems*. The pain systems include (1) peripheral neurons with a set of peripheral receptive elements, the nociceptors, (2) numerous central neuronal relay pathways, and (3) sets of integrative neurons that impose excitatory or inhibitory influences on nociceptive information at numerous levels of the neuraxis.

The initial reception of inputs perceived to be painful occurs on the peripheral terminations of the nociceptors transducing noxious mechanical, temperature, and chemical stimuli. Nociceptors transmit the information about noxious events to second-order neurons located in the appropriate spinal cord or brainstem level, that is, lumbar spinal cord for leg input, thoracic spinal cord for stomach lining input, and trigeminal spinal nucleus for face input. Nociceptive signals are then transmitted by projection neurons of the pain system to integration sites in the brainstem, with collateral input to other spinal cord levels. The primary integration site for sensory information is the thalamus. Further processing of the nociceptive information also occurs in numerous brain structures by integrative neuronal circuits activating excitatory and inhibitory mechanisms.

The central relay pathways alert spinal cord, brainstem, and higher brain integrative sites to internal or external stimuli which are distressing or damaging. A variety of coordinated pain reactions are generated, including protective somatic and autonomic reflexes, endocrine actions, emotional responses, learning and memory about the event, and cortical awareness of pain. In addition to pain and pain reactions, the brain centers that receive nociceptive information also provide either negative or positive feedback that reduces or accentuates pain and pain reactions. Negative feedback to the spinal cord circuitry is mediated by descending pathways that are often called the "endogenous analgesia system." The mechanism and pathways responsible for accentuation of pain and pain reactions, referred to as *central sensitization*, can involve increased responsivity at all levels of the pain system, including the peripheral nociceptors, the spinal cord, brainstem, and higher centers. The net effect of the positive and negative circuitry alterations leads to the perceptual experience "pain."

NOCICEPTORS

Peripheral Receptive Elements

The initial reception of noxious inputs perceived to be painful is by the specialized endings of primary afferent neurons known as *nociceptors*. Reception of noxious input occurs in functionally specialized free nerve endings of the skin, muscle, joints, viscera, and dura (Fig. 7–1). Nociceptor subtypes respond best to either mechanical (mechanical nociceptors), mechanical and thermal (mechanothermal nociceptors), or mechanical, thermal, and chemical stimuli (polymodal nociceptors).[5,6] Common types of cutaneous nociceptors are A-delta mechanoreceptors and C polymodal nociceptors that relay the transduced information about potentially harmful input via A-delta and C-fibers, respectively.[7,8] Nociceptive endings are also located in muscle,[9] the fascia and adventitia of blood vessels,[10] the knee joint,[11,12] the dura,[13] and viscera.[14,15] Glutamate receptors, as well as μ and δ-opiate, substance P, somatostatin, and vanilloid receptors, have been identified immunohistochemically on the peripheral endings of cutaneous nerve fibers.[16-20]

The axons that relay information about noxious input from the skin and other tissues to the central nervous system (CNS) fall characteristically into the

Pain Systems

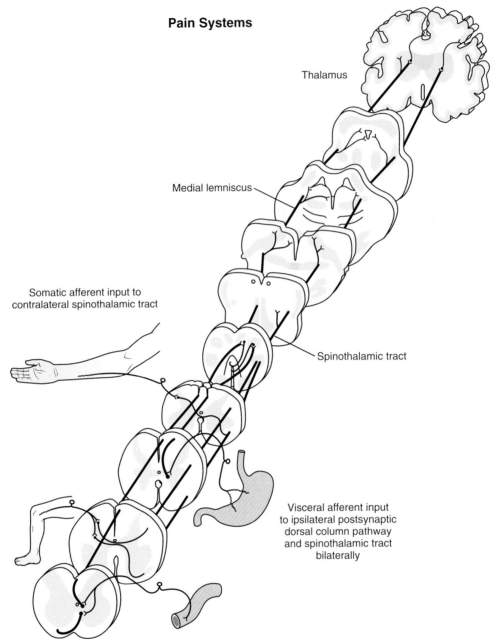

Thalamus

Medial lemniscus

Somatic afferent input to
contralateral spinothalamic tract

Spinothalamic tract

Visceral afferent input
to ipsilateral postsynaptic
dorsal column pathway
and spinothalamic tract
bilaterally

Figure 7–1. The pain systems convey input from somatic structures, as well as from viscera and other deep tissues via peripheral nerves. Afferent nerve fibers carrying nociceptive information have free nerve endings in the peripheral tissue and terminate in the spinal cord dorsal horn. Information about pain is relayed through at least one synapse to cells in the spinal cord dorsal horn. Two parallel ascending pathways provide the information to integration centers in the thalamus that provide the information to cortical regions. Input primarily from somatic structures is relayed to spinothalamic tract cells whose axons cross the midline and ascend in the lateral and ventrolateral spinal white matter as the spinothalamic tract. As the spinothalamic tract courses through the brainstem, collateral fibers innervate a variety of brainstem centers involved in providing responses to nociceptive input on its path to the thalamus. Nociceptive input arising from visceral structures is relayed by postsynaptic dorsal column cells whose axons course in the dorsal columns. After a synaptic relay in the dorsal column nuclei and crossing to the opposite side of the brainstem, the medial lemniscus carries nociceptive information to the thalamus. Both of these routes are somatotopically or viscerotopically arranged throughout their length.

range of small, unmyelinated fibers with conduction velocities less than 2.5 m/sec for the C-fiber (or group IV) nociceptors[21] (Fig. 7–2), and small fibers wrapped in a thin layer of myelin produced by Schwann cells with a conduction velocity of 4 to 30 m/sec in the case of the A-delta fibers (or group III).[22] Primary afferent C-fibers are more numerous than myelinated primary afferents in peripheral nerves. For example, in dorsal roots, the ratio of C-fibers to A-fibers is about 2.5:1[23] and in joint nerves (after sympathetic postganglionic axons are removed by sympathectomy) the ratio of C to A fibers is 2.3:1.[24]

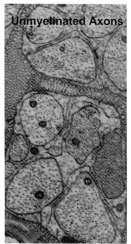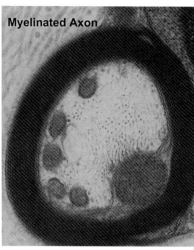

Figure 7–2. Peripheral nerves conveying information about pain are either small, slowly conducting fibers found unmyelinated in bundles or are medium-sized axons with thin myelin providing a higher conduction velocity.

Peripheral Nerves

Peripheral nerves have both sensory and motor functions. Sensory information is brought into the CNS by the primary afferent nerve fibers through the dorsal root. Motor commands are sent out to the periphery through the ventral root by large, rapidly conducting somatic efferent nerve fibers and small, slowly conducting autonomic motor fibers. Whereas the motor neurons are located in the ventral horn of the spinal cord or intermediate regions in the case of autonomic motor neurons, the sensory afferent fibers have their cell bodies in the dorsal root ganglia (or cranial nerve ganglia) located outside the spinal cord or brainstem. The primary afferent fiber type and site of its terminations centrally are relevant to its function. Incoming cutaneous non-noxious input important for discerning fine, discriminative touch, pressure, and position in space is transmitted by large, myelinated peripheral nerve fibers directly through the dorsal column of the spinal cord. The first synapse of these large, uncrossed ascending primary afferent fibers is in the dorsal column nuclei of the medulla. From there, cutaneous sensory information is transmitted as the decussated medial lemniscal pathway to the contralateral ventral posterolateral (VPL) nucleus of the thalamus, the primary sensory integrative relay of the sensory system. Similar information is relayed to the brainstem through several tracts whose cells of origin are within the spinal cord, including the tactile component of the postsynaptic dorsal column pathway, the spinocervical tract, and the lower limb proprioceptive pathway that projects to nucleus Z in the medulla.[7]

In contrast, noxious mechanical, temperature, and chemical (nociceptive) information are first relayed across a synapse located in the spinal cord before transmission to the brainstem sites (including VPL thalamus) (Fig. 7–3; see Fig. 7–1). The cutaneous and visceral nociceptive inputs are provided to spinal neurons in different spinal regions, have different ascending spinal projection pathways, and have different brainstem terminations.

Primary afferent fibers providing input to autonomic regions of the spinal cord from visceral structures and the vasculature travel with the sympathetic efferent nerves. They pass directly through the sympathetic trunk, however, to join other afferent fibers entering the dorsal horn of the spinal cord (see Fig. 7–3).

Cell Bodies in Dorsal Root Ganglia

All afferent fibers, whether they innervate cutaneous, deep, vascular, or visceral tissue, separate from the motor fibers near the spinal cord and join to form the dorsal root before entering the spinal cord on the dorsal surface. The cell bodies of the primary afferent nerve fibers, which compose the dorsal root ganglia (DRG), lie just outside the spinal column. As in many central neuronal circuits, glutamate is the primary neurotransmitter substance in primary afferent nociceptors and its action is modulated by neuropeptides coreleased at their terminal endings, such as calcitonin gene–related peptide (CGRP), substance P (SP), neurokinin A, adenosine triphosphate, adenosine, galanin, and somatostatin.[25,26] All of these substances have been identified in the dorsal root ganglia; however, they are produced and transported quickly to terminal endings in the spinal cord and thus may not necessarily be evident in the dorsal root ganglia without further manipulations. The dorsal root ganglia are composed of large, medium, and small cells with many of the small dorsal root ganglion cells belonging to the nociceptors.[25]

Spinal Cord Terminations

The afferent fibers enter the gray matter of the spinal cord through the dorsal root entry zone and primarily innervate regions of the spinal cord within the same spinal segment matching that spinal nerve. In general, large myelinated primary afferent fibers carrying sensory discriminative information (tactile, pressure, vibratory sense) enter in dorsal roots, traverse across the top of the dorsal horn of the spinal cord (Lissauer's tract), and turn to ascend uncrossed as the dorsal column. They provide only collateral input into the dorsal horn. The smaller myelinated and unmyelinated fibers carry information about temperature and nociceptive input perceived as pain in humans. The fibers enter Lissauer's tract, then innervate the gray matter core of the spinal cord where neuronal cell bodies and dendrites receive their arborized synaptic endings (Fig. 7–4; see Fig. 7–3). The afferent fibers may also ascend rostrally or descend caudally through Lissauer's tract, however. It is known that primary afferents labeled with CGRP can innervate up to 6 spinal segments above and below their level of entry.[27]

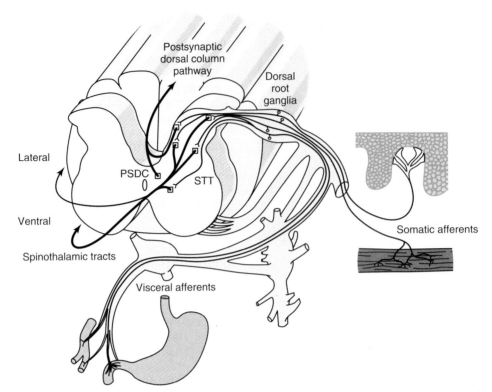

Figure 7–3. Nociceptive afferent nerve fibers have receptive free nerve endings in the dermal papillae of skin, in muscle, in the vasculature, and in visceral structures. Nerves carrying nociceptive information travel with other somatic and autonomic motor axons, even passing through the autonomic ganglia, but have their cell bodies in the dorsal root ganglia located in the spinal vertebral column. The central axonal projection of afferent nerve fibers then passes through the dorsal root to innervate the spinal cord dorsal horn. Nociceptive information is relayed across at least one synapse in the dorsal horn to alert cells with projections to higher centers. The spinothalamic tract (STT) cells in the superficial dorsal horn send an axonal projection across the midline to travel in the lateral spinothalamic tract. STT cells in the deep dorsal horn send axons across the midline to ascend in the ventral white matter. STT cells bring information about both somatic and visceral pain to thalamic levels. Postsynaptic dorsal column (PSDC) cells relay information about visceral pain through the ipsilateral dorsal column. After relay through the dorsal column, the medial lemniscus brings visceral pain information to the thalamus.

Because the sole source of CGRP in the dorsal horn of the spinal cord is primary afferents, this peptide serves as a marker for primary afferent terminal endings in the spinal cord (Fig. 7–5).[27-29] CGRP fibers extend extensive fiber terminations up and down the superficial spinal cord dorsal horn through numerous spinal levels upon entering at a particular spinal segment.[27] Numerous other neuropeptides have been localized in the dorsal horn.[26] Visceral afferents are rich in vasoactive intestinal polypeptide (VIP), bombesin, CGRP, and SP[8,25] and would account for some of the population of these peptides in the dorsal horn. Other neurotransmitters and neuromodulators will be discussed more thoroughly in the next chapter.

Whereas most primary afferent endings contain small, round, clear vesicles, the large, glomerular endings typically contain large, dense cored vesicles as well and are believed to contain peptides (Fig. 7–6). Glutamate is also localized in the glomerular endings.[30] CGRP receptors have been localized on postsynaptic membranes opposite glomerular, elongated, and dome-shaped synaptic endings in the superficial dorsal horn.[31] Increased release of glutamate and activation of dorsal horn neurons by glutamate is enhanced by the modulatory effects of neuropeptides, such as SP, CGRP, VIP, and cholecystokinin (CCK),[32-34] as in other sites of neural integration.

SPINAL CORD AND SPINAL TRIGEMINAL NUCLEUS

Spinal Cord Dorsal Horn

Noxious input from the body relayed by the primary afferent fibers is received by the dorsal horn of the spinal cord. The dorsal horn contains both local interneurons and the projection neurons, which provide the information to higher processing centers in the brain. Signals from nociceptors are relayed by at least one spinal neuron before arriving at higher brain regions (see Figs. 7–1 and 7–3).

The gray matter at the core of the spinal cord is a matrix of synaptic terminations and cells forming the first tier of processing and integration of sensory information. The gray matter of the spinal cord has been described topographically as 10 laminae by Rexed[35] based on histologic appearance (Fig. 7–7; see also Fig. 7–4 and reference 36). The gray matter of the dorsal horn includes laminae I to VI. Laminae VII to IX and lamina X are involved in somatic and

C-fiber Terminal Ending Arborizations

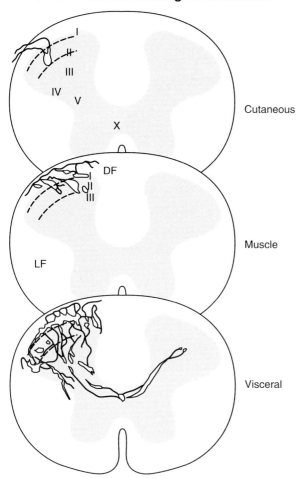

Figure 7–4. C-fiber terminal endings have been physiologically characterized and then filled with dye to reveal their terminal arborizations in the dorsal horn of the spinal cord. Examples of terminal arbors of axonal fibers with cutaneous, muscle, and visceral receptive fields are illustrated. The morphology of the cutaneous axonal ending would provide the anatomic substrate for precise point to point localization of a nociceptive insult on the cutaneous surface. Likewise, the diffuse widespread terminal arborization pattern for the visceral afferent nerve fiber would account for the poor localization of visceral nociceptive sensation that can be "referred" to other structures. Most visceral structures lie in the midline and some of the visceral fibers shown even cross the midline. The Roman numerals indicate Rexed's laminae. (From Sugiura Y, Terui N, Hosoya Y: Difference in distribution of central terminals between visceral and somatic unmyelinated [C] primary afferent fibers. J Neurophysiol 1989;62:834-840; and Ling LJ, Honda T, Shimada Y, et al: Central projection of unmyelinated (C) primary afferent fibers from gastrocnemius muscle in the guinea pig. J Comp Neurol 2003;461:140-150.)

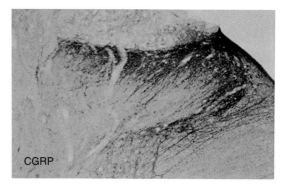

Figure 7–5. Calcitonin gene–related peptide (CGRP) is a good marker of the population of primary afferent nerve terminals innervating the dorsal horn.

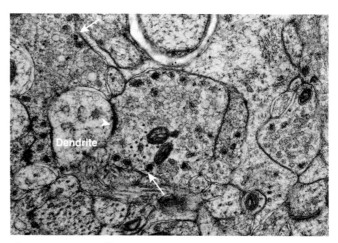

Figure 7–6. Many afferent nerve terminals in the spinal cord dorsal horn terminate with irregular, scalloped endings filled with both clear and dense core vesicles containing neurotransmitter substances. The scalloped endings (colored yellow) are formed as the endings contact numerous small dendrites of spinal neurons, such as the one shown containing the arrowhead marker. The arrowhead marker is directed toward a post-synaptic contact. Several of the dense core vesicles illustrated *(arrows)* in the terminal endings contain dense gold particles indicating immunolocalization of calcitonin gene–related peptide.

autonomic motor function, respectively. Some cells in deep laminae relay visceral nociceptive information to the brainstem.

The white matter encasing the gray matter is comprised of ascending and descending fiber bundles traveling longitudinally and connecting the spinal cord and the brain. Many of the axons are ensheathed in myelin formed by oligodendroglia. These myelin-producing glial cells are unique to the CNS. Other glial cells in the CNS include astrocytes and microglia.

Somatic C nociceptor afferent endings are distributed mainly to laminae I and II in the same and adjacent segments, whereas visceral C afferents can extend for more than five segments before they terminate. Somatic C nociceptors end rather focally in the spinal cord gray matter, whereas visceral C nociceptors are widely distributed in laminae I, II, V, X ipsilaterally as well as in laminae III and X contralaterally[37-39] (see Fig. 7–4). Cutaneous A-delta mechanical nociceptors terminate in the ipsilateral laminae I and V, and they may also have endings in lamina X and the contralateral dorsal horn.[40]

The outer marginal layer or lamina I of the dorsal horn contains afferent nerve fibers and the dendrites of cells that are longitudinally arranged along the length of the cord. Many of the cells are interneurons, but there are also lamina I cells that send axonal

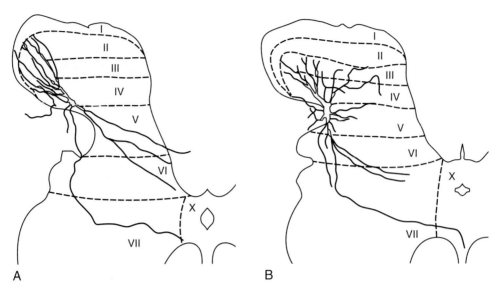

Figure 7–7. Spinal cord cells that were physiologically characterized were filled with a stainable dye and reconstructed over many spinal cord slices to provide details of their dendritic arborization. The cell in **A** was characterized as a high threshold cell in that it responded to intense stimulation in the digit of the hindlimb. The cell body is situated in lamina IV and its dendrites extend into all laminae. Dendrites extended almost 1 mm in the rostrocaudal direction. Its axon is bifurcated to cross the midline ventrally below lamina X as well as passing into the dorsal column. The cell in **B** was characterized as a "wide dynamic range cell" responding to a broader range of cutaneous inputs. The cell body is situated in lamina V and its dendrites extend radially in all directions including 1.2 mm in the rostrocaudal direction. The axon is seen crossing the midline in lamina X. The dashed line and Roman numerals indicate Rexed's laminae. (From Westlund KN, Carlton SM, Zhang D, et al: Direct catecholaminergic innervation of primate spinothalmic tract neurons. J Comp Neurol 1990;299:178-186.)

projections to the brainstem, hypothalamus, and the thalamus (for review, see reference 41). Most of the primary afferent endings heavily innervate the superficial dorsal horn of the spinal cord (laminae I and II) (see Figs. 7–4 and 7–5). In addition to the afferent endings, fiber terminations of the descending pathways and the local interneurons also heavily innervate the superficial dorsal horn, adding to the dense crescent of terminal endings when stained immunocytochemically for many neurotransmitters and receptors.

Typical of lamina II are the large glomerular synaptic complexes, sometimes referred to as *scalloped primary afferent endings,* which contact multiple dendrites of dorsal horn cells simultaneously[7,42-45] (see Fig. 7–6). Terminals that contain large, dense core vesicles identify them as neuropeptide-containing. Lamina II, or the substantia gelatinosa, also contains excitatory and inhibitory interneurons but few projection neurons. The interneurons take the form of stalked (limiting) cells and islet (central) cells.[46-48] Stalked cells project dorsally into lamina I. Islet cells are oriented longitudinally and their dendritic trees tend to be flattened so that they resemble slabs oriented in the dorsoventral plane. Lamina II interneurons synthesize either excitatory or inhibitory neurotransmitters, such as glutamate and gamma-aminobutyric acid (GABA), respectively.

Laminae III and IV contain interneurons and the large projection neurons of the spinocervical and postsynaptic dorsal column pathways relaying mechanotactile information and visceral nociceptive information. Laminae IV to VI contain interneurons and nociceptive projection neurons that distribute

input to the brainstem, thalamus, and hypothalamus. The projections of these cells form the spinoreticular, spinothalamic, and spinohypothalamic tracts. Noxious cutaneous input is relayed by lamina I, IV, and V projection neurons as the crossed spinothalamic tract (STT) pathway traveling to the ventral posterolateral nucleus of the thalamus.[2,49-53]

There is a visceral nociceptive processing area in the central region of the spinal cord, including lamina X and adjacent parts of laminae III, IV, V, and VII. In addition to interneurons, this area contains projection cells that send axons to the dorsal column nuclei, as well as to brainstem reticular formation, periaqueductal gray (PAG), hypothalamus, and thalamus, relaying information about visceral pain. These visceral nociceptive response cells are postsynaptic dorsal column, spinoreticular, spinohypothalamic, and spinothalamic cells. The visceral nociceptive input relayed by the postsynaptic dorsal column cells travels through the dorsal column midline from sacral levels and along the intermediate septum of the dorsal column from thoracic levels. The pathway remains uncrossed and then is relayed with the crossed medial lemniscal fibers to the thalamus[54-57] (see Fig. 7–1). Visceral pain information transmitted by the ventral STT is likely originating from cells also receiving convergent somatic nociceptive input. In fact, the early intermediate gene product c-Fos in cells in deeper laminae does not appear except after noxious visceral or prolonged pain states.[58]

Incoming sensory information received from the head, neck, and dura arrives via the trigeminal nerve afferent fibers. The terminal distribution in the dorsal horn of the spinal trigeminal nucleus in the caudal medulla is situated in a position equivalent to the spinal cord dorsal horn and appears very similar when stained for peptides. Glutamate and glutaminase have been found in spinal trigeminal neurons.[59] The projection neurons of the spinal trigeminal nucleus terminate in the ventromedial nucleus of the thalamus, relaying nociceptive information from the face and dura.

Spinal Interneurons

Most of the neurons in the dorsal horn are interneurons.[60] The neurons in the dorsal horn have been found to contain any of a large number of neuroactive substances that are presumably neurotransmitters or modulators. These substances include adenosine, choline acetyltransferase, cholecystokinin, corticotropin-releasing factor, dynorphin, enkephalin, galanin, GABA, glutamate, glycine, neurotensin, neuropeptide Y, somatostatin, SP, and thyrotropin-releasing hormone.[8] These substances are involved in excitatory or inhibitory nociceptive processing by the interneuronal circuits of the dorsal horn.

Inhibition of spinal transmission, by weak mechanical stimulation, for example, can occur either through activation of segmental or supraspinal circuitries. The events that can inhibit nociceptive transmission can occur by reducing neurotransmitter release from nociceptor terminals. While physiologists have conveniently explained "surround" type inhibition of dorsal horn synaptic transmission in terms of dorsal horn axo-axonic synaptic transmission, only a few anatomic figures of this type have been described for the dorsal horn.[48,61,62] Rather, the anatomic arrangement of synapses for the Gate Theory of Pain proposed by Melzack and Wall[63] is likely mediated through axodendritic arrangements of CGRP primary afferent terminals innervating the dendrites of GABA interneurons in lamina II and dendroaxonic synapses back onto the CGRP endings. Fine myelinated and unmyclinated CGRP-labeled afferent fibers are observed synapsing with GABAergic dendritic profiles (islet cells).[62] GABA interneurons are primarily the islet cells,[47] which are also found in laminae I and III and which have been stained for another inhibitory amino acid, glycine.[48] GABA interneurons are uniquely qualified to provide the "presynaptic" inhibition of nociceptive input either through contacts provided by their dendrites back onto CGRP primary afferent endings or through axonal contacts back onto primary afferent endings or onto other dorsal horn neurons. Other inhibitory neurons in the dorsal horn contain dynorphin and glycine. Likewise, an interposed excitatory interneuron, for example one containing glutamate, would provide an excitatory boost to spinal nociceptive processing. Interestingly, neurons in lamina II, the substantia gelatinosa, do not respond to release of substance P, because they lack NK1 (SP) receptors.[64] Substance P terminal endings are located on nocicep-

tive projection cells in both lamina I and the deep dorsal horn, including lamina I cells with NK1 receptors which rapidly internalize the receptors upon nociceptive stimulation.[65,66]

In the case of intense or prolonged nociceptive stimulation, the same anatomic arrangement of the dorsal horn circuitry providing the "presynaptic inhibition" can override the inhibition and result in sensitization.[67,68] Prolonged membrane hyperpolarization, using glutamatergic and GABA$_B$ receptors, alters the membrane conductance of the central primary afferent terminals to the point that the terminal endings themselves become depolarized. This generates an action potential that travels back toward the periphery. These "dorsal root reflexes" would release neurotransmitters such as glutamate and peptides from the axonal terminals into the damaged tissue and allow increased transmitter release at the central terminals in the dorsal horn. This sets up a reverberating positive feedback loop amplifying nociceptive input and resulting in both peripheral and central sensitization that can promote the establishment of chronic pain.

Thus, nociceptive information entering the spinal cord dorsal horn is modulated by both excitatory and inhibitory influences at the periphery and at the level of the spinal cord, before being relayed by projection neurons to higher centers. Modulation occurs not only through primary afferent nerve influences on the local interneuronal circuitry, but also through input provided to projection neurons by descending input from the brainstem. This modulatory input likely also involves the spinal interneuronal circuitry.

Projection Neurons

Several types of projection neurons in lamina I have been described by Lima and Coimbra that send their axon rostrally to the brainstem.[69-72] These cell types include fusiform (spindle-shaped), multipolar, flattened, and pyramidal neurons. Different subsets of these cells project their axons to the nucleus of the solitary tract; to the dorsal and lateral reticular nuclei in the medulla, pons, and midbrain; and to the thalamus. Neurons of the same morphologic types are found to stain for SP, enkephalin, dynorphin, or GABA,[73] although some of the cells may have been interneurons. Three morphologic types of lamina I STT cells have been described in cats and monkeys: fusiform, pyramidal, and multipolar.[74,75] Evidence has been provided that the fusiform and multipolar STT cells are nociceptive, whereas the pyramidal STT cells are thermoreceptive.[76] Consistent with this, most fusiform and multipolar lamina I STT neurons express NK1 receptors and most pyramidal STT cells do not.[64,77]

The projection cells that are found in deeper laminae of the dorsal horn are typically large, multipolar neurons with extensive dendritic arbors. The dendrites of the deep projection cells tend to arborize radially in the spinal cord dorsal horn, in contrast to the lamina I projection cells whose dendrites are longitudinally distributed along the dorsal surface of the spinal cord gray matter so that in the coronal plane they are barely visible. A radial dendrite arrangement provides for the convergent input encoded by the STT cells in the deeper laminae, as opposed to the superficial projection neurons situated to have ready access to specific incoming nociceptive and thermal input via the afferent nerve fibers. Some STT cells in deeper laminae do have dendrites that extend dorsally into lamina I and II (see Fig. 7–7). These STT cells receive direct synaptic connections from the terminals of nociceptors, ending in the superficial dorsal horn, and are particularly responsive to "high threshold" input.[53,78-80] Other STT cells identified as "wide dynamic range" cells respond to a variety of mechanical, thermal, and nociceptive inputs. They have dendrites that extend chiefly in the ventral direction and receive convergent input from afferents supplying both deep somatic and visceral structures.

The STT cells in laminae I, IV, and V express the early intermediate gene activation marker, c-Fos, in many pain models. The STT cells in the deeper laminae (III, V, VII, X) express c-Fos protein in response to sustained nociceptive activation, as in models of joint and visceral inflammation.[58] The STT neurons contain glutamate[80] and some also contain peptides, such as SP, enkephalin, dynorphin, or VIP.[81-83] Lamina X STT cells have been shown to contain CCK, bombesin, and galanin.[84,85] Synapses found on the cell bodies of STT neurons of deep layers of the dorsal horn have been shown to contain glutamate, GABA, glycine, SP, CGRP, vasopressin, norepinephrine, and serotonin,[65,80,86-92] indicating that these STT cells are affected by both excitatory and inhibitory events associated with nociceptive processing. The dorsally directed dendrites of many deep dorsal horn neurons contain NK1 (substance P) receptors,[64] and these are internalized following presumably painful stimulation occurring during inflammation.[93] Ultrastructural studies have revealed postsynaptic localization of glutamate receptor subunits NMDA R1, AMPA GluR1 and GluR2/3, and metabotropic mGluR1 and mGluR2/3 associated with terminals in contact with identified STT neurons.[94,95] The NMDA R1 and AMPA Glu R2/3 were also localized presynaptically on the terminals contacting STT neurons.

CENTRAL ASCENDING PATHWAYS

Nociceptive neurons in the spinal cord include neurons with axonal fiber projections to the many sensory processing regions in the brain including the dorsal column nuclei, dorsal and ventral reticular formation, parabrachial region, PAG, thalamus, anterior pretectal nucleus, hypothalamus, and amygdala (Fig. 7–8; see Fig. 7–1).

Spinothalamic Tract

STT neurons are the primary relay cells providing nociceptive input from the spinal cord to the thalamus, the main integration site of sensory information. Tactile information from the same body region

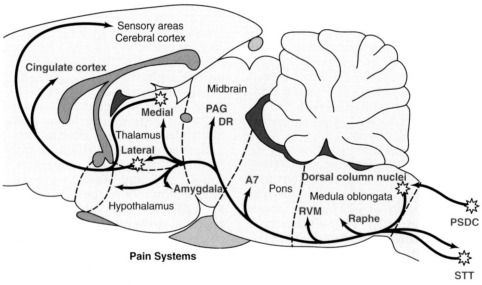

Figure 7–8. Pain systems include the spinothalamic tract and the postsynaptic dorsal column pathways. These parallel pain systems ascending from the spinal cord converge to course through the brainstem as the spinothalamic tract and the medial lemniscus. While the primary termination site for sensory integration is the thalamus, abundant collateral terminations are provided to integration sites throughout the brainstem. The ventral posterolateral nucleus of the thalamus is the principal somatosensory relay for information provided to the sensory areas of the cerebral cortex for localization of pain sensation. The intermediate and medial thalamus project to the anterior cingulate and orbital frontal cortex, respectively, providing input relevant to the affective responses to pain. Autonomic adjustments occur in response to input provided to the hypothalamus. A7, noradrenergic cell group; DR, dorsal raphe; PAG, periaqueductal gray; PSDC, postsynaptic dorsal column cell; RVM, rostral ventromedial medulla; STT, spinothalamic tract cell.

converges upon the same thalamic neurons. The point-to-point reception of information in the lateral thalamus provides somatotopic encoding for specific localization of the input onto the cortical representation of the specific body region. This provides the ability to locate precisely the origin of the nociceptive input. The STT cells receiving noxious cutaneous input are largely situated in lamina I and the lateral half of the neck of the dorsal horn in laminae IV and V.[49,50,52,53] Other STT neurons are scattered throughout the deep dorsal horn, intermediate region (including lamina X[96]) and even in laminae VII of the ventral horn. Many of these STT cells receive both cutaneous and visceral nociceptive information.

The axons of STT cells cross the midline of the spinal cord in the anterior white commissure[53] (see Figs. 7–1, 7–3, and 7–7) and ascend primarily in the contralateral (opposite) white matter in the lateral and ventrolateral funiculus.[97] The axons of STT cells terminate in the posterior complex, ventral posterior lateral, ventral posterior inferior, central lateral, subparafascicular, and other nuclei of the thalamus.[98] Lamina I STT neurons send their axonal projections in the middle of the lateral funiculus to terminate in the posterior part of the ventral medial nucleus of the thalamus as well as in the ventral posterior and medial dorsal nuclei.[99]

Postsynaptic Dorsal Column Pathway

In addition to the ascending axons of primary afferent neurons relaying touch, pressure, and vibratory sensation, the dorsal column contains the ascending axons of second order spinal cord projection neurons called *postsynaptic dorsal column neurons*. The cell bodies of many of these cells are located in laminae III and IV,[100] but are also described for lamina X.[54,56] The postsynaptic dorsal column cell neurons may respond to noxious visceral stimulation, although they may also respond to tactile stimulation. These cells send a direct projection to the dorsal column nuclei in the dorsal medulla.[54,57] Cells in sacral spinal levels terminate in the gracile nucleus, and cells in thoracic spinal levels terminate in both the gracile and cuneate nuclei. Postsynaptic dorsal column neurons transmit visceral nociceptive information to the thalamus, to converge on some of the same thalamic cells receiving nociceptive information from the skin and other somatic structures[55,57,101,102] (see Figs. 7–1 and 7–7).

Spinoreticular Pathways

Many projection axons from the spinal cord also provide collateral innervation to other regions of the brainstem involved in pain-related activities, including autonomic responsiveness, the alerting response, and escape responses. Collectively, these neurons are referred to as the *spinoreticular system* (see Figs. 7–1 and 7–8).

A dorsal spinomedullary pathway arises from cells in laminae I, IV, and X to terminate in the sub-nucleus reticularis dorsalis (SRD) of the medullary reticular formation, which is located just ventral to the cuneate and solitary nucleus of the dorsal medulla.[103] This nucleus is a brainstem site that is active in descending inhibition of nociceptive processes. The diffuse noxious inhibitory controls (DNIC) or inhibition of wide dynamic range neurons in the spinal cord by competing afferent input are dependent on a supraspinal loop through the SRD and a descending pathway.[104]

In the medulla, a major ascending lateral axonal projection relaying information about pain passes through and terminates in the reticular formation of the ventrolateral medulla (VLM).[71,105,106] This is part of a direct spinal projection pathway that traverses brainstem regions containing catecholaminergic neurons, including the C1, A1, A2, A5, A6, and A7 regions of both the pons and medulla.[107] Many fiber projections terminate in the parabrachial region. Small injections of retrograde tracer in the parabrachial nucleus confirm that this nucleus receives projections primarily from lamina I.[108] The catecholaminergic neurons of the brainstem are involved in diverse functions, including arousal and learning. Descending inhibitory input from this region to the spinal cord limits responses to painful stimulation.[109] Connections between the rostral ventromedial medulla and the catecholamine cells of the pons[110] and between brainstem serotonergic and catecholaminergic cells and the thalamus[111] have also been described that may assist in coordination of descending influences on pain perception.

Ascending pathways relaying information about pain also terminate in the PAG and midline midbrain reticular formation.[106,112-115] The PAG and the raphe magnus are the sources of input driving descending inhibition and facilitation known to impact the perception of pain. A direct neuronal projection from the central region of the spinal cord to nuclei in the midline, including the rostral ventromedial nucleus of the medulla and the midbrain raphe magnus, has been described as well.[56]

Another termination site receiving ascending pathways directly from the spinal cord and also receiving input from the dorsal column nuclei is the anterior pre-tectal nucleus.[116] The anterior pretectal nucleus is thought to be an important source of descending inhibition of nociceptive pathways. Evidence suggests that it sends axons to catecholaminergic neurons of the parabrachial region.[117]

Spinohypothalamic, Limbic, and Cortical Connections

Pain is often accompanied by motivational-affective responses, including suffering, anxiety, increased attention and arousal, increased heart rate and blood pressure, as well as by changes in endocrine and autonomic responses. The neural structures that relay these changes are likely to be parallel to those relaying information localizing the source of the noxious input on the body map. An interesting hypothesis is that a medial and a lateral pain pathway provide affective and epicritic (discriminative) pain sensation, respectively. The lateral and ventrolateral STTs clearly provide information for specific discrimination of pain and temperature, somatotopic localization, and intensity coding of cutaneous pain. Some of the pathways in unique positions to assume a role in affective pain awareness would include the spinoamygdalar pathway, spinal pathways relaying visceral pain through the postsynaptic medial dorsal column route and ventromedial STT projections to midline structures including the rostral ventromedial medulla, PAG, hypothalamus, and centrolateral and medial thalamus.[56,98] Interestingly, some thalamic cells in the centrolateral nucleus are activated only by noxious visceral stimulation.[118] The thalamic connections to the somatosensory (SI, SII) cortex have not been well studied. Centrolateral and medial thalamic projections to the anterior cingulate and frontal cortices, respectively, have been described.[119]

Spinohypothalamic and spinoamygdalar pathways that may be involved in autonomic and affective responses to pain have been described.[120-122] Ascending axonal projections of these pathways arise primarily from the spinal cord laminae I and X, as well as from the lateral reticular region of the spinal cord. Synapses are made in the lateral hypothalamus (LH) and the central nucleus of the amygdala (CA). Both of these regions are also involved in antinociceptive actions, as well as autonomic and affective responses to nociceptive input through connections with the thalamus and with other parts of the limbic system. Spinal projections to the VLM are conveniently located to relay to the paraventricular nucleus of the hypothalamus,[123] amygdala,[124] and medial preoptic region.[125] The direct route to the medial thalamus, amygdala, and the spino-parabrachial-amygdala pathways[126,127] are clearly involved. A spino-reticulo-thalamo-cortical pathway was originally proposed as a projection to the forebrain, relaying information about painful input presumably for subjective interpretation based on known anatomic projections of the reticular formation to higher brain centers.[128] Relays to the insular cortical structures have also been described.

DESCENDING PATHWAYS MODULATING PAIN

Descending inhibition of spinal nociceptive processes was initially described in behavioral experiments in which electrical stimulation of the PAG resulted in antinociception.[129] The antinociception was proposed, based on behavioral, electrophysiologic, and morphologic studies, to occur through a PAG relay to the rostral ventromedial medulla (RVM) and then to the spinal cord[130-139] (also see reviews in references 112 and 140 to 142). Subsequent findings suggest that the process is mediated through more complicated circuitry (Fig. 7–9).

It is now known that both inhibitory and excitatory influences on spinal cord nociceptive processing occur after activation of recurrent loops through

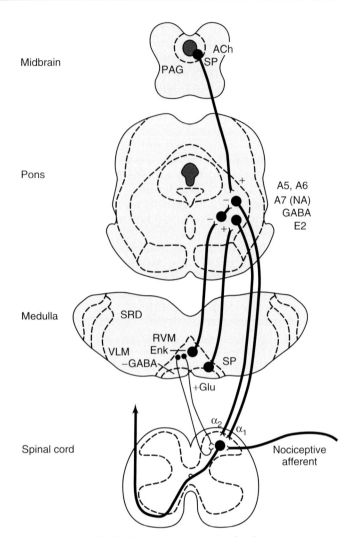

Figure 7–9. Multiple integration sites in the brainstem receive nociceptive input from the ascending pain systems. Complex brainstem circuitry provides both descending inhibitory and excitatory alterations of nociceptive responses at the level of the spinal cord. Cells are situated side by side in the rostral ventromedial medulla (RVM) that impose either excitatory or inhibitory influences. Cells in the RVM are both serotonergic (5HT) and nonserotonergic. They provide both a direct descending pathway to the spinal cord and a major input to the dorsolateral pons. The A5-A7 noradrenergic (NA) cell groups in the dorsolateral pons provide major inhibitory feedback to spinal cord. The periaqueductal gray (PAG) and the anterior pretectal nuclei provide inhibitory input to the spinal cord through connections with the descending pathways from the dorsolateral pons. Specific neurotransmitters within brainstem regions are noted, as are specific receptors impacting nociception in the spinal cord dorsal horn. ACh, acetylcholine; α1, noradrenergic receptor, alpha 1; α2, noradrenergic receptor, alpha 2; Enk, enkephalin; E2, adrenergic receptor 2; GABA, gamma-aminobutyric acid; Glu, glutamate; SP, substance P; SRD, nucleus reticularis dorsalis; VLM, ventrolateral medulla.

the brainstem activated by ascending pathways from the spinal cord. Extensive behavioral and electrophysiologic studies have found that bulbospinal facilitatory projections and in particular those descending from the RVM promote tactile and thermal hyperesthesias.[143-146] The RVM is responsible for the maintenance, although not the initiation, of neuropathic central[147-149] and visceral pain.[150] The RVM is composed of the midline raphe system and the adjacent ventral reticular formation. The raphe-spinal pathway is largely, but not entirely, serotonergic.[151-153] The component that originates from the nucleus raphe magnus (NRM) descending in the dorsolateral funiculus is primarily associated with inhibitory control and a ventrolateral descending pathway is typically attributed with facilitatory control of nociceptive responses. Excitatory substance P and inhibitory enkephalinergic connections between the RVM and the noradrenergic neurons of the dorsolateral pons are a major component of the descending control system that promotes both facilitatory and inhibitory influences modulating pain.[154,155] An additional supraspinal loop from the dorsal horn to the nucleus reticularis dorsalis (SRD) and back to the dorsal horn also mediates both descending inhibition and facilitation.[104]

Descending noradrenergic input to the spinal cord from the dorsolateral pons provides direct inhibitory modulation of spinal nociceptive mechanisms. The largest percentage of spinally projecting noradrenergic neurons have been identified in the locus coeruleus, subcoeruleus, parabrachial, and Kölliker-Fuse nuclei.[156-158] The noradrenergic A5 cell group in the ventrolateral pons/medulla and the adrenergic neurons of the VLM also send axonal projections to influence nociception in the spinal cord as well.[159]

The PAG in the midbrain makes descending connections not only with the RVM,[160] but also with the noradrenergic system of the dorsolateral pons.[161] A net inhibition of spinal nociceptive processing is initiated from the PAG through glutamate and substance P inputs to these brainstem regions with major descending axonal projections. The cholinergic neuronal system is another major reticular system of the midbrain and other portions of the brainstem that provides descending influences on nociception. The cholinergic mechanisms can reduce nociception as well as potentiate opiate analgesia.[162,163] These analgesic actions may also be mediated through presynaptic terminations of laminae III to V cholinergic interneurons reported to synapse directly onto primary sensory endings.[164]

The anterior pretectal nucleus has also been associated with inhibition of nociceptive somatosensory function.[116] The anterior pretectal region evokes antinociceptive responses in the tail flick, formalin, and paw pressure tests. However, this region has minor direct input from lamina I and X in the spinal cord, and direct innervation of the spinal cord by the anterior pretectal nucleus has not been reported. Indications are that these effects are mediated through anatomical connectivity with the dorsolateral pontine pathways.

Many hypothalamic nuclei, including the lateral hypothalamus, have descending connections with the PAG.[165-167] The hypothalamic input to the PAG is topographic, linking particular hypothalamic nuclei with particular regions of the PAG. Hypothalamic axons form the largest input to the PAG.[167]

Descending projections from several forebrain areas impact nociception, including the central nucleus of the amygdala and many parts of the cerebral cortex, including the infralimbic and prelimbic cortex medially, the anterior cingulate gyrus, the precentral medial cortex, and laterally the anterior and posterior insular cortex and perirhinal cortex.[165,168] Although less is known as yet about these systems, some evidence implies descending modulation through the circuitry of the dorsolateral pons.

The simplified schema of the supraspinal circuitry of the descending control systems imposing facilitative and inhibitory modulation of nociceptive processing is shown in Figure 7–9. Nociceptive insults, such as nerve damage or tissue inflammation, increase the tone of both modulatory events, shifting the balance toward facilitation. While increased activation of pain systems and increased descending facilitation predominate during pain states, descending inhibitory systems continue to damp the increasing nociceptive activation. Conversely, "stress-induced analgesia" would imply a shift in the balance favoring descending inhibitory pathway activation. In truth, it is the sum of the effects of this complex polysynaptic circuitry that establishes the level of perceived pain intensity.

CENTERS FOR HIGHER PROCESSING

Even though it is clear that the perception of pain requires the activity of higher cortical centers of the brain, the precise regional association has remained a mystery until the advent of positron emission tomography (PET) and functional magnetic resonance imaging (fMRI) studies in both animals and humans. These imaging studies have mapped areas of increased blood flow indicating regions of increased activity.[169-175] These studies implicate the thalamus, SI and SII somatosensory cortex, the anterior cingulate gyrus, the insula, the prefrontal cortex, lentiform nucleus, and the cerebellum as major players in the higher processing of pain (see Fig. 7–8). Many of these same regions were activated after noxious visceral stimulation.[176] The thalamus and the SI and SII cortex are known to be somatosensory processing regions, and evidence from the imaging studies is consistent with a sensory-discriminative role of these structures. The anterior cingulate cortex presumably is involved in the interpretation of the emotional significance of the painful input by the limbic system,[174] whereas the lentiform nucleus and cerebellum may be involved in the learning of reflexive motor responsiveness to painful input necessary to protect the individual. The insula, cerebellum, and frontal cortex may contribute to memory and learning of events related to painful stimuli, such as avoidance behavior.[177] (A more detailed discussion of this topic is in Chapter 10.)

SUMMARY

- Nociceptive information is brought to the spinal cord by fine unmyelinated C-fiber axons and thinly myelinated A-delta fibers traveling in the peripheral nerves.
- Spinal cord neurons receiving nociceptive information have highly arborized dendrites and are located in various laminae of the dorsal horn, depending on their function.
- Spinal neurons receiving cutaneous thermal information are located primarily in lamina I. Spinal neurons receiving cutaneous mechanical information are located primarily in laminae IV and V.
- Spinal neurons receiving information about visceral structures are located primarily in laminae III, VII, and X.
- There are two parallel pain system ascending pathways bringing nociceptive information to higher brain centers.
- The spinothalamic tract brings primarily cutaneous nociceptive information and sends its axons across the midline in the spinal cord before ascending to the thalamus.
- The postsynaptic dorsal column pathway brings primarily visceral nociceptive information. Uncrossed axons are sent up the dorsal column to synapse in the dorsal column nuclei, in the dorsal medulla midline. A crossed axonal projection from the dorsal column nuclei ascends as the medial lemniscus, bringing information about visceral pain to the thalamus.
- The ventral posterolateral nucleus of the thalamus is the principal sensory relay nucleus providing discriminative site-specific information about pain to the somatosensory cortex, SI, and SII.
- Other thalamic nuclei receive nociceptive information provided to frontal, insular, and anterior cingulate cortices for affective responses to pain, including nuclei of the medial and intralaminar thalamus.
- Descending modulatory systems impact nociceptive processing through complex brainstem circuitry.

References

1. Hardy JD, Wolff HG, Goodell H (eds): Pain Sensations and Reactions. New York: Hafner Publishing, 1967.
2. Willis WD: The Pain System; The Neural Basis of Nociceptive Transmission in the Mammalian Nervous System. Basel, Karger, 1985.
3. Willis WD, Westlund KN: Pain system. In Paxinos G, Mai JK (eds): The Human Nervous System, 2nd ed. New York, Elsevier, 2004, pp. 1125-1170.
4. Willis WD, Westlund KN, Carlton, SM. Pain System. In Paxinos G (ed): The Rat Nervous System, 3rd ed. New York, Elsevier, 2004, pp. 853-890.
5. Belmonte C, Cervero F (eds): Neurobiology of Nociceptors. Oxford: Oxford University Press, 1996.
6. Kumazawa T, Kruger L, Mizumura K (eds): The Polymodal Receptor—A Gateway to Pathological Pain. Progress in Brain Research, vol 113. Amsterdam, Elsevier, 1996.
7. Willis WD, Coggeshall RE: Sensory Mechanisms of the Spinal Cord, 2nd ed. New York, Plenum Press, 1991.
8. Willis WD, Coggeshall RE: Sensory Mechanisms of the Spinal Cord, vol 1, 3rd ed. New York, Plenum Press, 2004.
9. Mense S: Nociception from skeletal muscle in relation to clinical muscle pain. Pain 1993;54:241-289.
10. Stacey MJ: Free nerve endings in skeletal muscle of the cat. J Ant 1969;105:231-254.
11. Schaible HG, Grubb BD: Afferent and spinal mechanisms of joint pain. Pain 1993;55:5-54.
12. Heppelmann B, Messlinger K, Neiss WF, et al: Ultrastructural three-dimensional reconstruction of group III and group IV sensory nerve endings ("free nerve endings") in the knee joint capsule of the cat: Evidence for multiple receptive sites. J Comp Neurol 1990;292:103-116.
13. Messlinger K: Functional morphology of nociceptive and other fine sensory endings (free nerve endings) in different tissues. In Kumazawa T, Kruger L, Mizumura K (eds): The Polymodal Receptor—A Gateway to Pathological Pain. Progress in Brain Research, vol 113. Amsterdam, Elsevier, 1996, pp. 273-298.
14. Cervero F: Sensory innervation of the viscera: Peripheral basis of visceral pain. Physiol Rev 1994;74:95-138.
15. Ness TJ, Gebhart GF: Visceral pain: A review of experimental studies. Pain 1990;41:167-234.
16. Sato K, Kiyama H, Park HT, et al: AMPA, KA and NMDA receptors are expressed in the rat DRG neurones. NeuroReport 1993;4:1263-1265.
17. Carlton SM, Hargett GL, Coggeshall RE: Localization and activation of glutamate receptors in unmyelinated axons of rat glabrous skin. Neurosci Lett 1995;197:25-28.
18. Carlton SM, Zhou S, Coggeshall RE: Localization and activation of substance P receptors in unmyelinated axons of rat glabrous skin. Brain Res 1996;734:103-108.
19. Coggeshall RE, Carlton SM: Receptor localization in the mammalian dorsal horn and primary afferent neurons. Brain Res Rev 1997;24:28-66.
20. Coggeshall RE, Zhou S, Carlton SM: Opioid receptors on peripheral sensory axons. Brain Res 1997;764:126-132.
21. Gasser HS: Unmedullated fibers originating in dorsal root ganglia. J Gen Physiol 1950;3:651-690.
22. Boivie J, Perl ER: Neural substrates of somatic sensation. In: Hunt CC (ed): MTP International Review of Science, Physiology Series One, Neurophysiology, vol 3. Baltimore, University Park Press, 1975, pp 303-411.
23. Hulsebosch CE, Coggeshall RE: Quantitation of sprouting of dorsal root axons. Science 1981;213:1020-1021.
24. Langford LA, Schmidt RF: Afferent and efferent axons in the medial and posterior articular nerves of the cat. Anat Rec 1983;206:71-78.
25. Lawson SN: Peptides and cutaneous polymodal nociceptor neurones. In Kumazawa T, Kruger L, Mizumura K (eds): Progress in Brain Research. Elsevier, Amsterdam, 1996, pp. 369-385.
26. Chung K, Briner RP, Carlton SM, et al: Immunohistochemical localization of seven different peptides in the human spinal cord. J Comp Neurol. 1989;280:158-170.
27. Chung K, Lee WT, Carlton SM: The effects of dorsal rhizotomy and spinal cord isolation on calcitonin gene-related peptide containing terminals in the rat lumbar dorsal horn. Neurosci Lett 1988;90:27-32.
28. Carlton SM, McNeill DL, Chung K, et al: Organization of calcitonin gene-related peptide-immunoreactive terminals in the primate dorsal horn. J Comp Neurol 1988;276:527-536.
29. Harmann PA, Chung K, Briner RP, et al: Calcitonin gene-related peptide (CGRP) in the human spinal cord: A light and electron microscopic analysis. J Comp Neurol 1988;269:371-380.
30. Maxwell DJ, Christie WM, Short AD, et al: Central boutons of glomeruli in the spinal cord of the cat are enriched with L-glutamate-like immunoreactivity. Neuroscience 1990;36:83-104.
31. Ye Z, Wimalawansa SJ, Westlund KN: Receptor for calcitonin gene-related peptide: Localization in the dorsal and ventral spinal cord. Neuroscience 1999;92:1389-1397.
32. Murase K, Ryu PD, Randíc M: Excitatory and inhibitory amino acids and peptide-induced responses in acutely isolated rat spinal cord dorsal horn neurons. Neurosci Lett 1989;103:56-63.
33. Kangrgra I, Larew JS, Randíc M: The effects of substance P and calcitonin-gene-related peptide on the efflux of endogenous glutamate and aspartate from the rat spinal dorsal horn in vitro. Neurosci Lett 1990;108:155-160.

34. Dougherty PM, Willis WD: Enhancement of spinothalamic neuron responses to chemical and mechanical stimuli following combined micro-iontophoretic application of N-methyl-D-aspartic acid and substance P. Pain 1991;47: 85-93.
35. Rexed B: The cytoarchitectonic organization of the spinal cord in the cat. J Comp Neurol 1952;96:415-466.
36. Paxinos G (ed): The Rat Nervous System. San Diego, Academic Press, 1995.
37. Morgan MM, Fields HL: Pronounced changes in the activity of nociceptive modulatory neurons in the rostral ventromedial medulla in response to prolonged thermal noxious stimuli. J Neurophysiol 1994;72:1161-1170.
38. Sugiura Y: Spinal organization of C-fiber afferents related with nociception or non-nociception. In Kumazawa T, Kruger L, Mizumura K (eds): The Polymodal Receptor: A Gateway to Pathological Pain. Progress in Brain Research, vol 113. New York, Elsevier, 1996, pp 319-339.
39. Sugiura Y, Terui N, Hosoya Y: Difference in distribution of central terminals between visceral and somatic unmyelinated (C) primary afferent fibers. J Neurophysiol 1989;62:834-840.
40. Light AR, Perl ER: Spinal termination of functionally identified primary afferent neurons with slowly conducting myelinated fibers. J Comp Neurol 1979;186:133-150.
41. Willis WD, Westlund KN: Neuroanatomy of the pain system and of the pathways that modulate pain. J Clin Neurophysiol 1997;14:2-31.
42. Cruz F, Lima D, Coimbra A: Several morphological types of terminal arborizations of primary afferents in laminae I-II of the rat spinal cord, as shown after HRP labeling and Golgi impregnation. J Comp Neurol 1987;261:221-236.
43. Cruz F, Lima D, Zieglgänsberger W, et al: Fine structure and synaptic architecture of HRP-labeled primary afferent terminations in lamina IIi of the rat dorsal horn. J Comp Neurol 1991;305:3-16.
44. Ribeiro-da-Silva A., Coimbra A: Two types of synaptic glomeruli and their distribution in laminae I-III of the rat. J Comp Neurol 1982;209:176-186.
45. Ribeiro-da-Silva A, Tagari P, Cuello AC: Morphological characterization of substance P-like immunoreactive glomeruli in the superficial dorsal horn of the rat spinal cord and trigeminal subnucleus caudalis: A quantitative study. J Comp Neurol 1989;281:497-415.
46. Cajal SR: Histology of the Nervous System of Man and Vertebrates, vol 1. Swanson N, Swanson LW (Engl Trans). New York, Oxford University Press, 1995.
47. Gobel S: Neural circuitry in the substantia gelatinosa of Rolando: Anatomical insights. Adv Res Pain Ther 1979;3: 175-195.
48. Spike RC, Todd AJ: Ultrastructural and immunocytochemical study of lamina II islet cells in rat spinal dorsal horn. J Comp Neurol 1992;323:359-369.
49. Apkarian AV, Hodge CJ: Primate spinothalamic pathways: I. A quantitative study of the cells of origin of the spinothalamic pathway. J Comp Neurol 1989;288:447-473.
50. Burstein R, Dado RJ, Giesler GJ: The cells of origin of the spinothalamic tract of the rat: A quantitative reexamination. Brain Res 1990;511:329-337.
51. Granum SL: The spinothalamic system of the rat: I. Locations of cells of origin. J Comp Neurol 1986;247:159-180.
52. Hayes NL, Rustioni A: Spinothalamic and spinomedullary neurons in macaques: A single and double retrograde tracer study. Neuroscience 1980;5:861-874.
53. Willis WD, Kenshalo DR, Leonard RB: The cells of origin of the primate spinothalamic tract. J Comp Neurol 1979;188: 543-574.
54. Hirshberg RM, Al-Chaer ED, Lawand NB, et al: Is there a pathway in the posterior funiculus that signals visceral pain? Pain 1996;67:291-305.
55. Houghton AK, Wang C-C, Westlund KN: Do nociceptive signals from the pancreas travel in the dorsal column? Pain 2001;89:207-220.
56. Wang CC, Willis WD, Westlund KN: Ascending projections from the area around the spinal cord central canal: A *Phaseo-lus vulgaris* leucoagglutinin study in rats. J Comp Neurol 1999;415:341-367.
57. Willis WD, Al-Chaer ED, Quast MJ, et al: A visceral pain pathway in the dorsal column of the spinal cord. Proc Natl Acad Sci U S A 1999;96:7675-7679.
58. Abbadie C, Besson JM: c-fos expression in rat lumbar spinal cord during the development of adjuvant-induced arthritis. Neuroscience 1992;48:985-993.
59. Magnusson KR, Larson AA, Madl JE, et al: Co-localization of fixative-modified glutamate and glutaminase in neurons of the spinal trigeminal nucleus of the rat: An immunohistochemical and immunoradiochemical analysis. J Comp Neurol 1986;247:477-490.
60. Chung K, Kevetter GA, Willis WD, et al: An estimate of the ratio of propriospinal to long tract neurons in the sacral spinal cord of the rat. Neurosci Lett 1984;44:173-177.
61. Ralston HJ: Dorsal horn projections to dorsal horn neurons in the cat spinal cord. J Comp Neurol 1968;132:303-330.
62. Hayes ES, Carlton SM: Primary afferent interactions: Analysis of calcitonin gene-related peptide-immunoreactive terminals in contact with unlabeled and GABA-immunoreactive profiles in the monkey dorsal horn. Neuroscience 1992;47: 873-896.
63. Melzack R, Wall PD. Pain mechanisms: A new theory. Science 1965;150:971-979.
64. Brown JL, Liu H, Maggio JE, et al: Morphological characterization of substance P receptor-immunoreactive neurons in the rat spinal cord and trigeminal nucleus caudalis. J Comp Neurol 1995;356:327 344.
65. Carlton SM, LaMotte CC, Honda CN, et al: Ultrastructural analysis of substance P and other synaptic profiles innervating an identified primate spinothalamic tract neuron. Neurosci Abstr 1985;11:578.
66. Mantyh PW, DeMaster E, Malhotra A, et al: Receptor endocytosis and dendrite reshaping in spinal neurons after somatosensory stimulation. Science 1995;268:1629-1632.
67. Willis WD, Sluka KA, Rees H, et al: Cooperative mechanisms of neurotransmitter action in central sensitization. In Carli G, Zimmermann M (eds): Progress in Brain Research, Towards the Neurobiology of Chronic Pain, vol 110. New York, Elsevier, 1996, pp 151-166.
68. Willis WD, Sluka KA, Rees H, et al: A contribution of dorsal root reflexes to peripheral inflammation. In Rudomin P, Romo R, Mendell LM (eds): Presynaptic Inhibition and Neural Control. New York: Oxford University Press, 1998, pp 407-423.
69. Lima D, Coimbra A: The spinothalamic system of the rat: Structural types of retrogradely lablled neurons in the marginal zone (lamina I). Neuroscience 1988;27:215-230.
70. Lima D, Coimbra A: Morphological types of spinomesencephalic neurons in the marginal zone (lamina I) of the rat spinal cord, as shown after retrograde labelling with cholera toxin subunit B. J Comp Neurol 1989;279:327-339.
71. Lima D, Coimbra A: Structural types of marginal (lamina I) neurons projecting to the dorsal reticular nucleus of the medulla oblongata. Neuroscience 1990;34:591-606.
72. Lima D, Mendes-Ribeiro JA, Coimbra A: The spino-latero-reticular system of the rat: Projections from the superficial dorsal horn and structural characterization of marginal neurons. Neuroscience 1991;45:137-152.
73. Lima D, Avelino A, Coimbra A: Morphological characterization of marginal (lamina I) neurons immunoreactive for substance P, enkephalin, dynorphin and gamma-aminobutyric acid in the rat spinal cord. J Chemical Neuroanat 1993;6: 43-52.
74. Zhang ET, Craig AD: Morphology and distribution of spinothalamic lamina I neurons in the monkey. J Neurosci 1997;17:3274-3284.
75. Zhang ET, Han ZS, Craig AD: Morphological classes of spinothalamic lamina I neurons in the cat. J Comp Neurol 1996; 367:537-549.
76. Han ZS, Zhang E-T, Craig AD: Nociceptive and thermoreceptive lamina I neurons are anatomically distinct. Nat Neurosci 1998;1:218-225.

77. Yu XH, Zhang E-T, Craig AD, et al: NK-1 receptor immuno-reactivity in distinct morphological types of lamina I neurons of the primate spinal cord. J Neurosci 1999;19:3545-3555.

78. Willis WD, Coggeshall RE: Sensory Mechanisms of the Spinal Cord, vol 2, 3rd ed. New York, Plenum Press, 2004.

79. Surmeier DJ, Honda CN, Willis WD: Natural groupings of primate spinothalamic neurons based upon cutaneous stimulation. Physiological and anatomical features. J Neurophysiol 1988;59:833-860.

80. Westlund KN, Carlton SM, Zhang D, et al: Glutamate-immunoreactive terminals synapse on primate spinothalamic tract cells. J Comp Neurol 1992;322:519-527.

81. Battaglia G, Rustioni A: Substance P innervation of the rat and cat thalamus. II. Cells of origin in the spinal cord. J Comp Neurol 1992;315:473-486.

82. Coffield JA, Miletic V: Immunoreactive enkephalin is contained within some trigeminal and spinal neurons projecting to the rat medial thalamus. Brain Res 1987;425:380-383.

83. Nahin RL: Immunocytochemical identification of long ascending peptidergic lumbar spinal neurons terminating in either the medial or lateral thalamus in the rat. Brain Res 1988;443:133-138.

84. Ju G, Melander T, Ceccatelli S, et al: Immunohistochemical evidence for a spinothalamic pathway co-containing cholecystokinin- and galanin-like immunoreactivities in the rat. Neuroscience 1987;20:439-456.

85. Leah J, Menétrey D, De Pommery J: Neuropeptides in long ascending spinal tract cells in the rat: Evidence for parallel processing of ascending information. Neuroscience 1988;24:195-207.

86. Carlton SM, Westlund KN, Zhang D, et al: Calcitonin gene-related peptide containing primary afferent fibers synapse on primate spinothalamic tract cells. Neurosci Lett 1990;109:76-81.

87. Carlton SM, Westlund KN, Zhang D, et al: GABA-immunoreactive terminals synapse on primate spinothalamic tract cells. J Comp Neurol 1992;322:528-537.

88. LaMotte CC, Carlton SM, Honda CN, et al: Innervation of identified primate spinothalamic tract neurons: Ultrastructure of serotonergic and other synaptic profiles. Neurosci Abstr 1988;14:852.

89. Lekan H, Carlton SM: Glutamatergic and gabaergic input to rat spinothalamic tract cells in the superficial dorsal horn. J Comp Neurol 1995;361:417-428.

90. Westlund KN, Carlton SM, Zhang D, et al: Direct catecholaminergic innervation of primate spinothalamic tract neurons. J Comp Neurol 1990;299:178-186.

91. Westlund KN, Carlton SM, Zhang D, et al: Vasopressin innervation of monkey spinothalamic tract neurons. Abstract. VIth World Congress on Pain, Adelaide, Australia, 1990.

92. Ye Z, Westlund KN: Glycine-like Immunoreactive terminals contacting spinothalamic tract neurons in rat spinal cord. Soc Neurosci Abstr 1998;24:387.

93. Abbadie C, Trafton J, Liu H, et al: Inflammation increases the distribution of dorsal horn neurons that internalize the neurokinin-1 receptor in response to noxious and non-noxious stimulation. J Neurosci 1997;17:8049-8060.

94. Ye Z, Westlund KN: Ultrastructural localization of glutamate receptor subunits (NMDAR1, AMPA GluR1 and GluR2/3) and spinothalamic tract cells. NeuroReport 1996;7:2581-2585.

95. Ye Z, Westlund KN: Relationships of NMDA, AMPA, and metabotropic types of glutamate receptor subunits to spinothalamic tract cells: Light and EM studies. Neurosci Abstr 1996;22:868.

96. Honda CN, Perl ER: Functional and morphological features of neurons in the midline region of the caudal spinal cord of the cat. Brain Res 1985;340:285-295.

97. Applebaum AE, Beall JE, Foreman RD, et al: Organization and receptive fields of primate spinothalamic tract neurons. J Neurophysiol 1975;38:572-586.

98. Apkarian AV, Hodge CJ: Primate spinothalamic pathways: III. Thalamic terminations of the dorsolateral and ventral spinothalamic pathways. J Comp Neurol 1989;288:493-511.

99. Craig AD, Bushnell MC, Zhang ET, et al: A thalamic nucleus specific for pain and temperature sensation. Nature 1994;372:770-773.

100. Bennett GJ, Seltzer Z, Lu GW, et al: The cells of origin of the dorsal column postsynaptic projection in the lumbosacral enlargements of cats and monkeys. Somatosensory Res 1983;1:131-149.

101. Al-Chaer ED, Lawand NB, Westlund KN, et al: Pelvic visceral input into the nucleus gracilis is largely mediated by the postsynaptic dorsal column pathway. J Neurophysiol 1996;76:2675-2690.

102. Al-Chaer ED, Lawand NB, Westlund KN, et al: Visceral nociceptive input into the ventral posterolateral nucleus of the thalamus: A new function for the dorsal column pathway. J Neurophysiol 1996;76:2661-2674.

103. Raboisson P, Dallel R, Bernard JF, et al: Organization of efferent projections from the spinal cervical enlargement to the medullary subnucleus reticularis dorsalis and the adjacent cuneate nucleus: A PHA-L study in the rat. J Comp Neurol 1996;367:503-517.

104. Villanueva LD, Bouhassira D, Bing D, et al: Convergence of heterotropic nociceptive information onto subnucleus reticularis dorsalis neurons in the rat medulla. J Neurophysiol 1988;60:980-1009.

105. Menetrey D, Roudier F, Besson JM: Spinal neurons reaching the lateral reticular nucleus as studied in the rat by retrograde transport of horseradish peroxidase. J Comp Neurol 1983;220:439-452.

106. Chaouch A, Menétrey D, Binder D, et al: Neurons at the origins of the medial component of the bulbopontine spinoreticular tract in the rat: an anatomical study using horseradish peroxidase retrograde transport. J Comp Neurol 1983;214:309-320.

107. Westlund KN, Craig AD: Association of spinal lamina I projections with brainstem catecholamine neurons in the monkey. Exp Brain Res 1996;110:151-162.

108. Cechetto DF, Standaert DG, Saper CB: Spinal and trigeminal dorsal horn projections to the parabrachial nucleus in the rat. J Comp Neurol 1985;240:153-160.

109. Bernard, JM, Huang GF, Besson JM: The parabrachial area: Electrophysiological evidence for an involvement in visceral nociceptive processes. J Neurophysiol 1994;71:1646-1660.

110. Clark FM, Proudfit HK: Projections of noradrenergic neurons in the A5 catecholamine cell groups to the spinal cord in the rat: Anatomical evidence that A5 neurons modulate nociception. Brain Res 1993;616:200-210.

111. Westlund KN, Sorkin LS, Ferrington DG, et al: Serotoninergic and noradrenergic projections to the ventral posterolateral nucleus of the monkey thalamus. J Comp Neurol 1990;295:197-207.

112. Basbaum AI, Fields HL: Endogenous pain control systems: Brainstem spinal pathways and endorphin circuitry. Annu Rev Neurosci 1984;7:309-338.

113. Zhang D, Carlton SM, Sorkin LS, et al: Collaterals of primate spinothalamic tract neurons to the periaqueductal gray. J Comp Neurol 1990;296:277-290.

114. Craig AD: Distribution of brainstem projections from spinal lamina I neurons in the cat and the monkey. J Comp Neurol 1996;361:225-248.

115. Keay KA, Feil K, Gordon BD, et al: Spinal afferents to functionally distinct periaqueductal gray columns in the rat: An anterograde and retrograde tracing study. J Comp Neurol 1997;385:207-229.

116. Rees H, Roberts MHT: The anterior pretectal nucleus: A proposed role in sensory processing. Pain 1993;53:121-135.

117. Christensen M, Willis WD, Westlund KN: Anterior pretectal nucleus projections to pontine catecholamine cell regions. Neurosci Abstr 1997;23:157.

118. Ren Y, Lu Y, Yang H, et al: Responses of neurons in central lateral thalamic nucleus to visceral stimulation in rats. Soc Neurosci Abst 346.8/T3, 2006.

119. Hsu DT, Price JL: Midline and intralaminar thalamic connections with the orbital and medial prefrontal networks in macaque monkeys. J Comp Neurol 2007;504:89-111.

120. Cliffer KD, Burstein R, Giesler GJ: Distributions of spinothalamic, spinohypothalamic, and spinotelencephalic fibers revealed by anterograde transport of PHA-L in rats. J Neurosci 1991;11:852-868.

121. Burstein R, Potrebic S: Retrograde labeling of neurons in the spinal cord that project directly to the amygdala or the orbital cortex in the rat. J Comp Neurol 1993;335:469-485.

122. Newman HM, Stevens RT, Apkarian AV: Direct spinal projections to limbic and striatal areas: Anterograde transport studies from the upper cervical spinal cord and the cervical enlargement in squirrel monkey and rat. J Comp Neurol 1996;365:640-658.

123. Sawchenko PE, Swanson LW: The organization of noradrenergic pathways from the brainstem to the paraventricular and supraoptic nuclei in the rat. Brain Res 1982;257:275-325.

124. Petrov T, Krukoff TL, Jhamandas JH: Branching projections of catecholaminergic brainstem neurons to the paraventricular hypothalamic nucleus and the central nucleus of the amygdala in the rat. Brain Res 1993;609:81-92.

125. Saper CB, Levisohn D: Afferent connections of the median preoptic nucleus in the rat: Anatomical evidence for a cardiovascular integrative mechanism in the anteroventral third ventricle. Brain Res 1983;288:21-31.

126. Fallon JH, Koziel DA, Moore RY: Catecholamine innervation of the basal forebrain. II. Amygdala, suprarhinal cortex and entorhinal cortex. J Comp Neurol 1978;180:509-532.

127. Bernard JF, Dallel R, Raboisson P, et al: Organization of the efferent projections from the spinal cervical enlargement to the parabrachial area and periaqueductal gray: A PHA-L study in the rat. J Comp Neurol 1995;353:480-505.

128. Nauta HJM, Kuypers HGJM: Some ascending pathways in the brainstem reticular formation. In Jasper HH, Proctor LD, Knighton RS, et al (eds): Reticular Formation of the Brain. Boston, Little Brown, 1958, pp 3-30.

129. Reynolds DV: Surgery in the rat during electrical analgesia induced by focal brain stimulation. Science 1969;164:444-445.

130. Mayer DJ, Wolfe TL, Akil H, et al: Analgesia from electrical stimulation in the brain stem of the rat. Science 1971;174:1351-1354.

131. Liebeskind JC, Guilbaud G, Besson JM, et al: Analgesia from electrical stimulation of the periaqueductal gray matter in the cat: Behavioral observations and inhibitory effects on spinal cord interneurons. Brain Res 1973;50:441-446.

132. Oliveras JL, Besson JM, Guilbaud G, et al: Behavioral and electrophysiological evidence of pain inhibition from midbrain stimulation in the cat. Exp Brain Res 1974;20:32-44.

133. Oliveras JL, Woda A, Guilbaud G, et al: Inhibition of the jaw opening reflex by electrical stimulation of the periaqueductal gray matter in the awake, unrestrained cat. Brain Res 1974;72:328-331.

134. Oliveras JL, Redjemi F, Guilbaud G, et al: Analgesia induced by electrical stimulation of the inferior centralis nucleus of the raphe in the cat. Pain 1975;1:139-145.

135. Proudfit HK, Anderson EG: Morphine analgesia: Blockade by raphe magnus lesions. Brain Res 1975;98:612-618.

136. Basbaum AI, Clanton CH, Fields HL: Opiate and stimulus-produced analgesia: Functional anatomy of a medullospinal pathway. Proc Natl Acad Sci U S A 1976;73:4685-4688.

137. Basbaum AI, Clanton CH, Fields HL: Three bulbospinal pathways from the rostral medulla of the cat: An autoradiographic study of pain modulating systems. J Comp Neurol 1978;178:209-224.

138. Beall JE, Martin RF, Applebaum AE, et al: Inhibition of primate spinothalamic tract neurons by stimulation in the region of the nucleus raphe magnus. Brain Res 1976;114:328-333.

139. Willis WD, Haber LH, Martin RF: Inhibition of spinothalamic tract cells and interneurons by brain stem stimulation in the monkey. J Neurophysiol 1977;40:968-981.

140. Basbaum AI, Fields HL: Endogenous pain control mechanisms: Review and hypothesis. Ann Neurol 1978;4:451-462.

141. Willis WD: Control of nociceptive transmission in the spinal cord. In Ottoson D (ed): Progress in Sensory Physiology 3. Berlin, Springer-Verlag, 1982.

142. Besson JM, Chaouch A: Peripheral and spinal mechanisms of nociception. Physiol Rev 1987;67:67-186.

143. Morgan C, Nadelhaft I, De Groat WC: The distribution of visceral primary afferents from the pelvic nerve to Lissauer's tract and the spinal gray matter and its relationship to the sacral parasympathetic nucleus. J Comp Neurol 1981;201:415-440.

144. Urban MO, Jiang MC, Gebhart GF: Participation of central descending nociceptive facilitatory systems in secondary hyperalgesia produced by mustard oil. Brain Res 1996;737:83-91.

145. Zhuo M, Gebhart GF: Biphasic modulation of spinal nociceptive transmission from the medullary raphe nuclei in the rat. J Neurophysiol 1997;78:746-758.

146. Urban MO, Gebhart GF: Supraspinal contributions to hyperalgesia. Proc Natl Acad Sci U S A 1999;96:7687-7692.

147. Porreca F, Burgess SE, Gardell LR, et al: Inhibition of neuropathic pain by selective ablation of brainstem medullary cells expressing the mu-opioid receptor. J Neurosci 2001;21:5281-5288.

148. Burgess SE, Gardell LR, Ossipov MH, et al: Time-dependent descending facilitation from the rostral ventromedial medulla maintains, but does not initiate, neuropathic pain. J Neurosci 2002;22:5129-5136.

149. Vera-Portocarrero LP, Zhang ET, Ossipov MH, et al: Descending facilitation from the rostral ventromedial medulla maintains nerve injury-induced central sensitization. Neuroscience 2006;140:1311-1320.

150. Vera-Portocarrero LP, Xie J, Kowal J, et al: Descending facilitation from the rostral ventromedial medulla maintains visceral pain in rats with experimental pancreatitis. Gastroenterology 2006;130:2155-2164.

151. Oliveras JL, Guilbaud G, Besson JM: A map of serotoninergic structures involved in stimulation producing analgesia in unrestrained freely moving cats. Brain Res 1979;164:317-322.

152. Bowker RM, Steinbusch HWM, Coulter JD: Serotonergic and peptidergic projections to the spinal cord demonstrated by a combined retrograde HRP histochemical and immunocytochemical staining method. Brain Res 1981;211:412-417.

153. Bowker RM, Westlund KN, Coulter JD: Origins of serotonergic projections to the spinal cord in rat: An immunocytochemical-retrograde transport study. Brain Res 1981;226:181-199.

154. Yeoman DC, Proudfit HK. Projections of substance P-immunoreactive neurons located in the A7 catecholaminergic cell group of the rat. Pain 1990;48:1389-1397.

155. Holden JE, Proudfit HK: Enkephalin neurons that project to the A7 catecholamine cell group are located in nuclei that modulate nociception: Ventromedial medulla. Neuroscience 1998;83:929-947.

156. Stevens RT, Hodge CJ Jr, Apkarian AV: Kölliker-Fuse nucleus: The principal source of pontine catecholaminergic cells projecting to the lumbar spinal cord of cat. Brain Res 1982;239:589-594.

157. Westlund KN, Bowker RM, Ziegler MG, et al: Noradrenergic projections to the spinal cord of the rat. Brain Res 1983;263:15-31.

158. Clark FM, Proudfit HK: Projections of neurons in the ventromedial medulla to pontine catecholamine cell groups involved in the modulation of nociception. Brain Res 1991;540:105-115.

159. Carlton SM, Honda CN, Willcockson WS, et al: Descending adrenergic input to the primate spinal cord and its possible role in modulation of spinothalamic cells. Brain Res 1991;543:77-90.

160. Depaulis A, Bandler R (eds): The Midbrain Periaqueductal Gray Matter: Functional, Anatomical, and Neurochemical Organization. New York: Plenum Press, 1991.

161. Cameron AA, Khan IA, Westlund KN, et al: The efferent projections of the periaqueductal gray in the rat: A *Phaseolus*

vulgaris-leukoagglutinin study. II. Descending Projections. Neurosci Lett 1995;351:1-17.

162. Green PG, Kitchen I: Antinociception opioids and the cholinergic system. Progr Neurobiol 1986;26:118-146.

163. Bannon AW, Porsolt RD, Williams M, et al: Broad spectrum, non-opioid analgesic activity by selective modulation of neuronal nicotinic acetylcholine receptors. Science 1998;279:77-81.

164. Ribeiro-da-Silva A, Cuello AC: Choline acetyltransferase-immunoreactive profiles are pre-synaptic to primary sensory fibers in the rat superficial dorsal horn. J Comp Neurol 1990;295:370-384.

165. Beitz AJ: The organization of afferent projections to the midbrain periaqueductal gray of the rat. Neuroscience 1982;7:133-159.

166. Meller ST, Dennis BJ: Afferent projections to the periaqueductal gray in the rabbit. Neuroscience 1986;19:927-964.

167. Veening J, Buma P, Ter Horst GJ, et al: Hypothalamic projections to the PAG in the rat: Topographical, immuno-electromiscroscopical and functional aspects. In Depaulis A, Bandler R (eds): The Midbrain Periaqueductal Gray Matter: Functional, Anatomical, and Neurochemical Organization. NATO ASI Series A, Life Sciences, vol 213. New York, Plenum Press, 1991, pp 387-415.

168. Shipley MT, Ennis M, Rizvi TA, et al: Topographical specificity of forebrain inputs to the midbrain periaqueductal gray: Evidence for discrete longitudinally organized input columns. In Depaulis A, Bandler (eds): The Midbrain Periaqueductal Gray Matter: Functional, Anatomical, and Neurochemical Organization. NATO ASI Series A, Life Sciences, vol 213. New York, Plenum Press, 1991, pp 417-448.

169. Jones AKP, Brown WD, Friston KJ, et al: Cortical and subcortical localization of response to pain in man using positron emission tomography. Proc R Soc Lond B 1991;244:39-44.

170. Casey KL, Minoshima S, Berger KL, et al: Positron emission tomographic analysis of cerebral structures activated specifically by repetitive noxious heat stimuli. J Neurophysiol 1994;71:802-807.

171. Casey KL, Minoshima S, Morrow TJ, et al: Comparison of human cerebral activation pattern during cutaneous warmth, heat pain, and deep cold pain. J Neurophysiol 1996;76:571-581.

172. Coghill RC, Talbot JD, Evans AC, et al: Distributed processing of pain and vibration by the human brain. J Neurosci 1994;14:4095-4108.

173. Davis KD, Taylor SJ, Crawley AP, et al: Functional MRI of pain- and attention-related activations in the human. J Neurophysiol 1997;77:3370-3380.

174. Rainville P, Duncan GH, Price DD, et al: Pain affect encoded in human anterior cingulate but not somatosensory cortex. Science 1997;277:968-971.

175. Svensson P, Minoshima S, Beydoun A, et al: Cerebral processing of acute skin and muscle pain in humans. J Neurophysiol 1997;78:450-460.

176. Silverman DHS, Munakata JA, Ennes H, et al: Regional cerebral activity in normal and pathological perception of visceral pain. Gastroenterology 1997;112:64-72.

177. Friedman DP, Murray EA, O'Neill JB, et al: Cortical connections of the somatosensory fields of the lateral sulcus of macaques: Evidence for a corticolimbic pathway for touch. J Comp Neurol 1986;252:323-347.

CHAPTER
8   A Review of Pain-Processing Pharmacology

Tony L. Yaksh

In the early 1900s, Sir Charles Sherrington designated high-intensity stimuli that signaled a potential injury to the body as being nociceptive. The application of such stimuli to the body produces a discrete pain sensation referred to the site of stimulation, and the psychophysical magnitude of the report or response covaries with the intensity of the stimulus. Termination of the stimulus prior to injury will result in cessation of the sensation. Should the stimulus be of sufficient magnitude as to result in local injury (e.g., tissue disruption, plasma extravasation), a pain sensation will persist after removal of the stimulus and the injury will be accompanied by an increased sensitivity to subsequent stimuli applied to the injury site (primary hyperalgesia) and an enhanced sensitivity to stimuli applied at sites adjacent to the injury (e.g., secondary hyperalgesia).

These effects of a high-intensity, tissue-injuring stimulus reflect an initial activation of the primary afferents that project to the dorsal horn of the spinal cord, where there is a release of transmitters that activate a complex dorsal horn circuitry. Under normal circumstances, these spinal neurons respond maximally to input arising from the root projecting to the spinal segments in which the cell lies. However, whereas these afferents primarily activate these homosegmental neurons, they also send collaterals rostrally and caudally up to several spinal segments, where they make synaptic contact with neurons in adjacent segments (heterosegmental). These distal neurons are less efficiently activated than the homosegmental cells, and may not be activated sufficiently to generate an action potential, but together these homosegmental and heterosegmental cells form the real or potential dimension of the dermatome of that spinal segment. As will be shown later, if the excitability of these distal heterosegmental neurons is increased, cells that were not activated by a given input now become depolarized and the size of the dermatome of a given segment will be increased. These dorsal horn neurons then project by long tracts in the ventrolateral quadrant either directly to diencephalic sites (e.g., thalamus, hypothalamus) or indirectly though an intermediate synapse on neurons in the medulla, pons, or mesencephalon, which then project to various diencephalic and limbic forebrain sites. The anatomical details of these pathways have been previously discussed (see Chapter 7).

In general, the processes leading to a pain state secondary to a high-intensity peripheral stimulus reflect the frequency of traffic that appears in these spinofugal pathways. The activity in the spinofugal systems are primarily dependent on the intensity of the afferent stimulus but, as will be evident, various systems serve to increase the gain of the spinal input-output function whereas others serve to depress this gain. In the first case, we would anticipate that there would be an increased pain sensation associated with any given stimulus; in the second case, however, the pain sensation produced by a given stimulus would be diminished. This dynamic property of the input-output system represents an important characteristic of systems that process nociceptive stimuli. The following sections present a consideration of the transmitter pharmacology that defines these synaptic linkages.

PRIMARY AFFERENT SIGNALING

Acute Stimulation

The systems underlying this acute psychophysical experience start with the primary afferent. In the absence of a stimulus, most primary afferents show little if any ongoing activity. Physical stimuli activate specific populations of primary afferents. The nature of the sensory information encoded by a given primary afferent is dependent on the properties of the transduction channel or receptors expressed on the terminals of that axon. Thus, the intensity of the message is encoded by the specific population of primary afferents activated and the frequency of discharge. As reviewed elsewhere, large fast-conducting primary afferents (A-beta) are typically activated by low-intensity mechanical stimuli and many small myelinated (A-delta) or unmyelinated (C) fibers are activated by high-intensity thermal or mechanical stimuli, or both. The myelinated afferent axon therefore displays specialized terminals that are

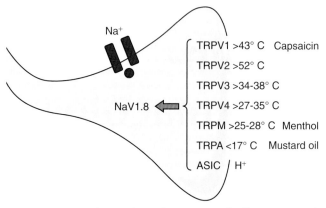

Figure 8–1. Transducer channels on a small-afferent terminal. Optimal stimulus intensities for channel activation and various chemicals that also activate these channels are indicated. Different terminals express different combinations of channels; these would define the response properties of that afferent channel activation, which leads to activation of voltage-sensitive sodium (NaV) channels. The NaV1.8 subtype of channels is frequently present only in unmyelinated axons (C-fibers). ASIC, acid-sensing channel.

particularly sensitive to mechanical distortion, leading to a local increase in sodium current depolarizing the axon. Unmyelinated afferent axons typically show "free nerve endings"—for example, they display no evident morphologic specialization. However, these terminals express specific transducer channels that are sensitive over ranges of stimulus intensities. When activated by the appropriate stimulus, these channels activate voltage-sensitive sodium (NaV) channels passing Na^+ and initiating action potentials (Fig. 8–1). As shown in the figure, some channels that transduce a physical stimulus may also be activated by various chemicals. In that case, these chemicals produce a sensation reflective of the physical stimulus transduced by that channel (e.g., the TRPV1 receptor is activated by capsaicin, which produces a painful burning sensation, but menthol activates a cold receptor, which initiates the sensation of a low temperature).

Tissue-injuring Stimuli

High-intensity stimuli may result in local tissue injury. Such injury will lead to cellular disruption and injury to local vascular integrity, resulting in plasma extravasation and a migration of inflammatory cells, such as macrophages and neutrophils, and giving rise to the release of various active factors (Box 8–1). These products act through eponymous receptors that are present on the terminals of many unmyelinated axons. Activation of these receptors initiates two events: (1) depolarization of the terminal, leading to afferent discharge, with the frequency of activation dependent on concentration; and (2) activation of intraterminal processes (phosphorylation of local membrane channels), which sensitizes the terminal

so that the degree of depolarization for a given stimulus is enhanced. Such effects produce spontaneous afferent activity and an enhanced response to a second stimulus applied to the injury site. These changes, in the milieu of the peripheral terminal, occur secondary to tissue damage and the accompanying extravasation of plasma because of an increased permeability of the capillary wall (see Box 8–1). These events are responsible for the triple response—reddening at the site of the stimulus reflecting local arterial dilation, local edema (increased capillary permeability), and regional reduction in the magnitude of the stimulus required to elicit a pain response (i.e., hyperalgesia).

Nerve Injury as a Stimulus

Following nerve injury arising from various insults, the organisms will over time frequently display the development of highly aversive spontaneous sensations. These ongoing sensations are believed to arise in part from afferent traffic. Sensory axons typically display little spontaneous activity in the absence of a stimulus; this is particularly true for small high-threshold afferents. However, after a chemical, immune, or mechanical injury to the nerve, afferent axons display (1) an initial bursting afferent activity, (2) electrical silence for an interval of hours to days, and (3) the appearance over hours to days of spontaneous bursting activity in myelinated and unmyelinated axons. This ongoing activity is a reflection of the initial dying back of the injured axon (retrograde chromatolysis) followed by the initiation of sprouting. Collections of these sprouts form neuromas. Recordings from the afferent axon indicate that the ongoing activity originates after an interval of days to weeks from the lesioned site (neuroma) and from the dorsal root ganglion (DRG) of the injured nerve. A number of changes occur, which can lead to prominent alterations in ongoing afferent activity.

Altered Channel Expression

Channels in the sensory afferent can modulate excitability. Two major classes are the sodium channel, which carries the primary current for axonal depolarization, and potassium channels. Activation of such potassium channels can reduce axon excitability. Clearly, an upregulation of sodium channels or a downregulation of potassium channels would have the net effect of increasing axon excitability.

Sodium Channels
A large increase in the expression of sodium channels occurs after nerve injury in the neuroma and the dorsal root ganglia. Several sodium channel variants exist in primary afferent neurons, including subtypes NaV1.6, NaV1.7, and NaV1.9. Those designated as resistant to the sodium channel blocker tetrodotoxin

BOX 8–1. AGENTS RELEASED BY TISSUE INJURY THAT DEPOLARIZE AND SENSITIZE SMALL PRIMARY AFFERENT TERMINALS

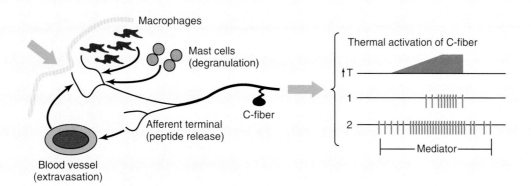

Mediators listed below are released by injury from macrophages, mast cells, and blood vessels. They evoke spontaneous activity in otherwise silent C-fibers and lower threshold to activation in response to a ramped thermal stimulus and enhance the response to any given stimulus (Right: 1 vs. 2). These interactions are mediated by eponymous receptors or channels that trasduce the presence of the product to a terminal depolarization.

1. Amines. Histamine (mast cells, basophils, and platelets) and serotonin (mast cells and platelets) are released by various stimuli, including mechanical trauma, heat, radiation, and certain products of tissue damage.
2. Kinin. Bradykinin is synthesized by cascade-triggered activation of factor XII by agents such as kallikrein and trypsin and by physical trauma. It acts via specific bradykinin receptors (B1, B2).
3. Lipidic acids. Tissue injury activates widely distributed phospholipases, which free arachidonic acid (AA). AA is a substrate for a large family of enzymes, such as cyclooxygenase, to synthesize lipid mediators, including prostaglandin E_2 (PGE_2), PGI_2, and thromboxane A_2 (TXA_2), all of which can facilitate the excitability of C-fibers through specific membrane receptors.
4. Cytokines. Cytokines such as tumor necrosis factor α and interleukins (e.g., interleukin-1β) are released by inflammatory cells (macrophages) and sensitize C-fibers through eponymous binding sites.
5. Proteinases. Thrombin or trypsin is released from inflammatory cells and activates specific receptors (e.g., proteinase-activated receptors).
6. Neurotrophic factors. Nerve growth factor (NGF) will activate primary afferent terminals by binding to tyrosine kinase A. NGF is released from fibroblasts and mast cells by injury and inflammation.
7. [H], [K]. Elevated H^+ (low pH) and high K^+ concentrations are found in injured tissue. Channels present on C-fibers (e.g., TRPV1, acid-sensing channels [ASICs]), are activated by H^+. Acid pH potentiates terminal activation by noxious heat and other chemical mediators. Many of these channels also respond to natural products. Thus, the TRPV1 receptor responds to capsaicin.
8. Primary afferent peptides. Calcitonin gene-related peptide and substance P are found in and released from the peripheral terminals of C-fibers. These peptides produce vasodilation, plasma extravasation, and degranulation of mast cells through their respective receptors. This leads to local reddening and swelling in skin innervated by the stimulated sensory nerve.

(TTX), NaV1.8, and Nav1.9 are found primarily in small DRG cells (C-fibers). These channels mediate slow-activating and slow-inactivating sodium currents. The importance of some of these in nerve injury pain states is suggested by knockdown studies, in which reduction of a sodium channel (e.g., Nav1.8) has no effect on baseline pain thresholds but reverses nerve injury–evoked pain states in animal models. In human and animal models, systemic lidocaine in plasma at concentrations with no effect on conduction will block ectopic activity and attenuate the hyperpathic state observed after nerve injury. Such results confirm the importance of these upregulated sodium channels in the post–nerve injury pain state.

Potassium Channels
Following nerve injury, potassium currents have been shown to be reduced, suggesting a downregulation of these channels. Potassium channel blockers can increase and potassium channel agonists can decrease ectopic firing after peripheral nerve injury.

Changes in Chemical Sensitivity of Neuroma and Dorsal Root Ganglion

Sprouted terminals of an injured axon display sensitivity to a number of humoral factors, such as prostanoids, catecholamines, and cytokines (e.g., tumor necrosis factor α [TNFα]). This sensitivity is involved in the appearance of ongoing activity, as shown by the following examples. These are though to contribute to the development of spontaneous afferent traffic after peripheral nerve injury. Such afferent input thus provides the basis for the origin of sensory experiences after nerve injury.

Cytokines

After nerve injury, the release of cytokines, particularly TNFα, is noted from local inflammatory cells. These cytokines directly activate the nerve and neuroma through eponymous receptors, which become expressed in the membrane after the nerve injury. The mechanism of the TNFα interactions are multiple and complicated. Acutely, TNFα decreases potassium conductance in neurons, whereas longer term effects may be initiated through the activation of various kinases (e.g., mitogen-activated protein kinases [MAPKs]). Behaviorally, application of TNFα to the nerve results in hyperalgesia, whereas systemic delivery of TNFα binding protein reduces free TNFα, thus decreasing pain behavior in neuropathic pain animal models.

Catecholamines

Following nerve injury, postganglionic sympathetic efferents sprout into the injury site. In response to the release of nerve growth factor (NGF) released from local Schwann cells and inflammatory cells, these postganglionic terminals locally release catecholamines. Physiologic studies have shown that following nerve injury, stimulation of postganglionic axons will excite the injured axon and DRG of the injured axon; this activation is blocked by α-adrenergic antagonism. After nerve injury, upregulation of the expression of α_1-adrenergic receptors has been demonstrated. Accordingly, increased catecholamine concentrations in the vicinity of the DRG or injured neuroma can translate to enhanced activity.

Prostaglandin Receptor

Prostanoids are released by inflammatory cells secondary to tissue injury. They can enhance the opening of NaV1.8 TTX-insensitive sodium channels by acting through eponymous receptors on the afferent terminal.

First-order Synapse

Primary afferents enter the spinal dorsal horn. Large afferents (A-beta) terminate deep to Rexed lamina 3 of the dorsal horn. A-delta afferent fibers terminate both superficially and in deeper laminae, whereas C-fibers generally terminate superficially in laminae I and II (marginal layer and substantia gelatinosa).

Primary Afferent Transmitters

It has been classically appreciated that primary afferent input results in a postsynaptic excitatory event, emphasizing that the primary afferent transmitters are uniformly excitatory. Generally, it appears that the principal primary afferent neurotransmitter evoking acute excitation is glutamate. It is contained in synaptic vesicles of most spinal afferent terminals and its synthetic enzymes have been identified in almost every primary afferent dorsal root ganglion cell body, regardless of size or state of myelination. These acute effects are mediated by the DL-α-amino-3-hydroxyl-5-methyl-4-isoxazole propionic acid (AMPA)-type glutamate ionophore present on the second-order neuron. This receptor produces a robust but short-lasting depolarization of the postsynaptic membrane by increasing sodium conductance (Table 8–1).

In addition to glutamate, populations of primary afferents may contain and release various neuropeptides, notably substance P (sP), calcitonin gene-related peptide (CGRP), and even certain growth factors, such as brain-derived nerve growth factor (BDNF). Given the complexity of the coding, it is likely that nociceptive information is processed by various transmitters. The transmitters in these small high-threshold afferents display several general properties:

1. Consistent with their location in small-afferent terminals, high levels of peptides are present in laminae I and II. These levels are reduced by rhizotomy and/or ganglionectomy, or by treatment with the small-afferent neurotoxin capsaicin. The sensitivity of these afferents to capsaicin indicates that one important characteristic of many, but not all, C-fibers is the expression of the TRPV1 (capsaicin) receptor. A second population of C-fibers that does not express the TRPV1 receptor typically expresses a second marker (IB4). These IB4-positive afferents typically project to the deeper layers of the dorsal horn and do not express neuropeptides.
2. Glutamate and many peptides are cocontained and coreleased (e.g., glutamate, sP, CGRP) in the same C-fiber terminal.
3. The release is dependent on the opening of the voltage-sensitive calcium channel and the magnitude of release is proportional to stimulus frequency.
4. Iontophoretic application onto the dorsal horn of glutamate and the peptides found in primary afferents will produce postsynaptic excitation. Amino acids produce a rapid, short-lasting depolarization, whereas peptides produce a delayed and long-lasting discharge (see Table 8–1).

Regulation of Dorsal Horn Excitability

As noted, the intensity of the pain stimulus is encoded in the projection to higher centers by the frequency of the output function. Accordingly, factors that

Table 8–1.   Summary of Primary Afferent Transmitter Organization

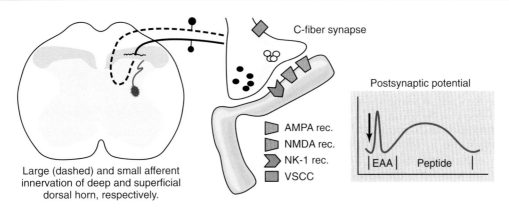

Large (dashed) and small afferent innervation of deep and superficial dorsal horn, respectively.

PRIMARY AFFERENT TRANSMITTER	RECEPTOR	POSTSYNAPTIC ACTION
Peptides		
Substance P	Neurokinin 1 (NK-1)	G protein–coupled; slow, long-lasting depolarization
CGRP	CGRP1	
Growth Factors		
BDNF	TRK B	Depolarizes, activates tyrosine kinase (TRK) cascade
Purine		
Adenosine triphosphate (ATP)	P2X receptor (P2X1-7)	Ligand-gated ion channels that differ in ion selectivity, gating properties
	P2Y receptor (P2Y1-14)	Metabotropic G protein–coupled receptors
Excitatory Amino Acids		
Aspartate, glutamate	AMPA receptor	Sodium ionophore; rapid, short-lasting depolarization; gates sodium A subtype of the AMPA receptor; can also gate calcium
	NMDA receptor	Calcium ionophore; slow onset, long- lasting; gates calcium

AMPA, DL-α-amino-3-hydroxyl-5-methyl-4-isoxazole propionic acid; BDNF, brain-derived nerve growth factor; CGRP, calcitonin gene-related peptide; EAA, excitatory amino acids; NMDA, *N*-methyl-D-aspartate; VSCC, voltage-sensitive calcium channel

enhance the excitability of spinal afferent terminals, leading to increased transmitter release, or of the dorsal horn projection neuron will increase the apparent magnitude of a given stimulus. Factors that diminish the excitability of the primary afferent or projection neurons will lead to a reduction in the apparent stimulus intensity. The following section will consider substrates that enhance and diminish the dorsal horn response to a given stimulus.

Facilitation of Dorsal Horn Excitability

Persistent small (C-fiber) but not large (A fiber) afferent activation of lamina I (marginal cell) and lamina V (wide dynamic range), as occurs with tissue injury and inflammation, has been shown to enhance the response to subsequent dorsal horn input and increase the receptive field of the activated neurons. Thus, the conditioning afferent input increases the receptive field size of the neurons, so that afferent input from dermatomal areas that previously did not activate the given neuron now evokes a prominent response. Moreover, low-threshold tactile stimulation also becomes increasingly effective in driving these neurons. The phenomena first described by

Lorne Mendell and Patrick Wall in the mid-1960s is broadly referred to as "windup."

These physiologic effects are believed to underlie the psychophysic correlates of tissue injury, wherein tissue injury leads to hyperalgesia and secondary hyperpathias (e.g., increased sensitivity to stimuli applied outside the area of injury). The relevance of this small-afferent–evoked facilitation to humans has been emphasized by psychophysical studies. Here, local activation of C-fibers by intradermal injection of capsaicin, an agent that uniquely activates populations of C-fibers possessing the TRPV1 receptor (see Fig. 8–1), leads to an initial pain report, followed for an extended period by a surrounding region showing enhanced mechanical and thermal sensitivity. This effect is blocked by a transient local anesthetic block of the nerves innervating the capsaicin-injected area. These observations emphasize that ongoing small-afferent input can initiate a central sensitization of pain processing.

Based on these studies, a reduction in C-fiber–evoked excitation in the dorsal horn produced by reducing the release of small-afferent transmitters or blocking the postsynaptic receptor (e.g., AMPA for glutamate) will diminish the magnitude of the afferent drive and, accordingly, diminish the facilitated processing evoked by protracted small-afferent input. The facilitated state, however, reflects more than the repetitive activation of a simple excitatory system.

Glutamate Receptors and Spinal Facilitation

The first actual demonstration of the unique pharmacology of the facilitated state showed that spinal windup is prevented by the spinal delivery of antagonists for the N-methyl-D-aspartate (NMDA) receptor, a glutamate ionophore composed of a number of subunits that is potently excitatory. When activated, it passes many Ca^{2+} and Na^+ currents. An important observation is that NMDA antagonists have no effect on acute evoked activity, but reduce windup evoked by repetitive C-fiber stimulation. Correspondingly, behavioral studies have revealed that such drugs had no effect on behavior evoked by acute noxious stimuli, but reduced the hyperalgesia observed after tissue injury and inflammation.

The absence of an effect of NMDA antagonism on the acute afferent–evoked activation or pain state reflects an important property of this receptor. At resting membrane potentials, the NMDA receptor displays a block of the channel by Mg^{2+}. Occupancy of the NMDA receptor by glutamate will not activate the ionophore in the presence of Mg^{2+}. In the presence of ongoing depolarization of the membrane, as produced during repetitive stimulation secondary to the activation of AMPA and sP receptors, the Mg^{2+} block is removed. If several allosteric binding sites on the NMDA ionophore are occupied (e.g., glycine, polyamine sites), glutamate may now activate the NMDA channel, permitting the passage of Ca^{2+} and Na^+ currents. This opening thus serves to depolarize the membrane further and, importantly, to increase intracellular Ca^{2+} concentration, which serves to initiate downstream components of the excitatory and facilitatory cascade (see later).

Downstream Cascades
Primary afferent C-fibers release peptide (e.g., sP, CGRP), purine (e.g., adenosine triphosphate, ATP), and excitatory amino acid (e.g., glutamine) products. These peptides and excitatory amino acids evoke excitation in second-order neurons. As noted for glutamate, direct monosynaptic excitation is mediated by AMPA receptors (i.e., acute primary afferent excitation of wide dynamic range [WDR] neurons is not mediated by the NMDA or neurokinin 1 [NK-1] receptor). This initial activation leads to enabling of the NMDA ionophore and complex cascades are consequently engaged, which reflects processes activated in the postsynaptic neuron. Several examples of such facilitatory cascades initiated by the repetitive small-afferent input are summarized here.

Local Neuronal Circuits. The best example of a cascade initiated by the small-afferent input is activation of the *NMDA receptor.* As noted, in the presence of ongoing membrane depolarization, the NMDA iono-

phore loses its Mg block and acts to allow the large increase in intracellular Ca^{2+} concentration.

Although the *AMPA receptor* is largely considered to be an ionophore that allows the acute passage of sodium, there are structural variants on the AMPA receptor that allow it to pass calcium. These calcium-permeable AMPA receptors are believed to participate with the NMDA receptor in various aspects of spinal facilitation.

Neurokinin 1 receptors are G protein–coupled receptors that are activated by substance P released from small primary afferents. Activation of these receptors leads to prolonged depolarization and a mobilization of intracellular calcium. The spinal delivery of agents that block the NK-1 site for substance P can diminish windup and significantly reduce the second-phase response to intradermal formalin injection.

Prostaglandin Cascade. The increase in the intracellular calcium concentration helps promote the transmigration of various phospholipases to the membrane, where they cleave arachidonic acid. Arachidonic acid serves as a substrate for cyclooxygenase to produce various prostanoids. All these enzymes have been found to be constitutively expressed in the spinal neurons and non-neuronal cells. This cascade leads to the release of a number of prostaglandins (PGs), which act on eponymous receptors located presynaptically on the primary afferent terminal and postsynaptically on the higher order neurons. The presynaptic effect has been shown to enhance the opening of voltage-sensitive calcium channels (VSCCs) that mediate vesicular mobilization and transmitter release. A postsynaptic mechanism of action has been shown that attenuates the activation of inhibitory glycine receptors. This leads to a loss of regulatory inhibition that otherwise limits the postsynaptic activation (Fig. 8–2).

Nitric Oxide Synthase. Small-afferent input also leads to the activation of nitric oxide synthase (NOS). Neuronal and inducible NOS are present in neurons and other cells. In the presence of arginine, there is the formation of nitric oxide (NO), which diffuses to act presynaptically (retrograde transmission) through cyclic glucose monophosphate (GMP) to enhance transmitter release (e.g., glutamate). These events can serve to increase terminal release and increase postsynaptic excitation (see Fig. 8–2).

Phosphorylation. Small-afferent input increases intracellular Ca^{2+} concentration in second-order neurons. This leads to the activation of a number of protein kinases (PKs), such as PKC and PKA, or MAPK (Fig. 8–3). There are many isoforms of these kinases, which act to phosphorylate consensus sites on various proteins. PKC has been shown to phosphorylate amino acids sites on NMDA and AMPA receptors, which tends to lower the threshold for activation, leading to greater membrane permeability. In the case of the NMDA ionophore, it acts to lower the threshold for the removal of the Mg block that otherwise prevents

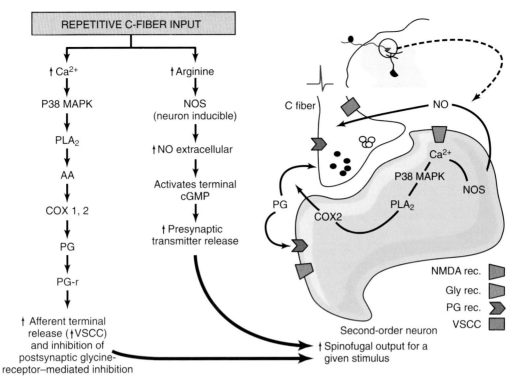

Figure 8–2. Small-afferent input activates second-order neurons, leading to increased intracellular calcium concentration, which initiates several intracellular cascades. In the left column, activation of phospholipase A_2 (PLA_2) increases free arachidonic acid (AA). This serves as a substrate for cyclooxygenase (COX1 and COX2), which leads to prostaglandin (PG) release. These act on eponymous prostanoid receptors located presynaptically on the primary afferent terminal and postsynaptically on the higher order neurons. See text for details. In the right column, activation of nitric oxide synthase (NOS) in the presence of arginine leads to the nitric oxide (NO) that diffuses to enhance transmitter release (e.g., glutamate). These events can serve to increase terminal release and increase postsynaptic excitability. cGMP, cyclic guanine monophosphate; Gly, glycine; NMDA, N-methyl-D-aspartate; P38 MAPK, P38 mitogen-activated protein kinase; rec., receptor; VSCC, voltage-sensitive calcium channel.

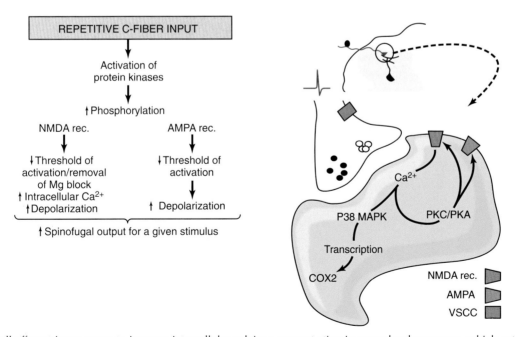

Figure 8–3. Small-afferent input serves to increase intracellular calcium concentration in second-order neurons, which activates a protein kinase (PK) such as PKC and PKA or a mitogen-activated protein kinase (MAPK), which acts to phosphorylate various proteins. Specifically, in this schematic, PKC, NMDA, and AMPA receptors are phosphorylated, leading to lower activation thresholds. P38 MAPK, when activated, phosphorylates phospholipase A_2 (PLA_2), leading to its activation (see Fig. 8–2); this also helps activate transcription factors that increase the synthesis of various proteins, such as cyclooxygenase (COX). AMPA, DL-α-amino-3-hydroxyl-5-methyl-4-isoxazole propionic acid; NMDA, N-methyl-D-aspartate; rec., receptor.

channel activation. P38 MAPK, when activated, phosphorylates phospholipase A$_2$ (PLA$_2$), leading to its activation (see Fig. 8–2); this activates various transcription factors, such as NFKβ, which acts to increase the synthesis of various proteins, such as cyclooxygenase (COX).

Bulbospinal Pathways. Of particular interest has been the growing appreciation that small-afferent input can initiate facilitated activation through spinobulbospinal linkages (Fig. 8–4). Thus, C-fibers make synaptic contact with superficial dorsal horn neurons (lamina I neurons). These project into the brainstem to make synaptic contact with medullary midline raphe spinal neurons, which are serotonergic. These cells project into the spinal dorsal horn and make synaptic contact with a number of neuronal populations but, importantly, those with cell bodies in the deep dorsal horn (lamina V). The serotonergic projections act through excitatory 5-hydroxytryptamine 3 (5-HT$_3$) receptors to enhance the firing of these lamina V neurons. These cells are noted for their ability to display a facilitated state—called windup block—of this bulbospinal linkage; the use of 5-HT$_3$ inhibitors has been reported to reduce this facilitated state.

Non-neuronal Cells

In the CNS, there are wide variety of non-neuronal cells. Among these are astrocytes and microglia; together with neurons, they form a complex network in which each can influence the excitability of the other (Fig. 8–5).

Transmitter Mediators of Non-neuronal Cell Activation. Primary afferents and intrinsic neuron transmitters (glutamate, ATP, sP) can overflow from the synaptic cleft to these adjacent non-neuronal cells and lead to their activation, which can result in the release of chemokines, such as fractalkine. Astrocytes may communicate with microglia by the release of a number of products, including glutamate, cytokines, and S-100 protein. These products have eponymous receptors that can produce changes in the biology of the astrocytes and microglial cells, leading to the extracellular movement of various neuroactive products, such as free radicals, cytokines (interleukin-1β [IL-1β] and TNFα), and lipid mediators (e.g., arachidonic acid, platelet-activating factor, prostaglandins, leukotrienes). Astrocytes have the well-known ability to regulate extracellular glutamate though an active uptake system. Conversely, during certain activation or stresses, these intracellular glutamate stores can be released, leading to significant increases in extracellular glutamate concentrations.

Gap Junctions. Astrocytes may communicate over a distance by the spread of excitation through local nonsynaptic contacts, referred to as gap junctions.

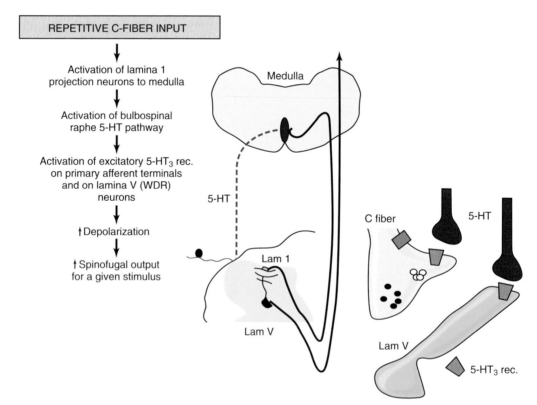

Figure 8–4. Small-afferent–evoked activation of lamina (lam) I neurons that project into the medullary raphe nuclei, exciting bulbospinal serotonin (5-hydroxytryptamine, 5-HT) pathways that activate excitatory 5-HT$_3$ receptors on lamina V neurons. This projection serves to facilitate the firing of these lamina V projection neurons and may underlie the phenomenon of windup. Rec., receptor; WDR, wide dynamic range.

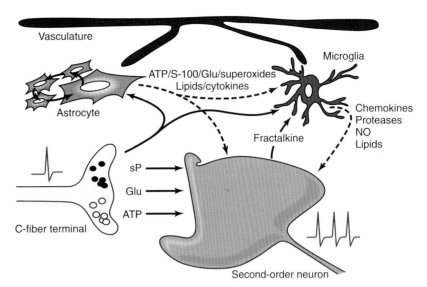

Figure 8–5. Complex assemblage relating astrocytes, microglia, and neurons. Products released from neurons can activate the release of active products from astrocytes and microglia. Astrocytes can activate other astrocytes through gap junctions, as well as microglia, and can induce the excitability of neurons by the release of active factors. As indicated, postsynaptic neuronal activation can lead to the release of chemokines, such as fractalkine, which can act on eponymous receptors on microglia. See text for details. ATP, adenosine triphosphate; Glu, glutamine; NO, nitric oxide; sP, substance P.

These junctions represent specialized proteins—hexagonal multimers made up of connexin macromolecules—that act to link the adjacent membranes of two cells. Through such linkages, local excitation in one astrocyte can lead to increased Ca^{2+} reversal of a glutamate transporter, increased extracellular ATP, which can depolarize local neuronal processes and produce local cerebrovascular constriction. While classically limited to astrocytes, it is presently evident that such linkages may also occur between astrocytes and neuron and microglia. The gap junctions thus represent a mechanism whereby a syncytium of cells can communicate local gradients' excitability to other non-neuronal cells, microvessels, and neurons.

Circulating Factors. Finally, after tissue injury and inflammation, circulating cytokines (e.g., IL-1β, TNFα) can activate perivascular astrocytes and microglia. As noted, microglia are brain-residing macrophages, and such activation can initiate changes in local neuronal excitability. These mechanisms are believed to provide an important linkage for the somatic sensations associated with systemic infections (e.g., as in the course of a common cold or the flu).

The relevance of the non-neuronal cell population to the facilitation process in pain processing after peripheral injury is supported by various observations. First, peripheral injury and inflammation will lead to the acute and chronic activation of microglia and astrocytes. Thus, P38 MAPK is present in microglia and shows activation within minutes after a peripherally injuring stimulus. Over longer periods of time, other markers of microglia (e.g., OX42) and astrocytes (e.g., glial fibrillary acidic protein [GFAP]) show a significant increase in expression. Drugs such as minocycline (a second-generation tetracycline) and pentoxifylline have been reported to block microglial activation and diminish hyperalgesic states. Similar metabolic inhibitors that block astrocyte activation (e.g., fluorocitrate) can similarly diminish hyperalgesia after nerve and tissue injury.

These agents, although not clinically implemented, suggest important directions in drug therapy development. The role of non-neuronal cells in regulating neuronal excitability has been increasingly cited in the past several years, but it should be noted that the importance of such glial-neuronal circuits in brain function was strongly argued by Robert Galambos in the early 1950s.

Importance of Facilitatory Systems to Injury-evoked Pain

The preceding section has reviewed a number of systems that act to increase the gain of the spinal transmission system. This facilitation has two interrelated functions. First, it helps explain in part the mechanisms whereby a peripheral injury, which leads to repetitive small-afferent input, can result in a potent hyperalgesic state (i.e., there is an enhanced response to any subsequent afferent stimulus). Second, following local injury, there is frequently the development of enlarged receptive fields that extend beyond the territory of the original injury. The dermatome for any given root is represented in part by spinal collaterals of afferents that project to neurons in an adjacent segment. When these cells undergo facilitation, the input from distal dermatomes becomes sufficient to drive activity in these cells. The receptive field of that cell consequently incorporates this distal body surface.

Therefore, it is not surprising that agents targeted at these facilitatory mechanisms can have profound effects on injury-induced pain states. Agents such as COX inhibitors are an important example for emphasizing the role of the facilitated state in the pain experience. COX inhibitors act to diminish hyperesthesia secondary to tissue injury. This reaction reflects on the important role of prostaglandins, released not only in the periphery but in the spinal cord, where they can act to facilitate the release of C-fiber transmitters, such as sP. Current evidence has suggested that COX1 and COX2 are important constitutive enzymes in the spinal systems. Spinal COX2 inhibitors appear particularly important in regulating injury-induced spinal facilitation. However, research has also indicated other facilitatory mechanisms that may also be useful targets in the development of future agents. The potency of NOS inhibitors on behavior suggests the importance of spinal NO release in facilitatory processes leading to hyperalgesia. Agents that inhibit microglial and astrocyte activation can also diminish hyperalgesic states, as mentioned earlier and, although not clinically useful or defined as safe after spinal delivery, could help in future studies for the development of drug therapies.

As a final caveat to this discussion of neuraxial facilitation, it is important to note that central facilitation studies examining the effects of repetitive C-fiber stimulation on dorsal horn neurons (see earlier) are typically carried out in animals that are under a surgical plane of anesthesia (usually isoflurane or halothane). It has been demonstrated that behavioral models of facilitation using a systemic anesthetic (e.g., barbiturate, volatile agent) show that the hyperalgesic state may be initiated in spite of the fact that the injury is carried out under anesthetic. The relevance of this observation to the performance of surgery on patients anesthetized with volatile anesthetics or barbiturates alone is clear. These agents, although preventing the ascending pain message, surprisingly do not appear to block the facilitatory processes initiated by small-afferent input, likely at the level of transmitter release at the first spinal synapse. This lack of anesthetic effect on primary afferent release is believed to represent the basis for the concept of preemptive analgesia, using such therapeutic approaches as regional anesthesia or opiates. As noted later, opiates have as a primary target the presynaptic terminal of the C-fiber primary afferent.

PHARMACOLOGY OF SPINAL INHIBITION

Second-order dorsal horn neurons (WDR neurons) receive excitatory input from large afferents as well as from excitatory interneurons. This input is typically mediated by glutamate. Output from the spinal dorsal horn evoked by such excitation is subject to an upregulation of excitability, but it has long been appreciated that these cells are also subject to mechanisms that downregulate local excitability. Here the pharmacology of such processes will be considered.

Local Inhibitory Circuits

These are systems that are local to the dorsal horn and that regulate local excitability.

Inhibitory Amino Acids

Based on the effects of various inhibitory amino acid antagonists, it appears that the excitatory effect of primary afferents, including small but especially large

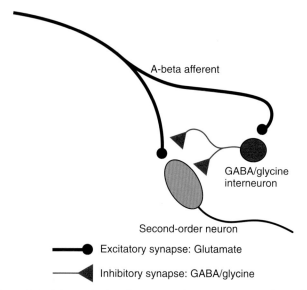

Figure 8–6. Schematic showing pre- and postsynaptic regulation by glycine and gamma-aminobutyric acid (GABA) interneurons of A-beta input onto a second-order dorsal horn neuron.

(A-beta) afferents, are subject to potent inhibition expressed by inhibitory gamma-aminobutyric acid (GABA) and glycine receptors, which are presynaptic on the primary afferent and postsynaptic on the second-order neuron. This relationship is indicated in Figure 8–6. Release of GABA and glycine from local interneurons will act on GABA A and GABA B receptors and glycine receptors, respectively. The GABA A and glycine receptors are ionophores that, when activated, help increase Cl^- conductance. Based on resting transmembrane Cl^- gradients, such an increase in permeability, leads to modest membrane hyperpolarization and an increase in shunting current. These effects serve to reduce the ability of an excitatory input to depolarize the cell. GABA B receptors are G protein–coupled receptors that are also inhibitory. The relevancy of this ongoing inhibitory organization to ongoing sensation is evidenced by the fact that local application of GABA A (bicuculline) or glycine (strychnine) receptor inhibitors will lead to powerful augmentation of the discharge of dorsal horn neurons evoked by large-afferent (A-beta) input.

Opioids

The potent analgesic effects of opiates reveal the efficient role played by opiate receptors in regulating pain transmission. Systematic studies have shown that opiate receptors that regulate the pain response are located at the spinal level and in several brain loci.

Spinal Opiate Action

The intrathecal delivery of opiate agonists will potently inhibit the injury-evoked discharge of superficial and deep dorsal horn neurons evoked by small high-threshold afferents (C-fiber). The deep dorsal

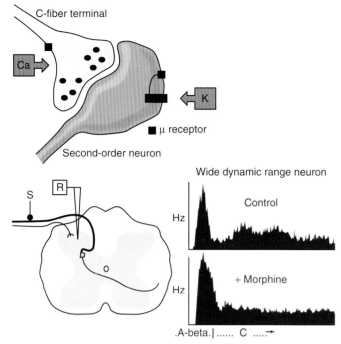

Figure 8–7. Opioid receptors are located pre- and postsynaptically on small primary afferents, terminating in the substantia gelatinosa. A local action of opioids in the spinal cord will selectively depress the discharge of spinal dorsal horn neurons activated by small (high-threshold, longer latency) but not large (low-threshold, short latency) afferents. C, C-fiber; R, recording electrode; S, stimulating electrode.

horn neurons also receive input from low-threshold large (A-beta) afferents; this evoked component is not usually blocked by opiates. These effects are mediated by an action on opioid receptors (typically characterized as μ-opioid receptors, based on the agonist and antagonist pharmacology). Location of these μ receptors has revealed them to be largely on C-fiber primary afferents that terminate in the superficial dorsal horn and on the dendrites and cell bodies of deeper dorsal horn neurons (Fig. 8–7).

Intrathecal administration will reliably attenuate the response of an animal to unconditioned somatic and visceral stimuli that otherwise evoke an organized escape behavior in all species. Confirmation of the presynaptic action has been provided by the observation that opiates reduce the release of primary afferent peptide transmitters, such as substance P, contained in small afferents. The presynaptic action corresponds to the ability of opiates to prevent the opening of voltage-sensitive Ca^{2+} channels, thereby preventing transmitter mobilization and release. A postsynaptic action is demonstrated by the ability of opiates to block the excitation of dorsal horn neurons evoked by glutamate, reflecting a direct activation of the dorsal horn. The activation of potassium channels leading to a membrane hyperpolarization is consistent with a direct postsynaptic inhibition.

Supraspinal Opiate Action

Direct injection of opiates into the brain has shown that opioid receptors that modulate pain behavior are found in several restricted brain regions, includ-

ing the amygdala and midline medulla, but the best characterized of these supraspinal sites is the mesencephalic periaqueductal gray (PAG). Microinjections of opiates into this region will block nociceptive responses in a naloxone-reversible fashion. Several mechanisms exist whereby opiates acting in the PAG may alter nociceptive transmission:

1. Activation of bulbospinal projection. In the PAG, opiate receptors are presynaptic on GABAergic terminals that inhibit projection to the medulla. Morphine acts to block GABA release, releasing the inhibitory control over PAG outflow. The PAG has excitatory projections into the medulla, which then activates bulbospinal noradrenergic and serotonergic pathways. The noradrenergic projection acts through spinal α_2 receptors to reduce dorsal horn excitation.
2. Opiate binding within the PAG. This may be preterminal on the ascending spinofugal projection. Such a preterminal action would inhibit input into the medullary and mesencephalic cores.
3. Outflow from the PAG. This can serve to act to increase excitability of the dorsal raphe and locus coeruleus–lateral tegmental nuclei from which ascending serotonergic and noradrenergic projections, respectively, originate to project to limbic forebrain. These projections are considered to modulate emotionality (see later). The mechanisms are summarized in Figure 8–8.

Endogenous Opiates

Opiate receptors are presumed to be targeted by endogenous compounds released from local interneurons. A number of such functionally qualified families of agents have been identified according to the family of prohormones from which they are derived—pro-enkephalin (enkephalins), prodynorphins (dynorphins), and pro-opiomelanocortins (β-endorphins). Other endogenous opioids have also been described, such as the endomorphins. These are all peptides that have been shown to have a significant affinity for one or more of the several identified opioid receptors. Enkephalins have been found in dorsal horn interneurons and in bulbospinal pathways. Such interneuronal systems are present throughout the brain. β-Endorphin is present in long projection pathways, which largely originate in the hypothalamus. Although opiate receptors can regulate spinal nociceptive processing, there is surprisingly little evidence to suggest that the endogenous systems have a robust effect on pain processing. Naloxone, an opioid antagonist, has modest effects on ongoing pain processing. Enkephalins, however, are rapidly metabolized by peptidases and peptidase inhibitors have been shown to alter pain thresholds in a naloxone-reversible fashion in animal models.

Bulbospinal Projection Systems

Various transmitters are known to be contained in and released from bulbospinal projecting pathways. Those that have been characterized best are the monoamines norepinephrine and serotonin.

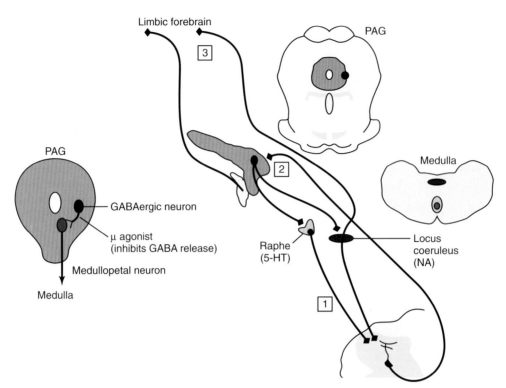

Figure 8–8. Lower left, Schematic of organization of opiate action within the periaqueductal gray. μ-Opioid actions block release of gamma-aminobutyric acid (GABA) from tonically active systems that otherwise regulate projections to the medulla, leading to an activation of periaqueductal gray (PAG) outflow. **1,** Excitatory outflow from the PAG activates bulbospinal projections, releasing serotonin and/or noradrenaline at the spinal level. **2,** Preterminal opioid binding within the PAG on the ascending spinofugal projection. **3,** Outflow from the PAG increases excitability of the dorsal raphe and locus coeruleus, from which ascending serotonergic and noradrenergic projections originate to project to the limbic forebrain. 5-HT, 5-hydroxytryptamine; NA, noradrenaline.

Bulbospinal Norepinephrine

Norepinephrine projections to the spinal cord arise from lateral medullary sites and the locus coeruleus, whereas the norepinephrine projections to the forebrain arise from the locus coeruleus (see Fig. 8–8). The rostral projections are believed to play the primary role in altering the affective components of behavior. The caudal adrenergic projections play a principal role in regulating spinal nociceptive processing through an action on spinal dorsal horn α_2 receptors, which are located pre- and postsynaptically to the primary afferent. The spinal delivery of α_2 adrenoceptor agonists such as clonidine and dexmedetomidine produce a significant analgesia. This spinal action of an α_2 agonist is mediated by a mechanism similar to that of spinal opiates, but the receptor is distinct: (1) α_2 binding is presynaptic on C fibers and postsynaptic on dorsal horn neurons; (2) α_2 receptors can depress the release of C-fiber transmitters; and (3) α_2 agonists can hyperpolarize dorsal horn neurons through a Gi-coupled potassium channel.

Bulbospinal Serotonin

Serotonin (5-HT) arises from the nucleus raphe magnus, which projects spinally, and the raphe dorsalis, which provides the principal source for forebrain 5-HT. As noted earlier, spinopetal 5-HT projections can have multiple effects, including excitation and inhibition. These complex effects suggest that under certain conditions, increasing spinal 5-HT tone may facilitate nociceptive processing.

Altering Terminal Monoamine Concentrations

Importantly, agents that regulate the extracellular concentrations of these monoamines can have pronounced effects on emotional tone and nociceptive transmission. Because extracellular levels depend not only on release but on reuptake, agents that block the reuptake transporter, such as the tricyclic antidepressants, can have analgesic properties. Current evidence suggests that the analgesic actions are largely mediated through the effect on norepinephrine, not on serotonin. This difference in their relative contributions to analgesic efficacy may reflect the several opposing effects associated with the action of serotonin.

PHARMACOLOGY OF FACILITATORY STATES SECONDARY TO NERVE INJURY

In the preceding sections, it was evident that events that occur following peripheral tissue injury can lead to a potent facilitation of neuraxial processing. Such facilitation results in large part from persistent small-afferent traffic that is seen with the local injury and inflammation. These changes reflect events in the injured nerve, with the alteration of protein expression leading to an upregulation of some proteins and a downregulation of others. The increased spontaneous activity arising from the neuroma and the DRG provides a tentative explanation for the ongoing dysesthesia associated with various nerve injury conditions. The prominent finding that low-threshold tactile stimulation acquires an aversive component (e.g., tactile allodynia) appears to present a more complex set of events. It is currently hypothesized that the allodynia is mediated by low-threshold mechanosensitive (A-beta) afferents. As reviewed elsewhere, A-beta afferents carry information initiated by low-intensity, non–tissue-injuring mechanical stimuli. These afferents project centrally to terminate in the deeper layers of the dorsal horn, deep to laminae receiving small-afferent input. The precise mechanism of this involvement of low-threshold afferents in pain initiation is unknown, although several possibilities have been considered.

Cross-talk between Large and Small Afferents

Following nerve injury, cross-talk mediated by ephaptic contacts may develop between afferents in the DRG and neuroma. Here, depolarizing currents in one axon or DRG cell would generate a depolarizing voltage in an adjacent quiescent axon or DRG cell. In this manner, a large low-threshold afferent would drive activity in an adjacent high-threshold afferent.

Large Afferent Sprouting

As reviewed previously, large myelinated (A-beta) afferents project into the spinal Rexed lamina III and deeper. Small afferents (C-fibers) tend to project into spinal laminae I and II, a region populated by neurons responding to this high-threshold input. Following peripheral nerve injury, it has been argued that the central terminals of myelinated afferents (A fibers) sprout into lamina II of the spinal cord. With this synaptic reorganization, stimulation of low-threshold mechanoreceptors (A-beta fibers) could produce excitation of these neurons and be perceived as painful. Although an inviting hypothesis, the degree to which this sprouting occurs is considerably less prominent than originally reported.

Loss of Intrinsic Inhibitory Control

A large number of small interneurons lie in the superficial dorsal horn, which contain and release GABA and glycine. These terminals are presynaptic to the large central afferent terminal complexes and form reciprocal synapses, whereas GABAergic axosomatic connections have been identified on second-order and projection neurons (see Fig. 8–6). Accordingly these transmitters exert a powerful inhibitory control over the activity of A-beta primary afferent terminals and second-order neurons in the spinal dorsal horn. As discussed earlier, the importance of this local inhibitory circuitry is indicated by the observation that intrathecal delivery of a GABA A (bicuculline) receptor or glycine (strychnine) receptor antagonist evokes a powerful tactile allodynia. Such observations led to the hypothesis that nerve injury may evoke a loss of GABAergic-glycinergic neurons. Although some data do support a loss of such neurons, this loss appears to be minimal. Recent observations now suggest a second alternative. After nerve injury, spinal neurons are altered so that GABA A and glycine receptor activation becomes excitatory.

These receptors are chloride ionophores. When these ionophores are activated, Cl^- moves according to its transmembrane gradient. The transmembrane gradient is maintained by cotransporters that import or export Cl^-. After nerve injury, there is reduced activity of the chloride exporter, leading to an increase in intracellular Cl^- concentration. With such an increase in extracellular Cl^- concentration, increasing membrane chloride conductance, as occurs with GABA A receptor activation, causes a net outward movement of negative charge, leading to a membrane depolarization. Thus, paradoxically, afferent input that activates GABA A–glycine channels may actually serve to *facilitate* membrane depolarization, leading to a much enhanced response to the A-beta drive (Fig. 8–9). As reviewed elsewhere (Chapter 7), A-beta input makes synaptic contact with lamina V projection neurons. The fact that A-beta drive normally does not initiate a pain state probably depends on the intrinsic inhibition discussed earlier. As noted, removing that intrinsic inhibition with local receptor blockers leads to a powerful allodynia. With the change in chloride transporter activity, the system has not simply lost an intrinsic inhibition, but conceivably every GABA A or glycine synapse that was inhibitory is now excitatory. Thus, A-beta input, which originally drove this intrinsic inhibition, now drives an intrinsic excitation.

Glutamate Release

Spinal glutamate release plays an important role in post–nerve injury pain states. There is a significant enhancement in resting spinal glutamate secretion after nerve injury. This release is in accord with increased spontaneous activity in the primary afferent and with the loss of intrinsic inhibition, which may help modulate resting glutamate secretion (see below). The significance of this release is emphasized by several observations:
1. Intrathecally delivered glutamate will evoke a powerful tactile allodynia and thermal hyperalgesia though the activation of spinal NMDA and non-NMDA receptors.
2. The spinal delivery of NMDA antagonists has been shown to attenuate the hyperpathic states arising in animal models of nerve injury. NMDA receptor activation mediates an important facilitation in neuronal excitability.

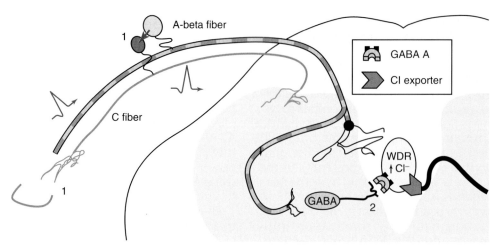

Figure 8–9. Two mechanisms believed to be associated with A-beta afferent–evoked pain processing. **1,** Cross-talk between large afferents and C-fibers. This cross-talk may occur at the level of the neuroma, the level of the dorsal root ganglion cell, or both. Afferent activity in the large A-beta axon or cell gives rise to depolarizing currents in the adjacent small axon. **2,** After nerve injury, there is a change in the activity of chloride exporters in dorsal horn neurons, which leads to an intracellular accumulation of chloride. This accumulation leads to a transmembrane distribution in which, when there is an increase in chloride conductance through the opening of a gamma-aminobutyric acid A (GABA A) or glycine receptor, the effect is not inhibition as it occurs normally, but depolarization. Thus, A-beta input becomes massively excitatory and the dorsal horn projection neurons are prominently activated. CI, chloride; WDR, wide dynamic range.

In addition, the NMDA receptor is a calcium ionophore, which, when activated, leads to prominent increases in intracellular calcium concentration. This initiates a cascade of events, including the activation of various enzymes (kinases), some of which phosphorylate membrane proteins (e.g., calcium channels and NMDA receptors) and others, such as MAPKs, help mediate intracellular signaling, which leads to the altered expression of various proteins and peptides (e.g., cyclooxygenase, dynorphin). Various factors have been shown to enhance glutamate release.

Spinal Dynorphin

Nerve injury leads to a prominent increase in spinal dynorphin expression. Intrathecal delivery of dynorphin can initiate the concurrent release of spinal glutamate and a potent tactile allodynia; the latter effect is reversed by NMDA antagonists. Although dynorphin is an endogenous opioid peptide, these effects appear to be independent of any action on an opiate receptor.

Altered Channel Expression

In the presence of nerve injury, there is an upregulation of sodium channels and a downregulation of potassium channels This assertion belies the enormous changes in channel expression associated with nerve injury. For example, it has been shown that after nerve injury there is a significant increase in the expression of the α^2-δ subunit. This subunit is found in the structures of several members of the VSCC family. At the spinal level, this binding site is densely present in the superficial dorsal horn in the substantia gelatinosa and DRG. The relevance of this increased expression is suggested by the potent anti-allodynic effects associated with the actions of gabapentin. This molecule appears to exert its effects by a highly selective binding to the α^2-δ subunit. N-type VSCCs also show an increase in expression, and the spinal delivery of N-type calcium channel blockers such as ziconotide also have potent antiallodynic effects.

Non-neuronal Cells and Nerve Injury

Astrocytes and microglia have been shown to play a powerful constitutive role in increasing synaptic excitability through the release of various active factors (see Fig. 8–5). After nerve injury, there is a significant activation of spinal microglia and astrocytes in the spinal segments receiving input from the injured nerves. This is manifested by morphologic changes in these cells, as well as by an increased expression of cellular markers for microglia (e.g., OX42, P38 MAPK) and GFAP for astrocytes. Of particular interest is that in the presence of pathology such as bone cancer, extravagant activation of these non-neuronal cells has been shown. Although the origin of this activation is not clear, it seems to involve increased afferent traffic and the release of excitatory transmitters, as well as products that appear to be increased secondary to nerve injury, such as growth factors. This activation of intracellular transcription factors acts to increase the spinal expression of COX, NOS, glutamate transporters, and proteinases and downregulate other systems, such as the chloride transporters discussed in the preceding section. Such biochemical components have been previously shown to play an important role in the facilitated state.

CONCLUSION

This chapter has focused on some aspects of the pharmacology of systems that regulate the processing of nociceptive stimuli. Broadly speaking, the output of this system is defined by the nature of the afferents that are activated and by the complex interplay between excitatory and inhibitory influences. Afferent transmitters are uniformly excitatory in nature and, for acute stimulation, the output is dependent on stimulus intensity. After tissue injury, the magnitude of the resulting pain state for any given stimulus reflects the development of spontaneous afferent traffic and sensitization of the peripheral terminal secondary to the release of local factors released from inflammatory cells, plasma extravasation, and injured cells. The output function is enhanced by a potent central (spinal) sensitization, which leads to an enhanced responsiveness of dorsal horn neurons that receive ongoing small-afferent traffic. This condition leads to an enhanced response to input from the injured receptive field and to an enlargement of the peripheral fields, which can now activate those neurons through originally ineffective subliminal input. This augmentation reflects not only local synaptic circuitry (glutamate, sP), but spinobulbospinal linkages (5-HT) and byproducts released from local non-neuronal cells. The afferent activation and sensitization are subject to regulation by systems such as those that regulate transmitter release from the primary afferent or that activate second-order or projection neurons.

In regard to events seen after nerve injury, it is evident that there are two principal elements—those that account for the spontaneous pain and those that lead to an alteration in the encoding of normally innocuous low-threshold mechanical stimuli. The spontaneous activity likely reflects the complex events that arise from channel expression and the inflammatory factors appearing after nerve injury that lead to ectopic activity. The alterations related to the facilitated response represent evident changes in dorsal horn function. The net effect appears to be an enhanced excitability that arises from increased expression of excitatory elements and a reduced inhibitory contribution. The change in chloride transporters and the activation of non-neuronal cells probably have a major role in the enhanced response displayed by the neuraxis after nerve injury. The increased excitation likely arises from a number of sources, including the activation of non-neuronal cells.

Importantly, agents that suppress the excitability of systems enhanced by injury or increase the inhibition that otherwise regulates this processing typically have predictable effects on the animal's response to a strong or injuring stimulus. Such covariation between pharmacology and pain behavior provides validation of the contribution of these respective mechanisms to the hypothesis that these systems regulate processing relevant to pain.

The discussion of the pharmacology of the substrates activated after tissue injury and nerve injury must be considered as a broad overview. More detailed considerations can be found in the reviews and texts listed below.

Suggested Readings

Dray A: Novel molecular targets in pain control. Curr Opin Anaesthesiol 2003;16:521-525.

McMahon SB, Jones NG: Plasticity of pain signaling: Role of neurotrophic factors exemplified by acid-induced pain. J Neurobiol 2004;61:72-87.

Suzuki R, Dickenson A: Spinal and supraspinal contributions to central sensitization in peripheral neuropathy. Neurosignals 2005;14:175-181.

Todd AJ: Anatomy of primary afferents and projection neurones in the rat spinal dorsal horn with particular emphasis on substance P and the neurokinin 1 receptor. Exp Physiol 2002; 87:245-249.

Watkins LR, Maier SF: Sickness responses to pathological pain. J Intern Med 2005;257:139-155.

Willis WD: Role of neurotransmitters in sensitization of pain responses. Ann N Y Acad Sci 2001;933:142-156.

Wood JN: Ion channels in analgesia research. Handb Exp Pharmacol 2007;177:329-358.

Yaksh TL: Central pharmacology of nociceptive transmission. In McMahon S, Koltzenburg M (eds): Wall and Melzack's Textbook of Pain, 5th ed. London, Churchill Livingstone, 2006, pp 371-414.

CHAPTER
9 Pain and Brain Changes

A. V. Apkarian

Change, alternatively referred to as reorganization or plasticity, is a fundamental property of the brain that enables it to adapt and thus enhance survival of the organism. It has been documented and studied across all the scales of the brain. The smallest unit of neural processing is the individual channel and its related receptor. Its efficacy can be modulated by various mechanisms, for example, changes in availability or concentration of various chemicals within the intracellular or extracellular environment. Such a change can lead to an increase either in the local resting membrane potential or, when it influences the excitability of the neuron, increased or decreased rate of firing. A change in either resting membrane potential or individual neuronal firing rate can in turn modulate individual synapse strengths, which can be experimentally demonstrated as phenomena called long-term potentiation (LTP) and long-term depression (LTD). Cumulative changes across these microscopic scales would in turn lead to reorganization of whole territories of the cortex in which one functional specialization may be abandoned and replaced by another. Several review articles highlight the recent excitement in the topic across multiple brain functional systems, from the single synapse to large-scale reorganization.[1-6] We now know that all of this happens in the human brain, perhaps more subtly in the adult than in the developing brain, and we also know that such events are fundamental to understanding the brain mechanisms of pain. We will revisit each of these mechanisms specifically in the context of pain perception.

Regarding pain, there has been a fundamental shift in our concepts of the functional role of the brain. Until about 15 years ago, most basic research in pain involved charting the "telephone lines" and the "code" for those lines. Basically most work in the field was an attempt to establish pain as a sensory modality with its unique pathways and presentation within the peripheral nervous system (PNS) and central nervous system (CNS). Chapter 7, on anatomy of pain systems, nicely demonstrates this knowledge and shows the distinct PNS and CNS components that participate in coding pain. This work has been highly successful in showing that unique receptors in the skin are involved in responding to mechanical, thermal, and chemical noxious stimuli. This information is transmitted through specialized myelinated and unmyelinated fibers to the spinal cord, where the nociceptive input converges on specific populations of cells, which in turn transmit the signal cephalad through multiple ascending pathways to give rise to the perception of pain. Descending modulatory pathways converge back on nociceptive neurons in the spinal cord and control their level of excitability based on environmental conditions. This is the "telephone line" view for pain perception, also known as the specificity theory for pain, which some researchers criticized for years as being too limited and simplistic in scope.[7-9] Its basic underlying assumption is a unidirectional information flow from the environment to the cortex through specific pathways, of which the disruption of any parts would break the telephone lines of communication and relieve pain. Within this viewpoint there is little space to accommodate some of the most debilitating clinical pain conditions, namely chronic pains, and in fact even the existence of these conditions was highly controversial for large portions of the past century. There remain hardcore scientists who still adhere to this notion[10]; however, the brunt of scientific evidence generated recently shows that plasticity of the brain and peripheral nerves is a fundamental component of pain, especially for clinical pains in general, and even more specifically for chronic pain. Recent studies have repeatedly uncovered that disruption of any of the PNS or CNS components of the network underlying pain perception, in most cases, results in exacerbation of pain behavior, rather than its diminution, in which the specific site and extent of injury result in mimicking, at least in part, various clinical pain conditions. Plasticity of PNS and CNS seems a universal consequence of persistent pain, the details of which depend on the types and extent of injury giving rise to the persistent pain, leading Woolf and Salter[11] to conclude: "All living organisms need to be able to react to noxious stimuli, and a major evolutionary drive for the development of a plastic nervous system might have been the acquisition of the capacity to detect and remember pain. (p. 1765)" This suggests the possibility that the ability of the brain to change was driven by its need to adapt to coping with pain, rather than the other way around.

ACUTE NOCICEPTION IN CONTRAST WITH PERSISTENT PAIN

Activation of the nociceptive system in the absence of PNS or CNS changes is supposed to happen only when short lasting stimuli (in the scale of a few seconds and not persisting for more than minutes) are applied that can evoke pain but do not cause inflammation or injury. Under such restricted conditions one expects to observe a primarily neuroelectric response, in which, depending on the stimulus, nerve endings of unmyelinated and small myelinated nociceptors are excited, in turn activating second-order spinal cord cells that project to multiple supraspinal sites. The best known and best characterized of these is the spinothalamic pathway, which has all the characteristics necessary for coding stimulus properties such as its location, intensity, and modality. The spinothalamic pathway also has classically been attributed with conveying the emotional properties of noxious stimuli,[12] although recent brain imaging studies are beginning to question this notion, at least in humans.[13,14] As soon as noxious stimuli increase in duration or intensity they are accompanied by inflammation or injury, which in turn results in a long list of PNS and CNS changes.

Definitions of General Pain Types

- **Nociceptive pain** refers to normal, acute pain perception evoked by short-lasting noxious stimuli in intact tissue, in the absence of peripheral or central sensitization.
- **Inflammatory pain** refers to pain following tissue injury but with no neural injury. Some group this under nociceptive, others under pathophysiologic pain. There is ample evidence of peripheral and central reorganization in such conditions; thus it cannot be regarded as normal pain.
- **Neuropathic pain** refers to pain after neural injury. Generally accepted as a pathophysiologic state, accompanied with peripheral and central reorganization.

Definitions of Abnormal Pain

- **Allodynia** is perception of pain by a stimulus that in the healthy organism is not painful.
- **Hyperalgesia** is an enhanced perception of pain for a stimulus that does evoke pain in the healthy organism but to a lesser extent.
- **Primary sensitization** is an enhanced sensation and related enhanced neuronal transmission within and around the site of injury, suggesting that the effect is a consequence of reorganization of neuronal signaling directly from the injury.
- **Secondary sensitization** is an enhanced sensation and neural transmission at body sites removed from the site of injury. This is usually attributed to changes in neuronal properties in the spinal cord where the end product of various changes leads to increased excitability of neurons involved in

transmitting nociceptive inputs cephalad. The process is assumed to be a result of reorganization of the spinal cord nociceptive circuitry.
- **Supraspinal sensitization** is the term used to distinguish between spinal and supraspinal changes in nociceptive coding. Such processes are assumed to change the cortical elements involved in pain perception. These in turn would modulate spinal cord processing of afferent nociceptive inputs through descending modulatory pathways.

INFLAMMATION AND RESPONSE CHANGES IN FREE-NERVE ENDINGS

Free-nerve endings terminating in the skin and viscera are the machinery for signaling local mechanical, thermal, and chemical changes[15,16] as well as modulating this local environment (Fig. 9–1). Thus even at the level of the afferent receptor, nociceptive afferents are involved in two-way communication. Moreover, these receptors undergo changes in their response properties that affect the trafficking of chemicals as well as sensitivity to local events. Free-nerve endings possess a long list of receptors (proteins that span the lipid bilayer membrane that separates extracellular and intracellular spaces) specialized for detecting the presence of specific chemicals or stimuli (Fig. 9–2) that act as agonists and by binding to the receptor either activate intracellular second messenger events or directly open the channel. To provide inflow of Na^+ ions, for example, the VR1 cation channel activates at around 43° C and is also sensitive to capsaicin and to acidity.[17,18] This process initiates a current that then generates an action potential that by propagating centrally into the spinal cord may in turn activate second-order neurons that transmit this information farther centrally. Injury or inflammation results in the local release of the "inflammatory soup," which includes peptides (bradykinin), neurotransmitters (serotonin), and neurotrophins (nerve growth factor). These factors interact with cell-surface receptors (see Fig. 9–2) activating the nociceptor. This, besides centrally transmitting the information, also initiates neurogenic inflammation by locally releasing various neurotransmitters, such as substance P and calcitonin gene-related peptide. Release of these substances by terminals of free endings of nociceptors induces local vasodilation and plasma extravasation, as well as activation of non-neuronal cells, like mast cells and neutrophils, all of which contribute to the inflammatory soup (Fig. 9–3) and further sensitize these peripheral nociceptors by binding to their respective receptors, thus enhancing intracellular processes.[11,19]

NEUROPATHIC PAIN AND PERIPHERAL CHANGES

Neuropathic pain is distinct from nociceptive and inflammatory pain conditions by the fact that the injury is itself neuronal, whereas inflammatory

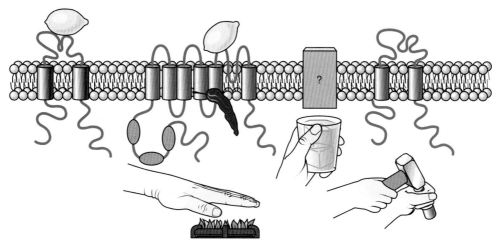

Figure 9–1. Nociceptors use a variety of signal-transduction mechanisms to transmit local mechanical, thermal, and chemical events. Change in local pH can be directly detected by a variety of types of receptors, while other receptors may be more specialized for mechanical deformation. The receptor for detecting cold pain remains controversial, although a number of candidates have been recently identified. The transient receptor potential vanilloid-1 (TRPV1) responds to noxious heat as well as to acidity, and to capsaicin, the pungent ingredient in chili pepper, and these three dimensions interact and enhance responses from each other. The large majority of free-nerve endings in the skin are called polymodal nociceptors because they contain multiple receptors and thus respond to various combinations of mechanical, heat, cold, and chemical stimuli. (Adapted from Julius D, Basbaum AI: Molecular mechanisms of nociception. Nature 2001;413:203-210, with permission.)

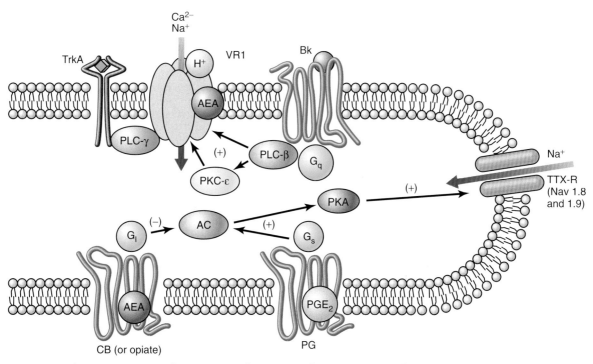

Figure 9–2. A variety of receptors spanning the nociceptive free-nerve ending interact intracellularly to either enhance or diminish excitability as a function of the extracellular milieu. If the nociceptor's environment changes as a result of inflammation or injury, its excitability is altered. The effect of such changes on the vanilloid receptor (VR1) and voltage-gated sodium channels (Nav 1.8 and 1.9) are illustrated. Extracellular increase in concentration for bradykinin (Bk) and nerve growth factor, acting through its own receptor (TrkA), shifts the excitability of VR1 to heat and to acidity through intracellular pathways. Similarly, inflammatory products like prostaglandin (PG) increase excitability of sodium channels through intracellular messengers, whereas cannabinoids or opiates (CB) counteract this effect. (Adapted from Julius D, Basbaum AI: Molecular mechanisms of nociception. Nature 2001;413:203-210, with permission.)

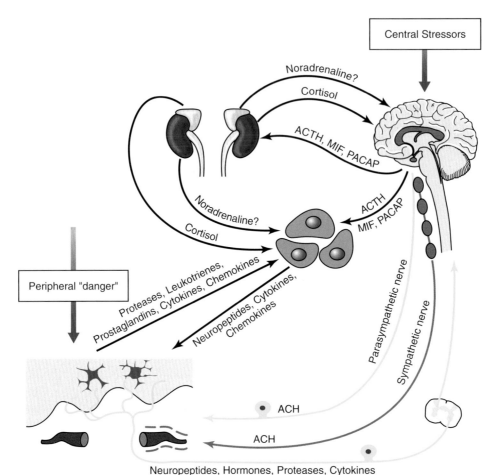

Figure 9–3. Inflammatory response at the skin is more complex than presented in the text. The figure illustrates the main components that influence local inflammatory responses in the skin. The skin is regarded as a neuroimmunoendocrine organ, and is associated with the peripheral nervous system (PNS), central nervous system (CNS), and autonomic nervous system. Stressors activate the hypothalamus/hypophysis in the CNS, releasing neuromediators such as adrenocorticotropic hormone (ACTH), as well as MIF and pituitary adenylate cyclase activating polypeptide (PACAP). They may stimulate either the release of norepinephrine and cortisol from the adrenal glands or directly stimulate leukocytes in the blood via CRH, MC, or PAC receptors, thereby modulating immune responses during inflammation. Norepinephrine and cortisol affect several immune cells including lymphocytes, granulocytes, and macrophages. Immune cells release cytokines, chemokines, and neuropeptides that modulate inflammatory responses in the skin. On stimulation, sensory nerves release neuromediators that modulate cutaneous inflammation and pain. Skin inflammation affects the activation of immune cells via cytokines, chemokines, prostaglandins, leukotrienes, nitric oxide, and melanocyte stimulating hormone (MSH), which may have a proinflammatory (for example, substance P), or anti-inflammatory effect (for example, calcitonin gene-related peptide), and PACAP by upregulating or downregulating inflammatory mediators such as cytokines. Autonomic nerves in the skin, mainly sympathetic cholinergic and rarely parasympathetic cholinergic nerves (ACH), innervate several cells in the skin, thereby maintaining skin homeostasis and regulating inflammation as well as host defense. CRH, corticotrophin releasing factor; MC, melanocortin; PAC, pituitary adenylate cyclase. (From Roosterman D, Goerge T, Schneider SW, et al: Neuronal control of skin function: The skin as a neuroimmunoendocrine organ. Physiol Rev 2006;86:1309-1379.)

injuries are caused by disease of non-neural tissue. Osteoarthritis is the prime example of a persistent (or chronic) non-neuropathic condition, whereas clinical conditions like postherpetic neuralgia and diabetic neuropathy are classic examples of neuropathic pain following metabolic disease or infection. When neuropathic pain is of central origin (e.g., after autoimmune disease, stroke, trauma, or cancer) it has been proposed that it occurs only if the central insult directly involves the nociceptive pathways.[20] The opposite does not seem to be true. That is, an injury of the nociceptive system does not imply the necessity of having pain. A partial lesion of a peripheral nerve commonly induces neuropathic pain.[21]

However, severing dorsal roots seems to have little chance of creating lasting pain.[22] Generally, neuropathic pain conditions are associated with abnormal neuronal activity at the site of the injury as well as with central sensitization.[23] Thus neuropathic pain is generally viewed as paradoxical because it involves severing portions of the nociceptive system, and thereby usually causing various types of sensory deficits, which rather than decreasing pain transmission results in long sustained increased pain as a result of reorganization of peripheral and central neural elements participating in pain perception.

When neuropathic pain is a consequence of injury to the PNS, the extent to which it depends on peripheral in contrast to central sensitization continues to be debated, with strong evidence provided for both views. Mechanisms underlying such conditions have been extensively studied and peripheral and central changes have been well characterized, primarily because of a number of animal models that have been advanced over the past 15 years. In contrast, central neural injury–induced pain remains less characterized and best studied following spinal cord injury.[24] Neuropathic as well as inflammatory pain conditions are commonly accompanied with tactile allodynia, heat or cold hyperalgesia, and spontaneous pain. The extent of the contribution of each of these abnormalities to specific clinical conditions varies with type of clinical condition; for example, postherpetic neuralgia shows a very high incidence of tactile allodynia, whereas chronic back pain is dominated by spontaneous pain. Consistent with this clinical picture, animal models of inflammatory pain that persist for different durations show distinct peripheral and central reorganization. Similarly, different animal models of neuropathic pain, in which sometimes the differences seem trivial (for example, different approaches used to induce partial sciatic nerve injuries), also show various reorganization differences.

In the intact healthy organism, nociceptive inputs are transmitted through A-delta and C-nociceptors. However, now there is very good evidence that following central sensitization caused by inflammation or neuropathic injury, peripheral inputs to the CNS through non-nociceptive, thickly myelinated, A-beta touch afferents may evoke pain.[25,26] The latter is clear evidence that the functional roles of afferent fibers can be disturbed, again providing evidence that notions regarding specificity of the pain pathway are tenuous.

Nerve injury provides a new source of afferent activity as a result of ectopic discharge from injured axons in contrast with the normal tissue in which electrogenesis is limited to excitation of free-nerve ending through transduction of noxious stimuli.[27] When an axon is severed, its proximal stump seals off and forms a terminal swelling or end bulb. In adults, axotomized cells survive and begin to regenerate from the proximal cut end. Many of these grow back and reinnervate peripheral target tissue. When growth is blocked as commonly occurs in most injury conditions, terminal end bulbs persist, turn back on themselves, and form a tangled mass, termed a neuroma. There is good evidence that neuromas generate spontaneous ectopic activity that directly contributes to perception of spontaneous pain. Neuromas are also sensitive to mechanical and chemical stimuli; their activity is exacerbated by temperature. Both A-fibers and C-fibers show ectopic activity, although the latter persist longer after injury; and sympathetic-sensory coupling may occur at the neuroma through noradrenergic sensitization.[27] Overall, these changes, which are a consequence of damage to peripheral nerves, are triggered by metabolic and functional responses of the sensory cell, rendering it hyperexcit-

able, contributing to the positive sensory symptoms of neuropathic pain as well as triggering and maintaining central sensitization. Nerve injury induces alterations at multiple sites along the neural axis. Abnormalities occur in the injured and uninjured afferents, accompanied with central sensitization at the spinal cord level coupled with cell death. Additionally, there are changes in the descending control system, and immune responses in the periphery and the spinal cord are observed. As described later, such changes are also accompanied by reorganization of cortical-subcortical circuitry involved in pain perception, in which immune responses as well as signs for cell death also have been observed. Generally, literature regarding central sensitization simply refers to the fact that spinal cord nociceptive information transmission is enhanced. Here, I argue that there is a specific cortical-subcortical reorganization that accompanies neuropathic pain, and perhaps also persistent inflammatory pain states. I label the latter "supraspinal sensitization."

Following is a summary of the evidence regarding the role of various sources of afferent inputs in neuropathic pain. (1) Systemic administration of a selective CB2 cannabinoid receptor agonist reverses mechanical and thermal hyperalgesia–related behavior in an animal model for peripheral neuropathy.[28] Because CB2 is only expressed in the periphery, the result is strong evidence for the role of peripheral afferents. (2) Similarly, decreasing efficacy of specific sodium channel subtypes in the periphery can decrease signs of mechanical hyperalgesia.[29] (3) In addition to the hyperexcitable injured afferents, there is also good evidence that neuropathic pain can develop in the absence of activity from the injured nerve.[30] (4) Spontaneous activity develops in uninjured, unmyelinated nociceptive afferents that innervate the same territory as the injured afferents, similar spontaneous activity develops following inflammatory injury, and in both the rate of this activity relates to spontaneous pain as assessed by frequency of lifting the injured limb.[31] (5) There also is evidence for sensitization of intact afferents that develop adrenergic sensitivity[32] and increased responsiveness to thermal and mechanical stimuli.[33] (6) The messenger ribonucleic acid (mRNA) for a variety of receptors is upregulated in cell bodies of dorsal root ganglion neurons for both injured and uninjured afferents, which are regulated by trophic factors transported from the site of injury to these cell bodies.[23] These contribute to changes in sensitivity to heat, cold, and mechanical stimuli for intact and injured afferents, as well as their responses to various modulatory inputs.

CENTRAL SENSITIZATION FOLLOWING INFLAMMATORY, NEUROPATHIC, OR CANCER PAIN

Glutamate is the dominant excitatory neurotransmitter in all nociceptors, and all primary nociceptors terminate and make synaptic contacts with second-order neurons in the dorsal horn gray matter of the

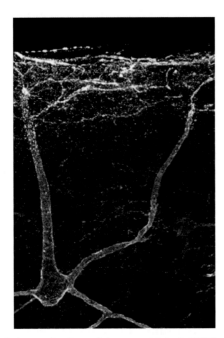

Figure 9–4. Internalization of the neurokinin-1 (NK1) receptor, a receptor that preferentially binds to substance P released from afferent terminals, in the spinal cord. The cell body is located in layers 3 and 4 of the dorsal horn, whereas its dendrites extend to layer 1. The highest concentration of NK1 receptors is in layer 1 and a noxious stimulus induces internalization of these receptors from the cell surface into intracellular compartments. Changes in location of expression and concentration of NK1 have been used to chart central sensitization processes. (Adapted from Hunt SP, Mantyh PW: The molecular dynamics of pain control. Nat Rev Neurosci 2001;2:83-91, with permission.)

spinal cord. Unlike the rest of the CNS, nociceptive afferents also contain a long list of neuropeptides that are coreleased from afferents and can modulate neurotransmission at longer distances than just at the synapse. Substance P is a peptide neurotransmitter that binds preferentially to the neurokinin-1 (NK1) receptor in the spinal cord. Changes in NK1 receptor expression and internalization can be used to identify the spatial and temporal effects of peripheral nociceptive in-puts on individual spinal cord neurons (Fig. 9–4). In animal models for both inflammatory and neuropathic injury there is ample evidence that second-order synaptic transmission becomes sensitized, although with distinct properties for each general type of injury.[23] Moreover, newer evidence shows that in animal models of cancer pain there is yet another set of distinct cellular and molecular signs of reorganization regarding the state of second-order neurons within the spinal cord.[34]

Inflammatory pain involves the sensitization of both primary afferent and spinal cord neurons. The neurochemical changes that contribute to inflammatory pain have been examined using expression and internalization of the NK1 receptor in the spinal cord (see Fig. 9–4) in acute, short-term, and long-term inflammatory pain states.[35] In acute inflammatory pain there is ongoing release of substance P as measured by NK1 internalization in layer 1 neurons

(neurons located at the marginal zone; these neurons send supraspinal projections to a variety of targets). Although there is no tonic release of substance P in short-term inflammatory pain, at 3 hours after injury, both noxious and non-noxious somatosensory stimulation induce NK1 internalization in neurons located in both layers 1, 3, and 4. This is significant because neurons in layers 3 and 4 are classically responsive only to innocuous stimuli and in the intact, healthy organism do not show NK1 internalization. In longer-term inflammatory pain models (3 weeks after initial injury) the same pattern of substance P release and NK1 activation occurs as in short-term inflammation, with the addition of a significant upregulation of NK1 in layer 1 neurons. These changes suggest that there are unique neurochemical signatures for acute, short-term, and long-term inflammatory pain, and given that NK1 internalization is associated with potentiation of glutamatergic neurotransmission, it is clear that the longer inflammatory conditions persist, the more spinal cord circuitry is recruited and associated with the behavior.

In inflammation, there is a significant upregulation of substance P and other neuropeptides, such as calcitonin gene-related peptide (CGRP), in the dorsal horn, whereas there is a downregulation of these same primary afferent neurotransmitters in neuropathic pain. In contrast, in a bone cancer pain model, there is no change in these peptidergic neurotransmitters. Likewise, galanin and neuropeptide Y are markedly upregulated in sensory neurons in neuropathic pain, with no change observed in these neurotransmitters in cancer pain. Even more marked are the different neurochemical changes induced by each pain state in the spinal cord. Whereas inflammation induces an increase in substance P and CGRP in layers 1 and 2 of the spinal cord, nerve injury induces a downregulation of these same markers in this area of the spinal cord with an additional upregulation of galanin and neuropeptide Y. In contrast, in cancer pain, the concentrations of these molecules or markers are not significantly changed. However, the greatest change observed in the spinal cord in response to metastatic bone cancer pain is the activation of astrocytes. These results imply that in inflammatory, neuropathic, or cancer pain, a unique and highly distinct set of neurochemical changes occur in the spinal cord and dorsal root ganglion (DRG).[36]

Central sensitization occurs following inflammation or neuropathic injury, and involves homo-synaptic and heterosynaptic mechanisms.[11,23] Homosynaptic mechanisms involve changes in response properties of second-order neurons with direct afferent inputs from the site of injury, whereas heterosynaptic mechanisms underlie spread of hyperexcitability to neurons with inputs from intact afferents. The latter accounts for the mechanisms of allodynia. In this case nociceptive inputs alter synaptic efficacy such that A-b mechanoreceptors acquire the capacity to activate second-order nociceptors. Additionally, uninjured nociceptors can acquire spontaneous activity after neuropathic injury, and this leads to enhanced excitability for spinal cord nociceptors supplied by these inputs. Sensitization, both homosynaptic and heterosynaptic, involves increased release of excitatory neurotransmitters, such as glutamate and substance P, or enhanced synaptic efficacy, altogether resulting in reduction in threshold for activation, increased responsiveness as measured by the number of action potentials generated for a given stimulus, and expansion of receptive fields of dorsal horn neurons.[11] There is a long list of mechanisms that can contribute to different extents toward this outcome, including (1) presynaptic changes, (2) postsynaptic changes, (3) interneuron changes, (4) changes in descending modulation, (5) immune and microglial mechanisms, and (6) cell death. Convincing evidence along all of these lines is only briefly outlined here.

1. Regarding presynaptic effects, the best evidence is for opioid receptors, which are downregulated in neuropathic pain and upregulated in inflammatory pain. As opioid receptors control presynaptic and postsynaptic neural transmission from nociceptive afferents, these changes in its expression result in modulating central nociceptive transmission by both mechanisms.[11,37]

2. There is ample evidence for postsynaptic mechanisms in central sensitization. Primarily release of substance P and other peptides open the NMDA glutamate-gated channel, leading to increased calcium entry, which in turn may also potentiate glutamate transmission through AMPA receptors.[38]

3. Inhibitory gamma-aminobutyric acid (GABA)–ergic interneurons control the overall excitability of neuronal transmission throughout the CNS, and play an important role in governing sensitivity of dorsal horn–projecting neurons. Decreased expression of inhibitory receptors is observed following nerve injury,[35] which decreases the inhibitory control on afferent inputs. Also nerve injury is accompanied with downregulation of the potassium-chloride (K-Cl) transporter, which reverses the effects of GABA release in which opening the Cl channel now leads to excitation rather than inhibition.[39]

4. Descending modulatory pathways seem to reorganize in neuropathic pain and play a critical role in associated behavior. The rostroventromedial medulla (RVM) receives inputs from the periaqueductal gray, which in turn receives convergent inputs from cortical, basal ganglia, and amygdala inputs. RVM projects to the spinal cord and has excitatory and inhibitory innervations within the dorsal horn. Many of RVM cells express opioid receptors, the ablation of which either before or after induction of neuropathic behavior eliminates hyperalgesic behavior.[29] This evidence is important from two viewpoints: first, the descending modulation must be substantially reorganized in neuropathic pain, and second, the supraspinal, including cortical, inputs interact with the spinal cord processing of nociceptive afferent inputs and play an important role in hyperalgesic behavior. Again this provides the view that pain behavior is the integrated output of ascending and descending signals throughout the CNS, and casts grave doubt on the unidirectional, dedicated telephone line model for pain perception.

5. Involvement of the immune system in peripheral inflammation is well established (see Fig. 9–3). There is now also good evidence for its role in neuropathic conditions.[40] Peripheral nerve damage evokes a cascade of peripheral immune responses, leading to macrophage infiltration, and increased expression of proinflammatory cytokines.[23] Knockout of proinflammatory IL-1 receptor and overexpression of IL-1 receptor antagonist decreases hyperalgesia and results in reduced spontaneous activity as recorded from dorsal root fibers.[41] Thus peripheral IL-1 clearly participates in neuropathic pain. There is recent evidence that central immune mechanisms are also essential in neuropathic pain, mediated through activation of microglia (Fig. 9–5).[42]

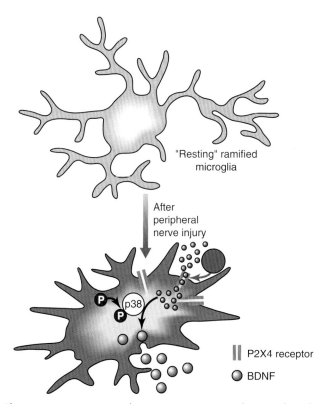

"Resting" ramified microglia

After peripheral nerve injury

P2X4 receptor

BDNF

Figure 9–5. Numerous changes occur to spinal microglia after peripheral nerve injury, resulting in the phenomenon of activation, leading to enhancement of central sensitization and mechanical allodynia. A critical factor in relation to neuropathic pain is the upregulation of expression of the P2X4 receptor. Calcium influx into the microglia through the P2X4 receptors results in an intracellular cascade involving phosphorylation (P), the result of which is the release of brain-derived neurotrophic factor (BDNF). BDNF then acts on neurons in the dorsal horn to drive the spinal hyperexcitability underlying neuropathic pain. (From Trang T, Beggs S, Salter MW: Purinoceptors in microglia and neuropathic pain. Pflügers Arch 2006;452:645-652, with permission.)

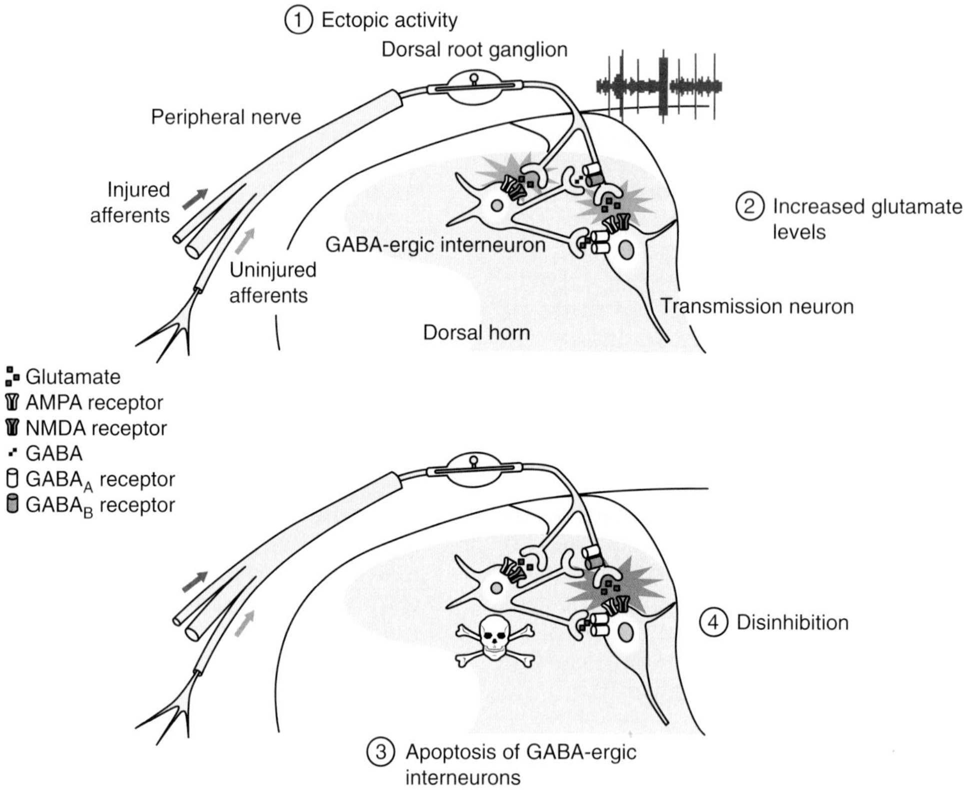

Figure 9–6. Mechanisms of neurodegeneration in the spinal cord following peripheral nerve injury. (1) Abnormal ectopic activity from injured and neighboring uninjured primary afferents generates increased extracellular glutamate levels in the dorsal horn. (2) Excess activation of N-methyl-D-aspartate (NMDA) glutamate α-amino-3-hydroxy-5-methylisoxazole-4-propionic acid (AMPA) receptors leads to a rising influx of Ca^{2+} into dorsal horn neurons, which over time exhausts the buffering capacity of mitochondria. (3) Apoptosis is induced in gamma-aminobutyric acid (GABA)–ergic interneurons. (4) As a result, the GABA-mediated pre- and postsynaptic inhibition of sensory transmission is diminished so that input from nociceptive and non-nociceptive afferents is conveyed without adequate control. Response to noxious stimulation becomes exaggerated (producing hyperalgesia) and normally innocuous stimuli begin to produce pain (allodynia). (From Apkarian AV, Scholz J: Shared mechanisms between chronic pain and neurodegenerative disease. Drug Disc Today Dis Mech 2006;3:319-326, with permission.)

6. Cell death has now been repeatedly documented to occur in the spinal cord following peripheral nerve injury.[43,44] It seems to have a limited time course, underlies apoptosis, and affects primarily GABA-ergic inhibitory interneurons (Fig. 9–6).

This summary of peripheral and spinal cord changes for persistent pains of various kinds highlights the main components involved. It also ignores or skims over much of the detail. In fact the literature on the subject is vast and rapidly growing. Here I have attempted to identify cellular, molecular, and structural changes that accompany persistent or chronic pain. This overview also sets the stage so that one can examine the literature regarding human brain activity for pain and its relationship to expected equivalences between supraspinal sensitization and peripheral and central sensitization.

NOCICEPTIVE SUPRASPINAL PROJECTIONS AND CORTICAL-SUBCORTICAL PAIN CIRCUITRY

There is a long list of pathways that convey nociceptive information from the spinal cord to higher brain centers (see chapter on anatomy of pain systems).

These can generally be subdivided into two groupings: pathways accessing the cortex through the thalamus, that is the spinothalamic pathway, and pathways that access the cortex more indirectly through synapses at the brainstem, amygdala, basal ganglia, as well as direct projections from the spinal cord to the prefrontal cortex. The relative size of these projections and response properties of spinal cord neurons that participate in different pathways have been studied relatively well in mammals but such information is mostly lacking for humans. It is quite possible that some of these pathways may be preferentially enhanced in humans as compared with other mammals. The spinothalamic pathway has been studied most extensively, and supraspinal circuitry regarding pain is usually cast within the anatomic framework of this pathway, ignoring the contribution of the others.

Conscious perception of external stimuli requires encoding by sensory organs, processing within the respective sensory system, and activation of the appropriate sensory cortical areas. Based on a small case series of infra- and supratentorial brain lesions in 1911, Head and Holmes[45] postulated that the sensation of pain is an exception to this rule and that its conscious perception occurs in the "essential organ of the thalamus" (p. 177). In spite of evidence to the contrary from clinical reports,[46,47] single unit recordings in animals,[48,49] and neuroanatomic tracings,[50] it was maintained for a long time that the cortical representation of pain was a negligible one.

This situation changed when the modern neuroimaging techniques (positron-emission tomography [PET] and functional magnetic resonance imaging [fMRI]) demonstrated systematic metabolic and perfusion changes in a large number of cortical areas following the application of painful stimuli.[51-54] These findings were supported by invasive and noninvasive electrophysiologic studies in humans, using magnetoencephalography (MEG), electroencephalography (EEG), and subdural and depth recordings. Meanwhile it has been recognized that painful stimuli activate a vast network of cortical (and subcortical) areas, including the primary and secondary somatosensory cortex (SI, SII), the insula, posterior parietal cortex, anterior and midcingulate cortex, and parts of the prefrontal cortex (Fig. 9–7). These areas are now presumed to be involved in the generation of pain perception as well as in the descending control of pain.[14,55,56] A recent meta-analysis examined the incidence of statistically significant activity across all brain imaging studies of pain in healthy subjects over the past 15 years, and indicated that in 68 studies incidence of activity across these regions was from 55% to 94%, with the lowest incidence seen for prefrontal cortex (55%) and highest for insula (94%).[14] Hence the nociceptive system converges with other systems for the generation of the conscious percept of pain. In that sense the nociceptive system is not different from, for example, the visual system. But it is still an open question as to what extent any cortical regions can be considered nociceptive specific.

Over the past 15 years or so, the cortical and subcortical areas (including thalamus, basal ganglia, amygdala, and brainstem) activated with pain in healthy subjects has been examined regarding the specific dimensions of pain that can be mapped within this network as well as its modifications with various cognitive and pharmacologic manipulations. Traditionally pain perception has been conceived to consist of sensory-discriminative, affective-motivational, and cognitive-evaluative dimensions.[57] The sensory-discriminative dimension includes intensity discrimination, pain qualities, stimulus localization, and timing discrimination; this dimension is traditionally thought to involve lateral thalamic nuclei and the somatosensory cortices SI and SII. The affective-motivational dimension includes perception of the negative hedonic quality of pain, autonomic nervous system manifestations of emotions,

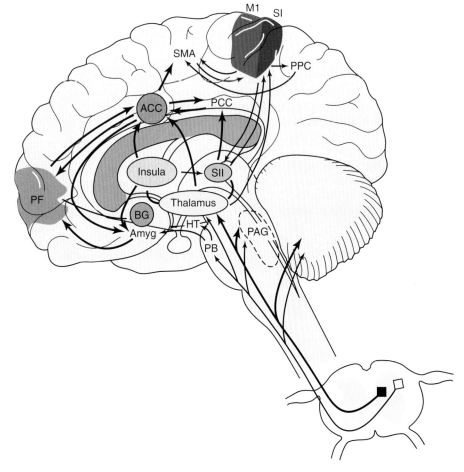

Figure 9–7. A cartoon of main cortical-subcortical brain regions implicated in pain. Multiple ascending pathways are shown transmitting nociceptive information cephalad. The spinothalamic pathway with connectivity between the thalamus, primary and secondary somatosensory cortex (SI, SII), insula, and anterior cingulate cortex (ACC) is supposed to provide both sensory and affective information to the cortex. However, nociceptive information flowing through pathways outside of the spinothalamic tract accesses the cortex through limbic and prefrontal pathways and may be more important in hedonic and emotional aspects of pain. The cartoon is misleading in that it emphasizes unidirectional flow of nociceptive information. As emphasized throughout the chapter, there is now very good evidence that the cortical-subcortical circuitry projects through the periaqueductal gray (PAG), parabrachial nucleus (PB), basal ganglia (BG), and rostro-ventromedial medulla (RVM) back to the spinal cord and affects afferent excitability. (From Apkarian AV, Bushnell MC, Treede RD, Zubieta JK: Human brain mechanisms of pain perception and regulation in health and disease. Eur J Pain 2005;9:463-484, with permission.)

and motivated behavioral responses; this dimension is traditionally thought to involve medial thalamic nuclei and the limbic anterior and medial cingulate cortices (ACC and MCC, respectively). The insula has an intermediate position in that concept, receiving input from lateral thalamus but projecting into the limbic system. The cognitive-evaluative dimension includes interaction with previous experience, cognitive influence on perceived pain intensity, and an overall evaluation of its salience; this dimension is traditionally thought to involve the prefrontal cortex. However, numerous neuroimaging studies have assessed various experimental paradigms derived from several psychological concepts that do not easily fit into the traditional three dimensions of pain. Therefore I discuss the evidence for involvement of cortical areas in specific functions instead of the dimensions of pain.

Location and Quality of Phasic Pain

Neuroimaging studies have examined brain regions activated by many types of painful stimulation, including noxious heat and cold, muscle stimulation, topical and intradermal capsaicin, colonic distention, rectal distention, gastric distention, esophageal distention, ischemia, cutaneous electric shock, ascorbic acid, laser heat, and the illusion of pain evoked by combinations of innocuous temperatures.[14,58] Despite the differences in sensation, emotion, and behavioral responses provoked by these different types of pain, individuals can easily identify each as being painful. Thus there appears to be a common construct of "pain" with an underlying network of brain activity in the areas described. Nevertheless, despite the similarities in pain experiences and similarities in neural activation patterns, each pain experience is unique. Subjects can usually differentiate noxious heat from noxious cold from noxious pressure. Given that there is ubiquitous convergence of information from cutaneous, visceral, and muscle tissue throughout the afferent nociceptive system,[59] differentiation of types of pain must be caused by feature extraction by interactions between neurons in the cortical-subcortical circuitry (Fig. 9–8). Although this has not yet been demonstrated, somatotopic organization for noxious stimuli has been shown in human brain imaging at least for SI, SII, basal ganglia, and electrophysiologically in non-human primates in the thalamus. Thus these regions can all play a part in localization of pain. Strigo and colleagues[60] directly compared brain activations produced by esophageal distention and cutaneous heat on the chest that were matched for pain intensity. They found that the two qualitatively different pains produced different primary loci of activation with insula, SI, and motor and prefrontal cortices. Such local differences in responses within the "nociceptive network" might subserve our ability to distinguish visceral and cutaneous pain as well as the differential emotional, autonomic, and motor responses associated with these different sensations.

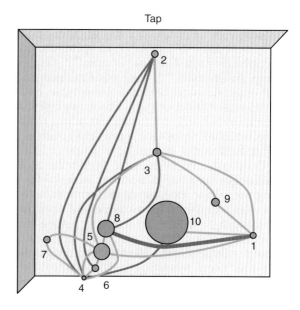

Tap

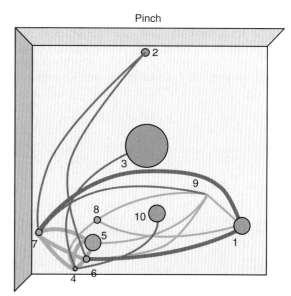

Pinch

Figure 9–8. Connectivity and firing rate changes in a group of 10 neurons, recorded within the lateral thalamus in an anesthetized monkey, in response to either tapping or pinching the skin. The 10 neurons are numbered and their mean firing rate is indicated by the size of each circle, and strengths of positive and negative functional connections are indicated by the colored connections (red and green lines of different thickness). The data demonstrate that functional connectivity between neighboring neurons in the thalamus shifts with the types of stimulus applied on the skin. (From Apkarian AV, Shi T, Bruggemann J, et al: Segregation of nociceptive and non-nociceptive networks in the squirrel monkey somatosensory thalamus. J Neurophysiol 2000;84:484-494, with permission.)

Representation in Time Domain

The dual pain sensation elicited by a single brief painful stimulus that is caused by the different conduction times in nociceptive A- and C-fibers (about 1 second difference) is reflected in two sequential brain activations in EEG and MEG recordings from SI, SII, and MCC.[61-64] Intracranial recordings[65,66] show that the earliest pain-induced brain activity originates in the vicinity of SII. These observations support the suggestion derived from anatomic studies that the SII region and adjacent insula are primary receiving areas for nociceptive input to the brain.[67,68]

Attention and Distraction Effects

Early human brain imaging studies examining the effects of attention and distraction show modulation of pain-evoked activity in a number of cortical regions, including sensory and limbic structures, as well as prefrontal areas.[69-71] Other studies extend these notions by showing that during distraction there is a functional interaction between pregenual ACC and frontal cortex exerting a top-down modulation on periaqueductal gray (PAG) and thalamus to reduce activity in cortical sensory regions and correspondingly decrease perception of pain.[72-74]

Anticipation and Expectation

Anticipation or expectation of pain can activate many of the cortical areas related to perception of pain in the absence of a physical pain stimulus.[75-78] Two studies have attempted to identify the circuitry for modulation of pain by expectation.[79,80] The results indicate that expectancy for high pain intensity is necessary for maximal activation of afferent pain circuitry and maximal perceived pain intensity, suggesting that cortical modulation by expectancy changes the gain for afferent inputs to the cortex. Generally there remains a strong need for systematic studies to identify brain elements that modulate pain responses because of expectation.

Empathy

A provocative study opened the field regarding the interaction between pain and empathy, in which the authors defined empathy as the ability to have an experience of another's pain. Using this definition and comparing brain activity for experiencing pain or knowing that a loved one, present in the same room, was experiencing the same pain, the authors showed many cortical regions similarly activated for both conditions.[81] These results were interpreted as evidence for the affective component of pain being active in both empathy and pain, and thus concluded that empathy for pain involves the affective component but not the sensory component of pain. The study induced a flurry of activity in attempting to understand the relationship between empathy and pain. Multiple groups have replicated the main finding and proposed different underlying mechanisms.[82-84] Even though these results are internally consistent, their interpretation remains problematic. Simple introspection casts doubt on the notion that empathy means actually experiencing another person's pain. Instead, what is called empathy may be the assessment of the magnitude of negative emotion that the other person may be experiencing, that is, a cognitive function of interpersonal communication. According to that concept, empathy may be conceived of as a psychological process using cognitive/evaluative and affective mechanisms that allow us to understand the personal experience of another person. A study in patients with congenital insensitivity to pain[85] reported a deficit in rating pain-inducing events, but normal inference of pain from facial expressions ("empathy"), indicating that empathy for pain does not require an intact pain percept.

Mood and Emotional States

Studies show that experimental procedures that improve mood generally reduce pain, whereas those that have a negative effect on mood increase pain. One study showed that looking at fearful faces increased the level of anxiety and discomfort, which also resulted in enhanced esophageal stimulation and evoked activity in limbic regions like the ACC and insula.[86]

Placebo

Placebo is a potent modulator of pain; it affects all clinical studies of pain pharmacology. Placebo effects have also been seen in depression and in Parkinson's disease, and recent brain imaging studies show a robust brain and subcortical reward circuitry's involvement in these.[87] The first neurochemical evidence for opiate involvement of placebo was demonstrated about 30 years ago by showing that placebo analgesia can be blocked by naloxone.[88] Consistent with this notion, changes in endogenous opiate release are shown to be involved in placebo-induced analgesia, in which prefrontal cortex (medial and lateral) as well as insula and ventral striatum seem to be involved, and in high-placebo responders increased opiate release in ventral striatum is positively correlated with pain ratings.[89] Results generally consistent with this brain response pattern have been demonstrated by a number of other groups[80,90,91]; the medial prefrontal/rostral ACC responses for placebo seem to recruit PAG and amygdala[92]; and involvement of PAG in placebo-induced analgesia is experimentally observed as well, which links opiate descending modulation with prefrontal cortical control of placebo analgesia. The correspondence between placebo analgesia and reward was directly studied, and the results show a strong correspondence between brain regions involved in each.[93]

PHARMACOLOGIC MODULATION OF PAIN

Opiates

Vast literature regards opiate descending modulation through the PAG and its effects on inhibitory interneurons in the spinal cord. Presence of large concentrations of opiate receptors at the cortical and subcortical level has also been known for decades, yet little effort has been devoted to understanding the role of the latter in pain. Recent studies of opiate responses in the brain have used two approaches: examination of metabolic function in response to pharmacologic agents and direct measurement of receptors. μ-Opioid agonist fentanyl on brain responses to painful stimuli has been explored, showing that most cortical responses to pain are reduced or eliminated, confirming analgesic effects of the opiate.[94,95] Changes in endogenous opioid system are studied using a selective μ-opioid radiotracer, showing activation of opiate neurotransmission in ACC, prefrontal cortex (PFC), insular cortex (IC), and subcortical areas during a tonic muscle pain.[96-98]

Dopamine

Dopamine is best known for its role in motor, motivation, and pleasure control; accumulating evidence suggests that dopamine primarily acting at the level of subcortical basal ganglia may also be involved in pain modulation. Human brain imaging studies document increased pain sensitivity associated with lower levels of endogenous dopamine,[99-101] and sustained experimental pain results in release of dopamine in the basal ganglia.[101] Moreover, abnormal levels of dopamine in the basal ganglia have been associated with chronic pain in burning mouth syndrome and atypical facial pain,[102-104] and perhaps in fibromyalgia.[105]

Estrogen

Women far outnumber men in susceptibility to many autoimmune disorders, fibromyalgia, and chronic pain. Differences in physiologic responses to stress may be an important risk factor for these disorders as physiologic responses to stress seem to differ according to sex, phase of menstrual cycle, menopausal status, and with pregnancy.[106] Some studies have documented that threshold and tolerance for pain is lower for women.[107,108]

The association of sex hormones with pain perception and pain memory was studied by Zubieta and colleagues.[97,101] These studies showed that more μ-opioid receptors were available in the presence of high estrogen levels, and women reported less pain in response to acute painful stimuli than when their estrogen levels were low. Moreover, estrogen-associated variations in the activity of μ-opioid neurotransmission correlated with individual ratings of the sensory and affective perceptions of pain and the subsequent recall of that experience. These data demonstrate a significant role of estrogen in modulating endogenous opioid neurotransmission and associated psychophysical responses to an acute pain stressor in humans.

OVERVIEW OF THE ROLE OF THE CORTEX IN ACUTE PAIN PERCEPTION

The preceding section describes the contribution of modern imaging studies to our understanding of the involvement of the cortex in pain perception. Cortical activity is demonstrated to possess properties necessary for involvement in pain perception, like somatotopic representation of painful stimuli, correlation with stimulus intensity, modulation with attention, modulation with expectation and other psychological variables, and distinct brain regions showing differential activity for sensory and affective dimensions of pain, as well as attenuation of responses with analgesic drugs. Thus human brain imaging studies have asserted the role of the cortex in acute pain.

However, because imaging studies identify brain responses in a correlative manner, they may all reflect secondary processes. Perception of pain automatically directs attention to the source of pain and results in autonomic responses, motor reflexes to escape from the pain, and other emotional and cognitive responses that undoubtedly are at least partially mediated through cortical processes. Therefore the role of the cortex in pain perception in contrast with its activity as a consequence of these secondary responses remains unclear and needs to be properly addressed in future studies.[109] In fact, unpublished data from the author's lab suggest that a large proportion of the brain network activated with acute pain may be responses that are commonly involved in general magnitude estimation for any sensory modality, and as a result are not specific for nociception, suggesting that the majority of cortical activity for acute pain is instead sensory, cognitive, emotional, and attentional responses to nociceptive inputs. Therefore the extent to which any given cortical region is necessary for acute pain needs further studies using multiple technologic approaches. For most parts of the nociceptive cortical network, as illustrated earlier, it is likely that they participate only partly in pain perception (by providing certain feature extraction functions) and also participate in other functions in different contexts.

CLINICAL PAIN

It should be emphasized that although the subjective phenomenon of being in pain can be considered an emergent phenomenon of cortical activity,[56] there is currently no measure of brain activity that would objectively show whether a person is in pain. Therefore neither electrical (EEG or MEG) nor imaging with fMRI or PET can be used to verify the presence of ongoing spontaneous pain in an individual. Neither fMRI nor PET allows clinical assessment of nociceptive pathways in individual cases because so far no activation paradigm has been developed that would reliably induce a particular cortical activation pattern in each and every healthy subject. Thus negative findings with these techniques are inconclusive.

For the study of pathologic nociceptive processing at the group level, however, fMRI and PET techniques are extremely powerful. These techniques have broadened our understanding of the pathophysiology of conditions with decreased pain perception such as afferent pathway lesions or borderline personality disorder, and conditions with increased pain perception such as neuropathic pain or fibromyalgia.[110-114] Nevertheless, there are also large gaps in our current knowledge regarding general clinical pain states. For example, we have yet to begin to understand how duration of pain in simple clinical states effects brain pain processing. Does a patient with tooth pain suffering for 24 hours versus another suffering for a week have similar or distinct brain responses? Clearly the animal data regarding spinal cord processing of inflammatory pain suggest that the two conditions should engage and excite more projecting neurons but the clinical data are missing. Similarly, we have little knowledge regarding inflammatory clinical pain states in general. However, chronic pain conditions have been studied more extensively, which is appropriate because these are the conditions that we understand the least and this knowledge may translate into new avenues for therapies.

CHRONIC PAIN

Studying Brain Activity in Chronic Pain with Nonspecific Painful Stimuli

Chronic pain might result from cortical processing of chronic nociceptive input according to the same mechanisms as in acute pain, or there might be specific changes in cortical processing of nociceptive input in patients with chronic pain. Such changes could then either be a causal factor for or a consequence of the chronicity of the pain condition. The primary expectation from animal model studies for persistent pain whether inflammatory or neuropathic is enhanced excitability of spinal cord nociceptive neurons, which would translate into a generally larger cortical activity throughout the brain regions activated with acute pain. This is exactly what has not been observed for a long list of chronic pain conditions. Pointing to an important disconnect between the animal models and the human studies, it is unclear whether the mismatch is a result of inadequate animal models or inappropriate explanation of the results seen in animal models.

A recent meta-analysis in fact shows that across some 100 studies one can establish statistically significant differences in incidence of different brain areas activated by experimental painful stimuli between acute and chronic pain conditions: prefrontal cortex shows a stronger activation in chronic pain patients, whereas other nociceptive cortical areas and the thalamus show a weaker response.[14] A simple interpretation of these findings is that nociceptive signal processing for experimental painful stimuli in chronic pain patients involves a reduced sensory discriminative component and an increased affective-motivational or cognitive-evaluational component. That interpretation also is consistent with the stronger affective component of clinical pain as compared

with experimental pain.[115] But there are further implications: Is the result a consequence of some trivial confounds or does it signify changes in the physiology of pain? One could construct a long list of confounds that may underlie the observation, from attentional shifts, to coping mechanisms, to effects of drug use, and heightened anxiety and depression.

The standard approach for studying brain activity for acute pain is to induce pain by a mechanical or thermal stimulus and determine brain regions modulated with the stimulus period and even with the various intensities used. Therefore it is natural to carry the same technology to the clinical arena and apply it to chronic pain patients. An example is one study that attempted to identify brain activity in patients with chronic regional pain syndrome (CRPS) using fMRI.[116] The design of the study was to examine brain activity for thermal stimuli applied to the body part where CRPS pain was present, and compare brain responses to this stimulus between CRPS and healthy subjects. Moreover, as the pain in CRPS patients with sympathetically maintained pain (SMP) may be modulated by a sympathetic block, it was reasoned that one could decrease the patients' ongoing pain and then reexamine brain activity responses to the same stimulus. The study was done in a small group of patients and this by itself is an important weakness, endemic throughout the clinical pain brain imaging studies. The main observation was that thermal stimuli in CRPS evoked more prefrontal cortical activity than usually seen in healthy subjects, and this was reversed (became more similar in pattern to normal subjects' brain activity to thermal stimuli) following sympathetic blocks. The introduction of sympathetic blocks necessitated the use of the same procedure in healthy subjects as well, and its effects were minimal. The study also observed that when a placebo block resulted in decreased pain perception, then the cortical response pattern changed similarly to that of effective blocks. These results show that brain activity may be distinct between CRPS and healthy subjects for thermal stimuli, but raised a number of unanswered questions, many of which challenge the validity of the approach. For example, the simple assumption that sympathetic blocks were only, or mainly, affecting the CRPS pain without interfering with afferent sensory transmission was unclear. The analysis was based on the idea that spontaneous pain per se would not affect subjects' ability to assess stimulus pain, which may not be true, and that contrasting sympathetic block effects in CRPS and healthy subjects is valid.

Clinical Pain Conditions Studied by Stimulation and the Role of the Cortex

A direct approach to studying clinical pain states is to provoke it and examine brain activity. This is feasible by drugs in headaches and in cardiac pain. As a result there is growing literature in both fields. There is also now good evidence that migraine with aura is accompanied with decreased blood flow and decreased activity in the occipital cortex, and migraine with or without aura is associated with increased cortical thickness in visual-cortical regions involved in motion detection.[117]

MIGRAINE

Migraine attacks are characterized by unilateral severe headache often accompanied by nausea, phonophobia, and photophobia. Activation of the trigeminovascular system (TGVS) is thought to be responsible for the pain itself, and cortical spreading depression (CSD) seems to underlie the aura symptoms. This view has been greatly advanced and substantiated by brain imaging studies. fMRI studies show CSD-typical cerebrovascular changes in the cortex of migraineurs while experiencing a visual aura.[118] The subsequent decrease in fMRI signal is temporally correlated with the scotoma that follows the scintillations. These fMRI signal changes develop first in the extrastriate cortex, contralateral to the visual changes. It then slowly migrates toward more anterior regions of the visual cortex, representing peripheral visual fields, in agreement with the progressive movement of the scintillations and scotoma from the center of vision toward the periphery. A recent study that analyzed visually triggered attacks showed hyperemia in the occipital cortex, independently of whether the headache was preceded by visual symptoms.[119] An alternative view considers migraine aura and headache as parallel rather than sequential processes, and proposes that the primary cause of migraine headache is an episodic dysfunction in brainstem nuclei that are involved in the central control of nociception.[120]

Cluster Headache

The pathophysiology of cluster headache is thought to involve multiple brain regions. Brain imaging studies imply that the associated excruciatingly severe unilateral pain is likely mediated by activation of the first (ophthalmic) division of the trigeminal nerve, whereas the autonomic symptoms are caused by activation of the cranial parasympathetic outflow from the seventh cranial nerve.

Using PET in cluster headache patients, significant activations ascribable to the acute cluster headache were observed in the ipsilateral hypothalamic gray matter and in multiple cortical areas including cingulate and prefrontal cortex. When compared with the headache-free state, only hypothalamic activity was distinct.[121] This highly significant activation was only observed in patients while they were experiencing an acute cluster headache attack. Newer magnetic resonance spectroscopy (MRS) results further substantiate this idea by showing reduced metabolites within the hypothalamus of cluster headache patients in contrast with healthy or migraine headache controls.[122] These data suggest that although primary headaches such as migraine and cluster headache

may share a common pain pathway (the trigeminovascular innervation) and activate similar cortical regions, the underlying pathogenesis may be quite different.

Cardiac Pain

Cardiac pain and its variants have been studied by brain imaging using various drugs that bring about these symptoms.[123-125] Overall, these studies imply that differences between different cardiac pain conditions are a result of central processing. Syndrome X, for example, is interpreted as a cortical pain syndrome, a "top-down" process, in contrast with the "bottom-up" generation of a pain percept caused by myocardial ischemia in coronary artery disease.

Irritable Bowel Syndrome

Irritable bowel syndrome (IBS) is a disorder of abdominal pain or discomfort associated with bowel dysfunction. Hypersensitivity to visceral but not somatic stimuli has been demonstrated in IBS. A number of groups have examined brain activity in this condition mainly by monitoring responses to painful and nonpainful rectal distentions, as well as responses to the anticipation of painful distentions. Two studies are interesting because both show in normal subjects a significant positive correlation between cingulate cortex activity and subjective rating of rectal distention pain, and in both studies this relationship completely disappears in IBS patients.[126,127]

More recent studies show a hint for sensitization in IBS patients because subliminal and supraliminal distentions of rectal distention seem to indicate small differences between IBS and healthy controls in the total cortical volume activated or in regional activity as a function of distention volume.[128,129] A study of IBS in contrast with healthy subjects examined thermal and visceral hyperalgesia and related brain activity.[130] This seems the only study in which, besides pain intensity and unpleasantness measures, the authors also document fear and anxiety and show that all are rated higher by IBS for both heat and rectal distention, and not surprisingly these increased sensations and emotions give rise to larger cortical activations in IBS. The latter is most likely a reflection of a perceptual magnitude mismatch between the groups and says little as to the IBS cortical activity abnormalities. Such mismatches at least for fear and anxiety most likely are common in the majority of studies of IBS. One assumes that the simple introduction of a rectal balloon in IBS would result in increased anxiety, which undoubtedly affects cortical activity to visceral and somatic pain, yet its specific contribution has remained unexplored.

In an elegant study, perception-related ratings were used during rectal distention to evoke either the urge to defecate or pain, and compared brain activity related to the ratings between IBS patients and healthy subjects.[131] The approach is similar to the technique used in mapping brain activity for spontaneous pain in chronic back pain and in postherpetic neuralgia.[132,133] The results show large differences between the two groups contrasted, with far more extensive brain activations in the healthy subjects. The results are complicated by the fact that the authors do not take into consideration the influence of spontaneous pain. Still, this is perhaps one of the best-controlled IBS studies and indicates distinct cortical areas involved in the urge and pain perceptions in each group.

Spontaneous Pain as a Confound in Assessing Brain Activity

A person who has lived for years in the presence of pain must have developed some coping mechanisms that aid in pursuing other everyday life interests. How does this affect the brain? Can one consider the brain of a patient in chronic pain as composed of a brain signaling pain together with a brain undertaking other tasks as in healthy subjects? Or does the presence of ongoing pain interact and affect other processes as well? There is now direct evidence of the modulation that ongoing pain imposes on brain activity in general.

A recent study reported brain activity for spontaneous pain in postherpetic neuralgia (PHN) patients before and after topical lidocaine treatment.[133] The PHN patients were imaged using fMRI before treatment, after 6 hours, then again after 2 weeks treatment with lidocaine. Behaviorally and based on questionnaires, most participants showed a modest but significant decrease in their ongoing pain. The patients were scanned while they were either rating their pain or rating a visual bar that varied in time in a pattern that mimicked their ratings of pain. Thus the latter is a control task that captures motor and cognitive parts of the task, but of course it does not reflect the pain. Brain activity for both tasks increased from the first to the third session. This observation is similar to earlier reports that decrease in clinical pain in many cases results in increased brain activity. In this case, however, the internal control was also changing in a manner parallel to the pain condition, hinting that the effects of decreased pain were modulating more than just pain-related circuitry.

To identify the role of spontaneous pain on brain activity in general, a correlation analysis was performed for both tasks with mean spontaneous pain. The result showed that brain activity for both tasks was influenced by the level of spontaneous pain, implying that pain intensity in general influences task performance. This is in line with previous studies showing that ongoing pain may interfere with cognitive function.[134] The finding indicates that the intensity of spontaneous pain affects brain activity for any task that the subject attempts to perform, enhancing some aspects and inhibiting others. Therefore the decreased brain activity reported for pain tasks in many clinical pain conditions is most likely a reflection of the presence of the spontaneous pain, and is not specific to the task being investigated. The fact that pain intensity seems to modulate brain activity in general has another powerful consequence. It suggests that simply studying brain activity in tasks unrelated to pain, one should be able to identify the presence of pain and study its effects on sensory/cognitive/motor/attentional processing, an exciting prospect that remains to be pursued.

Functional Magnetic Resonance Imaging of Spontaneous Pain

Spontaneous pain is highly prevalent in clinical pain conditions, and is usually the primary drive for patients seeking medical care. Thus understanding its related brain circuitry is scientifically as well as therapeutically imperative. Cortical responses to standard mechanical or thermal stimulation are of limited value for understanding these clinical pain conditions. Spontaneous pain fluctuates unpredictably in the time scale of seconds to minutes, and these fluctuations have characteristic properties that differentiate between different chronic pain conditions such as postherpetic neuralgia and chronic back pain.[135] This variability also can be observed in fMRI signals when such patients rate their spontaneous pain. Therefore this technique was applied to study brain activity in CBP and PHN patients[132,133] in relation to their subjective report of fluctuations of spontaneous pain.

The combination of relating brain activity to spontaneous pain and correcting for confounds by subtracting brain activity for visual bar lengths, provides a robust approach with which clinical pain may be studied directly. Note that in this case the brain activity is related to exactly the event about which the patient complains. With this approach, in CBP patients[132] it was shown that the brain regions activated when the pain was increasing correspond to brain regions seen for acute pain in normal subjects. In contrast, for times when the pain was high and sustained, the brain activity was mainly limited to medial prefrontal cortex, a region usually not activated for acute pain (Fig. 9-9). The resultant brain activity was strongly correlated to the patients' reported pain intensity at the time of the scan, specifically with medial prefrontal activity. Also the duration or chronicity of the pain was captured in the insular activity, a region activated only during increases in spontaneous pain. Thus two fundamental properties of CBP—its intensity and duration—were directly reflected in the brain activity identified in these patients (Fig. 9-10). By applying a thermal painful stimulus in the same patients (as well as in healthy subjects) the same study showed that brain regions reflecting the stimulus intensity were not related to that reflecting the intensity of spontaneous pain. In turn, the brain region that reflected spontaneous pain intensity was only activated for the latter and did not reflect thermal painful stimulus intensity. Therefore at least in the patient group studied spontaneous pain involved a different brain activity pattern than acute pain.

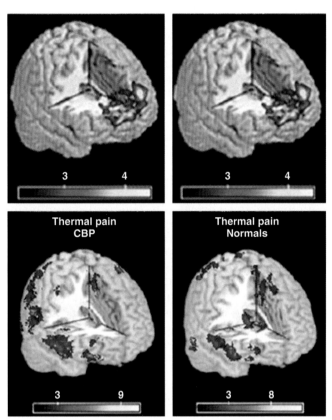

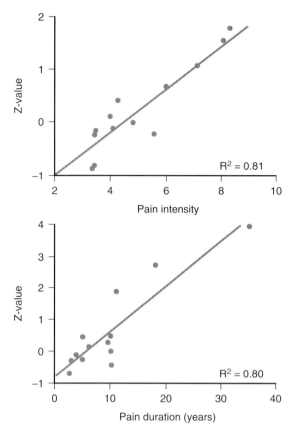

Figure 9–9. Brain activity for spontaneous pain in chronic back pain (CBP). *Top left panel:* Brain activity in chronic back pain patients specifically for spontaneous pain periods when it is rated as high intensity. Activity is limited to medial prefrontal cortex, a brain region involved in emotional assessment, especially in relation to the self. In contrast, when the pain is transitioning from low to high the brain activity is very different *(top right panel). Lower left panel:* Brain activity for thermal painful stimuli applied to the back in chronic back pain patients at a location where back pain was indicated to be most intense. *Lower right panel:* Brain activity for thermal painful stimuli applied to approximately the same back area in healthy normal subjects. Note that there is no difference between the two activity patterns, which shows that thermal pain responses are not different between chronic back pain and healthy subjects. Moreover, the brain activity shown in the low panels is similar to that shown in top right panel. Therefore the increases in spontaneous pain are most likely mediated through a nociceptive signal that invades the cortex, which is in turn sustained in the prefrontal cortex. (From Baliki MN, Chialvo DR, Geha PY, et al: Chronic pain and the emotional brain: Specific brain activity associated with spontaneous fluctuations of intensity of chronic back pain. J Neurosci 2006;26:12165-12173, with permission.)

Figure 9–10. Brain activity in chronic back pain reflects pain intensity and pain duration. Top panel shows that activity in the medial prefrontal cortex, for time periods when spontaneous pain was rated to be of high intensity, very strongly correlates with the intensity of pain that chronic back pain patients report at the time of scan. Each point on the graph represents an individual participant's pain, whereas the z-value is the intensity of brain activity extracted from the medial prefrontal cortex in each individual. Lower panel shows the relationship between the numbers of years each patient has had pain and activity in the insula, when the spontaneous pain was increasing. Again there is a very strong correlation between brain activity and pain duration in this case. These results demonstrate that by simply looking at brain activity at these two sites, one can predict at the individual level, pain intensity and pain duration with a very high confidence.

Neuropathic Pain

A magnetic resonance spectroscopy study showed a decrease in the level of *N*-acetyl-aspartate, a neuronal marker, in the thalami of patients with chronic neuropathic pain after spinal cord injury (SCI), when compared with patients with SCI but without pain.[136] Thus neurochemical brain imaging provides evidence for the occurrence of long-term changes in the brain chemistry and morphology of chronic neuropathic pain patients. Thalamic activity in neuropathic patients was also reported to increase after pain

relief,[137] and to be significantly negatively correlated with the duration of the condition in complex regional pain syndrome patients.[138] Thus the reduced activation of the thalamus also may be an altered functional state rather than an irreversible degeneration. Neuropathic pain patients in addition show a reduced availability of opioid receptor binding sites.[139] This reduction was symmetric in peripheral neuropathic pain, suggesting a possible release of endogenous opioids, but lateralized to the hemisphere contralateral to the pain in central pain patients, consistent with a loss of receptors.[140]

Brain activity differences between healthy subjects and patients in activation paradigms are difficult to interpret because they do not distinguish between brain activity specifically related to the clinical condition and abnormalities in sensory processing secondarily associated with the clinical state. Particularly in neuropathic pain, the accompanying sensory deficit may be reflected in the imaging results and not the pain. Reduced relevance of the acute stimulus to subjects who are already in pain may also account for much of the decreased regional brain activity in neuropathic pain. To overcome such nonspecific brain activity differences one needs to compare brain activity for stimuli in which perceptual evaluation has been equated between patients and normal healthy subjects.

A number of studies[76,116,133,137] have looked at the regions of the brain modulated by relief of chronic neuropathic pain. The brain regions modulated by these procedures were quite disparate. This heterogeneity is not surprising because pattern of brain activity may be specific to each neuropathic pain condition. The most recent study[133] illustrates how such therapeutic procedures can be used to functionally subdivide brain responses to areas related to acute changes with therapy and those that respond with longer-term treatment, and regions involved in sensory coding such as the thalamus seem associated with the former, while areas involved in emotions and hedonics like the ventral striatum and amygdala seem to respond to the longer-term treatment.

Low Back Pain and Fibromyalgia

As mentioned, brain activity of healthy subjects and patients with increased pain sensitivity should be compared in such a way that perceived intensity has been matched across the two groups. A recent study used such a design and showed generally heightened brain activity for mechanical painful stimuli of equivalent perceptual intensity both in fibromyalgia and chronic back pain patients as compared with healthy subjects.[111,141] Morphometric and neurochemical brain imaging studies provide evidence for the occurrence of long-term changes in the brain chemistry and morphology of chronic pain patients. The level of N-acetyl-aspartate, a neuronal marker, was decreased in the medial and lateral prefrontal cortex of chronic back pain patients compared with an age- and gender-matched control group.[142] A morphometric study in chronic pain showed also a decrease in gray matter density in the dorsolateral prefrontal cortex and the thalamus of chronic back pain patients when compared with matched controls.[109] Furthermore, these long-term chemical and morphologic changes are significantly correlated with different characteristics of pain such as pain duration,[13] pain intensity,[13,136,143-145] and sensory-affective components.[145] The morphometric and neurochemical studies imply an active role of the CNS in chronic pain, suggesting that supraspinal reorganization may be critical for chronic pain.

EVIDENCE FOR SUPRASPINAL NEURODEGENERATION IN CHRONIC PAIN

Neurodegeneration in the spinal cord, which changes the topography as well as the gain for nociceptive signal transmission, likely provokes parallel reorganizations in supraspinal pathways. Human brain imaging studies are beginning to address this question in relation to specific chronic pain conditions.

Thalamic Activity in Chronic Pain

In contrast with experimentally induced pain in normal subjects, chronic clinical pain conditions are consistently associated with decreased baseline activity or decreased stimulus-related activity in the thalamus.[14] Interpretations of these results though are hampered by inadequate controls. The most elegant study on the topic so far has been a single photon emission computed tomography (SPECT) blood flow experiment[138] showing a strong relationship between time of onset of CRPS and thalamic activity, suggesting that thalamic activity undergoes adaptive changes in the course of CRPS and indicating a transition from an acute to a chronic state. Unfortunately there are no biologic markers for pain that would define standard timelines for the transition from acute to chronic pain. This ambiguity complicates interpreting the thalamic adaptive changes seen in CRPS. Early hyperperfusion in the thalamus might be a consequence of central sensitization or spinal disinhibition as a result of the apoptosis of interneurons. Increased polysynaptic excitation after the removal of GABA-ergic inhibitory control may prompt a vicious circle, causing the degeneration of more dorsal horn neurons including nociceptive transmission neurons, which would explain long-term thalamic hypoperfusion.

Regional brain activation with experimental pain in humans is usually interpreted in relation to the spinothalamic pathway. Decreased thalamic signaling in chronic pain poses a puzzling dilemma from this viewpoint, suggesting that nociceptive pathways outside of this projection may be more important in chronic pain. Given the thalamic activity changes seen in CRPS,[138] one possible explanation is an early activation of the spinothalamic pathway, which at longer periods becomes hypoactive, compensated by enhanced activity in other nociceptive pathways, such as spino-parabrachial-amygdala, spino-basal ganglia, spino-prefrontal, and spino-hypothalamic pathways.

Decreased Metabolism in Thalamus and Cortex

In most human neurodegenerative conditions, such as Alzheimer's or Parkinson's disease, proton MRS shows decreased levels of brain metabolites, primarily of N-acetyl-aspartate (NAA) either in absolute terms or in relation to internal markers such as creatine, phosphocreatine, inositol, or choline. Because NAA is found mainly in neuronal cell bodies, it has become accepted as a parameter for neuronal density and a tool with which neurodegeneration can be studied noninvasively. Recent studies indicate that NAA levels discriminate between amyotrophic lateral sclerosis patients and healthy controls with 71% sensitivity and 93% specificity and predict survival outcomes in this population.[146,147] In Alzheimer's disease (AD), parietal lobe NAA levels are reported as predictive of positive treatment outcome, and its levels correlate with AD progression as strongly as the rate of ventricular expansion.[148,149]

In chronic pain, NAA decreases in the dorsolateral prefrontal cortex (DLPFC) of patients with chronic back pain.[142] The concentration of NAA in DLPFC correlated with the pain intensity as well as affective dimensions of back pain. In contrast, NAA in orbitofrontal cortex was not associated with particular pain descriptors but correlated with state and trait anxiety parameters.[143] The association of decreased thalamic NAA levels and pain intensity has also been observed in patients with central pain after spinal cord injury[136] and in patients with CRPS or postherpetic neuralgia.[150] Decreased concentrations of metabolites such as glucose or inositol have been found in the cerebrospinal fluid of patients with back pain caused by disk herniation or spinal stenosis.[151]

Reduction of Cerebral Gray Matter

Given the baseline activity pattern and metabolic changes in the brain that have been found in functional imaging studies, one would expect a decrease in neocortical gray matter volume and regional gray matter density in the thalamus and the DLPFC. Such changes were in fact the main observation of the first morphometric study contrasting the morphology of chronic back pain patients with sex- and age-matched healthy control subjects (Fig. 9–11).[13] Total neocortical gray matter volume was negatively correlated with the duration of chronic pain. Every year of living with the condition decreased the cortical volume by an additional 1.5 cm³ beyond the decrease in volume attributable to normal aging. The specificity of the outcome is corroborated by the fact that the magnitude of DLPFC gray matter changes in patients with spinal nerve root injury differed from that in patients with non-neuropathic back pain.

Furthermore, gray matter variability correlated with sensory and affective dimensions of back pain. A recent independent study replicated most of these results.[152] Specific changes in regional gray matter density also have been found in patients with tension headache,[152] and recently in fibromyalgia.[153] Details of the morphologic changes may be specific to particular chronic pain states, potentially providing biologic parameters that allow a differentiation of chronic pain conditions.

The results imply that chronic pain is accompanied by cerebral atrophy. Yet the mechanisms underlying this atrophy remain to be elucidated. Cortical neurodegeneration may occur secondarily to spinal cord neurodegeneration, or reflect stress impinging on neurons that are trying to cope with increased afferent input. Genetic factors may render subjects vulnerable to chronic pain either because they have genetically determined lower gray matter density in brain regions such as the DLPFC or because neurons in brain regions at risk of chronic pain-related degeneration are more susceptible to stress, such as increased excitatory input. Brain atrophy in chronic pain may be caused by an irreversible loss of neurons or volume changes that could recover when chronic pain is properly treated. The extent of reversibility of brain atrophy in chronic pain is a crucial issue and its relationship to successful therapy deserves to be investigated.

Increased Amygdala Excitability in Persistent Pain

As part of the limbic system the amygdala plays a key role in attaching emotional significance to sensory stimuli, emotional learning and memory, and affective states and disorders.[154] The amygdala also mediates conditioned and environmentally and morphine-induced analgesia suggesting a coupling to descending inhibition.[155] The amygdala is one of the higher brain centers with direct links to brainstem centers that are important for pain inhibition and facilitation.[156] Only recently, however, a systematic

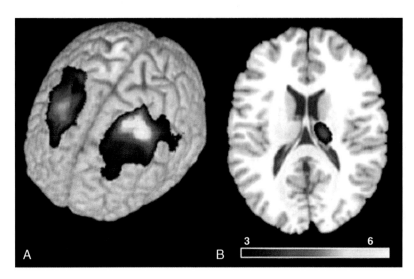

Figure 9–11. Brain regions that show reduced regional gray matter in chronic back pain patients in contrast with matched healthy control subjects. The regional atrophy is shown in increasing brightness; a brighter color indicates increased confidence that the region has reduced gray matter in the patient group. The main brain regions are bilateral dorsolateral prefrontal cortex (A) and unilateral thalamus (B). The result suggests that such patients undergo continued decrease in regional gray matter as long as they are living with their chronic pain. (Adapted from Apkarian AV, Sosa Y, Sonty S, et al: Chronic back pain is associated with decreased prefrontal and thalamic gray matter density. J Neuroscience 2004;24:10410-10415, with permission.)

analysis of pain processing and pain modulation in the amygdala was begun.[157] In these studies an arthritis model was used to show pain-related sensitization and synaptic plasticity of amygdala neurons and, as a consequence, increased nocifensive and affective pain behaviors.[158]

Neuroimaging pain studies using PET and fMRI have produced mixed results regarding pain-related amygdala function in humans. Some studies identified pain-related signal changes in the human amygdala. The experimental conditions included the application of brief noxious heat stimuli to the skin of humans,[159-161] noxious rectal distention in patients with irritable bowel syndrome,[162,163] and mechanical allodynia in neuropathic pain patients.[164] In these studies both activation and deactivation were measured. Importantly, a significant number of neuroimaging pain studies were unable to detect any signal changes in the amygdala in response to painful stimuli or in certain pain states.[157] Evidence from recent studies suggests a correlation between amygdala activity and spontaneous pain in patients with chronic back pain[132] or neuropathic pain,[133] in the absence of amygdala activity for acute thermal pain in chronic back pain or in healthy control subjects.[132] The latter, consistent with the animal studies, suggests that amygdala activity is increased in chronic pain at least in proportion of spontaneous pain.

Cytokines in the Brain and Thalamus

Role of proinflammatory cytokines has been extensively studied in the periphery, spinal cord, and hypothalamus, following peripheral inflammation. Recent results indicate that mice with IL-1 gene deficiency show reduced inflammatory and neuropathic injury responses. The authors conclude that IL-1 modulates both generation and maintenance of inflammatory and neuropathic pain.[165] Another study in rats with neuropathic pain indicates increased endogenous levels of the proinflammatory cytokine interleukin-1β only in the animals in whom there were clear behavioral signs for presence of pain.[166] The latter is proposed as a marker for brain regions undergoing synaptic plasticity because changes in neuronal activity can result in cytokine induction in the brain and in long-term potentiation of synaptic activity in the hippocampus.[167]

ROLE OF THE CORTEX IN CHRONIC PAIN PERCEPTION

In spite of a plethora of data there remains a host of uncertainties about their significance. Overall, the clinical brain imaging studies indicate reduced information transmission through the thalamus to the cortex, and increased activity in prefrontal cortex, coupled with regional atrophy. The number of studies remain small and hence our confidence as to the reproducibility of these changes remains minimal. Still, the observations regarding cortical and thalamic activity changes in chronic pain are in general consistent with the notion that chronic pain conditions preferentially engage brain areas involved in cognition/emotion and decreased activity in regions involved in sensory evaluation of nociceptive inputs.

Evidence has been presented that brain activity, chemistry, and morphology may be reorganized in chronic pain conditions. Does this evidence imply that there is supraspinal reorganization, above and beyond what is established in the periphery and spinal cord? That is, even if we establish a brain pattern of activity for some chronic pain condition, does this reflect some unique contribution of the brain to this state or is it simply a reflection of lower level reorganization? The answer is not straightforward. However, only by answering such questions will brain imaging be able to provide new information to myriad mechanisms described for peripheral and spinal cord reorganization in chronic pain. Overall, this evidence provides signs regarding the supraspinal sensitization and the long list of changes that may underlie this phenomenon, in which the primary or critical parameters that control these changes remain essentially unknown.

CONCLUSION

This chapter outlines peripheral and central events that accompany pain, emphasizing cellular, molecular, anatomical, and physiologic changes that accompany various types of pain conditions. The review also attempts to highlight the gaps that continue to become apparent as the field moves forward and unravels the large number of factors that shift in relation to pain. The gap between animal models for pain and human clinical conditions should be apparent. Yet in many cases there seems to be growing evidence from studies in both groups that similar and parallel changes accompany persistent pain. The animal studies provide convincing evidence for changes in receptor properties both in the periphery and the spinal cord, as well as changes in excitability and neurodegeneration, especially in the spinal cord. Human studies, however, provide better evidence for topographic changes in pain encoding between acute and chronic pain states, especially indicating that distinct portions of the cortex may be involved in each. The accumulating evidence for cortical neurodegeneration poses new questions regarding the driving forces for chronic pain, namely are the latter a consequence or predisposing events for such conditions? More important, the chapter indicates that pain perception cannot be viewed as a unidirectional information transmission from the periphery to the cortex, rather that pain is caused by the interaction between ascending and descending pathways that reorganize the system at all levels.

Images of brain activation by painful stimuli leave the impression that at least half of the brain participates in processing nociceptive information. At other times, many of the same areas participate in visual, motor, emotional, cognitive, or other signal processing. In that sense our current understanding of the nociceptive network in the brain is consistent with the current understanding of how the brain uses distributed processing for its many functions. It is not clear, however, to what extent any part of the cerebral cortex is specific for nociception. The best candidate region for such a function lies in the parasylvian cortex, in the vicinity of SI and SII, and portions of ACC. In chronic pain, nociceptive processing in the cerebral cortex is partly preserved and partly altered, in particular with respect to prefrontal cortex functions. This reorganization may be a neuroplastic response to the chronicity of pain, it may reflect activation of antinociceptive processes, or it may even represent a predisposing factor for the development of chronic pain.

References

1. Dancause N: Neurophysiological and anatomical plasticity in the adult sensorimotor cortex. Rev Neurosci 2006;17:561-580.
2. Karmarkar UR, Dan Y: Experience-dependent plasticity in adult visual cortex. Neuron 2006;52:577-585.
3. Jorntell H, Hansel C: Synaptic memories upside down: Bidirectional plasticity at cerebellar parallel fiber-Purkinje cell synapses. Neuron 2006;52:227-238.
4. Disterhoft JF, Oh MM: Learning, aging and intrinsic neuronal plasticity. Trends Neurosci 2006;29:587-599.
5. Dan Y, Poo MM: Spike timing-dependent plasticity: From synapse to perception. Physiol Rev 2006;86:1033-1048.
6. Johansen-Berg H: Structural plasticity: Rewiring the brain. Curr Biol 2007;17:R141-R144.
7. Melzack R, Wall PD: The Challenge of Pain. Harmondsworth, England, Penguin, 1986.
8. Hill A: Phantom limb pain: A review of the literature on attributes and potential mechanisms. J Pain Symptom Manage 1999;17:125-142.
9. Devor M: Centralization, central sensitization and neuropathic pain. Focus on "sciatic chronic constriction injury produces cell-type-specific changes in the electrophysiological properties of rat substantia gelatinosa neurons." J Neurophysiol 2006;96:522-523.
10. Craig AD: Pain mechanisms: Labeled lines versus convergence in central processing. Annu Rev Neurosci 2003;26:1-30.
11. Woolf CJ, Salter MW: Neuronal plasticity: Increasing the gain in pain. Science 2000;288:1765-1769.
12. Willis WD, Westlund KN: Neuroanatomy of the pain system and of the pathways that modulate pain. J Clin Neurophysiol 1997;14:2-31.
13. Apkarian AV: Cortical pathophysiology of chronic pain. Novartis Found Symp 2004;261:239-245.
14. Apkarian AV, Bushnell MC, Treede RD, Zubieta JK: Human brain mechanisms of pain perception and regulation in health and disease. Eur J Pain 2005;9:463-484.
15. Basbaum AI, Woolf CJ: Pain. Curr Biol 1999;9:R429-R431.
16. Julius D, Basbaum AI: Molecular mechanisms of nociception. Nature 2001;413:203-210.
17. Caterina MJ, Schumacher MA, Tominaga M, et al: The capsaicin receptor: A heat-activated ion channel in the pain pathway. Nature 1997;389:816-824.
18. Tominaga M, Caterina MJ, Malmberg AB, et al: The cloned capsaicin receptor integrates multiple pain-producing stimuli. Neuron 1998;21:531-543.
19. Bevan S: Nociceptive peripheral neurons: Cellular processes. In Wall PD, Melzack R (eds): Textbook of Pain, 3rd Ed. New York, Churchill Livingstone, 1999, pp 85-103.
20. Boivie J, Leijon G, Johansson I: Central post-stroke pain—A study of the mechanisms through analyses of the sensory abnormalities. Pain 1989;37:173-185.
21. Bennett GJ: An animal model of neuropathic pain: A review. Muscle Nerve 1993;16:1040-1048.
22. Li Y, Dorsi MJ, Meyer RA, Belzberg AJ: Mechanical hyperalgesia after an L5 spinal nerve lesion in the rat is not dependent on input from injured nerve fibers. Pain 2000;85:493-502.
23. Campbell JN, Meyer RA: Mechanisms of neuropathic pain. Neuron 2006;52:77-92.
24. Yezierski RP: Spinal cord injury: A model of central neuropathic pain. Neurosignals 2005;14:182-193.
25. Campbell JN, Raja SN, Meyer RA, Mackinnon SE: Myelinated afferents signal the hyperalgesia associated with nerve injury. Pain 1988;32:89-94.
26. Woolf CJ, Thompson SW: The induction and maintenance of central sensitization is dependent on N-methyl-D-aspartic acid receptor activation; implications for the treatment of post-injury pain hypersensitivity states. Pain 1991;44:293-299.
27. Devor M, Seltzer Z: Pathophysiology of damaged nerves in relation to chronic pain. In Wall PD, Melzack R (eds): Textbook of Pain, 3rd Ed. New York, Churchill Livingstone, 1999, pp 129-164.
28. Ibrahim MM, Deng H, Zvonok A, et al: Activation of CB2 cannabinoid receptors by AM1241 inhibits experimental neuropathic pain: Pain inhibition by receptors not present in the CNS. Proc Natl Acad Sci U S A 2003;100:10529-10533.
29. Porreca F, Lai J, Bian D, et al: A comparison of the potential role of the tetrodotoxin-insensitive sodium channels, PN3/SNS and NaN/SNS2, in rat models of chronic pain. Proc Natl Acad Sci U S A 1999;96:7640-7644.
30. Sheth RN, Dorsi MJ, Li Y, et al: Mechanical hyperalgesia after an L5 ventral rhizotomy or an L5 ganglionectomy in the rat. Pain 2002;96:63-72.
31. Djouhri L, Koutsikou S, Fang X, et al: Spontaneous pain, both neuropathic and inflammatory, is related to frequency of spontaneous firing in intact C-fiber nociceptors. J Neurosci 2006;26:1281-1292.
32. Sato J, Perl ER: Adrenergic excitation of cutaneous pain receptors induced by peripheral nerve injury. Science 1991;251:1608-1610.
33. Shim B, Kim DW, Kim BH, et al: Mechanical and heat sensitization of cutaneous nociceptors in rats with experimental peripheral neuropathy. Neuroscience 2005;132:193-201.
34. Mantyh PW: Cancer pain and its impact on diagnosis, survival and quality of life. Nat Rev Neurosci 2006;7:797-809.
35. Honore P, Wade CL, Zhong C, et al: Interleukin-1 alpha beta gene-deficient mice show reduced nociceptive sensitivity in models of inflammatory and neuropathic pain but not postoperative pain. Behav Brain Res 2005;167:355-364.
36. Hunt SP, Mantyh PW: The molecular dynamics of pain control. Nat Rev Neurosci 2001;2:83-91.
37. Kohno T, Ji RR, Ito N, et al: Peripheral axonal injury results in reduced mu opioid receptor pre- and post-synaptic action in the spinal cord. Pain 2005;117:77-87.
38. Yoshimura M, Yonehara N: Alteration in sensitivity of ionotropic glutamate receptors and tachykinin receptors in spinal cord contribute to development and maintenance of nerve injury-evoked neuropathic pain. Neurosci Res 2006;56:21-28.
39. Coull JA, Boudreau D, Bachand K, et al: Trans-synaptic shift in anion gradient in spinal lamina I neurons as a mechanism of neuropathic pain. Nature 2003;424:938-942.
40. Marchand F, Perretti M, McMahon S: Role of the immune system in chronic pain. Nat Rev Neurosci 2005;6:521-532.
41. Wolf G, Gabay E, Tal M, et al: Genetic impairment of interleukin-1 signaling attenuates neuropathic pain, autotomy, and spontaneous ectopic neuronal activity, following nerve injury in mice. Pain 2006;120:315-324.
42. Trang T, Beggs S, Salter MW: Purinoceptors in microglia and neuropathic pain. Pflugers Arch 2006;452:645-652.
43. Whiteside GT, Munglani R: Cell death in the superficial dorsal horn in a model of neuropathic pain. J Neurosci Res 2001;64:168-173.

44. Scholz J, Broom DC, Youn DH, et al: Blocking caspase activity prevents transsynaptic neuronal apoptosis and the loss of inhibition in lamina II of the dorsal horn after peripheral nerve injury. J Neurosci 2005;25:7317-7323.

45. Head H, Holmes G: Sensory disturbances from cerebral lesions. Brain 1911;34:102-254.

46. Marshall J: Sensory disturbances in cortical wounds with special reference to pain. J Neurol Neurosurg Psychiatry 1951;14:187-204.

47. Biemond A: The conduction of pain above the level of the thalamus opticus. AMA Arch Neurol Psychiatry 1956;75:231-244.

48. Kenshalo DR Jr, Isensee O: Responses of primate SI cortical neurons to noxious stimuli. J Neurophysiol 1983;50:1479-1496.

49. Kenshalo DR Jr, Chudler EH, Anton F, Dubner R: SI nociceptive neurons participate in the encoding process by which monkeys perceive the intensity of noxious thermal stimulation. Brain Res 1988;454:378-382.

50. Gingold SI, Greenspan JD, Apkarian AV: Anatomic evidence of nociceptive inputs to primary somatosensory cortex: Relationship between spinothalamic terminals and thalamocortical cells in squirrel monkeys. J Comp Neurol 1991;308:467-490.

51. Jones AK, Brown WD, Friston KJ, et al: Cortical and subcortical localization of response to pain in man using positron emission tomography. Proc R Soc Lond B Biol Sci 1991;244:39-44.

52. Talbot JD, Marrett S, Evans AC, et al: Multiple representations of pain in human cerebral cortex. Science 1991;251:1355-1358.

53. Apkarian AV, Stea RA, Manglos SH, et al: Persistent pain inhibits contralateral somatosensory cortical activity in humans. Neurosci Lett 1992;140:141-147.

54. Davis KD, Wood ML, Crawley AP, Mikulis D: fMRI of human somatosensory and cingulate cortex during painful electrical nerve stimulation. Neuroreport 1995;7:321-325.

55. Price DD: Psychological and Neural Mechanisms of Pain. New York, Raven Press, 1988, pp 18-49.

56. Treede RD, Apkarian AV, Bromm B, et al: Cortical representation of pain: Functional characterization of nociceptive areas near the lateral sulcus. Pain 2000;87:113-119.

57. Melzack R, Casey K: Sensory, motivational, and central control determinants of pain. In Kenshalo DR (ed): The Skin Senses. Springfield, Ill, Charles C Thomas, 1968, pp 423-443.

58. Bushnell MC, Apkarian AV: Representation of pain in the brain. In McMahon SB, Koltzenburg M (eds): Wall and Melzack's Textbook of Pain. London, Elsevier, 2006, pp 107-124.

59. Willis WD, Coggeshall RE: Sensory Mechanisms of the Spinal Cord. New York, Plenum Press, 1978.

60. Strigo IA, Duncan GH, Boivin M, Bushnell MC: Differentiation of visceral and cutaneous pain in the human brain. J Neurophysiol 2003;89:3294-3303.

61. Bromm B, Treede RD: CO$_2$ laser radiant heat pulses activate C nociceptors in man. Pflugers Arch 1983;399:155-156.

62. Bragard D, Chen AC, Plaghki L: Direct isolation of ultra-late (C-fibre) evoked brain potentials by CO2 laser stimulation of tiny cutaneous surface areas in man. Neurosci Lett 1996;209:81-84.

63. Magerl W, Ali Z, Ellrich J, et al: C- and A delta-fiber components of heat-evoked cerebral potentials in healthy human subjects. Pain 1999;82:127-137.

64. Iannetti GD, Truini A, Romaniello A, et al: Evidence of a specific spinal pathway for the sense of warmth in humans. J Neurophysiol 2003;89:562-570.

65. Lenz FA, Rios M, Chau D, et al: Painful stimuli evoke potentials recorded from the parasylvian cortex in humans. J Neurophysiol 1998;80:2077-2088.

66. Frot M, Rambaud L, Guenot M, Mauguiere: Intracortical recordings of early pain-related CO$_2$-laser evoked potentials in the human second somatosensory (SII) area. Clin Neurophysiol 1999;110:133-145.

67. Apkarian AV, Shi T: Squirrel monkey lateral thalamus. I. Somatic nociresponsive neurons and their relation to spinothalamic terminals. J Neurosci 1994;14:6779-6795.

68. Craig AD: How do you feel? Interoception: The sense of the physiological condition of the body. Nat Rev Neurosci 2002;3:655-666.

69. Bushnell MC, Duncan GH, Hofbauer RK, et al: Pain perception: Is there a role for primary somatosensory cortex? Proc Natl Acad Sci U S A 1999;96:7705-7709.

70. Longe SE, Wise R, Bantick S, et al: Counter-stimulatory effects on pain perception and processing are significantly altered by attention: An fMRI study. Neuroreport 2001;12:2021-2025.

71. Bantick SJ, Wise RG, Ploghaus A, et al: Imaging how attention modulates pain in humans using functional MRI. Brain 2002;125:310-319.

72. Petrovic P, Dietrich T, Fransson P, et al: Placebo in emotional processing—Induced expectations of anxiety relief activate a generalized modulatory network. Neuron 2005;46:957-969.

73. Tracey I, Ploghaus A, Gati JS, et al: Imaging attentional modulation of pain in the periaqueductal gray in humans. J Neurosci 2002;22:2748-2752.

74. Valet M, Sprenger T, Boecker H, et al: Distraction modulates connectivity of the cingulo-frontal cortex and the midbrain during pain—An fMRI analysis. Pain 2004;109:399-408.

75. Ploghaus A, Tracey I, Gati JS, et al: Dissociating pain from its anticipation in the human brain. Science 1999;284:1979-1981.

76. Hsieh JC, Stone-Elander S, Ingvar M: Anticipatory coping of pain expressed in the human anterior cingulate cortex: A positron emission tomography study. Neurosci Lett 1999;262:61-64.

77. Sawamoto N, Honda M, Okada T, et al: Expectation of pain enhances responses to nonpainful somatosensory stimulation in the anterior cingulate cortex and parietal operculum/posterior insula: An event-related functional magnetic resonance imaging study. J Neurosci 2000;20:7438-7445.

78. Porro CA, Baraldi P, Pagnoni G, et al: Does anticipation of pain affect cortical nociceptive systems? J Neurosci 2002;22:3206-3214.

79. Keltner JR, Furst A, Fan C, et al: Isolating the modulatory effect of expectation on pain transmission: A functional magnetic resonance imaging study. J Neurosci 2006;26:4437-4443.

80. Kong J, Gollub RL, Rosman IS, et al: Brain activity associated with expectancy-enhanced placebo analgesia as measured by functional magnetic resonance imaging. J Neurosci 2006;26:381-388.

81. Singer T, Seymour B, O'Doherty J, et al: Empathy for pain involves the affective but not sensory components of pain. Science 2004;303:1157-1162.

82. Morrison I, Lloyd D, di Pellegrino G, Roberts: Vicarious responses to pain in anterior cingulate cortex: Is empathy a multisensory issue? Cogn Affect Behav Neurosci 2004;4:270-278.

83. Botvinick M, Jha AP, Bylsma LM, et al: Viewing facial expressions of pain engages cortical areas involved in the direct experience of pain. Neuroimage 2005;25:312-319.

84. Jackson PL, Brunet E, Meltzoff AN, Decety: Empathy examined through the neural mechanisms involved in imagining how I feel versus how you feel pain. Neuropsychologia 2006;44:752-761.

85. Danziger N, Prkachin KM, Willer JC: Is pain the price of empathy? The perception of others' pain in patients with congenital insensitivity to pain. Brain 2006;129:2494-2507.

86. Phillips ML, Gregory LJ, Cullen S, et al: The effect of negative emotional context on neural and behavioural responses to oesophageal stimulation. Brain 2003;126:669-684.

87. Lidstone SC, Stoessl AJ: Understanding the placebo effect: Contributions from neuroimaging. Mol Imaging Biol 2007;9:258.

88. Levine JD, Gordon NC, Fields HL: The mechanism of placebo analgesia. Lancet 1978;2:654-657.

89. Zubieta JK, Bueller JA, Jackson LR, et al: Placebo effects mediated by endogenous opioid activity on mu-opioid receptors. J Neurosci 2005;25:7754-7762.

90. Wager TD, Rilling JK, Smith EE, et al: Placebo-induced changes in fMRI in the anticipation and experience of pain. Science 2004;303:1162-1167.

91. Benedetti F, Mayberg HS, Wager TD, et al: Neurobiological mechanisms of the placebo effect. J Neurosci 2005;25: 10390-10402.
92. Bingel U, Lorenz J, Schoell E, et al: Mechanisms of placebo analgesia: rACC recruitment of a subcortical antinociceptive network. Pain 2006;120:8-15.
93. Petrovic P, Petersson KM, Ghatan PH, et al: Pain-related cerebral activation is altered by a distracting cognitive task. Pain 2000;85:19-30.
94. Casey KL, Svensson P, Morrow TJ, et al: Selective opiate modulation of nociceptive processing in the human brain. J Neurophysiol 2000;84:525-533.
95. Petrovic P, Kalso E, Petersson KM, Ingvar M: Placebo and opioid analgesia—Imaging a shared neuronal network. Science 2002;295:1737-1740.
96. Zubieta JK, Smith YR, Bueller JA, et al: Regional mu opioid receptor regulation of sensory and affective dimensions of pain. Science 2001;293:311-315.
97. Zubieta JK, Smith YR, Bueller JA, et al: mu-Opioid receptor-mediated antinociceptive responses differ in men and women. J Neurosci 2002;22:5100-5107.
98. Zubieta JK, Ketter TA, Bueller JA, et al: Regulation of human affective responses by anterior cingulate and limbic mu-opioid neurotransmission. Arch Gen Psychiatry 2003;60:1145-1153.
99. Pertovaara A, Martikainen IK, Hagelberg N, et al: Striatal dopamine D2/D3 receptor availability correlates with individual response characteristics to pain. Eur J Neurosci 2004;20:1587-1592.
100. Martikainen IK, Hagelberg N, Mansikka H, et al: Association of striatal dopamine D2/D3 receptor binding potential with pain but not tactile sensitivity or placebo analgesia. Neurosci Lett 2005;376:149-153.
101. Scott DJ, Heitzeg MM, Koeppe RA, et al: Variations in the human pain stress experience mediated by ventral and dorsal basal ganglia dopamine activity. J Neurosci 2006;26:10789-10795.
102. Jaaskelainen SK, Rinne JO, Forssell H, et al: Role of the dopaminergic system in chronic pain—A fluorodopa-PET study. Pain 2001;90:257-260.
103. Hagelberg N, Forssell H, Aalto S, et al: Altered dopamine D2 receptor binding in atypical facial pain. Pain 2003;106: 43-48.
104. Hagelberg N, Forssell H, Rinne JO, et al: Striatal dopamine D1 and D2 receptors in burning mouth syndrome. Pain 2003;101:149-154.
105. Wood PB, Patterson JC, Sunderland JJ, et al: Reduced presynaptic dopamine activity in fibromyalgia syndrome demonstrated with positron emission tomography: A pilot study. J Pain 2007;8:51-58.
106. Kajantie E, Phillips DI: The effects of sex and hormonal status on the physiological response to acute psychosocial stress. Psychoneuroendocrinology 2006;31:151-178.
107. Wiesenfeld-Hallin Z: Sex differences in pain perception. Gend Med 2005;2:137-145.
108. Wilson JF: The pain divide between men and women. Ann Intern Med 2006;144:461-464.
109. Apkarian AV, Sosa Y, Sonty S, et al: Chronic back pain is associated with decreased prefrontal and thalamic gray matter density. J Neurosci 2004;24:10410-10415.
110. Gracely RH, Geisser ME, Giesecke T, et al: Pain catastrophizing and neural responses to pain among persons with fibromyalgia. Brain 2004;127:835-843.
111. Gracely RH, Petzke F, Wolf JM, Clauw DJ: Functional magnetic resonance imaging evidence of augmented pain processing in fibromyalgia. Arthritis Rheum 2002;46:1333-1343.
112. Schweinhardt P, Glynn C, Brooks J, et al: An fMRI study of cerebral processing of brush-evoked allodynia in neuropathic pain patients. Neuroimage 2006;32:256-265.
113. Garcia-Larrea L, Maarrawi J, Peyron R, et al: On the relation between sensory deafferentation, pain and thalamic activity in Wallenberg's syndrome: A PET-scan study before and after motor cortex stimulation. Eur J Pain 2006;10:677-688.
114. Schmahl C, Bremner JD: Neuroimaging in borderline personality disorder. J Psychiatr Res 2006;40:419-427.
115. Chen AC, Treede RD, Bromm B: Tonic pain inhibits phasic pain: Evoked cerebral potential correlates in man. Psychiatry Res 1985;14:343-351.
116. Apkarian AV, Thomas PS, Krauss BR, Szeverenyi NM: Prefrontal cortical hyperactivity in patients with sympathetically mediated chronic pain. Neurosci Lett 2001;311:193-197.
117. Granziera C, DaSilva AF, Snyder J, et al: Anatomical alterations of the visual motion processing network in migraine with and without aura. PLoS Med 2006;3:e402.
118. Hadjikhani N, Sanchez del Rio M, Wu O, et al: Mechanisms of migraine aura revealed by functional MRI in human visual cortex. Proc Natl Acad Sci U S A 2001;98:4687-4692.
119. Cao Y, Welch KMA, Aurora S, Vikingstad EM: Functional MRI-BOLD of visually triggered headache in patients with migraine. Arch Neurol 1999;56:548-554.
120. Goadsby PJ, Lipton RB, Ferrari MD: Migraine—Current understanding and treatment. N Engl J Med 2002;346: 257-270.
121. May A, Bahra A, Buchel C, et al: Hypothalamic activation in cluster headache attacks. Lancet 1998;352:275-278.
122. Wang SJ, Lirng JF, Fuh JL, Chen JJ: Reduction in hypothalamic 1H-MRS metabolite ratios in patients with cluster headache. J Neurol Neurosurg Psychiatry 2006;77:622-625.
123. Rosen SD, Paulesu E, Nihoyannopoulos P, et al: Silent ischemia as a central problem: Regional brain activation compared in silent and painful myocardial ischemia. Ann Intern Med 1996;124:939-949.
124. Rosen SD, Camici PG: The brain-heart axis in the perception of cardiac pain: The elusive link between ischaemia and pain. Ann Med 2000;32:350-364.
125. Rosen SD, Paulesu E, Wise RJ, Camici PG: Central neural contribution to the perception of chest pain in cardiac syndrome X. Heart 2002;87:513-519.
126. Silverman DH, Munakata JA, Ennes H, et al: Regional cerebral activity in normal and pathological perception of visceral pain. Gastroenterology 1997;112:64-72.
127. Mertz H, Morgan V, Tanner G, et al: Regional cerebral activation in irritable bowel syndrome and control subjects with painful and nonpainful rectal distention. Gastroenterology 2000;118:842-848.
128. Andresen V, Bach DR, Poellinger A, et al: Brain activation responses to subliminal or supraliminal rectal stimuli and to auditory stimuli in irritable bowel syndrome. Neurogastroenterol Motil 2005;17:827-837.
129. Lawal A, Kern M, Sidhu H, et al: Novel evidence for hypersensitivity of visceral sensory neural circuitry in irritable bowel syndrome patients. Gastroenterology 2006;130:26-33.
130. Verne GN, Himes NC, Robinson ME, et al: Central representation of visceral and cutaneous hypersensitivity in the irritable bowel syndrome. Pain 2003;103:99-110.
131. Kwan CL, Diamant NE, Pope G, et al: Abnormal forebrain activity in functional bowel disorder patients with chronic pain. Neurology 2005;65:1268-1277.
132. Baliki MN, Chialvo DR, Geha PY, et al: Chronic pain and the emotional brain: Specific brain activity associated with spontaneous fluctuations of intensity of chronic back pain. J Neurosci 2006;26:12165-12173.
133. Geha PY, Baliki MN, Chialvo DR, et al: Brain activity for spontaneous pain of postherpetic neuralgia and its modulation by lidocaine patch therapy. Pain 2007;128:88-100.
134. Lorenz J, Bromm B: Event-related potential correlates of interference between cognitive performance and tonic experimental pain. Psychophysiology 1997;34:436-445.
135. Foss JM, Apkarian AV, Chialvo DR: Dynamics of pain: Fractal dimension of temporal variability of spontaneous pain differentiates between pain states. J Neurophysiol 2006;95: 730-736.
136. Pattany PM, Yezierski RP, Widerstrom-Noga EG, et al: Proton magnetic resonance spectroscopy of the thalamus in patients with chronic neuropathic pain after spinal cord injury. AJNR Am J Neuroradiol 2002;23:901-905.
137. Hsieh JC, Belfrage M, Stoneelander S, et al: Central representation of chronic ongoing neuropathic pain studied positron emission tomography. Pain 1995;63:225-236.

138. Fukumoto M, Ushida T, Zinchuk VS, et al: Contralateral thalamic perfusion in patients with reflex sympathetic dystrophy syndrome. Lancet 1999;354:1790-1791.
139. Maarrawi J, Peyron R, Mertens P, et al: Differential brain opioid receptor availability in central and peripheral neuropathic pain. Pain 2007;127:183-194.
140. Willoch F, Tolle TR, Wester HJ, et al: Central pain after pontine infarction is associated with changes in opioid receptor binding: A PET study with 11C-diprenorphine. Am J Neuroradiol 1999;20:686-690.
141. Giesecke T, Gracely RH, Grant MA, et al: Evidence of augmented central pain processing in idiopathic chronic low back pain. Arthritis Rheum 2004;50:613-623.
142. Grachev ID, Fredrickson BE, Apkarian AV: Abnormal brain chemistry in chronic back pain: An in vivo proton magnetic resonance spectroscopy study. Pain 2000;89:7-18.
143. Grachev ID: Spectroscopic brain mapping the N-acetyl aspartate to cognitive-perceptual states in chronic pain. Mol Psychiatry 2001;6:124.
144. Grachev ID, Fredickson BE, Apkarian AV: Dissociating anxiety from pain: Mapping the neuronal marker N-acetyl aspartate to perception distinguishes closely interrelated characteristics of chronic pain. Mol Psychiatry 2001;6:256-258.
145. Grachev ID, Fredrickson BE, Apkarian AV: Brain chemistry reflects dual states of pain and anxiety in chronic low back pain. J Neural Transm 2002;109:1309-1334.
146. Kalra S, Hanstock CC, Martin WR, et al: Detection of cerebral degeneration in amyotrophic lateral sclerosis using high-field magnetic resonance spectroscopy. Arch Neurol 2006;63:1144-1148.
147. Kalra S, Vitale A, Cashman NR, et al: Cerebral degeneration predicts survival in amyotrophic lateral sclerosis. J Neurol Neurosurg Psychiatry 2006;77:1253-1255.
148. Jessen F, Traeber F, Freymann K, et al: Treatment monitoring and response prediction with proton MR spectroscopy in AD. Neurology 2006;67:528-530.
149. Kantarci K, Weigand SD, Petersen RC, et al: Longitudinal (1)H MRS changes in mild cognitive impairment and Alzheimer's disease. Neurobiol Aging 2006;28:1330-1339.
150. Fukui S, Matsuno M, Inubushi T, Nosaka S: N-Acetylaspartate concentrations in the thalami of neuropathic pain patients and healthy comparison subjects measured with (1)H-MRS. Magn Reson Imaging 2006;24:75-79.
151. Garseth M, Sonnewald U, White LR, et al: Metabolic changes in the cerebrospinal fluid of patients with lumbar disc herniation or spinal stenosis. J Neurosci Res 2002;69:692-695.
152. Schmidt-Wilcke T, Leinisch E, Straube A, et al: Gray matter decrease in patients with chronic tension type headache. Neurology 2005;65:1483-1486.
153. Kuchinad A, Schweinhardt P, Seminowicz DA, et al: Accelerated brain gray matter loss in fibromyalgia patients: Premature aging of the brain? J Neurosci 2007;27:4004-4007.
154. LeDoux JE: Emotion circuits in the brain. Annu Rev Neurosci 2000;23:155-184.
155. McGaraughty S, Heinricher MM: Microinjection of morphine into various amygdaloid nuclei differentially affects nociceptive responsiveness and RVM neuronal activity. Pain 2002;96:153-162.
156. Heinricher MM, McGaraughty S, Farr DA: The role of excitatory amino acid transmission within the rostral ventromedial medulla in the antinociceptive actions of systemically administered morphine. Pain 1999;81:57-65.
157. Neugebauer V, Li W, Bird GC, Han JS: The amygdala and persistent pain. Neuroscientist 2004;10:221-234.
158. Han JS, Li W, Neugebauer: Critical role of calcitonin gene-related peptide 1 receptors in the amygdala in synaptic plasticity and pain behavior. J Neurosci 2005;25:10717-10728.
159. Derbyshire SW, Jones AK, Gyulai F, et al: Pain processing during three levels of noxious stimulation produces differential patterns of central activity. Pain 1997;73:431-445.
160. Becerra LR, Breiter HC, Stojanovic M, et al: Human brain activation under controlled thermal stimulation and habituation to noxious heat: An fMRI study. Magn Reson Med 1999;41:1044-1057.
161. Bornhovd K, Quante M, Glauche V, et al: Painful stimuli evoke different stimulus-response functions in the amygdala, prefrontal, insula and somatosensory cortex: A single-trial fMRI study. Brain 2002;125:1326-1336.
162. Naliboff BD, Derbyshire SW, Munakata J, et al: Cerebral activation in patients with irritable bowel syndrome and control subjects during rectosigmoid stimulation. Psychosom Med 2001;63:365-375.
163. Bonaz B, Baciu M, Papillon E, et al: Central processing of rectal pain in patients with irritable bowel syndrome: An fMRI study. Am J Gastroenterol 2002;97:654-661.
164. Petrovic P, Ingvar M, Stone-Elander S, et al: A PET activation study of dynamic mechanical allodynia in patients with mononeuropathy. Pain 1999;83:459-470.
165. Honor P, Menning PM, Rogers SD, et al: Spinal substance P receptor expression and internalization in acute, short-term, and long-term inflammatory pain states. J Neurosci 1999;19:7670-7678.
166. Apkarian AV, Lavarello S, Randolf A, et al: Expression of IL-1 beta in supraspinal brain regions in rats with neuropathic pain. Neurosci Lett 2006;407:176-181.
167. Schneider H, Pitossi F, Balschun D, et al: A neuromodulatory role of interleukin-1 beta in the hippocampus. Proc Natl Acad Sci U S A 1998;95:7778-7783.

CHAPTER

10 History and Physical Examination of the Pain Patient

Irfan Lalani and Charles E. Argoff

The physical examination serves to further explore and confirm the findings on clinical history. Objective data obtained from the examination is essential to accurately diagnose the etiology of pain. This chapter provides an overview of a structured approach to the physical examination of the pain patient along with the anatomic and physiologic basis of the physical findings.

The key components of the physical examination include a general physical examination, a detailed neurologic examination, a detailed musculoskeletal examination, and an examination for cutaneous or trophic findings. The musculoskeletal examination includes inspection, palpation, percussion, auscultation, and provocative maneuvers.

GENERAL PHYSICAL EXAMINATION

Vital signs including temperature, heart rate, respiratory rate, blood pressure and weight should be noted at each visit. This information is useful in forming an impression of the overall health and comorbid conditions of the patient.

A few moments should be spent in observing and documenting the general appearance and gait of the patient. Attributes include how the patient dresses and personal hygiene. Pain behaviors, posture, and anatomic abnormalities such as contractures, amputation, and asymmetries should also be noted. Maladaptive postural dynamics play an important role in generating myofascial pain. Excessive lumbar lordosis places strain on the lumbar extensor muscles and results in low back pain. Similarly, forward flexion of the cervical spine with drooping of the shoulders strains the cervical paraspinous and scapular muscles, causing neck and upper back pain.

Gait evaluation includes assessment of the stride length, base, arm swing, and stability. An unsteady, wide-based ataxic gait can be seen in patients with cerebellar and proprioceptive disorders. In patients with hip and lower extremity pain, the stance phase is reduced in the affected limb, resulting in an antal-

gic gait pattern. The waddling gait is seen in patients with hip girdle muscle weakness, whereas the steppage gait occurs in patients with foot drop.[1]

NEUROLOGIC EXAMINATION

The components of the neurologic examination are the following:
1. Mental status examination
2. Cranial nerve testing
3. Motor strength examination
4. Deep tendon reflexes
5. Sensation
6. Coordination
7. Special tests

MENTAL STATUS EXAMINATION

A reasonable assessment of mental status can often be made as part of history taking and inquiry into activities of daily living and function. A basic mental status examination includes assessment of the level of consciousness, orientation to person, place, time and situation, registration and short-term memory, attention and concentration, and language assessment for aphasia. The Folstein Mini-Mental Status Examination is a useful screening tool for detecting cognitive deficits and dementia.

Assessment of mood, affect, suicidal and homicidal ideation, and neurovegetative symptoms such as sleep, appetite, and energy level should be inquired about routinely. This helps uncover comorbid psychiatric conditions (e.g., depression, anxiety, and psychosis), which can profoundly impact the treatment of pain patients.

CRANIAL NERVE TESTING

The cranial nerve examination localizes pathology primarily at the level of the brainstem. Central pain conditions associated with brainstem pathology (e.g., strokes, tumors, demyelinating disease, and vascular malformations) can be associated with cranial nerve deficits.[1]

Cranial Nerve I

Olfactory Nerve

Test one nostril at a time. Odors such as coffee, mint, or cloves can be used. Noxious odors such as ammonia should be avoided because they activate the trigeminal nerve receptors in the nasal passages.

The most common cause of smell dysfunction is nasal and sinus pathology. Dementia, neurodegenerative conditions, and basal frontal tumors can also cause smell dysfunction.

Cranial Nerve II

Optic Nerve

Visual acuity is determined using a Snellen chart. Visual fields are tested by the confrontation method at the bedside. More formal visual field testing with perimetry can be requested, if indicated. Pupillary reaction to light and accommodation tests the optic and ophthalmic nerves. Funduscopic examination is done to evaluate the optic disc and retina. Papilledema and enlargement of the blind spot can be seen in conditions with elevated intracranial pressure, including idiopathic intracranial hypertension, which is a relatively common cause of intractable headache.

Cranial Nerves III, IV, and VI

Ophthalmic, Trochlear, and Abducens Nerves

These nerves control eye movement and can be tested by asking the patient to track a moving object in the eight positions of cardinal gaze. Eyelid elevation and pupillary constriction are controlled by the third nerve and are assessed with the direct, consensual, and accommodation reflexes. Sympathetic fibers innervate pupillary dilator muscles. Horner's syndrome can be detected in several clinical conditions, including after stellate ganglion blockade. This syndrome includes ipsilateral ptosis, miosis, and anhydrosis. However, the mechanism of these changes involves sympatholysis and is independent of cranial nerve function.

Cranial Nerve V

Trigeminal Nerve

This nerve supplies sensory input to the face, mouth, tongue, and scalp up to the vertex. The mandibular division of the trigeminal nerve also supplies the muscles of mastication (i.e., temporalis, masseter, medial, and lateral pterygoid muscles).

Sensation along the ophthalmic, maxillary, and mandibular divisions of the trigeminal nerve can be tested with temperature, pinprick, and light touch. The trigeminal nerve also provides the afferent limb of the corneal blink reflex.

Peripheral lesions of the trigeminal nerve result in ipsilateral loss of facial sensation with weakness and atrophy of the ipsilateral jaw muscles.

Cranial Nerve VII

Facial Nerve

The facial nerve innervates the muscles of facial expression, submandibular, and lacrimal glands and taste to the anterior two thirds of the tongue. Testing is usually limited to checking facial motor function (e.g., forehead wrinkling, eye closure, smile, pursing lips, and corneal blink). Supranuclear lesions of the seventh nerve typically spare the forehead, whereas nuclear and infranuclear lesions do not.

Sensory testing for the facial nerve is not routinely performed. This can be accomplished by applying sweet, sour, and salt stimuli to the ipsilateral half of the anterior two thirds of the tongue.

Cranial Nerve VIII

Vestibulocochlear Nerve

The vestibulocochlear nerve mediates hearing and balance. Hearing can be assessed with a 512-Hz tuning fork. Rinne and Weber tests are commonly used to assess for sensorineural and conductive deafness.

In the Weber test, the base of a gently vibrating tuning fork is placed on the mid-forehead or the vertex. The patient is asked which ear hears the sound better. Normally the sound is heard equally in both ears. In unilateral sensorineural hearing loss, sound is heard better in the unaffected ear. In unilateral conductive hearing loss, sound is heard better in the affected ear.

The Rinne test is conducted by placing the base of a gently vibrating tuning fork on the mastoid bone behind the ear. When the patient can no longer hear the sound, the fork is quickly moved next to the patient's ear. In sensorineural deafness and normal hearing, air conduction is better than bone conduction. In conductive deafness, bone conduction is better than air conduction.

Nystagmus noted on eye movement testing may be a sign of vestibular dysfunction. In patients with complaints of episodic vertigo, the Dix-Hallpike maneuver is useful for making the diagnosis of benign paroxysmal positional vertigo.

Glossopharyngeal Nerve

The glossopharyngeal nerve subserves taste to the posterior one third of the tongue and sensation to the pharynx. It provides the afferent limb of the gag reflex.

Cranial Nerve X

Vagus Nerve

The vagus nerve innervates pharyngeal and laryngeal muscles and forms the efferent limb of the gag reflex. Symptoms of vagus nerve lesions include dysarthria and dysphagia.

Cranial Nerve XI

Accessory Nerve

The cranial segment of the accessory nerve supplies muscles of the larynx, while the spinal segment innervates the trapezius and sternocleidomastoid muscles. These are tested by ipsilateral shoulder shrug and contralateral head turn maneuvers.

Cranial Nerve XII

Hypoglossal Nerve

The hypoglossal nerve provides motor supply to the tongue. Testing is performed by tongue protrusion and pushing the tongue against the cheek on either side. Lesions in the hypoglossal nerve produce ipsilateral deviation on tongue protrusion.

MOTOR STRENGTH EXAMINATION

Manual muscle testing is performed by asking the patient to place each muscle in its position of maximal mechanical advantage. Muscle strength is commonly assessed with the Medical Research Council scale (Table 10–1). Grades 1 to 3 are relatively objective and less prone to interobserver variation. However, grades 4 and 5 are difficult to standardize among different examiners. Factors such as a patient's body habitus, age, and expected functional status contribute to the difficulty of grading muscle strength above grade 3.[2]

The screening muscle strength examination should correspond to a template that evaluates sequential nerve roots and peripheral nerves. Tables 10–2 and 10–3 provide a summary of the commonly tested muscles with their corresponding nerve root and peripheral nerve innervation.[3]

Table 10–1. Medical Research Council Grading

Grade 0	No movement
Grade 1	Flicker of movement
Grade 2	Movement only with gravity eliminated
Grade 3	Full range of movement against gravity
Grade 4	Full range of movement against some resistance
Grade 5	Full power against resistance

Table 10–2. Upper Extremity Muscles: Innervation and Action

MUSCLE	ACTION	NERVE ROOT	NERVE
Infraspinatus	Shoulder external rotation	C5-6	Suprascapular
Deltoid	Shoulder abduction, extension, and flexion	C5-6	Axillary
Biceps	Forearm flexion and supination	C5-6	Musculocutaneous
Triceps	Forearm extension	C7-8	Radial
Brachioradialis	Forearm flexion in the mid-prone position	C6	Radial
Extensor carpi radialis longus and brevis	Wrist extension	C6-7	Radial
Flexor carpi ulnaris	Wrist flexion with ulnar deviation	C8-T1	Ulnar
Flexor digitorum profundus	Flexion at distal interphalangeal joints	C7-8	Anterior interosseus branch of median nerve
Abductor pollicis brevis	Abduction of thumb	C8	Median
Adductor pollicis	Adduction of thumb	C8-T1	Ulnar

Table 10–3. Lower Extremity Muscles: Innervation and Action

MUSCLE	ACTION	NERVE ROOT	NERVE
Iliopsoas	Hip flexion	L2, 3, 4	Femoral
Adductor longus and brevis	Hip adduction	L2, 3, 4	Obturator
Gluteus maximus	Hip extension	L5, S1, S2	Inferior gluteal
Gluteus medius and minimus	Hip abduction	L5, S1, S2	Superior gluteal
Quadriceps femoris	Knee extension	L2, 3, 4	Femoral
Hamstrings (i.e., semitendinosus, semimembranosus, and biceps femoris)	Knee flexion	L5, S1	Sciatic
Tibialis anterior	Foot dorsiflexion	L4-5	Deep peroneal
Extensor hallucis longus	Extension of big toe	L5	Deep peroneal
Peroneus longus	Foot eversion	L5	Superficial peroneal
Gastrocnemius/soleus	Foot plantar flexion	S1, S2	Tibial
Tibialis posterior	Foot inversion and plantar flexion	L5, S1	Tibial

The muscle strength examination depends significantly on patient comprehension and effort. Suboptimal or volitional lack of effort may be apparent as "give-way weakness" where the patient gives intermittent resistance to the examiner interspersed with moments of near complete cessation of effort. The Hoover test is useful to detect psychogenic weakness of the lower extremities. The patient is examined while lying supine in bed and is asked to elevate the paretic leg. The examiner's hand should be placed underneath the contralateral heel. A positive Hoover test occurs if the patient fails to exert downward force on the examiner's hand. The Hoover sign is based on the crossed extensor reflex mediated by interneurons in the spinal cord. This reflex was first described by Sherrington and can be demonstrated in decorticate animals.[1]

REFLEX TESTING

Deep tendon reflexes are mediated by a monosynaptic arc. The afferent limb is provided by Ia sensory fibers, which innervate muscle spindles. These fibers project centrally toward the spinal cord and synapse with alpha motor neurons in the ventral horn. The alpha motor neurons comprise the efferent limb of the reflex arc. It is important to note that normal individuals can have diminished deep tendon reflexes. The Jendrassik maneuver can be used to elicit deep tendon reflexes in this situation. The patient is asked to interlock the fingers of both hands and pull them apart. Jaw clenching can also be used to achieve a similar effect. Lesions of the afferent limb or efferent limb of this arc can cause diminished or absent deep tendon reflexes. This includes conditions such as peripheral neuropathy and radiculopathy. However, patients with small fiber neuropathy have preserved deep tendon reflexes because the neural deficit spares large myelinated Ia fibers.

Deep tendon reflexes are best examined using a Queen square or Troemner hammer with the patient comfortably seated in the upright position. Table 10–4 explains grading of deep tendon reflexes. Table 10–5 reviews the important deep tendon reflexes and their corresponding nerve root level.

Upper motor neuron lesions cause hyperreflexia. The Babinski and Hoffman signs can be present in patients with upper motor neuron dysfunction. The Babinski sign is elicited by stroking the lateral aspect of the sole of the foot with a blunt object (e.g., a disposable wooden spatula). A positive sign is indicated by extension of the great toe (Fig. 10–1). Care should be taken not to stimulate the more medial aspect of the sole, which will evoke a withdrawal response. Hoffman's sign is elicited by briskly flicking the dorsal or volar aspect of the distal phalanx of the middle finger. Reflex flexion of the index finger and thumb constitutes a positive response.[4]

SENSATION

Sensory examination should include the modalities of temperature, pinprick, proprioception, and vibration. Pinprick and temperature are mediated by A-delta and C small fibers and are transmitted in the spinal cord by the lateral spinothalamic tract. Proprioception and vibration are mediated by A-beta large fibers and are carried by the dorsal columns in the spinal cord.

Pinprick testing can be performed using a clean disposable safety pin. A distal to proximal pattern of testing is useful in evaluating patients with length-

Table 10–4. Grading of Deep Tendon Reflexes

Grade 0	Absent
Grade 1+	Hypoactive
Grade 2+	Normal
Grade 3+	Spread of reflex contraction to muscles innervated by adjacent root level
Grade 4+	Sustained clonus

Table 10–5. Nerve Root Innervation of Deep Tendon Reflexes

MUSCLE TENDON	NERVE ROOT LEVEL
Biceps	C5-6
Brachioradialis	C6
Triceps	C7-8
Quadriceps femoris	L3-4
Gastrocnemius/achilles tendon	S1-2

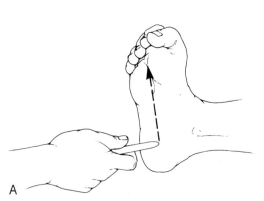
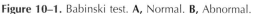
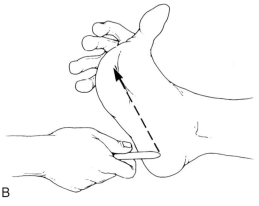

A   B

Figure 10–1. Babinski test. **A,** Normal. **B,** Abnormal.

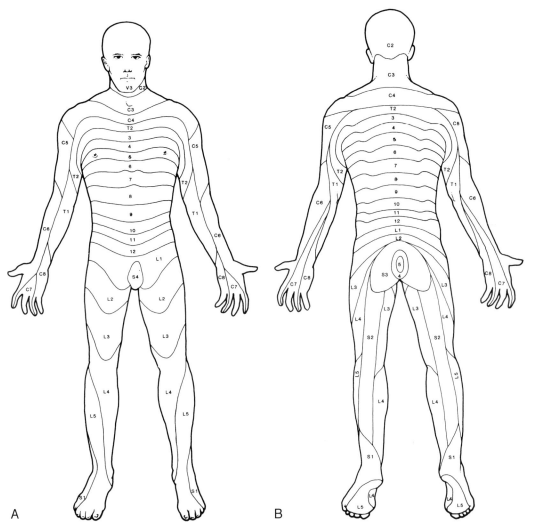

Figure 10–2. Anterior **(A)** and posterior **(B)** dermatomes of the body. (From Baker AB, Baker LH: Clinical Neurology, vol 1. New York, Harper & Row, 1983.)

dependent peripheral neuropathy. In patients with nerve root pathology, testing in a dermatomal pattern is recommended (Fig. 10–2). Temperature sensation can be assessed rapidly using the cold metal portion of a tuning fork and warm water in a test tube. The format for testing is identical to that for pinprick testing.

Proprioception is assessed at individual synovial joints. The most sensitive test for proprioception is at the interphalangeal joint of the big toe. The toe is grasped at its lateral margins between the thumb and index finger of the examiner's hand. The big toe is then abducted from the remaining toes and moved superiorly and inferiorly in increments of 5 degrees while the patient's eyes are closed. The patient is then asked to identify whether the toe is being moved up or down. If proprioception is impaired at the toe, the same test can be repeated at the ankle, knee, and distal interphalangeal joint of the index finger.

Vibration sense is usually examined by placing a vibrating 128-Hz tuning fork over a distal bony prominence. The dorsal surface of the interphalangeal joint of the big toe, medial malleolus, tibial tuberosity, and patella are the relevant lower extremity landmarks. The distal phalanx of the index finger, distal radius, and olecranon process of the ulna are the important sites for testing vibration in the upper extremity. Recently, the Rydel-Seiffer 64-Hz quantitative tuning fork has been shown to have a better correlation with sural nerve sensory nerve action potential and ankle reflex results than the traditional 128-Hz tuning fork.[5]

COORDINATION

Cerebellar function can be divided into midline/vermal and hemispheric functions. The vermis controls axial coordination and balance, whereas the hemispheres coordinate the limbs. Vermian function is assessed with observation of gait and standing balance. Hemispheric function is assessed by the finger to nose and heel to shin tests. Other tests include rapid alternating movements (e.g., sequential hand pronation and supination) and examination for motor tone, which is reduced in cerebellar disease. Chronic alcohol abuse and long-term use of medications such as phenytoin can cause acquired cerebellar degeneration.[4]

MUSCULOSKELETAL EXAMINATION

The musculoskeletal examination serves to evaluate integrated functioning of bones, joints, supporting ligaments, and muscular tissue. Information from the examination can be used to localize possible sources of pain in various structures including skin, subcutaneous tissue, tendons, joints, ligaments, or periosteum. The format of the musculoskeletal examination follows the steps of inspection, palpation, range of motion, and special tests. The components tested are the spine (cervical/thoracic/lumbar) and the extremities with their respective joints.

Spinal Examination

Inspection of the cervical and thoracolumbar spine provides information on posture and alignment. Abnormal kyphosis, lordosis, or scoliosis should be noted. Palpation of the spinous processes can reveal localized tenderness. This is seen in conditions including vertebral compression fractures, epidural tumor, or abscess. Step-off (i.e., sudden change in prominence of the spinous processes) is also indicative of a vertebral compression fracture with resultant height loss. Tenderness in the paraspinous regions can be seen in facet arthropathy and myofascial pain syndrome. Normal range of motion of the cervical spine is 60 degrees of forward flexion, 75 degrees of extension, 45 degrees of lateral flexion, and 80 degrees of lateral rotation. Range-of-motion testing should be performed with the patient in both supine and sitting positions. Improvement in the range of motion with the supine position suggests that muscle spasm is responsible for restricting cervical mobility. However there is no positional improvement in cervical range of motion with cervical arthropathy. Normal thoracolumbar spine range of motion is 90 degrees of forward flexion, 30 degrees of back extension, 25 degrees of lateral flexion, and 60 degrees of lateral rotation. Pain that is provoked by back extension and lateral rotation is suggestive of facet arthropathy in that these maneuvers result in zygapophysial joint loading. Pain that is provoked by back flexion is consistent with a discogenic or vertebral body source of pain because flexion causes axial loading. Lumbar discogenic pain is often restricted to the axial spine and is associated with sitting intolerance and pain provoked by coughing, sneezing, and Valsalva maneuvers. The Spurling maneuver is highly specific for confirming the diagnosis of cervical radiculopathy. The patient is asked to perform simultaneous lateral flexion and extension of the neck toward the symptomatic side. Provocation of ipsilateral neck and arm pain constitutes a positive Spurling sign.[6,7]

MYOFASCIAL EXAMINATION

Myofascial pain is caused by the presence of tender palpable bands of muscle called *trigger points*. Active myofascial trigger points are associated with complaints of spontaneous pain and restricted range of motion. Latent trigger points are tender and palpable upon direct examination but they do not produce spontaneous pain.

A myofascial examination should start with an assessment of posture and joint function to determine any underlying causes for regional myofascial pain. Myofascial trigger points can be identified by gentle palpation in the direction of muscle fibers. Trigger points can be felt as a ropelike region of nodularity. Palpation of trigger points is also exquisitely tender and produces local as well as referred pain. Commonly affected muscles include the trapezius, glutei, and cervical and lumbar paraspinous musculature but many others may be affected as well.[8]

EXAMINATION OF THE EXTREMITIES

Inspection and where indicated, measurement of the extremities reveals length discrepancies, deformities, and bulk. Range of motion can be demonstrated by asking the patient to perform specific tasks such as raising the hands above the head. The lower extremities can be assessed during the gait evaluation. The pattern of gait abnormality can direct the clinician to the underlying cause of dysfunction, such as foot drop, leg length discrepancy, or hip or knee pain.[6,7,9,10]

Upper Extremity

Shoulder Joint Examination

Inspection should evaluate for symmetry, bulk of the deltoid muscles, and posture. Palpation of the shoulder joint should include the sternoclavicular joint, clavicle, acromioclavicular joint, glenohumeral joint, and the scapular spine. Normal range of motion for the shoulder joint is 180 degrees of flexion/extension in the sagittal plane, 180 degrees of abduction and adduction in the frontal plane, 90 degrees of external rotation, and 40 degrees of internal rotation. Common etiologies of shoulder pain include glenohumeral arthritis, acromioclavicular arthritis, subacromial/subdeltoid bursitis, supraspinatus and bicipital tendinitis, and rotator cuff tears. A variety of special tests are used to diagnose these conditions. The tests most commonly used in clinical practice are described below.

Pain on shoulder abduction and elevation is seen in impingement syndrome. The etiology involves entrapment of soft tissue between the humeral head and the coracoacromial arch. Subacromial bursitis, supraspinatus tendinitis, and partial or complete tears of the rotator cuff tendons can be present at the same time. In case of a complete tear, the patient will be unable to abduct the arm. Untreated tears of the rotator cuff tendons result in disuse atrophy of the scapular muscles. The drop arm test is used to diagnose complete rotator cuff tears. The patient's arm is passively abducted to 90 degrees and then released. Failure to maintain shoulder abduction suggests a complete rotator cuff tear. The diagnosis can be investigated further with magnetic resonance imaging.

Adhesive Capsulitis

Frozen shoulder or adhesive capsulitis is characterized by diminished range of motion at the scapulothoracic and glenohumeral joints. There is progressive fibrosis of the shoulder joint capsule, which disrupts normal shoulder mobility. Normally the shoulder joint can be abducted to 180 degrees. The scapulothoracic motion begins at 90 degrees of shoulder abduction and there is a 2:1 ratio between glenohumeral and scapulothoracic motion. Adhesive capsulitis results in gradual loss of range of motion with little to no shoulder movement present in advanced cases.

Elbow Joint

Inspection of the elbow joint includes assessment of humeral and radial-ulnar symmetry. The carrying angle between the arm and forearm is measured with the patient standing with arms to the side and facing anteriorly. The normal carrying angle is 10 to 15 degrees for men and up to 18 degrees for women. Readily palpable landmarks of the elbow joint include the olecranon process and the medial and lateral epicondyles. Normal range of motion at the elbow is 30 degrees of extension and 180 degrees flexion at the humeroulnar joint and 170 degrees of pronation/supination at the radioulnar joint.

Lateral Epicondylitis

Overuse of the forearm extensor muscles results in inflammation of the common extensor tendon insertion at the lateral epicondyle. Patients report constant elbow pain that is worse with wrist movement. Bedside testing is performed by asking the patient to extend the wrist and resist forcible wrist flexion. Pain over the lateral epicondyle confirms the diagnosis of lateral epicondylitis.

Medial Epicondylitis

This condition is similar to lateral epicondylitis and results from overuse of forearm flexor muscles. Pain is experienced over the medial epicondyle and can be reproduced by forcibly extending the patient's flexed wrist.

Wrist Joint

Inspection and palpation of the wrist joint is used to evaluate joint symmetry. Range of motion is 60 degrees of extension, 70 degrees flexion, 20 degrees of abduction, and 30 degrees of adduction. The most common clinically encountered specific wrist joint pain disorder is the carpal tunnel syndrome. This entity is a result of entrapment of the median nerve at the wrist, with symptoms of wrist pain and numbness and weakness of the hand. The diagnosis of carpal tunnel syndrome is supported by the presence of Tinel's and Phalen's signs. In the Tinel sign, percussion of the proximal volar wrist crease produces paresthesias in the thumb, index, and middle fingers of the ipsilateral hand. To elicit the Phalen sign, the patient is asked to forcibly flex both wrists against each other for 1 minute. Dysesthesias in the thumb, index and middle fingers characterizes a positive Phalen's sign.

Evaluation of the Digits

Inspection evaluates symmetry and presence of any deformities. Heberden's nodes at the distal interphalangeal joint and Bouchard's nodes at the proximal interphalangeal joints can be seen in patients with osteoarthritis. Range of motion can be assessed by asking patients to open and close their fist. Normal range of motion in the sagittal plane is 90 degrees at the metacarpophalangeal joints, 120 degrees at the proximal interphalangeal joints, and 70 degrees at the distal interphalangeal joints. The first metacarpophalangeal joint has 50 degrees of motion in abduction, 50 degrees in adduction, and 35 degrees in opposition.

Evaluation of the Hip Joint

Inspection of the hip joint should pay attention to symmetry, muscle bulk, and surgical scars. Normal range of motion at the hip is 100 degrees of flexion, 30 degrees of extension, 20 degrees adduction, and 40 degrees abduction. With the hip joint in flexed position, range of motion is 45 degrees for internal rotation and 40 degrees for external rotation. Hip pain may result from pathology of the acetabulum, femoral neck or head, periosteum, or joint capsule. It may also result from abnormalities of a surrounding structure such as bursae or may be referred from the lumbar spine or sacroiliac joint. Hip joint pathology usually results in pain in the groin, anteromedial thigh, or laterally over the greater trochanter region.

Pain referral patterns alone are often insufficient to diagnose the etiology of hip pain and an appropriate imaging evaluation is helpful in this regard.

Trochanteric Bursitis

Patients report a deep, dull, aching pain with radiation to the lateral hip region. The pain is worse at night. Inflammation primarily involves the trochanteric bursa, which lies between the gluteus maximus and gluteus medius tendons. The diagnosis is supported by tenderness to palpation over the greater trochanter and pain on thigh extension.

Patrick's Test

Patrick's test evaluates hip and sacroiliac joint pathology. With the patient in the supine position, the examiner passively flexes, abducts, and externally rotates the hip. Pain in the groin suggests hip joint pathology, whereas sacroiliac pain indicates dysfunction of the sacroiliac joint (Fig. 10–3).

Straight-Leg Raise Test

With the patient in the supine position, the examiner passively elevates one leg by holding it at the ankle. The hip is flexed to an angle of 70 to 90 degrees with the knee extended (Fig. 10–4). A positive straight-leg raise test produces pain starting at the hip with radiation down to the ankle. Pain that remains localized to the posterior thigh is caused by tension on the hamstrings. A crossed straight-leg raise sign is present if testing the uninvolved leg produces contralateral symptoms. Both the straight and crossed straight-leg raise test place the lumbosa-

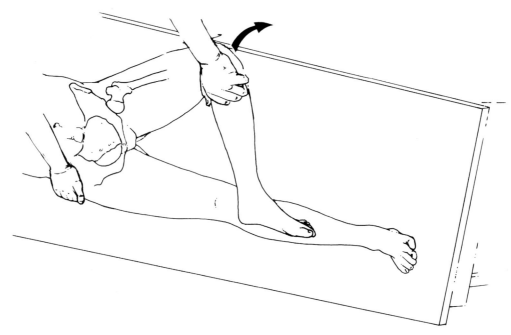

Figure 10–3. The Patrick or FABER test.

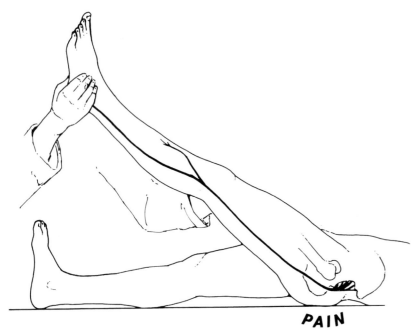

PAIN

Figure 10–4. Straight-leg raising test (Lasègue's sign).

cral nerve roots under tension and a positive test is suggestive of a lumbosacral radiculopathy.

Evaluation of the Knee

Inspection should assess symmetry, position of the patella, surgical scars, and bulk of the surrounding musculature, including the quadriceps femoris muscle. Valgus deformity of the knee is a result of medial compartment loss, whereas varus deformity is caused by lateral compartment loss. Bilateral genu valgum (knock knees), genu varum (bowed legs), or genu recurvatum (back knees) should be noted as well. Palpation should include surrounding bursae (i.e., the pes anserinus and prepatellar bursae) because these are common sources of pain. Normal range of motion at the knee joint is 150 degrees in the sagittal plane.

Special Tests

Drawer Sign
With the patient's knee in the flexed position, the examiner draws the tibia anteriorly. If the tibia moves in the forward direction, this constitutes a positive anterior drawer sign and suggests a tear of the anterior cruciate ligament. Similarly, if the tibia moves posteriorly when pulled backward, this is a positive posterior drawer sign and is caused by a torn posterior cruciate ligament (Fig. 10–5).

Patellar Femoral Grinding Test
Knee pain on rising to a standing position or while climbing stairs can occur in chondromalacia patellae. With the patient's knee extended, the examiner exerts downward pressure on the patella into the femoral groove. Patients with chondromalacia patellae will complain of pain with this maneuver.

Apley's Compression or Grinding Test
This test is used to evaluate for medial and lateral meniscal tears. With the patient in the prone position, the knee is flexed to 90 degrees, downward force is applied to the heel, and the tibia is rotated medially and laterally against the femur (Fig. 10–6). Pain provoked in the medial or lateral aspect of the knee indicates a tear in the respective collateral ligament.

Evaluation of the Ankle

Inspection should include evaluation of bony landmarks, symmetry, and edema. Normal range of motion of the ankle is 20 degrees of dorsiflexion, 40 degrees of plantar flexion, 30 degrees of inversion, and 15 degrees of eversion.

Pain and excessive motion on pulling the ankle joint anteriorly indicates a tear in the anterior talofibular ligament while similar findings on forced inversion occur in tears of the calcaneofibular ligament. The posterior talofibular ligament is usually damaged only if there is a significant history of preceding trauma.

Evaluation of the Foot

The functional assessment of the foot is targeted toward its anterior, middle, and posterior segments. The anterior segment comprises the five metatarsal and 14 phalangeal bones, the middle segment includes the navicular, cuboid, and three cuneiform bones, and the posterior segment includes the talus and calcaneus (Fig. 10–7).

The posterior segment of the foot transmits body weight to the ground. The middle segment provides flexibility and the ability to adapt gait to uneven surfaces. The anterior segment acts as a fulcrum to

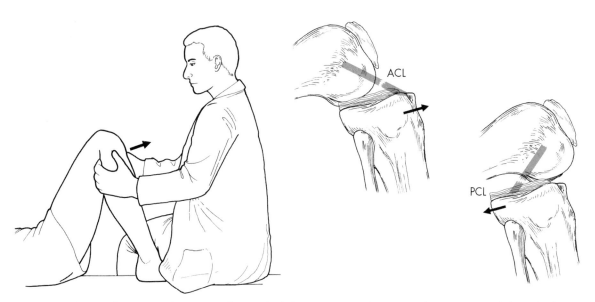

Figure 10–5. Drawer sign test for cruciate ligaments. The standard drawer sign test for cruciate ligaments immobilizes the foot and stresses the lower leg on the femur. Pulling the leg forward tests the anterior cruciate ligament (ACL) and posterior pressure tests the posterior cruciate ligament (PCL). (Redrawn from Calliet R: Knee Pain and Disability, ed. 3. Philadelphia, FA Davis, 1992, pp 1-69.)

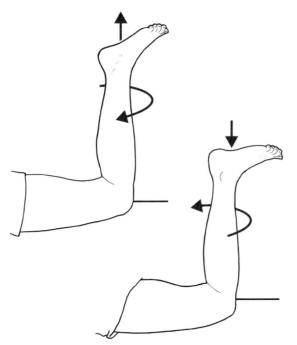

Figure 10–6. Examination of ligament injury, including the meniscus (Apley test). The Apley test checks the integrity of the knee ligamentous structures and of the menisci. It is performed in two aspects. *Left,* With the patient prone and the knee flexed to the right angle, downward pressure is put upon the lower leg. The leg is then rotated to test the menisci. This maneuver compresses the menisci between the femoral condyles and the tibial plateau, as in the McMurray test. With the lower leg internally rotated, the medial meniscus is tested. Grating, crepitation, limitation, and pain imply meniscal damage. From the same position, the leg is elevated (*right*), which places traction upon the ligaments. Excessive motion, deduced by a comparison to the contralateral side, indicates laxity or injury to the knee ligaments and capsule. (Redrawn from Calliet R: Knee Pain and Disability, ed. 3. Philadelphia, FA Davis, 1992, pp 1-69.)

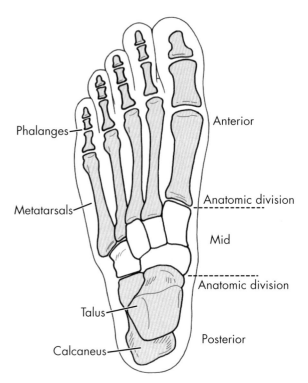

Figure 10–7. Anatomy of the foot with functional segmentation. (Redrawn from Abrams B, Glaser L: Painful conditions of the foot and ankle: Evaluation and treatment. Pain Diag 1997;7:351-363.)

provide forward thrust during ambulation. The impact of the foot against the ground is cushioned by its longitudinal and transverse arches.

Foot pain is a common presenting symptom for patients (Fig. 10–8). The more common pain syndromes that are diagnosed by physical examination are described below.

Tarsal Tunnel Syndrome

In the tarsal tunnel syndrome, the posterior tibial nerve is entrapped beneath the lancinate ligament, posterior to the medial malleolus. Patients present with pain and paresthesias affecting the toes and sole of the foot. Physical examination may demonstrate atrophy of the intrinsic foot muscles and hypoesthesia of the sole of the foot. Percussion posterior to the medial malleolus can provoke paresthesia in the ipsilateral sole and toes in patients with tarsal tunnel syndrome.

Morton's Neuroma

Morton's neuroma is characterized by pain between the metatarsal bones, usually between the third and fourth toes and less commonly between the second and third toes. The pain is reproducible on palpation of the space between the metatarsal heads. The etiology of Morton's neuroma is not well understood. It likely represents a form of interdigital neuritis. Interestingly, surgically resected specimens in patients with Morton's neuroma do not show any significant changes in nerve histology compared to control tissue obtained from cadavers.

Metatarsalgia

Pain in metatarsalgia occurs on weight bearing and localizes to the plantar aspect of the metatarsal heads. The pain occurs maximally over the first metatarsal head and can be reproduced by direct palpation. With foot inversion, weight is shifted to the heads of the second and third metatarsal bones and repetitive stress can result in pain over these sites as well. Patients can walk with a characteristic antalgic gait, holding the foot in the inverted position. This can serve as a useful clue to the diagnosis.

Foot Strain

Foot strain affects the middle segment of the foot. Repetitive patterns of overuse result in elongation of

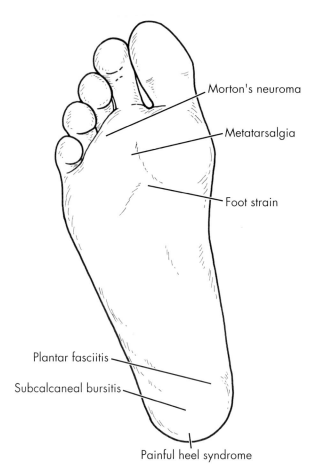

Morton's neuroma

Metatarsalgia

Foot strain

Plantar fasciitis

Subcalcaneal bursitis

Painful heel syndrome

Figure 10–8. Location of common painful conditions in the plantar foot. (Redrawn from Abrams B, Glaser L: Painful conditions of the foot and ankle: Evaluation and treatment. Pain Diag 1997;7: 351-363.)

the longitudinal arch with alteration of the normal alignment of the talus and calcaneus. Elongation of the longitudinal arch produces excessive strain on the plantar fascia, medial collateral ligament, and talocalcaneal ligament. Physical findings include flattening and pain on compression of the longitudinal arch.

Plantar Fasciitis

Plantar fasciitis is manifested by plantar foot pain on weight bearing. Patients often have a history of prolonged standing in footwear lacking arch support or on hard surfaces. Inflammation develops in the point of attachment of the plantar fascia to the calcaneus. Calcaneal bone spurs can develop from chronic strain in the plantar fascia. Clinically, tenderness to palpation can be elicited over the anterior portion of the calcaneus with radiation into the plantar fascia.

Painful Heel Syndrome

Painful heel syndrome is a result of degenerative changes in the weight bearing aspect of the calcaneus

and occurs primarily in morbidly obese individuals or those who stand or walk excessively. Pain is often worse in the morning on waking up or after prolonged rest. Examination is significant for tenderness to palpation over the posterior portion of the plantar aspect of the calcaneus.

TESTS FOR NONORGANIC ETIOLOGY OF PAIN

Waddell's Signs

Waddell's tests were intended to evaluate low back pain patients for functional overlay. There are five signs in total, and the presence of any three of these five signs in a patient was considered suggestive of a nonorganic pain etiology.[11]
1. Tenderness to palpation
   Widespread skin tenderness to light touch
   Tenderness upon deep palpation which is not restricted to a single anatomic area
2. Simulation
   Low back pain provoked by axial loading pressure on the skull of the standing patient, or rotation of shoulders and pelvis in the same plane resulting in increased low back pain
3. Distraction
   For example, a patient with positive response to the straight-leg raise test in the supine position, with no pain on the same test repeated in the sitting position
4. Regional disturbance in function
   Weakness involving multiple muscle groups in a nonmyotomal distribution with "give-way" effort
   Sensory loss in a segmental pattern (e.g., glove-stocking rather than a dermatomal distribution) observed in a patient for whom polyneuropathy is not an appropriate diagnosis
5. Overreaction
   Disproportionate facial or verbal behaviors (e.g., moaning and grimacing on light touch, posturing, and withdrawing from the examiner)
   However, there are several limitations of Waddell's signs. Widespread superficial tenderness is commonly found in patients with fibromyalgia, and tenderness to deep palpation is part of myofascial pain syndrome. Sensory loss in a glove and stocking distribution is present in peripheral polyneuropathy. Moreover, studies have not found a consistent relationship between the presence of Waddell's signs and subscale scores on the Minnesota Multiphasic Personality Inventory. In fact, recent data suggest that Waddell's signs cannot accurately distinguish between organic and nonorganic pain etiologies.[12]

The physical examination may be helpful in elucidating the etiology of a patient's pain complaints; however, used alone it has its limitations and the results of a physical examination need to be considered in the context of the patient's history as well as in the context of the results of diagnostic studies.

References

1. Brazis PW, Masdeu JC, Biller J: Localization in Clinical Neurology. Philadelphia, Lippincott Williams & Wilkins, 2001.
2. Bickley LS, Szilagyi PG: Bates' Guide to Physical Examination and History Taking. Philadelphia, Lippincott Williams & Wilkins, 2002.
3. Preston DC, Shapiro B: Electromyography and Neuromuscular Disorders: Clinical-Electrophysiologic Correlations. Philadelphia, Elsevier, 2005.
4. Bradley WG, Daroff RB, Fenichel G, et al: Neurology in Clinical Practice. Boston, Elsevier, 2003.
5. Pestronk A, Florence J, Levine T, et al: Sensory exam with a quantitative tuning fork: Rapid, sensitive and predictive of SNAP amplitude. Neurology 2004;62:461-464.
6. Waldman S: Physical Diagnosis of Pain. Philadelphia, Elsevier, 2005.
7. Raj PP: Practical Management of Pain, 3rd Edition. Philadelphia, Elsevier, 2000.
8. Simmons DG, Travell JG, Simons LS, et al: Travell and Simons' Myofascial Pain and Dysfunction: The Trigger Point Manual, vols 1 and 2. Philadelphia, Lippincott Williams & Wilkins, 1993.
9. Foley BS, Buschbacher RM: Sacroiliac joint pain: Anatomy, biomechanics, diagnosis, and treatment. Am J Phys Med Rehabil 2006;85:997-1006.
10. Malanga GA, Andrus S, Nadler SF, et al: Physical examination of the knee: A review of the original test description and scientific validity of common orthopedic tests. Arch Phys Med Rehabil 2003;84:592-603.
11. Waddell G, Bircher M, Finlayson D, et al: Symptoms and signs: Physical disease or illness behaviour? Br Med J 1984;289: 739-741.
12. Fishbain DA, Cutler RB, Rosomoff HL, et al: Is there a relationship between nonorganic physical findings (Waddell signs) and secondary gain/malingering? Clin J Pain 2004;20: 399-408.

11 Electromyography and Evoked Potentials

Bernard M. Abrams and Howard J. Waldman

Electrodiagnostic techniques such as electromyography (EMG) and evoked potentials (EPs) are very useful adjuncts to physical examination of the patient in pain. Conditions in which EMG or EPs may be of use include painful peripheral neuropathies, entrapment neuropathies, traumatic nerve injuries, radicular and multiradicular problems, lumbar spinal stenosis, arachnoiditis, and painful myopathies.

In recent years there has been increased reliance on anatomic measures such as intradermal nerve biopsy for small fiber neuropathy and magnetic resonance imaging (MRI) for larger neural structures. This "anatomic" approach fails to recognize the differences and respective advantages and shortcomings of physiologic versus anatomic testing and, above all, fails to recognize the inherent nature of pain, a subjective experience that can only be *correlated* with the clinical picture.

The problems inherent in applying electrodiagnostic techniques to pain diagnosis and management are no different from those encountered in history taking, physical examination, radiologic evaluation, and therapeutic diagnostic testing (e.g., nerve blocks). Pain is a subjective experience, often without an objective "litmus test," and the final diagnosis of the etiology and presumptive treatment of a pain syndrome is a *clinical* one that can be *supported* only by relevant data, including EMG findings.

Electrodiagnostic techniques can be applied virtually without complications to large portions of the body and hence the nervous system to gain an overall understanding of the distribution of abnormalities, if present, or relative normalcy if not. The distribution of abnormalities correlates strongly with the etiology of a disease process causing pain. Questions that can be posed and answered through the use of electrodiagnostic techniques include the following:

- Is there a disease of nerves present?
- If so, is it a mononeuropathy, polyneuropathy, or mononeuritis multiplex?
- Does the distribution of abnormalities suggest involvement at the nerve root, plexus, or nerve level?
- If there is a disease process involving a single (or multiple) nerve such as injury or compression, is it improving, worsening, or static?
- Is the nerve involved motor, sensory, or mixed?
- Is the process one of nerve, muscle, or both?
- Are small fibers selectively involved or is this mainly a large fiber disorder, or are both involved?
- Is there autonomic involvement as well as somatic involvement?
- Are more proximal structures, rather than distal structures, involved?
- Is the central nervous system involved?

These are the types of inquiries that add substantially to the diagnostic information about the etiology, severity, and prognosis of painful disorders. Although many painful disorders do not affect either the peripheral or central nervous systems, electrodiagnostic testing can often add reassuring negative results to the diagnostic picture.

Electrodiagnosis is an extremely useful investigative technique in evaluating the patient with pain because it satisfies two fundamental steps in the assessment of a neuropathic painful syndrome before any attempt at therapy: (1) rigorously establishing the presence or absence of a peripheral nervous system lesion and (2) determining the relevance of an established peripheral neuropathic lesion to the subjective clinical complaint.

ELECTROMYOGRAPHY

EMG is a method of testing both the physiologic state and the anatomic integrity of lower motor neuron structures (anterior horn cells, nerve roots, plexuses, peripheral nerves, neuromuscular junction and muscles), their sensory components, and some spinal and brainstem reflex pathways.[1] The term *electromyography* previously caused considerable confusion because, strictly speaking, it was the needle evaluation of muscle function but often was expanded to include nerve conduction velocity and other tests. However, its common usage has come to mean needle electromyography, nerve conduction velocity determinations, and, less frequently, testing such as the *H reflex* and *F response*, cranial nerve reflexes (e.g., the blink reflex), and studies of the neuromuscular junction. The all-inclusive term *EMG* is used here with an effort to avoid confusion among tests.

Longmire[2] pointed out the puzzling dichotomy in the medical literature on pain and electrodiagnostic testing. In standard textbooks on electrodiagnostic testing,[3-7] little or no reference is made to painful syndromes and their diagnosis despite their excellent discussions of physiology, technique, and clinical correlations. On the other hand, a perusal of pain textbooks[1,8,9] reveals cogent attempts to correlate neurophysiologic studies in pain management. The reason for the paucity of references appears to be at least in part the attitudes of pain specialists themselves, who point out that "large caliber afferent fibers are physiologically unrelated to pain, a submodality mediated by small caliber fibers. Additionally, the test is unable to explore the bases for positive sensory phenomena, generated by dysfunction even of large caliber afferent channels."[10]

Electrical Testing of Nerves and Muscles

Brief History

The existence of electricity resulting from muscular contractions was described by Galvani as early as 1791.[11] The first experimental work with EMG was performed by Lord Adrian in 1925. In 1928, Proebster first described the presence of "spontaneous irregular action potentials in denervated muscle."[11] In its progression to clinical application, EMG made a major step forward with the use of the cathode ray oscilloscope by Erlanger and Gasser as well as with the concentric needle electrode and loudspeaker.[12] Vast numbers of nerve injuries in World War II and later conflicts added further impetus to the study of nerve and muscle by electrodiagnostic technique.

The Electrodiagnostic Method

There are only four basic components to any electrical diagnostic measurement system[2]:
1. Electrodes
2. Stimulator
3. High-gain differential amplifier
4. Recording display or central processing device

The EMG apparatus amplifies and displays biologic information derived from either surface or needle electrodes. Electrical information may be recorded from muscles, nerves, or other nervous system structures and is displayed on an oscilloscope. In addition to the visual display on the oscilloscope, a permanent recording may be made, audio amplification may allow it to be heard over a loudspeaker, and analog-digital analysis of signals may be used. Electrical nerve stimulation is used to stimulate nerves to measure nerve conduction.

For nerve conduction studies, skin surface electrodes are used for recording compound muscle or nerve action potentials. For needle electromyography, needle electrodes are used with a strong trend toward disposable needles. For sensory testing, ring electrodes are used for measurement (Fig. 11–1). Modern EMG equipment is manufactured by numerous companies and is generally standardized to allow reliable and reproducible testing by different laboratories,[8] but normative data may differ among laboratories and require standardization by each laboratory.[6,13,14]

Precautions for testing include extra care with patients who are taking coumadin or other blood thinners, who have hemophilia or other blood dyscrasias, whose status is positive for human immunodeficiency virus, or who have a cardiac pacemaker or transcutaneous stimulator.[1] Beyond placing a needle through an infected site, there are probably no absolute but only relative contraindications for EMG. Extremely anxious patients and some children occasionally require some sedation. After-effects are

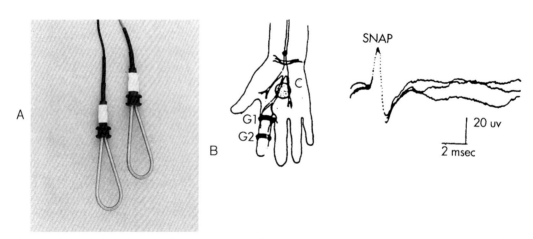

Figure 11–1. A, Commonly used ring electrodes for measurement of median and ulnar sensory nerve conduction studies. **B,** Placement of electrodes for median sensory nerve conduction studies and sensory nerve action potentials (SNAP) obtained on stimulation of median nerve at the wrist. G1, recording electrode; G2, reference electrode; C, ground electrode; uv, microvolts; msec, millisecond. (**A,** Courtesy of Oxford Instruments Medical, Inc., Hawthorne, NY.)

negligible with rare bruising, although occasionally a highly disturbed, suggestible, or litigious patient may complain vehemently of increased pain or disability.

Physiology

Physiologic Mechanisms in the Production of Muscle Potentials

When an impulse arrives at the region of the junction between nerve and muscle, the entire muscle fiber is thrown into an almost simultaneous contraction. This is brought about by a wave of excitation that moves rapidly along the fiber surface and stimulates the contractile substance as it passes over the fiber. The stimulus is transmitted along the fiber by an excitable membrane that surrounds the muscle fiber. The action potential results from the breakdown of the surface membrane potential, which is associated with critical changes in ionic permeability. In the resting muscle fiber, the potential difference across the surface membrane is 90 mV, with negative inside, positive outside. During excitation, the resting potential temporarily reverses to 40 mV, negative outside. This action potential travels along the muscle fiber at velocities ranging from 3.5 to 5 meters per second (m/sec) in different fibers.[15]

In recording extracellularly, as in EMG, the electrode picks up the action potential as it is conducted through the medium that surrounds the active fiber. The impedance of the external medium is small, compared with the impedance of the fiber interior, and hence the voltage of the extracellularly recorded potentials is maximally only 2% to 10% of the intracellularly recorded potential changes. The functional unit (Fig. 11–2) in reflex or voluntary activity is the *motor unit*; a motor unit is the group of muscle fibers innervated by a single anterior horn cell.

Conduction along the fine intramuscular branches of the anterior horn cell axon occurs so rapidly that all muscle fibers in a motor unit are activated nearly simultaneously. The number of muscle fibers per motor unit varies considerably from muscle to muscle; for example, in the gastrocnemius the motor unit consists of about 1600 muscle fibers, whereas in the small muscles of the eye there are only 5 to 10 fibers. The motor units in various muscles cover differing areas of muscle cross section (e.g., brachial biceps, 55 mm; rectus femoris, anterior tibial, and opponens pollicis, 8 to 9 mm). The distribution of fibers is such that fibers from several different motor units are intermingled, which is why four to six motor units can be identified by EMG from the same intramuscular recording point. In normal muscle, these single motor unit potentials can be differentiated only during weak voluntary effort.[13,16]

The potentials from different motor units are recognized by their frequency of discharge, which varies for each motor unit (some are more or less excitable). Moreover, the various potentials often differ in appearance because of the differential distance of the recording electrode from the individual fibers of the activated motor units and the differential distribution of the motor end plates in the several units within "range" of a concentric or single needle electrode in one position in the muscle. An upward deflection on the oscilloscope is considered electrically negative, and a downward deflection is considered electrically positive. In the immediate vicinity of a potential, there is an upward or a negative deflection.

Physiology of Nerve Conduction

The cell membrane (axolemma) of a nerve axon separates the intracellular axoplasm from the extracellular fluid.[6] The unequal distribution of ions between these fluids produces a potential difference across the cell membrane. This resting potential is about 70 mV and is negative on the inside with respect to the outside of the cell membrane. When a nerve fiber is stimulated, it causes a change in the membrane potential; a rapid but brief flow of sodium ions occurs through ionic channels inward across the cell membrane, giving rise to an action potential.

NORMAL AND ABNORMAL MOTOR UNITS

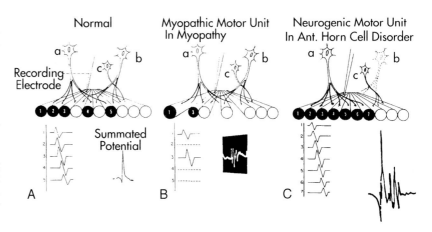

Figure 11–2. A, Schematic illustration of three normal motor units, "a," "b," and "c." *Note:* Muscle fibers of different motor units are normally intermingled. Below the motor units are action potentials of five individual muscle fibers of a motor unit and its summated motor unit potential. **B,** Myopathic motor unit changes in motor unit "a." Of original five muscle fibers, three have undergone degeneration, reducing the size of the motor unit. **C,** Neurogenic transformation of motor unit "a." Anterior horn cell "b" is shown undergoing degeneration and its two muscle fibers are not innervated by axons of anterior horn cell "a," thus leading to increase in territory and size of motor unit "a."

The way in which an action potential is conducted along an axon depends on whether the axon is myelinated or unmyelinated.[17] In a *myelinated* fiber, the action potential is regenerated only at the nodes of Ranvier, so that the resulting action potentials "jump" from node to node, yielding saltatory conduction. The velocity of nerve conduction depends on the diameter of the myelinated fiber. Small myelinated fibers may conduct as slowly as 12 m/sec, whereas large motor and sensory fibers conduct at a rate of 50 to 70 m/sec in humans. In an *unmyelinated* fiber in a human, the conduction rate is about 2 m/sec.

Several factors affect conduction velocity other than whether or not the axon is myelinated:
- Temperature of the limb[18]
- Age of the patient (infants have slow conduction velocities and older adults have increasingly slowed conduction velocities)
- Height of an individual; increased height may increase the internodal distances of the nodes of Ranvier[6]

Basic Electromyography Examination

EMG must be combined with the clinical examination of the patient by the electromyographer. This includes a grading of muscle strength. It is of prime importance for the electromyographer to personally correlate clinical data and those data obtained by EMG. Each examination must be planned individually. There is no "cookbook" formula to follow. Because the EMG examination is an extension of the clinical examination, the patient must be evaluated fully and the problem tentatively assigned to the portion of the anterior horn cell system that seems most likely to be involved. The electromyographer determines the segment or segments of the peripheral nervous system suspected to be involved, and the examination is planned to either substantiate or invalidate the presumptive clinical diagnoses.

Conducting the Examination

The needle examination of the patient is designed to determine the following:
1. Integrity of muscle and its nerve supply
2. Location of any abnormality
3. Any abnormalities of the muscle itself

The electrodes may be monopolar or concentric (Fig. 11–3). The examination proceeds through the following steps (Fig. 11–4):
1. Determination of activity of the muscle in the relaxed state[7,13]
2. Evaluation of any insertional activity that arises
3. Assessment of the activity seen on weak voluntary effort
4. Determination of the pattern seen on maximum voluntary effort. This is known as the *interference pattern* (there is interference with the discernment of individual muscle action potentials from the resting baseline).

MONOPOLAR

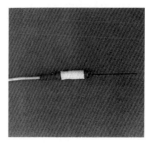

CONCENTRIC

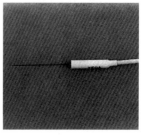

Figure 11–3. Commonly used monopolar and concentric needle electrodes. (Courtesy of Oxford Instruments Medical, Inc., Hawthorne, NY.)

Needle Findings in Normal Muscle

Insertional Activity

When the needle is inserted into a normal muscle, it evokes a brief burst of electrical activity that lasts no more than 2 to 3 msec, a little longer than the actual movement of the needle.[8] This activity is described as insertional activity and is generally 50 to 250 mV in amplitude (see Fig. 11–4A). These insertional potentials are believed to represent discharges from muscle fibers produced by injury, mechanical stimulation, or irritation of the muscle fibers.

Spontaneous Activity (Activity at Rest)

When the needle is stationary and the muscle is relaxed, there is no electrical activity present in normal muscle except when the needle is in the area of the end plate. Two types of end-plate "noise" are normal (see Fig. 11–4C): (1) low-amplitude and undulating, probably representing extracellularly recorded miniature end-plate potentials, and (2) high-amplitude intermittent spike discharges, probably representing discharges of single muscle fibers excited by intramuscular nerve terminals irritated by the needle. Any other spontaneous activity at rest is abnormal. An increase in duration of insertional activity may be seen in loss of innervation or primary disease of muscle fiber.[8] Reduction may occur in myopathies or more advanced degeneration in which muscle tissue has been replaced by fat or fibrous connective tissue.[19]

Voluntary Activity

Voluntary activity of the muscle is analyzed after the muscle is studied at rest (see Fig. 11–4D). Electrical activity (termed a *motor unit action potential*) is noted. As previously mentioned in the discussion of physiology, the motor unit refers to a number of muscle fibers supplied by one motor neuron and its axon. This varies from muscle to muscle and may be as few as 10 to more than 1000 muscle fibers. When a motor neuron discharges, it activates all the muscle fibers of the motor unit.

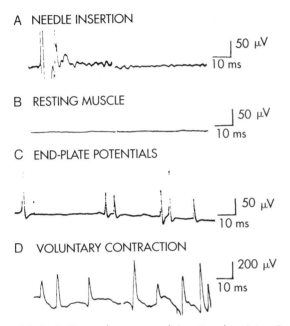

A NEEDLE INSERTION

50 μV
10 ms

B RESTING MUSCLE

50 μV
10 ms

C END-PLATE POTENTIALS

50 μV
10 ms

D VOLUNTARY CONTRACTION

200 μV
10 ms

Figure 11–4. A, Trace shows normal insertional activity. **B,** No spontaneous activity in a normal muscle at rest. **C,** Spontaneous end-plate potentials. **D,** Normal biphasic and triphasic motor unit potentials during weak voluntary contraction.

The force of contraction determines the number of motor units brought into play.[13,16] This begins with a single motor unit that fires and can be identified on the screen by its distinctive morphology. As the effort is increased, other motor units come into play, which can still be individually discerned and have their own individual morphology and audio representation on the loudspeaker. As the contraction increases, the firing rate of each individual motor unit action potential increases, and the action potential is subsequently joined by other motor unit action potentials whose firing rates also increase. This phenomenon is known as *recruitment* (Fig. 11–5). In normal muscles, the strength of a voluntary muscle contraction is directly related to the number of individual motor units that have been recruited and their firing rate.[16,20] Analysis of motor units includes (1) waveform, (2) amplitude, and (3) interference patterns.

Waveform

Most units are biphasic or triphasic. The number of phases is determined by the "baseline crossings." Motor units that cross the baseline or have more than five phases are called *polyphasic motor units*. While occasionally seen in healthy muscles, they do not exceed 15% of the total number of motor units. In some muscles, polyphasic motor units are more prevalent. Polyphasic potentials are a measure of fiber synchrony.

Amplitude

The amplitude depends on the number of fibers in the motor unit and the type of EMG needle used. Monopolar needles are associated with higher-amplitude potentials than bipolar or coaxial needles. Normal amplitude ranges from 1 to 5 mV. Because the motor unit is the sum of the action potentials of each muscle fiber of the unit, a large motor unit has a larger amplitude; conversely, a smaller motor unit has a smaller amplitude.

MOTOR UNIT INTERFERENCE PATTERNS

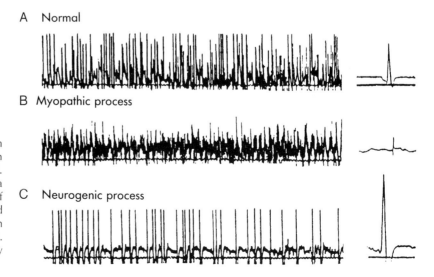

A Normal

B Myopathic process

C Neurogenic process

Figure 11–5. A, Full interference pattern on maximum effort in a normal muscle. **B,** Full interference pattern in a myopathic muscle on submaximal effort. Number of spikes is greater (each spike represents a motor unit) owing to an increase in firing rate of motor units with early recruitment. **C,** Reduced interference pattern in a denervated muscle on maximal effort resulting from loss of motor units. *Note:* The decreased number of spikes is evident by an increased gap between spikes.

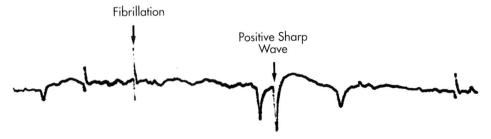

Fibrillation

Positive Sharp
Wave

Figure 11–6. Positive sharp wave and fibrillation potentials recorded from a denervated muscle.

Interference Patterns

With maximum voluntary effort, a large number of motor units are brought into play and their firing rate increases. They tend to "interfere" with each other, and they are not recognized further as individual units. This gives rise to the situation called an *interference pattern* (see Fig. 11–5). In a normal muscle, there is a "full" interference pattern.

Needle Findings in Abnormal Muscle

Various abnormalities may occur that indicate the presence of total denervation-neurogenic paresis, peripheral type, or neurogenic paresis, anterior horn cell type. In addition, myogenic paresis may be detected. Generally, on the basis of abnormal findings and with a well-determined examination, the presence of a radiculopathy, generalized neuropathy, focal or mononeuropathy, or plexopathy can be determined. The following are needle abnormalities in abnormal muscles:

1. Insertional activity (decreased or increased)
2. Spontaneous activity (fibrillations, positive sharp waves, or fasciculations) (Fig. 11–6)
3. Abnormalities of voluntary motor unit activity, especially recruitment (see Fig. 11–5)
4. Abnormal motor unit morphology (e.g., excessive or extreme polyphasia)

Nerve conduction studies are of value in the following cases:

1. Determining whether a disease of nerve is present
2. Determining the distribution of a neuropathy (e.g., mononeuritis, polyneuropathy, mononeuritis multiplex). This may be a valuable point in the differential diagnosis of the cause of a neuropathy.
3. Determining at what point in a nerve there is conduction block and locating an entrapment site
4. Studying the progress of disease of a peripheral nerve (e.g., Is it getting better? Worse? Staying the same?)
5. Seeing whether there is reinnervation of a previously sectioned nerve
6. Establishing in a disease of the myoneural junction (e.g., myasthenia gravis) the fact that conduction along the nerve is adequate or normal

Conduction velocity studies are carried out by the insertion of a needle electrode into a muscle innervated by the nerve under study or by the use of

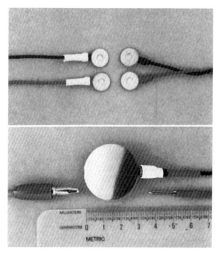

Figure 11–7. Disk surface electrodes (G1, G2) and ground electrode (C) is used in measurement of motor conduction velocity. (Courtesy of Oxford Instruments Medical, Inc., Hawthorne, NY.)

surface electrodes over that muscle (Fig. 11–7). For example, the first dorsal interosseous muscle may be examined to determine the function of the ulnar nerve (Fig. 11–8). The nerve is stimulated, in the case of the ulnar nerve, at the elbow, and the latency of the response is determined. The response is generally a spikelike large motor unit action potential. The ulnar nerve is then stimulated in the wrist or in the axillary region, or in both. The difference in latencies between the two points of stimulation and the distance between the two points of stimulation provide the basis for the calculation of the conduction velocity. The conduction velocity is given by the following formula:

$$MCV\,(m/sec) = \frac{DMM}{PML - DML}$$

where DMM is the distance between the two stimulus points in millimeters, PML is the proximal motor latency (in milliseconds), DML is the distal motor latency (in milliseconds), and MCV is the motor conduction velocity in meters per second.[1]

Textbooks of stimulation points and pickup points are readily available.[5,6] Normal values are usually established for each nerve in individual laboratories, but normal values for commonly tested sensory and motor nerves are generally available (Table 11–1).

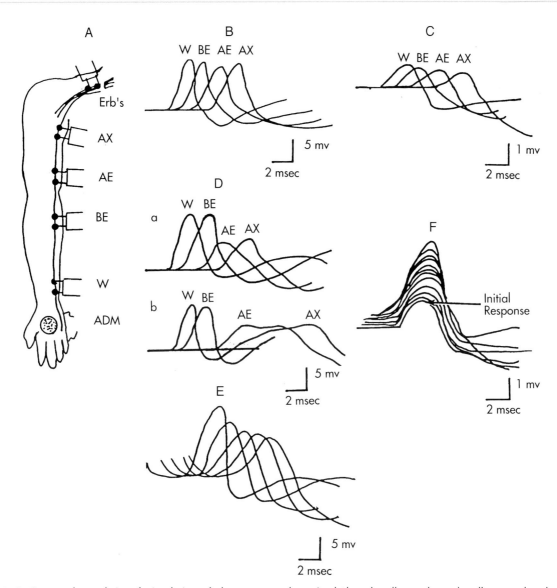

Figure 11–8. A, Commonly used site of stimulation of ulnar nerve at the wrist, below the elbow, above the elbow, and at the axilla. The ulnar nerve can also be stimulated at Erb's point in the supraclavicular fossa. **B,** Normal amplitude compound motor action potentials (CMAPs) recorded from the abductor digiti minimi manus (ADM) following stimulation of ulnar nerve at these various sites. **C,** Low-amplitude CMAPs in a patient with axonal neuropathy. All CMAPs are of the same amplitude but are much smaller than normal. **D,** Decremental response *(a)* and decremental and dispersed response *(b)* on stimulation above the elbow and the axilla and normal response on stimulation below the elbow and wrist. **E,** Repetitive nerve stimulation of the ulnar nerve at the wrist in myasthenia gravis. Note the initial normal response and subsequent decremental response at slow rate (3 pulses/sec). **F,** Repetitive nerve stimulation in Lambert-Eaton syndrome. On rapid rate (20 to 50 pulses/sec) a marked incremental response occurs. Note the very low initial response and the twofold to fourfold increase following the rapid rate of stimulation. AE, above the elbow; AX, axilla; BE, below the elbow; W, wrist.

Table 11–1.   Normal Values for Commonly Tested Sensory and Motor Nerves

NERVES	AMPLITUDE (AVG)	DISTAL LATENCY IN MILLISECONDS (AVG)*	CONDUCTION VELOCITY IN METERS/SEC (AVG)
Median (sensory)	10 to 85 µV (20)	2.0 to 3.7 (3.2)	
Ulnar (sensory)	5 to 70 µV (15)	1.6 to 3.2 (2.8)	
Radial (sensory)	10 to 60 µV (18)	1.7 to 2.8 (2.4)	
Median (motor)	5 to 25 mV (8)	2.0 to 4.0 (3.3)	48 to 69 (54)
Ulnar (motor)	5.5 to 20 mV (8)	1.6 to 3.1 (2.6)	50 to 69 (55)
Sural (sensory)	3 to 38 mV (8)	2.3 to 4.6 (4.1)	41 to 61 (46)
Peroneal (motor)	2.5 to 18 mV (4)	2.3 to 6.0 (4.1)	41 to 58 (45)
Posterior tibial (motor)	4 to 38 mV (11)	2.1 to 6.0 (4.3)	

*Distal latencies are based on standard distance: 13 cm for median (S); 11 cm for ulnar (S); 10 cm for radial (S): 14 cm for sural (S); 4 to 6 cm for median (M) and ulnar (M); 6 to 8 cm for peroneal (M); 8 to 12 cm for the posterior tibial (M) nerves.

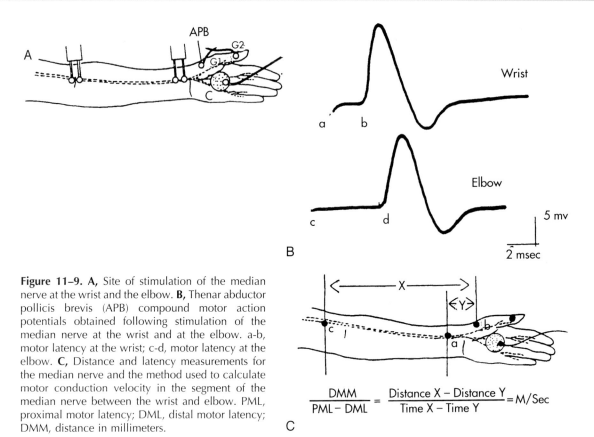

Figure 11–9. A, Site of stimulation of the median nerve at the wrist and the elbow. **B,** Thenar abductor pollicis brevis (APB) compound motor action potentials obtained following stimulation of the median nerve at the wrist and at the elbow. a-b, motor latency at the wrist; c-d, motor latency at the elbow. **C,** Distance and latency measurements for the median nerve and the method used to calculate motor conduction velocity in the segment of the median nerve between the wrist and elbow. PML, proximal motor latency; DML, distal motor latency; DMM, distance in millimeters.

$$\frac{DMM}{PML - DML} = \frac{\text{Distance X} - \text{Distance Y}}{\text{Time X} - \text{Time Y}} = M/Sec$$

Median nerve stimulation is comparable to ulnar nerve stimulation (Fig. 11–9).

F Wave

Definition

Motor conduction velocity along the whole axon, including proximal portions, can be studied by eliciting the F-wave response, a small, late muscle response that occurs from backfiring of anterior horn cells.[21-23] F waves may be obtained from almost any mixed nerve that can be stimulated, but the median, ulnar, peroneal, and posterior tibial nerves are the most commonly used (Fig. 11–10). If the standard distal motor conduction velocities are normal but the F-wave value is prolonged, slowing must be occurring somewhere more proximal to the distal normal segment. (The method used to determine the F-wave latency varies from laboratory to laboratory; the F-wave value with each successive shock stimulus shows variability of several milliseconds, with some examiners averaging 10, 30, or 50 responses and some taking the shortest of 10, 20, or more responses.) Limb temperature and arm or leg length also may be important to know. A comparison with the opposite limb may be most helpful if that limb is asymptomatic.

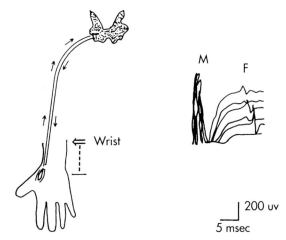

Figure 11–10. Consecutive tracing showing M responses and F waves recorded from the abductor pollicis brevis after stimulation of median nerve at the wrist.

Pitfalls and Comments

In addition to the variability of F waves and how they are obtained in different laboratories, many electromyographers overuse (or at least overperform) the F-wave study when proximal slowing in a nerve or nerve root is not even in the differential diagnosis.

The most accepted use of the study is in suspected early *Guillain-Barré syndrome*, when the usual studies are still normal—usually in the first 10 days of the illness. It is highly controversial in the evaluation of radiculopathies.[24,25]

Hoffman Reflex (H Reflex)

Definition

The H reflex is obtained by electrostimulation of the posterior tibial nerve in the popliteal space at a slow rate with long duration and submaximal electrical shock; it is recorded with surface electrodes over the gastrocnemius-soleus (Fig. 11–11). The impulse travels up the sensory fibers to the spinal cord, synapses with the alpha motor neuron, and returns down the motor fibers to the calf muscle. H-reflex latencies are therefore long, in the range of 40 to 45 msec. They are mostly carried in the S1 nerve root distribution and cannot be recorded consistently from other muscles. To determine a delay or an asymmetry, one should always study the opposite leg for comparison.[26-29]

Pitfalls and Comments

The H reflex is somewhat more useful than the F wave, but the main reason for the study can be seen in the evaluation of a suspected S1 radiculopathy in which the history or physical examination is suggestive but the EMG is normal.[30] Usually when an absent H reflex is noted, suggesting a problem with S1 nerve root conduction, an absent or depressed ankle reflex has already been noted in the physical examination, so the study is, for many, redundant. Pitfalls occur when the opposite leg is not studied to show a normal H reflex as a contrast. If the H reflex is bilaterally absent, it may reflect more generalized disease, for example, peripheral neuropathy. Older patients often do not have good H reflexes as a normal finding. In addition, a unilaterally absent H reflex with normal needle EMG examination does not indicate when the injury occurred; it may have been the result of a previous injury.

Quantitative Sensory Testing (Pseudomotor Axon Reflex Test)

Quantitative sensory testing takes various forms, including the quantitative somatosensory thermotest using a controlled ramp of ascending or descending temperature through a Peltier device.[31] Measurement of threshold for cold sensation reflects function of small caliber A-delta myelinated afferents. Threshold for warm sensation reflects function of warm-specific small unmyelinated afferent channels. Cold pain and heat pain thresholds test the function of unmyelinated C fiber, polymodal nociceptors, and, to a lesser extent, A-delta fiber nociceptors. Certain abnormal patterns are characteristic of dysfunction of small caliber peripheral nerve afferents.[32] To obtain maximal information from a quantitative somatosensory thermotest, it is necessary to test for cold, pain, and heat sensations, mandatory in the evaluation of painful syndromes.[33] Quantitative sensory testing performed at different sites along an extremity in cases of polyneuropathy yields useful information about the staging of the pathologic process along the extremity.

The quantitative pseudomotor axon reflex test (Q-sart) is a quantitative thermoregulatory sweat test. It has been used to detect postganglionic pseudomotor failure in neuropathies[34,35] and preganglionic neuropathies with presumed transsynaptic degeneration.[36] In patients with distal small fiber neuropathy, it is the most sensitive diagnostic test.[37] Various commercial devices have been used to differentiate axonal from demyelinating polyneuropathy.[38]

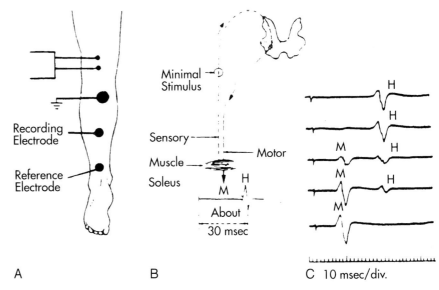

Figure 11–11. A, Placement of recording electrodes and site of stimulation of posterior tibial nerve for recording of Hoffman (H) reflex from the soleus muscle. **B,** H-reflex pathways. An electrical impulse generated on stimulation of the tibial nerve travels along with sensory axon (afferent), within the spinal cord and along the motor axon (efferent). **C,** Motor response (M) and H reflex (H). Five consecutive traces are shown. Starting from the top, each trace is obtained with increasing stimulus intensity. With minimal stimulus only, the H response is obtained. As the intensity of the stimulus is increased, the M response begins to appear and the H response begins to decrease, finally becoming unobtainable.

Clinical Correlations of Electromyographic Testing

Clinical correlations can be based on a careful history, clinical examination, and electrodiagnostic studies. Electrodiagnostic studies are best for separating neuropathy from myopathy and determining whether a neuropathy is generalized axonal, demyelinating, mixed, or focal, thus giving important clues as to the cause. Furthermore, nerve trauma can be followed up serially to determine recovery. In many instances, a diagnosis of plexopathy or radiculopathy can be made.

Nerve Trauma

Often after injury, such as a laceration, the nerve is completely severed. At rest, denervation potentials are recorded in the muscles supplied by that nerve in the form of positive sharp waves or fibrillation potentials, and on electromyography, no motor unit action potentials are seen. Sometimes, however, an injury is incomplete, and the type of nerve lesion is uncertain.

Neurapraxia
Neurapraxia is the mildest form of nerve injury. It consists of conduction loss without associated axonal structural changes. This form of conduction block often occurs with compressive or ischemic nerve injuries, such as mild entrapment syndrome or compression (e.g., "Saturday night palsy"). In neurapraxic injuries, focal demyelination occurs. Serial nerve conduction determinations along the course of the nerve enable one to locate the site of the conduction block. The prognosis for complete recovery is generally good, and healing occurs within days or weeks, barring further injury.

Axonotmesis
In axonotmesis, a more severe form of nerve injury, the axon is disrupted in its myelin sheath. The neural tube, consisting of the endoperineurium and epineurium, remains intact. The nerve undergoes wallerian degeneration, with fragmentation of the axon distal to the site of injury. Motor and sensory paralysis occurs with associated atrophy of supplied muscles and loss of reflexes. After about 4 to 5 days, the distal segments of the nerve become inexcitable. In 1 to 2 weeks, positive sharp waves are seen; fibrillations in involved musculature occur in 2 to 3 weeks. The intact neural tube forms a lattice for the regenerating axon, and the prognosis for recovery is generally good.

Neurotmesis
Neurotmesis is the most severe form of nerve injury and consists of severe disruption or transection of the nerve. Nerve regeneration and recovery are often incomplete and may require surgical reanastomosis. Neuromas may form and are commonly associated with pain. Only serial determinations over time can determine the difference between axonotmesis and neurotmesis.

Nontraumatic Neuropathies

In a patient with a nontraumatic neuropathy, segmental demyelination is generally associated with slowing of nerve conduction velocities and temporal dispersion of evoked responses. With axonal degeneration, however, reduction of the evoked response amplitudes with mild or minimal slowing of nerve conduction velocities is typical. An EMG provides early information regarding reinnervation before clinical recovery is evident. The earliest positive evidence of reinnervation is the appearance during voluntary effort of motor unit potentials that are of low amplitude in the beginning but are highly polyphasic ("nascent") units. They may be present several weeks before there is clinical evidence of functional recovery.

Polyneuropathy

EMG and nerve conduction evaluation are useful in diagnosing polyneuropathy and in determining whether a pathologic process is axonal and demyelinating. A diagnosis of polyneuropathy is made when abnormal nerve conduction and EMG findings are bilateral and symmetric.

Generalized peripheral neuropathies often associated with pain are noted in Box 11–1.[39-44] Electrodiagnostic findings characteristic of axonal neuropathy are as follows:

1. Abnormally low or absent sensory nerve action potentials and compound muscle action potential amplitudes

---

BOX 11–1. GENERALIZED PERIPHERAL NEUROPATHIES

Diabetes mellitus
Polyneuropathy associated with insulinoma
Polyneuropathy associated with nutritional deficiency
Alcohol-nutritional deficiency polyneuropathy
Vasculitis-associated neuropathy
Amyloidosis
Toxic (arsenic and thallium)
HIV-related distal symmetric polyneuropathy
Fabry's disease
Guillain-Barré syndrome (acute inflammatory demyelinating polyneuropathy)
Cryptogenic sensory, or sensorimotor neuropathy
Polyneuropathy due to neoplasm, including paraneoplastic syndromes, such as acute sensory neuropathy, or sensorimotor neuropathy associated with carcinoma

HIV, human immunodeficiency virus.

2. Normal distal latencies
3. Near-normal motor and sensory conduction velocities

If a disease process affects the large-diameter axons, some slowing of conduction occurs; the velocity is seldom reduced by more than 20% to 30% of normal. However, fibrillations and positive sharp waves are present in muscles innervated by affected nerves and are generally worse distally. The feet are more involved than the hand muscles, and the leg muscles are more involved than the arm muscles. Motor unit potentials are decreased in number with deficient recruitment and an incomplete interference pattern. Some motor units are of increased amplitude and duration.

In contrast, diffuse demyelinating neuropathy is characterized by reduction of conduction velocities, usually more than 40% of the normal range. Distal latencies are also prolonged. The sensory nerve action potentials and compound muscle action potentials usually have low amplitudes and temporal dispersion. A needle EMG shows no fibrillations or positive sharp waves unless there is secondary axonal degeneration. In a pure demyelinating neuropathy, there is no denervation of muscle fibers. Motor units are decreased in number; decreased recruitment is attributable to conduction block in some fibers. Usually, there is no significant change in the duration, amplitude, or morphology of motor units, but the number of polyphasic potentials may be increased if there is demyelination of terminal axons.

Once it has been determined electromyographically whether a neuropathy is primarily axonal or demyelinating, one can then consider clinically which neuropathies are diffusely axonal and which are demyelinating. Subacute and chronic diffuse axonal types include most toxic and nutritional neuropathies, uremia, diabetes, hypothyroidism, human immunodeficiency virus (HIV) infection, Lyme disease, paraneoplastic disease, dysproteinemia, and amyloidosis.

Demyelinating polyneuropathies include hereditary motor and sensory neuropathies, types 1 and 3, Refsum's disease, multifocal leukodystrophy, and Krabbe's disease. *Acute* nonuniform demyelinating diseases include Guillain-Barré syndrome, diphtheria, and acute arsenic intoxication, whereas *chronic* versions include inflammatory demyelinating peripheral neuropathy, idiopathic disease, and neuropathies accompanying HIV as well as various paraproteinemias, dysproteinemias, and osteosclerotic myeloma.[45]

Mononeuropathies and Entrapment Neuropathies

With an entrapment neuropathy, the most commonly involved nerves are the median, ulnar, radial, common peroneal, and tibial. Entities such as trauma, vasculitis, diabetes mellitus, leprosy, and sarcoidosis can affect any nerve in the body. Electrophysiologic studies are of great assistance in localizing the lesion in the individual nerve and in differentiating mononeuropathy from diffuse polyneuropathy, plexopathies, and radiculopathies.

Median Nerve

The median nerve is most commonly entrapped at the wrist as it passes through the carpal tunnel, but it may also be injured at the elbow where it passes between the two heads of the pronator teres or, less frequently, is compressed by a dense band of connective tissue (the ligament of Struthers immediately above the elbow) (see Fig. 11–9).[46,47] The median nerve is derived from C6 through T1 nerve roots (lateral and medial cords of the brachial plexus). The diagnosis of carpal tunnel syndrome is made by demonstrating localized slowing of sensory and motor conductions across the wrist as evidenced by prolonged sensory and motor distal latencies.[1] In addition, with late changes there may be denervation in the form of fibrillations, positive sharp waves, and reduced motor units with polyphasia in the median innervated hand muscles.

Pronator Teres and Anterior Interosseous Syndromes

The pronator teres and anterior interosseous syndromes are proximal compression or entrapment neuropathies of the median nerve. The pronator teres syndrome may also show a normal distal latency but no evidence of denervation in the median innervated hand and forearm muscles except for the pronator teres.[47] The anterior interosseous nerve is a motor branch of the median nerve with its origin just distal to the pronator teres.[47]

Ulnar Nerve

The ulnar nerve is derived from C8 and T1 cervical nerve roots (medial cord of the brachial plexus). It is usually injured at the elbow but occasionally at the wrist in the canal of Guyon or deep in the palm (silver beater's palsy). EMG helps differentiate C8 and T1 radiculopathies from plexopathy or more distal ulnar nerve palsy (see Fig. 11–8).[48,49] When the lesion is in the wrist at the canal of Guyon, usually both sensory and motor fibers are involved and the amplitude of the sensory nerve action potential and muscle action potential is reduced. Distal sensory and motor latency across the wrist is prolonged, and there is no focal slowing of motor conduction velocity or decrement of compound muscle action potential across the elbow. With a lesion in the deep palmar branch, there is no sensory abnormality and all of the changes are in the motor distribution distal to the lesion.[50] When the abnormality is at the elbow, there may be localized slowing of conduction velocity across the elbow, often as much as 25% to 40% below normal. Normal values may depend on the method used (arm straight versus arm bent). The sensory potential may be affected, as may the EMG of the ulnar hand muscles.

Radial Nerve

The radial nerve is a continuation of the posterior cord of the brachial plexus and receives fibers from C5 to C8 cervical roots. It is usually involved at the spiral groove of the humerus, often secondary to a humeral fracture. With a lesion at the spiral groove, the triceps muscle is spared on EMG, but all of the extensor muscles of the forearm are involved. An isolated superficial radial nerve palsy sometimes occurs at the wrist with the only abnormality in the radial sensory nerve action potential.

Posterior Interosseous Syndrome

The posterior interosseous nerve syndrome (sometimes known as *complicated lateral epicondylitis*) occurs from entrapment of this radial nerve branch at the arcade of Frohse between the two heads of the supinator. EMG shows involvement of the extensor carpi ulnaris, extensor digitorum longus, extensor pollicis longus, and extensor indicis while sparing the more proximal supinator and extensor carpi radialis longus and brevis.[51] Sensation is unaffected.

Common Peroneal Nerve

The common peroneal nerve is derived from L4 through S1 roots but is primarily from L5. It may be compressed at the head of the fibula. Peroneal nerve conduction studies show reduced compound action potentials, as recorded from the extensor digitorum brevis on stimulation above the fibular head and normal compound action potentials below the fibular head and at the ankle.

Posterior Tibial Nerve at the Ankle

The posterior tibial nerve is derived from L4 through S3 roots and may be compressed in the tarsal tunnel. Nerve conduction studies show prolongation of the distal motor and sensory latency of the tibial nerve.[52-54] There may be EMG changes in the appropriate foot muscles. This syndrome is relatively uncommon.

Sciatic Nerve

The sciatic nerve arises from the L4, L5, S1, S2, and S3 nerve roots. A controversial syndrome is entrapment by the piriformis muscle as it passes through the greater sciatic notch. A lesion of the sciatic nerve is defined and localized by detailed needle examination of muscle in the lower limb.[55]

Other Uncommon Neuropathies

There are numerous potential mononeuropathies, including those involving the long thoracic nerve, dorsal scapular nerve, suprascapular nerve, musculocutaneous nerves, and axillary nerves in the shoulder girdle and upper extremity; and those in the pelvic girdle, including the femoral, obturator, saphenous, lateral femoral cutaneous, genitofemoral, ilioinguinal, and superior and inferior gluteal nerves. Needle EMG reveals denervation changes in muscle innervated by individual nerves. Nerve conduction studies are rarely useful in their evaluation.[56]

Radiculopathies

Radiculopathies are diseases of the nerve roots and must be differentiated from plexopathies as well as from complex individual nerve root lesions. Roots are commonly involved by compression, especially in the cervical and lumbar region, but may also be involved by diseases such as diabetes mellitus, herpes zoster, carcinomatous infiltration, and lymphomatous infiltration of nerves as well as rare sarcoidosis and infectious processes. Motor and sensory nerve conductions are rarely useful because the lesion in a radiculopathy is proximal to the dorsal root ganglion and motor conduction studies are usually normal, although they may be reduced in amplitude if the lesion is severe enough to cause axonal loss. The H reflex is absent or latency-delayed when the S1 root is involved. Typically, nerve root lesions are identified by the abnormal needle examination results in the appropriate paraspinal and limb muscles.[57] Because most limb muscles are supplied by more than one nerve root (Tables 11–2 and 11–3), a normal study does not exclude the diagnosis of radiculopathy; however, when EMG findings are abnormal,

Table 11–2. Segmental Innervation of Commonly Tested Muscles in the Upper Extremity

MUSCLE	SPINAL SEGMENT	NERVE SUPPLY
Cervical paraspinal	C2 to C8	Corresponding cervical root
Trapezius	C2, C3, C4	Spinal accessory
Supraspinatus	C5, C6	Subscapular
Infraspinatus	C5	Subscapular
Deltoid (circumflex)	C5, C6	Axillary
Biceps brachii	C5, C6	Musculocutaneous
Brachioradialis	C6, C7	Radial
Flexor carpi radialis	C6, C7, C8	Median
Pronator teres	C6, C7	Median
Triceps brachii	C7, C8	Radial
Extensor digitorum communis	C7, C8	Radial
Extensor indicis	C7, C8	Radial
Flexor carpi ulnaris	C8, T1	Ulnar
Abductor pollicis brevis	C8, T1	Median
First dorsal interosseus	C8, T1	Ulnar
Abductor digiti minimi manus	C8, T1	Ulnar

Table 11–3. Segmental Innervation of Commonly Tested Muscles in the Lower Extremity

MUSCLE	SPINAL SEGMENT	NERVE SUPPLY
Lumbosacral paraspinal	L1 to S1	Corresponding roots
Iliacus	L2, L3, L4	Femoral
Adductors of thigh	L2, L3, L4	Obturator
Quadriceps femoris	L2, L3, L4	Femoral
Tibialis anterior	L4, L5	Deep peroneal
Gluteus medius	L4, L5, S1	Superior gluteal
Gluteus maximus	L5, S1	Inferior gluteal
Peroneus longus	L5, S1	Superficial peroneal
Biceps femoris—long head	L5, S1	Sciatic
Biceps femoris—short head	L5, S1	Sciatic
Flexor digitorum longus	L5, S1	Posterior tibial
Tibialis posterior	L5, S1	Posterior tibial
Extensor digitorum brevis	L5, S1	Deep peroneal
Gastrocnemius—lateral	L5, S1	Posterior tibial
Gastrocnemius—medial	S1, S2	Posterior tibial
Abductor hallucis	S1, S2	Posterior tibial
Abductor digiti quinti	S1, S2	Posterior tibial
Tensor fasciae latae	L5, S1	Superior gluteal

they provide objective evidence of impairment of function in the nerve root and localize the lesion to one or more roots in addition to revealing the severity of involvement.[1]

Plexopathies

In plexopathies, motor conduction studies are useful in excluding a peripheral nerve lesion; otherwise, findings are normal except that amplitudes of compound muscle action potentials may be reduced. Sensory nerve conductions are usually helpful in excluding other causes. Again, the needle examination is most helpful, requiring a knowledge of which muscles are supplied by which portions of the plexus.

Anterior Horn Cell Disease

Disorders of the anterior horn cell do not cause pain except for acute poliomyelitis (acute febrile stage).

Disorders of the Central Nervous System

EMG findings are almost always normal in diseases of the central nervous system.

Primary Muscle Disorders

One of the clearest applications of EMG is in differentiating myopathies from neuropathic processes.[58-60] The differentiation in EMG studies between myopathy and neuropathy should be obvious by needle examination. In myopathy, the potentials are reduced in amplitude and may be very polyphasic,

BOX 11–2. PAINFUL MYOPATHIES[58-60]

Dermatomyositis
Polymyositis
Toxic myopathies
  AZT,* lovastatin
  Unusual diseases showing muscle cramping, including stiff-man syndrome (Moersch-Woltman syndrome), simply show muscle contraction and spasms. Continuous muscle fiber activity (Isaacs-Mertens syndrome) shows continuous, low-amplitude, fibrillation-type potentials.

*Azidothymidine (zidovudine).
Data from Kuncl RW, Wiggins WW: Toxic myopathies. Neurol Clin 1988;6:593-619; Walton J, ed: Disorders of Voluntary Muscle, ed 4. New York, Churchill Livingstone, 1981, pp 478-584; and Roland LP, ed: Merritt's Textbook of Neurology, ed 9. Baltimore, Williams & Wilkins, 1995, pp 766-803.

recruit paradoxically (i.e., more potentials seen on the screen than would be expected for the corresponding amount of effort), and are accompanied by marked signs of irritability. In polymyositis and metabolic muscle disorders, sensory nerve conductions are always normal. The compound muscle action potential amplitude may be low, but otherwise motor conduction results are normal. EMG findings are commonly normal in myofascial pain syndromes and fibromyalgia, but in polymyositis and metabolic muscle disorders (e.g., glycogen and lipid storage disease) muscle pain, cramps, and weakness can occur. Box 11–2[58-60] lists the painful myopathies.

Usefulness and Limitations of Electromyography

EMG and nerve conduction studies are useful in localizing neuromuscular disease sites and in providing information about the nature of the process (demyelinating, axonal, primary muscular, radicular) but cannot give the cause (diabetes, Guillain-Barré syndrome, myositis, tumor, or ruptured disk). Figure 11–12 presents a summary of EMG findings in various conditions. In addition, a normal result does not mean the patient does not have pain. Electrodiagnostic studies in the EMG laboratory, as usually performed, measure only activity related to the motor nerve fibers, the larger sensory nerve fibers, and the muscles. Sympathetic and small unmyelinated nerve fiber functions are not evaluated except by quantitative sensory testing.

The timing of the EMG in relation to injury or onset of symptoms may be very important. Early after nerve injury (0 to 14 days), the EMG may show only electrical silence, which is not helpful. If any motor units are seen at that time, the nerve to that muscle is at least partially intact. Fibrillation potentials appear only after 2 to 3 weeks. If reinnervation is occurring, small, very polyphasic recovery or "nascent" units will be noted. Serial studies after nerve injury are more helpful than a single study.

Cost-containment issues have become extremely important, and Medicare and other insurers have

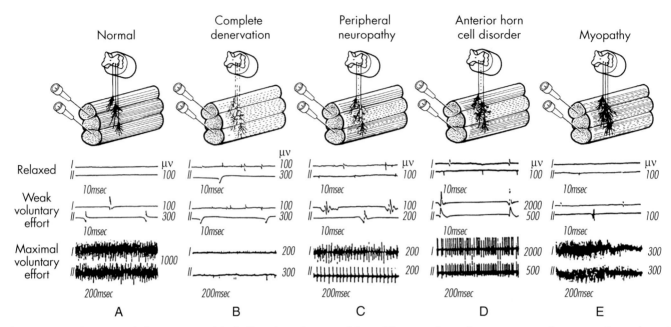

Figure 11–12. Summary of electromyographic findings in various conditions. Diagrams show electromyograms from normal muscle and from muscles with paresis of neurogenic and myogenic origin with a schematic presentation of the muscle fibers from three motor units (marked *solid circle, open circle,* or *x*; affected fibers are *dotted*). Two recording electrodes I and II and the corresponding recordings I and II. Up is negative. **A,** Normal. *At rest:* no action potentials. *Weak voluntary effort:* single motor unit potentials. *Maximal voluntary effort:* interference pattern; no synchronization. **B,** Total denervation. Diffuse atrophy of muscle fibers. *At rest:* diphasic and positive denervation potentials. *Voluntary effort:* no motor unit potentials. **C,** Peripheral neurogenic paresis. Patchy loss of muscle fibers. *At rest:* denervation potentials. *Voluntary effort:* often with increased action potential duration; polyphasic potentials. Pattern of single motor unit potentials or mixed pattern during maximal voluntary effort. No synchronization between various leads. **D,** Neurogenic paresis in diseases of the anterior horn cells. Patchy loss of muscle fibers. *At rest:* denervation potentials. *Voluntary effort:* increased action potential duration and voltage; polyphasic potentials. Single motor unit potentials with maximal voluntary effort, often synchronous in different leads. **E,** Myogenic paresis. Diffuse atrophy of muscle fibers. *At rest:* spontaneous discharges of short duration (in severe cases). *Voluntary effort:* diminished action potential duration; diminished action potential voltage; polyphasic potentials. Interference pattern with maximal effort; a short duration of the single spike potentials is often seen. (From Buchthal F: An Introduction to Electromyography. Copenhagen, Scandinavia University Books, 1957, p. 40.)

developed guidelines for when it is appropriate to test for various conditions. In response, the American Association of Electrodiagnostic Medicine (AAEM) has promulgated a proposed policy for electrodiagnostic medicine, including guidelines for each suspected entity (September 16, 1997).*

EVOKED POTENTIALS

Evoked potentials (EPs) are electrical responses of the nervous system to external sensory stimuli. It has been known for decades that these responses are present; however, their clinical usefulness did not become possible until the development of computerized averaging and advanced signal processing in the late 1960s.[61] Since then, the importance of EPs in diagnosing diseases of the peripheral nervous system and the central nervous system has undergone exponential growth.

The utility of EPs is based on their ability to provide objective and reproducible data concerning the status of the sensory nervous system. EP testing can dem-

---

* Available from AAEM Education and Marketing Department, telephone 507-228-0100.

onstrate abnormalities of the sensory system when clinical signs and symptoms are ambiguous. In addition, evidence of clinically unsuspected lesions may be provided when the history and physical examination are normal. EP testing may help delineate the anatomic distribution of nervous system lesions and help monitor their progression or regression; this testing may be used to demonstrate integrity of nervous system pathways placed at risk during surgery.[61,62]

General Principles

EP responses have very low amplitude (0.1 to 20 mV); consequently, they are obscured by random noise consisting primarily of spontaneous electroencephalographic activity, muscle artifact, and environmental interference. Extraction of the EP response is accomplished by signal averaging. This process summates the "time-locked" EP response, which occurs at the same interval after the stimuli and minimizes unwanted noise.

Although EPs can be elicited by a wide variety of stimuli, the most commonly used stimuli are visual, auditory, and somatosensory.[63] This gives rise to the *visual evoked potential* (VEP) test, the *brainstem auditory evoked potential* (BAEP) test, and the *somatosensory evoked potential* (SEP) test. In each of these tests, the EP response consists of a sequence of upward and downward deflections (e.g., peaks and waves). The characteristics to be evaluated are presence or absence, polarity, configuration, amplitude, latency, and interval between individual peaks (*interpeak latency* [IPL]).

Standardized nomenclature for identification of individual peaks or waves has not been universally established,[64,65] although some general principles for labeling have been agreed on.[66,67] Peaks or waves, or both, may be identified by their polarity and the latency at which they occur. For example, the positive peak occurring at 100 msec in the VEP is commonly designated *P100*. Labeling may also be based on the anatomic site at which the response is recorded (e.g., Erb's point), or the deflections may be simply numbered in sequence (e.g., waves I through V in the BAEP).

Normal values for the components of the EP response are affected by numerous factors, including the technique and equipment employed by different laboratories. Therefore each laboratory generally establishes its own normal values using 2.5 or 3 standard deviations from the mean to determine the limits of normality. Normal values are also influenced by subject factors, including gender, age, body size, and temperature. Clinical interpretation of the EP requires consideration of these factors.[61,68,69]

Equipment

Most laboratories use commercially available EP equipment that should meet the standards established by the American Association of Electrodiagnostic Medicine and by the American Electroencephalographic Society.[66,67,70] In simplest terms, recording the EP consists of attaching electrodes to the patient over specific areas of the extremities, spine, and scalp, depending on the type of test being performed. After the electrodes are attached to record the EP signals, repetitive stimuli timed with the recording process are presented to the patient. The EP signal is collected by the recording electrodes and amplified, filtered, averaged, and displayed for evaluation, printing, and storage. Careful application of the recording electrodes is critical to obtain an EP response of good quality.[64] The electrode site must be cleaned, and the electrode must be attached with a medium that conducts electricity. Standard metal electroencephalographic cup electrodes are commonly used, although other types of electrodes, including needles, may be used.

Placement of the electrodes on the scalp is standardized, following the International 10-20 System.[71] This system refers to placement of electrodes either 10% or 20% of the total distance between prominent landmarks on the skull (Fig. 11–13). The specific configuration of electrode placement for a given test is referred to as the *montage*.

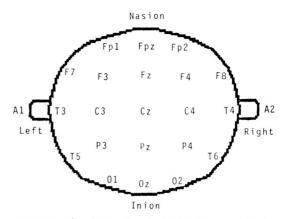

Figure 11–13. The International 10-20 System of electrode placement using 10% or 20% increments between bony skull landmarks to determine individual electrode locations.

Specific Tests of Evoked Potentials

The three tests of EPs that are used most often measure the visual, brainstem auditory, and the somatosensory pathways. Testing of cognitive function and transcranial[66] magnetic stimulation to determine central motor conduction may also be performed. In the patient with pain, SEP testing generally offers the greatest clinical utility and therefore is discussed here in the greatest detail.

Visual Evoked Potentials

VEPs are used to evaluate pathologic conditions affecting the visual pathways. VEPs are generated primarily in the visual cortex and may be affected by abnormalities anywhere along the visual pathway from the cornea to the occipital cortex.[64,72,73] Because the anterior visual pathway from the cornea to the retina may be evaluated directly by ophthalmologic examination, the VEP is mainly used to assess the optic pathway posterior to the retina.

The most common stimulus to elicit the VEP is a reversing checkerboard pattern, transmitted typically through a video monitor and producing checks that alternate from black to white and vice versa. This is referred to as a *pattern-reversal* VEP. Flashes of light also may be used to produce VEPs, but they result in greater variability of the response and are less sensitive to pathway abnormalities than pattern-reversal testing.[73]

Flash-elicited VEPs are used primarily when an individual cannot cooperate with pattern-reversal testing and a gross determination of visual pathway integrity is required (e.g., in infants or comatose patients and during general anesthesia).[62,68] A flash stimulus is also used to produce the electroretinogram, a specialized type of VEP that reflects the function of the retina and distal portion of the optic nerve.

During performance of the pattern-reversal VEP, each eye is tested separately to localize the lesion to the affected side. Because the visual pathways cross at the optic chiasm, evaluation of chiasmal and retrochiasmal pathology requires that the individual temporal and nasal portions of the visual fields of each eye be tested. This is referred to as *partial field stimulation,* whereas *full field stimulation* is used to evaluate prechiasmal lesions.[68]

For pattern-reversal VEP, the patient is seated comfortably in front of the video monitor producing the alternating checkerboard pattern. The distance of the patient from the monitor and the size of the checks are adjusted to produce a visual angle of 10 to 20 degrees. This stimulates the central retina, which is responsible for the greatest portion of the VEP response.[61,73] If the patient wears eyeglasses, they should be worn during the test because a decreased visual acuity will alter results. Recording electrodes are placed on the scalp, typically over the midline occiput, vertex, and forehead (Oz, Cz, and Fpz, respectively, in the International 10-20 System). Additional electrodes are placed laterally to the midline occipital electrode if partial field stimulation is performed. The eye not being tested is patched, and the patient is instructed to gaze at the center of the monitor screen. The checkerboard pattern reverses one to two times per second, generally requiring 100 reversals (trials) to produce a clearly defined response.

The test is repeated under identical conditions to demonstrate reproducibility of the response.

The VEP response consists of three peaks (Fig. 11–14). The primary peak of interest is positive with a latency of approximately 100 msec and is referred to as the *P100.* The remaining two peaks are negative, occurring at latencies of about 75 and 145 msec, respectively. They are more variable than the P100 and are of lesser clinical usefulness. Normal values vary among laboratories, although the upper limits of normal generally range from 117 to 120 msec, with latency differences between eyes of no more than 6 to 7 msec for the P100 response.

Clinical Utility

VEPs are used in the evaluation of many conditions affecting the visual system. In clinical settings, the VEP is used primarily in the diagnosis of multiple sclerosis. Numerous studies have shown that a high percentage of patients with multiple sclerosis exhibit VEP abnormalities, most commonly a prolongation of P100 latency.[61,74-76] As in conventional nerve conduction studies, conditions producing demyelination produce an increase in response latency, whereas axonal loss produces a reduction in response amplitude (Fig. 11–15). Of patients undergoing VEP for

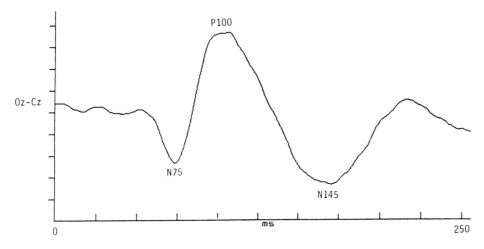

Figure 11–14. Normal visual evoked potential (VEP) response from one eye to pattern shift stimulation recorded from the mid-occiput. The typical response consists of three peaks designated N75, P100, and N145.

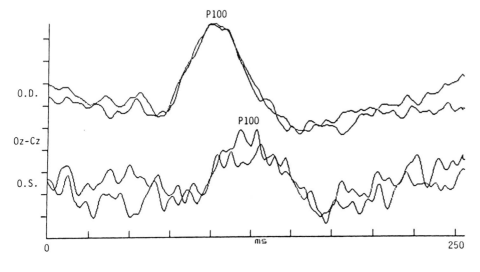

Figure 11–15. Abnormal visual evoked potential (VEP) response from a patient with multiple sclerosis demonstrating prolonged latency and reduced amplitude of the left eye (O.S.) P100 response. The response from the right eye (O.D.) is normal.

evaluation of multiple sclerosis, 63% have abnormal test results. Abnormality rates of at least 85% have been reported in patients known definitely to have multiple sclerosis.[61] Additionally, abnormalities have been found to persist for years after a single episode of optic neuritis, even if the individual remains free of symptoms.[72] The addition of BAEP and SEP testing improves the diagnostic yield over that of VEP alone.[68,77,78]

VEP abnormalities have been reported in patients with migraine headaches, with some researchers claiming the ability to classify the type of migraine.[79-82] Abnormalities may be more common if the VEP is performed soon after the migraine attack.[80] Flash-elicited VEPs may reveal a higher frequency of abnormality compared with pattern-reversal testing. Nevertheless, the use of VEPs in the diagnosis of migraine headache remains controversial.[81]

Diseases of the eye, such as cataracts, glaucoma, and diminished visual acuity, may produce VEP abnormalities, most frequently a decrease in P100 amplitude. Because a direct correlation exists between visual acuity and VEP amplitude, VEP testing may be used to determine visual acuity.[68,83] This is used primarily in patients who are unable to undergo conventional refraction, such as infants and patients with severe mental retardation.

Diseases affecting the anterior visual pathways, such as tumors and ischemia, may produce VEP abnormalities.[84,85] Tumors and infarctions in the posterior optic pathways may also produce VEP abnormalities, especially to partial field stimulation. Unfortunately, "masking" effects from the normal side in unilateral retrochiasmal lesions may result in normal VEPs. At present, the use of VEPs in retrochiasmal disease remains complicated and contentious.[61,64,68,83] Diseases associated with VEP abnormalities are listed in Box 11–3.

Monitoring visual pathway integrity during surgical procedures that jeopardize the visual system has become increasingly widespread. Various techniques using strobe lights, light-emitting diode goggles, and fiberoptic contact lenses have been developed to stimulate the optic system in the anesthetized patient. In addition to providing information concerning pathway integrity, VEPs can help identify optic nerve elements that may be embedded in tumor, thereby

---

BOX 11–3. DISEASES ASSOCIATED WITH ABNORMALITIES OF VISUAL EVOKED POTENTIALS

Multiple sclerosis
Optic pathway tumors
Spinocerebellar degeneration
Charcot-Marie-Tooth disease
Pernicious anemia
Retinopathy
Optic neuropathy
Glaucoma
Refraction errors

---

reducing the risk of accidentally disrupting these structures.[62,86]

Auditory Evoked Potentials

Just as visual stimuli are used to produce the VEP to evaluate the visual pathway, auditory stimuli may be used to assess the auditory pathway. The auditory pathway extends from the middle ear structures through the eighth cranial nerve, the brainstem, and into the auditory cortex. The *auditory evoked potential* (AEP) is produced by presenting auditory stimuli to each ear, which results in a sequence of waveforms that bear a close relationship to these auditory pathway structures and allows relatively specific localization of pathology in the auditory pathway, particularly in the eighth cranial nerve and the brainstem.

Although the AEPs parallel hearing, they do not test hearing per se; rather, they reflect a synchronous neural discharge in the auditory system.[87] Thus an individual may have a normal behavioral audiogram and a grossly abnormal AEP or, conversely, a normal AEP and central auditory deafness.

Brainstem Auditory Evoked Potential

The BAEP is one of several tests included under the general heading of "auditory evoked potentials" that are differentiated by recording techniques and latency of responses. Of these tests, the BAEP is most used clinically. The BAEP is also referred to as the *auditory brainstem response* (ABR) or the *brainstem auditory evoked response* (BAER).

Method
Recording the BAEP response is accomplished by presenting an auditory stimulus to each ear individually and recording the response from electrodes placed on the scalp and on or near each ear. Typically, a montage of four electrodes is used on the forehead, vertex, and each earlobe (Fpz, Cz, A1/A2, respectively). The auditory stimulus used most frequently consists of a brief (100 msec) electrical pulse referred to as a "click." Usually, these clicks are presented to the patient through standard audiologic earphones or insert earphones that fit into the ear canal. Clicks are presented normally at an intensity of 65 to 70 decibels (dB) above normal hearing level and at a rate of 10 to 50 clicks/sec. Averaging of 1000 to 2000 stimuli is usually necessary to produce a well-defined BAEP response.

The typical response consists of a series of seven positive waves numbered by Roman numerals I through VII (Fig. 11–16). For the purpose of clinical evaluation, the first five waves are used because waves VI and VII are not present consistently. The BAEP waveform occurs normally within the first 10 msec following stimulus presentation; the latency of each wave and the IPL among waves I, III, and V are mea-

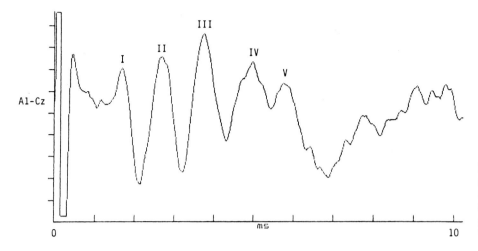

A1-Cz

0   ms   10

Figure 11–16. Normal brainstem auditory evoked potential (BAEP) response recorded from the left ear to click stimuli, demonstrating the five principal peaks. The peaks are labeled with Roman numerals I through V.

Table 11–4. Normative Parameters for Brainstem Auditory Evoked Potentials*

WAVE	NORMAL VALUE (MSEC)	STANDARD DEVIATION (MSEC)
I	1.7	0.2
II	2.8	0.2
III	3.8	0.2
IV	5.1	0.2
V	5.6	0.2
I-III	2.1	0.4
III-V	1.9	0.4
I-V	3.9	0.4

*Normative values from Waldman HJ, Leawood, Kansas.
Wave V/I amplitude ratio >1.0; wave V interaural latency difference = 0.4 msec.

sured (IPL or interpeak latency refers to the latency between each individual wave). Generally, the amplitude of the BAEP response varies too much to be clinically useful, but the amplitude ratio between waves I and V may be abnormal in demyelinating disease.[88]

Normal values for the waves and IPLs vary among laboratories, but average normal values are presented in Table 11–4. Many factors may affect the absolute latencies of the BAEP waves (e.g., peripheral hearing loss). The IPLs offer a more reliable measure of pathology in the auditory pathway, since they frequently remain constant despite changes in the absolute latencies of the waves themselves. Several technical factors, such as varying the stimulus rate or intensity, alter the BAEP. These must be considered when the obtained results are evaluated.

Because clinical use of the BAEP relies on the relationship between individual BAEP waves and the anatomic structures that produce them, identification of individual generator sources of the BAEP has been researched extensively. Some controversy remains,[61,62,68,87] particularly concerning waves IV and V, which appear to have multiple generator sources: Wave I is thought to be produced by the

auditory portion of the eighth cranial nerve; wave II, by the eighth cranial nerve and the cochlear nucleus, and wave III, by the lower pons (likely in the superior olivary complex); waves IV and V, in the upper pons and lower midbrain, possibly in the lateral lemniscus or inferior colliculus.

The status of the patient does not usually affect the ability to obtain a BAEP response. This response may even be obtained from patients who are under general anesthesia or are comatose.[62,89] Mild to moderate peripheral hearing loss may alter absolute wave latencies, although generally IPLs are not changed significantly, therefore allowing interpretation of the BAEP. Marked hearing loss, however, may make interpretation of the BAEP extremely difficult or impossible because of degradation of the response. If possible, behavioral audiometry should be performed before BAEP testing to allow more accurate interpretation of the results.[61,87]

Clinical Utility

BAEPs are useful in evaluating various disease states affecting the auditory pathways. In addition to their VEP abnormalities, patients with multiple sclerosis may demonstrate abnormal BAEPs.[87,88,90] Reported rates of abnormality range from 32% to 72%.

The most common BAEP abnormalities are increased IPLs and a decreased wave V–to–wave I amplitude ratio. Although the BAEP has been found useful in evaluation of patients with multiple sclerosis, most studies have found it the least sensitive diagnostically when compared with the VEP and SEP.[76,91,92] BAEPs are extremely useful in the diagnosis of acoustic neuromas and other cerebellopontine angle tumors. BAEP abnormality rates greater than 90% have been noted in most studies. Also, the BAEP was superior to routine audiometry and computed tomography in early detection of these lesions. Increase in wave I–to–wave III IPL is the most common BAEP abnormality (Fig. 11–17).[93-95]

Brainstem tumors and strokes frequently produce abnormalities of the BAEP if the areas involved lie in the auditory pathway. Prolongation of interpeak or

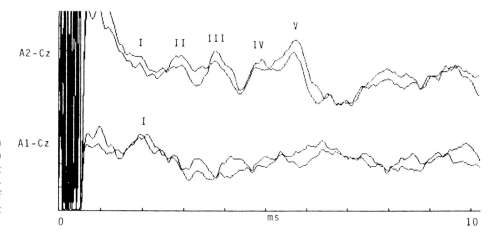

Figure 11–17. Abnormal brainstem auditory evoked potential (BAEP) response from a patient with a left acoustic neuroma. The left trace (A1-Cz) demonstrates only the presence of wave I with an absence of subsequent waves.

absolute latencies, or both, and absence of waves may be seen, depending on the anatomic site of the lesion.[68,72,91]

The BAEP aids evaluation of comatose and head-injured patients. Coma produced by toxic or metabolic causes generally does not produce BAEP abnormalities, whereas BAEPs are abnormal frequently in comas secondary to structural brainstem lesions. In patients with head injuries, BAEPs have been predictors of outcome; more severe BAEP abnormalities indicate poorer prognoses.[96,97] AEP abnormalities have also been described in patients with minimal head injuries, such as postconcussive syndrome.[98] Many other disorders have been associated with BAEP abnormalities,[61,68,99] including degenerative disorders such as Friedreich's ataxia, vertebrobasilar transient ischemic attacks, basilar migraine, and spasmodic torticollis.[100,101]

As with VEPs and the visual pathway, BAEPs may be used to monitor auditory pathway integrity during surgical procedures. BAEP operative monitoring has been used most frequently during resection of acoustic neuromas and tumors of the cerebellopontine angle.[62] The primary use of BAEPs has been to determine hearing sensitivity in patients who are unable to undergo behavioral audiometry (e.g., infants). Estimates of hearing sensitivity are usually obtained by progressively decreasing the intensity of the auditory stimulus until no discernible BAEP response is obtained. Because click stimuli are broad band with a frequency range between 1000 and 4000 Hz, filtered clicks and tone bursts with narrower frequency spectra have been employed to obtain better frequency specificity of hearing.[88,102,103]

Other Auditory Evoked Potentials

Although the BAEP is the most commonly used AEP, other AEPs have been developed to expand clinical utility. The electrocochleogram begins within the first 3 msec after the presentation of auditory stimuli and reflects electrical activity of the cochlear hair cells and the auditory nerve. This measurement has been used clinically to evaluate patients with Ménière's disease, to monitor damage caused by ototoxic drugs, and to evaluate sensorineural hearing loss.[104]

The 40-Hz, middle latency, and long latency AEPs occur later in latency than does the BAEP. They are thought to be generated primarily by structures above the brainstem and therefore may be useful in evaluating more central auditory disorders as well as in determining hearing sensitivity. These responses are less reliable and are more commonly affected by the patient's state than is the BAEP.[88,105]

Somatosensory Evoked Potentials

SEPs are evoked responses to stimulation of sensory nerves. Allowing assessment of somatosensory pathway function, SEPs have been obtained by stimulating sensory and mixed nerves in the upper and lower extremities, dermatomal sensory areas of the skin, and cranial nerves. Recording of the SEP response depends on stimulation of large, fast-conducting sensory fibers in the peripheral nerve. From the peripheral nerve, the SEP pathway enters the spinal cord through the dorsal root ganglion, ascending in the ipsilateral dorsal columns. The pathway crosses at the medial lemniscus, traveling to the contralateral ventroposterolateral nucleus of the thalamus, and then on to the primary sensory cortex.

The correlation between the SEP and disorders affecting joint and position sense is generally accepted. The SEP usually is normal in patients with abnormalities affecting only pain and temperature sensation.[61,64] Cortical evoked potentials have been recorded following noxious stimuli, although these pain-related potentials currently offer limited clinical usefulness.[68] Recent studies have suggested that in some individuals with altered pain-temperature sensation there may be abnormalities of pain-related EPs. Some disagree on whether this reflects abnormalities of spinothalamic function or whether these potentials are related to the cognitive processing of pain.[106-113]

Method

Numerous methods have been described to record SEPs with attempts at standardization occurring only recently.[114-116] Consequently, recording technique, waveform nomenclature, and normal values may vary between investigators.[64,65] Certain general principles, however, apply to most studies. The stimulus of choice for the SEP is electrical and consists of a square wave pulse delivered to the patient by surface or, less commonly, by needle electrodes. Stimulus duration is usually 100 to 200 msec at a rate of three to seven stimuli per second. Stimulus intensity is adjusted to the point of producing an observable muscle twitch for mixed nerves or 2.5 to 3 times sensory threshold for sensory nerve stimulation. When properly applied, the stimulus generally is not painful.

Unilateral stimulation is used routinely to permit lateralization of abnormalities, with bilateral stimulation often being reserved for intraoperative monitoring.[62] The site of stimulation depends on the nerve being studied. Typically, distal sites overlying the nerve are used (e.g., median nerve stimulation at the wrist).

The ascending SEP response is recorded by placing pairs of recording electrodes at different locations along the somatosensory pathway being studied. The placement of these recording electrodes depends on whether the nerve being evaluated is located in the upper or lower extremity and on the specific nerve being tested.

Upper Extremity Somatosensory Evoked Potential

Sites for recording electrodes to study nerves in the upper extremity generally include Erb's point in the supraclavicular fossa, the cervical spine (typically over the C2 or C5 spinous process), and the contralateral scalp overlying the area of the primary sensory cortex (corresponding to C3 or C4 of the International 10-20 System). Also, a reference electrode is placed on the forehead (Fz) and a ground electrode is placed proximal to the stimulation site. A noncephalic reference electrode also may be used to allow better visualization of subcortical potentials.

The median nerve has been the most extensively studied upper extremity nerve and is prototypical of an upper extremity SEP.[114,115] When the median nerve is stimulated at the wrist, expected responses are recorded at each electrode site (Fig. 11–18):

1. At Erb's point, a negative peak with a latency of about 9 msec (designated N9)
2. From the cervical spine, a negative peak at about 13 msec (designated N13)
3. From the scalp, a negative peak at about 20 msec (designated N20), followed by a positive peak at around 23 msec (designated P23)

The sources of these responses remain controversial, although N9 may be generated by fibers in the brachial plexus.[116] N13 is thought to be generated by the dorsal column nuclei, and N20 by the thalamocortical radiations and possibly the primary sensory cortex. Occasionally, a negative peak of approximately 11-msec latency (N11) precedes the N13 response and is believed to reflect activity in the posterior columns and the dorsal root entry zone of the spinal cord.[61,68,117]

Lower Extremity Somatosensory Evoked Potential

Recording the SEP from nerves situated in the lower extremity generally includes placement of recording electrodes on the lumbar spine over the L3 spinous process, on the lower thoracic spine at T12, and on the scalp over the primary sensory cortex (Cz). In studies of the extremity, SEP responses are difficult to record above the thoracic spine; thus cervical spine recording sites are usually not included.

As in upper extremity SEPs, a reference electrode and ground electrode are necessary. Like the median nerve in the upper extremity, the tibial nerve provides a characteristic SEP of the lower extremity.[115,118] When the tibial nerve is stimulated at the ankle, expected responses include the following (Fig. 11–19):

1. A negative peak with an approximate latency of 19 msec recorded at L3 (designated L3S)
2. At T11, a negative peak at about 21 msec (designated T11S)

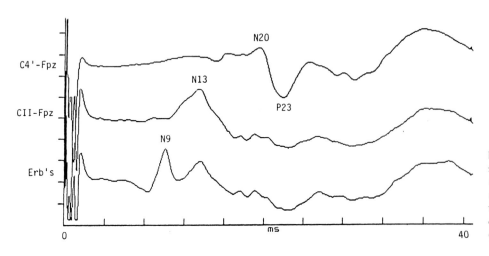

Figure 11–18. Normal upper extremity somatosensory evoked potential (SEP) response from stimulation of the left median nerve. Responses were recorded from Erb's point (N9), the second cervical vertebra (N13), and the cortex (N20-P23).

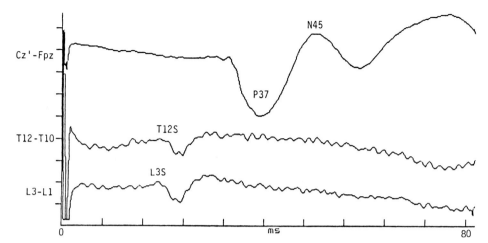

Figure 11–19. Normal lower extremity somatosensory evoked potential (SEP) response from stimulation of the left posterior tibial nerve. Responses were recorded from the third lumbar vertebra (L3S), the twelfth thoracic vertebra (T12S), and the cortex (P37-N45).

3. At the scalp, a positive peak at approximately 37 msec (designated P37), followed by a negative peak with a latency of about 45 msec (designated N45)

The L3S response is thought to reflect activity in the nerve roots of the cauda equina. The T11S response is thought to be generated by the dorsal fibers of the spinal cord, and the scalp potentials are considered reflections of thalamocortical activity.[61,115,117]

In general, cortical responses can be obtained easily, requiring as few as 100 to 200 stimuli. Lumbar and thoracic spinal responses are difficult to acquire and may be unrecordable in obese or uncooperative patients without the use of sedation. Frequently, 1000 to 2000 stimuli are required to obtain clearly defined responses.

Interpretation

Interpretation of SEP depends on the presence or absence of expected waves and, when present, their absolute and IPLs. Latencies beyond 2.5 to 3 standard deviations from the mean are considered abnormal. If the SEP is considered a wave traveling from the stimulation site at the peripheral nerve and ascending proximally through the various recording sites on its way to the cortex, it can be seen that a lesion along the ascending somatosensory pathway will result in normal responses distal to the lesion and abnormal responses proximally. Thus if the brachial plexus response (N9) is normal and the cervical spine potential (N13) is delayed or absent, a lesion is located central to the brachial plexus but below the lower medulla in the cervical root or cord. Similarly, if the brachial plexus potential (N9) is absent or prolonged, a lesion distal to the plexus in the peripheral nerve is likely.

Because diseases of the peripheral nerves that cause slowing of conduction velocity (e.g., demyelinating neuropathies) prolong the latencies of all peaks proximal to the nerve, IPLs are useful to confirm normal conduction through the central nervous system despite peripheral nerve abnormalities.[119] Conduction through the central nervous system is referred to as central conduction time and is measured from N13 to N20 in the upper extremity and from L3S to P37 in the lower extremity. Besides peripheral nerve disease, decreased body temperature and increased limb length result in prolongation of absolute peak latencies, making determination of central conduction time critical.[61,68,107]

Clinical Uses of Somatosensory Evoked Potentials

Peripheral Nerve Disease

The occurrence of central nervous system amplification of the peripheral nerve volley permits cortical SEPs to be recorded when sensory nerve responses are unrecordable by conventional techniques.[107,110,111] Therefore in cases of severe peripheral nerve disease in which conventional determination of nerve conduction is impossible, nerve conduction velocities may be calculated by stimulating a peripheral nerve at two sites and subtracting the latencies of the corresponding scalp-recorded SEPs. Similarly, conduction can be determined in cases of peripheral nerve entrapment in which conventional nerve conduction responses are difficult or impossible to obtain, as in the case of entrapment of the lateral femoral cutaneous nerve (meralgia paresthetica).[110]

Radiculopathy

Much has been published on the use of SEPs in the diagnosis of radiculopathy.[110,112-132] These studies have shown that SEPs recorded from nerves derived from several nerve roots (e.g., median and peroneal nerves) have limited value in diagnosing radiculopathies because abnormalities in a single involved root would be "overshadowed" by contributions from uninvolved roots supplying that nerve. To circumvent this problem, techniques to derive SEPs from single nerve roots have been investigated. This has been accomplished by stimulation of an area of skin derived from a single dermatome (e.g., the great and first toe web space innervated by the L5 nerve

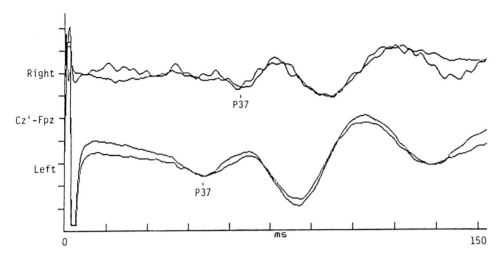

Figure 11–20. Abnormal cortically recorded somatosensory evoked potential (SEP) response from stimulation of the right sural nerve in a patient with a right lumbar radiculopathy. The P37 response demonstrates prolonged latency and reduced amplitude as compared with the normal left-sided response. ms = milliseconds.

root).[123-126] Another method has involved stimulation of segmentally innervated cutaneous sensory nerves (e.g., using the sural nerve to evaluate the S1 nerve root) (Fig. 11–20).[127]

Results from these "segmentally specific" techniques have ranged from excellent to "essentially useless," with reported abnormality rates in radiculopathy ranging from 7% to 92%.[128-131] Some of the controversy stems from differences in diagnostic criteria used to determine abnormality. Because any slowing of nerve conduction velocity from a focal lesion of an individual nerve root would be "diluted" by normal conduction along the remainder of the nerve, abnormalities of latency are found less often than is a reduction of amplitude. Because amplitude varies even among normal individuals, reduction of amplitude as an indication of abnormality is less reliable than are latency abnormalities.[77,117,122]

Abnormalities of latency were observed in some individuals, and diagnostic yield was improved when latency and amplitude values were compared with those of an opposite uninvolved extremity that was used as a control. Reports of using spinal rather than cortical SEPs after segmental sensory stimulation suggest a more reliable method for diagnosis of radiculopathies.[132]

Despite the controversy, some consensus exists regarding the usefulness of SEPs in diagnosing radiculopathies. They are purportedly useful in radiculopathies in which sensory symptoms predominate and diagnosis by other diagnostic techniques, for instance, electromyography (EMG) is difficult.[120,123,126,133] Nevertheless, EMG remains the "gold standard" for the electrodiagnostic evaluation of radiculopathies.

Thoracic Outlet Syndrome

Although ulnar nerve SEPs are controversial, they have been used in an attempt to identify thoracic outlet syndrome. In patients with suspected thoracic outlet syndrome who demonstrated no objective signs of neurologic involvement (e.g., weakness of the hand muscle, numbness, and abnormal EMG), ulnar nerve SEPs were generally normal.[134]

In neurogenic thoracic outlet syndrome, SEP abnormalities included prolonged, attenuated, or absent N9 or N13 peaks, or both, and an increased N9 to N13 IPL. Normal SEP studies of the median nerve in their involved extremity and side-to-side comparisons were also employed to confirm the diagnosis. In cases treated surgically, postoperative improvement in ulnar SEPs was reported.[135-138]

Brachial Plexopathy

Studies have shown that SEPs may provide useful information for the management of patients with brachial plexopathies.[119,120] The ability to record SEPs helps confirm axonal continuity and may help determine whether lesions are preganglionic or postganglionic. As in the case of radiculopathy, segmentally specific testing rather than stimulation of multisegmented nerves provides more specific and accurate information.[139,140]

SEPs are limited, in that they test the sensory portions of nerves, allowing only inference concerning motor function. Furthermore, when multiple lesions are present, SEP abnormalities may reflect only the most distal lesions. Therefore in the presence of a postganglionic lesion, a preganglionic lesion involving the same nerve fibers may go undetected.

Lumbar Spinal Stenosis and Cervical Spondylosis

SEPs have been useful in the diagnosis of lumbar and cervical spinal stenosis, with dermatomal SEPs reported to be superior to EMG in central and lateral recess lumbar stenosis.[136,141,142] SEP abnormalities have improved after surgical decompression of these lesions.[143] In central spondylosis, SEP abnormalities correlated well with the presence of myelopathy but not with radiculopathy alone.[144]

Spinal Cord Lesions

SEPs are frequently abnormal in spinal cord lesions affecting the posterior columns. Intramedullary and extramedullary tumors, traumatic spinal cord injury, and vascular lesions may produce these abnormalities. Complete spinal cord lesions generally abolish all recordable SEP responses above the lesion. Partial lesions may or may not produce SEP abnormalities, depending on the extent of posterior column involvement.[145-148] In traumatic spinal cord injury, good correlation between SEP results and the severity of spinal cord injury have been noted. Prognosis for recovery is better when the SEPs are normal in the early post-traumatic period.[149,150]

Trigeminal Nerve Lesions
SEPs recorded from the trigeminal nerve are reported to be abnormal in approximately 41% of patients with idiopathic and multiple sclerosis–related trigeminal neuralgia. In patients undergoing retrogasserian injection of glycerol, alteration in SEP waveforms correlated well with successful treatment measured by pain relief. Trigeminal SEPs have been successfully used in the diagnosis of parasellar and cerebellopontine angle tumors affecting the trigeminal nerve, even if involvement was subclinical. In addition, information concerning the site of the lesion along the trigeminal pathway can be obtained.[146,151-153]

Lesions of the Brainstem and Cerebral Hemisphere
Tumors, infarcts, and hemorrhages involving the somatosensory pathway of the brainstem and cerebrum generally produce SEP abnormalities.[61,68,149] SEPs may be particularly useful in patients with thalamic pain in whom abnormalities of N20 and P23 have been reported following median nerve stimulation. Thalamic lesions involving areas other than the ventroposterolateral nucleus are usually associated with normal SEPs.[146,154] Lesions involving the thalamocortical radiations or sensory cortex may present a normal N20 and an abnormal P23 response unless retrograde degeneration of the thalamic nuclei has occurred, which results in abnormalities in both responses.[68,149]

Median nerve SEPs have demonstrated prognostic value in patients with right hemiplegia. Abnormalities of N20 and P23 correlate with a poorer prognosis for functional recovery.[155] In cases of traumatic head injury and coma, SEPs have proved valuable in localizing lesions and as a predictor of both favorable and unfavorable outcomes.[96,97,156]

Multiple Sclerosis
SEPs are used frequently in conjunction with VEPs and AEPs to evaluate patients with suspected multiple sclerosis. The incidence of SEP abnormalities runs higher in patients with sensory symptoms. Furthermore, SEP abnormalities are more frequent in the lower extremities.[76,77,149] Sensitivity of SEPs in the diagnosis of multiple sclerosis has been comparable to that of VEP testing. Some studies have demonstrated SEPs to be equal to or better than magnetic resonance imaging for diagnosis of this disease.[121,157]

SEP abnormalities include prolongation of latencies and attenuation or absence of responses.

Monitoring during Surgery
SEPs have monitored somatosensory pathway integrity and cerebral status during various vascular and neurosurgical procedures, most notably carotid endarterectomy and scoliosis surgery. The use of SEP surgical monitoring has become routine in many communities, and its applications continue to expand.[62,158,159]

Other Uses
SEP abnormalities have been found in various degenerative, hereditary, and metabolic disorders. Abnormal SEPs have been reported in Friedreich's and other cerebellar ataxias, Huntington's chorea, motor neuron disorders, Guillain-Barré syndrome, Charcot-Marie-Tooth disease, vitamin B_{12} deficiency, diabetes, and hyperthyroidism.[61,68,107,160,161] SEPs have been used in conjunction with electroencephalography to determine brain death.[146,162] Pudendal nerve SEPs have been applied in evaluation of bladder and sexual dysfunction.[163-165]

Motor Evoked Potentials

Because of the inability of conventional nerve conduction studies to evaluate anatomically deep structures (e.g., cortical structures, lumbosacral plexus), alternate techniques were sought. EPs allowed evaluation of the sensory portions of anatomically deep structures, but the motor portions of these structures remained inaccessible. It had long been known that a high-voltage, short-duration electrical pulse could stimulate these remote structures, but the technique was painful and, in some cases, required direct electrical stimulation (e.g., via needle insertion or during surgical exposure of the structure).[73,166] It had also been known that a magnetic field was able to induce electric current flow in neuronal structures, but it was not until the 1980s that a practical technique was developed. Essentially, an extension of conventional nerve conduction studies, motor evoked potentials allow assessment of motor pathways in peripheral neuronal structures. Unlike conventional nerve conduction studies, assessment of central motor conduction pathways may also be performed. Stimulation may be electrical or magnetic, although magnetic stimulation is the most commonly used form because it is relatively painless.

Motor evoked potentials have found their greatest usefulness in determining central conduction through the motor structures of the brain and spinal cord. By recording from distant sites (e.g., muscles in the extremities), one can determine motor conduction throughout the entire motor pathway. This test is performed in a manner similar to that for SEPs, with the exception that the stimulus is applied centrally and recorded peripherally.[73,107,166,167]

Clinical Utility

Motor evoked potentials have found wide clinical utility in the diagnosis of disorders that affect central or peripheral motor pathways. Abnormalities of motor evoked potentials have been described in multiple sclerosis, Parkinson's disease, cerebrovascular accident, myelopathy in the cervical and lumbar spines, plexus lesions, and motor neuron disorders.[107,166-170] Cortical hyperexcitability has been demonstrated in migraine patients with transcranial magnetic stimulation.[171] Motor evoked potentials are also finding a role in intraoperative monitoring of neuronal structures placed at surgical risk.[107,166,167]

Event-Related Potentials

Unlike the previously discussed EPs, which are recorded from simple sensory or motor stimuli, event-related potentials record cortical activity evoked by a stimulus with cognitive significance. Various techniques have been developed to assess temporal aspects of cognitive processing. The most common technique uses the presentation of randomly occurring infrequent stimuli interspersed among more frequently occurring stimuli of a different type (i.e., an infrequent deep tone occurring randomly among more frequently occurring high-pitched tones). The subject is instructed to attend only to (or to count) the infrequent stimuli, which results in an evoked waveform with a latency of approximately 300 msec with a positive polarity. This waveform is referred to as the *P300 response*. Prolongation of the P300 response is associated with disorders that impair cognition, such as dementia, neurodegenerative disorders, schizophrenia, and autism.[61,68,172-174] It has also been used as a predictor of early outcome after emergence from traumatic coma.[175]

CONCLUSION

In conclusion, electrodiagnostic techniques such as electromyography and evoked potential testing remain useful techniques for the diagnosis of central and peripheral neuropathies. While their use has been found helpful in some central nervous system disorders,[8] they are much more useful in disorders of the nerve roots, plexus lesions, neuropathies, and disorders of the peripheral nerves and less frequently in painful myopathies. Neuromuscular junction disorders, amyotrophic lateral sclerosis, and other anterior horn cell disorders, except poliomyelitis in its acute stage, rarely produce pain.

Clinical use of electrodiagnostic techniques has expanded rapidly due to equipment improvements and increased standardization of techniques. Recent advances in magnetic stimulation are allowing evaluations of central motor pathways and deep peripheral nerves that were not possible previously with somatosensory evoked potentials and conventional nerve conduction techniques. Advancements in quantitative electroencephalographic and topographic brain mapping are being applied to evoked potentials and promise additional information beyond that provided currently by evoked potential testing alone.

Whereas electrodiagnostic techniques may find, confirm, and localize a nerve or muscle disease process, the relevance of the electrodiagnostic finding to the patient's pain symptomatology must be determined by the referring physician and the electromyographer, who should work together to assess all available history, physical examination, other laboratory tests, and imaging findings before finalizing the diagnosis and establishing a treatment plan.

References

1. Roongta S: Electromyography. In Raj PP (ed): Practical Management of Pain, ed 2. St. Louis, Mosby-Year Book, 1992, pp 137-154.
2. Longmire D: Tutorial 10: Electrodiagnostic studies in the assessment of painful disorders. Pain Dig 1993;3:116-122.
3. Aminoff MJ: Electromyography. In Aminoff MJ (ed): Electrodiagnosis in Clinical Neurology. New York, Churchill Livingstone, 1992, pp 249-281.
4. Daube JR, ed: Clinical Neurophysiology. Philadelphia, FA Davis, 1966, pp 199-330.
5. Dumitru D: Electrodiagnostic Medicine. Philadelphia, Hanley and Belfus, 1995.
6. Oh SJ: Clinical Electromyography: Nerve Conduction Studies, ed 2. Baltimore, Williams & Wilkins, 1993.
7. Brown WF, Bolton CF: Clinical Electromyography, ed 2. Boston, Butterworth-Heinemann, 1993.
8. Waldman HJ: Neurophysiologic testing in the evaluation of the patient in pain. In Waldman SD, Winnie AP (eds): Interventional Pain Management. Dannemiller Memorial Educational Foundation. Philadelphia, WB Saunders, 1996, pp 104-118.
9. Stolov WC: Electrodiagnostic evaluation of acute and chronic pain syndrome, ed 2. In Bonica JA (ed): The Management of Pain. Philadelphia, Lea & Febiger, 1990, pp 622-640.
10. Verdugo R, Ochoa JL: Use and misuse of conventional electrodiagnosis, quantitative sensory testing, thermography, and nerve blocks i n the evaluation of painful neuropathic syndromes. American Association of Electrodiagnostic Medicine, International Symposium on Neuropathic Pain, October 18, 1992, Charleston, SC.
11. McDermott JF, Modaff WL, Boyle RW: Electromyography. GP 27, January 1963.
12. Norris FH: The EMG. New York, Grune & Stratton, 1963.
13. Kimura J: Electrodiagnosis in Diseases of Nerve and Muscle: Principles and Practice. Philadelphia, FA Davis, 1983.
14. Sivak M, Ochoa J, Fernandez JM: Positive manifestations of nerve fiber dysfunction: Clinical, electrophysiologic, and pathologic correlates. In Brown WF, Bolton CF (eds): Clinical Electromyography, ed 2. Boston, Butterworth-Heinemann, 1993, pp 119-137.
15. Buchthal R: An Introduction to Electromyography. Copenhagen, Scandinavian University Books, 1957.
16. Wiechers DO: Normal and abnormal motor unit potentials. In Johnson EW (ed): Practical Electromyography, ed 2. Baltimore, Williams & Wilkins, 1988, pp 22-91.
17. Waxman SG: Conduction in myelinated, unmyelinated and demyelinated fibers. Arch Neurol 1977;34:585-589.
18. Bolton CF, Carter K, Koval JJ: Temperature effects on conduction studies of normal and abnormal nerve. Muscle Nerve 1982;5:S145-S147.
19. Ball RD: Basics of Needle Electromyography: An AAEE Workshop, Rochester, Minn, American Association of Electrodiagnosis and Electromyography, October 1985.
20. Jablecki C: Physiologic Basis of Electromyographic Activity: Standard Needle Electromyography of Muscles. American Association of Electromyography and Electrodiagnosis, 11th

Annual Continuing Education Course, San Diego, October 1988, pp 15-21.

21. Kimura J: F-wave velocity in the central segment of the median and ulnar nerves: A study in normal subjects and in patients with Charcot-Marie-Tooth disease. Neurology 1974;24:539-546.

22. Mayer RF, Feldman RG: Observations on the nature of the F-wave in man. Neurology 1967;17:147.

23. Magladery JW, McDougal DB: Electrophysiological studies and reflex activity in normal man. Identification of certain reflexes in the electromyogram and conduction velocity of peripheral nerve fiber. Bull Johns Hopkins Hosp 1950; 86:265.

24. Fisher MA: F-wave studies: Clinical utility. Muscle Nerve 1998;21:1098-1101.

25. Rivner MH: F-wave studies: Limitations. Muscle Nerve 1998;21:1101-1104.

26. Hoffmann P: Untersuchungen uber Bie Eigenreflexe (Sehnenre flexe) Nenschlicher Muskeln. Berlin, Springer, 1922.

27. Braddom RL, Johnson EW: Standardization of H-reflex and diagnostic use of S1 radiculopathy. Arch Phys Med Rehabil 1974;55:161-166.

28. Braddom RL, Johnson EW: H-reflex: Review and classification with suggested clinical uses. Arch Phys Med Rehabil 1974; 55:417-419.

29. Schuchmann JA: H-reflex: Latency and radiculopathy. Arch Phys Med Rehabil 1978;59:185-187.

30. Johnson EW: Electrodiagnosis of radiculopathy. In Johnson EW (ed): Practical Electromyography, ed 2. Baltimore, Williams & Wilkins, 1988, pp 229-245.

31. Fruhstorfer H, Lindblom U, Schmidt WG: Method for quantitative estimation for thermal thresholds in patients. J Neurol Neurosurg Psychiatry 1971;39:1071-1075.

32. Verdugo RJ, Ochoa JL: Quantitative somatosensory thermotest: A key method for functional evaluation of small caliber afferent channels. Brain 1992;115:893-913.

33. Ashbury AK, Porte D, Genuth SM, et al: Report and Recommendations of the San Antonio Conference on Diabetic Neuropathy, 1988.

34. Low PA, Caskey PE, Tuck RR, et al: Quantitative pseudomotor axon reflex test in normal and neuropathic subjects. Ann Neurol 1983;14:573-580.

35. Low PA, Zimmerman BR, Dyck PJ: Comparison of distal sympathetic with vagal function in diabetic neuropathy. Muscle Nerve 1986;9:592-596.

36. Cohen J, Low P, Fealey R, et al: Somatic and autonomic function in progressive autonomic failure and multiple system atrophy. Ann Neurol 1987;22:692-699.

37. Sandroni P, Ahlskog JE, Fealey RD, et al: Autonomic involvement in extrapyramidal and cerebellar disorder. Clin Auton Res 1991;1:147-155.

38. Menkes DL: Quantitative sensory testing distinguishes axonal from demyelinating polyneuropathies. Poster Session 1, No. 9, Abstracts, p. 70, 44th Annual Meeting of the American Association of Electrodiagnostic Medicine, San Diego, September 1997.

39. Schaumburg HH, Berger AR, Thomas PK: Disorders of Peripheral Nerves, ed 2. Contemporary Neurology Series. Philadelphia, FA Davis, 1992.

40. Barohn RJ: Approach to peripheral neuropathy and neuronopathy. Semin Neurol 1998;18:7-18.

41. Ropper AH, Gorson KC: Neuropathies associated with paraproteinemia. N Engl J Med 1998;338:1601-1607.

42. Cornblath DR, Melitts BD, Griffin JW, et al: Motor conduction studies in Guillain-Barré syndrome: Description and prognostic value. Ann Neurol 1988;23:354-359.

43. Pourmand R, Maybury B: American Association of Electrodiagnostic Medicine, Case Report No. 31, Paraneoplastic Sensory Neuropathy. Muscle Nerve 1996;19:1517-1528.

44. Albers JW, Donofrio PD, McGonagle TK: Sequential electrodiagnostic abnormalities in acute inflammatory demyelinating polyradiculopathy. Muscle Nerve 1985;8:528-539.

45. Bromberg MB: Comparison of electrodiagnostic criteria for primary demyelination in chronic polyneuropathy. Muscle Nerve 1991;14:968-976.

46. Stevens JC: Mini-monograph No. 26: The Electrodiagnosis of Carpal Tunnel Syndrome. Rochester, Minn, American Association of Electrodiagnostic Medicine, December 1997.

47. Rosenbaum RB, Ochoa JL: Carpal Tunnel Syndrome and Other Disorders of the Median Nerve. Boston, Butterworth-Heinemann, 1993.

48. Kincaid JC, Phillips LH, Daube JR: The evaluation of suspected ulnar neuropathy at the elbow. Normal conduction values. Arch Neurol 1986;43:44-47.

49. Miller RG: The cubital tunnel syndrome: Diagnosis and precise localization. Ann Neurol 1979;6:56-59.

50. Ebbling P, Gilliatt RW, Thomas PK: A clinical and electrical study of ulnar nerve lesions in the hand. J Neurol Neurosurg Psychiatry 1960;23:1-9.

51. Stuart JV: The radial nerve. In Stewart JV (ed): Focal Peripheral Neuropathy, ed 2. New York, Raven Press, 1993, pp 231-252.

52. DeLisa JA, Saed MA: American Association of Electrodiagnosis and Electromyography, Case Report No. 8, The tarsal tunnel syndrome. Muscle Nerve 1983;6:664-670.

53. Keck C: The tarsal tunnel syndrome. J Bone Joint Surg 1992;44:180-184.

54. Oh SJ, Sarala PK, Kuba T, et al: Tarsal tunnel syndrome, electrophysiological study. Ann Neurol 1979;5:327-330.

55. Stuart JD, ed: The sciatic nerve of gluteal, and pudendal nerves in the posterior cutaneous nerve of the thigh. In Stuart JD (ed): Focal Peripheral Neuropathies, ed 2. New York, Raven Press, 1993, pp 321-345.

56. Stuart JD: Focal Peripheral Neuropathies, ed 2. New York, Raven Press, 1993.

57. Tonvola RF, Ackil AA, Shahani BT, et al: Usefulness of electrophysiological studies in the diagnosis of lumbosacral root disease. Ann Neurol 1981;9:305-309.

58. Kuncl RW, Wiggins WW: Toxic myopathies. Neurol Clin 1088;6:593-619.

59. Walton J: Disorders of Voluntary Muscle (ed) 4. New York, Churchill Livingstone, 1981, pp 478-584.

60. Rowland LP: Myopathies. In Roland LP (ed): Merritt's Textbook of Neurology, ed 9. Baltimore, Williams & Wilkins, 1995, pp 766-803.

61. Chiappa K: Evoked Potentials in Clinical Medicine. New York, Raven Press, 1985.

62. Nuwer MR: Evoked Potential Monitoring in the Operating Room. New York, Raven Press, 1986.

63. Starr A: Natural forms of somatosensory stimulation that can evoke cerebral, spinal, and peripheral nerve potentials in man. American Association of Electromyography and Electrodiagnosis International Symposium on Somatosensory Evoked Potentials, Rochester, Minn, 1984.

64. Braddom R: Somatosensory, brain stem, and visual evoked potentials. In Johnson E (ed): Practical Electromyography, ed 2. Baltimore, Williams & Wilkins, 1988, pp 369-416.

65. Celesia G: Somatosensory evoked potentials: Nomenclature. American Association of Electromyography and Electrodiagnosis International Symposium on Somatosensory Evoked Potentials, Rochester, Minn, 1984.

66. American Electroencephalography Society: Clinical evoked potential guidelines. J Clin Neurophysiol 1984;1:6-52.

67. American Association of Electromyography and Electrodiagnosis: Guidelines for Somatosensory Evoked Potentials. Rochester, Minn, 1984.

68. Spehlmann R: Evoked Potential Primer. Boston, Butterworth, 1985.

69. Dorfman LJ, Robinson LR: American Association of Electrodiagnostic Medicine Mini-monograph No. 17: Normative Data in Electrodiagnostic Medicine. Rochester, Minn, American Association of Electrodiagnostic Medicine, 1997.

70. Gitter AJ, Stolov WC: American Association of Electrodiagnostic Medicine Mini-monograph No. 16: Instrumentation and Measurement in Electrodiagnostic Medicine. Rochester, Minn, American Association of Electrodiagnostic Medicine, 1995.

71. Jasper HH: The ten-twenty electrode system of the International Federation: Report of the Committee on Clinical

Examination in Electroencephalography. Electroencephalogr Clin Neurophysiol 1958;10:371-375.

72. Chiappa K, Ropper A: Evoked potentials in clinical medicine: Part I. N Engl J Med 1982;306:1140-1150.

73. Daube J: Clinical Neurophysiology. Philadelphia: FA Davis, 1996.

74. Halliday A: Visual evoked responses in the diagnosis of multiple sclerosis. Br Med J 1973;4:661-664.

75. Halliday A: Visual evoked potentials in demyelinating disease. In Waxman S, Ritchie J (eds): Demyelinating Disease: Basic and Clinical Electrophysiology. New York, Raven Press, 1981, pp 201-215.

76. Hume AL, Waxman SG: Evoked potentials in suspected multiple sclerosis: Diagnostic value and prediction of clinical course. J Neurol Sci 1988;83:191-210.

77. Aminoff M: American Association of Electromyography and Electrodiagnosis Mini-monograph No. 22: The Clinical Role of Somatosensory Evoked Potential Studies: A Critical Appraisal. Rochester, Minn, American Association of Electromyography and Electrodiagnosis, 1984.

78. Chiappa K, Ropper A: Evoked potentials in clinical medicine: Part II. N Engl J Med 19082;306:1205-1211.

79. Marsters JB, Good PA, Mortimer MJ: A diagnostic test for migraine using the visual evoked potential. Headache 1988;28:526-530.

80. Muller-Jensen A, Zschocke S: Pattern-induced visual evoked response in patients with migraine accompagnee. Electroencephalogr Clin Neurophysiol 1980;50:37.

81. Polich J, Maung A, Dalessio D: Pattern-shift visual evoked responses in cluster headache. Headache 1987;27:446-451.

82. Raudino F: Visual evoked potential in patients with migraine. Headache 1988;28:531-532.

83. Halliday A, Mushin J: The visual evoked potential in neuroophthalmology. Int Ophthalmol Clin 1980;20:155-183.

84. Halliday A, Halliday E, Kriss A, et al: The pattern-evoked potential in compression of the anterior visual pathways. Brain 1976;99:357-374.

85. Ikeda H, Tremain K, Sanders M: Neurophysiological investigation in optic nerve disease: Combined assessment of the visual evoked response and electroretinogram. Br J Ophthalmol 1978;62:227-239.

86. Harding G, Smith V, Yorke H: Visual evoked potential monitoring of orbital surgery using a contact-lens stimulator. In Barber C, Blum T (eds): Evoked Potentials III. Boston, Butterworth, 1987, pp 240-244.

87. Hood L, Berlin C: Auditory Evoked Potentials. Austin, Tex, Pro-Ed, 1986.

88. Soustiel JF, Hafner H, Chistyakov AV, et al: Brain-stem trigeminal and auditory evoked potentials in multiple sclerosis: Physiological insights. Electroencephalogr Clin Neurophysiol 1996;100:152-157.

89. Sanders R, Duncan P, McCullough D: Clinical experience with brain stem audiometry performed under general anesthesia. J Otolaryngol 1979;8:24-31.

90. Hammond S, Yiannikas C: The relevance of contralateral recordings and patient disability to assessment of brain stem auditory evoked potential abnormalities in multiple sclerosis. Arch Neurol 1987;44:382-387.

91. Donohoe C: Application of the brain stem auditory evoked response in clinical neurologic practice. In Owen J, Donohoe C (eds): Clinical Atlas of Auditory Evoked Potentials. New York, Grune & Stratton, 1988, pp 29-62.

92. Kirshner HS, Tsai SI, Runge VM, et al: Magnetic resonance imaging and other techniques in the diagnosis of multiple sclerosis. Arch Neurol 1985;42:859-863.

93. Deka R, Kacker S, Tandon P: Auditory brain stem evoked responses in cerebellopontile angle tumors. Arch Otolaryngol Head Neck Surg 1987;113:647-650.

94. Musiek F, Josey A, Glasscock M: Auditory brain stem response in patients with acoustic neuromas. Arch Otolaryngol Head Neck Surg 1986;112:186-189.

95. Raber E, Dort JC, Sevick R, et al: Asymmetric hearing loss: Toward cost-effective diagnosis. J Otolaryngol 1997;26:88-91.

96. Newton P, Greenberg R: Evoked potentials in severe head injury. J Trauma 1984;24:61-65.

97. Stone J, Ghaly R, Hughes J: Evoked potentials in head injury and states of increased intracranial pressure. J Clin Neurophysiol 1988;5:135-160.

98. Drake ME, Weate SJ, Newell SA: Auditory evoked potentials in postconcussive syndrome. Electromyogr Neurophysiol 1996;7-462.

99. Jewett D: Auditory evoked potentials: Overview of the field. In Barber C, Blum T (eds): Evoked Potentials III. Boston, Butterworth, 1987, pp 19-30.

100. Drake M: Brain stem auditory-evoked potentials in spasmodic torticollis. Arch Neurol 1988;4-175.

101. Yamada T, Dickins Q, Arensdorg K, et al: Basilar migraine: Polarity-dependent alteration of brain stem auditory evoked potentials. Neurology 1986;36:1256-1260.

102. Jerger J, Oliver T, Stack B: ABR testing strategies. In Jacobson J (ed): The Auditory Brain Stem Response. San Diego, College Hill Press, 1985, pp 371-388.

103. Watson DR, McClelland RJ, Adams DA: Auditory brainstem response screening for hearing loss in high risk neonates. Int J Pediatr Otorhinolaryngol 1996;36:147-183.

104. Ferraro J: Electrocochleography. In Owen J, Donohoe C (eds): Clinical Atlas of Auditory Evoked Potentials. New York, Grune & Stratton, 1988, pp 1-14.

105. Owen J: Clinical audiologic applications of acoustically elicited evoked responses. In Owen J, Donohoe C (eds): Clinical Atlas of Auditory Evoked Potentials. New York, Grune & Stratton, 1988, pp 15-28.

106. Nakashima K, Yokoyama Y, Shimoyama R, et al: Clinical usefulness of electrically-elicited pain-related evoked potentials. Electromyogr Clin Neurophysiol 1998;36:305-310.

107. Kanda M, Fujiwara N, Zu X, et al: Pain-related and cognitive components of somatosensory evoked potentials following CO_2 laser stimulation in man. Electroencephalogr Clin Neurophysiol 1996;100:103-114.

108. Swensson P, Beydoun A, Morrow TJ, et al: Non-painful and painful stimulation of human skin and muscle: Analysis of cerebral-evoked potentials. Electroencephalogr Clin Neurophysiol 1997;105:343-350.

109. Zaslllansky R, Sprecjer E, Katz Y, et al: Pain-evoked potentials: What do they really measure? Electroencephalogr Clin Neurophysiol 1996;100:384-392.

110. Lorenz J, Grasedyck K, Bromm B: Middle and long latency somatosensory evoked potentials after painful laser stimulation in patients with fibromyalgia syndrome. Electroencephalogr Clin Neurophysiol 1996;100:165-168.

111. Bertens A: Somatosensory evoked potentials in relation to nociception and anesthesia. Electromyogr Clin Neurophysiol 1985;25:3-33.

112. Dumitru D: Electrodiagnostic Medicine. Philadelphia: Hanley & Belfus, 1995.

113. Nielsen L, Bjerring P: Cortical response characteristics to noxious argon laser stimulation. Clin Evoked Potentials 1988;5:11-17.

114. Eisen A, Stevens J: Upper limb somatosensory evoked potentials. American Association of Electromyography and Electrodiagnosis Workshop. Rochester, Minn, undated monograph.

115. Kimura J: Somatosensory evoked potentials to median and tibial nerve stimulation in normal subjects. American Association of Electromyography and Electrodiagnosis Somatosensory Evoked Potentials, Sixth Annual Continuing Education Course, Rochester, Minn, 1983.

116. Halliday A: Current status of the SEP: American Association of Electromyography and Electrodiagnosis International Symposium on Somatosensory Evoked Potentials, Rochester, Minn, 1984.

117. Cracco R: Origin of potentials: Human studies. American Association of Electromyography and Electrodiagnosis International Symposium on Somatosensory Evoked Potentials, Rochester, Minn, 1984.

118. Baran E, Daube J: Lower extremity somatosensory evoked potentials. American Association of Electromyography and Electrodiagnosis Workshop, Rochester, Minn, 1984.

119. Jones S: Clinical applications of somatosensory evoked potentials: Peripheral nervous system. American Academy of Electromyography and Electrodiagnosis International Symposium on Somatosensory Evoked Potentials. Rochester, Minn, 1984.

120. Eisen A: SEP in the evaluation of disorders of the peripheral nervous system. In Cracco R, Bodis-Wollner I (eds): Evoked Potentials. New York, AR Liss, 1986, pp 409-417.

121. Aminoff M, Cutler J, Brant-Zawadzki M: The sensitivity of MR imaging and multimodality evoked potentials in the evaluation of patients with suspected multiple sclerosis. In Barber C, Blum T (eds): Evoked Potentials III. Boston, Butterworth, 1987, pp 405-407.

122. Aminoff M, Goodin D, Parry G, et al: Electrophysiologic evaluation of lumbosacral radiculopathies: Electromyography, late responses, and somatosensory evoked potentials. Neurology 1985;35:1514-1518.

123. Perlik S, Fisher M, Patel D, et al: On the usefulness of somatosensory evoked responses for the evaluation of lower back pain. Arch Neurol 1986;43:907-913.

124. Aminoff M, Goodin D, Barbara N, et al: Dermatomal somatosensory evoked potentials in unilateral lumbosacral radiculopathy. Ann Neurol 1985;17:171-176.

125. Katifi H, Sedgwick E: Dermatomal somatosensory evoked potentials in lumbosacral disk disease: Diagnosis and results of treatment. In Barber C, Blum T (eds): Evoked Potentials III. Boston, Butterworth, 1987, pp 285-292.

126. Katifi H, Sedgwick E: Evaluation of the dermatomal somatosensory evoked potential in the diagnosis of lumbosacral root compression. J Neurol Neurosurg Psychiatry 1987;50:1204-1210.

127. Eisen A, Hoirch M, Moll A: Evaluation of radiculopathies by segmental stimulation and somatosensory evoked potentials. Can J Neurol Sci 1983;10:178-182.

128. Machida M, Asai T, Sato K, et al: New approach for diagnosis in herniated lumbosacral disc. Spine 1986;11:380-384.

129. Rodriguez A, Kanis L, Rodriguez AA, et al: Somatosensory evoked potentials from dermatomal stimulation as an indicator of L5 and S1 radiculopathies. Arch Phys Med Rehabil 1987;6:366-368.

130. Scarff R, Dallmann D, Roleikis J: Dermatomal somatosensory evoked potentials in the diagnosis of lumbosacral root entrapment. Surg Forum 1981;32:489-491.

131. Schmid U, Hess C, Ludin H: Somatosensory evoked potentials following nerve and segmental stimulation do not confirm cervical radiculopathy with sensory deficit. J Neurol Neurosurg Psychiatry 1988;51:182-187.

132. Seyal M, Palma G, Sandhu L, et al: Spinal somatosensory evoked potentials following segmental sensory stimulation: A direct measure of dorsal root function. Electroencephalogr Clin Neurophysiol 1988;69:390-393.

133. Dumitru D, Dreyfuss P: Dermatomal/segmental somatosensory evoked potential evaluation of L5/S1 unilateral/unilevel radiculopathies. Muscle Nerve 1996;19:442-449.

134. Komanetsky RM, Novak CB, Mackinnon SE, et al: Somatosensory evoked potentials fail to diagnose thoracic outlet syndrome. J Hand Surg 1996;21a:662-666.

135. Machleder H, Moll F, Nuwer M, et al: Somatosensory evoked potentials in the assessment of thoracic outlet compression syndrome. J Vasc Surg 1987;6:177-184.

136. Oh SJ: Clinical electromyography: Nerve conduction studies. Baltimore, University Park Press, 1984.

137. Synek V: Diagnostic importance of somatosensory evoked potentials in the diagnosis of thoracic outlet syndrome. Clin Electroencephalogr 1986;17:112-116.

138. Yiannikas C, Walsh J: Somatosensory evoked responses in the diagnosis of thoracic outlet syndrome. J Neurol Neurosurg Psychiatry 1983;46:234-240.

139. Aminoff M: Use of somatosensory evoked potentials to evaluate the peripheral nervous system. J Clin Neurophysiol 1987;4:135-144.

140. Yiannikas C, Shahani B, Young R: The investigation of traumatic lesions of the brachial plexus by electromyography and short latency somatosensory evoked potentials evoked by stimulation of multiple peripheral nerves. J Neurol Neurosurg Psychiatry 1983;46:1014-1022.

141. Stolov W, Slimp J: Dermatomal Somatosensory Evoked Potentials in Lumbar Spinal Stenosis. American Association of Electromyography and Electrodiagnosis/American Electroencephalographic Society Joint Symposium of Somatosensory Evoked Potentials and Magnetic Stimulation, Rochester, Minn, 1988.

142. Yiannikas C, Shahani B, Young R: Short-latency somatosensory evoked potentials from radial, median, ulnar, and peroneal nerve stimulation in the assessment of cervical spondylosis. Arch Neurol 1986;43:1264-1271.

143. Gonzales E, Hajdu M, Bruno R, et al: Lumbar spinal stenosis: Analysis of pre- and post-operative somatosensory evoked potentials. Arch Phys Med Rehabil 1985;66:11-15.

144. Yu Y, Jones S: Somatosensory evoked potentials in cervical spondylosis. Brain 1985;108:273-300.

145. Baran E: Spinal and Scalp Somatosensory Evoked Potentials in Spinal Disorders. American Association of Electromyography and Electrodiagnosis Somatosensory Evoked Potentials, Sixth Annual Continuing Education Course, Rochester, Minn, 1983.

146. Chiappa K: Clinical applications of short latency somatosensory evoked potentials to central nervous system disease. American Association of Electromyography and Electrodiagnosis International Symposium on Somatosensory Evoked Potentials, Rochester, Minn, 1984.

147. Lehmkuhl L, Dimitrijevic M, Zidar J: Lumbosacral evoked potentials and cortical somatosensory evoked potentials in patients with lesions of the conus medullaris and cauda equina. Electroencephalogr Clin Neurophysiol 1988;71:161-169.

148. Miyoshi R, Kimura J: Short-latency somatosensory evoked potentials in patients with cervical compressive lesions: Morphological versus functional examination. Electromyogr Clin Neurophysiol 1996;36:323-332.

149. Oken B, Chiappa K: Somatosensory evoked potentials in neurological diagnosis. In Cracco RQ, Bodis-Wollner I (eds): Evoked Potentials. New York, AR Liss, 1986, pp 379-389.

150. Toleikis J, Sloan T: Comparison of major nerve and dermatomal somatosensory evoked potentials in the evaluation of patients with spinal cord injury. In Barber C, Blum T (eds): Evoked Potentials III. Boston, Butterworth, 1987, pp 309-316.

151. Buettner U, Rieble S, Altenmuller E, et al: Trigeminal somatosensory evoked potentials in patients with lesions of the mandibular branches of the trigeminal nerve. In Barber C, Blum T (eds): Evoked Potentials III. Boston, Butterworth, 1987, pp 299-302.

152. Iraguy V, Wiederholt W, Romine J: Evoked potentials in trigeminal neuralgia associated with multiple sclerosis. Arch Neurol 1986;43:444-446.

153. Leandri M, Parodi C, Favale E: Early trigeminal evoked potentials in tumors of the base of the skull and trigeminal neuralgia. Electroencephalogr Clin Neurophysiol 1988;71:114-124.

154. Robinson R, Richey E, Kase C, et al: Somatosensory evoked potentials in pure sensory stroke and related conditions. Stroke 1985;16:818-823.

155. La Joie W, Reddy N, Melvin J: Somatosensory evoked potentials: Their predictive value in right hemiplegia. Arch Phys Med Rehabil 1982;63:223-226.

156. Anderson D, Bundlie S, Rockswold G: Multi-modality evoked potentials in closed head trauma. Arch Neurol 1984;41:369-374.

157. Giesser B, Kurtzberg D, Baughan H, et al: Trimodal evoked potentials compared with magnetic resonance imaging in the diagnosis of multiple sclerosis. Arch Neurol 1987;44:281-284.

158. Maccabee P: Intraoperative spinal monitoring. American Association of Electromyography and Electrodiagnosis Somatosensory Evoked Potentials, Sixth Annual Continuing Education Course, Rochester, Minn, 1983.

159. Schramm J, Romstock J, Watanabe E: Cortical versus spinal recordings in intraoperative monitoring of space-occupying spinal lesions. In Barber C, Blum T (eds): Evoked Potentials III. Boston, Butterworth, 1987, pp 328-336.

160. Georgesco M, Salerno A, Camu W: Somatosensory evoked potentials elicited by stimulation of lower-limb nerves in amyotrophic lateral sclerosis. Electroencephalogr Clin Neurophysiol 1997;104:333-342.

161. Sivri A, Hascelik Z, Celiker R, et al: Early detection of neurological involvement in systemic lupus erythematosus patients. Electromyogr Clin Neurophysiol 1995;35:195-199.

162. Buchner H, Ferbert A, Hacke W: Serial recording of median nerve somatosensory evoked potentials before brain death: Subcortical SEPs and their significance in the diagnosis of brain death. In Barber C, Blum T (eds): Evoked Potentials III. Boston, Butterworth, 1987, pp 323-327.

163. Haldeman S, Bradley W, Bhatia N, et al: Pudendal evoked responses. Arch Neurol 1982;34:280-283.

164. Lin J, Bradley W: Penile neuropathy in insulin-dependent diabetes mellitus. J Urol 1985;133:213-215.

165. Susset J, Ghoniem G: Rapid cystometry and sacral-evoked response in the diagnosis of peripheral bladder and sphincter denervation. J Urol 1984;132:704-707.

166. Eisen AA, Shtybel W: AAEM Minimonograph 35: Clinical Experience with Transcranial Magnetic Stimulation. Rochester, Minn: American Association of Electrodiagnostic Medicine, 1990.

167. Chiappa KH. Transcranial motor evoked potentials. Electromyogr Clin Neurophysiol 34:15-21, 1994.

168. Kalita J, Misra UK: Motor and sensory evoked potential studies in brainstem strokes. Electromyogr Clin Neurophysiol 1997;37:379-383.

169. Andersson T, Siden A, Persson A: A comparison of motor evoked potentials and somatosensory evoked potentials in patients with multiple sclerosis and potentially related conditions. Electromyogr Clin Neurophysiol 1995;35:17-24.

170. Salerno A, Carlander B, Camu W, et al: Motor evoked potentials (MEPs): Evaluation of the different types of responses in amyotrophic lateral sclerosis and primary lateral sclerosis. Electromyogr Clin Neurophysiol 1996;36:361-368.

171. Can der Kamp W, VanDenBrink AM, Ferrari MD, et al: Interictal cortical hyperexcitability in migraine patients demonstrated with transcranial magnetic stimulation. J Neurol Sci 1996;139:106-110.

172. Aotsuka A, Weate SJ, Drake ME, et al: Event-related potentials in Parkinson's disease. Electromyogr Clin Neurophysiol 1996;36:215-220.

173. Boutros N, Nasrallah H, Leighty R, et al: Auditory evoked potentials: Clinical vs. research applications. Psychiatr Res 1997;69:183-195.

174. Rosler KM, Magistris MR, Glocker FX, et al: Electrophysiological characteristics of lesions in facial palsies of different etiologies: A study using electrical and magnetic stimulation techniques. Electroencephalogr Clin Neurophysiol 1995;97:155-168.

175. Kane NM, Curry SH, Rowlands CA, et al: Event-related potentials-neurophysiological tools for predicting emergence and early outcome from traumatic coma. Intensive Care Med 1996;22:39-46.

CHAPTER

12 Radiologic Assessment of the Patient with Spine Pain

Timothy P. Maus

Imaging is integral to the evaluation of the patient with spine pain. There have been revolutionary advances in spine imaging in the past decade, allowing an unprecedented ability to display spine anatomy and pathology. Imaging also, however, contributes significantly to the massive cost of evaluating and treating back pain; it must be used with restraint and reason. Despite advances, there remain significant sensitivity and specificity challenges that must be understood to use imaging wisely. Recommendations, including sensitivity and specificity caveats, for the use of imaging are discussed. The strengths and weaknesses of various modalities are explored. Imaging characteristics of degenerative spine disease, traumatic lesions, infectious disease of the spine, noninfectious inflammatory disease, and neoplastic involvement of the spine are discussed. Imaging of degenerative spine disease is emphasized, because it is the dominant pathologic process causally associated with spine pain syndromes.

APPROPRIATENESS OF IMAGING

Low back pain is the most common and most expensive reason for work disability in the United States.[1] The direct and indirect costs of low back pain evaluation and management are estimated to range up to $100 billion annually in the United States.[2] This does not include the cost of thoracic and cervical pain. Back pain is, however, usually benign in nature, transient, and self-limiting. The primary diagnostic task, in which imaging plays a key role, is to distinguish the 95% of patients with uncomplicated back pain from the 5% or fewer patients who have significant underlying systemic disease or neurologic compromise requiring intervention.[1] This must be done in a cost-efficient fashion.

Studies dating to the 1980s have questioned the utility of early imaging in back pain. A review by Scavone of 1000 lumbar spine radiographs in patients presenting with acute low back pain showed that

75% of the studies provided no useful information.[3] Liang and Komaroff in 1982 concluded that the radiation risks and costs did not justify plain radiographs of the spine at the time of an initial visit for back pain.[4] A cost analysis by Jarvik and Deyo demonstrated that plain films of the lumbar spine performed on the initial visit for acute low back pain in the absence of signs of systemic disease will ultimately cost approximately $2000 (1982 dollars) to alleviate a single day of pain.[1] This was carried a step further in a United Kingdom study randomizing patients who had experienced back pain for 6 weeks to further clinically guided care or lumbar radiographs.[5] At 9 months follow-up, there were no significant differences in clinical outcome. Patients who received radiographs did, however, have a higher degree of satisfaction with their care, presumably related to reassurance. A study by Gilbert[6] evaluated the early use of advanced imaging (computed tomography [CT] or magnetic resonance imaging [MRI]). Patients were randomized between advanced imaging as soon as possible following presentation for low back pain versus imaging only when a clear clinical indication developed. Early imaging had no effect on therapy as measured by hospital admissions or utilization of surgery or injections. There was a slightly greater improvement in outcomes measures in the group receiving early imaging, likely due to reassurance, but the difference was of questionable clinical significance. Costs were significantly higher in the early imaging group.

The American College of Radiology does not consider imaging appropriate in acute low back pain in the absence of complicating (red flag) features: significant recent trauma, unexplained weight loss, fever, immunosuppression, history of neoplasm, intravenous drug use, steroid use, osteoporosis, or age older than 70 years. The Agency for Healthcare Research and Quality (AHRQ) guidelines similarly suggest no imaging in patients younger than 50 years of age in the absence of systemic disease until pain persists for at least 6 weeks.[1] Imaging becomes a part of the clinical evaluation when one of the "red flags" is present or when pain is prolonged and unremitting, when pain is radicular in nature accompanied by motor dysfunction, or when there is evidence of cauda equina syndrome or myelopathy.

In the presence of clinical red flags, imaging may help to identify neoplasm, unsuspected trauma, or infection as underlying causes of the back pain. These conditions are uncommon in the population of patients presenting with back pain to a primary care provider. In this population, only 0.7% of patients will have metastatic cancer; 0.01% will have spine infections, 4% will have osteoporotic compression fractures, and 0.3% will have ankylosing spondylitis.[1] The imperfect sensitivity and specificity of all imaging studies makes accuracy problematic given the low pretest probability of disease. According to Jarvik and Deyo, there are three essential questions that must be answered for the patient with back pain: (1) Is there evidence of underlying systemic disease? (2) Is there neurologic impairment requiring surgical intervention? (3) Are there social/psychological factors exacerbating the pain.[1] Imaging may help identify systemic disease and anatomic neural impingement, but its role should not be overstated. An elegant study by Jarvik and colleagues noted that depression is a more significant predictor of new low back pain than MRI findings.[7]

Positive findings on spine imaging may lead to intervention. This was demonstrated in the study by Jarvik, in which early imaging (MRI) resulted in more surgical interventions with no measurable differences in patient pain or disability profiles, compared with patients who did not have MRI examinations.[8] Many of the surgical and nonsurgical interventions performed for axial and radicular back pain have only modest, if any, literature support of efficacy. Open diskectomy for radiculopathy has been considered the standard of care for decades. In the SPORT trial, patients with radiculopathy and correlative imaging findings were randomized to standard open diskectomy or individualized nonoperative care.[9] Considerable patient crossover between the treatment groups complicated analysis, but there were no statistically significant differences in the primary outcomes measures (SF-36 bodily pain and physical function scales and the Oswestry Disability Index) in the operated versus conservatively treated groups at three months, six months, one year, and two years of follow-up. A secondary outcome measure, the Sciatica Bothersomeness Index, favored the surgical group. Similarly, the 10-year results of the Maine lumbar spine study showed only a modest additional benefit in relief of leg pain, improvement in function, and patient satisfaction for surgical diskectomy versus nonsurgical therapy in patients with radiculopathy.[10] Work and disability status were comparable among surgically treated and nonsurgically treated groups at 10 years. Improvement in the patients' predominant symptoms was similar in both surgical and nonsurgical groups.[10] Atlas and colleagues[11] also studied 8- to 10-year outcomes of surgical and nonsurgical man-

agement of spinal stenosis; surgical decompression in this setting is generally considered standard of care. Surgical intervention for spinal stenosis has increased significantly in recent years, although there are wide variations (up to 12-fold) among regions of the United States. Regional differences in use of CT and MRI are thought to account for much of this variation in surgical rates.[12] There is always a temptation to treat the image rather than the patient. In the Atlas study, low back pain relief, predominant symptom improvement, and satisfaction with current state were not significantly different in surgical and nonsurgical patients. Leg pain relief and functional status favored surgically treated patients.[11]

Imaging findings may also provoke unproven invasive therapies. Three randomized controlled trials have addressed fusion for discogenic pain versus nonoperative rehabilitation. There was no evidence for superiority of fusion over nonoperative care in the trials of Brox, Fairbanks, and colleagues.[13,14] The trial of Fritzell and associates suggested a greater benefit for surgery.[15] Despite the lack of consensus support for operative intervention for discogenic pain, there has been an explosion in the rate of surgical interventions for axial back pain in recent years. Lumbar fusions were performed at a rate of 19.1 operations per 100,000 adults in 1990; the rate in 2001 was 61.1 operations per 100,000 adults.[16] There was a significant acceleration in this curve in 1996 after the introduction of cage fusion devices. Given the absence of reports of expanded indications for lumbar fusion or increased efficacy to support this dramatic acceleration in fusion rates, Deyo and coworkers speculated that marketing of the new devices alone has led to increases in fusion surgery.[16] This is also likely the case for minimally invasive therapies. In an imperfect medical marketplace, imaging itself may be a risk factor.

Imaging is costly. Low back pain resulted in excess of $25 billion in direct medical care costs in 1995 in the United States.[17] In the United Kingdom, direct health care costs for back pain were estimated to be 1.62 billion pounds in 1998; imaging accounted for approximately 5% of direct costs.[18] Given easier access to MRI, imaging likely accounts for a significantly higher percentage of direct costs in the United States. The Medicare imaging reimbursements in the Midwest in 2007 were as follows: lumbar spine radiographs: $40; lumbar spine CT with contrast: $262; MRI lumbar spine with and without contrast: $1,192; CT myelogram: $447. Typical nominal fees are generally 2.5 to 3.5 times the Medicare reimbursements. These expenditures must be incurred wisely with due consideration of the contextual features noted above.

Significant specificity caveats must be applied to all spine imaging, from plain radiographs to MRI. Even extensive anatomic abnormalities may be asymptomatic. An autopsy study demonstrated a 30% prevalence of posterior radial annular tears in patients 50 to 60 years of age; 75% of patients 60 to 70 years of age exhibited tears.[19] Hitselberger and Witten[20] found that 24% of 300 patients asymptomatic for low back pain had significant lumbar disk abnormalities on myelography. A CT-based study found that 35% of asymptomatic volunteers have abnormal lumbar scans. In volunteers 20 to 39 years of age, 19.5% exhibited disk herniation; in volunteers older than 40 years, 50% had significant abnormalities: disk herniation, spinal stenosis, or facet arthropathy.[21] Using MRI, Boden and colleagues[22] noted that asymptomatic patients younger than 60 years had a 20% rate of disk herniation; those older than 60 years showed abnormalities 57% of the time, with 36% exhibiting disk herniation and 21% exhibiting spinal stenosis. Weishaupt and colleagues[23] studied 60 asymptomatic patients with MRI and found that 67% had disk bulges or protrusions; annular tears were seen in 33%, while disk extrusions were present in only 18%. Boos and colleagues[24] noted that only direct evidence of neural compression allowed differentiation of symptomatic patients from asymptomatic controls. Jarvik and colleagues' large study[25] also identified moderate to severe stenosis, extrusions, and direct neural compressions as critical features that stand out against a background of asymptomatic degenerative disease, which includes disk protrusions, facet degeneration, and spondylolisthesis.

Imaging therefore demonstrates significant abnormalities in the lumbar spine in one third to two thirds of asymptomatic patients. Annular fissures or tears, bulges, facet degeneration, mild spondylolisthesis, and disk protrusions are common. The prevalence of such asymptomatic abnormalities increases with age. Disk extrusion, frank neural compression, and severe central canal stenosis are uncommon in asymptomatic patients. These findings are more likely to be significant given appropriate correspondence with the clinical syndrome. There must be a clear concordance of clinical pain syndrome and imaging to suggest a causal relationship; confirmation with provocative or anesthetic procedures may be necessary to provide a basis for therapy decisions.

There is also a basic sensitivity flaw in advanced imaging as it is most commonly performed. Most patients with neuroclaudicatory pain syndromes report exacerbation of symptoms with extension and weight bearing. It is well known that the cross-sectional area of the central spinal canal, lateral recess, and neural foramina are maximized with flexion positioning; the dimensions of these structures diminish with extension positioning and axial load. Intradiskal pressures are significantly lower in a recumbent position than when sitting or standing. Schmid and colleagues[26] noted a 40 mm^2 reduction in cross-sectional area of the dural sac at the L3/4 level in moving from flexion to extension. They also reported a 23% reduction in neural foraminal cross-sectional area in moving from an upright neutral to an upright extended position. Danielson and Willen[27] studied asymptomatic volunteers and noted a significant decrease in the dural sac cross-sectional area with axial loading in 56% of the subjects, most commonly at L4/5. This finding was more common with increasing age. Decrease in dural sac area with loading was less frequent in normal volunteers than

in a population of patients with neuroclaudicatory symptoms.[28] In Willen and coworkers' study, 80% of symptomatic patients crossed the threshold of relative (100 mm^2) or absolute (75 mm^2) lumbar central canal stenosis with axial loading.[28] Kimura and associates[29] have also demonstrated decreased dural sac cross-sectional area in the cervical spine with axial loading.

Despite strong evidence for the effects of extension positioning and axial loading on neural element compression, the vast majority of advanced imaging (CT and MRI) is performed in a supine position, without axial load and with legs slightly elevated, relaxing the psoas muscles and reducing lumbar extension. This positioning is adopted to make the patient comfortable and better able to tolerate the study, but this ultimately compromises the sensitivity of these examinations. It has been suggested that when the dural cross-sectional area in the lumbar region is 130 mm^2 or less and there is clinical suspicion of neural compromise, imaging with axial loading should be considered.[28] There are two current methodologies that can be employed to achieve this. The simplest is a loading device as described by Danielson and Willen.[27,28] This uses tension bands applied between a shoulder harness and footplate to apply axial load and pull the lumbar spine into slight extension. A load of 50% of body weight applied for 5 minutes before imaging is used. Such devices can be used with CT or high field (1.5 or 3 Tesla) MRI. A second strategy is to employ uniquely built MRI scanners in which the patient may either sit or stand; dynamic motion studies can then also be performed. The drawback of the current generation of such scanners is their lower field strength (0.6 T) and lessened image quality. They do have potential for higher sensitivity to neural compression seen only under axial load or in specific positions.[30,31] As with many new devices, a unique terminology is emerging: *pMRI* refers to positional or upright MRI with load bearing, and *kMRI* refers to kinetic or dynamic MRI in which the spine can be studied in motion. The ultimate utility of these devices remains to be determined.

OVERVIEW OF IMAGING

When red flags are present at patient presentation, or when spine pain persists for 6 to 7 weeks despite conservative measures, imaging should commence with plain films of the relevant spinal segment. A primary motivation for plain radiographs is the detection of clinically occult neoplasm, infection, or fracture. Plain radiographs should be performed in an upright position, with weight bearing, to best assess alignment in a physiologic setting.[5] Only frontal and lateral views of the lumbar spine are indicated; the traditionally obtained oblique views and lateral spot view of the lumbosacral junction cannot be justified—these views rarely provide additional clinical information and double the gonadal radiation dose.[1] Oblique views to evaluate for spondylolysis should only be obtained in the setting of clinical suspicion and when no advanced imaging is contemplated.

Table 12–1. Estimated Accuracy of Imaging Technique for Lumbar Spine Conditions*

TECHNIQUE	SENSITIVITY	SPECIFICITY	POSITIVE LIKELIHOOD RATIO	NEGATIVE LIKELIHOOD RATIO
Plain radiography				
Cancer	0.6	0.95-0.995	12-120	0.40-0.42
Infection	0.82	0.57	1.9	0.32
Ankylosing spondylitis	0.26-0.45	1	ND	0.55-0.74
Computed tomography				
Herniated disk	0.62-0.9	0.7-0.87	2.1-6.9	0.11-0.54
Stenosis	0.9	0.8-0.96	4.5-22	0.10-0.12
Magnetic resonance imaging				
Cancer	0.83-0.93	0.90-0.97	8.3-31	0.07-0.19
Infection	0.96	0.92	12	0.04
Ankylosing spondylitis	0.56			
Herniated disk	0.6-1.0	0.43-0.97	1.1-33	0-0.93
Stenosis	0.9	0.72-1.0	3.2-ND	0.10-0.14
Radionuclide scanning				
Cancer				
Planar imaging	0.74-0.98	0.64-0.81	3.9	0.32
SPECT	0.87-0.93	0.91-0.93	9.7	0.14
Infection	0.90	0.78	4.1	0.13
Ankylosing spondylitis	0.26	1.0	ND	0.74

*Estimated ranges are derived from multiple studies described in the text.
ND, not defined; SPECT, single photon emission computed tomography.
Permission to republish granted from Annals of Internal Medicine. Jarvik JG, Deyo R: Diagnostic evaluation of low back pain with emphasis on imaging. Ann Intern Med 2002;137:586-597.

Plain radiographs reveal vertebral body height, integrity, alignment, and enumeration. Vertebral enumeration should not be considered trivial, and any advanced imaging should be correlated with plain films to be certain of the level of pathology before surgical or percutaneous intervention. Disk space height as an indicator of disk degeneration can be observed. The sensitivity and specificity of plain films and other imaging techniques is summarized in Table 12–1 from Jarvik and Deyo[1] Plain films have modest sensitivity for the detection of neoplasm or infection. Metastatic neoplasm is far more common than primary bone tumors. Metastatic disease may be lytic, blastic, or mixed in character; there must be destruction of at least 50% of trabecular bone for lytic disease to be visible on radiographs. Plain film findings of osteomyelitis/diskitis lag weeks behind clinical presentation. Plain films allow detection of fractures with loss of vertebral body height, but often cannot characterize them as acute or chronic. Radiographs can detect noninfectious inflammatory disease such as ankylosing spondylitis, but with lower sensitivity than MRI or nuclear medicine techniques. Plain films also reveal numerous findings such as vertebral osteophytes, facet arthropathy, Schmorl's nodes, and mild scoliosis, which are not likely clinically significant.

When plain film findings are not explanatory of the patient's persistent pain, advanced imaging may be considered; this includes CT, MRI, and nuclear medicine techniques. CT has undergone enormous technical advancement in the past decade. Multislice acquisition has given CT the capability of scanning extremely rapidly; a lumbar spine study can be accomplished in a matter of seconds, within a single breath-hold. CT is better tolerated and is more readily accessible than MRI. It is much less costly. Current scanners can rapidly generate reconstructed images in sagittal, coronal, and more complex planes with spatial resolution equal to that of the axial images, thus eliminating an advantage previously enjoyed by MRI. CT provides superior evaluation of cortical and trabecular bone when compared to MRI. It can demonstrate soft tissue anatomy, including root compression in the lateral recess and foramen, but lacks the sensitivity of MRI for evaluation of intrathecal structures, bone marrow infiltration, and soft tissue lesions that do not alter structural contours. CT does deliver a significant radiation dose.

CT is more sensitive than plain radiographs in the detection of spinal neoplasm, infection, and inflammatory conditions, but is exceeded in sensitivity by MRI in these conditions. In evaluating for root compressive degenerative disease, without strong clinical concern for neoplasm or infection, CT likely exceeds MRI in cost effectiveness and patient acceptance. In a clinical setting of potential systemic disease, MRI may be a better choice. New comparative studies are needed. CT myelography exceeds MRI in spatial resolution; it remains definitive in the cervical spine, in MRI-incompatible patients, and has a lumbar problem-solving role. CT myelography excels at the discrimination between bone and soft tissue intrusion into the cervical foramina, a distinction difficult with MRI. CT myelography remains operator dependent and carries a small risk from its delivery of intrathecal contrast material.

Over the past decade, MRI has become the premier imaging modality for evaluation of the spine due to its superior contrast resolution and improving spatial resolution. With the use of fat-saturated postgadolinium images or heavily T2-weighted sequences (short τ inversion recovery, STIR), MRI can assess active inflammatory processes of a degenerative or infectious nature. It has superior sensitivity in the detection of infection or tumor, including marrow infiltration. It can characterize the chronicity of fractures. It allows discrimination of postoperative granulation tissue from recurrent disk material. MRI poses no known risks to the MRI-compatible patient. MRI does not image cortical bone well; CT may be necessary to characterize primary bone tumors. MRI is burdened by its significant cost, substantial imaging time, claustrophobic imaging environment, and difficulty in patient access.

Nuclear medicine techniques, including technetium, gallium, and positron emission tomography (PET) scanning, may be used in evaluation of the patient with spine pain. Technetium scanning with SPECT may be used to evaluate the whole body burden of metastatic disease with good sensitivity and moderate specificity. Technetium can also assess fractures for metabolic activity (acuity). Technetium in combination with gallium scanning offers high sensitivity in the detection of diskitis/osteomyelitis, comparable to that of MRI. It does not, however, provide the anatomic information regarding central canal compromise or epidural abscess that may be necessary in clinical decision making. Technetium scanning with SPECT can also identify noninfectious inflammatory disease in the sacroiliac and facet joints. PET scanning and PET/CT fusion studies are assuming an ever increasing role in whole body evaluation for metastatic disease.

NORMAL IMAGING ANATOMY

Sacrum

The sacrum consists of five fused segments pieced by four Y-shaped foramina. The stem of the Y is the anterior foramen; the two posterior limbs are the dorsal foramen and the intervertebral foramen communicating with the central sacral canal. Superiorly the sacrum articulates with the L5 vertebral body via the lumbosacral disk and the L5/S1 facet joints. The lumbosacral junction represents the most abrupt change in alignment of the vertebral column, resulting in significant sheer stresses at this level. The sacrum is bound to the lumbar spine by the anterior and posterior longitudinal ligaments, interspinous and supraspinous ligaments, and the iliolumbar ligament. Inferiorly the sacrum articulates with the coccyx, consisting of three to five rudimentary segments usually fused in the adult. The sacrococcygeal junction consists of an oval facet surrounded by ventral, dorsal, and lateral sacrococcygeal ligaments. This joint is often obliterated with age; a moveable synovial joint is rare in adulthood.[32]

The sacroiliac joint is a large irregular synovial joint lined by thick hyaline cartilage on its sacral surface and thinner fibrocartilage on its ileal surface. Only the inferior one half to two thirds of the radio-graphically perceived joint is synovial; its superior aspect is ligamentous. The posterior surface of the joint is covered by thick interosseous and dorsal sacroiliac ligaments. There is minimal movement of the joint, except during the hormonal influences of pregnancy. The synovial portion of the joint is uniformly present in young adults, with a cartilage thickness of 2 to 5 mm; the synovial space may be obliterated in older adults by fibrous adhesions.[32] Potential communications between the synovial space and the dorsal sacral foramina, the L5 epiradicular sheath, and the ventrally situated lumbosacral plexus have been observed.[33] These could explain radicular pain associated with sacroiliac joint dysfunction. Innervation of the sacroiliac joint is complex. Recent anatomic studies have suggested an exclusive or dominant innervation from the L5 and S1 to S4 dorsal rami, with little if any ventral contribution.[34,35] This innervation has been targeted with radiofrequency neurotomy, although the inconsistent anatomic course of these contributors makes this challenging.[36]

Lumbar Spine

The lumbar spine consists of five rectangular lumbar vertebrae above the five fused sacral segments. The vertebrae are separated by the intervertebral disk; the height of normal disks increases with caudal progression from L1 through L4. The L5 disk space height is variable and may be normally diminished relative to upper lumbar interspaces. On axial images, the normal L1 through L4 disks are concave posteriorly. The L5 disk can normally be rounded in contour and convex posteriorly. The interpedicular distance in the lumbar region increases slightly as one descends caudally. The shape of the lumbar canal is triangular in up to 90% of patients; it is less frequently oval. A normal cross-sectional area of the lumbar canal is generally considered to be greater than 1.45 cm², with a minimum normal AP dimension of 11.5 mm, and interpedicular diameter of more than 16 mm.

On MRI, the appearance of normal vertebral body marrow is age dependent (Fig. 12–1). With progression from childhood through adolescence, functional red marrow is replaced by fatty yellow marrow. On T1-weighted images, this results in increased signal due to the fat within the marrow space. Normal adult marrow should always be brighter than the adjacent intervertebral disks on T1-weighted images. A modest degree of heterogeneity of marrow signal is normal in adults and may be more pronounced in older adults. Normal adult marrow shows mild uniform enhancement with gadolinium. The marrow space is demarcated by a crisp dark line of cortical bone, which blends imperceptibly with the low signal anterior and posterior longitudinal ligaments. The posterior longitudinal ligament is bound to the vertebral body only at the disk/end plate level. It is separated from the posterior vertebral body by the ventral epidural space, which is variably divided into right- and left-sided compartments by a midline septum.

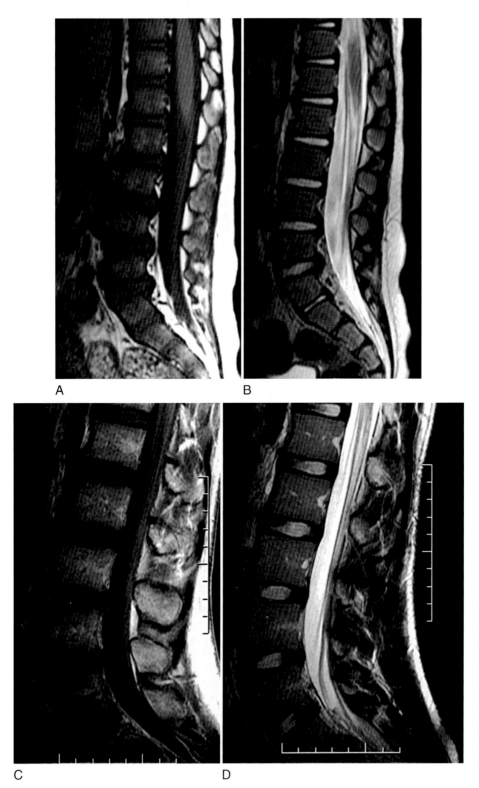

A   B

C   D

Figure 12–1. Disk and marrow change with aging. **A** and **B,** Normal juvenile spine (age 2). **C** and **D,** Normal young adult spine (age 18). In juvenile spine, note low signal hematopoietic marrow minimally brighter than disk in T1 image **(A).** On T2-weighted image **(B),** nucleus occupies vast majority of disk volume. By early adulthood, the marrow has accrued more fat and is brighter than disk on T1 image **(C).** On T2-weighted image **(D),** nucleus is bright and well defined but reduced in volume. Faint intranuclear clefts are present.

The intervertebral disk is well demonstrated on MRI; the central high T2 signal zone of the disk on MRI consists of the nuclear compartment plus the inner annulus. The nuclear compartment seen on discography thus is smaller than the MRI-perceived nucleus. In childhood, the nuclear compartment of the disk comprises a high percentage of its total volume, and has high signal on T2-weighted images (see Fig. 12–1). The surrounding fibrous annulus is of diminished T2 signal. There is little discrimination between the nuclear and annular compartments on T1-weighted images. In adolescence and early adulthood, a normal fibrous horizontal band appears within the nuclear compartment of the disk, the intranuclear cleft. This dark line bisects the high T2 signal nucleus and is a normal aging phenomenon. The annulus becomes proportionately larger and the nuclear compartment smaller at maturity.

The pars interarticularii and facet joints can be demonstrated on oblique plain films or axial CT and MRI. Normal facet joints have a dominant parasagittal orientation in the upper lumbar region (resisting axial rotation) and become more coronal/oblique in orientation in the low lumbar region (restricting AP translation). CT or MRI best displays the articular surfaces of the facet joints. On axial images, the superior articular processes are situated anterior and lateral to the inferior articular processes. The joint surface is curved, a critical determinant of its appearance on fluoroscopic observation. The posterior ligamentous complex consists of the interspinous ligaments, ligamentum flavum, and the facet joint capsules. These are only well demonstrated on MRI.

The tip of the conus is typically seen at the L1 or L2 level. The lower sacral roots of the cauda equina are found centrally in the dorsal aspect of the thecal sac with lumbar roots situated more anterolaterally. As each segmental root leaves the common thecal sac, it is encased in a root sleeve of variable length. It enters the lateral recess or subarticular space that is bounded anteriorly by the vertebral body, laterally by the pedicle, and posteriorly by the superior articular process. The lateral recesses are best evaluated with axial CT or MRI. The minimum AP dimension of the lateral recess is variably placed at 3 or 4 mm. The nerve root continues to pass lateral and inferior, entering the intervertebral foramen. The teardrop-shaped neural foramen is widest superiorly. It is bounded superiorly and inferiorly by the pedicles, posteriorly by the facet and ligamentum flavum, and anteriorly by the disk and posterior vertebral body. Foramina can be evaluated on lateral and/or oblique plain films, sagittal MRI images, or sagittal CT reconstructions. The nerve root, surrounded by fat, exits the spinal canal immediately under the pedicle in the widest portion of the neural foramen. There are five lumbar roots, which exit under the like-numbered pedicle.

The lumbosacral junction is a common site of bony anomaly, with the frequent presence of transitional segments, which in part resemble lumbar vertebrae, but also have sacral characteristics. There may be pseudoarticulations, potential pain generators, between enlarged transverse processes of a transitional segment and the sacral ala. Of even greater importance are the potential for transitional segments to cause confusion in vertebral body numbering and the correlation between findings on MRI and plain films. MRI findings should always be correlated with plain films before initiating percutaneous or surgical interventions.

Another commonly observed anomaly is the limbus type vertebrae. This represents an intravertebral disk displacement typically at the anterosuperior margin of a vertebral body. This separates a fragment of the ring apophysis, which remains distinct from the vertebral end plate. It is seen as a well-corticated ossicle contiguous with an anterior vertebral end plate, which has a corresponding defect. It invites confusion with a fracture, but is a developmental variant without clinical consequence. It is most common in the mid-lumbar or mid-cervical region.

Thoracic Spine

The thoracic spine consists of 12 rectangular vertebral bodies that gradually increase in size with caudal progression. The intervertebral disks are uniformly thin relative to their lumbar counterparts. The nuclear compartment is small, with a thicker annulus fibrosis. The interpedicular distance diminishes from T1 through T6 and then increases to the T12 level. The facet joints lie in the coronal plane. The spinal cord in the thoracic region has a uniform round to oval cross section, which expands normally at the conus. There are 12 thoracic roots, which exit under the like-numbered pedicle. There may be transitional segments at the cervicothoracic junction and the thoracolumbar junction, although with lesser frequency than at the lumbosacral junction.

Cervical Spine

The C1 and C2 vertebral bodies are unique. C1 consists of a bony ring without a discrete vertebral body; its lateral masses articulate with the occipital condyle superiorly and the articular pillar of C2 caudally. The vertebral body of C2 is marked by the cephalad extension of the dens, which articulates superiorly with the C1 ring. The transverse ligament, as well as subsidiary ligaments, tightly bind it to C1. Primary rotation of the cervical spine occurs at this level. Primary flexion/extension motion of the cervical spine occurs at the C4/5 level. The C3 through C7 vertebral bodies are more conventional, rectangular, and of increasing size as one progresses caudally. They are, however, unique in the presence of the uncinate processes, bony flanges, which extend superiorly at the lateral aspect of the superior end plate to articulate with the vertebra above. These uncovertebral joints may be true synovial joints or simply filled with loose connective tissue. Bony spurring arising from the uncovertebral joint may extend laterally and posteriorly to compromise the adjacent neural foramen.

The cervical intervertebral disks differ structurally from the lumbar disk. The cervical disks are thicker anteriorly than posteriorly and have a less well-defined nuclear/annular structure. There is no discrete annulus at the posterior disk margin. Cervical facet joints are situated in the coronal plane, with significant inferior angulation. The cervical central canal is triangular in shape. The lower limit of normal AP dimension of the cervical canal is 12 mm in the low cervical region, with a lower limit of 15 mm at the C1/2 level. The cervical neural foramina are best seen on oblique plain films or MRI images. In contrast to the lumbar region, the exiting root is found in the inferior portion of the neural foramen. There are eight cervical roots; the roots exit immediately above the like-numbered pedicle. The C8 root exits at the C7/T1 intervertebral foramen. The round upper cervical cord becomes more clearly oval at the normal cervical expansion, maximal at the C5 level.

The vascular supply to the spinal cord is complex and inconsistent, but of great significance to the spine interventionalist. The primary arterial supply to the cord occurs via the anterior spinal artery, situated on the midline ventral surface of the cord. This supplies the anterior two thirds of the cord, including the ventral horns, spinothalamic tracts, and corticospinal tracts. The smaller paired posterior spinal arteries are situated on the dorsal aspect of the cord, supplying the posterior one third of the cord, primarily the dorsal columns. The anterior spinal artery arises from the intradural vertebral arteries. The vertebral artery ascends in the neck via the foramen transversaria, at the anterior margin of the cervical intervertebral foramina. This relationship is well demonstrated on axial CT or MRI images; it should be scrutinized before intervention in the foraminal region. The ascending and deep cervical arteries may also contribute to the anterior spinal artery; the ascending cervical may supply contributors at the C3 or C4 levels, and the deep cervical at the C5, C6, or C7 levels. These small segmental vessels have been shown to enter the intervertebral foramen inferiorly and posteriorly, and hence may be at risk during interventions within the foramen.[37] They cannot be reliably imaged with CT or MRI. There is no right/left preference. The posterior spinal arteries arise from the vertebral or posterior inferior cerebellar arteries. They are reinforced by three to four tiny segmental feeders in the cervical region.

In the thoracic region, the anterior spinal artery is reinforced by two to three segmental vessels, usually from the left, via intercostal arteries. The dominant segmental contributor is the artery of Adamkiewicz; this originates from the left in 73% of cases. It arises from the T6 to T8 levels in 12%, the T9 to T12 levels in 62%, and in the lumbar region (primarily L1 and L2) in 26%. It is recognized at angiography by its characteristic intradural hairpin turn. The posterior spinal arteries are reinforced by 9 to 12 tiny segmental contributors, with no right/left preference. There are very rare additional contributors to the anterior spinal artery from the low lumbar or iliac arteries.

LUMBAR DEGENERATIVE DISEASE

Low back pain is usually benign in nature, transient, and self-limiting. Only approximately 1% of patients who present with acute low back pain have radicular symptoms. As noted above, plain film imaging should occur at presentation only when red flag conditions are present. Advanced imaging with CT or MRI may occur when plain films fail to explain a clinical scenario of progressive pain or neurologic dysfunction or there is clinical suspicion of systemic disease. Degenerative spine disease is the single most common entity that will provoke advanced imaging.

One of the confounding features in any discussion of degenerative spine disease imaging has been a lack of standardized nomenclature. Through years of effort, a combined task force of the North American Spine Society (NASS), American Society of Spine Radiology (ASSR), and the American Society of Neu-

roradiology (ASNR) has recently published a lexicon of lumbar disk pathology.[38] This nomenclature has been endorsed by the American Association of Neurologic Surgeons (AANS), the Congress of Neurologic Surgeons (CNS), and the American Academy of Orthopedic Surgeons (AAOS). This terminology is used herein.

Numerous morphologic changes are seen in the disk and adjacent end plates/marrow space as the spine ages. It remains controversial whether these changes are a normal aging phenomenon or a unique pathologic entity. Spondylosis deformans describes those changes thought to be due to normal aging (Fig. 12–2). This reflects predominantly outer annular degeneration and evolution of anterior and laterally situated osteophytes. The nuclear compartment of the disk is transformed with aging from a highly hydrated, proteoglycan rich, mucoid matrix to a more fibrous structure. The boundary between the nuclear and anular compartments becomes blurred as fibrosis occurs. This transformation of nuclear structure may occur with preservation of disk space height and normal cartilaginous end plate and subchondral marrow. MRI imaging shows loss of the normal intranuclear cleft and mild to moderately diminished T2 signal within the disk. Small concentric and transverse annular tears may be seen in spondylosis; radial tears are not considered a normal aging phenomenon. There may be small amounts of gas present within the disk that may be detected on plain films.

Clearly pathologic disk degeneration is termed intervertebral osteochondrosis (Fig. 12–3). This includes radial and large circumferential tears or fissures within the disk extending from the nuclear compartment through the annulus. These are predominantly situated posteriorly and posterolaterally. On MRI such fissures are seen as foci of high T2 signal (high intensity zones, HIZ) within the dark degenerated disk; they exhibit gadolinium enhancement due to the presence of vascularized granulation tissue. They may be accompanied by the development of posterior osteophytes that encroach on the central canal. In addition to posterior osteophytes, plain film manifestations of intervertebral osteochondrosis include large amounts of gas within the interspace, loss of disk space height, and end plate irregularity. On T2-weighted MRI images, the disk is of markedly diminished signal intensity. An irregular disk contour which bulges beyond the end plate apophysis and disk herniations are common.

Intravertebral disk displacements (cartilaginous or Schmorl's nodes) are also frequent in patients with early onset disk degeneration. Their role in the pathogenesis of disk degeneration is unclear. They are commonly the result of rests of embryonic notochordal tissue, but subclinical end plate fractures are indistinguishable. Intravertebral disk displacements are generally thought to be individually asymptomatic. In rare circumstances, an acute or subacute lesion may be implicated in axial pain. In these circumstances there may be marrow edema (low T1, high T2 signal)

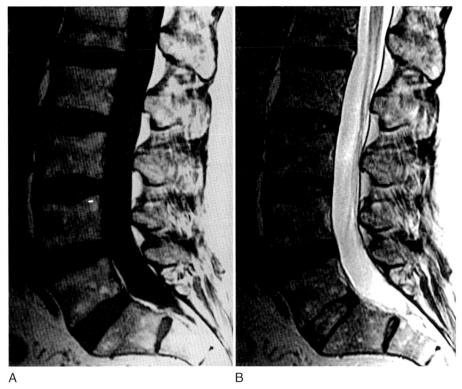

A   B

Figure 12–2. Spondylosis deformans in a 77-year-old woman. Sagittal T1- **(A)** and T2- **(B)** weighted MRI images show loss of normal signal in lumbar disks with preservation of disk space height. There is no osteophyte formation. Note normal heterogeneity of marrow in the elderly.

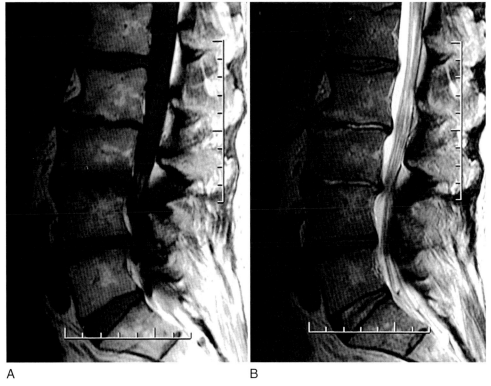

A   B

Figure 12–3. Intervertebral osteochondrosis in a 71-year-old man with back pain. Sagittal T1- **(A)** and T2- **(B)** weighted MRI images show extensive loss of disk space height at L2, L3, and L4. Type I marrow changes about L2 and L3 levels. End plate irregularity. Note potential confusion with diskitis at L2 and L3 levels in this noninfected patient.

with gadolinium enhancement at the periphery of the defect in the vertebral end plate. There is typically no enhancement within the displaced disk material itself; such enhancement should raise concern for a more sinister lesion.

The functional unity of the disk/end plate structure is emphasized by degenerative marrow changes (Modic changes) which accompany intervertebral osteochondrosis[39] (Fig. 12–4). Type I degenerative change reflects the ingrowth of fibrovascular tissue into the subchondral marrow. This is seen as diminished T1 and elevated T2 signal with gadolinium enhancement. Type II degenerative change may occur subsequent to type I change and consists of fatty infiltration of the marrow. This is seen as elevated T1 and T2 signal with or without enhancement. Type III changes are sclerosis with diminished T1 and T2 signal on MRI.

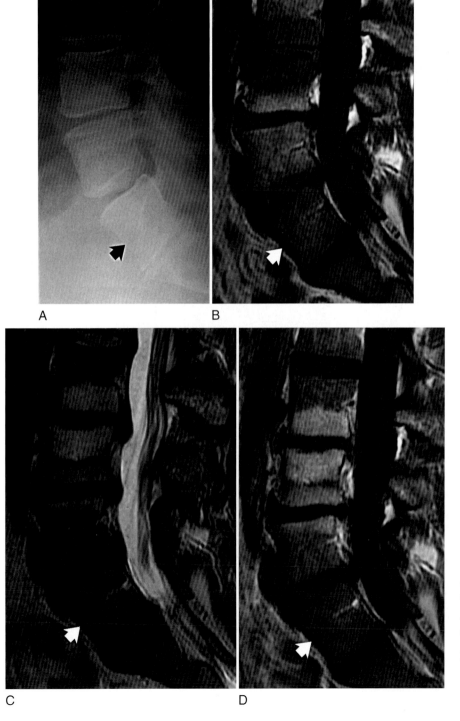

Figure 12–4. Degenerative (Modic) marrow changes. Lateral plain radiograph (**A**) shows a transitional lumbosacral segment, considered S1 (*arrows* in **A** to **D**). Modest narrowing of L3 and L4 disk spaces. Sagittal T1 (**B**), T2 (**C**), and gadolinium-enhanced T1 (**D**) images show type I marrow changes about L3 interspace with low T1 and high T2 signal with enhancement. Type II marrow changes are present at the L4 interspace with high T1 and high T2 signal. Disk extrusions are present at L3 and L4.

Disk Herniations: Nomenclature

Herniation is the inclusive term for localized displacement of nucleus, cartilage, annular material, or fragmented apophyseal bone beyond the normal intervertebral disk space[38] (Fig. 12–5). Herniation by definition involves less than 50% of the circumference of the disk. Generalized displacement of disk material (greater than 50% of its circumference) is a disk bulge. Disk herniations may be subdivided into protrusions and extrusions, based upon the shape of the displaced disk material. A protrusion is extension of disk material beyond the disk space where the distance between the edges of the displaced disk material is always less than the distance between the edges of the base of this process. A broad-based protrusion involves 25% to 50% of the circumference of the disk; a focal protrusion involves less than 25% (Fig. 12–6). An *extrusion* is a herniation where in any plane, the distance between the edges of the displaced disk material is greater than the distance between the edges of the base, or where there is no continuity with the parent disk (Fig. 12–7). This complete loss of continuity with the parent disk is also termed *sequestration*.

Migration describes displacement of disk material away from its disk of origin, regardless of continuity. Herniations may also be characterized as contained or noncontained, dependent on whether the outer annular fibers/posterior longitudinal ligaments remain intact. Integrity of the annulus/ligamentous complex may not be determinable by CT, myelography, or MRI. Discography may demonstrate the uncontained nature of a herniation when contrast extravasates into the epidural space. The volume of displaced disk material into the central canal is quantified in a three-part classification. Mild canal compromise involves less than one third of the cross-

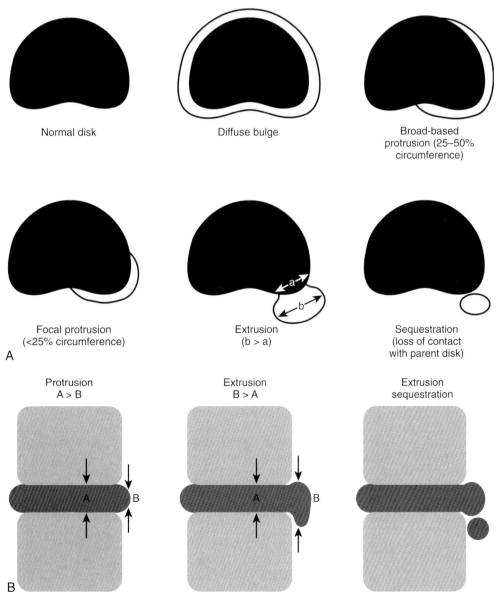

Normal disk

Diffuse bulge

Broad-based protrusion (25–50% circumference)

Focal protrusion (<25% circumference)

Extrusion (b > a)

Sequestration (loss of contact with parent disk)

A

Protrusion A > B

Extrusion B > A

Extrusion sequestration

B

Figure 12–5. Schematic representation of disk herniations in the axial plane **(A)** and sagittal plane **(B)**.

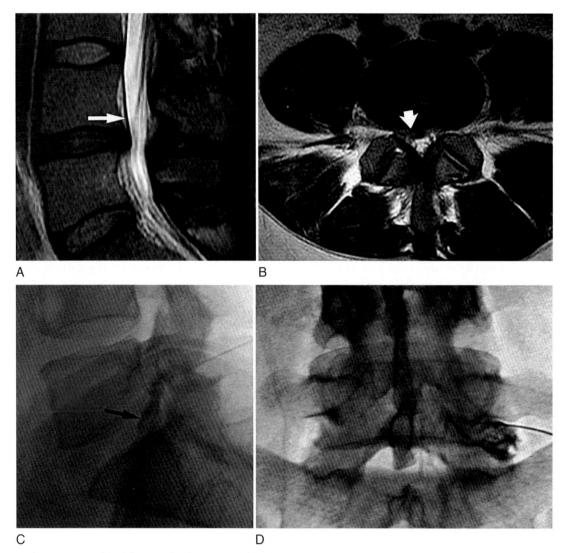

Figure 12–6. Right L4 protrusion. Right L5 radicular pain. Sagittal T2 image **(A)** and axial T2 image **(B)** at L4 interspace. Right central and subarticular disk protrusion at L4 interspace (*arrow* in **B**) encroaches on traversing L5 root. Note posterior longitudinal ligament displacement (*arrow* in **A**). Treated with right L5 transforaminal epidural steroid injection **(C, D).** Note contrast flow along L5 root (*arrow* in **C**).

sectional area of the central canal, moderate compromise involves one third to two thirds, and severe compromise involves more than two thirds of the central canal.

Description of displaced disk material (Fig. 12–8) in the axial plane is defined by zones: the central zone, defined by the medial margins of the facets; the subarticular zone extending from the medial facet margin to the medial pedicle margin; the foraminal zone extending from the medial to lateral margins of the pedicle; and the extraforaminal zone, peripheral to the lateral pedicle margin. A right-sided focal disk herniation may therefore be described as right central, right subarticular, right foraminal, or right extraforaminal. Similarly, location in the sagittal plane (superoinferior) is defined by levels, in relationship to the vertebral end plate and pedicle margins. Extending from superior to inferior, the designations include the disk level, suprapedicular level, pedicle level, infrapedicular level, and the subsequent

disk level. Even though an element of subjectivity remains inherent in any usable system of terminology, careful adherence to the above descriptors should allow more coherent discussion of disk pathology.

Disk Herniation: Natural History

Whereas extensive morphologic abnormalities may be clinically asymptomatic, it has also become apparent that disk disease that causes radicular pain or radiculopathy is a dynamic phenomenon. Teplick and Haskin initially reported spontaneous resolution of disk herniation on CT images.[40] Saal and associates subsequently described 11 patients with disk extrusions and clinical radiculopathy treated with conservative therapy.[41] Nearly half of these underwent a greater than 75% reduction in size of the disk extrusion on follow-up imaging. Maigne and coworkers, in a CT-based study of 48 patients with acute radicu-

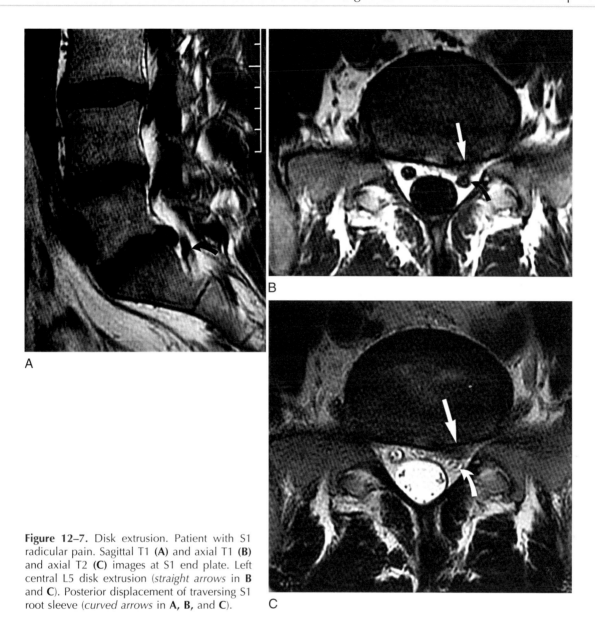

A

B

C

Figure 12–7. Disk extrusion. Patient with S1 radicular pain. Sagittal T1 (**A**) and axial T1 (**B**) and axial T2 (**C**) images at S1 end plate. Left central L5 disk extrusion (*straight arrows* in **B** and **C**). Posterior displacement of traversing S1 root sleeve (*curved arrows* in **A, B,** and **C**).

lopathies treated conservatively, demonstrated that 65% of this population underwent a 75% to 100% reduction in volume of the disk herniation.[42] The largest herniations showed the greatest tendency to resolve. The studies by Delauche-Cavalier and Bozzao and colleagues supported spontaneous resolution of large disk herniations.[43,44] Bush and associates studied 165 patients with radiculopathy treated conservatively.[45] Seventy-six percent of patients with disk herniation or sequestrations underwent complete or partial resolution on follow-up imaging. In contrast, 74% of patients with annular bulges showed no change on follow-up imaging. Those patients with the greatest reduction in volume of disk herniation tended to be younger, have shorter duration of symptoms, and highly positive straight leg raising. Disk herniations, therefore, frequently resolve spontaneously. Larger protrusions and extrusions are most likely to resolve. Diffuse bulges tend to be stable.

Disk Herniation: Imaging

Plain films should be the starting point for any imaging evaluation. There is relative consensus in the imaging community that MRI is the preeminent imaging tool for evaluation of lumbar degenerative disease (Fig. 12–9). This is based primarily on the superior contrast resolution of MRI, its multiplanar capabilities, and its noninvasive nature. Thornbury and coworkers, however, demonstrated little difference in the accuracy of MRI, CT myelography, or CT alone in assessment of herniated disk–related root compressive disease.[46] A study by van Rijn, Klemetso, and colleagues compared two-slice spiral CT with MRI in evaluation of radicular pain syndromes.[47] There was no evidence that CT was inferior to MRI in evaluation of disk herniation. There was more interobserver variability with CT than MRI in assessing nerve root compression. There are no compara-

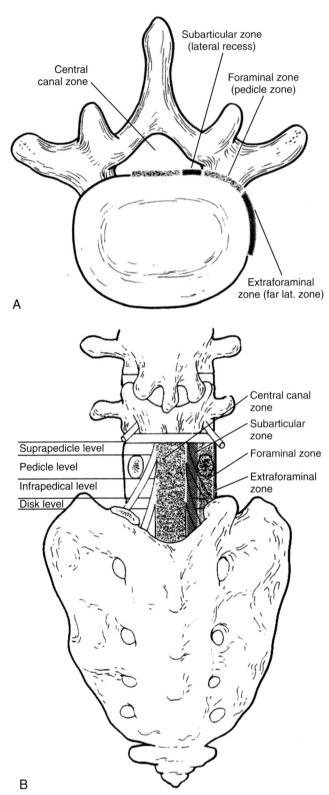

A

Central canal zone

Subarticular zone (lateral recess)

Foraminal zone (pedicle zone)

Extraforaminal zone (far lat. zone)

Central canal zone

Subarticular zone

Foraminal zone

Extraforaminal zone

Suprapedicle level

Pedicle level

Infrapedical level

Disk level

B

Figure 12–8. Schematic representations of zones in the axial plane (**A**) and levels in the coronal plane (**B**) for description of location of displaced disk material. (From Fardon DF, Milette PC: Nomenclature and classification of the lumbar disc pathology: Recommendations of the combined task forces of the North American Spine Society, American Society of Spine Radiology, and American Society of Neuroradiology. Spine 2001;26:E102-E103.)

tive studies with current generation scanners. CT myelography primarily has a problem-solving role in the lumbar region due to its invasive character. It is superior in discriminating bone from soft tissue (Fig. 12–10). It can be extremely useful when MRI does not explain the clinical findings (Fig. 12–11). Plain CT can provide high sensitivity in the detection of root compressive lesions and is inexpensive and readily accessible. It is most important that the individual clinician evolve an algorithm that works in the setting of their available imaging capabilities and the needs of their surgical colleagues. The availability of multiple imaging modalities may unfortunately result in their additive rather than selective use, driving up diagnostic costs.

Approximately 90% of lumbar disk herniations occur at the L4/5 and L5/S1 levels. The clinical syndrome, if any, caused by the disk herniation depends on its relationship to neural elements. Disk herniations resulting in radicular pain or radiculopathy most commonly occur at the posterolateral aspect of the disk; here they impinge on the ventral-lateral aspect of the thecal sac and the traversing nerve root (L4 disk herniation causing L5 radiculopathy). Laterally situated disk extrusions, often associated with a degree of cephalad migration, may affect the exiting nerve root within the neural foramina (Fig. 12–12). Typical MRI examinations of the spine consist of T1- and T2-weighted sagittal and axial images. The deformity of disk contour is most evident on the T2-weighted images where the dark annulus fibrosis is seen in relief against the bright cerebrospinal fluid (CSF) of the thecal sac (Fig. 12–13). On T1-weighted images the intermediate signal intensity of the disk may blend with that of the thecal sac. Its marginal boundary or its effacement of epidural or intraforaminal fat then identifies disk herniation.

Disk Herniation: Gadolinium

Gadolinium contrast enhancement is not routinely used in the absence of previous surgery but can be beneficial in selected cases of disk herniation. Although disk material is classically said not to enhance, there have been numerous cases of acute herniation with enhancement of the herniated material. In more subacute and chronic herniations, there may be a substantial epidural mass of disklike material on noncontrast images. With gadolinium enhancement, it may be demonstrated that the actual disk material (which does not enhance) is quite small, with a surrounding halo of enhancing granulation tissue (Fig. 12–14). Gadolinium has also been advocated as a means of detecting enhancing nerve roots, equating a clinical radiculopathy with blood–nerve barrier breakdown and root enhancement. Jinkins demonstrated good correlation of enhancing roots with clinical radiculopathies.[48] This finding has been challenged; in some instances enhancement along the course of the nerve root may reflect a prominent perineural vein rather then a pathologic process within the root itself.[49]

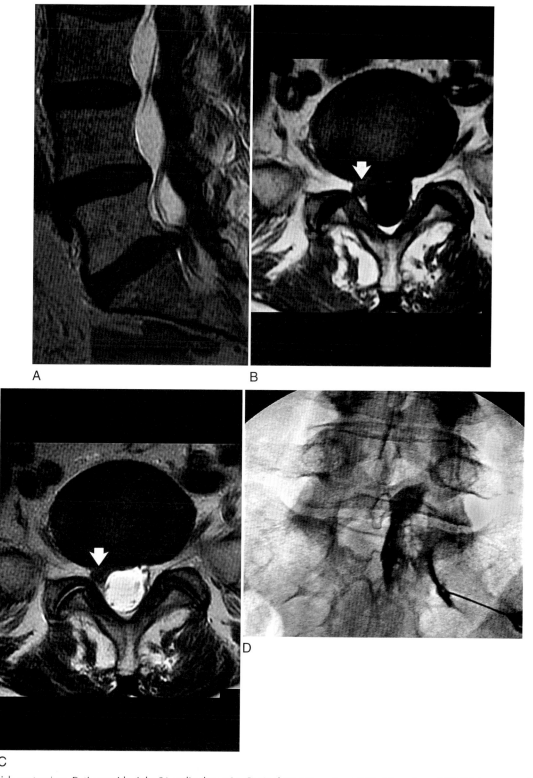

Figure 12–9. Disk protrusion. Patient with right S1 radicular pain. Sagittal T2 **(A)** and axial T1 **(B)** and axial T2 **(C)** images at L5 disk level. Right L5 subarticular focal disk protrusion (*arrows* in **B** and **C**). Note greater conspicuity on T2 image. Patient treated with S1 transforaminal steroid injection **(D).**

Gadolinium-enhanced MRI does have a well-defined role in the evaluation of the postoperative patient. Plain films, CT, and CT myelography are relatively uninformative in the postoperative patient, in that they cannot reliably distinguish recurrent disk herniation from epidural fibrosis/scar. Following diskectomy, there are extensive anatomic changes that evolve over time, confounding imaging interpretation. Great caution must be used in interpretation of MRI within 6 weeks of surgery.[50] In this time

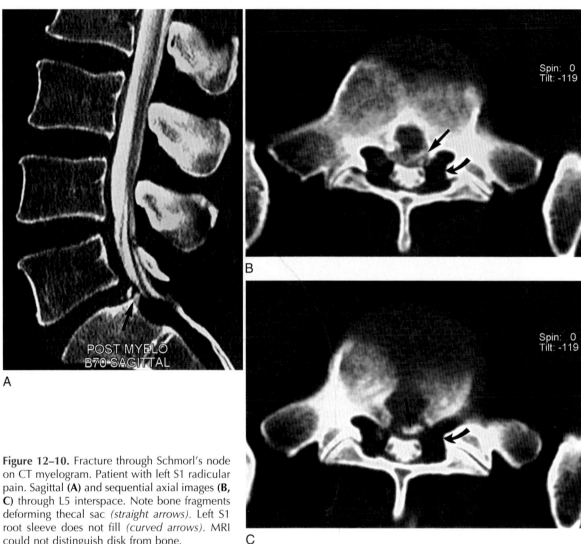

Figure 12–10. Fracture through Schmorl's node on CT myelogram. Patient with left S1 radicular pain. Sagittal **(A)** and sequential axial images **(B, C)** through L5 interspace. Note bone fragments deforming thecal sac *(straight arrows)*. Left S1 root sleeve does not fill *(curved arrows)*. MRI could not distinguish disk from bone.

frame, MRI is most useful in evaluation for hemorrhage, pseudomeningocele, or diskitis; evaluation for recurrent disk herniation is tenuous. The diagnosis of postoperative diskitis is also complicated by the normal linear enhancement that may be seen in the postoperative disk.[51] As postoperative tissue disruption and edema stabilize, MRI with gadolinium enhancement has been reported to be 96% to 100% accurate in distinguishing recurrent disk herniation from scar.[50] Scar or epidural fibrosis enhances rapidly and uniformly following gadolinium administration; disk material does not enhance for the first 20 to 30 minutes. Early postgadolinium images in the postoperative patient show recurrent disk herniation as a nonenhancing zone; enhancing epidural fibrosis may surround this. Extensive scar or epidural fibrosis is in itself a negative prognostic sign, associated with an increased incidence of postoperative radiculopathy.[52] In the postoperative setting, the thecal sac should be examined for evidence of arachnoiditis. In this condition, the roots of the cauda equina are either clumped together or adherent to the dural tube. The dural tube may even appear empty of roots, which

are smoothly scarred to its wall. Roots may exhibit enhancement in this condition.

Central Canal Stenosis

Spinal stenosis describes a syndrome characterized by neurogenic claudication with exertion. This is a clinical diagnosis; imaging identifies its anatomic substrate. Patients with a narrowed central spinal canal without symptoms do not suffer from spinal stenosis. Central canal stenosis can be congenital or acquired. Congenital spinal stenosis constitutes 10% to 15% of stenosis cases. This is generally idiopathic in nature, consisting of developmental hypoplasia of the posterior arch with short, thick pedicles that narrow the AP dimension of the central canal. The central canal may have a trefoil shape in cross section. Less common causes of congenital central canal stenosis include achondroplasia, Morquio's syndrome, and other bony dysplasias.

Degenerative central canal stenosis constitutes the great majority of clinical spinal stenosis. This includes mild cases of idiopathic congenital central canal nar-

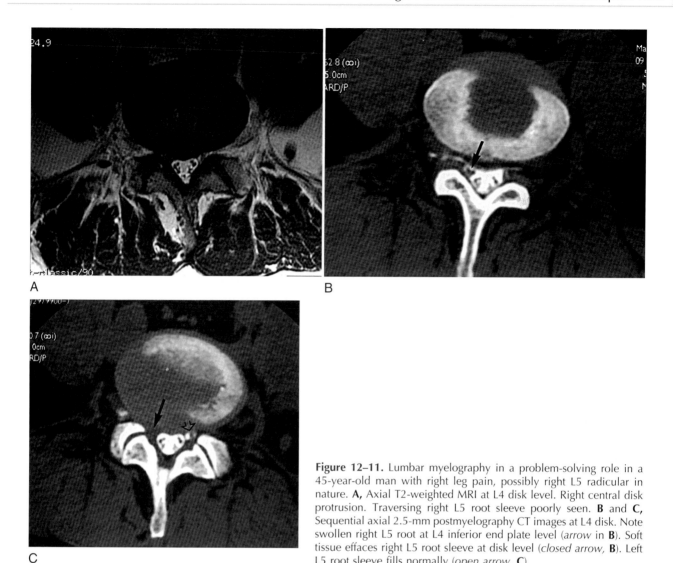

Figure 12–11. Lumbar myelography in a problem-solving role in a 45-year-old man with right leg pain, possibly right L5 radicular in nature. **A,** Axial T2-weighted MRI at L4 disk level. Right central disk protrusion. Traversing right L5 root sleeve poorly seen. **B** and **C,** Sequential axial 2.5-mm postmyelography CT images at L4 disk. Note swollen right L5 root at L4 inferior end plate level (*arrow* in **B**). Soft tissue effaces right L5 root sleeve at disk level (*closed arrow,* **B**). Left L5 root sleeve fills normally (*open arrow,* **C**).

rowing which, with the addition of degenerative change, become clinically significant (Fig. 12–15). Encroachment upon the central canal may occur anteriorly by disk bulge, herniation, or end plate hypertrophy. Posterolaterally, osteoarthritis involving the facet joints or associated synovial cysts may exert mass effect upon the central canal. The ligamentum flavum is crucial in the genesis of spinal stenosis. With loss of disk space height, the ligamentum flavum will buckle centrally into the spinal canal. There is controversy whether the ligamentum flavum undergoes true hypertrophy with advancing age and degeneration. It has, however, been demonstrated that with axial load, the ligamentum flavum will thicken by up to 3 mm in radial dimension.[53] The combination of facet and ligamentum flavum degeneration may also lead to instability. Where the pars interarticularis remains intact, slip of a more cephalad vertebral body will carry the posterior elements forward resulting in a significant reduction in central canal cross-sectional area at the disk level.

In epidural lipomatosis, excess epidural fat may cause or contribute to central canal stenosis (Fig.

12–16). This may accompany exogenous steroid therapy, endocrine abnormalities with increased endogenous steroid production, or generalized obesity. This is best demonstrated on MRI, wherein sagittal images show enlargement and continuity of the typically segmented dorsal epidural fat pads. On axial CT or MRI, the prominent dorsal and lateral epidural fat will encroach on the thecal sac, with convex medial borders.

Pathophysiology of spinal stenosis is multifactorial. The neurologic syndrome likely results from a combination of direct local trauma to the nerve roots, ischemic injury, transient demyelination, obstruction of axonal transport, and the gross anatomic observation that nerve roots in zones of stenosis become stretched and redundant. This redundancy is readily visible on MRI. The presence of multilevel stenosis on imaging significantly increases the likelihood of the clinical syndrome of spinal stenosis.

Plain films can demonstrate the short pedicles of congenital stenosis as well as degenerative processes including posterior osteophytes, facet hypertrophy,

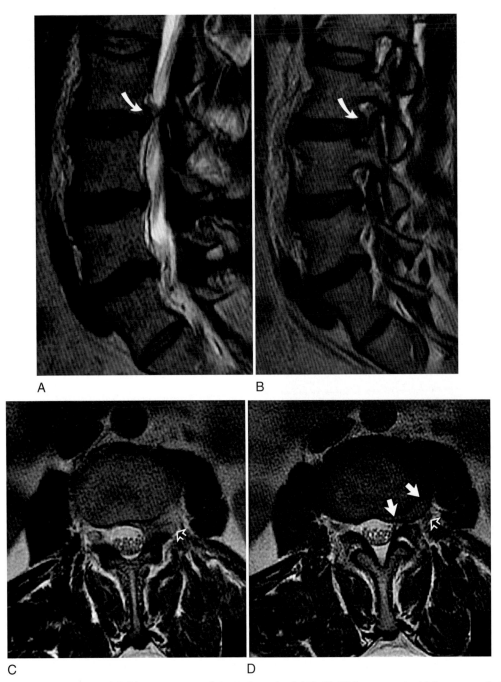

Figure 12–12. Disk extrusion. Patient with left hip pain. Sagittal T2 (**A, B**) and axial T2 (**C, D**) images at the L3 interspace. Left L3 subarticular, foraminal, and extraforaminal disk extrusion (*white arrows* in **A, B,** and **D**), impinging on exiting L3 root. Note posterior displacement of the L3 dorsal root ganglion and spinal nerves (*open arrows* in **C** and **D,** respectively).

or segmental instability. With CT, the effects of disk pathology, end plate hypertrophs, facet degeneration, and ligamentum flavum buckling/hypertrophy on the cross-sectional area of the canal can be directly viewed. The poor soft tissue contrast of CT may cause difficulty in resolving the disk/thecal sac or thecal sac/ligamentum flavum interface. The addition of intrathecal myelographic contrast material resolves this; CT myelography provides excellent spatial and soft tissue resolution for evaluation of central canal stenosis. The addition of intrathecal contrast allows the addition of a dynamic imaging component. The cross-sectional area of the dural sac diminishes with extension and axial load bearing; standing views in flexion/extension can demonstrate this effect. Axial load bearing has been shown to diminish the measured AP dimension of the central canal by as much as 3 mm on plain myelographic images.[54] The excellent soft tissue contrast of T2-weighted MRI images allows noninvasive evaluation of central canal stenosis (Fig. 12–17).

Early authors relied on AP measurements of the dural sac, with 10 mm being considered absolute spinal stenosis and 12 mm indicative of relative ste-

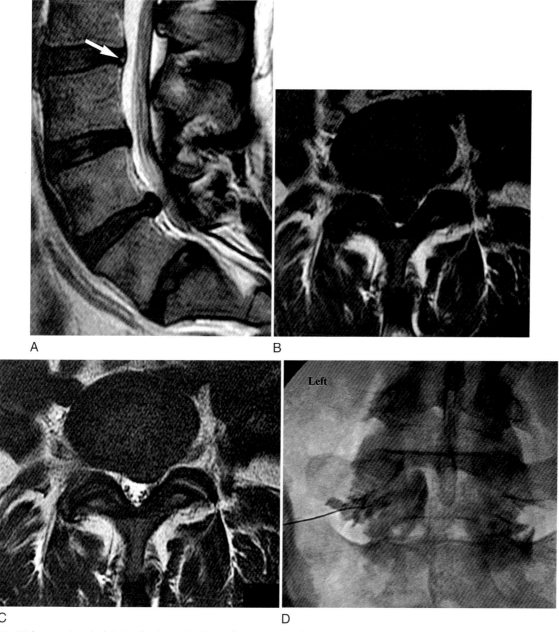

Figure 12–13. Disk extrusion. Left L5 radicular pain. Sagittal T2 **(A)** MRI demonstrates L4 disk extrusion. Note HIZ in posterior annulus L2 *(arrow)*. Axial T1 and T2 images at L4 disk space **(B, C)** illustrate the greater conspicuity of disk/CSF interface on T2 image. Patient treated with left L5 epidural steroid injection.

nosis.[55] Early CT studies placed 145 to 150 mm^2 as the lower limits of normal cross-sectional area at the mid lumbar level.[32] Subsequent studies with pressure measurements have shown that a cross-sectional area of 75 mm^2 in the dural sac at the L3 level is the threshold at which there is measurable increase in pressure among the roots of the cauda equina.[56] A 100-mm^2 cross-sectional area is considered to be relative stenosis.

Static measurements performed on a supine patient without axial loading may not reflect clinical reality, as noted above. Axial loading of the spine by means of a compression device designed to provide a load similar to that experienced in an upright position will reduce the measured cross-sectional area of the spinal canal. In the studies by Willen and colleagues,[27,28] axial loading with the spine in slight extension reduced the cross-sectional area of the mid-lumbar spine by up to 40 mm^2. Fifty percent of studied levels showed a statistically significant reduction in cross-sectional area with axial loading and extension. This suggests that our standard supine imaging may be relatively insensitive to the detection of physiologically significant degrees of spinal stenosis.

Quantitation of spinal canal dimensions remains largely an academic exercise and is not applied frequently in routine clinical practice. In most circumstances, a qualitative judgment of mild, moderate, or severe spinal stenosis is given, based on reduction in cross-sectional area of the dural sac by thirds.

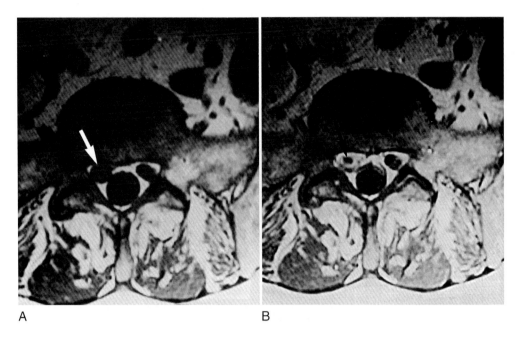

A   B

Figure 12–14. Enhancing granulation tissue about disk extrusion. Right S1 radiculopathy. Axial T1 MRI at S1 level **(A).** Apparent right S1 root sleeve is prominent *(arrow)*. Postgadolinium axial T1 MRI **(B)** at same level shows an enhancing collar of granulation tissue about non-enhancing sequestered disk fragment *(arrow)*. S1 root sleeve is completely effaced.

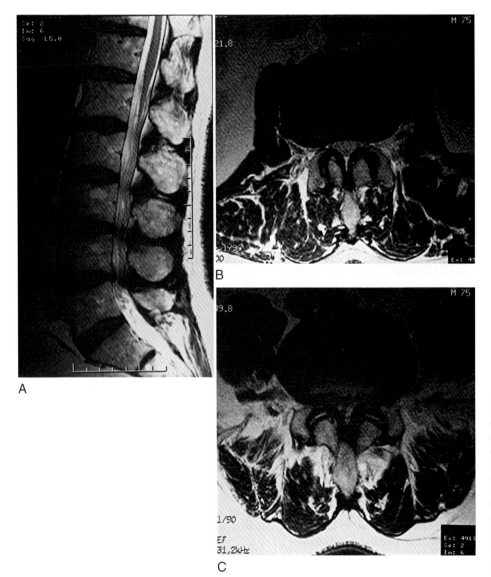

A

B

C

Figure 12–15. Central canal stenosis. Neurogenic claudication. Sagittal T2-weighted MRI shows congenital narrowing of anterior-posterior dimension of lumbar canal. Annular bulge at L4. Note redundant, undulating nerve roots. Axial T2-weighted images at L3 and L4 (**B** and **C,** respectively). There is moderate central canal narrowing at L3 **(B)** due to short pedicles, facet arthropathy, and ligamentous thickening. Severe central canal stenosis at L4 **(C)** is due to facet arthropathy, ligamentous thickening, and the annular bulge.

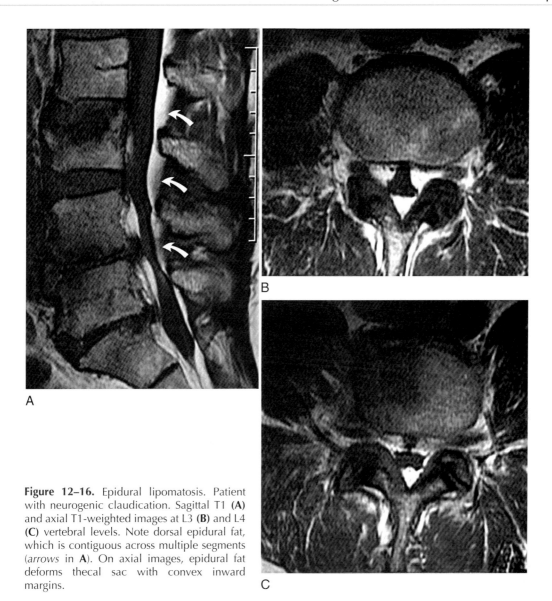

Figure 12–16. Epidural lipomatosis. Patient with neurogenic claudication. Sagittal T1 (**A**) and axial T1-weighted images at L3 (**B**) and L4 (**C**) vertebral levels. Note dorsal epidural fat, which is contiguous across multiple segments (*arrows* in **A**). On axial images, epidural fat deforms thecal sac with convex inward margins.

Lateral Recess Stenosis

As the nerve root exits the common dural sac into its root sleeve, it leaves the central canal, passing caudally and laterally into the lateral recess or subarticular zone. Lateral recess stenosis is primarily a product of facet joint osteoarthritis with overgrowth of the superior articular process. This encroaches on the posterior aspect of the lateral recess, impinging on the exiting nerve root. This is best demonstrated on axial MRI or CT myelographic images (Fig. 12–18). These images should be scrutinized to be certain that the nerve root in question is indeed entrapped within the lateral recess rather than simply displaced medially into the central canal. The minimum normal AP dimensions of the lateral recess have been variably reported as 3 to 4 mm.[32] The lumbar level most commonly involved with lateral recess stenosis is the L4/5 interspace level.

Foraminal Stenosis

As the exiting nerve root continues to progress caudally and laterally under its similarly numbered lumbar pedicle, it enters the foraminal zone. The intervertebral foramen is a teardrop shaped orifice; the exiting root is situated in the most superior aspect of the foramen. An annular bulge may intrude into the inferior portion of the neural foramen without causing neural compression. A disk extrusion with cranial migration of disk material into the foramen may compress the exiting root. Other degenerative phenomena causing foraminal stenosis include osteophytes arising from the posterior margin of the vertebral body or superior articular process, synovial cysts, or abnormalities of vertebral alignment, including the concavity of a scoliotic curve or spondylolisthesis due to spondylolysis or facet arthropathy. Foraminal stenosis is best demonstrated on sagittal

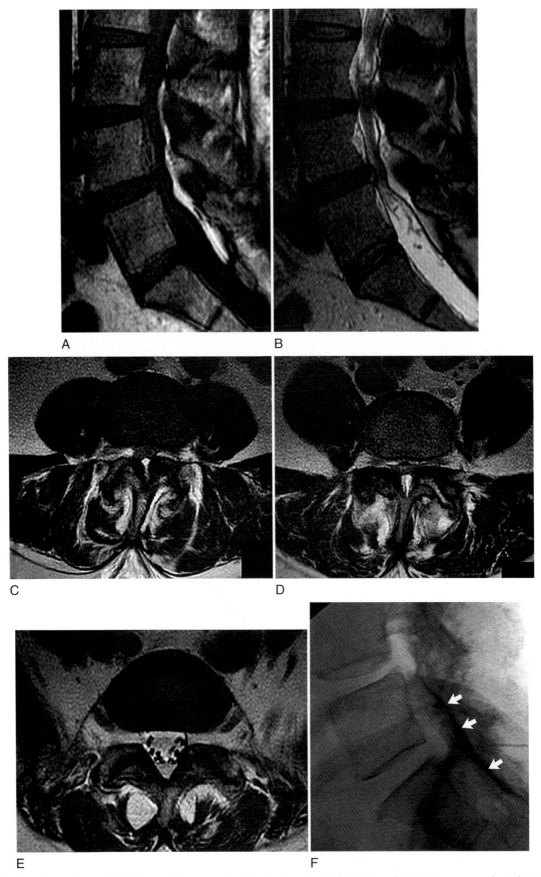

Figure 12–17. Central canal stenosis. Patient with neurogenic claudication. Sagittal T1 **(A)** and T2 **(B)** images, and axial T2 images at the L3, L4, and L5 levels **(C to E).** Note severe compression of thecal sac at L3 **(C)** and L4 **(D)** levels due to facet arthropathy, epidural lipomatosis, and disk bulge at L4. Interlaminar epidural steroid injection at L5-S1 level **(F).** Note contrast *(arrows)* conforming to dorsal epidural fat seen on sagittal MRI.

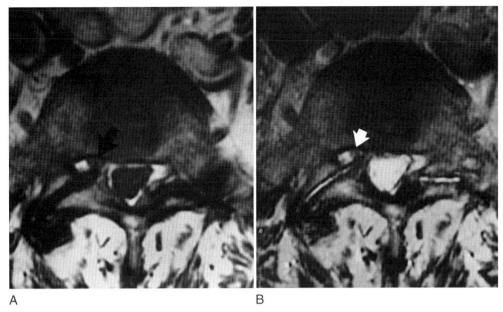

A   B

Figure 12–18. Lateral recess stenosis in an 80-year-old woman with right S1 radiculopathy. Axial T1 **(A)** and T2 **(B)** MRI images at L5 level demonstrate degenerated, asymmetric facets (facet tropism). Osteophyte from right-sided facet impinges upon S1 root in lateral recess *(arrow).*

MRI images (Fig. 12–19). The low signal nerve root and accompanying small veins should always be surrounded by high-signal fat on T1- or T2-weighted sagittal MRI images. Axial MRI images may also demonstrate foraminal stenosis, although to less advantage.

DISCOGENIC PAIN AND DISCOGRAPHY

The preceding discussion of imaging lumbar degenerative disease has focused on neural compressive lesions resulting in radicular pain, radiculopathy, or myelopathy. We turn now to axial somatic pain produced by the degenerative disk itself, usually referred to as *discogenic pain.* The concept of discogenic pain, and its diagnosis, is entwined with the history of discography. The literature of discogenic pain and discography is extensive, contradictory, and controversial. Its summarization here will be concise. More exhaustive reviews may be found in the North American Spine Society position paper on lumbar discography,[57] and the practice guidelines publication of the International Spine Intervention Society (ISIS).[58] Procedural recommendations here are intended to reflect ISIS standards.

Discography was initially described by Lindblom in 1948 as a means of evaluating disk morphology. Radiopaque material was injected into the disk and radiographs obtained. At a time when cross-sectional imaging did not exist, this provided the only means of imaging the nuclear compartment of the disk, displacement of nuclear material, and the integrity of the bounding annulus. As a morphologic imaging test, it fell prey to the specificity shortcomings of all purely anatomic spine imaging: asymptomatic degenerative changes are common and increase in prevalence with age. A causal relationship cannot be established between abnormal discographic mor-

phology alone and axial lumbar pain.[59] Observations regarding reproduction of a patient's typical axial pain during discography, combined with evolving histologic evidence of disk innervation, have resulted in the current concept of provocation discography, an anatomic and functional diagnostic study that seeks to identify a painful disk.

Discographic observations contributed to the evolution of the concept of discogenic pain, that is, somatic axial pain originating in the disk itself. The pathoanatomic basis of discogenic pain rests on the description of innervation of the outer third of the annulus fibrosis by nociceptors, whose afferent expression occurs via the sinuvertebral nerve, the grey rami communicans, the sympathetic plexus, and the lumbar ventral rami.[60-62] The degenerative disk may also acquire innervation via ingrowth of unmyelinated nociceptors into the deeper aspects of the annulus, accompanying granulation tissue within annular fissures. Inflammatory peptides such as substance P, vasoactive intestinal peptide (VIP), and calcitonin-gene related peptide (CGRP) have been identified in degenerative disks[63]; such peptides, as well as nuclear proteoglycans, may sensitize disk nociceptors. This is postulated to result in pain generation from within the disk itself under normal physiologic loads seen in daily life.

The requirement of pain provocation similar in character and location (concordant) to the patient's typical pain, during pressurization of a morphologically abnormal disk, brought reasonable specificity to the discographic study. Walsh and colleagues demonstrated this in their 1990 study in which concordant pain provocation in a morphologically abnormal disk was used to define a positive discogram. Using this criteria, normal disks in asymptomatic volunteers were not painful and only morphologically abnormal disks were painful in back pain patients.[64]

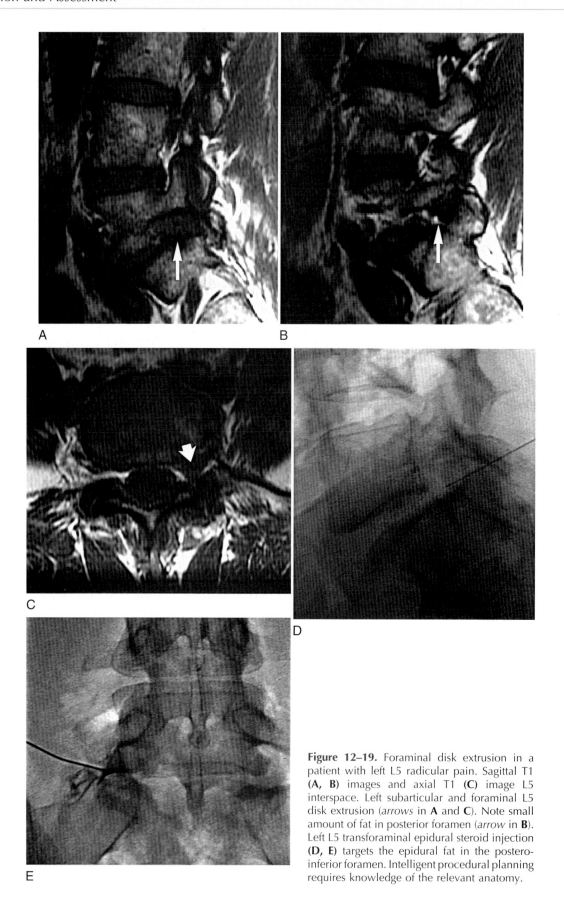

Figure 12–19. Foraminal disk extrusion in a patient with left L5 radicular pain. Sagittal T1 (**A, B**) images and axial T1 (**C**) image L5 interspace. Left subarticular and foraminal L5 disk extrusion (*arrows* in **A** and **C**). Note small amount of fat in posterior foramen (*arrow* in **B**). Left L5 transforaminal epidural steroid injection (**D, E**) targets the epidural fat in the postero-inferior foramen. Intelligent procedural planning requires knowledge of the relevant anatomy.

Vanharanta and coworkers subsequently demonstrated that pain reproduction correlated with the degree of annular disruption,[65] and Moneta and associates showed that discogenic pain did not correlate with aging or degenerative change, but was associated with annular fissures or tears.[66] Derby and colleagues incorporated pressure measurements into the discographic procedure; concordant pain provocation at low pressures of injection was a better predictor of favorable surgical outcome than pain provocation at higher pressures.[67]

Despite evolving support for provocation discography as a means of identifying a clinically painful disk, well-considered challenges to its validity persist. Carragee and colleagues performed discograms on patients without a history of back pain but with focal discomfort related to iliac crest bone graft donor sites; 37.5% of this small patient group reported reproduction of their typical pain with pressurization of a morphologically abnormal disk.[68] Disk stimulation may reproduce symptoms arising from an extraspinal source that is innervated by the same or an adjacent segmental level. Psychosocial factors may predispose to false-positive discograms; in a small study, Carragee and associates noted false-positive discograms in 10% of asymptomatic individuals, in 20% of patients with no lumbar pain but a history of chronic pain elsewhere, and in 75% of patients with established somatization disorders.[69] Provocation discography is also hampered by its subjective nature; despite attempts to quantify or score outcomes, there re-mains an undeniable art to its performance and interpretation.

ISIS suggests lumbar provocation discography as an investigation in patients with axial back pain to determine whether one or more demonstrably abnormal lumbar disks are the source of the pain. Patients should have undergone prior evaluation to eliminate other potential sources of axial pain, such as the facet or sacroiliac joints. If there is no need to establish the specific pain source, for example, the patient is not a candidate for therapies directed at the disk, then discography is of questionable value. It is not indicated in acute or subacute axial pain. In the face of intractable axial pain unresponsive to conservative measures, wherein surgical intervention or intradiscal electrothermal therapy (or new minimally invasive intradiskal interventions, which stand the test of a randomized controlled trial) is contemplated, provocation discography may serve to target the intervention, and evaluate adjacent levels for disk structural integrity and pain generation. NASS also considers discography indicated in the assessment of patients who have failed to respond to surgical intervention and there is concern for a painful pseudarthrosis or a symptomatic disk in a posteriorly fused segment.[57] Contraindications to discography include an inability to assess patient pain response to the procedure, pregnancy, local or systemic infection, coagulation disorders, and allergic response to the contrast agent, local anesthetics, or antibiotics used in the procedure.

Criteria for discogenic pain are well described by ISIS. Pressurization of the target disk must reproduce the patient's pain, and injection of adjacent disk(s) does not reproduce pain. Diagnosis of discogenic pain requires a control level, that is, disk pressurization of an adjacent normal disk that does not produce pain. If all disks injected are painful, discogenic pain cannot be diagnosed. Concordant pain should be reproduced at significant intensity; pain that is rated as 7 on a 10-point pain intensity scale is required for diagnosis. Concordant pain production is more significant when reproduced at low pressures of injection; discography should be controlled with manometry. By convention, the pressure at which contrast is first seen to enter the disk is "opening pressure." Concordant pain provocation at pressures less than 15 PSI above opening pressure is considered clearly positive. A disk that is painful at 15 to 50 PSI above opening is an indeterminate response, and may or may not be positive. Pain production at greater than 50 PSI is not considered significant.

The diagnosis of discogenic pain requires concordant pain production in a morphologically abnormal disk, with a tear extending to the outer third of the annulus. In discography, disk pressurization must occur via injection of the nucleus pulposus; contrast injection into the annulus may be painful in normal disks and invalidates the procedure. In the normal disk, contrast material injected in the nucleus remains confined in the spherical or rectangular nuclear compartment. This contrast-opacified nucleus may be bisected horizontally by a fibrous band, the intranuclear cleft. This is a normal phenomenon of aging, also seen on T2-weighted MRI images. With pathologic disk degeneration, clefts or fissures of varying width appear in the annulus, extending outward from the nuclear compartment in a radial fashion. Radially oriented fissures may terminate in circumferential accumulations of contrast as the fissure extends between annular lamellae. An uncontained or complete fissure shows contrast leaking into the epidural space or paraspinal tissues. These changes are best seen on axial CT images obtained immediately after the discography procedure (Fig. 12–20).

The Dallas discography classification is used to categorize morphologic disk degeneration seen on postdiscography CT: Grade 0 is a normal disk with contrast confined to the nuclear compartment; grades 1 to 3 describe radial tears reaching the inner, middle, and outer third of the annulus, respectively. Grade 4 describes circumferential extension of the fissure in the outer annulus over 30 degrees of arc. Grade 5 has been used by some authors to describe an uncontained fissure leaking into the epidural space. For a detailed description of appropriate discographic procedure, refer to the published ISIS guidelines. This describes general procedural requirements and needle placement, and elaborates on discography interpretation, including quantitative scoring.

Risks of discography include disk space infection, nerve root injury, CSF leak with headache, meningitis, arachnoiditis, intrathecal hemorrhage, and disk

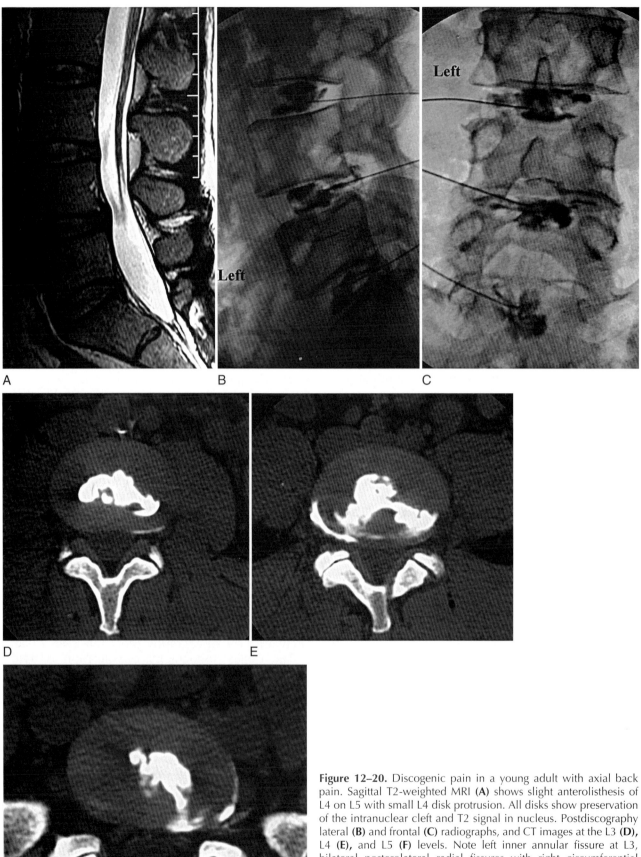

Figure 12–20. Discogenic pain in a young adult with axial back pain. Sagittal T2-weighted MRI **(A)** shows slight anterolisthesis of L4 on L5 with small L4 disk protrusion. All disks show preservation of the intranuclear cleft and T2 signal in nucleus. Postdiscography lateral **(B)** and frontal **(C)** radiographs, and CT images at the L3 **(D),** L4 **(E),** and L5 **(F)** levels. Note left inner annular fissure at L3, bilateral posterolateral radial fissures with right circumferential fissure at L4, and left posterolateral radial fissure with circumferential component and epidural extravasation at L5. Patient experienced concordant pain provocation at L4 only. Discography frequently shows internal disk derangement when the MRI appearance of the disks is normal.

injury. The primary concern is pyogenic diskitis due to direct contamination of the disk by the pressurizing needle. Meticulous asepsis is mandatory. Intradiskal or intravenous antibiotics (or both) are necessary. A double needle technique may reduce the incidence of infection. With appropriate precautions, diskitis should be rare (<0.1%).[57] Needle placement must be directed to the inferior portion of the disk, passing immediately anterior to the superior articular process of the facet, to avoid contact with the nerve root. Needle advancement when near the root must be slow and controlled. During needle placement, care must be taken not to violate the thecal sac and incur the potential risks of spinal headache, meningitis, arachnoiditis, or intrathecal hemorrhage. This requires inspection of CT or axial MRI images before discography to note the shape of the central canal and the angles of approach to the disk that are permissible without encountering the thecal sac. Use of fluoroscopic targeting alone, without an understanding of the three-dimensional structure of the central canal and disk from cross-sectional imaging, invites complications. Discography is not thought to injure the disk when appropriately performed.[57] Disk herniation induced by disk pressurization has been reported.[57] Manometric devices used in discography can generate very high instantaneous pressures; they must be used with care.

FACET (ZYGAPOPHYSIAL) JOINT DEGENERATION

We now move to imaging of potential somatic axial pain generators in the posterior column of the spine. The supporting structure of the posterior column of the spine includes the paired facet joints with their associated capsules, ligamentum flavum, the intraspinous and supraspinous ligaments joining the spinous processes, and the intertransverse ligamentous structures. The facet joints or zygapophysial joints are paired synovial joints whose articular surfaces are lined with hyaline articular cartilage and are bounded by a fibrous joint capsule approximately 1 mm in thickness. This capsule attaches to the superior and inferior articular processes approximately 2 mm peripheral to the articular margins.[70] The synovial space has an anteriorly situated superior recess and a posteriorly directed inferior recess. These recesses contain fibrous menisci, which may serve to protect the articular cartilage. The facet joints are biplane (curved) joints, with both a sagittal oriented component and a coronal oriented component. The joints tend to become more C-shaped or tightly curved with age.[71] The sagittal component of the joint is dominant in the upper lumbar spine and limits axial rotation; the coronal component of the joint is dominant at the lumbosacral level, limiting flexion and AP translation. The inferior articular process of the facet joint faces anteriorly and is convex in configuration; on axial images (CT, MRI) the inferior articular process is the more posterior component of the joint. The superior articular process (SAP) has a concave articular surface that faces posteriorly and medially; on axial images it appears as the anterior component of the joint. In addition to restricting rotation and translation motion, the facets participate in axial load bearing. In an erect standing position, the lumbar facets bear approximately 16% of the compressive load; in a flexed sitting position they bear essentially no load.[71] In the presence of degenerative disk disease with loss of disk space height, the lumbar facet joints bear proportionally more axial load.

The lumbar facet joints have been implicated as a source of axial low back pain for decades. The facet syndrome was initially described by Ghormley in 1933. It fell into neglect shortly thereafter with the description of the herniated disk as a cause of sciatica by Mixter and Barr. The disk dominated the literature for the next half century. In recent decades there has been renewed interest in the facet joint as a cause of axial pain.

The fibrous joint capsule has been demonstrated to be richly innervated by nociceptors and proprioceptive fibers.[72,73] There is up to 5 to 7 mm of sliding motion across the facet joint with physiologic motion. Maximal stretch of the joint capsule occurs when the lumbar spine is at the limit of physiologic extension.[73] In a normal state, nociceptors such as those seen in the facet capsule have a high threshold and would not be expected to fire unless loads are supraphysiologic. However, in the presence of pathologic joint inflammation, chemical mediators may sensitize these nociceptors and supraphysiologic levels of stress may no longer be required to stimulate pain.[73] Such inflammatory chemical mediators (substance P, bradykinin, PLA_2) have been detected in the facet joint capsule.[73,74] Substance P–sensitive nerve fibers have also been noted in the subchondral bone of degenerative lumbar facets.[75]

The facet capsule and subchondral bone of the facet joint are known to be innervated, and inflammatory chemical mediators may sensitize these nociceptors. Afferent innervation of the facet joint has been described by Bogduk and associates at the University of Newcastle in a series of landmark anatomic papers, most recently summarized by Lau and colleagues.[76] Each lumbar facet joint has afferent innervation from the like-numbered medial branch of the dorsal ramus, as well as descending innervation from the immediate supra-adjacent dorsal ramus. This medial branch of the dorsal ramus is fixed at two anatomic sites: (1) as it passes through a foramen in the intertransverse ligament just cephalad to the junction of the superior articular process and the transverse process, and after passing caudally across the base of the superior articular process, and (2) as it passes underneath the mamilloaccessory ligament. Although the medial branch dorsal ramus is too small to be directly visualized with current imaging techniques, the mamilloaccessory groove can be identified with cross-sectional imaging.[77] At the lumbosacral level, the dorsal ramus lies within a groove formed by the junction of the sacral ala and the root of the S1 superior articular process.

There is therefore a pathoanatomic basis for facet joint pain, particularly in the presence of inflammatory mediators within the facet joint, most commonly present in osteoarthritis. Osteoarthritis of the facet joint is a common phenomenon, present in greater than 50% of patients 40 yeas of age or older.[71] On plain films, osteoarthritis may be manifested as joint space narrowing with associated sclerosis of the facet articular surfaces as well as the development of marginal osteophytes. These changes are better displayed with CT, which can also identify subchondral erosions and cysts as well as synovial cysts, outpouchings of the synovial space. MRI can directly visualize the loss of joint cartilage and the presence of joint effusion, sometimes with widening of the joint. Use of fat-saturated T2-weighted images or postgadolinium fat-saturated T1-weighted images can elegantly display the inflammatory response within the joint, synovium, adjacent subchondral bone, and the extension of the inflammatory process peripheral to the joint capsule in the adjacent multifidus musculature. MRI also may show marrow edema or fatty replacement in the articular processes of arthritic joints and in the adjacent pedicle. Cross-sectional imaging has shown that the bony changes of osteoarthritis are more pronounced in the superior articular process. There is frequently enlargement of the medial aspect of the superior articular process, which may encroach on the lateral recess with resultant neural compression. Marginal osteophytes at the posterior aspect of the facet joint are more prominent on the superior articular process, often covering the posterior joint margin and complicating access to the synovial space of the joint for percutaneous intervention.

With the pathoanatomic basis of facet-mediated pain identified and with the ability of imaging to depict the most common inflammatory condition of the facet joint (osteoarthritis), it would seem that imaging would play a key role in identification of patients with facet joint pain. Reality is more complex. There are no specific symptoms or physical signs that allow a clinical diagnosis of facet joint pain.[78,79] The diagnosis of facet-mediated pain relies upon response to controlled local anesthetic blocks; controlled blocks with multiple anesthetic agents are critical in that there is a very high, in excess of 30%, rate of false-positive results from single anesthetic blocks.[78,79] Using dual blocks, Schwarzer and colleagues suggested there is a 15% prevalence of facet joint pain in young injured workers.[79] In an older population (average age 59 years), prevalence of facet-mediated pain was 40%.[77] In another study using 90% pain relief as a positive threshold, controlled blocks demonstrated a 34% prevalence of facet-mediated pain in an older population.[78] Provocation of pain during joint injection does not correlate well with pain relief by differential blocks.[80]

Unfortunately, with the diagnosis of facet-mediated pain dependent on differential blocks, no association can be shown between the degree of morphologic facet joint degeneration seen on plain films or CT and the response to such blocks.[81] Facet joints that show no significant morphologic degeneration may be painful, and degenerative joints depicted by imaging are most commonly asymptomatic. Although imaging of joint morphology has not been helpful, the detection of inflammation may be more useful. Technetium scanning with SPECT has shown a correlation between radionuclide uptake in the facet joints and response to intra-articular injections.[82] In this study there was no significant association between positive SPECT study and radiographically identified morphologic changes of degeneration. The MRI detection of inflammation using fat-saturated T2-weighted or STIR images or postgadolinium fat-saturated T1-weighted images has not been studied systematically, but holds promise for identification of painful joints (Fig. 12–21).

Despite the lack of utility of morphologic facet degeneration in identification of the painful joint, several authors have proposed classifications to grade the degree of facet joint degeneration. A meta-analysis of these grading systems by Kettler and colleagues[83] advocated the CT-based grading system of Pathria, a 0 to 3 grading system in which grade 0 is a normal joint; grade 1 shows joint space narrowing; grade 2 is joint space narrowing plus sclerosis or hypertrophic change; grade 3 is joint space narrowing plus sclerosis and hypertrophic change. The study also advocated the MRI-based classification of Weishaupt: grade 0 is normal, with a joint space of 2 to 4 mm; grade 1 equals joint space narrowing to less than 2 mm with small osteophytes; grade 2 equals joint space narrowing plus moderate osteophytes or subarticular erosions; grade 3 equals joint space narrowing with large osteophytes, hypertrophy of the superior articular process, and/or erosions or subchondral cysts.

SYNOVIAL CYSTS

Synovial cysts may accompany facet osteoarthritis, and may be a cause of radicular pain, neurogenic claudication, and may be associated with axial low back pain. Synovial cysts are thought to originate with a degenerative or traumatic defect in the fibrous facet joint capsule, with subsequent herniation of synovial membrane through the defect. Expansion of the synovial outpouching, no longer constrained by the joint capsule, results in a cystic lesion that may impinge on adjacent neural structures or simply serve as an imaging marker of capsular pathology. Synovial cysts may retain or potentially lose their communication with the facet joint. Ganglion cysts may have a similar gross appearance, but histologically lack a synovial lining; they may be indistinguishable on imaging studies.[85]

Although relatively unusual, synovial cysts are not rare: the series of Doyle and colleagues[86] demonstrated a prevalence of nearly 10% in a population of patients undergoing MRI for back or leg pain. In this series, anterior or intraspinal cysts, often arising from the superior recess, had a prevalence of 2.3%; poste-

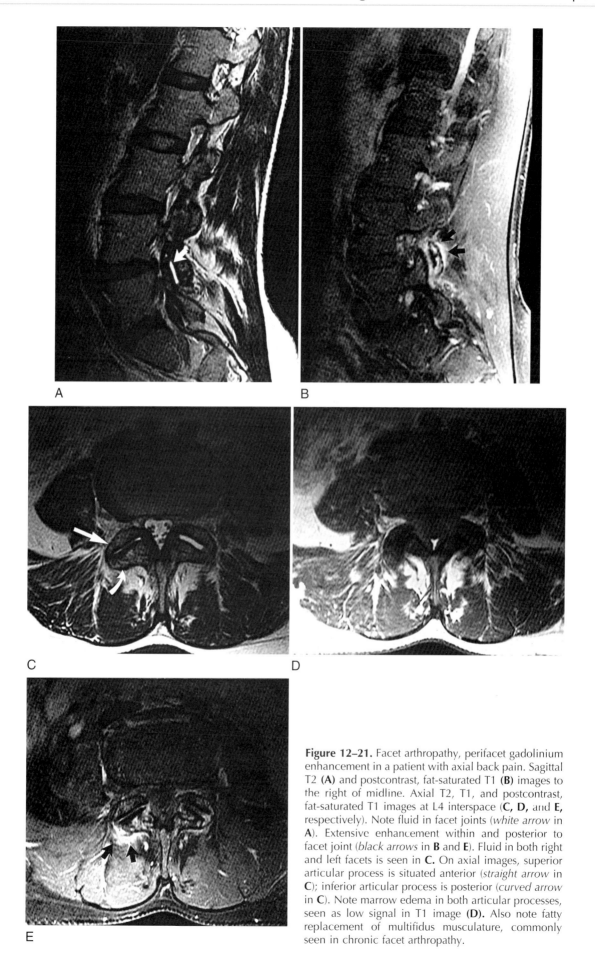

Figure 12–21. Facet arthropathy, perifacet gadolinium enhancement in a patient with axial back pain. Sagittal T2 (**A**) and postcontrast, fat-saturated T1 (**B**) images to the right of midline. Axial T2, T1, and postcontrast, fat-saturated T1 images at L4 interspace (**C, D,** and **E,** respectively). Note fluid in facet joints (*white arrow* in **A**). Extensive enhancement within and posterior to facet joint (*black arrows* in **B** and **E**). Fluid in both right and left facets is seen in **C.** On axial images, superior articular process is situated anterior (*straight arrow* in **C**); inferior articular process is posterior (*curved arrow* in **C**). Note marrow edema in both articular processes, seen as low signal in T1 image (**D).** Also note fatty replacement of multifidus musculature, commonly seen in chronic facet arthropathy.

rior or extraspinal cysts were more common with a 7.3% prevalence.[86] Most previous series had reported only anterior intraspinal cysts. Synovial cysts are detected in a relatively elderly population, with an average age of 63 years in Metellus and coworkers' study,[87] 61 in Apostalaki and associates'[85] study population, and 66 years in the large surgical series of Lyons and colleagues.[88] Reported male-female ratios are inconsistent, varying from a 1:1 ratio in the Lyons series to 1.2:1 in the Metellus series to 1:2 in the Apostalaki study; Doyle noted a female predominance in posterior cysts only. Synovial cysts are far more common in the lumbar region than in the thoracic or cervical spine. The literature has consistently shown that 60% to 70% of lumbar synovial cysts will be at L4/5 level, followed in relative order by L5/S1, L3/4, and L2/3. Anterior or intraspinal synovial cysts most commonly occur posterolateral to the thecal sac,[85-87] in close association to the facet joint. They may be embedded in the ligamentum flavum. Uncommonly, cysts may be located directly dorsal to the thecal sac,[85] laterally within the neural foramen,[85] or in a far lateral or extraforaminal site.[89,90]

Synovial cysts often arise from significantly degenerated facet joints with sclerosis, hypertrophy, and increased joint fluid, although most degenerated joints do not produce cysts. Segmental hypermobility is postulated as an underlying cause of synovial cysts. This is supported by the strong association with the most mobile lumbar segment (L4/5) and the frequent (42% to 65%) association with degenerative spondylolisthesis.[85] Degenerative disk disease is also commonly present at the level of the cyst. Metellus also noted that most cysts arise from joints with a predominant sagittal orientation; such orientation is also associated with segmental instability.

Synovial cysts may be detected by CT, CT myelography, or MRI; MRI is thought to be most sensitive (Fig. 12–22). Calcified cysts may rarely be seen on

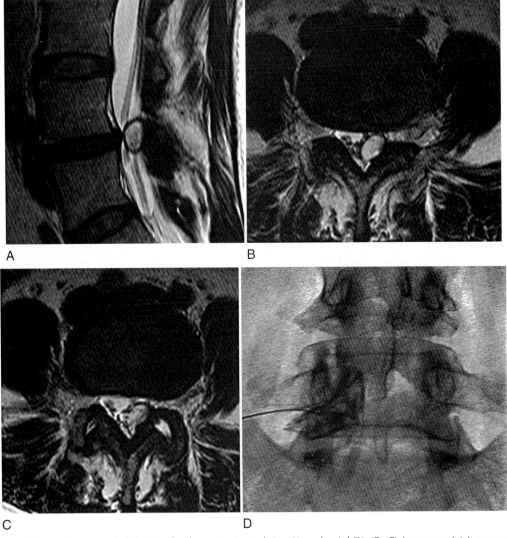

A   B

C   D

Figure 12–22. Synovial cyst. Patient with left L5 radicular pain. Sagittal T2 **(A)** and axial T2 **(B, C)** images at L4 interspace. Synovial cyst arising from left L4-5 facet joint deforms thecal sac and compresses traversing L5 root. Bulging L4 disk. Patient treated with aspiration of cyst via joint, intra-articular steroid injection, and left L5 transforaminal epidural steroid injection **(D).** Note low T2 signal capsule about synovial cyst. Also note widened facet joint space in fluoroscopic image **(D)** reflecting joint effusion.

plain radiographs. Synovial cysts have great variation in their histology, with corresponding variety in their imaging appearance. Synovial cysts may be thin-walled collections of pure synovial fluid or be complicated by varying degrees of chronic or acute hemorrhage and inflammation. Pure cysts have high T2 signal, equal to or exceeding that of CSF, with a thin, low signal wall. With chronic hemorrhage, cyst contents may develop high T1 signal (methemoglobin) and variable T2 signal; the wall often enhances with gadolinium. In the presence of chronic inflammation and calcification, the wall may become quite thick with very low T1 and T2 signal. On CT, calcification is variably seen and cyst contents range from hypodense to slightly hyperdense relative to muscle. Degenerative changes in the adjacent facet joint are typical, including abnormal marrow signal in the articular processes and pedicle.[91] A direct communication with the facet joint is not always demonstrable on either CT or MRI. The imaging differential diagnosis includes conjoined nerve root sleeves, sequestered disk fragments, cystic nerve sheath tumors, and degenerative cysts of other origins, such as pseudobursa in Baastrup's disease.

Anterior or intraspinal synovial cysts will often present as lesions causing unilateral radicular pain or contributing to neurogenic claudication. Anterior synovial cysts may cause focal neural compression in the lateral recess, foramen or extraforaminal space, or contribute to central canal stenosis. Posterior cysts do not cause neural compression, but may be associated with axial pain and be an imaging sign of facet capsular disease. Synovial cysts may regress spontaneously.[92] Radicular pain due to synovial cysts may be treated by injection of corticosteroid into the facet joint bearing the cyst, with a transforaminal epidural steroid injection at the same procedural setting. Such a strategy was successful in avoiding surgical intervention in 50% of patients in a series by Sabers and colleagues.[93] Other nonoperative therapies have included aspiration, fenestration, or rupture of cysts under CT or fluoroscopic guidance. Surgical resection of synovial cysts generally has a favorable outcome, but may require facetectomy and laminectomy.

DEGENERATIVE SPONDYLOLISTHESIS

Spondylolisthesis refers to the abnormal anterior or posterior displacement of one vertebral body relative to another. Displacement due to defects in the pars interarticularis (spondylolytic spondylolisthesis) is discussed later. Degenerative anterolisthesis is the anterior displacement of a vertebral body relative to the body immediately caudal to it. The etiology of degenerative anterolisthesis is primarily facet joint degeneration, often with a relative sagittal orientation of the facets. Disk degeneration is also necessary. Degenerative anterolisthesis may be present in 4% to 14% of elderly patients.[33,94] Anterolisthesis is most frequent at the L4 level, with less common occurrence at L5, followed by L3. It is significantly more common in women than men.[94] Radiographic findings of degenerative anterolisthesis include the obvious displacement itself, joint space narrowing and sclerosis in the associated facets, and findings of intervertebral osteochondrosis, including loss of disk space height, gas within the disk, and subchondral sclerosis.

Degenerative retrolisthesis describes the posterior displacement of the vertebral body relative to that below it; the primary causative process is intervertebral osteochondrosis. As there is loss of disk space height, the oblique orientation of the facet results in the more superior vertebral body gliding posterior relative to its inferior counterpart. Degenerative retrolisthesis is most commonly seen at the L2 interspace level, with less common occurrence at L1, followed by L3. There is no significant gender difference. Radiographic findings include the displacement as well as the aforementioned changes of intervertebral osteochondrosis.

Degenerative spondylolisthesis may be associated with axial low back pain. The Kauppila and colleagues study showed that patients with degenerative spondylolisthesis had a higher prevalence of daily low back symptoms.[94] There was, however, no increased disability in spondylolisthesis patients relative to controls. In this study the overall incidence of degenerative spondylolisthesis approached 20%. Degenerative spondylolisthesis carries with it the risk of neural element compromise with secondary central canal stenosis, lateral recess stenosis, or foraminal compromise.

Baastrup's Syndrome

Baastrup's syndrome describes an imaging finding in which lumbar spinous processes contact in extension, with radiographically evident sclerosis and flattening of the opposing bony surfaces and pseudarthrosis formation, which may be accompanied by formation of a pseudobursa. Such pseudobursa may have a synovial membrane[95] and can communicate with facet joints or pars defects via the retrodural space.[96] This is also likely the interfacet communication described by Okada.[97] The pseudobursa may extend anteriorly through a midline cleft in the ligamentum flavum and present on MRI or CT as a midline posterior epidural cyst, causing neural compression.[98] It may be mistaken for a synovial cyst of facet origin, but is distinguished by its midline posterior location, the relative absence of facet degeneration, a cystic pseudobursa, and inflammatory change in the interspinous ligament.

More commonly, Baastrup's syndrome is invoked to explain midline axial pain, which is exacerbated by extension, and may be relieved by local anesthetic and/or corticosteroid injection in the interspinous ligament. The posterior element findings often occur in association with disk degeneration and segmental instability; axial pain in this setting may be multifactorial.[98] Midline posterior element activity on technetium SPECT scans may suggest the diagnosis.[99] On MRI, we have observed marrow edema or sclerosis of

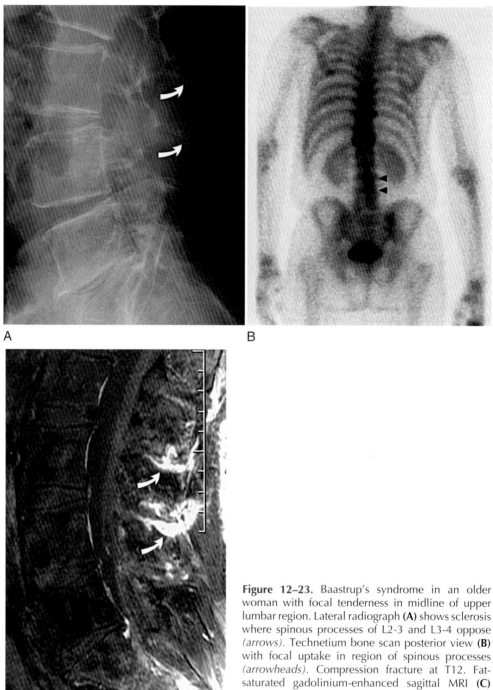

A

B

C

Figure 12–23. Baastrup's syndrome in an older woman with focal tenderness in midline of upper lumbar region. Lateral radiograph **(A)** shows sclerosis where spinous processes of L2-3 and L3-4 oppose *(arrows)*. Technetium bone scan posterior view **(B)** with focal uptake in region of spinous processes *(arrowheads)*. Compression fracture at T12. Fat-saturated gadolinium-enhanced sagittal MRI **(C)** demonstrates inflammatory enhancement at opposed spinous processes *(arrows)*. Patient responded well to interspinous injections.

the spinous processes, pseudobursae, and gadolinium enhancement in the interspinous ligament, particularly on fat-saturated images (Fig. 12–23).

Bertolotti's Syndrome

Bertolotti's syndrome describes the controversial association of transitional lumbosacral segments with mechanical back pain. It does not imply a specific mechanism of pain production. Transitional lumbosacral segments occur in 6% of the general population; such segments were seen in 7% of a population imaged due to axial and/or radicular pain.[100] Tini and coworkers found no correlation between the presence of a transitional segment and low back pain.[101] The disk at the level of the transitional segment is often rudimentary, with little nuclear material; disk herniations seldom occur at this level.[101] Rather, stresses may be accentuated at the supra-adjacent disk level, where accelerated disk degeneration and an increased incidence of disk herniations has been reported.[100]

Axial low back pain in the presence of a transitional segment has also been attributed to abnormal

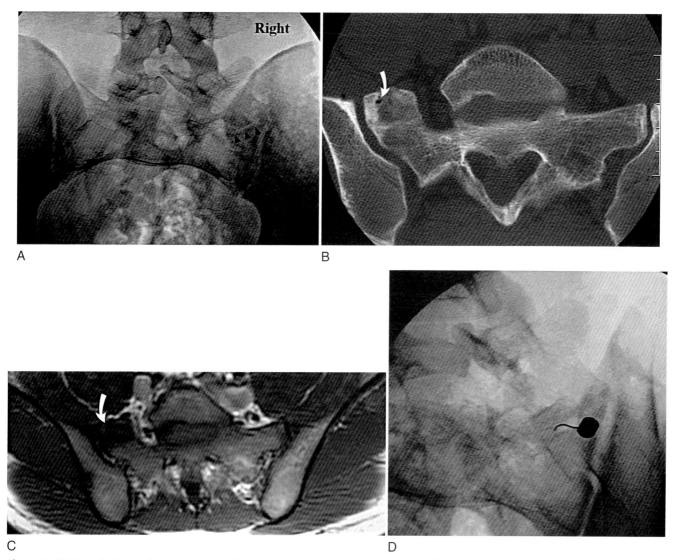

Figure 12–24. Bertolotti's syndrome in a young female patient with low back pain. Prone fluoroscopic image **(A)** shows transitional segment with pseudoarticulation with sacral ala on right *(arrowheads)*. Axial CT **(B)** demonstrates degenerative gas in pseudoarticulation *(arrow)*. Axial T1-weighted MRI **(C)** shows marrow edema (low signal) at pseudoarticulation *(arrow)*. Prone fluoroimage **(D)** shows needle in pseudoarticulation. Bupivacaine injection relieved pain completely.

or asymmetric motion at this level, with the neo-articulation of the transverse process with the sacral ala (Fig. 12–24) or the contralateral facet as the specific pain generator. Jonsson and associates reported 11 cases of mechanical pain attributed to the neoarticulation despite normal bone scans. Nine of 11 patients obtained pain relief with local anesthetic injection in the neoarticulation; a similar proportion of patients had improvement in pain with resection of the neoarticulation.[102] Brault and colleagues reported a case of an adolescent athlete with focal mechanical pain consistently relieved by intra-articular injection of the facet contralateral to the neoarticulation. Interestingly, bone scan showed increased uptake at the neoarticulation, but not at the contralateral facet. Surgical resection of the neoarticulation resulted in complete relief of the contralateral pain at 1 year.[103] This may represent a case of pain generated by excessive facet capsular stresses caused by the asymmetric motion at this

level, without detectable facet arthritis. The only other surgical series is that of Santavirta and associates. This patient group was heterogeneous in presentation and had mixed results from surgical intervention.[104]

Transitional lumbosacral segments therefore may be associated with axial mechanical pain, most likely related to the neoarticulation, but possibly due to the contralateral facet. Pain generation, as defined by pain relief with single local anesthetic blocks or positive response to surgical resection, may occur despite negative bone scan or lack of radiographic evidence of osteoarthritis (see Fig. 12–24). No studies of MRI-detected inflammation (STIR or fat-saturated gadolinium-enhanced imaging) have been performed. Recall that transitional segments also may cause confusion in vertebral numbering and the location of more cephalad pathology; always explicitly state assumptions in vertebral numbering and correlate plain films with cross-sectional imaging.

SACROILIAC, COCCYGEAL DEGENERATIVE DISEASE

Osteoarthritis of the sacroiliac joints may be seen in pathologic specimens of young adults, but is not generally appreciable radiographically until middle age. Changes of cartilage degeneration are more prominent on the iliac side of the joint. Beyond age 40 years, many patients have detectable narrowing of the sacroiliac joint, especially in its inferior portion. This may be accompanied by subchondral sclerosis and osteophyte formation, most prominent anteriorly and inferiorly. A vacuum phenomenon may be seen. The joint may undergo fibrous ankylosis over time. Intra-articular bony ankylosis is unusual as a manifestation of osteoarthritis; it is more typical of the inflammatory spondyloarthropathies. Osteoarthritic changes are evident on plain films; CT or MRI is more sensitive. It is unclear, however, that detection of typical changes of osteoarthritis radiographically is useful in identifying patients with a sacroiliac pain syndrome.

There is no gold standard for the diagnosis of sacroiliac joint pain. Medical history and physical examination provocative maneuvers have not been capable of consistently identifying painful sacroiliac joints.[105] Diagnostic blocks with local anesthetic are frequently cited as a means of identifying the painful sacroiliac joint, but, as in the lumbar facets, there may be a significant placebo effect. Maigne and colleagues[106] noted a 17% false-positive rate for single blocks, when compared with a double block technique. Intra-articular sacroiliac blocks may also be technically challenging, with not infrequent extra-articular spill of injectate and loss of specificity of the procedure. Attempts to establish the prevalence of sacroiliac pain have largely used response to intra-articular blocks as the means of diagnosis. Schwarzer and colleagues[107] studied patients with chronic low back pain experienced below the lumbosacral junction. Using response to single blocks as the diagnostic criteria for sacroiliac pain yielded a prevalence of 30%. Requiring a positive block and a ventral capsular tear on postarthrographic CT yielded a prevalence of 21%; adding pain provocation with joint distention to the criteria lowered prevalence to 16%. The Maigne study using double blocks suggested a prevalence of 18.5%.[106] An older series using clinical diagnostic end points suggested a 22.5% prevalence of sacroiliac pain among patients with chronic low back pain.[108]

The prevalence of sacroiliac pain among patients with chronic axial low back pain is thus probably between 15% and 25%,[105] but history, physical examination, and plain radiographs are not very helpful in making this diagnosis. The most commonly used gold standard (intra-articular blocks) is known to be flawed. It is not too surprising that advanced imaging has not leant clarity to the issue. Radionuclide bone scans have been shown to have sensitivities of 46% and 13%, although with high specificity, in the studies of Maigne and Slipman and colleagues,

respectively.[109,110] Elgafy and coworkers showed CT imaging to have a sensitivity of 58% and a specificity of 69%.[111] MRI-based studies have primarily focused on active inflammatory disease in the spondyloarthropathies. Given the paucity of supporting literature, it is difficult to suggest advanced imaging of the pelvis to detect sacroiliac osteoarthritis or manifestations of sacroiliac dysfunction. The primary purpose of imaging in this setting is to exclude the more sinister pathology of tumor, inflammatory spondyloarthropathy, or sacral insufficiency fracture. These are discussed later in the chapter.

The radiographic evaluation of the sacrococcygeal region in patients with coccydynia remains controversial. This largely female pain syndrome is probably multifactorial in origin with contributions by somatic and neuropathic pain.[112] A single lateral view of the coccyx to evaluate for destructive bony lesions is a reasonable screening study. Maigne and associates have described a dynamic radiographic study to more fully evaluate the mobility of the coccyx.[113] This consists of a lateral radiograph with the patient standing for 10 minutes to visualize the coccyx without load, followed by a sitting lateral view, with the patient altering the pelvic position to that which stimulates their usual pain. Maigne and colleagues have studied coccygeal mobility, and suggested that a normal coccyx may undergo from 5 to 25 degrees of angulation in moving from a standing to a sitting position. Flexion of the coccyx by more than 25 degrees with sitting, or posterior subluxation of the coccyx with sitting and reduction with standing, are considered pathologic and may be the anatomic basis of coccydynia.[113,114] Aggressive treatment decisions based on this evaluation are controversial. Advanced imaging has little role in this setting unless there is clinical suspicion of underlying systemic disease.

THORACIC DEGENERATIVE DISEASE

Symptomatic thoracic disk disease is uncommon; operation for symptomatic thoracic disk disease constitutes less than 1% to 2% of disk surgeries.[115] As noted in the discussion of lumbar degenerative disease, there also is a high rate of asymptomatic degenerative disk disease in the thoracic region. Wood and coworkers studied 90 asymptomatic patients with MRI.[116] In this population, 73% of the patients had positive thoracic imaging findings; 37% had disk herniations, 53% demonstrated disk bulges, 58% exhibited annular tears, and asymptomatic cord deformity was present in 29%. In a follow-up study the same authors reexamined a subgroup of their asymptomatic patients.[117] This showed that there was little demonstrable change over time in the size of asymptomatic disk herniations. There was a nonstatistically significant trend for small herniations to increase in size and for large herniations to diminish. New asymptomatic herniations appeared within the follow-up interval; no herniations became symptomatic.

The majority of symptomatic thoracic degenerative disk disease occurs in the mid and lower thoracic

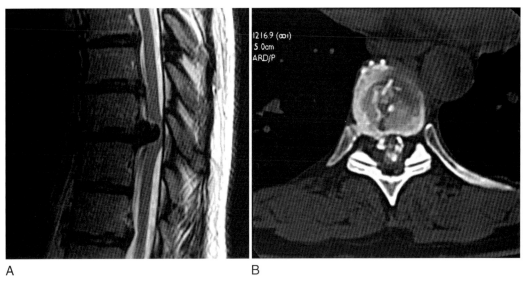

Figure 12–25. Thoracic disk extrusion in a 56-year-old woman with progressive thoracic myelopathy. Sagittal T2-weighted MRI **(A)** shows large T8 disk extrusion. Very low signal suggests calcification. Smaller T7 disk extrusion. Calcified disk extrusion confirmed on CT image at T8 level **(B).** At surgery the T8 extrusion had perforated the dura, but it was successfully resected.

spine. In the surgical series of Levi and colleagues, T6 and T7 were the most common levels of operation.[115] In the larger series of Stillerman and associates (82 patients), the T8 through T11 levels most commonly required intervention.[118] In this series, 76% of patients presented with pain, 61% with either motor or sensory dysfunction, and 24% with bladder dysfunction. Nearly two thirds of the disk herniations showed evidence of calcification on CT imaging (Fig. 12–25). At surgery, 7% showed intradural extension. Thoracic disk herniations at the level of the conus or high cauda equina can mimic lumbar radicular disease.[119] For this reason, it may be wise to include the conus on lumbar MRI examinations.

Imaging of thoracic degenerative disk disease is the province of MRI or CT myelography. As the central canal and vertebral bodies diminish in size in the thoracic region, spatial and contrast resolution become more critical. CT myelography has the greatest spatial resolution and may better demonstrate the presence of calcification within thoracic disks. MRI is noninvasive and can detect signal abnormality within the cord, which may serve as a marker of cord edema or venous hypertension, verifying the physiologic significance of a disk herniation. All imaging evaluation for thoracic disk disease must include careful enumeration of the segmental level involved. If a lesion that may require surgical or percutaneous intervention is detected, the imaging study should be extended to include sagittal images from the sacrum or skull base (or both) to the thoracic lesion. Communication between radiologist and surgeon or spine interventionalist is critical.

Posterior column degenerative disease involving the facet and costovertebral joints in the thoracic spine has not been well studied. Patterns of paraspinal pain provoked by thoracic facet capsule distention have been described, along with techniques for intra-articular injection.[120,121] There is little literature specifically addressing imaging of painful thoracic facets. Resnick and colleagues note that osteoarthritis of thoracic facets is dominant in the upper and mid-thoracic spine, and is similar in nature to lumbar disease with cartilage degeneration leading to joint space narrowing, sclerosis of subchondral bone, and osteophyte formation.[33] The coronal orientation of thoracic facets makes these osteoarthritic changes difficult to detect on plain radiographs. Such findings would be detected with greater sensitivity on axial or sagittal images obtained by CT or MRI. MRI may demonstrate marrow edema in the articular processes or joint effusion. It is reasonable to believe, however, that a similar lack of correlation between a painful joint and morphologic degenerative change exists in the thoracic spine, as has been well demonstrated in the lumbar spine. Nuclear medicine technetium scanning, and STIR or postgadolinium fat-saturated MRI images, can demonstrate active inflammatory disease in the thoracic facets and costovertebral joints in the clinical experience of the author.

Costovertebral and costotransverse joints are synovial joints and may also undergo degenerative change. They have been shown to have nociceptive innervation.[122] Degenerative changes of joint space narrowing, sclerosis, and osteophytes are especially prevalent at the T11 and T12 levels.[33] These changes may progress to bony ankylosis. Costovertebral and costotransverse degeneration is difficult to appreciate on plain films, and will be detected with greater sensitivity on CT, MRI, or technetium scanning. The use of advanced imaging in the detection of costovertebral-mediated pain has not been studied.

CERVICAL DEGENERATIVE DISEASE

As in the lumbar region, asymptomatic degenerative disease in the cervical spine increases with increasing age. Matsumoto and coworkers studied nearly 500 asymptomatic patients with MRI; he noted cervical disk degeneration in 12% to 17% of patients in their 20s, but in 86% to 89% of patients older than 60 years of age.[123] Asymptomatic cervical cord compression was seen in 7.6% of patients, mostly older than age 50 years. Similarly, Boden and colleagues studied 63 asymptomatic patients with MRI and noted disk degeneration in 25% of those younger than 40, and in excess of 60% of patients older than 40 years.[124] Patients older than 40 years of age had a 5% rate of disk herniations and a 20% rate of foraminal stenosis. Teresi and associates studied 100 asymptomatic patients with MRI and noted asymptomatic cervical cord compression in 7% and either disk protrusion or annular bulge in 57% of patients older than 64 years of age.[125] Humphreys and coworkers studied the cervical neural foramen in patients age 20 to 60 years using MRI.[126] Foraminal height changes little with age. Foraminal width diminishes with age due to hypertrophy of the superior articular process, decreasing the foraminal cross-sectional area and rendering the exiting root more susceptible to compression.

The natural history of cervical disk herniations parallels that of the lumbar region. Cervical disk herniations may undergo spontaneous regression, a finding that correlates with improvement in patients' symptoms.[127] As in the lumbar region, extrusions, migrated disk material, and laterally situated disk herniations are more likely to undergo spontaneous regression.[128]

Imaging evaluation of the cervical region is in evolution. CT myelography has traditionally been the gold standard for evaluation of the cervical canal and the cervical neural foramina due to its excellent spatial resolution and its ability to distinguish bone from soft disk (Fig. 12–26). Improved multiplanar capability of multislice CT scanners has negated advantages previously held by MRI. MRI has acknowledged superior soft tissue contrast, is noninvasive, and is the most common initial advanced imaging modality at this time. Because of the evolving nature of the technology, older studies in the literature are of limited value. In a recent study by Bartlett and coworkers, a gold standard of the combined imaging information from the CT myelogram and complete MRI examination was used.[129] With this as the reference, the CT myelogram and the MRI examination each yielded an approximately 90% accuracy rate. MRI was less effective than CT in distinguishing between encroachment on neural structures due to bone or disk. Shafaie and associates found only moderate agreement between CT myelography and MRI in the characterization of cervical central canal and foraminal stenosis.[130] The examinations were viewed as complementary.

The noninvasive character of MRI and its relatively high accuracy in the detection of significant central canal and foraminal compromise suggests its use as the primary imaging tool in suspected root compressive degenerative disease of the cervical spine (Fig. 12–27). MRI is clearly the imaging tool of choice for suspected intrinsic cord disease. CT myelography should be brought to bear when there are discrepancies between the clinical syndrome and the morphology demonstrated on MRI, or when discrimination of bone versus soft tissue impingement may change an operative approach.

In evaluation of cervical central canal stenosis, studies by Singh[131] and Wada[132] have suggested that measured cross-sectional area of the cord at the site of maximal compression is an imaging feature providing correlation with severity of the clinical myelopathy. It is also an indicator of ultimate recovery following decompression. MRI detection of elevated T2 signal within the cord at the site of compression is also an important imaging finding for clinically significant cord compression. There is discrepancy in the literature as to whether this is a positive or negative predictive factor for ultimate outcome. Increased T2 signal in the cord likely reflects a spectrum of pathologic change ranging from reversible edema to fixed cystic myelomalacia or syrinx formation. When low T1 cord signal is present accompanying elevated T2 signal, the prognosis for improvement with surgical decompression is poor, suggesting this signal pattern represents irreversible injury.[133,134] In those cases with only increased T2 cord signal, this is likely reversible edema or demyelination when the signal abnormality is faint and poorly marginated, whereas clearly demarcated, intense T2 cord signal abnormality is more likely to reflect irreversible injury such as cystic necrosis.[135] Multilevel T2 signal abnormality within the cord is a significant negative prognostic sign for outcome.[132] Metabolic imaging with FDG PET scanning has been shown to correlate strongly with neurologic dysfunction and may play a role in selecting patients for decompression in the future.[136]

The presence of congenital narrowing of the bony cervical spinal canal will also exacerbate symptoms in patients with soft disk protrusions. A study by Debois and coworkers noted that the degree and severity of neurologic symptoms associated with soft disk herniations was inversely related to the sagittal diameter and the area of the bony cervical canal.[137] Patients with motor dysfunction had significantly smaller sagittal canal dimensions than did patients with pain only.[137]

The cervical spine is also a dynamic biomechanical entity. In an MRI study using a device allowing graded flexion and extension, there was a significant increase in central canal stenosis in the extension position in 48% of patients and in the flexion position in 24% compared with neutral positioning.[138] Cord compromise was identified in 20% of patients in extension and 11% in flexion. It is also known that the cervical neural foraminal dimensions diminish with extension but increase slightly in flexion. Routine dynamic imaging is only now becoming readily available, and the indications for its use have not been clearly established.

Axial pain in the cervical spine may arise from the anterior or posterior columns and may have somatic referral patterns that mimic radicular pain. Posterior column pain arising from the cervical facet joints has been well studied by numerous investigators, primarily Bogduk and colleagues at University of Newcastle.

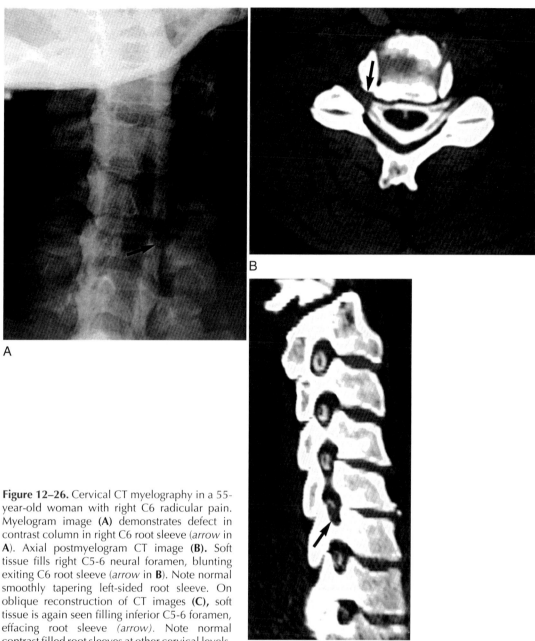

Figure 12–26. Cervical CT myelography in a 55-year-old woman with right C6 radicular pain. Myelogram image **(A)** demonstrates defect in contrast column in right C6 root sleeve (*arrow* in **A**). Axial postmyelogram CT image **(B).** Soft tissue fills right C5-6 neural foramen, blunting exiting C6 root sleeve (*arrow* in **B**). Note normal smoothly tapering left-sided root sleeve. On oblique reconstruction of CT images **(C),** soft tissue is again seen filling inferior C5-6 foramen, effacing root sleeve (*arrow*). Note normal contrast filled root sleeves at other cervical levels. Soft disk filled inferior foramen at surgery.

Cervical intra-articular injections, medial branch blocks, and radiofrequency neurotomy are discussed elsewhere. As in the lumbar spine, imaging plays only a modest role in identifying painful cervical facets. Cervical facet osteoarthritis is seen on plain radiographs as sclerosis and osteophyte formation in the lateral and frontal views. CT detects these findings with greater sensitivity, but the specificity caveat persists: most degenerative findings are asymptomatic. On MRI, facet degenerative disease can be seen as increased fluid in the joint space, marrow edema (low T1 and high T2 signal) in the articular processes, and intrafacet and perifacet gadolinium enhancement, best seen on fat-saturated images. High T2 signal on STIR images and facet enhancement may provide a means of identifying the painful facet in the authors' experience, but this has not been well studied. High metabolic activity localized to a facet on SPECT technetium scanning may also mark a painful facet, but this is not well validated against medial branch blocks.

Cervical discogenic pain, as in the lumbar region, is best identified with provocation discography. Plain films, CT, and MRI will all identify cervical disk degeneration in asymptomatic patients. MRI evidence of disk degeneration does not correlate well with positive provocation discography; in Zheng and colleagues' study, only 63% of disks showing uniform low T2 signal had positive discography.[139] Disks with heterogeneous signal were positive on provocation discography in only 45%. Disks that were normal on MRI were also identified as pain generators. In this series, MRI had a false-positive rate of 51% and a false-negative rate of 27% relative to discography. This

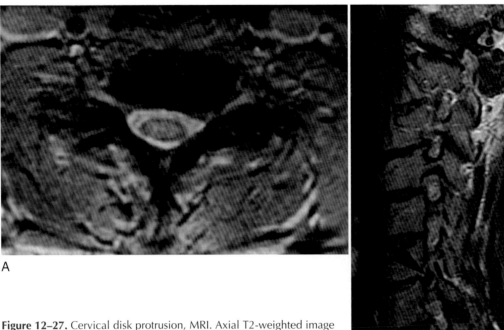

Figure 12–27. Cervical disk protrusion, MRI. Axial T2-weighted image **(A)** at C6 interspace suggests bilateral foraminal narrowing. Oblique T2-weighted image **(B)** more definitively demonstrates left C6/7 foraminal compromise due to disk and/or cartilaginous capping of end plate hypertrophy *(arrow)*. Patient was treated conservatively.

corroborates older studies.[140] Reproduction of concordant pain on provocation discography is the best existing, albeit imperfect, means of targeting disks for operative therapy or, perhaps more importantly, disqualifying patients from surgical intervention when several disks are pain generators. Cervical provocation discography is more technically demanding than its lumbar analog due to the proximity of the carotid sheath, esophagus, and larynx. One small series reported a complication rate of 13%[141]; larger series by Grubb[142] and Guyer and associates[143] reported 2.3% and 2.5% complication rates, respectively. Meticulous needle placement, prophylactic antibiotics, and careful patient selection are mandatory. ISIS guidelines may be consulted for specific recommendations regarding patient selection and procedural issues.

The fluoroscopic or CT images obtained in cervical discography are of less diagnostic value than in the lumbar region; the primary utility is to verify nuclear injection. The cervical disk has no posterior annulus; the nuclear compartment is essentially in contact with the posterior longitudinal ligament. Extravasation of contrast material from the disk occurred in nearly 50% of disks in asymptomatic volunteers in Schellhas and coworkers' study.[140] Such phenomena are likely simply age-related changes. Available evidence provides no good correlation between discographic appearance and pain provocation. Demonstration of disk fissuring or contrast extravasation is immaterial; only concordant pain provocation is of diagnostic value.

As in the lumbar region, provoked concordant pain must be of significant intensity. ISIS guidelines require a pain intensity of 7 on a 10-point scale for diagnosis. Evoked concordant pain of 7/10 intensity is only useful in the presence of nonpainful adjacent disks; controls must be used. A study by Bogduk and Aprill suggested that patients cannot discriminate between discogenic pain and facet-mediated pain at the same segmental level.[144] Therefore facet-mediated pain should by excluded by medial branch blocks before cervical discography.

Cervical discogenic pain is often multilevel. Grubb and Kelly[142] noted three or more discographically positive levels in 47% of patients in their large series; they recommend study of all accessible levels. Recognizing the potential increased risks of this practice, ISIS recommends injection of four cervical levels. The C2/3 level should be assessed when occipital headache is a major part of the pain syndrome. Similarly, the recent study by Slipman and colleagues[145] maps pain syndromes by segmental level, potentially allowing a more focused, and safer, discography study.

In summary, identifying cervical discogenic pain, and the targeting of its therapy, cannot be guided by anatomic imaging alone. Provocation discography is imperfect and subjective, and carries not insignificant risk. It is, however, the only means of directing operative therapy for discogenic pain, or avoiding futile operation in the patient with extensive multilevel disease.

INFLAMMATORY SPINE DISEASE

Noninfectious inflammatory disease of the spine includes rheumatoid arthritis (RA) and the seronegative spondyloarthropathies (SpA). Ankylosing spondylitis is the SpA prototype; this group also includes psoriatic arthritis, Reiter's syndrome, the spondyloarthritis of inflammatory bowel disease, and the SAPHO syndrome (synovitis, acne, pustulosis, hyperostosis, and osteitis). These diverse entities have spine involvement in common and may present with axial back pain. This discussion is limited to their spinal manifestations.

Rheumatoid arthritis is most common in the cervical spine, sometimes referred to as the fifth limb in RA patients. Symptoms and signs of cervical spine involvement are present in 60% to 80% of RA patients.[32] The most frequent site of involvement is the atlantoaxial articulation. Inflammatory pannus may be seen on MRI as a low T1, high T2 signal, enhancing mass posterior to the dens. This may cause central canal stenosis with compression of the cervicomedullary junction. The inflammatory change may destroy the transverse and alar ligaments resulting in atlantoaxial instability in 20% to 25% of RA patients.[32] A distance of greater than 2.5 to 3 mm between the posterior arch of C1 and the cortical surface of the dens on radiographs is abnormal; this is most evident in flexion views. The destruction of supporting structures at the craniocervical junction may also result in cranial settling, a vertical migration of the dens into the foramen magnum, with possible compression of C1 and C2 cranial nerves, the medulla, and vertebral arteries. There may also be lateral subluxation of the dens relative to C1 and erosion of the dens itself.

The cervical spine below the C1/C2 articulation demonstrates erosive arthritis in the uncovertebral and facet joints in RA patients. The inflammatory change can be demonstrated on MRI as increased T2 signal on STIR sequences and as gadolinium enhancement on fat-saturated T1 sequences. This results in multilevel instability, with anterior subluxation of successive vertebral bodies in flexion, the so-called "step ladder" cervical spine, seen in up to 30% of RA patients.[146] Disk space narrowing and end plate sclerosis are common, but this may be a secondary phenomenon to the posterior element instability.[32]

Involvement of the thoracic and lumbar spine in RA is uncommonly seen on imaging. Synovitis and erosive change may be present in the facet and costovertebral joints, but it is inconstant and not well demonstrated. Discovertebral changes may be present, but it is again unclear if these are primary inflammatory lesions or a response to facet instability. The sacroiliac joints may show inflammatory change, but with much less frequency and severity than in ankylosing spondylitis patients.

Ankylosing spondylitis is the prototypical seronegative spondyloarthropathy; imaging is integral to its diagnosis. The modified New York criteria require imaging evidence of sacroiliitis for diagnosis.[146] Ankylosing spondylitis has a prevalence of up to 0.1% in the general population; a very high percentage of these people are HLA B27 positive.[32] Males dominate by 4:1. The disease involves synovial and cartilaginous joints and entheses (ligament and tendon insertions on bone) with a strong predilection for the axial skeleton. The most common presentation is low back pain with inflammatory features (Calin criteria, 4 out of 5 of the following: insidious onset, age younger than 40 years, 3 months persistence, morning stiffness, and pain improved by exercise). Radiating pain mimicking sciatica may be seen in up to 50% of patients.[32]

Imaging findings in ankylosing spondylitis include sacroiliitis, ultimately bilaterally symmetric (although its initial presentation may be asymmetric in 10%), and multiple manifestations of spondylitis (Fig. 12–28). Sacroiliitis is the initial imaging finding in 99% of cases.[147] Early plain film findings of sacroiliitis are blurring of the subchondral cortex and small erosions, predominantly on the iliac side of the joint. As the erosions coalesce, the joint space appears widened and ill-defined; sclerotic reaction develops in the trabecular bone about both sides of the joint. Over time the joint undergoes ankylosis via direct bony bridging; the joint space is no longer visible and the sclerosis resolves. Plain films can detect these structural changes (erosions, sclerosis, ankylosis) with a sensitivity equal to MRI.[148] MRI, however, can detect inflammation in and about the sacroiliac joint in symptomatic patients with normal plain films.[148] Inflammation can be reliably identified with low interobserver variability as high T2 signal on STIR sequences or gadolinium enhancement on fat-saturated T1 images.[149] In patients with recent onset axial low back pain with inflammatory clinical characteristics, sacroiliac joint inflammation may be detected by MRI in one third of patients and structural changes in one sixth of patients.[149] Inflammation is initially seen in the iliac side of the joint at its caudal and dorsal aspects, and in the adjacent dorsal entheses.[150] STIR sequences may have equal or greater sensitivity to inflammatory changes than gadolinium enhancement[151,152]; avoiding contrast will reduce cost and imaging time. Baraliakos and associates, however, noted better interobserver variability with gadolinium-enhanced studies.[151]

The spine findings in ankylosing spondylitis include osteitis, syndesmophyte formation, diskovertebral lesions, and inflammation leading to ankylosis of facet and costovertebral joints. Osteitis is seen at the anterior margins of the diskovertebral junction, termed the *Romanus lesion*.[153] On plain films, sclerosis at these sites leads to increased density of the anterior corners of the vertebra, termed the "shiny corners" sign.[32] Remodeling of the anterior margin of the vertebral body due to osteitis straightens the normally concave anterior vertebral margin, termed "squaring" of the vertebra. These findings are most evident in the lumbar region. MRI is more sensitive to the early detection of osteitis, seen as diminished T1 and increased T2 signal and enhancement at the anterior vertebral corners.[153] Osteitis at the margins of the diskovertebral junctions leads to reactive bone formation in the outer annulus fibrosis, which ultimately bridges the margins of adjacent vertebrae.

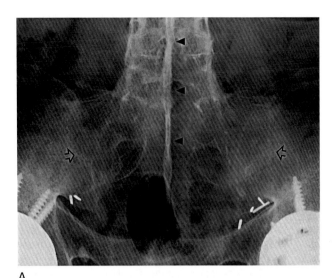

A

Figure 12–28. Ankylosing spondylitis in an older man with longstanding back pain and stiffness. In **A,** frontal view of pelvis shows fusion of sacroiliac joints *(open arrows)*. Note syndesmophytes bridging lumbar bodies and osseous bridging of interspinous ligament *(arrowheads)*. Frontal **(B)** and lateral **(C)** chest films show syndesmophytes bridging entire thoracic spine. In coronal CT reconstruction **(D),** vertically oriented syndesmophytes are well seen *(arrowheads)*. Note typical osteopenia in all images; on the CT image, marrow is of lower density than disks.

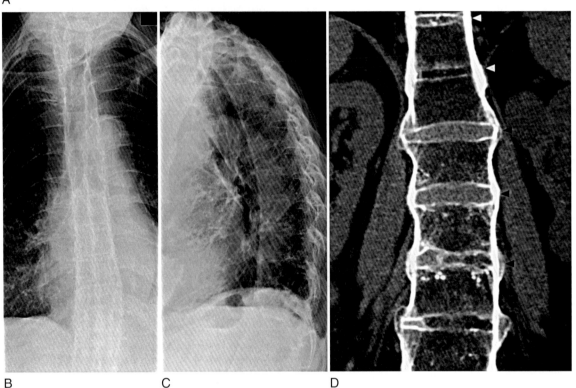

B   C   D

These vertically oriented bony struts are syndesmophytes. They are distinguished from osteophytes by their vertical orientation and gracile nature; osteophytes are oriented in the horizontal plane and are bulkier. Syndesmophytes are most common at the anterior and lateral aspects of the vertebral body; when long-standing, the ossification may involve the anterior longitudinal ligament.

Erosions at the diskovertebral junction are termed "Andersson" lesions; they are categorized as type I when focal and central, type II when focal and marginal, and type III when extensive, involving the entire diskovertebral junction. They represent inflammatory destruction of portions of the vertebral end plate and intravertebral disk displacement; type III lesions may be pseudarthroses. End plate destruction is seen on plain films; MRI demonstrates structural and inflammatory change. The inflammatory change will undergo evolution similar to that seen in Modic degenerative end plate change: initial high T2 and low T1 signal with gadolinium enhancement followed by fatty marrow replacement with high T1 and high T2 signal.[146] Over time there is sclerosis and transdiskal ossification leading to ankylosis. The facet and costovertebral joints show similar findings, with initial periarticular erosions followed by sclerosis and ankylosis. These findings may be difficult to appreciate on plain films; they are more evident on CT or MRI. Enthesitis of the posterior interspinous and supraspinous ligament attachments ultimately leads to ossification of these structures, seen as a vertical midline bony band on frontal radiographs, the so-called dagger sign.[32]

The inflammatory spinal lesions are most common in the midthoracic (T7/8) spine and in the mid-lumbar region (L2/3).[152] Spine disease burden in ankylosing spondylitis may be quantitated on plain films by the modified Stoke Ankylosing Spondylitis Spine Score (mSASS). Structural and inflammatory disease on MRI may be measured by the Ankylosing Spondylitis spine MRI chronicity (ASspi MRI-c) and the Ankylosing Spondylitis spine MRI acuity (ASspiMRI-a) scales respectively.[153] The MRI scoring systems may be used to monitor therapy with anti-tumor necrosis factor α agents (etanercept and inflix-imab). Use of the ASspiMRI-a scale documented diminished spine inflammation paralleling clinical improvement in patients treated with etanercept.[154]

Ankylosing spondylitis may also produce changes at the atlantoaxial articulation. Synovitis may result in erosive changes in the dens, although the extent of inflammatory change seldom reaches that seen in RA. Atlantoaxial subluxation may be present. The extensive ankylosis seen in patients with longstanding ankylosing spondylitis leads to flattening of the lumbar lordosis and exaggeration of the thoracic kyphosis. The rigidity places these patients at risk for catastrophic fracture-dislocations with modest trauma, most commonly with a hyperextension mechanism. The cervical spine is most frequently involved; neurologic deficits are common. Plain film evaluation is difficult due to the osteopenia typical of these patients; the three-column nature of these fractures is best appreciated with CT or MRI. The threshold for use of advanced imaging in the AS patient with trauma should be low. Three-column fractures that do not cause acute neurologic injury or go undetected may be a cause of chronic focal pain as a pseudarthrosis (type III diskovertebral lesion). MRI shows a linear zone of inflammatory change, often through a disk space with extension through the posterior elements. The cortical disruption may be best appreciated on CT. Finally, some ankylosing spondylitis patients have findings of dural ectasia. (Fig. 12–29). The thecal sac is abnormally capacious with diverticular-like outpouchings; there is associated bony erosion in the posterior elements, and medial margins of the pedicles and the posterior vertebral body. Such patients may present with a cauda equina syndrome, perhaps related to arachnoiditis.

Psoriatic arthritis is far less common than ankylosing spondylitis; it affects 5% to 8% of all patients with psoriasis.[147] Approximately 10% to 25% of patients with moderate to severe skin disease will have abnormal sacroiliac joint radiographs. Spondylitis is present in a roughly similar proportion, but

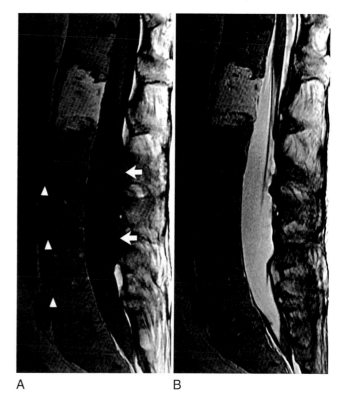

A   B

Figure 12–29. Dural ectasia in a patient with ankylosing spondylitis. Hemangioma L1. Sagittal T1 (**A**) and T2 (**B**) images of lumbar spine. Note expanded dural sac with irregular erosion of posterior elements of L2 through L4 (*arrows* in **A**). Note bridging syndesmophytes throughout the lumbar region with loss of normal dark cortical line at anterior margins of vertebral end plates (*arrowheads*). Hemangioma at L1 extends into perceived disk spaces; disk spaces have been replaced by marrow in this ankylosed spine. Note the hemangioma has characteristic elevated T1 and T2 signal due to fat content.

may or may not coexist with sacroiliitis.[32] Males and females are equally affected.[147] The sacroiliitis is usually bilateral but asymmetric, with a lesser tendency to progress to bony ankylosis. Erosions and foci of reactive sclerosis tend to be larger and more discrete than in ankylosing spondylitis. The spondylitis in psoriatic arthritis is characterized by asymmetric, coarse paravertebral ossification more resembling osteophytes than syndesmophytes. Vertebral squaring and shiny corners are absent. Facet involvement is infrequent. Cervical spine involvement exceeds that of the thoracic or lumbar spine. Atlantoaxial instability is common.

Reiter's syndrome describes an inflammatory arthropathy, primarily in males, that may affect the spine in association with the urethritis and conjunctivitis. Sacroiliitis is very common, affecting up to 75% of patients with chronic disease. It is more commonly unilateral or asymmetric than is ankylosing spondylitis, but less likely to result in ankylosis.[32] Spine involvement is less frequent than in ankylosing spondylitis or psoriatic arthritis and most frequently resembles the latter in its character. The

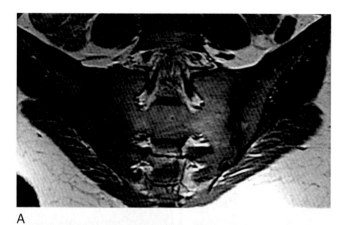

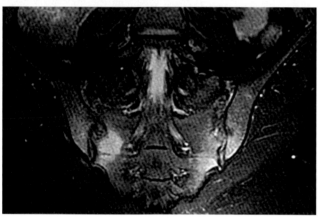

Figure 12–30. Sacroiliitis in a young female patient with low back and buttock pain. Coronal T1-weighted MRI (**A**) shows low signal on both sacral and iliac sides of both sacroiliac joints. Coronal fat-saturated T2-weighted MRI (**B**) shows corresponding high signal about both sacroiliac joints. Findings are consistent with marrow edema of inflammatory sacroiliitis.

thoracolumbar junction is most frequently involved; cervical involvement in uncommon.

Spondyloarthropathies may also be seen in association with ulcerative colitis, Crohn's disease, and Whipple's disease. The initial presentation of back pain may precede symptoms of gastrointestinal disease. The spondylitis and sacroiliitis seen in association with these conditions are indistinguishable from classic ankylosing spondylitis (Fig. 12–30). Sacroiliitis is usually bilaterally symmetric, progressing to ankylosis; spondylitic findings of vertebral squaring, diskovertebral lesions, syndesmophytes, and involvement of the facet joints are typical.

The SAPHO syndrome describes the association of synovitis, acne, pustulosis, hyperostosis, and osteitis. The skin lesions of palmar and plantar pustulosis are distinctive. Considered by some to be a multifocal infectious process due to *Propionibacterium acnes,* it may be the adult expression of the pediatric syndrome of chronic recurrent multifocal osteomyelitis (CRMO). The anterior chest wall is most frequently involved in the SAPHO syndrome, with synovitis and hyperostosis involving the sternoclavicular, cos-

tosternal, and manubriosternal junctions. Spine involvement is that of a spondylodiskitis, most commonly in the thoracic region. Plain films show end plate and vertebral corner erosions, sclerosis of vertebral bodies, disk space narrowing, osteophyte or syndesmophyte formation, and paravertebral ossification.[155] On MRI, elevated T2 and decreased T1 signal and enhancement is seen adjacent to vertebral end plates, within disks, and in paravertebral soft tissues[156] (Fig. 12–31). The imaging findings may closely resemble granulomatous (tubercular) spondylodiskitis. The sacroiliac joints are commonly involved, with extensive sclerosis on the iliac side of the joint.[155]

SPINE TRAUMA: SPONDYLOLYSIS

It is beyond the scope of this chapter to address imaging of all facets of spine trauma. We discuss spondylolysis, compression fractures, sacral insufficiency fractures, and pseudarthroses as lesions most frequently encountered in pain management. Isthmic spondylolysis describes a defect in the pars interarticularis, which may be unilateral or bilateral. It is considered a fatigue fracture occurring within a deficient pars; the deficiency may be related to the distribution of ossification centers within the posterior neural arch.[156] Spondylolysis has a familial predisposition; it is known to be more common in the Japanese, Inuit, and white populations. There is a 2-4:1 male-to-female predominance.[32] The incidence of isthmic spondylolysis has been estimated at 7% in the U.S. population.[157] Isthmic spondylolysis is frequently asymptomatic, but it is a particular clinical issue in adolescent athletes. A retrospective study of lumbar radiographs in more than 4000 athletes demonstrated a 13.9% rate of spondylolysis with concomitant spondylolisthesis in 47%.[158] Spondylolysis occurs most commonly at the L5 level (67%) followed by the L4 level (15% to 20%), and L3 (1% to 2%). It is unusual in the cervical region, where it is most often seen at the C6 level. Spondylolysis is extremely rare in the infant population but appears to develop in childhood or adolescence, with no significant change in its incidence beyond age 20.[32]

Although considered a fatigue fracture, it is unusual in that there is seldom an effective healing response, and the bony defect is persistent. The pars defect is frequently a synovial-lined pseudoarthrosis. Shipley and Beukes demonstrated that injection of the facet immediately superiorly to a pars defect showed communication with the pars defect cavity in 30 of 32 facets, with communication to the next most inferior facet in 20 of 32 facets.[159] The presence of synovial fluid in the defect likely contributes to its diminished capacity to heal.

Radiographic findings of isthmic spondylolysis are often evident on lateral or oblique plain films in which a radiolucent band can be directly visualized across the pars interarticularis, with or without a sclerotic margin. There is seldom callus present. CT allows direct visualization of the pars defect immedi-

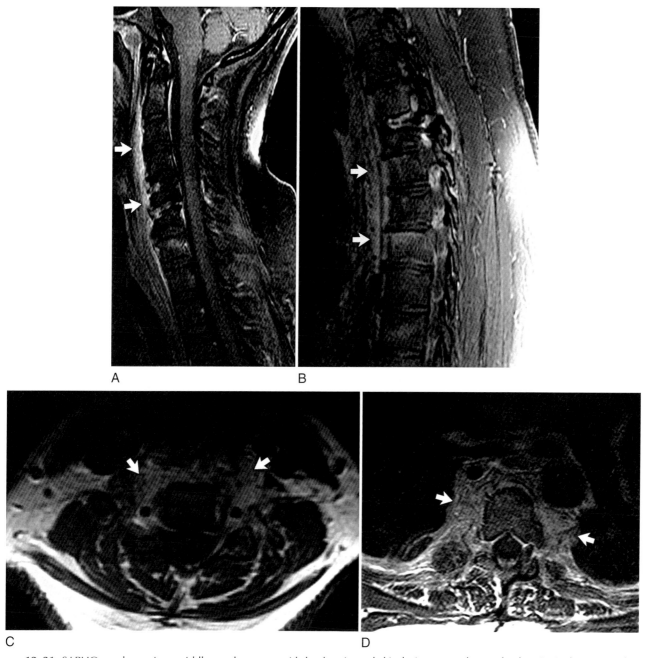

Figure 12–31. SAPHO syndrome in a middle-aged woman with back pain and skin lesions on palms and soles. Sagittal **(A, B)** and axial **(C, D)** postcontrast fat-saturated T1 images of cervical and thoracic spine. Extensive enhancement (high signal) at vertebral end plates, within multiple disks, and in paraspinal tissues *(arrows)*. The findings are those of a spondylodiskitis. Differential diagnosis would include pyogenic or tubercular infection and inflammatory spondyloarthropathies. Clinical context is key to the diagnosis.

ately superior to the closely associated facet on axial images (Fig. 15–32). Sagittal reconstructions make the defect more obvious. Care must be taken to distinguish between a true pars defect and a badly degenerated facet. The defect in the pars interarticularis can be directly visualized on sagittal MRI images, although normal intact pars are sometimes difficult to identify, leading to a potential false-positive diagnosis of spondylolysis. Several ancillary signs have been described on MRI, including (1) an increase in the sagittal diameter of the central canal at the level of the pars defect, (2) reactive marrow changes within

the adjacent pedicle, and (3) wedging of the posterior aspect of the associated vertebral body, usually L5.[160] Reactive marrow changes in a vertebral pedicle are not specific for the presence of spondylolysis and may be seen in the presence of adjacent facet disease.[161] The defect in the pars is frequently associated with a fibrocartilaginous mass; Major and colleagues described fibrocartilaginous masses associated with 90% of pars defects.[157] In 20% of patients, the fibrocartilaginous mass was of sufficient size to cause thecal sac compression requiring surgical intervention. Although adult isthmic spondylolysis is often

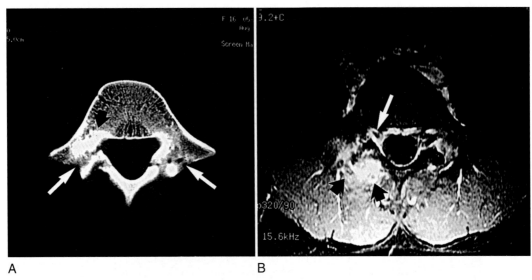

A   B

Figure 12–32. Spondylolysis in a 16-year-old female patient with right L5 radicular pain. Axial CT image at L5 **(A)** shows bilateral pars defects *(white arrows)*. Note sclerotic reaction in right pedicle *(black arrow)*. Gadolinium-enhanced fat-saturated axial MRI at L5 **(B)** demonstrates enhancing inflammatory mass *(black arrows)* about right pars defect. Inflammatory enhancement surrounds right L5 root entering neural foramen *(white arrow)*.

asymptomatic, there is a tendency to develop significant disk degeneration at the level of the pars defect which may result in late progression of the degree of vertebral displacement and neural element compromise due to central canal or more commonly foraminal stenosis.[162] The neural compromise can generally be well demonstrated with MRI (Fig. 15–33). Spondylolysis patients may then experience axial pain due to the inflammatory change about the pars defect, discogenic pain from the failed disk, or radicular pain from secondary foraminal compromise.

SPINE TRAUMA: VERTEBRAL COMPRESSION FRACTURES

There are estimated to be in excess of 700,000 osteoporotic vertebral compression fractures in the United States per year. There is a lesser, though still substantial, number of vertebral metastatic lesions. Imaging is frequently called upon to differentiate benign from malignant compressions. Plain films and CT are of little benefit in the absence of gross destruction; the distinction may be challenging with technetium bone scan. MRI is of greatest utility in characterizing fracture etiology.

Benign osteoporotic compression fractures may be asymptomatic. Wedge fractures are most commonly located in the midthoracic spine; central end plate fractures are more commonly seen at the thoracolumbar junction and in the upper lumbar spine. Chronic benign compression fractures exhibit marrow signal similar to that of adjacent normal vertebral bodies on T1-weighted images. Acute or early subacute fractures, however, may exhibit diminished T1 signal similar to that seen in metastatic lesions. Several MRI findings have been described to attempt

differentiation of acute benign fracture versus malignant lesions.[163,164]

Malignant lesions are much more likely to exhibit diminished T1 signal throughout the entire vertebral body. Extension of diminished T1 signal to the vertebral pedicles or posterior elements is also relatively specific for malignancy. Paravertebral or epidural mass associated with a fracture is more common in malignant lesions. Posterior bowing of the vertebral body is strongly suggestive of malignancy (Fig. 15–34). Gadolinium enhancement to a level greater than that seen in normal marrow suggests a malignant lesion. Associated disk rupture or retropulsion of a bony fragment without bowing of the posterior margin of the vertebral body are features suggesting a benign lesion. Discrete cystic lesions with high T2 signal within the vertebrae are also commonly associated with benign compression fractures.

Use of these MRI findings allows accurate classification of the majority of vertebral compression fractures as benign or malignant. Myeloma remains substantially difficult to classify because vertebral compression fractures in myeloma patients may exhibit benign MRI appearances.[165] Diffusion-weighted MRI imaging may be useful in further characterization of questionable lesions. Earlier reports have been promising, although the process remains in evolution.[166,167] Where clinical concern remains, image-guided biopsy of spinal lesions provides a minimally invasive means to a histologic diagnosis.

SPINE TRAUMA: PELVIC INSUFFICIENCY FRACTURES

Pelvic insufficiency fractures are increasingly recognized as a cause of axial and somatic referred pain experienced in the low back, pelvis, groin, and proxi-

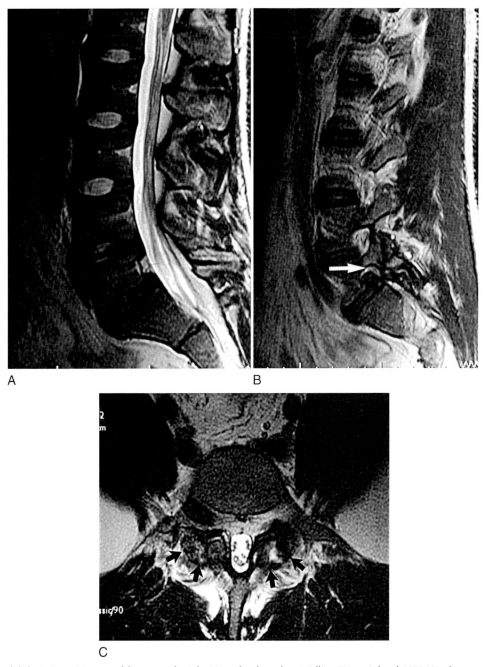

Figure 12–33. Spondylolysis in a 23-year-old man with right L5 radiculopathy. Midline T2-weighted MRI **(A)** shows anterior subluxation of L5 on the sacrum. Degenerated L4 and L5 disks. Note widened central canal at L5 and posterior wedging of L5 body, suggesting spondylolysis. Right parasagittal T1-weighted image **(B)** shows right L5 foraminal stenosis *(arrow)* due to subluxation and foraminal disk extrusion. Axial T2-weighted image **(C)** shows fibrocartilaginous masses *(arrows)* about the pars defects.

mal lower extremities. Insufficiency fractures are, by definition, fractures that occur in structurally inadequate bone, which fails when exposed to repeated normal physiologic loads. Postmenopausal osteoporosis is the dominant risk factor, along with pelvic radiation, corticosteroid use, rheumatoid arthritis, and osteomalacia. The role of osteoporosis is emphasized by the marked female predominance of these lesions, with a reported female-to-male ratio of 9:1.[168] Patients are typically in their sixth decade or older.

There is often significant morbidity associated with insufficiency fractures. Taillandier and colleagues[168] noted that 50% of their patients did not recover their former level of independence, and in 25% the insufficiency fracture precipitated institutionalization in their elderly study population. Sacral insufficiency fractures are the most common expression of this condition; pubic ramus fractures, parasymphyseal fractures, and para-acetabular fractures have also been described.

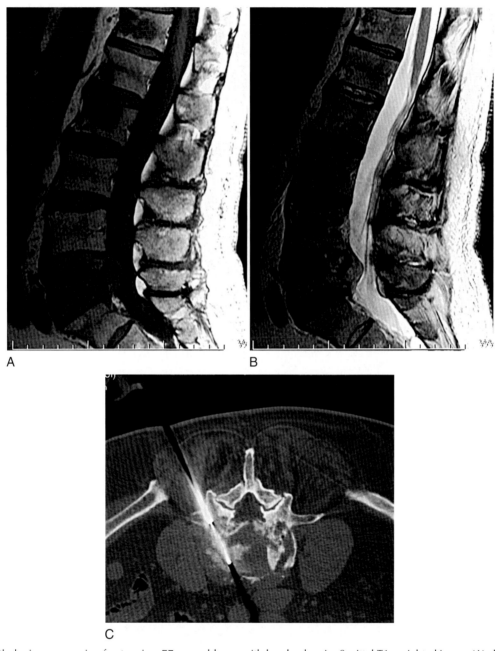

Figure 12–34. Pathologic compression fracture in a 77-year-old man with low back pain. Sagittal T1-weighted image **(A)** shows compression of L5 with bulging of its posterior wall suggesting a malignant lesion. Additional lesions in T12, L1, and L2. Sagittal T2-weighted image **(B)** better demonstrates the central canal stenosis due to expansion of the L5 body and epidural tumor extension. CT-guided biopsy **(C)** revealed B cell lymphoma.

Sacral insufficiency fractures were first described by Lourie in 1982.[169] Plain radiographs of the pelvis are relatively insensitive. The most common radiographic finding is a vertical sclerotic band in the sacral ala paralleling the sacroiliac joint representing trabecular compression and callous formation.[170] Less commonly one may see cortical disruption at the superior or inferior margins of the sacrum or directly visualize a fracture line. These are difficult findings to appreciate in the setting of osteoporotic bone and overlying bowel gas. In Grangier and colleagues' series,[170] only 25% of patients had typical plain film findings. CT is more sensitive in detecting cortical

disruption and the sclerotic margins of the fracture. Axial CT demonstrates the vertical component of the fracture. There is often a horizontal fracture line extending through the sacral body, which may be missed on axial images and which is better seen on coronal CT images.[171] Vacuum phenomenon may also be seen within the fracture.[172]

Technetium bone scan also represents a sensitive means of insufficiency fracture detection. The classic finding is the so-called Honda sign. Increased metabolic activity in bilateral vertical sacral ala fracture lines are bridged by a horizontal line representing a fracture through the sacral body, resulting in a representation of the letter H, or the insignia of the automaker. In Fujii and associates' series,[173] 63% of patients with sacral insufficiency fractures exhibited this sign in toto, with 35% showing a variant thereof such as two vertical lines without a crossbar, or a single vertical and horizontal line. In this series, the Honda sign taken with its variants had a 96% sensitivity and 92% positive predictive value for sacral insufficiency fracture. One patient with a sacral metastatic lesion did exhibit this sign. In Peh's series,[171] the complete Honda sign was not present in a majority of patients and incomplete variants were more common.

MRI is more sensitive than CT in the early detection of insufficiency fractures; MRI reveals marrow edema (low T1, high T2 signal with gadolinium enhancement) in a pattern typical of insufficiency fracture (Honda sign) before sclerosis or a fracture line can be visualized with CT.[170] Imaging in the coronal plane is preferred. Detection of increased T2 signal is improved with fat-saturated or STIR sequences (Fig. 15–35). In Grangier and colleagues' series, marrow edema was seen in all cases as early as 18 days after symptom onset.[170] Over time, the fracture line becomes visible within the zone of marrow edema as a line of diminished T1 and T2 signal. Peh[171] noted that fluid (very high, homogeneous T2 signal) may be detected within insufficiency fractures. The confidence in the diagnosis of sacral insufficiency fracture is increased by the presence of similar bone lesions in the pubic rami, immediately about the pubic symphysis, and in the para-acetabular region, also typical sites of insufficiency fracture.[171] Pubic insufficiency fractures accompanying sacral fractures were particularly common in Peh's series.[171] Detection of sacral and other pelvic insufficiency fractures is more significant now that these fractures may be successfully treated by image-guided injection of polymethylmethacrylate into the fracture and adjacent trabecular bone. In limited initial experience, this has resulted in significant rapid pain relief.[174-176]

SPINE TRAUMA: PSEUDARTHROSIS

Spinal fusions are performed for trauma, infection, neoplasm, and increasingly for degenerative disorders causing axial pain. Despite advances in surgical technique and fixation hardware, fusion remains an imperfect procedure. Pseudarthrosis is defined as the failure to achieve a solid bony fusion 1 year after attempted surgical fusion. It is manifested as persistent motion at the segment and absence of bony trabeculae bridging the vertebrae. Approximately 15% of lumbar spinal fusions result in pseudarthrosis; the range of successful reported technical and clinical outcomes spans 16% to 95%.[177]

The risk of pseudarthrosis relates to local and systemic factors. Local factors increasing the risk of pseudarthrosis include previous surgery, instability, deficient bone graft quality and quantity, surgical technique, and the number of levels fused.[177] Rates of pseudarthrosis increased with increasing number of fused levels.[178] For posterolateral lumbar fusion, reported successful fusion rates are 90.3% for single level, 77.2% for two level, and 65.2% for three level surgeries.[178] Systemic factors increasing the risk of pseudarthrosis include inadequate nutrition, comorbidities including diabetes and cardiovascular disease, medications such as corticosteroids, nonsteroidal anti-inflammatory agents, and chemotherapy, and nicotine intake. Nicotine can have a dramatic effect; Brown's study of L4 to S1 fusions showed a pseudarthrosis rate of 40% in smokers and 8% in nonsmokers.[179]

Detection of pseudarthrosis with imaging is of significance, in that it is a cause of persistent or recurrent pain following surgery. The correlation is not

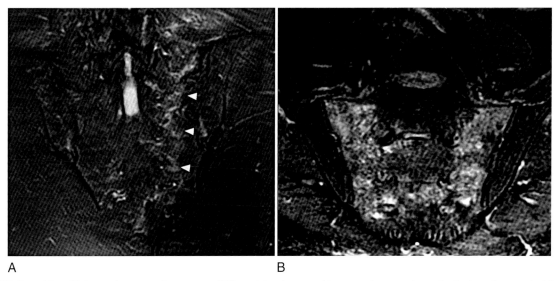

A   B

Figure 12–35. Sacral insufficiency fractures. Fat-saturated T2-weighted coronal images of two patients. In **A,** there is a vertical band of high signal in the left sacral ala *(arrowheads)* consistent with insufficiency fracture. In a second patient **(B),** there is much more extensive signal abnormality involving both sacral ala and crossing the S3 segment horizontally to complete the "Honda" sign.

exact; patients with radiographic pseudarthrosis may be pain-free and patients with solid fusions by all imaging techniques may have persistent pain arising from other factors. The clinical questions therefore are twofold: is a pseudarthrosis present, and, if so, is it the cause of persistent or recurrent pain? The ultimate gold standard for fusion is surgical exploration; even this is not foolproof, because patients who have had hardware removal after intraoperative evaluation of stability have subsequently gone on to develop progressive deformity.[180]

It may take 6 to 9 months for a solid fusion to be evident on plain films; remodeling of the fusion mass will continue for up to 2 years.[181] Plain film evaluation of fusion should include flexion and extension views to evaluate for motion across the fused segment by direct inspection and measurement of Cobb angles. Measurement of the distance between the tips of the spinous processes on flexion-extension views of the cervical spine has also been suggested as a means of detecting subtle motion.[182] Hardware failure may be seen as fracture of the metal components, migration of components, and lucency/bone resorption about pedicle screws or intervertebral cages. Bone graft should be inspected for adequate mass and any evidence of lucent fractures lines, linear sclerosis, or fragmentation. Plain films are relatively insensitive to subtle changes. Multislice CT scanners with isotropic voxels can provide reformatted images with equal spatial resolution in any plane. This should provide greater sensitivity to the detection of pseudarthrosis; there are no studies to verify this. Newer scanners also have improved means of suppressing the artifact from metal fixation hardware. Ideally, to verify solid fusion, one would like to be able to confirm the presence of continuous bony trabeculae across the site of fusion. In patients with intervertebral cage devices, bony trabeculae should be seen bridging the interspace through the cage and external to the cage.

Technetium bone scans with SPECT may be helpful. The fusion mass will be metabolically active for a prolonged period after surgery and increased tracer uptake diffusely in the fusion mass is expected for several months. In normal healing, studies with serial bone scans have shown a steady decrease in tracer uptake after 3 months, with only minimal increased uptake at 1 year.[183] Increased uptake within the fusion mass beyond 1 year after surgery, or new increased uptake not present on prior studies, should raise concern for pseudarthrosis. On MRI, solid bone graft should exhibit signal characteristics of normal marrow. Focal zones of low T1 signal, elevated T2 signal, and gadolinium enhancement may indicate a site of pseudarthrosis with ongoing motion and inflammation. This requires careful inspection.

Interventional techniques may also be of value. Discography may be useful in identifying painful segments even in the presence of cage fusion devices, in the author's experience. Fixation hardware may be painful at its interface with surrounding soft tissues even though the fusion is solid. If careful palpation localizes pain to prominent hardware and if infiltration of the metal–soft tissue interface with local anesthetics relieves the patient's typical pain, then hardware removal may be indicated.

The clinician and imager must also be aware of adjacent segment disease as a cause of recurrent pain in the post-fusion patient. Although controversial, this likely occurs at a rate of approximately 3% per year following lumbar fusion.[184] A similar rate has been associated with cervical fusion.[185] The imaging findings will be those of disk degeneration and facet arthropathy as has been previously discussed. Radiographic evidence of adjacent segment disease may or may not be clinically symptomatic.

Pseudarthrosis and adjacent segment disease are two primary causes of pain in the postoperative patient, sometimes labeled the "failed back." Although conventionally considered a dread diagnosis, recent studies have shown that careful clinical evaluation, augmented by high-quality imaging and provocation and anesthetic interventions can identify the specific cause of pain in the vast majority of cases. Waguespack and Slipman and coworkers have each published large series of patients with so-called failed back syndrome.[186,187] A specific diagnosis identifying the pain generator was achieved in more than 90% of patients in both of these series. The most common diagnoses were foraminal stenosis (>20%), discogenic pain (20%), pseudarthroses (14%), neuropathic pain (10%), and recurrent disk herniation (7% to 12%) with lesser contributions from facet and sacroiliac joints. All of these morphologic lesions have been individually addressed in preceding sections. The imaging challenge is to systematically evaluate each segmental level for these potential pain generators despite the confusion of the surgically altered anatomy.

SPINE INFECTION

Extradural spinal infections are primarily the result of arterial seeding. In children, the disk and end plate have a rich blood supply; infection occurs initially in the disk itself. In the adult, the disk is avascular; an infection develops in the anterior subchondral vertebral body with secondary spread to the disk, adjacent vertebrae, and subligamentous space. Most disk space infections involve two adjacent lumbar vertebrae. Spread from contiguous infection or direct inoculation of the disk (surgery, discography) are much less common.

Pyogenic disk space infection involves men much more commonly than women (2-3:1) in the fifth to seventh decades of life.[33] Clinical symptoms may precede radiographic findings by 1 to 8 weeks. Clinical signs of elevated sedimentation rate, white cell count, and C-reactive protein are usually present. Plain films reveal early rarefaction of anterior subchondral bone, followed by loss of disk space height (at 1 to 3 weeks) with subsequent destructive changes in the vertebral end plates. Late changes include variable amounts of sclerosis, kyphotic deformity from vertebral collapse, and ankylosis. CT in pyogenic diskitis shows early hypodensity in the disk, moth-eaten destruction of the vertebral end plates, inflammatory changes in paravertebral soft tissues, and epidural mass. Scattered gas formation may be seen. Extensive gas formation in the central portion of the disk is more typical of intervertebral osteochondrosis.

MRI is the preferred imaging modality for the evaluation of diskitis, with a greater than 90% sensitivity and specificity in disease detection.[188-191] It also provides critical anatomic information. Early marrow changes are elevated T2 signal (best seen with fat saturation), diminished T1 signal, and gadolinium enhancement (Fig. 12–36). There is loss of the crisp dark cortical line of the vertebral end plate. Within the disk, the intranuclear cleft is lost and foci of elevated T2 signal develop, as well as gadolinium enhancement. The paravertebral and epidural soft tissues show diffuse enhancement (phlegmon) or frank abscess formation with zones of hypoenhancement and increased T2 signal. The imaging differential diagnosis consists of Modic type I degenerative change, atypical cartilaginous (Schmorl's) nodes, adjacent metastatic lesions, osteomalacia secondary to osteodystrophy, pseudoarthroses in patients with ankylosing spondylitis, or a Charcot spine.

MRI abnormalities lag behind the clinical syndrome. Imaging may be minimally abnormal early in the disease process, and remain quite dramatic even after a gratifying clinical response to antibiotics.

In following the short-term efficacy of antibiotic therapy, erythrocyte sedimentation rate, C-reactive protein, and white cell count will be more useful then frequently repeated imaging. Follow-up imaging should be reserved for patients in whom there is a clinical concern for continued infection with central canal compromise.

Nuclear medicine scans using gallium-67 citrate and technetium-99m diphosphonate are considered by some to be the primary imaging modality for suspected spondylodiskitis. Technetium and gallium scans are complementary, with the combination of the two scans exhibiting greater sensitivity than either alone.[191] A recent series reported by Hadjipavlou and colleagues demonstrated 100% sensitivity, specificity, and accuracy for the combination of gallium and technetium scans when compared with surgical biopsy results; others have reported similar results.[191] Gallium may be useful in following resolution of the infection. Indium-labeled white blood cell scans are highly specific, but lack sensitivity.[192] All nuclear medicine techniques lack anatomic information; they are unable to define the extent of epidural or paraspinal disease or central canal compromise.

Tuberculosis (TB) remains the most common cause of spinal infection worldwide, and is of increasing incidence in industrialized societies. Clinical symptoms are usually insidious. While 90% to 100% of patients will have back pain, only 50% will have

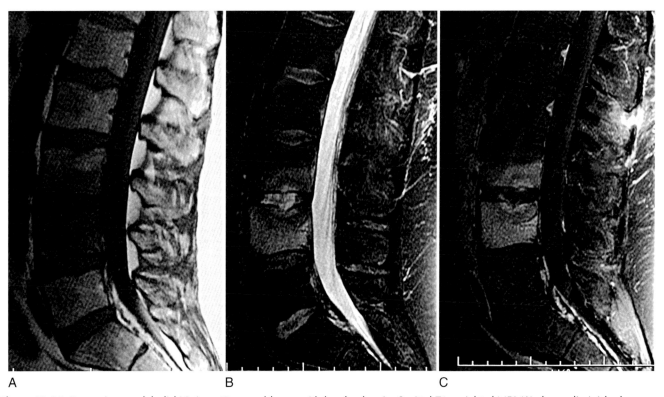

A   B   C

Figure 12–36. Pyogenic spondylodiskitis in a 48-year-old man with low back pain. Sagittal T1-weighted MRI **(A)** shows diminished marrow signal in L3 and L4 vertebral bodies, about the L3 disk. Fat-saturated T2-weighted image **(B)** demonstrates high signal edema in L3 and L4 marrow space. Note disruption of superior end plate of L4. Enhancement in L3 disk and adjacent vertebral bodies are seen on fat-saturated, enhanced T1 image **(C).** Image-guided biopsy yielded *Staphylococcus aureus.*

constitutional symptoms or fever. Tuberculous spondylitis arises from hematogenous (arterial) spread of tuberculous bacilli, usually from a pulmonary source. Initial infection occurs in the anterior subchondral bone. There is early anterior subligamentous extension and then spread to adjacent vertebrae, often multiple, as well as spread across the disk. Neurologic deficit occurs in a moderate number of patients due to epidural extension. Posterior elements tend to be spared. Extensive anterior destruction with gibbus deformity is characteristic.

Tuberculous spondylitis with diskitis shows disk space narrowing, vertebral osteolysis with collapse, and gibbus deformity on plain films. L1 is most frequently affected, with less frequent involvement as one ascends the thoracic or descends the lumbar spine.[32] Plain films may not be abnormal until 2 to 5 months after the onset of infection. Paraspinal soft tissue masses due to subligamentous spread, particularly with calcification, are characteristic. CT demonstrates the osteolytic changes of spinal tuberculosis earlier than plain films. It more readily demonstrates epidural involvement, particularly when calcification or bone fragments are seen in the epidural space. Paraspinal involvement is also well demonstrated.

MRI is the primary imaging procedure for detection of spinal TB.[188,193] Early changes of tuberculous spondylitis with diskitis are very similar to pyogenic disk space infection, with marrow and disk inflammatory changes consisting of elevated T2 signal, diminished T1 signal, and enhancement. Extensive subligamentous spread of disease suggests TB. Paraspinal abscesses, granulomas, and epidural involvement are common. Epidural involvement may be seen in 60% to 80% of cases.[193]

A second pattern of tuberculous infection is spondylitis without diskitis[193] (Fig. 12–37). This describes lytic lesions in the central portions of the vertebral bodies, often multiple, without disk involvement. This pattern of involvement was present in approximately 50% of patients in a recent large series. The spondylitis without diskitis pattern is particularly common in the sub-Saharan African population.

Imaging findings consist of discrete, destructive vertebral body lesions. Plain films show well-defined lytic lesions, often multifocal, and with more frequent posterior element and cervical involvement than is seen in tuberculous diskitis. Lytic lesions may exhibit marginal sclerosis on CT. Such lesions typically enhance peripherally on MRI, often with a cystic central cavity. There may be cortical destruction with an adjacent paravertebral abscess. Due to the greater frequency of multiple lesions, this entity must be distinguished from metastasis, myeloma, or lymphoma.

MRI imaging has significantly advanced the diagnosis of spinal infection, allowing this to be suggested as a likely diagnosis before destructive changes evolve. The MRI findings remain unspecific, however, and accurate diagnosis and therapy requires tissue sampling for histology and culture. Image-guided percutaneous aspiration/biopsy with large-caliber bone cutting needles can provide minimally invasive tissue sampling.

SPINAL DURAL ARTERIOVENOUS FISTULA

Spinal dural arteriovenous fistulas (AVFs) are the most common form of vascular malformation involving the spine. This lesion merits description in that it may present with pain and progressive neurologic deficit, mimicking spinal stenosis; it frequently remains undiagnosed for prolonged periods. In Atkinson and coworkers' series, the mean delay from symptom onset to diagnosis was 23 months.[194] When diagnosed, it is treatable with arrest of the progressive neurologic deficit.

Spinal dural AVFs are an acquired lesion, with a fistulous communication within the dura of a root sleeve and intrathecal venous drainage to the venous plexus surrounding the cord. This results in venous hypertension within the cord and ultimately cord dysfunction. The fistula is most commonly in the low thoracic or lumbar spine. It is a lesion of older men. Gilbertson and associates' series[195] had a mean age of 62 years, with a range from 37 to 81 years; Atkinson and colleagues' series[194] reported a 4:1 male predominance. Pain was a reported symptom in 53% of patients, many of whom describe a burning, dysesthetic pain in the lower extremities. Fifteen percent had low back pain when erect, which worsened with use of the lower extremities. This is typically accompanied by a slowly progressive or stepwise worsening myelopathy, manifest as lower extremity fatigue and weakness. Atkinson and associates' series[194] reported 69% of patients with upper and lower motor neuron signs; 30% had only lower motor neuron signs.

Imaging findings of dural AVFs are well described. On CT myelogram, abnormally prominent tortuous vessels are present in 100% of cases; this may give the cauda equina a beaded appearance. On MRI, there is increased T2 signal in the cord in nearly 100% of cases (Fig. 12–38). This typically extends over multiple vertebral segments and may be accompanied by cord enlargement in 45%. There may be patchy cord enhancement; these findings may raise concern for tumor. A differentiating finding is the presence of prominent flow voids or intravascular enhancement due to the dilated veins, particularly on the dorsal surface of the cord. The T2 signal change in the cord usually involves the low thoracic cord and conus; this does not predict the site of the fistula. Magnetic resonance angiography (MRA) may be useful in predicting the site of the fistula,[196] but definitive diagnosis depends on spinal angiography. The fistula then may be disconnected surgically or by an endovascular approach.

SPINE NEOPLASM

Spinal neoplasms are classified by the anatomic compartment from which they arise: extradural, intradural-extramedullary, or intramedullary. Extradural

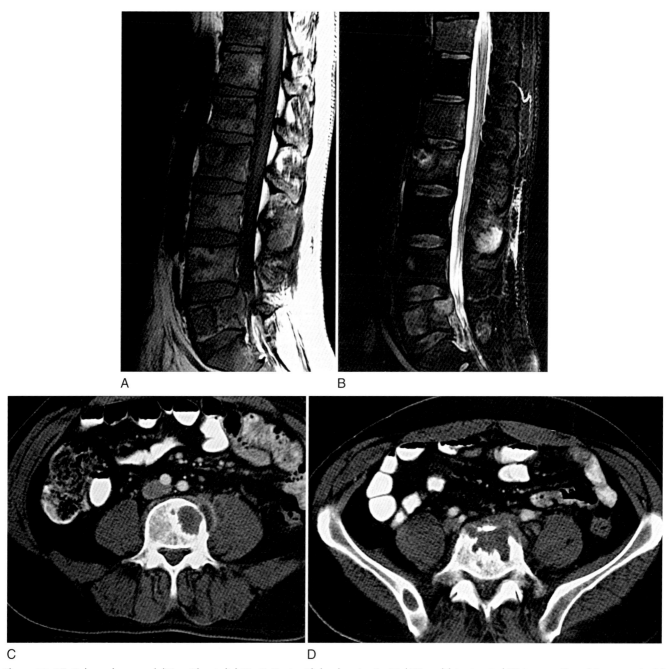

Figure 12–37. Tubercular spondylitis without diskitis. Patient with back pain. Sagittal T1 and fat-saturated T2 images (**A** and **B,** respectively) demonstrated multiple lesions in vertebral bodies and posterior elements. Disks are normal. CT images of lumbar region (**C** and **D**) show destructive lesions with reactive, sclerotic margins in vertebral bodies and pelvis. Lesion in **C** extends to left psoas muscle. CT-guided biopsy revealed granulomatous inflammation on histology; culture grew *Mycobacterium tuberculosis*. Multiple lesions of tuberculosis spondylitis can mimic metastases.

neoplasms arise from the vertebral bodies, within the paravertebral soft tissues or within the epidural space. These include metastatic lesions, hematologic malignancies, and primary osseous or cartilaginous tumors. Intradural-extramedullary lesions arise within the dural tube, but are extrinsic to the spinal cord itself. Lesions in this category include meningiomas, Schwannomas, neurofibromas, and leptomeningeal metastatic disease. Intramedullary lesions are those that arise primarily from the spinal cord or filum

terminale. Astrocytomas, ependymomas, and hemangioblastomas make up the vast majority of these lesions.

Extradural neoplasms are common. MRI provides the best combination of lesion detection, morphologic characterization, and assessment of neural compromise. Nuclear medicine techniques such as technetium bone scan and PET scanning provide high sensitivity to lesion detection and excellent body-wide assessment of tumor burden (Fig. 12–39).

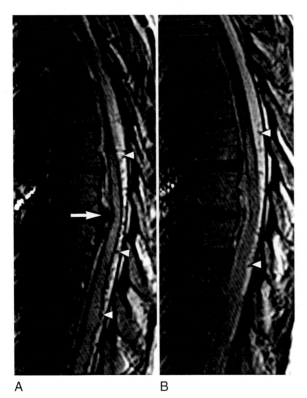

A   B

Figure 12–38. Dural arteriovenous fistula in an older man with progressive myelopathy. **A** and **B** are contiguous sagittal T2-weighted images of midthoracic spine. Note increased signal within the cord, which extends to conus, due to venous hypertension. Multiple small signal voids *(arrowheads)* on the dorsal surface of cord are enlarged veins draining the fistula, which was located in the root sleeve of T6 on the left at angiography. The disk protrusion *(arrow)* is purely incidental and not a factor in the patient's myelopathy. Beware of distraction by obvious but insignificant findings.

Nuclear medicine studies do not provide anatomic information regarding compression of neural elements. CT is less sensitive than MRI in lesion detection; plain films are far less sensitive.

Extradural neoplasms may narrow the subarachnoid space (cerebrospinal fluid) as they extrinsically intrude into the spinal canal. They exhibit diminished T1 signal, elevated T2 signal, and gadolinium-enhancement on MRI. The unenhanced T1 image is the mainstay of lesion detection. Fat-saturated fast spin echo T2-weighted images and STIR images provide high sensitivity to lesion detection with less morphologic information. Fat-saturated postgadolinium images also display extradural neoplasm with high sensitivity. Images should be assessed for osseous involvement, cortical destruction (loss of the dark cortical line), and paravertebral or epidural extension. On axial images, compression of the thecal sac or exiting nerve roots can be directly displayed. CT and plain films play a role in characterizing primary bone and cartilaginous tumors including malignant lesions such as osteosarcoma, chondrosarcoma, chordoma, and the benign tumors, including hemangioma, osteoid osteoma, giant cell tumor, and aneurysmal bone cyst.

Metastases are the most common extradural spine tumor, and the spinal column is the most common site of osseous metastases. An overwhelming majority of spine metastases are due to prostate, lung, and breast cancer. The thoracic spine is most commonly involved (70%), followed by the lumbar and cervical segments. Involvement of the vertebral body is most common (85%), with less frequent spread to the paravertebral tissues or epidural space. The disks, dura, and anterior longitudinal ligament are resistant to invasion by metastatic tumor; the posterior longitudinal ligament is more readily involved, in that it is penetrated by numerous venous channels. Vertebral body metastases may be blastic (bone forming), lytic (destructive), or mixed. Blastic lesions are seen as ill defined areas of increased density on plain films or CT; on MRI blastic lesions have low T1 and T2 signal with enhancement. Common primary tumors are prostate, carcinoid, or bladder cancer. Lytic metastases show destruction on plain films and CT, low T1, and variable T2 signal with enhancement on MRI. Lytic metastases are most commonly produced by breast, lung, renal, and thyroid neoplasms. Mixed lytic and blastic lesions are seen in lung, breast, cervical, and ovarian primaries.

Hemangiomas are the most common spine tumor, present in up to 10% to 12% of adults (Fig. 12–40). They are frequently multiple. Typical hemangiomas are benign and of no clinical significance; they are identified by their fatty content on MRI (high T1 and high T2 signal) and a corduroy appearance on plain films or CT. This is due to sparse, thickened trabeculae surrounded by fat; on axial images, this results in a polka dot appearance.

Osteoid osteomas occur in patients younger than age 30 years and typically present with pain, often nocturnal (Fig. 12–41). Pain is usually relieved by aspirin or nonsteroidal anti-inflammatory drugs. The lesion consists of a small nidus, less than 1.5 cm in diameter, surrounded by a larger zone of sclerotic reaction and/or soft tissue inflammation, visible on plain films or CT. The nidus is intensely enhancing on CT, MRI, or bone scan. Ten percent of osteoid osteomas occur in the spine, almost exclusively in the posterior neural arch. The lumbar spine is involved in 59% of spinal osteoid osteomas, the cervical region in 27%, and the thoracic spine in 12%. Lesions larger than 1.5 cm are considered osteoblastomas.

Aneurysmal bone cysts are benign expansile neoplasms seen in young patients (80% are younger than 20). The most common presentation is pain. These lesions arise in the posterior elements but frequently expand into the vertebral body. They are multilocular. Fluid-fluid levels of blood products on MRI are characteristic. The plain film and CT appearance is that of an expansile lesion, with thinning cortical bone and fine internal septations. The lesion may compromise the central canal and cause neural compression.

Giant cell tumors are benign but locally aggressive destructive lesions that present in the third to fifth

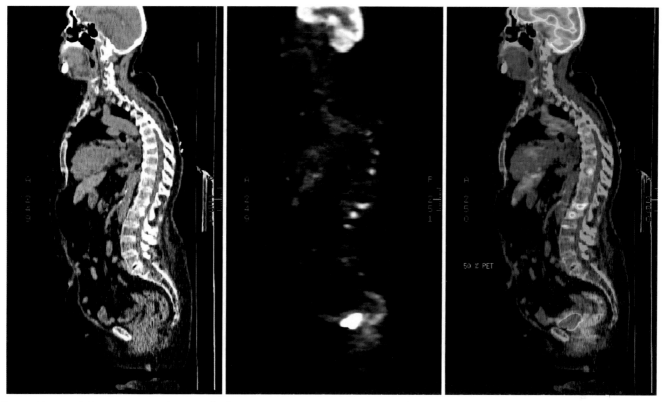

Figure 12–39. FDG-PET CT scan shows multiple spine metastases in a patient with breast cancer. Three panels of the image, from left to right, show simultaneously obtained CT, PET, and fused PET-CT images. High metabolic activity in multiple thoracic and lumbar vertebrae are consistent with metastases. (Courtesy of Dr. Mark Nathan.)

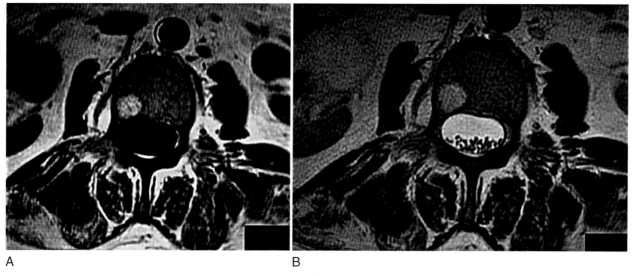

A   B

Figure 12–40. Hemangioma. T1-weighted MRI **(A)** shows high signal lesion in right side of vertebral body. Lesion also has high T2 signal in **(B).** Well-circumscribed lesion with high T1 and T2 signal is typical of benign hemangioma.

decades with back pain of insidious onset. The lesion is seen as a lytic zone without marginal sclerosis in a vertebral body or the sacrum. There may be cortical destruction. There may be heterogeneous enhancement on CT or MRI with central necrosis.

Myeloma is the most common malignant primary tumor of bone; it presents with bone pain in 75% of patients. It is often widespread at presentation. Its imaging appearance can range from discrete destructive lesions to diffuse loss of bone density indistinguishable from osteoporosis on plain films. CT is better able to resolve the discrete destructive lesions in trabecular or cortical bone. The MRI appearance is variable, with diminished T1 marrow signal and

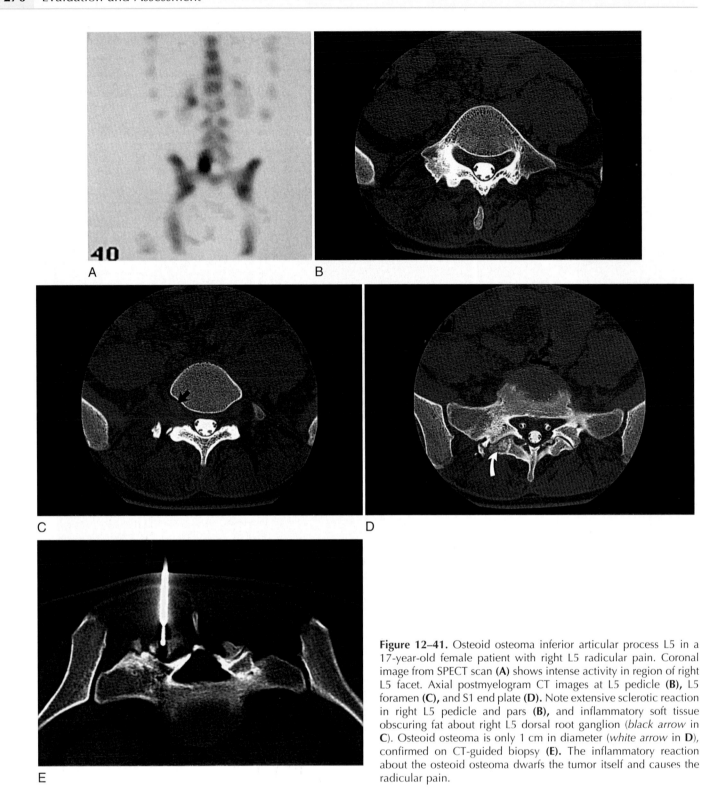

Figure 12–41. Osteoid osteoma inferior articular process L5 in a 17-year-old female patient with right L5 radicular pain. Coronal image from SPECT scan **(A)** shows intense activity in region of right L5 facet. Axial postmyelogram CT images at L5 pedicle **(B)**, L5 foramen **(C),** and S1 end plate **(D).** Note extensive sclerotic reaction in right L5 pedicle and pars **(B),** and inflammatory soft tissue obscuring fat about right L5 dorsal root ganglion (*black arrow* in **C**). Osteoid osteoma is only 1 cm in diameter (*white arrow* in **D**), confirmed on CT-guided biopsy **(E).** The inflammatory reaction about the osteoid osteoma dwarfs the tumor itself and causes the radicular pain.

gadolinium enhancement in a multifocal or diffuse pattern. Compression fractures are common and may be indistinguishable from benign osteoporotic fractures. Single focal lesions (plasmacytomas) are expansile and lytic on imaging.

Leukemia may present with spine pain in the setting of diffuse marrow involvement and associated compression fractures. The most common imaging finding is that of diffuse marrow replacement, with osteopenia on plain films and CT, and generalized loss of the normal intermediate T1 signal of marrow (Fig. 12–42). Focal extraosseous soft tissue masses of leukemic tissue may be present and are termed *chloromas.*

Lymphoma is the great mimic. It can present in the spine as vertebral lesions indistinguishable from

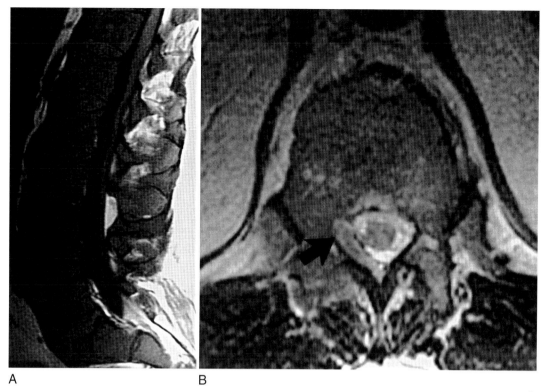

A   B

Figure 12–42. Leukemia in a 47-year-old man with back pain. Sagittal T1-weighted image of lumbar spine **(A)** shows diffuse decreased T1 signal in marrow indicating an infiltrative process. Marrow is similar in signal intensity to disk; it should always be brighter than the disk on a normal T1 image. Infiltration of the right lateral epidural space *(arrow)* by leukemic cells (chloroma) on axial T2-weighted MRI **(B).**

metastases, as an epidural soft tissue mass without bone involvement, as a diffuse leptomeningeal process, and as a primary intramedullary lesion.

Chordomas are malignant extradural tumors arising from notochord remnants. They may present in late–middle-aged men with pain or neurologic dysfunction due to mass effect. Chordomas occur in or near the midline, most commonly in the clivus-sacrum-vertebral body. Chordomas, along with chondrosarcomas, are among the few neoplastic lesions that cross the disk space and involve two adjacent vertebrae. The plain film and CT appearance is a destructive lesion with an associated soft tissue mass. The MRI appearance can be characteristic, with a lobular, septated lesion of very high T2 signal and heterogeneous enhancement. The lesion is extremely prone to local recurrence; any attempt at image-guided biopsy of a suspected chordoma should occur in consultation with the orthopedic surgeon to ensure that the biopsy tract can be excised in the resection.

Intradural-extramedullary neoplasms are situated within the dural sac, widening the subarachnoid space as they displace the cord or cauda equina. Meningiomas typically exhibit a broad base against the dural surface and enhance uniformly. Schwannomas and neurofibromas are indistinguishable on imaging. They may enhance uniformly or show central zones of cystic degeneration. The classic "dumb-bell" neurofibroma may issue through and

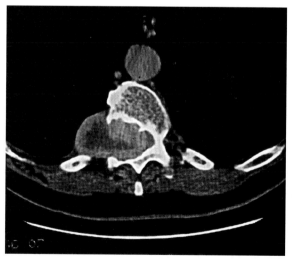

Figure 12–43. Neurofibroma in an older man with right thoracic radiculopathy. Enhanced CT image shows an intradural and extradural extramedullary lesion expanding the right neural foramen. Central cystic degeneration. Note sclerotic bone about remodeled foramen indicating an indolent process.

widen a neural foramen (Fig. 12–43). They may also occur entirely within the dural sac or in a paravertebral location. Leptomeningeal metastatic disease is most typically seen as enhancement on the surface of the cord or within the roots of the cauda equina (Fig. 12–44). In some cases more discrete small masses

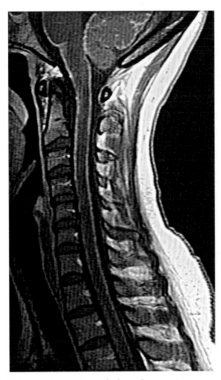

Figure 12-44. Leptomeningeal lymphoma in a woman with progressive headaches, neck pain, and cognitive dysfunction. Sagittal gadolinium-enhanced T1-weighted image shows diffuse enhancement over pial surface of cord and brainstem. Large cell lymphoma cells were recovered from spinal fluid.

may be seen within the cauda equina. CSF cytology remains more sensitive than MRI in the detection of leptomeningeal metastatic disease.

Intramedullary neoplasms are rare entities, but may present with pain or dysfunction that can mimic degenerative disease (Fig. 12–45). Ependymomas arise from the ependymal cells lining the central canal of the cord. Ependymomas are the most common intramedullary tumor in adults; they are most frequently located in the conus medullaris and filum terminale (myxopapillary ependymoma). Because of their slow growth, they may cause bony erosion and scalloped enlargement of the central canal. MRI demonstrates an enlarged cord or filum terminale with elevated T2 signal and heterogeneous enhancement. Small cysts or hemorrhage are frequent. Astrocytomas are typically low-grade neoplasms, more commonly seen in young patients and in the cervical region. They typically extend over multiple vertebral segments within the cord with poorly defined margins. The cord is enlarged with heterogeneous enhancement. The entire cross section of the cord is typically involved. Considerable edema within the white matter of the cord extends cephalad and caudal to the enhancing neoplasm itself. There may be peritumoral cysts present. Hemangioblastomas are rare lesions that typically occur in the cervical and thoracic spine. An intensely enhancing vascular nodule adjacent to the pial surface, often associated with an intramedullary cyst, is typical.

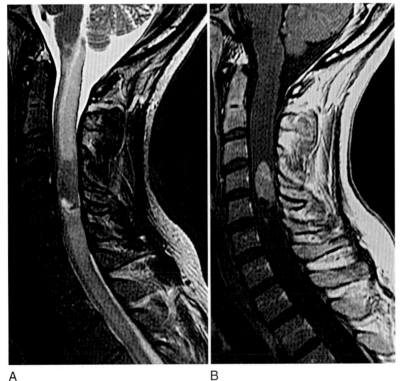

A B

Figure 12-45. Neck pain and myelopathy in an adult woman. Sagittal T2-weighted image **(A)** shows intermediate signal intramedullary mass at the C4 level. High signal edema extends cephalad to medulla, caudal to thoracic cord. Note cord expansion, effacing CSF of subarachnoid space. Sagittal gadolinium-enhanced T1 image **(B)** demonstrates enhancing tumor at C4 level. Radiographic differential is ependymoma or astrocytoma. Well-demarcated enhancement favors the former. Ependymoma was resected at surgery.

About one third of patients with hemangioblastomas have von Hippel-Lindau syndrome.

CONCLUSION

Imaging plays a crucial role in the evaluation of the patient with spine pain. It is also generally overused and contributes to the enormous costs of this medical condition. It must be used wisely, with full realization of its sensitivity and specificity limitations. It cannot stand alone, but can only contribute in the context of the individual patient's pain syndrome. Ultimate diagnosis must be a combination of clinical acumen, imaging morphology, and physiologic testing. The best care of the patient will be achieved through close cooperation and communication among clinician, imaging specialist, and surgeon.

SUMMARY

- Imaging of back pain is expensive; it must be used wisely.
- No imaging is indicated in acute back pain in the absence of "red flag" signs or symptoms suggesting systemic disease.
- All imaging demonstrates asymptomatic degenerative changes; the prevalence of such findings increases with increasing age.
- Only a clear correlation between the imaging findings and pain syndrome, preferably augmented by anesthetic or provocative procedures, allows establishment of a cause-and-effect relationship.
- Treat the patient, not the images.
- When imaging commences, it should start with plain radiographs.
- Imaging may be insensitive to the detection of neural compression without axial loading.
- Close communication among imaging physician, pain clinician, interventionalist, and surgeon is critical to the best care of the patient.

References

1. Jarvik JG, Deyo R: Diagnostic evaluation of low back pain with emphasis on imaging. Ann Intern Med 2002;137: 586-597.
2. Data-driven effort standardizes low back pain outcomes. Data strategies and benchmarks. National Health Information LLC 1997;1:49-64.
3. Scavone JC, Latshaw RF, Rohrar GV: Use of lumbar spine films: Statistical evaluation at a teaching hospital. JAMA 1981;246:1105-1108
4. Liang M, Komaroff AL: Roentgenograms in primary care patients with acute low back pain: A cost-effective analysis. Arch Intern Med 1982;142:1108-1112.
5. Simmons ED, Guyer RG, Graham-Smith A, et al: Radiograph assessment for patients with low back pain. Spine J 2003;3: 3S-5S.
6. Gilbert FJ, Grant AM, Gillan MG, et al: Low back pain: Influence of early MR imaging or CT on treatment and outcome—Multicenter randomized trial. Radiology 2004;231:343-351.
7. Jarvik JG, Hollingworth W, Heagerty PJ, et al: Three-year incidence of low back pain in an initially asymptomatic cohort: Clinical and imaging risk factors. Spine 2005;30: 1541-1548.
8. Jarvik JG, Hollingworth W, Martin B, et al: Rapid magnetic resonance imaging vs radiographs for patients with low back pain. JAMA 2003;289:2810-2818.
9. Weinstein J, Tosteson T, Lurie J, et al: Surgical vs. nonoperative treatment for lumbar disk herniation. The Spine Patient Outcomes Research Trial (SPORT): A randomized trial. JAMA 2006;296:2441-2450.
10. Atlas SJ, Keller RB, Wu UA, et al: Long-term outcomes of surgical and nonsurgical management of sciatica secondary to a lumbar disc herniation: 10 years results from the Maine lumbar spine study. Spine 2005;30:927-935.
11. Atlas SJ, Keller RB, Wu YA, et al: Long-term outcomes of surgical and nonsurgical management of lumbar spinal stenosis: 8 to 10 year results from the Maine lumbar spine study. Spine 2005. 30(8):936-943.
12. Lurie JD, Birkmeyer NJ, Weinstein JN: Rates of advanced spinal imaging and spine surgery. Spine 2003;28:616-620.
13. Brox JI, Sorensen R, Friis A, et al: Randomized clinical trial of lumbar instrumented fusion and cognitive intervention and exercise in patients with chronic low back pain and disc degeneration. Spine 2003;28:1913-1921.
14. Fairbank J, Frost H, Wilson-MacDonald J, et al: Randomised controlled trial to compare surgical stabilization of the lumbar spine with an intensive rehabilitation programme for patients with chronic low back pain: The MRC spine stabilisation trial. BMJ 2005;28:330(7502):1233.
15. Fritzell P, Hagg O, Wessberg P, et al: 2001 Volvo award winner in clinical studies: Lumbar fusion versus nonsurgical treatment for chronic low back pain: A multicenter randomized controlled trial from the Swedish Lumbar Spine Study Group. Spine 2001;26(23):2521-2532
16. Deyo RA, Gray DT, Kreuter W, et al: United States trends in lumbar fusion surgery for degenerative conditions. Spine 2005;30:1441-1445.
17. Carey TS, Garrett J, Jackman A, et al: The outcomes and costs of care for acute low back pain among patients seen by primary care practitioners, chiropractors, and orthopedic surgeons. The North Carolina Back Pain Project. N Engl J Med 1995;333:913-917.
18. Maniadakis N, Gray A: The economic burden of back pain in the UK. Pain 2000;84:95-103.
19. Hirsch C, Schajowikz F: Studies on structural changes in the lumbar annulus fibrosus. Acta Orthop Scand 1952;22:185-231.
20. Hitselberger WE, Witten RM: Abnormal myelograms in asymptomatic patients. J Neurosurg 1968;28:204-206.
21. Wiesel SW, Tsourmas N, Feffer HL, et al: A study of computer-assisted tomography. I. The incidence of positive CAT scans in an asymptomatic group of patients. Spine 1984;9:549-551.
22. Boden SD, Davis DO, Dina TS, et al: Abnormal magnetic-resonance scans of the lumbar spine in asymptomatic subjects. J Bone Surg Am 1990;72:403-408.
23. Weishaupt D, Zanetti M. Hodler J, et al: MR imaging of the lumbar spine: Prevalence of intervertebral disc extrusion and sequestration, nerve root compression, end plate abnormalities, and osteoarthritis of the facet joint in asymptomatic volunteers. Radiology 1998;209:661-666.
24. Boos N, Rieder R, Schade V, et al: Volvo Award in clinical sciences: The diagnostic accuracy of magnetic resonance imaging, work perception, and psychosocial factors in identifying symptomatic disc herniation. Spine 1995;20:2613-2625.
25. Jarvik JJ, Hollingworth W, Heagert P, et al: The longitudinal assessment of imaging and disability of the back (LAID Back) study. Spine 2001;26:1158-1166.
26. Schmid MR, Stucki G, Duewell S, et al: Changes in cross-sectional measurements of the spinal canal and intervertebral foramina as a function of body position: In vivo studies on an open-configuration MR system. AJR Am J Roentgenol 1999;172:1095-1102.
27. Danielson B, Willen J: Axially loaded magnetic resonance image of the lumbar spine in asymptomatic individuals. Spine 2001;26:2601-2606.
28. Willen J, Danielson B, Gaulitz A, et al: Dynamic effects on the lumbar spinal canal. Spine 1997;22:2968-2976.

29. Kimura S, Hesselink JR, Gargin SR, et al: Axial load-dependent cervical spinal alterations during simulated upright posture: A comparison of healthy controls and patients with cervical degeneration disease. J Neurosurg Spine 2005;2:13744.

30. Jinkins JR, Dworkins JS, Dmadian RV: Upright, weight-bearing, dynamic-kinetic MRI of the spine: Initial results. Euro Radiol 2005;15:1815-1825.

31. Weishaupt D, Boxheimer L: Magnetic resonance imaging of the weight-bearing spine. Semin Musculoskel Radiol 2003;7:277-286.

32. Resnick D, et al: Diagnosis of Bone and Joint Disorders, 4th ed. Philadelphia, WB Saunders, 2002.

33. Fortin JD, Washington WJ, Falco FJ: Three pathways between the sacroiliac joint and neural structures. AJNR Am J Neuroradiol 1999;20:1429-1434.

34. Grob KR, Neuhuber WL, Kissling RO: Innervation of the sacroiliac joint of the human. Z Rheumatol 1995;54:117-122.

35. Fortin JD, Kissling RO, O'Connor BL, et al: Sacroiliac joint innervation and pain. Am J Orthop 1999;28:687-690.

36. Yin W, Willard F, Carreiro J, et al: Sensory stimulation guided sacroiliac joint radio frequent neurotomy: Technique based on neuroanatomy of the dorsal sacral plexus. Spine 2003;28:2419-2425.

37. Huntoon MA: Anatomy of the cervical intervertebral foramina: Vulnerable arteries and ischemic neurologic injuries after transforaminal epidural injections. Pain 2005;117:104-111.

38. Fardon DF, Milette PC: Nomenclature and classification of the lumbar disc pathology: Recommendations of the combined task forces of the North American Spine Society, American Society of Spine Radiology, and American Society of Neuroradiology. Spine 2001;26:E93-E113.

39. Modic MT, Steinberg PM, Ross JS, et al: Degenerative disk disease: Assessment of changes in vertebral body marrow with MR imaging. Radiology 1988;166(1 Part 1):193-199.

40. Teplick JG, Haskin ME: Spontaneous regression of herniated nucleus pulposus. AJNR Am J Neuroradiol 1985;145:371-375.

41. Saal JA, Saal JS, Herzog RJ: The natural history of lumbar intervertebral disc extrusions treated nonoperatively. Spine 1990;15:683-686.

42. Maigne J, Rime R, Delignet B: Computed tomographic follow-up study of forty-eight cases of nonoperatively treated lumbar intervertebral disc herniation. Spine 1992;17:1071-1074.

43. Delauche-Cavalier MC, Budet C, Laredo JD: Lumbar disc herniation: Computed tomography scan changes after conservative treatment of nerve root compression. Spine 1992;17:927-933.

44. Bozzao A, Gallucci M. Masciocchi C, et al: Lumbar disk herniation: MR imaging assessment of natural history in patients treated without surgery. Radiology 1992;185:135-141.

45. Bush K, Cowan N, Katz D, et al: The natural history of sciatica associated with disc pathology: A prospective study with clinical and independent radiologic follow-up. Spine 1992;17:1208-1212.

46. Thornbury JR, Fryback DC, Turski PA, et al: Disk-cased nerve compression in patients with acute low-back pain: Diagnosis with MR, CT myelography, and plan CT. Radiology 1993;186:731-738.

47. Van Rijn J, Klemetso N, et al: Observer variation in the evaluation of lumbar discs and root compression: Spiral CT compared with MRI. BJR 2006;79:372-377.

48. Jinkins JR: MR of enhancing nerve root in the unoperated lumbosacral spine. AJNR Am J Neuroradiol 1993;14:193-202.

49. Lane JL, Koeller KK, Atkinson JD: MR imaging of the lumbar spine: Enhancement of the radicular veins. AJR Am J Roentgenol 1996;166:181-185.

50. Ross JS: MR imaging of the postoperative lumbar spine. MRI Clin North Am 1999;7:513-524.

51. Ross JS, Zepp R, Modie MT: The postoperative lumbar spine: Enhanced MR evaluation of the interventional disk. AJNR Am J Neuroradiol 1996;17:323-331.

52. Ross JS, Robertson JT, Frederickson RC, et al: Association between peridural scar and recurrent radicular pain after lumbar discectomy: Magnetic resonance evaluation. ADCON-L European Study Group. Neurosurgery 1996;38:855-861; discussion, 861-863.

53. Schonstrom NSR, Hansson TH: Thickness of the human ligamentum flavum as a function of load: An in vitro experimental study. Clin Biomechanics 1991;76:19-24.

54. Schumacher D: Die Belastungsmyelographic. Fortschr Rontgensrt 1986;145:642-648.

55. Verbiest J: Neurogenic intermittent claudication in cases with absolute and relative stenosis of the lumbar vertebral canal (ASLC and RSLC), in cases with narrow lumbar intervertebral foramina, and in cases with both entities. Clin Neurosurg 1973;20:204-214.

56. Schonstrom NSR, Hansson TH: Pressure changes following constriction of the cauda equina: An experimental study in situ. Spine 1988;12:1385-1388.

57. Guyer RD, Ohnmeiss DD: Lumbar discography. Spine J 2003;3:11S-27S.

58. Bogduk N, ed: Practice Guidelines for Spinal Diagnostic and Treatment Procedures. San Francisco, International Spine Intervention Society, 2004.

59. Holt EP: The question of lumbar discography. J Bone Joint Surg 1968;50A:720-725.

60. Bogduk N, Tynan W, Wilson AS: The nerve supply to the human lumbar intervertebral discs. J Anat 1981;132:39-56.

61. Yoshizawa H, O'Brien JP, Thomas-Smith W, et al: The neuropathology of intervertebral discs removed for low-back pain. J Pathol 1980;132:95-104.

62. Groen GJ, Baljet B, Drukker J: Nerves and nerve plexuses of the human vertebral column. Am J Anat 1990;188:282-296.

63. Konttinen YT, Gronblad M, Antti-Poika I, et al: Neuroimmunohistochemical analysis of peridiscal nociceptive neural elements. Spine 1990;15:383-386.

64. Walsh TR, Weinstein JN, Spratt KF, et al: Lumbar discography in normal subjects. J Bone Joint Surg 1990;72A:1081-1088.

65. Vanharanta H, Sachs BL, Spivey MA, et al: The relationship of pain provocation to lumbar disc deterioration as seen by CT/discography. Spine 1987;12:295-298.

66. Moneta GB, Videman T, Kaivanto K, et al: Reported pain during lumbar discography as a function of anular ruptures and disc degeneration. A re-analysis of 833 discograms. Spine 1994;17:1968-1974.

67. Derby R, Howard MW, Grant JM, et al: The ability of pressure-controlled discography to predict surgical and nonsurgical outcomes. Spine 1999;24:364-371.

68. Carragee EJ, Tanner CM, Yang B, et al: False-positive findings on lumbar discography: Reliability of subjective concordance assessment during provocative disc injection. Spine 1999;24:2542-2547.

69. Carragee EJ, Tanner CM, Khurana S, et al: The rates of false-positive lumbar discography in select patients without low back symptoms. Spine 2000;25:1373-1381.

70. Dreyfuss PH, Dreyer SJ: Lumbar zygapophysial (facet) joint injections. Spine 2003;3:50-59.

71. Sowa G: Facet-mediated pain. Dis Mon 2005;Jan:18-33.

72. Ashton IK, Ashton BA, Gibson SJ, et al: Morphological basis for back pain: The demonstration of nerve fibers and neuropeptides in the lumbar facet joint capsule but not in ligamentum flavum. J Orthop Res 1992;10:72-79.

73. Cavanaugh JM, Ozaktay AC, Yamashita HT, et al: Lumbar facet pain: Biomechanics, neuroanatomy, and neurophysiology. J Biomechanics 1996;29:1117-1129.

74. Igarashi A, Kikuchi S, Konno S, et al: Inflammatory cytokines released from the facet joint tissue in degenerative lumbar spinal disorders. Spine 2004;29:2091-2095.

75. Beaman DN, Graziano GP, Glover RA, et al: Substance P innervation of lumbar spine facet joints. Spine 1993;15;18:1044-1049.

76. Lau P, Mercer S, Govind J, et al: The surgical anatomy of lumbar medial branch neurotomy (facet denervaton). Pain Med 2004;5:289-298.

77. Demondion X, Vidal C, Glaude E, et al: The posterior lumbar ramus: CT-anatomic correlation and propositions of new sites of infiltration. AJNR Am J Neuroradiol 2005;26:692.

78. Bogduk N: A narrative review of intra-articular corticosteroid injections for low back pain. Am Acad Pain Manage. 2005;4:287-296.

79. Schwarzer AC, Aprill CN, Derby R, et al: Clinical features of patients with pain stemming from the lumbar zygapophysial joints. Is the lumbar facet syndrome a clinical entity? Spine 1994;19:1132-1137.

80. Schwarzer AC, Derby R, Aprill CN, et al: The value of the provocation response in lumbar zygapophysial joint injections. Clin J Pain 1994;10:309-313.

81. Schwarzer AC, Wang SC, O'Driscoll D, et al: The ability of computed tomography to identify a painful zygapophysial joint in patients with chronic low back pain. Spine 1995;20:907-912.

82. Dolan AL, Ryan PJ, Arden NK, et al: The value of SPECT scans in identifying back pain likely to benefit from facet joint injection. Br J Rheumatol 1996;35:1269-1273.

83. Kettler A, Wilke HJ: Review of existing grading systems for cervical or lumbar disc and facet joint degeneration. Eur Spine J 2006;15:705-718.

84. Thalgott JS, Albert TJ, Vaccaro AR, et al: A new classification system for degenerative disk disease of the lumbar spine based on magnetic resonance imaging, provocative discography, plain radiographs, and anatomic considerations. Spine J 2004;4:167S-172S.

85. Apostolaki E, Davies AM, Evans, et al: MR imaging of lumbar facet joint synovial cyst. Eur Radiol 2000;10,615-623.

86. Doyle AJ, Merrilees M: Synovial cysts of the lumbar facet joints in a symptomatic population. Spine 2004;29:874-878.

87. Metellus P, Fuentes S, Adetchessi T, et al: Retrospective study of 77 patients harbouring lumbar synovial cysts: Functional and neurological outcome. Acta Neurochir 2006;148:147-154.

88. Lyons MK, Atkinson JLD, Wharen RE, et al: Surgical evaluation and management of lumbar synovial cysts: The Mayo Clinic experience. J Neurosurg 2000;93:53-57.

89. Phuong LK, Atkinson JL, Thielen KR: For lateral extraforaminal lumbar synovial cyst: report of two cases. Neurosurgery 2002;51:505-507.

90. Salmon BL, Deprez MP, Stevenaert AE, et al: The extraforaminal juxtafacet cyst as a rare cause of L5 radiculopathy: A case report. Spine 2003;28:E405-E407.

91. Tillich M, Trummer M, Lindbichler F, et al: Symptomatic intraspinal synovial cysts of the lumbar spine: Correlation of MR and surgical findings. Neuroradiology 2001;43:L1070-L1075.

92. Swartz PG, Murtagh FR: Spontaneous resolution of an intraspinal synovial cyst. Am J Neuroradiol 2003;24:1261-1263.

93. Sabers SR, Ross SR, Grogg BE: Procedure-based nonsurgical management of lumbar zygapophysial joint cyst induced radicular pain. Arch Phys Med Rehabil 2005;86:1767-1771.

94. Kauppila LI, Eustace S, Kiel D, et al: Degenerative displacement of lumbar vertebrae: A 25-year follow-up study in Framingham. Spine 1998;23:1868-1873.

95. Bywaters EG, Evans S: The lumbar interspinous bursae and Basstrup's syndrome: An autopsy study. Rheumatol Int 1982;2:87-96.

96. Chen CK, Yeh L, Resnick R, et al: Intraspinal posterior epidural cysts associated with Baastrup's disease: Report of 10 patients. AJR 2004;183:191-194.

97. Okada K: Studies on the cervical facet joints using arthrography of the cervical facet joint (author's transl). Nippon Seikeigeka Gakkai Zasshi 1981;55:563-580.

98. Rajasekaran S, Pithwa YK: Baastrupo's disease as a cause of neurogenic claudication. Spine 2003;28:273-275.

99. Hamlin LM, Delaplain CB: Bone SPECT in Baastrup's disease. Clin Nucl Med 1994;19:640-641.

100. Elster AD: Bertolotti's syndrome revisited: Transitional vertebrae of the lumbar spine. Spine 1989;14:1373-1377.

101. Tini PG, Wieser C, Zinn WM: The transitional vertebra of the lumbosacral spine: Its radiological classification, incidence, prevalence, and clinical significance. Rheumatol Rehabil 1977;16:180-185.

102. Jonsson B, Stromqvist B, Egund N: Anomalous lumbosacral articulations and low back pain: Evaluation and treatment. Spine 1989;14:831-834.

103. Brault JS, Smith J, Currier BL: Partial lumbosacral transitional vertebra resection for contralateral facetogenic pain. Spine 2001;26:226-229.

104. Santavirta S, Tallroth K, Ylinen P: Surgical treatment of Bertolotti's syndrome. Follow-up of 16 patients. Arch Orthop Trauma Surg 1993:112:82-87.

105. Cohen SP: Sacroiliac joint pain: A comprehensive review of anatomy, diagnosis, and treatment. Anesth Analg 2005; 101:1440-1453.

106. Maigne JY, Alivaliklis A, Pfefer F: Results of sacroiliac joint double block and value of sacroiliac pain provocation tests in 54 patients with low back pain. Spine 1996;21:1889-1892.

107. Schwarzer AC, April CN, Bogduk N: The sacroiliac joint in chronic low back pain. Spine 1995;20:31-37.

108. Bernard TN, Kirkaldy-Willis WH: Recognizing specific characteristics of nonspecific low back pain. Clin Orthop 1987; 217:266-280.

109. Maigne JY, Boulahdour H, Chatellier G: Value of quantitative radionuclide bone scanning in the diagnosis of sacroiliac joint syndrome in 32 patients with low back pain. Euro Spine J 1998;4:328-331.

110. Slipman CW, Sterenfeld EB, Chou LH, et al: The value of radionuclide imaging the diagnosis of sacroiliac joint syndrome. Spine 1996;21:2251-2254.

111. Elgafy H, Semaan HB, Ebraheim NA, et al: Computed tomography findings in patients with sacroiliac pain. Clin Orthop 2001;382:112-118.

112. DeAndres J, Chaves S: Coccygodynia: A proposal for an algorithm for treatment. J Pain 2003;4:257-266.

113. Maigne JY, Lagauche D, Doursounian L: Instability of the coccyx in coccydynia. J Bone Joint Surg 2000:82B:1038-1041.

114. Maigne JY, Tamalet B: Standardized radiological protocol for the study of common coccygodynia and characteristics of the lesions observed in the sitting position: Clinical elements differentiating subluxation, hypermobility and normal mobility. Spine 1996;21:2588-2593.

115. Levi N, Gjerris F, Dons K: Thoracic disc herniation: Unilateral transpedicular approach in 35 consecutive patients. J Neurosurg Sci 1999;43:37-42.

116. Wood KB, Garvey TA, Gundrey C, et al: Magnetic resonance imaging of the thoracic spine: Evaluation of asymptomatic individuals. J Bone Joint Surg Am 1995;77:1631-1638.

117. Wood KB, Blair JM, Aepple DM, et al: The natural history of asymptomatic thoracic disc herniations. Spine 1997;22:525-529.

118. Stillerman CB, Chen TC, Douldwell WE, et al: Experience in the surgical management of 82 symptomatic herniated thoracic discs and review of the literature. J Neurosurg 1998;88:623-633.

119. Lyu RK, Chang HS, Tang LM, et al: Thoracic disc herniation mimicking acute lumbar disc disease. Spine 1999;24:416-418.

120. Dreyfuss P, Tibiletti P, Dreyer SJ: Thoracic zygapophysial joint pain patterns: A study in normal volunteers. Spine 1994;19:807-811.

121. Dreyfuss P, Tibiletti P, Dreyer SJ: Thoracic zygapophysial joint pain: A review and description of an intra-articular block technique. Pain Digest 1994;4:46-54.

122. Erwin WM, Jackson PC, Homonki DA: Innervation of the human costovertebral joint: Implications for clinical back pain syndromes. J Manip Physiol Ther 2000;23:531.

123. Matsumoto M, Fujimura Y, Suzuki N, et al: MRI of cervical intervertebral discs in asymptomatic subjects. J Bone Joint Surg Br 1998:80:19-24.

124. Boden SD, McCowin PR, Davis DO, et al: Abnormal magnetic-resonance scans of the cervical spine in asymptomatic subjects: a prospective investigation. J Bone Joint Surg Am 1990;72:1178-1184.

125. Teresi LM, Lufin RB, Reicher MA, et al: Asymptomatic degenerative disc disease and spondylolysis of the cervical spine: MR imaging. Radiology 1987;164:82-88.

126. Humphreys SC, Hodges SC, Patwardhan A, et al: The natural history of the cervical foramen in symptomatic and asymptomatic individuals aged 20-60 years as measured by magnetic resonance imaging. Spine 1998;23:2180-2184.

127. Bush K, Chaudhuri R, Hillier S, et al: The pathomorphologic changes that accompany the resolution of cervical radicu-

lopathy: A prospective study with repeat magnetic resonance imaging. Spine 1997:22:183-186.

128. Mochida K, Komori H, Okawa A, et al: Regression of cervical disc herniation observed on magnetic resonance images. Spine 1998;23:990-997.

129. Bartlett RJ, Hill CR, Gardiner E. A comparison of T2 and gadolinium enhanced MRI with CT myelography in cervical radiculopathy. Br J Radiol 1998;71:11-19.

130. Shafaie FF, Wippold FJ II, Gado M, et al: Comparison of computed tomography, myelography, and magnetic resonance imaging in the evaluation of cervical spondylotic myelopathy and radiculopathy. Spine 1999;24:1781-1785.

131. Singh A, Crockard HA, Platts A, et al: Clinical and radiological correlates of severity and surgery-related outcome in cervical spondylosis. J Neurosurg 1994;94(Suppl 2):189-198.

132. Wada E, Yonenobu K, Suzuki S, et al: Can intramedullary signal change on magnetic resonance imaging predict surgical outcome in cervical spondylotic myelopathy? Spine 1999;24:455-461.

133. Morio Y, Teshima R, Nagashima H, et al: Correlation between operative outcomes of the cervical compression myelopathy and MRI of the spinal cord. Spine 2001;26:1238-1245.

134. Suri A, Chabbra R, Mehta V, et al: Effect of intramedullary signal changes on the surgical outcome of patients with cervical spondylotic myelopathy. Spine J 2003;3:33-45.

135. Chen CJ, Lyu RK, Lee ST, et al: Intramedullary high signal intensity on T2-weighted MR images in cervical spondylotic myelopathy: Prediction of prognosis with type of intensity. Radiology 2001;221:789-794.

136. Uchida K, Kobayashi S, Yayama T, et al: Metabolic neuroimaging of the cervical spinal cord in patients with compressive myelopathy: A high-resolution positron emission tomography study. J Neurosurg Spine 2004;1:72-79.

137. DeBois V, Herz R, Berghmans D, et al: Soft cervical disc herniation: Influence of cervical spinal canal measurements on development of neurologic symptoms. Spine 1999;24:1996-2002.

138. Muhle C, Weinert D, Falliner A, et al: Dynamic changes of the spinal canal in patients with cervical spondylosis at flexion and extension using magnetic resonance imaging. Invest Radiol 1998;33:444-449.

139. Zheng Y, Liew SM, Simmons ED: Value of magnetic resonance imaging and discography in determining the level of cervical discectomy and fusion. Spine 2004;29:2140-2145.

140. Schellhas KP, Smith MD, Gundry CR, et al: Cervical discogenic pain: Prospective correlation of magnetic resonance imaging and discography in asymptomatic subjects and pain sufferers. Spine 1996;21:300-311.

141. Connor PM, Darden BV II: Cervical discography complications and clinical efficacy. Spine 1993;18):2035-2038.

142. Grubb SA, Kelly CK: Cervical discography: Clinical implications from 12 years of experience. Spine 2000;25:1382-1389.

143. Guyer RD, Ohnmeiss DD, Mason SL, et al: Complications of cervical discography: Findings in a large series. J Spinal Disord 1997;10:95-101.

144. Bogduk N, Aprill C: On the nature of neck pain, discography, and cervical zygapophysial joint blocks. Pain 1993;54:213-217.

145. Slipman CW, Plastaras C, Patel R, et al: Provocative cervical discography symptom mapping. Spine J 2005;5:381-388.

146. Hermann K, Bollow M: Magnetic resonance imaging of the axial skeleton in rheumatoid disease. Best Pract Res Clin Rheumatol 2004;18:881-907.

147. Bennett D, Ohashi K, El-Khoury E: Spondyloarthropathies: Ankylosing spondylitis and psoriatic arthritis. Radiol Clin N Am 2004;42:121-134.

148. Heuft-Dorenbosch L, Landewe R, Weijers R, et al: Combining information obtained from MRI and conventional radiographs in order to detect sacroiliitis in patients with recent onset inflammatory back pain. Ann Rheum Dis 2006;65:804-808.

149. Heuft-Dorenbosch L, Weijers R, Landewe R, et al: Magnetic resonance imaging changes of sacroiliac joints in patient with recent-onset inflammatory back pain: Inter-reader reli-

ability and prevalence of abnormalities. Arthrit Res Ther 2006,9:R11.

150. Bollow M, Hermann K, Biedermann T, et al: Very early spondyloarthritis: Where the inflammation in the sacroiliac joints starts. Ann Rheum Dis 2005;64:1644-1646.

151. Baraliakos X, Hermann K, Landewe R, et al: Assessment of acute spinal inflammation in patients with ankylosing spondylitis by magnetic resonance imaging: A comparison between contrast enhanced T1 and short tau inversion recovery (STIR) sequences. Ann Rheum Dis 2005;64:1141-1144.

152. Baraliakos X, Landewe R, Hermann K, et al: Inflammation in ankylosing spondylitis: A systematic description of the extent and frequency of acute spinal changes using magnetic resonance imaging. Ann Rheum Dis 2005;64:730-734.

153. Levine DS, Forbat SM, Saifuddin A: MRI of the axial skeletal manifestations of ankylosing spondylitis. Clin Radiol 2004;59:400-413.

154. Rudwaleit M, Baraliakos Z, Listing J, et al: Magnetic resonance imaging of the spine and the sacroiliac joints in ankylosing spondylitis and undifferentiated spondyloarthritis during treatment with etanercept. Ann Rheum Dis 2005;64:1305-1310.

155. Earwaker J, Cooton A: SAPHO: syndrome or concept? Imaging findings. Skeletal Radiol 2003;32:311-327.

156. Nachtigal A, Cardinal E, Bureau N, et al: Vertebral involvement in SAPHO syndrome: MRI findings. Skeletal Radiol 1999;28:163-183.

157. Major NM, Helms CA, Richardson WJ: MR imaging of the fibrocartilaginous masses arising on the margins of spondylolysis defects. AJR 1999;173:673-676.

158. Rossi F, Dragoni S: The prevalence of spondylolysis and spondylolisthesis in symptomatic elite athletes: Radiographic findings. Radiology 2001;7:37-42.

159. Shipley JA, Beukes CA: The nature of the spondylolytic defect: Demonstration of a communicating synovial pseudoarthrosis in the pars interarticularis. J Bone Joint Surg Br 1998;80:662-664.

160. Ulmer JL, Mathews VP, Elster AD, et al: MR imaging of lumbar spondylolysis: The importance of ancillary observations. AJR 1997;169:233-239.

161. Morrison JL, Kaplan PA, Dussault RG, et al: Pedicle marrow signal intensity changes in the lumbar spine: A manifestation of facet degenerative joint disease. Skeletal Radiol 2000;29:703-707.

162. Floman Y: Progression of lumbosacral isthmic spondylolisthesis in adults. Spine 2000;25:342-344.

163. Yuh WT, Zachar CK, Barloon TJ, et al: Vertebral compression fractures: Distinction between benign and malignant causes with MR imaging. Radiology 1989;172:215-219.

164. Ca C, Laredo JD, Chevret S, et al: Acute vertebral collapse due to osteoporosis or malignancy; appearance on unenhanced gadolinium-enhanced MR images. Radiology 1996;199:541-549.

165. Lecouvet FE, Vande Berg BC, Maldague BE, et al: Vertebral compression fractures in multiple myeloma. Part I. Distribution and appearance at MR imaging. Radiology 1997;204:195-199.

166. Spuentrup E, Bueker A, Adam G, et al: Diffusion-weighted MR imaging for differentiation of benign fracture edema and tumor infiltration of the vertebral body. AJR 2001;176:351-358.

167. Baur A, Stabler A, Bruning R, et al: Diffusion-weighted MR imaging for differentiation of benign versus pathologic compression fractures. Radiology 1998;207:349-356.

168. Taillandier J, Langue F, Alemanni M, et al: Mortality and functional outcomes of pelvic insufficiency fractures in older patients. Joint Bone Spine 2003;70:287-289.

169. Lourie H: Spontaneous osteoporotic fracture of the sacrum: An unrecognized syndrome of the elderly. JAMA 1982:248:715-717.

170. Grangier C, Garcia J, Howarth N, et al: Role of MRI in the diagnosis of insufficiency fractures of the sacrum and acetabular roof. Skeletal Radiol 1997;26:517-524.

171. Peh W: Intrafracture fluid: a new diagnostic sign of insufficiency fractures of the sacrum and ilium. Br J Radiol 2000; 73:895-898.
172. Stabler A, Beck R, Schmidt D, et al: Vacuum phenomena in insufficiency fractures of the sacrum. Skeletal Radiol 1995;24:31-35.
173. Fujii M, Abe K, Hayashi K, et al: Honda signs and variants in patients suspected of having a sacral insufficiency fracture. Clin Nucl Med 2005;30:165-169.
174. Pommersheim W, Huang-Hellinger F, Maker M, et al: Sacroplasty: A treatment for sacral insufficiency fractures. Am J Neuroradiol 2003;24:1003-1007.
175. Butler CL, Given CA 2nd, Michel SJ, et al: Percutaneous sacroplasty for the treatment of sacral insufficiency fractures. AJR 2005;184:1956-1959.
176. Brook AL, Mirsky DM, Bellow JA: Computerized tomography guided sacroplasty: A practical treatment for sacral insufficiency fracture: A case report. Spine 2005;30: E450-E454.
177. Etminan M, Girardi FP, Khan SN, et al: Revision strategies for lumbar pseudoarthrosis. Orthop Cin N Am 2002;33: 381-392.
178. Cleeland M, Bosworth DM, Thompson FR: Pseudoarthrosis in the lumbosacral spine. J Bone Joint Surg 1948;30:301-312.
179. Brown CW, Orme TJ, Richardson HD. The rate of pseudoarthrosis (surgical nonunion) in patients who are smokers and patients who are non-smokers: A comparison study. Spine 1986;11:942-943.
180. Deckey JE, Court C, Bradford DS: Loss of sagittal plane correction after removal of spinal implant. Spine 2000;25: 2453-2460.
181. Foley MJ, Calenoff L, Hendrix RW, et al: Thoracic and lumbar spine fusion: Postoperative Radiologic evaluation. AJR 1983;141:373-380.
182. Cannada LK, Scherping SC, Yoo JU, et al: Pseudoarthrosis of the cervical spine: A comparison of radiographic diagnostic measures. Spine 2003;28:46-51.
183. Gates GF, McDonald RJ: Bone SPECT of the back after lumbar surgery. Clin Nucl Med 1999;24:395-403.
184. Ghiselli G, Wang JC, Bjatia NN, et al: Adjacent segment degeneration in the lumbar spine. J Bone Joint Surg Am 2004;86A:1497-1503.
185. Hilibrand AS, Carlson GD, Palumbo MA, et al: Radiculopathy and myelopathy at segments adjacent to the site of a previous anterior cervical arthrodesis. J Bone joint Surg Am 1999;81:519-528.
186. Waguespack A, Schofferman J, Slosar P, et al: Etiology of long-term failures of lumbar spine surgery. Pain Med 2002;3:18-22.
187. Slipman CW, Shin CH, Patel RK, et al: Etiologies of failed back surgery syndrome. Pain Med 2002;3:200-214, discussion 214-217.
188. Perronne C, Saba J, Behloul Z, et al: Pyogenic and tuberculous spondylodiscitis (vertebral osteomyelitis) in 80 adult patients. Clin Infect Dis 1994;19:746-750.
189. Modic MT, Feiglin DH, Piraino DW: Vertebral osteomyelitis: Assessment using MR. Radiology 1985;157:157-166.
190. Maiuri F, Iaconetta G, Gallicchio B, et al: Spondylodiscitis: Clinical and magnetic resonance diagnosis. Spine 1997;22: 1741-1746.
191. Hadjipavlou AG, Cesani-Vazquez F, Villaneuva-Meyer J: The effectiveness of gallium citrate Ga 67 radionuclide imaging in vertebral osteomyelitis revisited. Am J Orthop 1998;27: 179-183.
192. Whalen JL, Brown ML, McLeod R, et al: Limitations of indium leukocyte imaging for diagnosis of spine infections. Spine 1991;16:193-197.
193. Pertuiset E, Beaudreuil J, Liote F: Spinal tuberculosis in adults: A study of 103 cases in a developed country, 1980-1994. Medicine (Baltimore) 1999;78:309-320.
194. Atkinson JLD, Miller GM, Krauss WE, et al: Clinical and radiographic features of dural arteriovenous fistula, a treatable cause of myelopathy. Mayo Clin Proc 2001;76: 1120-1130.
195. Gilbertson JR, Miller GM, Goldman MS, et al: Spinal dural arteriovenous fistulas: MRI and myelographic findings. AJNR Am J Neuroradiol 1995;16:2049-2057.
196. Luetmer PH, Lane JI, Gilbertson JR, et al: Preangiographic evaluation of spinal dural arteriovenous fistulas with elliptic centric contrast-enhanced MR angiography and effect on radiation dose and volume of iodinated contrast material. AJNR Am J Neuroradiol 2005;26:711-718.

CHAPTER
13 Psychological and Behavioral Assessment

Alicia Heapy and Robert D. Kerns

Chronic pain presents two broad challenges to proper assessment; the inherently subjective nature of pain complaints and the wide-ranging influence of chronic pain on patient functioning. These challenges necessitate a systematic assessment approach that employs standardized assessment of multiple domains of functioning using several assessment techniques, including questionnaires, behavioral observation, psychophysiologic measurement, diary data, and reports of significant others. This chapter begins with a brief discussion of the clinical goals of psychological and behavioral assessment of the patient with persistent pain, provides a rationale and context for the use of psychological assessment in the practice of pain medicine, articulates recommendations for the core domains of assessment, and provides an overview of the psychological assessment process. The remainder of the chapter provides specific information about some of the most commonly employed psychological and behavioral assessment strategies.

CLINICAL OBJECTIVES

Psychological and behavioral assessment of pain serves several clinical goals. First, information gathered in the assessment process provides important information about patients' pain experiences, their pain treatment histories, their current and past emotional and physical functioning, and their beliefs about pain. A thorough assessment of the multidimensional nature of the patients' pain experiences not only informs clinicians' treatment planning by identifying problems and intervention targets, but also reinforces the multidimensional nature of pain to patients, which may enhance engagement in future treatment modalities. Second, assessment allows the clinician to identify an individual's strengths and weaknesses and the factors that contribute to the development and maintenance of problems in physical, social, and emotional functioning. This information can direct the selection of the treatment modality that is most likely to correspond to the patient's assets and the intervention targets most related to the individual's specific functional deficits. Third, comorbid psychiatric or behav-

ioral conditions that may interfere with pain coping and overall adjustment can be identified and treated. Fourth, assessment can determine whether individuals are psychologically appropriate and likely to benefit from surgical or invasive procedure if they are medically indicated. Finally, a thorough assessment of a patient's pain complaint and functioning at baseline provides an important benchmark against which the efficacy of future treatments can be measured. Assessment should not stop after the initial visit but should be ongoing throughout the treatment process. This allows for the identification of new problems, quantifies progress across domains, and facilitates the refinement or revision of treatment if necessary. Posttreatment assessment is imperative to assess the overall success of the treatment, as well as the differential success of the treatment across various domains of functions such as pain intensity, social, emotional, and physical functioning.

Use of Psychological Assessment in the Practice of Pain Medicine

A request for a psychological evaluation or the report of the psychologist to a multidisciplinary pain team assists the treating provider or team in several ways. As noted, this multidimensional assessment is vital to proper treatment planning and subsequent evaluation of treatment outcomes. Psychological assessment may also reveal the need for adjunctive psychological treatment for the individual for treatment of preexisting or emerging psychosocial difficulties that may interfere with medical treatments for their painful condition. Psychological assessment can provide information about the individual's motivation and readiness to engage in treatment and the individual's treatment preferences. Finally, psychological assessment can provide data about a patient's suitability for surgical or other invasive procedures under consideration.

When making a request for a psychological or behavioral assessment, it is necessary to explicitly state the reasons for the request. It is helpful for the psychologist to understand what question the physician or team is trying to answer about a patient in order to do a thorough evaluation and provide meaningful feedback. Although any psychological or behavioral assessment should be multidimensional and include all relevant domains of function, the specific measures used and the areas of most intense focus will differ depending on the consultation question.

OVERVIEW OF THE PSYCHOLOGICAL ASSESSMENT PROCESS

Psychological and behavioral assessment of the patient with chronic pain should follow a hypothesis generating and testing approach. The assessment should begin broadly, and as problems are identified, contributing and maintaining mechanisms are hypothesized. The assessment process will be increasingly focused and behaviorally oriented as the hypothesized mechanisms are investigated. Generally the assessment process begins with a standardized interview that assesses the pain complaint as well as the individual's physical, emotional, social, and occupational functioning. It is essential to determine the individual's past and present level of functioning and the temporal association of any changes in functioning to the pain complaint. In addition to the information gained in the interview, questionnaires, diaries, behavioral observations, significant other reports, and medical record information may be used as adjunct sources of information. Use of multiple adjunct measures helps avoid the biases or error associated with reliance on a single assessment strategy. Hypotheses about the factors that initiated and maintain adjustment and functioning problems are generated and refined throughout the assessment process. Ultimately, the validity of the hypotheses is tested by examining the individual's response to treatment.

For example, anxiety and fear of pain have been shown to contribute to unfavorable outcomes for persons with chronic pain complaints.[1] Significant functional disability can be associated with fear of pain and further injury. These fears may lead to behavioral avoidance, muscle deconditioning due to reduced activity, muscle hyperreactivity to stress, negative and distorted cognitions about the adverse effects of activity, and psychological distress secondary to restricted access to pleasant and rewarding activities. Thus when an initial interview provides evidence of a significant decline in physical functioning and the presence of anxiety, the above described process becomes a reasonable hypothesis and avenue for more targeted assessment through the use of specific questionnaires, diaries, or significant other reports. Ultimately, the assessment process should result in a model that describes the individual's specific pain experience, explicates how that individual's beliefs, experiences, strengths, and weaknesses have resulted in their current level of functioning across domains, and provide an individualized treatment that uses these hypotheses to target specific factors for intervention.

DOMAINS OF FUNCTIONING

The multidimensional nature of chronic pain necessitates a broad assessment of multiple domains of functioning in order to provide a valid snapshot of the patient's unique pain experience and to meaningfully guide intervention strategies. A useful guide for the assessment process is the Initiative on Methods, Measurement, and Pain Assessment in Clinical Trials (IMMPACT) group consensus statement regarding the core outcome domains that should be assessed, and recommended instruments for measuring those domains, when evaluating the efficacy of a pain treatment.[2-4]

These recommendations, though originally generated to aid researchers in increasing comparability across randomized controlled studies of pain treatments, can be useful to the clinician in guiding assessment. The IMMPACT group consists of approximately 35 members from academia, government agencies, and the pharmaceutical industry. They recommend assessing the following chronic pain domains: pain, physical functioning, emotional functioning, patient ratings of improvement and satisfaction with treatment, treatment-related symptoms and adverse events, and patient disposition. Additionally, through literature review and expert consensus, the group has provided recommendations regarding specific assessment instruments within each domain that are applicable across a diverse range of pain complaints. Most recently, this same group has provided recommendations for future development of patient-oriented outcome measures that may provide more sensitive and efficient assessment of the key outcome domains relevant to a comprehensive assessment of persons with pain.

OVERVIEW OF ASSESSMENT STRATEGIES

Multiple strategies can be used to determine pain intensity, pain-related disability, and distress. Interviews, standardized questionnaires, diaries, behavioral observation, psychophysiologic assessment, and assessment of family members and significant others are commonly used to investigate and quantify pain experience and concomitant physical and emotional functioning. The use of multiple standardized assessment measures is encouraged to obtain comprehensive, valid, and reliable information.

The well-conducted *clinical interview* can be a rich source of information regarding a patient's pain and pain treatment history as well as the resulting physical, emotional, behavioral, and cognitive responses.[5,6] The interview also provides an opportunity for clinicians to interact with patients, to establish rapport, and to develop an impression of a patient's receptivity to rehabilitation and treatment efforts. Interviews may be standardized or "unstandardized." Even when conducting an unstandardized interview, it is useful to systematically investigate a prespecified set of domains. (Table 13–1 is an example of an interview

Table 13–1. Clinical Interview Template

CPMC Pain Assessment Template

Demographics:
Age, marital status, race, etc.

Referral Source:
Referring MD and service, reason for referral

Behavioral Observations:
Noteworthy pain behaviors or behaviors indicative of psychiatric disturbance, otherwise, state 'unremarkable'

Pain Complaints and Treatment History:
Please ask patient location of pain sites, then copy and paste questions 1 through 7 for each pain site. If patient describes a pain site as running through the leg, knee, and foot, check all sites below but evaluate as one pain site. Thus, for a patient who identifies 3 pain sites: lower back, right hip and leg, and hands, record 3 pain sites here, then complete 1–7 three times, each time identifying a different pain location "lower back," "hip and leg," and "hand." Qualify when necessary (e.g., left leg only, write this in).

1. Location of Pain
   [ ] Head/face [ ] neck [ ] shoulder [ ] arm [ ] hands
   [ ] stomach/abdomen [ ] upper back [ ] lower back [ ] hip
   [ ] leg
   [ ] knee [ ] foot [ ] anal [ ] genital
   [ ] whole body [ ] other sites (specify)

2. Intensity of Pain
   The patient rates their present level of pain as follows:

   0—1—2—3—4—5—6—7—8—9—10
   No Pain   Worst Possible Pain

   Worst pain gets: Best pain gets: Average pain rating:

3. Quality of Pain
   Don't prompt; use patient's own words when possible
   [ ] dull [ ] stabbing [ ] hot-burning [ ] shooting [ ] aching
   [ ] piercing [ ] tingling [ ] numb [ ] squeezing [ ] throbbing
   [ ] pulling [ ] sharp [ ] cramping [ ] gnawing [ ] heavy
   [ ] tender [ ] radiating [ ] deep
   [ ] other (specify)

4. Onset/Duration:
   Approximate time pain started:

5. Variations/Patterns/Rhythms:
   The pain is [ ] constant [ ] [ ] intermittent [ ] episodic/recurring
   [ ] other (specify)

6. What Relieves the Pain?
   [ ] sitting [ ] lying down [ ] standing [ ] heat [ ] cold [ ] rest
   [ ] distraction [ ] exercises [ ] movement
   [ ] other (specify)

7. What Causes or Increases Pain?
   [ ] sitting [ ] lying down [ ] standing [ ] heat [ ] cold [ ] rest
   [ ] exercises
   [ ] movement
   [ ] other (specify)

8. Effects of Pain
   Other associated symptoms: [ ] nausea [ ] vomiting
   [ ] dyspnea
   [ ] confusion [ ] weakness [ ] numbness
   [ ] other (specify)

   The pain affect the patient's
   [ ] sleep [ ] movement [ ] energy
   [ ] lifestyle [ ] personal relationships [ ] work [ ] emotions
   [ ] concentration [ ] appetite [ ] motivation [ ] ADLs
   [ ] IADLs
   [ ] other (specify)

9. Patient's Pain Goal
   Check any appropriate boxes, if appropriate, add brief descriptors of patient goals regarding reduced level of pain intensity, goals related to function, ADLs, quality of life, etc.):
   [ ] sleep comfortably [ ] comfort at rest
   [ ] comfort with movement
   [ ] stay alert [ ] perform activity (specify)
   [ ] other (specify)

   Acceptable level of pain (0–10 scale):

10. Pain Medications
    During interview, determine current use, dosage, and general effectiveness of pain medications to determine patient perception of effectiveness. For the report and CPMC rounds, cut and paste the complete list of current medications from medical chart in CPRS (1) click on "Templates" tab; (2) click on "Shared Templates," (3) scroll down and click on "Patient Data Objects"; when the cursor is in the correct place in the report, double click on "Active Medications."

11. Non-Pharmacologic Methods of Pain Relief and Effectiveness
    For each method patient has used, note which pain sites involved, past or present use, and effectiveness [yes/no]:
    [ ] Physical Therapy
    [ ] Surgical Interventions
    [ ] Psychotherapy
    [ ] Relaxation
    [ ] Biofeedback
    [ ] Manual Treatments
    [ ] TENS
    [ ] Heat Application
    [ ] Cold Application
    [ ] Occupational Therapy
    [ ] Distraction
    [ ] Exercises [ ] Stretching
    [ ] Other (specify)

Relevant Medical History
Significant recent medical history

Psychosocial History and Present Status:
Significant mental health and substance abuse history
Current employment status, current living arrangements

---

structure used in the author's [RK] comprehensive pain management clinic.)

Questionnaires and inventories provide opportunities for focused assessment of specific domains of functioning and quantifying patient responses. Because published questionnaires have typically met standards for reliability and validity, greater confidence can be placed in the information provided by this means. Questionnaires typically permit quantification of important dimensions of the experience of pain that allows for evaluation of within-person change over time. The concurrent administration of measures of multiple domains of functioning can assist in the identification of a person's relative strengths and weaknesses across these domains, such as the identification of the person who reports low levels of disability and distress despite an apparently severe level of pain intensity. Questionnaires with normative data offer the added benefit of providing a comparison point for evaluating the status of the respondent relative to others with similar painful conditions or within similar demographic (i.e., age, race/ethnicity, gender) groups. Ultimately, they may provide a more efficient and cost-effective option to more intensive and time-consuming interviews. Following this brief overview of the types of psychological and behavioral assessment strategies, a number of questionnaires and inventories that are frequently used in the assessment of persons with pain in the clinical setting are reviewed.

Diaries offer two advantages to other assessment methods. Diaries allow for the recording of prospective, day to day, or even more frequent, information about pain, sleep, and physical and emotional function, thereby eliminating distortion associated with memory and retrospective recall.[7] Additionally, diaries allow for the recording of the temporal association between pain and other factors. For example, many sleep diaries collect information about pain intensity scores before sleep as well as sleep quality and duration.[8] This allows for the investigation of the relationship between pain and functioning as opposed to examining either factor in isolation. The composition of diaries can vary from those designed to assess a single domain such as pain intensity to those that are much more comprehensive and multidimensional. The use of innovative technologies such as the personal digital assistant (PDA) and interactive voice response systems are increasingly being promoted as more efficient strategies for collection of prospective information.[9]

Although pain is a private, subjective experience, it is possible to observe signs that a person is experiencing pain by direct *behavioral observation*. Individuals can communicate that they are experiencing pain and the intensity of the pain through facial expressions, crying, moaning, limping, guarding, and rubbing affected areas. Behavioral observation of patients with chronic pain can provide valuable adjunct information beyond that gathered using a self-report format and is crucial to the evaluation of patients with cognitive or physical limitations that interfere with verbal communication. Behavioral observation methods have been developed for the assessment of persons with a range of painful medical conditions, including cancer pain,[10] rheumatoid arthritis,[11] osteoarthritis,[12] and low back pain.[13] Recently, Prkachin and colleagues[14] reported on a method for assessment of pain behaviors in the context of a clinical evaluation of persons with low back pain. These methods have also been developed and used in studies of pain-relevant communication in partner dyads.[15] In order to obtain reliable and valid behavioral observation data, it is necessary to have a systematic plan for behavioral observation, coding, and interpretation of the data; as such, the use of these methods requires considerable technologic sophistication and expense.[16] However, the use of behavioral observation methods is commonly limited to the clinical research setting due to the time-intensive and costly nature of these methods.

Psychophysiologic assessment methods are used to quantify the influence of psychological factors on physical processes that initiate and maintain chronic pain symptoms.[17] Evidence of the contribution of both psychological and physiologic factors to chronic pain argues for the inclusion of these methods in a comprehensive assessment of patients with chronic pain.[18] In the clinical setting, psychophysiologic assessment may serve several useful purposes. For example, demonstration of the relationship between experiences of personal and mental stress and psychophysiologic processes may be quite compelling in helping patients understand the importance of these relationships and the potential value of engaging in psychological interventions targeting the experience of stress.[19] Flor and Birbaumer[20] have proposed that psychophysiologic data may be used to tailor treatment, especially when incorporating the use of biofeedback. Psychophysiologic assessment data may be particularly valuable in monitoring response to treatment. Examples of psychophysiologic assessment measures are electromyography recordings, skin temperature and conductance readings, and heart rate and blood pressure values. Most recently, investigators have begun to employ neuroimaging and neurophysiologic methods such as electroencephalography, functional magnetic resonance imaging, and positron emission tomography to more explicitly examine the role of specific brain structures in central processing of pain and in the development and maintenance of persistent pain.[21] Flor[17] encourages research that may lead to better integration of these largely laboratory-based methods for the assessment of central functioning with peripheral psychophysiologic methods in the assessment of clinical pain conditions.

The *reports of families and significant others* in the assessment of pain has been strongly encouraged. Contemporary models of pain, particularly Fordyce's operant conditioning model[22] and Turk's cognitive-behavioral model[23] have specifically encouraged this focus given hypothesized roles of social contingencies in the perpetuation, if not etiology, of persistent pain and disability and the awareness of the frequent negative impact of persistent pain on significant others. In particular, the role of solicitousness in the development and maintenance of pain-related disability has been a topic of a great deal of research. Operant principles specify that when spouses provide solicitous responses to pain behaviors, the pain behaviors are more likely to be emitted in the future, even in the absence of continued nociception. Examples of solicitous behavior examined in the literature include expressions of sympathy or concern for the spouse, physical assistance or performance of a task and encouraging rest and discouraging activity. A recent review summarized evidence of relationships between marital functioning and chronic pain.[24] In addition to global measures of family and marital relationships, numerous questionnaires and inventories,[25-27] diaries,[28] and behavioral observation methods[15] have been developed specifically for the assessment of pain-relevant communication and the impact of pain on family members and significant others.

SPECIFIC PSYCHOLOGICAL AND BEHAVIORAL ASSESSMENT STRATEGIES

Standardized assessment instruments, often in the form of questionnaires or inventories are frequently used in the assessment of persons with pain (Table 13–2). Questionnaires allow for a focused examination of a specific domain, such as pain intensity, physical and emotional functioning, or coping beliefs, and provide quantitative data that can be used to understand the patient's functioning relative to the general population or other persons experiencing pain.

Pain Intensity

A primary objective in assessing persons experiencing pain is to determine their level of pain intensity. Change in pain intensity from baseline to posttreatment is often the primary outcome measure used in evaluating the efficacy of a given treatment. The following measures attempt to quantify the private experience of perceived pain. The three most commonly used measures of pain intensity are the *numeric rating scale (NRS)*, the *verbal rating scale (VRS)*, and the *visual analogue scale (VAS)*.[29]

The *NRS* is a single-item rating scale of pain intensity that can be administered in an oral or written format. Patients are asked to specify their pain on a scale from 0 to 10 with 0 representing "no pain" and 10 representing "the worst pain imaginable" or extreme pain. Although a 0 to 10 scale is the most commonly used, ranges of 0 to 20 or 0 to 100 are also used. Farrar and colleagues[30] have suggested that a decrease of 2 points on the 0 to 10 NRS may be indicative of clinically important change in pain intensity. Other advantages of the NRS include ease of administration and scoring, and high rates of completion by respondents.[29]

The *VRS* contains a list of pain descriptors that typically range in intensity from "no pain" to "severe pain." The number of descriptors can range from 4 to 15. Patients are asked to select the descriptor that best characterizes their level of pain. The descriptors are then assigned a number value based on intensity level (i.e., no pain = 0, mild = 1, moderate = 2, and severe = 3). Like the NRS, the VRS has demonstrated validity through significant correlations with other measures of pain intensity.[29] Strengths of this measure include ease of administration and scoring and high completion rate by respondents. Weaknesses include difficulty responding for persons with limited vocabularies or command of English and the possibility that the available descriptor choices do not adequately describe the respondent's pain, especially when the four-descriptor format is used.[29]

The *VAS* uses a 10-cm long line with end points denoting "no pain" at one end and "pain as bad as it could be" at the other. Respondents place a mark on the line that best characterizes their pain intensity. A pain intensity score is calculated based on the distance from the "no pain" end point to the respondent's mark.

A review by Jensen and Karoly found that all of the above mentioned measures demonstrated validity through significant correlations to other pain intensity measures and have comparable responsiveness with changes in pain in response to pain treatment.[29] Evidence suggests that respondents may prefer the VRS and NRS instruments over the VAS, and VAS instruments are more likely than NRS measures to result in missing or incomplete data, possibly due to cognitive or motor disabilities.[31] For these reasons, the consensus statement of the IMMPACT committee's review of core measures for chronic pain clinical trials recommends using the 11-point NRS scale to assess pain intensity and the VRS as an adjunct.[2] Although these recommendations were developed for use by clinical researchers, the importance of consistent use of valid, reliable, and understandable measures in clinical practice should not be ignored, and the guidelines provide valuable information for all users of these measures.

The *McGill Pain Questionnaire* (MPQ)[32] is a more lengthy measure designed to assess the quality of the pain experience, not simply pain intensity. Respondents choose the descriptors that best characterize their pain from a list of 78 potential descriptors that fall into 20 pain categories. These descriptors assess four pain domains: sensory, affective, evaluative, and miscellaneous. Within each category the individual descriptors reflect varying degrees of intensity and are assigned corresponding numeric values that reflect this difference. Respondents also indicate the location of their pain on a figure drawing and provide information about the factors that increase and decrease their pain intensity. The MPQ generates four scores: (1) the Pain Rating Index-Mean Scale Values, which is the sum of all words chosen in the available categories; (2) the Pain Rating Index-Rank Values, which is the sum of the value of each descriptor; (3) Number of Words Chosen, score that reflects the number of words chosen from each of the four categories; and (4) the Present Pain Intensity, a rating of current pain on a scale from 1 (mild) to 5 (excruciating). The MPQ has been widely used in a variety of pain studies and has been translated into several languages.[31] A 15-item short version of the MPQ (SF-MPQ) is also available.[33]

A recent review of the literature found that the MPQ scales have demonstrated validity through their association with perceived quality of life, pain medication use, and sensitivity to the effects of pain treatment.[31] The affective scale of the MPQ has been shown to be more strongly associated with measures of psychological distress than measure of pain intensity, which demonstrates the validity of this scale.[10] The MPQ scale scores have not shown a consistent association with pain intensity ratings, and a recent review concludes that there is not strong support to show that the MPQ scales measure the same construct as other pain intensity measures and may be less sensitive than "pure" measures of pain intensity

Table 13–2. Overview of Assessment Measures

MEASURE	DOMAIN	MEASURE DETAILS	ADVANTAGE/DISADVANTAGES
Numeric rating scale (NRS)*	Pain Intensity	Single item, written or oral	Demonstrated validity, easy to administer, high completion rate
Verbal rating scale (VRS)		Collection of pain descriptors	Demonstrated validity, easy to administer, high completion rate; may be difficult for persons with poor command of English
Visual analogue scale (VAS)		10-cm line with descriptive end points	Demonstrated validity, easy to administer; more likely to be incomplete than NRS or VRS
McGill Pain Questionnaire (MPQ)*	Pain Quality	Collection of pain descriptors; also assesses location of pain, and exacerbating and ameliorating factors	Demonstrated validity; not consistently associated with pain intensity but associated with psychological distress
Minnesota Multiphasic Personality Inventory (MMPI)	Personality	567 true-false items	Most widely used personality measure; uses normative data in scoring; high response burden; differences between pain and nonpain populations likely due to disease status rather than psychological functioning
Millon Behavioral Health Inventory (MBHI)		150 true-false items	Developed specifically for use with persons with medical conditions, demonstrated validity and reliability; not predictive of outcomes in treatment studies of persons with chronic pain
Multidimensional Pain Inventory (MPI)* (interference subscale)	Psychosocial Impact	52 items; assesses multiple domains	Demonstrated validity and reliability; useful with a variety of pain complaints; widely used
Sickness Impact Profile (SIP)		136 items and 24-item brief version for persons with chronic back pain	Demonstrated validity and reliability; responsive to change
Pain Disability Index (PDI)	Physical/Social Role Function	49 items; assesses perceived disability in 7 areas	Demonstrated validity and reliability; can identify specific areas of perceived disability
Brief Pain Inventory (BPI)*		32-items; short form has 15 items	Demonstrated validity and reliability; brief, easy to administer
Oswestry		10-item, multiple choice; measures degree of disability in 10 categories	Widely used, non-English versions available; can be used only for persons with low back pain
Beck Depression Inventory (BDI)*	Emotional Function	21 items; measures depression	Demonstrated reliability and validity, sensitive to change; possible bias for certain populations
Center for Epidemiologic Studies Depression Scale (CES-D)		20 items; measures depression	Demonstrated reliability and validity in a wide variety of ethnic populations; non-English version available; lacks sensitivity and specificity without psychiatric interview
Geriatric Depression Scale (GDS)		30 yes-no questions; measures depression in older adults	Demonstrated reliability and validity; good sensitivity and specificity; has not yet been widely used in chronic pain samples
Pain Anxiety Symptom Scale (PASS)		53 items; assesses pain-related fear	Demonstrated validity; poor prediction of pain-related disability
Spielberger State-Trait Anxiety Inventory (STAI)		20-item measure of state and trait anxiety	Acceptable psychometric properties; widely used; sensitive to change
Profile of Mood States (POMS)		65-item measure of several dimensions of emotional functioning	Strong psychometric properties; sensitive to change; captures negative and positive dimensions of emotional functioning
Symptom Checklist-90 Revised (SCL-90R)		90-item measure assesses numerous areas of psychological functioning	Demonstrated reliability and validity; normed on psychiatric patients and may not be valid for use with persons with chronic pain
Medical Outcomes Study Short Form Health Survey (SF-36)		36-item measure of perceived physical and emotional health	Psychometrically sound; widely used; has not yet been widely used in chronic pain samples
Survey of Pain Attitudes (SOPA)	Pain Beliefs and Coping	57-item measure of pain-related beliefs; brief forms also available	Psychometrically sound; scores correlated with treatment outcomes and physical and emotional functioning
Pain Stages of Change Questionnaire (PSOCQ)		30-item measure of readiness to change	Demonstrated reliability and validity; predicts completion of treatment; changes in PSOCQ predict changes in "readiness"; may not be predictive of treatment outcomes
Chronic Pain Coping Inventory (CPCI)		64-item measure to assess use of pain coping strategies	Psychometrically sound, patient coping strategies found to be associated with outcomes

*Measure was selected by the IMMPACT panel as the preferred measure within a domain.
From Dworkin RH, Turk DC, Farrar JT, et al: Core outcome measures for chronic pain clinical trials: IMMPACT recommendations. Pain 2005;113:9-19.

like the NRS and VRS.[31] The SF-MPQ demonstrated high correlations with the pain rating indices of the MPQ and was sensitive to change produced by epidural blocks and analgesic drugs in patients with pain.[33] The IMMPACT committee recommends the use of the SF-MPQ as a measure of pain quality and the affective component of pain because these aspects of the pain experience may respond differently to treatment than pain intensity.[2]

Personality

The *Minnesota Multiphasic Personality Inventory* (MMPI)[34] is by far the most commonly used objective measure of personality, and it is similarly the most commonly employed measure for the evaluation of psychological functioning of persons with pain. A recently revised version, known as the MMPI-2, is comprised of 567 true-false items that are used to derive scores on 10 clinical scales, 3 validity scales, and 15 new content scales.[35] The 10 clinical scales are the most commonly examined scales in clinical settings. These scales are named Hypochondriasis, Depression, Hysteria, Psychopathic Deviate, Masculinity-Femininity, Paranoid, Psychesthenia, Schizophrenia, Mania, and Social Isolation. Respondent scores on these scales are converted into standard T-scores so that they may be compared to normative data. The revised version of the measure is thought to be more culturally sensitive and advantageous relative to the original version because the validation samples were more representative of the population of the United States.

Nevertheless, significant concerns have been raised about the appropriateness of either the MMPI or the MMPI-2 for use in the assessment of persons with chronic pain.[36] Observed differences on the clinical scales between pain and nonpain samples have been demonstrated to more likely reflect disease status rather than psychological functioning.[37] An extensive research effort has focused on the identification of reliable subgroups of patients with chronic pain based on their MMPI profiles. The sum of this literature suggests that, although reliable subgroups can be identified, and despite evidence that the subgroups differ in terms of behavioral correlates of the experience of pain, it has yet to be demonstrated in a compelling fashion that the MMPI has value in characterizing patterns of coping with chronic pain over and above data derived from pain-specific measures.[36] This is particularly notable given the high response burden required for completion of the MMPI. In addition, inconsistent results from several studies challenge support for the value of the MMPI profiles as reliable predictors of pain treatment responsiveness.[38-40] Two studies stand in contrast to these relatively disappointing findings. In one study, Clark[41] reported that the negative treatment indicators (NTI) content scale from the MMPI-2 reliably predicted male patients' improvement in depressive symptom severity and physical capacity evaluations after multidisciplinary treatment. A study by Vendrig and colleagues[42] demonstrated that scores on several MMPI-2 scales reliably predicted posttreatment changes on measures of pain intensity and disability. Interestingly, in contrast to the Clark study findings, MMPI-2 scores did not predict posttreatment change on a similar measure of physical capacity.

The *Millon Behavioral Health Inventory* (MBHI)[43] was developed to assess the psychological functioning of individuals with medical conditions. This 150-item measure contains eight scales designed to assess the respondent's interaction style with medical professions (e.g., cooperation), six scales that assess the respondent's response to illness (e.g., pain treatment responsivity), and six scales that assess the presence of psychosocial stressors (e.g., social alienation). Questions are posed in a true/false format. Respondent's answers are scored by comparison with the base rate in the normative sample, which consisted of patients with a variety of medical illnesses.

The MBHI has been demonstrated to have substantial reliability and validity indices. It may have advantages relative to the MMPI-2 for use in the assessment of persons with pain conditions as a function of its relative brevity and the fact that it was developed and normed on medical, as opposed to psychiatric, populations. However, to date, studies have failed to demonstrate the predictive validity of the scale in studies of psychological interventions,[44] surgical interventions,[45] or multidisciplinary treatment[46] of persons with chronic pain.

Assessment of Psychosocial Impact

The *West Haven-Yale Multidimensional Pain Inventory* (WHYMPI)[47] is designed to measure psychosocial and behavioral aspects of chronic pain, and is useful across a variety of pain complaints. It is a 52-item multidimensional self-report instrument that employs 7-point Likert scales. The instrument consists of three sections. Section one includes six scales measuring pain-related interference across several domains including work and leisure activities as well as interpersonal relationships; perceived support from spouse or significant other; pain severity and suffering; perceived life control; and negative mood. Section 2 assesses patients' perception of their significant others' responses to their overt expressions of pain, classifying responses as solicitous, distracting, or negative. Section 3 measures the frequency with which patients engage in four clusters of everyday activities including household chores, social activities, outdoor work, and activities away from home. The WHYMPI takes approximately 10 to 15 minutes to complete and is written at a fifth grade reading level. Test-retest reliability over 2 weeks ranges from 0.62 to 0.91 and internal reliability coefficients range from 0.70 to 0.90.[47] Several investigative teams have generally replicated the factor structure and psychometric properties of the WHYMPI.[48] Turk and colleagues have proposed an empirically derived taxonomy of the

WHYMPI that includes three reliable profiles of persons with persistent pain labeled as Dysfunctional, Interpersonally Distressed, and Adaptive Copers[49]; these investigators and several other groups have replicated these findings in numerous samples of persons with various pain conditions.[50] The measure has been used in numerous empirical studies, including clinical trials of psychological and pharmacologic interventions, studies of the psychosocial impact of pain, and studies examining the role of psychosocial factors as contributors to the development and maintenance of persistent pain. Recently, a consensus group of academic, industry, and government experts (the IMMPACT group) recommended the use of the Interference Scale of the WHYMPI for use as an outcome measure in pain clinical trials.[2] The second section of the measure that focuses on significant other responses has been particularly valuable in evaluating the role of such responses as predictors of severity of pain and pain-related disability and distress.[51]

Three additions to the original version of the scale have enhanced its overall reliability, validity, and clinical utility. Rudy[52] added two items to the Life Control and Interference scales, Okifuji and colleagues[53] proposed alternative instructions for the significant other response section to reduce missing observations, and Bruehl and colleagues[54] developed a scale to detect random responding and malingering. A significant other version of the measure has also been published.[25]

The *Sickness Impact Profile* (SIP)[55] measures degree of disability across 12 domains of functioning. One hundred and thirty-six items are used to derive measures of sleep and rest, eating, work, home management, recreation and pastimes, ambulation, mobility, body care and movement, social interaction, alertness behavior, emotional behavior, and communication. These domain scores are combined to produce Physical, Psychosocial, and Total Disability scores. The SIP can be self-administered or administered by an interviewer in about 20 to 30 minutes.

An extensive period of development and testing and reports on these efforts support the reliability and validity of the measure. It has been found to be responsive to change during treatment for chronic pain.[56] A brief version consisting of 24 items has been developed specifically for use with persons with chronic low back pain,[57] and this measure has also been shown to have strong evidence of reliability, validity, and responsiveness to change as a function of psychological interventions.[58]

Physical and Social Role Functioning

Assessment of physical functioning has been recommended as a core outcome domain in pain clinical trials,[3] and others have suggested that it should perhaps be considered as the primary outcome in such trials.[59] Measurement of physical and social role functioning represents a challenge to the field given the broad range of levels of functioning, for example, the range from activities of daily living to the broader

domain of health-related quality of life. A variety of strategies have been developed to assess these varying dimensions, and selection of the appropriate measure in the research or clinical setting should take into account the specific population being assessed (e.g., unexplained chronic low back pain, frail elderly) and the purpose of the assessment (e.g., responsivity to change during treatment, comparison with population norms). Three of the most commonly used measures of this domain for the assessment of persons with painful medical conditions are briefly reviewed.

The *Pain Disability Index* (PDI)[60] is a brief measure of pain-related interference with role functioning. The PDI includes seven items assessing perceived disability in each of seven areas of functioning: family/home responsibilities, recreation, social activity, occupation, sexual behavior, self-care, and life-support activity. Each item is rated on a 10-point Likert scale (0 = no disability to 10 = total disability).

The PDI has demonstrated internal consistency values of 0.85 to 0.86 and excellent test-retest reliabilities.[61] Validity has been demonstrated through its association with the Oswestry Disability Questionnaire,[62] physical functioning tests,[63] and measures of pain intensity.[62]

The *Brief Pain Inventory* (BPI)[64] was originally developed to measure pain intensity and interference in patients with cancer pain, although it has been widely used to assess noncancer pain. A short form of the BPI containing 15 items is also available. The short form of the BPI has been found to have high internal consistency scores ranging from 0.82 to 0.95 for the Severity and Interference scales in a sample of patients with arthritis and lower back pain.[65] Demonstrations of its responsivity to change as a function of treatment for chronic pain, its brevity and ease of administration, and its availability in multiple languages have contributed to it being recommended by IMMPACT for use as a measure of physical functioning in pain clinical trials.[2]

The *Oswestry Disability Questionnaire* (ODQ)[66] was developed to measure functional status in persons with low back pain. Respondents are asked to indicate, using a multiple choice format, the degree of interference they experience in 10 functional categories (e.g., sleep, lifting, traveling) as a result of pain. This measure is widely used and has been translated in nine languages.[67] The ODQ has been recommended for use in functional evaluations[68] and spinal fusion outcomes assessment.[69] The major drawback of this measure is that it is specifically written for and validated in patients with low back pain and cannot be used in persons with other types of pain complaints.

Emotional Functioning

Assessment of the emotional functioning of persons experiencing chronic pain should be conducted in the context of any pain-relevant intervention. The high prevalence of emotional distress among persons with chronic pain conditions, the negative effects of emotional distress on pain and pain-related disability, the inflated health care costs associated with emotional distress among persons with chronic pain, and the influence of emotional distress on pain treatment participation provides the rationale for this recommendation.[2] The following brief review considers just a few of the many standardized measures of depressive symptom severity, anxiety, and anger, the three most commonly cited and studied emotional concomitants of the experience of persistent pain.

The *Beck Depression Inventory* (BDI) was developed to measure the behavioral manifestations of depression in adolescents and adults and to standardize the assessment of depressive symptom severity in order to monitor change over time.[70] In its original form, the BDI consisted of 21 groups of four to five statements describing symptoms in each cluster from low to high. Respondents were instructed to endorse the single item in each group that best described how they were feeling "right now." The original version was designed to be used in an interview format, but subsequent versions have more commonly been used in a self-report questionnaire format. In 1978, the full scale was revised to eliminate redundancy among some of the items and the time frame for assessment was altered to "during the last week, including today." Only four possible responses for each symptom cluster are now included, so that scores on the measure range from 0 to 63. In 1996, the BDI-II was published and included revisions to some items and the time frame for assessment to be consistent with the *Diagnostic and Statistical Manual of Mental Disorders IV* (DSM-IV). Although the BDI-II has advantages in terms of the content of the items and consistency with current diagnostic nomenclature, concerns have been raised about its sensitivity to change during brief periods of time.[71] The 21-item version of the BDI takes about 5 to 10 minutes to complete.

The reliability and several dimensions of validity of the measure have been extensively reported. In a review of 25 years of research with the BDI, Beck and colleagues reported on 25 studies that reported on the internal consistency of the measure.[72] Across psychiatric, healthy, and medically ill samples, indices of internal consistency (alphas) ranged from 0.73 to 0.95. Stability estimates (i.e., test-retest correlations) have consistently been high as well, typically varying in the 0.80 to 0.90 range depending on the assessment interval and sample. Validity estimates for psychiatric patients have been assessed by examining the correlation between BDI scores, and clinical ratings of depression (e.g., using the Hamilton Rating Scale for Depression) average about 0.72. For nonpsychiatric patients, the average validity estimate is 0.60. In a review of eight studies of sensitivity to change, Moran and Lambert[73] found that the BDI was sensitive to change as a function of psychotherapy and pharmacotherapy outcome studies. Some evidence suggests a reporting bias for certain populations,

including women, adolescents, and older adults, although the robustness of these observations is not clear.

The BDI has been used extensively in studies designed to evaluate the efficacy of pharmacologic and nonpharmacologic treatments for chronic pain,[74-85] and there is ample evidence of its sensitivity to change. Results of most studies provide compelling support for the use of the BDI in assessing improvements in depressive symptom severity as a function of pain treatment, and it has been recommended as one of the core outcome measures for assessment in pain clinical trials.[2]

The *Center for Epidemiologic Studies Depression Scale* (CES-D) was developed to screen for the presence of depressive illness and to measure levels of symptoms of depression in community samples.[86] The scale's 20 items were selected from existing scales (e.g., BDI, MMPI Depression scale, Zung Self-Rating Depression Scale) to represent the major components of depression on the basis of clinical and empirical studies. Respondents are asked to rate the frequency of a given symptom on a 0 (rarely or none of the time) to 3 (most or all of the time) scale with reference to the past week. Four items are worded in the positive direction to partially control for response bias. The CES-D takes about 5 minutes to complete.[87]

Indices of internal consistency (Cronbach's alpha) have been reported to be 0.85 for community samples and 0.90 in psychiatric samples. Split-half reliabilities are also high, ranging from 0.77 to 0.92. Test-retest correlations over a 6- to 8-week period range from 0.51 to 0.67.[87] Roberts[88] reported that studies of African American and Mexican American respondents revealed similar reliability estimates. The reliability and validity of the measure have also been examined in numerous ethnic populations,[89] and it has been translated into several languages.[87] Overall, high levels of internal consistency have been reported across numerous samples from the general population and patient samples, regardless of age, gender, race, and geographic location. In a sample of chronic pain patients, the level of internal consistency was found to be 0.90.[89] Indices of criterion-related validity have generally been reported to be moderate to high. For example, correlations between the CES-D and the Depression scale of the SCL-90 for samples of psychiatric patients have been reported to range from 0.73 to 0.90. Correlations with the Hamilton Rating Scale for Depression for similar samples have ranged from 0.49 to 0.85. Studies in older adult samples have revealed somewhat lower validity estimates.

Investigators have challenged the diagnostic sensitivity of the CES-D.[90-94] Investigators in the pain field have called for modifications of the measure in terms of item content[95,96] or scale cutoffs for the diagnosis of depression.[97,98] Ultimately, it is fair to say that the measure lacks the sensitivity and specificity for supporting its use in clinical diagnosis without concurrent use of a psychiatric interview. The CES-D has increasingly been used for the assessment of outcome following pain interventions, and in numerous cases, the measure has been demonstrated to be sensitive to change.[99,100]

The *Geriatric Depression Scale* (GDS)[101] was specifically developed to assess depressive symptom severity among older adults and was encouraged by observations that all of the other self-report measures of the construct were developed and validated with medically healthy younger adults. These measures suffer from the criticism that they include numerous somatic symptoms that are common among nondepressed older persons and that their format for responding may be difficult for some older persons.

The GDS consists of 30 "yes" versus "no" questions; 10 are negatively keyed and 20 are positively keyed. Questions are ordered with more "acceptable" items presented first. A 15-item short form is also available.[102]

In the original publication, indices of internal consistency (0.94) and split-half reliability (0.94) were extremely high. Correlations with the Zung SDS (0.84) and HAM-D (0.83) were also reported to be high, and the GDS was successful in discriminating mild from severe depressed groups in this same study and depressed older persons with arthritis from nondepressed persons with arthritis. Brink and colleagues[103] reported a high degree of sensitivity and specificity in discriminating depressed from nondepressed persons in a separate sample.

This measure seems to have substantial advantages for the assessment of depressive symptom severity among older persons. However, additional research with chronic pain samples will be necessary before its use in pain treatment outcome research can be supported.

The *Pain Anxiety Symptom Scale* (PASS)[104] was designed to assess the cognitive, physiologic, and behavioral domains of pain-related fear. It includes 53 items distributed across four subscales measuring Fear of Pain, Cognitive Anxiety, Somatic Anxiety, and Escape and Avoidance. Respondents use 0 (never) to 6 (always) scales to endorse the frequency of each of the symptoms. The PASS has been demonstrated to have adequate internal consistency[104] with indices of internal consistency ranging from 0.81 to 0.89 for each of the four scales and 0.94 for the total scale. Good predictive validity[105] and acceptable validity[106] have also been demonstrated. The PASS has been criticized for its poor prediction of disability relative to other pain-related fear measures,[107] and its factor structure has also been challenged.[108]

The *Spielberger State-Trait Anxiety Inventory* (STAI)[109] was designed to identify and quantify both situational anxiety (state) and dispositional anxiety (trait). The STAI consists of two 20-item self-report inventories of each of these constructs. Respondents rate the degree of agreement to brief statements (e.g., "I feel calm") on 4-point scales ranging from "not at all" to "very much so" in terms of both their present state (state version) and their frequency over time (trait version). There is a high concordance between pain and anxiety as measured by the STAI,[110] and it has

been widely used in the pain literature. It has acceptable psychometric properties,[111] and it is sensitive to change in anxiety as a function of pain treatment.[74,76,82,99,112]

The *Profile of Mood States* (POMS)[113] is a self-report measure comprised of a list of 65 mood-related adjectives that requires respondents to report the degree to which each feeling or mood state has applied to them over the past week using a 0 (not at all) to 4 (extremely) Likert scale. The scale assesses six dimensions of mood: Tension-Anxiety, Depression-Dejection, Anger-Hostility, Fatigue-Inertia, Vigor-Activity, and Confusion-Bewilderment. Because of its capacity for briefly assessing the multiple dimensions of emotional functioning of persons with pain, its strong psychometric properties including evidence of its responsiveness to change especially in analgesic medication trials, and its availability in multiple languages, it has been recommended for use in pain clinical trials.[2]

Indices of internal consistency (alphas) for the six mood scales ranged from 0.84 for Confusion-Bewilderment to 0.95 for Depression-Dejection. Stability estimates (test-retest reliability correlations) ranged from 0.65 for Vigor-Activity to 0.74 for Depression-Dejection. Concurrent validity was examined via correlations with MMPI-2 scales. Correlations between scales of the POMS and analogous scales from the MMPI-2 were largely in the expected direction and significant, with coefficients ranging from −0.58 to 0.69. The POMS requires only about 3 to 5 minutes to administer. The POMS has been used extensively in the pain treatment literature and has been shown to be sensitive to change as a function of pain treatment.[114,115] Advantages of the POMS include its ease of administration, its brevity, its development on nonpsychiatric populations, and its design to capture both negative and positive dimensions of emotional functioning. In particular, because the POMS has scales for anxiety, depression, and anger, three of the most important dimensions of emotional distress among persons with pain, the scale has an explicit advantage over any alternative scale. Within each of these three negative emotions, there is also an intuitive appeal to some of the items that are used to capture the construct for use with persons with chronic pain. For example, the Tension-Anxiety scale incorporates items that reflect both somatic and cognitive distress. The Depression-Dejection scale includes mood descriptors other than sadness that have been observed to be present in a large proportion of persons with chronic pain who meet criteria for current major depressive disorder but who otherwise deny feelings of depression. The inclusion of an Anger-Hostility scale is particularly novel and potentially an advantage of the POMS relative to any other comparable instrument. The Vigor-Activity scale represents a relatively unique opportunity to assess improvements in this key dimension of emotional functioning rather than relying on a reduction in negative mood and symptoms of emotional distress. The Fatigue-Inertia scale provides an opportunity to measure this common concomitant of the experience of chronic pain, especially when assessing pain treatment among persons with clinical pain conditions in which fatigue is particularly prevalent (e.g., pain in multiple sclerosis). The opportunity to attempt to discriminate effects of a pain intervention on fatigue and anergia, on the one hand, and other symptoms of emotional distress, on the other, may have particular utility in certain cases. Finally, given concerns about the effects of certain pain medications on cognitive functioning, the Bewilderment-Confusion scale may also have some benefit.

The *Symptom Checklist-90 Revised* (SCL-90R)[116] requires respondents to rate the extent to which they have been bothered by each of 90 physical or mental health symptoms in the past week. Responses are used to derive nine specific standardized indices of psychological disturbance labeled as Somatization, Obsessive-Compulsive, Interpersonal Sensitivity, Depression, Anxiety, Hostility, Phobic Anxiety, Paranoid Ideation, and Psychoticism. A Global Severity Index may also be derived. The reliability and validity of the SCL-90R for the evaluation of psychiatric patients have been extensively reported in a manual for the instrument[116] and by others.[117]

Like the MMPI-2, the appropriateness of this measure for use in the assessment of persons with chronic pain has numerous critics. For example, Shutty and colleagues[118] were able to identify only five, rather than nine, reliable factors from the SCL-90R in a sample of chronic pain patients. These investigators also challenged the validity of evaluating patients with chronic pain by using norms developed from samples of psychiatric patients.[119] On the other hand, Jamison and colleagues[120] identified three reliable subgroups of patients with chronic pain using the SCL-90R. These investigators demonstrated that patients with elevations on the subscales of the measure, relative to those with a profile consistent with normative data, reported significantly higher levels of disability, sleep disturbance, and emotional distress. Several other investigators have largely replicated these findings. Unfortunately, no data have been published in support of the ability of these subgroups or the individual scales to predict pain treatment response.[36] Finally, the sensitivity of the SCL-90R to change as a function of treatment has not been adequately demonstrated.

The *Medical Outcomes Study Short Form Health Survey* (SF-36)[121] was developed as a general measure of perceived health status and is generally self-administered. The measure contains 36 items that are combined to form eight scales: Physical Functioning, Physical Role Functioning, Bodily Pain, General Health, Vitality, Social Functioning, Emotional Role Functioning, and Mental Health. Respondents use "yes-no" or 5- or 6-point scales to endorse the presence of degree of specific symptoms, problems, and concerns. Scores on the scales range from 0 to 100 with higher scores indicating better health status and functioning. The measure takes about 10 to 15

minutes to complete. The SF-36 has been extensively validated with large samples from the general population and across several demographic subgroups, including samples of healthy persons older than age 65 years.[122] However, the SF-36 has only recently begun to be studied in chronic pain populations, including use as an outcome measure in pain intervention trials.[123]

Estimates of internal consistency (alphas) for most samples range from 0.62 to 0.94 for the subscales, with most estimates ranging to more than 0.80. Test-retest coefficients ranged from 0.43 to 0.81 for a 6-month period, and from 0.60 to 0.81 for a 2-week period.[124] The SF-36 has been shown to correlate reasonably well with other criterion measures including the Sickness Impact Profile and the Duke Health Profile, measures of ability to work and utilization of health care resources, and other such clinically meaningful criteria such as "burden of care."[125,126] Factor analytic studies have supported the presence of two distinct factors labeled Physical Health and Mental Health Functioning that account for 82% of the measure's variance.[127,128]

The SF-36 has only recently begun to be studied in chronic pain populations, including use as an outcome measure in pain intervention trials.[114,115,123] In one recent multisite trial of cognitive-behavior therapy, exercise, and their combination for persons with Gulf War illness that included chronic diffuse musculoskeletal pain as a primary feature, each of these treatments was found to be associated with improvements in the Mental Health Functioning component score.[129] On a more negative note, Rogers and colleagues reported that the SF-36 lacked reliability for the assessment of outcomes following multidisciplinary pain treatment and they questioned aspects of the measure's validity in discriminating dimensions of functional limitations.[130] Similar concerns about the sensitivity of the SF-36 to change have also been raised.[131] Continued examination of the sensitivity of the SF-36 Mental Health Functioning component to change as a function of pain interventions is indicated.

Pain Beliefs and Coping

The *Survey of Pain Attitudes* (SOPA)[132] was developed to measure beliefs about chronic pain and included five domains: perceived ability to control pain (Control), perceived level of pain-related disability (Disability), belief in medical cures for pain (Medical Cures), belief that others should be solicitous toward them when they are in pain (Solicitude), and the important of medication as a treatment for pain (Medication). The measure was later expanded to include two new dimensions: belief in the influence of emotions on pain (Emotions) and belief that pain indicates underlying physical damage that necessitates the limiting of physical activity (Harm).[133,134] The final version of the SOPA has 57 items and uses a 0 (this is very untrue for me) to 4 (this is very true for me) scale for responding. The SOPA is grounded in cognitive behavioral theory, which specifies that a person's beliefs about their pain influence important pain-related outcomes including emotional and physical functioning. A 30-item brief form of the SOPA (the SOPA-B)[135] and a 35-item short version (the SOPA-R)[136] are also available.

Internal consistency alphas for the 57-item SOPA scales are good, ranging from 0.71 (Control) to 0.81 (Disability), and test-retest stability ranged from 0.63 to 0.81.[134] The shorter version of the SOPA, the SOPA-B, has demonstrated a seven-factor structure consistent with the original measure, adequate internal consistency (ranging from 0.56 ([Medication] to 0.83 [Solicitude]), and strong correlations with the corresponding SOPA scales (0.79 to 0.97).[135] The original factor structure of the SOPA-R has largely been confirmed by other investigators and the measure has demonstrated good internal consistency (0.65 to 0.84) with the exception of the Medication scale (0.49).[137]

The main strength of the various versions of the SOPA is their correlation with clinical treatment outcomes. The Disability scale of the SOPA (belief that one is disabled) has demonstrated significant correlations with physical and emotional functioning[134,138,139] The Harm scale showed significant association with reported physical disability and the Medication scale was associated with treatment utilization.[134]

The most frequently used measure of the construct of "pain readiness to change" is the *Pain Stages of Change Questionnaire* (PSOCQ).[140] The PSOCQ measures persons' beliefs about their degree of personal responsibility for pain control and their interest in making behavioral changes to cope with pain. The measure is a 30-item self-report comprised of four distinct scales. The Precontemplation scale measures the degree to which a person endorses little personal responsibility for pain control and no interest in making behavioral changes. Contemplation represents an increasing recognition of personal responsibility for pain control and interest in behavioral changes that support pain management. The Action scale measures the extent to which a person believes that he or she is actively learning pain management skills. The Maintenance scale quantifies a person's degree of commitment to using self-management strategies in daily life and a high degree of personal responsibility for pain management.

A recent review of the empiric literature documents the reliability and the criteria and concurrent validity of the measure.[141] Internal consistencies of the four scales range from 0.77 to 0.86, and stability indices range from 0.74 to 0.88. The utility of the PSOCQ, however, hinges on its ability to predict important treatment process variables. Thus far, research has been encouraging. For example, PSOCQ subscales (i.e., Precontemplation, Contemplation, Action, and Maintenance) predict completion of outpatient[142] and inpatient[143] self-management treatment programs and improvements in pain coping during treatment.[137] Furthermore, changes in PSOCQ during treatment consistent with increased readiness to change or "forward stage movement" are associ-

ated with improvements in pain and physical and emotional functioning.[142,144] The readiness to change model, however, has not been without critics. For example, Strong and colleagues[145] challenged the external validity of the PSOCQ and demonstrated that a measure of self-efficacy had greater predictive validity than the PSOCQ.

The *Chronic Pain Coping Inventory* (CPCI)[146] is a 64-item questionnaire designed to assess an individual's use of pain coping strategies. Thus unlike other measures in this category, the CPCI focuses on behavioral strategies as opposed to cognitive strategies. The questions contained in the scale fall into three broad categories and comprise eight subscales: wellness-focused coping strategies (Exercise, Relaxation, Task Persistence, Coping Self-Statements), illness-focused coping strategies (Guarding, Asking for Assistance, Resting), and neutral coping strategies (Seeking Social Support). Respondents are asked to report the number of days in the last week that they used each strategy.

In the initial validation, the CPCI subscales demonstrated good internal consistency (0.74 to 0.91) and test-retest reliability (0.65 to 0.90).[146] Spouse report of patient disability and activity level was significantly associated with CPCI scales.[146] Other studies have largely confirmed the initially specified eight-subscale factor structure.[147,148]

Studies have found various associations between CPCI subscales and patient adjustment and outcomes, but overall, illness-focused coping strategies were found to be significantly associated with poorer patient adjustment and outcomes, and wellness-focused strategies were significantly associated with better patient adjustment and outcomes.[147-149] An exception is Relaxation with some studies showing a counterintuitive association between Relaxation and higher affective distress and lower pain control[147,150] and another showing no associations between Relaxation and any patient adjustment or outcome variable examined.[149] Importantly, even after controlling for pain severity and demographic factors, CPCI subscales were significant predictors of patient-reported pain-related interference, depressive symptoms severity, disability, and activity level.[148] A 6-month longitudinal study of persons on leave from work following a work accident producing lower back pain demonstrated that Higher Guarding scores were predictive of prolonged leave from work.[150]

CONCLUSION

This chapter provides an overview of the role of psychological and behavioral assessment in the context of the provision of comprehensive and integrative care to persons with painful medical conditions. Discussion of more general principles that can be used to guide decisions regarding psychological assessment of pain in the clinical setting is followed by a more detailed consideration of the some of the most commonly used standardized psychological assessment strategies. This review is designed to serve as a general guide to providers who are compelled by the value of more thorough consideration of psychosocial factors in the assessment of persons with pain that may be used to guide and evaluate pain care. Having acknowledged the potential value of such an approach, several relevant issues that may serve as cautionary notes and targets for future research and clinical investigation may be highlighted.

Of particular note are the overall limitations of this field with regard to consideration of the influence of cultural, racial, ethnic, and other aspects of diverse society on the reliability and validity of existing psychological and behavioral assessment methods. Few standardized measures have been specifically evaluated for their use with specific populations. Given a growing awareness and empirical evidence of reliable differences in the experience of pain among persons of differing racial/ethnic backgrounds, gender, and age, among other relevant variables,[151] caution is encouraged when employing most of the reviewed assessment strategies, and specific consideration of culturally specific norms for the measures is important.

Already emphasized throughout this chapter is the fact that several measures that are frequently used in this field were not originally developed for use with persons with painful conditions, and as a result, the validity of these methods is still subject to concern. The continued development and evaluation of psychological and assessment methods designed specifically for persons with painful conditions, and the further evaluation of the psychometric properties of these measures is clearly indicated. With increasing appreciation of differences in the experience of pain and its impact among persons with different conditions, specific examination of the psychometric properties among persons with similar disorders is encouraged. Consistent with this observation, the IMMPACT group, for example, although providing recommendations for the use of specific measures in the assessment of pain treatment effects, has encouraged the selection of measures that were developed and normed for a specific population (e.g., osteoarthritis patients) when such instruments are available.

Another area for continued work is the importance of developing patient-oriented outcome measures. One recent example is work that helped identify the types of pain coping strategies that are commonly used among older adults living in the community.[152] Using a more qualitative approach, these investigators have collected information that may be useful in developing an age-appropriate quantitative measure of pain coping that may be more valid than existing coping measures for this population. Several other investigator groups are working on the development and validation of more comprehensive measures for assessing patient-oriented outcomes, and the future availability of these methods promises to provide alternatives to existing methods that may have increased sensitivity to important and meaningful changes in pain and its impact, at least from the patient's perspective.

One particularly challenging area of ongoing research is the development of reliable and valid strategies for the assessment of pain among persons who are significantly cognitively impaired or otherwise unable to communicate. In the absence of existing reliable methods, clinical scholars have encouraged the use of an array of methods including reliance on systematic observation and reports from significant others. With a growing population of older persons with significant dementia and younger persons with significant brain injuries, efforts designed to develop reliable and valid strategies for pain assessment among persons with cognitive impairment will continue to be a high priority for clinical investigation.

Having cited a broad array of existing methods and measures for the psychological and behavioral assessment of persons with pain, it is critical to acknowledge some of the pragmatic issues related to their use in the clinical setting. Response burden is a critically important factor to consider when selecting measures for use in the clinical setting. Providers are encouraged to consider specific objectives of the assessment and the importance of reaching a balance between the desire for more thorough assessment and patient burden. Measurement precision, brevity, and costs of the assessment process are critical to consider in making decisions about the use of psychological assessment strategies. As already emphasized, the clinical interview and examination remain the core, or essential, methods for clinical assessment, and should not be displaced by the use of questionnaires, diaries, and other methods. Finally, managed care reimbursement methodologies are, of course, critical to consider in most clinical settings.

In closing, the potential value of incorporating assessment methods that permit a more comprehensive evaluation of the psychological and behavioral aspects of the experience of pain has been emphasized. As in most similar contexts, the "devil is in the details," and providers and investigators alike are encouraged to consider a range of important issues when designing an assessment approach consistent with their goals and objectives.

References

1. Vlaeyen JW, Linton SJ: Fear-avoidance and its consequences in chronic musculoskeletal pain: A state of the art. Pain 2000;85:317-332.
2. Dworkin RH, Turk DC, Farrar JT, et al: Core outcome measures for chronic pain clinical trials: IMMPACT recommendations. Pain 2005;113:9-19.
3. Turk DC, Dworkin RH, Allen RR, et al: Core outcome domains for chronic pain clinical trials: IMMPACT recommendations. Pain 2003;106:337-345.
4. Turk DC, Dworkin RH, Burke LB, et al: Developing patient-reported outcome measures for pain clinical trials: IMMPACT recommendations. Pain 2006;125:208-215.
5. Jamison RN: Mastering chronic pain: A professional's guide to behavioral treatment. Professional Resource Press. Sarasota, FL, 1996.
6. Heaton RK, Lehman RAW, Getto CJ: A manual for the psychosocial pain inventory. Odessa, FL, Psychological Assessment Resources, 1985.

7. Kerns RD, Finn PE, Haythornthwaite J: Self-monitored pain intensity: Psychometric properties and clinical utility. J Behav Med 1988;11:71-82.

8. Haythornthwaite JA, Hegel MT, Kerns RD: Development of a sleep diary for chronic pain patients. J Pain Symptom Manage 1991;6:65-72.

9. Heapy A, Sellinger J, Higgins D, et al: Using interactive voice response to measure pain and quality of life. Pain Med 2007;8:S145-S154.

10. Ahles TA, Coombs DW, Jensen L, et al: Development of a behavioral observation technique for the assessment of pain behaviors in cancer patients. Behav Ther 1990;21:449-460.

11. Anderson KO, Bradley LA, McDaniel LK, et al: The assessment of pain in rheumatoid patients: Validity of a behavioral observation method. Arth Rheum 1987;30:36-43.

12. Keefe FJ, Caldwell DS, Queen RT, et al: Osteoarthritic knee pain: A behavioral analysis. Pain 1987;28:309-321.

13. Keefe FJ, Block AR: Development of an observation method for assessing pain behavior in chronic low back pain patients. Behav Ther 11982;3:363-375.

14. Prkachin KM, Hughes E, Schultz I, et al: Real-time assessment of pain behavior during clinical assessment of low back pain patients. Pain 2002;95:23-30.

15. Romano JM, Turner JA, Friedman LS, et al: Observational assessment of chronic pain patient-spouse behavioral interactions. Behav Ther 1991;22:549-567.

16. Keefe FJ, Williams DA, Smith SJ: Assessment of pain behaviors. In Turk DC, Melzack R, (eds): Handbook of Pain Assessment. New York, The Guilford Press, 2001.

17. Flor H: Psychophysiological assessment of the patient with chronic pain. In Turk DC, Melzack R, (eds): Handbook of Pain Assessment. New York, The Guilford Press, 2001.

18. Flor H, Birbaumer N, Turk DC: The psychobiology of chronic pain. Adv Behav Res Ther 1990;12:47-84.

19. Flor H, Turk DC, Birbaumer N: Assessment of stress-related psychophysiological reactions in chronic back pain patients. J Consult Clin Psych 1985;53:354-4364.

20. Flor H, Birbaumer N: Comprehensive assessment and treatment of chronic back pain patients without physical disabilities. In Bond M, (ed): Proceedings of the VIth World Congress on Pain. Amsterdam, Elsevier, 1991.

21. Flor H, Elbert T, Knecht S, et al: Phantom limb pain as a perceptual correlate of cortical reorganization. Nature 1995; 357:482-484.

22. Fordyce W: Behavioral methods for chronic pain and illness. St Louis, CV Mosby, 1976.

23. Turk DC, Meichenbaum D, Genest M: Pain and behavioral medicine: A cognitive-behavioral perspective. New York, Guilford Press, 1983.

24. Leonard MT, Cano A, Johansen AB: Chronic pain in a couples context: A review and integration of theoretical models and empirical evidence. J Pain 2006;7:377-390.

25. Kerns RD, Rosenberg R: Pain relevant responses from significant others: Development of a significant other version of the WHYMPI scales. Pain 1995;61:245-249.

26. Schwartz L, Jensen MP, Romano JM: The development and psychometric evaluation of an instrument to assess spouse responses to pain and well behavior in patients with chronic pain: The Spouse Response Inventory. J Pain 2005;6:243-252.

27. Sharp TL, Nicholas MK: Assessing the significant others of chronic pain patients: The psychometric properties of significant other questionnaires. Pain 2000;88:135-144.

28. Flor H, Kerns RD, Turk DC: The role of spouse reinforcement, perceived pain, and activity levels of chronic pain patients. J Psychosom Res 1987;31:251-259.

29. Jensen MP, Karoly P: Self-report scales and procedures for assessing pain in adults. In Turk DC, Melzack R, (eds): Handbook of Pain Assessment. New York, Guilford Press, 2001.

30. Farrar JT, Portenoy RK, Berlin JA, et al: Defining the clinically important difference in pain outcome measures. Pain 2000;88:287-294.

31. Jensen MP: The validity and reliability of pain measures for use in clinical trials in adults. Presented at the second meeting of the Initiative on Methods, Measurement, and Pain Assessment in Clinical Trials (IMMPACT-II). Available at www.immpact.org/meetings.html.

32. Melzack R: The McGill Pain Questionnaire: Major properties and scoring methods. Pain 1975;1:277-299.

33. Melzack R: The Short-Form McGill Pain Questionnaire. Pain 1987;30:191-197.

34. Hathaway SR, McKinley J: The Minnesota Multiphasic Personality Inventory. Minneapolis, University of Minnesota Press, 1943.

35. Hathaway SR, McKinley JC, Butcher JN, et al: Minnesota Multiphasic Personality Inventory-2: Manual for administration. Minneapolis, University of Minnesota Press, 1989.

36. Bradley LA, McKendree-Smith NL: Assessment of psychological status using interviews and self-report instruments. In Turk DC, Melzack R, (eds): Handbook of Pain Assessment, 2nd ed. New York, Guilford Press, 2001.

37. Pincus T, Callahan LF, Bradley LA, et al: Elevated MMPI scores for hypochondriasis, depression, and hysteria in patients with rheumatoid arthritis reflect disease rather than psychological status. Arthritis Rheum 1986;29:1456-1466.

38. Guck TP, Meilman PW, Skultety M, et al: Pain-patient Minnesota Multiphasic Personality Inventory subgroups: Evaluation of long-term treatment outcome. J Behav Med 1988; 11:159-169.

39. McCreary C: Empirically derived MMPI profile clusters and characteristics of low back pain patients. J Consult Clin Psychol 1985;53:558-560.

40. Moore JE, Armentrout DP, Parker JC, et al: Empirically-derived pain-patient MMPI subgroups: Prediction of treatment outcome. J Behav Med 1986;9:51-63.

41. Clark ME: MMPI-2 Negative treatment indicators content and content component scales: Clinical correlates and outcome prediction for men with chronic pain. Psychol Assess 1996;8:32-38.

42. Vendrig AA, Derksen JL, deMey HR: Utility of selected MMPI-2 scales in the outcome prediction for patients with chronic back pain. Psychol Assess 1999;11:381-385.

43. Millon T, Green C, Meagher R: Millon Behavioral Health Inventory Manual, 3rd ed. Minneapolis, MN, National Computer Systems, 1983.

44. Gatchel RJ, Deckel AW, Weinberg N, et al: The utility of the Millon Behavioral Health Inventory in the study of chronic headaches. Headache 1985;25:49-54.

45. Herron L, Turner JA, Eersek M, et al: Does the Millon Behavioral Health Inventory (MBHI) predict lumbar laminectomy outcome? A comparison with the Minnesota Multiphasic Personality Inventory (MMPI). J Spin Disord 1992;5:188-192.

46. Gatchel RJ, Mayer TG, Capra P, et al: Millon Behavioral Health Inventory: Its utility in predicting physical function in patients with low back pain. Arch Phys Med Rehabil 1986;6:878-882.

47. Kerns RD, Turk DC, Rudy TE: The West Haven-Yale Multidimensional Pain Inventory (WHYMPI). Pain 1985;23:345-356.

48. Riley JL III, Zawacki TM, Robinson ME, et al: Empirical test of the factor structure of the West Haven-Yale Multidimensional Pain Inventory. Pain 1999;15:24-30.

49. Turk DC, Rudy TE: Toward an empirically derived taxonomy of chronic pain patients: Integration of psychological assessment data. J Couns Clin Psych 1988;56:233-238.

50. Turk DC, Rudy TE: The robustness of an empirically derived taxonomy of chronic pain patients. Pain 1990;43:27-36.

51. Kerns RD, Haythornthwaite JA, Southwick S, et al: The role of marital interaction in chronic pain and depressive symptom severity. J Psychosom Res 1990;34:401-408.

52. Rudy TE: Multiaxial assessment of pain: Multidimensional Pain Inventory. Computer program users' manual. Version 2.1. Pittsburgh, PA, Pain Evaluation and Treatment Institute, 1989.

53. Okifuji A, Turk DC, Eveleigh DJ: Improving the rate of classification of patients with the Multidimensional Pain Inventory (MPI): Clarifying the meaning of "significant other." Clin J Pain 1999;15:290-296.

54. Bruehl S, Lofland KR, Sherman JJ, et al: The Variable Responding Scale for detecting random responding on the Multidimensional Pain Inventory. Psychol Assess 1999;10:3-9.
55. Bergner M, Bobbitt RA, Carter WB, et al: The Sickness Impact Profile: Development and final revision of a health status measure. Med Care 1981;19:787-805.
56. Sanders SH, Brena SF: Empirically derived chronic pain patient subgroups: The utility of multidimensional clustering to identify differential treatment effects. Pain 1983;54:51-56.
57. Roland M, Morris R: A study of the natural history of back pain: Part I. Development of a reliable and sensitive measure of disability in low-back pain. Spine 1983;8:141-144.
58. Klein RG, Eek BC: Low-energy laser treatment and exercise for chronic low back pain: Double blind controlled trial. Arch Phys Med Rehabil 1990;71:34-37.
59. Kerns RD: Psychosocial factors: Primary or secondary outcomes? In Campbell JN, Mitchell MJ, (eds): Pain treatment centers at a crossroads: A practical conceptual reappraisal. Seattle, IASP Press, 1996.
60. Pollard CA: Preliminary validity study of the pain disability index. Percept Mot Skills 1984;59:974.
61. Tait RC, Pollard CA, Margolis RB, et al: The Pain Disability Index: Psychometric and validity data. Arch Phys Med Rehabil 1987;68:438-441.
62. Gronblad M, Hupli M, Wennerstrand P, et al: Intercorrelation and test-retest reliability of the Pain Disability Index (PDI) and the Oswestry Disability Questionnaire (ODQ) and their correlation with pain intensity in low back pain patients. Clin J Pain 1993;9:189-195.
63. Gronblad M, Jarvinen E, Hurri H, et al: Relationship of the Pain Disability Index (PDI) and the Oswestry Disability Questionnaire (ODQ) with three dynamic physical tests in a group of patients with chronic low-back and leg pain. Clin J Pain 1994;10:197-203.
64. Cleeland CS, Ryan KM: Pain assessment: Global use of the brief pain inventory. Ann Acad Med 1994;23:129-138.
65. Keller S, Bann CM, Dodd SL, et al: Validity of the brief pain inventory for use in documenting the outcomes of patients with noncancer pain. Clin J Pain 2004;20:309-318.
66. Fairbank JC, Couper J, Davies JB, et al: The Oswestry low back pain disability questionnaire. Physiotherapy 1980;66:271-273.
67. Roland M, Fairbank J: The Roland-Morris Disability Questionnaire and the Oswestry Disability Questionnaire. Spine 2000;25:3115-3124.
68. Deyo R, Battie M, Beurskens A, et al: Outcome measures for low back research: A proposal for standardized use. Spine 1998;23:2003-2013.
69. Blount K J, Krompinger WJ, Maljanian R, et al: Moving toward a standard for spinal fusion outcomes assessment. J Spin Disord Tech 2002;15:16-23.
70. Beck AT, Ward CH, Mendelsohn M, et al: An inventory for measuring depression. Arch Gen Psychiatry 1961;4:561-571.
71. Yonkers KA, Samson J: Mood disorders measures. In American Psychiatric Association Handbook of Psychiatric Measures. Washington, DC, American Psychiatric Association, 2000.
72. Beck AT, Steer RA, Garbin MG: Psychometric properties of the Beck Depression Inventory: Twenty-five years of evaluation. Clin Psychol Rev 1988;8:77-100.
73. Moran PW, Lambert MJ: A review of current assessment tools for monitoring changes in depression: In Lamber MD, Christiensen ER, Dejolie SS, (eds): The Assessment of Psychotherapy and Outcomes. New York, Wiley, 1983.
74. Applebaum KA, et al: Cognitive-behavioral therapy of a veteran population with moderate to severe RA. Behav Ther 1988;19:489-502.
75. Burns JW, Johnson BJ, Mahoney N, et al: Cognitive and physical capacity process variables predict long-term outcome after treatment for chronic pain. J Consult Clin Psychol 1998;66:434-439.
76. Kerns RD, Turk DC, Holzman AD, et al: Comparison of cognitive-behavioral and behavioral approaches to the out-patient treatment of chronic pain. Clin J Pain 1986;1:195-203.
77. Khatami M, Rush AJ: A one-year follow-up of the multimodal treatment for chronic pain. Pain 1982;14:45-52.
78. Kleinke CL: How chronic pain patients cope with pain: Relation to treatment outcome in a multidisciplinary pain clinic. Cognit Ther Res 1992;16:669-685.
79. Marhold C, Linton SJ, Melin L: A cognitive-behavioral return-to-work program: Effects on pain patients with a history of long-term versus short-term sick leave. Pain 2001;91:155-163.
80. Nicholas MK, Wilson PH, Goyen J: Operant-behavioral and cognitive-behavioral treatment for chronic low back pain. Pain 1991;48:339-347.
81. Philips HC: The effects of behavioral treatment on chronic pain. Behav Res Ther 1987;25:365-377.
82. Richardson IH, Richardson PH, Williams AC de C, et al: The effects of a cognitive-behavioural pain management programme on the quality of work and employment status of severely impaired chronic pain patients. Disabil Rehabil 1994;16:26-34.
83. Taenzer P, Melzack R, Jeans ME: Influence of psychological factors on postoperative pain, mood, and analgesic requirements. Pain 1986;24:331-342.
84. Turner JA: Comparison of group progressive-relaxation and cognitive-behavioral group therapy for chronic low back pain. J Consult Clin Psychol 1982;50:757-765.
85. Williams AC de C, Richardson PH, Nicholas MK, et al: Inpatient vs. outpatient pain management: Results of a randomized controlled trial. Pain 1996;66:13-22.
86. Radloff LS: The CES-D Scale: A self-report depression scale for research in the general population. Appl Psychol Measure 1977;1:385-401.
87. Radloff LS, Locke BZ: Center for Epidemiologic Studies Depression Scale (CES-D). In Handbook of Psychiatric Measures. Washington, DC, American Psychiatric Association, 2000.
88. Roberts RE: Reliability of the CES-D in different ethnic contexts. Psychiatry Res 1980;12:125-134.
89. Arnstein P, Caudill M, Mandle CL, et al: Self efficacy as a mediator of the relationship between pain intensity, disability and depression in chronic pain patients. Pain. 1999;80:483-491.
90. Boyd JH, Weissman MM, Thompson WD, et al: Screening for depression in a community sample: Understanding the discrepancies between depression symptom and diagnostic scales. Arch Gen Psychiatry 1982;39:1195-1200.
91. Breslau N: Depressive symptoms, major depression, and generalized anxiety: A comparison of self-reports on CES-D and results from diagnostic interviews. Psychiatry Res 1985;15:219-229.
92. Fechner-Bates S, Coyne JC, Schwenk TL: The relationship of self-reported distress to depressive disorders and other psychopathology. J Consul Clin Psychol 1994;62:550-559.
93. Myers JK, Weissman MM: Use of a self-report symptom scale to detect depression in a community sample. J Psychiatry 1980;137:1081-1084.
94. Roberts RE, Vernon SW: The Center for Epidemiological Studies-Depression Scale: Its use in a community sample. Am J Psychiatry 1983;140:41-46.
95. Blalock SJ, DeVellis RF, Brown GK, et al: Validity of the Center for Epidemiological Studies Depression Scale in arthritis populations. Arthrit Rheum 1989;32:991-997.
96. Brown GK: A causal analysis of chronic pain and depression. J Abnorm Psychol 1990;99:127-137.
97. Magni G, Caldieron C, Rigatti-Luchini S, et al: Chronic musculoskeletal pain and depressive symptoms in the general population: An analysis of the 1st National Health and Nutrition Examination Survey data. Pain 1990;43:299-307.
98. Turk DC, Okifuji A: Detecting depression in chronic pain patients: Adequacy of self-reports. Behav Res Ther 1994;32:9-16.
99. Nielsen WR, Walker C, McCain GA: Cognitive-behavioral treatment of fibromyalgia: Preliminary findings. J Rheumatol 1992;19:98-103.

100. Turner JA, Clancy S, McQuade KJ, et al: Effectiveness of behavioral therapy for chronic low back pain: A component analysis. J Consult Clin Psychol 1990;58:573-579.

101. Yesavage JA, Brink TL: Development and validation of a geriatric depression screening scale: A preliminary report. J Psychiatr Res 1983;17:37-49.

102. Sheikh JI, Yesavage JA: Geriatric Depression Scale (GDS): Recent evidence and development of a shorter version. Clin Gerontol 1986;5:165-173.

103. Brink TA, Yesavage JA, Lum O, et al: Screening tests for geriatric depression. Clin Gerontol 1982;1:37-43.

104. McCracken LM, Zayfert C, Gross RT: The Pain Anxiety Symptoms Scale: Development and validation of a scale to measure fear of pain. Pain 1992;50:67-73.

105. McCracken LM, Faber SD, Janeck AS: Pain-related anxiety predicts nonspecific physical complaints in persons with chronic pain. Behav Res Ther 1998;34:927-933.

106. McCracken LM, Gross RT, Aikens J, et al: The assessment of anxiety and fear in persons with chronic pain: A comparison of instruments. Behav Res Ther 1996;34:927-933.

107. Crombez G, Vlaeyen JWS, Heuts PHTG, et al: Pain-related fear is more disabling than pain itself: Evidence on the role of pain-related fear in chronic back pain disability. Pain 1999;80:329-339.

108. Larsen DK, Taylor S, Asmundson GJG: Exploratory factor analysis of the Pain Anxiety Symptoms Scale in patients with chronic pain complaints. Pain 1997;69:27-34.

109. Spielberger CD, Gorsuch RL, Lushene R: Manual for the State-Trait Anxiety Inventory. Palo Alto, CA, Consulting Psychologists Press, 1970.

110. Polatin PB, Kinney RK, Gatchel RJ, et al: Psychiatric illness and chronic low-back pain. The mind and the spine—Which goes first? Spine 1993;18:66-71.

111. Spielberger CD, Gorsuch RL, Lushene R, et al: Manual for the State-Trait Anxiety Inventory (Form Y). Palo Alto, CA, Consulting Psychologists Press, 1983.

112. Bradley LA, Young LD, et al: Effects of psychological therapy on pain behavior of RA patients: Treatment outcome and six month follow-up. Arthritis Rheum 1987;30:1105-1114.

113. McNair DM, Lorr M, Droppleman LF: Manual for the profile of mood states. San Diego, CA, Educational and Industrial Testing Service, 1971.

114. Backonja M, Beydoun A, Edwards KR, et al, for the Gabapentin Diabetic Neuropathy Study Group: Gabapentin for the symptomatic treatment of painful neuropathy in patients with diabetes mellitus. JAMA 1998;280:1831-1836.

115. Rowbotham M, Harden N, Stacey B, et al, for the Gabapentin Postherpetic Neuralgia Study Group. Gabapentin for the treatment of postherpetic neuralgia. JAMA 1998;280:1837-1842.

116. Derogatis L: The SCL-90R manual-II: Administration, scoring and procedures. Towson, MD, Clinical Psychometric Research, 1983.

117. Peveler RC, Fairburn CG: Measurement of neurotic symptoms by self-report questionnaire: Validity of the SCL-90R. Psych Med 1990;20:873-870.

118. Shutty MS, DeGood DE, Schwartz DP: Psychological dimensions of distress in chronic pain patients: A factor analytic study of Symptom Checklist-90 responses. J Consult Clin Psychol 1986;54:836-842.

119. Buckalew SP, DeGood DE, Schwartz DP, et al: Cognitive and somatic item response patterns of pain patients, psychiatric patients, and hospital employees. J Clin Psychol 1986;42:852-860.

120. Jamison RN, Rock DL, Parris WCV: Empirically derived Symptom Checklist 90 subgroups of chronic pain patients: A cluster analysis. J Behav Med 1988;11:147-158.

121. Ware JE, Sherbourne CD: The MOS 36-item Short-Form Health Survey (SF-36), I: Conceptual framework and item selection. Med Care 1992;30:473-483.

122. Kazis LE, Miller DR, Clark J, et al: Health related quality of life in patients served by the Department of Veterans Affairs: Results from the Veterans Health Study. Arch Intern Med 1998;158:626-632.

123. Katz JN, Harris TM, Larson MG, et al: Predictors of functional outcomes after arthroscopic partial meniscectomy. J Rheumatol 1992;19:1938-1942.

124. McHorney CA, Ware JE, Lu JFR, et al: The MOS 36-item Short-Form Health Survey (SF-36), III: Tests of data quality, scaling assumptions, and reliability across diverse patient groups. Med Care 1994;32:40-66.

125. McHorney CA, Ware J, Raczek AE: The MOS 36-item Short-Form Health Survey (SF-36), II: Psychometric and clinical tests of validity in measuring physical and mental health constructs. Med Care 1993;31:247-263.

126. Ware JE Jr: SF-36 health survey update. Spine 2000;25:3130-3139.

127. Kazis LE, Skinner K, Rogers W, et al: Health status and outcomes of veterans: Physical and mental component summary scores (SF-36V). 1998 National Survey of Ambulatory Care Patients. Mid-year executive report. Washington, DC, and Bedford, Office of Performance and Quality, Health Assessment Project, Center for Health Quality Outcomes and Economic Research, HSR&D Service, Veterans Administration, 1998.

128. Ware JE, Kosinski M, Keller SD: SF-36 physical and mental health summary scales: A user's manual. Boston, Health Assessment Lab, New England Medical Center, 1994.

129. Donta ST, Clauw DJ, Engel CC, et al: A randomized, multi-center trial of cognitive behavioral therapy and aerobic exercise for Gulf War veterans' illnesses: A Veterans Affairs cooperative study (CSP #470). JAMA 2003;289:1396-1404.

130. Rogers WH, Wittink H, Wagner A, et al: Assessing individual outcomes during outpatient multidisciplinary chronic pain treatment by means of an augmented SF-36. Pain Med 2000;1:44-54.

131. McHorney C, Tarlov A: Individual-patient monitoring in clinical practice: Are available health status surveys adequate? Qual Life Res 1995;4:293-307.

132. Jensen MP, Karoly P, Huger R: The development and preliminary validation of an instrument to assess patients' attitudes toward pain. J Psychosom Res 1987;31:393-400.

133. Jensen MP, Karoly P, O'Riordan EF, et al: The subjective experience of acute pain: An assessment of the utility of 10 indices. Clin J Pain 1989;5:153-159.

134. Jensen MP, Turner JA, Romano JM, et al: Relationship of pain-specific beliefs to chronic pain adjustment. Pain 1994;57:301-309.

135. Tait RC, Chibnall JT: Development of a brief version of the Survey of Pain Attitudes. Pain 1997;70:229-235.

136. Jensen MP, Turner JA, Romano JM: Pain belief assessment: A comparison of short and long versions of the Survey of Pain Attitudes. J Pain 2000;1:138-150.

137. Strong J, Ashton R, Chant D: The measurement of attitudes towards and beliefs about pain. Pain 1992;48:227-236.

138. Strong J, Ashton R, Chant D: Pain intensity measurement in chronic low back pain. Clin J Pain 1990;7:209-218.

139. Jensen MP, Karoly P: Control beliefs, coping efforts, and adjustment to chronic pain. J Consult Clin Psych 1991;59:431-438

140. Kerns RD, Rosenberg R, Jamison RN, et al: Readiness to adopt a self-management approach to chronic pain: The Pain Stages of Change Questionnaire (PSOCQ). Pain 1997;72:227-234.

141. Kerns RD, Habib S: A critical review of the Pain Readiness to Change Model. J Pain 2004;5:357-367.

142. Kerns RD, Rosenberg R: Predicting responses to self-management treatments for chronic pain: Application of the pain stages of change model. Pain 2000;51:49-55.

143. Biller N, Arnstein P, Caudill M, et al: Predicting completion of a cognitive-behavioral pain management program by initial measures of a chronic pain patient's readiness for change. Clin J Pain 2000;16:352-359.

144. Glenn B, Burns J: Pain self-management in the process and outcome of multidisciplinary treatment of chronic pain: Evaluation of a stage of change model. J Behav Med 2003;26:417-433.

145. Strong J, Westbury K, Smith G, et al: Treatment outcome in individuals with chronic pain: Is the Pain Stages of Change Questionnaire (PSOCQ) a useful tool? Pain 2002;97:65-73.

146. Jensen MP, Turner JA, Romano JM, et al: The Chronic Pain Coping Inventory: Development and preliminary validation. Pain 1995;60:203-216.

147. Hadjistavropoulos HD, MacLeod FK, Asmundson GJG: Validation of the Chronic Pain Coping Inventory. Pain 1999;80:471-481.

148. Tan G, Nguyen Q, Anderson KO, et al: Further validation of the Chronic Pain Coping Inventory. J Pain 2005;6:29-40.

149. Jensen MP, Nielson WR, Kerns RD: Toward the development of a motivational model of pain self-management. J Pain 2003;4:477-492.

150. Truchon M, Cote D: Predictive validity of the Chronic Pain Coping Inventory in subacute low back pain. Pain 2005;116:205-212.

151. Otis J, Cardella L, Kerns RD: The influence of family and culture on pain. In Dworkin RH, Breitbart WS, (eds). Psychosocial and psychiatric aspects of pain: A handbook for health care providers, vol 27. Seattle, WA, International Association for the Study of Pain Press, 2003.

152. Barry LC, Gill TM, Kerns RD, et al: Identification of pain-reduction strategies used by community-dwelling older persons. J Gerontol Med Sci 2005;60:1569-1575.

PART IV

Clinical Conditions

H. T. Benzon and C. Wu

14 Postoperative Pain and Other Acute Pain Syndromes

Brian A. Williams, Krystof J. Neumann, Shiv K. Goel, and Christopher L. Wu

Providing analgesia in the setting of moderate to severe pain, especially in the setting of surgery or trauma, is an important ethical responsibility of the medical profession. Anesthesiologists are uniquely positioned to understand and apply principles and techniques of meaningful analgesia. No single analgesic technique is fool-proof, or free from potential side effects or complications. Cautious selection and careful administration remains a central guiding principle. Certain traditional analgesic strategies are known to have analgesic ceilings, whether due to pharmacologic thresholds that cannot be exceeded, or side effects, which prohibit dose escalation. Traditional analgesics such as opioids are also known to have side effects that can occur even at lower doses, and escalating or sustained use of opioids may contribute to a recently described phenomenon called *opioid-induced hyperalgesia*. The prospects of worsening long-term outcome by using traditional methods to treat acute pain should be unsettling to the conscientious practitioner.

Emerging analgesic pharmacotherapies and techniques indeed require extensive literature review, as well as formal training (e.g., in the case of procedures such as peripheral nerve block techniques). Although no pharmaceutical agent and no procedure is risk-free, interventions such as peripheral nerve blocks and multimodal techniques may prove to be associated with fewer complications with improved long-term outcomes, pending further research. However, at this time, no comprehensive recommendations can be made favoring particular single-treatment or multimodal strategies.

An escalating societal demand for rapid delivery of medical care with minimized postoperative convalescence forces the practitioner of acute pain management to reconsider almost every therapeutic option available in the anesthetic and analgesic milieu. Intraoperative anesthetic choices may also need to be thoroughly reexamined, because some mechanisms that are presently thought to have no effect on postoperative pain may ultimately prove to be associated with adverse postoperative analgesic outcomes.

Therefore, as of this writing, the individual encounter between physician and patient carries important implications for quality outcomes in analgesic care. Patient care should be individualized; practitioners can no longer ignore important emerging literature on the modalities covered in this chapter if they want to provide "individualized patient care." The simplest traditional analgesic strategy in the short term may prove to be harmful in the long term. Careful consideration of patient-specific factors, including planned procedure, medical/social/surgical history, and preoperative baseline pain scores are starting points that should be considered in earnest, in a health care system laden with increasing productivity pressures.

TREATMENT OPTIONS

Systemic Analgesics

Opioid Analgesics

Traditionally, opioid analgesics are the foundation for the treatment of postoperative and acute pain (Table 14–1). Opium and its derivatives have been used for centuries as analgesics, and opioids continue to be one of the most commonly used analgesic agents in modern times. There are many advantages of opioid analgesics for the treatment of acute postoperative pain, including that there is theoretically no analgesic ceiling, and opioids may be administered via a number of routes (e.g., subcutaneous, oral, intravenous [IV], intramuscular [IM], and neuraxial). These features enhance the versatility of opioids as a therapeutic agent. For the treatment of moderate to severe postoperative pain, opioids are typically

Table 14–1. Systemic Opioid and Non-opioid Analgesic Options

AGENT	DELIVERY	ANALGESIC CEILING	SIDE EFFECTS	COMMENTS
Opioids	PO; IV/PCA; IM; SQ; NA; PNB; TD (including TD PCA)	No	Induced hyperalgesia, nausea, vomiting, sedation, respiratory depression, pruritus, constipation, urinary retention	Side effects limit full analgesic potential.
Tramadol	PO, IV	Yes (comparable to ibuprofen 400 mg)	Dizziness, drowsiness, sweating, nausea, vomiting, dry mouth, headache	Also inhibits serotonin reuptake. Caution/contraindication in patients taking MAOI, having seizure history, or with increased ICP. Appears to lack side effects of respiratory depression, major organ toxicity, constipation, and dependence.
Acetaminophen	PO; parenteral preparations available outside of US	Yes	Hepatotoxicity	Coadministration with opioids appears to provide opioid-sparing analgesia, but may not reduce opioid-related side effects.
NSAIDs	PO, IV, IM	Yes	Renal; GI Platelet inhibition Inhibition of bone healing Inhibition of osteogenesis Cardiovascular	Coadministration with opioids appears to provide opioid-sparing analgesia, but may not reduce opioid-related side effects.
COX-2 inhibitors	PO	Yes	Renal Cardiovascular Inhibition of bone healing Inhibition of osteogenesis	Coadministration with opioids appears to provide opioid-sparing analgesia, but may not reduce opioid-related side effects.
Ketamine ("low-dose")	IV	Yes	No cognitive impairments and psychotomimetic effects seen with dosing of 0.25 mg/kg	May attenuate both postoperative pain and chronic pain; may attenuate opioid-induced hyperalgesia.
Gabapentin and pregabalin	PO	Unknown	Dizziness, somnolence, ataxia, memory impairment, weight gain, edema, altered vision	May be useful for acute analgesia and chronic antihyperalgesia, pending further study. Possible interaction (increasing somnolence) in combination with low circulating levels of local anesthetics (e.g., epidural).

COX, cyclooxygenase; ICP, intracranial pressure; IM, intramuscular; IV, intravenous; MAOI, monoamine oxidase inhibitor; NA, neuraxial; NSAID, non-steroidal anti-inflammatory drug; PCA, patient-controlled analgesia; PNB, peripheral nerve block; PO, per-oral; SQ, subcutaneous; TD, transdermal; US, United States.

administered parenterally (IV, IM), although there may be wide intersubject and intrasubject variability in the relationship between opioid dose, serum concentration, and analgesic response in the treatment of postoperative pain. Oral administration of opioids (possibly as part of a combination product that includes an adjuvant such as acetaminophen) is generally used for the treatment of mild or moderate postoperative pain or when inpatients have successfully initiated oral intake.

Opioids exert their analgesic effect typically through the μ-opioid receptors located in both the central and peripheral nervous systems.[1] Although the δ and κ receptor subtypes are also present in addition to the μ receptor subtype, the therapeutic benefits (and side effects) of morphine, the prototypic opioid analgesic agent, are mediated predominantly via activation of opioid μ receptors.[2] Although opioid analgesics theoretically do not exhibit an analgesic ceiling per se, the analgesic efficacy of opioids is limited by the development of side effects. One study

determined that every morphine equivalent of 3 mg per 24-hour period corresponds to one additional symptom, side effect, or hospital-related complication.[3] Common opioid-related side effects include nausea, vomiting, bowel dysfunction (constipation or ileus), and pruritus, although sedation or significant respiratory depression may also occur. Opioid receptor physiology is complex, not completely understood, and regulated by multiple mechanisms, which may play a role in the development of opioid receptor tolerance and desensitization, which may not only contribute to a short-term decrease in analgesic efficacy (e.g., paradoxical hyperalgesia) but also to long-term changes in receptor sensitivity.[2,4,5]

Intravenous Patient-Controlled Analgesia
Intravenous patient-controlled analgesia (IV PCA) is considered the gold standard by which systemic opioids are delivered postoperatively. Unlike that seen for traditional "as needed" PRN analgesic

regimens, IV PCA allows the clinician to compensate for several factors, including the wide interpatient and intrapatient variability in analgesic needs, variability in serum drug levels, and administrative delays, which might result in inadequate postoperative analgesia. By incorporating a negative feedback loop into the device itself (presence of pain leads to self-administration of opioid, whereas there should be no demands with the absence of pain), the IV PCA device per se has a safety device integrated into its design, although when the negative feedback loop is violated, excessive sedation or respiratory depression may occur.[6,7] The majority of the problems related to IV PCA usage result from user or operator errors, and are not attributable to the device itself.[6]

The variables that can be programmed into an IV PCA device include the demand or bolus dose, lockout interval, and background infusion. The optimal settings for IV PCA administration of opioids for postoperative pain management are not known; however, there are general principles that may promote effective postoperative analgesia. The demand or bolus dose should be set such that there is not an insufficient demand dose (which may result in inadequate analgesia) nor an excessive demand dose (which may result in side effects such as respiratory depression).[8] For opioid-naïve patients, a commonly used demand dose for *morphine* is 1 mg, and that for *fentanyl* is 10 to 20 µg.[6,8] The lockout interval should be set such that the patient may evaluate the full analgesic effect of the previous dose before self-administration of a subsequent dose. A lockout interval that is too short may contribute to an increase in medication-related side effects whereas one that is too long may result in inadequate analgesia. Commonly used lockout intervals range from 5 to 10 minutes and varying the interval within this range appears to have no effect on analgesia or side effects.[6,9] The final variable is the continuous or background infusion. Although the use of a background infusion was initially thought to provide improved analgesia especially during sleep, the routine use of continuous or background infusions in IV PCA in adult opioid-naïve patients is not recommended due to the increased incidence of side effects such as respiratory depression.[10,11] Use of a background infusion, even if limited to nighttime, in opioid-naïve patients does not improve analgesia or sleep patterns.[10,12,13] However, a background infusion for opioid-tolerant or pediatric patients may be more appropriate.

Use of IV PCA when compared to traditional PRN analgesic regimens may be associated with improved patient outcomes including superior postoperative analgesia, improved patient satisfaction, and possibly a decreased risk of pulmonary complications.[14,15] At least two meta-analyses have been conducted in comparing IV PCA to PRN administration of opioids. Both meta-analyses suggest improved analgesia with IV PCA compared to PRN administration of opioids. An early meta-analysis of 15 randomized trials compared PRN IM dosing versus IV PCA but without a significant decrease in opioid consumption.[14,15] There

was no obvious economic benefit for IV PCA, although one meta-analysis demonstrated a decreased risk of pulmonary complications with IV PCA.[14] In addition, patients tended to prefer IV PCA,[14,15] which may result in greater patient satisfaction.[14-17] In terms of opioid-related side effects, the incidence of these, including respiratory depression (<0.5%), from IV PCA does not appear to differ significantly from that administered via other routes (e.g., IV, IM, or subcutaneous).[11,14,17,18]

Patient-Controlled Transdermal Fentanyl

Although IV PCA administration of opioids is generally effective, IV PCA may fail in up to 25% of patients due to technical issues or side effects.[19] Transdermal delivery of fentanyl (as a continuous passive dose) is already an option for the treatment of chronic or cancer pain; however, a recent technologic development has added the process of iontophoresis to substantially increase dermal penetration capacity to allow in essence a "PCA fentanyl patch." This credit card–sized transdermal PCA system can be applied like the traditional fentanyl patch and uses a low-intensity current to transfer fentanyl upon patient activation across the skin into the systemic circulation. The extent of iontophoretic fentanyl delivery is directly related to the magnitude of the current applied to the system.[20] Although this system is in the final stages of development, preliminary indications suggest that it will be designed to deliver a preprogrammed amount of fentanyl over 10 minutes, for a total of 80 doses, or for 24 hours, whichever occurs first.[21] Absorption of clinically significant levels of drug occurs only on patient activation of the system and the decline in serum fentanyl concentrations is similar to that delivered intravenously.[20]

Clinical studies have shown iontophoretic patient-controlled transdermal fentanyl to be superior to placebo and comparable to IV PCA morphine for the treatment of acute postoperative pain.[19,22] Two prospective randomized trials, not surprisingly, demonstrated that the iontophoretic fentanyl patient-activated transdermal system was superior to placebo for acute postoperative pain management.[22,23] In another prospective, randomized, controlled, multi-center trial, patients were randomly assigned to IV PCA morphine (1 mg bolus every 5 minutes) or iontophoretic fentanyl hydrochloride (40-µg infusion over 10 minutes) via a patient-controlled transdermal system. There was neither any difference in pain ratings after 24 hours of treatment nor any incidence of opioid-related adverse events.[19] Further studies are required to elucidate the role of the new device in the management of postoperative pain.

Tramadol

Tramadol is a centrally acting, synthetic analgesic agent that is structurally related to codeine and morphine. Tramadol is composed of two enantiomers: (+)tramadol inhibits serotonin reuptake and is a weak µ-opioid receptor, whereas (−)tramadol inhibits norepinephrine reuptake.[24] Thus tramadol produces its analgesic effects mainly through central mechanisms, although it may exhibit peripheral local anesthetic properties.[25] With a mean elimination half-life of approximately 6 hours, tramadol and its metabolites are primarily excreted through the kidneys.[24] Tramadol is typically used to treat moderate postoperative pain[26,27] and has an analgesic efficacy comparable to aspirin 650 mg with codeine 60 mg or ibuprofen 400 mg.[27] The use of tramadol for postoperative analgesia may confer several advantages compared to traditional opioids, including the relative lack of respiratory depression, major organ toxicity, constipation, and dependence.[26,28] Common side effects of tramadol include dizziness, drowsiness, sweating, nausea, vomiting, dry mouth, and headache.[26,27] Tramadol should be used with caution in certain populations including persons with a history of seizures, those with increased intracranial pressure, or those taking monoamine oxidase inhibitors.[27]

Non-opioid Analgesics

Nonsteroidal Anti-inflammatory Agents and Acetaminophen

Nonsteroidal anti-inflammatory agents (NSAIDs) and acetaminophen are traditionally used as an adjunct agent for the treatment of acute postoperative pain. For mild to moderate pain, NSAIDs and acetaminophen generally provide effective analgesia as the sole analgesic agent or may be combined with an opioid as a combination analgesic. In these cases, it is important to remember that the amount of combination product that may be administered may be limited by the NSAID or acetaminophen, which exhibits an analgesic ceiling and has potentially toxic dose-dependent side effects. For moderate to severe pain, NSAIDs are typically used as an adjunct to opioids, although some single-dose quantitative systematic reviews suggest that the analgesic efficacy of NSAIDs, either alone or in combination with opioids, may be greater than previously thought.

Although NSAIDs and acetaminophen exhibit an analgesic ceiling, these agents are valuable in the management of postoperative pain in that they may be administered either orally or parenterally. These agents are commonly used as part of a "multimodal" analgesic regimen with the perception that combining two or more analgesic agents with a different mechanism of analgesic action may produce at least additive analgesia and decrease the incidence of side effects associated with each analgesic agent (especially opioid analgesics) by reducing the dosage used of each individual analgesic agent. However, the concurrent use of NSAIDs and acetaminophen with IV PCA may not be as beneficial as previously thought. Several meta-analyses suggest that use of NSAIDs, COX-2 inhibitors, or acetaminophen in combination with IV PCA does result in an opioid-sparing effect. However, the use of acetaminophen and COX-2 inhibitors does not appear to decrease the relative risk of opioid-related side effects (e.g., postoperative nausea and vomiting [PONV], sedation, pruritus, urinary retention) or adverse events (respiratory depression), whereas the use of nonspecific NSAIDs only appears to decrease the relative risk of some opioid-related side effects (e.g., PONV, sedation).[29-33] In terms of pain control, the addition of NSAIDs (multiple dose or infusion only) and COX-2 inhibitors, but not acetaminophen or single-dose NSAIDs, result in significantly lower pain scores postoperatively.[29-33]

NSAIDs and acetaminophen, a diverse group of analgesic compounds that exhibit different pharmacokinetic properties, produce analgesia presumably through the inhibition of the cyclooxygenase (COX) and subsequent synthesis of prostaglandins, which are important mediators of peripheral and central nervous system (CNS) hyperalgesia.[34] There are at least two isoforms of cyclooxygenase (COX-1: constitutive; COX-2: inducible) with different functions. The COX-1 enzyme is always present and mediates platelet aggregation, hemostasis, and gastric mucosal protection. The COX-2 enzyme is upregulated during inflammation, and may play a role in nociception. More recently, it has been recognized that the COX-2 enzyme may play an important role in cardioprotection via prostacyclin I2 (PGI2).[35]

Although NSAIDs are an integral part of postoperative pain management, their use is limited by several adverse effects (e.g., gastrointestinal bleeding, impaired renal function, inhibition of platelet aggregation, and inhibition of bone healing and osteogenesis). These adverse effects are the result of inhibition of COX, and subsequent formation of prostaglandins that mediate many physiologic processes. Inhibition of platelet dysfunction and decreased perioperative hemostasis results from NSAID inhibition of thromboxane A2 (COX-1), a mediator of platelet aggregation and vasoconstriction,[36,37] although the available evidence on the effect of NSAIDs on perioperative bleeding is equivocal.[37-39] High-risk surgical patients (e.g., hypovolemia, abnormal renal function, or abnormal serum electrolytes) may be at risk for NSAID-induced renal dysfunction. Prostaglandins dilate renal vascular beds, and NSAIDs may inhibit these beneficial diuretic and natriuretic renal effects,[40] although euvolemic patients with normal renal function are unlikely to be affected.[41] NSAIDs may also have an adverse effect on bone healing[42] and may be associated with a higher incidence of gastrointestinal bleeding[39] as a result of NSAID-inhibition of cytoprotective gastric mucosal prostaglandins (COX-1).[36]

Traditional NSAIDs block both COX-1 and COX-2 enzymes, and the development of "selective" COX-2 inhibitors was based on the premise that selective inhibition of COX-2 would theoretically provide analgesia without the side effects associated with COX-1 inhibition. Although COX-2 inhibitors are associated with a lower incidence of GI complications,[43] and they exhibit minimal platelet inhibition even when administered in supratherapeutic doses,[44] recent data indicate that COX-2 inhibitors are associated with a higher incidence of cardiovascular events such as myocardial infarction.[45] Because COX-2 inhibitors inhibit PGI2, these agents may actually promote coronary thrombosis via the unopposed action of thromboxane A2.[35] A meta-analysis of rofecoxib trials indicated that administration of rofecoxib is associated with an increased risk (2.3 times greater) of cardiovascular events.[45] Unlike rofecoxib, celecoxib was not removed from the market, although some data also suggested that celecoxib was associated with a higher incidence of cardiovascular events.[46-48]

Ketamine

Ketamine is an *N*-methyl-D-aspartate (NMDA) receptor antagonist and has been generally used as an intraoperative anesthetic agent. Because of its NMDA antagonistic properties, which may attenuate central sensitization (chronic postsurgical pain) and opioid tolerance, ketamine has been reexamined for its potential use for postoperative analgesia.[49] The perioperative administration of low-dose ketamine may be integrated in a multimodal analgesic regimen or used as an adjunct to opioids and local anesthetics to enhance postoperative analgesia and potentially reduce opioid-related side effects.[49-52] A systematic review revealed that perioperative administration of ketamine (versus control) resulted in lower pain scores and a significantly decreased morphine consumption over 24 hours, with no difference in morphine-related adverse effects between the groups.[53] However, use of ketamine as an adjunct to IV PCA may not improve postoperative analgesia.[54] Low-dose ketamine infusions do not appear to cause hallucinations or cognitive impairment, and in patients undergoing general anesthesia (GA), the incidence of hallucinations appears low and may be independent of benzodiazepine premedication.[53,55,56] Reports of epidural and intrathecal ketamine have been published,[57,58] but the use of neuraxial ketamine is discouraged until further safety and neurotoxicity data are available. Although the intraoperative administration of IV subanesthetic ketamine as part of a general anesthetic may attenuate acute postoperative pain and potentially chronic postsurgical pain, the role of low-dose ketamine for postoperative analgesia remains unclear.[53,59] In addition, it is unclear at this time whether perioperative use of ketamine will result in better long-term recovery or improved functional outcome, and there is insufficient evidence to show a clear benefit of S(+) ketamine compared with racemic ketamine.[59]

Gabapentin and Pregabalin

Gabapentin and pregabalin are analogous in molecular structure to gamma-aminobutyric acid. Their use in acute pain models has provided promising preliminary evidence for potential routine use.[60] Their role in preempting chronic hyperalgesia is uncertain.[61] Five studies have shown benefit in acute pain management when a preoperative oral dose of 1200 mg gabapentin was administered,[62-66] and one of these studies also incorporated a limited postoperative dosing course (for 10 days after breast surgery, with resultant lower opioid requirements and pain scores with movement).[63] After abdominal hysterectomy, gabapentin use (400 mg four times a day for 1 day preoperatively and 5 days postoperatively) led to lower pain scores 1 month after surgery, but not in the immediate postoperative period.[67] Somnolence from single-dose gabapentin pretreatment was only described when epidural analgesia was coadministered,[65] leading to the possibility that the interaction of gabapentin and local anesthetics may augment sedative effects. Pregabalin, to date, has only been shown to be effective in humans in dental pain models,[68] with no other human studies available at the time of this writing regarding pregabalin and acute pain.[60]

Neuraxial Analgesia

Single-Dose Neuraxial (Spinal, Epidural) Opioids

A single-injection of neuraxial (spinal or epidural) opioid may provide effective postoperative analgesia. These agents may be administered alone or as an adjuvant analgesic agent. The degree of lipophilicity/hydrophilicity is probably the most important determinant of the analgesic onset and duration of a specific opioid. Because hydrophilic opioids (e.g., morphine and hydromorphone) tend to remain within the cerebrospinal fluid (CSF) after neuraxial administration, these agents tend to produce a delayed but longer duration of analgesia (along with a higher incidence of side effects due to cephalad CSF spread) unlike lipophilic opioids (e.g., fentanyl and sufentanil), which tend to provide a more rapid but shorter duration of analgesia due to their relatively rapid clearance from the CSF. For postoperative analgesia, the limited cephalic spread of lipophilic opioids may limit development of certain side effects such as delayed respiratory depression. Although it appears that hydrophilic opioids provide analgesia via a primarily spinal mechanism, whether single-dose neuraxial lipophilic opioids produce analgesia via a spinal or systemic mechanism is not as clear.[69,70]

One can use the differences between lipophilic and hydrophilic opioids to tailor a patient's postoperative analgesic regimen. For instance, a single shot of hydrophilic opioid (e.g., morphine or hydromorphone) will provide analgesia at a location far from its injection site (due to cephalic CSF migration of opioid) and as such may provide effective postoperative analgesia for thoracic and upper abdominal surgery even when injected at a lumbar interspace, although lower doses of opioids may be prudent for older patients.[71] For clinical situations in which a rapid but shorter duration of analgesia is warranted to minimize risk of respiratory depression, a single-shot neuraxial administration of a lipophilic opioid may be appropriate.[72] For clinical situations in which a longer duration of analgesia is required (e.g., following inpatient surgery), a single-shot neuraxial

Table 14–2. Neuraxial Analgesic Options and Considerations

TECHNIQUE	EXAMPLES	CONSIDERATIONS AND COMMENTS
Intrathecal lipophilic opioid	Fentanyl, sufentanil	Limited rostral spread after intrathecal injection. Spinal analgesic mechanism. Unlikely respiratory depression, but possible pruritus.
Intrathecal hydrophilic opioid	Morphine, hydromorphone	Rostral spread after intrathecal injection. Spinal and/or systemic analgesic mechanism. Postoperative respiratory monitoring recommended. Respiratory depression and pruritus common.
Epidural hydrophilic opioid	Morphine, hydromorphone	Rostral spread after epidural injection via intrathecal diffusion. Spinal and/or systemic analgesic mechanism. Postoperative respiratory monitoring recommended. Respiratory depression and pruritus common. Limited analgesic mechanism (24 hours). Safely combined with local anesthetics.
Extended-release epidural morphine		Not to be coadministered with local anesthetics. Caution with vials during preparation. Up to 48 hours of analgesia. Dose-dependent side effects (respiratory depression/desaturation).
Continuous epidural analgesia	Combinations of low-concentration local anesthetics and opioids	Fixed rate infusion, patient-controlled boluses, or combinations of both. More efficacious analgesia than IV PCA. Clonidine and epinephrine have been reported as useful adjuvants. May lose popularity with increasing use of perioperative anticoagulation.

IV PCA, intravenous patient-controlled analgesia.

administration hydrophilic opioid may provide effective postoperative analgesia in an appropriately monitored setting (Table 14–2).[73]

Extended-Release Epidural Morphine

Traditionally available morphine for neuraxial administration may provide up to 24 hours of analgesia but may not be adequate in that postoperative pain is often most intense during the first 2 to 3 days after surgery.[74] Although epidural catheter analgesia or IV PCA may provide adequate analgesia, technical problems (e.g., early dislodgment, concurrent anticoagulation) may limit the duration or analgesic efficacy of these techniques. The development of an extended-release epidural morphine incorporates new technology wherein microscopic particles, consisting of numerous vesicles containing morphine with each vesicle separated from adjacent chambers by naturally occurring lipid membranes, provide a longer duration of postoperative analgesia compared to traditionally available formulations but without the need for indwelling epidural catheters.[75] Preliminary randomized controlled trials indicate that extended-release epidural morphine provides significant postoperative analgesia for up to 48 hours after hip and abdominal surgery.[75,76] For patients undergoing cesarean section, the 10- and 15-mg single-dose extended-release epidural morphine may provide lower pain scores at rest and with activity than traditional epidural morphine group for 24 to 48 hours after surgery.[75] There appears to be a dose-dependent relationship for decreased oxygen saturation, with the 20- and 25-mg doses associated with higher rates of desaturation.[75] Based on available studies, the safety profile of extended-release epidural morphine is generally consistent with that reported for other epidurally administered opioid analgesics[75]; however,

clinicians should not freeze, aggressively agitate, or shake the extended-release epidural morphine vials (gently invert the vial before use). In addition, one should not administer any other agents epidurally around the time of extended-release epidural morphine administration (particularly local anesthetics), because this may result in an increased peak serum concentrations of morphine.

Continuous Epidural Analgesia

One of the disadvantages of single-injection neuraxial opioid is the limited duration of analgesia (less than 24 hours for traditional agents and less than 48 hours with extended-release morphine). Continuous epidural analgesia may provide a longer duration of effective analgesia compared to single-shot neuraxial opioids and superior analgesia compared to systemic opioids.[74] Although continuous epidural analgesia may provide effective postoperative analgesia,[77] the efficacy of this technique is in part dependent on the many factors (e.g., analgesic solution; opioid versus local anesthetic; catheter insertion location; duration of analgesia; adjuvant agents) that comprise its insertion and management.

There are many options for analgesic agents used for postoperative epidural analgesia; however, the most common options include local anesthetics and opioids, either alone or in combination. Although either agent (local anesthetic or opioid) can be used as a sole agent for postoperative epidural analgesia, the overall analgesia may not be as effective as a combination of local anesthetic with opioid.[77-79] There may be certain clinical situations in which a single epidural analgesic agent may be preferable. Epidural infusions of local anesthetic alone may be used to decrease opioid-related side effects; epidural infusions of opioids alone may be used if avoidance of motor block or hypotension from sympathetic blockade is a concern.[77]

Clinically, the most commonly used epidural regimen is a combination of both a local anesthetic and opioid, which may confer advantages over using either agent alone. When compared to opioid alone, a local anesthetic-opioid combination provides superior postoperative analgesia.[78] When compared to local anesthetic alone, a local anesthetic-opioid combination provides equivalent postoperative analgesia but with fewer side effects.[78] Continuous or patient-controlled epidural infusions of a local anesthetic-opioid combination also provide superior analgesia when compared to IV PCA with opioids,[78] although it is unclear whether the analgesic effect of the local anesthetic and opioid in the epidural analgesia is additive or synergistic.

There is no consensus as to the optimal choice of local anesthetic or opioid for postoperative epidural analgesia. Generally, a local anesthetic (e.g., bupivacaine, ropivacaine, or levobupivacaine at analgesic concentrations) with a longer duration of action and preferential clinical sensory blockade with minimal impairment of motor function is used.[80] With regard to the choice of opioid, a lipophilic opioid (e.g., fentanyl or sufentanil), which allows for relatively rapid titration of analgesia, is generally used,[77,81] although hydrophilic opioids (e.g., morphine or hydromorphone) may also be used for postoperative analgesia.[81]

Although there are a number of adjuvants that may be added to epidural infusions, none are widely used clinically. Two potentially useful adjuvants are clonidine and epinephrine. Through activation of the descending noradrenergic pathway, clonidine may enhance postoperative analgesia; however, the clinical usefulness is typically limited by the presence of hypotension, bradycardia, and sedation.[82,83] Epinephrine has been shown to improve epidural analgesia and increase sensory block in the postoperative setting.[84]

Postoperative epidural analgesia may be delivered as a fixed rate or continuous infusion (CEI) or patient-controlled device (PCEA). Based on the principles of patient-controlled analgesia, PCEA would theoretically confer benefits of individualization of postoperative analgesic requirements, lower drug use, greater patient satisfaction, and superior analgesia. Although CEI may provide superior analgesia compared to PCEA, patients with CEI appear to have a higher incidence of side effects such as motor block, nausea, and vomiting.[78] When compared to IV PCA, both CEI and PCEA provide superior analgesia.[78] Observational data suggest that PCEA is a safe and effective technique for postoperative analgesia.[85,86] Although the optimal PCEA analgesic solution and delivery parameters (i.e., demand dose, lockout interval) are unknown, it does appear that a continuous/background infusion (in addition to the demand dose) may provide superior analgesia than a demand

dose alone.[87] As discussed earlier, probably the most common PCEA regimens incorporate a low-concentration local anesthetic-opioid combination.[74]

Summary

Neuraxial analgesic agents, either as a single-shot or continuous epidural analgesia, provide effective postoperative analgesia (see Table 14–2). The choice of a particular technique should be made based on the clinical situation, patient preferences, and skills of the practitioner. The use of these techniques should be evaluated on an individual basis, weighing both the risks and benefits of a particular neuraxial technique for a particular patient. Many of the benefits and complications (including epidural hematoma, epidural abscess, and medication-related side effects) from neuraxial analgesia are discussed in Chapter 69.

Peripheral Analgesia

Peripheral analgesia has gained increasing popularity in recent years. The extent to which anesthesia and analgesia achieved with peripheral mechanisms has the greatest potential benefit is when these techniques are able to reduce or eliminate the use of volatile anesthetics and opioids. In North America and many parts of the world, increasing numbers of patients are undergoing surgery on an outpatient basis. With the goals of same-day discharge and length-of-stay reductions, avoidance of anesthetic and analgesic agents (and their side effects of PONV and somnolence) forces practitioners to routinely employ multimodal peripheral analgesic techniques. Volatile agents lead to higher rates of PONV (when compared with the use of anesthetic maintenance with propofol).[88-90] Volatile agents have also been associated with increased incidence of postoperative pain and unplanned admission (e.g., after invasive outpatient orthopedic surgery).[91-95] Awareness and routine implementation of peripheral multimodal analgesic techniques will likely lead to the increase of patient eligibility for same-day discharge and/or length-of-stay reduction. In addition, other efficiencies can be gained when postoperative multimodal peripheral analgesia and systematic avoidance of GA-associated side effects are implemented as a comprehensive anesthesia care plan.[96] Further importance to seeking alternative strategies to systemic opioid use has become evident for two reasons. First, escalating doses of opioids produce a dose-dependent increase in side effects and hospital-related complications[3]; second, opioids induce postoperative hyperalgesia.[97]

Continuous Subcutaneous Infusions of Local Anesthetics

Compared to systemic opioids, continuous epidural and peripheral nerve infusions of local anesthetics provide superior analgesia[78,98]; however, these analgesic modalities are labor intensive, expensive, and a certain percentage will become dislodged prematurely. The relatively simple technique of infusion of local anesthetic into the surgical wound site via a catheter placed directly by the surgeon at the end of the procedure may be an effective method for postoperative analgesia. The advantages of a continuous subcutaneous infusion of local anesthetics are that this technique can be widely and easily used, may provide effective analgesia for mild postoperative pain, may potentially reduce the need for opioids, and may be used for several days, possibly on an ambulatory basis.[99] Although a one-time infiltration of local anesthetic into the wound may provide effective postoperative analgesia, the duration of analgesia is typically limited by the properties of the local anesthetics used (i.e., generally less than 6 to 8 hours of analgesia).

A systematic review of randomized trials examining use of continuous wound catheters in multiple surgical procedures consistently demonstrated analgesic efficacy in terms or reduced pain scores and opioid use for all surgical subgroups examined.[100] A total of 39 randomized controlled trials (1761 patients) were included in the final analysis. Overall, when compared to placebo, local anesthetic infusions resulted in a significant decrease in pain scores by approximately 33% both at rest and with activity. Subgroup analysis confirmed decreased pain scores in all types of surgical procedures with the exception of subjects undergoing abdominal surgery. Compared to subjects taking placebo, subjects who were randomized to receive subcutaneous infusions of local anesthetics demonstrated a reduction in the need for opioid rescue and daily consumption of opioids, which may have contributed to a reduction in the incidence of nausea in the continuous wound catheter group (21% vs. 39%, odds ratio = 0.42; 95% CI = 0.27 to 0.67).

There are several mechanisms by which direct application of local anesthetic to surgical wounds may provide analgesia, including blockade of nociceptive transmission from afferents from the wound surface, local anesthetic inhibition of local inflammatory response to surgical injury,[101,102] which might sensitize nociceptive receptors that contribute to pain and hyperalgesia, and suppression of peripheral nociceptive afferents or spinal cord suppression from systemic absorption of local anesthetics.[103] It is recognized that administration of continuous subcutaneous infusion of local anesthetics will result in nontoxic blood levels of local anesthetic.[104] Thus the use of continuous subcutaneous infusion of local anesthetics may be an attractive option for postoperative analgesia and may reduce overall opioid consumption compared to placebo.

Extremity Blocks

In addition to the analgesic benefits of peripheral nerve blocks (PNBs) described in this section, there are other potential benefits to advancing the quality of anesthesia care. These advances are achieved when used in the context of ambulatory surgery, and when hospital length-of-stay is reduced. PNBs reduce operating room time when a regional anesthesia (RA) induction room is used.[91,105] In addition, use of RA results in bypass of "phase 1" recovery (postanesthesia care unit [PACU] bypass).[91-94] Hospital cost savings appear to be achievable when PACU bypass, same-day discharge, and length-of-stay criteria are standardized and uniformly applied.[94,105-108] RA techniques are important in facilitating cost savings in ambulatory surgery, because GA techniques (including airway devices, volatile agents, and opioids, without RA use) do not reduce postoperative nursing workload when PACU bypass criteria are used.[109] Therefore high-volume RA practice, in combination with modern "milestone criteria" for the entire recovery-to-discharge period, appears necessary to achieve hospital cost savings.

Several case series,[92-94,110-113] reviews,[114,115] meta-analyses,[98,116] accompanying editorials,[117,118] and a recent randomized clinical trial[119] have reported improved analgesic outcomes in orthopedic patients receiving techniques either incorporating [92-94,110-113] or exclusively consisting of [92-94,119] RA.

Upper Extremity Blocks

Upper extremity nerve blocks can be performed at various levels along the course of the brachial plexus, at the level of the individual nerves, or as an IV regional (Bier) block. Nerve conduction in the brachial plexus can be interrupted at various levels, with specific advantages for anesthesia and postoperative pain relief for specific surgical procedures of the upper extremity (Table 14–3).

IV (Bier) Block. The mechanism of IV RA is generally accepted to involve diffusion from veins to small nerves and nerve endings after exsanguination. There is minimal block at the nerve trunk (i.e., peripheral nerve) level. Because the small nerves and nerve endings are the site of action of the local anesthetic injection, it is generally accepted that epinephrine should not be included in the IV regional anesthetic mixture. IV regional blocks are well described in the upper extremity, using a proximal arm tourniquet or double-tourniquet, and have been reviewed in the lower extremity as well.[120] Traditional IV regional techniques for the lower extremity using single- or double-tourniquet techniques may carry a high failure rate,[121] requiring supplementation by the surgeon or conversion to GA. Of potential interest, however, is an intercuff technique for IV RA for knee surgery that has been developed in an effort to produce better localization and reduce overall dosing requirements.[122,123]

Local anesthetics administered alone in IV regional blocks are not expected to provide meaningful postoperative analgesia. Low doses of *muscle relaxants* are known to improve motor block,[124] but should be used with caution to avoid adverse respiratory depression upon tourniquet release. *Neostigmine* was shown

Table 14–3. Upper Extremity Block Considerations

TECHNIQUE	AGENTS	CONSIDERATIONS AND COMMENTS
IV regional (Bier)	Lidocaine (0.5%) or ropivacaine (0.1% to 0.2%)	Local anesthetic selected does not influence postoperative analgesia. Additives may be very useful in prolonging tourniquet tolerance and prolonging postoperative analgesia (e.g., ketamine 0.1 mg/kg, ketorolac 20 mg, clonidine 1 µg/kg, dexamethasone 8 mg). Caution with allowing sufficient inflated tourniquet time before deflating.
Interscalene single-injection	Ropivacaine or levo-bupivacaine (0.5% to 0.67%)	Additives may be very useful in prolonging postoperative analgesia when ropivacaine is used (e.g., clonidine 1 mcg/kg, buprenorphine ≤300 mcg). Ipsilateral phrenic nerve block is expected, but may be less common with variant procedures (cervical paravertebral, supraclavicular). Risk epidural spread/vertebral artery injection.
Interscalene continuous infusion	Ropivacaine 0.2% or levobupivacaine 0.125%	Ipsilateral phrenic nerve block possible. Additives not considered useful in continuous infusions. Stimulating and nonstimulating catheters have been studied. Analgesic gold standard for arthroplasty procedures and open rotator cuff repairs.
Axillary single-injection and variants	Ropivacaine or levo-bupivacaine (0.5% to 0.67%)	Additives may be very useful in prolonging postoperative analgesia when ropivacaine is used (e.g., clonidine 1 µg/kg, buprenorphine ≤300 µg). Paracoracoid/infraclavicular approaches may reduce total number of injections, while midhumeral approach may reduce total local anesthetic volume requirements. Cutaneous block required via individually blocking musculocutaneous nerve, intercostobrachial nerves, medial brachial cutaneous nerve, and medial antebrachial cutaneous nerve.
Axillary (and variant) continuous infusion	Ropivacaine 0.2% or levobupivacaine 0.125%	Additives not considered useful in continuous infusions. Most stable catheter placement likely via paracoracoid/infraclavicular approaches. Incidence of moderate to severe pain after outpatient hand surgery may prove to be surprisingly high, pending further study.

to produce analgesic benefit when 0.5 mg was added to the injectate,[125] but this finding was refuted when 1 mg of neostigmine was used.[126] Opioids (other than meperidine 30 mg or more) are generally considered nonbeneficial when given via the IV regional technique[124]; systemic side effects of *meperidine* manifested at the 30-mg threshold. *Tramadol* 100 mg administered as an IV regional technique with lidocaine is associated with a self-limited rash below the tourniquet, and did not necessarily confer analgesic benefits.[127] In addition, tramadol has not been shown to improve block or postoperative analgesic quality when coadministered with ropivacaine.[128]

Less controversial additives to IV RA appear to have potential in providing intraoperative tourniquet tolerance, postoperative analgesia, or both. *Ketorolac* is successful in achieving both end points when the tourniquet is applied to both the upper arm[129] and lower arm,[130] and the use of ketorolac for this purpose is generally accepted, with no basis at this time to exceed a 20-mg dose in adults.[124] *Clonidine* is considered successful for improving tourniquet tolerance and reducing postoperative analgesic requirements, and side effects are minimized while still achieving these benefits at a 1-µg/kg dose.[124] *Dexmedetomidine* (0.5 mg/kg) has also shown benefit.[131] *Ketamine,* at the dose of 100 µg/kg, has also been shown to improve tourniquet tolerance and reduce postoperative analgesic requirements, in a manner that appears to be more potent than clonidine at the 1-µg/kg dose.[132] When compared with plain lidocaine, *dexamethasone* (8 mg) was recently shown to reduce postoperative

analgesic requirements during the first 24 hours after surgery.[133] Given the multiple mechanisms contributing to postoperative pain, the logical future study would involve a step-function assessment of serial additives and combinations, with the additives to be considered including *ketorolac, clonidine or dexmedetomidine, ketamine,* and *dexamethasone.* The coadministered local anesthetic (lidocaine 0.5% vs. ropivacaine 0.1% to 0.2%) is unlikely to influence results with respect to duration of postoperative analgesia beyond the recovery room period.[134]

Brachial Plexus Blocks
Interscalene block. The most proximal approach to the brachial plexus (at the level of the roots), the interscalene block is typically performed at the level of C6, where the roots of the brachial plexus pass between the anterior and middle scalene muscles. It provides good block for the upper (C5-6) and the middle trunks (C7), but the lower trunk (C8-T1) is often blocked incompletely. Diffusion of local anesthetic leads to partial blockade of the superficial cervical plexus, providing cutaneous anesthesia and analgesia for the shoulder. Consequently, the interscalene block is a good block for shoulder or upper arm surgeries, but is not suited for surgeries on the forearm or the hand. This block can also be used for elbow procedures, but supplemental blocks (ulnar, intercostobrachial, medial brachial cutaneous, and medial antebrachial cutaneous) are typically required.

Interscalene block is considered by many to be the gold standard in postoperative analgesia for shoulder surgeries. The superior pain relief by this technique is well documented when compared with opioid analgesia. Greater than 50% reduction in the verbal pain scale (VPS) scores,[135-137] delayed time to first analgesic use,[136] and reduced total opioid requirement[135-138] have been reported. Interscalene blocks can be performed either as a single injection block for postoperative pain relief, typically lasting between 12 to 20 hours, or as a continuous catheter insertion with a continuous infusion of local anesthetic leading to more consistent and prolonged analgesia. The benefit of continuous interscalene catheters for shoulder arthroplasty and rotator cuff repair is well documented.[139-145]

Although logic would indicate similar effectiveness for less invasive procedures, there is little evidence at this time to indicate that interscalene brachial plexus catheters would be similarly useful for patients undergoing "less invasive" shoulder operations such as shoulder stabilization procedures, distal clavicle resection and/or acromioplasty, subacromial decompression, biceps tenodesis and/or tenotomy, or even routine debridement inside the glenohumeral joint, when compared with single-injection nerve blocks and perioperative multimodal oral analgesia. Thus, studies are needed to show the benefit of continuous nerve blocks (vs. single injection), and single-injection blocks (vs. no blocks) for a wide variety of shoulder procedures that produce an uncertain magnitude of postoperative pain. A review by Chelly and colleagues[146] provides an overview that may guide practitioners for categories of postoperative shoulder pain, until more definitive evidence is available. In this review, shoulder procedures are clustered into a "catheter-eligible" category if the following procedures are involved: shoulder arthroplasty, rotator cuff repair, Bankart repair, and open reduction/internal fixation of the humerus.

One important safety feature to consider in the postoperative recovery of patients receiving interscalene analgesia is adequate ventilatory function. It is generally accepted that most patients undergoing brachial plexus nerve blocks for shoulder surgery will encounter simultaneous block of the phrenic nerve, which is responsible for proper function of the diaphragm.[147-149] Borgeat and colleagues measured respiratory function during use of a continuous nerve block (CNB) technique that included both a continuous infusion (ropivacaine 0.2%, 5 mL/hr) and a CNB bolus function (3 to 4 mL with a 20-minute lockout).[150] In this study, all patients received a preoperative bolus injection of ropivacaine 0.75%, 30 mL, and all patients underwent major shoulder surgery (rotator cuff repair, n = 26; arthroplasty, n = 7). The control group consisted of patients receiving IV PCA consisting of IV opioids. Patients in the CNB group had better pain relief for up to 24 hours after surgery, when compared with patients who were randomized to receive IV PCA. Overall respiratory function was also better in the CNB group versus the IV PCA group. Forced respiration (i.e., movement in the diaphragm on the nonoperated side) was better in the CNB

group at 24 and 48 hours when compared with the PCA group. The rationale for this finding was that the pain control was better in the CNB group and that there were fewer opioid-related side effects (e.g., respiratory depression) in the CNB group, facilitating patients' forced respiratory efforts. Interestingly, forced diaphragmatic excursion on the side of surgery was not significantly different between the CNB and PCA groups at 24 and 48 hours after surgery. This study showed that forced respiratory effort was improved up to 48 hours after surgery in the CNB group, which when combined with better analgesia in the CNB group, provided an important safety validation in the evolution of same-day discharge of patients with CNB catheters and appropriate infusion devices after shoulder surgery.

Supraclavicular block. This block is associated with the greatest blockade of the brachial plexus with a single injection of the local anesthetic, primarily because the plexus is the most compact at this level. The plexus is blocked at the level of the trunks and divisions. However, the supraclavicular block misses the dorsal scapular nerve arising from the root of C5 and also misses the superficial cervical plexus. Hence this block may be inadequate for shoulder surgery, but provides adequate block for upper arm surgeries. As with interscalene block, supplemental blocks are required for elbow procedures (i.e., intercostobrachial). The supraclavicular block has the highest risk of pneumothorax amongst all brachial plexus blocks, especially when done with the traditional "plumb bob" technique, making this an unpopular block in practice. Despite some attractive advantages of this block, for example, rapidity of onset and broad upper extremity coverage, this block remains the least common brachial plexus block to be performed for postoperative analgesia, and recent literature on this approach is sparse.

Infraclavicular block. Like the supraclavicular block, this block also approaches the brachial plexus where it is most compact, at the level of divisions and proximal cords. This block is akin to performing a proximal axillary block; can be used for procedures involving the elbow, forearm, or hand; and is especially useful in patients unable to abduct their shoulders to allow access to the axilla. A single injection or a continuous catheter placed using this technique provides effective analgesia.[146,151-153] This approach also provides the most secure catheter insertion site of all brachial plexus blocks. There are two main approaches to this block—the traditional perivascular infraclavicular approach and the coracoid approach,[154] both of which provide similar results, but the coracoid approach is associated with the least risk of pneumothorax among the approaches to brachial plexus mentioned above. That said, Franco and Vieira demonstrated the safety and efficacy of the perivascular approach with no incidences of pneumothoraces or neurologic deficits in a series of 1001 blocks.[151]

For outpatient wrist and hand surgery, Hadzic and colleagues addressed this patient population comparing chloroprocaine infraclavicular nerve block with GA with volatile agents (GAVA), showing that GAVA use led to increased PACU admissions (vs. phase 1 recovery bypass), higher reports of postoperative pain, longer time to ambulation, and longer time to same-day discharge.[153] Chelly and coworkers state that PNB catheters are likely indicated for implantation procedures after trauma, as well as for open reduction and internal fixation of the hand and/or digits,[146] although a prospective randomized trial to definitively verify this intuitive concept may be difficult to achieve. Ilfeld and colleagues have shown that a continuous infraclavicular brachial plexus catheter (when compared with placebo catheter infusion) resulted in less postoperative dynamic pain and opioid consumption, and fewer sleep disturbances.[152] The surgical procedures performed included open reduction and internal fixation (elbow, radius, or ulna), bony/capsular wrist procedures (carpectomy, capsulodesis, fusion, or shrinkage), metacarpal arthroplasty, suspension plasty, and ulnar nerve transposition.

Axillary block. This is the most distal approach to the still-compact brachial plexus, at the level of the terminal branches as they surround the axillary artery. This is the most commonly performed PNB in the United States,[155,156] likely because of the ease of performance and a low incidence of side effects. It produces the most effective block for all surgical procedures on the elbow and distal to it, but requires supplementation for the tourniquet (intercostobrachial, medial brachial cutaneous, and medial antebrachial cutaneous) if it is to be used as a surgical block. Axillary block leads to a greater than 50% reduction in the pain scores postoperatively and decreases the total in-hospital opioid requirement with longer time to the first analgesic dose.[157,158] The axillary sheath at this level is often discontinuous, and the block should be performed as a series of multiple injections using the nerve stimulator to block all the individual components and obtain a consistently effective block.[159-161] The traditional transarterial and the single injection techniques can often miss the musculocutaneous nerve (from C5-6); therefore that nerve should be specifically sought and blocked.

Axillary brachial plexus catheters with continuous infusions have further increased the duration of effective analgesia after painful forearm and hand procedures.[162,163] However, maintaining a clean catheter site and avoiding catheter dislodgment from this very mobile area is a challenge for clinicians and patients.

Outpatient hand surgery has the potential to create not insignificant postoperative pain, with at least one study showing that patient pain scores reach or exceed 5 (out of 10),[164] while myriad studies of shoulder surgery patients have usually shown pain scores well exceeding 5 out of 10 postoperatively. Retrospective reviews and prospective studies have demonstrated uniformly that patients receiving PNBs (wrist blocks, Bier blocks, and brachial plexus blocks) have dramatically improved outcomes on the day of

surgery when compared with patients receiving GAVA. For shoulder surgery, the use of continuous brachial plexus catheters is sufficiently substantiated to recommend their routine placement (by trained practitioners) for "invasive" shoulder surgery. These findings also encourage the routine use (by trained practitioners) of all peripheral and regional techniques for upper extremity surgery, although further research is needed to determine outcome benefits of continuous versus single-injection nerve blocks in the days and weeks following "mildly-to-moderately invasive" shoulder and distal upper extremity surgery. The usefulness of intra-articular and incisional infusions after simple arthroscopic procedures of the shoulder has been documented, but these articular and incisional infusions do not appear to confer sufficient analgesia after more invasive, open shoulder surgery.[165,166]

Lower Extremity Blocks

The nerve supply to the lower extremity comes from two nerve plexuses arising from the ventral rami of the spinal nerve roots of the lower spinal cord—the lumbar plexus (L1-4) and the sacral plexus (L4-5, S1-3). The lumbar plexus gives rise to the femoral nerve (L2-4), the obturator nerve (L2-4), the lateral femoral cutaneous nerve (L2-3), and three other branches supplying the inguinal and the genital area. The sacral plexus gives rise to the sciatic nerve (L4-5, S1-3), as well as providing branches that supply the musculature around the hip and pelvis. By interrupting the nerve conduction at the level of the plexus (i.e., lumbar plexus block) and along the course of the individual nerves arising from these plexuses, anesthesia and postoperative analgesia can be effectively provided for specific surgical procedures of the lower extremities (Table 14-4).

Lumbar Plexus Block. This is the only reliable block for the femoral, the lateral femoral cutaneous, and the obturator nerves with a single injection. While performing this block it is necessary to obtain the optimal twitch response with the nerve stimulator— the rectus femoris twitch with proximal patellar excursion; this twitch is a guide to proper needle placement. If the needle is too far medial, as is the case with an obturator (hip adduction) or a sciatic (dorsiflexion/plantar flexion) twitch, the needle is probably too close to the dural sleeve, and there is a possibility of epidural or even intrathecal spread of the local anesthetic. Using the same logic and in our clinical experience, the dose of the local anesthetic should be limited to 0.5 mL/kg, with a maximum injected volume of 30 mL in the average adult population. Dosing reductions are likely beneficial for older patients being considered for this block.

Because the main nerves supplying the hip joint are the femoral and the obturator, this block (either single shot or continuous) provides adequate postoperative analgesia for any procedures involving the hip joint, including total joint replacement and hip fractures. Turker and colleagues compared in a ran-

Table 14–4. Lower Extremity Block Considerations

TECHNIQUE	AGENTS	CONSIDERATIONS AND COMMENTS
Parasacral sciatic	Ropivacaine or levo-bupivacaine (0.5% to 0.67%)	Complex surrounding anatomy, this block is logically reserved for hip-specific procedures. Additives may be very useful in prolonging postoperative analgesia when ropivacaine is used (e.g., clonidine 1 mcg/kg, buprenorphine ≤300 µg).
Other proximal sciatic approaches	Ropivacaine or levo-bupivacaine (0.5% to 0.67%)	Approaches include gluteal (e.g., Labat), subgluteal, lateral, and anterior. Additives may be very useful in prolonging postoperative analgesia when ropivacaine is used (e.g., clonidine 1 mcg/kg, buprenorphine ≤300 µg). Logically reserved for knee surgery, or procedures where a thigh tourniquet is planned. Produces unwanted hamstring weakness if used for foot-ankle surgery. Catheter techniques have been successfully described; additives to low-concentration local anesthetics not considered useful in continuous infusions.
Distal sciatic approaches	Ropivacaine or levo-bupivacaine (0.5% to 0.67%)	Approaches include posterior popliteal and lateral popliteal. Additives may be very useful in prolonging postoperative analgesia when ropivacaine is used (e.g., clonidine 1 µg/kg, buprenorphine ≤300 µg). Logically reserved for foot/ankle surgery, or procedures where a calf tourniquet is planned. Avoids hamstring weakness. Catheter techniques have been successfully described; probably most useful for bony surgery; additives to low-concentration local anesthetics not considered useful in continuous infusions.
Lumbar plexus block in the psoas compartment	Ropivacaine or levo-bupivacaine (0.5% to 0.67%)	Most reliable way to block femoral, lateral femoral cutaneous, and obturator nerves with a single injection. Ensure quadriceps twitch without foot twitch and without obturator (hip adduction) twitch, to reduce chances of unwanted epidural spread. Volume dosing limits may reduce risk of unwanted epidural spread (e.g., 0.5 mL/kg up to 30 mL in adults, 0.4 mL/kg up to 20 to 25 mL in the elderly). Additives may be very useful in prolonging postoperative analgesia when ropivacaine is used (e.g., clonidine 1 mcg/kg, buprenorphine ≤300 µg). Added epinephrine (1:200,000) may be associated with unwanted tachycardia, via systemic absorption. Catheter techniques have been successfully described; additives to low-concentration local anesthetics are not considered useful in continuous infusions.
Femoral	Ropivacaine or levo-bupivacaine (0.5–0.67%)	Efficacious and well-documented analgesic technique for moderately-complex (e.g., ACL) and most complex (e.g., TKR) knee surgery, commonly combined with sciatic single-injection or catheter techniques. Commonly insufficient for surgical anesthesia due to unreliable coverage of lateral femoral cutaneous and obturator nerves. Additives may be very useful in prolonging postoperative analgesia when ropivacaine is used (e.g., clonidine 1 µg/kg, buprenorphine ≤300 µg). Catheter techniques have been successfully described; additives to low-concentration local anesthetics are not considered useful in continuous infusions. The extent to which "deep threading" of a femoral nerve block catheter (e.g., under nerve stimulator guidance with stimulating catheter) in producing a "3-in-1" block requires study.
Saphenous block using the femoral approach	Bupivacaine 0.5%, volume limited to 10 mL	Vastus medialis twitch is the proxy twitch response for saphenous nerve proximity. Do not confuse vastus medialis twitch for sartorius twitch; avoid cephalad aim of injection needle. Avoid other quadriceps twitch responses, to better avoid unwanted quadriceps weakness. Logically used for foot-ankle surgery when a calf tourniquet is planned, or when the saphenous nerve distribution is encroached surgically.

ACL, anterior cruciate ligament reconstruction; TKR, total knee replacement.

domized clinical trial patients receiving continuous lumbar plexus catheter (n = 15) versus epidural catheter (n = 15) for patients undergoing hip hemiarthroplasty under GA and found that lumbar plexus catheter patients (1) had less motor block, (2) ambulated sooner, and (3) had significantly fewer overall complications.[167] Stevens and colleagues reported that patients undergoing total hip arthroplasty receiving lumbar plexus single-injection blocks had less pain for up to 6 hours after surgery and less blood loss during and for up to 48 hours after surgery.[168] Naja and associates reported (retrospectively) that older hip fracture patients receiving lumbar plexus and parasacral blocks (vs. GA) encountered significantly less hypotension during surgery, less likely intensive care unit admission after surgery (0/30 vs.

11/30), and shorter length of hospital stay (7 vs. 14 days).[169]

Lumbar plexus block also provides excellent postoperative analgesia for most invasive knee procedures such as anterior cruciate ligament (ACL) reconstruction, multiligament reconstruction, or total knee arthroplasty (TKA). Matheny and colleagues found 89% lower opioid requirements after arthroscopic ACL reconstruction in the group receiving continuous lumbar plexus block versus those who had IV PCA.[170] Similarly, Luber and associates reported more comfortable recovery after TKA for patients with lumbar plexus and sciatic nerve blocks compared with IV PCA.[171] However, femoral nerve block in the groin is a much simpler and easier to perform block than lumbar plexus block, while providing equally efficacious analgesia for invasive knee procedures[172] in which obturator nerve coverage is not relevant. Femoral nerve block, with or without sciatic block, appears to be the block of choice at most centers providing meaningful postoperative analgesia after invasive knee surgeries; however, further studies of surgical procedure subtype and approach are needed to better delineate or predict pain mediated by the obturator nerve distribution.

Femoral Nerve Block. The femoral nerve block is relatively noninvasive, very safe, and technically simple to perform. The femoral nerve block (single-injection or continuous) is one of the most commonly performed nerve blocks for lower extremity surgery. Like the lumbar plexus block, the femoral nerve block provides excellent postoperative analgesia for all invasive procedures around the knee. Unlike with the lumbar plexus block, the femoral nerve block preserves hip adduction and psoas-mediated hip flexion. By increasing the volume of the local anesthetic and applying pressure distal to the point of injection, one can attempt to spread the local anesthetic along the fascia iliaca to cover the obturator and the lateral femoral cutaneous nerves (the "3-in-1" block). However, the results are often inconsistent, and it is generally accepted that all three nerves are more consistently covered in a single injection with the lumbar plexus block and not with a femoral nerve block in the groin. Femoral nerve block can provide optimal analgesia for patellar surgeries, knee arthroscopies, meniscal surgeries, knee ligament surgeries, and the like. However, supplementing the femoral block with a single shot or continuous sciatic nerve block is often needed for procedures such as TKA[173] or ACL reconstruction using hamstring autograft.[93]

In the late 1990s, two important studies from Europe examined rehabilitation outcomes after total knee replacement when a continuous femoral catheter was used (vs. epidural catheter, or control group IV PCA device). These studies were predicated on the notion that continuous femoral nerve block analgesia (when compared with IV PCA) leads to not only better pain relief but also significantly better knee flexion, faster achievement of ambulation goals, and overall faster convalescence.[174,175] Studies by Capdevila and colleagues and Singelyn and associates showed that total knee replacement patients undergoing GA with either continuous epidural analgesia or continuous femoral nerve block analgesia made faster progress meeting rehabilitation objectives, and were discharged from the inpatient rehabilitation unit sooner than were patients receiving IV PCA. Patients receiving femoral nerve catheter infusions experienced fewer side effects than did epidural patients in both studies, and continuous femoral catheter patients were discharged home from inpatient rehabilitation units 20% sooner in the femoral catheter versus IV PCA groups.[174,175]

In the United States, a similar anesthetic treatment method was applied by Chelly and colleagues to total knee replacement patients.[108] All patients received GA and were randomized to receive IV PCA, epidural infusion, or single-injection femoral-sciatic blocks followed by a continuous femoral infusion. Continuous femoral patients (vs. IV PCA patients) had an associated reduction of postoperative bleeding by 72% (P < 0.05), achieved better performance on continuous passive motion, had a 90% decrease in serious complications (including less blood loss), ambulated sooner (2.5 vs. 3.5 days), and had a 20% decrease in the length of hospitalization (4 vs. 5.5 days).[108] Duration of hospitalization did not include postoperative long-term rehabilitation (which is usually done on an outpatient basis in the United States) as did the two previously listed European studies,[174,175] although early postoperative rehabilitation was described as aggressive.[108]

Sciatic Nerve Block. The sciatic nerve has three distinct anatomic and functional parts—the posterior femoral cutaneous nerve, the tibial nerve, and the common peroneal nerve. The sciatic nerve is the main innervation to the posterior thigh, including the hamstring muscles, and major sensory and complete motor innervation to the lower extremity below the knee, including the foot and ankle. The sciatic nerve can be blocked at various sites along its course. Most proximally, it is blocked before it comes out of the greater sciatic notch (the parasacral approach). Around the hip, the sciatic nerve is blocked using different approaches (the classical or the gluteal approach, the lateral approach, the subgluteal approach, and the anterior approach). Distally, it is blocked in the popliteal fossa (posteriorly or laterally). Proximal sciatic nerve blocks are most often used as an adjunct to femoral or lumbar plexus blocks for painful procedures around the hip or the knee as discussed above,[93] but can also provide excellent analgesia for all major foot and ankle procedures (especially when a thigh tourniquet is planned). In studies examining subgluteal continuous sciatic nerve blockade for orthopedic ankle and foot surgeries, significantly decreased visual analogue pain scores have been reported.[176,177]

Similarly, significant analgesic benefit with continuous sciatic nerve block is proven for patients undergoing below-knee amputation.[178] The use of proximal sciatic nerve block for distal foot and ankle procedures is often limited by concerns of hamstring muscle weakness.[179]

Knee surgery block selection based on surgical invasiveness. Williams and associates have provided detailed insights on the allocation of femoral with or without sciatic nerve blocks, also considering the selection of single-injection techniques versus continuous nerve blocks, for outpatient knee surgery (Table 14–5). These reports were based on assessing the need for postoperative nursing interventions for parenteral analgesia after (1) a survey of 1200 outpatient knee surgery patients,[93] (2) a survey of 948 outpatients undergoing ACL reconstruction,[94] and (3) a prospective randomized trial involving 270 patients undergoing ACL reconstruction.[119] The allocation scheme has been summarized in a review.[180] To summarize, (1) patients in whom postoperative pain (exceeding

a verbal pain score of 3 out of 10) in a specific nerve distribution is likely to last 24 hours or less, single-injection femoral with or without sciatic nerve blocks are recommended; and (2) patients in whom postoperative pain (exceeding a verbal pain score of 3 out of 10) in a specific nerve distribution is likely to last greater than 24 hours, femoral with or without sciatic nerve block catheters are recommended. Special considerations are necessary for knee surgery patients who present with preoperative baseline verbal pain scores of 3 out of 10 or higher,[119,181] in that catheters may be indicated where single injections would have been originally planned (in the absence of preoperative pain).

Popliteal fossa sciatic nerve block. The sciatic nerve divides into the tibial and the common peroneal nerves in the popliteal fossa. The popliteal fossa sciatic nerve block is performed as cephalad as possible in the popliteal fossa, due to varying bifurcation

---

Table 14–5. Recommended Allocation of Analgesic Nerve Blocks for Knee Surgery

Category I (Mild)
• No blocks unless unanticipated postoperative pain occurs

Category II (Moderate)—Postoperative Pain Mediated Primarily by the Femoral Nerve
• Single-injection femoral nerve block recommended (anticipated moderate-severe pain duration ≤24 hours):
Arthrotomy, synovectomy, deep hardware removal, meniscal repair with fibrin clot injection, osteochondral allograft/autologous transfer system (OATS) procedure; microfracture, mosaicplasty/chondroplasty, quadriceps or patellar tendon repair, ACL allograft
  • Femoral bolus: *30 to 40 mL ropivacaine 0.5%, with additives*
  • *No sciatic block unless unanticipated pain (4 out of 10 or higher) refractory to femoral block*
• Continuous catheter recommended (anticipated moderate-severe pain duration ≥24 hours):
ACL patellar tendon autograft, femur osteotomy
  • Femoral catheter initial bolus: *20 to 30 mL 0.33% ropivacaine*
  • Femoral catheter infusion: *5 mL/hr 0.2% ropivacaine*
  • *No sciatic block unless unanticipated pain refractory to femoral block*

Category III (Severe)—Postoperative Pain Mediated by Both Femoral and Sciatic Nerves

PROCEDURE	FEMORAL NERVE BLOCK	SCIATIC NERVE BLOCK
Most Invasive Category III (Test for Dorsiflexion Postoperatively before Ablating Sciatic Nerve Motor Response)		
Total knee replacement High tibial osteotomy Multiligament reconstruction *(including PCL, LCL, MCL, POL)* Posterolateral corner reconstruction Meniscal reconstruction Unicompartmental knee arthroplasty	Continuous femoral catheter Initial bolus: *20 to 30 mL* *0.2% to 0.33% ropivacaine* Catheter dose: *5 mL/hr 0.2% ropivacaine*	Continuous sciatic catheter Initial postoperative bolus: *5 to 10 mL 0.2% ropivacaine, titrated to achieve desired analgesia and motor sparing* Catheter dose (postoperatively): *3 mL/hr 0.2% ropivacaine*
Moderately Invasive Category III		
ACL hamstring autograft ACL double-bundle allograft Chondrocyte transplant	Continuous femoral catheter Initial bolus: *20 mL 0.2% ropivacaine* Catheter dose: *5 mL/hr 0.2% ropivacaine*	Single-injection sciatic: *20 to 25 mL 0.33% to 0.5% ropivacaine, with additives*
Less Invasive Category III		
Complex meniscal repairs with anterior and posterior meniscal suturing Distal patella realignment	Single-injection femoral: *30 to 40 mL 0.5% ropivacaine, with additives*	Single-injection sciatic: *20 to 25 mL 0.33% to 0.5% ropivacaine, with additives*

Algorithm for the use of nerve block additives with ropivacaine:
—If a catheter is to be used, additives are not included.
—If no catheter is used, clonidine and buprenorphine are recommended.
—Buprenorphine dose should be restricted to a total of 200-300 µg per adult patient in order to prevent nausea, vomiting, and pruritus associated (anecdotally) with higher doses.
—Clonidine dose should be restricted to 1.0 to 1.2 µg/kg per adult patient in order to prevent systemic side effects associated with higher doses.

ACL, anterior cruciate ligament; LCL, lateral collateral ligament; MCL, medial collateral ligament; PCL, posterior cruciate ligament; POL, posterior oblique ligament.
Modified from Williams BA, Spratt D, Kentor ML: Continuous nerve blocks for outpatient knee surgery. *Techn Reg Anesth Pain Manage* 2004;8:76-84.

points 5 to 12 cm proximal to the popliteal crease.[182] The posterior approach is often preferred, although the lateral approach can be used whenever there are concerns regarding patient positioning.[183,184] Popliteal fossa block provides effective postoperative analgesia for all foot and ankle procedures. It also preserves hamstring function, facilitating ambulation.[179]

The effectiveness of the popliteal sciatic block for outpatient foot and ankle procedures was demonstrated by McLeod and colleagues.[184,185] They compared the lateral popliteal fossa block with ankle block,[185] and with subcutaneous infiltration of local anesthetics.[183] The popliteal fossa block provided 1080 minutes of postoperative analgesia, significantly longer than either the ankle block (690 minutes) or subcutaneous infiltration (373 minutes). Provenzano and associates reported a significant reduction in postoperative opioid requirements in patients with a successful popliteal fossa block, when compared with 367 patients who did not receive the block.[186]

Continuous popliteal sciatic nerve catheters have gained popularity in recent years. This technique was first introduced by Singelyn and colleagues, who described a challenging Seldinger (catheter-over-guidewire) technique for catheter placement, and achieved a 92% success rate.[187] Since then, authors have repeatedly found that continuous infusion nerve blocks lead to excellent analgesic outcomes when compared with single-injection blocks (or placebo catheters).[188-190] At this time, there are no definitive guidelines for the selection of single-injection versus continuous popliteal/sciatic techniques based on anticipated surgery, with the exception of recommendations implied by the myriad findings reported above, and the recommendation of Chelly and colleagues,[146] stating that for hardware removal of the foot and ankle, a single-injection block is likely to be sufficient, whereas for most other foot and ankle procedures, the use of a continuous sciatic catheter is likely to be a reasonable choice. Another rational approach, pending further studies, is to use the single-injection technique for soft tissue surgery and surgery of tendons and ligaments, and to use CNB for bony procedures of the foot and ankle.

Current Concepts in Analgesic Additives for Single-Injection Peripheral Nerve Blocks

Three analgesic adjuncts will be summarized in this section: buprenorphine, clonidine, and dexamethasone. All three have been shown to be efficacious at prolonging single-injection PNB duration when used in isolation, and to our knowledge, no combination perineural adjunct therapy studies have been reported. Perineural adjuncts for single-injection nerve blocks are important to consider because studies have shown that ropivacaine administered alone in PNBs can only yield 10 to 12 hours of analgesic duration.[191-193] Ropivacaine is now the most commonly used long-duration local anesthetic for the indication of single-injection and continuous PNB.[194] The local anesthetic levobupivacaine, is no longer available in the United States, but is accepted to provide analgesia of a similar duration as equivalently dosed racemic bupivacaine.

Buprenorphine and Clonidine. Buprenorphine is an opioid agonist-antagonist. Original studies of buprenorphine in brachial plexus blocks used this adjunct with a local anesthetic mixture consisting of mepivacaine and tetracaine,[195,196] and prolonged analgesia from 5 to 6 hours (local anesthetics alone) to 17 to 22 hours (with buprenorphine added). *Clonidine* has been shown to prolong brachial plexus analgesia by 3 hours when added to ropivacaine.[197,198] Clonidine has not been shown to prolong perineural analgesia provided by bupivacaine or levobupivacaine.[199,200]

Dexamethasone. Dexamethasone has rarely been studied as an additive to single-injection PNBs.[201] The first reports of the use of dexamethasone for this purpose were based on the incorporation of dexamethasone into local anesthetic microspheres, which contained the free-base of bupivacaine. Curley and colleagues found that sciatic nerve blocks in rats with bupivacaine microspheres did not experience motor or sensory block beyond 1 day. Meanwhile, rats receiving the same microspheres including dexamethasone experienced 8- to 13-fold prolongation of sensory and motor block.[201] Drager and associates found that intercostal nerve blocks for sheep with aqueous bupivacaine hydrochloride 0.25% lasted 12 hours.[202] Meanwhile, bupivacaine microcapsules provided 48 hours of analgesia, and bupivacaine microcapsules with dexamethasone (0.05%) provided 4 to 14 days of analgesia.[202] Kohane and colleagues, using the rat hindpaw/sciatic nerve pain model, found that bupivacaine microspheres yielded 6.2 to 8.5 hours of sensory-motor block (respectively), versus 31.3 to 45.1 hours when dexamethasone was included in the microsphere ($P = 0.03$).[203]

Holte and colleagues found that in human volunteers receiving subcutaneous injections, the "area under the curve" analgesic benefits from 1 to 7 days after a 10-mL subcutaneous injection were significantly better for the treatment group receiving dexamethasone.[204] In this study, dexamethasone comprised 0.04% of microsphere weight, and a dose of 50-μg dexamethasone was injected.[204] Kopacz and colleagues found that in human volunteers receiving intercostal nerve blocks, participants receiving dexamethasone-laden bupivacaine microspheres had block durations ranging from 18 to 30 hours versus shorter durations in the nondexamethasone microsphere group (8 to 16 hours) and aqueous injection group (5 to 7 hours).[205]

In the first human trial of the coadministration of dexamethasone with aqueous local anesthetic (lidocaine), Movafegh and associates recently reported that nerve block duration was increased by 2.4-fold (98 to 130 minutes with plain lidocaine vs. 242 to 310 minutes with added dexamethasone, for sensory-motor blocks, respectively).[206] The dexamethasone dose selected by these authors was 8 mg, which is consistent with the parenteral dose for the prevention of postoperative nausea, and is certainly much greater than the 50-μg dose given in the study by Holte and colleagues.[204] The study by Movafegh and associates did not have a treatment group that included parenteral (instead of perineural) dexamethasone dosing. There have been no reports of the coadministration of dexamethasone with ropivacaine and appropriate perineural safety studies are needed.

Intra-articular Analgesia

Myriad reports in the literature have evaluated single-agent intra-articular injections, as well as combination therapies. Opioids have been extensively studied, with morphine studied most commonly, based on the breakthrough report from Stein and colleagues[207] and subsequent works from that research team.[1,208-213] Intra-articular morphine (as a sole agent or in combination therapy) is not reviewed in this chapter; there have been extensive reviews (with intra-articular doses of 1 to 5 mg) elsewhere.[214,215] Instead, we focus on two reports from Soderlund and colleagues who used intra-articular meperidine[216,217] and then on other analgesic modalities that have been reported regarding intra-articular knee surgery (NSAIDs, neostigmine, and clonidine).

It is important to note that the extent of surgical trespass may be a predictor of intra-articular analgesic efficacy of local anesthetics versus opioids. Local anesthetics are considered effective short-term postoperative analgesics, with opioids conferring more sustained intra-articular analgesia. This was illustrated in a study by Marchal and colleagues (2003), in which "low inflammatory surgery" showed greater short-term (4 to 8 hours) benefit with intra-articular bupivacaine (vs. morphine 5 mg); while "high inflammatory surgery" showed greater long-term (24 hours) ben-efit after intra-articular morphine 5 mg versus intra-articular bupivacaine.[218] The timing of intra-articular dosing (preoperatively vs. postoperatively) may not necessarily bring any additional clinical benefits after the first 2 hours in the recovery room.[219]

Intra-articular Meperidine. Soderlund and colleagues compared three intra-articular opioids with saline controls, along with "route of administration" (IM) opioid controls. The doses that were administered were morphine (1 mg), meperidine (10 mg), and fentanyl (10 μg).[217] Of importance, no other preoperative or intraoperative opioids were permitted by protocol. The study had seven treatment groups of 10 patients each, and was powered to detect treatment group differences in patients receiving intra-articular versus IM opioids. The surprising element of this study with this limited sample size was that intra-articular meperidine patients showed a trend ($P = 0.06$) of improved analgesia (at rest and with movement) when compared with all other treatment groups (including the groups with intra-articular morphine and fentanyl). These authors postulated that the dual local anesthetic effect of meperidine

likely conferred these additional analgesic benefits.[217] The author of this textbook section (BAW) has used this study as basis for switching the standard intra-articular opioid from morphine to meperidine. Morphine[214] and meperidine in escalating intra-articular doses may produce a histamine-releasing hyper-algesic effect; meperidine's local anesthetic properties may offset potential histamine-induced hyperalgesia in the joint capsule. Unfortunately, no further studies have been done (to our knowledge) investigating morphine versus meperidine when used intra-articularly.

Soderlund and colleagues followed up on this report with a comparison of escalating doses of intra-articular meperidine (50 mg vs. 100 mg vs. 200 mg) in comparison with prilocaine for providing surgical anesthesia for diagnostic knee arthroscopy.[216] All meperidine patients had lower pain scores than prilocaine patients, but the meperidine 50-mg patients more likely required conversion to GA. There were no side effects (nausea, vomiting, somnolence) reported in the meperidine 50- to 100-mg treatment group. The meperidine 200-mg treatment group had a higher incidence of side effects (nausea, vomiting, and somnolence), which also corresponded with higher circulating concentrations of normeperidine, attributed to rapid demethylation of meperidine by, and systemic uptake of normeperidine from, the synovium.[216]

Intra-articular NSAIDs. Both ketorolac and tenoxicam have shown efficacy when delivered via the intra-articular route. Reuben and Connolly showed improved analgesia with intra-articular bupivacaine and ketorolac versus either drug used alone.[220] This finding was confirmed by Gupta and associates studying morphine with or without ketorolac,[221] and Rao and Rao studying bupivacaine with or without ketorolac; both studies showed improved analgesia and ambulation in patients receiving combination therapy.[222] Vintar and associates showed that a continuous intra-articular infusion of ropivacaine, morphine, and ketorolac led to lower pain scores and analgesics consumed after ACL reconstruction than did the continuous mixture excluding ketorolac.[223] Tenoxicam 20 mg has been used successfully both as a sole intra-articular analgesic and as an adjunct in combination therapy.[224-230]

Intra-articular Neostigmine and Clonidine. Neostigmine (0.5 mg intra-articularly) was shown by Yang and colleagues to be more efficacious than morphine 2 mg.[231] Neostigmine (0.5 mg) has not been shown to increase postoperative nausea/vomiting when given intra-articularly.[232] Neostigmine (0.5 mg) and clonidine (1 μg/kg) as sole analgesics have been shown to be superior to tenoxicam (20 mg), and all three single agents were superior to the single agents morphine (2 mg) and bupivacaine (100 mg).[225] Clonidine (1 μg/kg) coadministered with bupivacaine has improved analgesic benefits when compared with either agent used alone.[233] The combination of clonidine (150 μg) and neostigmine (0.5 mg) was no more effective than either agent given alone, but all intra-articular treatment groups had lower pain scores than did intra-articular placebo groups.[234] Clonidine (150 μg) was compared with morphine (2 mg) and found to be equivalent and superior to placebo, but the combination or clonidine and morphine provided no additional benefit.[235] The analgesic benefits of intra-articular clonidine have been shown to be unrelated to vascular uptake.[236]

To summarize, bupivacaine or ropivacaine can be logically combined with neostigmine (0.5 mg) or clondine (1 μg/kg) to achieve quality analgesia after arthroscopic procedures. Neostigmine may be preferable due to lower costs, when applicable; however, the combination of local anesthetic with neostigmine has not been studied (whereas the combination of local anesthetic with clonidine has produced positive results). The NSAIDs ketorolac and tenoxicam have shown benefit in combination with local anesthetics, opioids, or both, but may be less effective than clonidine and neostigmine. Meperidine may prove to be a more logical choice as an intra-articular opioid adjunct than morphine, pending further study.

Thorax and Abdominal Blocks

Although epidural analgesia is commonly used for the treatment of postoperative thoracic and upper abdominal surgical pain, there are a number of alternate analgesic techniques that can also be used. These techniques include interpleural (intrapleural) analgesia, paravertebral (extrapleural) blocks, and intercostal blocks. The most effective technique appears to be the paravertebral (extrapleural) block, which may be used for thoracic, breast, and upper abdominal surgery and treatment of rib fracture pain.[237] The paravertebral block provides analgesia presumably via direct somatic nerve, sympathetic nerve, or epidural blockade.[237] The paravertebral (extrapleural) block can be administered as a single injection or continuous infusion through a catheter, and may be inserted by either the anesthesiologist or surgeon (under direct vision at the conclusion of surgery). Paravertebral catheters provide superior analgesia compared to placebo and may provide equal analgesia when compared to thoracic epidural analgesia.[238] A systematic review of six trials (152 subjects received extrapleural/paravertebral analgesia; 149 subjects received epidural analgesia) indicated that extrapleural/paravertebral catheters provided equivalent analgesia compared to thoracic epidural analgesia at 8 to 12 hours postoperatively.[239]

Conversely, the analgesic efficacy of interpleural analgesia is not as compelling as extrapleural/paravertebral catheters. The mechanism of analgesic action from interpleural analgesia is not clear, and may be related to sensory or sympathetic blockade. Compared to epidural or paravertebral analgesia, interpleural analgesia provides inferior pain control and does not preserve lung function after thoracotomy, nor reduce the incidence of postoperative pulmonary complications.[240] A systematic review of eight trials (141 subjects received intrapleural analgesia; 134 subjects received saline placebo) indicated that intrapleural catheters did not provide significantly superior analgesia even versus placebo.[241]

Intercostal blocks may be another option for postoperative analgesia for thoracic pain. These blocks may be administered by the surgeon at the end of the open thoracic procedure but only provide short-term postoperative analgesia limited to the duration of the local anesthetic injected. Intercostal blocks may be repeated postoperatively but at the risk of increasing the incidence of pneumothorax: 1.4% per nerve blocked with an overall incidence of 8.7% per patient.[242] Intercostal blocks have not been shown to reduce the incidence of pulmonary complications postoperatively compared to systemic opioids.[242]

Summary

The rational use of peripheral analgesic techniques largely depends on allocation of the time, effort, and relevant acquisition costs of drugs and supplies to perform the analgesic procedures. Myriad techniques described above are logically included before and/or during surgical procedures known to create postoperative pain that would exceed the "mild" threshold (i.e., pain scores above 3 out of 10). Any peripheral or regional analgesic technique that has the potential to create risks that may exceed analgesic benefits (for the most minimally invasive and nonpainful surgery) should be reserved until a need is demonstrated postoperatively (e.g., pain scores at or exceeding 4 out of 10). Avoiding routine nerve blocks, for example, for patients that probably do not need them (or providing single-injection nerve blocks when a continuous catheter is not likely needed) will avail time for the practitioner to perform analgesic procedures for patients that do need them. This strategy allows the skilled practitioner to dedicate time to the performance of analgesic procedures for both outpatients and inpatients. However, the risks of opioid-induced hyperalgesia[97] seem likely to promote more use of multiple peripheral analgesic procedures. From the perspective of public health, allowing patients to encounter pain at or above the moderate threshold (e.g., pain scores at or above 4 out of 10 if there was zero preoperative pain) may soon prove to be unacceptable.

SPECIAL POPULATIONS

Trauma

Trauma is a major source of morbidity and mortality in the United States, as well as throughout the world. For the patient, the burden of trauma results from multiple factors, including loss of function due to limb, spine, or neurologic injury, economic losses due to time lost from work, as well as from pain and suffering during all phases of care. With respect to

Table 14–6. Pain Management Options in the Acute Trauma Setting

PATIENT CHARACTERISTIC	THERAPY	CONSIDERATIONS AND COMMENTS
Primary survey complete, patient is hemodynamically stable	Short-acting IV opioid (fentanyl)	Goals to improve patient cooperation, improve detection of unrecognized injuries. Risk for decreased sympathetic tone, with possible vasodilation and hemodynamic decompensation.
Patient conscious, hemodynamically unstable	Ketamine, tramadol	Ketamine risks: dysphoria, agitation, airway secretions. Tramadol risks: sedation especially if coadministered with other CNS depressants. Not recommended in head trauma patients.
Head trauma, need for neurologic assessment	Ultra-short acting opioids (remifentanil)	Allows for rapid neurologic evaluation. Only effective as an infusion.
Pain related to specific interventions (IV access, DPL, fracture manipulation)	Short-acting and ultra-short acting opioids, ketamine, dexmedetomidine, nitrous oxide	Opioids are generally more readily available. Dexmedetomidine may cause vasodilation and hypotension with initial bolus. Nitrous oxide is contraindicated in the setting of potential pneumothorax or bowel obstruction.
Concern for respiratory depression	Ketamine, dexmedetomidine	Both maintain respiratory drive; ketamine may be a better choice if patient is hypovolemic or hemodynamically unstable. Ketamine's dissociative effects may be dose-limiting.
Pain likely to exceed 2 days' duration	Perineural catheterization	May need to be accompanied by an intracompartmental pressure monitor (i.e., evaluate for developing compartment syndrome). Possible infection risk if sterile field is disrupted or systemic sepsis ensues.
Desire for amnesia related to painful procedures	Midazolam, scopolamine	If analgesic intervention not possible due to hemodynamic decompensation, inducing amnesia is still commonly indicated.

CNS, central nervous system; DPL, diagnostic peritoneal lavage; IV, intravenous.

pain, numerous reports point to the inadequacy of pain management in trauma patients, particularly during the evaluation and resuscitation phase of care (Table 14–6).[243-248]

Several reasons have been proposed to account for this observation. These include inadequate evaluation of pain, late or improper administration of analgesics, concerns about hemodynamics, fear that analgesia may interfere with the accurate diagnosis of injuries, the misconception that sleep automatically indicates the absence of pain, unfounded concerns that opioid use in the management of acute pain leads to addiction, and beliefs that trauma patients do not remember painful events.[245,249-251]

Evidence indicates that pain has a negative impact on the physiologic stress response to injury, and can contribute to the incidence of complications such as pulmonary dysfunction, thromboembolic phenomena, myocardial infarction, decreased immune function, and immobility.[250,252-254] Furthermore, there is evidence that acute pain may lead to secondary hyperalgesia, allodynia, and chronic pain by inducing changes in the way pain signals are transmitted and processed within the CNS.[255-257] Finally, there are reports of post-traumatic stress disorder (PTSD) resulting directly from uncontrolled pain.[258]

In light of this information, current recommendations are for early and aggressive analgesic therapy for postsurgical and trauma patients.[250] To this end, pain is now considered the "fifth vital sign" in the clinical setting, underlining the importance of frequent and accurate pain assessment, the first step toward adequate analgesia in the trauma setting.

Primary and Secondary Surveys, and Evaluation of Analgesic Needs in the Trauma Patient

The prehospital and emergency department evaluation and resuscitation phase of trauma care is a period of severe physiologic stress for the victim. The primary therapeutic goals during this time are to maintain a patent airway, ensure adequate oxygenation and ventilation, support the circulation, and assess global neurologic function.[259,260] The assessment and management of life-threatening injuries takes priority above all else, but the treatment of pain is not necessarily contraindicated. During this period, the patient is likely to experience severe generalized pain in the setting of multiple trauma, as well as localized pain at specific sites of injury. Furthermore, the patient is likely to undergo painful procedures that may include peripheral and central venous cannulation, chest tube placement, diagnostic peritoneal lavage (DPL), tracheostomy, or the manipulation of extremity fractures.

Once the primary survey has been completed, and the patient has been determined to have a stable or hyperdynamic circulation, careful use of short-acting IV opioids such as *fentanyl* is indicated. Often a patient will become more cooperative once adequate analgesia is achieved, facilitating further evaluation and the detection of previously unrecognized injuries. This is particularly important during the evaluation of cervical spine injuries, wherein distracting injuries can contribute to late or missed diagnoses.[261,262] In rare cases, the stress response to pain and associated elevations in catecholamine levels may contribute to the patient's hemodynamic stability; alleviation of pain may result in hemodynamic decompensation. In such cases, even though analgesic administration may be the proximal cause of the decompensation, the actual cause is generally related to blood loss and hypovolemia, which is responsive to rapid but careful fluid resuscitation.

In a study evaluating the use of *fentanyl* during air medical transport for trauma, only 4 out of 177 patients (2.2%) demonstrated systolic blood pressure (SBP) reductions below 90 mm Hg following fentanyl administration, with the lowest in this study being 81 mm Hg. In all cases, the SBP returned to or above 90 mm Hg within 3 to 10 minutes.[263] This indicates that fentanyl is a safe and effective analgesic in the prehospital setting and that analgesia should not be withheld because of concerns regarding hemodynamic instability in patients who are otherwise stable.

In patients who are conscious but hemodynamically unstable, *ketamine* or *tramadol* have been shown to be useful alternatives.[264,265] *Nitrous oxide* may be available in some clinical settings for the management of pain related to specific procedures, such as establishment of IV access, DPL, or manipulation of extremity fractures. Nitrous oxide should not be used in patients with pneumothorax.[266,267] If respiratory depression is of concern, *dexmedetomidine,* a centrally acting α_2-adrenergic agonist without respiratory effects, has been shown to provide effective analgesia and sedation with minimal hemodynamic changes, when given as an infusion without an initial bolus.[268] If the ability to rapidly evaluate a patient's neurologic status is of primary concern, one can consider an infusion of *remifentanil,* an ultrashort-acting opioid.[269] Finally, in patients for whom none of the above options are available due to hemodynamic instability, drug allergy, or institutional drug availability, the use of an adjuvant agent such as *scopolamine* or *midazolam* alone, may be useful to promote amnesia and minimize the psychological impact that is associated with uncontrolled pain without further compromising hemodynamic stability.[270]

Inpatient Hospitalization of Trauma Patients and Evaluation of Analgesic Needs

Following the initial assessment and stabilization of life-threatening injuries, a period of inpatient care usually ensues. The patient may be in the intensive care unit or on a surgical patient ward. During this time, additional invasive and noninvasive diagnostic studies are performed to identify and further characterize the patient's injuries. Operative management of second priority injuries such as eye and facial trauma, musculoskeletal and spine injuries, as well as vascular or visceral trauma may be undertaken at this time.[259,260] The patient will continue to have generalized pain, as well as regional or localized pain specific to the sites of injury. This can be characterized as background pain with frequent episodes of break-through pain. The patient will also experience acute pain related to any operative, diagnostic, and therapeutic interventions, as well as that due to routine nursing care such as dressing changes.[271]

Use of Opioids in Trauma Patients

Systemic opioids will likely continue to be the mainstay of pain therapy for generalized and regionalized pain. Intermediate-acting agents such as *morphine, hydromorphone,* and *meperidine* are useful to achieve a stable level of analgesia for background pain, although meperidine is logically avoided due to toxicities associated with its metabolite normeperidine, which can accumulate especially in the context of renal failure (with acute renal failure being a common complication in trauma). IV PCA is a very useful mode of delivery, because it can be programmed to treat both background and breakthrough pain.[6,272] Later during hospitalization, IV PCA opioids will often be converted to an oral preparation, when the patient begins to tolerate oral intake of food. As the patient's baseline opioid requirement is established, longer-acting or sustained-release opioids are added to the pain regimen to specifically treat background pain. These sustained-release opioids may include *controlled-release morphine* or *oxycodone, methadone,* or *transdermal fentanyl.* Breakthrough pain treatments can include either short-acting oral or IV opioids that are available upon patient request. Patients should be encouraged to anticipate painful activities by requesting additional pain medication in advance. Sometimes patients will undergo procedures or dressing changes where the pain is very intense compared to the baseline level of background pain. Such pain may not be adequately covered by the typical doses available for standard breakthrough pain. A plan must be in place to provide additional analgesia for these pain exacerbations. Often, a period of brief and intense analgesia is required, with minimal sedation and respiratory depression afterwards. IV or oral opioid analgesics are commonly used, depending on the severity of the pain. In special cases, other adjuncts such as *propofol,* with *fentanyl, ketamine,* or *midazolam* may be used to provide adequate analgesia and sedation, or even GA.[273]

The Use of Neuraxial Techniques in Trauma Patients

Spinal or epidural analgesia can be very useful for the treatment of postoperative pain in the trauma patient, after procedures such as laparotomy, thoracotomy, or reduction of lower extremity fractures.[274] Continuous epidural analgesia has been shown to provide superior analgesia following intra-abdominal surgery when compared to IV PCA.[275] The potential hemodynamic impact of the sympathetic blockade associated with these techniques must be carefully considered. IV crystalloid administration during the placement of a spinal anesthetic has been shown to decrease hemodynamic changes.[276]

Depending on the mechanism of injury, one should confirm definitive spine clearance before proceeding with a neuraxial technique. Another consideration, depending on the nature and extent of the patient's injuries, is that patient positioning may factor into the feasibility of these techniques. Finally, one should be alert for the presence of coagulopathy in patients with polytrauma, which would be a contraindication for neuraxial techniques.

Use of Peripheral Regional Analgesia in the Trauma Patient

Select peripheral regional analgesic techniques may be useful for the management of pain related to specific sites of injury. For example, paravertebral blocks may be indicated for pain related to rib fractures.[277] Isolated PNBs may also be useful in the management of extremity injuries. These may include femoral and sciatic nerve blocks for knee injuries, popliteal sciatic nerve and saphenous nerve blocks for lower leg injuries, and brachial plexus blocks for upper extremity injuries.[278-281] The use of continuous perineural catheters should be considered in patients with more extensive trauma where the duration of severe pain is expected to be longer than 1 to 2 days.

Peripheral regional techniques not only improve pain and patient satisfaction and decrease side effects related to systemic opioids, but they also facilitate participation in physical therapy as well as the examination of painful injured extremities.[175,281,282] As the patient's severity of pain begins to decline as the initial inflammation related to the injury begins to subside and healing begins, neuraxial and peripheral catheters are often converted to multimodal systemic analgesics during this period, unless specific surgical interventions affecting the affected extremity are planned. The ongoing benefit of perineural catheters, as healing begins to take place, must be weighed against the small but real potential for infection if catheters are left in place for prolonged durations.[283]

Analgesia in the Trauma Setting for the Alcohol-intoxicated Patient

There is a strong association between alcohol consumption and trauma,[284,285] both accident-related and violence-related. According to the Insurance Institute for Highway Safety, alcohol is a contributing factor in 50% of all trauma deaths. Patients who are not accustomed to regularly using alcohol are subject to higher risk of an injury immediately after alcohol consumption, when compared with patients who drink more heavily.[286] Furthermore, alcohol abuse is associated with an increased risk of readmission for new trauma.[287]

During the acute phase of injury, the intoxicated patient is at risk for increased CNS and respiratory depression with the administration of sedative or opioid medications, due to additive effects with alcohol. However, once the acute effects of alcohol intoxication have worn off, the chronic alcoholic patient will demonstrate tolerance to sedative medications, as well as cross-tolerance to opioids. As a result, much higher doses of opioids may be necessary to achieve adequate analgesia. This may be particularly problematic if the patient's alcohol abuse history is undocumented, and generally adequate doses of opioids are proving to be ineffective. In patients with alcoholic cirrhosis and advanced liver disease, altered metabolism and excretion of drugs will alter the dosing of hepatic-metabolized medications, including opioid analgesics. In cases of end-stage liver disease, coagulopathy may contraindicate the use of neuraxial and some PNB techniques for pain control. In alcoholics receiving disulfiram, potentiation of CNS depressants may occur secondary to the ability of disulfiram to inhibit the metabolism of drugs other than alcohol.[249] Patients with a history of chronic alcohol abuse are also at a twofold increased risk of complications, particularly pneumonia, infection, prolonged hospitalization, and respiratory failure.[288] Pain control in the setting of abdominal and thoracic trauma becomes particularly important in these patients in order to promote deep breathing and appropriate pulmonary toilet. Given the increased risk of pneumonia, and the known respiratory depressant effects of opioids, one may consider neuraxial or regional techniques in alcoholic patients who undergo exploratory laparotomy or thoracotomy, as long as coagulopathy has been ruled out. Paravertebral nerve blocks can also be considered for the same reasons in chronic alcoholic patients with rib fractures.

Analgesia in the Setting of Head Trauma

Acute pain management of head trauma patients presents several unique considerations. First, it is difficult to assess the level of pain in patients with an altered mental status. Patients who are unable to voice their pain may be mistakenly believed to not have pain. There are also concerns that the sedating effects of opioids could interfere with adequate neurological assessment. As a result, trauma patients with head injuries are less likely to receive opioids than patients with comparable injuries who have not sustained head trauma.[251] Whether pain results directly from head trauma or, more likely, as a result of other injuries, it is important to tailor the analgesic regimen to facilitate ongoing neurological assessment. Analgesic treatments include the use of nonsedating analgesic agents and opioid-reducing strategies wherever possible, to minimize the sedating effects of opioids. *Acetaminophen* is a good choice for mild-to-moderate pain for patients able to tolerate oral intake or in whom a nasogastric tube is inserted (assuming lack of a commercially available parenteral equivalent of acetaminophen in many centers). NSAIDs such as *ibuprofen* and *ketorolac* are best avoided in any patient at risk for intracranial bleeding due to the platelet-inhibiting effects of this drug class. For moderate-to-severe pain, shorter-acting opioids such as *fentanyl,* or *remifentanil* (as an infusion), can be used for the management of background and breakthrough pain in the acute period. IV PCA is a good choice in sufficiently alert patients. A continuous background infusion can be added via IV PCA to provide baseline analgesic requirements. *Morphine* and *hydromorphone* have longer half-lives than fentanyl, and can be used in many cases, but sedating effects may persist longer than analgesic effects, possibly impeding neurological evaluation. In the critical care setting, continuous brief infusions of *fentanyl, alfentanil, or sufentanil,* or ultrashort-acting *remifentanil* can be used.[289] These infusions can be temporarily stopped, allowing for rapid neurological assessment due to their shorter half-lives. Both *morphine* and *fentanyl* have prolonged context-sensitive half-lives following extended infusions, prolonging recovery after their termination.[290] Longer-acting or sustained-release preparations should be started only after intracranial injury has been definitively excluded, or the patient's neurologic status has stabilized.

Regional anesthetic techniques can have an important role in the management of head-injured patients, because regional techniques can significantly reduce the use of opioids (and their sedating side effects). In patients with thoracic trauma concomitant with head injury, adequate management of thoracic pain gains greater importance. Chest analgesia reduces pulmonary morbidity (outlined in the next section) and decreases hypoventilation due to poor respiratory mechanics, splinting, and resultant atelectasis. Hypoventilation and resultant hypercarbia can lead to increased intracranial pressure in patients with traumatic brain injury.

Paravertebral blocks may be a better alternative to epidural analgesia in this setting because of the small but real risk of dural puncture associated with epidurals. Dural puncture could result in the expansion of an intracranial hematoma or uncal herniation. Continuous nerve block techniques should be considered for the management of coexisting extremity injuries to further reduce opioid requirements.

Analgesia in the Setting of Blunt Thoracic Trauma

Injuries typically categorized under this heading (Table 14–7) include rib fractures, flail chest, pulmonary and cardiac contusions, disruption of thoracic vessels, hemothorax, pneumothorax, and soft tissue

Table 14–7. Analgesic Modalities in Blunt Chest Trauma

THERAPY	PROS	CONS	COMMENTS
Opioids	Effective Simple administration Readily available	CNS/respiratory depression, impaired cough reflex, risks for hypoxia, hypoventilation	Patients with multiple rib fractures may have opioid-induced sedation before analgesic efficacy is achieved NSAIDs may improve analgesia and decrease opioid requirement
Continuous epidural analgesia	Better analgesia than IV PCA Improved respiratory function	Hypotension Nausea, pruritus, constipation Technical difficulties (placement, maintenance) Caution with anticoagulation	Advise against simultaneous opioid dosing via epidural and IV PCA in trauma setting
Paravertebral nerve blocks	Improved respiratory function Greater hemodynamic stability and spirometry compared to thoracic epidural Ability to use percutaneous catheter for continuous analgesia	Technical difficulties (placement, maintenance) Caution with anticoagulation Risk of pneumothorax	Excellent alternative to thoracic epidural, especially in unilateral chest trauma
Intercostal nerve blocks	Comparable analgesia with epidural Improved respiratory function	Risk of pneumothorax Multiple blocks often required Risk of local anesthetic toxicity due to large volumes used and increased systemic uptake Limited duration may require repeated injections for single shot techniques High rate of misplaced catheters due to technical difficulties	Patients may not tolerate palpation of fractured ribs and multiple injections in the setting of multiple rib fractures
Interpleural catheter analgesia	May be useful when other techniques contraindicated	Requires supine position for adequate spread, negatively impacting respiratory mechanics Risk of pneumothorax	Conflicting evidence regarding efficacy

CNS, central nervous system; IV, intravenous; NSAIDs, nonsteroidal anti-inflammatory drugs; PCA, patient-controlled analgesia.

trauma. Motor vehicle accidents and falls account for the majority of these injuries.[291] Thoracic injuries significantly contribute to morbidity and mortality arising from trauma, leading to 25% of trauma deaths.[292] Rib fractures are the most common injury, and are seen in 10% of all trauma patients.[293] Thoracic injuries can impair respiratory function directly though physiologic and mechanical changes, such as those seen with pneumothorax, flail chest, and pulmonary contusions. Thoracic injuries can also have indirect effects via increased pain with respiration, commonly seen with multiple rib fractures. These factors lead to splinting during respiration increasing atelectasis, decreases in functional residual capacity, impairments of coughing ability, and predispositions to pneumonia. Furthermore, these effects can lead to changes in pulmonary ventilation-perfusion matching (V/Q mismatch), resulting in hypoxia. Because of these latter pain-related sources of morbidity, adequate pain control is of obvious importance, particularly in patients who are breathing spontaneously.

Opioids in the Setting of Chest Trauma

Multiple options exist for the management of pain in the setting of blunt thoracic trauma. Traditionally, systemic opioids have been the primary means of controlling pain in these patients. They offer the advantage of simplicity of administration and are readily available, are easily titrated, and are effective, particularly when administered via IV PCA.[6] Their primary disadvantage is that opioids cause CNS and respiratory depression, and opioids impair the cough reflex. These factors lead to hypoxemia and further impairment in ventilation. Patients suffering from multiple fractures who are treated only with IV opioids tend to be excessively sedated, but when aroused, will often report unacceptable pain levels. The addition of NSAIDs to opioid analgesia can reduce opioid dose required to achieve adequate pain relief.

Continuous Epidural Analgesia in the Setting of Chest Trauma

CEIs of a local anesthetic combined with a low-dose opioid have been shown to confer superior pain relief when compared with IV PCA, resulting in increased tidal volume and inspiratory force.[294,295] The CEI can be combined with a patient-administered bolus via patient-controlled epidural analgesia (PCEA), to give patients a similar degree of control over their pain management as seen with IV PCA. Hypotension is the most common side effect seen with epidural infusions and is related to local anesthetic-mediated effects on the sympathetic nervous system. Good analgesic results have also been reported with continuous epidural opioid infusions.[296] As with IV opioids, nausea, pruritus, and constipation are frequently seen with epidural opioids. In some cases, excessive sedation and respiratory depression are seen. If these findings occur while using a combined local anesthetic/opioid epidural infusion, one can

change to a local anesthetic only–epidural infusion, adding an opioid IV PCA for more precise control of the opioid dose.

Paravertebral Nerve Blocks in the Setting of Chest Trauma

Paravertebral blocks provide an alternative to epidural analgesia in the setting of unilateral thoracic trauma, which commonly presents in side-impact motor vehicle accidents and in falls. Paravertebral blocks involve the injection of local anesthetic into the paravertebral space and produce an ipsilateral block at multiple dermatomes. A catheter can also be inserted percutaneously, or by the surgeon under direct vision during thoracotomy, to provide continuous analgesia.[297] Paravertebral analgesia has been shown to provide effective pain relief in patients with multiple rib fractures, as well as improved respiratory parameters and oxygenation.[277] Paravertebral techniques have been considered technically easier to perform than epidural techniques,[237] making the paravertebral block a better choice in patients who are able to cooperate in a limited manner due to pain. Furthermore, paravertebral blocks can be safely performed in anesthetized or sedated patients.[237,298]

There is a low incidence of complications with paravertebral blocks. These include failure, inadvertent vascular puncture, hypotension, hematoma, epidural or intrathecal spread, pleural puncture, and pneumothorax.[299] Paravertebral blocks are an excellent choice in patients who already have chest tubes inserted on the side of the planned block. Because the sympatholytic effects of paravertebral blocks are typically unilateral, hypotension occurs much less frequently when compared to patients receiving continuous epidural analgesia, provided the patient is adequately fluid resuscitated.[277,300]

Intercostal Nerve Blocks in the Setting of Blunt Chest Trauma

Intercostal nerve blocks are another effective option for the management of pain associated with chest trauma and rib fractures. These blocks have been shown to improve oxygenation and respiratory mechanics, and offer pain relief that is comparable to that of epidural analgesia.[301,302] The intercostal block technique involves the palpation of the ribs, and injection of local anesthetic proximally to the fracture site. Because of overlapping innervation, the intercostal nerves above and below the fracture site should be blocked as well. The need to palpate fractured ribs, combined with the need for multiple injections, may make this a difficult technique to perform in patients with multiple rib fractures, or in those experiencing significant pain. The technique is also limited by the relatively large doses of local anesthetic required, and relatively high intravascular uptake from the intercostal space, increasing risk of local anesthetic toxicity. The most common complication associated with this technique is pneumothorax (occurring with an incidence of 1.4% per individual nerve block and in 5.6% of patients with multiple blocks for multiple rib fractures).[242] The duration of analgesia is only 6 to 12 hours, which often necessitates multiple daily injections.[277] Even though percutaneously placed intercostal nerve block catheters can deliver effective continuous analgesia, their placement is technically difficult and results in a high rate of misplaced catheters.[303]

Interpleural Catheter Analgesia in the Setting of Blunt Chest Trauma

Local anesthetics can be delivered via a catheter into the interpleural space; the local anesthetics then diffuse through the parietal pleura to block the intercostal nerves. The local anesthetic spreads in a gravity-dependent manner within the interpleural space, and patients are maintained in a supine position following the injection to facilitate spread to the proximal portions of the intercostal nerves. However, the supine position can have an adverse impact on respiratory mechanics. One study shows this technique to be comparable to systemic opioids in efficacy,[304] while another shows no difference when compared to placebo.[305] Interpleural blocks may or may not be as effective as epidural blocks in the setting of rib fractures,[306,307] or after thoracotomy.[308,309] Catheter insertion may be technically difficult and can result in catheter misplacement either into the pleura or the chest wall. Pneumothorax is the most common complication of interpleural catheters. Despite these limitations, this technique may be useful in patients in whom other techniques are contraindicated. However, a systematic review has indicated that intrapleural catheters do not provide significantly superior analgesia even versus placebo.[241]

Analgesia in the Setting of Burn Injury

Burn injuries (Table 14–8) often cause very severe pain associated with the injury itself, as well as with the multiple interventions that follow. This results in a combination of background pain, exacerbated by short periods of severe pain associated with wound care, including dressing changes and debridements. The level of pain is difficult to predict, however. Full-thickness burns involve the destruction of nerve fibers, and thus do not result in pain. Patients with extensive full-thickness burns will experience pain only from tissues at the margins of the burned areas. Patients with partial-thickness burns will have damaged but functioning nerve fibers that are exposed at the surface of the skin. These nerve fibers can transmit severe pain, particularly in response to surface contact. Furthermore, activation of nociceptive and inflammatory mediators can alter the response to further stimulation resulting in hyperalgesia and temporal summation.[310] Pain can persist well beyond the healing period, resulting in impaired function and psychological problems. It is thus imperative to aggressively manage burn pain.

Table 14–8. Analgesic Modalities in Burn Patients

THERAPY	PROS	CONS	COMMENTS
Opioids	Effective for background pain Short-acting opioids (fentanyl, remifentanil) effective for dressing changes	Tolerance develops	Once adequate baseline established, can be converted to continuous IV infusion or long-acting oral therapy Transdermal absorption is variable due to alterations in tissue perfusion
NSAIDs	Useful adjunct to opioid therapy	Risk of peptic ulcers in already predisposed patients	Ibuprofen may improve tissue perfusion and decrease hypermetabolic response
Ketamine	Provides analgesia while maintaining hemodynamic and respiratory function Multiple available routes of administration May suppress secondary hyperalgesia	Dissociative effects may be unpleasant Agitation	Suitable for repetitive administration (e.g., dressing changes) Dissociative effects attenuated by midazolam, propofol
Clonidine	No respiratory depression	Possible hypotension, sedation	Synergistic effects with opioids
Local anesthetics	Significant opioid-sparing effect when given IV Decreases inflammation at burn sites No respiratory depression	Variable systemic absorption when applied topically Potential for cardiac and CNS toxicity	
Regional analgesia	Useful for management of pain at graft donor sites Effective analgesia Opioid-sparing effects	Risks associated with techniques	Regional analgesic techniques are often not practical in burn patients because the skin overlying the site of the block must be intact, and the burn must be contained in the neural distribution of the block

CNS, central nervous system; IV, intravenous; GI, gastrointestinal; NSAIDs, nonsteroidal anti-inflammatory drugs.

Opioids in the Setting of Burn Injury

Opioids continue to be the primary therapy used for the management of background and procedural pain. Despite the enhanced potency of opioids following acute burn injury,[311] opioid requirements can be quite high. Even though burns cause significant changes in metabolism and protein binding, the pharmacokinetics of IV opioids remain unaltered.[249] Therapy is initiated with small IV boluses, which are titrated to effect. To this end, IV PCA has been shown to be safe and effective.[312] The absorption of IM and transdermal opioids is variable due to decreased tissue perfusion and uptake, making these routes unsuitable in this patient population. Gastrointestinal absorption and emptying appear to be unchanged, however.[313] Once an adequate baseline opioid requirement is established for the management of background pain, opioids can be given via continuous IV infusion or by equianalgesic enteral formulations of long-acting or sustained-release opioids.

Dressing changes and wound debridements result in a brief but exquisite period of pain. Opioids again are the principal therapy, with preference given to *fentanyl* or short-acting opioids including *alfentanil* and *remifentanil.* These can be administered by a provider or by the patient via IV PCA. Opioids with effects lasting longer than the duration of the procedure can result in excessive sedation and respiratory depression once the intervention is completed.

Non-opioid Analgesics in the Setting of Burn Injury

NSAIDs are a useful adjunct to opioids, decreasing inflammation and opioid requirements. Ibuprofen may improve tissue perfusion following burn injury,[314] and may decrease the hypermetabolic response.[315] However, one should be wary of NSAIDs' gastrointestinal side effects, including gastric ulcers, particularly in a patient population already predisposed to stress gastritis. In addition, NSAIDs have been implicated as a contributing cause in renal impairment following burn injury.[316] *Acetaminophen* may be a better alternative for mild pain in burn patients with normal hepatic function.

Local anesthetics have been used in a variety of ways for burn patients. Efficacy has been demonstrated with topical application for the treatment of post-burn pain[317] and of pruritus.[318] There is however, an increased risk of rapid systemic uptake and local anesthetic toxicity when applied to nonintact skin, potentially resulting in seizures,[319] or in dysrhythmias. *Lidocaine,* when given by IV infusion, has significant opioid-reducing effects[320] and acts to decrease inflammation at the burn site.[321] Local anesthetics, both topical and by local infiltration, have also been used successfully to decrease pain associated with skin grafting.[322,323]

Ketamine, a dissociative anesthetic, has the advantage of providing analgesia while maintaining stable hemodynamic function with minimal respiratory depression. Studies also suggest that ketamine may suppress burn-induced secondary hyperalgesia.[324] Ketamine can be administered via IV or IM injection, as well as via oral, rectal, or nasal administration. The primary clinical use of ketamine has been to provide sedation and analgesia during wound dressing changes and debridements, particularly in children. Ketamine by infusion has also been used successfully for long-term sedation and analgesia in a burn patient, with remarkable opioid-sparing effects.[325] Its dissociative effects can be unpleasant for patients, however, and can lead to emergence delirium. Delirium may be attenuated by preemptive or rescue doses of *midazolam* or *propofol.*[326-328]

Clonidine, an α_2 adrenoreceptor agonist, exerts sedative and analgesic effects via action on the CNS. Clonidine has been used as an adjunct in the management of postoperative pain, demonstrating synergistic effects with opioids.[329] Several case studies report its successful use in burn patients.[330,331] Clonidine has the benefit of not causing respiratory depression, and its opioid-sparing effect can be used to decrease side-effects associated with their use. One should avoid clonidine in hemodynamically unstable or hypovolemic patients because of the risk of hypotension.

Peripheral Regional Analgesic Techniques in the Setting of Burn Injury

Patients with burn injuries are generally poor candidates for regional techniques. In most cases, the duration of pain following burn injury is far longer than is practical to maintain an indwelling perineural catheter. Also, the skin overlying the proposed peripheral block site must be intact to reduce the risk of infection in patients already at increased risk of infection and sepsis. In addition, many burns are not limited to the distribution of one or two peripheral nerves that are easily blocked. This limits the usefulness of these techniques to cases of mild isolated extremity burns. One area where nerve blocks have been successful is in the management of pain at graft donor sites.[332]

Psychological Support after Burn Injury

Burn trauma can be a devastating injury, not only physically, but psychologically as well. Patients can become depressed or have high levels of fear and anxiety, particularly if the degree of injury or disability is severe, or if hospitalization is lengthy. The anxiety often revolves around the repeated painful wound treatments that patients undergo. Evidence demonstrates a relationship between patients' levels of depression and anxiety, and the level of pain reported by patients.[333] Burn patients frequently have difficulty sleeping.[334] In one study looking at predictors of posttraumatic stress disorder following burn injury, as many as 25% of patients developed this complication.[335] Predictors included anxiety measures, female gender, and severity of injury.

Effective anxiolysis with benzodiazepines including *midazolam, diazepam,* and *lorazepam* has proven to reduce pain in the treatment of burns,[336,337] as well as in other surgical areas.[338,339] Low doses of antidepressants including *serotonin specific reuptake inhibitors* and *tricyclic antidepressants* have also been shown to potentiate the analgesic effects of opioids.[340,341] Other therapeutic interventions including hypnosis, acupuncture, auricular electrical stimulation, massage therapy, biofeedback, mental imagery, and relaxation training have all been employed to reduce pain scores in burn patients with mixed results.[249,342,343]

Older Adults

Older patients constitute an ever-growing proportion of the American population. According to the U.S. census bureau, currently more than 12% of Americans are 65 years of age or older. This number is projected to increase to over 20% by the year 2020. As their numbers grow, there will continue to be an increase in the number of patients presenting for the management of acute pain relating to surgery as well as trauma. Persons 65 years of age and older are leading more active lifestyles today, which places them at increased risk for injury. In one study, older adults accounted for 24% of all trauma admissions.[344] Older adults are likely more predisposed to trauma due to common physiologic effects that are associated with aging: decreasing visual and hearing acuity, impaired coordination and proprioception, dementia, degenerative joint disease, and weakness.

Pain management in the elderly population is complicated by a number of factors (Table 14–9). The assessment of pain is often difficult due to cognitive impairment and difficulties in communication.[345] There is also an association between depression and pain complaints in the elderly,[346] with those suffering from depression reporting higher pain scores than nondepressed patients.[347] This is significant, in that 24% of community-living and 47% of nursing home residents suffer from depression.[348] It is important to screen for and treat depression, while simultaneously managing pain. The duration of action of many medications is prolonged, and the incidence of drug-related side-effects and toxicity are increased as a result of age-related changes in medication uptake, changes in body composition and distribution, and slowing of drug metabolism and elimination. Potentially adverse medication effects are further complicated by the fact that most patients older than 65 have at least one chronic condition, with more than 90% taking at least one medication and many taking multiple medications.[349] "Polypharmacy" combined with decreased cognitive ability contribute to patient noncompliance. Twenty-five percent to 50% of those living in the community and 50% to 80% living in nursing homes suffer from chronic pain.[350-352] Consequently, a large proportion of these patients will already be taking pain medication on a regular basis, contributing to side effects and medication tolerance. Adequate management of pain in the elderly is particularly important, because pain can contribute to other conditions such as malnutrition, gait disturbances, and delayed rehabilitation.[353]

The goal of pain management in older adults is to maximize function and quality of life while minimizing side effects. To this end, non-opioid analgesics such as *acetaminophen* and *NSAIDs* are the first-line

Table 14–9. Options for Pain Management in the Older Adults

THERAPY	TYPE OF PAIN	BENEFITS	SIDE EFFECTS	COMMENTS
Non-opioid analgesics (NSAIDs, acetaminophen)	Mild to moderate	First-line agents since neither impairs cognitive function	NSAIDs—GI/renal COX-2 inhibitors may cause cardiovascular events	Acetaminophen first choice in patients without hepatic impairment
Opioids	Moderate to severe	Should *not* be withheld if non-opioids are ineffective	Cognitive impairment, sedation, respiratory depression, constipation, urinary retention, nausea/vomiting Tolerance usually develops to all side effects, except constipation (use stool softener)	Start opioids with low dose of short-acting agent, and titrate upward to minimize side effects Once therapeutic dose achieved, convert to longer-acting preparation Simplify regimen with once/twice daily dosing Avoid meperidine—increased risk of sedation and falls
Regional anesthesia (neuraxial blocks, peripheral nerve blocks)	Focal	Minimizes systemic opioid use Increased patient satisfaction	Procedural risks Potential for cardiac and CNS toxicity with large volumes of local anesthetics	Requires technical proficiency and nursing support for successful implementation
Nonpharmacologic interventions (physical therapy, massage, alternating heat/cold, TENS, acupuncture)	Adjuvant	May stimulate release of endogenous opioids, allowing dose reduction in opioid medications	Modality- and patient-specific	

COX, cyclooxygenase; NSAID, nonsteroidal anti-inflammatory drug; TENS, transcutaneous electrical nerve stimulation.

agents, because neither impairs cognitive function. Given the adverse gastrointestinal and renal effects of NSAIDs and the recent association between COX-2 inhibitors and cardiovascular events,[354] *acetaminophen* is probably the agent of choice for the treatment of mild to moderate pain in older patients without hepatic impairment. *Opioids* are effective for the treatment of moderate to severe pain and should not be withheld from patients for whom non-opioid medications have proven to be ineffective. However, opioid side effect profiles are particularly troubling in this population. These side effects include cognitive effects, sedation, respiratory depression, constipation, urinary retention, and nausea/vomiting. Fortunately, tolerance to most of these symptoms (except constipation) generally develops over time. Because of these effects, as well as slowed drug metabolism, one should start opioid therapy with a low dose of a short-acting agent and titrate upward while monitoring for side effects. This allows for prompt adjustment of therapy in case undesirable effects are noted. Of note, *meperidine* should be avoided in the older population because of an unacceptable side effect profile that includes an increased risk of sedation and falls. Once an adequate therapeutic dose is established for an agent with acceptable side effects, the opioid can be converted to a regularly scheduled longer-acting preparation. A stool softener or promotility agent should also be prescribed when initiating opioid therapy. Attention should be given to simplifying the dosing regimen whenever possible by favoring drugs with once- or twice-daily dosing intervals.

Measures to decrease the use of opioids, such as adding adjuvant non-opioid medications and using regional nerve block techniques with local anesthetic drugs for postoperative pain control, should be employed whenever practical. Nonpharmacologic interventions such as physical therapy, massage, alternating heat and cold compresses, transcutaneous electrical nerve stimulation, and acupuncture may also be beneficial by stimulating the release of endogenous opioids.[355] Furthermore, the use of cognitive-behavioral approaches may improve patients' coping strategies thus further reducing the use of opioid medications.[356]

Opioid-Tolerant Patients

Patients with opioid tolerance pose unique challenges with respect to acute pain management. These include patients who use opioids legitimately for the treatment of chronic pain problems, those who illicitly obtain opioid medications, as well as those who abuse heroin. The opioid-tolerant patient will be encountered in the acute pain setting as a result of routine operative care as well as following trauma. There is a high incidence of drug use among trauma victims with studies showing that as many as 50% of all trauma victims test positive for drugs other than alcohol.[357,358] Opiates are one of the most common drug classes detected, with an incidence of 10% to 24%, ranking second only to marijuana.[357-360] Furthermore, opiates have been independently associated with nonviolent injuries and burns.[361] There are data to suggest that patients with substance use disorders are more likely to have chronic pain conditions, further complicating acute pain management.[362,363] Even though there are concerns regarding physicians contributing to patients' opioid addiction, physical dependence, increased tolerance, and opportunities for drug diversion, the overriding treatment principle remains to provide adequate analgesia. This is obviously important for patient's rights, as well as from an ethical perspective. However, appropriate opioid analgesic treatments are also important, because undertreated pain can lead to drug-seeking behavior known as *pseudoaddiction*.[364] Undertreatment of pain in such patients can result in the loss of trust between patient and caregivers, impeding adequate pain therapy.

The attainment of adequate analgesia can be more difficult in opioid-dependent patients, because they are likely to demonstrate cross-tolerance to all opioids. They will sometimes require substantially higher doses to achieve adequate analgesia, when compared with patients not dependent on opioids. The exact degree of tolerance is difficult to predict in advance, and is dependent on multiple patient factors. In addition, patients who abuse opiates are not typically forthcoming about the magnitude of their opioid use history. It is generally recommended that any long-acting opioid therapy such as methadone or transdermal fentanyl (that the patient had been on before the trauma or preoperatively) be continued after the event, or resumed as soon as possible. In patients who are unable to take oral medications, this will necessitate having to convert oral medications to parenteral dosing either in the form of transdermal patches, scheduled nurse-administered IV or IM doses, or a baseline continuous IV infusion. When converting from oral to parenteral dosing, the dose is usually decreased because parenteral administration bypasses gastrointestinal absorption variables and first-pass hepatic effects.[365,366] Caution is needed to avoid placing a patient on a continuous therapy that causes excessive CNS and respiratory depression. Frequent assessment of the patient is recommended, especially during the early phase of therapy before a stable dose has been reached. In alert patients, IV PCA is a very useful tool to help the physician safely determine the dose of opioids required to adequately treat pain. One can see how much a patient has used via the PCA in the first 24 hours, and can subsequently convert a portion of that dose to continuous therapy in the form of a baseline infusion. This calculation is often necessary in patients who require frequent dosing via the PCA to maintain an adequate level of analgesia. These patients are at risk for having their opioid blood concentration drop below their therapeutic level when they fall asleep and they may not be able to catch up given the dosing parameters programmed into the PCA pump. Another alternative to continuous baseline infusion in this setting is to allow for a larger nurse-administered bolus that the patient can request in the event that the patient has "fallen behind" in self-administration.

A treatment involving multimodal analgesia can be used to decrease the total amount of opioid medication that is administered. The use of non-opioid analgesics, including *acetaminophen* and *NSAIDs,* can help to decrease the pain from inflammation and subsequently the use of opioids. *Ketorolac* is particularly useful because it is available in IV form, and has been shown to decrease the morphine use and morphine-related side effects.[367] The use of ketorolac must be weighed against an increased risk for bleeding and potential impairment of bone fracture healing, especially in the early postoperative period.[368,369] NMDA receptor antagonists such as *ketamine* potentiate the analgesic effects of opioids and may decrease opioid tolerance.[370-373]

In addition to providing a more stable level of analgesia and better control of background pain, long-acting opioids and continuous IV infusions have the benefit of decreasing the required dose of short- and intermediate-acting opioids that have a higher abuse potential. The use of opioid agonist/antagonists such as *buprenorphine* and *nalbuphine* should be avoided as it may potentiate acute opioid withdrawal reactions.[374,375]

Other ways to decrease the amount of overall opioid use is through the use of single shot and continuous *regional nerve blocks* and *neuraxial techniques* such as spinal and epidural infusions. Opioids can be added to both single and continuous neuraxial blocks, and will further decrease the requirements for short- and intermediate-acting opioids. The additive effects and differing pharmacokinetics of opioids administered via different routes must be considered carefully. One common example is the delayed onset of respiratory depression caused by intrathecal and epidural morphine administration.[376,377] In most cases, opioids should logically be administered via the neuraxial route or intravenously, but not both. Finally, another way to decrease the use of opioids is the infiltration of surgical wounds with long-acting local anesthetics.

Obesity and Obstructive Sleep Apnea

The interaction of obstructive sleep apnea and postoperative analgesia has been termed a "potentially dangerous combination."[378] Physiologic and airway management issues have been reviewed recently,[379] although this review does not address postoperative pain management. Primary principles of pain management include the preferential avoidance of sedating medications, meaning that systemic opioids should not be used as a first choice. Neuraxial opioids may seem to be an attractive first choice in analgesia, when compared with systemic opioids,[380] but in these high-risk patients, neuraxial opioids can prolong the need for critical care management including intubation and mechanical ventilation.[381] Therefore, regional analgesics consisting of local anesthetics may be preferable to any opioid use.[381,382] There are

no reports of whether low doses of circulating local anesthetics (delivered via incisional, perineural, or neuraxial techniques) may inhibit respiratory drive in these patients. However, IV lidocaine has been shown to depress the ventilatory response to hypoxia in healthy subjects.[383]

In the setting of patients who are overweight (body mass index of 25 to 30 kg/m^2), or obese (body mass index of 30 kg/m^2 or higher), PNBs may be critical components in providing postoperative pain relief. This concept was reviewed by Nielsen and colleagues, who prospectively collected observational data on almost 7000 patients receiving 9000 nerve blocks.[111] This report indicated that block failure rate was higher in obese patients (1.62 times more likely, P = 0.04), and that the unadjusted rate of acute complications was higher in obese patients (P = 0.001). However, when compared with patients with a normal BMI, postoperative pain at rest, unanticipated hospital admissions, and overall satisfaction were similar in overweight and obese patients.[111] Therefore nerve blocks in overweight and obese patients will likely be more technically complicated with a higher risk of block failure, but PNBs (in the hands of experienced practitioners) are the logical first choice of analgesic technique, pending further study. Additional study is needed to determine potential risks of inhibited hypoxic ventilatory drive when PNB single-injections and continuous infusions are used in patients with sleep apnea.

SUMMARY

- Postoperative pain continues to be a public health problem.
- Systemic opioids have been the traditional foundation for the treatment of acute and postoperative pain.
- Systemic non-opioid analgesics now have a sufficient body of evidence to assume a primary role in attenuating moderate-to-excruciating acute and postoperative pain, and should likely be coadministered with opioids.
- All systemic analgesics have analgesic ceilings, which are modulated by pharmacologic factors, side effects, or both.
- Although neuraxial analgesia has established an important role in acute and postoperative analgesia, the incompatibility of these techniques with modern anticoagulation methods may significantly restrict their use.
- Peripheral analgesia, including subcutaneous local anesthetics, PNBs, and intra-articular techniques, when applicable, are gradually emerging as the new gold standard for analgesia. However, this new standard is limited by variability in the skills and experiences of practitioners that may have not received formal training in these techniques.
- All peripheral analgesic techniques have potential risks and complications, some of which remain independent of the skills and experience of the practitioner.
- Analgesic needs warrant special considerations for patients having undergone trauma or burn injury, or in patients who are older, obese, or opioid tolerant.

References

1. Stein C: The control of pain in peripheral tissue by opioids. N Engl J Med 1995;332:1685-1690.
2. Borgland SL: Acute opioid receptor desensitization and tolerance: Is there a link? Clin Exp Pharmacol Physiol 2001;28:147-54.
3. Zhao SZ, Chung F, Hanna DB, et al: Dose-response relationship between opioid use and adverse effects after ambulatory surgery. J Pain Symptom Manage 2004;28:35-46.
4. von Zastrow M: Opioid receptor regulation. Neuromolecular Med 2004;5:51-58.
5. Taylor DA, Fleming WW: Unifying perspectives of the mechanisms underlying the development of tolerance and physical dependence to opioids. J Pharmacol Exp Ther 2001;297:11-18.
6. Macintyre PE: Safety and efficacy of patient-controlled analgesia. Br J Anaesth 2001;87:36-46.
7. Wakerlin G, Larson CP Jr: Spouse-controlled analgesia. Anesth Analg 1990;70:119.
8. Camu F, Van Aken H, Bovill JG: Postoperative analgesic effects of three demand-dose sizes of fentanyl administered by patient-controlled analgesia. Anesth Analg 1998;87:890-895.
9. Ginsberg B, Gil KM, Muir M, et al: The influence of lockout intervals and drug selection on patient-controlled analgesia following gynecological surgery. Pain 1995;62:95-100.
10. Smythe MA, Zak MB, O'Donnell MP, et al: Patient-controlled analgesia versus patient-controlled analgesia plus continuous infusion after hip replacement surgery. Ann Pharmacother 1996;30:224-227.
11. Looi-Lyons LC, Chung FF, Chan VW, et al: Respiratory depression: An adverse outcome during patient controlled analgesia therapy. J Clin Anesth 1996;8:151-156.
12. Parker RK, Holtmann B, White PF: Patient-controlled analgesia. Does a concurrent opioid infusion improve pain management after surgery? JAMA 1991;266:1947-1952.
13. Parker RK, Holtmann B, White PF: Effects of a nighttime opioid infusion with PCA therapy on patient comfort and analgesic requirements after abdominal hysterectomy. Anesthesiology 1992;76:362-367.
14. Walder B, Schafer M, Henzi I, et al: Efficacy and safety of patient-controlled opioid analgesia for acute postoperative pain: A quantitative systematic review. Acta Anaesth Scand 2001;45:795-804.
15. Ballantyne JC, Carr DB, Chalmers TC, et al: Postoperative patient-controlled analgesia: Meta-analyses of initial randomized control trials. J Clin Anesth 1993;5:182-193.
16. Chumbley GM, Hall GM, Salmon P: Why do patients feel positive about patient-controlled analgesia? Anaesthesia 1999;54:386-389.
17. Etches RC: Respiratory depression associated with patient-controlled analgesia: A review of eight cases. Can J Anaesth 1994;41:125-132.
18. Sidebotham D, Dijkhuizen MR, Schug SA: The safety and utilization of patient-controlled analgesia. J Pain Symptom Manage 1997;14:202-209.
19. Viscusi ER, Reynolds L, Chung F, et al: Patient-controlled transdermal fentanyl hydrochloride vs intravenous morphine pump for postoperative pain: A randomized controlled trial. JAMA 2004;291:1333-1341.
20. Viscusi ER, Witkowski TA: Iontophoresis: The process behind noninvasive drug delivery. Reg Anesth Pain Med 2005;30:292-294.
21. Sinatra R. The fentanyl HCl patient-controlled transdermal system (PCTS): An alternative to intravenous patient-controlled analgesia in the postoperative setting. Clin Pharmacokinet 2005;1:1-6.
22. Viscusi ER, Reynolds L, Tait S, et al: An iontophoretic fentanyl patient-activated analgesic delivery system for postoperative pain: A double-blind, placebo-controlled trial. Anesth Analg 2006;102:188-194.
23. Chelly JE, Grass J, Houseman TW, et al: The safety and efficacy of a fentanyl patient-controlled transdermal system for acute postoperative analgesia: A multicenter, placebo-controlled trial. Anesth Analg 2004;98:427-433.
24. Grond S, Sablotzki A. Clinical pharmacology of tramadol. Clin Pharmacokinet 2004;43:879-923.
25. Pang WW, Huang PY, Chang DP, et al: The peripheral analgesic effect of tramadol in reducing propofol injection pain: A comparison with lidocaine. Reg Anesth Pain Med 1999;24:246-249.
26. Scott LJ, Perry CM: Tramadol: A review of its use in perioperative pain. Drugs 2000;60:139-176.
27. Edwards JE, McQuay HJ, Moore RA: Combination analgesic efficacy: Individual patient data meta-analysis of single-dose oral tramadol plus acetaminophen in acute postoperative pain. J Pain Symptom Manage 2002;23:121-130.
28. Budd K, Langford R: Tramadol revisited. Br J Anaesth 1999;82:493-495.
29. Marret E, Kurdi O, Zufferey P, et al: Effects of nonsteroidal antiinflammatory drugs on patient-controlled analgesia morphine side effects: Meta-analysis of randomized controlled trials. Anesthesiology 2005;102:1249-1260.
30. Remy C, Marret E, Bonnet F: Effects of acetaminophen on morphine side-effects and consumption after major surgery: Meta-analysis of randomized controlled trials. Br J Anaesth 2005;94:505-513.
31. Elia N, Lysakowski C, Tramer MR: Does multimodal analgesia with acetaminophen, nonsteroidal antiinflammatory drugs, or selective cyclooxygenase-2 inhibitors and patient-controlled analgesia morphine offer advantages over morphine alone? Meta-analyses of randomized trials. Anesthesiology 2005;103:1296-304.
32. Straube S, Derry S, McQuay HJ, et al: Effect of preoperative COX-II-selective NSAIDs (coxibs) on postoperative outcomes: A systematic review of randomized studies. Acta Anaesthesiolog Scand 2005;49:601-613.
33. Kranke P, Morin AM, Roewer N, et al: Patients' global evaluation of analgesia and safety of injected parecoxib for postoperative pain: A quantitative systematic review. Anesth Analg 2004;99:797-806.
34. Vanegas H, Schaible HG: Prostaglandins and cyclooxygenases in the spinal cord. Prog Neurobiol 2001;64:327-363.
35. Howard PA, Delafontaine P: Nonsteroidal anti-inflammatory drugs and cardiovascular risk. J Am Coll Cardiol 2004;43:519-525.
36. FitzGerald GA: Cardiovascular pharmacology of nonselective nonsteroidal anti-inflammatory drugs and coxibs: Clinical considerations. Am J Cardiol 2002;89:21.
37. Schafer AI: Effects of nonsteroidal anti-inflammatory therapy on platelets. Am J Med 1999;106:31.
38. Souter AJ, Fredman B, White PF: Controversies in the perioperative use of nonsteroidal antiinflammatory drugs. Anesth Analg 1994;79:1178-1190.
39. Strom BL, Berlin JA, Kinman JL, et al: Parenteral ketorolac and risk of gastrointestinal and operative site bleeding. A postmarketing surveillance study. JAMA 1996;275:376-382.
40. Whelton A: Nephrotoxicity of nonsteroidal anti-inflammatory drugs: Physiologic foundations and clinical implications. Am J Med 1999;106:31.
41. Lee A, Cooper MG, Craig JC, et al: The effects of nonsteroidal anti-inflammatory drugs (NSAIDs) on postoperative renal function: A meta-analysis. Anaesth Intensive Care 1999;27:574-580.
42. Maxy RJ, Glassman SD: The effect of nonsteroidal anti-inflammatory drugs on osteogenesis and spinal fusion. Reg Anesth Pain Med 2001;26:156-158.
43. Laine L: Gastrointestinal safety of coxibs and outcomes studies: What's the verdict? J Pain Symptom Manage 2002;23(4S):S5-S10.
44. Leese PT, Hubbard RC, Karim A, et al: Effects of celecoxib, a novel cyclooxygenase-2 inhibitor, on platelet function in healthy adults: A randomized, controlled trial. J Clin Pharmacol 2000;40:124-132.
45. Juni P, Nartey L, Reichenbach S, et al: Risk of cardiovascular events and rofecoxib: Cumulative meta-analysis. Lancet 2004;364:2021-2029.

46. Solomon SD, McMurray JJ, Pfeffer MA, et al: Cardiovascular risk associated with celecoxib in a clinical trial for colorectal adenoma prevention. N Engl J Med 2005;352:1071-1080.

47. Okie S: Raising the safety bar—The FDA's coxib meeting. N Engl J Med 2005;352:1283-1285.

48. Wright JM: The double-edged sword of COX-2 selective NSAIDs. Can Med Assoc J 2002;167:1131-1137.

49. Schmid RL, Sandler AN, Katz J: Use and efficacy of low-dose ketamine in the management of acute postoperative pain: A review of current techniques and outcomes. Pain 1999;82: 111-125.

50. Tverskoy M, Oren M, Vaskovich M, et al: Ketamine enhances local anesthetic and analgesic effects of bupivacaine by peripheral mechanism: A study in postoperative patients. Neurosci Lett 1996;215:5-8.

51. Suzuki M, Tsueda K, Lansing PS, et al: Small-dose ketamine enhances morphine-induced analgesia after outpatient surgery. Anesth Analg 1999;89:98-103.

52. Menigaux C, Guignard B, Fletcher D, et al: Intraoperative small-dose ketamine enhances analgesia after outpatient knee arthroscopy. Anesth Analg 2001;93:606-612.

53. Elia N, Tramer MR: Ketamine and postoperative pain—A quantitative systematic review of randomised trials. Pain 2005;113:61-70.

54. Subramaniam K, Subramaniam B, Steinbrook RA: Ketamine as adjuvant analgesic to opioids: A quantitative and qualitative systematic review. Anesth Analg 2004;99:482-495.

55. Krystal JH, Karper LP, Bennett A, et al: Interactive effects of subanesthetic ketamine and subhypnotic lorazepam in humans. Psychopharmacology 1998;135:213-229.

56. Sethna NF, Liu M, Gracely R, et al: Analgesic and cognitive effects of intravenous ketamine-alfentanil combinations versus either drug alone after intradermal capsaicin in normal subjects. Anesth Analg 1998;86:1250-1256.

57. Wong CS, Liaw WJ, Tung CS, et al: Ketamine potentiates analgesic effect of morphine in postoperative epidural pain control. Reg Anesth 1996;21:534-541.

58. Hawksworth C, Serpell M: Intrathecal anesthesia with ketamine. Reg Anesth Pain Med 1998;23:283-288.

59. Himmelseher S, Durieux ME: Ketamine for perioperative pain management. Anesthesiology 2005;102:211-220.

60. Dahl JB, Mathiesen O, Møiniche S: "Protective premedication": An option with gabapentin and related drugs? A review of gabapentin and pregabalin in the treatment of postoperative pain. Acta Anaesthesiol Scand 2004;48:1130-1136.

61. White PF: The changing role of non-opioid analgesic techniques in the management of postoperative pain. Anesth Analg 2005;101:S5-S22.

62. Menigaux C, Adam F, Guignard B, et al: Preoperative gabapentin decreases anxiety and improves early functional recovery from knee surgery. Anesth Analg 2005;100:1394-1399.

63. Fassoulaki A, Patris K, Sarantopoulos C, et al: The analgesic effect of gabapentin and mexiletine after breast surgery for cancer. Anesth Analg 2002;95:985-991.

64. Dirks J, Fredensborg BB, Christensen D, et al: A randomized study of the effects of single-dose gabapentin versus placebo on postoperative pain and morphine consumption after mastectomy. Anesthesiology 2002;97:560-564.

65. Turan A, Kaya G, Karamanlioglu B, et al: Effect of oral gabapentin on postoperative epidural analgesia. Br J Anaesth 2005;16:16.

66. Rorarius MG, Mennander S, Suominen P, et al: Gabapentin for the prevention of postoperative pain after vaginal hysterectomy. Pain 2004;110:175-181.

67. Fassoulaki A, Stamatakis E, Petropoulos G, et al: Gabapentin attenuates late but not acute pain after abdominal hysterectomy. Eur J Anaesthesiol 2006;23:136-141.

68. Hill CM, Balkenohl M, Thomas DW, et al: Pregabalin in patients with postoperative dental pain. Eur J Pain. 2001;5:119-124.

69. Cooper DW: Can epidural fentanyl induce selective spinal hyperalgesia? Anesthesiology 2000;93:1153-1154.

70. Bernards CM: Rostral spread of epidural morphine: The expected and the unexpected. Anesthesiology 2000;92:299-301.

71. Ready LB, Chadwick HS, Ross B: Age predicts effective epidural morphine dose after abdominal hysterectomy. Anesth Analg 1987;66:1215-1218.

72. Liu SS, McDonald SB: Current issues in spinal anesthesia. Anesthesiology 2001;94:888-906.

73. Gwirtz KH, Young JV, Byers RS, et al: The safety and efficacy of intrathecal opioid analgesia for acute postoperative pain: Seven years' experience with 5969 surgical patients at Indiana University Hospital. Anesth Analg 1999;88:599-604.

74. Block BM, Liu SS, Rowlingson AJ, et al: Efficacy of postoperative epidural analgesia: A meta-analysis. JAMA 2003;290: 2455-2463.

75. Viscusi ER, Martin G, Hartrick CT, et al: Forty-eight hours of postoperative pain relief after total hip arthroplasty with a novel, extended-release epidural morphine formulation. Anesthesiology 2005;102:1014-1022.

76. Carvalho B, Riley E, Cohen SE, et al: Single-dose, sustained-release epidural morphine in the management of postoperative pain after elective cesarean delivery: Results of a multicenter randomized controlled study. Anesth Analg 2005;100:1150-1158.

77. Wheatley RG, Schug SA, Watson D: Safety and efficacy of postoperative epidural analgesia. Br J Anaesth 2001;87:47-61.

78. Wu CL, Cohen SR, Richman JM, et al: Efficacy of postoperative patient-controlled and continuous infusion epidural analgesia versus intravenous patient-controlled analgesia with opioids: A meta-analysis. Anesthesiology 2005;103: 1079-1088.

79. Kopacz DJ, Sharrock NE, Allen HW: A comparison of levobupivacaine 0.125%, fentanyl 4 microg/mL, or their combination for patient-controlled epidural analgesia after major orthopedic surgery. Anesth Analg 1999;89:1497-1503.

80. Zaric D, Nydahl PA, Philipson L, et al: The effect of continuous lumbar epidural infusion of ropivacaine (0.1%, 0.2%, and 0.3%) and 0.25% bupivacaine on sensory and motor block in volunteers: A double-blind study. Reg Anesth 1996;21:14-25.

81. de Leon-Casasola OA, Lema MJ: Postoperative epidural opioid analgesia: What are the choices? Anesth Analg 1996;83:867-875.

82. Curatolo M, Schnider TW, Petersen-Felix S, et al: A direct search procedure to optimize combinations of epidural bupivacaine, fentanyl, and clonidine for postoperative analgesia. Anesthesiology 2000;92:325-337.

83. Paech MJ, Pavy TJ, Orlikowski CE, et al: Postoperative epidural infusion: A randomized, double-blind, dose-finding trial of clonidine in combination with bupivacaine and fentanyl. Anesth Analg 1997;84:1323-1328.

84. Sakaguchi Y, Sakura S, Shinzawa M, et al: Does adrenaline improve epidural bupivacaine and fentanyl analgesia after abdominal surgery? Anaesth Intensive Care 2000;28:522-526.

85. Liu SS, Allen HW, Olsson GL: Patient-controlled epidural analgesia with bupivacaine and fentanyl on hospital wards: Prospective experience with 1,030 surgical patients. Anesthesiology 1998;88:688-695.

86. Wigfull J, Welchew E: Survey of 1057 patients receiving postoperative patient-controlled epidural analgesia. Anaesthesia 2001;56:70-75.

87. Komatsu H, Matsumoto S, Mitsuhata H, et al: Comparison of patient-controlled epidural analgesia with and without background infusion after gastrectomy. Anesth Analg 1998;87: 907-910.

88. Sinclair DR, Chung F, Mezei G: Can postoperative nausea and vomiting be predicted? Anesthesiology 1999;91:109-118.

89. Sneyd JR, Carr A, Byrom WD, et al: A meta-analysis of nausea and vomiting following maintenance of anaesthesia with propofol or inhalational agents. Eur J Anaesthesiol 1998;15: 433-445.

90. Apfel CC, Korttila K, Abdalla M, et al: A factorial trial of six interventions for the prevention of postoperative nausea and vomiting. N Engl J Med 2004;350:2441-2451.

91. Williams BA, Kentor ML, Williams JP, et al: Process analysis in outpatient knee surgery: Effects of regional and general

anesthesia on anesthesia-controlled time. Anesthesiology 2000;93:529-538.

92. Williams BA, Kentor ML, Williams JP, et al: PACU bypass after outpatient knee surgery is associated with fewer unplanned hospital admissions but more phase II nursing interventions. Anesthesiology 2002;97:981-988.

93. Williams BA, Kentor ML, Vogt MT, et al: Femoral-sciatic nerve blocks for complex outpatient knee surgery are associated with less postoperative pain before same-day discharge: A review of 1200 consecutive cases from the period 1996-1999. Anesthesiology 2003;98:1206-1213.

94. Williams BA, Kentor ML, Vogt MT, et al: The economics of nerve block pain management after anterior cruciate ligament reconstruction: Significant hospital cost savings via associated PACU bypass and same-day discharge. Anesthesiology 2004;100:697-706.

95. Kentor ML, Williams BA: Antiemetics in outpatient regional anesthesia for invasive orthopedic surgery. Int Anesth Clin 2005;43:197-205.

96. Williams BA: Potential economic benefits of regional anesthesia for acute pain management: The need to study both inputs and outcomes. Reg Anesth Pain Med 2006;31:95-99.

97. Wilder-Smith OHG, Arendt-Nielsen L: Postoperative hyperalgesia: Its clinical importance and relevance. Anesthesiology 2006;104:601-607.

98. Richman JM, Liu SS, Courpas G, et al: Does continuous peripheral nerve block provide superior pain control to opioids? A meta-analysis. Anesth Analg 2006;102:248-57.

99. Ilfeld BM, Morey TE, Enneking FK: New portable infusion pumps: Real advantages or just more of the same in a different package? Reg Anesth Pain Med 2004;29:371-376.

100. Liu SS, Richman JM, Thirlby RC, et al: Efficacy of local anesthetic infusions on postoperative pain: A meta-analysis (abstract). Postgraduate Assembly, New York, December 2005.

101. Hollmann MW, Durieux ME: Local anesthetics and the inflammatory response: A new therapeutic indication? Anesthesiology 2000;93:858-875.

102. Hahnenkamp K, Theilmeier G, Van Aken HK, et al: The effects of local anesthetics on perioperative coagulation, inflammation, and microcirculation. Anesth Analg 2002;94:1441-1447.

103. Koppert W, Weigand M, Neumann F, et al: Perioperative intravenous lidocaine has preventive effects on postoperative pain and morphine consumption after major abdominal surgery. Anesth Analg 2004;98:1050-1055.

104. Bianconi M, Ferraro L, Ricci R, et al: The pharmacokinetics and efficacy of ropivacaine continuous wound instillation after spine fusion surgery. Anesth Analg 2004;98:166-172.

105. Chelly JE, Greger J, Al Samsam T, et al: Reduction of operating and recovery room times and overnight hospital stays with interscalene blocks as sole anesthetic technique for rotator cuff surgery. Minerva Anesth 2001;67:613-619.

106. Williams BA: For outpatients, does regional anesthesia truly shorten the hospital stay, and how should we define postanesthesia care unit bypass eligibility? Anesthesiology 2004;101:3-6.

107. Hadzic A, Williams BA, Karaca PE, et al: For outpatient rotator cuff surgery, nerve block anesthesia provides superior same-day recovery over general anesthesia. Anesthesiology 2005;102:1001-1007.

108. Chelly JE, Greger J, Gebhard R, et al: Continuous femoral blocks improve recovery and outcome of patients undergoing total knee arthroplasty. J Arthroplasty 2001;16:436-446.

109. Song D, Chung F, Ronayne M, et al: Fast-tracking (bypassing the PACU) does not reduce nursing workload after ambulatory surgery. Br J Anaesth 2004;93:768-774.

110. Klein SM, Nielsen KC, Greengrass RA, et al: Ambulatory discharge after long-acting peripheral nerve blockade: 2382 blocks with ropivacaine. Anesth Analg 2001;94:65-70.

111. Nielsen KC, Guller U, Steele SM, et al: Influence of obesity on surgical regional anesthesia in the ambulatory setting: An analysis of 9,038 blocks. Anesthesiology 2005;102:181-187.

112. Capdevila X, Pirat P, Bringuier S, et al: Continuous peripheral nerve blocks in hospital wards after orthopedic surgery: A multicenter prospective analysis of the quality of postoperative analgesia and complications in 1,416 patients. Anesthesiology 2005;103:1035-1045.

113. Auroy Y, Benhamou D, Bargues L, et al: Major complications of regional anesthesia in France: The SOS Regional Anesthesia Hotline Service. Anesthesiology 2002;97:1274-1280.

114. Ilfeld BM, Enneking FK: Continuous peripheral nerve blocks at home: A review. Anesth Analg 2005;100:1822-1833.

115. Klein SM, Evans H, Nielsen KC, et al: Peripheral nerve block techniques for ambulatory surgery. Anesth Analg 2005;101:1663-1676.

116. Liu SS, Strodtbeck WM, Richman JM, et al: A comparison of regional versus general anesthesia for ambulatory anesthesia: A meta-analysis of randomized controlled trials. Anesth Analg 2005;101:1634-1642.

117. Hadzic A: Is regional anesthesia really better than general anesthesia? Anesth Analg 2005;101:1631-1633.

118. Klein SM. Continuous peripheral nerve blocks: Fewer excuses. Anesthesiology 2005;103:921-923.

119. Williams BA, Kentor ML, Vogt MT, et al: Reduction of verbal pain scores after anterior cruciate ligament reconstruction with two-day continuous femoral nerve block: A randomized clinical trial. Anesthesiology 2006;104:315-327.

120. Singelyn FJ: Single-injection applications for foot and ankle surgery. Best Pract Res Clin Anaesth 2002;16:247-254.

121. Kim DD, Shuman C, Sadr B: Intravenous regional anesthesia for outpatient foot and ankle surgery: A prospective study. Orthopedics 1993;16:1109-1113.

122. Al-Metwalli R, Mowafi HA: A modification of the inter-cuff technique of IVRA for use in knee arthroscopy. Can J Anaesth 2002;49:687-689.

123. Hannington-Kiff JG: Bier's block revisited: Intercuff block. J R Soc Med 1990;83:155-158.

124. Choyce A, Peng P: A systematic review of adjuncts for intravenous regional anesthesia for surgical procedures. Can J Anaesth 2002;49:32-45.

125. Turan A, Karamanlyoglu B, Memis D, et al: Intravenous regional anesthesia using prilocaine and neostigmine. Anesth Analg 2002;95:1419-1422.

126. McCartney CJ, Brill S, Rawson R, et al: No anesthetic or analgesic benefit of neostigmine 1 mg added to intravenous regional anesthesia with lidocaine 0.5% for hand surgery. Reg Anesth Pain Med 2003;28:414-417.

127. Alayurt S, Memis D, Pamukcu Z: The addition of sufentanil, tramadol or clonidine to lignocaine for intravenous regional anaesthesia. Anaesth Intensive Care 2004;32:22-27.

128. Sakirgil E, Gunes Y, Ozbek H, et al: Comparison of ropivacaine, ropivacaine plus tramadol and ropivacaine plus morphine in patients undergoing minor hand surgery. Agri Dergisi 2005;17:52-58.

129. Reuben SS, Steinberg RB, Kreitzer JM, et al: Intravenous regional anesthesia using lidocaine and ketorolac. Anesth Analg 1995;81:110-113.

130. Reuben SS, Steinberg RB, Maciolek H, et al: An evaluation of the analgesic efficacy of intravenous regional anesthesia with lidocaine and ketorolac using a forearm versus upper arm tourniquet. Anesth Analg 2002;95:457-460.

131. Memis D, Turan A, Karamanlioglu B, et al: Adding dexmedetomidine to lidocaine for intravenous regional anesthesia. Anesth Analg 2004;98:835-840.

132. Gorgias NK, Maidatsi PG, Kyriakidis AM, et al: Clonidine versus ketamine to prevent tourniquet pain during intravenous regional anesthesia with lidocaine. Reg Anesth Pain Med 2001;26:512-517.

133. Bigat Z, Boztug N, Hadimioglu N, et al: Does dexamethasone improve the quality of intravenous regional anesthesia and analgesia? A randomized, controlled clinical study. Anesth Analg 2006;102:605-609.

134. Atanassoff PG, Ocampo CA, Bande MC, et al: Ropivacaine 0.2% and lidocaine 0.5% for intravenous regional anesthesia in outpatient surgery. Anesthesiology 2001;95:627-631.

135. Brown AR, Weiss R, Greenberg C, et al: Interscalene block for shoulder arthroscopy: Comparison with general anesthesia. Arthroscopy 1993;9:295-300.

136. Al-Kaisy A, McGuire G, Chan VW, et al: Analgesic effect of interscalene block using low-dose bupivacaine for outpatient arthroscopic shoulder surgery. Reg Anesth Pain Med 1998; 23:469-473.

137. Kinnard P, Truchon R, St-Pierre A, et al: Interscalene block for pain relief after shoulder surgery: A prospective randomized study. Clin Orthop 1994;304:22-24.

138. Arciero RA, Taylor DC, Harrison SA, Snyder et al: Interscalene anesthesia for shoulder arthroscopy in a community-sized military hospital. Arthroscopy 1996;12:715-719.

139. Klein SM, Grant SA, Greengrass RA, et al: Interscalene brachial plexus block with a continuous catheter insertion system and a disposable infusion pump. Anesth Analg 2000; 91:1473-1478.

140. Borgeat A, Schappi B, Biasca N, et al: Patient-controlled analgesia after major shoulder surgery: Patient-controlled interscalene analgesia versus patient-controlled analgesia. Anesthesiology 1997;87:1343-1347.

141. Borgeat A, Tewes E, Biasca N, et al: Patient-controlled interscalene analgesia with ropivacaine after major shoulder surgery: PCIA vs PCA. Br J Anaesth 1998;81:603-605.

142. Borgeat A, Ekatodramis G, Kalberer F, et al: Acute and non-acute complications associated with interscalene block and shoulder surgery: A prospective study. Anesthesiology 2001; 95:875-880.

143. Ilfeld BM, Morey TE, Wright TW, et al: Continuous interscalene brachial plexus block for postoperative pain control at home: A randomized, double-blinded, placebo-controlled study. Anesth Analg 2003;96:1089-1095.

144. Ilfeld BM, Morey TE, Wright TW, et al: Interscalene perineural ropivacaine infusion: A comparison of two dosing regimens for postoperative analgesia. Reg Anesth Pain Med 2004;29:9-16.

145. Singelyn FJ, Seguy S, Gouverneur JM: Interscalene brachial plexus analgesia after open shoulder surgery: Continuous versus patient-controlled infusion. Anesth Analg 1999;89: 1216-1220.

146. Chelly JE, Ben-David B, Williams BA, et al: Anesthesia and postoperative analgesia: Outcomes following orthopedic surgery. Orthopedics 2003;26:s865-s871.

147. Urmey WF, Gloeggler PJ: Pulmonary function changes during interscalene brachial plexus block: Effects of decreasing local anesthetic injection volume. Reg Anesth. 1993;18:244-249.

148. Urmey WF, McDonald M: Hemidiaphragmatic paresis during interscalene brachial plexus block: Effects on pulmonary function and chest wall mechanics. Anesth Analg 1992;74: 352-357.

149. Urmey WF, Talts KH, Sharrock NE: One hundred percent incidence of hemidiaphragmatic paresis associated with interscalene brachial plexus anesthesia as diagnosed by ultrasonography. Anesth Analg 1991;72:498-503.

150. Borgeat A, Perschak H, Bird P, et al: Patient-controlled interscalene analgesia with ropivacaine 0.2% versus patient-controlled intravenous analgesia after major shoulder surgery: Effects on diaphragmatic and respiratory function. Anesthesiology. 2000;92:102-108.

151. Franco CD, Vieira ZE: 1,001 subclavian perivascular brachial plexus blocks: Success with a nerve stimulator. Reg Anesth Pain Med 2000;25:41-46.

152. Ilfeld BM, Morey TE, Enneking FK: Continuous infraclavicular brachial plexus block for postoperative pain control at home: A randomized, double-blinded, placebo-controlled study. Anesthesiology 2002;96:1297-1304.

153. Hadzic A, Arliss J, Kerimoglu B, et al: A comparison of infraclavicular nerve block versus general anesthesia for hand and wrist surgery in day-case surgery. Anesthesiology 2004;101: 127-132.

154. Desroches J: The infraclavicular brachial plexus block by the coracoid approach is clinically effective: An observational study of 150 patients. Can J Anaesth 2003;50:253-257.

155. Hadzic A, Vloka JD, Kuroda MM, et al: The practice of peripheral nerve blocks in the United States: A national survey. Reg Anesth Pain Med 1998;23:241-246.

156. Klein SM, Pietrobon R, Nielsen KC, et al: Peripheral nerve blockade with long-acting local anesthetics: A survey of the Society for Ambulatory Anesthesia. Anesth Analg 2002;94: 71-76.

157. Chan VW, Peng PW, Kaszas Z, et al: A comparative study of general anesthesia, intravenous regional anesthesia, and axillary block for outpatient hand surgery: Clinical outcome and cost analysis. Anesth Analg 2001;93:1181-1184.

158. McCartney CJ, Brull R, Chan VW, et al: Early but no long-term benefit of regional compared with general anesthesia for ambulatory hand surgery. Anesthesiology 2004;101:461-467.

159. Koscielniak-Nielsen ZJ, Hesselbjerg L, Fejlberg V: Comparison of transarterial and multiple nerve stimulation techniques for an initial axillary block by 45 mL of mepivacaine 1% with adrenaline. Acta Anaesthesiol Scand 1998;42:570-575.

160. Koscielniak-Nielsen ZJ, Stens-Pedersen HL, Lippert FK: Readiness for surgery after axillary block: Single or multiple injection techniques. Eur J Anaesthesiol 1997;14:164-71.

161. Coventry DM, Barker KF, Thomson M: Comparison of two neurostimulation techniques for axillary brachial plexus blockade. Br J Anaesth 2001;86:80-83.

162. Mezzatesta JP, Scott DA, Schweitzer SA, et al: Continuous axillary brachial plexus block for postoperative pain relief. Intermittent bolus versus continuous infusion. Reg Anesth 1997;22:357-362.

163. Bergman BD, Hebl JR, Kent J, et al: Neurologic complications of 405 consecutive continuous axillary catheters. Anesth Analg 2003;96:247-252.

164. Rawal N, Allvin R, Axelsson K, et al: Patient-controlled regional analgesia (PCRA) at home: Controlled comparison between bupivacaine and ropivacaine brachial plexus analgesia. Anesthesiology 2002;96:1290-1296.

165. Singelyn FJ, Lhotel L, Fabre B: Pain relief after arthroscopic shoulder surgery: A comparison of intraarticular analgesia, suprascapular nerve block, and interscalene brachial plexus block. Anesth Analg 2004;99:589-592.

166. Laurila PA, Lopponen A, Kanga-Saarela T, et al: Interscalene brachial plexus block is superior to subacromial bursa block after arthroscopic shoulder surgery. Acta Anaesthesiol Scand 2002;46:1031-1036.

167. Turker G, Uckunkaya N, Yavascaoglu B, et al: Comparison of the catheter-technique psoas compartment block and the epidural block for analgesia in partial hip replacement surgery. Acta Anaesthesiol Scand 2003;47:30-36.

168. Stevens RD, Van Gessel E, Flory N, et al: Lumbar plexus block reduces pain and blood loss associated with total hip arthroplasty. Anesthesiology 2000;93:115-121.

169. Naja Z, el Hassan MJ, Khatib H, et al: Combined sciatic-paravertebral nerve block vs. general anaesthesia for fractured hip of the elderly. Mid East J Anesth 2000;15:559-568.

170. Matheny JM, Hanks GA, Rung GW, et al: A comparison of patient-controlled analgesia and continuous lumbar plexus block after anterior cruciate ligament reconstruction. Arthroscopy 1993;9:87-90.

171. Luber MJ, Greengrass R, Vail TP: Patient satisfaction and effectiveness of lumbar plexus and sciatic nerve block for total knee arthroplasty. J Arthroplasty 2001;16:17-21.

172. Kaloul I, Guay J, Cote C, Fallaha M: The posterior lumbar plexus (psoas compartment) block and the three-in-one femoral nerve block provide similar postoperative analgesia after total knee replacement. Can J Anaesth 2004;51:45-51.

173. Ben-David B, Schmalenberger K, Chelly JE: Analgesia after total knee arthroplasty: Is continuous sciatic blockade needed in addition to continuous femoral blockade? Anesth Analg 2004;98:747-749.

174. Capdevila X, Barthelet Y, Biboulet P, et al: Effects of perioperative analgesic technique on the surgical outcome and duration of rehabilitation after major knee surgery. Anesthesiology 1999;91:8-15.

175. Singelyn FJ, Deyaert M, Pendeville E, et al: Effects of intravenous patient-controlled analgesia with morphine, continuous epidural analgesia, and continuous three-in-one block on postoperative pain and knee rehabilitation after unilateral total knee arthroplasty. Anesth Analg 1998;87:88-92.

176. di Benedetto P, Casati A, Bertini L: Continuous subgluteus sciatic nerve block after orthopedic foot and ankle surgery:

Comparison of two infusion techniques. Reg Anesth Pain Med 2002;27:168-172.

177. di Benedetto P, Casati A, Bertini L, et al: Postoperative analgesia with continuous sciatic nerve block after foot surgery: A prospective, randomized comparison between the popliteal and subgluteal approaches. Anesth Analg 2002;94:996-1000.

178. Smith BE, Fischer HB, Scott PV: Continuous sciatic nerve block. Anaesthesia 1984;39:155-157.

179. Evans H, Steele SM, Nielsen KC, et al: Peripheral nerve blocks and continuous catheter techniques. Anesthesiol Clin North Am 2005;23:141-162.

180. Williams BA, Spratt D, Kentor ML: Continuous nerve blocks for outpatient knee surgery. Techn Reg Anesth Pain Manage 2004;8:76-84.

181. Henderson RC, Campion ER, DeMasi RA, et al: Postarthroscopy analgesia with bupivacaine. A prospective, randomized, blinded evaluation. Am J Sports Med 1990;18:614-617.

182. Vloka JD, Hadzic A, April E, et al: The division of the sciatic nerve in the popliteal fossa: Anatomical implications for popliteal nerve blockade. Anesth Analg 2001;92:215-217.

183. McLeod DH, Wong DH, Claridge RJ, et al: Lateral popliteal sciatic nerve block compared with subcutaneous infiltration for analgesia following foot surgery. Can J Anaesth 1994;41:673-676.

184. Shah S, Tsai T, Iwata T, et al: Outpatient regional anesthesia for foot and ankle surgery. Int Anesthesiol Clin 2005;43:143-51.

185. McLeod DH, Wong DH, Vaghadia H, et al: Lateral popliteal sciatic nerve block compared with ankle block for analgesia following foot surgery. Can J Anaesth 1995;42:765-769.

186. Provenzano DA, Viscusi ER, Adams SB Jr., et al: Safety and efficacy of the popliteal fossa nerve block when utilized for foot and ankle surgery. Foot Ankle Int 2002;23:394-399.

187. Singelyn FJ, Aye F, Gouverneur JM: Continuous popliteal sciatic nerve block: An original technique to provide postoperative analgesia after foot surgery. Anesth Analg 1997;84:383-386.

188. White PF, Issioui T, Skrivanek GD, et al: The use of a continuous popliteal sciatic nerve block after surgery involving the foot and ankle: Does it improve the quality of recovery? Anesth Analg 2003;97:1303-1309.

189. Ilfeld BM, Morey TE, Wang RD, et al: Continuous popliteal sciatic nerve block for postoperative pain control at home: A randomized, double-blinded, placebo-controlled study. Anesthesiology 2002;97:959-965.

190. Chelly JE, Greger J, Casati A, et al: Continuous lateral sciatic blocks for acute postoperative pain management after major ankle and foot surgery. Foot Ankle Int 2002;23:749-752.

191. Casati A, Fanelli G, Cappelleri G, et al: A clinical comparison of ropivacaine 0.75%, ropivacaine 1% or bupivacaine 0.5% for interscalene brachial plexus anaesthesia. Eur J Anaesthesiol 1999;16:784-789.

192. Casati A, Fanelli G, Albertin A, et al: Interscalene brachial plexus anesthesia with either 0.5% ropivacaine or 0.5% bupivacaine. Minerva Anest 2000;66:39-44.

193. Klein SM, Greengrass RA, Steele SM, et al: A comparison of 0.5% bupivacaine, 0.5% ropivacaine, and 0.75% ropivacaine for interscalene brachial plexus block. Anesth Analg 1998;87:1316-1319.

194. Simpson D, Curran MP, Oldfield V, et al: Ropivacaine: A review of its use in regional anaesthesia and acute pain management. Drugs 2005;65:2675-2717.

195. Candido KD, Franco CD, Khan MA, et al: Buprenorphine added to the local anesthetic for brachial plexus block to provide postoperative analgesia in outpatients. Reg Anesth Pain Med 2001;26:352-356.

196. Candido KD, Winnie AP, Ghaleb AH, et al: Buprenorphine added to the local anesthetic for axillary brachial plexus block prolongs postoperative analgesia. Reg Anesth Pain Med 2002;27:162-167.

197. Casati A, Magistris L, Fanelli G, et al: Small-dose clonidine prolongs postoperative analgesia after sciatic-femoral nerve block with 0.75% ropivacaine for foot surgery. Anesth Analg 2000;91:388-392.

198. Casati A, Magistris L, Beccaria P, et al: Improving postoperative analgesia after axillary brachial plexus anesthesia with 0.75% ropivacaine. A double-blind evaluation of adding clonidine. Minerva Anest 2001;67:407-412.

199. Mannion S, Hayes I, Loughnane F, et al: Intravenous but not perineural clonidine prolongs postoperative analgesia after psoas compartment block with 0.5% levobupivacaine for hip fracture surgery. Anesth Analg 2005;100:873-878.

200. Duma A, Urbanek B, Sitzwohl C, et al: Clonidine as an adjuvant to local anaesthetic axillary brachial plexus block: A randomized, controlled study. Br J Anaesth 2005;94:112-116.

201. Curley J, Castillo J, Hotz J, et al: Prolonged regional nerve blockade: Injectable biodegradable bupivacaine/polyester microspheres. Anesthesiology 1996;84:1401-1410.

202. Drager C, Benziger D, Gao F, et al: Prolonged intercostal nerve blockade in sheep using controlled-release of bupivacaine and dexamethasone from polymer microspheres. Anesthesiology 1998;89:969-979.

203. Kohane DS, Smith SE, Louis DN, et al: Prolonged duration local anesthesia from tetrodotoxin-enhanced local anesthetic microspheres. Pain 2003;104:415-421.

204. Holte K, Werner MU, Lacouture PG, et al: Dexamethasone prolongs local analgesia after subcutaneous infiltration of bupivacaine microcapsules in human volunteers. Anesthesiology. 2002;96:1331-1335.

205. Kopacz DJ, Lacouture PG, Wu D, et al: The dose response and effects of dexamethasone on bupivacaine microcapsules for intercostal blockade (T9 to T11) in healthy volunteers. Anesth Analg. 2003;96:576-582.

206. Movafegh A, Razazian M, Hajimaohamadi F, et al: Dexamethasone added to lidocaine prolongs axillary brachial plexus blockade. Anesth Analg 2006;102:263-267.

207. Stein C, Comisel K, Haimerl E, et al: Analgesic effect of intraarticular morphine after arthroscopic knee surgery. N Engl J Med 1991;325:1123-1126.

208. Khoury GF, Chen AC, Garland DE, et al: Intraarticular morphine, bupivacaine, and morphine/bupivacaine for pain control after knee videoarthroscopy. Anesthesiology 1992;77:263-266.

209. Stein C. Peripheral mechanisms of opioid analgesia. Anesth Analg 1993;76:182-191.

210. Likar R, Kapral S, Steinkellner H, et al: Dose-dependency of intra-articular morphine analgesia. Br J Anaesth 1999;83:241-244.

211. Likar R, Mousa SA, Philippitsch G, et al: Increased numbers of opioid expressing inflammatory cells do not affect intra-articular morphine analgesia. Br J Anaesth 2004;93:375-380.

212. Stein A, Yassouridis A, Szopko C, et al: Intraarticular morphine versus dexamethasone in chronic arthritis. Pain 1999;83:525-532.

213. Lehrberger K, Stein C, Hassan A, et al: Opioids as novel intra-articular agents for analgesia following arthroscopic knee surgery. Knee Surg Sports Traumatol Arthrosc 1994;2:174-175.

214. Gupta A, Bodin L, Holmstrom B, et al: A systematic review of the peripheral analgesic effects of intraarticular morphine. Anesth Analg 2001;93:761-770.

215. Kalso E, Smith L, McQuay HJ, et al: No pain, no gain: Clinical excellence and scientific rigour–lessons learned from IA morphine. Pain. 2002;98:269-275.

216. Soderlund A, Boreus LO, Westman L, et al: A comparison of 50, 100 and 200 mg of intra-articular pethidine during knee joint surgery, a controlled study with evidence for local demethylation to norpethidine. Pain 1999;80:229-238.

217. Soderlund A, Westman L, Ersmark H, et al: Analgesia following arthroscopy—A comparison of intra-articular morphine, pethidine and fentanyl. Acta Anaesthesiol Scand 1997;41:6-11.

218. Marchal JM, Delgado-Martinez AD, Poncela M, et al: Does the type of arthroscopic surgery modify the analgesic effect of intraarticular morphine and bupivacaine? A preliminary study. Clin J Pain 2003;19:240-246.

219. Rosaeg OP, Krepski B, Cicutti N, et al: Effect of preemptive multimodal analgesia for arthroscopic knee ligament repair. Reg Anesth Pain Med 2001;26:125-130.

220. Reuben SS, Connelly NR: Postoperative analgesia for outpatient arthroscopic knee surgery with intraarticular bupivacaine and ketorolac. Anesth Analg 1995;80:1154-1157.

221. Gupta A, Axelsson K, Allvin R, et al: Postoperative pain following knee arthroscopy: The effects of intra-articular ketorolac and/or morphine. Reg Anesth Pain Med 1999;24:225-230.

222. Rao SK, Rao PS: Comparison of intra-articular analgesics for analgesia after arthroscopic knee surgery. Med J Malaysia 2005;60:560-562.

223. Vintar N, Rawal N, Veselko M: Intraarticular patient-controlled regional anesthesia after arthroscopically assisted anterior cruciate ligament reconstruction: Ropivacaine/morphine/ketorolac versus ropivacaine/morphine. Anesth Analg 2005;101:573-578.

224. Guler G, Karaoglu S, Velibasoglu H, et al: Comparison of analgesic effects of intra-articular tenoxicam and morphine in anterior cruciate ligament reconstruction. Knee Surg Sports Traumatol Arthrosc 2002;10:229-232.

225. Alagol A, Calpur OU, Usar PS, et al: Intraarticular analgesia after arthroscopic knee surgery: Comparison of neostigmine, clonidine, tenoxicam, morphine and bupivacaine. Knee Surg Sports Traumatol Arthrosc 2005;24:24.

226. Talu GK, Ozyalcin S, Koltka K, et al: Comparison of efficacy of intraarticular application of tenoxicam, bupivacaine and tenoxicam: Bupivacaine combination in arthroscopic knee surgery. Knee Surg Sports Traumatol Arthrosc 2002;10:355-360.

227. Elhakim M, Fathy A, Elkott M, et al: Intra-articular tenoxicam relieves post-arthroscopy pain. Acta Anaesthesiol Scand 1996;40:1223-1226.

228. Elhakim M, Nafie M, Eid A, Hassin M: Combination of intra-articular tenoxicam, lidocaine, and pethidine for outpatient knee arthroscopy. Acta Anaesthesiol Scand 1999;43:803-808.

229. Cook TM, Tuckey JP, Nolan JP: Analgesia after day-case knee arthroscopy: Double-blind study of intra-articular tenoxicam, intra-articular bupivacaine and placebo. Br J Anaesth 1997;78:163-168.

230. Colbert ST, Curran E, O'Hanlon DM, et al: Intra-articular tenoxicam improves postoperative analgesia in knee arthroscopy. Can J Anaesth 1999;46:653-657.

231. Yang LC, Chen LM, Wang CJ, et al: Postoperative analgesia by intra-articular neostigmine in patients undergoing knee arthroscopy. Anesthesiology 1998;88:334-339.

232. Williams BA, Vogt MT, Kentor ML, et al: Nausea and vomiting after outpatient ACL reconstruction with regional anesthesia: Are lumbar plexus blocks a risk factor? J Clin Anesth 2004;16:276-281.

233. Reuben SS, Connelly NR: Postoperative analgesia for outpatient arthroscopic knee surgery with intraarticular clonidine. Anesth Analg 1999;88:729-733.

234. Gentili M, Enel D, Szymskiewicz O, et al: Postoperative analgesia by intraarticular clonidine and neostigmine in patients undergoing knee arthroscopy. Reg Anesth Pain Med 2001;26:342-347.

235. Gentili M, Houssel P, Osman M, et al: Intra-articular morphine and clonidine produce comparable analgesia but the combination is not more effective. Br J Anaesth 1997;79:660-661.

236. Gentili M, Juhel A, Bonnet F: Peripheral analgesic effect of intra-articular clonidine. Pain 1996;64:593-596.

237. Karmakar MK: Thoracic paravertebral block. Anesthesiology 2001;95:771-780.

238. Kaiser AM, Zollinger A, De Lorenzi D, et al: Prospective, randomized comparison of extrapleural versus epidural analgesia for postthoracotomy pain. Ann Thorac Surg 1998;66:367-372.

239. Andrew R, Hurley RW, Hanna M, et al: Analgesic efficacy of extrapleural catheters versus placebo postoperative pain control: Systematic review/meta-analysis [abstract]. American Society of Regional Anesthesia, 31st Annual Meeting, Palm Springs, CA, April 2006.

240. Ballantyne JC, Carr DB, deFerranti S, et al: The comparative effects of postoperative analgesic therapies on pulmonary outcome: Cumulative meta-analyses of randomized, controlled trials. Anesth Analg 1998;86:598-612.

241. Hobelmann JT, Hurley RW, Bolka J, et al: Analgesic efficacy of intraapleural catheters versus placebo postoperative pain control: Systematic review/meta-analysis (abstract). American Society of Regional Anesthesia, 31st Annual Meeting, Palm Springs, CA, April 2006.

242. Shanti CM, Carlin AM, Tyburski JG: Incidence of pneumothorax from intercostal nerve block for analgesia in rib fractures. J Trauma 2001;51:536-539.

243. Hostetler MA, Auinger P, Szilagyi PG: Parenteral analgesic and sedative use among ED patients in the United States: Combined results from the National Hospital Ambulatory Medical Care Survey (NHAMCS) 1992-1997. Am J Emerg Med 2002;20:139-143.

244. Silka PA, Roth MM, Geiderman JM: Patterns of analgesic use in trauma patients in the ED. Am J Emerg Med 2002;20:298-302.

245. Zohar Z, Eitan A, Halperin P, et al: Pain relief in major trauma patients: An Israeli perspective. J Trauma 2001;51:767-772.

246. Selbst SM, Clark M: Analgesic use in the emergency department. Ann Emerg Med 1990;19:1010-1013.

247. Whipple JK, Lewis KS, Quebbeman EJ, et al: Analysis of pain management in critically ill patients. Pharmacotherapy 1995;15:592-599.

248. Lewis LM, Lasater LC, Brooks CB: Are emergency physicians too stingy with analgesics? South Med J 1994;87:7-9.

249. Cohen SP, Christo PJ, Moroz L: Pain management in trauma patients. Am J Phys Med Rehabil 2004;83:142-161.

250. Silka PA, Roth MM, Moreno G, et al: Pain scores improve analgesic administration patterns for trauma patients in the emergency department. Acad Emerg Med 2004;11:264-270.

251. Neighbor ML, Honner S, Kohn MA: Factors affecting emergency department opioid administration to severely injured patients. Acad Emerg Med 2004;11:1290-1296.

252. Lewis KS, Whipple JK, Michael KA, et al: Effect of analgesic treatment on the physiological consequences of acute pain. Am J Hospital Pharmacy 1994;51:1539-1554.

253. Puntillo K, Weiss SJ: Pain: its mediators and associated morbidity in critically ill cardiovascular surgical patients. Nurs Res 1994;43:31-36.

254. Liebeskind JC: Pain can kill. Pain 1991;44:3-4.

255. Jabbur SJ, Saade NE: From electrical wiring to plastic neurons: Evolving approaches to the study of pain. Pain Suppl 1999;6:87-92.

256. Dickenson AH: Central acute pain mechanisms. Ann Med 1995;27:223-227.

257. Coderre TJ, Katz J, Vaccarino AL, et al: Contribution of central neuroplasticity to pathological pain: Review of clinical and experimental evidence. Pain 1993;52:259-285.

258. Schreiber S, Galai-Gat T: Uncontrolled pain following physical injury as the core-trauma in post-traumatic stress disorder. Pain 1993;54:107-110.

259. Krettek C, Simon RG, Tscherne H: Management priorities in patients with polytrauma. Langenbecks Arch Surg 1998;383:220-227.

260. Tscherne H, Regel G: Care of the polytraumatised patient. J Bone Joint Surg Br 1996;78:840-852.

261. Heffernan DS, Schermer CR, Lu SW: What defines a distracting injury in cervical spine assessment? J Trauma 2005;59:1396-1399.

262. Holmes JF, Panacek EA, Miller PQ, et al: Prospective evaluation of criteria for obtaining thoracolumbar radiographs in trauma patients. J Emerg Med 2003;24:1-7.

263. Thomas SH, Rago O, Harrison T, et al: Fentanyl trauma analgesia use in air medical scene transports. J Emerg Med 2005;29:179-187.

264. Porter K: Ketamine in prehospital care. Emerg Med J 2004;21:351-354.

265. Vergnion M, Degesves S, Garcet L, et al: Tramadol, an alternative to morphine for treating posttraumatic pain in the prehospital situation. Anesth Analg 2001;92:1543-1546.

266. Old S: Management of trauma. Nitrous oxide dangerous in pneumothorax. Br Med J 1993;306:5.

267. Johnson JC, Atherton GL: Effectiveness of nitrous oxide in a rural EMS system. J Emerg Med 1991;9:45-53.

268. Ickeringill M, Shehabi Y, Adamson H, et al: Dexmedetomidine infusion without loading dose in surgical patients requiring mechanical ventilation: Haemodynamic effects and efficacy. Anaesth Intensive Care 2004;32:741-745.

269. Soltesz S, Biedler A, Silomon M, et al: Recovery after remifentanil and sufentanil for analgesia and sedation of mechanically ventilated patients after trauma or major surgery. Br J Anaesth 2001;86:763-768.

270. Izquierdo I: Mechanism of action of scopolamine as an amnestic. Trends Pharmacol Sci 1989;10:175-177.

271. Hollinworth H: The management of patients' pain in wound care. Nurs Stand 2005;20:65-66.

272. Grass JA: Patient-controlled analgesia. Anesth Analg 2005; 101:44-61.

273. Godambe SA, Elliot V, Matheny D, et al: Comparison of propofol/fentanyl versus ketamine/midazolam for brief orthopedic procedural sedation in a pediatric emergency department. Pediatrics 2003;112:116-123.

274. Mandabach MG: Intrathecal and epidural analgesia. Crit Care Clin 1999;15:105-118.

275. Werawatganon T, Charuluxanun S: Patient controlled intravenous opioid analgesia versus continuous epidural analgesia for pain after intra-abdominal surgery. Cochrane Database Syst Rev 2005;1:CD004088.

276. Mojica JL, Melendez HJ, Bautista LE: The timing of intravenous crystalloid administration and incidence of cardiovascular side effects during spinal anesthesia: The results from a randomized controlled trial. Anesth Analg 2002;94: 432-437.

277. Karmakar MK, Critchley LA, Ho AM, et al: Continuous thoracic paravertebral infusion of bupivacaine for pain management in patients with multiple fractured ribs. Chest 2003;123:424-431.

278. Bishop JY, Sprague M, Gelber J, et al: Interscalene regional anesthesia for shoulder surgery. J Bone Joint Surg Am 2005; 87:974-979.

279. Kim CW, Hong JP: Lower extremity reconstruction under popliteal sciatic nerve (tibioperoneal trunk) and saphenous nerve block. Plast Reconstr Surg 2005;115:563-566.

280. Fuzier R, Fuzier V, Albert N, et al: The infraclavicular block is a useful technique for emergency upper extremity analgesia. Can J Anaesth 2004;51:191-192.

281. Rooks M, Fleming LL: Evaluation of acute knee injuries with sciatic/femoral nerve blocks. Clin Orthop 1983;179:185-188.

282. Singelyn FJ, Ferrant T, Malisse MF, et al: Effects of intravenous patient-controlled analgesia with morphine, continuous epidural analgesia, and continuous femoral nerve sheath block on rehabilitation after unilateral total-hip arthroplasty. Reg Anesth Pain Med 2005;30:452-457.

283. Du Pen SL, Peterson DG, Williams A, et al: Infection during chronic epidural catheterization: Diagnosis and treatment. Anesthesiology 1990;73:905-909.

284. Cherpitel CJ, Ye Y, Bond J: Attributable risk of injury associated with alcohol use: Cross-national data from the emergency room collaborative alcohol analysis project. Am J Public Health 2005;95:266-272.

285. Rehm J, Room R, Monteiro M, et al: Alcohol as a risk factor for global burden of disease. Eur Addict Res 2003;9: 157-164.

286. Borges G, Cherpitel C, Mittleman M: Risk of injury after alcohol consumption: A case-crossover study in the emergency department. Soc Sci Med 2004;58:1191-1200.

287. Rivara FP, Koepsell TD, Jurkovich GJ, et al: The effects of alcohol abuse on readmission for trauma. JAMA 1993;270: 1962-1964.

288. Jurkovich GJ, Rivara FP, Gurney JG, et al: The effect of acute alcohol intoxication and chronic alcohol abuse on outcome from trauma. JAMA 1993;270:51-56.

289. Karabinis A, Mandragos K, Stergiopoulos S, et al: Safety and efficacy of analgesia-based sedation with remifentanil versus standard hypnotic-based regimens in intensive care unit patients with brain injuries: A randomised, controlled trial. Crit Care 2004;8:R268-R280.

290. Shapiro BA, Warren J, Egol AB, et al: Practice parameters for intravenous analgesia and sedation for adult patients in the intensive care unit: An executive summary. Society of Critical Care Medicine. Crit Care Med 1995;23:1596-1600.

291. Mayberry JC, Trunkey DD: The fractured rib in chest wall trauma. Chest Surg Clin N Am 1997;7:239-261.

292. Yamamoto L, Schroeder C, Morley D, et al: Thoracic trauma: The deadly dozen. Crit Care Nurs Q 2005;28:22-40.

293. Ziegler DW, Agarwal NN: The morbidity and mortality of rib fractures. J Trauma 1994;37:975-979.

294. Wu CL, Jani ND, Perkins FM, et al: Thoracic epidural analgesia versus intravenous patient-controlled analgesia for the treatment of rib fracture pain after motor vehicle crash. J Trauma 1999;47:564-567.

295. Moon MR, Luchette FA, Gibson SW, et al: Prospective, randomized comparison of epidural versus parenteral opioid analgesia in thoracic trauma. Ann Surg 1999;229:684-691.

296. Mackersie RC, Karagianes TG, Hoyt DB, et al: Prospective evaluation of epidural and intravenous administration of fentanyl for pain control and restoration of ventilatory function following multiple rib fractures. J Trauma 1991; 31:443-449.

297. Sabanathan S, Richardson J, Shah R: 1988: Continuous intercostal nerve block for pain relief after thoracotomy. Updated in 1995. Ann Thorac Surg 1995;59:1261-1263.

298. Richardson J, Lonnqvist PA: Thoracic paravertebral block. Br J Anaesth 1998;81:230-238.

299. Naja Z, Lonnqvist PA. Somatic paravertebral nerve blockade: Incidence of failed block and complications. Anaesthesia 2001;56:1184-1188.

300. Hultman JL, Schuleman S, Sharp T, et al: Continuous thoracic paravertebral block. J Cardiothorac Anesth 1989;3(Suppl 1):54.

301. Concha M, Dagnino J, Cariaga M, et al: Analgesia after thoracotomy: Epidural fentanyl/bupivacaine compared with intercostal nerve block plus intravenous morphine. J Cardiothorac Vasc Anesth 2004;18:322-326.

302. Osinowo OA, Zahrani M, Softah A: Effect of intercostal nerve block with 0.5% bupivacaine on peak expiratory flow rate and arterial oxygen saturation in rib fractures. J Trauma 2004;56:345-347.

303. Mowbray A, Wong KK, Murray JM: Intercostal catheterisation: An alternative approach to the paravertebral space. Anaesthesia 1987;42:958-961.

304. Short K, Scheeres D, Mlakar J, et al: Evaluation of intrapleural analgesia in the management of blunt traumatic chest wall pain: A clinical trial. Am Surg 1996;62:488-493.

305. Schneider RF, Villamena PC, Harvey J, et al: Lack of efficacy of intrapleural bupivacaine for postoperative analgesia following thoracotomy. Chest 1993;103:414-416.

306. Shinohara K, Iwama H, Akama Y, et al: Interpleural block for patients with multiple rib fractures: Comparison with epidural block. J Emerg Med 1994;12:441-446.

307. Luchette FA, Radafshar SM, Kaiser R, et al: Prospective evaluation of epidural versus intrapleural catheters for analgesia in chest wall trauma. J Trauma 1994;36:865-869.

308. Brockmeier V, Moen H, Karlsson BR, et al: Interpleural or thoracic epidural analgesia for pain after thoracotomy: A double blind study. Acta Anaesthesiol Scand 1994;38:317-321.

309. Bachmann-Mennenga B, Biscoping J, Kuhn DF, et al: Intercostal nerve block, interpleural analgesia, thoracic epidural block or systemic opioid application for pain relief after thoracotomy? Eur J Cardiothorac Surg 1993;7:12-18.

310. Pedersen JL, Andersen OK, Arendt-Nielsen L, et al: Hyperalgesia and temporal summation of pain after heat injury in man. Pain 1998;74:189-197.

311. Silbert BS, Lipkowski AW, Cepeda MS, et al: Enhanced potency of receptor-selective opioids after acute burn injury. Anesth Analg 1991;73:427-433.

312. Choiniere M, Grenier R, Paquette C: Patient-controlled analgesia: A double-blind study in burn patients. Anaesthesia 1992;47:467-472.

313. Hu OY, Ho ST, Wang JJ, et al: Evaluation of gastric emptying in severe, burn-injured patients. Crit Care Med 1993;21:527-531.

314. Barrow RE, Ramirez RJ, Zhang XJ: Ibuprofen modulates tissue perfusion in partial-thickness burns. Burns 2000;26:341-346.

315. Cone JB, Wallace BH, Olsen KM, et al: The pharmacokinetics of ibuprofen after burn injury. J Burn Care Rehabil 1993;14:666-669.

316. Jonsson CE, Ericsson F: Impairment of renal function after treatment of a burn patient with diclofenac, a non-steroidal antiinflammatory drug. Burns 1995;21:471-473.

317. Brofeldt BT, Cornwell P, Doherty D, et al: Topical lidocaine in the treatment of partial-thickness burns. J Burn Care Rehabil 1989;10:63-68.

318. Kopecky EA, Jacobson S, Bch MB, et al: Safety and pharmacokinetics of EMLA in the treatment of postburn pruritus in pediatric patients: A pilot study. J Burn Care Rehabil 2001;22:235-242.

319. Wehner D, Hamilton GC: Seizures following topical application of local anesthetics to burn patients. Ann Emerg Med 1984;13:456-458.

320. Cassuto J, Tarnow P: Potent inhibition of burn pain without use of opiates. Burns 2003;29:163-166.

321. Mattsson U, Cassuto J, Tarnow P, et al: Intravenous lidocaine infusion in the treatment of experimental human skin burns—Digital colour image analysis of erythema development. Burns 2000;26:710-715.

322. Fischer CG, Lloyd S, Kopcha R, et al: The safety of adding bupivacaine to the subcutaneous infiltration solution used for donor site harvest. J Burn Care Rehabil 2003;24:361-364.

323. Jellish WS, Gamelli RL, Furry PA, et al: Effect of topical local anesthetic application to skin harvest sites for pain management in burn patients undergoing skin-grafting procedures. Ann Surg 1999;229:115-120.

324. Warncke T, Stubhaug A, Jorum E: Ketamine, an NMDA receptor antagonist, suppresses spatial and temporal properties of burn-induced secondary hyperalgesia in man: A double-blind, cross-over comparison with morphine and placebo. Pain 1997;72:99-106.

325. Edrich T, Friedrich AD, Eltzschig HK, et al: Ketamine for long-term sedation and analgesia of a burn patient. Anesth Analg 2004;99:893-895.

326. Kudoh A, Katagai H, Takazawa T: Anesthesia with ketamine, propofol, and fentanyl decreases the frequency of postoperative psychosis emergence and confusion in schizophrenic patients. J Clin Anesth 2002;14:107-110.

327. Nakao S, Nagata A, Miyamoto E, et al: Inhibitory effect of propofol on ketamine-induced c-Fos expression in the rat posterior cingulate and retrosplenial cortices is mediated by GABAA receptor activation. Acta Anaesthesiol Scand 2003;47:284-290.

328. Nagata A, Nakao S, Miyamoto E, et al: Propofol inhibits ketamine-induced c-fos expression in the rat posterior cingulate cortex. Anesth Analg 1998;87:1416-1420.

329. Viggiano M, Badetti C, Roux F, et al: Controlled analgesia in a burn patient: Fentanyl sparing effect of clonidine. Ann Fr Anesth Reanim 1998;17:19-26.

330. Kariya N, Shindoh M, Nishi S, et al: Oral clonidine for sedation and analgesia in a burn patient. J Clin Anesth 1998;10:514-517.

331. Lyons B, Casey W, Doherty P, et al: Pain relief with low-dose intravenous clonidine in a child with severe burns. Intensive Care Med 1996;22:249-251.

332. Cuignet O, Mbuyamba J, Pirson J: The long-term analgesic efficacy of a single-shot fascia iliaca compartment block in burn patients undergoing skin-grafting procedures. J Burn Care Rehabil 2005;26:409-415.

333. Choiniere M, Melzack R, Rondeau J, et al: The pain of burns: Characteristics and correlates. J Trauma 1989;29:1531-1539.

334. Jaffe SE, Patterson DR: Treating sleep problems in patients with burn injuries: Practical considerations. J Burn Care Rehabil 2004;25:294-305.

335. Van Loey NE, Maas CJ, Faber AW, et al: Predictors of chronic posttraumatic stress symptoms following burn injury: Results of a longitudinal study. J Trauma Stress 2003;16:361-369.

336. Patterson DR, Ptacek JT, Esselman PC: Management of suffering in patients with severe burn injury. West J Med 1997;166:272-273.

337. Patterson DR, Ptacek JT, Carrougher GJ, et al: Lorazepam as an adjunct to opioid analgesics in the treatment of burn pain. Pain 1997;72:367-374.

338. Pud D, Amit A: Anxiety as a predictor of pain magnitude following termination of first-trimester pregnancy. Pain Med 2005;6:143-148.

339. Ng EH, Miao B, Ho PC: Anxiolytic premedication reduces preoperative anxiety and pain during oocyte retrieval. A randomized double-blinded placebo-controlled trial. Hum Reprod 2002;17:1233-1238.

340. Pick CG, Paul D, Eison MS, et al: Potentiation of opioid analgesia by the antidepressant nefazodone. Eur J Pharmacol 1992;211:375-381.

341. Stoddard FJ: Psychiatric management of the burned patient. In Martyn JAJ (ed): Acute Management of the Burned Patient. Philadelphia, Saunders, 1990, pp 256-272.

342. Gallagher G, Rae CP, Kinsella J: Treatment of pain in severe burns. Am J Clin Dermatol 2000;1:329-335.

343. Pal SK, Cortiella J, Herndon D: Adjunctive methods of pain control in burns. Burns 1997;23:404-412.

344. Zautcke JL, Coker SB Jr, Morris RW, et al: Geriatric trauma in the State of Illinois: Substance use and injury patterns. Am J Emerg Med 2002;20:14-17.

345. Kaasalainen S, Crook J: An exploration of seniors' ability to report pain. Clin Nurs Res 2004;13:199-215.

346. Landi F, Onder G, Cesari M, et al: Pain and its relation to depressive symptoms in frail older people living in the community: An observational study. J Pain Symptom Manage 2005;29:255-262.

347. Tsai YF, Wei SL, Lin YP, et al: Depressive symptoms, pain experiences, and pain management strategies among residents of Taiwanese public elder care homes. J Pain Symptom Manage 2005;30:63-69.

348. Meldon SW, Emerman CL, Schubert DS, et al: Depression in geriatric ED patients: Prevalence and recognition. Ann Emerg Med 1997;30:141-145.

349. Klarin I, Fastbom J, Wimo A: A population-based study of drug use in the very old living in a rural district of Sweden, with focus on cardiovascular drug consumption: Comparison with an urban cohort. Pharmacoepidemiol Drug Saf 2003;12:669-678.

350. Weiner D, Peterson B, Keefe F: Chronic pain-associated behaviors in the nursing home: Resident versus caregiver perceptions. Pain 1999;80:577-588.

351. Davis GC: Chronic pain management of older adults in residential settings. J Gerontol Nurs 1997;23:16-22.

352. Sengstaken EA, King SA: The problems of pain and its detection among geriatric nursing home residents. J Am Geriatr Soc 1993;41:541-544.

353. Horgas AL: Pain management in elderly adults. J Infusion Nursing 2003;26:161-165.

354. Bresalier RS, Sandler RS, Quan H, et al: Cardiovascular events associated with rofecoxib in a colorectal adenoma chemoprevention trial. N Engl J Med 2005;352:1092-1102.

355. Gloth FM 3rd: Principles of perioperative pain management in older adults. Clin Geriatr Med 2001;17:553-573.

356. Gibson SJ, Helme RD: Cognitive factors and the experience of pain and suffering in older persons. Pain 2000;85:375-383.

357. Walsh JM, Flegel R, Atkins R, et al: Drug and alcohol use among drivers admitted to a Level-1 trauma center. Accid Anal Prev 2005;37:894-901.

358. Walsh JM, Flegel R, Cangianelli LA, et al: Epidemiology of alcohol and other drug use among motor vehicle crash victims admitted to a trauma center. Traffic Inj Prev 2004;5:254-260.

359. Soderstrom CA, Ballesteros MF, Dischinger PC, et al: Alcohol/drug abuse, driving convictions, and risk-taking dispositions among trauma center patients. Accid Anal Prev 2001;33:771-782.

360. Carrigan TD, Field H, Illingworth RN, et al: Toxicological screening in trauma. J Accid Emerg Med 2000;17:33-37.

361. Blondell RD, Dodds HN, Looney SW, et al: Toxicology screening results: Injury associations among hospitalized trauma patients. J Trauma 2005;58:561-570.

362. Rosenblum A, Joseph H, Fong C, et al: Prevalence and characteristics of chronic pain among chemically dependent patients in methadone maintenance and residential treatment facilities. JAMA 2003;289:2370-2378.

363. Jamison RN, Kauffman J, Katz NP: Characteristics of methadone maintenance patients with chronic pain. J Pain Sympt Manage 2000;19:53-62.

364. Weissman DE, Haddox JD: Opioid pseudoaddiction—An iatrogenic syndrome. Pain 1989;36:363-366.

365. Mitra S, Sinatra RS: Perioperative management of acute pain in the opioid-dependent patient. Anesthesiology 2004;101: 212-227.

366. Pereira J, Lawlor P, Vigano A, et al: Equianalgesic dose ratios for opioids: A critical review and proposals for long-term dosing. J Pain Sympt Manage 2001;22:672-687.

367. Cepeda MS, Carr DB, Miranda N, et al: Comparison of morphine, ketorolac, and their combination for postoperative pain: Results from a large, randomized, double-blind trial. Anesthesiology 2005;103:1225-1232.

368. Tornkvist H, Lindholm TS, Netz P, et al: Effect of ibuprofen and indomethacin on bone metabolism reflected in bone strength. Clin Orthop 1984;187:255-259.

369. Allen HL, Wase A, Bear WT: Indomethacin and aspirin: Effect of nonsteroidal anti-inflammatory agents on the rate of fracture repair in the rat. Acta Orthop Scand 1980;51:595-600.

370. Chow LH, Huang EY, Ho ST, et al: Dextromethorphan potentiates morphine-induced antinociception at both spinal and supraspinal sites but is not related to the descending serotoninergic or adrenergic pathways. J Biomed Sci 2004;11:717-725.

371. Weinbroum AA, Rudick V, Paret G, et al: The role of dextromethorphan in pain control. Can J Anaesth 2000;47:585-596.

372. Clark JL, Kalan GE: Effective treatment of severe cancer pain of the head using low-dose ketamine in an opioid-tolerant patient. J Pain Sympt Manage 1995;10:310-314.

373. Trujillo KA, Akil H: Inhibition of morphine tolerance and dependence by the NMDA receptor antagonist MK-801. Science 1991;251:85-87.

374. Hartree C: Caution with nalbuphine in patients on long-term opioids. Palliat Med 2005;19:168.

375. Jacobs EA, Bickel WK: Precipitated withdrawal in an opioid-dependent outpatient receiving alternate-day buprenorphine dosing. Addiction 1999;94:140-141.

376. Sjostrom S, Tamsen A, Persson MP, et al: Pharmacokinetics of intrathecal morphine and meperidine in humans. Anesthesiology 1987;67:889-895.

377. Nordberg G, Hedner T, Mellstrand T, et al: Pharmacokinetics of epidural morphine in man. Eur J Clin Pharmacol 1984;26:233-237.

378. Cullen DJ: Obstructive sleep apnea and postoperative analgesia—A potentially dangerous combination. J Clin Anesth 2001;13:83-85.

379. Loadsman JA, Hillman DR: Anaesthesia and sleep apnoea. Br J Anaesth 2001;86:254-266.

380. Pellecchia DJ, Bretz KA, Barnette RE: Postoperative pain control by means of epidural narcotics in a patient with obstructive sleep apnea. Anesth Analg 1987;66:280-282.

381. Wiesel S, Fox GS: Anaesthesia for a patient with central alveolar hypoventilation syndrome (Ondine's Curse). Can J Anaesth 1990;37:122-126.

382. Williams BA, Green JM, Stapelfeldt WH: Snoring and obstructive sleep apnea as risk factors for perioperative postobstructive pulmonary edema. Am J Anesthesiol 1997;24:89-93.

383. Gross JB, Caldwell CB, Shaw LM, et al: The effect of lidocaine infusion on the ventilatory response to hypoxia. Anesthesiology 1984;61:662-665.

15 Preemptive Analgesia and Prevention of Chronic Pain Syndromes after Surgery

Fred Perkins and Tabitha Washington

Chronic pain as an outcome of surgery is an area of investigation that has received more attention over the last decade.[1-4] Previous reviews have emphasized the prevalence of chronic pain following a few specific surgical procedures. In this chapter we will try to address the extent of the problem of chronic pain following surgery in general, the factors that can or may influence the prevalence of chronic pain following surgery, and interventions that may be of benefit. Among the questions that we will address are:

- Can patients at increased risk of developing chronic pain be identified before surgery or in the immediate postoperative period?
- Are there interventions that can be initiated in the preoperative, intraoperative, or postoperative period to minimize the probability of chronic pain?
- What are the surgical factors that come into play?

To discuss these questions in an effective manner, it is necessary to agree on the definitions of the terms used in the discussion. Table 15–1 is a list of definitions of important terms used in this chapter. The term *preemptive analgesia* has been used by different authors to mean different things. Depending on the definition used and the population studied, authors have come to differing conclusions. In a recent meta-analysis of preemptive analgesia, Ong and colleagues[5] found evidence that preemptive epidural analgesia had a moderate effect size, but preemptive opioids yielded equivocal results at best. They used a broad definition of *preemptive* that allowed the intervention to be continued in the postoperative period. A previous meta-analysis[6] did not find evidence that epidural analgesia had a preemptive effect, but those authors had excluded studies in which the prestimulus intervention was continued into the postopera-

tive period. We use a broad definition for *preemptive analgesia* in that a number of surgeries are associated with intense nociceptive stimulation for a length of time that is longer than the operative procedure.

The concept of preemptive analgesia originated with a paper by Clifford Woolf in 1983.[7] This study, when combined with evidence for what is known as *wind-up*,[8] gave rise to the hope that interventions that decrease nociceptive input, or block central sensitization, would have lasting analgesic benefit. It should be noted that central sensitization and wind-up are different phenomena,[9] and it is primarily sensitization that would be of importance clinically. How a pain experience progresses from acute nociceptive pain, to subacute pain, to chronic pain has been reviewed by Devor[10] incorporating both animal model data and clinical data. In brief, acute pain is pain associated with a nociceptive stimulus to tissues that results in activation of nociceptive neurons. The pain that persists immediately following cessation of the nociceptive stimulus has been referred to as *subacute pain,* which is usually thought of as a transition in the peripheral and central nervous systems that leads to the continued perception of pain. There is continued firing of some nociceptors during the period when patients experience subacute pain and there is also incident pain with movement. At the same time, stimulation of nociceptors that have been sensitized and stimulation of other nerves, which before injury had not been nociceptors, both lead to increased pain. For most surgical procedures tissue trauma and nociceptive stimulation goes on for most if not all of the procedure. Thus during a thoracotomy the initial stimulation from skin incision would have changed to a subacute pain while the ongoing nociceptive stimulation of the pleura is generating an acute pain (if the patient were awake to experience the phenomenon). Thus before a major surgical procedure is completed, there should be both peripheral sensitization and central sensitization. The peripheral sensitization can be blocked to some extent by nonsteroidal anti-inflammatory agents (NSAIDs), while the central sensitization may be blocked by local anesthetics that prevent the nociceptive information from getting to the spinal cord or by N-methyl-D-aspartate (NMDA) blockers that can decrease or eliminate the central sensitization. The extent to which data from experimental pain in humans or data gathered from animal experiments can be extrapolated to clinical situations is less than clear.

Table 15–1. Definitions

TERM	DEFINITION
Central sensitization	Persistent postinjury changes in the central nervous system that result in pain hypersensitivity.
Chronic pain	Pain that lasts for more than 3 months.
Pain	An unpleasant sensory and emotional experience associated with actual or potential tissue damage, or described in terms of such damage.
Peripheral sensitization	A lowering of the threshold for a stimulus to be felt as painful.
Preemptive analgesia	An intervention that is initiated before a nociceptive stimulus, and the intervention either lasts or is continued until nociceptive stimulus has abated. The intervention needs to significantly decrease or eliminate the usual immediate effect of the nociceptive stimulus (e.g., pain, central sensitization).
Preincisional	An intervention that is started before an initial surgical incision.

FACTORS INFLUENCING THE PREVALENCE OF CHRONIC PAIN

There are numerous factors related to the surgery that appear to be of importance. First among these is the surgical procedure. Previous reviews have documented that the prevalence of chronic pain varies with the type of surgery,[1] with some surgical procedures such as lower extremity amputation and posterolateral thoracotomy having a high prevalence of chronic pain (greater than 50%). Table 15–2 is an attempt to try to summarize the prevalence of chronic pain following many common surgical procedures. Table 15–2 shows that chronic pain is infrequent following some surgical procedures such as cataract extraction, but chronic pain is prevalent following other surgical procedures such as thoracotomy. Additionally the prevalence of pain may decrease following certain surgeries (hip arthroplasty, lumbar laminectomy for herniated disk), while increasing following other surgeries (thoracotomy, breast surgery).

Within a given type of operation, the surgical approach may have a number of options. For thoracotomy, an anterior approach appears to have less acute and chronic pain than the classic posterolateral approach.[1] Additionally there may be less acute and chronic pain with visually aided thoracoscopic surgery than with the same operation performed as an open procedure.[11] Likewise laparoscopic inguinal hernia repair is associated with less acute pain and may be associated with less chronic pain than open inguinal hernia repair.[12,13] Thus there are data to support the hypothesis that minimally invasive surgical procedures are associated with less chronic pain than the same operations performed as open procedures.

Another factor may be what has been referred to as *volume-dependent outcome*. Database studies[14,15] demonstrated that for a number of major, high-risk surgeries, outcome is worse when the procedure is

Table 15–2. Prevalence of Chronic Pain and Pre-procedure Pain

SURGICAL PROCEDURE	PREVALENCE OF CHRONIC PAIN	PREVALENCE OF PRE-OP PAIN
Amputation, lower extremity[1]	Phantom pain 70% Stump pain 62%	Very common, chronic, continuous ischemic pain
Arthroplasty, hip[55]	20%	Common, chronic, incident arthritic pain
Cataract with lens implant[56]	<1%	Uncommon
Cesarean section[57]	6%	Common, intermittent, acute labor pain
Cholecystectomy[1]	26%	Common, variable, from acute cholecystitis to chronic vague abdominal pain
Colectomy[39]	28%	Infrequent
Hernia repair, inguinal[1]	12%	Common, incident pain with peritoneal stretch
Lumbar spine surgery for herniated disk[58]	44%	Very common, primary reason for surgery
Mastectomy[1]	30%	Infrequent
Mastectomy + axillary dissection[1]	50%	Infrequent
Prostatectomy, radical[38]	30%	
Sternotomy, CABG[59]	30%	Common, intermittent, exertional angina
Sternotomy, valve[60]	32%	Infrequent
Thoracotomy, posterolateral[1]	50%	Infrequent
Thoracotomy, VATS[61]	31%	Infrequent
Vasectomy[62]	20%	Rare

CABG, coronary artery bypass graft; VATS, video-assisted thoracoscopic surgery.

performed in a low-volume institution and that a large part of the risk can be attributed to low-volume surgeons. We had previously noted that in the case of hernia repair, the lowest prevalence of chronic pain is reported by high-volume hernia centers.[1] The incidence of complications including chronic pain following laparoscopic hernia repair has been noted to be greater early in the experience of surgeons.[16,17] This may be analogous to the observation that patients of surgical trainees have a higher incidence of hernia recurrence and chronic pain than those of experienced surgeons.[18]

The extent of the surgical procedure also has an influence. When a thoracotomy is associated with a chest wall resection, both the extent of acute pain and the probability of chronic pain are increased.[19] Surgical procedures associated with nerve damage appear to have a higher probability of chronic pain.[4,20,21] A trend to a decreasing prevalence of neuropathic pain following breast surgery with axillary dissection has been noted and has been attributed to more careful handling of the intercostal-brachial nerves during axillary node dissection. Likewise sentinel node biopsy is associated with less chronic arm pain than axillary dissection.[22]

Adjuvant treatments are associated with a number of surgical procedures for cancer. In particular, radiation therapy for women undergoing breast and axillary surgery is associated with an increased probability of chronic pain.[23] Whether this will also be the case for other cancer surgeries has not yet been determined.

It should be clearly stated that patients vary in their sensitivity to pain and other factors that may predict the evolution of acute pain to chronic pain. This has been an area of research for many years, with Lasagna and Beecher[24] finding that a third of patients following surgery did not experience significant pain relief with commonly used dosages of morphine. Likewise in subsequent studies, Weis and colleagues continued to find significant patient variability to surgery and opioids,[25] and that patient report of pain sensitivity did not predict either the extent of pain or the response to opioids. Katz and colleagues[26] did not find that pressure pain sensitivity, preoperative depression, or preoperative anxiety predict the extent of acute or chronic pain following thoracotomy. More recently Werner and colleagues[27] applied a 2.5- × 5.0-cm first-degree burn to the contralateral calf of patients scheduled for elective arthroscopic repair of the anterior cruciate ligament. The extent of pain measured during the burn had a significant correlation with the extent of immediate postoperative pain (0 to 2 days) and intermediate postoperative pain (3 to 10 days) with movement. Likewise the extent of pain following cesarean section can be predicted by thermal pain sensitivity.[28] These differences in pain sensitivity among individuals may be of great significance because there are multiple studies demonstrating that more severe acute pain is a robust predictor of chronic pain (see reference 29 for a general review). This is discussed in

more detail later. As an aside, Gary Bennett (personal communication) has noted that his model of neuropathic pain is reproducible using Wistar rats from a certain breeder, but the model is less successful in producing chronic pain behaviors with other strains and breeds of rats.

There are also psychological factors, other than pain sensitivity, that appear to predispose certain individuals to experiencing pain. Psychological vulnerability has been found to be a predictor of long-term pain and symptoms following cholecystectomy.[30] Gatchel and colleagues[31] have noted a set of psychosocial risk factors for acute back pain to evolve into chronic back pain. From our review it appears that the strongest predictors involve deficits in coping ability, neuroticism, and somatization, although depression and anxiety may add a small component.

The intensity of pain in the postoperative period has been a reproducible predictor of chronic pain following a number of surgeries including lower extremity amputation, thoracotomy, mastectomy, cholecystectomy, and inguinal hernia surgery.[1] Usually pain intensity is measured directly using some instrument, but analgesic consumption is also frequently measured as a surrogate algometer. When looking at studies of interventions aimed to decrease the intensity of acute pain and decrease the prevalence or intensity of chronic pain there are a number of factors that we believe should be considered.

- What intervention was implemented?
- When was it initiated relative to the initial nociceptive stimulus?
- How long was the intervention continued?
- Was the intervention effective at decreasing acute pain or acute opioid consumption?
- Were the doses of medication used in a clinically reasonable range?
- Was there a systematic evaluation of pain and symptoms both acutely and chronically?
- What chronic pain was assessed?
- Was there adequate randomization and blinding to eliminate investigator bias?

We review studies for some selected surgical procedures here and identify how some of these factors may have influenced the observed outcome.

Clinical Studies, Epidural

Lower Extremity Amputation

There are a number of pain problems that have been described following lower extremity amputation, most commonly stump pain and phantom limb pain. Epidural analgesia and anesthesia have been advocated as a means of decreasing both acute pain and chronic phantom limb pain.[32] There are two prospective, randomized studies of epidural analgesia. One study[33] compared preoperative (18 hours) plus intraoperative epidural analgesia with bupivacaine and morphine (n = 29) to a control group that had an epidural catheter placed and dosed with saline (n = 31). Both groups received general anesthesia for the amputation and subsequently epidural bupivacaine and morphine postoperatively for a minimum of 2 days. The randomization was not really random in that assignment to treatment group was by alternating assignment (stratified for preoperative pain intensity). Blinding was less than complete. Effective preoperative analgesia was achieved in the epidural group (median Visual Analogue Scale [VAS] = 0) compared to the control group (median VAS = 31). The median postoperative VAS pain scores (stump pain) for the preoperative epidural group was 16 (8-25) and for the control group 15 (10-23). Median daily opioid consumption during the first postoperative week was 80 mg for both groups. There were no significant differences in the prevalence of pain at 12 months (75% vs. 69%). The second study[34] compared epidural 0.17% bupivacaine + diamorphine (0.1 mg/mL) to perineural 0.25% bupivacaine. The epidural group had epidural analgesia for 24 hours preoperatively and intraoperatively, while the perineural catheter was placed intraoperatively and dosed with bupivacaine at the end of the operation. All patients received general anesthesia for the operation. The study was not blinded and the method of randomization was not specified. Postoperative pain scores were lower in the epidural group (median = 1, 0-6) than the perineural group (median = 4, 0-10) using a 0 to 10 VAS scale. Postoperative opioid consumption was not significantly different between the groups, epidural 34 mg (0-143 mg), perineural 20 mg (5-42 mg) in morphine equivalents (time period not specified). There was no difference in the prevalence of phantom limb pain at 12 months (38% vs. 50%).

Both of these studies have problems in that blinding is incomplete or nonexistent, and it is not clear that effective epidural anesthesia was achieved in a significant number of patients. This is evident from both the pain scores and the dosage of opioids used in the postoperative period. The concentration of bupivacaine used (0.25% or 0.17%) is probably not sufficient to achieve a degree of neural blockade necessary to suppress intraoperative central sensitization. Somatosensory evoked potentials remain following higher doses of bupivacaine (see reference 35 for review), and it may be inferred that low-dose bupivacaine may not block sensitization.

Thoracotomy

Epidural anesthesia and analgesia has also been advocated as a technique to decrease acute pain following thoracotomy, and the influence of perioperative epidural analgesia on chronic pain has been assessed in at least two studies. Obata and colleagues[36] randomized patients to either intraoperative and postoperative epidural analgesia with 1.5% mepivacaine (4 mL initial dose followed by 4 mL/hr) or postoperative epidural analgesia with the same medication. Patients received indomethacin suppositories for break-

through pain. The group receiving intraoperative mepivacaine had lower VAS scores during the acute postoperative period. There was not a significant difference in indomethacin usage. The group receiving intraoperative mepivacaine also had a significantly lower pain prevalence at 3 months and 6 months. The prevalence of pain at 6 months for the intraoperative epidural group was 33% while for the postoperative epidural group it was 67%. A subsequent study by Senturk and colleagues[37] used a similar design, but with an additional control group (that did not receive an epidural catheter or epidural analgesics) that received patient-controlled analgesia (PCA) morphine for pain control. These investigators used 0.1% bupivacaine with 0.1 mg/mL morphine (10 mL) as an initial dose either 30 minutes before induction of anesthesia or starting in the postoperative period. The group that had the epidural dosed before surgery received an infusion of 7 mL/hr during the surgery. Both epidural groups received an epidural PCA regimen using 0.1% bupivacaine + 0.05 mg/mL morphine at 5 mL/hr, and patients could administer a 3-mL bolus every 30 minutes. The group receiving intraoperative epidural medication had less acute pain than either the postoperative epidural group or the PCA group. They also had less chronic pain than the PCA group. The prevalence of chronic pain (at 6 months) was 45% for the intraoperative epidural group, 63% for the postoperative epidural group, and 78% for the PCA group.

These studies both found a benefit of initiating epidural analgesia prior to skin incision. The Obata study appears to have been appropriately blinded. They used a relatively higher concentration of local anesthetic, and whether this contributed to their lower (33%) prevalence of chronic pain in their intraoperative epidural group at 6 months compared to Senturk's 45% cannot be ascertained.

Radical Prostatectomy

Gottschalk and colleagues[38] randomized 100 patients scheduled for radical prostatectomy under combined epidural and general anesthesia to one of three treatment groups: postoperative epidural analgesia only, preoperative epidural fentanyl (4 µg/kg) plus supplemental fentanyl (0.75 µg/kg) every 2 hours, or preoperative epidural bupivacaine (0.5% in 5-mL increments) to achieve a sensory level at the fourth thoracic dermatome plus supplemental bupivacaine every two hours or more if necessary by the anesthesia team. All patients received a standard general anesthetic plus 5 mg of epidural morphine at the start of fascial closure. In the postanesthesia care unit, all patients received a patient-controlled epidural infusion of 0.05% bupivacaine with 0.1 mg/mL morphine at 5 mL/hr plus 3 to 5 mL every 20 minutes as needed through the PCA mode. Mean postoperative pain scores were satisfactory (control 21, fentanyl 16, and bupivacaine 12) as assessed with the 100-mm VAS scale. The bupivacaine and fentanyl groups had significantly less postoperative pain than the control group, and the bupivacaine group used less supplemental opioid analgesics. At about 10 weeks follow-up, the control group had a significantly higher prevalence of pain (53%) compared to fentanyl and bupivacaine groups (14%). Blinding was not adequate, and a number of patients were lost to follow-up by 10 weeks.

Colon Resection

Lavand'homme and colleagues[39] randomized 85 patients scheduled for colectomy to one of four groups where the intraoperative and postoperative analgesic regimens were specified: intravenous-intravenous, intravenous-epidural, epidural-epidural, or epidural-intravenous. The intraoperative intravenous regimen consisted of lidocaine, clonidine, and sufentanil; the postoperative intravenous regimen consisted of lidocaine, clonidine, and morphine; the intraoperative epidural regimen consisted of bupivacaine, clonidine, and sufentanil; the postoperative epidural regimen consisted of bupivacaine, clonidine, and sufentanil. The intravenous-intravenous group had significantly more postoperative pain and significantly more tactile hyperalgesia. At 12 months' follow-up the prevalence of pain was as follows: intravenous-intravenous 28%, intravenous-epidural 11%, epidural-epidural 0%, and epidural-intravenous 0%. All patients received intraoperative ketamine at a dose that should suppress hyperalgesia. The study was adequately, but less than completely blinded, and an adequate dose of 0.5% bupivacaine was used intraoperatively. If this study can be replicated in other surgical procedures, then a combination of high-dose (0.5% bupivacaine, up to 20 mL) epidural local anesthesia before surgical incision combined with intraoperative ketamine could be advocated to decrease the prevalence of chronic postoperative pain.

CLINICAL STUDIES, OTHER LOCAL ANESTHETIC BLOCKS

Paravertebral block has been shown to achieve at least as effective postoperative analgesia as epidural analgesia following thoracotomy,[40] but studies of chronic pain are lacking. Katz and colleagues,[26,41] in a small study, were not able to decrease the prevalence of chronic pain using a multimodal set of interventions—intercostal nerve blocks with 0.5% bupivacaine plus indomethacin suppository plus intramuscular morphine. Paravertebral block has been shown to decrease pain following breast cancer surgery,[42] but long-term follow-up studies have not been published. Similarly, thoracic epidural analgesia can decrease postoperative pain following radical mastectomy,[43] but long-term outcome studies are lacking. Anesthetic technique has not had a significant effect on long-term outcome following inguinal hernia repair.[1,44]

Adjuvant Medications

Gabapentin

Gabapentin has been shown to decrease hyperalgesia following experimental pain in humans.[45] Oral gabapentin (400 mg, three times per day) started the night before surgery decreases postoperative systemic analgesic consumption without significantly altering VAS pain scores,[46] and burning pain at 3 months' follow-up is significantly less prevalent. In a follow-up study,[47] the combination of gabapentin and EMLA cream started preoperatively and continued postoperatively plus intraoperative use of ropivacaine resulted in less postoperative pain, less postoperative analgesic consumption, and less pain at 6 months' follow-up (57% vs. 30%). Dirks and colleagues[48] administered 1200 mg of gabapentin before mastectomy and found significantly less pain with movement and less PCA opioid consumption in the postoperative period. There are two recent meta-analyses of gabapentin as an adjuvant analgesic to decrease acute pain.[49,50] Both reviews concluded that gabapentin decreased pain and opioid consumption. Whether this can be generalized to a longer term effect as found by Fassoulaki and colleagues[46] remains to be seen.

Venlafaxine

Although antidepressants are used commonly in the management of chronic pain, there are surprisingly few studies using them to prevent chronic pain. Reuben and colleagues[51] randomized patients scheduled for mastectomy to placebo or venlafaxine for 2 weeks starting the night before surgery. At 6 months, the venlafaxine group had significantly less chest wall pain (55% vs. 19%), arm pain (45% vs. 17%), and axillary pain (51% vs. 19%). Postoperative pain scores and analgesic consumption were not different between the treatments.

Dextromethorphan

NMDA receptor blockers have been shown to inhibit central sensitization in animal models, and may be of benefit in humans. Dextromethorphan is a weak NMDA receptor blocker. In one randomized controlled study,[52] it decreased postoperative opioid consumption following radical mastectomy, but no significant differences in worst pain experienced were noted. Long-term follow-up data were not included.

Ketamine

In a very small study (n = 16), Sano and colleagues[53] reported that patients undergoing thoracotomy randomized to intravenous preoperative ketamine (1 mg/kg) plus a continuous intraoperative infusion

Table 15–3. Clinical Points

1. Chronic pain following surgery is not rare and should be discussed as a risk before surgery.
2. Minimally invasive surgery, performed by experienced surgeons, appears to decrease the risk of chronic pain.
3. For patients undergoing posterolateral thoracotomy, intraoperative plus postoperative epidural analgesia with local anesthetics decreases the prevalence of chronic pain.
4. Adjuvant analgesics have not been adequately studied, but gabapentin and venlafaxine use has been associated with a lower prevalence of chronic pain.
5. Patients vary in their sensitivity to pain and probably in psychological factors that will alter the individual's risk of developing chronic pain.

(1 mg/kg/hr) had less pain on postoperative day 1 and at 4 weeks' follow-up. No long-term follow-up data were provided. Ozyalcin and colleagues,[54] in patients undergoing thoracotomy, compared epidural ketamine to intramuscular ketamine to placebo and found less postoperative epidural patient-controlled epidural analgesic use in the epidural ketamine group. At 1 month follow-up, brush allodynia was less in the ketamine group, but pain scores at that time were not reported.

SUMMARY

From the above studies we come to a number of conclusions (Table 15–3).
- Chronic pain following surgery is far from rare.
- The use of minimally invasive surgical techniques by experienced surgeons should decrease the prevalence of chronic pain.
- For thoracotomy performed by the posterolateral approach, intraoperative combined with postoperative epidural analgesia can decrease the prevalence of chronic pain while also decreasing the extent of postoperative pain. When epidural anesthesia and analgesia are employed, higher concentrations of local anesthetics used intraoperatively appear to have a greater probability of decreasing chronic pain prevalence.
- Adjuvant medications (alpha-blockers, anticonvulsants, antidepressants, NMDA receptor blockers) have not been adequately studied. Recommendations regarding their dosing, route of administration, or duration of treatment need to be determined.
- Individual patient factors are important. These include both pain sensitivity (as measured by thermal pain sensitivity) and personality factors such as neuroticism and somatization.

References

1. Perkins FM, Kehlet H: Chronic pain as an outcome of surgery. Anesthesiology 2000;93:1123-1133.
2. Macrae WA: Chronic pain after surgery. Br J Anaesth 2001:87:88-98.
3. Eisenach JC: Treating and preventing chronic pain: A view from the spinal cord—Bonica Lecture, ASRA Annual Meeting, 2005. Reg Anesth Pain Med 2006;31:146-151.
4. Kehlet H, Jensen TS, Woolf CJ: Persistent postsurgical pain: Risk factors and prevention. Lancet 2006;367:1618-1625.
5. Ong CKS, Lirk P, Seymour RA, et al: The efficacy of preemptive analgesia for acute postoperative pain management: A meta-analysis. Anesth Analg 2005;100:757-773.
6. Møiniche S, Kehlet H, Dahl JB: A qualitative and quantitative systematic review of preemptive analgesia for postoperative pain relief. Anesthesiology 2002;96:725-741.
7. Woolf CJ: Evidence for a central component of postinjury pain hypersensitivity. Nature 1983;308:386-388.
8. Mendell LM, Wall PD: Responses of single dorsal cord cells to peripheral cutaneous unmyelinated fibres. Nature 1965;206:97-99.
9. Woolf CJ: Windup and central sensitization are not equivalent [editorial]. Pain 1996;66:105-108.
10. Devor M, Seltzer Z: Pathophysiology of damaged nerves in relation to chronic pain. In Wall PD, Melzack R, (eds): Textbook of Pain, 4th ed. Edinburgh, Churchill Livingstone, 1999, pp 129-164.
11. Landreneau RJ, Mack MJ, Hazelrigg SR, et al: Prevalence of chronic pain after pulmonary resection by thoracotomy or video-assisted thoracic surgery. J Thorac Cardiovasc Surg 1994;107:1079-1085.
12. Aasvang E, Kehlet H: Chronic postoperative pain: The case of inguinal herniorrhaphy. Br J Anaesth 2005;95:69-76.
13. Neumayer L, Giobbie-Hurder A, Jonasson O, et al: Open mesh versus laparoscopic mesh repair of inguinal hernia. N Engl J Med 2004;350:1819-1827.
14. Birkmeyer JD, Siewers AE, Finlayson EVA, et al: Hospital volume and surgical mortality in the United States. N Engl J Med 2002;346:1128-1137.
15. Birkmeyer JD, Stukel TA, Siewers AE, et al: Surgeon volume and operative mortality in the United States. N Engl J Med 2003;349:2117-2127.
16. Gillion JF, Fagniez PL: Chronic pain and cutaneous sensory changes after inguinal hernia repair: Comparison between open and laparoscopic techniques. Hernia 1999;3:75-80.
17. Dirksen CD, Beets GL, Go PM, et al: Bassini repair compared with laparoscopic repair for primary inguinal hernia: A randomised controlled trial. Eur J Surg 1998;164:439-447.
18. Deysine M, Grimson RC, Soroff HS: Inguinal herniorrhaphy: Reduced morbidity by service standardization. Arch Surg 1991;126:628-630.
19. Kanner R, Martini N, Foley KM: Nature and incidence of post-thoracotomy pain. Proc Am Soc Clin Oncol 1982;1:152-159.
20. Benedetti F, Amanzio M, Casadio C, et al: Postoperative pain and superficial abdominal reflexes after posterolateral thoracotomy. Ann Thorac Surg 1997;64:207-210.
21. Benedetti F, Vighetti S, Ricco C, et al: Neurophysiologic assessment of nerve impairment in posterolateral and muscle-sparing thoracotomy. J Thorac Cardiovasc Surg 1998;115:841-847.
22. Veronesi U, Paganelli G, Viale G, et al: A randomized comparison of sentinel-node biopsy with routine axillary dissection in breast cancer. N Engl J Med 2003;349:546-553.
23. Tasmuth T, Kataja M, Blomqvist C, et al: Treatment-related factors predisposing to chronic pain in patients with breast cancer—a multivariate approach. Acta Oncol 1997;36:625-630.
24. Lasagna L, Beecher HK: The optimal dose of morphine. JAMA 1954;156:230-234.
25. Weis OF, Sriwatanakul K, Alloza JL, et al: Attitudes of patients, housestaff, and nurses toward postoperative analgesic care. Anesth Analg 1983;62:70-74.
26. Katz J, Jackson M, Kavanagh BP, et al: Acute pain after thoracic surgery predicts long-term post-thoracotomy pain. Clin J Pain 1996;12:50-55.
27. Werner MU, Duun P, Kehlet H: Prediction of postoperative pain by preoperative nociceptive responses to heat stimuli. Anesthesiology 2004;100:115-119.
28. Pan PH, Coghill R, Houle TT, et al: Multifactorial preoperative predictors of postcesarean section pain and analgesic requirements. Anesthesiology 2006;104:417-425.
29. Poleschuck EL, Dworkin RH: Risk factors for chronic pain in patients with acute pain and their implications for prevention, psychosocial aspects of pain. In Dworkin RH, Breitbart WS,

(eds): A Handbook for Health Care Providers. Seattle, IASP Press, 2003, pp 589-606.

30. Jorgensen T, Teglbjerg JS, Wille-Jorgensen P, et al: Persisting pain after cholecystectomy: A prospective investigation. Scand J Gastroenterol 1991;26:124-128.

31. Gatchel RJ, Polatin PB, Mayer TG: The dominant role of psychosocial risk factors in the development of chronic low back pain. Spine 1995;20:2702-2709.

32. Bach S, Noreng MF, Tjellden NU: Phantom limb pain in amputees during the first 12 months following limb amputation, after preoperative lumbar epidural blockade. Pain 1988;33: 297-301.

33. Nikolajsen L, Ilkjaer S, Christensen JH, et al: Randomised trial of epidural bupivacaine and morphine in prevention of stump and phantom pain in lower-limb amputation. Lancet 1997; 350:1353-1357.

34. Lambert AW, Dashfield AK, Cosgrove C, et al: Randomized prospective study comparing preoperative epidural and intraoperative perineural analgesia for the prevention of postoperative stump and phantom pain following major amputation. Reg Anesth Pain Med 2001;26:316-321.

35. Lund C: Somatosensory evoked potentials in the assessment of neural blockade. Danish Med Bull 1993;40:266-272.

36. Obata H, Saito S, Fujita N, et al: Epidural block with mepivacaine before surgery reduces long-term post-thoracotomy pain. Can J Anaesth 1999;46:1127-1132.

37. Senturk M, Ozcan PE, Talu GK, et al: The effect of three different analgesia techniques on long-term postthoracotomy pain. Anesth Analg 2002;94:11-15.

38. Gottschalk A, Smith DS, Jobes DR, et al: Preemptive epidural analgesia and recovery from radical prostatectomy. JAMA 1998;279:1076-1082.

39. Lavand'homme P, De Kock M, Waterloos H: Intraoperative epidural analgesia combined with ketamine provides effective preventive analgesia in patients undergoing major digestive surgery. Anesthesiology 2005;103:813-820.

40. Davies RG, Myles PS, Graham JM: A comparison of the analgesic efficacy and side-effects of paravertebral vs epidural blockade for thoracotomy—A systematic review and meta-analysis of randomized trials. Br J Anaesth 2006;96:418-426.

41. Kavanagh BP, Katz J, Sandler AN, et al: Multimodal analgesia before thoracic surgery does not reduce postoperative pain. Br J Anaesth 1994;73:184-189.

42. Kairaluoma PM, Bachman MS, Korpinen AK, et al: Single-injection paravertebral block before general anesthesia enhances analgesia after breast cancer surgery with and without associated lymph node biopsy. Anesth Analg 2004; 99:1837-1843.

43. Doss NW, Ipe J, Rajpal S, et al: Continuous thoracic epidural anesthesia with 0.2% ropivacaine versus general anesthesia for perioperative management of modified radical mastectomy. Anesth Analg 2001;92:1552-1557.

44. Bay-Nielsen M, Perkins FM, Kehlet H: Pain and functional impairment 1 year after inguinal herniorrhaphy: A nationwide questionnaire study. Ann Surg 2001;233:1-7.

45. Werner MU, Perkins FM, Holte K, et al: Effects of gabapentin in acute inflammatory pain in humans. Reg Anesth Pain Med 2001;26:322-328.

46. Fassoulaki A, Patris K, Sarantopoulos C, et al: The analgesic effect of gabapentin and mexiletine after breast surgery. Anesth Analg 2002;95:985-991.

47. Fassoulaki A, Triga A, Melemeni A, et al: Multimodal analgesia with gabapentin and local anesthetics prevents acute and chronic pain after breast surgery for cancer. Anesth Analg 2005;101:1427-1432.

48. Dirks J, Fredensborg BB, Christensen D, et al: A randomized study of the effects of single-dose gabapentin versus placebo on postoperative pain and morphine consumption after mastectomy. Anesthesiology 2002;97:560-564.

49. Seib RK, Paul JE: Preoperative gabapentin for postoperative analgesia: A meta-analysis. Can J Anaesth 2006;53:461-469.

50. Hurley RW, Cohen SP, Williams K, et al: The analgesic effects of gabapentin on postoperative pain: A meta-analysis. Reg Anesth Pain Med 2006; 31:237-247506.

51. Reuben SS, Makari-Judson G, Lurie SD: Evaluation of efficacy of the perioperative administration of venlafaxine XR in the prevention of postmastectomy pain syndrome. J Pain Sympt Manage 2004;27:133-139.

52. Wong C-S, Wu C-T, Yu J-C, et al: Preincisional dextromethorphan decreases postoperative pain and opioid requirement after modified radical mastectomy. Can J Anaesth 1999; 46:1122-1126.

53. Sano M, Inaba S, Yamamoto T, et al: Intra-operative ketamine administration reduced the level of post-thoracotomy pain. Masui-Jpn J Anesth 2005;54:19-24.

54. Ozyalcin NS, Yucel A, Camlica H, et al: Effect of pre-emptive ketamine on sensory changes and postoperative pain following thoracotomy: Comparison of epidural and intramuscular routes. Br J Anaesth 2004;93:356-361.

55. Nikolajsen L, Brandsborg B, Jensen TS, et al: Chronic pain following total hip arthroplasty: A nationwide questionnaire study. Acta Anaesth Scand 2006;50:495-500.

56. Snellingen T, Evans JR, Ravilla T, et al: Surgical interventions for age-related cataract. Cochrane Database Syst Rev 2006; 1:1-28.

57. Nikolajsen L, Sorensen HC, Jensen TS, et al: Chronic pain following caesarean section. Acta Anaesth Scand 2004;48:111-116.

58. Atlas SJ, Keller RB, Wu YA, et al: Long-term outcomes of surgical and nonsurgical management of sciatica secondary to a lumbar disc herniation: 10-year results from the Maine lumbar spine study. Spine 2005;30:927-935.

59. Bruce J, Drury N, Poobalan AS, et al: The prevalence of chronic chest and leg pain following cardiac surgery: A historical cohort study. Pain 2003;104:265-273.

60. Jensen MK, Andersen C: Can chronic poststernotomy pain after cardiac valve replacement be reduced using thoracic epidural analgesia? Acta Anaesth Scand 2004;48:871-874.

61. Hutter J, Miller K, Moritz E: Chronic sequels after thoracoscopic procedures for benign disease. Eur J Cardiothorac Surg 2000;17:687-690.

62. Macrae WA, Davies HTO: Chronic postsurgical pain. In Crombie IK, Croft PR, Linton SJ, et al, (eds): Epidemiology of Pain. Seattle, IASP Press, 1999, pp 125-142.

16 Chronic Pain Management in Children

Santhanam Suresh, Brenda C. McClain, and Sally Tarbell

Chronic pain in children is one of the most ignored and undertreated symptoms of disease. Over the last decade, there have been numerous studies in the literature that have addressed pain in children and its measurement and management.[1,2] In this chapter, we will discuss common chronic pain syndromes in children and their management. Recurrent or persistent pain is seen in 5% to 10% of children sampled at random. One study has demonstrated that 96% of children aged 9 to 13 years experience some type of chronic pain in the past month, with 78% experiencing headaches, 57% experiencing some degree of recurrent pain, and 6% experiencing chronic persistent pain.[3] The most common diagnoses of pediatric pain patients include headache, abdominal pain, chest pain, neuropathic pain, back pain, pelvic pain, and cancer-related pain (Box 16–1).

ASSESSMENT OF CHRONIC PAIN IN CHILDREN

Assessment of chronic pain in childhood starts with a biopsychosocial perspective to take into account the multiple factors that can influence the child's pain experience. Multidimensional models elaborate various biologic, developmental, temperamental, cognitive-behavioral, affective, social, and situational factors that may shape the child's pain experience, and the pathways by which they exert their effects.[4-6] Each domain may become a target of assessment and intervention. Several developmentally sensitive validated instruments are now available to measure the physiologic, sensory, affective, behavioral, interpersonal, and social aspects of children's pain[7] (Table 16–1).

Two standardized interviews for school-age and adolescent children and their parents provide comprehensive yet practical evaluations of the child's chronic pain—the Children's Comprehensive Pain Questionnaire (CCPQ)[8] and the Varni-Thompson Pediatric Pain Questionnaire (VTPPQ).[9] These interviews separately assess the child's and parents' experience of the pain problems with open-ended questions, checklists, and quantitative pain rating scales. Additionally, the Pain Behavior Observation Method is a 10-minute observational pain behavior measure that can be used with children with chronic pain who may have difficulty with self-report measures because of age or cognitive limitations.[10] Recently, there has been promising research on the use of electronic versus paper pain diaries for children with chronic pain: it was found that electronic diaries are feasible[11] and result in greater compliance and accuracy in diary recording as compared with traditional paper diaries in children with recurrent pain.[12]

The well-documented comorbidity between pediatric chronic pain and psychiatric disorders,[13,14] particularly internalizing disorders such as depression and anxiety,[15-18] obligate the clinician to screen for these disorders. The Children's Depression Inventory (CDI)[19] is a widely used self-report questionnaire to assess depression in children aged 7 to 17 years. The Beck Depression Inventory-II can be used with

BOX 16–1. CHRONIC PAIN IN CHILDREN: COMMON DIAGNOSES

Neuropathic pain
  Reflex sympathetic dystrophy
  Peripheral nerve injuries
  Postamputation pain
  Deafferentation pain
Headache
Chest pain
Chronic illness
  Sickle cell crisis
  Cystic fibrosis
  Collagen vascular disease (e.g., juvenile rheumatoid arthritis, systemic lupus erythematosus)
Recurrent abdominal pain
Pelvic pain
Back pain
Cancer-related pain

Table 16-1. Methods for Assessment of Chronic Pain in Children and Adolescents

PAIN MEASURE	DISABILITY OR QUALITY OF LIFE	STRESS AND COPING	ANXIETY	DEPRESSION	FAMILY AND PARENTAL FUNCTIONING	OTHER BEHAVIORAL MEASURES
Varni-Thompson Pediatric Pain Questionnaire (PPQ) Ages: 5-18	Functional Disability Inventory (FDI) Ages: 8-17 +Parent Form	Children's Hassles Scale (CHS) Ages: 8-17	Multidimensional Anxiety Scale for Children (MASC)[80] Ages: 8-19	Children's Depression Inventory (CDI) Ages: 7-17	Family Environment Scale (FES) Ages: Adult	Children's Somaticization Inventory (CSI) Ages: 8-18 (plus parent form)
Children's Comprehensive Pain Questionnaire (CCPQ) Ages: 5-19	Child Health Questionnaire (CHQ)[107] Ages: 5+ (plus parent)	Response to Stress Questionnaire (RSQ) Ages: 11+ (plus parent form)	Self-Report for Childhood Anxiety-Related Disorders (SCARED) Ages: 9-18 (plus parent form)	Beck Depression Inventory-II[156] Ages: 13+	Family Adaptation and Cohesion Scale, II (FACES-II) Ages: Adult	Harter Scales of Perceived Competence for Children Ages: 4-12
Pain diary (written, electronic) Ages: 8+	Pediatric Quality of Life Inventory Generic Core Scales (PedsQL 4.0) Ages: 5-18 (plus parent report ages 2-18)	Pain Coping Questionnaire (PCQ) Ages: 8-18	Spence Children's Anxiety Scale (SCAS) Ages: 8-12 (plus parent form)		Family Crisis-Oriented Personal Evaluation Scales (F-COPES) Ages: Adult	
Pain Behavior Observation Method Ages: 6-17	Quality of Life Pain-Youth (QLP-Y) Ages: 12-18	Pain Response Inventory (PRI)[90] Ages: 8-18	Revised Children's Manifest Anxiety Scale (RCMAS)[81] Ages: 6-19		Symptom Checklist-90-Revised (SCL-90-R) Ages: 13+	
Non-Communicating Children's Pain Checklist (NCCPC-R) Ages: 2-adult	Pediatric Migraine Disability Assessment Scale (PedMIDAS) Ages: 6-18	Pain Catastrophizing Scale (PCS) Ages: 8-16	State-Trait Anxiety Scale for Children (STAIC) Ages: 9-12		Medical Outcomes Survey-Short Form 36 (MOS-SF-36) Ages: Adult	
	Children's Activity Limitations Scale (CALI) Ages: 8-16		Childhood Anxiety Sensitivity Index (CASI) Ages: 7-12			
			Pain-Anxiety Symptoms Scale (PASS) Ages: 8-adult			

adolescents,[20] because some items on the CDI may be less age-appropriate for older adolescents. It is essential also to assess for anxiety symptoms, because pain-related disability has been associated with anxiety sensitivity, a stable predisposition toward fear of anxiety-related sensations,[21] and pain-related fears and avoidance behaviors in both adults and children with chronic pain.[22-24] The Children's Anxiety Sensitivity Index (CASI)[25] is the only instrument thus far developed to assess this characteristic in children, and the Pain-Anxiety Symptoms Scale (PASS)[26] was developed for adults to assess fear of pain, but has been used in children as young as 8 years of age.[24]

There are several well-validated self-report questionnaires that assess anxiety in children (see Table 16–1). Two of the more recently developed instruments, the Self-Report for Child Anxiety Related Disorders (SCARED)[27] and the Spence Children's Anxiety Scale (SCAS),[28] include subscales that distinguish among specific Diagnostic and Statistical Manual of Mental Disorders-IV (DSM-IV) anxiety disorders. The Multidimensional Anxiety Scale for Children (MASC)[29] and the Revised Children's Manifest Anxiety Scale (RCMAS)[30] include subscales that focus on other dimensions of anxiety. These include physical symptoms, social and separation anxiety, and harm avoidance (the MASC), and physiologic symptoms, worry and oversensitivity, and concentration factors (the RCMAS); both also include social desirability items to detect inconsistency or randomness in reporting. The SCAS and SCARED provide both a child and parent form of the instrument, allowing for examination of the convergence or lack thereof between the child's and parent's assessment of the child's anxiety symptoms. The State-Trait Anxiety Inventory for Children (STAIC)[31] provides a state version, which measures situation specific anxiety, and a trait form, which assesses anxiety symptoms that are stable across situations. This particular instrument provides a summary score only.

Factors that have been closely linked with a child's ability to function with chronic pain, such as perceived stress[32-34] and coping,[35-37] can assist in the planning of behavioral interventions. The Pain Coping Questionnaire (PCQ),[38] Pain Response Inventory (PRI),[39] and Pain Catastrophizing Scale for Children (PCS-C)[40] assess pain-specific coping strategies. The Response to Stress Questionnaire (RSQ) has been used to assess coping with abdominal pain, but also has other versions that target other stressors, such as social stress.[41] The identification and modification of maladaptive coping responses constitute core elements of cognitive-behavioral approaches for treating pediatric chronic pain. For example, if the child endorses a catastrophizing coping style, an established risk factor for poor adaptation to chronic pain,[42-44] then this coping style can become a target of treatment.

The ability to function at tasks of daily living is a critically important outcome to assess in the treatment of chronic pain in children and adolescents.

Often, pain cannot be completely relieved and the child must learn to accept, cope, and adapt to the pain so that he or she can participate in normal developmental activities and tasks, such as going to school, participating in extracurricular activities, and developing and sustaining social relationships. Several measures have been developed to assess the child's functional abilities as well as quality of life. A measure that specifically assesses disability associated with chronic pain in children has been developed to assess headache-related disability, the Pediatric Migraine Disability Scale (PedMIDAS).[45] This six-question tool assesses school, recreational, and social areas of participation and/or disability, domains relevant to all children with chronic pain. The Child Activity Limitations Interview (CALI)[46] assesses the impact of recurrent pain on children's daily activities as a way to identify appropriate targets for treatment. Additionally, the Functional Disability Inventory (FDI),[47,48] developed to assess illness-related disability in children and adolescents, is a useful tool in evaluating the functional status of pediatric patients with chronic pain, a particularly important concern in children with pain disorders associated with psychological factors and pain-associated disability syndrome (PADS).[49] Pain-related disability has been found to increase with age,[50] and there is a gender difference that emerges in adolescence, with more girls than boys reporting pain-related functional disability.[50]

Quality of life can also be used in the initial comprehensive assessment of children and adolescents with chronic pain and as an index of treatment progress,[51-53] with one study finding that the quality of life of children with recurrent headaches is similar to that of children with rheumatoid arthritis or cancer.[54] The Quality of Life Pain–Children (QLP-Y)[55] was developed to address quality of life issues particular to chronic pain. The Child Health Questionnaire, both child (CHQ-CF87) and parent report (CHQ-50),[56] as well as the PedsQL[57] are measures that may be used to assess more general quality of life in children with chronic pain, and have the advantage that the scores obtained on these instruments can be compared with standardization samples of scores obtained by children with other medical illnesses.

Other instruments that may further elucidate the psychological factors contributing to the child's behavioral adaptation to chronic pain include the Children's Somatization Inventory (CSI),[58] which measures the child's propensity toward somatization, and the Harter Scales of Perceived Competence,[59-61] which assess the child's judgment about his or her capabilities in important domains such as school performance, peer relationships, and athletic abilities. The child's own judgment of his or her competencies in these domains can be useful in understanding other factors that may contribute to the child's functioning.[62] For example, a child with chronic pain who rates herself or himself as low on social and academic competency may have multiple reasons to avoid returning to school.

Parental or family issues that could impede or support the child's progress with treatment are also important to assess. The Family Environment Scale (FES)[63] and the Family Adaptation and Cohesion Scales II (FACES II)[64] have been used to assess family characteristics, whereas the Family Crisis-Oriented Personal Evaluation Scale (F-COPES)[65] assesses the family's problem solving and coping efforts in relation to a challenging situation, such as having an ill child. At times, the parents themselves may need to be referred for rehabilitation or psychiatric treatment to assist them in their efforts to help their child's rehabilitation. The Symptom Checklist 90-Revised (SCL-90-R)[66] is a useful screen for parental psychiatric symptoms, and the Medical Outcomes Survey, Short Form-36,[67] can be used for assessing parental adaptive functioning as well as disabilities.

Recently, Scharff and colleagues[68] have attempted to identify specific subgroups of pediatric chronic pain patients. Identifying subgroups of adults with chronic pain has proven useful in identifying patients' coping efforts and in determining the most appropriate psychological interventions for them. For example, the West Haven–Yale Multidimensional Pain Inventory (WHYMPI)[69] has been used to identify clinical subgroups of adult chronic pain patients—"adaptive copers," who have good coping and supportive relationships, "dysfunctional copers," who have poor coping skills and are highly stressed, and "interpersonally distressed," who have inadequate social support.[70] These three subgroups have been found in diverse adult populations with chronic pain and are associated with different outcomes for behaviorally based pain treatment programs. Although all three groups were found to benefit from a behavioral intervention, the dysfunctional copers benefited the most, with lower pain scores, decreased impact of the pain on their lives, and decreased depression and negative thoughts.[71] Scharff and colleagues[68] have identified similar subgroups in a population of 117 children with various types of chronic pain conditions: a high-functioning group, a disabled and low-functioning group, and a group with family dysfunction. These strongly resemble the subgroups identified by Turk and Rudy[70] in adult chronic pain patients. Although findings from this study were preliminary and need to be interpreted cautiously, such efforts to distinguish subgroups of children with chronic pain should serve to provide targeted treatments to improve the care of pediatric patients with chronic pain.

Therefore, thorough baseline and ongoing assessment is essential for guiding intervention for chronic pain and evaluating the child's response to treatment. Core assessment elements include the comprehensive evaluation of the child's pain problem and screens for psychiatric comorbidity and functional status (Box 16–2). More intensive screening of the child's perceived stress, competencies, and the parents' and family's functioning add valuable information to treatment planning, especially in the child with long-standing pain problems that have not responded to prior treatment efforts.

BOX 16–2. PEDIATRIC QUESTIONNAIRE COMPONENTS

1. Developmental level
2. Understanding of pain
3. Pain and medical treatment history
4. Interactions with others in relation to pain
5. Affect and behavior
6. Impact of pain on functional abilities
7. Family environment and stresses
8. Coping skills
9. History of psychiatric illness
10. Medical problems

Psychological Methods

A rehabilitative approach that emphasizes improving the child's and family's ability to cope with a chronic condition characterizes the course of most chronic pain treatment programs for children. The focus shifts from the narrow goal of pain reduction that might be used in the treatment of acute pain and broadens to include decreasing pain-related emotional and behavioral disability, thereby increasing the child's functional status.[49,72,73] Psychological pain management methods are directed toward increasing the child's and family's understanding of the child's pain and its treatment, including factors that may reduce or exacerbate the child's pain, and enhancing cognitive-behavioral coping skills so that pain-related discomfort and disability are reduced. Research on the use of psychological therapies has been limited primarily to clinical trials in children with headache.[74] In a meta-analysis conducted to evaluate the efficacy of behavioral intervention for pediatric chronic pain, Eccleston and coworkers[74] have concluded that "There is strong evidence that psychological treatment, primarily relaxation and cognitive behavioural therapy, are highly effective in reducing the severity and frequency of chronic pain in children and adolescents."

A few promising psychological treatments have also been used for children with disease-related chronic pain, including sickle cell disease,[75-77] recurrent abdominal pain,[78-81] complex regional pain syndrome, type I,[82] musculoskeletal pain,[83,84] and juvenile primary fibromyalgia syndrome,[85,86] and further support the likely efficacy of cognitive-behavioral approaches to pediatric pain management. Although there is evidence to support the use of single behavioral treatment modalities in the treatment of pediatric chronic pain, as in the use of thermal biofeedback and relaxation for recurrent pediatric headache,[87] most treatment programs include a diverse array of techniques that treat chronic pain by modifying children's cognitive, affective, and sensory experiences of pain, their behavior in response to pain, and environmental and social factors that influence the pain experience. Education about chronic pain and problem solving for improving the child's functional status is central to the child's and family's assuming an active role in managing chronic pain. Cognitive techniques are targeted at modifying the child's thoughts about the pain, in particular to increase his or her sense of predictability and control over the pain, to alter memories about painful experiences,[88] and to reduce negative cognitions about pain, especially "catastrophizing."[89] Decreasing somatic preoccupation, pain-related rumination[90] and passive coping, and learning to accept that the pain may persist[91] are also key interventional goals in the psychological management of pain.[37]

Techniques to alter the sensory aspects of chronic pain can include relaxation training, biofeedback, imagery, and hypnosis. Interventions aimed at modifying situational factors that exacerbate chronic pain and disability include contingency or behavioral management methods, modification of activity and rest cycles, and exposure to situations previously avoided because of pain.[72,91] Few component analyses have been conducted to determine which psychological therapies may be most essential in the management of pediatric chronic pain, but it is likely that for most chronic pain conditions, a combination of modalities will provide the best opportunity to effect desired change. Changes in the emphasis of various behavioral components may present the opportunity to individualize treatment for the specific child, taking into account developmental, psychological, parental, and family factors, which may provide a way to tailor treatment to the specific child.

There is growing acknowledgment of the parents' crucial role in successful rehabilitation of children with chronic pain and thus they are increasingly becoming involved as active partners in their child's treatment.[72,79,92] Parental interactions with their child related to pain and family characteristics of children with chronic pain that may be associated with the development of maladaptive coping with pain are areas of active research.[93-95] Particular parent behaviors have been identified as influencing the child's coping with pain. For example, parental attention has been found to be associated with increased symptom complaints in children with recurrent abdominal pain.[96] Walker and colleagues[96] found that girls with functional abdominal pain are more vulnerable than boys to the symptom-reinforcing effects of parental attention. Interestingly, although the children with pain rated the parental distraction strategy as helpful, their patients rated distraction as having greater potential for a negative impact on their child than attention. Such findings help inform the behavioral intervention with children with chronic pain and their families, because the parents' beliefs in the most effective pain management strategies would need to be targeted in any intervention designed to increase the functional abilities of children with chronic functional abdominal pain.

Several methods for the delivery of psychological interventions for recurrent or chronic pain in children have been shown to be effective, including those that involve intensive inpatient[92,97] or outpatient treatment,[72,78] those that are self-administered,[98] school-based,[99,100] Internet-based,[101] or CD-ROM–based,[102] and those that involve minimal clinic contact with home-based practice.[103,104] The variety of methods for the delivery of these interventions offer opportunities to reach a broad population of children with chronic pain, thus increasing the potential to reach many more children than can be treated in specialized pediatric pain treatment centers. Optimally, the child's school and other caretakers are included in the treatment team to ensure a consistent and comprehensive approach to the child's pain and disability. For example, if a child's pain management involves strategies to cope with stress and headache pain at school, then the school nurse can prompt the child to use these strategies, rather than defaulting to having parents pick the child up from school to rest at home (see Brown[105] for a review of school issues related to pediatric pain). Complementary therapies such as occupational and physical therapies, massage, and acupuncture are increasingly available to children seen in chronic pain clinics, but there is limited literature thus far to document the efficacy of these treatments in pediatric patients.[106]

The complex nature of chronic pain in children creates many challenges in regard to its assessment and treatment, but this same complexity can be exploited to provide the most efficacious methods for pain control and functional rehabilitation. Multidimensional assessment provides the foundation for optimal pain management and functional rehabilitation of chronic pain in children. Psychological interventions include a diverse array of techniques that treat chronic pain by modifying children's cognitive, affective, and sensory experiences of pain, their behavior in response to pain, and environmental and interactional factors that influence the pain experience. Without addressing the factors that may contribute to pain and pain-related disability, medical treatment of a child's chronic pain may result in poorer outcomes. Research informed by multidimensional models of pediatric chronic pain can guide investigators in efforts to identify effective pain treatments as well as the individual children for whom they work best. Finally, the lessons learned about optimal management of pain in children need to be practiced to the fullest extent possible so that the incidence of their suffering and disability may be diminished. For further reviews of psychological interventions for pediatric chronic pain, see McGrath and Holahan,[107] Hillier and McGrath,[108] and Eccleston and coworkers.[74]

CHRONIC PAIN SYNDROMES

We will briefly discuss the diagnosis and management of some common chronic pain syndromes diagnosed in pediatric patients who are referred to the Chronic Pain Clinic for management. Prior to their visit, a questionnaire is sent to all patients by e-mail or regular mail. The pain clinic staff, prior to the appointment, reviews the questionnaire and results of imaging studies so that the need for additional services that may be needed on the first appointment can be assessed. This has also reduced the need for multiple visits prior to a treatment game plan because of the failure to bring images to the initial visit.

Complex Regional Pain Syndrome Type I (CRPS I or Reflex Sympathetic Dystrophy)

Neuropathic conditions are those that are associated with injury, dysfunction, or altered excitability of portions of the peripheral or central nervous system. Complex regional pain syndrome, type I (CRPS I), or reflex sympathetic dystrophy (RSD), is defined by the International Association for the Study of Pain (IASP) as "A continuous pain in a portion of an extremity after trauma, which may include fracture but does not involve major nerve lesions and is associated with sympathetic hyperactivity." This is often seen with any traumatic injury and presents as pain and discoloration in a swollen extremity. The incidence of neuropathic pain is higher in teenage girls than in boys.[82,109] Because of the underdiagnosis of this syndrome in children, the general incidence in the pediatric population is often underreported compared with adults. Although RSD has been reported in a 2½-year-old girl,[110] it is generally seen in children older than 9 years and is more frequently seen in girls 11 to 13 years old.[82,109] RSD is seen in girls of middle-class families, commonly overachievers who often participate in competitive athletic programs. This explanation underscores the psychological contribution to this disease state. Pain often persists, despite the absence of ongoing tissue injury or inflammation.

The mechanisms that generate neuropathic pain are varied and complex. Injuries to peripheral nerves may involve crush, transection, compression, demyelination, axonal degeneration, inflammation, ischemia, or other processes. The primary loci of increased irritability following peripheral nerve injury may be at several levels in the nervous system including axonal sprouts or neuroma, the dorsal root ganglia, the dorsal horn of the spinal cord, or sites more rostral in the central nervous system.[111,112] Central neural causes and peripheral small-fiber neuropathy have been implicated in the mechanisms leading to neuropathic pain. Although neuropathic pain has generally been regarded as psychogenic in children, it is also important to understand that neuropathic pain rarely keeps the subject from harm because it involves erroneous generation of impulses.

Evaluation of Neuropathic Pain

History
A detailed history of the nature of injury, type and duration of pain, relieving and aggravating factors, and dependence on medications is mandatory prior to the evaluation.

Physical Evaluation
A *thorough and systematic neurologic examination* should be performed. A complete evaluation of motor, sensory, cerebellar, cranial nerve, reflex, cognitive, and emotional functioning is important. A concerted effort must be made to rule out the rare, but possible, malignancy or central degenerative disorder.

Sympathetically mediated pain is often diagnosed using clinical and diagnostic criteria based on responses to sympathetic blocks. However, the diagnosis of sympathetically mediated pain cannot be based on responses to sympathetic blocks alone.

The *strength* of the extremity should be evaluated on several occasions. It is important to compare the strength in the contralateral extremity, because CRPS I can occur in both extremities at the same time.

Allodynia is pain that can be produced by innocuous stimuli such as stroking, which elicits excruciating pain (e.g., stroking the skin with a feather). This is very characteristic of neuropathic pain. Tactile allodynia in the absence of skin problems signifies the presence of neuropathic pain. This is a classic diagnostic criterion for neuropathic pain.

Hyperalgesia means that a patient has a decreased threshold to pain. Hyperalgesia to cold is seen more frequently than to warmth. The distribution is generally not restricted to particular dermatomes, as in an adult, and is along a glove-and-stocking distribution.

Nerve conduction studies may provide some insight into the location and type of nerve injury.[113] However, the use of invasive electromyography (EMG) may not be acceptable to children.

Quantitative sensory testing (QST) with thermal and vibration sensations and thermal pain detection thresholds in the affected limbs can be compared with data from normal healthy children. The patient's rating of pain and quality of pain can be assessed. Mechanical static allodynia and dynamic allodynia can be measured. Quantitative thermal and vibration detection thresholds can be measured. Although this involves cumbersome equipment, bedside QST may have a greater role in diagnosis of CRPS I in children and adolescents.[114]

Bone scans may be helpful in the diagnosis of CRPS I. Although there are not enough data on their diagnostic accuracy in children, they are nevertheless performed in children and adolescents with CRPS I. A decrease in isotope uptake is noticed with CRPS I.[115]

Diagnosis
Diagnosis is made usually on the basis of symptoms and signs (Box 16-3). The characteristics of pain, sensory, motor, and sudomotor changes may vary among patients[82]; also, there are differences that can be noted between neuropathic and nociceptive pain (Table 16-2). The diagnosis in children is made using physical signs and symptoms. A test with phentolamine has been used to confirm the diagnosis and to predict the response to a sympathetic blockade.[116]

Bone scans may offer some information about CRPS I. Disturbed vascular scintigraphy with increased pooling in the initial phase and hyperfixation on bone scintigraphy may denote the presence of CRPS I. The IASP criterion for CRPS I is applicable to children and adolescents (see Box 16–3). Classic signs and symptoms of the various stages of CRPS I are presented in Table 16–3.[117]

Treatment of Neuropathic Pain

The management of neuropathic pain (Box 16–4) can be frustrating for the caregiver as well as the patient. There is no single therapy that can uniformly provide relief to these patients. Much of the management

---

BOX 16–3. INTERNATIONAL ASSOCIATION FOR THE STUDY OF PAIN DIAGNOSTIC CRITERIA FOR COMPLEX REGIONAL PAIN SYNDROME

1. The presence of an initiating noxious event or cause of immobilization
2. Continuous pain, allodynia, or hyperalgesia in which the pain is disproportionate to any known inciting event
3. Evidence at some time of edema, changes in blood flow, or abnormal sudomotor activity in the region of pain
4. Diagnosis excluded by the existence of other conditions that would otherwise account for the degree of pain and dysfunction

Adapted from Bruehl S, Harden RN, Galer BS, et al: External validation of IASP diagnostic criteria for complex regional pain syndrome and proposed research diagnostic criteria. International Association for the Study of Pain. Pain 1999;81:147-154.

BOX 16–4. MANAGEMENT OF NEUROPATHIC PAIN

Nonpharmacologic Treatment
Offered to all patients
Hypnosis, biofeedback, visual guided imagery (psychologist)
TENS; physical therapy, occupational therapy
Individual and family therapy (day program if required)

Pharmacologic Therapy
Acetaminophen, NSAIDs
Tricyclic antidepressants (e.g., amitriptyline, nortriptyline, doxepin); start at low doses, 0.1 mg/kg, and advance slowly
Anticonvulsant (gabapentin, pregabalin, carbamazepine, phenytoin, clonazepam), systemic local anesthetics (mexiletine, lidocaine)
Opioids (morphine, methadone given PO or IV or via regional technique [intrathecal] especially in cancer patients)

Regional Blockades for Chronic Pain
Epidural, subarachnoid and sympathetic plexus, peripheral catheter blockade
Sympathetic blockade for RSD
    Longer than 6 yr under sedation
    Less than 6 yr under general anesthesia
    Continuous catheter techniques may be used for 5-7 days
    Epidural and subarachnoid block for cancer patients: left in place for longer periods by tunneling subcutaneously
    Neurolytic blockade for cancer

NSAIDs, nonsteroidal anti-inflammatory drugs; RSD, reflex sympathetic dystrophy; TENS, transcutaneous electrical nerve stimulation.

Table 16–2. Differences between Neuropathic and Nociceptive Pain

CHARACTERISTIC	NEUROPATHIC PAIN	NOCICEPTIVE PAIN
Description of pain	Burning, lancinating; pins and needles	Varied
Tactile allodynia	Present	Absent
Duration and intensity of pain	Increases with duration	Decreases
Opioid-resistant	Present	Absent
Use of tricyclic antidepressants	Useful	Not useful

Table 16–3. Symptoms and Changes in Stages of Chronic Regional Pain Syndrome, Type I

CHARACTERISTIC	ACUTE	DYSTROPHIC	ATROPHIC
Pain	Hyperpathic, burning	Chronic	
Blood flow	Increased	Decreased	No change
Temperature	Increased	Decreased	No change
Hair and nail growth	Increased	Decreased	Chronic change
Sweating	Decreased	Increased	No change
Edema	None	Brawny edema	Wasted muscles, atrophic skin
Color	Red	Cyanotic	Atrophic

depends on the response to various clinical measures. The titration of medications is limited by the presence of side effects and complications. One of the main goals is to return the child to a functional state and to school. Definitive resolution of the pain is not always possible. Most management techniques have been extrapolated from work done in adult patients.[118] It is important to gain the trust of the patient and parents. Family dynamics are important, because the added burden of familial disharmony or parental abuse can increase the symptoms. There seems to be a greater propensity for enmeshment in these families. The algorithm shown in Figure 16–1 is used by our pain clinic.[119]

Psychological and Behavioral Therapy

Behavioral measures are extremely useful in the management of neuropathic pain. Family therapy is helpful for the family to cope with the situation.[120] We generally advocate a consultation with a medical psychologist on their first visit to the pain clinic. We have used a number of techniques, including biofeedback, visual guided imagery, and structured counseling regarding coping skills. The introduction of a day program for acute psychological intervention has been valuable for some of our patients, who may have significant psychiatric illness. See earlier for complete explanations of various psychological interventions.

Physical Therapy

Physical therapy is an integral part of management of these patients. TENS is widely used and its efficacy has been studied in adults as well as children; therapeutic benefits with the TENS unit in children with RSD have been reported by Kesler and colleagues.[121] We use TENS units extensively in our practice, along with physical therapy. Physical therapy consists of active and passive physical modalities. The program of physical therapy is geared toward individual patients and the goal is to allow the child to participate in as many activities as possible. It may be necessary to have input from a pediatric physical therapist or an occupational therapist for adequate management. Other modalities commonly used include desensitization, warm and cold baths, massage therapy, and heat therapy. We have used these therapies for most children with CRPS I. A dedicated physical therapist–occupational therapist who works with our pain management team has been essential for continued care of these children.

Medical Therapy

Most of the work in children has been extrapolated from the experience in adults. It is best to start with nonsteroidal anti-inflammatory drugs (NSAIDs) in moderate doses, followed by other medications (see Box 16–4). There are certain differences between adult and pediatric patients:

1. Neuropathic pain may differ in children than in adults in its presenting symptoms.
2. There may be a difference in the response to medication.
3. There may be unrecognized toxicity to medications.

Tricyclic Antidepressants. Adults are frequently placed on tricyclic antidepressants (TCAs) for the management of neuropathic pain.[122] Despite the lack of adequate controlled studies in pediatric patients, TCAs are widely prescribed for several forms of neuropathic pain.[123] The choice of agents depends on the side effects. If the patient is unable to sleep at night, amitriptyline may be a good choice. On the other hand, if the patient experiences anticholinergic side effects, such as dry mouth and morning sleepiness, an agent such as nortriptyline or desipramine can be used. A thorough examination of the cardiovascular system is necessary prior to instituting TCA treatment because of associated tachydysrhythmias and other conduction abnormalities of the heart, particularly prolonged Q-T syndrome.[124,125]

Anticonvulsants. Some children seem to benefit from the use of anticonvulsants for the management of neuropathic pain.[126] Gabapentin, pregabalin, carbamazepine, clonazepam, and phenytoin are the most commonly used. Regular monitoring of drug levels, blood counts, and liver function is recommended for these patients. Carbamazepine and gabapentin have been shown to be useful in neuropathic pain.[127-131]

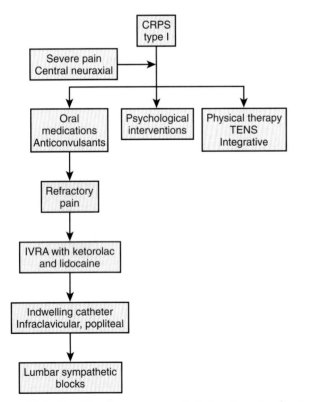

Figure 16–1. Algorithm for management of chronic regional pain syndrome (CRPS) type I. IVRA, Intravenous Regional Anesthesia; TENS, transcutaneous electrical nerve stimulation.

The use of gabapentin has been shown to be effective for the management of neuropathic pain.[128-131] More recently, although controlled trials are not available in children, pregabalin has been used in our practice and has been a welcome addition for the management of chronic pain in children.[132]

Opioids. Opioids can be helpful in the management of neuropathic pain, especially for cancer-related neuropathic pain (see later). Arner[116] has shown that there are several types of neuropathic pain resistant to the effects of opioids and that opioids reduce the emotional rather than the sensory aspect of pain. It is optimal to titrate the narcotic in a graded fashion to optimize the effect. Sedation is a side effect that may be desirable, especially in cancer-related neuropathic pain and, in some cases, may need to be antagonized with the addition of amphetamines.[133] For children with noncancer neuropathic pain, it is desirable to try nonopioid techniques, including behavior modification, prior to starting on opioids. We prefer using oral opioids such as morphine, hydromorphone, methadone, and oxycodone, with the doses titrated individually to each patient.

Systemic Vasodilators. Several patients with RSD have benefited from the use of vasodilators such as prazosin, nifedipine, or phenoxybenzamine.[134] However, overwhelming adverse effects of orthostatic hypotension often offset the efficacy of this therapy.

Sympathetic Blocks. The most common treatment for these syndromes is to provide interruption of the apparent pathologic reflexes by sympathetic blocks (Box 16–5). Although relief of pain after a sympathetic block may demonstrate the presence of sympathetic-mediated pain, the nonresponse may only suggest sympathetically independent pain and may still be a presentation of CRPS I. With serial blocks, the patient should notice pain relief that increases with each block and prevents the pain from returning to its original level. Concurrent physical therapy is indicated to improve range of motion and improve function. We institute physical therapy at the time

of provision of a block to enhance patient experience with therapy (see Fig. 16–1).

We prefer intravenous regional Bier blocks for the management of pain in RSD.[119] Using mild sedation, and after venous drainage of the extremity, a tourniquet is placed on the proximal end of the extremity. Intravenous local anesthetic with ketorolac is injected into a distal vein. The tourniquet is kept inflated for about 30 minutes and then slowly released. A single block has provided total pain relief for some patients in our pain clinic.

An alternate approach to the management of the peripheral manifestations of neuropathic pain is to use adrenergic blocking drugs such as guanethidine[135] or bretylium[136] as an intravenous regional technique. Occasionally, in the patient with upper extremity RSD, a stellate ganglion block[137] may be necessary to alleviate pain. Lumbar sympathetic blocks[138] and epidural blocks[139] with local anesthetics are used if the initial Bier block with local anesthetic and ketorolac is not effective. We have used an epidural analgesia at the time of diagnosis in certain cases with severe refractory pain to initiate physical therapy. There have been reports of the use of intrathecal analgesia to treat refractory CRPS I.[140,141] Several sympathetic blocks at intervals of 1 to 2 weeks may be necessary to see improvement in symptoms. Peripheral nerve block catheters have been used successfully to treat patients with CRPS I.[142] The management of pain secondary to physical therapy is the main goal for placement of these catheters. Although there are no prospective randomized trials in children to evaluate the efficacy of sympathetic blocks, we believe that they have a role in the management of pediatric CRPS I. The use of sympathetic blocks may be ineffective in the management of CRPS I.

Prognosis

Varni and colleagues[143] have reported uniform improvement in their series of patients in a prolonged course of physical therapy and inpatient rehabilitation programs. Ashwal and associates[144] have concluded that the prognosis of childhood RSD is more favorable than that of adult RSD. Neuropathic pain can be puzzling and frustrating and requires a strong alliance with the family and the patient. A multidisciplinary algorithmic management approach using available techniques can be helpful. The use of physical therapy and psychological management must be stressed while managing these patients.

BOX 16–5. REGIONAL ANESTHESIA FOR COMPLEX REGIONAL PAIN SYNDROME TYPE I

IV regional anesthesia—guanethidine, bretylium, lidocaine-ketorolac
Epidural analgesia (continuous)
Intrathecal analgesia
Sympathetic chain blocks
  Stellate ganglion blocks
  Lumbar sympathetic blocks
Indwelling regional anesthesia catheters
  Brachial plexus catheters
  Sciatic nerve catheters

Headaches in Children

Few physicians discussed headaches in children until 1873, when William Henry Day, a British pediatrician, devoted a chapter to the subject of headaches in his book, *Headaches in Children: Essays on Diseases in Children.*[145] In 1967, Freidman published available data in *Headaches in Children*.[146] These have provided impetus to the many subsequent papers dealing with headaches in children. Each year, at least 80% of the population will suffer from headaches. However, many child care providers do not believe that children have an appreciable number of headaches. In a study of 9000 children in Sweden, Bille[147] reported migraine headaches in 3.9% of children younger than 12 years and an incidence of 6.8% of nonmigrainous headaches daily. This translates to a greater number of days lost in school from absenteeism because of the debilitating nature of the headaches. A more recent study by the same group has demonstrated that almost 40% of these children with headaches in childhood progress to a headache-free state in adulthood.[148] Boys seemed to have a greater possibility of experiencing a decreased incidence of headaches in adulthood compared with girls.

Chronic daily headache is classified as headaches that occur at least 15 times monthly for a period of 3 months. The headaches can last for more than 4 hours daily.[149] Chronic daily headaches may be present for 24 hours, with waxing and waning of the pain symptoms. The difficulty for the physician arises from the fact that the headache may be functional.

Examination

A thorough physical examination helps determine the nature of the headache. Physical examination, including a thorough neurologic examination and blood pressure measurement, is mandated for children with headaches. Neuroimaging may be needed in some cases and a lumbar puncture may be advised for some patients. In children with chronic intracranial hypertension caused by pseudotumor cerebri, magnetic resonance imaging (MRI) may be indicated to rule out sinus thrombosis, which may lead to increased intracranial pressure. It appears that patients with chronic daily headaches or migraine are prone to developing postmeningeal puncture headaches; hence, the need for lumbar punctures should be judiciously advised.[149]

Pathophysiology

A headache is modulated by extracranial as well as intracranial structures (Box 16–6).

Classification

The classification of headaches is based on the presumed location of the abnormality, its origin, its pathophysiology, or the symptom complex with which the patient presents. The International Headache Society has recently updated its classification. By plotting the severity of a headache over time, headaches can be classified into five major categories (Box 16–7).

BOX 16–6. PATHOPHYSIOLOGY OF HEADACHE

Pain-sensitive headache
  Extracranial
    Skin
    Subcutaneous tissue
    Muscles
    Mucous membrane
    Teeth
    Larger vessels
  Intracranial
    Vascular sinuses
    Larger veins
    Dura surrounding the veins
    Dural arteries
    Arteries at the base of the brain
Pain-insensitive headache
  Brain
  Cranium
  Most of the dura
  Ependyma
  Choroid plexus

BOX 16–7. CLASSIFICATION OF HEADACHES: DIFFERENTIAL DIAGNOSIS

Acute headache
  Systemic illness
  Subarachnoid hemorrhage
  Trauma
  Toxins such as lead or carbon monoxide
  Electrolyte imbalances
  Hypertension
Acute recurrent headache
  Migraine
Chronic progressive headaches
  Organic brain disease
  Ventriculoperitoneal shunt malfunction
Chronic nonprogressive headache
  Functional in quality
Mixed headache

Evaluation

A detailed questionnaire should be routinely used to evaluate headaches in children. A thorough physical examination and history taking should be carried out, including blood pressure measurements. Neuroimaging and occasionally lumbar puncture may need to be performed in certain cases. If pseudotumor cerebri is a consideration, a venous angiogram may be needed to rule out sinus thrombosis. Benign intracranial hypertension or idiopathic intracranial hypertension is a constellation of symptoms and signs that includes headaches, diplopia, tinnitus, and eye pain. These usually have normal imaging results.[149] Although a diagnostic lumbar puncture may be needed in some settings, patients with chronic daily headaches may be prone to postlumbar puncture headaches.[149]

Comorbid symptoms coexist with headaches. The most common comorbidity is sleep deprivation. Delayed sleep is a common disorder seen in children with headaches. Many also have symptoms of dizziness, which may be associated with postural hypotension and tachycardia (postural orthostatic tachycardia syndrome [POTS]).[150] Orthostatic hypotension should be treated by increasing fluid intake and, in some cases, a beta blocker may be needed. Other specific questions about neurologic symptoms such as ataxia, lethargy, seizures, or visual impairment should be part of the screening for children with headaches. Important medical problems such as hypertension, sinusitis, and other emotional disturbances have to be evaluated. A history of a severe headache without a previous history of headache, pain that awakens a child from sleep, headaches associated with straining, change in chronic headache patterns, or the presence of a headache with associated symptoms such as nausea or vomiting suggests a more pathologic origin to the headache and has to be carefully evaluated (Box 16–8).

BOX 16–8. EVALUATION FOR HEADACHE

General Physical Examination
Blood pressure, postural hypotension
Careful skin exam for café au lait spots, adenoma sebaceum, hypopigmented lesions, petechiae

Neurological Examination
Cranial circumference measurement
Bruit on auscultation of the cranium
Tenderness in the sinuses or presence of occult trauma indicating a battered child
Funduscopic examination—optic atrophy, papilledema
Cranial nerve examination for the presence of damage
Mental status
Alteration in language skills
Alteration in the gait
Cranial nerve examination

Laboratory Tests
Electroencephalography—very nonspecific
CT scan especially with contrast—may be useful in determining vascular abnormalities
MRI—best for delineating abnormalities in the sella turcica, posterior fossa, temporal lobes
Lumbar puncture helpful in determining acute infectious causes
Psychological tests to determine whether there is psychological basis for the headache
Tilt test—if postural hypotension is present (postural orthostatic tachycardia syndrome)
Angiography (venous or arterial) if intracranial pathology is suspected.

It is imperative to evaluate all images prior to the patient's appointment to the pain clinic. We routinely review the patient's clinical status and computed tomography (CT) and MRI scans with the neurosurgeon and neuroradiologist. Once it has been established by the neurosurgical service that the headaches are not related to increased intracranial pressure, we schedule the patient for a visit to the Chronic Pain Clinic. The following information is obtained:

1. Neurologic status, including a complete neurologic examination
2. Physical status of the patient (i.e., Is the patient actively mobile?)
3. Does the headache prevent the child from performing normal activities (e.g., interacting with others, participating in sports)?
4. Is there a history of school absenteeism?
5. What is the child's interaction with the parents and siblings at home?
6. Are there any relieving factors for the headache?
7. Has the child been placed on any medications for pain? Has there been any improvement at all in the clinical characteristics of the pain?
8. Are there any postural changes with headaches? Is there diurnal variation with the headaches?
9. Family history is crucial in these children; a family history of migraine is suggestive of childhood migraine.

Having answered some or all of these questions, we then offer various modalities in a stepwise fashion based on the pain status. We use the algorithm shown in Figure 16–2 for the management of headaches.

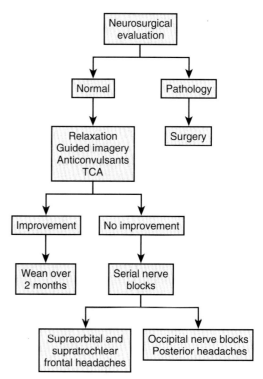

Figure 16–2. Algorithm for headache management. If the patient experiences nausea, vomiting, and/or other signs of increased intracranial pressure, neurosurgical consultation should be obtained. TCA, tricyclic antidepressants.

We have treated several patients who had been debilitated because of headaches and have now resumed normal activity. Most of these children also have musculoskeletal problems. Hence, the addition of physical therapy has been shown to increase muscle strength and help in the recovery of these patients. We have recently added complementary medicine as part of our treatment algorithm; we routinely offer acupuncture as well as massage therapy for all our patients with headaches. Most of these children have significant neck and back problems, which predispose them to a continuum of pain, so this early intervention helps many of them return to their normal activities. The intervention of our medical psychologist proficient in pain management has been vital to recovery. This not only helps when dealing with family dynamics but also helps in the management of pain by teaching the patient coping mechanisms, visual guided imagery, and biofeedback techniques.

Functional Abdominal Pain

The term *recurrent abdominal pain syndrome* (RAPS) has been altered to functional abdominal pain (FAP) and recurrent abdominal pain (RAP), two different entities with similar presenting signs and symptoms. The most important aspect of managing recurrent abdominal pain is to rule out pathology. Once this has been done, and the patient has had daily pain for 3 months lasting for at least 3 hours, a diagnosis of recurrent abdominal pain syndrome is established. FAP syndrome is frequently associated with psychological changes that may overwhelm the family. A recent study has compared the association of irritable bowel syndrome and loose stools and found the presence of altered family dynamics associated with FAP to be more common than with RAP.[151] Functional abdominal pain responds well to small doses of the TCA amitryptyline.[152,153] A thorough psychological profile, along with interventions including biofeedback and guided imagery, has been very effective in managing these patients. We have recently included the use of massage and acupuncture in the management of these children, with increasing success.

Chest Pain

The presence of chest pain or chest wall pain is seen commonly in adolescents. They usually present to the emergency room with acute exacerbation of pain symptoms. In a study conducted in Belgium, patients were 3 to 15 years of age, with a greater preponderance of males.[154]

Causes

The most common causes of chest pain include chest wall pain (64.5%) and cardiac (5%), respiratory (13%),

Table 16–4. Causes of Chest Pain

CAUSE	MANIFESTATIONS
Chest wall pain	Musculoskeletal chest wall pain, costochondritis, Tietze's syndrome
Respiratory disease	Pneumonia, pleuritis, asthma, upper respiratory infection
Psychogenic	Anxiety, depression, hyperventilation
Traumatic	Soft tissue injury, pneumothorax
Cardiac	Carditis, arrhythmia, mitral valve prolapse, ischemia
Digestive	Esophagitis, gastritis
Miscellaneous	Sickle cell disease, cystic fibrosis–related

gastrointestinal (3%), psychological (9%), and traumatic causes (5%). Younger children were more likely to have respiratory problems and older children were more likely to have psychogenic problems. Each has similar presenting symptoms, although the diagnostic workup may be different based on physical findings (Table 16–4).

Chest Wall Pain
This is most commonly seen in teenagers and presents with acute pain along the costal margin. The most common chest wall pain is costochondritis. The diagnosis is made by eliciting pain along the costochondral margin with deep pressure. Other chest wall pain syndromes include Tietze's syndrome[155] and slipping rib cage syndrome.[155] Management usually consists of the use of NSAIDs. We have had several patients with slipping rib cage syndrome who have not had relief, despite resection of the slipping rib. In addition, we use alternative therapies, including acupuncture and massage therapy, for these children.

Pulmonary Causes
The most common respiratory emergency presenting with acute chest wall pain is in children with acute asthma attacks who may have primarily chest pain, without actual respiratory embarrassment. Other common causes include bronchial pneumonia and respiratory illnesses, including severe lower respiratory tract illnesses. Management includes treating the respiratory illness with antibiotics or anticholinergics and inhaled bronchodilators.

Cardiac Causes
Cardiac reasons for pain are probably the most compelling reasons for a good diagnostic workup. The most common causes of chest pain include mitral valve prolapse and the presence of dysrhythmias. Workup may include echocardiography, electrocardiography and, in some cases, Holter monitoring for diagnosis. It is important to address the pain in an expeditious manner.

Abdominal Causes
Gastroesophageal reflux is the most common cause of continued chest pain in children. In addition, the presence of eosinophilic esophagitis should be ruled

out by upper endoscopy, because this can usually be treated.

Psychogenic Causes

Usually there is a family history of intercurrent cardiac illness, including a recent myocardial infarction in an older family member or possibly the death of a family member from cardiac causes that can lead to chest wall pain. In most cases, adequate family therapy should be offered. With increasing diagnostic methodologies available, the diagnosis is far more accurate in these children than several decades ago.

Back Pain

Back pain is a common problem in adults and is now becoming a serious health problem in children.[156-159] With high-impact sports that involve a greater degree of stress to the back muscles, such as gymnastics, children seem to have a higher degree of injuries to their backs. Common back problems include spondylolysis,[160] spondylolisthesis, disk degeneration, disk herniation,[161,162] tumors of the spinal cord, and other diseases, including sickle cell disease. Classic symptoms of herniation may be seen, including radicular symptoms (see Chapters 17–19, 55–62, and 70 for more detailed discussion of back pain and its treatment). Management in children is usually conservative, with an emphasis on exercise for the back. We have found that a small segment of these children may require a lumbar epidural steroid injection. Alternative medicine, including the use of massage therapy and acupuncture, is used extensively for pain management in children and adolescents with back pain.

Pelvic Pain

Pelvic pain is often reported in female adolescents. A thorough history has to be obtained, including a history of sexual activity. Children who have a history of sexual abuse have a greater preponderance for developing chronic pelvic pain.[163] Although not common, there is a subpopulation of these adolescent females with a history of endometriosis. This could lead to severe pelvic pain and may have to be treated more aggressively than the occasional pelvic pain. Alteration of the ovulatory cycles using birth control pills, as well as the use of strong NSAIDs, should be prescribed for these patients. We have had success with the use of active massage therapy and physical therapy as adjuncts for the management of these patients.

Cancer-Related Pain

The 5-year survival rate from childhood cancer has improved from 20% in 1954 to over 80% in 2000 for children 0 to 14 years of age. However, cancer remains the second leading cause of death in children. Over 12,000 children are diagnosed annually with cancer and 2,200 children die each year from this disease.[164]

Pain is a common symptom during different phases of cancer treatment. The incidence of cancer-related pain in children at the time of diagnosis is estimated to be 75%, with ongoing pain affecting 50%.[165,166] However, the incidence of pain at the terminal phase of disease is likely to be greater than 89%.[167] Pain caused by treatment and procedural pain are cited as the most frequent types of pain experienced by children with cancer.[168] Although more than 90% of pain complaints can be managed by the implementation of the World Health Organization (WHO) cancer pain ladder paradigm, there is a significant number of children who may require additional therapies and/or techniques for pain management because of escalating or intractable pain. Only novel allopathic techniques are discussed in this section. The pediatric doses for most medications are off-label recommendations; dosing is based on the current pediatric clinical literature.

Oral Medications

Most pain management is achieved with oral maintenance dosing. Around-the-clock scheduling is supplemented with as-needed analgesic doses for breakthrough pain. Novel oral techniques include sublingual and transmuscosal applications for breakthrough and procedural pain.

Application of sublingual morphine is as effective as intravenous morphine for pediatric postoperative pain.[169] Because sublingual administration avoids hepatic first-pass dosing, it is comparable with intravenous administration. Sublingual morphine may be a suitable alternative to intravenous morphine for pain control in children with cancer-related pain if enteral tolerance or intravenous access is limited. Sublingual buprenorphine, 5 to 7 µg/kg/dose, has demonstrated similar analgesic efficacy in comparison with intravenous morphine, 150 µg/kg.[170] Oxycodone concentrate prepared as 20 mg/mL is appropriate for sublingual application, but small volume changes can mean large dose changes. Using this concentrated formulation, an increment of 0.1 mL, from 0.2 to 0.3 mL, is a 50% increase in dose; an additional 0.1-mL increase, from 0.2 to 0.4 mL, represents a 100% increase or doubling of the dose administered. Thus, to prescribe dosing increments of less than 5 mg may result in variation in the actual amount of oxycodone concentrate delivered. Oxycodone concentrate is not recommended for use in small children.

Intravenous preparations administered by the transmucosal route have been tried with some success. Oral administration of the intravenous formulation of fentanyl can achieve a pharmacokinetic distribution similar to that of oral transmucosal fentanyl citrate (OTFC) lozenges, but there is much interpatient variability. OTFC lozenges have been used for breakthrough pain and procedural pain in children. Oral mucositis pain treated with 200 µg OTFC lozenges is tolerated but ineffective in adult cancer patients.[171] The effective oral dosage range is 10 to 15 μg/kg for buccal application in postoperative pain management.[172] Schechter and colleagues[173] found 15 to 20 μg/kg of OTFC to be effective for pediatric procedural pain but one third of the children experienced vomiting. Transmucosal oxycodone 200 μg/kg provides relief similar to 10 μg/kg of OTFC for procedure-related pain.[174]

Tablets designed for buccal delivery aim to enhance bioavailability and drug uptake and speed onset of pain relief. Hepatic first-pass effects are avoided.[175] Studies on fentanyl effervescent buccal tablets have revealed pain relief onset times of 10 to 15 minutes. The efficacy of the system is pH-dependent because higher plasma levels are achieved at a lower pH. Another benefit of the technique is its discrete nature, because the tablets are held between the cheek and gum without telltale evidence of drug intake. The buccal tablet is designed for faster onset than oral or transmucosal delivery, so it is particularly useful in the management of breakthrough pain and may be helpful in cases of anticipated incident pain or potentially noxious activity. This formulation may be an alternative form of administration for those with an inability to swallow medications because of dysphagia or a history of pill aversion.

Integumentary Applications

Transdermal Delivery Systems

Transdermal delivery systems of analgesics and adjuvants can be effective for chronic pain. Ideal characteristics of a transdermal delivery system include low molecular weight, lipophilicity, high potency, and reliable patch adhesion.[176] The drug's solubility in the adhesive, diffusion coefficient, and permeability coefficient also play major roles in time to steady state release into the skin.[177] Release rates of the agent are dependent on the drug concentration and type of matrix used. A steady-state skin flux is required to yield consistent rates of drug release at zero order kinetics. Several transdermal systems are available for opioids, α_2 agonists, and anesthetics.[178]

Fentanyl. Transdermal fentanyl was approved for use in children in 2002.[178,179] A prospective study has cited improvement in pain and quality of life for children 2 to 16 years of age who had established opioid requirements for cancer and chronic noncancer pain.[179] In pediatric oncology studies, 75% to 90% have reported that transdermal fentanyl therapy is "good" or "very good" for relief of cancer-related pain. These findings suggest that transdermal fentanyl is effective and acceptable for children and their families.[179,180]

Buprenorphine. Transdermal buprenorphine has been used for treatment of nociceptive and neuropathic pain. Buprenorphine is a long-acting partial μ agonist, with antagonist action at κ-opioid and δ-opioid receptors. Reversal of respiratory depression and sedation from this mixed agonist-antagonist is difficult to achieve with naloxone.[181,182] Patients with previous opioid use have experienced up to a 30% dose reduction in analgesic requirements. Pediatric tolerance shows marked ventilatory reduction with buprenorphine in comparison with morphine and would warrant close observation for the initial 24 hours of use.[183]

Clonidine. Transdermal application of clonidine has been the most studied mode of delivery of α_2 agonists. Transdermal clonidine is well studied in adults but it is difficult to employ use modality for the management of acute or chronic pain. Although neuraxial clonidine has a place in cancer and chronic pain management, transdermal clonidine has limited evidence of analgesic efficacy or opioid sparing.[184] However, transdermal application does appear to increase the release of enkephalin-like substances and therefore may be an agent enhancer in balanced analgesia techniques.[185]

Lidoderm Patch

The 5% lidocaine patch is a topical peripheral analgesic and is approved by the U.S. Food and Drug Administration (FDA) for the treatment of postherpetic neuralgia.[186] It has been used for nociceptive and neuropathic pain in noncancer patients. This technique may be of use in malignancy-induced peripheral nerve disease. Unlike other transdermal delivery systems, which work by systemic uptake, the lidocaine contained in the patch penetrates the skin to act locally on damaged or dysfunctional nerves and soft tissue under the skin.[186] Each 10- × 14-cm 5% lidocaine patch contains 700 mg of lidocaine in an aqueous base. It should be applied to intact skin only because of the risk of possible systemic uptake. The patch is applied directly on or beside the area of pain. Patches can be cut before removal of the release liner to fit the targeted area. The recommended use is a 12 hours on–, 12 hours–off dosing schedule. It should be used with caution in patients taking oral local anesthetic antiarrhythmic drugs, such as mexiletine, to prevent additive effects. Patients sensitive to amide local anesthetics, such as bupivacaine or ropivacaine, should not use the lidocaine patch. The 5% lidocaine patch has not been studied in children.

Topical Local Anesthetic

Eutectic Mixture of Local Anesthetics. Four percent tetracaine gel and a eutectic mixture of local anesthetics (EMLA)—lidocaine and prilocaine—as a cream or patch have proven to be effective in relieving pain in children undergoing cancer-related procedures.[187,188] Studies in children 3 to 21 years old have shown benefit of these commercial preparations in diminishing pain associated with lumbar puncture, venipuncture, and central port accessing.[189] These preparations should not be used in premature infants because of risks of local anesthetic toxicity. Plasma levels of lidocaine and prilocaine were well below toxicity for each agent. Moderate plasma lidocaine levels (4.5 to 7.5 µg/mL) may cause restlessness, dizziness, blurred vision, or tremors. At high levels (more than 7.5 µg/mL), lidocaine can produce generalized tonic-clonic seizures.[190] Buccal application of EMLA has not led to local anesthetic toxicity. A study in 12 subjects showed peak concentrations at 40 minutes for lidocaine and prilocaine; the maximum concentration measured in any subject was 418 ng/mL for lidocaine and 223 ng/mL for prilocaine, each below toxic plasma levels.[191] Methemoglobinemia from prilocaine has been reported from application of EMLA onto newly regenerated postburn or abraded skin.[192] An occlusive dressing was also used in both cases. Methemoglobin levels below 3% are nontoxic, but skin cyanosis may occur. Levels above 3% can be associated with agitation and levels higher than 50% result in coma, seizures, arrhythmias, and acidosis.[193] Adverse effects of EMLA include transient skin blanching, erythema, urticaria, allergic contact dermatitis, irritant contact dermatitis, hyperpigmentation, and purpura.

Liposome-Encapsulated Lidocaine. Another option for topical pain control before venipuncture is 4% liposomal lidocaine (L-M-X4), an over-the-counter topical local anesthetic that poses no risk of methemoglobinemia because it does not contain prilocaine. Both 4% tetracaine gel and 4% liposomal lidocaine are effective within 30 minutes of application.

Compounding Topicals
Creams and gels applied topically to the skin target the primary site of pain and discomfort. Pluronic lecithin organogel (PLO) is a poloxamer used in topical delivery, with a bioavailability of 10% to 60%.[194] The advantage to using topical medications is the high concentration of drug deposited exactly where it is needed, and purportedly little drug that is taken up systemically. This would reduce or eliminate the usual side effects of these medications when taken orally. With a prescription, compounding pharmacies can locally prepare select agents into topical preparations not currently available on the open market. However, variation in concentration, sterility, and lack of FDA regulatory control requires caution in the use of these agents. Death has resulted from the use of PLO preparations.[194] Commonly compounded agents for topical application include NSAIDs (e.g., aspirin, ketoprofen), membrane stabilizers (e.g., amitriptyline, clonidine, gabapentin, lidocaine), muscle relaxants (e.g., cyclobenzaprine [Flexeril], baclofen), and antibiotics (e.g., amoxicillin, clavulanate). Topical application of clonidine has been shown to be beneficial for a child with cancer. Successful use of topical clonidine ointment in a child post–bone marrow transplantation with herpetic neuralgia relieved the associated pain, pruritus, and insomnia.[195]

Parenteral Medications

Subcutaneous Infusions
Subcutaneous infusions are considered equivalent to intravenous infusions once a plasma steady state is achieved. Up to 5 mL/hr can be absorbed by subcutaneous infusion, making this route of delivery feasible for pediatric cancer pain management.[196] This technique should be considered when oral management is not practical but long-term opioid requirements have been substantiated. The success of this technique is dependent on patient selection, ongoing home health care support, and choice of analgesic drug. Highly concentrated solutions are well tolerated and allow lower infusion rates. Opioid concentrations up to 30 mg/mL have been used in adults and tolerated for up to 7 days, with rotation of site of delivery every 72 hours.[197] Patient-controlled analgesia (PCA) can be delivered via subcutaneous infusion if intravenous access is not possible. Access via small-caliber needles, such as a 27-gauge butterfly needle, or as large as a 22-gauge tunneled intravenous catheter can be maintained in situ for the infusion. Combined techniques of subcutaneous and intravenous infusions may be indicated when venous access is limited but titration of individual agents is needed.

Intravenous Infusions
Outpatient use of intravenous opioids and adjuvants is indicated in the presence of gastroenteric intolerance, escalating pain inadequately controlled with adjusted oral medications, or intolerable side effects from oral agents. Intravenous access via peripheral catheters or central ports and catheters are often used in situ for chemotherapy or nutrition. Because of limited access, coadministration of analgesics with parenteral nutrition should be considered to limit interruption of access for infection risk control. Trissel and coworkers[198] have studied the compatibility of parenteral nutrition solutions with selected drugs during simulated Y-site administration. They reported that parenteral nutrition solutions are compatible with many agents, including opioids, for 4 hours at 23° C. Morphine, fentanyl, hydromorphone, and oxymorphone are compatible via a filter with total parenteral nutrition. Despite visual compatibility testing, admixtures of analgesics into nutritive solutions are not advised. Delivery of the analgesic drug at a Y site of the central catheter system is best.

Neuraxial Delivery System
The World Health Organization (WHO) has advocated a three-step ladder approach designed to provide adequate analgesia for most adults with cancer-related pain; however, only 60% of adults have satisfactory pain control. Children with solid tumor disease compounded by extension of the neoplasm to peripheral nerves or nerve roots at the neuraxis are more likely to require massive opioid doses

than children with nonsolid tumors (e.g., leukemia).[199] It is proposed that hyperalgesia and neuropathic pain are associated with reduced opioid antinociception and contribute to massive dose requirements. Systemic morphine doses as high as 518 mg/kg/hr have been cited in the pediatric literature.[200] The use of neuraxial (epidural and intrathecal) analgesia is indicated for the management of cancer pain when other routes are impractical or yield intolerable side effects. Retrospective reviews from adult and pediatric populations suggest that neuraxial (epidural or intrathecal) infection is a rare occurrence. The review by Strafford and colleagues[201] revealed no serious complications in 1620 general pediatric subjects who underwent short-term epidural catheterization. Bacterial colonization of caudal and lumbar epidural catheters in children has been studied prospectively. Kost-Byerly and associates[202] found a 35% colonization rate of epidural catheters and an 11% occurrence of local inflammatory change when catheters remained in situ for up to 5 days (mean duration, 3 days). No clinical evidence of epidural abscess was found, but no reports in the literature have identified the risk factors for epidural infection.[63,203] Fine and coworkers[204] have noted that epidural infection is rare in the adult immunocompromised cancer patient.

Long-standing epidural analgesia is effective and safe in the spectrum of cancer-related pain as well as in the terminally ill patient, but proper management of infection risks and strict catheter care are imperative. Tunneling of epidural catheters is done to decrease the likelihood of infection, improve catheter stability, and aid patient mobility during prolonged administration of neuraxial analgesia. One case report noted a 15-year-old child who received 5 months of effective analgesia until his disease-related demise.[205] A percutaneously inserted tunneled catheter connected to an externalized pump is a feasible technique for prolonged care (Figs. 16–3 to 16–6). Use of a 0.2-μ filter, regular changing of the pump tubing, and weekly or biweekly dressing site care performed using sterile technique may decrease risks of infection.[206] In a retrospective pediatric study of 25 children, the externalized catheters remained in place for up to 240 days without the occurrence of epidural abscess or meningitis.[207] The duration of tunneled catheter use by region was 22 days for thoracic (3 catheters), 240 days for lumbar (12 catheters), and 42 days for caudal (10 catheters).

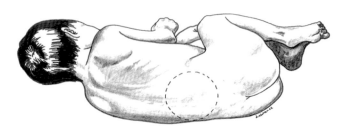

Figure 16–3. Positioning for epidural placement in a child.

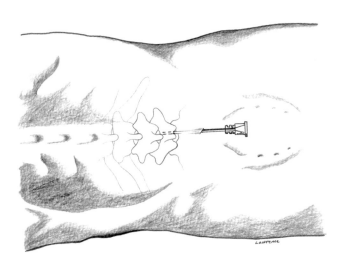

Figure 16–4. Percutaneous placement of epidural.

Tunneled epidural catheters placed in patients with cancer and coexisting neuropathic pain may have a higher likelihood of infection. Patients with noncancer-related neuropathic pain appear to have a higher rate of neuraxial infection than patients with chronic noncancer pain. Hayek and colleagues[208] have reviewed 260 accounts of tunneled epidural use in 218 adult patients with neuropathic or nociceptive pain. Because of superficial infection or suspected infection, 34 catheters were removed; 33 of those removed were in the neuropathic pain group. Also, 24 patients had epidural space infections confirmed by positive catheter tip cultures or epidural fluid lavage; 23 of these patients were in the neuropathic pain group.[208] The duration of catheter use was not ruled out as a contributing factor because those with neuropathic pain had their catheters indwelling for a significantly longer time (28 days) than those in the somatic pain group (16.5 days).

The risks and benefits of tunneled epidural analgesia in patients with cancer and coexisting neuropathic pain should be closely weighed. It is recommended that totally implanted systems be considered for patients with neuropathic pain.[208] The signs and symptoms of epidural infection include fever, escalating back pain, back or neck ache, MRI evidence of inflammation, and elevated sedimentation rate, C-reactive protein level, and white count.[208] Superficial infection may include local tenderness, erythema, subcutaneous phlegmon, and exudates at the exit site. The presence of an epidural abscess is confirmed by aspiration of exudates, an epidurogram with dye loculation at the catheter tip and/or retrograde flow, positive culture of the catheter tip, or positive culture of epidural lavage.[208] Removal of the epidural catheter is indicated for fever of 39° C or higher and if any of the above signs and symptoms are present.[202] Superficial infections are treated with a 7- to 14-day course of antibiotics. Epidural abscess management includes 6 weeks or more of intravenous antibiotics, with or without neurosurgical drainage of the epidural abscess.[202,208]

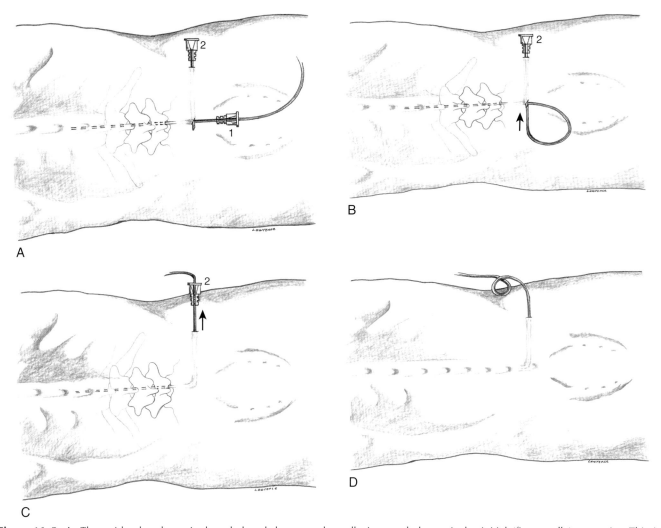

Figure 16–5. A, The epidural catheter is threaded and the second needle is tunneled to exit the initial (first needle) entry site. This is performed before removal of the first needle to avoid shearing of the catheter. **B,** The second needle acts as a trocar. This step can be repeated for a longer tunneled section that can be brought to the anterior. **C,** The first needle is removed and the catheter is threaded in a retrograde fashion into the tip of the second needle and exits the hub. **D,** The second needle is then withdrawn.

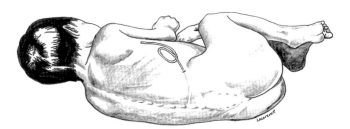

Figure 16–6. The externalized catheter can be connected to a balloon-type pump or patient-controlled analgesia apparatus.

Analgesia via the neuraxial route is associated with less sedation and fewer adverse effects because significantly smaller doses of opioids are used. Spinal opioids provide selective pain blockade without sympathetic nervous system blockade.[209] The more hydrophilic or hydrophobic opioids have limited uptake in the epidural fat and its vasculature and yield greater rostral spread in the cerebrospinal fluid (CSF) than hydrophobic lipophilic opioids such as fentanyl. Intrathecal opioids bypass the bloodstream and have direct CSF spread. The onset of intrathecal morphine is 15 to 45 minutes.[209] Delayed respiratory depression is a concern with spinal opioids. Gregory and co-workers[210] noted peak morphine levels in the medulla coincided with peak ventilatory depression 6 hrs after lumbar intrathecal injection. Nichols and colleagues[211] injected 0.020 mg/kg morphine into the intrathecal space at the L4-L5 interspace; this showed greatest depressed ventilatory response to carbon dioxide at 6 hours that persisted for up to 18 hours, and infants 4 to 12 months of age responded similarly to children 2 to 15 years old. Other side effects do not appear to be dose-dependent and include nausea, vomiting, pruritus, and urinary retention. However, side effects are worse with intrathecal than epidural opioids.[212] The incidence of nausea and vomiting in cancer patients is lower when repeated epidural dosing is used.[212]

The more commonly used adjuvants to improve pain and decrease opioid requirements include local anesthetics and α_2 agonists. The literature has consistently documented appreciable pain control when clonidine is administered by the intravenous and neuraxial routes as an adjuvant to opioid or local anesthetics.[213] The benefits of clonidine as an adjuvant include the following: (1) reduction in the amount of opioid required for analgesia and thus a likely decrease in the side effects because of opioids; (2) titrated sedation and anxiolysis without additive respiratory depression when given in combination with opioids; and (3) vasodilation and improved circulation of cerebral, coronary, and visceral vascular beds.[213]

Continuous infusion of intravenous clonidine has been cited as a safe adjuvant for pain control in adult and pediatric populations but the question of long-term impact on neurobehavioral function has been raised. The amount of opioid required by patients experiencing procedural pain was found to be reduced by 30%. Hemodynamic stability was maintained within normal limits because patients experienced less than a 10% change in mean blood pressure. Clonidine has the further advantage of producing sedation associated with only small reductions in minute ventilation and has no effect on hypercapnic or hypoxic respiratory drive.[214,215]

PAIN IN TERMINAL ILLNESS

There has recently been a surge in treatment modalities for pain and the treatment for children is now part of a cure-oriented and technology-based heath care system. Recently, with the involvement of facilities such as hospices, the care of terminally ill children has been based on the same philosophy as that for adults.[216,217] Pain can be a significant problem in children who require terminal care. When some children with a life-threatening illness have a significant setback, there may be no firm criteria to stop treatment and direct palliative care.

Alternate novel methods for providing analgesia have been used by our pain service in children who do not have intravenous access. Nebulized opioids[218] or the use of transdermal delivery systems have been used to offset pain in children with intractable pain. The adverse effects associated with the long-term use of opioids include tolerance and withdrawal. Careful rotation of opioids, along with the judicious use of other adjuvants such as N-methyl-D-aspartate (NMDA) receptor antagonists, should be considered in the care of children and adolescents.

Several approaches to pain management can be taken based on the state of the patient, involvement of the disease process, and general state of the caregivers. Patient-controlled analgesia (PCA) has been widely used in our institution for homebound patients with terminal cancer. Smaller, more user-friendly pumps have been devised for easy programming and less frequent changing. In patients who do not have venous access, we recommend the use of subcutaneous PCA. Other drugs are useful for the terminally ill child. NSAIDs and steroids are particularly useful in the management of bone pain from metastasis. Carbamazepine, gabapentin, pregabalin, and TCA are useful for the management of neuropathic pain. TCAs can be used for the management of neuropathic pain. Hypnosis, biofeedback, and distraction techniques can be used effectively in children who are not heavily sedated.

A child's view of death is very different from that of an adult. There is a consistent progression of the conceptual aspects of death in the child as he or she grows older. The school-age child finally understands the permanence of death. Home care may be useful for the family to cope with the grief and sorrow. It also allows other siblings to spend some time with the loved one. A home care coordinator should be available for the management of any adverse conditions. Knowing the family helps the coordinator understand the goals of the family. One basic tenet of hospice care is to enable the patient to lead a full life, of the best quality, for whatever time is remaining. Cooperation between the family and caregiver should allow the child to die with as much dignity as possible. It is the responsibility of the home coordinator to provide the caregivers with enough information about the management of pain.

Targeted and titrated delivery of antinociception is becoming a reality as more receptor-specific agents are devised. More pediatric studies are needed to substantiate the use of the agents and techniques discussed for the management of cancer-related pain in children and adolescents. Regardless of how creative advancements in pain management may become, patient safety must be first. Novel applications of older agents have broadened the armamentarium of pediatric anesthesiologists and pain management specialists.

References

1. Anand KJ: The stress response to surgical trauma: From physiological basis to therapeutic implications. Prog Food Nutr Sci 1986;10:67-132.
2. McGrath PA: Pain in the pediatric patient: Practical aspects of assessment. Pediatr Ann 1995;24:26-128.
3. van Dijk M, de Boer JB, Koot HM, et al: The reliability and validity of the COMFORT scale as a postoperative pain instrument in 0- to 3-year-old infants. Pain 2000;84:367-377.
4. McGrath PA, Seifert CE, Speechley KN, et al: A new analogue scale for assessing children's pain: An initial validation study. Pain 1996;64:435-443.
5. Varni JW, Rapoff MA, Waldron SA, et al: Chronic pain and emotional distress in children and adolescents. Dev Behav Pediatr 1996;17:154-161.
6. McGrath PA, Hillier LM: Modifying the psychologic factors that intensify children's pain and prolong disability. In Schecter NL, Berde CB, Yaster M (eds): Pain in Infants, Children, and Adolescents, 2nd ed. Baltimore, Lippincott Williams & Wilkins, 2003, pp 85-104.
7. Finley GA, McGrath PJ: Measurement of Pain in Infants and Children: Progress in Pain Research and Management. Seattle, IASP Press, 1998.
8. McGrath PJ, Beyer J, Cleeland C, et al: American Academy of Pediatrics Report of the Subcommittee on Assessment and

Methodologic Issues in the Management of Pain in Childhood Cancer. Pediatrics 1990;86(5 Pt 2):814-817.

9. Varni JW, Thompson KL, Hanson V: The Varni/Thompson Pediatric Pain Questionnaire. I. Chronic musculoskeletal pain in juvenile rheumatoid arthritis. Pain 1987;28:27-38.

10. Jaworski TM, Bradley LA, Heck LW, et al: Development of an observation method for assessing pain behaviors in children with juvenile rheumatoid arthritis. Arthritis Rheum 1995; 38:1142-1151.

11. Stinson JN, Petroz GC, Tait G, et al: e-Ouch: Usability of an electronic chronic pain diary for adolescents with arthritis. Clin J Pain 2006;22:295-305.

12. Palermo TM, Valenzuela D, Stork PP: A randomized trail of electronic versus paper pain diaries in children: Impact on compliance, accurary, and acceptability. Pain 2004;107: 213-219.

13. Konijnenberg AY, de-Graeff-Meeder ER, van der Hoeven J, et al: Psychiatric morbidity in children with medically unexplained chronic pain: Diagnosis from the pediatrician's perspective. Pediatrics 2006;117:889-897.

14. Vaalamo I, Pulkkinin L, Kinnunen T, et al: Interactive effects of internalizing and externalizing problem behaviors on recurrent pain in children. J Pediatr Psychol 2002;27: 245-257.

15. Dorn LD, Campo JC, Thato S, et al: Psychological comorbidity and stress reactivity in children and adolescents with recurrent abdominal pain and anxiety disorders. J Am Acad Child Adolesc Psychiatry 2003;42:66-75.

16. Martin-Herz SP, Smith MS, McMahon RJ: Psychosocial factors associated with headache in junior high school students. J Pediatr Psychol 1999;24:13-23.

17. Anttilla P, Sourander A, Metsååhonkala L, et al: Psychiatric symptoms in children with primary headache. J Am Acad Child Adolesc Psychiatry 2004;43:412-419.

18. Campo JV, Comer DM, Jansen-Mcwilliams L, et al: Recurrent pain, emotional distress, and health service use in childhood. J Pediatr 2002;141:76-83.

19. Kovacs M: Rating scales to assess depression in school-aged children. Acta Paedopsychiatrica 1981;46:437-457.

20. Beck AT, Steer RA, Brown GK: The Beck Depression Inventory-II. San Antonio, Tex, The Psychological Corporation, 1996.

21. Silverman WK, Goedhart AW, Barrett P, et al: The facets of anxiety sensitivity represented in the Childhood Anxiety Sensitivity Index: Confirmatory analyses of factor models from past studies. J Abnorm Psychol 2003;112:364-374.

22. Nash JM, Williams DM, Nicholson R, et al: The contribution of pain-related anxiety to disability from headache. J Behav Med 2005;29:61-67.

23. Peterson CC, Palermo TM: Parental reinforcement of recurrent pain: The moderating impact of child depression and anxiety on functional disability. J Pediatr Psychol 2004;29: 331-341.

24. Martin A, McGrath PA, Brown S, et al: Anxiety sensitivity, fear of pain and pain-related disability in children and adolescents with chronic pain. Pain Res Manage 2006;11(suppl B):64b.

25. Silverman WK, Fleisig W, Rabian B, et al: Childhood Anxiety Sensitivity Index. J Clin Child Psychol 1991;20:162-168.

26. McCracken LM, Zayfert C, Gross RT: The Pain Anxiety Symptom Scale: Development and validation of a scale to measure fear of pain. Pain 1992;50:67-73.

27. Birmaher B, Brent D, Chiapetta L: Psychometric properties of the Screen for Child Anxiety-Related Emotional Disorders (SCARED): A replication study. J Am Acad Child Adolesc Psychiatry 1999;38:230-1236.

28. Spence SH: A measure of anxiety symptoms among children. Behav Res Ther 1998;36:545-566.

29. March JS, Parker JD, Sullivan K, et al: The Multidimensional Anxiety Scale for Children: Factor structure, reliability, and validity. J Am Acad Child Adolesc Psychiatry 1997;36: 554-565.

30. Reynolds CR, Richmond BO: What I think and feel: A revised measure of children's manifest anxiety. J Abnorm Child Psychol 1978;6:271-280.

31. Spielberger C, Edwards C, Lushene R, et al: The State-Trait Anxiety Inventory for Children. Palo Alto, Cal, Consulting Psychologists Press, 1973.

32. Varni JW, Rapoff MA, Waldron SA, et al: Effects of perceived stress on pediatric chronic pain. J Behav Med 1996;19: 515-528.

33. von Weiss RT, Rapoff MA, Varni JW, et al: Daily hassles and social support as predictors of adjustment in children with pediatric rheumatic disease. J Pediatr Psychol 2002;27: 155-165.

34. Walker LS, Garber J, Smith CA, et al: The relation of daily stressors to somatic and emotional symptoms in children with and without recurrent abdominal pain. J Consult Clin Psychol 2001;69:85-91.

35. Eccleston C, Crombez G, Scotford A, et al: Adolescent chronic pain: Patterns and predictors of emotional distress in adolescents with chronic pain and their parents. Pain 2004;108: 221-229.

36. Thomsen AH, Compas BE, Colletti RB, et al: Parent reports of coping and stress responses in children with recurrent abdominal pain. J Pediatr Psychol 2002;27:215-226.

37. Walker LS, Smith CA, Garber J, et al: Testing a model of pain appraisal and coping in children with chronic abdominal pain. Health Psychol 2005;24:364-374.

38. Reid GJ, Gilbert CA, McGrath PJ: The Pain Coping Questionnaire: Preliminary validation. Pain 1998;76:83-96.

39. Walker SM, Cousins MJ: Complex regional pain syndromes including "reflex sympathetic dystrophy" and "causalgia." Anaesth Intens Care 1997;25:113-125.

40. Crombez G, Bijttebier P, Eccleston C, et al: The child version of the pain catastrophizing scale (PCS-C): A preliminary validation. Pain 2003;104:639-646.

41. Connor-Smith JK, Compas BE, Wadsworth ME, et al: Responses to stress in adolescence: Measurement of coping and involuntary stress responses. J Consult Clin Psychol 2000;68:976-992.

42. Thorn BE, Boothby JL, Sullivan MJL: Targeted treatment of catastrophizing for the management of chronic pain. Cogn Behav Pract 2002;9:127-138.

43. Keefe FJ, Crisson J, Urban BJ, et al: Analyzing chronic low back pain: The relative contribution of pain coping strategies. Pain 1990;40:293-301.

44. Vervoort T, Goubert L, Eccleston C, et al: Catastrophic thinking about pain is independently associated with pain severity, disability, and somatic complaints in schoolchildren and children with chronic pain. J Pediatr Psychol 2006;31: 674-683.

45. Hershey AD, Powers SW, Bentti AL, et al: Characterization of chronic daily headaches in children in a multidisciplinary headache center. Neurology 2001;56:1032-1037.

46. Palermo TM, Witherspoon D, Valenzuela D, et al: Development and validation of the Child Activities Limitations Interview: A measure of pain-related functional impairment in school-age children and adolescents. Pain 2004;109: 461-470.

47. Walker L, Greene J: The Functional Disability Inventory: Measuring a neglected dimension of child health status. J Pediatr Psychol 1991;16:39-58.

48. Claar RL, Walker LS: Functional asssessment of pediatric pain patients: Psychometric properties of the Functional Disability Inventory. Pain 2006;121:77-84.

49. Bursch B, Joseph MH, Zeltzer LK: Pain-associated disability syndrome. In Schecter NL, Berde CB, Yaster M (eds): Pain in Infants, Children and Adolescents, 2nd ed. Baltimore, Lippincott Williams & Wilkins, 2003, pp 841-848.

50. Roth-Isigkeit A, Thyen U, Stoven H, et al: Pain among children and adolescents: Restrictions in daily living and triggering factors. Pediatrics 2005;115:e152-e162.

51. Varni JW, Seid M, Knight TS, et al: The PedsQL 4.0 Generic Core Scales: Sensitivity, responsiveness, and impact on clinical decision-making. J Behav Med 2002;25:175-193.

52. Sawyer MG, Carbone JA, Whitham JN, et al: The relationship between health-related quality of life, pain, and coping strategies in juvenile arthritis—a one-year prospective study. Qual Life Res 2005;14:1585-1598.

53. Hunfeld JA, Perquin CW, Duivenvoorden HJ, et al: Chronic pain and its impact on quality of life in adolescents and their families. J Pediatr Psychol 2001;26:145-153.
54. Powers SW, Patton SR, Hommel KA, et al: Quality of life in childhood migraines: Clinical impact and comparison to other chronic illnesses. Pediatrics 2003;112:e1-e5.
55. Hunfeld JA, Perquin CW, Hazebroek-Kampschreur AA, et al: Physically unexplained chronic pain and its impact on children and their families: The mother's perception. Psychol Psychother 2002;75:251-260.
56. Langraf JL, Abetz L, Ware JE: The Child Health Questionnaire Manual. Boston, The Health Institute, New England Medical Center, 1996.
57. Varni JW, Seid M, Rode CA: The PedsQL: Measurement model for the Pediatric Quality of Life Inventory. Medical Care 1999;37:126-139.
58. Garber J, Walker LS, Zeman J: Somatization symptoms in a community sample of children and adolescents: Further validation of the Children's Somatization Inventory. Psychol Assess 1991;3:588-595.
59. Harter S: The Perceived Competence Scale for Children. Child Dev 1982;53:87-97.
60. Harter S: The Self-Perception Profile for Adolescents. Denver, University of Denver, 1988.
61. Harter S, Pike R: The Pictorial Scale of Perceived Competence and Social Acceptance for Young Children. Child Dev 1985;55:1969-1982.
62. Walker LS, Claar RL, Garber J: Social consquences of children's pain: When do they encourage symptom maintenance? J Pediatr Psychol 2002;27:689-698.
63. Moos RH, Moos BS: Family Environment Scale Manual, 3rd ed. Palo Alto, Cal, Consulting Psychologists Press, 1994.
64. Olson DH, Portner J, Bell R: FACES II: Family Adaptability and Cohesion Evaluations Scales. St. Paul, Minn, Family Social Science, University of Minnesota, 1982.
65. McCubbin HI, Olson D, Larsen A: Family Crisis-Oriented Personal Scales (F-COPES). In McCubbin HI, Thompson AI, McCubbin MA (eds): Family Assessment: Resiliency, Coping and Adaptation—Inventories for Research and Practice. Madison, Wis, University of Wisconsin System, 1996, pp 455-507.
66. Derogatis LR: Symptom Checklist-90-R (SCL-90-R). Minneapolis, National Computer Systems, 1993.
67. Ware JF: SF-36 Health Survey: Manual and Interpretation Guide. Boston, Medical Outcomes Trust, 1993.
68. Scharff L, Langan N, Rotrer N, et al: Psychological, behavioral and family characteristics of pediatric patients with chronic pain. Clin J Pain 2005;21:8.
69. Turk DC, Rudy TE: The West Haven–Yale Multidimensional Pain Inventory (WHYMPI) Pain 1985;23:345-356.
70. Turk DC, Rudy TE: Toward an empirically derived taxonomy of chronic pain patients: Integration of psychological assessment data. J Consult Clin Psychol 1988;56:233-238.
71. Rudy TE, Turk DC, Kubinski JA, et al: Diffferential treatment responses of TMD patients as a function of psychological characteristics. Pain 1995;61:103-112.
72. Wicksell RK, Melin L, Olsson GL: Exposure and aceptance in the rehabilitation of adolescents with idiopathic chronic pain—a pilot study. Eur J Pain 2007;11:267-274.
73. McGrath PJ, Dunn-Geier J, Cunningham SJ, et al: Psychological guidelines for helping children cope with chronic benign intractable pain. Clin J Pain 1986;1:229-233.
74. Eccleston C, Morley S, Williams A, et al: Systematic review of randomised controlled trials of psychological therapy for chronic pain in children and adolescents, with a subset meta-analysis of pain relief. Pain 2002;99:157-165.
75. Powers SW, Mitchell MJ, Graumlich SE, et al: Longitudinal assessment of pain, coping, and daily functioning in children with sickle cell disease receiving pain management skills training. J Clin Psychol Med Settings 2002;9:109-119.
76. Gil KM, Anthony KK, Carson JW, et al: Daily coping practice predicts treatment effects in children with sickle cell disease. J Pediatr Psychol 2001;26:163-173.
77. Chen E, Cole SW, Kato PM: A review of empirically supported psychosocial interventions for pain and adherence outcomes in sickle cell disease. J Pediatr Psychol 2004;29:197-209.
78. Sanders MR, Shepherd RW, Cleghorn G, et al: The treatment of recurrent abdominal pain in children: A controlled comparison of cognitive-behavioral family intervention and standard pediatric care. J Consult Clin Psychol 1994;62:306-314.
79. Robins PM, Smith SM, Glutting JJ, et al: A randomized controlled trial of a cognitive-behavioral family intervention for pediatric recurrent abdominal pain. J Pediatr Psychol 2005;30:397-408.
80. Blanchard EB, Scharff L: Psychosocial aspects of assessment and treatment of irritable bowel syndrome in adults and recurrrent abdominal pain in children. J Consult Clin Psychol 2002;70:725-738.
81. Janicke DM, Finney JW: Empirically supported treatments in pediatric psychology: Recurrent abdominal pain. J Pediatr Psychol 1999;24:115-127.
82. Lee BH, Scharff L, Sethna N, et al: Physical therapy and cognitive-behavioral treatment for complex regional pain syndromes. J Pediatr 2002;141:135-140.
83. Walco GA, Illowite NT: Cognitive-behavioral intervention for juvenile primary fibromyalgia syndrome. J Rheumatol 1992;19:1617-1619.
84. Lavigne JV, Ross CK, Berry SL, et al: Evaluation of a psychological treatment package for treating pain in juvenile rheumatoid arthritis. Arthritis Care Res 1992;5:101-110.
85. Kashikar-Zuck S, Swain NF, Jones BA, et al: Efficacy of cognitive-behavioral intervention for juvenile primary fibromyalgia syndrome. J Rheumatol 2005;32:1594-1602.
86. Degotardi PJ, Klass ES, Rosenberg BS, et al: Development and evaluation of a cognitive-behavioral intervention for juvenile rheumatoid arthritis. J Pediatr Psychol 2006;31:714-723.
87. Holden EW, Deichmann MM, Levy JD: Empirically supported treatments in pediatric psychology: Recurrent pediatric headache. J Pediatr Psychol 1999;24:91-109.
88. Chen E, Zeltzer LK, Craske MG, et al: Alteration of memory in the reduction of children's distress during repeated aversive medical procedures. J Consult Clinical Psychol 1999;67:481-490.
89. Schanberg LE, Lefebvre JC, Keefe FJ, et al: Pain coping and the pain experience in children with juvenile rheumatoid arthritis. Pain 1997;73:181-189.
90. Zeltzer LK, Bush JP, Chen E, et al: A psychobiologic approach to pediatric pain: Part I. History, physiology and assessment strategies. Curr Prob Pediatr 1997;27:225-253.
91. Wicksell RK, Dahl J, Magnusson B, et al: Using acceptance and commitment therapy in the rehabilitation of an adolescent female with chronic pain: A case example. Cogn Behav Pract 2005;12:415-423.
92. Eccleston C, Malleson PN, Clinch J, et al: Chronic pain in adolescents: Evaluation of a programme of interdisciplinary cognitive behaviour therapy. Arch Dis Child 2003;88:881-885.
93. Palermo TM, Chambers CT: Parent and family factors in pediatric chronic pain and disability: An integrative approach. Pain 2005;119:1-4.
94. Logan DE, Scharff L: Relationships between family and parent characteristics and functional abilities in children with recurrent pain syndromes: An investigation of moderating effects on the pathway from pain to disability. J Pediatr Psychol 2005;30:698-707.
95. Reid GJ, Lang BA, McGrath PJ: Primary juvenile fibromyalgia: Psychological adjustment, family functioning, coping, and functional disability. Arthritis Rheum 1997;40:752-760.
96. Walker LS, Williams SE, Smith CA, et al: Parent attention versus distraction: Impact on symptom complaints by children with and without chronic functional abdominal pain. Pain 2006;122:43-52.
97. Eccleston C, Jordan AL, Crombez G: The impact of chronic pain on adolescents: A review of previously used measures. J Pediatr Psychol 2006;31:684-697.

98. McGrath PJ, Humphreys P, Keene D, et al: The efficacy and efficiency of a self-administered treatment for adolescent migraine. Pain 1992;49:321-324.

99. Osterhaus SO, Passchier J, van der Helm-Hylkema H, et al: Effects of behavioral psychophysiological treatment on students with migraine in a nonclinical setting: Predictors and process variables. J Pediatr Psychol 1993;18:697-715.

100. Larsson B, Carlsson J: A school-based, nurse-administered relaxation training for children with chronic tension-type headache. J Pediatr Psychol 1996;21:603-614.

101. Hicks CL, Rapoff MA, Thompson N, et al: Online psychological treatment for pediatric recurrent pain: A randomized evaluation. J Pediatr Psychol 2006;31:724-736.

102. Connelly M, Rapoff MA, Thompson N, et al: A pilot study of a CD-ROM intervention for recurrent pediatric headache. J Pediatr Psychol 2006;31.

103. Rowan AB, Andrasik F: Efficacy and cost-effectiveness of minimal therapist contact treatments of chronic headaches: A review. Behav Ther 1996;27:207-234.

104. Scharff L, Marcus DA, Masek BJ: A controlled study of minimal-contact thermal biofeedback in the treatment of children with migraine. J Pediatr Psychol 2002;27:109-119.

105. Brown RT: Managing pediatric pain in school. In Finley GA, McGrath PJ, Chambers CT (eds): Bringing Pain Relief to Children. Totowa, NJ, Humana Press, 2006, pp 113-129.

106. Tsao JCI, Meldrum M, Zeltzer LK: Efficacy of complementary and alternative medicine approaches for pediatric pain. In Finley GA, McGrath PJ, Chambers CT (eds): Bringing Pain Relief to Children. Totowa, NJ, Humana Press, 2006, pp 131-158.

107. McGrath PA, Holahan A-L: Psychological interventions with children and adolescents: Evidence for their effectiveness in treating chronic pain. In Lebovits AH (ed): Seminars in Pain Medicine. Philadelphia, WB Saunders, 2003, pp 99-109.

108. Hillier LM, McGrath PA: A cognitive-behavioral program for treating recurrent headache. In Hillier LM, McGrath PA (eds): The Child with Headache: Diagnosis and Treatment. Seattle, IASP Press, 2001, pp 183-219.

109. Wilder RT, Berde CB, Wolohan M, et al: Reflex sympathetic dystrophy in children: Clinical characteristics and follow-up of seventy patients. J Bone Joint Surg Am 1992;74:910-919.

110. Guler-Uysal F, Basaran S, Geertzen JH, et al: A 2½-year-old girl with reflex sympathetic dystrophy syndrome (CRPS type I): Case report. Clin Rehabil 2003;17:224-227.

111. Konen A: Measurement of nerve dysfunction in neuropathic pain. Curr Rev Pain 2000;4:388-394.

112. Nicholson B: Taxonomy of pain. Clin J Pain 2000;16:S114-S117.

113. Kurvers HA: Reflex sympathetic dystrophy: Facts and hypotheses. Vasc Med 1998;3:207-214.

114. Sethna NF, Meier PM, Zurakowski D, et al: Cutaneous sensory abnormalities in children and adolescents with complex regional pain syndromes. Pain 2007;131:153-161.

115. Sarikaya A, Sarikaya I, Pekindil G, et al: Technetium-99m sestamibi limb scintigraphy in post-traumatic reflex sympathetic dystrophy: Preliminary results. Eur J Nucl Med 2001;28:1517-522.

116. Arner S: Intravenous phentolamine test: Diagnostic and prognostic use in reflex sympathetic dystrophy. Pain 1991;46:17-22.

117. Bruehl S, Harden RN, Galer BS, et al: External validation of IASP diagnostic criteria for complex regional pain syndrome and proposed research diagnostic criteria. International Association for the Study of Pain. Pain 1999;81:147-154.

118. Harden RN, Cole PA: New developments in rehabilitation of neuropathic pain syndromes. Neurol Clin 1998;16:937-950.

119. Suresh S, Wheeler M, Patel A: Case series: IV regional anesthesia with ketorolac and lidocaine: Is it effective for the management of complex regional pain syndrome 1 in children and adolescents? Anesth Analg 2003;96:694-695.

120. Karakaya I, Coskun A, Agaoglu B, et al: Psychiatric approach in the treatment of reflex sympathetic dystrophy in an adolescent girl: A case report. Turk J Pediatr 2006;48:369-372.

121. Kesler RW, Saulsbury FT, Miller LT, et al: Reflex sympathetic dystrophy in children: Treatment with transcutaneous electric nerve stimulation. Pediatrics 1988;82:728-732.

122. Tollison CD, Kriegel ML: Selected tricyclic antidepressants in the management of chronic benign pain. South Med J 1988;81:562-564.

123. Richeimer SH, Bajwa ZH, Kahraman SS, et al: Utilization patterns of tricyclic antidepressants in a multidisciplinary pain clinic: A survey. Clin J Pain 1997;13:324-329.

124. Burgess CD, Montgomery S, Wadsworth J, et al: Cardiovascular effects of amitriptyline, mianserin, zimelidine and nomifensine in depressed patients. Postgrad Med J 1979;55:704-708.

125. Prensky A: Childhood migraine headache syndromes. Curr Treat Options Neurol 2001;3:257-270.

126. Tong HC, Nelson VS: Recurrent and migratory reflex sympathetic dystrophy in children. Pediatr Rehabil 2000;4:87-89.

127. Ross EL: The evolving role of antiepileptic drugs in treating neuropathic pain. Neurology 2000;55:S41-S46.

128. Wheeler DS, Vaux KK, Tam DA: Use of gabapentin in the treatment of childhood reflex sympathetic dystrophy. Pediatr Neurol 2000;22:220-221.

129. Rusy LM, Troshynski TJ, Weisman SJ: Gabapentin in phantom limb pain management in children and young adults: Report of seven cases. J Pain Symptom Manage 2001;21:78-82.

130. Rosner H, Rubin L, Kestenbaum A: Gabapentin adjunctive therapy in neuropathic pain states. Clin J Pain 1996;12:56-58.

131. Lauder GR, White MC: Neuropathic pain following multilevel surgery in children with cerebral palsy: A case series and review. Paediatr Anaesth 2005;15:412-420.

132. Freynhagen R, Strojek K, Griesing T, et al: Efficacy of pregabalin in neuropathic pain evaluated in a 12-week, randomised, double-blind, multicentre, placebo-controlled trial of flexible- and fixed-dose regimens. Pain 2005;115:254-263.

133. Yee JD, Berde CB: Dextroamphetamine or methylphenidate as adjuvants to opioid analgesia for adolescents with cancer. J Pain Symptom Manage 1994;9:122-125.

134. Muizelaar JP, Kleyer M, Hertogs IA, et al: Complex regional pain syndrome (reflex sympathetic dystrophy and causalgia): Management with the calcium channel blocker nifedipine and/or the alpha-sympathetic blocker phenoxybenzamine in 59 patients. Clin Neurol Neurosurg 1997;99:26-30.

135. Kaplan R, Claudio M, Kepes E, Gu XF: Intravenous guanethidine in patients with reflex sympathetic dystrophy. Acta Anaesthesiol Scand 1996;40:1216-1222.

136. Ford SR, Forrest WH, Eltherington L: The treatment of reflex sympathetic dystrophy with intravenous regional bretylium. Anesthesiology 1988;68:137-140.

137. Forouzanfar T, van Kleef M, Weber WE: Radiofrequency lesions of the stellate ganglion in chronic pain syndromes: Retrospective analysis of clinical efficacy in 86 patients. Clin J Pain 2000;16:164-168.

138. Irazuzta JE, Berde CB, Sethna NF: Laser Doppler measurements of skin blood flow before, during, and after lumbar sympathetic blockade in children and young adults with reflex sympathetic dystrophy syndrome. J Clin Monit 1992;8:16-19.

139. Pariente GM, Lombardi AV Jr, Berend KR, et al: Manipulation with prolonged epidural analgesia for treatment of TKA complicated by arthrofibrosis. Surg Technol Int 2006;15:221-224.

140. Lundborg C, Dahm P, Nitescu P, et al: Clinical experience using intrathecal (IT) bupivacaine infusion in three patients with complex regional pain syndrome type I (CRPS-I). Acta Anaesthesiol Scand 1999;43:667-678.

141. Farid IS, Heiner EJ: Intrathecal local anesthetic infusion as a treatment for complex regional pain syndrome in a child. Anesth Analg 2007;104:1078-1080.

142. Dadure C, Motais F, Ricard C, et al: Continuous peripheral nerve blocks at home for treatment of recurrent complex regional pain syndrome I in children. Anesthesiology 2005;102:387-391.

143. Varni JW, Walco GA, Wilcox KT: Cognitive-biobehavioral assessment and treatment of pediatric pain. In Gross AM, Drabman RS (eds): Handbook of Clinical Behavioral Pediatrics: Applied Clinical Psychology. New York, Plenum Press, 1990, pp 83-97.

144. Ashwal S, Tomasi L, Neumann M, et al: Reflex sympathetic dystrophy syndrome in children. Pediatr Neurol 1988;4: 38-42.

145. Day WH: Headaches in Children: Essays on Diseases of Children. London, J&A Churchill, 1873.

146. Freidman AP: Headaches in Children. Springfield, Ill, Charles C Thomas, 1967.

147. Bille BS: Migraine in school children: A study of the incidence and short-term prognosis, and a clinical, psychological and electroencephalographic comparison between children with migraine and matched controls. Acta Paediatr 1962;51: 1-51.

148. Bille B: A 40-year follow-up of school children with migraine. Cephalalgia 1997;17:488-491.

149. Mack KJ: An approach to children with chronic daily headache. Dev Med Child Neurol 2006;48:997-1000.

150. Meier PM, Alexander ME, Sethna NF, et al: Complex regional pain syndromes in children and adolescents: Regional and systemic signs and symptoms and hemodynamic response to tilt table testing. Clin J Pain 2006;22:399-406.

151. Shulman RJ, Eakin MN, Jarrett M, et al: Characteristics of pain and stooling in children with recurrent abdominal pain. J Pediatr Gastroenterol Nutr 2007;44:203-208.

152. Hislop IG: Psychological significance of the irritable colon syndrome. Gut 1971;12:452-457.

153. Hyams JS, Hyman PE: Recurrent abdominal pain and the biopsychosocial model of medical practice. J Pediatr 1998;133: 473-478.

154. Massin MM, Bourguignont A, Coremans C, et al: Chest pain in pediatric patients presenting to an emergency department or to a cardiac clinic. Clin Pediatr (Phila) 2004;43: 231-238.

155. Saltzman DA, Schmitz ML, Smith SD, et al: The slipping rib syndrome in children. Paediatr Anaesth 2001;11:740-743.

156. Mohseni-Bandpei MA, Bagheri-Nesami M, Shayesteh-Azar M: Nonspecific low back pain in 5000 Iranian school-age children. J Pediatr Orthop 2007;27:126-129.

157. Cardon GM, de Clercq DL, Geldhof EJ, et al: Back education in elementary schoolchildren: The effects of adding a physical activity promotion program to a back care program. Eur Spine J 2007;16:125-133.

158. Reneman MF, Poels BJ, Geertzen JH, et al: Back pain and backpacks in children: Biomedical or biopsychosocial model? Disabil Rehabil 2006;28:1293-1297.

159. Ippolito E, Versari P, Lezzerini S: The role of rehabilitation in juvenile low back disorders. Pediatr Rehabil 2006;9: 174-184.

160. McCleary MD, Congeni JA: Current concepts in the diagnosis and treatment of spondylolysis in young athletes. Curr Sports Med Rep 2007;6:2-6.

161. Korovessis P, Zacharatos S, Koureas G, et al: Comparative multifactorial analysis of the effects of idiopathic adolescent scoliosis and Scheuermann kyphosis on the self-perceived health status of adolescents treated with brace. Eur Spine J 2007;16:537-546.

162. Sachs B, Bradford D, Winter R, et al: Scheuermann kyphosis: Follow-up of Milwaukee-brace treatment. J Bone Joint Surg (Am) 1987;69:50-57.

163. Champion JD, Piper JM, Holden AE, et al: Relationship of abuse and pelvic inflammatory disease risk behavior in minority adolescents. J Am Acad Nurse Pract 2005;17: 234-241.

164. Houlahan KE, Branowicki PA, Mack JW, et al: Can end of life care for the pediatric patient suffering with escalating and intractable symptoms be improved? J Pediatr Oncol Nurs 2006;23:45-51.

165. Miser AW, McCalla J, Dothage JA, et al: Pain as a presenting symptom in children and young adults with newly diagnosed malignancy. Pain 1987;29:85-90.

166. Miser AW, Dothage JA, Wesley RA, et al: The prevalence of pain in a pediatric and young adult cancer population. Pain 1987;29:73-83.

167. Wolfe J, Grier HE, Klar N, et al: Symptoms and suffering at the end of life in children with cancer. N Engl J Med 2000;342:326-333.

168. Ljungman G, Kreuger A, Gordh T, et al: Pain in pediatric oncology: Do the experiences of children and parents differ from those of nurses and physicians? Ups J Med Sci 2006;111:87-95.

169. Engelhardt T, Crawford M: Sublingual morphine may be a suitable alternative for pain control in children in the postoperative period. Paediatr Anaesth 2001;11:81-83.

170. Maunuksela EL, Korpela R, Olkkola KT: Comparison of buprenorphine with morphine in the treatment of postoperative pain in children. Anesth Analg 1988;67:233-239.

171. Shaiova L, Lapin J, Manco LS, et al: Tolerability and effects of two formulations of oral transmucosal fentanyl citrate (OTFC; ACTIQ) in patients with radiation-induced oral mucositis. Support Care Cancer 2004;12:268-273.

172. Binstock W, Rubin R, Bachman C, et al: The effect of premedication with OTFC, with or without ondansetron, on postoperative agitation, and nausea and vomiting in pediatric ambulatory patients. Paediatr Anaesth 2004;14:759-767.

173. Schechter NL, Weisman SJ, Rosenblum M, et al: The use of oral transmucosal fentanyl citrate for painful procedures in children. Pediatrics 1995;95:335-339.

174. Sharar SR, Carrougher GJ, Selzer K, et al: A comparison of oral transmucosal fentanyl citrate and oral oxycodone for pediatric outpatient wound care. J Burn Care Rehabil 2002;23:27-31.

175. Portenoy RK, Taylor D, Messina J, et al: A randomized, placebo-controlled study of fentanyl buccal tablet for breakthrough pain in opioid-treated patients with cancer. Clin J Pain 2006;22:805-811.

176. Roy SD, Gutierrez M, Flynn GL, et al: Controlled transdermal delivery of fentanyl: Characterizations of pressure-sensitive adhesives for matrix patch design. J Pharm Sci 1996;85: 491-495.

177. Kogan A, Garti N: Microemulsions as transdermal drug delivery vehicles. Adv Colloid Interface Sci 2006;123-126: 369-385.

178. Finkel JC, Finley A, Greco C, et al: Transdermal fentanyl in the management of children with chronic severe pain: Results from an international study. Cancer 2005;104: 2847-2857.

179. Hunt A, Goldman A, Devine T, et al: Transdermal fentanyl for pain relief in a paediatric palliative care population. Palliat Med 2001;15:405-412.

180. Noyes M, Irving H: The use of transdermal fentanyl in pediatric oncology palliative care. Am J Hosp Palliat Care 2001;18:411-416.

181. Likar R, Kayser H, Sittl R: Long-term management of chronic pain with transdermal buprenorphine: A multicenter, open-label, follow-up study in patients from three short-term clinical trials. Clin Ther 2006;28:943-952.

182. Lewis JW, Husbands SM: The orvinols and related opioids—high-affinity ligands with diverse efficacy profiles. Curr Pharm Des 2004;10:717-732.

183. Olkkola KT, Leijala MA, Maunuksela EL: Paediatric ventilatory effects of morphine and buprenorphine revisited. Paediatr Anaesth 1995;5:303-305.

184. Owen MD, Fibuch EE, McQuillan R, et al: Postoperative analgesia using a low-dose, oral-transdermal clonidine combination: Lack of clinical efficacy. J Clin Anesth 1997;9:8-14.

185. Nakamura M, Ferreira SH: Peripheral analgesic action of clonidine: Mediation by release of endogenous enkephalin-like substances. Eur J Pharmacol 1988;146:223-228.

186. Gammaitoni AR, Alvarez NA, Galer BS: Safety and tolerability of the lidocaine patch 5%, a targeted peripheral analgesic: A review of the literature. J Clin Pharmacol 2003;43:111-117.

187. Lander JA, Weltman BJ, So SS: EMLA and amethocaine for reduction of children's pain associated with needle insertion. Cochrane Database Syst Rev 2006;(3):CD004236.

188. Holdsworth MT, Raisch DW, Winter SS, et al: Pain and distress from bone marrow aspirations and lumbar punctures. Ann Pharmacother 2003;37:17-22.
189. Miser AW, Goh TS, Dose AM, et al: Trial of a topically administered local anesthetic (EMLA cream) for pain relief during central venous port accesses in children with cancer. J Pain Symptom Manage 1994;9:259-264.
190. Naguib M, Magboul MM, Samarkandi AH, et al: Adverse effects and drug interactions associated with local and regional anaesthesia. Drug Saf 1998;18:221-250.
191. Vickers ER, Marzbani N, Gerzina TM, et al: Pharmacokinetics of EMLA cream 5% application to oral mucosa. Anesth Prog 1997;44:32-37.
192. Kopecky EA, Jacobson S, Bch MB, et al: Safety and pharmacokinetics of EMLA in the treatment of postburn pruritus in pediatric patients: A pilot study. J Burn Care Rehabil 2001;22:235-242.
193. Brisman M, Ljung BM, Otterbom I, et al: Methaemoglobin formation after the use of EMLA cream in term neonates. Acta Paediatr 1998;87:1191-1194.
194. Perrin JH: Hazard of compounded anesthetic gel. Am J Health Syst Pharm 2005;62:1445-1446.
195. Hagihara R, Meno A, Arita H, et al: [A case of effective treatment with clonidine ointment for herpetic neuralgia after bone marrow transplantation in a child]. Masui 2002; 51:777-779.
196. Coyle N, Cherny NI, Portenoy RK: Subcutaneous opioid infusions at home. Oncology (Huntingt) 1994;8:21-27.
197. Bruera E, MacEachern T, Macmillan K, et al: Local tolerance to subcutaneous infusions of high concentrations of hydromorphone: A prospective study. J Pain Symptom Manage 1993;8:201-204.
198. Trissel LA, Gilbert DL, Martinez JF, et al: Compatibility of parenteral nutrient solutions with selected drugs during simulated Y-site administration. Am J Health Syst Pharm 1997;54:1295-1300.
199. Collins JJ, Grier HE, Kinney HC, et al: Control of severe pain in children with terminal malignancy. J Pediatr 1995;126:653-657.
200. Collins JJ: Intractable pain in children with terminal cancer. J Palliat Care 1996;12:29-34.
201. Strafford MA, Wilder RT, Berde CB: The risk of infection from epidural analgesia in children: A review of 1620 cases. Anesth Analg 1995;80:234-238.
202. Kost-Byerly S, Tobin JR, Greenberg RS, et al: Bacterial colonization and infection rate of continuous epidural catheters in children. Anesth Analg 1998;86:712-716.
203. Du Pen SL, Peterson DG, Williams A, et al: Infection during chronic epidural catheterization: Diagnosis and treatment. Anesthesiology 1990;73:905-909.
204. Fine PG, Hare BD, Zahniser JC: Epidural abscess following epidural catheterization in a chronic pain patient: A diagnostic dilemma. Anesthesiology 1988;69:422-424.
205. Galloway KS, Yaster M: Pain and symptom control in terminally ill children. Pediatr Clin North Am 2000;47:711-746.
206. D'Arcy Y: Using tunneled epidural catheters to treat cancer pain. Nursing 2003;33:17.
207. Aram L, Krane EJ, Kozloski LJ, et al: Tunneled epidural catheters for prolonged analgesia in pediatric patients. Anesth Analg 2001;92:1432-1438.
208. Hayek SM, Paige B, Girgis G, et al: Tunneled epidural catheter infections in noncancer pain: Increased risk in patients with neuropathic pain/complex regional pain syndrome. Clin J Pain 2006;22:82-89.
209. Cousins MJ, Mather LE: Intrathecal and epidural administration of opioids. Anesthesiology 1984;61:276-310.
210. Gregory MA, Brock-Utne JG, Bux S, et al: Morphine concentration in brain and spinal cord after subarachnoid morphine injection in baboons. Anesth Analg 1985;64:929-932.
211. Nichols DG, Yaster M, Lynn AM, et al: Disposition and respiratory effects of intrathecal morphine in children. Anesthesiology 1993;79:733-738.
212. Martin R, Salbaing J, Blaise G, et al: Epidural morphine for postoperative pain relief: A dose-response curve. Anesthesiology 1982;56:423-426.
213. Sung CS, Lin SH, Chan KH, et al: Effect of oral clonidine premedication on perioperative hemodynamic response and postoperative analgesic requirement for patients undergoing laparoscopic cholecystectomy. Acta Anaesthesiol Sin 2000; 38:23-29.
214. Eisenach JC, De Kock M, Klimscha W: alpha(2)-adrenergic agonists for regional anesthesia: A clinical review of clonidine (1984-1995). Anesthesiology 1996;85:655-674.
215. Ambrose C, Sale S, Howells R, et al: Intravenous clonidine infusion in critically ill children: Dose-dependent sedative effects and cardiovascular stability. Br J Anaesth 2000;84:794-796.
216. Strassels SA, Blough DK, Hazlet TK, et al: Pain, demographics, and clinical characteristics in persons who received hospice care in the United States. J Pain Symptom Manage 2006; 32:519-531.
217. Feudtner C, Feinstein JA, Satchell M, et al: Shifting place of death among children with complex chronic conditions in the United States, 1989-2003. JAMA 2007;297:2725-2732.
218. Cohen SP, Dawson TC: Nebulized morphine as a treatment for dyspnea in a child with cystic fibrosis. Pediatrics 2002;110: e38.

CHAPTER
17 Low Back Pain

Khalid Malik and Honorio T. Benzon

Low back pain (LBP) is the most common source of pain and disability in modern society; the costs related to the disorders that cause spinal pain amount to billions of dollars each year.[1] Pathologic lesions responsible for spinal pain are protean. Pain can originate not only from the various components of the spinal column, such as the intervertebral disks (IVDs), vertebral bodies, facet joints, spinal nerve roots, surrounding muscles and ligaments, but can also be referred from adjacent structures including the abdominal or pelvic viscera. The symptoms and signs produced by these disorders are frequently similar, and these disorders are often concomitantly present. Diagnostic tools that may be nonspecific and show abnormalities in asymptomatic individuals further complicate the problem. It is therefore crucial that a thorough clinical evaluation be accompanied by appropriate diagnostic testing to elucidate the cause of LBP. In this chapter, we discuss causes of LBP that are pertinent mostly to a pain medicine physician: lumbar radicular syndrome (LRS), herniated disk (HD), spinal stenosis, internal disk disruption, facet syndrome, and sacroiliac joint (SIJ) syndrome. Other significant causes of LBP, including myofascial syndrome, spondylosis, spondylolisthesis, and spinal instability, are discussed elsewhere.

LUMBAR RADICULAR SYNDROME

Definition and Terminology

The origin of radicular symptoms of pain, paresthesias and numbness in a typical dermatomal distribution in the presence of objective signs of weakness, diminished reflexes, and positive straight-leg raise test (SLR) lies in the pathology or dysfunction of the sensory spinal nerve roots (SSNR) and dorsal root ganglia (DRG).[2] Often present in conjunction with LBP, this pain syndrome by its nature, etiology, and treatment is distinct from syndromes causing axial back symptoms. Although the term *lumbar radiculopathy* is often used to describe this clinical entity, it inappropriately implies the presence of objective signs of nerve root (NR) damage—loss of sensation, muscle weakness, and diminished reflexes.[2] *Lumbar radiculitis* is another term commonly used; however, it incorrectly suggests inflammatory processes being solely responsible for the causation of radicular signs

and symptoms. The term *lumbar radicular pain* mistakenly assumes pain as the predominant symptom. The descriptive term *lumbar radicular syndrome* may be the most accurate in that it correctly suggests a constellation of clinical signs and symptoms of variable etiology secondary to pathology or dysfunction of the NR or DRG. Although the term *sciatica* is often used synonymously for LRS, this term is more suited to describe the pain in the distribution of sciatic nerve.[3]

Prevalence

The epidemiologic studies of LBP and lower extremity pain are often inexact, in that the conditions producing these symptoms are often nonhomogeneous and poorly defined. Although the prevalence and lifetime incidences of LBP are reported variably, their overall occurrence ranges from 13.8%[4] to 31%[5] and the health care costs related to these disorders amount to billions of dollars each year.[6] The incidence of radicular symptoms in patients with back pain has been reported from 12%[3] to 40%.[4]

Etiology and Differential Diagnosis

The pathologic involvement of the SSNRs and DRGs generates ectopic impulses at these locations, which are perceived as pain, numbness, and tingling in the areas innervated by the affected axons, that is, a radicular distribution.[2] Pathologic processes that can affect the SSNRs and DRGs are diverse; lesions of the IVDs and degenerative spinal disorders (DSDs), however, are the most prevalent. Neoplastic, infectious, traumatic, metabolic, and vascular lesions involving the SSNR, the DRG, the spine itself, and the lumbosacral plexuses can also produce radicular signs and symptoms.[7] The list of conditions that can produce LBP—with or without LRS—is exhaustive and includes causes as diverse as spinal metastasis, vertebral body fractures, abdominal aortic aneurysm, and chronic pancreatitis. Pathologic lesions and entrapment neuropathies involving the sciatic nerve (e.g., piriformis muscle and ischial tunnel syndromes) can generate pain and paresthesias in its distribution and often involve multiple dermatomes.[7] Pain originating in the IVDs and in the sacroiliac and facet joints, and pain of myofascial origin can also refer to the lower extremities. This somatic referred pain is due to interneuronal convergence within the spinal cord. It is nondermatomal, has deep aching quality, rarely radiates below the knees, and lacks the objective signs of NR involvement.[2]

Clinical Features

Although pain is the predominant symptom, other symptoms of radicular involvement include paresthesias, and numbness and weakness in the territory of the involved NR. Radicular pain typically travels along a narrow band and has a sharp, shooting, and lancinating quality.[8] Objective signs of gait disturbances, loss of sensation, reduced muscle strength, and diminished reflexes involve appropriate dermatomal distribution. Herniated disk (HD) and the DSD commonly involve the lower lumbar NRs, whereas other, often more sinister causes of LRS, involve higher NRs with greater frequency.[9] The following are characteristic features of various lumbar and sacral NR involvements:

- S1 NR involvement results in pain, paresthesia, and numbness of the posterior thigh, calf, and plantar surface of the foot; there may be associated difficulty in toe walking, weakness of plantar flexion, and loss of plantar reflex.
- L5 NR involvement is indicated by similar symptoms involving the buttock, anterolateral leg, dorsal foot, and great toe, with possible difficulty in heel walking (steppage gait) and weakness of ankle and toe extension.
- L4 radicular involvement typically involves the anterior thigh, knee, and upper-medial leg, with weakness of knee extension and diminished patellar tendon reflex.
- L3 and L2 NRs tend to produce symptoms and sensory alterations involving the groin and inner thigh areas.
- Involvement of lower sacral NRs produces decreased sensation in the buttock and perineal areas (i.e., saddle anesthesia) and autonomic dysfunction, indicated by bowel and bladder dysfunction, typically urinary retention and constipation followed by incontinence, and sexual dysfunction presenting as loss of erection in men and vaginal anesthesia in women.[10,11]

Clinical Tests of Nerve Root Irritation

Several tests confirm the presence of NR irritation (Box 17-1). A positive straight-leg raise test (SLR) or Lasegue test is suggestive of radicular pathology of lower lumbar NRs (L4, L5, and S1). Passive SLR and ankle dorsiflexion of the extended lower extremity causes traction of the lower lumbar NRs by pulling them caudally between 1.4 and 4 mm.[12] The radicular nature of the pain is suggested by worsening pain in the radicular distribution caused by such a maneuver. Radicular pain in the affected leg when the contralateral asymptomatic leg is lifted is a positive crossed straight-leg raise test (X-SLR). Although a

---

BOX 17–1. TESTS TO CONFIRM THE PRESENCE OF NERVE ROOT IRRITATION

- Straight leg raise (SLR)
- SLR and ankle dorsiflexion of the extended lower extremity
- Crossed straight leg raise
- Tripod test
- Femoral stretch test

---

positive SLR is highly sensitive, X-SLR is more specific for lumbar NR irritation.[13] Increase in back pain during SLR is typically attributed to lumbar spinal movement and indicates the mechanical nature of LBP.[14] Centrally HDs, however, can also generate LBP on SLR due to tensioning of the anterior theca.[15] The tripod test is a maneuver to confirm a positive SLR test when the patient is sitting. The femoral stretch test places the L2 and L3 NRs under tension and indicates irritation of these NRs: this is tested by bending the knee and extending the hip with the patient in prone position.

"Red Flags" in the Medical History

The list of causes of LRS with or without LBP is daunting. The majority of patients, however, suffer from musculoskeletal conditions that are self-limiting and their symptoms usually resolve within 4 to 6 weeks.[16] The Agency for Health Care Policy and Research (AHCPR) developed guidelines to identify signs and symptoms, or "red flags," that indicate the presence of conditions that pose significant threat to life or neurologic function. These include tumors, infections, fractures, and cauda equina syndrome (CES), and require further diagnostic testing.[16] Indiscriminate diagnostic workup is not only expensive, but it may also yield no diagnostic information or yield findings that are unrelated and misleading. Following is the list of red flags proposed by the Agency for Health Care Policy and Research (AHCPR) Publication 95-0643, published in 1994.[16]

- Age younger than 20 or older than 50 years: Patients younger than 20 years of age have a higher incidence of congenital and developmental anomalies and those older than 50 years of age are prone to neoplasms, pathologic fractures, serious infections, and life-threatening extraspinal processes as a cause of their low back and radicular symptoms.[7]
- Duration of symptoms: The AHCPR guidelines consider symptoms of less than 3 months' duration as acute and subacute LBP. Chronic pain, or pain greater than 3 months' duration, indicates symptoms of less serious etiology.
- History of trauma: A history of trauma in older patients and in patients with serious medical conditions may result in bony injury and require further workup.

- Constitutional symptoms: A history of fever, chills, malaise, night sweats, and unexplained weight loss should raise a red flag.
- Systemic illness: History of cancer, recent bacterial infections such as serious respiratory or urinary tract infections, intravenous drug abuse, immunosuppression (e.g., infection with human immunodeficiency virus), transplant recipients, and corticosteroid use increase the risk of pathologic fractures, epidural and vertebral body abscesses, and metastasis.
- Unrelenting pain: Pain of benign etiology is typically relieved with rest and in supine position, especially at night. Unrelenting pain from serious pathologic conditions is often worse at night and is unresponsive to analgesics.
- Cauda equina syndrome: CES is caused by acute compression of spinal NRs comprising the cauda equina. Symptoms similar to CES may be produced by spinal cord compression at higher levels and constitute about 10% of patients presenting with CES.[17] Although rare, with a prevalence of approximately 4/10,000 in patients with LBP and LRS,[18] it is a neurosurgical emergency requiring emergent decompressive surgery.[18] Massive midline disk herniation[10,11] or a smaller disk herniation in a previous stenotic spine[19] is the most frequent cause of CES. Rare causes of CES include spinal metastases, spinal hematoma, epidural abscess, traumatic compression, acute transverse myelitis, and abdominal aortic dissection. Most patients with CES (70%) have a history of chronic LBP (CLBP), while the rest present with CES as their primary manifestation.[19] Patients often present within 24 hours of the onset of their symptoms, typically with bilateral radicular pains, although one leg pain is often worse than the other, and less frequently with back pain. The pain is often accompanied by weakness in both feet, gait disturbances due to pain and weakness, and abdominal discomfort due to urinary retention that may be followed by overflow urinary incontinence. The objective signs include motor and sensory deficits, diminished reflexes, and positive SLR in both lower extremities. Of particular importance is diminished sensation in the buttocks and perineum—saddle anesthesia, diminished sphincter tone, and evidence of urinary bladder retention. Imaging of the entire spine, with magnetic resonance imaging (MRI) being the gold standard, is indicated due to the possibility of spinal cord compression at higher levels.[17] Once the diagnosis is made, treatment involves high-dose intravenous steroids and urgent decompressive surgery to reduce permanent neurologic disability.[19]

Diagnostic Studies

Diagnostic studies are not recommended for symptoms of less than 4 to 6 weeks' duration.[16,20] This is due to the favorable natural history of conditions that commonly cause LRS and LBP and the often sponta-

neous resolution of symptoms in the absence of red flags. In addition, the frequent presence of abnormal diagnostic findings in asymptomatic individuals[21-23] makes the interpretation of these test results difficult. Diagnostic testing should be used to corroborate the clinical findings and to determine the site of surgical or minimally invasive spinal interventions. Ordering tests selectively and correlating the results with clinical presentation should prevent inappropriate diagnosis, treatment, and poor outcomes.[16]

Imaging Studies

- Magnetic resonance imaging: MRI is considered the gold standard in determining the etiology of LRS. It offers the best resolution of the spinal canal, spinal cord, neural foramina, NRs, and disk spaces, and allows evaluation of the entire spine. In patients with a history of previous spine surgery, a contrast-enhanced MRI scan is recommended to differentiate between scar tissue and recurrent disk herniation. The limitations of MRI include lengthy examination time, claustrophobia, and its effects on metallic objects. It is contraindicated in patients with pacemakers, mechanical heart valves, aneurysm clips, and intraocular foreign bodies.
- Computed tomography: Computed tomography (CT) scanning is superior to MRI in evaluating bony details of the spine, particularly the facet joints and lateral recesses. When combined with myelography (CT myelogram), the results are comparable to those of MRI in diagnosing spinal canal lesions. It can therefore be used as a substitute when MRI is contraindicated.[24] CT without myelography cannot distinguish between HD and other intradural lesions, such as tumors, and its routine use is therefore discouraged.[24]
- Plain radiography: The anteroposterior and lateral spinal films are the simplest and most readily available tests. Although spine fractures and deformities are easily appreciated, the findings of lumbar lordosis, transitional vertebra, disk space narrowing, and spondylolisthesis are common in asymptomatic individuals.[23] Routine spine roentgenograms are therefore not recommended.[25] Flexion and extension films are used to reveal segmental instability as a source of pain; however, there is little correlation between abnormal motion and pathologic instability.[26]
- Myelography: Myelography without CT scan is useful in detecting lesions in the spinal canal when other studies yield conflicting information, are not available, or are contraindicated.

Electrodiagnostic Studies

In contrast to imaging studies, electromyography (EMG)/nerve conduction studies (NCS) have high diagnostic specificity.[27] They are useful in establishing the radicular nature of symptoms when physical examination is inconclusive and in distinguishing LRS from symptoms of peripheral neuropathy. These tests, however, give no information regarding the etiology of LRS and correlate poorly with the anatomic level of the radicular lesions; their routine use is therefore not recommended.[20] The use of somatosensory evoked potentials is typically limited to identifying nerve injury intraoperatively because the test cannot pinpoint the exact location of nerve dysfunction.

OTHER DIAGNOSTIC TESTS

Various other diagnostic and laboratory tests are useful when spinal tumors, infections, and rheumatologic disorders are suspected. These include bone scan, complete blood count, urinalysis, erythrocyte sedimentation rate, C-reactive protein, rheumatoid factor, antinuclear antibodies, and HLA-B27 antigen.

In this chapter, we review the two most common causes of LRS: the HD and the DSD. Entrapment neuropathies of the sciatic nerve such as piriformis syndrome are discussed elsewhere.

HERNIATED LUMBAR DISK

History and Epidemiology

Although radicular symptoms were known in ancient times, Goldthwait in 1911 first attributed these symptoms to posterior displacement of the disk.[28] The incidence of symptomatic HD has been estimated to be 1% to 2%[4] in the general population, for which approximately 200,000 lumbar diskectomies are performed each year.[29]

Terminology

Disk herniation may be defined as displacement of the disk material beyond the confines of the IVD space.[30] Although nucleus pulposus (NP) is the predominant component of the herniated material, other disk parts (e.g., cartilage, bone, and annular tissue) are frequently present.[31] Various terms such as *herniated nucleus pulposus, ruptured disk,* and *prolapsed disk* have been used to describe this entity. The term *herniated disk* seems most appropriate, in that it conveys the image of displacement of any disk component regardless of the cause.[30] HD is variably classified, based on the morphology of the herniated material.[30] A *protruded disk* is present if the neck of the herniated material, that is, the distance between the edges of the base, is wider than the widest disk diameter in any given plane. *Disk extrusion* is the opposite of the disk protrusion; the neck is shorter than the widest disk diameter in any given plane. *Disk sequestration* is a type of disk extrusion, wherein no continuity exists between the herniated material and the parent disk. In contrast to *noncontained* herniation, the term *contained* herniation is used when the displaced portion is covered by an intact annulus. However, with currently available diagnostic modalities such as CT, MRI, and discography, the details of

the integrity of the annulus are often unknown, and these distinctions therefore are arbitrary. The terms *disk desiccation, disk fibrosis, disk narrowing, disk bulging, disk fissuring,* and *disk sclerosis* are often used; these, however, suggest degenerative disk processes and do not reflect disk herniation.[30]

Pathophysiology

Since Mixter and Barr first reported alleviation of the lumbar radicular pain after removal of the HD material in 1934,[32] HD is thought to be the most common cause of LRS. Although degenerated disk bulging and protrusions are common in asymptomatic individuals,[21] disk extrusions are uncommon in patients with LRS.[22] Mechanical compression of the NRs by the herniated material has been assumed to be the primary factor inducing radicular symptoms. Data from animal studies indicate that compression of the NRs impairs their nutrition and can lead to NR ischemia and injury.[33,34] Deformation of the NRs by the HD is also often seen on diagnostic imaging in patients with radicular symptoms. There is, however, no direct evidence of increased mechanical pressure created by an HD. Clinical studies demonstrate that only NRs, which are exposed to HD material for a long time, produce pain on mechanical deformation. Similar deformation of NRs not exposed to HD material produces no pain, suggesting mechanisms other than mechanical pressure in the causation of LRS.[8,35] The presence of inflammatory mediators in the HD material, retrieved from patients at diskectomy, has been demonstrated.[36,37] In animal models, the application of the NP to the NR, and not the epidural fat, produced the physiologic and anatomic evidence of radiculopathy.[38] The presence of clinical and electromyographic evidence of radiculopathy in patients with normal spinal imaging has also been shown.[39] The above observations suggest that factors other than mechanical compression may contribute to LRS and bioactive molecules may play a major role.

Natural History

The natural history of HD is favorable in that the majority of patients (60%) experience significant resolution of their symptoms within the first few months of their onset. In a smaller percentage of patients (20% to 30%), however, the symptoms fail to improve over time.[40] Clinical improvement is usually accompanied by resolution of HD on spinal imaging.[41] Large extruded disks have a higher tendency to decrease in size than small disk protrusions and disk bulges.[42] Spontaneous regression is thought to be caused by the phagocytic process, predominated by macrophages, which is most prominent in the outermost layers of the HD material.[43]

Clinical Correlations

Most lumbar disk herniations occur at lower lumbar levels with L4/5 HD being the most common (59%), followed by L5/S1 (30%) and L3/4 (9%) disks.[19] Herniation at these levels produces typical radicular signs and symptoms in the affected dermatomes described earlier. Central HDs may, however, produce primarily LBP, which is exacerbated by SLR.[15]

Nonoperative Treatments for Herniated Disks

Due to favorable natural history, in the absence of progressive neurologic deficit and red flags in the clinical history, expectant and symptomatic treatment is recommended.[16,20] Opioids, muscle relaxants, and neuroleptics are routinely used for the symptomatic treatment, although there is minimal data in the literature to support their use. Only nonsteroidal anti-inflammatory drugs (NSAIDs) have been shown to have some efficacy in the management of acute radicular symptoms.[44] A wide array of nonoperative treatments are available and each has claimed success.

- Systemic corticosteroids: Corticosteroids are often prescribed orally and sometimes parenterally in the treatment of acute disk herniation; there is, however, little in the literature to support this practice.[45,46]
- Bed rest: Strict bed rest was traditionally recommended for acute HD. Because of the potentially harmful effects of prolonged bed rest,[47] continuation of activities, within the limits permitted by the pain, is reported to result in more rapid recovery.[48]
- Bracing: Bracing is another method of immobilizing the painful spine; there is limited evidence in support of the use of lumbar braces compared to no treatment.[49]
- Traction: Once a mainstay of treatment, traction either in its continuous or intermittent forms, remains an unproven treatment of HD.[50] Vertebral axial decompression (VAX-D) is a newer modality based on traction principles; it also remains untested in the treatment of HD.
- Acupuncture: There are case reports of the effectiveness of acupuncture; its efficacy exists in the treatment of CLBP. The literature does not support its use in the treatment of acute LBP.[51]
- Chiropractic manipulations, massage, magnets, transcutaneous electrical nerve stimulation, and ultrasound: These modalities are often used in the treatment of HD; their use, however, remains unproven.
- Behavioral therapy, biofeedback, and other psychological treatments: Although psychological treatment modalities have been shown to have some efficacy in patients with CLBP, their role in the treatment of HD remains unknown.[52]
- Physical therapy: Physical therapy techniques for acute LBP and LRS include active and passive exercises. Although active exercises are claimed to be more effective,[53] the overall role of physical therapy in the treatment of acute HD remains questionable.[54]

Intraspinal Injections

Epidural steroid injections (ESIs) have been performed for HD for more than 40 years. Traditionally, a posterior interlaminar (IL-ESI) approach is used. The injectate reaches the site of HD anteriorly by flowing around the thecal sac. More recently, fluoroscopically guided transforaminal injections (TF-ESI) have been performed. These have the theoretical advantage of delivering the injectate directly into the anterior epidural space. Fluoroscopic guidance significantly improves the precision with which the injectate is deposited in the epidural space.[55] The literature is replete with case series and uncontrolled studies, both in support of and against the efficacy of ESIs. A review of the literature on randomized control trials (RCTs) of IL-ESIs for sciatica showed four such trials: ESIs were found to be more beneficial than control treatments, especially in the short term.[56] Although no long-term RCTs exists for TF-ESIs, they were found to have superior results than IL-ESIs in one study.[57]

Percutaneous Disk Decompression

Percutaneous disk decompression (PDD) was developed following the success of intradiskal injection of chymopapain. Although still used in many countries, chymopapain injections are rarely performed in the United States because of complications from unintentional injections into the subarachnoid space and the rare occurrence of severe allergic reactions. The endoscopes used initially to remove NP and HD materials were based on the principles of joint endoscopy, were large in size (7 mm), and cumbersome to operate. The added risk of removal of normal tissue and trauma to the disk annulus curbed the initial enthusiasm for these techniques. The technique of automated percutaneous lumbar diskectomy (APLD) was then introduced wherein a smaller introducer cannula (2.5 mm) was used and nuclear material removed by suction and cutting technique. A variety of lasers has also been used to vaporize the nuclear material, including YAG, KTP, holmium, argon, and CO_2 lasers. The various percutaneous laser disk decompression (PLDD-LASE) devices use cannulas less than 3 mm in diameter and often include a fiberoptic channel for viewing. The technique of disk nucleoplasty uses a 1.5-mm (17-G) introducer needle and bipolar radiofrequency (RF) energy to create small channels in the disk, removing finite amounts of nuclear material. The proponents of this technique claim that the procedure provides localized ablation with minimal damage to the surrounding tissue. Percutaneous diskectomy probe (DeKompressor) uses 1.5-mm and 1.0-mm (19-G) outer cannulas, and when activated the probe rotates to remove disk material. Modified intradiskal electrothermal therapy (IDET) catheter (Acutherm) is also available and is claimed to cause localized thermal lesioning and shrinkage at the base of the HD material.

Diskectomy procedures are traditionally applied to directly remove the HD material causing the radicular irritation. Removal of normal nuclear tissue, in the presence of intact annulus (contained HD), in small disk herniations (>4 mm) has been postulated to reduce intradiskal pressure and allow implosion of the herniated fragment.[58] MRI scans of patients, however, before and after APLD, showed no measurable difference in the size of HD at 6 weeks.[59] Although animal[60] and cadaver studies[61] showed reduction of disk pressures after PDD, there is no evidence of either high intradiskal pressures in patients with HDs or its reduction after disk decompressive procedures. The amount of nuclear material removed ranges from 4 to 5 g for APLD, and 1 g for nucleoplasty and DeKompressor devices; it varies greatly for various PLDD devices and is unknown for the Acutherm device. There are no studies that correlate either disk pressures or eventual outcomes with the amount of nuclear material removed. Removing large amounts of disk material has been correlated to disk collapse and may lead to accelerated disk degeneration.[62] It is therefore prudent to remove the least amount of disk material to achieve beneficial results. Removing nuclear contents from within the protrusion using a more lateral percutaneous approach has also been recommended.[58] Use of smaller gauge introducer cannulas limits the annular damage and should be preferred. Discography followed by a postdiscography CT scan can be used to assess the size and the location of the HD and the integrity of the disk annulus. Use of discography before PDD has been linked to improved clinical results.[63]

Claims of efficacy of various PDD procedures are based mostly on retrospective studies and case reports. Two randomized trials of APLD showed success rates of 29%[64] and 33%.[65] There are no randomized trials supporting the use of PLDD. Minimal literature is available on nucleoplasty, DeKompressor, and Acutherm, and their use is based mostly on anecdotal reports and remains experimental.

Outcome Predictors for Nonoperative Treatment

There are several predictors of a favorable outcome of conservative treatment (Box 17–2); these include a negative X-SLR, absence of leg pain with spine extension, absence of stenosis on spine imaging, favorable response to ESIs, return of any neurologic deficits within 12 weeks, a motivated physically fit patient with more than 12 years of education, no worker's compensation claims, and a normal psychological profile.[53]

Operative Treatments for Herniated Disk

Although surgery for HD is commonly performed,[29] there remains little high-quality evidence to support this practice. A prospective, randomized study of operative treatment for HD was published in 1983.[66] It demonstrated that during the first year, surgically

---

BOX 17–2. PREDICTORS OF FAVORABLE OUTCOMES OF CONSERVATIVE TREATMENT FOR HERNIATED DISK

- Negative crossed straight leg raise
- Absence of leg pain on extension of spine
- Return of neurologic function within 12 weeks of onset
- Absence of stenosis on spine imaging
- Favorable response to epidural steroid injections
- Patient has 12 years of education
- Patient is motivated and physically fit
- Patient has a normal psychological profile
- Absence of worker's compensation claim

---

treated patients had significantly better results (92%) compared with nonsurgically treated patients (61%). The results of surgery deteriorated over time and the difference became statistically insignificant at 4 years; there was no difference between the two groups at 10 years. Even this study was criticized for the lack of careful randomization, lack of blinding, the large number of crossovers to the surgically treated group, the insensitive outcome measures, and the small sample size.[67] The other major prospective study of operative treatment for HD was nonrandomized and observational,[68] and reported results similar to the previous study at 1 and 5 years. At 10 years, however, the results of surgical treatment were slightly better (56% vs. 40%, $P = 0.006$), but the incidence of work and disability status remained the same.[68]

A recently published study showed the efficacy of both surgical and nonoperative treatments for lumbar disk herniation. The Spine Patient Outcomes Research Trial (SPORT)[69] showed between-group differences in improvements to be consistently in favor of surgery for all the observation periods but the differences were small and not statistically significant for their primary outcomes. The patients in both groups were satisfied with their care, with the main benefit of surgery appearing to be a more rapid resolution of their disabling pain. The decision with regard to surgery depends on how urgently a patient wishes to achieve pain relief in the next 2 to 4 months.[70]

The need for surgery in the presence of CES is absolute,[19] and surgical treatment in the presence of progressive motor deficits is generally agreed upon. Other indications for surgery are relative and include intractable pain and poor response to conservative therapy.[71] The lack of consensus and the variability with which these indications are adhered to is supported by a nearly 20-fold difference in surgery rates in otherwise demographically similar populations within the United States.[72] For decades, the standard surgical technique has been open diskectomy. The newer minimally invasive technique of microdiskectomy focuses on minimizing surgical trauma in order to limit the potential for NR injury and epidural scarring. Microdiskectomy has been reported to have results superior to traditional diskectomy.[73] Although patients with sciatica of more than 12 months' duration have been shown to have less favorable results after surgery,[74] the effects of potential delay in operative treatment by nonsurgical treatments remain unknown.

LUMBAR SPINAL STENOSIS

Terminology and Etiology

Although recognized for some time, the modern descriptions of the clinical syndrome and pathological lesions of lumbar spinal stenosis (LSS) first appeared in 1954.[74] LSS is defined as a clinical syndrome of neurogenic claudication and/or radicular pain secondary to the narrowing of the spinal or NR canal and compression of its neural elements.[75] Traditionally classified into congenital and acquired types, it is the degenerative variety of the acquired type that is most prevalent. Developmental LSS is either idiopathic in nature or due to rare developmental bone dysplasias such as achondroplasia. Aside from the degenerative type, less common causes of acquired spinal stenosis include metabolic disorders such as Paget's disease, post-traumatic, postsurgical, spinal tumors, and spinal deformity. Anatomically, classification of LSS is comprised of central canal stenosis or central stenosis, and lateral recess and neural foraminal stenosis or lateral stenosis.[75]

Pathophysiology

Degeneration of the IVD with bulging and loss of disk height in conjunction with facet joint hypertrophy, thickening and redundancy of the ligamentum flavum, and osteophyte formation are the typical lesions seen in LSS.[76] These abnormalities are most common at the disk level, and one or several vertebral motion segments may be effected. Central stenosis causes compression of the NRs of the cauda equina, while lateral stenosis typically causes compression of exiting spinal NRs. The L5 NR is most commonly involved (75%), followed by L4 (15%), L3 (5.3%), and L2 (4%) NRs.[77] The capacity of lumbar spinal canal is significantly larger during flexion than during extension; the symptoms of LSS therefore are typically worse with lumbar extension.[78] Degenerative changes of LSS are prevalent in older adults[79] and have been shown to be frequently asymptomatic.[20,21] Direct compression or ischemia of the neural structures is thought to be primarily responsible for the clinical manifestations.[80] In contrast to HD, the role played by inflammation in the causation of symptoms due to LSS is less clear. Degenerative changes that result in spinal stenosis can also result in spinal instability (degenerative spondylolisthesis) and spinal deformities (degenerative scoliosis) and can contribute to further spinal narrowing and deformity. These changes typically result in axial LBP and deformity.

Clinical Considerations

- Neurogenic claudication: The typical manifestations of neurogenic claudication include pain radiating to both lower extremities at the posterolateral aspects of the thighs and legs. This is worse with walking and with lumbar extension, and is relieved by sitting down. The pain is often associated with numbness, and with heaviness or weakness in the lower extremities. It is crucial to distinguish these symptoms from claudication of vascular origin, and this possibility must be entertained in the presence of any sign of vascular insufficiency.[81] In contrast to vascular claudication, the pain of neurogenic claudication continues to be present with standing and is eased by walking in flexed position, such as pushing a walker or a shopping cart.[82]
- Radicular pain: Unilateral radicular symptoms unrelated to any activity reflect the involvement of NRs, and can be present with or without symptoms of neurogenic claudication.[83]
- Axial pain: Axial pain is more reflective of disk, facet joint, or sacroiliac joint pathology, or it may be due to spinal instability. It is unlikely a symptom of LSS.[84]
- Clinical signs: Patients with LSS tend to walk with stooped forward gait, often maintain this position while standing (i.e., a "stooped posture") with loss of lumbar lordosis and decreased range of lumbar extension. Due to the slow onset and chronic nature of the symptoms, SLR is infrequently positive. In a clinical study of patients with LSS, sensory motor deficits in the LE were seen in 30% of patients, most commonly in the L5 NR distribution. A decreased or absent Achilles reflex was seen in 43% (patellar reflex in 18%) of the patients, while the SLR was positive only 10% to 23% of the time.[85]

Diagnosis

MRI is the most common imaging technique used to detect the pathologic lesions of LSS. It provides the best visualization of IVDs, ligamentum flavum, central canal, and neural foraminae.[86] CT scan provides better imaging of the bony details, especially facet pathology, and superior visualization of the lateral recesses. Lumbar myelography followed by CT scan (CT myelogram) is the imaging technique of choice when MRI is contraindicated or not available. The value of EMG/NCS and plain radiologic films in LSS are similar to their applications in other types of LRS and is discussed earlier. Because of the frequent presence of radiologic abnormalities of LSS in asymptomatic individuals[21,22] and their common occurrence in older adults,[79] it is crucial to correlate the radiologic abnormalities with the clinical findings in order to make this diagnosis.

Natural History and Treatment Options

Initially thought to be unrelentingly progressive,[87] the natural history of LSS, although interspersed by intermittent flare-ups, remains relatively unchanged over time.[88,89] Because of its perceived progressive nature and poor prognosis, LSS was typically treated by early surgical intervention in the past.[87] Nonsurgical treatment modalities have been shown to be effective and can prevent progression of patient's symptoms.[89,90] Surgical treatments for LSS typically provide superior control of symptoms initially,[91] but this benefit declines over time.[92] The prevalence of this condition in older adults, with the frequent presence of other comorbidities, often make these patients unsuitable for invasive treatments. Delaying surgery for a trial of nonsurgical treatment, even in the presence of severe stenosis, has been shown to have minimal detrimental effect on the final surgical outcome.[93] In conclusion, in the absence of progressive neurologic deficits or CES (which is rare in LSS), surgical treatment is prudent in patients who have failed an appropriate trial of nonoperative treatment.

Nonoperative Treatments

Nonoperative treatment modalities are particularly useful for the acute flare-ups of LSS and include medications, activity modification, bracing, physical therapy, and ESIs.

- Medications: Acetaminophen and NSAIDs are often helpful in providing symptomatic relief. Because this condition is chronic, however, the use of narcotic pain medications should be limited to the acute flare-ups.[94] Calcitonin has been found to be beneficial in spinal stenosis and is particularly effective for LSS resulting from Paget's disease.[95]
- Activity modification: Avoidance of aggravating activities and relative rest are suggested during acute flare-ups. Because of the potential for deconditioning, strict bed rest is no longer advocated in the treatment of LSS.[94]
- Bracing: Rigid lumbar braces extend the lumbar spine and may be detrimental. Lumbar binders reduce loads across the lumbar spine and may be helpful; they may be worn for short periods of time only to avoid deconditioning.
- Physical therapy: Flexion-based exercises (e.g., stationary bicycle and inclined treadmill) increase the cross-sectional area of the spinal canal and improve the microcirculation of the neural elements. These allows patients to tolerate the exercise program better and help improve weight loss and cardiovascular fitness.[96] Aquatic therapy is also useful; it stretches the hip flexors and hamstrings and strengthens the abdominal and trunk muscles.
- Epidural steroid injections: Interlaminar ESIs have been shown to be effective especially in the short term and may provide symptomatic control of acute exacerbations of neurogenic claudication.[97]

Fluoroscopically directed transforaminal ESIs appear to be better suited for radicular symptoms secondary to LSS and have been shown to have both short-[98] and long-term efficacy.[99]

Operative Treatments

Wide laminectomy, performed at the stenotic levels, is the standard procedure for the surgical decompression for LSS.[100] This procedure involves removal of the spinal laminae and the ligamentum flavum, extending laterally from pedicle to pedicle. Extensive removal of posterior spinal elements can result in spinal instability; this can be avoided by preservation of the pars interarticularis and the lateral 50% portion of the facet joints. Extensive decompressive surgery is indicated in the presence of complex stenosis and degenerative spondylolisthesis or deformity. In conjunction with postdecompressive fusion, with or without instrumentation, surgery avoids ensuing spinal instability.[100] Surgical techniques involving minimal decompression—laminotomy, fenestration, laminoplasty—are aimed at preserving spine stability. However, they have been shown to be associated with higher rates of restenosis. Surgical treatments are discussed in more detail in Chapter 18.

INTERNAL DISK DISRUPTION

Although the role of HD as a cause of pain is well established, pain originating from the disk itself—varyingly termed *discogenic pain, internal disk disruption (IDD), painful degenerative disk disease (DDD)*—is poorly understood and is shrouded with controversy.[101]

Normal Disk Physiology

The IVD is grossly compartmentalized into the nucleus pulposus (NP) and annulus fibrosus (AF). This distinction is most obvious at the lumbar levels compared with cervical levels and decreases with advancing age. Cells that maintain disk integrity populate both the NP and AF. Chondrocyte-like cells often found in clusters sparsely populate the NP, while cells in the AF have fibrocyte-like features.[102] The matrix composition in which these cells are suspended also differs significantly. The matrix is jelly-like in the NP and has a high concentration of water and proteoglycans, whereas the matrix in AF is high in collagen that is arranged as interlacing lamellae, firmly attached to the adjacent vertebral bodies.[102] A healthy IVD is able to sustain a substantial amount of physical strain.[103] These compressive forces are borne directly by the NP and are equally distributed to the AF as a tensile force.[104] Incompressibility exhibited by a normal NP is largely due to its high water content, maintained by the hydrostatic pressure generated by its proteoglycans.[102] A delicate balance between the anabolic activities of the cells in NP and catabolic activities of the matrix metalloproteinases (MMPs) maintain the normal nuclear proteoglycan content. The state of hydration and thus compressibility of the NP can therefore be affected by a variety of factors that influence the metabolic activities within the disk.[105]

The IVD is the largest avascular structure in the body: its nerves are mostly mechanoreceptors, and the blood vessels are typically found only in the outer third of the AF.[102,106] The innervation of the IVD is by plexuses along the anterior and posterior longitudinal ligaments. The posterior plexus receives its input from the sinuvertebral nerve and gray rami communicans; the latter also mainly contribute to the anterior plexus. The sinuvertebral nerve receives its contributions from the ventral rami and gray rami communicans.[107] A normal disk has rich autonomic connections, which may contribute to the hyperalgesia exhibited by a chronically painful disk. The metabolic requirements of the cells in the NP and inner AF are met almost entirely by diffusion from and to the capillary plexuses in the adjacent vertebral bodies and outer AF.[108] This arrangement is tenuous at best and cells in the NP function in a precarious anaerobic environment.[109] The IVD also lacks scavenger cells and degradative products of disk macromolecules accumulate over time, which can alter normal cell matrix interactions.[110]

Pathophysiology of Degenerative Disk Disease

Degenerative changes in the IVDs are commonly seen in older asymptomatic individuals[111] and may be regarded as a physiologic consequence of aging. Certain disks however can undergo progressive degeneration early in life and this process may be pathologic in nature.[112] A host of factors predispose to early and progressive DDD (Box 17–3).[113-117] Dysfunction and decline in the viable cells,[118] coupled with enhanced MMP activity[119] and an increase in the cytokines and proinflammatory mediators[120] within the disk, can start a vicious cycle resulting in the reduction in the nuclear proteoglycan content. The loss of the hydrostatic pressure and the water content follows, making the NP compressible and exposing the AF to direct compression.[104]

The AF also undergoes degenerative changes similar to those seen in the NP resulting in the loss of annular collagen. These changes, along with direct annular compression, lead to annular failure and development of fissures that spread outward toward the periphery.[121] These structural changes affect the biomechanical properties of the disk causing it to shrink

---

BOX 17–3. FACTORS PREDISPOSING TO DEGENERATIVE DISK DISEASE

- Diminished blood supply
- Genetic predisposition
- Increased mechanical stress
- End plate injury
- Vascular disease
- Obesity

---

and become less mobile.[122] Changes in the disk dynamics increase stress on adjacent structures and may lead to sclerosis and hypertrophic new bone formation in the adjacent vertebral bodies, that is, Modic changes,[123] accelerated degeneration of adjacent disks, hypertrophy and arthritis of the facet joints, sacroiliac joint dysfunction (SIJD), and paraspinal myofascial syndrome.[124] Stenotic changes in the spinal canal and intervertebral foraminae may follow and can cause NR and spinal cord compressive symptoms.[125] Although spinal degenerative changes are seen commonly in patients with spinal pain, they are also frequently seen in asymptomatic individuals[111] and their presence correlates poorly with the pain experienced by the patients.[126] It is likely that only certain types of degenerative changes at certain times produce pain.

Pathology of Internal Disk Disruption and Discogenic Pain

Although subjective and potentially confounded by a host of psychosocial and somatization influences,[127] the pain of positive discographic evaluation is linked to the pathologic lesions of internal disk disruption (IDD).[128-135] Whether IDD is a distinct disease entity or it is painful, early and progressive DDD is not clear and often these terms are used interchangeably. It is likely that factors that predispose to early and progressive DDD also lead to the pathologic changes of IDD. Although innervation and vascularity of a normal disk is limited to the outer one third of the AF,[102,106,107] disks from patients with pain on discographic evaluation (those with concordant pain), show zones of vascularized granulation tissue that extend from the NP to outer AF.[133-135] These granulation tissue zones correlate with annular tears seen on post-discography CT scans[133] and high intensity zones seen on MRI.[134] Two types of nerve fibers that are found mainly along the zones of granulation tissue have been identified in these disks.[133] Nerve fibers that accompany the neovascularization are possibly vasoregulatory, and free nerve endings that are high in substance P and penetrate deep into the inner AF and NP are most likely nociceptors.[129,130] These zones of granulation tissue also show abundant mononuclear cell infiltration and strong expression of nerve growth factors that may contribute to nerve in-growth and accelerate disk degeneration.[132,135] These disks also produce significant amounts of proinflammatory mediators,[131] which can sensitize the neonociceptors and maintain a state of hyperalgesia within the affected disk. These hyperalgesic disks can cause chronic pain, worse with mechanical stress (axial loading), and produce a painful response with minimal stimulation on discography (i.e., a chemically sensitized disk).[136] The presence of annular tears, nociceptive innervation of the inner AF and NP, and presence of proinflammatory mediators and inflammatory cells, along with the abundance of sympathetic connections at the spinal cord level, provide a ready substrate for the origin of discogenic pain.

Historical Background

The concept of IVD as a source of pain is not new and was espoused as early as 1947.[137] The term *internal disk disruption*, however, was not introduced until 1986[138] and was based on the observation that disks that produced pain on discography often appeared morphologically intact. These disks therefore appear normal on spinal imaging studies, and the diagnosis of IDD was based primarily on a subjective pain response during provocative discography. However, the validity of pain on discography was seriously challenged in a study published by Holt in 1968 showing a false-positive rate of 37%.[139] Although the methodology of Holt's study was later seriously criticized[140] and a study by Walsh showed a false-positive rate of 0%,[141] Carragee and colleagues[127] have continued to criticize the diagnostic significance of pain of discography. More stringent criteria for positive discograms were adopted to reduce the false-positive rates. These included concordant pain response, presence of at least one disk level with no pain on disk provocation—"control disk," and the evidence of disk disruption on postdiscography CT scan, that is, tears extending to the outer annulus.[142] Pressure manometry during discography is often used, and it can identify disks that are painful with minimal stimulation and may increase the specificity of discography.[143] No test, however, is available to date that can objectively detect the pathologic lesions of IDD.

Clinical Presentation

A study performed by Schwarzer and colleagues[144] showed that in a group of patients with axial CLBP, when all the criteria of IDD suggested by the International Spine Intervention Society (ISIS)[142] were satisfied, the incidence of IDD was as high as 40%. The authors also claimed that their study population represented the general population. In another study by Hyodo and associates,[145] 73% of patients with severe acute LBP obtained greater than 70% relief of their pain by intradiskal injection of local anesthetic, suggesting that the pain was discogenic in origin. Pain originating from the disk can therefore be either acute or chronic and it may be due to either an acute tear of the disk or the chronic lesions of IDD. In both studies, the incidence of discogenic pain was highest in patients who were younger than 40 years of age. The pain is located primarily in the low back and buttocks region.[145] It is often precipitated by a torsion injury to the low back and exacerbated by axial loading such as occurs with prolonged sitting and standing. Radiation of the pain to the lower extremities has also been reported.[146]

Diagnosis

Spinal imaging frequently shows degenerative disk changes in asymptomatic individuals[111,126] and are, therefore, of limited value in the diagnosis of IDD.

IDD is frequently referred to as "black disk disease,"[147] which is due to loss of signal intensity on T2-weighted MR images and signifies desiccation of NP. However, it is a change representative of early DDD and may not be painful. A high-intensity zone (HIZ) in the posterior annulus, most prominent on T1-weighted MR images, indicates the presence of a tear in the posterior annulus and correlates closely with the pain of discography and pathologic lesions of IDD.[134] Several studies have attempted to correlate the results of discography with the radiologic features of DDD, and concordance has ranged from 55%[148] to almost 100%.[149] Concordant pain response to disk provocation, in the presence of a nonpainful or nonconcordant response at another disk level, coupled with morphologic abnormalities seen on postdiscography CT scan (i.e., tears extending to the outer one third of the AF) currently remain the only means of diagnosing IDD.

Treatments

To date, treatments of IDD and painful DDD remain palliative. Intradiskal electrothermal therapy (IDET) is a minimally invasive procedure that involves thermal lesioning of the posterior disk annulus by a percutaneously placed heating coil.[150] Based on studies of joint capsular collagen,[151] the mechanism of IDET action is hypothesized as shrinkage of the annular collagen and coagulation of the neonociceptive fibers. The true nature of its reported benefits, however, remain unknown.[152] Outcome studies for IDET are also mixed with efficacy measurements ranging from minimal benefit[153] to success rates approaching 80%.[150] The removal of the painful disk and arthrodesis of the adjacent vertebral bodies—spinal fusion—should theoretically relieve the pain of discogenic origin. The results of spinal fusion are mixed and serious doubts have been raised regarding its efficacy.[154] Disk arthroplasty was introduced to obviate some of the problems associated with spinal fusion, such as loss of mobility and adjacent disk degeneration. The initial outcome studies of disk arthroplasty showed that results were no better than spinal fusion and several unanswered questions regarding device longevity, complication rates, and long-term effects remain.[155] Currently available treatments for discogenic pain are therefore symptomatic therapies with questionable efficacy and possible associated complications; they also are unable to restore or prevent further deterioration of disk architecture and function.

Future Directions

The future for the diagnosis and treatment of pain of discogenic origin is promising. The understanding of the pathologic processes responsible for discogenic pain has increased in recent years. A better knowledge of differences between a normal and a painful disk should allow their distinction and may make the objective and early diagnosis of IDD a reality. Biologic treatments such as gene therapy,[156] tissue engineering, and stem cell transplantation[157] are currently being investigated. Successful and early application of these modalities may retard further disk degeneration and prevent development of related spinal syndromes, ultimately reducing the incredible costs and suffering from the disorders that cause spinal pain.

LUMBAR FACET SYNDROME

Anatomy

Lumbar facet joints (LFJs) or zygapophyseal joints are synovial joints with cartilaginous articular surfaces, synovial membranes, fibroadipose meniscoids, and fibrous capsule.[158] These paired joints are located dorsally at the junction of lamina, pedicle, and base of the transverse process. Each joint is comprised of two articular processes, superior and inferior, stemming from the corresponding vertebrae. The orientation of facet joints is distinct at lumbar, thoracic, and cervical levels. The medial branch (MB) of the posterior primary ramus courses over the base of the superior articular processes (SAP) at its junction with the transverse process (TP), to innervate the facet joint at the same vertebral level and the vertebral level below—each facet joint therefore receives innervation from the MB at the same vertebral level and from the vertebral level above. The course of the MB is relatively fixed as it originates from the dorsal ramus, proximally at the base of SAP, and as it passes under the mamilloaccessory ligament, at the caudal edge of the SAP.[159] The L5 dorsal ramus passes over the sacral ala at the base of the sacral SAP.[159] The fibrous capsule and the synovium of the facet joints are richly innervated by the nociceptive fibers.[160]

Historical Background

Goldthwait first proposed LFJs as a potential source of pain in the early 1900s[28] and the term *facet syndrome* was introduced by Ghormley as early as 1933.[161] Several investigators have since reproduced pain in the low back and the proximal leg by injecting hypertonic saline (a physiologic irritant) into the facet joints.[162-164] Relief of pain in patients with CLBP by intra-articular injections of local anesthetic and steroids was first reported by Mooney and Robertson in 1976.[163]

Pathophysiology

The exact nature of pathologic lesions responsible for the pain originating from the LFJs remains unknown (Box 17–4). Systemic inflammatory arthritides (e.g., rheumatoid arthritis and ankylosing spondylitis), villonodular synovitis, synovial cysts, and infections are rare causes of pain originating from LFJs.[165] Microtrauma, including microfractures, and capsular and cartilaginous tears, have been observed on postmortem studies, which are undetected by routine imaging studies[166]; the role of these injuries in causing CLBP,

---

BOX 17–4. PATHOLOGIC LESIONS THAT CAN CAUSE LUMBAR FACET SYNDROME

- Systemic inflammatory arthritides
  - Rheumatoid arthritis
  - Ankylosing spondylitis
- Degenerative arthritic changes
- Villonodular synovitis
- Synovial cysts
- Infections
- Microtrauma
  - Microfractures
  - Capsular and cartilaginous tears
- Meniscoid and synovial entrapment
- Joint subluxation

BOX 17–5. CLINICAL FEATURES OF LUMBAR FACET SYNDROME

- Low back pain
- Referred pain to groin, hip, posterior thigh rarely below the knee
- Pain exacerbated by twisting or arching movements, prolonged sitting or standing
- Pain relieved by forward flexion, rest, and walking
- Pain on back extension
- Localized tenderness over facet joints
- No neurologic deficits
- Normal straight leg raise

---

however, remains unknown. Meniscoid and synovial entrapment and joint subluxation have also been proposed as potential causes.[167] Degenerative arthritic changes are commonly observed, both in asymptomatic individuals and in patients with CLBP, and are often presumed to be a frequent source of lumbar facet syndrome (LFS). Their correlation with the diagnostic facet injections, however, is poor.[168] The degenerative arthritic changes in the facet joints frequently accompany degenerative changes in the disks and neural canals, and their contribution to patients' overall pain often remains undetermined.

Diagnosis

The clinical features of LFS have been varyingly described. The typical features described include unilateral or bilateral LBP, which frequently refers to the groin, hip, or thighs but infrequently below the knee joints (Box 17–5).[169] The pain is often exacerbated by arching or twisting movements and prolonged standing or sitting, and is reportedly relieved by forward flexion, rest, and walking. Painful limitation of back extension, lack of neurologic findings, negative SLR, and localized tenderness over the facet joints, have all been described as typical findings on physical examination. Other investigators, however, report lack of consistent clinical findings in patients who respond positively to the diagnostic facet joint injections.[170] Although correlation between arthritic findings on imaging studies and pain relief from diagnostic injections has been suggested,[171] no imaging findings or radionuclide scans reliably predict facet joints as a source of pain.[172] Although controversial, analgesic response to targeted, low-volume, intra-articular local anesthetic injections or MB blocks (MBBs), remain currently the only accepted standard for diagnosing the pain originating from the LFJs.[169,170,173]

Diagnostic Facet Injections

The suspected painful joints injected are either the most tender joints on palpation and, in the absence of any localizing signs, the lower most joints, L5/S1 and L4/5, because these joints are most commonly affected.[170] Fluoroscopic guidance using coaxial needle insertion technique is deemed essential for intra-articular needle placement. The injectate volume is kept less than 2 mL; larger injectate volumes can cause capsular rupture and leakage into the neural foraminae and epidural space, losing diagnostic specificity. Injection of a small volume of contrast medium (0.2 to 0.3 mL) delineating the joint space and indicating correct needle tip location is highly recommended. MBBs are performed by injecting a small volume (<1 mL) of local anesthetic at the junction of TP and SAP (the "eye of the scottie dog") and have been shown to have equal diagnostic sensitivity.[170] Injection of a small volume of contrast medium is often used before injection of local anesthetic for MBB to confirm correct needle placement and to rule out intravascular needle tip location. MBBs are especially useful if joint entry cannot be obtained, as is often the case in severely degenerated joints and in postspinal surgery patients. MBBs are also preferred diagnostic injections before radiofrequency MB rhizotomy, because they allow direct testing of the nerves targeted for subsequent neurotomy. Avoidance or use of only short-acting systemic analgesics and resumption of routine activities after the diagnostic injection facilitates the evaluation of pain response from the procedure. The use of local anesthetics of different duration on two separate occasions provides double comparative blocks. The patient who reports pain relief that corresponds with the duration of the local anesthetic used indicates a positive response. The prevalence of LFS among patients with CLBP using a single set of diagnostic injections has been variably reported and ranges between 7.7% to as high as 75%.[173] The wide variation in prevalence rates may reflect variations in technique and subsets of patients with LBP that were studied. Placebo response rates of almost 40% are reported with single diagnostic blocks.[174] Prevalence rates of 15% to 40% have been reported using more stringent double comparative blocks.[173] The latter is highly recommended for appropriate diagnosis of LFS and to avoid an unacceptably high false-positive response rate obtained with single blocks.

Therapeutic Lumbar Facet Joint Injections

Therapeutic lumbar intra-articular facet joint injection (TLFJIs) of steroids, often mixed in local anesthetic solution, is one of the most commonly performed pain management procedures. Based on the practice of intra-articular injection of steroids into painful knee and shoulder joints, intra-articular injection of steroids into LFJ was first performed by Mooney and Robertson in 1976.[163] There are, however, no scientific studies documenting capsular inflammation in painful LFJ, and their use along with the typical dosage used (20 to 30 mg of methylprednisolone per joint) remains empiric. Although confirmation of LFS by diagnostic facet injections before facet denervation is also recommended, it is rarely practiced clinically; clinicians tend to do diagnostic MBBs rather than facet joint injections before rhizotomy.[175] Observational studies report long-term (greater than 6 months) success rates of TLFJI in the range of 18% to 63%.[173] Long-term pain relief, however, is also reported after intra-articular facet injections of local anesthetics and saline.[176] The few prospective controlled trials conducted on this topic have been seriously criticized[173] and failed to show the efficacy of TLFJIs.[173,176]

Facet Denervation

Facet denervation, rhizotomy, neurotomy, or ablation is accomplished by lesioning of the MB at the same vertebral level and one vertebral level above. Although chemical neurolysis and cryoablation have been used, RF ablation (RFA) is the most frequently used technique. Because the distal circumferential radius is shorter than the more proximal circumferential radius of the thermal lesion generated, RFA lesioning is performed by placing the RFA electrode along the path of the nerve (i.e., along the base of the SAP).[177] Optimal electrode position is confirmed radiologically and by sensory and motor testing before the creation of the lesion. The size of the electrodes used vary from 22 to 18 gauge, with temperatures ranging between 80° and 90° C and the duration of RF lesioning varying from 60 to 90 seconds in different reports. Larger probe size and longer duration of lesion creation tend to produce larger size lesions with greater likelihood of thermal injury to the target nerve. The routine use of 18-gauge electrodes with a 1-cm exposed tip with RF lesioning for 120 seconds at 80° C, have been recommended.[178] Aside from several observational studies reporting the efficacy of LFJ RFA, three randomized controlled trials of its efficacy are available. Two of those demonstrate improvement in CLBP following the RFA treatments while the third showed no benefit.[178]

SACROILIAC JOINT DYSFUNCTION

Epidemiology

The SIJ was first described as a source of pain in 1905.[179] Of the various potential sources of pain in the SIJ area, SIJ dysfunction (SIJD) appears to be the most frequent and is thought to be the primary source of pain in 10% to 25% of patients with low back problems.[180,181] SIJD is especially common in women and during pregnancy, when the incidence can be as high as 20% to 80%.[182]

Etiology

Factors predisposing to SIJD are myriad (Box 17–6): abnormal stress across the joint by conditions such as leg length discrepancy, spinal deformity, previous surgery,[183,184] and painful conditions of adjacent structures (e.g., IVDs and facet joints) can all predispose to SIJD. Patients with SIJD often report a history of minor trauma,[185] while ligament laxity may explain its predisposition during pregnancy and in women.[186] Ligaments and musculature immediately outside the SIJ can also become painful, and pain from IVDs and facet joints can refer to the SIJ area. These conditions often coexist and one condition may predispose to the development of the other; for example, painful conditions of IVDs may lead to facet and sacroiliac joint pain. Because it is a synovial joint, the SIJ can become painful from a variety of pathologic processes that affect other synovial joints in the body. These disorders include inflammation (ankylosing spondylitis), degenerative disease (osteoarthritis), metabolic dysfunction (gout and pseudogout), traumatic injuries, infections, and tumors.[187] The origin of pain in the SIJ area can therefore be complex and its diagnosis challenging.

Diagnosis

The term *sacroiliac joint dysfunction* was first described in the osteopathic medicine and physical therapy literature as a functional disorder manifested by hypomobility and pain in the SIJ area without recognizable pathologic lesions.[188,189] Imaging and laboratory studies in SIJD should therefore be normal. In addition to pain, hypomobility, and normal laboratory and imaging studies, one or two diagnostic local anesthetic injections have been recommended as a part of the diagnostic criteria.[190] Painful pathologic conditions of the SIJ other than SIJD, can often be diagnosed by a typical history, physical examination, and appropriate laboratory and imaging studies.

Clinical Features

Pain originating in SIJ and surrounding structures is typically located in the lower back with greatest intensity in the region of the affected SIJ and medial buttock.[191] The pain may radiate to the groin, posterior thigh, and only occasionally below the knee joint.[192] Physical examination often reveals tenderness over the affected sacroiliac sulcus, most obvious in the prone position, reduction in the joint mobility, and reproduction of the pain when the affected SIJ is stressed.

Clinical Tests for Sacroiliac Joint Dysfunction

Tests based on movement dysfunction show inadequate interexaminer reliability[193] and are infrequently conducted. A battery of SIJ stress tests, however, is available. Performed individually these tests may not be reliable, although the diagnostic sensitivity and specificity can be greatly enhanced by using multiple tests in various combinations.[194]

The most commonly used tests for SIJD include the Faber Patrick, Gaenslen's, Yeoman's, sacroiliac shear, and Gillet tests. The tests are performed by the following maneuvers.[195]

Faber Patrick Test (Left Sacroiliac Joint Dysfunction) (Fig. 17–1)

- Patient is supine
- Left leg, near the ankle, is placed in front of the right thigh above the knee. Physician places one hand over the right iliac crest while the other hand pushes over the medial aspect of the left knee.
- Positive test: pain over left SIJ region (also back, buttock, groin)
- Comment: Test stresses the SI and hip joints.

Gaenslen's Test (Left Sacroiliac Joint Dysfunction) (Fig. 17–2)

- Patient is supine. Left lower thigh and leg hang over the examination table.
- Examiner flexes right hip and right knee (i.e., hip joint is maximally flexed).
- Examiner presses downward over the left thigh (hip joint is hyperextended).
- Positive test: pain in the left SIJ
- Comments: Test stresses both SIJs simultaneously by counterrotation at the extreme range of motion of the joint. Test also stresses the hip joint and stretches the femoral nerve.

BOX 17–6. FACTORS PREDISPOSING TO SACROILIAC JOINT SYNDROME

- Trauma
- Leg length discrepancy
- Spinal deformity
- Previous surgery
- Disk pathology
- Lumbar facet syndrome
- Pregnancy
- Inflammation of the joint (ankylosing spondylitis)
- Degenerative disease of the joint (osteoarthritis)
- Metabolic dysfunction affecting the joint (gout)
- Infection
- Tumor

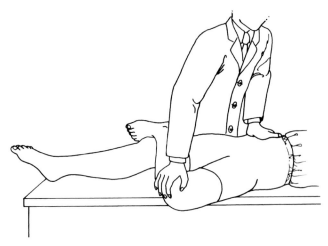

Figure 17–1. Faber Patrick test. (From Benzon HT: Pain originating from the buttock: Sacroiliac joint dysfunction and piriformis syndrome. In Benzon HT, Raja SN, Molloy RE, et al [eds]: Essentials of Pain Medicine and Regional Anesthesia, 2nd ed. Philadelphia, Elsevier, 2005.)

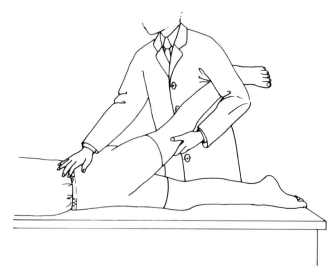

Figure 17–3. Yeoman's test (also called extension test). (From Benzon HT: Pain originating from the buttock: Sacroiliac joint dysfunction and piriformis syndrome. In Benzon HT, Raja SN, Molloy RE, et al [eds]: Essentials of Pain Medicine and Regional Anesthesia, 2nd ed. Philadelphia, Elsevier, 2005.)

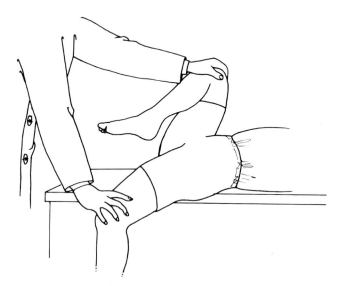

Figure 17–2. Gaenslen's test. (From Benzon HT: Pain originating from the buttock: Sacroiliac joint dysfunction and piriformis syndrome. In Benzon HT, Raja SN, Molloy RE, et al [eds]: Essentials of Pain Medicine and Regional Anesthesia, 2nd ed. Philadelphia, Elsevier, 2005.)

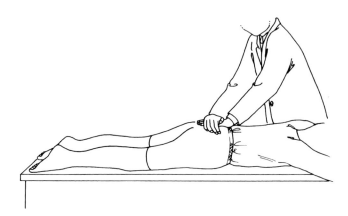

Figure 17–4. Sacroiliac shear test. (From Benzon HT: Pain originating from the buttock: Sacroiliac joint dysfunction and piriformis syndrome. In Benzon HT, Raja SN, Molloy RE, et al [eds]: Essentials of Pain Medicine and Regional Anesthesia, 2nd ed. Philadelphia, Elsevier, 2005.)

Sacroiliac Shear Test (Fig. 17–4)

- Patient is prone.
- Palm of examiner's hand is placed over the posterior iliac wing.
- Shear thrust is directed inferiorly producing a shearing force across the SIJ.
- Positive test: pain in dysfunctional SIJ.

Gillet's Test (Fig. 17–5)

- Patient is standing.
- One of examiner's thumbs is placed on the second sacral spinous process; the other thumb is placed on the posterior superior iliac spine (PSIS).

Yeoman's Test, Also Called Extension Test (Fig. 17–3)

- Patient is prone.
- Examiner places one hand above the anterior knee and elevates it slightly; the other hand presses downward over the crest of the ilium.
- Positive test: pain over the posterior SIJ.
- Comments: The hip is extended and the ipsilateral ilium is rotated. Test stresses the SIJ, extends the lumbar spine, and stresses the femoral nerve. Considered to be the most specific and reliable test.

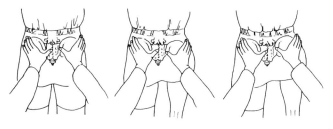

Normal Gillet's Test   Abnormal Gillet's Test

Figure 17–5. Gillet's test. (From Benzon HT: Pain originating from the buttock: Sacroiliac joint dysfunction and piriformis syndrome. In Benzon HT, Raja SN, Molloy RE, et al [eds]: Essentials of Pain Medicine and Regional Anesthesia, 2nd ed. Philadelphia, Elsevier, 2005.)

- Normal SIJ: When the patient maximally flexes the hip, the PSIS moves inferior to the S2 spinous process.
- Dysfunctional or fixed SIJ: PSIS remains at the level of the S2 spinous process or moves superior to the sacrum.

Diagnostic Sacroiliac Joint Injection

The diagnostic SIJ injection typically involves placement of a needle under radiologic imaging into the most caudal aspect of the joint. Intra-articular position of the needle is further confirmed by the appropriate spread of contrast medium into the joint.[196] Adequate needle positioning is followed by injection of a small volume of long- or short-acting local anesthetic. Pain intensity at rest or with activities that typically provoke patients' pain is compared to pre-injection pain levels. Concordant pain relief coinciding with the duration of local anesthetic indicates a positive response, that is, pain of SIJ origin. Criteria for positive response vary and range from 75%[181] to 90%[197] on a visual analogue scale score. Either a single injection[181,192] or double comparative blocks[180] are performed to minimize the placebo response. More stringent criteria add to diagnostic specificity but may also reduce the sensitivity of the test. Although not validated, diagnostic injection of the SIJ, using fluoroscopic guidance, currently remains the gold standard for the diagnosis of the pain of SIJ origin.[181] Poor technique, pain originating from structures immediately outside the SIJ, and extravasation of local anesthetic, especially anteriorly to the sciatic nerve, may reduce the validity of the diagnostic SIJ injection.

Treatment

The modalities available for the treatment of SIJD include physical therapy, manipulations, intra-articular steroid injections, RF denervation, and surgical fusion. Physical therapy[198] and chiropractic manipulations[199] are used extensively for the treatment of SIJD, but there is no large outcome study validating their use. The technique of therapeutic SIJ injection is similar to the diagnostic SIJ block, with a single needle placed into the caudal aspect of the joint and with the addition of depot steroids to the local anesthetic. Some practitioners prefer a two-needle technique: an additional needle is placed into the upper pole of the joint, in addition to the needle in the lower pole, to facilitate the spread of injectate into the superior half of the joint and the sacroiliac ligament. Intra-articular steroid injections of the SIJ have been shown to be effective[200]; however pain relief is typically short-term and no prospective controlled studies support their use. Surgical fusion of the SIJ for SIJD is also claimed to be successful[201]; however, all outcome studies of SIJ fusion are either small case series or are retrospective in nature.

Radiofrequency Denervation of the Sacroiliac Joint

RF denervation (RFD) of the SIJ is an attractive proposition that is expected to provide prolonged pain relief for SIJD. The goal of the RFD is to ablate the sensory nerves carrying painful signals from the affected SIJ. The nerve supply of the SIJ is complex and variable, making this treatment modality difficult to apply. Earlier literature suggests the sensory innervation of the SIJ by the ventral and dorsal rami of both lumbar and sacral NRs.[202] Recent reports have demonstrated a predominantly dorsal innervation from the L5 dorsal ramus and lateral branches of the S1 to S4 dorsal rami.[203,204] RFD of the SIJ is accomplished either by RF lesioning of these nerves as they emanate from the dorsal sacral foramina[205,206] or as they enter the SIJ along its posterior border.[207] A combination of these two techniques has also been described.[208] All studies pertaining to RFD of the SIJ have been either retrospective[205-207] or small and observational in nature.[208] The success rates of various RFD techniques quoted in these studies range from 50% to 70%.

Techniques for Radiofrequency Lesioning of the Sacroiliac Joint

Sacroiliac Joint Dorsal Border Radiofrequency Lesioning

Bipolar RF lesions are created along the dorsal border of the SIJ in a "leapfrog" manner.[207] In this leapfrog technique, two needles are used at less than 1 cm distance to create a bipolar "strip" lesion.[207] The lower needle is moved less than 1 cm cephalad to the other needle and another RF lesion is created. The process is repeated, creating a "strip" RF lesion along the joint. The ideal distance between the two needles was investigated by Pino and colleagues[209] who concluded that the needles should be placed between 4 and 6 mm apart to create a contiguous "strip" lesion and that the treatment duration should be between 120 to 150 seconds with electrode heated to 90° C.

Lateral Branch Radiofrequency Lesioning

Typically the dorsal rami of L4 and L5 or L5 alone, along with the lateral branches of the dorsal rami of S1 to S3 are lesioned. The L4 dorsal ramus is located at the junction of the superior articular process and the transverse process of the L5. The L5 dorsal ramus is located at the junction of the superior articular process of the S1 and the sacral ala. The lateral branches are located at the respective sacral foramina between the 2- and 6-o'clock positions on the right side and between the 6- and 10-o'clock positions on the left side.[206] Proximity to the target nerves is facilitated by sensory stimulation at frequencies of 50 Hz and by concordant pain reproduction at lowest possible voltage (<0.6 V). The RF needles range in size from 23 G[208] to 20 G[206] and have 5-mm[205,208] to 10-mm[206] active tips. The lesions are made for 60 to 90 seconds at 80 to 90° C.

The efficacy of lesioning the lateral branches has been questioned because the innervation of the ventral aspect of the SIJ is not lesioned.[210] However, Yin and colleagues[206] previously noted the predominant dorsal innervation of the SIJ.

A retrospective study showed the efficacy of monopolar thermal RF lesioning of the L4/S3 lateral branches in the treatment of SIJ pain.[205] Nine of 13 patients underwent RF lesioning of the L5/S3 lateral branches; 8 of the 9 patients experienced greater than 50% relief that persisted for at least 9 months.[205] In another study wherein monopolar RF lesioning of the S1-S3 lateral branches was performed,[206] 9 of 14 (64%) patients experienced a successful outcome (defined as greater than 60% patient-perceived improvement with concurrent greater than 50% decrease in visual analogue pain score for 6 months) while 5 patients (36%) had complete relief at 6 months. A recent study showed *bipolar strip* RF lesions at the lateral dorsal S1-S3 periforaminal areas to be effective in relieving SIJ pain.[211]

CONCLUSION

Low back pain (LBP) is a major source of pain and disability in modern society. The low back syndromes commonly encountered by a pain physician include radicular pain secondary to an HD or spinal stenosis, internal disk disruption, facet syndrome, sacroiliac joint dysfunction, and myofascial pain syndrome. Although various other causes of LBP (e.g., spinal deformities and spondylolisthesis) are not discussed in this chapter, the syndromes discussed here form the bulk of patients with LBP. In addition to the chronicity and concurrent presence of these syndromes, the complexity of LBP is contributed to by the psychosocial issues and the lack of adequate diagnostic tests and available treatments. The incredibly high toll from LBP can be reduced by appropriate diagnoses and treatments of the conditions discussed here. A thorough clinical evaluation to recognize specific signs and symptoms and their correlation with the findings from the available diagnostic tests, in combination with the application of proven therapeutic interventions, should help achieve this goal.

SUMMARY

- Numerous structural abnormalities, including HD and spinal stenosis, have been noted in asymptomatic patients.
- The symptoms of NR irritation include pain, paresthesia, and weakness and numbness in the territory of the affected NR. The involvement of the L2 and L3, L4, L5, and S1 nerve results in characteristic clinical features. Certain tests confirm the presence of NR irritation.
- The clinician should be aware of the red flags in the patient's medical history that may indicate tumor, infection, fracture, or CES.
- There are nonoperative treatments for HD, many of which have little proven efficacy. Newer studies showed the long-term efficacy of operative and nonoperative treatments for HD not to be significantly different.
- Similar to that for HD, the efficacy of surgery for spinal stenosis seems to decrease over time.
- IDD is diagnosed mostly by discography: (1) concordant pain response to disk provocation; (2) presence of a nonpainful or nonconcordant response at another disk level; and (3) morphologic abnormalities seen on postdiscography CT scan, that is, tears extending to the outer one third of the AF.
- Facet syndrome is characterized by pain in the lower back, paraspinal tenderness, back pain on extension and lateral flexion/rotation, absence of neurologic deficits, and a normal SLR.
- A diagnostic MBB, if it relieves the patient's back pain, is usually followed by a thermal facet rhizotomy.
- The tests to confirm the presence of SIJ pain include the Patrick Faber, Gaenslen's, Yeoman's, posterior shear, and Gillet's tests.
- The interventional treatment for SIJD includes injection of local anesthetic and steroid into the SIJ, thermal RF of the posterior SIJ, and RF of the lateral branches of the L5/S3 dorsal rami.

References

1. Frymoyer JW, Cats-Baril WL: An overview of the incidence and costs of low back pain. Orthop Clin N Am 1991;22:263-271.
2. Govind J: Lumbar radicular pain. Aust Fam Physician 2004;33:409-412.
3. Merskey H, Bogduk N: Classification of Chronic Pain. Description of Chronic Pain Syndromes and Definitions of Pain Terms, 2nd ed. Seattle, WA: IASP Press, 1994.
4. Deyo RA, Tsui-Wu YJ: Descriptive epidemiology of low back pain and its related medical care in United States. Spine 1987;12:264-268.
5. Svensson HO, Andersson GBJ: Low back pain in 40- to 47-year old men: Work history and work environment factors. Spine 1983;8:272-276.
6. Frymoyer JW, Cats-Baril WL: An overview of the incidence and costs of low back pain. Orthop Clin North Am 1991;22:263-271.
7. Filler AG, Haynes J, Jordan SE, et al: Sciatica of nondisc origin and piriformis syndrome: Diagnosis by magnetic resonance neurography and interventional magnetic resonance imaging with outcome study of resulting treatment. J Neurosurg Spine. 2005;2:99-115.

8. Smyth MJ, Wright V: Sciatica and the intervertebral disc: An experimental study. J Bone Joint Surg (Am) 1958;40:1401-1418.

9. Kleiner JB, Donaldson WF, Curd JG, et al: Extraspinal causes of lumbosacral radiculopathy. J Bone Joint Surg (Am) 1991;73(6):817-821.

10. Jennett W: A study of 25 cases of compression of the cauda equina by prolapsed intervertebral disc. J Neurol Neurosurg Psychiatr 1956;19:109-116.

11. Shapiro S: Cauda equina syndrome secondary to lumbar disc herniation. Neurosurgery 1993;32:743-747.

12. Goddard MP, Reid JD: Movement induced by straight leg raising in the lumbo-sacral roots, nerves and plexus, and in the intrapelvic section of the sciatic nerve. J Neurol Neurosurg Psychiatr 1965;28:12-18.

13. Frymoyer J: Back pain and sciatica. N Engl J Med 1988;318:291-300.

14. O'Connell JER: Sciatica and the mechanism of the production of clinical syndrome in protrusions of the lumbar intervertebral discs. Br J Surg 1943;30:315-317.

15. Xin SQ, Zhang QZ, Fan DH: Significance of the straight-leg-raising test in the diagnosis and clinical evaluation of the lower intervertebral-disc protrusion. J Bone Joint Surg (Am) 1987;69:517-522.

16. Bigos S, Bowyer O, Braen G, et al: Acute low back problems in adults. In Clinical Practice Guideline, Quick Reference Guide Number 14. AHCPR Pub. No. 95-0643, December 1994.

17. Portenoy RK, Lipton RB, Foley KM: Back pain in the cancer patient: An algorithm for evaluation and management. Neurology 1987;37:134-138.

18. Deyo R, Rainville J, Kent D: What can the history and physical examination tell us about low back pain: JAMA 1992;286:760-765.

19. Dinning T, Schaeffer H: Discogenic compression of the cauda equina: A surgical emergency. Aust N Z J Surg. 1993;63:927-934.

20. Anderson GBJ, Brown MD, Dvorak J, et al: Consensus summary on the diagnosis and treatment of lumbar disc herniation. Spine 1996;21(Suppl 24S):75S-78S.

21. Boden SD, Davis DO, Dina TS, et al: Abnormal magnetic-resonance scans of the lumbar spine in asymptomatic subjects: A prospective investigation. J Bone Joint Surg (Am) 1990;72:403-408.

22. Jensen MC, Brant-Zawadzki MN, Obuchowski N, et al: Magnetic resonance imaging of the lumbar spine in people without back pain. N Engl J Med. 1994;331:69-73.

23. Scavone JG, Latshaw RF, Rohrer GV: Use of lumbar spine films: Statistical evaluation of a university teaching hospital. JAMA 1981;246:1105.

24. Deen HG: Diagnosis and management of lumbar disc disease. Mayo Clin Proc 1996;71:283-287.

25. Rockey PH, Tompkins RK, Wood RW, et al: The usefulness of x-ray examinations in the evaluation of patients with low back pain. J Fam Pract 1978;7:455.

26. Hayes MA, Howard TC, Gruel CR, et al: Roentgenographic evaluation of lumbar spine flexion-extension in asymptomatic individuals. Spine 1989;14:327.

27. Robinson LR: Electromyography, magnetic resonance imaging and radiculopathy: It's time to focus on specificity. Muscle Nerve 1999;22:149-150.

28. Goldthwait JE: The lumbosacral articulations: An explanation of many cases of "lumbago," "sciatica," and paraplegia. Bost Med Surg J 1911;164:365.

29. Taylor VM, Deyo RA, Cherkin DC, et al: Low back pain hospitalization: Recent United States trends and regional variations. Spine 1994;19:1207-1213.

30. Fardon DF, Milette PC: Nomenclature and classification of lumbar disc pathology. Spine 2001;26:E93-E113.

31. Brock M, Patt S, Mayer H: The form and structure of the extruded disc. Spine 1992;17:1457-1461.

32. Mixter WJ, Barr JS: Rupture of the intervertebral disc with involvement of the spinal canal. N Engl J Med. 1934;211:210.

33. Rydevik BL, Myers RR, Powell HC: Pressure increase in the dorsal root ganglion following mechanical compression: Closed compartment syndrome in nerve roots. Spine. 1989;14:574-576.

34. Olmarker K, Rydevik B, Hansson T, et al: Compression-induced changes of the nutritional supply to the porcine cauda equina. J Spinal Disord 1990;3:25-29.

35. Kuslich SD, Ulstrom CL, Michael CJ: The tissue origin of low back pain and sciatica: A report of pain response to tissue stimulation during operations on lumbar spine using local anesthesia. Orthop Clin North Am. 1991;22:181-187.

36. Kang JD, Georgescu HI, McIntyre-Larkin L, et al: Herniated lumbar intervertebral discs spontaneously produce matrix metalloproteinases, nitric oxide, interleukin-6, and prostaglandin E2. Spine 1996;21:271-277.

37. Miyamoto H, Saura R, Doita M, et al: The role of cyclooxygenase-2 in lumbar disc herniation. Spine 2002;27:2477-2483.

38. Olmarker K, Rydevik B, Nordborg C: Autologous nucleus pulposus induced neurophysiologic and histologic changes in porcine cauda equine nerve roots. Spine 1993;18:1425-1432.

39. Slipman CW, Isaac Z, Lenrow DA, et al: Clinical evidence of chemical radiculopathy. Pain Physician 2002;5:260-265.

40. Benoist M: The natural history of the lumbar disc herniation and radiculopathy. Joint Bone Spine 2002;69:155-160.

41. Teplick JG: Spontaneous regression of herniated nucleus pulposus. AJR 1985;145:371-375.

42. Ahn SH, Ahn MW, Byun WM: Effect of the transligamentous extension of lumbar disc herniation on their regression and the clinical outcome of sciatica. Spine 2000;25:475-480.

43. Doita M, Kanatani T, Harada T, et al: Immunohistologic study of the ruptured intervertebral disc of lumbar spine. Spine 1996;21:235-241.

44. Van Tulder MW, Scholten RJ, Koes BW, et al: Nonsteroidal anti-inflammatory drugs for low back pain: A systemic review within the frame work of Cochrane Collaboration Back Review Group. Spine 2000;25:2501-2513.

45. Haimovic IC, Beresford HR: Dexamethasone is not superior to placebo for treating lumbosacral radicular pain. Neurology 1986;36:1593-1594.

46. Porsman O, Friis H: Prolapsed lumbar disc treated with intra-muscularly administered dexamethasone phosphate: A prospectively planned, double-blind, controlled clinical trial in 52 patients. Scand J Rheumatol 1979;8:142-144.

47. Hagen KB, Hilde G, Jamtvedt G, et al: The Cochrane review of bed rest for acute low back pain and sciatica. Spine 2000;25:2932-2939.

48. Malmivaara A, Hakkinen U, Aro T, et al: The treatment of acute low back pain—Bed rest, exercises, or ordinary activity? N Engl J Med 1995;332:1786.

49. Van Tulder MW, Jellema P, Van Poppel MN, et al: Lumbar supports for prevention and treatment of low back pain. Cochrane Database Syst Rev 2000;(3):CD001823.

50. Clarke JA, Van Tulder MW, Blomberg SE, et al: Traction for low-back pain with or without sciatica. Cochrane Database Syst Rev 2005;(4):CD003010.

51. Van Tulder MW, Cherkin DC, Berman B, et al: The effectiveness of acupuncture in the management of acute and chronic low back pain: A systematic review within the framework of Cochrane Collaboration Back Review Group. Spine 1999;24:1113-1123.

52. Van Tulder MW, Ostelo R, Vlaeyen JW, et al: Behavioral treatments for chronic low back pain: A systematic review within the framework of Cochrane Collaboration Back Review Group. Spine 2000;25:2688-2699.

53. Saal JA: Natural history and nonoperative treatment of lumbar disc herniation. Spine 1996;21(24S):2S-9S.

54. Van Tulder MW, Malmivaara A, Esmail R, et al: Exercise therapy for low back pain. Cochrane Database Syst Rev 2000;(2):CD000335.

55. Renfrew DL, Moore TE, Kathol ME, et al: Correct placement of epidural steroid injections: Fluoroscopic guidance and contrast administration. Am J Neuroradiol 1991;12:1003-1007.

56. Vroomen PC, de Krom MC, Slofstra PD, et al: Conservative treatment of sciatica: A systematic review. J Spinal Disord. 2000;13:463-469.

57. Schaufele M, Hatch L: Interlaminar versus transforaminal epidural injections in the treatment of symptomatic lumbar intervertebral disc herniations. Arch Phys Med Rehabil 2002;83:1661.

58. Singh V, Derby R: Percutaneous lumbar disc decompression. Pain Physician 2006;9:139-146.

59. Delamarter RB, Howard MW, Goldstein T, et al: Percutaneous lumbar discectomy: Preoperative and postoperative magnetic resonance imaging. J Bone Joint Surg Am 1995;77:578-584.

60. Yonezawa T, Onomura T, Kosaka R, et al: The system and procedures of percutaneous intradiscal laser nucleotomy. Spine 1990;15:1175-1185.

61. Choy D, Altman P: Fall of intradiscal pressure with laser ablation. Spine State Art Rev 1993;7:23-29.

62. Castro WH, Halm H, Rondhuis J: The influence of automated percutaneous lumbar discectomy (APLD) on the biomechanics of the intervertebral disc: An experimental study. Acta Orthop Belg 1992;58:400-405.

63. Ohnmeiss DD, Guyer RD, Hochschuler SH: Laser disc decompression: The importance of proper patient selection. Spine 1994;19:2054-2058.

64. Chatterjee S, Foy PM, Findlay GF: Report of a controlled clinical trial comparing automated percutaneous lumbar discectomy in the treatment of contained lumbar disc herniations. Spine 1995;20:734-738.

65. Revel M, Payan C, Vallee C, et al: Automated percutaneous lumbar discectomy versus chemonucleolysis in the treatment of sciatica: A randomized multicenter center trial. Spine 1993;18:1-7.

66. Weber H: Lumbar disc herniation: A controlled, prospective study with ten years of observation. Spine 1983;8:131-140.

67. Bessette L, Liang MH, Lew RA, Weinstein JN: Classics in spine: Surgery literature revisited. Spine 1996;21:259-263.

68. Atlas SJ, Keller RB, Wu YA, et al: Long-term outcomes of surgical and nonsurgical management of sciatica secondary to a lumbar disc herniation: 10 year results from the Maine lumbar spine study. Spine 2005;30:927-935.

69. Weinstein JN, Tosteson TD, Lurie JD, et al: Surgical versus nonoperative treatment for lumbar disc herniation. JAMA 2006;296:2441-2450.

70. Carragee E: Surgical treatment of lumbar disk disorders. JAMA 2006;296:2485-2487.

71. McCulloch JA: Focus issue on lumbar disc herniation: Macro- and microdiscectomy. Spine 1996;21:45S-56S.

72. Taylor VM, Deyo RA, Cherkin DC, et al: Low back pain hospitalization: Recent United States trends and regional variations. Spine 1994;19:1207-1213.

73. Andrews DW, Lavyne MH: Retrospective analysis of microsurgical and standard lumbar discectomy. Spine 1990;15:329-335.

74. Verbiest H: A radicular syndrome from developmental narrowing of the lumbar vertebral canal. J Bone Joint Surg. 1954;36:230-237.

75. Arnoldi CC, Brodsky AE, Crock HV: Lumbar spinal stenosis and nerve root entrapment syndromes: Definitions and classification. Clin Orthop 1976;115:4-5.

76. Schonstrom NSR, Bolender NF, Spengler DM: The pathomorphology of spinal stenosis as seen on CT scans of the lumbar spine. Spine 1985;10:806-811.

77. Jenis LG, An HS: Spine update. Lumbar foraminal stenosis. Spine 2000;25:389-394.

78. Dai LY, Yu YK, Zhang WM, et al: The effect of flexion-extension motion of the lumbar spine on the capacity of the spinal canal. An experimental study. Spine 1989;14:523-525.

79. Sasaki K: Magnetic resonance imaging findings of the lumbar nerve root pathway in patients over 50 years old. Eur Spine J 1995;4:71-76.

80. Ooi Y, Mita F, Satoh Y: Myeloscopic study on lumbar spinal canal stenosis with special reference to intermittent claudication. Spine 1990;15:544-549.

81. Hawkes CH, Roberts GM: Neurogenic and vascular claudication. J Neurol Sci 1978;38:337-345.

82. Katz JN, Dalgas M, Stucki G, et al: Degenerative lumbar spinal stenosis. Diagnostic value of the history and physical examination. Arthritis Rheum 1995;38:1236-1241.

83. Johnson B, Stromqvist B: Symptoms and signs in degeneration of the lumbar spine: A prospective, consecutive study of 300 operated patients. J Bone Joint Surg 1993;75-B:381-385.

84. Katz JN, Lipson SJ, Brick GW, et al: Clinical correlates of patient satisfaction after laminectomy for degenerative lumbar spinal stenosis. Spine 1995;20:1155-1160.

85. Hall SJ, Bartleson JD, Onofrio BM, et al: Lumbar spinal stenosis: Clinical features, diagnostic procedures, and results of surgical treatment in 68 patients. Ann Intern Med 1985;103:271-275.

86. Postacchini F, Amatruda A, Morace GB, et al: Magnetic resonance imaging in the diagnosis of lumbar spinal canal stenosis. Italian J Orthop Traumat 1991;17:327-337.

87. Wiltse LL, Kirkaldy-Willis WH, McIvor GWD: The treatment of spinal stenosis. Clin Orthop 1976;115:83-91.

88. Johnsson DE, Rosen I, Uden A: The natural course of lumbar spinal stenosis. Clin Orthop 1992;279:82-86.

89. Benoist M: The natural history of lumbar degenerative spinal stenosis. Joint Bone Spine 2002;69:450-457.

90. Houedakor J, Cabre P, Pascal-Moussellard H, et al: Rehabilitation treatment in lumbar canal stenosis: Intermediate results of a prospective study (Telemar). Ann Readapt Med Phys 2003;46:227-232.

91. Turner JA, Ersek M, Herron L, Deyo R: Surgery for lumbar spinal stenosis: Attempted meta-analysis of the literature. Spine 1992;17:1-8.

92. Jonsson B, Annertz M, Sjoberg C, et al: A prospective and conservative study of surgically treated lumbar spinal stenosis. Part II: Five-year follow-up by an independent observer. Spine 1997;22:2938-2944.

93. Amundsen T, Weber H, Nordal HJ, et al: Lumbar spinal stenosis: Conservative or surgical management? A prospective 10-year study. Spine 2000;25:1424-1436.

94. Zdeblick TA: The treatment of degenerative lumbar disorders: A critical review of the literature. Spine 1995;20:126S-137S.

95. Eskola A, Pohjolainen T, Alaranta H, et al: Calcitonin treatment in lumbar spinal stenosis: A randomized, placebo-controlled, double blind, cross-over study with one year follow-up. Calcif Tissue Int 1992;50:400-403.

96. Bodack MP, Monteiro M: Therapeutic exercise in the treatment of patients with lumbar spinal stenosis. Clin Orthop 2001;384:144-152.

97. Benzon HT: Epidural steroid injections for low back pain and lumbosacral radiculopathy. Pain 1986;24:277-295.

98. Schmid G, Vetter S, Gottmann D, et al: CT-guided epidural/perineural injections in painful disorders of the lumbar spine: short—and extended-term results. Cardiovasc Intervent Radiol 1999;22:493-498.

99. Riew KD, Yin Y, Gilula L, et al: The effect of nerve-root injections on the need for operative treatment of lumbar radicular pain: A prospective, randomized, controlled, double-blind study. J Bone Joint Surg (Am) 2000;82:1589-1593.

100. Yuan PS, Albert TJ: Nonsurgical and surgical management of lumbar spinal stenosis. J Bone Joint Surg (Am) 2004;2320-2330.

101. Lee KS, Doh JW, Bae HG, et al: Diagnostic criteria for the clinical syndrome of internal disc disruption: Are they reliable? Br J Neurosurg 2003;17:19-23.

102. Buckwalter JA, Mow VC, Boden SD, et al: Intervertebral disk structure, composition, and mechanical function. In Buckwalter JA, Einhorn TA, Simon SR (eds): Orthopaedic Basic Science-Biology and Biomechanics of the Musculoskeletal System. Rosemont, IL: American Academy of Orthopaedic Surgeons 2000:548-555.

103. Cholewicki J, McGill SM, Norman RW: Lumbar spine loads during the lifting of extremely heavy weights. Med Sci Sports Exerc 1991;23:1179-1186.

104. Adams MA, McNally DS, Dolan P: Stress distribution inside intervertebral discs: The effects of age and degeneration. J Bone Joint Surg (Br) 1996;78B:965-972.

105. Buckwalter JA: Aging and degeneration of the human intervertebral disc. Spine 1995;20:1307-1314.

106. Ashton IK, Roberts S, Jaffray DC, et al: Neuropeptides in the human intervertebral disc. J Orthop Res 1994;12:186-192.

107. Bogduk N, Tynan W, Wilson AS: The nerve supply to the human lumbar intervertebral discs. J Anat 1981;132:39-56.
108. Holm S, Maroudas A, Urban JP, et al: Nutrition of the intervertebral disc: Solute transport and metabolism. Connect Tissue Res 1981;8:101-109.
109. Ohshima H, Urban JP: The effects of lactate and pH on the proteoglycan and protein synthesis rates in the intervertebral disc. Spine 1992;17:1079-1082.
110. Yasuma T, Arai K, Suzuki F: Age-related phenomena in the lumbar intervertebral discs: Lipofuscin and amyloid deposition. Spine 1992;17:1194-1198.
111. Boden SD, McCowin PR, Davis DO: Abnormal magnetic-resonance scans of the cervical spine in asymptomatic subjects: A prospective investigation. J Bone Joint Surg (Am) 1990;72:1178-1184.
112. Boos N, Weissbach S, Rohrbach H, et al: Classification of age-related changes in lumbar intervertebral discs. Spine 2002;27:2631-2644.
113. Sambrook PN, MacGregor AJ, Spector TD: Genetic influences on cervical and lumbar disc degeneration: A magnetic resonance imaging study in twins. Arthritis Rheum 1999;42: 366-372.
114. Sandover J: Dynamic loading as a possible source of low-back disorders. Spine 1983;8:652-658.
115. Adams MA, Freeman BJC, Morrison HP, et al: Mechanical initiation of intervertebral disc degeneration. Spine 2000;25: 1625-1636.
116. Kauppila LI, McAlindon T, Evans S, et al: Disc degeneration/back pain and calcification of the abdominal aorta: A 25-year follow-up study in Framingham. Spine 1997;22:1642-1647.
117. Böstman OM. Body mass index and height in patients requiring surgery for lumbar intervertebral disc herniation. Spine 1993;18:851-854.
118. Buckwalter JA: Aging and degeneration of the human intervertebral disc. Spine 1995;20:1307-1314.
119. Roberts S, Caterson B, Menage J: Matrix metalloproteinases and aggrecanase: Their role in disorders of the human intervertebral disc. Spine 2000;25:3005-3013.
120. Kang JD, Georgescu HI, McIntyre-Larkin L: Herniated lumbar intervertebral discs spontaneously produce matrix metalloproteinases, nitric oxide, interleukin-6, and prostaglandin E2. Spine 1996;21:271-277.
121. Berlemann U, Gries NC, Moore RJ: The relationship between height, shape and histological changes in early degeneration of the lower lumbar discs. Eur Spine J 1998;7:212-217.
122. Mimura M, Panjabi MM, Oxland TR, et al: Disc degeneration affects the multidirectional flexibility of the lumbar spine. Spine 1994;19:1371-1380.
123. Modic MT, Masaryk TJ, Ross JS: Imaging of degenerative disk disease. Radiology 1988;168:177-186.
124. Adams MA, Dolan P, Hutton WC, et al: Diurnal changes in spinal mechanics and their clinical significance. J Bone Joint Surg (Br) 1990;72:266-270.
125. Postacchini F, Gumina S, Cinotti G, et al: Ligamenta flava in lumbar disc herniation and spinal stenosis: Light and electron microscopic morphology. Spine 1994;19:917-922.
126. Borenstein DG, O'Mara JW, Boden SD: The value of magnetic resonance imaging of the lumbar spine to predict low-back pain in asymptomatic subjects: A seven year follow-up study. J Bone Joint Surg (Am) 2001;83-A:1306-1311.
127. Carragee EJ, Tanner CM, Khurana S, et al: The rates of false-positive lumbar discography in select patients without low back symptoms. Spine 2000;25:1373-1380.
128. Moneta GB, Videman T, Kaivanto K, et al: Reported pain during lumbar discography as a function of anular ruptures and disc degeneration. A re-analysis of 833 discograms. Spine 1994;19:1968-1974.
129. Freemont AJ, Peacock TE, Goupille P, et al: Nerve ingrowth into disease intervertebral disc in chronic back pain. Lancet 1997;350:178-181.
130. Coppes MH, Marani E, Thomeer RT, et al: Innervation of "painful" lumbar discs. Spine 1997;22:2342-2349.
131. Burke JG, Watson RW, McCormack D, et al: Intervertebral discs which cause low back pain secrete high levels of proinflammatory mediators. J Bone Joint Surg (Br) 2002;84-B:196-201.
132. Freemont AJ, Watkins A, LeMaitre C, et al: Nerve growth factor expression and innervation of the painful intervertebral disc. J Pathol 2002;197:286-292.
133. Peng B, Wu W, Hou S, et al: The pathogenesis of discogenic low back pain. J Bone Joint Surg (Br) 2005;87-B:62-67.
134. Peng B, Hou S, Wu W, et al: The pathogenesis and clinical significance of a high-intensity zone (HIZ) of lumbar intervertebral disc on MR imaging in the patients with discogenic low back pain. Eur Spine J 2006;15:583-587.
135. Peng B, Hao J, Hou S, et al: Possible pathogenesis of painful intervertebral disc degeneration. Spine 2006;31:560-566.
136. Derby R, Howard MW, Grant JM, et al: The ability of pressure-controlled discography to predict surgical and nonsurgical outcomes. Spine 1999;24:364-372.
137. Inman VT, Saunders JBM: Anatomicophysiological aspects of injuries to the intervertebral disc. J Bone Joint Surg (Am) 1947;29:461-468.
138. Crock HV: Internal disc disruption: A challenge to disc prolapse fifty years on. Spine 1986;11:650-653.
139. Holt EP: The question of lumbar discography. J Bone Joint Surg (Am) 1968;50:720-726.
140. Simmons JW, April CN, Dwyer AP, et al: A re-assessment of Holt's data on "The question of lumbar discography." Clin Orthop 1998;237:120-124.
141. Walsh TR, Weinstein JN, Spratt KF, et al: Lumbar discography in normal subjects: A controlled, prospective study. J Bone Joint Surg (Am) 1990;72:1081-1088.
142. Endres S, Bogduk N: Practice guidelines and protocols: Lumbar disc stimulation. Presented at The International Spine Intervention Society 9th Annual Scientific Meeting, Boston, MA, Sept 14-16, 2001, pp 56-57.
143. Derby R, Lee SH, Kim BJ, et al: Pressure-controlled lumbar discography in volunteers without low back symptoms. Pain Med 2005;6:213-221.
144. Schwarzer AC, Aprill CN, Derby R, et al: The prevalence and clinical features of internal disc disruption in patients with chronic low back pain. Spine 1995;20:1878-1883.
145. Hyodo H, Sato T, Sasaki H, et al: Discogenic pain in acute nonspecific low-back pain. Eur Spine J 2005;14:573-577.
146. Ohnmeiss DD, Vanharanta H, Ekholm J: Degree of disc disruption and lower extremity pain. Spine 1997;22:1600-1605.
147. Rengachary SS, Blabhadra RSV: Black disc disease: A commentary. Neurosurg Focus 2002;13:1-4.
148. Simmons JW, Emery SF, McMillin JN, et al: Awake discography: A comparison study with magnetic resonance imaging. Spine 1991;16:S216-S221.
149. Schneiderman G, Flannigan B, Kingston S, et al: Magnetic resonance imaging in the diagnosis of disc degeneration: Correlation with discography. Spine 1987;12:276-281.
150. Saal JS, Saal JA: Management of chronic discogenic low back pain with a thermal intradiscal catheter: A preliminary report. Spine 2000;25:382-388.
151. Hayashi K, Thabit G, Bogdanske JJ, et al: The effect of non-ablative laser energy on the ultrastructure of joint capsular collagen. Arthroscopy 1996;12:474-481.
152. Freeman BJ, Walters RM, Moore RJ, et al: Does intradiscal electrothermal therapy denervate and repair experimentally induced posterolateral annular tears in an animal model? Spine 2003;28:2602-2608.
153. Spruit M, Jacobs WC: Pain and function after intradiscal electrothermal treatment (IDET) for symptomatic lumbar disc degeneration. Eur Spine J 2002;11:589-593.
154. Gibson JN, Waddell G, Grant IC: Surgery for degenerative lumbar spondylosis. Cochrane Database Syst Rev 2000;(2): CD001352.
155. German JW, Foley KT: Disc arthroplasty in the management of the painful lumbar motion segment. Spine 2005;30(16S): 60-67.
156. Wallach CJ, Gilbertson LG, Kang JD: Gene therapy applications for intervertebral disc degeneration. Spine 2003;28(15S): 93-98.
157. Risbud MV, Shapiro IM, Vaccaro AR, et al: Stem cell regeneration of the nucleus pulposus. Spine J 2004;4:348S-353S.

158. Bogduk N, Engel R: The menisci of the lumbar zygapophyseal joints: A review of their anatomy and clinical significance. Spine 1984;9:454-460.
159. Bogduk N, Long DM: The anatomy of the so-called "articular nerves" and their relationship to facet denervation in the treatment of low-back pain. J Neurosurg 1979;51:172-177.
160. Ashton IK, Ashton BA, Gibson SJ: Morphological basis for back pain: The demonstration of nerve fibers and neuropeptides in the lumbar facet joint capsule but not in the ligamentum flavum. J Orthop Res 1992;10:72-78.
161. Ghormley RK: Low back pain with special reference to the articular facet, with presentation of an operative procedure. JAMA 1933;101:1773-1777.
162. Hirsch D, Ingelmark B, Miller M: The anatomical basis for low back pain. Acta Orthop Scand 1963;33:1-17.
163. Mooney V, Robertson J: Facet joint syndrome. Clin Orthop. 1976;115:149-156.
164. McCall IW, Park WM, O'Brien JP: Induced pain referral from posterior lumbar elements in normal subjects. Spine 1979;4:441-446.
165. Jayson MIV: Degenerative disease of the spine and back pain. Clin Rheumatol Dis 1976;2:557-584.
166. Twomey LT, Taylor JR, Taylor MM: Unsuspected damage to the lumbar zygapophyseal (facet) joints after motor vehicle accidents. Med J Aust 1989;151:210-217.
167. Bogduk N, Jull G: The theoretical pathology of the acute locked back: A basis for manipulative therapy. Manual Medicine 1985;1:78-82.
168. Schwarzer AC, Wang S, O'Driscoll D, et al: The ability of computed tomography to identify a painful zygapophyseal joint in patients with chronic low back pain. Spine 1995;20:907-912.
169. Destouet JM, Murphy WA: Lumbar facet block: Indications and technique. Orthop Rev 1985;14:57-65.
170. Schwarzer AC, April CN, Derby R, et al: Clinical features of patients with pain stemming from the lumbar zygapophyseal joints: Is the lumbar facet syndrome a clinical entity? Spine 1994;19:1132-1137.
171. Helbig T, Lee CK: The lumbar facet syndrome. Spine 1988;13:61-64.
172. Revel ME, Listrat VM, Chevalier XJ, et al: Facet joint block for low back pain: Identifying predictors of good response. Arch Phys Med Rehabil 1992;73:824-828.
173. Dreyfuss PH, Dreyer SJ: Lumbar zygapophysial (facet) joint injections. Spine J 2003;3:50S-59S.
174. Schwarzer AC, April CN, Derby R, et al: The false positive rate of uncontrolled diagnostic blocks of the lumbar zygapophysial joints. Pain 1994;58:195-200.
175. Bogduk N: A narrative review of intra-articular corticosteroid injections for low back pain. Pain Med 2005;6:287-296.
176. Carette S, Marcoux S, Truchon R, et al: A controlled trial of corticosteroid injections into the facet joints for chronic low back pain. N Engl J Med 1991;325:1002-1007.
177. Goldberg SN, Gazelle GS, Dawson SL, et al: Tissue ablation with radiofrequency: Effect of probe size, gauge, duration and temperature on lesion volume. Acad Radiol 1995;2:399-404.
178. Hooten WM, Martin DP, Huntoon MA: Radiofrequency neurotomy for low back pain: Evidence-based procedure guidelines. Pain Med 2005;6:129-138.
179. Goldthwaite GE, Osgood RB: A consideration of the pelvic articulations from an anatomical, pathological, and clinical standpoint. Boston Med Surg J 1905;152:593-601.
180. Maigne JY, Aivaliklis A, Pfefer F: Results of sacroiliac joint double block and value of sacroiliac pain provocation tests in 54 patients with low back pain. Spine 1996;21:1889-1892.
181. Schwarzer AC, April CN, Bogduk N: The sacroiliac joint in chronic low back pain. Spine 1995;20:31-37.
182. Ostgaard HC, Andersson GJ, Karlsson K: Prevalence of back pain in pregnancy. Spine 1991;16:549-552.
183. Schuit D, McPoil TG, Mulesa P: Incidence of sacroiliac joint malalignment in leg length discrepancies. J Am Podiatr Med Assoc 1989;79:380-383.
184. Katz V, Schofferman J, Reynolds J: The sacroiliac joint: A potential cause of pain after lumbar fusion to the sacrum. J Spinal Disord Tech 2003;16:96-99.
185. Chou LH, Slipman CW, Bhagia SM, et al: Inciting events initiating injection-proven sacroiliac joint syndrome. Pain Med 2004;5:26-32.
186. Larsen EC, Wilken-Jensen C, Hansen A, et al: Symptom-giving pelvic girdle relaxation in pregnancy: I. Prevalence and risk factors. Acta Obstet Gynecol Scand 1999;78:105-110.
187. Bernard TN, Cassidy JD: The sacroiliac joint syndrome: Pathophysiology, diagnosis, and management. In Frymoyer JW (ed): The Adult Spine: Principles and Practice. New York, Raven Press, 1991, pp 2107-2130.
188. Mitchell FL, Moran PS, Pruzzo NA: An evaluation and treatment manual of osteopathic muscle energy technique procedures. Valley Park, MO, Mitchell, Moran, and Pruzzo Associates, 1979, pp 207-225.
189. DonTigny R: Anterior dysfunction of the sacroiliac joint as a major factor in the etiology of idiopathic low back pain syndrome. Phys Ther 1990;70:250-262.
190. Merskey H, Bogduk N: Classifications of Chronic Pain: Descriptions of Chronic Pain Syndrome and Definitions of Pain Terms, 2nd ed. Seattle, WA: IASP Press, 1993, pp 190-191.
191. Slipman CW, Jackson HB, Lipetz JS, et al: Sacroiliac joint pain referral zones. Arch Phys Med Rehabil 2000;81:334-338.
192. Fortin JD, Dwyer AP, West S, et al: Sacroiliac joint: Pain referral maps upon applying a new injection/arthrography technique. Part I: Asymptomatic volunteers. Spine 1994;19:1475-1482.
193. Potter NA, Rothstein JM: Intertester reliability for selected clinical tests of the sacroiliac joint. Phys Ther 1985;65:1671-1675.
194. Lasletta M, Aprill CN, McDonald B, et al: Diagnosis of sacroiliac joint pain: Validity of individual provocation tests and composites of tests. Manual Therapy 2005;10:207-218.
195. Benzon HT: Pain originating from the buttock: Sacroiliac joint dysfunction and piriformis syndrome. In Benzon HT, Raja SN, Molloy RE, et al (eds): Essentials of Pain Medicine and Regional Anesthesia, 2nd ed. New York, Elsevier, 2005, pp 358-359.
196. Hendrix RW, Lin PJ, Kane WJ: Simplified aspiration or injection technique for the sacro-iliac joint. J Bone Joint Surg (Am) 1982;64A:1249-1252.
197. Dreyfuss PH, Michaelsen M, Pauza K, et al: The value of history and physical examination in diagnosing sacroiliac joint pain. Spine 1996;21:2594-2602.
198. Prather H: Sacroiliac joint pain: Practical management. Clin J Sports Med 2003;13:252-255.
199. Osterbauer PJ, De Boer KF, Widmaier R, et al: Treatment and biomechanical assessment of patients with chronic sacroiliac joint syndrome. J Manipul Physiol Ther 1993;15:82-90.
200. Slipman CW, Lipetz JS, Plastaras CT, et al: Fluoroscopically guided therapeutic sacroiliac joint injections for sacroiliac joint syndrome. Am J Phys Med Rehabil 2001;80:425-432.
201. Waisbrod H, Krainick JU, Gerbershagen HU: Sacroiliac joint arthrodesis for chronic lower back pain. Arch Orthop Trauma Surg 1987;106:238-240.
202. Ikeda R: Innervation of the sacroiliac joint: Macroscopic and histological studies. J Nippon Med School 1991;58:587-596.
203. Grob K, Neuhuber W, Kissling R: Innervation of the sacroiliac joint of the human. Z Rheumatol 1995;54:117-122.
204. Fortin J, Kissling R, O'Connor B, et al: Sacroiliac joint innervation and pain. Am J Orthop 1999;28:687-690.
205. Cohen SP, Abdi S: Lateral branch blocks as a treatment for sacroiliac joint pain: A pilot study. Reg Anesth Pain Med 2003;28:113-119.
206. Yin W, Willard F, Carreiro J, et al: Sensory stimulation guided sacroiliac joint radiofrequency neurotomy: Technique based on neuroanatomy of the dorsal sacral plexus. Spine 2003 28:2419-2425.

207. Ferrante FM, King LF, Roche EA, et al: Radiofrequency sacro-iliac joint denervation for sacroiliac syndrome. Reg Anesth Pain Med 2001;26:137-142.

208. Gavargez A, Groenemeyer D, Schirp S, et al: CT-guided per-cutaneous radiofrequency denervation of the sacroiliac joint. Eur Radiol 2002;12:1360-1365.

209. Pino CA, Hoeft MA, Hofsess C, et al: Morphologic analysis of bipolar radiofrequency lesions: Implications for treatment of the sacroiliac joint. Reg Anesth Pain Med 2005;30:335-338.

210. Manchikanti L, Boswell MV, Singh V, et al: Sacroiliac joint pain: Should physicians be blocking lateral branches, medial branches, dorsal rami, or ventral rami? Reg Anesth Pain Med.2003;28:488-490.

211. Burnham RS, Yasui Y: An alternate method of radiofrequency neurotomy of the sacroiliac joint: A pilot study of the effect on pain, function, and satisfaction. Reg Anesth Pain Med 2007;32:12-19.

CHAPTER
18 Surgical Treatment of Lumbar Spinal Disorders

Matthew D. Hepler and Michael F. Schafer

The surgical treatment of lumbar spinal disorders has made substantial advances in the last two decades. Rigid instrumentation systems, minimally invasive techniques, recombinant DNA, and joint replacement are just a few technologies that are rapidly changing what and how we treat spinal pathology. With these advances has come a corresponding increase in the rates of spine surgery—as high as 8.6/1000 Medicare enrollees in some regions.[1] Although many of these patients benefit immensely, there is a definitive complication rate that must be carefully weighed against potential benefits when considering surgical intervention. Validated outcome measures and randomized trials must be applied to these new techniques to accurately assess both their effectiveness and inherent risks.

The most common spinal disorders manifest themselves as pain secondary to neural compression or mechanical dysfunction. As a result, treatment usually necessitates neural decompression or spinal fusion respectively. More recently arthroplasty (disk replacement) has demonstrated encouraging results and may, as it has in the peripheral skeleton, become an alternative to arthrodesis. This chapter reviews some of the more common surgical treatments for lumbar spinal disorders and is organized by the underlying treatment principle rather than specific diagnosis: decompression, pars repair, fusion, arthroplasty, and reconstruction. It is important to emphasize that each patient has a unique combination of pathology and expectations for treatment. Successful surgical management requires a detailed clinical evaluation with confirmatory imaging studies to accurately identify the symptomatic pathology, a careful assessment of the risks and benefits associated with any procedure, and a strict adherence to orthopedic principles while implementing treatment.

DECOMPRESSIONS

Herniated Disk

Acute low back pain is the fifth most common complaint leading to physician visits, and the vast majority of these complaints relate to disk degeneration and herniation.[2] The classic disk herniation most commonly occurs between the third and sixth decades of life with a peak at age 40 years. Back pain is the predominant complaint and is thought to be the result of stimulation of local nerve endings along the posterior disk by inflammatory cytokines.[3] Approximately 90% to 95% of these painful episodes abate within months while a fraction go on to develop chronic disabling back pain. The surgical management of this group is discussed in a later section for fusion procedures.

Another segment of this acute back pain population will progress within days, months, or years to include *predominant* "sciatic" leg pain. Symptoms typically include pain, numbness, paresthesias, or weakness in a dermatomal distribution secondary to nerve root compression and local inflammation.[4] About 95% of herniations occur at the L4-5 or L5-S1 levels and affect the exiting or traversing nerve roots depending upon the specific location and direction of the herniation. Although the sciatic pain may be quite severe, it typically improves within 1 to 3 weeks and mostly resolves within 3 months in most patients.[5] Nonoperative treatment, including nonsteroidal anti-inflammatory drugs (NSAIDs), physical therapy, and injections, may be helpful in reducing pain and time of recovery.[6,7]

Surgical treatment is an excellent alternative for those patients who have continued pain in that it definitively removes the neurologic compression and inflammatory nidus. In the only randomized comparison of nonoperative and operative treatment, surgical patients were significantly better at 1 year (with 26% crossover of nonoperative patients) although these differences disappeared at 10-year follow-up.[5] Surgery should be considered for all patients with acute and dense motor deficits and is emergently necessary in the presence of bowel and bladder dysfunction (cauda equina syndrome). Since Mixter and Barr's classic report in 1934,[8] open disk excision has become the most commonly performed spinal surgery and remains the gold standard with high (90%) patient satisfaction.

Microdiskectomy using magnification loupes or a microscope was popularized in the late 1970s. It involves a smaller exposure with less soft tissue dissection, and studies have shown faster recovery and return to work with improved patient outcomes.[9,10] Indicating factors include predominant leg pain, a positive straight leg raise, and imaging studies confirming compression at the symptomatic level. The principles of surgical treatment are decompression and mobilization of the affected neural elements and removal of the herniated fragment. This typically includes release of the ligamentum flavum, partial laminotomy, and medial facetectomy. The neurologic structures are dissected off the disk with a Penfield elevator, exposing the underlying noncontained herniation, which is then removed. Contained herniations require an annulotomy before the disk fragment can be identified and removed.

More recently, endoscopic techniques have allowed diskectomy to be performed safely and effectively as an ambulatory procedure with results superior to those of other outpatient therapies (chemonucleolysis, percutaneous diskectomy, and thermal coagulation). The endoscopic technique allows a limited exposure through an 18-mm tubular retractor with an average length of stay of $3\frac{1}{2}$ hours (Fig. 18–1). Results compare favorably to those for microdiskectomy, with 72% of patients experiencing complete relief and 20% experiencing minimal discomfort

requiring no further treatment.[11] Complications include infection, durotomy, nerve root injury, recurrent disk herniation, and chronic back or leg pain. Rarely, patients develop far lateral compression of the nerve root in the foramen, which may be approached directly through a lateral approach as described by Wiltse and colleagues.[12]

Spinal Stenosis

Stenosis is defined as narrowing of the cross-sectional area of the spinal canal as a result of congenital or acquired factors. Acquired stenosis is far more common and usually the result of degenerative changes such as disk bulges/herniations, facet arthropathy, osteochondral spurs, ligament hypertrophy, and spondylolisthesis. Symptomatic lumbar stenosis usually presents between the fifth and seventh decade of life with an incidence of 2% to 10%.[13] Symptoms typically include low back and leg pain aggravated by standing and walking and must be differentiated from vascular claudication. Although the degenerative process and associated symptoms may gradually worsen with time, natural history studies show little risk for severe worsening.[14] Nonoperative treatment includes physical therapy,

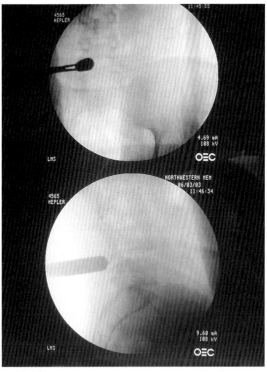

A

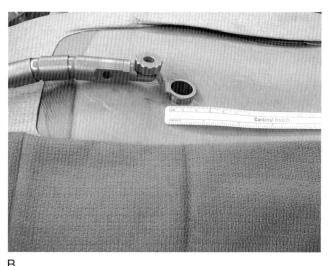

B

Figure 18–1. Patient undergoing endoscopic diskectomy. **A,** AP and lateral fluoroscopic image demonstrating placement of the endoscope at the left L4-5 intralaminar level. **B,** METRx endoscope locked in position with flexible arm assembly. (From Jabri RS, Hepler M, Benzon HT: Overview of low back pain disorders. In Benzon HT, Raja SN, Molloy RE, et al [eds]: Essentials of Pain Medicine and Regional Anesthesia, 2nd ed. Philadelphia, Elsevier, 2005.)

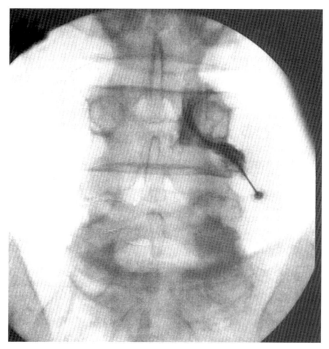

Figure 18–2. Fluoroscopic image of right-sided L4-5 transforaminal steroid injection. Dye injection prior to steroid injection demonstrates proper position and backflow along L4 nerve root sheath. (From Jabri RS, Hepler M, Benzon HT: Overview of low back pain disorders. In Benzon HT, Raja SN, Molloy RE, et al [eds]: Essentials of Pain Medicine and Regional Anesthesia, 2nd ed. Philadelphia, Elsevier, 2005.)

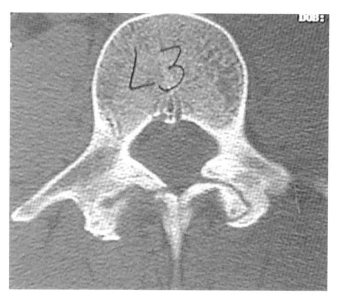

Figure 18–3. Note the chronic lytic lesions bilaterally characterized by their sclerotic margins. The defect itself is filled with fibro-cartilaginous tissue, which prevents healing and must be removed.

NSAIDs, and steroid injections, although there are no controlled studies supporting their use. Selective nerve root blocks are helpful diagnostically as well as therapeutically because they identify symptomatic levels and may help predict response to surgical decompression (Fig. 18–2).

Patients who fail to improve with nonoperative treatment are candidates for surgical decompression. This typically involves laminotomy or laminectomy for central stenosis, partial medial facetectomy for lateral recess stenosis, and foraminotomies for foraminal stenosis or any combination thereof. Success depends upon an accurate determination of clinically significant pathologic lesions and careful correlation with appropriate confirmatory imaging studies. One randomized prospective study comparing operative versus nonoperative management demonstrates substantially better outcome at 1 year for the surgical group (89% vs. 64%) although this difference tended to fade with time.[15] In addition, a significant number of patients crossover from nonoperative to operative treatment groups and those with more severe symptoms appear to do better with surgery. A number of nonrandomized studies also support the efficacy of surgical management.[16-18] Patients with predominant back pain or instability (spondylolisthesis or more than 50% of the facet joints resected) may require fusion in addition to decompression, which

is discussed in a later section under spine fusion procedures.

Although surgical decompression remains the gold standard for treating symptomatic lumbar stenosis, other surgical techniques have been introduced. Interspinous process decompression with X-STOP has recently been gaining increased publicity for treating symptomatic stenosis. The authors propose that insertion of the X-STOP device between the spinous processes will reduce stenosis in extension and thereby reduce pain. Although the report concluded that the X-STOP had better outcome compared to the nonoperative control group, the device is "not approvable" by the Food and Drug Administration and results have not been corroborated by independent examiners.[19,20]

PARS REPAIR (SPONDYLOLYSIS)

Spondylolysis is a common pathologic lesion present in 5% to 7% of individuals in the U.S. population[21,22] (Fig. 18–3). Many of these may be asymptomatic, whereas others may interfere with sporting activities, work, or activities of daily living. Many individuals with acutely painful spondylolytic lesions will improve with nonoperative management, including activity restriction, NSAIDs, and bracing, and frequently return to full activity.[23] Others may require surgical treatment for continued pain and occasional neurologic symptoms. Many more may improve with cessation of high school sports/vigorous activities only to return decades later with worsening low back pain and accompanying disk degeneration and or progression to spondylolisthesis.[24] Various techniques have been described to surgically treat spondylolysis, including bone graft repair with internal fixation

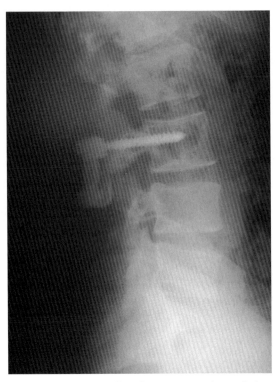

Figure 18–4. Lateral x-ray film demonstrating the pedicle screw-laminar hook (claw) construct.

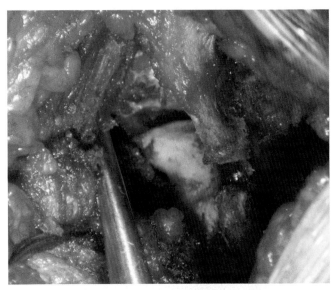

Figure 18–5. The stress fracture on the left has been debrided of fibrocartilaginous debris and the remaining defect is seen. The right stress fracture has not yet been debrided and is characterized by an inflammatory pannus of tissue overlying the fracture itself. This inflammatory tissue must be removed before the margins of the fracture can be visualized and debrided.

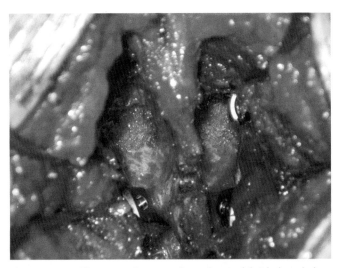

Figure 18–6. The stress fractures have been debrided and then packed with autologous bone graft. The surrounding posterior elements (lamina, pars, base of pedicle, and transverse process) have been decorticated.

(wires, screws, and hook screw constructs).[25-27] Each of these methods has been affected by technical difficulties and high complication rates including construct loosening and nonunion. Others treat spondylolysis with posterior fusion, which sacrifices the motion segment and leads to higher levels of stress and degeneration at the adjacent levels.[28] We recently reported our results treating the pars defect with rigid fixation using a pedicle screw-hook (claw) construct[29] (Fig. 18–4). We prospectively evaluated the clinical and radiologic results of pars repair of nine lesions in eight consecutive patients who failed nonoperative treatment including bracing. Surgical technique included debridement of the pseudoarthrosis, bone grafting (iliac crest autograft), and rigid stabilization with a pedicle screw–sublaminar hook (claw) construct (Figs. 18–5 and 18–6). Concomitant diagnosis included an adjacent spondylolysis,[2] spondylolisthesis,[3] and degenerative disk disease/ herniated nucleus pulposus.[4] Postoperative treatment included thoracolumbosacral orthosis (TLSO) bracing for 3 months, physical therapy (aerobic conditioning and core strengthening) at 3 months, and sport-specific rehabilitation thereafter. Outcome measures demonstrated an improvement from preoperative to 1 year postoperative in Oswestry 2.0 (5.2 to 1), Roland Morris (7.4 to 0), Visual Analogue Scale (VAS) (8.3 to 0), and SF-36 measures. Flexion/extension x-ray studies and computed tomography scan demonstrated solid pars repair in 10/10 lesions (Fig. 18–7). All patients returned to a full level of activity including contact sports within 6 months (two football players had bone morphogenic protein (BMP) to increase rate of healing and permit competition within 6 months). We strongly recommend primary repair and rigid fixation of spondylolysis in patients who fail to heal with nonoperative treatment because this therapy has excellent clinical results and fusion rates, restores physiologic motion and biomechanics, and permits early return to full activity level (including contact sports), even in the presence of other lumbar pathology.

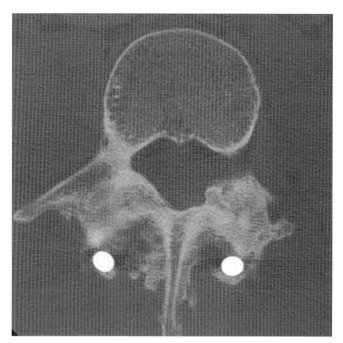

Figure 18–7. Axial computed tomography scan through the level of the pars 6 months postoperatively demonstrating complete bony healing of the lytic defect. At this point the patient, a Division I college tight end, returned to complete the full season without limitation or back pain.

FUSION

Fusion procedures have been used successfully for more than 100 years but have been much more frequently performed over the last 10 to 15 years. The most common indication is disabling mechanical low back pain secondary to an underlying disorder (spondylolysis, spondylolisthesis, degenerative arthritis, and scoliosis). Lumbar spine fusion is a salvage procedure in which pain-generating degenerative joints are removed and motion segments stabilized. Results vary with specific pathology but many reports demonstrate good to excellent outcomes in as many as 94% of patients[30,31] (Fig. 18–8).

Discogenic Back Pain

The relief of back pain attributed to "discogenic disk disease" remains far more controversial, with most studies demonstrating clinical improvement closer to 63% and return to work rates of 36%.[32] The actual fusion rates also vary and range from as low as 40% in posterolateral fusions to 100% with circumferential (360 degrees) fusions.[33,34] Although achieving fusion does not always correlate with clinical improvement, patients with nonunions are more likely to have a worse outcome. In addition, patients with degenerative disk disease tend to have greater clinical improvement when the pain-generating disk itself is removed. This can be accomplished with anterior stand-alone interbody fusion with good clinical success and fusion rates, but patients must not have any posterior pathology, which is relatively uncommon.[35] An anterior-posterior spinal fusion and instrumentation has been the standard for treating discogenic back pain with posterior lesions, demonstrating good clinical results and 95% to 100% fusion rates (Fig. 18–9). More recently, posterior approaches such as the transforaminal lumbar interbody fusion provide the advantages of a circumferential fusion through a lower risk posterior approach (Fig. 18–10). Clinical studies demonstrate equal or superior results with lower complication rates.[36] Various devices can be placed in the interbody space, including cylindrical cages, carbon fiber devices, and bone. The highest fusion rates and clinical outcomes occur when following basic biomechanical principles including restoring lumbar lordosis and loading bone under compression. Most recently, recombinant human bone morphogenic protein has been shown to have similar clinical outcomes and equal or superior fusion rates in various studies.[37] This may be a useful alternative to autologous bone grafting but future studies are needed to assess effectiveness in larger populations, including multilevel cases and patients with various other risk factors.

DISK REPLACEMENT ARTHROPLASTY

Although spinal fusion has been beneficial in many patients, it remains a salvage procedure that compromises joint function and increases stresses and consequently accelerates degeneration at adjacent levels. Disk replacement has been advocated since the 1950s because it removes the painful and dysfunctional disk and restores physiologic motion. However, it was not until the early 1980s that a viable design began demonstrating encouraging results. Since then, various implants have emerged including ProDisk (semiconstrained device manufactured by Spine Solutions), Maverick (nonconstrained device by Medtronic Sofamor Danek), and Flexcore. The Link SB Charite III is the most commonly used prosthesis with as many as 5000 implanted worldwide. It is a nonconstrained design consisting of two cobalt-chrome end plates with a sliding polyethylene core (Fig. 18–11). The implant is anchored to the vertebral bodies by teeth and a bony ingrowth on the end plate surface. Biomechanical studies demonstrate increased motion in flexion and extension, mobility in torsion, and relative immobility in lateral bending. The essential indication is disabling low back pain secondary to discogenic disk disease that has failed to improve with at least 6 months of adequate nonoperative treatment. The accurate diagnosis of discogenic back pain and identification of the symptomatic level is best confirmed by MRI and concordant pain on discography. Exclusion criteria include nerve root compression and facet arthropathy. Clinical results are good in properly selected patients with as many as 79% of patients reporting substantial improvement and 87% returning to work.[38] The postoperative rehabilitation encourages early, controlled, progressive

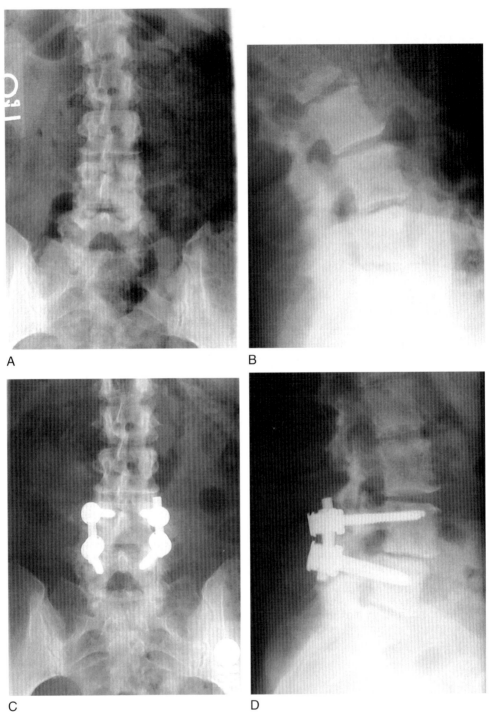

A   B

C   D

Figure 18–8. Anteroposterior **(A)** and lateral lumbar **(B)** spine radiographs demonstrating grade I spondylolisthesis in a 47-year-old woman with disabling back and leg pain refractory in nonoperative treatment. **C** and **D,** Postoperative radiographs demonstrating stable fusion 1 year following posterior decompression and fusion with supplemental instrumentation. Note the robust fusion mass bridging transverse processes laterally. The patient is pain-free and has returned to full level of activity including participating in triathlons and skiing. (From Jabri RS, Hepler M, Benzon HT: Overview of low back pain disorders. In Benzon HT, Raja SN, Molloy RE, et al [eds]: Essentials of Pain Medicine and Regional Anesthesia, 2nd ed. Philadelphia, Elsevier, 2005.)

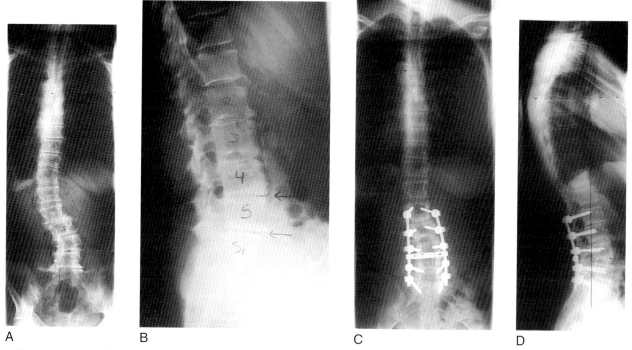

A   B   C   D

Figure 18–9. A 64-year-old woman with degenerative scoliosis and disabling low back and radicular leg pain. **A,** Anteroposterior radiograph demonstrates severe lateral listhesis at L2-3 and L3-4 resulting in symptomatic compressive neuropathy. **B,** Lateral radiograph demonstrating severe disk degeneration and consequent loss of lumbar lordosis. She was treated with anterior-posterior fusion, instrumentation, and decompression. **C,** Anteroposterior radiograph demonstrates correction of lateral listhesis and tilt. **D,** Lateral film show excellent restoration of lumbar lordosis with structural interbody allograft. (From Jabri RS, Hepler M, Benzon HT: Overview of low back pain disorders. In Benzon HT, Raja SN, Molloy RE, et al [eds]: Essentials of Pain Medicine and Regional Anesthesia, 2nd ed. Philadelphia, Elsevier, 2005.)

spinal motion and rapid functional recovery compared to prolonged rehabilitation in fusion patients. It is hoped that long-term studies will demonstrate continued clinical improvement and implant survivability with motion preservation and decreased adjacent degeneration. These remain hypothetical advantages and to date fusion procedures remain the gold standard to which arthroplasty must compare.

SPINAL RECONSTRUCTION

Spinal reconstruction is necessary when a disease process destroys the structural integrity of the spine or produces a deformity, which alters normal spinal balance and biomechanics. The most common conditions requiring spinal reconstruction include trauma, infection, tumor, scoliosis, kyphosis, and increasingly iatrogenic causes from failed spinal surgery. The principles of reconstruction include resection and soft tissue release to allow realignment, anterior column support with structural grafting, rigid fixation, and biologic fusion. There are various surgical techniques employed to effect reconstruction, some of which are described below.

Reconstruction frequently requires resection of diseased tissue and release of soft tissues in malaligned segments of the spine. Anteriorly, this is accomplished with vertebral body resection (corpectomy) or diskectomy. Once a corpectomy is performed, the anterior column must be reconstructed with structural support. This can be accomplished with implants such as mesh cages or structural allograft or autograft. It is essential that the spine be realigned after release to restore physiologic cervical and lumbar lordosis and thoracic kyphosis, and that the appropriate graft length be selected to maintain sagittal balance (Fig. 18–12). Most structural grafts require some form of internal fixation to maintain stability until fusion is successfully achieved. In severe cases of spinal deformity, such as scoliosis exceeding 90 degrees, the rib cage itself may become ankylosed and also require release in the form of rib head resections to effect realignment (Fig. 18–13).[39] Such reconstruction will similarly require posterior releases. These may include chevron osteotomies, which can correct sagittal and coronal malalignment,[40] rib resection or osteotomy, and pedicle subtraction osteotomy[41] (Fig. 18–14).

Once a spinal segment is properly realigned, it must be rigidly fixed to maintain alignment and effect successful fusion. Modern instrumentation systems include hooks, sublaminar cables, and most frequently pedicle screws connected by rods. These

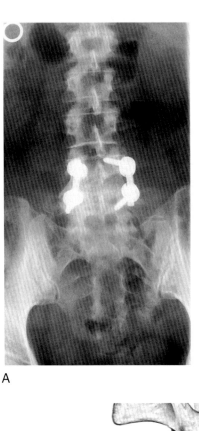

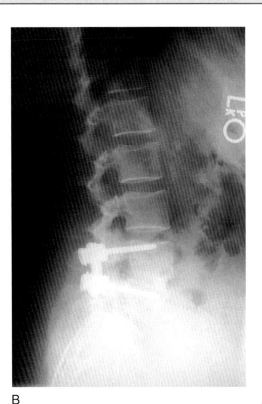

A   B

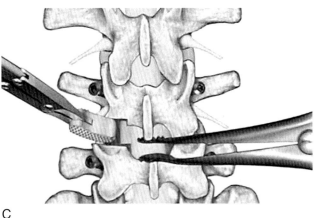

C

Figure 18–10. A 51-year-old man with recurrent L4-5 disk herniation with disabling back and leg pain treated with revision diskectomy and transforaminal lumbar interbody fusion at L4-5. **A,** Circumferential fusion avoids exposure and fusion of transverse processes and resulting denervation of paraspinal muscles. **B,** The lateral radiograph demonstrates excellent interbody support and trabeculating bone. **C,** Technique of inserting structural AlloGrip through transforaminal approach. (From Jabri RS, Hepler M, Benzon HT: Overview of low back pain disorders. In Benzon HT, Raja SN, Molloy RE, et al [eds]: Essentials of Pain Medicine and Regional Anesthesia, 2nd ed. Philadelphia, Elsevier, 2005.)

"segmental" instrumentation systems allow much greater correction than earlier systems and have substantially increased management options for spinal deformity over the last 20 years. Nonetheless, they are subject to fatigue failure and will fracture if the spine does not go on to a solid union.

Spinal fusion remains the goal of most reconstruction procedures for long-term stability and function. In effect, it requires resection of articulations (disk space and facet joints), rigid stabilization, and a biologic fusion bed. Bone fusion requires the presence of precursor cells capable of transformation into bone forming osteoblasts, osteoconductive materials (which serve as scaffolds for formation of new bone), and osteoinductive materials, which contain growth factors that promote differentiation of progenitor cells into osteoblasts. Autologous bone graft contains all three materials and remains the gold standard against which all other products must be compared. Limitations in the amount of graft available and morbidity associated with harvesting have led to use of various other products including allograft, ceramics, collagen, demineralized bone matrix, and more recently bone morphogenic protein: BMP-2 (Infuse) and BMP-7 (OP-1). Although preliminary clinical studies have demonstrated promising results, these products must be validated by prospective randomized trials and they do not replace the need for following well-established biomechanical and biologic principles.

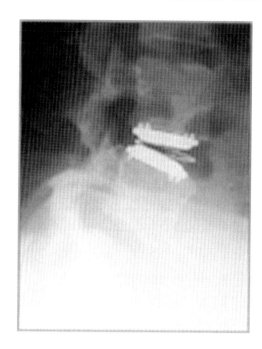

Figure 18–11. Lateral radiograph of patient treated for degenerative disk disease with Link SB Charite III at L4-5. (From Jabri RS, Hepler M, Benzon HT: Overview of low back pain disorders. In Benzon HT, Raja SN, Molloy RE, et al [eds]: Essentials of Pain Medicine and Regional Anesthesia, 2nd ed. Philadelphia, Elsevier, 2005.)

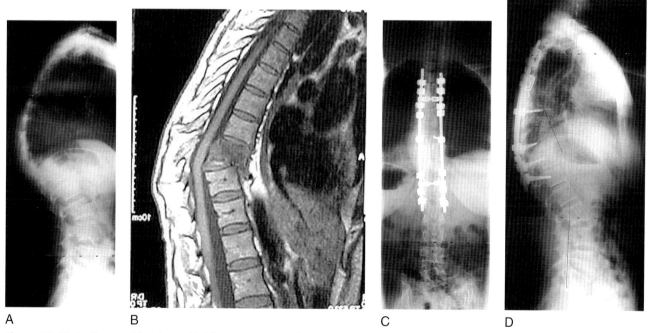

A   B   C   D

Figure 18–12. A 43-year-old patient with blastomycosis involving T9 and T10 with progressive collapse **(A)** and lower extremity weakness secondary to neurologic compromise **(B). C** and **D,** Reconstruction involved T9 and T10 vertebrectomies and anterior column support with fibular allograft and vascularized rib autograft, followed by posterior fusion and instrumentation. The patient had resolution with full functional and motor recovery. (From Jabri RS, Hepler M, Benzon HT: Overview of low back pain disorders. In Benzon HT, Raja SN, Molloy RE, et al [eds]: Essentials of Pain Medicine and Regional Anesthesia, 2nd ed. Philadelphia, Elsevier, 2005.)

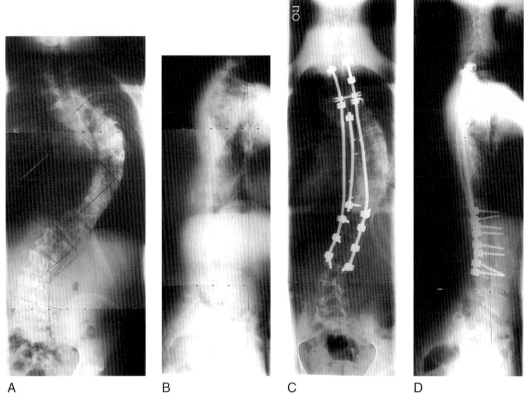

A B C D

Figure 18–13. A, A 22-year-old man with progressive idiopathic scoliosis, stiff right thoracic curve measuring 97 degrees, decompensation, and forced vital capacity 37%. **B,** Lateral radiograph demonstrates thoracic lordosis and positive sagittal balance measuring 5 cm. The patient was treated with T9 vertebrectomy, internal thoracoplasties, and posterior osteotomies to release safely the stiff deformity and stabilization with fusion and instrumentation from T2 to L3. **C,** Two-year follow-up demonstrates excellent correction of scoliosis and restoration of balance in both coronal and sagittal planes. **D,** Spondylolisthesis remains asymptomatic with progression. (From Jabri RS, Hepler M, Benzon HT: Overview of low back pain disorders. In Benzon HT, Raja SN, Molloy RE, et al [eds]: Essentials of Pain Medicine and Regional Anesthesia, 2nd ed. Philadelphia, Elsevier, 2005.)

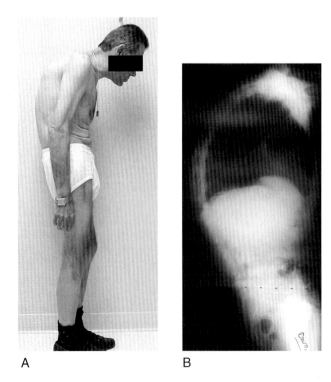

A B

Figure 18–14. A, A 42-year-old man with ankylosing spondylitis and progressive kyphotic deformity. **B,** Lateral radiographs demonstrated kyphosis involving primarily the lumbar spine.

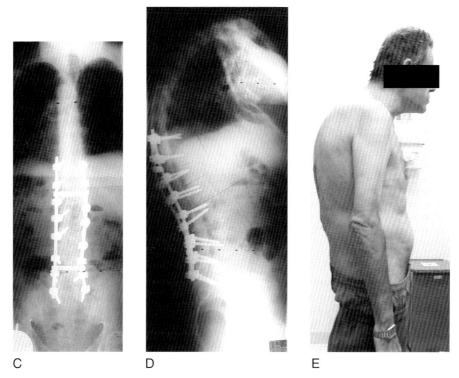

C   D   E

Figure 18–14, cont'd. C and **D,** Anteroposterior and lateral radiographs following a pedicle subtraction osteotomy of L3. **E,** Note the substantial improvement in forward gaze and neutralization of C-7 plumbline. (From Jabri RS, Hepler M, Benzon HT: Overview of low back pain disorders. In Benzon HT, Raja SN, Molloy RE, et al [eds]: Essentials of Pain Medicine and Regional Anesthesia, 2nd ed. Philadelphia, Elsevier, 2005.)

CONCLUSION

There have been tremendous advances in both the understanding and treatment of lumbar spinal disorders over the last two decades.[42] These advances have dramatically increased our ability to manage various spinal disorders with a corresponding increase in rates of surgery and devices used. Although many patients obtain substantial benefit, there are inherent and quantifiable risks that must be carefully assessed before considering surgical treatment. The injudicious use of surgery and spinal devices exposes patients to unnecessary risks and society to excessive costs. As a result, there has already been a call for restraint in the performance of such procedures.[43]

Disorders of the lumbar spine are extremely common and increase with the age and activity of the population. Fortunately, the vast majority of these patients improve with appropriately guided low-risk nonoperative care. For the small group of patients who fail to improve, there is now a wide array of surgical options available. By thoroughly evaluating each patient's unique condition, carefully balancing the risks and benefits of various interventions, and employing well-established treatment principles, we ensure the best chance for a satisfactory outcome.

References

1. Lurie JD, Birkmeyer NJ, Weinstein JN: Rates of advanced spinal imaging and spine surgery. Spine 2003;28:616-620.
2. Hart LG, Deyo RA, Cherkin DC: Physician office visits for low back pain: Frequency, clinical evaluation, and treatment patterns from a U.S. national survey. Spine 1995;20:11-19.
3. Kuslich SD, Ulstrom CL, Michael CJ: The tissue origin of low back pain and sciatica: A report of pain response to tissue stimulation during operations on the lumbar spine using local anesthesia. Orthop Clin North Am 1991;22:181-187.
4. Olmarker K, Rydevik B, Nordborg C: Autologous nucleus pulposus induces neurophysiologic and histologic changes in porcine cauda equina nerve roots. Spine 1993;18:1425-1432.
5. Weber H: Lumbar disc herniation: A controlled, prospective study with ten years of observation. Spine 1983;8:131-140.
6. Riew KD, Yin Y, Gilula L, et al: The effect of nerve-root injections on the need for operative treatment of lumbar radicular pain: A prospective, randomized, controlled, double-blinded study. J Bone Joint Surg 2000;82-A(11):1589-1593.
7. Simotas AC, Dorey FJ, Hansraj KK, et al: Nonoperative treatment for lumbar spinal stenosis. Spine 2000;25:197-209.
8. Mixter WJ, Barr JS: Rupture of the intervertebral disc with involvement of the spinal canal. N Engl J Med 1934;211:210-215.
9. Caspar W: A new surgical procedure for lumbar disc herniation causing less tissue damage through microsurgical approach. Adv Neurosurg 1977;4:74-79.
10. Williams RW: Microlumbar discectomy: A conservative surgical approach to the virgin herniated lumbar disc. Spine 1978;3:175-182.

11. Hilton DL: Microdiscectomy with minimally invasive tubular retractor. Outpatient Spinal Surgery 2002;171-195.

12. Wiltse LL, Bateman JG, Hutchinson RH, et al: The paraspinal sacro-spinalis approach to the lumbar spine. Clin Orthop 1964;35:80.

13. De Villiers PD, Boysen EL: Fibrous spinal stenosis: A report on 850 myelograms with a water-soluble contrast medium. Clin Orthop 1976;115:4-5.

14. Johnsson KE, Rosen I, Uden A: The natural course of lumbar spinal stenosis. Clin Orthop Rel Res 1992;279:82-86.

15. Amundsen T, Weber H, Nordal HJ, et al: Lumbar spinal stenosis: Conservative or surgical management? A prospective 10 year study. Spine 2000;25:1424-1436.

16. Atlas SJ, Deyo RA, Keller RB, et al: The Maine lumbar spine study, Part III. Spine 1996;21:1787-1794.

17. Atlas SJ, Keller RB, Wu YA, et al: Long term outcomes of surgical and nonsurgical management of lumbar stenosis: 8 to 10 year results from the Maine Lumbar spine study. Spine 2005;30:936-943.

18. Verbiest H: Results of surgical treatment of idiopathic developmental stenosis of the lumbar vertebral canal: A review of twenty-seven years of experience. J Bone Joint Surg 1977;59-B:181-188.

19. Andersen PA, Tribus CB, Kitchel SH: Treatment of neurogenic claudication by interspinous decompression: Application of the X STOP device in patients with lumbar degenerative spondylolisthesis. J Neurosurgery 2006;4:463-471.

20. Weiner BK: Re: Zucherman JF, Hsu KY, Hartjen CA, et al: A multicenter, prospective, randomized trial evaluating the X STOP interspinous process decompression system for the treatment of neurogenic intermittent claudication: Two-year follow-up results (letter to editor). Spine 2005;30:2846-2847.

21. Sales DeGauzt J, Vadier F, Cahuzac JP: Repair of lumbar spondylolysis using Morscher material: 14 children followed for 1-5 years. Acta Orthop Scand, 2000;71:292-296.

22. Fredrickson BE, Baker D, McHolick WJ, et al: The natural history of spondylolysis and spondylolisthesis. J Bone Joint Surg Am 1984;66:699-707.

23. Sys J, Michielsen J, Bracke P, et al: Nonoperative treatment of active spondylolysis in elite athletes with normal X-ray findings: Literature review and results of conservative treatment. Eur Spine J 2001;10:498-504.

24. Saraste H: Long term clinical, radiological follow-up of spondylolysis, spondylolisthesis. J Pediatr Orthop 1987;7:631-638.

25. Buck JE: Direct repair of the defect in spondylolisthesis: Preliminary report. J Bone Joint Surg 1970;52-B(3):432-437.

26. Scott JHS: The Edinburgh repair of isthmic (group II) spondylolysis. In Proceedings of of the British Orthopaedic Association. J Bone Joint Surg 1987;69-B(3):491.

27. Heft F, Seelig W, Morscher E: Repair of spondylolysis with a hook-screw. Int Orthop 1992;16:81-85.

28. Mihara H, Onari K, Cheng BC, et al: The biomechanical effects of spondylolysis and its treatment. Spine 2003;28:235-238.

29. Hepler MH, Walker MT: Pars repair with rigid fixation. International Meeting on Advanced Spinal Techniques July 12, 2006 Athens, Greece.

30. L'Heureux EA, Perra JH, Pinto MR, et al: Functional outcome analysis including preoperative and postoperative SF-36 for surgically treated adult isthmic spondylolisthesis. Spine 2003;28:1269-1274.

31. Shapiro GS, Gaku T, Ohenaba B-A: Results of surgical treatment of adult idiopathic scoliosis with low back pain and spinal stenosis: A study of long term clinical radiographic outcomes. Spine 2003;28:358-363.

32. Fritzell P, Hagg O, Wessberg P, et al: Lumbar fusion versus nonsurgical treatment for chronic low back pain. Spine 2001;26:2521-2534.

33. Boden SD, Kang J, Sandhu H, et al: Use of recombinant human bone morphogenetic protein-2 to achieve posterolateral lumbar spine fusion in humans: A prospective, randomized clinical pilot trial: 2002 Volvo award in clinical studies. Spine 2002;27:2662-2673.

34. Vaccaro AR, Anderson G, Patel T, et al: Comparison of OP-1 putty (rhBMP-7) to iliac crest autograft for posterolateral lumbar arthrodesis. Spine 2005;30:2709-2716.

35. Boden SD, Zdeblick TA, Sandhu HS, et al: The use of rhBMP-2 in interbody fusion cages: Definitive evidence of osteoinduction in humans: A preliminary report. Spine 2000;25:376-381.

36. Hee HT, Castro FP, Majd ME, et al: Anterior/posterior fusion versus transforaminal lumbar interbody fusion: Analysis of complications and predictive factors. J Spinal Dis 2001;14:533-540.

37. Boden SD, Kang J, Sandhu H, et al: Use of recombinant human bone morphogenetic protein-2 to achieve posterolateral lumbar spine fusion in humans: A prospective, randomized clinical pilot trial: 2002 Volvo award in clinical studies. Spine 2002;27:2662-2673.

38. Lemaire JP, Skalli W, Lavaste F, et al: Intervertebral disc prosthesis: Results and prospects for the year 2000. Clin Orthop Rel Res 1997;337:64-76.

39. Bradford DS, Tribus CB: Vertebral column resection for the treatment of rigid coronal decompensation. Spine 1997;22:1590-1599.

40. Voos K, Boachie-Adjei O, Rawlins BA: Multiple vertebral osteotomies in the treatment of rigid adult spinal deformities. Spine 2001;26:526-533.

41. Thiranont N, Netrawichien P: Transpedicular decancellation closed wedge vertebral osteotomy for treatment of fixed flexion deformity of spine in ankylosing spondylitis. Spine 1993;18:2517-2522.

42. Lipson SJ: Spinal-fusion surgery—Advances and concerns. N Engl J Med 2004;350:643-645.

43. Deyo RA, Nachemson A, Mirza SK: Spinal-fusion surgery—The case for restraint. N Engl J Med 2004;350:722-726.

19 Neurosurgical Management of Pain

Michael D. Sather and Kenneth A. Follett

Neurosurgical techniques for the management of pain include anatomic, augmentative, and ablative types of procedures. Anatomic techniques address structural abnormalities that result in pain. They generally encompass spinal decompressive or reconstructive procedures, which may be performed to treat pain, neurologic deficit, or alignment abnormalities. Augmentation therapy, also referred to as neuromodulation, has largely replaced ablative procedures as the treatment of choice for chronic pain. However, ablative procedures may be appropriate for certain patients. There is some overlap in the use of these techniques among physicians of different parent medical specialties who practice pain management, and some therapies discussed in this chapter will be described in more detail elsewhere in this text. Regardless, all pain medicine specialists should be aware of the broad spectrum of pain therapies available and refer patients for specialized procedures, when indicated, if the specialist does not personally provide the therapy.

PATIENT SELECTION FOR SURGERY

Surgical treatment of intractable pain is not usually the first treatment option. In general, the treatment of intractable pain should follow a rational process, whereby the simplest and safest methods are employed first, while reserving interventional therapy for later.[1] A simple way of picturing this approach is to imagine a pain treatment ladder, similar to that proposed by the World Health Organization for analgesic use.[2] The simplest and safest methods rest on the bottom rung. Each additional rung upward reflects a more invasive treatment, which often entails greater risk. Even though this is a good guideline to follow, an element of flexibility should be maintained and the treatment should be tailored to the individual patient. For some individuals, this may mean surgical intervention earlier rather than later in the course of therapy.

A challenge to any physician managing pain is to determine whether pain signifies an underlying disorder that should be treated directly, or whether pain is chronic (in which case it may become the primary disorder) and best treated with medication, surgical or interventional pain therapies, cognitive-behavioral strategies, or other pain management approaches. In general, surgical treatment of intractable pain is appropriate for individuals in whom more conservative therapies have not provided adequate pain relief, or in whom other treatments are associated with unacceptable side effects (e.g., medication side effects) or risks. Except in patients being considered for surgical correction of anatomic/structural abnormality in the hope of relieving pain, further direct treatment of the underlying cause of pain should not be possible or practical, or may be inappropriate.[1] For example, an individual with radicular leg pain from lumbar spinal stenosis can be treated with decompressive lumbar laminectomy; however, in the setting of severe coronary artery disease, spinal cord stimulation might be a safer and more appropriate treatment.[3] There should be no medical contraindications to surgery.

The pain should have a definable organic cause. This is important especially in the setting of chronic pain of nonmalignant origin because it reduces the likelihood that significant psychological dysfunction exists. Psychological dysfunction can be common in chronic pain disorders, and may preclude good outcomes to surgical treatment. Formal psychological evaluation may be appropriate for most individuals being considered for surgical treatment of intractable pain.[4] Overt dysfunction such as active psychosis, suicidal or homicidal behavior, major uncontrolled depression or anxiety, serious alcohol or drug abuse, and serious cognitive deficits contraindicate surgical intervention.[4] Other psychological factors may be viewed as "risk factors." Potential psychological risk factors include somatization disorders, personality disorders (e.g., borderline or antisocial), history of serious abuse, major issues of secondary gain, nonorganic signs on physical examination, unusual pain ratings (e.g., 12 on a 10-point scale), inadequate social support, unrealistic outcomes expectations, and, in the case of implantable augmentative devices, an inability to understand the device or its use.[4] Patients with psychological risk factors are not necessarily precluded from surgical treatment, but the treatment program should address the psychological issues to facilitate good outcomes.[4]

NEUROSURGICAL THERAPIES FOR INTRACTABLE PAIN

Neurosurgical modalities for the treatment of intractable pain include a wide variety of anatomic, neuroaugmentive, and neuroablative techniques (Table 19–1).[5] Augmentative therapies have largely replaced ablative techniques as procedures of choice for pain management and are generally preferred as initial surgical treatments because of their relative safety and reversibility. Nevertheless, ablative therapies still have a role in the treatment of certain pain syndromes. The specific treatment offered to a patient, whether correction of structural deformity, ablative, or augmentative, should be tailored to meet the needs of each individual patient and the skills of the treating physician. Specific interventions vary in their appropriateness as treatments for pain in specific body regions (Boxes 19–1 to 19–4). Patient-related factors that must be taken into consideration when selecting a therapy include the pain etiology (cancer-related versus nonmalignant), pain distribution and characteristics (nociceptive or neuropathic), patient life expectancy, and psychological, social, and economic issues relevant to the pain complaint. The relative advantages and disadvantages of anatomic, augmentative, and ablative therapies should be weighed in view of these factors, and a choice between these general approaches should be made. A specific intervention can then be tailored from one of these general approaches. Successful outcomes are facilitated by selecting the right treatment for the right patient at the right time.

Anatomic Therapies

Anatomic techniques address abnormalities in the structures surrounding the central or peripheral nervous system that result in pain. The surgical treatments may address a variety of conditions including spondylolisthesis, traumatic vertebral compression or burst fractures, cervical or lumbar spinal stenosis, cervical or lumbar disk herniation, nerve entrapment syndromes, trigeminal or glossopharyngeal neural-

---

BOX 19–1. PROCEDURES FOR TREATMENT OF PAIN OF THE HEAD/NECK

- Augmentative
  - Peripheral nerve stimulation
  - Intraventricular analgesic administration
  - Deep brain/motor cortex stimulation
- Ablative
  - Cranial/cervical rhizotomy/ganglionectomy
  - Caudalis dorsal root entry zone
  - Trigeminal tractotomy
  - Mesencephalotomy
  - Medial thalamotomy
  - Cingulotomy

BOX 19–2. PROCEDURES FOR TREATMENT OF PAIN OF THE UPPER TRUNK/SHOULDER/ARM

- Augmentative
  - Peripheral nerve stimulation
  - Spinal cord stimulation
  - Intraspinal/intraventricular analgesic administration
  - Deep brain/motor cortex stimulation
- Ablative
  - Sympathectomy
  - Neurectomy
  - Ganglionectomy/rhizotomy
  - Spinal dorsal root entry zone
  - Mesencephalotomy
  - Thalamotomy
  - Cingulotomy
  - Hypophysectomy

Table 19–1. Neurosurgical Pain Therapies

ANATOMIC	ABLATIVE	AUGMENTATIVE
Correction of structural deformity	Neurectomy	*Stimulation*
	Sympathectomy	Peripheral nerve
	Ganglionectomy	Spinal cord
	Rhizotomy	Thalamus
	Spinal dorsal root entry zone lesion	Motor cortex
	Cordotomy	
	Myelotomy	*Neuraxial Drug Infusion*
	Nucleus caudalis dorsal root entry zone	Intrathecal/epidural
	Trigeminal tractotomy	Intraventricular
	Mesencephalotomy	
	Thalamotomy	
	Cingulotomy	
	Hypophysectomy	

Modified from R. North, personal communication, 1998.

BOX 19–3. PROCEDURES FOR TREATMENT OF PAIN OF THE LOWER TRUNK/LEG

- Augmentative
  - Peripheral nerve stimulation
  - Spinal cord stimulation
  - Intraspinal/intraventricular analgesic administration
  - Deep brain/motor cortex stimulation
- Ablative
  - Sympathectomy
  - Neurectomy
  - Ganglionectomy/rhizotomy
  - Spinal dorsal root entry zone
  - Cordotomy
  - Myelotomy
  - Thalamotomy
  - Cingulotomy
  - Hypophysectomy

BOX 19–4. PROCEDURES FOR TREATMENT OF DIFFUSE PAIN

- Augmentative
  - Intraspinal/intraventricular analgesic administration
- Ablative
  - Thalamotomy
  - Cingulotomy
  - Hypophysectomy

gia, syringomyelia, and intracranial or intraspinal neoplasms. The surgical interventions for these conditions may consist of spinal fusion, spinal decompression, diskectomy, vertebroplasty or kyphoplasty, carpal tunnel release, ulnar nerve transposition, and microvascular decompression. Detailed discussion of each of these disorders is beyond the scope of this text but several warrant brief consideration.

Approximately 84% of vertebral compression fractures are associated with pain.[6] Most fractures heal within a few months and the pain abates along with the healing. However, in some instances pain persists for an extended period, or conservative management fails in the short term. Vertebroplasty was first introduced in France in 1987 for the treatment of painful vertebral hemangiomas.[7] It is now a widely accepted treatment for persistent pain related to osteoporotic compression fractures.[8-10] Vertebroplasty has been shown to be beneficial for the relief of pain associated with vertebral compression fractures; in one study, 96% of patients experienced pain relief that persisted for 21 months with dramatic improvement in pain scores (numeric pain rating decreased from 8.9 to 2 on a 10-point scale).[10] The mechanism by which vertebroplasty alleviates pain relates to the increased strength and stiffness of the vertebral body.[11,12]

Microvascular decompression is an important technique for the treatment of trigeminal neuralgia, glossopharyngeal neuralgia, and nervus intermedius neuralgia.[13,14] The primary indication is for treatment of classic neuralgia (paroxysmal, lancinating pain) that is refractory to pharmacologic treatment. It is most appropriate for healthy patients, generally younger than 65 years of age. The rationale of the surgery is to eliminate compression of the cranial nerve by a blood vessel (usually small artery), generally occurring near the entry of the nerve into brainstem. The advantage of microvascular decompression compared to percutaneous (e.g., radiofrequency rhizotomy for trigeminal neuralgia) or open ablative procedures for cranial neuralgias is the absence of postoperative sensory deficit, which is an obligate outcome of most ablative procedures. Pain relief is achieved in more than 95% of patients. Pain may recur over months or years in some patients but is maintained in most patients.[13,14]

Augmentation Therapy

An augmentative therapy is one that supplements the body's own intrinsic pain-relieving systems. The two broad categories of augmentative therapies are neurostimulation and neuraxial drug infusion. Neurostimulation consists of spinal cord stimulation, peripheral nerve stimulation, motor cortex stimulation, and deep brain stimulation. Neuraxial drug infusion locations include either intrathecal or intraventricular.

In comparison to ablative therapies, there are both advantages and disadvantages to augmentative therapy. Augmentative therapies offer the advantages of relative safety, reversibility, and adjustability. For example, intraspinal analgesic infusion can be adjusted to meet the changing needs of a patient who has progressively worsening cancer pain. Major disadvantages of augmentative therapies, however, are their greater cost (initial device costs and upkeep), the need for maintenance (e.g., refilling of infusion pumps, replacement of stimulation system battery packs), and the potential for device-related complications. General indications for augmentative therapies are those for neurosurgical pain treatment in general. In addition (especially for treatment of cancer pain), estimated patient life expectancy should be sufficient to warrant implantation of a neuroaugmentive device (e.g., greater than 3 months for a cancer patient being considered for implantation of a drug delivery system).

Stimulation

Stimulation therapies approved currently for use in the United States include spinal cord stimulation (SCS) and peripheral nerve stimulation (PNS). Other stimulation therapies in clinical use include deep brain stimulation and motor cortex stimulation. SCS leads may be implanted percutaneously or surgically.

Surgical ("laminotomy," "plate," or "paddle") leads offer the advantages of increased patient-reported pain coverage area, greater long-term pain relief, decreased stimulation amplitude requirements, and longer pulse generator battery life.[15,16] In addition, SCS adjustment that is patient-interactive provides better pain relief and longer battery life.[17]

Spinal cord stimulation is appropriate for the treatment of neuropathic pain. Pain should be relatively focal (e.g., localized to one or two extremities or focal on the trunk) and static in nature. The prototypical indication for SCS is for treatment of neuropathic pain in an extremity. Common applications for extremity pain include treatment of persistent radicular pain associated with failed back surgery syndrome,[18-21] neuropathic pain related to complex regional pain syndrome ("reflex sympathetic dystrophy"),[22-24] diabetic and peripheral neuropathies,[25] root injury, phantom limb pain[22] (in contrast, post-amputation stump pain does not improve consistently with SCS), and ischemic extremity pain due to peripheral vascular disease.[26,27] In the failed back surgery syndrome population, the success rate (defined typically as greater than 50% reduction in pain) is approximately 60% at 5 years.[3,19-22] Patients with complex regional pain syndromes have similar outcomes, although success rates as high as 70% to 100% have been reported.[22-24]

Neuropathic pain affecting the trunk (e.g., post-herpetic neuralgia, or some types of post-thoracotomy pain) may improve with SCS. In addition, SCS is gaining acceptance as a treatment for refractory angina pectoris[28,29] and interstitial cystitis, but is not approved currently by the United States Food and Drug Administration for these indications.

The indications for peripheral nerve stimulation (PNS) are similar to those for spinal cord stimulation, except that the distribution of pain should be limited to the territory of a single peripheral nerve.[30] For example, peripheral nerve stimulation via a percutaneously implanted lead can be very effective for the treatment of occipital neuralgia or cranial post-herpetic neuralgia.[31] Sacral nerve stimulation can be beneficial for the treatment of pelvic pain associated with interstitial cystitis, with average pain reduction of 73% reported.[32,33] Early studies have shown improved symptoms and decreased disability with C1 to C3 PNS for disabling transformed migraine.[34] Some overlap exists between applications of SCS and PNS. Extremity pain that might be appropriate for PNS can sometimes be treated equally well with SCS, and many physicians find it easier to implant an SCS lead (which can be done percutaneously) than to implant a PNS lead (which often requires an open procedure).

Intracranial stimulation therapies include focal deep brain stimulation (DBS) of the somatosensory thalamus and periventricular-periaqueductal gray,[35-38] and direct stimulation of the motor cortex.[39-42] These therapies are used primarily for treating pain of nonmalignant origin, such as pain associated with failed back surgery syndrome, neuropathic pain following central or peripheral nervous system injury (post-stroke, phantom limb pain), or trigeminal pain.[43,44] Recent positron emission scanning and functional magnetic resonance imaging (MRI) have demonstrated activation of the posterior hypothalamus in attacks of cluster headaches, which have led to successful hypothalamic DBS in refractory cases of chronic cluster headaches.[45,46] Neither DBS nor motor cortex stimulation is currently approved by the United States Food and Drug Administration for the treatment of pain, although DBS has been used clinically for more than 20 years.

Targets for deep brain stimulation include the ventrocaudal nucleus (Vc) of the thalamus (nucleus ventroposterolateralis [VPL] and ventroposteromedialis [VPM]), and the periventricular-periaqueductal gray (PVG-PAG). Recent diffusion tractography imaging has elucidated the connections of the PVG-PAG to include ascending fibers to the thalamus and frontal lobe and descending projections to the spinal cord and cerebellum.[47] This suggests that stimulation not only activates endogenous opiates, as previously suggested, but that it may also modulate central pain networks as well. Stimulation sites for DBS are chosen generally on the basis of the pain characteristics. Nociceptive pain and paroxysmal, lancinating, or evoked neuropathic pain (e.g., allodynia, hyperpathia) tend to respond best to PVG-PAG stimulation, which may activate endogenous opioid systems. Continuous neuropathic pain responds most consistently to paresthesia-producing stimulation of the sensory thalamus (nucleus ventrocaudalis).[38] Because many pain syndromes (e.g., cancer pain, failed back surgery syndrome) have mixed components of nociceptive and neuropathic pain, some physicians prefer to place electrodes in both regions, subject the patient to a trial of stimulation using externalized leads, and internalize the electrode that provides the best pain relief. Patients may be given a morphine-naloxone test to clarify the extent of nociceptive and neuropathic pain components to facilitate selection of the best stimulation target.[36]

Success rates of DBS for the treatment of intractable pain are difficult to determine from the literature because patient selection, techniques, and outcomes assessments vary substantially among studies. A review of DBS for the treatment of pain concluded that it is ineffective.[48] However, interest in the therapy remains because some individual reports suggest efficacy for the treatment of otherwise refractory pain. In general, the literature suggests that approximately 60% to 80% of patients undergoing a screening trial with DBS will have pain relief sufficient to warrant implantation of a permanent stimulation system. Approximately 50% to 60% of those who receive a permanent stimulation system will have acceptable long-term pain relief,[35] although results vary between 25% and 80%.[35-38] Overall, approximately 25% to 35% of individuals undergoing a trial of DBS have good long-term pain relief,[35,38] although success rates as high as 80% have been reported.[35-38] Patients with pain related to cancer,[38] failed back surgery syndrome, peripheral neuropathy, and trigeminal neuropathy (not anesthesia dolorosa)[35,36,38] tend to respond to DBS more favorably than patients with central pain syndromes (e.g., thalamic pain, spinal cord injury pain, anesthesia dolorosa, post-herpetic neuralgia, or phantom limb pain).[35,36,38] The incidence of serious complications of DBS is generally low, but the combination of morbidity, mortality, and technical complications can approach 25% to 30%.[35,38]

Finally, motor cortex stimulation has received attention lately as an alternative to thalamic and PAG-PVG stimulation.[39-42] It is used primarily for treatment of localized neuropathic pain syndromes and may be particularly effective for certain varieties of intractable facial pain (e.g., trigeminal neuropathic pain).[42] Pain localized to the face and arm is most amenable to treatment with motor cortex stimulation because the appropriate topographic regions of motor cortex are accessible for placement of a stimulation electrode, while pain localized to the trunk and legs is technically challenging because of the difficulty with positioning the electrode over the appropriate region of the motor cortex. Approximately 50% of patients undergoing motor cortex stimulation have good long-term pain relief. As with DBS, motor cortex stimulation appears most effective when used in the absence of anesthesia in the distribution of pain being treated. Compared to DBS, complications may be less serious because the electrode is placed epidurally rather than within the brain parenchyma. Motor cortex stimulation is a promising therapy but its long-term efficacy has not been determined. It is under active investigation at several centers.

Neuraxial Analgesic Infusion

Neuraxial analgesic infusion has become a popular interventional treatment for intractable pain.[49-54] It is well-accepted in the treatment of cancer-related pain; in contrast, the use of this therapy for chronic nonmalignant pain has been more controversial.[55] In part, this reflects concern that neuropathic pain (common in chronic nonmalignant pain syndromes) may be relatively opioid-nonresponsive. The authors' preference is to reserve neuraxial analgesic administration for the treatment of pain syndromes with a significant nociceptive pain component (e.g., cancer-related pain). However, neuropathic pain may improve also with intrathecal analgesic administration.[51,54] In fact, the most common indication for intrathecal analgesic administration is for management of pain related to failed back surgery syndrome, which typically includes neuropathic (extremity) pain as well as nociceptive (low back) pain. In general, approximately 60% to 80% of patients achieve good long-term relief of pain with intrathecal analgesics. Despite controversy about the use of this therapy for noncancer pain, outcomes are similar (degree of pain relief, patient satisfaction, and dose requirements) for patients with cancer-related and noncancer pain.[50,51] Serious complications are uncommon.

The key advantage of neuraxial analgesic administration over other pain treatments is its versatility. It has a wide range of indications, including nociceptive and mixed nociceptive/neuropathic pain syndromes. It can be used to treat focal or diffuse pain (e.g., pain related to diffuse metastatic bone lesions), and can be used to treat axial or extremity pain. It is used commonly to treat pain below cervical levels but can be effective for head and neck pain, especially if analgesic agents are delivered intraventricularly.[56,57] Neuraxial analgesics can be used in the setting of changing pain (e.g., in a patient with progressive cancer, whose sites or intensity of pain are expected to change over time). Significant disadvantages include the device costs, medication costs, and need for maintenance (e.g., refilling and, in the case of programmable pumps, replacement when the battery becomes depleted).

Ablative Therapies

Augmentative pain therapies are becoming increasingly common techniques for pain management but ablative therapies still have an important role in the treatment of some types of intractable pain. Generally, ablative therapies are viewed as the top and final rung on the pain treatment ladder (i.e., the last resort); however, in some instances, they are the procedure of choice and should be offered earlier rather than later. For instance, phantom limb pain in the setting of root avulsion, or "end-zone" pain arising from spinal cord injury, can be treated effectively by dorsal root entry zone (DREZ) lesioning. A patient with cancer-related pain and short life expectancy might be treated more appropriately with cordotomy rather than intrathecal analgesic administration via implanted infusion system. Therapy must be tailored to meet the needs of each individual patient.

Ablative therapies have been developed that target almost every level of the peripheral and central nervous system. Peripheral techniques interrupt or alter nociceptive input into the spinal cord (e.g., neurectomy, ganglionectomy, rhizotomy). Spinal interventions alter afferent input or rostral transmission of nociceptive information (e.g., DREZ lesioning, cordotomy, myelotomy). Supraspinal intracranial procedures can interrupt transmission of nociceptive information (e.g., mesencephalotomy, thalamotomy) or influence perception of painful stimuli (e.g., cingulotomy).

As with augmentation techniques, a successful outcome requires that the appropriate patient and appropriate intervention be selected. Ablative therapies tend to be most appropriate for the treatment of nociceptive pain rather than neuropathic pain. Improvement in neuropathic pain treated with ablative therapies is limited primarily to intermittent, paroxysmal, or evoked (allodynia, hyperpathia) neuropathic pain, whereas continuous neuropathic pain remains relatively unchanged in long-term follow-up.[58]

Sympathectomy

Sympathectomy is beneficial in the management of visceral pain associated with certain types of cancer.[59,60] It can also be an effective treatment for some types of noncancer pain, such as pain associated with vasospastic disorders or sympathetically maintained pain (when sympathetic blocks reliably relieve the pain). However, results of sympathectomy in the treatment of nonmalignant pain have been inconsistent, making it a less viable option.[59-62] In addition, some data suggest that SCS provides a better long-term outcome with lower morbidity.[63] SCS may, therefore, replace sympathectomy in the treatment of sympathetically maintained pain of noncancer origin affecting an extremity.

Neurectomy

In a select group of patients with pain following peripheral nerve injury, including that associated with limb amputation, neurectomy may be a useful procedure. The resection of an identifiable, pain-generating neuroma can provide significant relief.[64] Neurectomy, however, is not useful for the management of nonspecific stump pain after amputation, nor is it generally useful for the treatment of other nonmalignant peripheral pain syndromes. The utility of neurectomy is limited because pain arising from a pure sensory nerve is not common, and mixed sensory motor nerves cannot be sectioned without risk of functional impairment. There are a few specific exceptions to this general rule. For example, section of the lateral femoral cutaneous nerve may provide good long-lasting relief of meralgia paresthetica,[65] and section of the ilioinguinal or genitofemoral nerves may provide good relief of some inguinal pain syndromes (e.g., post-herniorrhaphy pain) in properly selected individuals.[66]

Dorsal Rhizotomy/Ganglionectomy

Dorsal rhizotomy and ganglionectomy serve similar purposes in denervating somatic or visceral tissues but ganglionectomy may produce more complete denervation than can be accomplished by dorsal rhizotomy alone. This is because some of the afferent fibers enter the spinal cord through the ventral root even though the cell bodies are located in the dorsal root ganglion.[67] Dorsal rhizotomy does not affect these ventral root afferent fibers, whereas ganglionectomy eliminates their input by removing the cell bodies. Rhizotomy and ganglionectomy can be used to treat pain in axial regions, such as the neck, trunk, and abdomen. These procedures are applicable in the extremities only when the limb is functionless because both procedures eliminate proprioceptive input and produce a useless limb. Limited denervation (e.g., one or two levels) does not usually provide adequate pain relief, probably because of overlap of segmental innervation of dermatomes. These procedures are most appropriate for the treatment of cancer-related pain, because noncancer pain does not improve consistently.[68,69] In the cancer setting, rhizotomy and ganglionectomy can be useful for thoracic and abdominal wall pain, perineal pain in patients with impaired bladder, bowel, and sex function, and for the treatment of pain in a functionless extremity.[70] Multiple sacral rhizotomies can be performed (e.g., to treat pelvic pain from cancer) by passing a ligature around the thecal sac below S1.[71]

Cranial Nerve Rhizotomy

In contrast to its limited utility in treating pain elsewhere in the body, rhizotomy is quite useful as a treatment for cranial neuralgias, especially trigeminal and glossopharyngeal neuralgia.[72,73] Classic trigeminal and glossopharyngeal neuralgias are unique among neuropathic pain syndromes in their uniformly good response to ablation. In contrast, atypical facial pain syndromes (constant, dysesthetic, burning pain) do not improve with ablative techniques and may be worsened by denervation procedures. Percutaneous trigeminal rhizotomy can be accomplished with radiofrequency (RF) ablation, glycerol injection, and balloon compression. These techniques are performed on an outpatient basis, are well tolerated, and have high success rates in relieving paroxysmal pain of cranial neuralgias.[73] Open rhizotomy (i.e., via craniotomy or craniectomy) is usually reserved for the treatment of glossopharyngeal and nervus inter-medius neuralgia, but may be required for treatment of some trigeminal neuralgias.

Stereotactic radiosurgery rhizotomy for the treatment of trigeminal neuralgia is an alternative to percutaneous rhizotomy, open rhizotomy, or microvascular decompression in some individuals.[74] However, unlike other surgical treatments for trigeminal neuralgia, pain relief does not occur typically for several weeks following radiosurgical treatment. Therefore, radiosurgery is not appropriate for individuals with severe acute exacerbation of pain that cannot be controlled adequately with medications because it does not provide immediate pain relief. In contrast, early pain relief is achieved in more than 95% of patients undergoing percutaneous or open rhizotomy. Pain may recur over months or years in some patients but relief is maintained in the majority of patients.[72,73]

C2 Ganglionectomy

C2 ganglionectomy is useful for the treatment of occipital neuralgia. It is especially effective for individuals with post-traumatic occipital neuralgia who have no migraine component to their headache.[75] Long-term pain relief is achieved in most patients. Pain relief may be comparable to that achieved with occipital nerve stimulation but without the need for implanted devices and long-term follow-up.

Dorsal Root Entry Zone Lesioning

DREZ lesioning of the spinal cord (for trunk or extremity pain)[76-78] or nucleus caudalis (for facial pain)[77,79,80] can provide significant pain relief. Improvement in pain is reported at greater than 70% to 80% in properly selected individuals. The rationale of DREZ lesioning is to disrupt input into and outflow from the superficial layers of the spinal cord dorsal horn, which are the sites of termination of afferent nociceptive fibers, and sites of origin of some of the nociceptive fibers ascending within the spinal cord. DREZ lesioning disrupts the spontaneous abnormal activity and hyperactivity which often develops within the spinal cord dorsal horn neurons in the setting of neuropathic pain. These techniques are best reserved for localized pain. The most successful applications are related to treatment of neuropathic pain arising from root avulsions (cervical or lumbosacral), which can result in phantom limb pain, and "end-zone" or "boundary" pain following spinal cord injury. These pain syndromes sometimes respond adequately to spinal cord stimulation or intrathecal drug infusion but DREZ lesioning can provide pain relief without the need for long-term maintenance of an augmentative device. DREZ lesioning has been used for the treatment of other neuropathic pain syndromes such as post-herpetic neuralgia, but good pain relief is not achieved consistently. Nucleus caudalis lesioning seems most useful for deafferentation pain affecting the face (including post-herpetic neuralgia), and less helpful for facial pain of peripheral origin (e.g., traumatic trigeminal neuropathy). Certain types of cancer pain can be treated effectively with DREZ lesioning (e.g., neuropathic arm pain associated with Pancoast's tumor). As with other ablative procedures, DREZ is most effective for relieving paroxysmal rather than continuous neuropathic pain.[78]

Cordotomy

Cordotomy is especially valuable for the control of pain related to malignancy, particularly for individuals with relatively short life expectancies, for whom it is difficult to justify the costs of implantation of drug infusion systems. Whereas intrathecal analgesic administration has largely replaced cordotomy for the treatment of cancer pain, cordotomy offers several advantages. As a one-time procedure, it requires no long-term follow-up or maintenance. This is especially important for individuals who may find it difficult to return to a medical facility for refilling of an infusion system or for whom costs of ongoing medical care become burdensome.

The rationale of cordotomy is to disrupt the nociceptive afferent fibers ascending in the spinothalamic tract in the anterolateral quadrant of the spinal cord. It can be performed as an open[81] or closed (percutaneous)[82,83] procedure. Percutaneous techniques are less invasive, but open techniques remain viable options because some surgeons lack the expertise and equipment required for percutaneous procedures. In general, the level of analgesia produced by cordotomy falls over time such that within 3 weeks after the procedure the level has fallen three to six spinal levels and by 6 months the level may have fallen six to eight segments. Consequently, the procedure is best for pain below mid to low cervical dermatome levels.[81,82] In addition, loss of pain relief overall tends to occur over time. Approximately one third of patients have recurrent pain in 3 months, half at 1 year, and two thirds at longer follow-up intervals.[70,84,85] However, cordotomy does provide good pain relief in approximately 60% to 80% of patients.[82,85]

Cordotomy is used most commonly for the treatment of cancer-related pain. It is used less frequently for management of noncancer pain because of concern about the potential loss of pain relief over time, the occurrence of postcordotomy dysesthesias, and the risk of neurologic complication.[81] In addition, pulmonary complications may ensue following cordotomy. The risk of respiratory depression subsequent to a unilateral high cervical procedure mandates that pulmonary function be acceptable on the contralateral side. For example, a patient who has undergone previous pneumonectomy for lung cancer should not be subject to cordotomy that would compromise pulmonary function on the side of the remaining lung.[82]

Pain relief varies with pain characteristics and location. Lancinating, paroxysmal, neuropathic pain and evoked (allodynic or hyperpathic) pain that sometimes occurs following spinal cord injury or as part of peripheral neuropathic pain syndromes can improve following cordotomy, but continuous neuropathic pain does not improve.[82] Laterally located pain responds better than midline or axial pain (e.g., visceral pain). Midline and axial pain may require bilateral procedures to achieve pain relief. However, bilateral cordotomies carry significantly greater risks of complication including weakness, bladder, bowel, and sexual dysfunction, and respiratory depression (if the procedure is performed bilaterally at cervical levels).[81,82] Bilateral percutaneous cervical cordotomies are usually staged at least 1 week apart to reduce the likelihood of serious complication.

Myelotomy

Myelotomy has also fallen into disfavor subsequent to the advent and popularity of intrathecal drug infusion therapy. Myelotomy is used very rarely but can provide good pain relief in properly selected patients, including some who fail treatment with intrathecal analgesics.[86] Commissural myelotomy was developed to provide the benefit of bilateral cordotomy without the risk of lesioning both of the anterior quadrants of the spinal cord.[86-88] This is accomplished by sectioning spinothalamic tract fibers as they decussate in the anterior commissure. The advantage compared to cordotomy is that bilateral and midline pain can be treated with a single operative procedure, with lower morbidity and mortality.

Subsequently, it was observed that a limited midline myelotomy[89] or high cervical myelotomy[85,90] could be as effective as classic commissural myelotomy. Limited midline myelotomy involves a lesion a few millimeters in length, compared to a few centimeters in commissural myelotomy. Furthermore, recent identification of a dorsal column visceral pain pathway has lead to the development of punctate midline myelotomy for the treatment of abdominal and pelvic pain.[88]

Similar to cordotomy, these procedures are indicated primarily for the treatment of cancer-related pain. Myelotomy is most useful for pain in the abdomen, pelvis, perineum, and legs. In this regard, myelotomy is comparable to bilateral cordotomy but with potentially fewer risks. The procedure is most effective for nociceptive rather than neuropathic pain. Early complete pain relief is achieved in more than 90% of patients but pain tends to recur over time, such that approximately 50% to 60% of patients have good long-term pain relief.[85] The risk of complications of bladder, bowel, and sexual dysfunction are less than that associated with bilateral cordotomy but still remains sufficiently high, limiting these procedures to patients with cancer-related pain who have pre-existing dysfunction.[70]

Mesencephalotomy

Mesencephalotomy is indicated for the treatment of intractable pain involving the head, neck, shoulder, and arm.[58,91] It can be viewed as a supraspinal version of cordotomy,[42] because the nociceptive fibers ascending in the brainstem are disrupted. This procedure is not in widespread use, in part because relatively few patients require such interventions and because relatively few neurosurgeons have the expertise to perform these interventions. As with other ablative procedures, however, this technique can provide benefit to carefully selected patients. Most commonly, the procedure is used for the treatment of pain related to cancer and provides satisfactory long-term pain relief in about 85% of patients.[85] It does not provide consistent good long-term relief of central neuropathic pain.[91] Side effects and complications can be frequent, especially oculomotor dysfunction.[58,85,91] As with most ablative procedures, the utility of mesencephalotomy has diminished subsequent to the advent of neuraxial analgesic administration. Intraventricular morphine infusion can provide good pain relief but with a lower incidence of complications. However, mesencephalotomy may be preferable for some individuals. For example, patients with short life expectancy and individuals who find the costs and long-term follow-up of neuraxial analgesics burdensome may be appropriate candidates.

Thalamotomy

Thalamotomy can be useful for individuals who are not candidates for cordotomy, such as those with pain above the C5 dermatome or with pulmonary dysfunction.[92] It has been used for the treatment of both cancer-related and noncancer-related pain.[93] In the setting of cancer, thalamotomy is most appropriate for individuals who have widespread pain (e.g., from diffuse metastatic disease), or who have midline, bilateral, or head/neck pain, for which other procedures may not be likely to provide relief.[93] The success rate of thalamotomy in relieving pain is slightly lower that achieved with mesencephalotomy, but importantly, the incidence of complications is also lower.[92]

Thalamotomy can be accomplished by either stereotactic radiofrequency[58,85,92,94,95] or radiosurgical[96] techniques. The lateral thalamus (nucleus ventrocaudalis) is not considered an acceptable target for ablation due to the risk of dysesthesias and sensory loss,[58] but the subjacent parvicellular ventrocaudal nucleus, which is thought to be a relay site for spinothalamic afferents, has been used as a target. Results of thalamotomy directed to this structure may be similar to those accomplished with cordotomy.[94]

Medial thalamotomy appears most effective for treating nociceptive pain (e.g., cancer pain), with acceptable long-term pain relief obtained in approximately 30% to 50% of patients.[58,93,95] Overall, neuropathic pain syndromes respond less consistently to thalamotomy, with only about one third of patients improving long term.[58,95] Patients with paroxysmal, lancinating neuropathic pain or neuropathic pain with elements of allodynia and hyperpathia may improve significantly following thalamotomy, whereas those with continuous neuropathic pain tend not to benefit.[58]

Cingulotomy

Cingulotomy is used less commonly for treatment of intractable pain than for management of psychiatric disorders. It is applied most commonly to the treatment of cancer pain, but has been used for noncancer pain as well.[85,97,98] Approximately 50% to 75% of patients benefit from the procedure, at least in the short term; generally, pain relief is maintained at least 3 months in the cancer population. In contrast, the utility of cingulotomy for chronic noncancer pain is less apparent, with some studies indicating relatively good long-lasting pain relief[85,98] and others indicating only 20% long-term success.[93] Cingulotomy may be a reasonable option for individuals with cancer-related pain in whom other treatments have failed. Because cingulotomy is sometimes performed for treatment in psychiatric disease, it carries the stigma of "psychosurgery" and may warrant formal review by institutional ethics committees if this procedure is being considered as a treatment for intractable pain.

Hypophysectomy

Hypophysectomy (surgical, chemical, or radiosurgical) can provide good relief of cancer-related pain. The mechanism of pain relief is unknown.[85,94,99,100] It is particularly beneficial in the case of hormonally responsive cancers (e.g., prostate, breast cancer), but may relieve pain associated with other tumors as well. Hypophysectomy is primarily used in the treatment of individuals with widespread disease and diffuse pain. Pain is alleviated in 45% to 95% of patients and occurs independent of tumor regression.

CONCLUSION

Surgical intervention is not generally the first treatment option for the management of pain. Typically it is reserved for patients in whom more conservative treatments have failed or are associated with unacceptable side effects. Nevertheless, the management of chronic pain requires an element of flexibility, and some individuals may be surgical candidates earlier in the course of therapy. Successful outcomes require that candidates for neurosurgical treatment be selected carefully, with full recognition of chronic pain as a biopsychosocial disorder and consideration of all the factors that contribute to a pain complaint.

Pain management physicians should be familiar with the variety of surgical techniques available for the treatment of pain, their general indications, and their general outcomes, and incorporate these treatments in the care of their patients when appropriate. They should understand that pain may result from structural abnormalities that are anatomically correctable, and have some ability to distinguish it from the pain that may respond better to augmentative or ablative therapies. Finally, pain management specialists should also be aware of the typical indications for both augmentation and ablation. As more attention is focused on augmentative therapies for the treatment of intractable pain, ablative therapies that might be appropriate for some individuals may be overlooked as treatment options.

Outcome of augmentation therapy in properly selected patients is good and the risk of serious or permanent complication is low, making neuromodulation therapy the first choice for many patients. For the most part, augmentative therapies have supplanted ablative therapies for the surgical treatment of most pain disorders. Augmentation techniques, especially the stimulation therapies such as SCS, are superior to ablative techniques for the treatment of neuropathic pain with a continuous, dysesthetic component.[58,94] On the other hand, ablative therapies may be more appropriate for some individuals, for example, individuals with cancer-related pain and short life expectancies. Patients with a predominant nociceptive component of pain, and those with neuropathic pain with paroxysmal or evoked components, can also benefit from ablative techniques.

SUMMARY

- Chronic pain patients being considered for treatment via surgical intervention should be evaluated by a multidisciplinary team that includes a neuropsychological assessment to facilitate good outcomes.
- Anatomic neurosurgical techniques address structural abnormalities causing pain and may include spinal procedures, vertebroplasty, nerve entrapment release, and microvascular decompression.
- Stimulation therapies include spinal cord stimulation, peripheral nerve stimulation, motor cortex stimulation, and deep brain stimulation. These therapies have been used for a large variety of indications, including persistent radicular pain, post-herpetic neuralgia, post-stroke pain, phantom limb pain, ischemic peripheral vascular disease, refractory angina pectoris, complex regional pain syndrome, peripheral neuropathy, headache disorders, and interstitial cystitis.
- Neuraxial analgesic administration is particularly useful in patients with a significant nociceptive pain component, including cancer pain and chronic back pain.
- The advantage of neuraxial drug infusion compared to pain therapies is its versatility; the disadvantage is the associated maintenance required for pump adjustments and refills.
- Ablative neurosurgical procedures target every level of the central and peripheral nervous system and include peripheral and spinal interventions that alter rostral transmission (ganglionectomy, DREZ lesioning, cordotomy, myelotomy) and supraspinal interventions that interrupt transmission (mesencephalotomy, thalamotomy) or alter pain perception (cingulotomy).
- Ablation therapies are most beneficial for cancer pain and patients with neuropathic pain that has paroxysmal or evoked components.

References

1. Krames ES: Intraspinal opioid therapy for chronic nonmalignant pain: Current practice and clinical guidelines. J Pain Symptom Manage 1996;11:333-352.
2. World Health Organization Expert Committee: Cancer pain relief and palliative care. World Health Organization Technical Report Series 1990;804:1-73.
3. North RB, Kidd DH, Lee MS, et al: A prospective, randomized study of spinal cord stimulation versus reoperation for failed back surgery syndrome: Initial results. Stereotact Funct Neurosurg 1994;62:267-272.
4. Doleys DM, Olson K: Psychological Assessment and Intervention in Implantable Pain Therapies, Minneapolis, MN, Medtronic Inc, 1997.
5. North RB, Levy RM: Consensus conference on the neurosurgical management of pain (review). Neurosurgery 1994;34:756-761.
6. Cooper C, Atkinson EJ, O'Fallon WM, et al: Incidence of clinically diagnosed vertebral fractures: A population based study in Rochester, Minnesota, 1985-1989. J Bone Miner Res 1992;7:221-227.
7. Galibert P, Deramond H, Rosat P, et al: Preliminary note on the treatment of vertebral angioma by percutaneous acrylic vertebroplasty. Neurochirurgie 1987;33:166-168.
8. Barr JD, Barr MS, Lemley TJ, et al: Percutaneous vertebroplasty for pain relief and spinal stabilization. Spine 2000;25:923-928.

9. Legroux-Gerot I, Lormeau C, Boutry N, et al: Long-term follow-up of vertebral osteoporotic fractures treated by percutaneous vertebroplasty. Clin Rheumatol 2004;23:310-317.

10. McGraw JK, Lippert JA, Minkus KD, et al: Prospective evaluation of pain relief in 100 patients undergoing percutaneous vertebroplasty: Results and follow-up. J Vasc Interv Radiol 2002;13:883-886.

11. Dean JR, Ison KT, Gishen P: The strengthening effect of percutaneous vertebroplasty. Clin Radiol 2000;55:471-476.

12. Botrom MP, Lane JM: Future directions. Augmentation of osteoporotic vertebral bodies. Spine 1997;22(suppl 24):S38-S42.

13. Barker FG II, Janetta PJ, Bissonette DJ, et al: The long-term outcomes of microvascular decompression for trigeminal neuralgia. N Engl J Med 1996;334:1077-1083.

14. Kasam PA, Horowitz M, Chang YF: Microvascular decompression in the management of glossopharyngeal neuralgia: Analysis of 217 cases. Neurosurgery 2002;50:705-710.

15. North RB, Kidd DH, Olin JC, et al: Spinal cord stimulation electrode design: Prospective, randomized, controlled trial comparing percutaneous and laminectomy electrodes-part I: Technical outcomes. Neurosurgery 2002;51:381-389.

16. Villavicencio AT, Leveque JC, Rubin L: Laminectomy versus percutaneous electrode placement for spinal cord stimulation. Neurosurgery 2000;46:399-405.

17. North RB, Calkins SK, Campbell DS, et al: Automated, patient-interactive, spinal cord stimulator adjustment: A randomized controlled trial. Neurosurgery 2003;52:572-580.

18. Deer TR: The role of neuromodulation by spinal cord stimulation in chronic pain syndromes: Current concepts. Techniques in Regional Anesthesia and Pain Management 1998;2:161-167.

19. North RB, Kidd DH, Zahurak M, et al: Spinal cord stimulation for chronic, intractable pain: Experience over two decades. Neurosurgery 1993;32:384-395.

20. Turner J, Loeser J, Bell K: Spinal cord stimulation for chronic low back pain: A systematic literature synthesis. Neurosurgery 1995;37:1088-1096.

21. Burchiel KJ, Anderson VC, Brown FD, et al: Prospective, multicenter study of spinal cord stimulation for relief of chronic back and extremity pain. Spine 1996;21:2786-2794.

22. Spiegelmann W: Spinal cord stimulation: A contemporary series. Neurosurgery 1991;28:65-70.

23. Barolat G, Schwartzman R, Woo R: Epidural spinal cord stimulation in the management of reflex sympathetic dystrophy. Stereotact Funct Neurosurg 1989;53:29-37.

24. Kumar K, Nath R, Toth C: Spinal cord stimulation is effective in the management of reflex sympathetic dystrophy. Neurosurgery 1997;3:503-508.

25. Kumar K, Nath R: Spinal cord stimulation for chronic pain in peripheral neuropathy. Surgical Neurology 1996;46:363-364.

26. Kumar K, Toth C, Nath R, et al: Improvement of limb circulation in peripheral vascular disease using epidural spinal cord stimulation: A prospective study. J Neurosurg 1997;86:662-669.

27. Huber S, Vaglienti R, Midcap M: Enhanced limb salvage for peripheral vascular disease with the use of spinal cord stimulation. W V Med J 1996;92:89-91.

28. Sanderson JE, Ibrahim B, Waterhouse D, et al: Spinal electrical stimulation for intractable angina—Long-term clinical outcome and safety. Eur Heart J 1994;15:810-814.

29. De Jongste MJL, Hautvast RWM, Hillege HL, et al: Efficacy of spinal cord stimulation as adjuvant therapy for intractable angina pectoris: A prospective, randomized clinical study. J Am Coll Cardiol 1994;23:1592-1597.

30. Hassenbusch SJ, Stanton-Hicks M, Schoppa D, et al: Long-term results of peripheral nerve stimulation for reflex sympathetic dystrophy. J Neurosurg 1996;84:415-423.

31. Weiner RL, Reed KL: Peripheral neurostimulation for control of intractable occipital neuralgia. Neuromodulation 1999;2:217-221.

32. Comiter CV: Sacral neuromodulation for the symptomatic treatment of refractory interstitial cystitis: A prospective study. J Urol 2003;169:1369-1373.

33. Maher CF, Carey MP, Dwyer PL, et al: Percutaneous sacral nerve root neuromodulation for intractable interstitial cystitis. J Urol 2001;165:884-886.

34. Popeney CA, Alo KM: Peripheral neurostimulation for the treatment of chronic, disabling transformed migraine. Headache 2003;43:369-375.

35. Levy RM, Lamb S, Adams JE: Treatment of chronic pain by deep brain stimulation: Long term follow-up and review of the literature. Neurosurgery 1987;21:885-893.

36. Kumar K, Toth C, Nath RK: Deep brain stimulation for intractable pain: A 15-year experience. Neurosurgery 1997;40:736-747.

37. Richardson DE: Deep brain stimulation for the relief of chronic pain. Neurosurg Clin N Am 1995;6:135-144.

38. Tasker RR, Filho OV: Deep brain stimulation for the control of intractable pain. In Youmans JR (ed): Neurological Surgery. Philadelphia, WB Saunders, 1996, pp 3512-3527.

39. Nguyen J-P, Lefaucheur J-P, Decq P, et al: Chronic motor cortex stimulation in the treatment of central and neuropathic pain: Correlations between clinical, electrophysiological and anatomical data. Pain 1999;82:245-251.

40. Ebel H, Rust D, Tronnier V, et al: Chronic precentral stimulation in trigeminal neuropathic pain. Acta Neurochir (Wien) 1996;138:1300-1306.

41. Tsubokawa T, Katayama Y, Yamamoto T, et al: Chronic motor cortex stimulation in patients with thalamic pain. J Neurosurg 1993;78:393-401.

42. Meyerson BA, Linderoth B, Lind G, et al: Motor cortex stimulation as a treatment of trigeminal neuropathic pain. Acta Neurochir (Wien) (Suppl) 1993;58:150-153.

43. Owen SL, Green AL, Stein JF, et al: Deep brain stimulation for the alleviation of post-stroke neuropathic pain. Pain 2006;120(1-2):202-206.

44. Bittar RG, Otero S, Carter H, et al: Deep brain stimulation for phantom limb pain. J Clin Neurosci 12005;2:399-404.

45. Leone M, Franzini A, Broggi G, et al: Hypothalamic deep brain stimulation for intractable chronic cluster headache: A 3-year follow-up. Neurol Sci 2003;24(suppl 2):S143-145.

46. Leone M, May A, Franzini A, et al: Deep brain stimulation for intractable chronic cluster headache: Proposals for patient selection. Cephalalgia 2004;24:934-937.

47. Sillery E, Bittar RG, Robson MD, et al: Connectivity of the human periventricular-periaqueductal gray region. J Neurosurg 2005;103:1030-1034.

48. Coffey RJ: Deep brain stimulation for chronic pain: Results of two multicenter trials and a structured review. Pain Med 2001;2:183-192.

49. Follett KA, Hitchon PW, Piper J, et al: Response of intractable pain to continuous intrathecal morphine: A retrospective study. Pain 1992;49:21-25.

50. Paice JA, Penn RD, Shott S: Intraspinal morphine for chronic pain: A retrospective, multicenter study. J Pain Symptom Manage 1996;11:71-80.

51. Winkelmüller M, Winkelmüller W: Long-term effects of continuous intrathecal opioid treatment in chronic pain of nonmalignant etiology. J Neurosurg 1996;85:458-467.

52. Schuchard M, Krames ES, Lanning R: Intraspinal analgesia for nonmalignant pain. A retrospective analysis for efficacy, safety, and feasibility in 50 patients. Neuromodulation 1998;1:46-56.

53. Hassenbusch SJ, Pillay PK, Magdinec M, et al: Constant infusion of morphine for intractable cancer pain using an implanted pump. J Neurosurg 1990;73:405-409.

54. Hassenbusch SJ, Stanton-Hicks M, Covington EC, et al: Long-term intraspinal infusions of opioids in the treatment of neuropathic pain. J Pain Symptom Manage 1995;10:527-543.

55. Maron J, Loeser JD: Spinal opioid infusions in the treatment of chronic pain of nonmalignant origin (review). Clin J Pain 1996;12:174-179.

56. Dennis GC, DeWitty RL: Long-term intraventricular infusion of morphine for intractable pain in cancer of the head and neck. Neurosurgery 1990;26:404-408.

57. Karavelis A, Foroglou G, Selviaridis P, et al: Intraventricular administration of morphine for control of intractable cancer pain in 90 patients. Neurosurgery 1996;39:57-62.
58. Tasker RR: Stereotactic surgery. In Wall PD, Melzack R (eds): Textbook of Pain, 3rd ed. Edinburgh, Churchill Livingstone, 1994, pp 1137-1158.
59. Hardy RW Jr, Bay JW: Surgery of the sympathetic nervous system. In Schmidek HH, Sweet WH (eds): Operative Neurosurgical Techniques: Indications, Methods, and Results, 3rd ed. Philadelphia, WB Saunders, 1995, pp 1637-1646.
60. Wilkinson HA: Sympathectomy for pain. In Youmans JR (ed): Neurological Surgery, Philadelphia, WB Saunders, 1996, pp 3489-3499.
61. Johnson JP, Obasi C, Hahn MS, et al: Endoscopic thoracic sympathectomy. J Neurosurg (Spine 1) 1999;91:90-97.
62. Schwartzman RJ, Liu JE, Smullens SN, et al: Long-term outcome following sympathectomy for complex regional pain syndrome type I (RSD). J Neurol Sci 1997;150: 149-152.
63. Kumar K, Nath RK, Toth C: Spinal cord stimulation is effective in the management of reflex sympathetic dystrophy. Neurosurgery 1997;40:503-509.
64. Burchiel KJ, Johans TJ, Ochoa J: The surgical treatment of painful traumatic neuromas. J Neurosurg 1993;78:714-719.
65. Van Eerten PV, Polder TW, Broere CAJ: Operative treatment of meralgia paresthetica: Transection versus neurolysis. Neurosurgery 1995;37(1):63-65.
66. Starling JR, Harms BA: Diagnosis and treatment of genitofemoral and ilioinguinal neuralgia. World J Surg 1989;13: 586-591.
67. Hosobuchi Y: The majority of unmyelinated afferent axons in human ventral roots probably conduct pain. Pain 1980;8:167-180.
68. Onofrio BM, Campa HK: Evaluation of rhizotomy: Review of 12 years' experience. J Neurosurg 1972;36:751-755.
69. North RB, Kidd DH, Campbell JN, et al: Dorsal root ganglionectomy for failed back surgery syndrome: A 5-year follow-up study. J Neurosurg 1991;74:236-242.
70. Taha JM, Favre J, Burchiel KM: Management of malignant chronic pain. In Grossman RG, Loftus CM (eds): Principles of Neurosurgery, 2nd ed. Philadelphia, Lippincott-Raven, 1999, pp 435-442.
71. Saris SC, Silver JM, Vieira JFS, et al: Sacrococcygeal rhizotomy for perineal pain. Neurosurgery 1986;19:789-793.
72. Tew JM Jr, Taha JM: Percutaneous rhizotomy in the treatment of intractable facial pain (trigeminal, glossopharyngeal, and vagal nerves). In Schmidek HH, Sweet WH (eds): Operative Neurosurgical Techniques: Indications, Methods, and Results, 3rd ed. Philadelphia, WB Saunders, 1995, pp 1469-1484.
73. Taha JM, Tew JM Jr: Comparison of surgical treatments for trigeminal neuralgia: Reevaluation of radiofrequency rhizotomy. Neurosurgery 1997;38:865-871.
74. Maesawa S, Salame C, Flickinger JC, et al: Clinical outcomes after stereotactic radiosurgery for idiopathic trigeminal neuralgia. J Neurosurg 2001;94:14-20.
75. Lozano AM, Vanderlinden G, Bachoo R, et al: Microsurgical C-2 ganglionectomy for chronic intractable occipital pain. J Neurosurg 1998;89:359-365.
76. Rath SA, Seitz K, Soliman N, et al: DREZ coagulations for deafferentation pain related to spinal and peripheral nerve lesions: Indication and results of 79 consecutive procedures. Stereotact Funct Neurosurg 1997;68(1-4 Pt 1):161-167.
77. Nashold JRB, Nashold BS Jr: Microsurgical DREZotomy in treatment of deafferentation pain. In Schmidek HH, Sweet WH (eds): Operative Neurosurgical Techniques: Indications, Methods, and Results, 3rd ed. Philadelphia, WB Saunders, 1995, pp 1623-1636.
78. Sindou MP: Microsurgical DREZotomy. In Schmidek HH, Sweet WH (eds): Operative Neurosurgical Techniques: Indica-
tions, Methods, and Results, 3rd ed., Philadelphia, WB Saunders, 1995, pp 1613-1621.
79. Bullard DE, Nashold BS Jr: The caudalis DREZ for facial pain. Stereotact Funct Neurosurg 1997;68(1-4 Pt 1):168-174.
80. Gorecki JP, Nashold BS: The Duke experience with the nucleus caudalis DREZ operation. Acta Neurochir (Suppl) 1995;64:128-131.
81. Poletti CE: Open cordotomy and medullary tractotomy. In Schmidek HH, Sweet WH (eds): Operative Neurosurgical Techniques: Indications, Methods, and Results, 3rd ed. Philadelphia, WB Saunders, 1995, pp 1557-1571.
82. Tasker RR: Percutaneous cordotomy. In Schmidek HH, Sweet WH (eds): Operative Neurosurgical Techniques: Indications, Methods, and Results, 3rd ed. Philadelphia, WB Saunders, 1995, pp 1595-1611.
83. Kanpolat Y, Akyar S, Caglar S, et al: CT-guided percutaneous selective cordotomy. Acta Neurochir 1993;123(1-2):92-96.
84. Rosomoff HL, Papo I, Loeser JD, et al: Neurosurgical operations on the spinal cord. In Bonica JJ (ed): The Management of Pain, 2nd ed. Philadelphia, Lea & Febiger, 1990, pp 2067-2081.
85. Gybels JM, Sweet WH: Neurosurgical Treatment of Persistent Pain: Physiological and Pathological Mechanisms of Human Pain. Basel, Karger, 1989.
86. Watling CJ, Payne R, Allen RR, et al: Commissural myelotomy for intractable cancer pain: Report of two cases. Clin J Pain 1996;12:151-156.
87. King RB: Anterior commissurotomy for intractable pain. J Neurosurg 1977;47:7-11.
88. Nauta HJW, Hewitt E, Westlund KN, et al: Surgical interruption of a midline dorsal column visceral pain pathway. Case report and review of the literature. J Neurosurg 1997;86: 538-542.
89. Hirshberg RM, Al-Chaer ED, Lawand NB, et al: Is there a pathway in the posterior funiculus that signals visceral pain? Pain 1996;67:291-305.
90. Hitchcock ER: Stereotactic cervical myelotomy. J Neurol Neurosurg Psychiatry 1970;33:224-230.
91. Bullard DE, Nashold BS Jr: Mesencephalatomy and other brain stem procedures for pain. In Youmans JR (ed): Neurological Surgery. Philadelphia, WB Saunders, 1996, p 3477.
92. Tasker RR: Thalamotomy. Neurosurg Clin N Am 1990;1: 841.
93. Jannetta PJ, Gildenberg PL, Loeser JD, et al: Operations on the brain and brain stem for chronic pain. In Bonica JJ (ed): The Management of Pain, 2nd ed. Philadelphia, Lea & Febiger, 1990, pp 2082-2103.
94. Tasker RR: Intracranial ablative procedures for pain. In Tindall TG, Cooper PR, Barrow DL (eds): The Practice of Neurosurgery. Baltimore, Williams & Wilkins, 1996, pp 3115-3128.
95. Tasker RR: Thalamic stereotaxic procedures. In Schaltenbrand G, Walker AE (eds): Stereotaxy of the Human Brain: Anatomical, Physiological and Clinical Applications. Stuttgart, Germany, Georg Thieme Verlag, 1982, pp 484-497.
96. Young RF, Vermeulen SS, Grimm P, et al: Gamma knife thalamotomy for the treatment of persistent pain. Stereotact Funct Neurosurg 1995;64(suppl 1):172-181.
97. Hassenbusch SJ, Pillay PK, Barnett GH: Radiofrequency cingulotomy for intractable cancer pain using stereotaxis guided by magnetic resonance imaging. Neurosurgery 1990;27(2): 220-223.
98. Bouckoms AJ: Limbic surgery for pain. In Wall PD, Melzack R (eds): Textbook of Pain, 3rd ed. Edinburgh, Churchill Livingstone, 1994, p 1171.
99. Levin AB, Katz J, Benson RC, et al: Treatment of pain of diffuse metastatic cancer by stereotactic chemical hypophysectomy: Long term results and observations on mechanism of action. Neurosurgery 1980;6:258-262.
100. Ramirez LF, Levin AB: Pain relief after hypophysectomy. Neurosurgery 1984;14:499-504.

CHAPTER
20 Cancer Pain

Oscar de Leon-Casasola and Anthony Yarussi

Cancer pain is the result of cancer growth in human tissues or the pain produced by any of the therapies implemented to treat it. Ideal management starts with a thorough assessment via history and physical examination, as well as the judicious use of diagnostic testing to try to define the pathophysiologic components involved in the expression of pain to implement optimal analgesic therapy. Adequate pain control can be achieved in the great majority of patients with aggressive pharmacologic treatment using opioids and adjuvants.[1,2] With the implementation of these strategies, 90% to 95% of the patients may achieve adequate pain control.[3] Consequently, 5% to 10% of patients will need some form of invasive therapy. Thus, when following specific guidelines, most patients with cancer-related pain may expect adequate pain control. Control of pain and related symptoms is a cornerstone of cancer treatment, because it promotes an enhanced quality of life, improved functioning, better compliance, and a means for patients to focus on what gives meaning to their lives.[4] In addition to its salutary effects on quality of life, mounting evidence suggests that good pain control influences survival.[5,6]

EPIDEMIOLOGY OF CANCER PAIN

Approximately 6.35 million new cases of cancer are annually diagnosed worldwide, and 50% of those originate in developing nations,[7] with 1.04 million occurring in the United State alone.[8] The mortality is very high; one of five deaths in the United States is the result of cancer, amounting to about 1400 cancer-related deaths every day.[9,10] The morbidity is equally concerning, because up to 50% of patients undergoing treatment for cancer and up to 90% of patients with advanced cancer have pain.[11] Most cancer pain (65%) is the result of tumor involvement of organic structures, notably bone, neural tissue, and viscera. Up to 25% of cancer pain is caused by therapy, including chemotherapy, radiotherapy, or surgery, and the rest of "cancer pain" is accounted for by common chronic pain syndromes, including back pain and headaches, which might have been exacerbated by the ongoing growth or treatment of cancer.[12] As new therapeutic regimens are introduced for cancer treatment, it is expected that cancer patients will be living longer, potentially experienc-ing pain caused by the cancer disease itself or by treatment modalities implemented for its control for longer periods.

Anorexia, fatigue, and pain are the most common symptom associated with cancer.[13,14] Significant pain is present in up to 25% of patients in active treatment and in up to 90% of patients with advanced cancer.[11,15-19] According to several studies, including a survey of oncologists in the Eastern Cooperative Oncology Group (ECOG) and a survey of 1103 consecutive admissions to a U.S. tertiary care cancer hospital, 73% of patients in active treatment admitted to pain, with 38% reporting severe pain.[20] Despite the availability of simple, cost-effective treatments,[21] inadequately controlled pain remains a significant problem. This is important because of the negative influence of pain on patients' performance status.

Performance status, as measured by the ECOG and Karnofsky scales (Table 20–1), is a global rating of patients' overall functional status. When performance status is low, as is often the case when pain is severe, patients may find it difficult to tolerate recommended chemotherapy; indeed, they may not be considered candidates for chemotherapy. Further benefits of good pain management often include improvements in nutrition, rest, and mood, all of which contribute to quality of life and have the potential to influence the outcome of antineoplastic therapy.

ASSESSMENT OF PAIN INTENSITY

Questionnaires have been used to aid in standardizing patients' assessment. Ideally, this assessment is completed by the patient prior to evaluation. The Wisconsin Brief Pain Inventory (BPI)[22] and the Memorial Pain Assessment Card[23] are becoming increasingly well accepted. The BPI is a 15-minute questionnaire that can be self-administered. It includes several questions about the characteristics of the pain, including its origin and effects of prior treatments. It incorporates two valuable features of the McGill Pain Questionnaire—a graphic representation of the location of pain and groups of qualitative descriptors. Severity of pain is assessed by a series of the Visual Analogue Scales (VAS) that score pain at its best, worst, and on average. The perceived level of interference with normal function is also quanti-

Table 20–1. Methods of Assessing Performance Status

Eastern Cooperative Oncology Group (ECOG)*		Karnofsky†	
SCORE	PERFORMANCE STATUS	SCORE	PERFORMANCE STATUS
0	Fully active; able to carry on all predisease performance without restriction	100	Normal; no complaints, no evidence of disease
1	Restricted in physically strenuous activity but ambulatory and able to carry out light or sedentary work (e.g., light housework, office work)	90	Able to carry on normal activity; minor signs or symptoms of disease
2	Ambulatory and capable of all self-care but unable to work; up and about more than 50% of waking hours	80	Normal activity with effort; some signs or symptoms of disease
3	Capable of only limited self-care; confined to bed or chair more than 50% of waking hours	70	Cares for self; unable to carry on normal activity or do active work
4	Completely disabled; cannot carry out any self-care; totally confined to bed or chair	60	Requires occasional assistance but able to care for most needs
5	Dead	50	Requires considerable assistance and frequent medical care
		40	Disabled; requires special care and assistance
		30	Severely disabled; hospitalization indicated; death not imminent
		20	Very sick; hospitalization necessary; active supportive treatment necessary
		10	Moribund; fatal processes; progressing rapidly
		0	Dead

*Oken MM, Creech RH, Tormey DC, et al: Toxicity and response criteria of the Eastern Cooperative Oncology Group. Am J Clin Oncol 1982;5:649-655.
†Schag CC, Heinrich RL, Ganz PA: Karnofsky performance status revisited: Reliability, validity, and guidelines. J Clin Oncol 1984;2:187-193.

fied with the VAS. Preliminary evidence has suggested that the BPI is cross-culturally valid and is useful, particularly when patients are not fit to complete a more thorough or comprehensive questionnaire.

The Memorial Pain Assessment Card is a simple, efficient, and valid instrument that provides rapid clinical evaluation of the major aspects of pain experienced by cancer patients.[23] It is easy to understand and use and can be completed by experienced patients in 20 seconds. It consists of a two-sided 8.5- × 11-inch card that is folded into four equal parts of separate measures—scale, intended for the measurements of pain intensity, pain relief, mood, and a set of descriptive adjectives.

The Edmonton Staging System is performed by health care providers. It was developed to predict the likelihood of achieving effective relief of pain in cancer patients[24,25] The system's originators have provided validation that treatment outcome can be accurately predicted according to five clinical features, neuropathic pain, movement-related pain, recent history of tolerance to opioids, psychological distress, and a history of alcoholism or drug abuse) Staging requires only 5 to 10 minutes and no special skills are needed to complete it. Its value lies in prospective identification of potentially problematic patients, further legitimizing clinical research on symptom control by introducing better standardization and improving the ability to assess critically the results of various therapeutic interventions in large populations of patients.

Often, pain is assessed on an 11-point numerical rating scale from 0 (no pain) to 10 (worst pain imaginable) using the Numerical Pain Rating Scale (NRS) or VAS. The VAS is a 10-cm line without markings from no pain to worst pain; the patient marks his or her pain score and the measurement in centimeters defines the level of pain.

Pain evaluation should be integrated with a detailed oncologic, medical, and psychosocial assessment. The initial evaluation should include an evaluation of the patient's feelings and attitudes about the pain and disease, family concerns, and premorbid psychological history. A comprehensive but objective approach to assessment instills confidence in the patient and family that will be valuable throughout treatment.

Pediatric cancer pain assessment includes use of the Beyer Oucher, Eland Color Scale-Body Outline, Hester Poker Chip Tool, and McGrath Faces Scale.[26-29]

EVALUATION OF THE PATIENT WITH CANCER PAIN

A comprehensive evaluation of the patient with cancer pain should include all the components detailed in this section. The reason for the visit is determined to ensure appropriate triage (e.g., a patient with severe pain caused by a bowel obstruction may need to be sent to the emergency center for urgent treatment).

History

The oncologic history is obtained to gain knowledge of the context of the pain problem. The oncologic history includes diagnosis and stage of disease, history of implemented therapies, including a list of the chemotherapeutic agents used, types of surgery, site of radiotherapy, outcome (including side effects), and the patient's understanding of the disease process and prognosis.

The pain history should include a description of any premorbid chronic pain. For each new pain site, the following information should be obtained: onset and evolution, site and radiation areas, pattern (constant, intermittent, or unpredictable), intensity (best, worst, average, current; rating on a 0 to 10 scale), quality, exacerbating and relieving factors, pain interference with usual activities, neurologic and motor abnormalities (including bowel and bladder continence), vasomotor changes, current and past analgesics (use, efficacy, side effects). Prior analgesic use, efficacy, and side effects should be catalogued. Prior treatments for pain should be noted (e.g., radiotherapy, nerve blocks, physiotherapy).

Review of the patient's medical record and radiologic studies should be thorough. Many treatments for cancer may cause pain themselves (e.g., chemotherapy, radiotherapy-induced neuropathy, postoperative pain syndrome, post-thoracotomy pain syndrome, postmastectomy pain syndrome), and many specific cancers may cause well-established pain patterns because of known likely sites of metastasis: (1) breast cancer to long bones, spine, chest wall, brachial plexus, and spinal cord; (2) colon cancer to pelvis, hips, lumbar plexus, sacral plexus, and spinal cord; and (3) prostate cancer to long bones, pelvis, hips, lung, and spinal cord.

Psychosocial history should include marital and residential status, employment history and status, educational background, functional status, activities of daily living, recreational activities, support systems, health and capabilities of spouse or significant other, and past history of (or current) drug or alcohol abuse.

Medical history (independent of oncologic history) should include coexisting systemic disease, exercise intolerance, allergies to medications, current medications, prior illness and surgery, and a thorough review of systems, including the following:

- General (including anorexia, weight loss, cachexia, fatigue, weakness, insomnia)
- Neurologic (including sedation, confusion, hallucination, headache, motor weakness, altered sensation, incontinence)
- Respiratory (including dyspnea, cough, pneumonia)
- Gastrointestinal (including dysphagia, nausea, vomiting, dehydration, constipation, diarrhea)
- Psychological (including irritability, anxiety, depression, dementia)
- Genitourinary (including urgency, hesitancy, hematuria)

Physical Examination

The physical examination must be thorough, although at times it is appropriate to perform a focused problem examination. In patients with spinal pain and known or suspected metastatic disease, a complete neurologic examination is mandatory. Gonzales and colleagues have found new evidence of metastatic disease in 64% of patients; this resulted in antitumor therapy for 18% of patients evaluated by their pain service.[30] Box 20–1 lists considerations that should be included in a thorough physical examination.

BOX 20–1. PHYSICAL EXAMINATION FOR CANCER PAIN

Arrange a meeting of the entire care team, if applicable.

Determine the need for further studies.

Formulate a clinical impression (diagnosis). Multiple diagnoses usually apply and it is best to use the most specific known diagnosis (e.g., somatic pain from a vertebral metastasis with severe pain in a patient with metastatic non–small cell carcinoma of the lung, neuropathic pain from a paravertebral mass invading the nerve root as it exits the vertebral foramen, nausea and vomiting with severe weight loss and fatigue, and constipation).

Formulate recommendations (plan) and alternatives for each problem. Related to the list of problems above, these could include the following:

- Performing MRI of the spine, with addition of a controlled-release opioid daily and transmucosal fentanyl citrate for breakthrough pain
- Implementation of therapy with a combination of a tricyclic antidepressant and anticonvulsant, with titration instructions
- Administration of an antiemetic prior to meals, as needed for nausea
- Administration of a bowel stimulant and bulk-forming compound twice daily for constipation
- Evaluation in 2 weeks to determine need for short course of steroid therapy

Call oncologist and/or primary care provider, if applicable. Have a discussion with the referring physician, primary care provider, and/or oncologist to establish short-term and long-term plans.

Conduct an exit interview:

- Explain the probable cause of symptoms in terms the patient can understand.
- Discuss prognosis for symptom relief, management options, and specific recommendations. In addition to writing prescriptions, oral and written instructions must be provided.
- Provide educational material regarding medications, pain management strategies, and procedures. Discuss potential side effects and their management.

Arrange for follow-up, with clinic contact information.

Dictate summary to referring and consulting physicians.

CLASSIFICATION OF CANCER PAIN

Cancer pain may be classified according to time of onset, intensity, pathophysiology, and other temporal aspects.

Classification According to Time of Onset

Acute Pain

This is frequently associated with sympathetic hyperactivity and heightened distress.[31] It is often temporally associated with the onset or recrudescence of primary or metastatic disease, and its presence should motivate the clinician to seek its cause and adjust the pharmacologic therapeutic scheme aggressively.

Subacute Pain

Some patients experience pain for 4 to 6 weeks after a major surgical procedure. This type of pain is largely undertreated and deserves special attention, because it may affect the patient's ability to perform activities of daily living after being discharged from the hospital.

Chronic Pain

Treating pain of a chronic nature mandates a combination of palliation, adjustment, and acceptance. With time, a biologic and behavioral adjustment to symptoms occurs, and hopefully associated symptoms are blunted. Chronic pain with superimposed episodes of acute pain (breakthrough pain) is probably the most common pattern observed in patients with ongoing cancer pain.

Classification According to Intensity

The consistent use of measurements of pain intensity aids in following a patient's progress and may serve as a basis for interpatient comparisons. High pain scores may alert the clinician to the need for more aggressive treatment, hospitalization for rapid symptom control via IV patient-controlled analgesia, antineuropathics with a rapid titration protocol, or a combination of these.

Classification According to Pathophysiology

A mechanistic approach is useful when formulating the initial treatment plan, as suggested in the example above.

Somatic pain is described as a constant, well-localized pain, often characterized as aching, throbbing, sharp or gnawing. It tends to be responsive to opioids and nonsteroidal anti-inflammatory drugs (NSAIDs) and cyclooxygenase-2 (COX-2) inhibitors and amenable to relief by interruption of proximal pathways by neural blockade when indicated.

Visceral pain originates from injury to organs. This pain is transmitted via fibers that travel along the sympathetic nervous system.[32] Visceral pain is characteristically vague in distribution and quality and is often described as a deep, dull, aching, dragging, squeezing, or pressure-like sensation. When acute, it may be paroxysmal and colicky and can be associated with nausea, vomiting, diaphoresis, and alterations in blood pressure and heart rate. Mechanisms of visceral pain include abnormal distention or contraction of the smooth muscle walls (hollow viscera), rapid capsular stretch (solid viscera), ischemia of visceral muscle, serosal or mucosal irritation by algesic substances and other chemical stimuli, distention and traction or torsion on mesenteric attachments and vasculature, and necrosis.[33] The viscera are, however, insensitive to simple manipulation, cutting, and burning.[32] Visceral involvement often produces referred pain (e.g., shoulder pain of hepatic origin).[34,35]

Neuropathic pain is defined as pain caused by injury or irritation to some element(s) of the nervous system. Examples of neuropathic pain syndromes include tumor growth around nerve structures, postsurgical pain syndromes such as post-thoracotomy, postmastectomy, post–radical neck dissection, and posthepatectomy pain, or pain induced by chemotherapeutic agents affecting peripheral nerve structures. Chemotherapeutic agents associated with this problem include vinca alkaloids (vincristine, vinblastine), cisplatinum, paclitaxel (Taxol), docetaxel (Taxotere), vinorelbine (Navelbine), and bortezomib (Velcade). Neuropathic pain is often resistant to standard analgesic therapies and often requires an approach using combinations of opioids, tricyclic antidepressants, anticonvulsants, oral or topical local anesthetics, corticosteroids, N-methyl-D-aspartate (NMDA) blockers, and others.

Temporal Aspects of Pain

Constant pain is most amenable to drug therapy administered around the clock, contingent on time rather than symptoms. It is best managed by long-acting analgesics or, in selected cases, infusion of analgesics.

Breakthrough pain related to a specific activity, such as eating, defecation, socializing, or walking, is referred to as *incident pain*. It is best managed by supplementing the preventive around-the-clock regimen with analgesics having a rapid onset of action and short duration. Once a pattern of incident pain is established, escape or rescue doses of analgesics can be administered in anticipation of the pain-provoking activity. Breakthrough pain that occurs consistently prior to the next scheduled dose of around-the-clock opioids is called end of dose failure (the plasma concentration falls below the minimum effective analgesic concentration [MEAC]) and is ideally managed by reducing the intervals between doses. In contrast, increasing the doses of the long-acting opioids, under these circumstances, may increase the incidence of side effects. Under a strict definition, breakthrough pain is the pain that may occur at any time during the day, increases to a high intensity very rapidly, and has a duration of 30 to 45 minutes. Consequently, it is important to recognize the differences among these three types of breakthrough pain to implement adequate therapy.

Intermittent pain is very unpredictable and can be best managed by administration of as-needed potent analgesics of rapid onset and short duration.

SPECIFIC CANCER PAIN SYNDROMES

Metastases

Bone tumor infiltration or bone metastases are cited as the most common cause of cancer pain,[36] and is most often seen in stage IV carcinoma of the prostate, breast, thyroid, lung, or kidney.[36,37] The pain is usually constant, dull, achy or deep, and often intense with movement or weight-bearing. Approximately 25% of patients with bone metastasis experience pain. Pressure and chemical irritation of nerve endings in the periosteum may cause pain.[38,39] It is noteworthy that more than 50% decalcification must occur before osseous lesions are visible on plain radiographs.[40] Thus, a bone scan (isotope scanning, scintigraphy) is preferred for detecting most bone metastases.[36] Nonetheless, in primary bone tumors, thyroid cancer, and multiple myeloma, plain films are considered to be more sensitive.[41] Neoplastic changes must be differentiated from changes related to infection, trauma, or degeneration, because treatment differs, even in the patient with cancer.

Prostaglandin E_2 (PGE_2) and other cytokines are elaborated by osseous metastasis. These cytokines are believed to contribute to pain by sensitization of peripheral nociceptors. NSAIDs and steroids are postulated to reduce pain from bony metastasis via inhibition of the COX pathway of arachidonic acid breakdown, thus decreasing the formation of PGE_2. As deposits enlarge, stretching of the periosteum, pathologic fracture, and perineural invasion contribute to pain, and requirements for analgesics increase. Palliative radiation is successfully used to relieve pain emanating from bony metastasis. However, pain relief may not be seen in all cases. Thus, other forms of therapy may need to be implemented.

Vertebral body metastases are associated with carcinoma of the lung, breast, and prostate. Localized paraspinal, radicular, or referred pain within the dermatomal distribution of the affected nerve structure is usually the first sign of metastasis to the spine. It often presents as severe local, dull, steady, aching pain, and is often exacerbated by movement and weight-bearing. In the physical evaluation, local midline tenderness may be present, along with corresponding neurologic changes associated with nerve compression or epidural-spinal cord compression. Invasion of the second cervical vertebra may result in referred pain to the occiput, and C7-T1 invasion may produce interscapular pain.[42]

Metastases involving the skull base usually present with headache and a spectrum of neurologic findings, especially when involving cranial nerves. Symptomatic metastasis to the skull is usually but not always a late finding.[43] Plain radiography, scintigraphy, and CT scanning are helpful for diagnosis of bony disease, whereas magnetic resonance imaging (MRI) and lumbar puncture are useful to evaluate soft tissues and detect leptomeningeal disease, respectively.[44]

Musculoskeletal pain in the form of myofascial pain is frequently seen in cancer patients.[45] Patients with bone metastases and those with post–radical neck dissection syndrome are frequently affected by this condition. Stress, anxiety, muscle overuse to compensate for the lack of bone support, or the absence or other muscles resected during the cancer surgery may play an important role in the development of this condition. Thus, treatment should be multidisciplinary and include pharmacologic therapy, trigger point injections, and physical rehabilitation with the use of orthotic devices as needed.

Leptomeningeal metastasis and meningeal carcinomatosis are frequently seen with primary malignancies of breast and lung, lymphoma, and leukemia; these are secondary to diffuse infiltration of the meninges. About 40% of patients have headache or back pain, presumably caused by traction on the pain-sensitive meninges, cranial, and spinal nerves, increased intracranial pressure, or both.[46,47] Headache is the most common presenting complaint, characteristically unrelenting, and may be associated with nausea, vomiting, nuchal rigidity, and mental status changes.[47] Neurologic abnormalities may include seizures, cranial nerve deficits, papilledema, hemiparesis, ataxia, and cauda equina syndrome. The diagnosis may be suggested by the T2 phase of the MRI and is usually confirmed via lumbar puncture and cerebrospinal (CSF) analysis that typically shows elevated protein and decreased glucose levels as well as malignant cells.[48] The natural history of patients with leptomeningeal metastasis is gradual decline and death over 4 to 6 weeks, although survival is often extended to 6 months or longer when treatment with radiation therapy, intrathecal chemotherapy, or both are instituted.[49] Steroids may be useful in the management of headache[44] as well as the neuropathic pain associated with spinal cord and nerve involvement.

Spinal Cord Compression and Plexopathies

Spinal cord compression is usually heralded by pain in the presence of neurologic changes. An urgent radiologic workup is mandatory in the face of neurologic deficits, particularly motor weakness, bandlike encircling pain, or incontinence. Prompt treatment in the form of radiotherapy or spinal stabilization and high-dose IV steroids may limit neurologic morbidity.[50]

Plexopathies are the result of tumor growth around the nerve plexi in the upper or lower extremity. Cervical plexopathy is most commonly caused by local invasion of head and neck cancers. Symptoms include aching preauricular, postauricular, or neck pain. Brachial plexopathy is most commonly caused by upper lobe lung cancer (Pancoast syndrome or superior sulcus syndrome), breast cancer, or lymphoma. Pain is an early symptom, usually preceding neurologic findings by up to 9 months.[51,52] The lower cord of the plexus (C8-T1) is affected most frequently, and pain is usually diffuse and aching, radiating down the arm, often to the elbow and medial (ulnar) aspect of the hand.[53,54] When the upper trunk is involved (C5-6), pain is usually in the shoulder girdle and upper arm, radiating to the thumb and index finger. Horner's syndrome, dysesthesias, progressive atrophy, and neurologic impairment (weakness and numbness) may occur. Brachial plexus invasion may be associated with contiguous spread to the epidural space.[50,55-57] Lumbosacral plexopathy may be caused by local soft tissue invasion or compression from tumors of the rectum, cervix, breast, sarcoma, and lymphoma; pain is usually the presenting symptom in 70% of patients.[58] The pain is usually described as aching or pressure-like and only rarely dysesthetic.[58] Depending on the level involved, pain is referred to the low back, abdomen, buttock, or lower extremity.[58,59] This medical problem must be differentiated from spinal cord invasion or cauda equina syndrome, in which urgent diagnosis and treatment are mandatory. Clinical experience has shown that brachial plexopathies respond better to medical therapy with opioids, tricyclic antidepressants, and anticonvulsants, whereas lumbosacral plexopathies may require early intervention with intrathecal opioid–bupivacaine–clonidine therapy.

Pain Associated with Cancer Treatment

Oral mucositis usually occurs within 1 to 2 weeks of the initiation of chemotherapy. This condition is most common with the use of methotrexate, doxorubicin, daunorubicin, bleomycin, etoposide, 5-fluorouracil, and dactinomycin.[60] Mucositis is often most severe when chemotherapy is combined with radiation treatments to the head and neck region. Treatment may require hospitalization for IV patient-controlled analgesia (PCA) opioid therapy. Ambulatory care may need transdermal opioids, local anesthetic, or doxepin swishes.

Painful polyneuropathy occurs most commonly with vincristine (motor and sensory involvement); vinblastine; paclitaxel; docetaxel, the platinum derivative of cisplatinum carboplatinum (predominantly sensory involvement); vinorelbine; and bortezomib.[61] Symptoms commonly include burning dysesthetic pain in the hands and feet. Most of these patients will respond to medical therapy with opioids, tricyclic antidepressants, and anticonvulsants. However, the small number of patients who do not achieve adequate pain control with this strategy will usually have a significant response to the use of spinal cord stimulation.

Postsurgical chronic pain syndromes are most common after mastectomy, thoracotomy, radical neck dissection, nephrectomy, and amputation.[62] The clinical characteristics usually include aching, shooting, or tingling pain in the distribution of peripheral nerves (e.g., intercostobrachial, intercostals, cervical plexus), with or without skin hypersensitivity. One study has suggested that the incidence of postmastectomy pain is higher after conservative surgery than modified radical mastectomy (33% versus 17%).[63] In this same study, 25% of patients experienced postoperative phantom breast pain. The exact incidence of postsurgical pain syndromes is unclear, but appears to be in the 25% to 50% range by some estimates.[62] Medical therapy with opioids, tricyclic antidepressants, and anticonvulsants is successful in the great majority of patients. Those who fail pharmacologic therapy will benefit from intrathecal therapy (post-thoracotomy, postmastectomy syndromes), spinal cord stimulation (post-thoracotomy, postmastectomy syndromes), or even peripheral subcutaneous nerve stimulation (post–radical neck dissection, post-thoracotomy syndromes).

Headache is present in 60% of patients with a primary or metastatic brain tumor, and 50% of these patients classified it as their primary complaint.[64] It is typically steady, deep, dull, and aching with moderate intensity and is rarely rhythmic or throbbing. It is usually intermittent and may be worse in the morning and with coughing or straining. Symptoms often improve with radiation therapy, NSAIDs, or corticosteroids.[65-67]

Cervicofacial pain syndromes are most common in patients with head and neck cancers. The head and neck are richly innervated by contributions from cranial nerves V, VII, IX, and X and upper cervical nerves, so pain varies in character. When cranial nerves are involved, symptoms represent those of trigeminal, glossopharyngeal, and/or intermittent neuralgia, with sudden, severe lancinating pain radiating to the face, throat, or ear, respectively. Pain may be accompanied by dysesthesias, trigger points, impaired swallowing, breathing, and phonation. Pharmacologic therapy with opioids, tricyclic antidepressants, and anticonvulsants is useful in the great majority of these patients. In those for whom pharmacologic therapy fails, radiofrequency lesioning of the sphenopalatine or gasserian ganglion may be useful.

Radiation therapy may be associated with acute and chronic pain syndromes. Acutely, mucositis and cutaneous burns may be seen. Chronically, post-radiation syndromes include osteoradionecrosis, myelopathy, plexopathy, soft tissue fibrosis, and the emergence of new secondary neurogenic tumors.

MANAGEMENT OF CANCER-RELATED PAIN

The goal of cancer pain treatment is to relieve pain by modifying its source, interrupting its transmission, or modulating its influence at brain or spinal cord sites. This can be achieved with monotherapy or combinations of the several types of available treatment modalities (Box 20–2).

Antineoplastic treatment
Pharmacologic management
- NSAIDs
- Opioids
- Adjuvant analgesics (antidepressants, anticonvulsants, oral local anesthetics, corticosteroids, N-methyl-D-aspartate antagonists, α_2-adrenergic antagonists, topical analgesics)

Interventional pain management
- Continuous parenteral infusion of opioids
- Neuraxial analgesia (epidural or intrathecal infusions)
- Vertebroplasty or kyphoplasty
- Nerve blocks (local anesthetic nerve blocks, neurolytic nerve blocks)
- Spinal cord stimulation, peripheral nerve stimulation, or peripheral subcutaneous nerve stimulation

Behavioral pain management techniques
Other interventions (aromatherapy, relaxation, herbal medications)
Home-based and hospice care

Antineoplastic Treatment

The most effective form of treatment of any cancer-related pain is treatment of the cancer itself, which in most cases will reduce or eliminate the pain. Once diagnosed, the pathologic process responsible for pain can often be altered with surgical resection, external beam radiation therapy (targeted fractionated or single-dose therapy, hemibody or whole-body irradiation),[68,69] radionuclides (e.g., strontium 89, samarium Sm 153 lexidronam), chemotherapy,[70] hormonal treatment,[71] and even whole-body or limb hyperthermia.[72] Most patients require some form of primary analgesia, even when undergoing antitumor therapy.

Pharmacologic Management

The control of pain involves three basic principles—modifying the source of the pain, altering the central perception of pain, and blocking the transmission of the pain to the central nervous system. In addition, any new pain in a patient with cancer is assumed to be disease progression or recurrence until proven otherwise.

Oral analgesics are the mainstay of therapy for patients with cancer pain. An estimated 70% to 95% of patients can be rendered relatively free of pain when straightforward guidelines-based principles are applied in a thorough and careful manner.[1,2,73]

The World Health Organization (WHO) has developed a three-step ladder approach to cancer pain management that relies exclusively on the administration of oral agents, and is usually effective.[18,73,74]

However, this approach lacks the mechanistic approach that may be more effective by decreasing the side effects from drugs that may not necessarily relieve some types of pain, such as NSAIDs or opioids as first-line agents for neuropathic pain syndromes. When more conservative therapies produce inadequate results, doses should be escalated or alternative therapies sought. The role of more invasive forms of analgesia, ranging from parenteral analgesics to neural blockade, or neuromodulation, should be considered judiciously.

Before initiation of therapy, assessing problems and setting realistic goals that are acceptable to the patient should be initiated, along with a treatment plan and contingencies. The noninvasive route should be maintained as long as possible for reasons that include simplicity, maintenance of independence and mobility, convenience, and cost. Treatment should be directed toward relief of pain and suffering, which includes consideration of all aspects of function (e.g., disturbance of sleep, appetite, mood, activity, posture, sexual activity), and attention should be paid not only to physical but also to emotional, psychological, and spiritual aspects of suffering.

For an in-depth discussion of the different agents that may be used for pharmacologic noninvasive therapy, see Chapters 31 to 35.

Interventional Techniques for Pain Management

When a comprehensive trial of pharmacologic therapy fails to provide adequate analgesia or leads to unacceptable side effects, consideration should be given to alternative modalities.

Continuous Subcutaneous Infusion of Opioids
This was frequently used in the past and proved to be effective.[75,76] However, the advent of IV PCA therapy and long-term IV lines such as the peripherally inserted central catheter (PICC) line have made it somehow obsolete in this population of patients.

Intravenous Infusion of Opioids with Patient-Controlled Analgesia Devices
The most frequent indication for this form of therapy is severe pain and the need to titrate opioids rapidly to effect in the hospital setting to achieve adequate pain control. Moreover, in the ambulatory setting, this modality is indicated for patients in whom the oral route is not available because of gastrointestinal (GI) obstruction, malabsorption, uncontrolled nausea and vomiting, dysphagia, or when the requirement for opioids is high because of tolerance. Some modifications in the implementation of this therapy can be used once the patient is no longer able to control the device; nurse- or family-controlled analgesia is an acceptable alternative under these circumstances. Consequently, patients will need to be treated in a controlled environment such as hospice or at home with the help and monitoring of family members, in which case visiting nurse services will be required.

Intraspinal Analgesia

Neuraxial analgesia is achieved by the epidural or intrathecal administration of an opioid alone (very rarely) or in combination with other agents such as bupivacaine, clonidine, or ziconotide. With the use of neuraxial analgesia, pain relief is obtained in a highly selective fashion without motor, sensory, and sympathetic effects, making these modalities highly adaptable to the home care environment.[77-81] At its inception, the principle of neuraxial opioid therapy was that introducing minute quantities of opioids in close proximity to their receptors (substantia gelatinosa of the spinal cord) achieves high local concentrations.[78,82] Thus, analgesia was potentially superior to that achieved when opioids were administered by other routes and, because the total amount of drug administered is reduced, side effects were minimized. Currently, the biggest advantage is the ability to use multiple agents to target neuropathic, somatic, and visceral components.

In general, patients with a survival expectancy longer than 3 months are candidates for intrathecal therapy with a permanent intraspinal catheter and an implanted subcutaneous pump. Conversely, those patients with survival expectancy less than 3 months will require epidural therapy with an implanted system (long-term epidural catheter [Du Pen] or epidural Port-A-Cath, which connects to an external pump with PCA capabilities). Either way, patients will need a trial with an epidural catheter placed at the site where nociception is being processed in the spinal cord.

We conduct the epidural trial on an outpatient basis. If successful, we then implant the permanent device. Catheter position is dermatome-specific under fluoroscopic guidance. Total volume should not exceed 600 mL, with basal infusion of 2 mL/hr, no bolus during the first 72 hours, and then 2 mL every 10 minutes.

The drugs, concentrations, and doses we use are the following[83]: (1) opioids—morphine, 0.1 to 0.2 mg/mL (1.0 to 20 mg/day) or hydromorphone, 0.03 to 0.12 mg/mL (0.5 to 25 mg/day); (2) sufentanil, 10 to 100 μg/day; (3) bupivacaine, 1 to 2 mg/mL (6 to 20 mg/day); and (4) clonidine, 3 to 5 μg/mL (250 to 2000 μg/day). Epidural opioid doses are determined as follows: (1) if the patient is receiving more than 300 μg/hr of fentanyl, 1200 mg/day of morphine sulfate (MS), 600 mg/day of oxycodone, or 160 mg/day of methadone—hydromorphone, 0.12 mg/mL; (2) if the patient is receiving 100 to 300 μg/hr of fentanyl or equivalent dose—hydromorphone, 0.06 mg/mL; and (3) if the patient is receiving less than 100 μg/hr of fentanyl or equivalent dose—hydromorphone, 0.03 mg/mL.

The trial is conducted for 7 days on an outpatient basis. The goal is to determine patient requirements. If the patient has had a successful trial, defined as a reduction in pain more than 80%, then we proceed to implant an intrathecal system if indicated by the survival expectancy. The following clinical pearls increase success rates in our practice:

1. Place the tip of the intrathecal catheter in the dermatome corresponding to the area of nociception.
2. For severe somatic pain, a combination of local anesthetics and an opioid is needed.
3. For neuropathic pain, place the tip of the catheter below L3-4 for initial therapy with opioid plus clonidine, or place the tip of the catheter above L1-2 for initial therapy with opioid plus bupivacaine.

Compounding by a trained pharmacist is needed. The goal is to concentrate these drugs to twice the daily dose, so that the pump may be programmed to deliver 0.5 mL/hr. This way the patient needs a pump refill monthly and does not have to make frequent office visits. The steps that we use to implement the therapy are as follows: (1) opioid + bupivacaine (MS, 3 to 25 mg/day or hydromorphone, 0.5 to 15 mg/day; 25 mg of MS/day = 4 mg of hydromorphone/day; bupivacaine, 6 to 20 mg/day) or opioid + clonidine (clonidine, 250 to 2000 μg/day); (2) opioid + bupivacaine + clonidine; or (3) ziconotide.

If the patient's insurance does not pay for hydromorphone, bupivacaine, or clonidine, the use of morphine plus ziconotide may be an alternative. However, this approach has its limitations in that ziconotide cannot be administered in the epidural space, so the trial can only be conducted with the implanted system in place. Also, patients may not tolerate a titration protocol lasting 4 to 6 weeks. To implement ziconotide therapy, rinse the pump with 2 mL of the 25-μg/mL solution three times. Initiate therapy at a dose of 2.4 μg/day (0.1 μg/hr) and titrate to patient response. Titration increments should not be more than 2.4 μg/day and ideally every week, because slower titration is better tolerated. The maximum recommended dose is 19.2 μg/day (0.8 μg/hr). Therapeutic effects are not usually seen until a dose of 10 μg/day is reached.

If triple therapy with an opioid, bupivacaine, and clonidine at optimal doses is not working, troubleshoot for pump- or catheter-related problems. In pump analysis, desired and actual volume should be within 10%; otherwise, pump or system failure (e.g., obstruction) should be suspected. For a suspected catheter problem, a myelogram should be performed to determine whether there is obstruction and the position of the catheter tip. When performing a myelogram through the diagnostic port of the pump, remember that this only accommodates a 25-gauge Huber needle. Also, consider the dead space of the catheter when injecting the contrast medium, and the need for a bolus dose after the study is completed.

A multicenter prospective randomized clinical trial[84] has compared intrathecal therapy with continued medical management and revealed a slight, albeit not statistically significant, trend toward better analgesia in the intrathecal group, but also an improved side effect profile and increased survival in the intrathecal group. Another study has reported significant improvement in pain scores and reduced oral opioid intake using epidural and intrathecal analgesia.[85]

The cost of implementing intrathecal therapy is initially high because of equipment acquisition cost; however, the cost of implementing long-term epidural therapy is low. Two studies have evaluated the cost of implementing therapy with these two modalities, showing a break-even point at approximately 3 months.[86,87] Thus, epidural therapy becomes very expensive after 3 months, and is one reason to limit its use in patients with survival expectation less than 3 months.

A consensus panel has published current practice data on intrathecal medication management, a survey of 413 physicians managing 13,342 patients.[88] It showed a variety of medications used in the intrathecal pump, including morphine (48%), morphine-bupivacaine (12%), hydromorphone (8%), morphine-clonidine (8%), hydromorphone-clonidine (8%), morphine-clonidine-bupivacaine (5%), morphine-baclofen (3%), and others (less than 3%). Other drugs included fentanyl, sufentanil, ziconotide, meperidine, methadone, ropivacaine, tetracaine, ketamine, midazolam, neostigmine, droperidol, and naloxone.

Nerve Blocks

Local anesthetic injections can be used for diagnostic or therapeutic purposes, or both.[89-98] Diagnostic blocks help characterize the underlying mechanism of pain (e.g., nociceptive, neuropathic, sympathetically mediated) and discern the anatomic pathways involved in pain transmission. Their main indication is as a preliminary intervention conducted prior to a therapeutic nerve block or other definitive therapy. This helps the clinician determine the potential for subsequent neurolysis, if indicated. Although results often have good predictive value, they are not entirely reliable.

Therapeutic injections of local anesthetics, with or without corticosteroid, into trigger points may provide lasting relief of myofascial pain.[93] They are unlikely to provide long-lasting relief for neuropathic pain of neoplastic origin. However, they do produce significant analgesia in patients who may not tolerate rapid titration of antineuropathic medications.

Local anesthetic injections administered in sympathetic ganglia may contribute to lasting pain relief in patients with complex regional pain syndrome (CRPS) type II, a condition frequently seen in cancer patients.[94-96] This condition may arise as a result of tumor invasion of nervous system structures (e.g., brachial or lumbosacral plexopathy), postsurgical pain syndromes, or chemotherapy-induced peripheral neuropathy. The use of local anesthetic blockade of the stellate ganglion or lumbar sympathetic chain has been used with some success to relieve pain in these patients temporarily.

Neurolytic Procedures

Neurolytic blocks have played an important role in the management of intractable cancer pain. This modality should be offered when pain persists despite the implementation of aggressive comprehensive medical management or when drug therapy produces unwanted and uncontrollable side effects. Patient selection is important. Some important variables to consider include the following: (1) the severity of the pain; (2) pain that is expected to persist despite chemotherapy or radiation therapy; (3) pain that cannot be modified by less invasive or risky means; (4) a clinical picture indicating that pain is somatic or visceral in origin; and (5) patients with a short life expectancy.

Alcohol and phenol are the two agents commonly used to produce chemical neurolysis. Ethyl alcohol is a pungent colorless solution that can be readily injected through a small-bore needle and that is hypobaric with respect to CSF. For peripheral and subarachnoid blocks, alcohol is generally used undiluted (referred to as 100% alcohol, dehydrated alcohol, or absolute alcohol), whereas a 50% solution is used for celiac plexus block. It should not be exposed to the air for a long period because absorbed moisture dilutes it. Alcohol injection is typically followed by intense burning pain and occasionally erythema along the targeted nerve distribution.

Phenol is fairly unstable at room temperature. Its shelf half-life is about 1 year when refrigerated and kept away from light. Phenol can be used in a 3% to 15% concentration with saline, water, and glycerol or radiologic contrast. It is relatively insoluble in water and, as a result, concentrations in excess of 6.7% will result in a suspension at room temperature without adding glycerin to increase its solubility in water. Phenol with glycerin is hyperbaric in CSF but is so dense that even when warmed, it is difficult to inject through needles smaller than 20 gauge. Phenol has a biphasic action—its initial local anesthetic action produces subjective warmth and numbness that usually gives way to chronic denervation over 24 hours. Hypoalgesia after phenol is not as dense as after alcohol, and the quality and extent of analgesia may fade slightly within the first 24 hours of administration, particularly when used for epidural neurolysis.

The use of subarachnoid (intrathecal) injections of alcohol or phenol has significantly decreased in the United States for the management of intractable cancer pain since polypharmacy intrathecal analgesia was implemented. Because alcohol and phenol destroy nervous tissue indiscriminately, careful attention to the selection of the injection site, volume and concentration of injectate, and selection and positioning of the patient are essential to avoid neurologic complications,[99,100] a risk that is responsible for the decrease in its use. Most agree that neither alcohol nor phenol offers a clear advantage, except in regard to variations in baric properties that may facilitate positioning of the patient.[101,102] With the exception of perineal pain treatment, alcohol is usually preferred for intrathecal neurolysis, because most patients are unable to lie on their painful side, as is required for intrathecal phenol neurolysis. In an analysis of 13 published series documenting intrathecal rhizolysis treatment of more than 2500 patients,

Swerdlow has reported that 58% of patients obtain "good" relief, "fair" relief in an additional 21%, and "little or no relief" in 20%.[101] Average duration of relief was estimated at 3 to 6 months, with a wide range of distribution. Reports of analgesia persisting 1 to 2 years are fairly common.[103] In representative series using alcohol ($n = 252$) and phenol ($n = 151$), a total of 407 and 313 blocks were performed, respectively.[104,105] In these two series, neither motor weakness nor fecal incontinence occurred and, of eight patients with transient urinary dysfunction, incontinence persisted only in one.

Subarachnoid neurolysis can be performed at any level up to the midcervical region, above which the risk of drug spread to medullary centers and the potential for cardiorespiratory collapse increase.[106] Hyperbaric phenol saddle block is relatively simple and is particularly suitable for many patients with colostomy and urinary diversion.

Until recently, epidural neurolysis was performed infrequently. Results were inferior to those obtained with subarachnoid blockade, presumably because the dura acts as a barrier to diffusion, resulting in limited contact between the drug and targeted nerves.[103,107]

Peripheral and Cranial Nerve Blocks

Peripheral nerve blockade has a limited role in the management of cancer pain.[98] Blockade of the ganglion of Gasser, within the foramen ovale at the base of skull or its branches, may be beneficial for facial pain.[108] However, the indications in tumor-related pain are truly minimal, because there is usually a neuropathic pain component. Thus, the risk of deafferentation pain is significantly increased with chemical neurolysis. Again, the use of intraspinal therapy by means of an implanted cervical epidural catheter or intraventricular opioid therapy has become a better option for these patients.[109,110]

Vertebroplasty

Many cancer patients with metastatic vertebral compression fractures (VCFs) or osteoporotic VCFs present with movement-related back pain. Percutaneous vertebroplasty (PV) is a minimally invasive procedure involving the injection of bone cement (usually polymethylmethacrylate [PMMA]) into the fractured vertebral body to alleviate the pain and hopefully enhance structural stability. This procedure is performed by placing needles under biplanar fluoroscopic guidance with a uni- or bipedicular approach. PMMA mixed with sterile barium is injected in a carefully controlled manner to avoid unintended cement spread into the spinal canal or into the veins within the affected vertebra. Injection is stopped as soon as cement starts approaching the posterior third of the vertebral body. PV has been shown to be efficacious in treating VCF-related pain in cancer patients.[111]

Spinal Cord Stimulation

This technique has been successfully used for refractory neuropathic chronic pain—chronic nononco-

logic pain. There is a lack of studies evaluating its use in cancer pain states. However, at Roswell Park Cancer Institute, we have successfully used it in patients with CRPS type II, such as postsurgical pain syndromes, chemotherapy-induced peripheral neuropathy, and postradiation nerve injury. Patient selection is important in the cancer population, because MRI at this point is contraindicated after the device is placed; medical oncologists rely on this radiologic study to follow the progress of disease in these patients.

Neurosurgical Palliative Techniques

Neurosurgical palliative techniques have fallen out of favor as more medications and reversible, titratable, lower risk techniques have largely replaced such procedures. Pituitary ablation entails destruction of the gland by injection of a small quantity of alcohol through a needle positioned transnasally under light general anesthesia. This technique is effective in relieving pain originating from disseminated bony metastases, particularly secondary to hormone-dependent tumors such as breast and prostate cancers.[112] Commissural myelotomy has been reported to be efficacious in cancer pain refractory to more conservative therapy.[113] Percutaneous cordotomy produces a thermal lesion in the substance of the spinal cord and reliably relieves unilateral truncal and lower limb pain.[114] As with pituitary ablation, it necessitates a high degree of skill and expertise, but pain relief is often profound and the rigors of a major neurosurgical procedure are avoided.

Behavioral Pain Management Techniques

Several behavioral pain management techniques have been used in patients with cancer, including hypnosis, relaxation, biofeedback, sensory alteration, guided imagery, and cognitive strategies.[115] Relaxation and imagery training significantly reduce Visual Analogue Scale scores in patients who have mucositis after bone marrow transplantation.[116] This training is probably most effective for patients who have no significant psychological or psychiatric problems[117] and for insightful psychology-minded patients.

Home-based and Hospice-based Pain Management

For many years, hospice has been regarded as a place where terminally ill patients "go to die," but in its purest form, hospice care represents a philosophy of care that is "a blend of clinical pharmacology and applied compassionate psychological care."[118,119] In the United States, hospice care has been developed primarily as a home-based service, with a minority of institutions offering short inpatient stays to stabilize refractory symptoms and provide respite for overwhelmed families.

The principles of home-based pain management are in most respects similar to those that apply to ambulatory and inpatient pain management. Differences generally relate to the recognition that further curative therapy is futile rather than that care is being provided at home. No compromise in quality of care based on where it is delivered is justified.

Hospice care is comfort-oriented, focusing specifically on alleviating symptoms rather than necessarily treating the underlying cause(s). Factors that influence the selection of home treatment are advanced incurable disease, realization and acceptance of the appropriateness of palliative care (care directed at preserving comfort and the quality of life rather than curing the tumor and extending life), and a desire to die in familiar surroundings. Many difficulties associated with providing intensive palliative care at home can be reconciled by education and orientation of the family. This can be accomplished by coordination with health care institutions and home care nursing, laboratory, and pharmacy services.

CONCLUSION

The occurrence of acute and chronic pain is highly prevalent in cancer patients. Inadequate assessment and treatment of pain and other distressing symptoms may interfere with antitumor therapy and markedly detract from the quality of life. Although a strong focus on pain control is important and independent of disease stage, it is a special priority in patients with advanced disease who are no longer candidates for potentially curative therapy.

Although rarely eliminated, pain can be controlled in the vast majority of patients with the implementation of aggressive and comprehensive medical management. In the small but significant proportion of patients whose pain is not readily controlled with noninvasive analgesics, various alternative invasive and noninvasive measures, when selected carefully, are also associated with a high degree of success. To this end, it is reassuring to conclude that we have the appropriate tools for adequate management of cancer-related pain in almost all patients.

References

1. American Pain Society: Principles of Analgesic Use in the Treatment of Acute Pain and Chronic Cancer Pain, 3rd ed. Skokie, Ill, American Pain Society, 1992.
2. Jacox A, Carr DB, Payne R, et al: Management of Cancer Pain: Clinical Practice Guideline 9. (ACHPR Publication No. 94-0592). Rockville, Md, Agency for Health Care Policy and Research, 1994.
3. Zech DFG, Grong S, Lynch J, et al: Validation of the World Health Organization guidelines for cancer pain relief: A 10-year prospective study. Pain 1996;63:65-76.
4. Ferrell BR, Wisdon C, Wenzl C: Quality of life as an outcome variable in management of cancer pain. Cancer 1989;63:2321-2327.
5. Liebeskind JC: Pain can kill. Pain 1991;44:3-4.
6. Lillemoe KD, Cameron JL, Kaufman HS, et al: Chemical splanchnicectomy in patients with unresectable pancreatic cancer. Ann Surg 1993;217:447-457.
7. Bonica JJ, Ekstrom JL: Systemic opioids for the management of cancer pain: An updated review. Adv Pain Res Ther 1990;14:425-446.
8. Silverberg E, Boring CC, Squires TS: Cancer statistics, 1990. CA Cancer J Clin 1990;40:9-26.
9. American Cancer Society: Cancer Facts and Figures: 1994. Atlanta, American Cancer Society, 1994.
10. American Cancer Society: Cancer Facts and Figures: 1989. Atlanta, American Cancer Society, 1989.
11. Cleeland CS, Gonin R, Hatfield AK, et al: Pain and its treatment in outpatients with metastatic cancer. N Engl J Med 1994;330:592-596.
12. Higginson IJ: Innovation in assessment: Epidemiology and assessment of pain in advanced cancer. In Janson TS, Turner JA, Wiesenfeld-Hallin Z (eds): Proceedings of the 8th World Congress of Pain; Progress in Pain Research and Therapy. Seattle, IASP Press, 1997, pp 707-716.
13. Walsh TD: Oral morphine in chronic cancer pain. Pain 1984;18:1-11.
14. Bruera E: Malnutrition and asthenia in advanced cancer. Cancer Bull 1991;43:387.
15. Bonica JJ: Management of cancer pain. Recent Results Cancer Res 1984;89:13-27.
16. Daut RL, Cleeland CS: The prevalence and severity of pain in cancer. Cancer 1982;50;1913-1918.
17. Mumford JW, Mumford SP: The care of cancer patients in a rural South Indian hospital. Palliat Med 1988;2:157-158.
18. World Health Organization: Cancer Pain Relief. Geneva, World Health Organization, 1986.
19. Portenoy RK: Cancer pain: Epidemiology and syndromes. Cancer 1989;63:2298-2307.
20. Brescia FJ, Adler D, Gray G, Ryan MA: A profile of hospitalized advanced cancer patients. J Pain Symptom Manage 1990;5:221-227.
21. Swerdlow M, Stjernsward J: Cancer pain relief: An urgent problem. World Health Forum 1982;3:325-330.
22. Daut RL, Cleeland CS, Flannery RC: Development of the Wisconsin Brief Pain Questionnaire to access pain in cancer and other diseases. Pain 1983;17:197-210.
23. Fishman B, Pasternak S, Wallenstein S, et al: The Memorial Pain Assessment Card: A valid instrument for the evaluation of cancer pain. Cancer 1987;60:1151-1158.
24. Bruera E, MacMillan K, Hanson J, et al: The Edmonton Staging System for cancer pain: Preliminary report. Pain 1989;37:203-209.
25. Bruera E, Schoeller T, Wenk R, et al: A prospective multicenter assessment of the Edmonton Staging System for cancer pain. J Pain Symptom Manage 1995;10:348-355.
26. Beyer J, Aradine C: Content validity of an instrument to measure young children's perceptions of the intensity of their pain. J Pediatr Nurs 1986;1:386-395.
27. Eland J: Eland color scale. In McCaffery M, Beebe A (eds): Pain: Clinical Manual for Nursing Practice. St. Louis, Mosby, 1989, pp 27-35.
28. Hester N, Foster R, Kristensen K: Measurement of pain in children: Generalizability and validity of the pain ladder and the poker chip tool. In Tyler D, Krane E (eds): Advances in Pain Research and Therapy: Pediatric Pain, vol 1. New York, Raven Press, 1990, pp 79-87.
29. McGrath PA: Pain in Children: Nature, Assessment and Treatment. New York, Guilford Press, 1990.
30. Gonzales GR, Elliott KJ, Portenoy RK, et al: The impact of a comprehensive evaluation in the management of cancer pain. Pain. 1991;47:141-144.
31. Sternbach RA: Pain: A Psychophysiologic Analysis. New York, Academic Press, 1968.
32. Newman PP: Visceral Afferent Functions of the Nervous System. London, Arnold, 1974.
33. Procacci P, Maresca M, Cersosimo RM: Visceral pain: Pathophysiology and clinical aspects. Adv Exp Med Biol 1991;298:175-181.
34. Kellgren JH: Somatic simulating visceral pain. Clin Sci 1939;4:303.
35. Cervero F: Visceral pain. In Dubner R, Gebhart GF, Bond MR (eds): Proceedings of the Sixth World Congress on Pain. Amsterdam, Elsevier, 1988, pp 216-238.
36. Galasko CSB: Skeletal metastases. London, Butterworths, 1986, pp 99-108.
37. Enneking WF, Conrad EU III: Common bone tumors. Clin Symp 1989;41:1-32.

38. Front D, Schneck SO, Frankel A, et al: Bone metastasis and bone pain in breast cancer: Are they closely associated? JAMA 1979;242:1747-1748.

39. Bennett A: The role of biochemical mediators in peripheral nociception and bone pain. Cancer Surv 1998;7:55-67.

40. Foley KM: Pain syndromes in patients with cancer. Adv Pain Res Ther 1979;2:59-63.

41. Merriman A: Uganda: Status of cancer pain and palliative care. J Pain Sympt Manage 1996;12:141-143.

42. Payne R: Pharmacologic management of bone pain in the cancer patient. Clin J Pain 1989;5(5 Suppl 2):S43-S49.

43. Greenberg HS, Deck MDF, Vikram B, et al: Metastases to the base of the skull: Clinical findings in 43 patients. Neurology 1981;31:530-537.

44. Elliot K, Foley KM: Neurologic pain syndromes in patients with cancer. Crit Care Clin 1990;6:393-420.

45. Abrams SE: The role of non-neurolytic blocks in the management of cancer pain. In Abrams SE (ed): Cancer Pain. Boston, Kluwer, 1989, pp 67-78.

46. Olson ME, Chernik NL, Posner JB. Infiltration of the leptomeninges by systemic cancer: A clinical and pathologic study. Arch Neurol 1930;2:122-125.

47. Wasserstrom WR, Glass JP, Posner JB: Diagnosis and treatment of leptomeningeal metastases from solid tumor: Experience with 90 patients. Cancer 1982;49:759-772.

48. Schild SC, Wasserstrom WR, Fleischer M, et al: Cerebrospinal fluid biochemical markers of central nervous metastases. Ann Neurol 1980;8:597-604.

49. Glass JP, Foley KM: Carcinomatous meningitis. In Harris JR, Hellman S, Henderson IC, et al (eds): Breast Diseases. Philadelphia, JB Lippincott, 1987, pp 497-502.

50. Gokaslan ZL: Spine surgery for cancer. Curr Opin Oncol 1996;8:178-181.

51. Foley KM: Brachial plexopathy in patients with breast cancer. In Harris JR, Hellman S, Henderson IC, et al (eds) Breast Diseases. Philadelphia, JB Lippincott, 1987, pp 202-215.

52. Scott JF: Carcinoma invading nerve. In Wall PD, Melzack R (eds): Textbook of Pain, 2nd ed. Edinburgh, Churchill Livingstone, 1989, pp 598-607.

53. Kori SH, Foley KM, Posner JB: Brachial plexus lesions in patients with cancer: 100 cases. Neurology 1981;31:45-50.

54. Batzdorf U, Brechner VL: Management of pain associated with the Pancoast syndrome. Am J Surg 1979;137:638-646.

55. Cascino TL, Kori S, Krol G, et al: CT scan of the brachial plexus in patients with cancer. Neurology 1983;33:1553-1557.

56. Kanner RM, Martini N, Foley KM: Epidural spinal cord compression in Pancoast syndrome (superior pulmonary sulcus tumor): Clinical presentation and outcome. Ann Neurol 1981;10:77-82.

57. Foley KM: Overview of cancer pain and brachial and lumbosacral plexopathy. In Foley KM (ed): Management of Cancer Pain. New York, Memorial Sloan Kettering Cancer Center, 1985, pp 25-32.

58. Jaekle KA, Young DF, Foley KM: The natural history of lumbosacral plexopathy in cancer. Neurology 1985;35:8-15.

59. Pettigrew LC, Glass JP, Maor M, et al: Diagnosis and treatment of lumbosacral plexopathy in patients with cancer. Arch Neurol 1984;41:1282-1285.

60. Shubert MM, Sullivan KM, Morten TH, et al: Oral manifestations of chronic graft-versus-host disease. Arch Intern Med 1984;144:1591-1595.

61. Young DF, Posner JB: Nervous system toxicity of chemotherapeutic agents. In Vinken PJ, Bruyn GW (eds): Handbook of Clinical Neurology, vol 9. Neurologic Manifestations of Systemic Diseases, Part II. Amsterdam, North Holland, 1989, pp 91-97.

62. Perkins FM, Kehlet H: Chronic pain as an outcome of surgery: A review of predictive factors. Anesthesiology 2000;93:1123-1133.

63. Tasmuth T, von Smitten K, Kalso E, et al: Pain and other symptoms during the first year after radical and conservative surgery for breast surgery. Br J Cancer 1996;74:2024-2031.

64. Rushton JG, Rooke ED: Brain tumor headache. Headache 1962;2:147-152.

65. Zimm S, Wampler GL, Stablein D, et al: Intracerebral metastases in solid tumor patients: Natural history and results of treatment. Cancer 1981;48:384-394.

66. Black P: Brain metastasis: Current status and recommended guidelines for management. Neurosurgery 1979;5:617-631.

67. Guitin PH: Corticosteroid therapy in patients with brain tumor. Natl Cancer Inst Monogr 1977;46:151-156.

68. Mauch PM, Drew MA: Treatment of metastatic cancer to bone. In Devita VT (ed): Cancer: Principles and Practice of Oncology, 2nd ed. Philadelphia, JB Lippincott, 1985, pp 2132-2141.

69. Salazar OM, Da Motta NW, Bridgman SM, et al: Fractionated half-body irradiation for pain palliation in widely metastatic cancers: Comparison with single dose. Int J Radiat Oncol Biol Phys 1996;36:49-60.

70. Estes NC, Morphis JG, Hornback NB, et al: Intraarterial chemotherapy and hyperthermia for pain control in patients with recurrent rectal cancer. Am J Surg 1986;152:597-601.

71. Mellette SJ: Management of malignant disease metastatic to the bone by hormonal alterations. Clin Orthop 1970;73:73-78.

72. Faithfull NS, Reinhold HS, Van Den Berg AP, et al: The effectiveness and safety of whole body hyperthermia as a pain treatment in advanced malignancy. In Erdmann W, Oyama T, Pernak MJ (eds): Pain Clinic. Utrecht, Holland, VNU Science, 1985, pp 85-97.

73. Foley KM: Treatment of cancer pain. N Engl J Med 1985;313:84.

74. Grond S, Zech D, Diefenbach C, et al: Assessment of cancer pain: A prospective evaluation in 2266 patients referred to a pain service. Pain 1996;64:107-114.

75. Bruera E: Subcutaneous administration of opioids in the management of cancer pain. In Foley K, Ventafridda V (eds): Recent Advances in Pain Research, vol 16. New York, Raven Press, 1990, pp 203-218.

76. Bruera E, Ripamonti C: Alternate routes of administration of narcotics. In Patt RB (ed): Cancer Pain. Philadelphia, JB Lippincott, 1993, pp 161-169.

77. Cousins MJ, Mather LE: Intrathecal and epidural administration of opioids. Anesthesiology 1984;61:276-310.

78. Yaksh TL: Spinal opiates: A review of their effect on spinal function with an emphasis on pain processing. Acta Anaesthesiol Scand 1987;31(Suppl 85):25-36.

79. Smith DE: Spinal opioids in the home and hospice setting. J Pain Symptom Manage 1990;5:175-182.

80. Boersma FP, Buist AB, Thie J: Epidural pain treatment in the northern Netherlands: Organizational and treatment aspects. Acta Anaesthesiol Belg 1987;38:213-216.

81. Crawford ME, Andersen HB, Augustenborg G, et al: Pain treatment on outpatient basis using extradural opiates: Danish multicenter study comprising 105 patients. Pain 1983;16:41-47.

82. Snyder SH: Opiate receptors in the brain. N Engl J Med 1977;296:266-271.

83. Du Pen S, Kharasch ED, Williams A, et al: Chronic epidural bupivacaine-opioid infusion in intractable cancer pain. Pain 1992;49:293-300.

84. Smith TJ, Staats PS, Deer T, et al: Randomized clinical trial of an implantable drug delivery system compared with comprehensive medical management for refractory cancer pain: Impact on pain, drug-related toxicity, and survival. J Clin Oncol 2002;20:4040-4049.

85. Burton AW, Rajagopal A, Shah HN, et al: Epidural and intrathecal analgesia is effective in treating refractory cancer pain. Pain Med 2004;5:239-247.

86. Bedder MD, Burchiel KJ, Larson A: Cost analysis of two implantable narcotic delivery systems. J Pain Symptom Manage 1991;6:368-373.

87. Hassenbusch SJ, Bedder M, Patt RB, et al: Current status of intrathecal therapy for nonmalignant pain management: Clinical realities and economic unknowns. J Pain Symptom Manage 1997;14:S36-S48.

88. Hassenbusch SJ, Portenoy RK: Current practices in intraspinal therapy: A survey of clinical trends and decision making. J Pain Symptom Manage 2000;20:S4-S11.

89. Bonica JJ: Management of Pain. Philadelphia, Lea & Febiger, 1953.
90. Cousins MJ: Anesthetic approaches in cancer pain. Adv Pain Res Ther 16;1990:249-273.
91. Raj P, Ramamurthy S: Differential nerve block studies. In Raj PP (ed): Practical Management of Pain. Chicago, Year Book, 1986, pp 173-177.
92. Abram SE: The role of non-neurolytic nerve blocks in the management of cancer pain. I. In Abram SE (ed): Cancer Pain. Amsterdam, Kluwer, 1989, pp 67-75.
93. Travel JG, Simons DG: Myofascial Pain and Dysfunction: The Trigger Point Manual. Baltimore, Williams & Wilkins, 1983.
94. Payne R: Neuropathic pain syndromes, with special reference to causalgia and reflex sympathetic dystrophy. Clin J Pain 1986;2:59-73.
95. Gerbershagen HU: Blocks with local anesthetics in the treatment of cancer pain. In Bonica JJ, Ventafridda V (eds): Advances in Pain Research and Therapy, vol 2. New York, Raven Press, 1979, pp 311-323.
96. Warfield CA, Crews DA: Use of stellate ganglion blocks in the treatment of intractable limb pain in lung cancer. Clin J Pain 1987;3:13.
97. Evans PJD: Cryoanalgesia. Anaesthesia 1981;36:1003-1013.
98. Doyle D: Nerve blocks in advanced cancer. Practitioner 1982;226:539-544.
99. Peyton WT, Semansky EJ, Baker AB: Subarachnoid injection of alcohol for relief of intractable pain with discussion of cord changes found at autopsy. Am J Cancer 1937;30:709.
100. Smith MC: Histologic findings following intrathecal injections of phenol solutions for relief of pain. Br J Anaesth 1963;36:387-406.
101. Swerdlow M: Intrathecal neurolysis. Anaesthesia 1978;33:733-740.
102. Katz J: The current role of neurolytic agents. Adv Neurol 1974;4:471-476.
103. Swerdlow M: Subarachnoid and extradural blocks. Adv Pain Res Ther 2;1979:325-337.
104. Hay RC: Subarachnoid alcohol block in the control of intractable pain. Anesth Analg 1962;41:12-16.
105. Stovner J, Endresen R: Intrathecal phenol for cancer pain. Acta Anaesthesiol Scand 1972;16:17-21.
106. Holland AJC, Youssef M: A complication of subarachnoid phenol blockade. Anaesthesia 1979;34:260-262.
107. Racz GB, Heavner J, Haynsworth R: Repeat epidural phenol injections in chronic pain and spasticity. In Lipton S, Miles J (eds): Persistent Pain, vol 5. Orlando, Fla, Grune & Stratton, 1985, pp 157-179.
108. Madrid JL, Bonica JJ: Cranial nerve blocks. In Bonica JJ, Ventafridda V (eds): Advances in Pain Research and Therapy, vol 2. New York, Raven Press, 1979, pp 463-468.
109. Waldman SD, Feldstein GS, Allen ML, et al: Cervical epidural implantable narcotic delivery systems in the management of upper body pain. Anesth Analg 1987;66:780-782.
110. Lobato RD, Madrid JL, Fatela LV, et al: Intraventricular morphine for intractable cancer pain: Rationale, methods, clinical results. Acta Anaesthesiol Scand 1987;31:68-74.
111. Shah H, et al: Neurolytic blockade of the splanchnic nerves effectively relieves refractory pain associated with upper abdominal malignancy. ASA Abstract 2003.
112. Lahuerta J, Lipton S, Miles J, et al: Update on percutaneous cervical cordotomy and pituitary alcohol neuroadenolysis: An audit of our recent results and complications. In Lipton S, Miles J (eds): Persistent Pain, vol 5. New York, Grune & Stratton, 1985, pp 197-223.
113. Watling CJ, Payne R, Allen RR, Hassenbusch S: Commissural myelotomy for intractable cancer pain: Report of two cases. Clin J Pain 1996;12:151-156.
114. Lipton S: Percutaneous cordotomy. In Wall PD, Melzack R (eds): Textbook of Pain. Edinburgh, Churchill Livingstone, 1984, pp 632-638.
115. Mount BM: Psychologic and social aspects of cancer pain. In Wall PD, Melzack R (eds): Textbook of Pain. Edinburgh, Churchill Livingstone, 1984, pp 460-471.
116. Syrjala KL, Donaldson GW, Davis MW, et al: Relaxation and imagery and cognitive-behavioral training reduce pain during cancer treatment: A controlled clinical trial. Pain 1995;63:189-198.
117. Angarola RT, Wray SD: Legal impediments to cancer pain treatment. Adv Pain Res Ther 1989;11:213-216.
118. Smith JL: Care of people who are dying: The hospice approach. In Patt R (ed): Cancer Pain Management: A Multidisciplinary Approach. Philadelphia, JB Lippincott, 1993, pp 543-552.
119. Doyle D: Education and training in palliative care. J Palliat Care 1987;2:5-7.

21 Neuropathic Pain Syndromes

*Kayode A. Williams, Robert W. Hurley,
Elaina E. Lin, and Christopher L. Wu*

Neuropathic pain comprises a wide range of hetero-geneous conditions with many different etiologies of pain. Different types of neuropathic pain may have different pathophysiologic etiologies and present with different clinical signs and symptoms. Despite the diversity in many conditions that are labeled as "neuropathic pain," many of these conditions may potentially share common underlying mechanisms of nociception including neuronal hyperexcitability. This may in part explain why certain analgesic agents are relatively effective for a wide range of neuro-pathic pain states. Although there are many types of neuropathic pain states, this chapter focuses on some of the more common states (complex regional pain syndrome [CRPS], post-herpetic neuralgia [PHN], dia-betic neuropathy, and HIV-sensory neuropathy).

COMPLEX REGIONAL PAIN SYNDROME

For more than a century, CRPS types I and II (for-merly known as reflex sympathetic dystrophy [RSD] and causalgia, respectively) have been clearly iden-tified as debilitating disorders. In 1864, S. Weir Mitchell made the observation that Civil War sol-diers with peripheral nerve damage resulting from gunshot wounds developed persistent burning pain, coining the term "causalgia." In 1900, Sudek observed muscle atrophy and bone rarefaction secondary to nerve injury. In 1947, Evans used the term *reflex sympathetic dystrophy* to reflect the belief that the sympathetic nervous system was involved in the abnormal activity in the periphery.

The presence of an inhomogeneous set of signs and symptoms in patients presenting with RSD/CRPS has engendered the need for consensus amongst physi-cians charged with the care of this devastating clini-cal problem and challenging patient population. The lack of evidence for a reflex mechanism, variable presence of dystrophy, and the absence of sympa-thetic involvement in a subset of these patients led to the term *complex regional pain syndrome*, coined by the Special Consensus Group of the International Association for the Study of Pain (IASP). The term,

complex regional pain syndrome, is broad enough to allow inclusion of patients who may demonstrate varying levels of sympathetic nervous system involve-ment in maintaining pain throughout the course of the disease process, hence the terms *sympathetically mediated pain (SMP)* or *sympathetically independent pain (SIP)*.[1]

Epidemiology

There is minimal epidemiologic data on CRPS. This may reflect the prior lack of consensus regarding signs, symptoms, and presentation of this patient population as well as the absence of outcomes studies. Although the true incidence is unknown, CRPS occurs more commonly in females than males with a ratio of 2.3:3.[1] A prospective study by Veldman and colleagues reviewed 829 patients, 628 of whom were female (76%).[2] The age ranged from 9 to 85 years (median age of 42 years) with only 12 patients younger than 14 years of old.[2] Several other authors have attempted to examine epidemiologic variables in patient populations. Raja and colleagues exam-ined multiple variables (risk factors) including patient sociodemographic factors, which resulted in a recent web-based survey of 1359 study patients.[3] The study concluded that CRPS commonly occurs among younger females and frequently results from surgery or work-related traumatic injuries. The survey also demonstrated that CRPS is associated with sleep disturbance, functional impairment, and suicidal ideation.[3]

In a retrospective study, Allen and associates reviewed the epidemiologic data from 134 CRPS patients at a university-based tertiary pain center. The mean duration for the CRPS symptoms before presentation was 30 months.[4] Furthermore, most patients had seen on average 4.8 physicians before referral, whereas 17% had pending lawsuits and 54% had a worker's compensation claim related to the CRPS.[4] Although half the patients received a bone scan, only 53% of the bone scans were consis-tent with a diagnosis of CRPS.[4] Most (56%) had a myofascial component, and the duration of CRPS and involvement of the upper extremity was significantly associated with the presence of myofascial dysfunction.[4] This was the first study to identify the types of occupation CRPS patients were employed in while injured. People in service occupations, such as restaurant workers and police officers, suffered almost twice as often from CRPS than did persons in other occupations. These findings may be related to the physical demands of these jobs.[4]

Other associated features that may also affect the onset and progression of the disease include psychological factors (presence of social stressors) and poor coping mechanisms. For example, 80% of patients with upper extremity CRPS experienced a significant social stressor within 2 months before or 1 month after the inciting event, compared to a 20% incidence in the control group.[1] Despite these findings, no specific psychological factors or personality trait predisposes subjects to developing CRPS.[5] Further epidemiologic studies are necessary to determine the incidence and true female-to-male ratio, risk factors, natural history, relationship between certain clinical signs, disease onset, and progression.[6]

Pathophysiology

The two known types of CRPS are type I and type II. They differ based upon the underlying pathophysiology (see review in reference 7). Pain remains the hallmark of CRPS type I, which commonly manifests as spontaneous pain, hyperalgesia, and allodynia. In addition, trophic, sudomotor, vasomotor abnormalities, and active and passive movement disorders characteristically develop following minor or major injuries with little or no nerve injury in the limb involved. Infrequently, it may develop after trauma in the visceral region or following a central nervous system (CNS) lesion (e.g., cerebrovascular accident). A consistent feature of CRPS I is that there is typically a discrepancy between the severity of the symptoms and severity of the inciting injury. In addition, there is a propensity for the symptoms to spread in the affected limb in a pattern not restricted to the area of innervation of a specific nerve. Even though the pathophysiology is not clearly defined, several underlying mechanisms have been postulated based on clinical observations. Clinical trials in human subjects and animal models indicate that the syndrome may be mainly a systemic disease involving the central and peripheral nervous system,[7,8] yet the specific interaction between the central and the peripheral mechanisms is unclear.[8] The postulated mechanisms include abnormalities of the somatosensory, sensory pathways, and sympathetically mediated pain.

Somatosensory Abnormalities

The main focus of investigations has been on the sudomotor and vasomotor abnormalities in CRPS,

hence the interest in sympathetically mediated pain (SMP). This led to an emphasis on the nociceptive system and its peripheral and central connections to the sympathetic nervous system. Clinical observations, however, suggest that in CRPS I, pain is commonly projected into the deep somatic tissues and many patients with CRPS I do not have SMP clinically (i.e., absence of allodynia and lack of reduction in pain following sympathetic blocks).[7] Up to 5% of patients with CRPS have more discrete evoked pain rather than the typical spontaneous pain.[7] Functional imaging suggests that chronic pain patients with nondermatomal hyperesthesia have deactivation of the S1 and S2 somatosensory cortical areas.[9] Results from magnetoencephalography studies in CRPS patients indicate somatosensory cortical reorganization proportional to the amount of pain,[10] which was reversed following pain relief.[11] Thus there is increasing data that indicate that the pain associated with CRPS alters somatosensory processing, or that pain and the susceptibility to cortical reorganization predisposes a patient to develop CRPS after an injury.[12]

Sensory Pathways

Most patients with CRPS I typically present with a burning pain in the extremity involved. Animal studies demonstrate that spontaneous pain, hyperalgesia, and allodynia are thought to result from peripheral and central sensitization.[13] Examination of the extent of sensory impairment in 24 CRPS I patients revealed that up to half of patients with chronic CRPS I develop hyperesthesia to temperature and pinprick on the affected side of the body or in the upper quadrant of the ipsilateral side.[14] Patients were also found to have a higher incidence of mechanical allodynia and hyperalgesia in addition to motor impairment.[14] These sensory changes and associated motor impairment suggest that the CNS may be involved in the widespread alteration in sensory perception and in the pathophysiology of CRPS in this group of patients.[14]

Sympathetically Mediated Pain

Coupling between the sympathetic noradrenergic neurons in the periphery and primary afferent neurons has clearly been shown to be the underlying mechanism of SMP in patients with CRPS I. However, CRPS II clinical studies support the notion that cutaneous nociceptors may become more sensitive to catecholamines after nerve injury. This is particularly evident in studies where intradermal application of epinephrine into an affected skin area causes a return of spontaneous pain with allodynia, which had previously been relieved by sympathetic blockade.[15,16] The return of the spontaneous pain may be relieved by a subsequent infusion of phentolamine.[15] Coupling of sympathetic neurons may occur to not only nociceptive afferents but also non-nociceptive mechanosensitive or cold-sensitive neurons. Other mechanisms for coupling between the sympathetic system and afferent nociceptive neurons have been suggested.[17,18]

Clinical Features

The definition of standardized diagnostic consensus-based criteria for CRPS by the IASP was a significant milestone in the classification of regional disorders with sudomotor or vasomotor instability.[19] The criteria are shown in Table 21–1. Even though the CRPS diagnostic criteria was intended to improve clinical recognition and facilitate outcomes research, there is no consensus with regard to how many of the different signs and symptoms described in the IASP criteria are needed for accurate diagnosis. Reinders and colleagues examined the use of the IASP criteria defined in 1994 in publications between 1996 and 2000, and found that none of the original publications met all the IASP criteria and the use of the diagnostic criterion pain was reported in only 38% of the publications reviewed.[20] Internal and external validation research suggests that CRPS may have been overdiagnosed.[21] Including "motor and trophic signs and symptoms" in addition to separating vasomotor signs and symptoms from sudomotor category improved the specificity without losing sensitivity. A suggested diagnostic algorithm has been proposed to enhance sensitivity and specificity (see review by Baron and colleagues, reference 22).

The distinction between CRPS I and II lies in the presence of a definable nerve lesion (CRPS II only). The signs and symptoms for both conditions are clinically indistinguishable and include sensory changes (allodynia, hyperalgesia, and hypoalgesia), edema, abnormalities of temperature, and sweating. Pain is the principal feature for both CRPS I and II. In CRPS I, the pain and associated clinical signs are typically out of proportion to the inciting injury. Patients describe a burning deep-seated ache that may be shooting in nature with associated allodynia or hyperalgesia.[23] Pain occurs in 81.1% of patients

meeting the CRPS criteria.[24] Patients also frequently complain of sensory abnormalities such as hyperesthesia in response to typical mechanical stimuli encountered in day to day activities, such as clothing on the affected limb.

In CRPS II (i.e., CRPS with associated major nerve injury), patients often report hyperethesia in the territory of the injured nerve in the presence of electrical sensations, shooting pain, and allodynia. Symptoms indicative of vasomotor autonomic abnormalities (including color changes) occurred in 86.9% of patients with temperature instability occurring in 78.7%.[24] Sudomotor symptoms of hyperhidrosis/hypohidrosis were reported in 52.9% as were trophic changes in skin (24.4%), nail (21.1%), or hair (18%) pattern.[24] Edema was reported in 79.7%, with decreased range of motion in 80.3% and motor weakness in 74.6%.[24]

Diagnosis

The current diagnostic criteria for CRPS types I and II are mainly based on the patient's history and physical examination. Studies on the external and internal validity of the IASP criteria suggest that patients should have (1) at least one symptom in each of the following general categories: sensory (hyperesthesia-increased sensitivity to a sensory stimulation), vasomotor (temperature abnormalities or skin color changes), sudomotor-fluid balance (sweating abnormalities or edema), or motor (decreased range of movement, weakness, tremor, or neglect); and (2) at least one sign within two or more of the following categories: sensory (allodynia or hyperalgesia) vasomotor (objective temperature abnormalities or skin color changes), sudomotor-fluid balance (sweating abnormalities or objective edema), or motor (objective decreased range of motion, weakness, tremor, or neglect).[21] A thorough history, vascular, and neurologic examination will help rule out the more common conditions that could mimic CRPS such as diabetic and small-fiber neuropathies, entrapment syndromes, discogenic disease, and thoracic outlet

Table 21–1. International Association for the Study of Pain Diagnostic Criteria for CRPS I and CRPS II

CRPS I (REFLEX SYMPATHETIC DYSTROPHY)*	CRPS II (CAUSALGIA)†
1. The presence of an initiating noxious event, or a cause of immobilization.	1. The presence of continuing pain, allodynia, or hyperalgesia after a nerve injury, not necessarily limited to the distribution of the injured nerve.
2. Continuing pain, allodynia, or hyperalgesia with which the pain is disproportionate to any inciting event.	2. Evidence at some time of edema, changes in skin blood flow, or abnormal sudomotor activity in the region of the pain.
3. Evidence at some time of edema, changes in skin blood flow, or abnormal sudomotor activity in the region of the pain.	3. This diagnosis is excluded by the existence of conditions that would otherwise account for the degree of pain and dysfunction.
4. This diagnosis is excluded by the existence of conditions that would otherwise account for the degree of pain and dysfunction.	

*Criteria 2 to 4 must be satisfied.
†All three criteria must be satisfied.
From Baron R, Binder A, Lugwig J, et al: Diagnostic tools and evidence-based treatment of complex regional pain syndrome. Pain 2005, an updated review. Seattle, IASP Press, 2005, pp 293-306.

syndrome. Vascular conditions to be considered in the differential diagnosis include deep vein thrombosis, cellulitis, vascular insufficiency, lymphedema, and erythromelalgia.[1]

There is neither a diagnostic gold standard nor an objective test for CRPS. However, some diagnostic tests do add important information that may help confirm the diagnosis even though a normal result does not rule out the possibility of CRPS diagnosis. The following tests may add diagnostic value:

Quantitative sensory testing. This includes the use of standardized psychophysical tests of the thermal, thermal pain, and vibratory thresholds to assess the function of large-fiber, myelinated small-fiber, and unmyelinated small afferent fibers. Static, dynamic allodynia, pinprick allodynia, heat and mechanical hyperalgesia, and temporal summation may be abnormal in patients with CRPS.[22] Although no specific sensory pattern has been associated with CRPS, quantification of individual signs may provide a valuable means of documenting response to therapy.

Autonomic function tests. These include infrared thermometry and thermography, the quantitative sudomotor axon reflex test (QSART), the thermoregulatory sweat test (TST), and the laser Doppler flowmetry.[22]

Temperature measurement. Infrared thermometry/infrared thermography has been used to assess skin temperature differences. A difference of more than 2.2° C between the sides of the body achieves a sensitivity of 76% and specificity of 100%.[25] However, temperature measurement under controlled thermoregulation cannot be achieved under clinical conditions. Therefore, temperature measurements should be made under conditions that allow the most accurate detection of temperature difference between sides. The duration of the disease may influence the direction of the temperature difference. Early in the disease process, the affected limb may show elevated temperatures while chronic stages of the disease may demonstrate lower temperatures compared to the unaffected side.[25]

Vascular abnormalities. Vascular reflex responses may be assessed using laser Doppler flowmetry. In patients with disease of less than 4 months, the affected extremity may exhibit higher skin perfusion.[26] In patients with a mean duration of disease of 15 months, the skin perfusion was either higher or lower, while in patients with a mean duration of disease of at least 28 months, the affected limb had lower skin perfusion and ultimately lower skin temperatures.[26]

Trophic changes. Three-phase bone scintigraphy can provide valuable information. A pathologic uptake in the metacarpophalangeal or metacarpal bones is thought to be highly sensitive and specific for CRPS.[22] The most significant changes are seen in the first year of the disease.[27] X-ray bone densitometry may have a high sensitivity and specificity for the diagnosis of CRPS.[22]

Treatment

Limited understanding of the pathophysiologic mechanisms involved in the development of CRPS and absence of clear objective diagnostic criteria impede progress with clinical trials of treatment modalities. As a result, only a select number of evidence-based treatment modalities are available thus far. Clinical therapies in the management of patients with CRPS are based on evidence from studies in other neuropathic states. With continued progress in defining pathophysiologic mechanisms (partly driven by the development of innovative preclinical models for CRPS I[28]), more mechanism-based treatment concepts are expected to emerge. In the interim, the current treatment philosophy centers on multimodal, multidisciplinary approaches involving effective pain control, functional restoration, and psychological interventions.

Pharmacologic Therapy

Nonsteroidal anti-inflammatory drugs (NSAIDs). NSAIDs have not been extensively investigated in the treatment of CRPS; however, clinical experience indicates that orally administered NSAIDs can provide mild to moderate pain control.[22] A retrospective study that examined the usefulness of intravenous regional anesthesia (IVRA) containing ketorolac demonstrated that up to 69% of patients had partial to complete resolution of pain.[29]

Antidepressants. No controlled trial is currently available for the use of antidepressants in CRPS. However, antidepressants have been extensively studied in other neuropathic pain states.[30-32] Norepinephrine and serotonin reuptake blockers (e.g., amitriptyline, 10 to 75 mg/day typically at night[30]) and selective norepinephrine blockers (e.g., desipramine) may exert their effect by enhancing the noradrenergic and serotonergic descending inhibitory pathways. Selective serotonin reuptake inhibitors have not been shown conclusively to be as effective. The balanced and selective serotonin and norepinephrine reuptake inhibitor duloxetine has been shown to be effective in painful diabetic neuropathy (suggested dose range 60 mg once a day to 60 mg twice a day[32,33]). These agents also may provide the added benefit of improving mood as a direct effect and enhancement of sleep as a side effect in selected patients. Although amitriptyline has been more widely studied because of the side effect profile, patients older than age 65 years may experience more side effects, and desipramine or nortriptyline is better tolerated with regard to side effects by most patients (Table 21–2).

Anticonvulsants. Gabapentin and more recently pregabalin[34] have been shown to be effective in painful diabetic neuropathy and PHN, and studies in patients with CRPS have demonstrated analgesic effect of gabapentin.[35] Carbamazepine is approved by the Food and Drug Administration for trigeminal neuralgia and may be considered as a second-tier

Table 21–2. Dosages of Commonly Used Analgesics for the Treatment of CRPS

AGENT	DOSE RANGE	FREQUENCY	COMMON SIDE EFFECTS
Antidepressants			
Amitriptyline	10-75 mg/day	Once a day (at night)	Sedation, anticholinergic effects
Nortriptyline	10-75 mg	Once a day (at night)	Sedation, anticholinergic effects
Desipramine	10-75 mg/day	Once a day (at night)	Least sedative/anticholinergic effects
Venlafaxine	37.5-340 mg/day	2-3 times per day	
Anticonvulsants			
Gabapentin	900-3600 mg/day	3 times per day	Somnolence, memory impairment, tremors
Pregabalin	150-600 mg/day	2-3 times per day	Dizziness, somnolence, peripheral edema
Carbamazepine	100-1000 mg/day	2-4 times per day	Ataxia, sedation, nausea, liver damage, skin rash, bone marrow
Opioids			
Morphine (extended release)	15-30 mg	2-3 times per day	Nausea, vomiting, constipation, sedation, pruritus
Oxycodone (extended release)	10-40 mg	2-3 times per day	As for morphine
Methadone	5-10 mg	2-3 times per day	As for morphine

option. Oxcarbazepine, a new analogue of carbamazepine without the side effects of liver and bone marrow toxicity, is currently under investigation with early reports of efficacy.

Opioid analgesics. There have been no long-term studies of oral opioid analgesics for the treatment of neuropathic pain states in general or in CRPS in particular. Raja and colleagues[30] demonstrated that patients with PHN demonstrated a preference for opioids (54%) over tricyclic antidepressant agents (30%) with marginally greater pain relief of the former. Opioids may be used as a part of a comprehensive treatment program if other agents do not provide sufficient analgesia.[31,33,36]

Calcium-regulating drugs. The mode of action of calcium-regulating drugs in CRPS is unknown; however, intranasally administered calcitonin may provide significant pain reduction in patients with CRPS.

Free radical scavengers. Topically applied dimethyl sulfoxide (DMSO) 50%, or oral N-acetylcysteine (NAC) were used in a placebo-controlled trial. Both were found to be effective in CRPS type I.[37]

Interventional Treatment

Intravenous regional anesthesia. Studies to date have yet to provide conclusive evidence to support the use of IVRA for sympatholysis. No difference was found between guanethidine and prilocaine versus placebo after four blocks,[22] while stellate ganglion blocks with bupivacaine and regional blocks with guanethidine showed a significant improvement compared with baseline, with both treatments providing similar effects.[22] Hord and colleagues demonstrated that IVRA with bretylium and lidocaine provided longer lasting pain relief than lidocaine alone.[38] However, it has been suggested that well-performed sympathetic ganglion blocks should be used rather than IVRA.[32]

Sympathetic nerve blocks. Price and colleagues in a double-blind crossover study evaluated the diagnostic and therapeutic value of local anesthetics compared with saline.[39] They found that an immediate effect on pain and mechanical allodynia (lasting a few hours) was similar in both groups, although the local anesthetic group showed prolonged effects beyond 24 hours (3 to 5 days).[39] They surmised that the immediate effect may be due to nonspecific effects. However, the local anesthetic block clearly outlasted the duration of action of the local anesthetic. Although sympatholysis may be important in prolonging the duration of pain relief for CRPS patients who respond to sympathetic blocks,[39] the primary utility of sympathetic blocks currently is still to differentiate between SMP and SIP. However, it is difficult to define "successful" sympathetic blockade due in part to the controversy and variability in use of various signs such as Horner's syndrome, increased skin blood flow, temperature, and reduced skin resistance in defining a "successful" sympathetic block. However, potential analgesia provided by these blocks in the patients will allow institution of physical therapy to enhance functional restoration.

Spinal cord stimulation. Limited available evidence suggests that spinal cord stimulation (SCS) is effective in the management of patients with CRPS who do not respond to conservative medical management.[40] However, the mechanism for producing analgesia, specific stimulation parameters or patterns, criteria for a successful trial, and effects on the natural course of the disease are questions that remain unanswered by the currently available literature. Thus more robust studies are required to provide conclusive evidence that place SCS in the management of CRPS.[40]

POST-HERPETIC NEURALGIA

PHN is a complication of herpes zoster (shingles) that may be difficult to successfully treat. PHN can be extremely debilitating for patients and may interfere with quality of life and functional status. There are certain risk factors for not only the development of herpes zoster but also PHN. Understanding the pathophysiology of PHN will provide rationale for an analgesic regimen for the treatment of PHN pain. There are several analgesic and interventional options for the treatment of PHN pain.

Epidemiology and Risk Factors

Although the actual incidence of PHN is not certain, depending in part on the precise definition of PHN applied (generally considered significant pain or dysesthesia present 3 to 6 months after herpes zoster),[41] approximately 9% to 34% of all patients with herpes zoster develop PHN.[42] The incidence of herpes zoster in the community has been reported at 2 to 3 per 1000 with approximately 500,000 new cases of zoster annually in the United States alone.[43] The key risk factor for development of herpes zoster is increasing age: the incidence is approximately 12 per 1000 in persons older than 65 years of age.[43] Other risk factors for the development of herpes zoster include administration of immunosuppressive therapy (e.g., chemotherapy, radiotherapy) and reduced immunity (e.g., lymphoma, leukemia, acquired immunodeficiency syndrome [AIDS]).[43]

Once herpes zoster occurs, there are risk factors for the development of PHN (Box 21–1). Older patients are at higher risk of developing not only herpes zoster but also PHN with the severity and duration of PHN being age-related.[44] Increased severity of acute pain, greater extent of rash, and presence of a prodrome of dermatomal pain during herpes zoster disease will correlate with increased severity of PHN pain.[43] Presence of these risk factors may increase the risk of development of PHN as much as 50% to 75%.[43] Use of antiviral agents such as famciclovir or valacyclovir may decrease the severity and duration of acute herpes zoster pain and as a result may decrease the incidence and severity of PHN with an odds ratio of 0.54 (95% confidence interval = 0.36-0.81) for the development of PHN after antiviral therapy.[43,45] A randomized controlled trial demonstrated that the administration of a zoster vaccine significantly decreased the incidence of both acute herpes zoster and PHN in adults older than 60 years of age.[46]

Pathophysiology

Following resolution of a primary infection with varicella (chickenpox), residual virus particles become dormant in the dorsal root or cranial nerve ganglia.[43,44] Although this virus most likely is often reactivated

---

BOX 21–1. RISK FACTORS FOR INCREASED SEVERITY OF PAIN OF POST-HERPETIC NEURALGIA

- Older patients
- Increased severity of acute pain
- Greater extent of rash
- Presence of a prodrome of dermatomal pain during herpes zoster

---

afterward, clinical manifestation of the disease is not apparent as a result of cellular-mediated immunity.[43] However, a decline in cellular-mediated immunity (as might occur with increasing age and presence of immunosuppressive agents or disease states) may result in a symptomatic reactivation (see Clinical Presentation below). This reactivation is recognized as acute herpes zoster (shingles) and is associated with viral replication and destruction of dorsal horn and peripheral sensory neurons.[44]

The neural degeneration associated with virus reactivation contributes to two primary pathophysiologic mechanisms of PHN pain: sensitization (hyperexcitability) and deafferentation.[42] Following neuronal injury, both peripheral nociceptors and central neurons may become sensitized (e.g., lower threshold for neuron activation, exaggerated responses to stimuli, spontaneous discharge activity, expansion of receptive fields) such that the hyperexcitability may result in allodynia without sensory loss.[42] With deafferentation pain, neuronal destruction from viral reactivation and the subsequent inflammatory response causes loss of afferent neurons, leading to spontaneous activity centrally and resulting in pain in areas of sensory loss. Neural sprouting (large-fiber mechanoreceptors) to reconnect with former C-fiber receptors results in hyperalgesia and allodynia.[42] Although sensitization and deafferentation appear to be the primary two mechanisms of PHN pain, other possibilities exist including coupling of the sympathetic nervous system to primary afferents, abnormal neuronal sprouting and neuroma formation, and reinnervation of denervated areas by neighboring axons.[42]

Clinical Presentation

The onset of acute herpes zoster is marked by a prodrome of pain in the affected dermatome, most commonly in the thoracic or lumbar region, although cervical (e.g., ophthalmic) dermatomes may also be affected. Eventually, the characteristic unilateral dermatomal rash will result in maculopapular vesicles, which in turn will crust over in approximately 1 to 2 weeks. Patients may experience acute pain from neuritis, which is characterized by a burning, stabbing pain.[47] For patients who develop PHN, pain may be constant (burning, throbbing) or intermittent (shooting, stabbing), with some also experiencing stimulus-evoked pain (allodynia).[47]

Treatment Options

PHN pain may be difficult to treat and may be resistant to many treatment options. Typically, treatment options are categorized as either analgesics (e.g., opioids, membrane stabilizers, and antidepressants) or interventional procedures (e.g., sympathetic blocks, intrathecal injections, or surgical interventions). Although more randomized controlled trials on treatment of PHN pain have been published within the past few years, several treatment options still have a relatively low number of subjects studied and a definitive statement regarding the analgesic efficacy of these interventions may be premature.

Analgesic Therapy

Although there are a number of different analgesic agents that have been used for the treatment of PHN pain, there are adequate data available on only a few agents to demonstrate analgesic efficacy for providing pain relief from PHN (Table 21–3). Other analgesic agents are either ineffective or lack the presence of adequate randomized controlled trials to allow for a definitive determination of their analgesic efficacy for the treatment of PHN pain.

Gabapentin/pregablin. Although originally developed as an anticonvulsant, gabapentin has been shown to be an effective analgesic for the treatment of inflammatory and neuropathic pain, including PHN.[48] The mechanism of analgesic action of gabapentin, a structural analogue of the inhibitory neurotransmitter gamma-aminobutyric acid (GABA), is unclear but most likely gabapentin acts at the alpha$_2$-delta$_1$ subunits of voltage-dependent Ca^{2+} channel to decrease calcium influx and thereby inhibit the release of neurotransmitters (e.g., glutamate) in the spinal cord.[49,50] Several clinical studies have established the analgesic efficacy of gabapentin for the treatment of PHN pain (see later). A quantitative systematic review of randomized controlled trials indicated that the pooled numbers-needed-to-treat (NNT) for gabapentin was approximately 4.4.[51] One of the earliest randomized, double-blind, placebo-controlled trials evaluated a total of 229 PHN subjects who received up to a maximum dosage of 3600 mg/day of gabapentin or placebo over a 4-week titration period.[48] Subjects who received gabapentin had a statistically significant reduction in average daily pain score from 6.3 to 4.2 points (vs. 6.5 to 6.0 points for placebo) but experienced a higher incidence of somnolence, dizziness, ataxia, peripheral edema, and

infection. Another large randomized, double-blind, placebo-controlled trial examined a total of 334 PHN subjects who received gabapentin 1800 or 2400 mg/day or placebo over a 7-week study period.[52] Patients who received gabapentin had a significantly greater improvement in pain scores from week 1 with the most common side effects noted as dizziness and somnolence.[52] Although the optimal dosing schedule for gabapentin is still not clear, a systematic review suggested that gabapentin treatment should be started at a dose of 900 mg/day (300 mg/day on day 1, 600 mg/day on day 2, and 900 mg/day on day 3) with additional titration to 1800 mg/day recommended for greater efficacy and occasionally doses up to 3600 mg/day needed for some patients.[53]

By binding to the alpha$_2$-delta$_1$ subunit of voltage-gated calcium channels to reduce the release of excitatory neurotransmitters, pregabalin has been shown to possibly have greater analgesic activity than gabapentin for the treatment of neuropathic pain. When compared to placebo, oral pregabalin at 150 to 600 mg/day was superior in providing pain relief and improving pain-related sleep interference in three randomized, double-blind, placebo-controlled trials in 776 patients with PHN.[54] The most common side effects of pregabalin in these studies were dizziness, somnolence, and peripheral edema.[54-56] Patients may notice a reduction in pain even after the first full day of treatment and side effects are generally mild to moderate in intensity.[55] Both a flexible- and fixed-dose pregabalin regimen appears to be effective for treatment of PHN pain.[56] Finally, concomitant use of gabapentin with an opioid such as morphine may provide superior analgesia at lower doses than either as administered as a single agent.[57]

Lidocaine patch. A topical lidocaine patch, an adhesive patch containing 5% lidocaine (700 mg), has been used for the treatment of PHN pain and presumably exerts its analgesic effects by blocking neuronal sodium channels.[58] Clinical trials in PHN patients with allodynia have demonstrated the analgesic efficacy of this modality in reducing pain from PHN, which is associated with few side effects, the most frequent being mild skin irritation at the site of application.[58] There is minimal systemic absorption from the lidocaine patch 5% with average maximum plasma concentrations suggesting a minimal risk for systemic toxicities or drug-drug interactions, even with continuous application of up to four patches/day.[59,60]

Thus the lidocaine patch 5% has demonstrated relief of pain and tactile allodynia in patients with PHN. There appears to be minimal risk of systemic adverse effects or drug-drug interactions and some have advocated the use of the lidocaine patch 5% as a first-line therapy for the treatment of PHN pain.[60] In an open-label, nonrandomized, prospective study, the lidocaine patch 5%, which was applied to the area of maximal pain, reduced the intensity of moderate-to-severe PHN pain as assessed by the Neuropathic Pain Scale.[61] Another open-label, nonrandomized study applied up to three lidocaine

Table 21–3. Efficacy of Analgesic Options for the Treatment of Post-herpetic Neuralgia

ANALGESIC OPTION	NUMBERS-NEEDED-TO-TREAT (NNT)*
Gabapentin	4.4 [3.3-6.1]
Lidocaine patch	2 [1.4-3.3]
NMDA antagonists	23.9 [n/a]
Opioids	2.7 [2.1-3.8]
Pregabalin	4.9 [3.7-17.3]
Topical capsaicin	2.3 [1.4-6.1]
Tramadol	4.8 [2.6-27.0]
Tricyclic antidepressants	2.6 [2.1-3.5]

*Data presented as mean NNT [95% confidence intervals].
n/a, not available; NMDA, N-methyl-d-aspartate.
Data from Hempenstall K, Nurmikko TJ, Johnson RW, et al: Analgesic therapy in postherpetic neuralgia: A quantitative systematic review. PLoS Med 2005;2:e164.

5% patches to area of greatest PHN pain for 12 hours per day for 28 days.[62] Use of the lidocaine patch was associated with a reduction in pain intensity and interference with quality of life (QOL) as assessed with the Brief Pain Inventory Short Form and global pain assessments.[62] In a randomized, crossover study, lidocaine patches were strongly preferred compared to a placebo patch (78.1% vs. 9.4%) with no significant difference noted between the active and placebo treatments with regard to side effects.[63] Thus the topical lidocaine 5% patch appears to be an effective analgesic treatment for PHN and is associated with minimal side effects when used.

Opioid analgesics. Although opioids have been a standard treatment for pain in general, their efficacy for the treatment of neuropathic pain such as PHN is considered to be uncertain and controversial. There appear to be some interindividual differences in opioid responsiveness[64]; a higher dose of opioid may be necessary to decrease neuropathic pain compared to nociceptive pain,[65] and a number of high-quality studies have shown that both intravenous and oral opioids (e.g., morphine, fentanyl, levorphanol) are effective in relieving neuropathic pain overall.[66-70] In terms of the use of opioids for treatment of PHN, both intravenous and oral opioids (morphine, oxycodone, levorphanol) have been shown to provide significant pain relief.[67,71] In a double-blind, placebo-controlled, randomized, controlled trial, intravenous infusions of morphine decreased PHN pain and there was a significant association between serum level of morphine and decrease in pain.[67] A PHN subgroup in another randomized controlled trial examining the use of opioids for neuropathic pain noted a greater reduction in pain with a higher rather than a lower dose of opioid.[68] Patients in the high-strength dose group had a 42% reduction in pain intensity from baseline compared to only 10% for the low-strength group. Thus, available randomized controlled trials suggest opioids may be efficacious for the treatment of PHN pain, and the NNT has been reported as low as 2.7 for use of opioids in PHN pain.[69] Although there is technically no analgesic ceiling for opioid analgesics, opioid-related side effects typically are the limiting factor in the dose that can be given.

Tricyclic antidepressants. Tricyclic antidepressants (TCAs) have been used for the treatment of a wide variety of neuropathic pain states including PHN. TCAs exert their analgesic effects presumably through blockade of primarily norepinephrine reuptake with other mechanisms possibly including blockade of serotonin reuptake and sodium channels.[72] A recent quantitative systematic review of analgesic therapy in PHN noted that there was a significant analgesic benefit with TCAs in the treatment of PHN pain, with the pooled data showing an NNT of 2.6 (95% confidence interval = 2.1-3.5).[51] An earlier quantitative systematic analysis of the efficacy of antidepressant drugs for the treatment of PHN pain revealed that the NNT for antidepressants was 2.1.[73,74] An individual randomized, double-blind, crossover trial of tricyclic antidepressants in PHN patients noted a higher

NNT of 3.7 with a lack of correlation in the analgesic responsiveness between TCAs and opioids (i.e., some patients who did not have pain relief with TCA experienced significant relief with opioids).[69] Although amitriptyline has been the most commonly studied TCA for the treatment of PHN pain, other TCAs (e.g., nortriptyline) appear to be equally efficacious,[51] although one study noted that desipramine might be more likely to provide clinically meaningful pain relief in antidepressant-naïve PHN patients.[72] Addition of fluphenazine to amitriptyline did seem to improve pain relief in PHN pain compared to amitriptyline alone.[75]

Interventional Therapy

Interventional treatment options for PHN include a diverse range of choices including sympathetic and other nerve blocks, intrathecal injections, and SCS. Although generally not considered a first-line choice, interventional treatment options should be considered in context of a comprehensive strategy for the treatment of PHN.

Sympathetic nerve blocks. Although sympathetic nerve blocks have traditionally been used for the treatment of pain from PHN, the analgesic efficacy of sympathetic nerve blocks for this indication is controversial. There are possible benefits of sympathetic blockade in attenuating potential pathophysiology from PHN (e.g., abnormal activation of the α-adrenergic receptors, neuronal regeneration and sprouting following nerve injury and tissue trauma, indirect neurovascular interactions, or other links between sympathetic nervous system activity and PHN pain).[76,77] Systematic reviews examining the analgesic efficacy of sympathetic nerve blocks for PHN do not demonstrate any significant benefit for these interventions[42] despite the fact that some retrospective studies and case series suggested a potential analgesic benefit.[78-80] There are many methodologic issues (e.g., lack of double-blind, randomized, controlled trials, inadequate assessments of pain severity, lack of control for other important covariates, and varying definitions for PHN) present that contribute to the controversial nature of sympathetic nerve blocks for the treatment of PHN pain.[81,82]

Despite the uncertainty of the analgesic efficacy of sympathetic nerve blocks for PHN pain, there may be a role for sympathetic nerve blocks in the treatment of acute herpes zoster pain, which would theoretically prevent the development of PHN. Nonrandomized data suggest that the administration of sympathetic nerve blocks may reduce the duration of acute herpes zoster pain.[78,79,83] A small prospective, randomized trial also indicated that sympathetic blocks (four sympathetic nerve blocks once a day for 4 consecutive days) might decrease the incidence of acute herpes zoster pain.[84] One theoretical advantage of sympathetic nerve block administration for the treatment of acute herpes zoster pain is its potential to decrease the incidence of PHN as severity of acute herpes zoster pain is an established risk factor for the development of PHN.[85] Despite similar data from the postoperative period suggesting that the severity of acute postoperative pain correlates with a higher incidence of long-term chronic postsurgical pain[86] and that preemptive analgesia may attenuate the severity of subsequent postoperative pain,[87] there are no similar high-quality data currently available that demonstrate a reduction in the incidence or severity of PHN with sympathetic blocks for treatment of acute herpes zoster pain.

Epidural nerve blocks. The evaluation of epidural block for the treatment of PHN has not been thoroughly evaluated, although there are several reports of epidural blockade for the treatment of acute herpes zoster pain.[88-90] Some prospective observational trials[88,90] indicate that this modality may be effective for the treatment of acute herpes zoster pain in that epidural blockade may shorten the total duration and decrease the overall severity of pain. There is also a report that high thoracic epidural block may be a viable alternative to sympathetic stellate ganglion block for the treatment of acute herpes zoster pain.[89]

Intrathecal methylprednisolone. One of the most intriguing and promising treatment options for PHN pain is the injection of intrathecal methylprednisolone. Because postmortem studies of PHN patients noted spinal cord inflammation[91] and PHN patients may have high levels of interleukin-8 within the cerebrospinal fluid (CSF),[92,93] intrathecal administration of a corticosteroid (methylprednisolone) might theoretically decrease proinflammatory mediators (which may contribute to central sensitization), neuraxial inflammation, and PHN pain as a result.[94] A randomized controlled trial in PHN patients with long-lasting pain refractory to conventional therapy demonstrated that intrathecal injection of methylprednisolone (vs. lidocaine alone or no treatment/control) resulted in a significant decrease in PHN pain relief (for both burning and lancinating pain), diclofenac use, and areas of maximal pain and allodynia.[93] CSF concentrations of interleukin-8 were significantly decreased in subjects who received intrathecal methylprednisolone with the amount of decrease correlating with the extent of global pain relief.[93] Intrathecal administration of methylprednisolone appears to provide superior pain relief and lower CSF interleukin-8 levels compared to that of methylprednisolone given epidurally.[92] Although this one study[93] provides promising data for the treatment of PHN pain, additional studies are needed to confirm these data and to examine the safety of intrathecal administration of methylprednisolone, which has been associated with neurologic complications such as adhesive arachnoiditis.[93,95,96]

Spinal cord stimulation. The mechanism of analgesic action of SCS is unclear and may include myelinated A-beta fiber interference with transmission of nociceptive information from unmyelinated C and myelinated A-delta fibers and GABAergic interneurons inhibiting nociceptive processing.[97,98] SCS is a recognized interventional treatment option and is effective in the management of certain types of neuropathic pain[99] with long-term pain relief in up to 60% to 80% of patients.[97] The scant data examining the use of SCS for the treatment of PHN pain indicate that this modality may be beneficial in up to approximately 80% of PHN patients who had pain of more than 2 years' duration that was refractory to medical therapy.[98] Further trials, including cost-effectiveness data, are needed to determine the role of SCS for the treatment of PHN pain.

Conclusion

PHN pain may be difficult to treat and the treatment options available may not be completely effective. Randomized controlled trials and systematic reviews of these trials indicate that opioid therapy, tricyclic antidepressants, gabapentin/pregablin, and tramadol are effective therapies for the treatment of PHN pain.[51] Of the interventional therapies, intrathecal methylprednisolone holds the most promise, although additional data are needed on the spinal neurotoxicity of this agent. Sympathetic blocks do not appear to be efficacious for the treatment of PHN pain, although there may be a role for this modality in the treatment of acute herpes zoster pain. SCS is a possible interventional therapy but further randomized trials are needed to confirm the analgesic efficacy of this modality and to determine its role in the overall treatment of patients with PHN pain.

DIABETIC NEUROPATHY

Epidemiology and Risk Factors

The diabetic neuropathies are heterogeneous diseases, affecting many components of the nervous system and presenting with diverse clinical manifestations (Box 21–2). They can be classified into two main categories: generalized neuropathies and focal/multifocal neuropathies. Generalized neuropathies include acute sensory, chronic sensorimotor distal polyneuropathy (DPN), and autonomic. Focal and multifocal neuropathies include cranial, truncal, focal limb, proximal motor (amyotrophy), and chronic inflammatory demyelinating polyneuropathy (CIDP).[100]

BOX 21–2. TYPES OF DIABETIC NEUROPATHIES

- Sensory neuropathy
  - Acute sensorimotor neuropathy
  - Chronic sensorimotor distal polyneuropathy
- Focal and multifocal neuropathies
- Autonomic neuropathies
  - Cardiovascular
  - Gastrointestinal
  - Genitourinary

The World Health Organization estimated that 150 million people had diabetes in the year 2000 and this number was expected to increase to 366 million by the year 2030.[101] Peripheral neuropathy may be present by objective testing in approximately 65% of patients with insulin-dependent diabetes mellitus (IDDM).[102] Of the neuropathies associated with diabetes mellitus, distal symmetric polyneuropathy may be the most common (54%), followed by median nerve mononeuropathy at the wrist (33%), and visceral autonomic neuropathy (7%).[102] For non–insulin-dependent diabetes mellitus (NIDDM), neuropathy may be present in approximately 60% with distal symmetric polyneuropathy being most common (45%), followed by median mononeuropathy (35%), and visceral autonomic neuropathy (5%).[102] Incidence of diabetic neuropathy increases with duration of diabetes, age, and degree of hyperglycemia.[101,103] Neuropathies generally develop after persistence of hyperglycemia for several years and, as such, it is generally a late finding in type 1 diabetes, but may already exist at the time of type 2 diabetes presentation due to delayed diagnosis.[104,105]

Pathophysiology

There are three main theories explaining the pathophysiology of diabetic neuropathy: the polyol pathway, the microvascular, and the glycosylation end-product theories. The three mechanisms probably act simultaneously and there may be some overlap.[103] In addition, neurotrophic factors and neuronal membrane ion channel dysfunction have also been shown to play a role in the development of DPN.[102]

In the *polyol pathway theory*, high blood glucose levels lead to high nerve glucose concentrations. The glucose is converted to sorbitol via the polyol pathway through a series of reactions involving aldose reductase with fructose levels also elevated. High sorbitol and fructose levels decrease expression of the sodium/myoinositol cotransporter leading to decreased myoinositol and phosphoinositide levels, which in turn decreases Na/K ATPase activity. Activation of the aldose reductase depletes cofactor nicotinamide adenine dinucleotide phosphate (NADPH) leading to a decrease in levels of nitric oxide and glutathione, which typically buffer against oxidative injury. A decrease in nitric oxide also results in inhibition of vasodilation, contributing to chronic ischemia.[103]

In the *microvascular theory*, capillary basement membrane thickening and endothelial cell hyperplasia lead to neuronal ischemia and infarction.[103]

Finally, the *glycosylation end-product theory* proposes that chronic hyperglycemia leads to generation of advanced glycosylation end products, which deposit within and around peripheral nerves and interfere with axonal transport, leading to decreased nerve conduction velocities. End products can also deplete NADPH by activation of NADPH oxidase, contributing to hydrogen peroxide formation and further increasing oxidative stress.[103] Neurotrophic factors

are essential for repair of nerve structure and function after an injury. Low levels of nerve growth factor and insulin-like growth factors have been shown to correlate with severity of diabetic neuropathy in animal models.[103] Abnormal calcium channel activity may also contribute to cellular injury and death. Increased activity of voltage-dependent calcium channels has been demonstrated in diabetic neuropathy and may lead to tissue injury. In addition, sodium channel dysfunction also plays a role in the genesis of painful neuropathy.[103]

Clinical Presentation

Acute sensorimotor neuropathy is rare and usually occurs in association with periods of poor metabolic control such as ketoacidosis or sudden changes in glycemic control.[100] Chronic sensorimotor distal polyneuropathy (DPN) is the most common type of diabetic neuropathy.[102] Up to 50% of patients may experience symptoms such as burning pain, electrical or stabbing sensations, paresthesias, hyperesthesias, and deep aching pain, which are generally worse at night.[100] The symptoms typically start in the toes and feet and ascend in the lower limb, typically over several years; however, upper limb involvement is rare.[100] Examination of the lower limbs generally shows sensory loss of vibration, pressure, pain, and temperature perception and absent ankle reflexes.[100] Loss of touch and pin sensation generally occurs before loss of proprioception and vibration, and gait ataxia may occur with severe neuropathy.[103] In addition, signs of peripheral autonomic dysfunction can be seen, including a warm or cold foot, distended dorsal foot veins, dry skin, and calluses under pressure-bearing areas.[100] Sensory loss may lead to complications such as nonhealing ulcers and Charcot joints.[103] DPN is a diagnosis of exclusion and nondiabetic causes such as vitamin B_{12} deficiency, hypothyroidism, and uremia should be considered.[100,103]

Autonomic neuropathy is common and often underreported.[103] Autonomic neuropathies may affect many organ systems but are most notable in the cardiovascular, gastrointestinal, and genitourinary systems. Clinical manifestations include resting tachycardia, orthostatic hypotension, distal anhidrosis, erectile dysfunction, female sexual dysfunction, bladder dysfunction, and gastrointestinal dysfunction with dysmotility syndrome, severe constipation, and diarrhea.[100,103,104]

Multifocal neuropathies comprise a wide spectrum of neuropathies including diabetic amyotrophy, truncal neuropathies, cranial neuropathies, and mononeuropathies. Mononeuropathies most commonly involve the median, ulnar, and common peroneal nerves although cranial neuropathies are extremely rare.[100] These neuropathies most likely result from nerve ischemia because diabetic nerves are more susceptible to compressive injury.[103] Electrophysiologic studies are helpful in identifying blocks in conduction at entrapment sites. Diabetic amyotrophy generally occurs in type 2 diabetics; diabetic anyotrphy is a subacute disease associated with pain and asymmetric weakness and atrophy of proximal lower limb muscles, although distal lower extremity muscles and rarely upper limb muscles may also be involved.[103] Sensory deficits are minimal, but pain is usually severe and there may be loss of the patellar reflex.[103,104]

Treatment Options

With our increasing knowledge of the possible pathophysiologic processes contributing to the neuropathic pain of diabetic neuropathy, we can identify many other potential analgesic agents in addition to those traditionally used for the treatment of neuropathic pain by recognizing potential new pharmacologic targets related to oxidative stress, advanced glycation end products, protein kinase C, and the polyol pathway.[106] Since there is no available treatment that can repair nerve function from damaged nerves, long-term pharmacologic therapy in conjunction with tight glycemic control provides the basis for the successful treatment of diabetic neuropathy (Table 21–4). Details of the mechanisms of action of individual classes of agents are provided elsewhere in this book.

Anticonvulsants. Anticonvulsant agents, such as carbamazepine and gabapentin, have traditionally been used for the treatment of neuropathic pain due to their membrane-stabilizing capabilities. Several systematic reviews indicate that anticonvulsants are very effective for the treatment of pain from diabetic neuropathy. One systematic review examined seven randomized controlled trials (four placebo-controlled, three active control) examining the analgesic efficacy of gabapentin for neuropathic pain.[107] The authors noted that the combined NNT for gabapentin versus placebo in the treatment of pain from diabetic neuropathy was 2.9 (95% CI = 2.2-4.3) with 64% of patients improved on gabapentin versus 28% on placebo.[107] Another systematic review also indicated that gabapentin was effective on a wide variety of neuropathic pain states including diabetic neuropathy.[108] A newer anticonvulsant, pregabalin, has also been shown to be effective for the treatment of pain from diabetic neuropathy in a number of studies.[109-112] The analgesic efficacy of gabapentin may be enhanced when combined with another agent such as morphine.[113]

Table 21–4. Efficacy of Analgesic Options for the Treatment of Diabetic Neuropathy

ANALGESIC OPTION	NUMBERS-NEEDED-TO-TREAT (NNT)*
Anticonvulsants	2.9 [2.2-4.3] [reference 67]
Antidepressants	1.3 [1.2-1.5] [reference 74]
	3.4 [2.6-4.7] [reference 75]
Opioids/Tramadol	2.6 [n/a] [references 85, 86]

*Data presented as mean NNT [95% confidence intervals].
n/a, not available.

Antidepressants. Like anticonvulsant agents, antidepressant agents (specifically the TCAs) have been used for the treatment of neuropathic pain. There have been several systematic reviews examining the analgesic efficacy of TCAs for the treatment of pain from diabetic neuropathy. Both systematic reviews indicate that TCAs are extremely effective to relieve pain of diabetic neuropathy with an NNT of 1.3 (95% CI = 1.2-1.5) from five randomized trials,[114] although one systematic review revealed a higher NNT (less efficacy) of 3.4 (95% CI = 2.6-4.7) from 16 trials.[115] There appears to be little difference in the overall incidence of minor adverse reaction between antidepressants and anticonvulsants, and the analgesic efficacy between the two classes of agents also appears to be similar.[116] Other antidepressant agents, particularly the selective serotonin reuptake inhibitors (SSRIs), are not as effective in relieving pain from diabetic neuropathy.[116]

Local anesthetics. Although intravenous lidocaine has been used to treat pain from diabetic neuropathy, the duration of analgesia and the need for repeated infusions makes this modality of local anesthetic administration impractical.[117] Mexiletine, an oral analogue of lidocaine, has been used for the treatment of diabetic neuropathic pain with mixed success.[118-120] One of the limiting factors for the use of mexiletine is the presence of dose-dependent side effects, which limits its overall analgesic efficacy. Lidocaine can also be administered transdermally as a 5% lidocaine patch and at least one randomized trial indicates that this may be an effective treatment for pain from diabetic neuropathy.[121]

NMDA receptor antagonists. Since the NMDA receptor plays a central role in nociceptive processing and chronic pain, it would be reasonable to expect that NMDA receptor antagonists may attenuate neuropathic pain. There are only a few clinically available forms of NMDA receptor antagonists with dextromethorphan being one of the most commonly available. There are only a few studies examining the analgesic efficacy of NMDA receptor antagonists for diabetic neuropathic pain and as such it is difficult to draw any definitive conclusions regarding the analgesic efficacy of this class of agents for this indication.[122] Dextromethorphan may provide pain relief in some subjects (reduction of pain intensity by 24% to 33%) and may provide greater analgesia with higher doses.[123,124]

Opioids and tramadol. Although opioids have traditionally been viewed as ineffective for the treatment of neuropathic pain, opioids are now recognized as an important and effective analgesic option for the treatment of neuropathic pain. The few studies examining the analgesic efficacy of opioids in diabetic neuropathy suggest that opioids will provide effective analgesia for patients with diabetic neuropathy with an NNT of 2.6 (for at least 50% pain relief).[125,126] Tramadol, an agent that provides analgesia primarily via inhibition of noradrenergic and serotonergic mechanisms, may also provide effective analgesia for diabetic neuropathy.[126]

Other. Because the pathophysiology of diabetic neuropathy is different from that for other types of neuropathic pain, different treatment options are available for the treatment of diabetic neuropathy that may not be effective for other neuropathic pain states. Because oxidative stress may play an important role in the pathogenic mechanisms of diabetic neuropathy, use of antioxidants such as alpha-lipoic acid may have some beneficial effect for the treatment of diabetic neuropathy. A meta-analysis of alpha-lipoic acid for diabetic neuropathy (four trials) demonstrated that administration of alpha-lipoic acid may significantly decrease pain, burning, and numbness from diabetic neuropathy. [127] By interfering with the polyol pathway, which plays a key role in the pathogenesis of the microvascular complications of diabetic neuropathy, aldose reductase inhibitors have been used for the treatment of diabetic neuropathy, although a meta-analysis of available trials did not indicate any benefit with regard to pain control.[128]

AIDS-RELATED PAIN SYNDROMES

With the development and widespread use of highly active antiretroviral therapy (HAART) and the resultant decrease in opportunistic infections of the CNS, polyneuropathy has become the most prevalent neurologic complication associated with human immunodeficiency virus (HIV) infection.[129] Although symptomatic neuropathy occurs in 10% to 35% of those seropositive for HIV, pathologic abnormalities exist in almost all of those with end-stage AIDS.[129,130] There are numerous types of the HIV-associated neuropathy classified by onset, putative etiology, pathology of nerve damage, and motor or sensory involvement (see reference 131 for review). The sensory neuropathies associated with HIV (HIV-SNs) include distal sensory polyneuropathy (DSP) due to the viral infection itself and antiretroviral toxic neuropathy (ATN) due to the medical treatment of the viral illness. DSP represents the more common of the two disorders.

Although these disorders of HIV-SN may represent two distinct entities,[132] the clinical syndrome and pathophysiologic manifestations of the two disorders are practically indistinguishable. The time course of the illness and, in the case of ATN, temporal relation to the commencement of antiretroviral therapy represents the primary differentiating characteristic. The onset of DSP can occur in either the subacute or chronic phases, or following the development of an AIDS-defining illness. The clinical manifestation of ATN can appear within the first week to 6 months of the initiation of antiretroviral therapy and may subside after its cessation.

The clinical features of HIV-SN are dominated by painful dysesthesia, allodynia, and hyperalgesia. Onset is often gradual and most commonly beginning with bilateral lower extremity involvement. The neuropathy progresses in a length-dependent fashion with a worsening gradient of disease from distal structures to those more proximal. The dysesthesias commonly first involve the soles of the feet and progress proximally; when the symptoms encompass the dermatomes of the knee, the patient will often report finger involvement. The first symptoms noted are often a numbness or burning sensation following a diurnal cycle with the pain worse at night. Shortly thereafter, patients will report allodynia (a stimulus previously not found to be noxious is perceived as painful) and hyperalgesia (a lower pain threshold) of the involved structures. As a result, wearing shoes and walking become painful and the patient's gait becomes antalgic. There is minimal subjective or objective lower extremity motor involvement and is generally limited to the intrinsic muscles of the foot. Physical examination reveals a diminution or loss of ankle reflexes in addition to the sensory findings.

Serum and CSF laboratory examinations are unrevealing. Electrophysiologic studies, although primarily testing large myelinated fibers, show an axonal, length-dependent, sensory polyneuropathy. Skin biopsies of the distal lower extremity reveal decreased intraepidermal nerve density indicative of loss of small, unmyelinated fibers[133,134] and later wallerian degeneration of myelinated fibers similar to autonomic neuropathy of diabetes mellitus. Dorsal root ganglion (DRG) neuronal loss has been reported, although the reduction is more modest than that of the distal axon loss.[135]

The pathogenesis of DSP axonal loss or DRG loss has not been fully elucidated. It may represent both direct peripheral nerve damage by the virus or the indirect consequences of the infection resulting in an aberrant inflammatory response from the activation cytokines and other inflammatory mediators. Likewise, the pathogenesis of pain in DSP is not fully explained by the direct action of the virus or the multifocal inflammatory response. Gp120, the viral coat protein of HIV, has been found to produce pain in rats when administered epineurally to the sciatic nerve[136] and intradermally into the paw.[137] It also directly stimulates small neurons of the DRG,[137] suggesting HIV can directly activate peripheral nerves and result in pain. The indirect causes of DSP pain are both thought to be mediated inflammatory injury.[131] These can be divided into a peripheral and a central mechanism. The peripheral hypothesis is that the pain results from spontaneous activity of uninjured pain-transmitting or C fibers after the injury of adjacent fibers. These fibers may be further sensitized by inflammatory mediators released by macrophages. The central hypothesis involves alteration in ion channels in the DRG combined with changes in the spinal cord dorsal horn resulting in "central sensitization."

The pathogenesis of ATN is directly related to the use of nucleoside reverse transcriptase inhibitors (NRTIs). In the past decade, the incidence of HIV-SN has increased with the introduction and increased use of NRTIs. The NRTIs (ddC, ddI, d4T) are known to be neurotoxic and in phase I clinical trials of ddC, ATN was found to be a dose- and duration-related phenomenon.[138] ddI and d4T are less neurotoxic when administered alone; however, the combination of the two along with other HIV medications increases the risk of development of ATN considerably.[139] Toxicity of NRTIs is thought to be mediated by mitochondrial dysfunction, resulting in lactic acidosis, mitochondrial DNA depletion, and cellular death. Unfortunately the damage is not always reversible; cessation of NRTI therapy results in improvement of symptoms in only one third of patients.

Treatment of HIV-SN is symptomatic because there are no therapies proven to restore the underlying pathology to the preinjured state. Treatment begins with optimization of the patient's metabolic and nutritional status and exclusion of alternate explanations for the neurologic symptoms. In some patients with presumed ATN, drug cessation or dose reduction of NRTIs can be beneficial. However, the symptoms of ATN can worsen for up to 2 months after cessation of therapy. A number of studies have been performed to investigate the efficacy of some therapies in the control of neuropathic pain symptoms of HIV-SN. Unfortunately, therapies commonly applied in patients with non–HIV-SN–related neuropathic pain including amitriptyline, mexiletine, or topical capsaicin did not show any benefit in double-blind, randomized, placebo-controlled trials (RCTs).[140-142] Less traditional therapies including acupuncture and peptide T treatment were also without benefit.[142,143] An 18-week RCT found treatment with nerve growth factor (NGF) (0.1 to 0.3 mg/kg) produced a significant improvement in pain in patients with HIV-SN.[144] In two RCTs, lamotrigine (300 mg/day) was found to significantly reduce pain in DSP but not ATN[145] and in a larger trial in ATN as well.[146] Most recently, the evidence for the effectiveness of gabapentin in the treatment of pain associated with HIV-SN, which had previously been solely derived from case reports and open label trials,[147,148] has now been supported by a properly conducted RCT.[149] In this study, after 4 weeks of gabapentin therapy (1200 to 3600 mg/day), pain and sleep interference scores were significantly lower in the gabapentin group as compared to the placebo group. Adverse events were minimal; the only statistically significant side effect was increased somnolence.

HIV-SN is now the most prevalent neurologic consequence of HIV infection. Although the advent of NRTI has produced an enormous morbidity and mortality benefit for those suffering with HIV, it has also increased the incidence of HIV-SN directly and indirectly. The incidence and prevalence of HIV-SN are substantial, and as other morbidities associated with HIV infection are lessened by aggressive pharmacotherapy, the need for effective treatment of this neuropathic pain becomes imperative.

CONCLUSION

Despite the diversity of conditions and pathophysiologies categorized as neuropathic pain, many of the underlying options for the treatment of these diverse conditions are comparable. Traditional systemic analgesic agents, such as antidepressants, anticonvulsants, local anesthetics, and opioids, are typically the mainstay of treatment for neuropathic pain, although the efficacy of individual classes of agents vary by specific type of neuropathic pain. Fewer high-quality trials are available for interventional options for the treatment of neuropathic pain, and clinicians should be aware that there is a paucity of high-quality trials to support the use of traditional interventional options in some cases.

SUMMARY

- The current IASP criteria results in the overdiagnosis of CRPS; a modification of the criteria has been proposed to increase sensitivity for clinicians and specificity for researchers.
- No laboratory test currently provides a gold standard for the diagnosis of CRPS. Following a thorough history and examination, tests such as those testing for difference in skin temperature help to confirm diagnosis.
- Evidence from studies on neuropathic pain suggests that anticonvulsants and antidepressants should be considered first line. Opioids should be used as second-line treatment to enhance pain control.
- Available evidence suggests that SCS is effective in patients who do not respond to conservative management. Further research is required to define mechanisms of pain relief and to provide more robust evidence for efficacy.
- The severity of acute pain during herpes zoster is an important risk factor for the development of PHN and clinicians should be aggressive in treating pain of herpes zoster.
- Although opioid therapy, tricyclic antidepressants, gabapentin/pregablin, and tramadol are effective therapies for the treatment of PHN pain, very few interventional therapies have been shown to be as effective, although additional trials are needed on intrathecal methylprednisolone.
- Diabetic neuropathy is a common complication from diabetes mellitus and although traditional analgesic agents (e.g., antidepressants, anticonvulsants, opioids) are effective for the treatment of pain from diabetic neuropathy, other agents may also be effective, reflecting the different pathophysiologic mechanisms underlying diabetic neuropathy.
- HIV-SN is the most common neurologic complication of HIV infection. Treatment of HIV-SN is symptomatic and the typical agents used for the treatment of neuropathic pain (e.g., antidepressants, local anesthetic, capsaicin) may not be effective for this type of neuropathic pain.

References

1. Raja SN, Grabow TS: Complex regional pain syndrome I (reflex sympathetic dystrophy). Anesthesiology 2002;96:1254-1260.
2. Veldman PH, Reynen HM, Arntz IE, et al: Signs and symptoms of reflex sympathetic dystrophy: Prospective study of 829 patients. Lancet 1993;342:1012-1016.

3. Shefali A, Broatch J, Raja SN: Web-based epidemiological survey of complex regional pain syndrome-1 (poster). The American Society of Anesthesiologists, New Orleans, 2005.

4. Allen G, Galer BS, Schwartz L: Epidemiology of complex regional pain syndrome: A retrospective chart review of 134 patients. Pain 1999;80:539-544.

5. Lynch ME: Psychological aspects of reflex sympathetic dystrophy: A review of the adult and pediatric literature. Pain 1992;49:337-347.

6. Kemler MA, de Vet HCW: Health-related quality of life in chronic refractory reflex sympathetic dystrophy (complex regional pain syndrome type I). J Pain Symptom Manage 2000;20:68-76.

7. Janig W: Pathophysiology of complex regional pain syndrome. Pain 2005 an updated review. Seattle, IASP Press, 2005, pp 307-316.

8. Janig W, Baron R: Complex regional pain syndrome is a disease of the central nervous system. Clin Auton Res 2002;12:150-164.

9. Mailis-Gagnon A, Giannoylis I, Downar J, et al: Altered central somatosensory processing in chronic pain patients with hysterical anesthesia. Neurology 2003;60:1501-1507.

10. Maihofner C, Handwerker HO, Neundofer B, et al: Patterns of cortical reorganization in complex regional pain syndrome. Neurology 2003;61:1707-1715.

11. Maihofner C, Handwerker HO, Neundofer B, et al: Cortical reorganization in during recovery from complex regional pain syndrome. Neurology 2004;63:693-701.

12. Schwenkreis P, Janssen F, Rommel O, et al: Bilateral motor cortex disinhibition in complex regional pain syndrome (CRPS) type I of the hand. Neurology 2003;61:515-519.

13. Woolf CJ, Mannion RJ: Neuropathic pain: Aetiology, symptoms, mechanisms, and management. Lancet 1999;353:1959-1964.

14. Rommel O, Gehling M, Dertwinkel R, et al: Hemisensory impairment in patients with complex regional pain syndrome. Pain 1999;80:95-101.

15. Torebjork E, Wahren L, Wallin G, et al: Noradrenalin-evoked pain in neuralgia. Pain 1995;63:11-20.

16. Ali Z, Raja SN, Wesselmann U, et al: Intradermal injection of norepinephrine evokes pain in patients with sympathetically maintained pain. Pain 2000;88:161-168.

17. Janig W, Baron R: Complex regional pain syndrome: Mystery explained? Lancet Neurology 2003;2:687-697.

18. Woolf CJ, Ma QP, Poole S: Peripheral cell types contributing to the analgesic action of nerve growth factor in inflammation. J Neurosci 1996;16:6-23.

19. Stanton-Hicks M, Jänig W, Hassenbusch S, Haddox JD, et al: Reflex sympathetic dystrophy: Changing concepts and taxonomy. Pain 1995;63:127-133.

20. Reinders M, Geertzen J, Dijkstra PU: Complex regional pain syndrome type I: Use of the International Association for the Study of Pain diagnostic criteria defined in 1994. Clin J Pain 2002;18:207-215.

21. Bruehl S, Harden RN, Galer BS, et al: External validation of IASP diagnostic criteria for complex regional pain syndrome and proposed research diagnostic criteria. Pain 1999;81:147-154.

22. Baron R, Binder A, Lugwig J, et al: Diagnostic tools and evidence-based treatment of complex regional pain syndrome. Pain 2005 an updated review. Seattle, IASP Press, 2005, pp 293-306.

23. Schurmann M, Gradl G, Andress HJ, et al: Assessment of peripheral sympathetic nervous function for diagnosing early post-traumatic complex regional pain syndrome type I. Pain 1999;80:149-159.

24. Harden RN, Bruehl S, Galer BS, et al: Complex regional pain syndrome: Are the IASP diagnostic criteria valid and sufficiently comprehensive? Pain 1999;83:211-219.

25. Wasner G, Schattschneider J, Baron R: Skin temperature side differences—A diagnostic tool for CRPS? Pain 2002;98:19-26.

26. Wasner G, Schattschneider J, Heckmann K, et al: Vascular abnormalities in reflex sympathetic dystrophy (CRPS): Mechanism and diagnostic value. Brain 2001;124:587-599.

27. Gellman H, Keenan MA, Stone L, et al: Reflex sympathetic dystrophy in brain-injured patients. Pain 1992;51:307-311.

28. Coderre TJ, Xanthos DN, Francis L, et al: Chronic post-ischemia pain (CPIP): A novel animal model of complex regional pain syndrome-type I (CRPS-I; reflex sympathetic dystrophy) produced by prolonged hindpaw ischemia and reperfusion in the rat. Pain 2004;112:94-105.

29. Connelly NR, Reuben S, Brull SJ: Intravenous regional anesthesia with ketorolac-lidocaine for the management of sympathetically-mediated pain. Yale J Biol Med 1995;68:95-99.

30. Raja SN, Haythornthwaite JA, Pappagallo et al: Opioids versus antidepressants in postherpetic neuralgia: A randomised, placebo-controlled trial. Neurology 2002;59:1015-1021.

31. Max MB, Culnane M, Schafer SC, et al: Amitriptyline relieves diabetic neuropathy pain with normal or depressed mood. Neurology 1987;37:589-596.

32. Goldstein DJ, Lu Y, Detke MJ, et al: Duloxetine vs. placebo in patients with painful diabetic neuropathy. Pain 2005;116:109-118.

33. Westanmo AD, Gayken J, Haight R: Duloxetine: A balanced and selective norepinephrine- and serotonin-reuptake inhibitor. Am J Health Syst Pharm 2005;62:2481-2490.

34. Freynhagen R, Strojek K, Griesing T, et al: Efficacy of pregabalin in neuropathic pain evaluated in a 12-week, randomised, double-blind, multicentre, placebo-controlled trial of flexible- and fixed-dose regimens. Pain 2005;115:254-263.

35. van de Vusse AC, Stomp-van den Berg SG, Kessels AH, et al: Randomised controlled trial of gabapentin in complex regional pain syndrome type 1. BMC Neurol 2004;29:4-13.

36. Becker WJ, Ablett DP, Harris CJ, et al: Long term treatment of intractable reflex sympathetic dystrophy with intrathecal morphine. Can J Neurol Sci 1995;22:153-159.

37. Perez RS, Zuurmond WW, Bezemer PD, et al: The treatment of complex regional pain syndrome type I with free radical scavengers: A randomized controlled study. Pain 2003;102:297-307.

38. Hord AH, Rooks MD, Stephens BO, et al: Intravenous regional bretylium and lidocaine for treatment of reflex sympathetic dystrophy: A randomized, double-blind study. Anesth Analg 1992;74:818-821.

39. Price DD, Long S, Wilsey B, et al: Analysis of peak magnitude and duration of analgesia produced by local anesthetics injected into sympathetic ganglia of complex regional pain syndrome patients. Clin J Pain 1998;14:216-226.

40. Grabow TS, Tella PK, Raja SN: Spinal cord stimulation for complex regional pain syndrome: An evidence-based medicine review of the literature. Clin J Pain 2003;19:371-383.

41. Johnson RW, Whitton TL: Management of herpes zoster (shingles) and postherpetic neuralgia. Expert Opin Pharmacother 2004;5:551-559.

42. Opstelten W, van Wijck AJ, Stolker RJ: Interventions to prevent postherpetic neuralgia: Cutaneous and percutaneous techniques. Pain 2004;107:202-206.

43. Johnson RW, Dworkin RH: Treatment of herpes zoster and postherpetic neuralgia. BMJ 2003;326:748-750.

44. Argoff CE, Katz N, Backonja M: Treatment of postherpetic neuralgia: A review of therapeutic options. J Pain Symptom Manage 2004;28:396-411.

45. Jackson JL, Gibbons R, Meyer G, et al: The effect of treating herpes zoster with oral acyclovir in preventing postherpetic neuralgia: A meta-analysis. Arch Intern Med 1997;157:909-912.

46. Oxman MN, Levin MJ, Johnson GR, et al: A vaccine to prevent herpes zoster and postherpetic neuralgia in older adults. N Engl J Med 2005;352:2271-2284.

47. Schmader K: Herpes zoster in older adults. Clin Infect Dis 2001;32:1481-1486.

48. Rowbotham M, Harden N, Stacey B, et al: Gabapentin for the treatment of postherpetic neuralgia: A randomized controlled trial. JAMA 1998;280:1837-1842.

49. Bennett MI, Simpson KH: Gabapentin in the treatment of neuropathic pain. Palliat Med 2004;18:5-11.

50. Maneuf YP, Gonzalez MI, Sutton KS, et al: Cellular and molecular action of the putative GABA-mimetic, gabapentin. Cell Mol Life Sci 2003;60:742-750.
51. Hempenstall K, Nurmikko TJ, Johnson RW: Analgesic therapy in postherpetic neuralgia: A quantitative systematic review. PLoS Med 2005;2:e164.
52. Rice AS, Maton S, Postherpetic Neuralgia Study Group: Gabapentin in postherpetic neuralgia: A randomised, double blind, placebo controlled study. Pain 2001;94:215-224.
53. Backonja M, Glanzman RL: Gabapentin dosing for neuropathic pain: Evidence from randomized, placebo-controlled clinical trials. Clin Ther 2003;25:81-104.
54. Frampton JE, Foster RH: Pregabalin: In the treatment of postherpetic neuralgia. Drugs 2005;65:111-118.
55. Freynhagen R, Strojek K, Griesing T, et al: Efficacy of pregabalin in neuropathic pain evaluated in a 12-week, randomised, double-blind, multicentre, placebo-controlled trial of flexible- and fixed-dose regimens. Pain 2005;115:254-263.
56. Dworkin RH, Corbin AE, Young JP Jr, et al: Pregabalin for the treatment of postherpetic neuralgia: A randomized, placebo-controlled trial. Neurology 2003 22;60:1274-1283.
57. Gilron I, Max MB: Combination pharmacotherapy for neuropathic pain: Current evidence and future directions. Expert Rev Neurother 2005;5:823-830.
58. Comer AM, Lamb HM: Lidocaine patch 5%. Drugs 2000;59:245-249.
59. Gammaitoni AR, Alvarez NA, Galer BS: Safety and tolerability of the lidocaine patch 5%, a targeted peripheral analgesic: A review of the literature. J Clin Pharmacol 2003;43:111-117.
60. Davies PS, Galer BS: Review of lidocaine patch 5% studies in the treatment of postherpetic neuralgia. Drugs 2004;64:937-947.
61. Argoff CE, Galer BS, Jensen MP, et al: Effectiveness of the lidocaine patch 5% on pain qualities in three chronic pain states: Assessment with the neuropathic pain scale. Curr Med Res Opin 2004;20(suppl 2):S21-28.
62. Katz NP, Gammaitoni AR, Davis MW, et al: Lidocaine patch 5% reduces pain intensity and interference with quality of life in patients with postherpetic neuralgia: An effectiveness trial. Pain Med 2002;3:324-332.
63. Galer BS, Rowbotham MC, Perander J, et al: Topical lidocaine patch relieves postherpetic neuralgia more effectively than a vehicle topical patch: Results of an enriched enrollment study. Pain 1999;80:533-538.
64. Dellemijn P: Are opioids effective in relieving neuropathic pain? Pain 1999;80:453-462.
65. Benedetti F, Vighetti S, Amanzio M, et al: Dose-response relationship in nociception and neuropathic postoperative pain. Pain 1998;74:205-211.
66. Wu CL, Tella P, Staats PS, et al: Analgesic effects of intravenous lidocaine and morphine on postamputation pain: A randomized double-blind, active placebo-controlled, crossover trial. Anesthesiology 2002;96:841-848.
67. Rowbotham MC, Reisner-Keller LA, Fields HL, et al: Both intravenous lidocaine and morphine reduce the pain of postherpetic neuralgia. Neurology 1991;41:1024-1028.
68. Rowbotham MC, Twilling L, Davies PS, et al: Oral opioid therapy for chronic peripheral and central neuropathic pain. N Engl J Med 2003;348:1223-1232.
69. Raja SN, Haythornthwaite JA, Pappagallo M, et al: Opioids versus antidepressants in postherpetic neuralgia: A randomized, placebo-controlled trial. Neurology 2002;59:1015-1021.
70. Dellemijn PL, Vanneste JA: Randomised double-blind active-placebo-controlled crossover trial of intravenous fentanyl in neuropathic pain. Lancet 1997;349:753-758.
71. Watson CP, Babul N: Efficacy of oxycodone in neuropathic pain: A randomized trial in postherpetic neuralgia. Neurology 1998;50:1837-1841.
72. Rowbotham MC, Reisner LA, Davies PS, et al: Treatment response in antidepressant-naive postherpetic neuralgia patients: Double-blind, randomized trial. J Pain 2005;6:741-746.
73. Sindrup SH, Jensen TS: Efficacy of pharmacological treatments of neuropathic pain: An update and effect related to mechanism of drug action. Pain 1999;83:389-400.
74. Collins SL, Moore RA, McQuay HJ, et al: Antidepressants and anticonvulsants for diabetic neuropathy and postherpetic neuralgia: A quantitative systematic review. J Pain Symptom Manage 2000;20:449-458.
75. Graff-Radford SB, Shaw LR, et al: Amitriptyline and fluphenazine in the treatment of postherpetic neuralgia. Clin J Pain 2000;16:188-192.
76. Janig W, Levine JD, Michaelis M, et al: Interactions of sympathetic and primary afferent neurons following nerve injury and tissue trauma. Prog Brain Res 1996;113:161-184.
77. Choi B, Rowbotham MC: Effect of adrenergic receptor activation on post-herpetic neuralgia pain and sensory disturbances. Pain 1997;69:55-63.
78. Colding A: The effect of regional sympathetic blocks in the treatment of herpes zoster. Acta Anaesthesiol Scand 1969;13:133-141.
79. Colding A: Treatment of pain: organization of a pain clinic: Treatment of acute herpes zoster. Proc R Soc Med 1973;66:541-543.
80. Winnie AP, Hartwell PW: Relationship between time of treatment of acute herpes zoster with sympathetic blockade and prevention of post-herpetic neuralgia: Clinical support for a new theory of the mechanism by which sympathetic blockade provides therapeutic benefit. Reg Anesth 1993;18:277-282.
81. Kingery WS: A critical review of controlled clinical trials for peripheral neuropathic pain and complex regional pain syndromes. Pain 1997;73:123-139.
82. Hogan QH, Abram SE: Neural blockade for diagnosis and prognosis. Anesthesiology 1997;86:216-241.
83. Yanagida H, Suwa K, Corssen G: No prophylactic effect of early sympathetic blockade on postherpetic neuralgia. Anesthesiology 1987;66:73-76.
84. Tenicela R, Lovasik D, Eaglstein W: Treatment of herpes zoster with sympathetic blocks. Clin J Pain 1985;1:63-67.
85. Dworkin RH, Boon RJ, Griffin DR, et al: Postherpetic neuralgia: Impact of famciclovir, age, rash severity, and acute pain in herpes zoster patients. J Infect Dis 1998;178(suppl 1):S76-80.
86. Perkins FM, Kehlet H: Chronic pain as an outcome of surgery. A review of predictive factors. Anesthesiology 2000;93:1123-1133.
87. Kissin I: Pre-emptive analgesia. Anesthesiology 2000;93:1138-1143.
88. Ahn HJ, Lim HK, Lee YB, et al: The effects of famciclovir and epidural block in the treatment of herpes zoster. J Dermatol 2001;28:208-216.
89. Higa K, Hori K, Harasawa I, et al: High thoracic epidural block relieves acute herpetic pain involving the trigeminal and cervical regions: Comparison with effects of stellate ganglion block. Reg Anesth Pain Med 1998;23:25-29.
90. Hwang SM, Kang YC, Lee YB, et al: The effects of epidural blockade on the acute pain in herpes zoster. Arch Dermatol 1999;135:1359-1364.
91. Watson CP, Deck JH, Morshead C, et al: Post-herpetic neuralgia: Further post-mortem studies of cases with and without pain. Pain 1991;44:105-117.
92. Kikuchi A, Kotani N, Sato T, et al: Comparative therapeutic evaluation of intrathecal versus epidural methylprednisolone for long-term analgesia in patients with intractable postherpetic neuralgia. Reg Anesth Pain Med 1999;24:287-293.
93. Kotani N, Kushikata T, Hashimoto H, et al: Intrathecal methylprednisolone for intractable postherpetic neuralgia. N Engl J Med 2000;343:1514-1519.
94. Cunha FQ, Lorenzetti BB, Poole S, et al: Interleukin-8 as a mediator of sympathetic pain. Br J Pharmacol 1991;104:765-767.
95. Nelson DA: Intraspinal therapy using methylprednisolone acetate: Twenty-three years of clinical controversy. Spine 1993;18:278-286.
96. Wilkinson HA: Intrathecal Depo-Medrol: A literature review. Clin J Pain 1992;8:49-56.

97. Krames E: Implantable devices for pain control: Spinal cord stimulation and intrathecal therapies. Best Pract Res Clin Anaesthesiol 2002;16:619-649.

98. Harke H, Gretenkort P, Ladleif HU, et al: Spinal cord stimulation in postherpetic neuralgia and in acute herpes zoster pain. Anesth Analg 2002;94:694-700.

99. Turner JA, Loeser JD, Deyo RA, et al: Spinal cord stimulation for patients with failed back surgery syndrome or complex regional pain syndrome: A systematic review of effectiveness and complications. Pain 2004;108:137-147.

100. Boulton AJ, Viink AI, Arezzo JC, et al: Diabetic neuropathies: A statement by the American Diabetes Association. Diabetes Care 2005;28:956-962.

101. Rathur HM, Boulton AJ: Recent advances in the diagnosis and management of diabetic neuropathy. J Bone Joint Surg Br 2005;87:1605-1610.

102. Gooch C, Podwall D: The diabetic neuropathies. Neurologist 2004;10:311-322.

103. Kelkar P: Diabetic neuropathy. Semin Neurol 2005;25:168-173.

104. Aring AM, Jones DE, Falko JM: Evaluation and prevention of diabetic neuropathy. Am Fam Physician 2005;71:2123-2128.

105. Sinnreich M, Taylor BV, Dyck PJ: Diabetic neuropathies: Classification, clinical features, and pathophysiological basis. Neurologist 2005;11:63-79.

106. Rathur HM, Boulton AJ: Recent advances in the diagnosis and management of diabetic neuropathy. J Bone Joint Surg Br 2005;87:1605-1610.

107. Wiffen PJ, McQuay HJ, Edwards JE, et al: Gabapentin for acute and chronic pain. Cochrane Database Syst Rev 2005;(3): CD005452.

108. Mellegers MA, Furlan AD, Mailis A: Gabapentin for neuropathic pain: systematic review of controlled and uncontrolled literature. Clin J Pain 2001;17:284-295.

109. Lesser H, Sharma U, LaMoreaux L, et al: Pregabalin relieves symptoms of painful diabetic neuropathy: A randomized controlled trial. Neurology 2004;63:2104-2110.

110. Freynhagen R, Strojek K, Griesing T, et al: Efficacy of pregabalin in neuropathic pain evaluated in a 12-week, randomised, double-blind, multicentre, placebo-controlled trial of flexible- and fixed-dose regimens. Pain 2005;115: 254-263.

111. Richter RW, Portenoy R, Sharma U, et al: Relief of painful diabetic peripheral neuropathy with pregabalin: A randomized, placebo-controlled trial. J Pain 2005;6:253-260.

112. Frampton JE, Scott LJ: Pregabalin: In the treatment of painful diabetic peripheral neuropathy. Drugs 2004;64:2813-2820.

113. Gilron I, Bailey JM, Tu D, et al: Morphine, gabapentin, or their combination for neuropathic pain. N Engl J Med 2005;352:1324-1334.

114. Saarto T, Wiffen PJ: Antidepressants for neuropathic pain. Cochrane Database Syst Rev 2005;(3):CD005454.

115. Collins SL, Moore RA, McQuayHJ, et al: Antidepressants and anticonvulsants for diabetic neuropathy and postherpetic neuralgia: A quantitative systematic review. J Pain Symptom Manage 2000;20:449-458.

116. Adriaensen H, Plaghki L, Mathieu C, et al: Critical review of oral drug treatments for diabetic neuropathic pain-clinical outcomes based on efficacy and safety data from placebo-controlled and direct comparative studies. Diabetes Metab Res Rev 2005;21:231-240.

117. Kastrup J, Petersen P, Dejgard A, et al: Intravenous lidocaine infusion—A new treatment of chronic painful diabetic neuropathy? Pain 1987;28:69-75.

118. Stracke H, Meyer UE, Schumacher HE, et al: Mexiletine in the treatment of diabetic neuropathy. Diabetes Care 1992;15:1550-1555.

119. Wright JM, Oki JC, Graves L 3rd: Mexiletine in the symptomatic treatment of diabetic peripheral neuropathy. Ann Pharmacother 1997;31:29-34.

120. Oskarsson P, Ljunggren JG, Lins PE: Efficacy and safety of mexiletine in the treatment of painful diabetic neuropathy.

The Mexiletine Study Group. Diabetes Care 1997;20: 1594-1597.

121. Barbano RL, Herrmann DN, Hart-Gouleau S, et al: Effectiveness, tolerability, and impact on quality of life of the 5% lidocaine patch in diabetic polyneuropathy. Arch Neurol 2004;61:914-918.

122. Criner TM, Perdun CS: Dextromethorphan and diabetic neuropathy. Ann Pharmacother 1999;33:1221-1223.

123. Nelson KA, Park KM, Robinovitz E, et al: High-dose oral dextromethorphan versus placebo in painful diabetic neuropathy and postherpetic neuralgia. Neurology 1997;48: 1212-1218.

124. Sang CN, Booher S, Gilron I, et al: Dextromethorphan and memantine in painful diabetic neuropathy and postherpetic neuralgia: Efficacy and dose-response trials. Anesthesiology 2002;96:1053-1061.

125. Watson CP, Moulin D, Watt-Watson J, et al: Controlled-release oxycodone relieves neuropathic pain: A randomized controlled trial in painful diabetic neuropathy. Pain 2003;105:71-78.

126. Gimbel JS, Richards P, Portenoy RK: Controlled-release oxycodone for pain in diabetic neuropathy: A randomized controlled trial. Neurology 2003;60:927-934.

127. Ziegler D, Nowak H, Kempler P, et al: Treatment of symptomatic diabetic polyneuropathy with the antioxidant alpha-lipoic acid: A meta-analysis. Diabet Med 2004;21:114-121.

128. Airey M, Bennett C, Nicolucci A, et al: Aldose reductase inhibitors for the prevention and treatment of diabetic peripheral neuropathy. Cochrane Database Syst Rev 2000;(2): CD002182.

129. Verma A: Epidemiology and clinical features of HIV-1 associated neuropathies. J Peripher Nerv Syst 2001;61:8-13.

130. Schifitto G, McDermott MP, McArthur JC, et al: Incidence of and risk factors for HIV-associated distal sensory polyneuropathy. Neurology 2002;5812:1764-1768.

131. Keswani SC, Pardo CA, Cherry CL, et al: HIV-associated sensory neuropathies. AIDS 2002;1616:2105-2117.

132. Luciano CA, Pardo CA, McArthur JC: Recent developments in the HIV neuropathies. Curr Opin Neurol 2003;163: 403-409.

133. McCarthy BG, Hsieh ST, Stocks A, et al: Cutaneous innervation in sensory neuropathies: Evaluation by skin biopsy. Neurology 1995;4510:1848-1855.

134. Polydefkis M, Yiannoutsos CT, Cohen BA, et al: Reduced intraepidermal nerve fiber density in HIV-associated sensory neuropathy. Neurology 2002;581:115-119.

135. Bradley WG, Shapshak P, Delgado S, et al: Morphometric analysis of the peripheral neuropathy of AIDS. Muscle Nerve 1998;219:1188-1195.

136. Herzberg U, Sagen J: Peripheral nerve exposure to HIV viral envelope protein gp120 induces neuropathic pain and spinal gliosis. J Neuroimmunol 2001;1161:29-39.

137. Oh SB, Tran PB, Gillard SE, et al: Chemokines and glycoprotein 120 produce pain hypersensitivity by directly exciting primary nociceptive neurons. J Neurosci 2001;2114: 5027-5035.

138. Berger AR, Arezzo JC, Schaumburg HH, et al: 2′,3′-dideoxy-cytidine (ddC) toxic neuropathy: A study of 52 patients. Neurology 1993;432:358-362.

139. Moore RD, Wong WM, Keruly JC, et al: Incidence of neuropathy in HIV-infected patients on monotherapy versus those on combination therapy with didanosine, stavudine and hydroxyurea. AIDS 2000;143:273-278.

140. Kieburtz K, Simpson D, Yiannoutsos C, et al: A randomized trial of amitriptyline and mexiletine for painful neuropathy in HIV infection. AIDS Clinical Trial Group 242 Protocol Team. Neurology 1998;516:1682-1688.

141. Paice JA, Ferrans CE, Lashley FR, et al: Topical capsaicin in the management of HIV-associated peripheral neuropathy. J Pain Symptom Manage 2000;191:45-52.

142. Shlay JC, Chaloner K, Max MB, et al: Acupuncture and amitriptyline for pain due to HIV-related peripheral neuropathy: a randomized controlled trial. Terry Beirn Community Programs for Clinical Research on AIDS. JAMA 1998;28018: 1590-1595.

143. Simpson DM, Dorfman D, Olney RK, et al: Peptide T in the treatment of painful distal neuropathy associated with AIDS: results of a placebo-controlled trial. The Peptide T Neuropathy Study Group. Neurology 1996;475:1254-1259.

144. McArthur JC, Yiannoutsos C, Simpson DM, et al: A phase II trial of nerve growth factor for sensory neuropathy associated with HIV infection. AIDS Clinical Trials Group Team 291. Neurology 2000;545:1080-1088.

145. Simpson DM, Olney R, McArthur JC, et al: A placebo-controlled trial of lamotrigine for painful HIV-associated neuropathy. Neurology 2000;5411:2115-2119.

146. Simpson DM, McArthur JC, Olney R, et al: Lamotrigine for HIV-associated painful sensory neuropathies: A placebo-controlled trial. Neurology 2003;609:1508-1514.

147. La Spina I, Porazzi D, Maggiolo F, et al: Gabapentin in painful HIV-related neuropathy: A report of 19 patients, preliminary observations. Eur J Neurol 2001;81:71-75.

148. Newshan G: HIV neuropathy treated with gabapentin. Aids 1998;122:219-221.

149. Hahn K, Arendt G, Braun JS, et al: A placebo-controlled trial of gabapentin for painful HIV-associated sensory neuropathies. J Neurol 2004;25110:1260-1266.

CHAPTER
22   Phantom Limb Pain

Richard W. Rosenquist and Naeem Haider

Ambroise Paré (1510-1590), a barber surgeon, is credited with the first documented account of phantom limb pain in the medical literature (Fig. 22–1).[1,2] Further accounts by Descartes, Lemos, and Bell, documented over the centuries, led to the use of the term *phantom* by surgeon Silas Weir Mitchell (1871) in his report on amputees returning from the American Civil War.[1] Despite major advances in the understanding of pain physiology and improved treatment in recent decades, persistent pain following the loss of a body part (phantom pain) continues to produce disabling consequences in many patients. Phantom pain has been described involving limbs, digits, eyes, nose, teeth, tongue, breasts, bladder, anus, and genital organs.[3] Out of the many treatments available, few have undergone rigorous critical investigation. An understanding of events occurring in both the peripheral and central nervous system may assist in the development of more effective means to prevent and treat phantom pain. This chapter describes the clinical presentation of phantom limb pain, postulated pathophysiologic mechanisms underlying its development, and current views on treatment aimed at prevention or resolution of symptoms associated with the disorder.

CLASSIFICATION

Phantom limb pain, as described by Nikolajsen and Jensen,[4] is one of three possible presentations following amputation:
1. Phantom pain: painful sensation referred to the phantom limb
2. Phantom sensation: any sensation, other than pain, in the phantom limb
3. Stump pain: pain localized to the stump

Patients with phantom limb sensations readily distinguish unpleasant or annoying sensations from those they regard as painful. Phantom pain is often described as intense normal exteroceptive sensations. Some patients offer bizarre descriptors, such as "my foot is being crushed by a bar rolling over it and my toes are twisted." Amputees often describe their pain as burning, tingling, cramping, shocking, shooting, or a feeling of "pins and needles." The characteristic of the phantom pain often mimics the preamputation pain state of the affected extremity.[5,6]

Virtually all amputees experience phantom sensations.[7,8] Nonpainful sensations do not usually pose a clinical problem. This is not the case with phantom limb pain. Nonpainful phantom sensations may be divided into three types. Kinetic sensations (movement) that may be perceived as if spontaneous or willed. Kinesthetic perceptions are those of the size, shape, and position of the body part, which may be normal or distorted. Exteroceptive perceptions of touch, pressure, temperature, itch, and vibration may be troubling to patients to a greater degree than painful sensations. It is common for patients to report more intense sensations in the distal phantom limb or in the nipple of the phantom breast. Phantom visceral organs may be associated with functional sensations such as the urge to urinate or defecate. Phantom sensations have been studied in healthy subjects using a combination of acute pain to the hand, followed by non-noxious tactile stimulation of the ipsilateral lip.[9] During stimulation, 2 out of 6 subjects reported phantom-like sensations in the hand, leading to the conclusion that even in the absence of deafferentation that accompanies amputation, pain can lead to a representational reorganization.

INCIDENCE

The incidence and severity of significant phantom pain is much higher than many physicians recognize. In surveys of 11,000 amputee veterans, 80% of respondents reported having significant phantom pain.[10,11] The high incidence with which this phenomenon occurs makes it a significant medical problem. In another study, amputees were asked to rate pain intensity on a scale from 0 to 10. The average intensity of phantom pain was 5.3, the worst was 7.7 and the least was 2.9.[12] Onset of pain may be immediate, but commonly occurs within the first few days following amputation.[11,13] In 10% to 33% of patients, pain may be delayed for more than a year and cases have been reported to have been delayed as long as 30 years.[14] Late onset pain may be gradual or sudden and its time course is variable in its resolution. Reactivation of phantom limb pain may occur during times of emotional stress or the development of a new pain site unrelated to the phantom pain.[14] There is little information to outline the incidence of phantom pain following amputation in malignant disease. Large surveys of postmastectomy patients reveal that at least 10% of patients experience chronic phantom breast pain beyond the first year.[15] A pro-

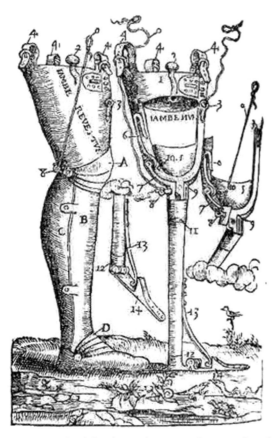

Figure 22–1. Artificial leg by Ambroise Paré. (Reproduced with permission from the "John Martin Rare Book Room," Hardin Medical Library, University of Iowa.)

spective study conducted over a 6-year period by Kroner and colleagues concluded that persistent phantom pain after mastectomy may be more common than usually expected and that persistence of pain in the scar seems higher than generally expected.[16] Studies to outline the incidence of phantom visceral pain have not been performed. Cortical phenomena related to the onset and maintenance of visceral phantoms have been described with multiple visceral organs having the propensity to present as phantoms following removal.[17,18]

Phantom pain in children has been poorly documented. It was once thought that young children did not experience phantom pain.[19,20] However, more recent reports have documented that phantom pain affects the majority of young children who have undergone transplantation.[21] The absence of data reflects our relatively primitive assessment methodology and persistent myths about the type of pain experienced by children. Boyle and colleagues reported that 7 years after amputation in childhood or adolescence, 70% to 75% of the individuals continued to experience phantom pain, but none reported the pain to be severe.[22] Krane and Heller retrospectively looked at 24 cases of amputations conducted in childhood; 92% of the subjects reported phantom pain.[13] The pain persisted for months to years in all subjects. The children described the pain

as uncomfortable, sharp, a feeling of pins and needles, tingling, tickling, stabbing, and itching. They found that the majority of children who had phantom pain reported having preamputation pain. Phantom pain was documented in only half of the medical records of children that were identified as having experienced continued pain following amputation. Some of the difficulty in evaluating pediatric phantom pain may reflect the lack of good evaluation tools. Wilkins and associates conducted a prospective diary based study on a sample of 14 children and adolescent amputees reporting phantom limbs.[21] Thirteen respondents reported having 104 nonpainful phantom sensations over a 1-month period; 8 amputees reported 53 incidents of phantom limb pain, averaging 6.43 on a 10-point pain scale. Girls reported more psychological triggers than boys, whereas physical triggers were more commonly reported by boys, leading to the conclusion that differences in activities, awareness, attribution, and willingness to report psychosocial triggers exist across the sexes.

TIME COURSE

Nonpainful and painful phantoms change in character and location over time. In a survey of 5000 veteran amputees, it was determined that 50% indicated that phantom pain decreased with time, whereas the other 50% reported no change or an increase in pain over time. Among those reporting current phantom pain, 27% felt it for at least 20 days per month, 10% for 11 to 20 days, and 14% for 1 day per month.[23] The rate of occurrence of phantom limb pain drops with time after surgery.

Patients frequently describe "telescoping" or shortening of the phantom limb (Fig. 22–2). In many cases, patients perceive only the distal portion of the limb attached to the stump. Others describe a gradual fading of the phantom. In a study by Shukla and colleagues, telescoping was reported by nearly two thirds of 72 amputees.[24] A clinical correlation that remains to be proven is a correlation between telescoping of the stump and resolution of phantom pain. It may be that a phantom limb remains distinct when pain persists. Although the majority of patients report immediate onset of phantom pain, late-appearing phantom pain has been reported.

Flor and associates, in an experimental case control study, demonstrated the influence of sensory discrimination training on reduction in phantom pain.[25] Cortical reorganization may provide insight into treatment modalities that influence the time course of the disease, leading to effective acceleration of the resolution of phantom limb pain.[26]

ETIOLOGY

Patients may experience both nonpainful and painful phantom sensations, stump pain, and involuntary motor activity. The location and character of pain is of importance in determining the best course of treatment. These experiences vary widely between

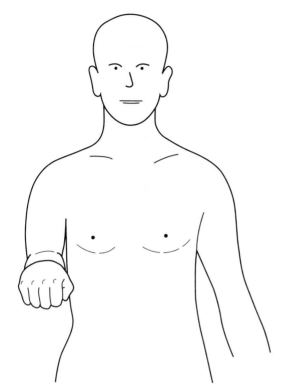

Figure 22–2. Telescoping of the phantom extremity. (Reproduced with permission from Nikolajsen L, Jensen TS: Phantom limb pain. Br J Anaesth 2001;87:107-116.)

Table 22–1. Factors That May Modulate the Experience of Phantom Pain

INTERNAL FACTORS	EXTERNAL FACTORS
Genetic predisposition	Weather change
Anxiety/emotional distress	Touching the stump
Attention/distraction	Use of prosthesis
Urination/defecation	Spinal anesthesia
Other disease (cerebral hemorrhage, prolapsed intervertebral disk)	Rehabilitation Treatment

Reproduced with permission from Nikolajsen L, Jensen TS: Phantom limb pain. Br J Anaesth 2001;87:107-116.

individuals and cannot be predicted reliably. As a result, it is important in taking a history to differentiate between nonpainful and painful phantom sensation and stump pain.

Following amputation, wound pain is expected to resolve as tissue healing occurs. Stump pain may be due to circulatory disturbance, infection, tumor, or other lesions involving skin, soft tissue, bone, or nerves. Prolonged stump pain is usually related to local factors such as delayed wound healing, surgical complications, tumor recurrence, or a poor fitting prosthetic. Neuromas that develop at the end of a severed peripheral nerve may contribute to stump pain and may act as a trigger for phantom pain.[27] The development of intermittent involuntary rhythmic movements (tremors) of a stump may produce discomfort for the patient. They may experience painful spasms of residual portions of muscle that may be accompanied by an associated paroxysm of stump or phantom pain. The characteristics, intensity, frequency, and duration of postamputation sensations and pain as well as the exacerbating and relieving factors vary widely among individuals (Table 22–1). The experience of nonpainful phantom sensation is almost universal, but this is not the case with painful phantom limb sensation.

The natural history of phantom limb pain has been studied in trauma patients and those undergoing surgical amputation for malignant and nonmalignant conditions.[8,10,28] The reported incidence of phantom limb pain varies widely due to a number of factors, including the cause of amputation. Weiss and Lindell reviewed the relationship between phantom limb pain and both the etiology of amputation (blood clots, nonclot diabetes, and miscellaneous) and the occurrence of gangrene and/or infection in 92 unilateral lower extremity amputees who were seen sequentially. There were 55 above-knee and 37 below-knee amputations in 61 men and 31 women. The blood clot etiology had the highest levels of phantom pain both before and after and after rehabilitation, the longest time interval between amputation and prosthetic fitting had the greatest number of medical conditions. The nonclot diabetes and miscellaneous etiologies followed in order.

A history of gangrene and/or infection was associated with higher levels of pain and longer time interval between amputation and prosthetic fitting.[29] Ehde and colleagues reported the results of a retrospective study designed to evaluate the characteristics of phantom limb sensation, phantom limb pain, and residual limb pain, and to evaluate pain-related disability associated with phantom limb pain.[30] The study consisted of a retrospective cross-sectional survey using an amputation pain questionnaire in 255 subjects 6 or more months after lower limb amputation. Of the respondents, 79% reported phantom limb sensations, 72% reported phantom limb pain, and 74% reported residual limb pain. Many described the phantom limb and residual limb pain as episodic and not particularly bothersome. Most participants with phantom limb pain were classified into the two low pain-related disability categories: grade I, low disability/low pain intensity (47%) or grade II, low disability/high pain intensity (28%). Many participants reported having pain in other anatomic locations, including the back (52%). They concluded that phantom limb and residual limb pain are common after lower limb amputation. For most, the pain is episodic and not particularly disabling. However, for others, the pain may be quite disabling.

MECHANISMS

Peripheral

Early theories grounded in the specificity theory of pain relied on peripheral mechanisms to explain phantom limb pain. Phantom limb pain is more frequent in patients with long-term stump pain.[12,31] Neuromas at peripheral nerve endings have been implicated in the development of phantom pain. This was initially inferred from the alteration of phantom limb pain following stimulation of the presumed neuroma within the stump. Nystrom and colleagues demonstrated the increase in C fiber activity associated with tapping of transected nerves in amputees and correlated that with an increase in pain sensation.[27] Sodium channel activation in amputees' stumps has been shown to increase pain sensation.[32] Lidocaine, a sodium channel blocker, in contrast blocks phantom pain.[32] Despite the clear association of neuroma to phantom limb pain, surgical removal of neuromas has not shown much promise in limiting phantom limb pain in amputees.[33]

Central

As early as 1943, involvement of abnormal spinal internuncial neuron firing was postulated to play a role in the development of phantom limb pain.[34] Sympathetic ganglionic block was shown to eliminate pain in one third of 36 patients treated by Livingston. Carlen and colleagues proposed that spinal and peripheral mechanisms alone are responsible for the onset and maintenance of phantom limb pain, citing the relative absence of phantom pain in paraplegics where cortical descending pathways are uninhibited by ascending sensory input.[35] More recent studies of cortical reorganization point toward a role for supraspinal involvement.[36-38] Development of new synaptic contacts from neuronal synaptic growth resulting in formation of new cortical connections has been proposed as one mechanism for cortical reorganization in amputees.[39] Neuronal plasticity may lead to reorganization of the sensory and motor systems in multiple levels of the central nervous system, including the spinal cord, brainstem, thalamus, and cortex.[40] An understanding of such mechanisms may lead to improved treatment programs leading to functional improvement.

Psychological

The loss of any body part is accompanied by psychological adjustment that may include a grief reaction.[41] Associated with the intensity of pain is psychological distress commonly manifested as depression. This has been determined to occur in 20% to 60% of amputees attending surgical or rehabilitation clinics.[42,43] In a telephone survey of phantom pain, residual limb pain, and back pain in amputees, conducted by Ephraim and associates, one third of the patients were found to have depressive symptoms.[44] Depression was associated with an increased level of intensity and interference with daily activities. For patients with significant depressive symptoms, 32.9% reported needing mental health service but not receiving any.[45] Attempts to explain the origin of phantom pain as a reflection of the personality type

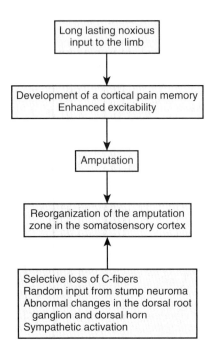

Figure 22–3. Flow chart incorporating the main factors thought to be relevant for the development of phantom limb pain. (Adapted with permission from Flor H: Phantom-limb pain: Characteristics, causes, and treatment. Lancet Neurol 2002;1:182-189.)

of the amputee have failed to produce a convincing argument.[46] Major personality disorders are no more prevalent among amputees reporting pain than among those not reporting it.[47]

Figure 22–3 lists the main factors thought to be relevant for development of phantom limb pain in the form of a schematic.[48] Phantom pain should be viewed from a broad perspective that considers other anatomic sites as well as the impact of pain on function.[49] Although studies have provided us with greater insight into postamputation pain, the number of studies is relatively small and many of the studies use only small numbers of patients. In some studies, no differentiation has been made for phantom sensation versus phantom pain. In many cases, patients may be reluctant to report their phantom sensations and pain. In a 1985 survey, 69% of 2700 veterans responded that their physician had directly stated or implied that phantom pain was "just in their heads."[49] Many physicians continue to believe that this syndrome is psychologically based. This viewpoint affects the willingness of prescribers to provide medical management of this type of pain with opiates or other medications. The lack of treatment may produce increased disability and decrease overall function. Disability that accompanies loss of limb has been reported to have a greater influence on depression in this population of patients.[46]

PREVENTION

The high incidence of phantom limb pain following amputation, whether traumatic or elective, has led to attempts to limit or eliminate phantom pain. In the case of planned amputation, psychological counseling may be useful in decreasing psychological distress.[50,51] A variety of surgical techniques for handling the severed nerve and vasculature have been proposed, although none have been proven to reduce postamputation pain.[52] Postoperative compression wrapping or hard casting to reduce stump edema may facilitate rehabilitation, but it is not certain that this reduces pain. Use of an immediate postoperative prosthesis has been shown to facilitate rehabilitation in 86% of a group of 167 patients studied retrospectively by Folsom and colleagues.[53] The impact on the incidence of postamputation pain was not reported. Epidural infusions of morphine and bupivacaine alone or in combination have been demonstrated to prevent phantom limb pain in patients with preexisting limb pain.[54] In addition, clonidine has been shown to be effective as an analgesic when applied epidurally.[55]

Jahangiri and colleagues reported on the use of a perioperative epidural infusion of diamorphine, bupivacaine, and clonidine to prevent phantom limb pain in patients with preexisting limb pain.[55] The authors set out to mitigate the potentially serious side effects of all these drugs by studying their combined efficacy in preventing phantom limb pain in a prospective controlled study of 24 patients undergoing lower limb amputation. In the study group (n = 13), an epidural infusion containing bupivacaine 75 mg, clonidine 150 mg, and diamorphine 5 mg in 60 mL normal saline was given at 1 to 4 mL/hr for 24 to 48 hours preoperatively and maintained for at least 3 days postoperatively. The control group (n = 11) received on-demand opioid analgesia. Pain was assessed by Visual Analogue Scale at 7 days, 6 months, and 1 year. At 1-year follow-up, one patient in the study group and eight patients in the control group had phantom pain, and two patients in the study group versus eight patients in the control group had phantom limb sensation. There was no improvement in stump pain.

In one study of patients amputated for nonmalignant disease, a threefold reduction in the incidence of phantom pain 1 year after amputation was demonstrated after preoperative treatment with an epidural infusion of opioid and local anesthetic.[54] A more recent investigation failed to replicate these results.[56,57] Investigation of pharmacologic means of preventing postamputation pain is ongoing. Enneking and colleagues reported on the use of local anesthetic infusion (0.25% bupivacaine) through nerve sheath catheters for analgesia following upper extremity amputation in six patients.[58] Complete analgesia was achieved in all patients by postoperative day 2. Narcotic usage was low. Three of six patients reported phantom limb pain during follow-up evaluation. They concluded that continuous local anesthetic perfusion of amputated nerves via a catheter placed under direct vision provided excellent postoperative analgesia. The incidence of phantom limb pain for cancer patients did not differ from that

previously reported, but was easily managed pharmacologically. In a follow-up study, Morey and associates retrospectively analyzed the effect of nerve sheath catheter analgesia after amputation and determined that there was a reduction in the incidence of postamputation phantom limb pain from 80% to 67%.[59] The incidence was not affected by the use of general anesthesia versus regional anesthesia as the primary anesthetic for the case. A similar trial by Pinzur and associates found that perineural infusions of local anesthetic provided effective relief of postoperative pain, but did not prevent residual or phantom limb pain in patients undergoing lower extremity amputation secondary to ischemic changes produced by peripheral vascular disease.[60]

Use of N-methyl-D-aspartate (NMDA) antagonists has been proposed to reduce the incidence of phantom limb pain. The results of randomized controlled trials have not been consistent. Perioperative infusion of ketamine has been evaluated for prevention of postamputation pain, based on the hypothesis that blockade of central sensitization at the time of amputation would reduce the incidence of postamputation pain.[61] The incidence of phantom pain was 47% in the ketamine group, compared to 71% in the placebo group. This did not reach statistical significance. Multiple trials of memantine (an NMDA antagonist) have not demonstrated benefit in the prevention of phantom limb pain.[62-64] Despite limited success in previous trials, Schley and colleagues successfully reduced the prevalence and intensity of phantom limb pain at 4 weeks and 6 months, but not 12 months, in a randomized, double-blind, controlled trial of 19 patients with acute traumatic amputation of the upper extremity.[65]

The preoperative application of opioids, local anesthetics, alpha-agonists, and excitatory amino acid receptor antagonists to prevent central nervous system consequences of amputation is being tested in animal models and humans. Both preamputation pain and immediate postamputation pain can lead to an increased incidence of phantom limb pain.[66] Further research is needed to assist in designing perioperative analgesic protocols that may be beneficial in reducing the incidence of postamputation phantom limb pain.

TREATMENT

The successful treatment of phantom limb pain remains challenging and a variety of methods, both pharmacologic and nonpharmacologic, have been used with varying degrees of success. When phantom limb pain resists treatment for greater than 6 months, the prognosis for spontaneous improvement is poor.[67]

Pharmacologic

A review of phantom limb treatment by Sherman and associates in 1980 found 68 treatment methods, none of which were uniformly successful.[68] More current reviews have found a similar lack of uniform success.[67,69-71] Halbert and colleagues, identifying the gap between practice and research in the treatment of phantom limb pain, reported that no trials in their review examined commonly recommended medications, such as membrane stabilizers or antidepressants.[67] Treatments have been directed at nociceptive, neuropathic, and psychologic elements of postamputation pain. As with any pharmacologic treatment for pain, the efficacy of pharmacologic agents varies widely between individuals. As a result, each patient must be treated in a systematic fashion to balance efficacy with side effects.

A very small number of patients are capable of achieving good pain control with opiates alone in widely varying doses. There are few published studies evaluating the efficacy of opiates in the treatment of postamputation pain. Wu and associates compared the effects morphine against intravenous lidocaine in a randomized, double-blind, placebo-controlled study.[72] Morphine was effective at reducing both phantom limb pain and stump pain. In contrast, intravenous lidocaine was only effective in reducing stump pain, suggesting that the mechanisms and pharmacologic sensitivity of stump pain and phantom limb pain are different.

In most patients with significant postamputation pain, treatment modalities directed at neuropathic pain are more effective. The data for treatment with this class of drugs is also quite limited. Rusy and colleagues reported the successful use of gabapentin to treat phantom limb pain in seven children and young adults.[73] Phantom limb pain resolved in six patients within 2 months. One patient still had symptoms to a lesser degree. The mean follow-up time was 1.74 years. Bone and colleagues conducted a prospective, randomized, placebo-controlled, crossover study of the effect of gabapentin on phantom limb pain.[74] Gabapentin was titrated from 300 mg to 2400 mg per day as tolerated by the patients. Nineteen patients were randomized to treatment, out of which 14 completed both arms of the study. After 6 weeks, gabapentin monotherapy was determined to be superior to placebo, with minimal side effects.

Antidepressants have been used to treat postamputation pain, although there are limited data to attest to their success in treating this type of pain. They are often chosen because of their efficacy in treating other types of neuropathic pain, but not because there are extensive data to support their use in phantom pain. Bartusch and colleagues reported the successful use of clonazepam to control lancinating phantom limb pain in two patients followed up for more than 6 months.[75] It should be noted that the use of sedatives and hypnotics is extremely limited due to the lack of any controlled data evaluating efficacy as well as the potential for addiction, increased depression, and altered sleep patterns.

NMDA receptor activation has been postulated to play a role in the maintenance of phantom limb pain. Pharmacologic agents targeting NMDA receptors have been used with success in both cancer and noncancer amputees. Dextromethorphan, in doses ranging from 120 to 270 mg per day, has been shown to reduce postamputation phantom limb pain, minimizing sedation, in comparison to the pretreatment condition of the patients.[76,77] Further clinical trials are needed to identify the optimal dosage and patient selection for this pharmacologic treatment modality.

Intravenous calcitonin has been described as a means of treating phantom limb pain in the early postoperative period, in a very small number of patients without any form of controlled trial.[78,79] Jaeger and Maier conducted a double blind study of the effects of calcitonin on 21 phantom limb patients.[80] One week after treatment, 90% of patients had greater than 50% pain relief, 76% were pain free, and 71% never experienced phantom limb pain again at the 2-year follow-up. Observations from this study led to the conclusion that calcitonin should be administered early in the course of treatment to obtain good results. Calcitonin can be readministered if patients report an increase in phantom limb pain.

Nonpharmacologic

Nonpharmacologic treatment has shown promise in the treatment of phantom limb pain. Therapies in use include stimulation via electrical, visual, thermal, and mechanical means. Transcutaneous electrical nerve stimulation has been demonstrated to produce faster stump healing, but did not affect postoperative pain or chronic phantom pain in a randomized trial of 51 patients.[81] Early studies on spinal cord stimulation (dorsal column stimulation) were successful in providing prolonged benefit in some instances.[82] Nielson and colleagues reported good to excellent relief of pain in 5 of 6 patients following dorsal column stimulation, with pain relief reported from 7 to 25 months.[82] More recent studies evaluating spinal cord stimulation have failed to produce consistent results in the treatment of phantom limb pain.[83,84] Thermal biofeedback sessions over the course of 4 to 6 weeks have demonstrated 30% pain reduction in a small pilot study conducted by Harden and colleagues[85] Further evaluation of this technique is needed to determine its role.

Visual stimulation is provided by means of a mirror box, designed to superimpose the reflection of the patients intact extremity over the space that would have been occupied by the missing extremity (Fig. 22–4).[86] Brodie and associates studied 80 amputees with one application of the mirror technique in a randomized controlled study and concluded that phantom limb pain and sensation were not reduced to a greater degree than in a control group that attempted phantom limb movements in the absence of the mirror box.[87]

Some patients are refractory to common treatments for phantom limb pain. Electroconvulsive therapy (ECT) has been used successfully in the treatment of patients with a variety of pain syndromes occurring along with depression. Rasmussen and colleagues

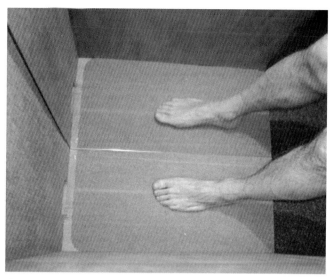

Figure 22–4. Mirror box in use, providing an example of an intact and mirrored extremity from the patient's perspective. (Reproduced with permission from Brodie EE, Whyte A, Niven CA: Analgesia through the looking-glass? A randomized controlled trial investigating the effect of viewing a "virtual" limb upon phantom limb pain, sensation and movement. Eur J Pain 2007;11:428-436.)

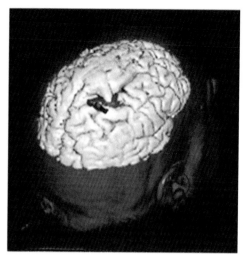

Figure 22–5. Three-dimensional image with superimposed functional magnetic resonance imaging (fMRI) data recorded by an infrared-based frameless stereotactic device. fMRI can detect the central sulcus as well as the exact locations of the stump area at which the electrode can be positioned. (Reproduced with permission from Roux FE, et al: Chronic motor cortex stimulation for phantom limb pain: A functional magnetic resonance imaging study: Technical case report. Neurosurgery 2001;48:681-688.)

reported on the successful use of ECT in two patients with severe phantom limb pain refractory to multiple therapies without concurrent psychiatric disorder.[88] Both patients enjoyed substantial pain relief. In one case, phantom pain was still in remission 3.5 years after ECT.

Recent limited reports of motor cortex stimulation for phantom limb pain are more encouraging.[89] Precise location of motor cortex electrodes can be determined using superimposed functional magnetic resonance imaging information on three-dimensional imaging of the motor cortex (Fig. 22–5).[90] Motor cortex stimulation has been attempted by Carroll and colleagues in patients with refractory phantom limb pain.[89] Two out of three patients reported greater than 50% relief of pain that was maintained for a period of 21 to 23 months. The third patient experienced technical difficulties with the device and did not receive a course of therapy. Patients that showed an initial response to the trial continued to experience long-term relief.

Deep brain stimulation also holds promise for patients with phantom limb pain resistant to treatment. Areas of interest for deep brain stimulation include the periaqueductal gray, periventricular gray (PVG), and the ventroposterior nucleus of the thalamus. Ascending pathways from the PVG may be involved in pain relief in addition to modifying the patient's emotional response to pain. The ventral posterior nucleus of the thalamus regulates sensory input to the cortex. It is divided into the ventroposterolateral nucleus (VPL) receiving input from the trunk and limbs, and the ventroposteromedial nucleus (VPM) receiving input from the head, neck, and face. Bittar and colleagues studied three patients with application of electrical stimulation in the PVG.[91]

Two out of three achieved optimal relief of pain, whereas the third required the use of thalamic stimulation. At follow-up (mean 13.3 months), pain was reduced by 62% (range 55% to 70%).[91] Yamamoto and colleagues successfully used long-term deep brain stimulation to reduce the visual analogue pain score in greater than 60% in 8 of 11 amputees.[92] Inhibition of spinothalamic neurons, restoration of the original receptive field representation, and modulation of thalamocortical rhythmic oscillations were proposed to play important roles in a possible mechanism for the treatment of postamputation pain.[92]

A variety of surgical procedures have been attempted to treat postamputation pain. These include dorsal root entry zone (DREZ) lesions, dorsal column tractotomy, anterolateral cordotomy, sympathectomy, thalamotomy, and cortical resection. Of the available surgical ablative procedures, DREZ lesioning has the greatest chance of success.[93,94] However, the basis on which to select patients to improve success remains unclear. The performance of any type of neuroablative procedure to treat phantom limb pain should be carefully considered due to the risk of delayed deafferentation pain.

The phenomenon of phantom limb pain remains poorly understood and is frequently underappreciated. At the present time, successful treatment is possible in some patients, but others will continue to experience significant pain and disability despite aggressive treatment. Careful and systematic application of available treatment methods will help to improve success without causing significant morbidity related to misapplied treatments. Ongoing research in the laboratory and clinical settings will continue to improve our understanding of this complex pain phenomenon and improve treatment in the future.

References

1. Finger S, Hustwit MP: Five early accounts of phantom limb in context: Pare, Descartes, Lemos, Bell, and Mitchell. Neurosurgery 2003;52:675-686.
2. Keil G: (So-called initial description of phantom pain by Ambroise Pare. "Chose digne d'admiration et quasi incredible": the "douleur es parties mortes et amputees"). Fortschr Med 1990;108:62-66.
3. Woodhouse A: Phantom limb sensation. Clin Exp Pharmacol Physiol 2005;32(1-2):132-134.
4. Nikolajsen L, Jensen TS: Phantom limb pain. Br J Anaesth 2001;87:107-116.
5. Katz J, Melzack R: Pain "memories" in phantom limbs: Review and clinical observations. Pain 1990;43:319-336.
6. Nikolajsen L, Ilkjaer S, Kroner K, et al: The influence of pre-amputation pain on postamputation stump and phantom pain. Pain 1997;72:393-405.
7. Jensen TS, Krebs B, Nielsen J, Rasmussen P: Non-painful phantom limb phenomena in amputees: Incidence, clinical characteristics and temporal course. Acta Neurol Scand 1984;70:407-414.
8. Steinbach TV, Nadvorna H, Arazi D: A five year follow-up study of phantom limb pain in post traumatic amputees. Scand J Rehabil Med 1982;14:203-207.
9. Knecht S, Sörös P, Gürtler S, et al: Phantom sensations following acute pain. Pain 1998;77:209-213.
10. Sherman RA, Sherman CJ, Parker L: Chronic phantom and stump pain among American veterans: Results of a survey. Pain 1984;18:83-95.
11. Sherman RA, Sherman CJ: Prevalence and characteristics of chronic phantom limb pain among American veterans: Results of a trial survey. Am J Phys Med 1983;62:227-238.
12. Jensen TS, Krebs S, Nielsen J, et al: Immediate and long-term phantom limb pain in amputees: Incidence, clinical characteristics and relationship to pre-amputation limb pain. Pain 1985;21:267-278.
13. Krane EJ, Heller LB: The prevalence of phantom sensation and pain in pediatric amputees. J Pain Sympt Manage 1995;10:21-29.
14. Schott GD: Delayed onset and resolution of pain: Some observations and implications. Brain 2001;124(Pt 6):1067-1076.
15. Kroner K, Krebs B, Skov J, et al: Immediate and long-term phantom breast syndrome after mastectomy: Incidence, clinical characteristics and relationship to pre-mastectomy breast pain. Pain 1989;36(3):327-334.
16. Kroner K, Knudsen UB, Lundby L, et al: Long-term phantom breast syndrome after mastectomy. Clin J Pain 1992;8:346-350.
17. Tichy J: (Somatognosis, body schema and the phenomena of somatic and visceral phantoms and phantom pain). Cas Lek Cesk 2003;142:331-334.
18. Humphreys S, Campbell W: Augmentation of phantom limb pain by normal visceral function. Ulster Med J 2001;70:142-144.
19. Easson WM: Body image and self-image in children: Phantom phenomenon in a 3-year-old child. Arch Gen Psychiatry 1961;4:619-621.
20. Kolb LC, Brodie HKH: Modern Clinical Psychiatry, 10th ed. Philadelphia, Saunders, 1982.
21. Wilkins KL, McGrath PJ, Finley GA, et al: Prospective diary study of nonpainful and painful phantom sensations in a preselected sample of child and adolescent amputees reporting phantom limbs. Clin J Pain 2004;20:293-301.
22. Boyle M, Tebbi CK, Mindell ER, et al: Adolescent adjustment to amputation. Med Pediatr Oncol 1982;10:301-312.
23. Sherman RA, Bruno GM: Concurrent variation of burning phantom limb and stump pain with near surface blood flow in the stump. Orthopedics 1987;10:1395-1402.
24. Shukla GD, Sahu SC, Tripathi RP, et al: A psychiatric study of amputees. Br J Psychiatry 1982;141:50-53.
25. Flor H, Denke C, Schaefer M, et al: Effect of sensory discrimination training on cortical reorganisation and phantom limb pain. Lancet 2001;357(9270):1763-1764.
26. Flor H: (Visualisation of phantom- and back pain using imaging techniques. Implication for treatment). Orthopade 2004;33:553-557.
27. Nystrom B, Hagbarth KE: Microelectrode recordings from transected nerves in amputees with phantom limb pain. Neurosci Lett 1981;27:211-216.
28. Wartan SW, Hamann W, Wedley JB, et al: Phantom pain and sensation among British veteran amputees. Br J Anaesth 1997;78:652-659.
29. Weiss SA, Lindell B: Phantom limb pain and etiology of amputation in unilateral lower extremity amputees. J Pain Sympt Manage 1996;11:3-17.
30. Ehde DM, Czerniecki JM, Smith DG, et al: Chronic phantom sensations, phantom pain, residual limb pain, and other regional pain after lower limb amputation. Arch Phys Med Rehabil 2000;81:1039-1044.
31. Kooijman CM, Dijkstra PU, Geertzen JH, et al: Phantom pain and phantom sensations in upper limb amputees: An epidemiological study. Pain 2000;87:33-41.
32. Chabal C, Jacobson L, Russell LC, et al: Pain responses to perineuromal injection of normal saline, gallamine, and lidocaine in humans. Pain 1989;36:321-325.
33. Sturm V, Kroger M, Penzholz H: (Problems of peripheral nerve surgery in amputation stump pain and phantom limbs). Chirurg 1975;46:389-391.
34. Hill A: Phantom limb pain: A review of the literature on attributes and potential mechanisms. J Pain Symptom Manage 1999;17:125-142.
35. Carlen PL, Wall PD, Nadvorna H, et al: Phantom limbs and related phenomena in recent traumatic amputations. Neurology 1978;28:211-217.
36. Flor H: Cortical reorganisation and chronic pain: Implications for rehabilitation. J Rehabil Med 2003;41(suppl):66-72.
37. Flor H: The modification of cortical reorganization and chronic pain by sensory feedback. Appl Psychophysiol Biofeedback 2002;27:215-227.
38. Flor H, Elbert T, Mühlnickel W, et al: Cortical reorganization and phantom phenomena in congenital and traumatic upper-extremity amputees. Exp Brain Res 1998;119:205-212.
39. Cohen LG, Bandinelli S, Findley TW, et al: Motor reorganization after upper limb amputation in man. A study with focal magnetic stimulation. Brain 1991;114(Pt 1B):615-627.
40. Chen R, Cohen LG, Hallett M: Nervous system reorganization following injury. Neuroscience 2002;111:761-773.
41. Horgan O, MacLachlan M: Psychosocial adjustment to lower-limb amputation: A review. Disabil Rehabil 2004;26(14-15):837-850.
42. Shukla GD, Sahu SC, Tripathi RP, et al: Phantom limb: A phenomenological study. Br J Psychiatry 1982;141:54-58.
43. Kashani JH, Frank RG, Kashani SR, et al: Depression among amputees. J Clin Psychiatry 1983;44:256-258.
44. Ephraim PL, Wegener ST, MacKenzie EJ, et al: Phantom pain, residual limb pain, and back pain in amputees: Results of a national survey. Arch Phys Med Rehabil 2005;86:1910-1919.
45. Darnall BD, Ephraim P, Wegener ST, et al: Depressive symptoms and mental health service utilization among persons with limb loss: Results of a national survey. Arch Phys Med Rehabil 2005;86:650-658.
46. Whyte AS, Niven CA: Psychological distress in amputees with phantom limb pain. J Pain Sympt Manage 2001;22:938-946.
47. Sherman RA, Sherman CJ, Bruno GM: Psychological factors influencing chronic phantom limb pain: An analysis of the literature. Pain 1987;28:285-295.
48. Flor H: Phantom-limb pain: Characteristics, causes, and treatment. Lancet Neurol 2002;1:182-189.
49. Sherman RA, Sherman CJ: A comparison of phantom sensations among amputees whose amputations were of civilian and military origins. Pain 1985;21:91-97.
50. Desmond DM, MacLachlan M: Affective distress and amputation-related pain among older men with long-term, traumatic limb amputations. J Pain Sympt Manage 2006;31:362-368.
51. Hanley MA, Jensen MP, Ehde DM, et al: Psychosocial predictors of long-term adjustment to lower-limb amputation and phantom limb pain. Disabil Rehabil 2004;26(14-15):882-893.

52. Chiodo CP, Stroud CC: Optimal surgical preparation of the residual limb for prosthetic fitting in below-knee amputations. Foot Ankle Clin 2001;6:253-264.

53. Folsom D, King T, Rubin JR: Lower-extremity amputation with immediate postoperative prosthetic placement. Am J Surg 1992;164:320-322.

54. Bach S, Noreng MF, Tjellden NU: Phantom limb pain in amputees during the first 12 months following limb amputation, after preoperative lumbar epidural blockade. Pain 1988;33:297-301.

55. Jahangiri M, Jayatunga AP, Bradley JW, et al: Prevention of phantom pain after major lower limb amputation by epidural infusion of diamorphine, clonidine and bupivacaine. Ann R Coll Surg Engl 1994;76:324-326.

56. Katz J: Phantom limb pain. Lancet 1997;350(9088):1338-1339.

57. Nikolajsen L, Ilkjaer S, Christensen JH, et al: Randomised trial of epidural bupivacaine and morphine in prevention of stump and phantom pain in lower-limb amputation. Lancet 1997;350(9088):1353-1357.

58. Enneking FK, Scarborough MT, Radson EA: Local anesthetic infusion through nerve sheath catheters for analgesia following upper extremity amputation. Clinical report. Reg Anesth 1997;22:351-356.

59. Morey TE, Giannoni J, Duncan E, et al: Nerve sheath catheter analgesia after amputation. Clin Orthop Relat Res 2002;397:281-289.

60. Pinzur MS, Garla PG, Pluth T, et al: Continuous postoperative infusion of a regional anesthetic after an amputation of the lower extremity: A randomized clinical trial. J Bone Joint Surg Am 1996;78:1501-1505.

61. Hayes CA, Armstrong-Brown, Burstal R: Perioperative intravenous ketamine infusion for the prevention of persistent postamputation pain: A randomized, controlled trial. Anaesth Intensive Care 2004;32:330-338.

62. Maier C, Dertwinkel R, Mansourian N, et al: Efficacy of the NMDA-receptor antagonist memantine in patients with chronic phantom limb pain—Results of a randomized double-blinded, placebo-controlled trial. Pain 2003;103:277-283.

63. Nikolajsen L, Gottrup H, Kristensen AG, et al: Memantine (a N-methyl-D-aspartate receptor antagonist) in the treatment of neuropathic pain after amputation or surgery: A randomized, double-blinded, cross-over study. Anesth Analg 2000;91:960-966.

64. Wiech K, Kiefer RT, Töpfner S, et al: A placebo-controlled randomized crossover trial of the N-methyl-D-aspartic acid receptor antagonist, memantine, in patients with chronic phantom limb pain. Anesth Analg 2004;98:408-413.

65. Schley M, Töpfner S, Weich K, et al: Continuous brachial plexus blockade in combination with the NMDA receptor antagonist memantine prevents phantom pain in acute traumatic upper limb amputees. Eur J Pain 2006;11:299-308.

66. Hanley MA, Jensen MP, Smith DG, et al: Preamputation pain and acute pain predict chronic pain after lower extremity amputation. J Pain 2007;8:102-109.

67. Halbert J, Crotty M, Cameron ID: Evidence for the optimal management of acute and chronic phantom pain: A systematic review. Clin J Pain 2002;18:84-92.

68. Sherman RA, Sherman CJ, Gall N: A survey of current phantom limb pain treatment in the United States. Pain 1980;8:85-99.

69. Loeser JD, Bonica JJ: Bonica's Management of Pain, 3rd ed. Philadelphia, Lippincott Williams & Wilkins, 2001, pp 412-423.

70. Wall PD, Melzack R, Bonica JJ: Textbook of Pain, 3rd ed. New York: Churchill Livingstone, 1994.

71. Davis RW: Phantom sensation, phantom pain, and stump pain. Arch Phys Med Rehabil 1993;74:79-91.

72. Wu CL, Tella P, Staats PS, et al: Analgesic effects of intravenous lidocaine and morphine on postamputation pain: A random-

73. Rusy LM, Troshynski TJ, Weisman SJ: Gabapentin in phantom limb pain management in children and young adults: Report of seven cases. J Pain Sympt Manage 2001;21:78-82.

74. Bone M, Critchley P, Buggy DJ: Gabapentin in postamputation phantom limb pain: A randomized, double-blind, placebo-controlled, cross-over study. Reg Anesth Pain Med 2002;27:481-486.

75. Bartusch SL, Sanders BJ, D'Alessio JG, Jernigan JR: Clonazepam for the treatment of lancinating phantom limb pain. Clin J Pain 1996;12:59-62.

76. Ben Abraham R, Marouani N, Kollender Y, et al: Dextromethorphan for phantom pain attenuation in cancer amputees: A double-blind crossover trial involving three patients. Clin J Pain 2002;18:282-285.

77. Ben Abraham R, Marouani N, Weinbroum AA: Dextromethorphan mitigates phantom pain in cancer amputees. Ann Surg Oncol 2003;10:268-274.

78. Wall GC, Heyneman CA: Calcitonin in phantom limb pain. Ann Pharmacother 1999;33:499-501.

79. Fiddler DS, Hindman BJ: Intravenous calcitonin alleviates spinal anesthesia-induced phantom limb pain. Anesthesiology 1991;74:187-189.

80. Jaeger H, Maier C: Calcitonin in phantom limb pain: A double-blind study. Pain 1992;48:21-27.

81. Finsen V, Persen L, Løvlien M, et al: Transcutaneous electrical nerve stimulation after major amputation. J Bone Joint Surg Br 1988;70:109-112.

82. Nielson KD, Adams JE, Hosobuchi Y: Phantom limb pain: Treatment with dorsal column stimulation. J Neurosurg 1975;42:301-307.

83. Kumar K, Toth C, Nath RK, et al: Epidural spinal cord stimulation for treatment of chronic pain—Some predictors of success. A 15-year experience. Surg Neurol 1998;50:110-121.

84. Garcia-March G, Sánchez-Ledesma MJ, Diaz P, et al: Dorsal root entry zone lesion versus spinal cord stimulation in the management of pain from brachial plexus avulsion. Acta Neurochir Suppl (Wien) 1987;39:155-158.

85. Harden RN, Houle TT, Green S, et al: Biofeedback in the treatment of phantom limb pain: A time-series analysis. Appl Psychophysiol Biofeedback 2005;30:83-93.

86. Ramachandran VS, Rogers-Ramachandran D: Synaesthesia in phantom limbs induced with mirrors. Proc Biol Sci 1996;263(1369):377-386.

87. Brodie EE, Whyte A, Niven CA: Analgesia through the looking-glass? A randomized controlled trial investigating the effect of viewing a "virtual" limb upon phantom limb pain, sensation and movement. Eur J Pain 2007;11:428-436.

88. Rasmussen KG, Rummans TA: Electroconvulsive therapy for phantom limb pain. Pain 2000;85(1-2):297-299.

89. Carroll D, Joint C, Maartens N, et al: Motor cortex stimulation for chronic neuropathic pain: A preliminary study of 10 cases. Pain 2000;84(2-3):431-437.

90. Roux FE, Ibarrola D, Lazorthes Y, et al: Chronic motor cortex stimulation for phantom limb pain: A functional magnetic resonance imaging study: technical case report. Neurosurgery 2001;48:681-688.

91. Bittar RG, Kar-Purkayastha I, Owen SL, et al: Deep brain stimulation for phantom limb pain. J Clin Neurosci 2005;12:399-404.

92. Yamamoto T, Katayama AY, Obuchi T, et al: Thalamic sensory relay nucleus stimulation for the treatment of peripheral deafferentation pain. Stereotact Funct Neurosurg 2006;84:180-183.

93. Siegfried J: (Neurosurgical treatment of pain). Schweiz Med Wochenschr 1981;111:1954-1959.

94. Meyerson BA: Neurosurgical approaches to pain treatment. Acta Anaesthesiol Scand 2001;45:1108-1113.

CHAPTER

23 Myofascial Pain Syndrome and Fibromyalgia Syndrome

I. Jon Russell

And a woman spoke, saying, "Tell us of pain."
And he said: "Your pain is the breaking of the
shell that encloses your understanding. And
could you keep your heart in wonder of the daily
miracles of your life, your pain would not seem
less wondrous than your joy."

THE PROPHET, KAHLIL GIBRAN (1923)

The focus of this chapter will be on two clinical soft tissue pain (STP) disorders, specifically the myofascial pain syndrome (MPS) and the fibromyalgia syndrome (FMS). They have separately struggled for recognition in the medical arena, despite being fairly common in every contemporary society and exacting a moderately severe toll on the patients who suffer from them. The explanations for this situation are varied, but may relate as much to obscure belief systems on the part of physicians as to the nature of the conditions themselves. Both are painful and impair the ability of the affected person to function normally. Both are assessed subjectively, with some semiobjective clinical signs. Both can be associated with patient behaviors that make clinicians worry that something is being missed. Neither has a laboratory test that unequivocally defines the condition, separating it from all other painful disorders. Both seek simple instruments that are robust to change, with clinical improvement. Until recently, neither has a medication approved by the U.S. Food and Drug Administration (FDA) specifically indicated for treatment of its symptoms.* Neither condition causes death nor prostration on a grand scale, so the populace has no reason to fear it enough to give it top billing on the national research agenda.

Despite their many similarities, these conditions are easily distinguished from each other on the basis of medical history, examination, and even some laboratory findings. Therefore, it is even possible to

*In July 2007, the U.S. FDA approved Lyrica (pregabalin) as indicated for the treatment of FMS.

identify patients who have both conditions at the same time. This chapter will attempt to summarize the current status of these disorders with respect to their clinical presentations, epidemiology, pathogenesis, and management.

CLASSIFICATION OF SOFT TISSUE PAIN DISORDERS

Box 23–1 provides a useful contemporary classification of STPs.[1] The main subheadings divide STPs into localized, regional, and generalized categories. Most of the localized conditions are believed to result from repetitive mechanical injury to inadequately conditioned tissues. They tend to be named anatomically and are disclosed by a typical history plus the exquisite tenderness elicited by digital palpation of the affected structure. There is usually not much controversy about the disorders in this category.

Regional STP conditions are limited in anatomic scope to a region or body quadrant. This category includes the following:

- Various examples of MPSs, which can involve almost any muscle of the body but tend to be clinically apparent in a relatively discrete number of patterns
- Myofascial pain dysfunction syndrome, MPDS, physiologically similar to MPS in other regions of the body but limited to muscles of mastication
- Complex regional pain syndrome, CRPS, with its new definition as types 1 and 2 CRPS, (taking the place of reflex sympathetic dystrophy and causalgia, respectively)
- Nerve entrapment syndromes—visceral referral to musculoskeletal structures
- Senile "aches and pains"

The generalized category implies a systemic process that affects the musculoskeletal system more globally. The FMS is properly listed in this category, as is chronic fatigue syndrome (CFS) when pain is a symptomatic component of that disorder. The hyper-

455

mobility syndrome tends to be generalized when symptomatic. It can present with regional symptoms such as low back pain, chronic knee pain, recurrent ankle sprain, or pes planus, depending on where the greatest strain is on tendons or ligaments, with a genetic variant admixture of elastic and the more rigid collagen fibers. The inclusion of polymyalgia rheumatica among the generalized STPs will certainly be controversial because, in contrast with the other conditions in this class, it is inflammatory (elevated erythrocyte sedimentation rate, ESR), can be accompanied by an erosive oligoarthritis, and is usually responsive to glucocorticoids. It is included to remind the clinician about its apparent similarity to FMS on initial presentation. Finally, statin-induced myalgia is included because of the growing importance of this condition in the differential diagnosis of STP with the widespread use of these drugs in medical practice.

MYOFASCIAL PAIN SYNDROME

Diagnostic Criteria

The early work by Travell[2] would likely have been informed by a knowledge of the experiments of Kellgren,[3] who injected distinct skeletal muscles with hypertonic saline and mapped the locations of the resulting zones of pain reference. The extensive discussions by Simons and Travell[4,5] have provided proposed criteria for the diagnosis of the MPS (Box 23–2). It is described as a painful regional syndrome characterized by the presence of an active trigger point (TrP) in a skeletal muscle. The implications of the active TrP are that the examiner should expect to find spot tenderness with deep palpation over the TrP, leading to the patient's recognition of the induced discomfort as a familiar pain, and concomitant referral of pain to a zone of reference that is fairly predictable for irritation within the affected muscle. A latent TrP has been defined as one for which there is no current experience of spontaneous pain, but pain is still inducible by manipulation of the TrP. Manipulation of the TrP—by digital pressure,

BOX 23–3. VALIDITY OF EXAMINATION FINDINGS FOR DOCUMENTING THE MYOFASCIAL PAIN SYNDROME*

The strongest examination findings were:
- A tender spot (trigger point) in an affected muscle
- Referral of pain to a zone of reference
- Reproducing the patient's usual pain

Poorer reliability was associated with:
- Eliciting local tenderness
- Palpating a taut band
- Documenting the local twitch response

*When experienced clinicians standardized their examination techniques and their approach to interpretation of the findings, before participating in a blinded examination.

Adapted from Gerwin RD, Shannon S, Hong CZ, et al: Interrater reliability in myofascial trigger point examination. Pain 1997;69:65-73.

a flick across the muscle, or penetration by a needle—typically induces a twitch response, which can be felt as a palpable taut band, and restricts normal excursion of the affected muscle.

The problem for investigators trying to validate MPS diagnostic criteria has been that experienced clinicians have not been able to demonstrate a high level of agreement when applying the Simons and Travell criteria to serially blinded patients versus disease controls or healthy controls.[6-10] It appears that even experienced clinicians need to standardize their examination techniques and their approach to interpretation of the findings. When that was done immediately before performing blinded examinations, the results were much more reproducible.[11] The most reproducible clinical features from among the Simons and Travell criteria were finding a tender spot (the TrP) in the proximal or distal third of an affected skeletal muscle, referral of pain to a zone of reference, and reproducing the patient's usual pain. Much poorer reliability was associated with eliciting local tenderness, palpating a taut band, and documenting the local twitch response. These findings are summarized in Box 23–3.

A telling series of two tables has been provided by Simons and colleagues.[4] The first table summarizes the interrater reliability kappa values from four clinical studies for various critical examination procedures used in diagnosing MPS. The second compares the relative difficulty of performing or interpreting those test procedures versus the relative importance of those tests to diagnosing MPS confidently. The tests considered more important to making the diagnosis are also the ones most difficult to perform or interpret.

Part of the problem may have been that there are so many muscles in the body that have the potential to be affected by MPS; examination techniques need to be adapted for each muscle. Clinicians who are skilled in diagnosing MPS must have a phenomenal knowledge of neuromuscular anatomy and function,

plus a remarkable level of manual dexterity and trained sensory discrimination in their hands. In addition, these skills must account for the common distortions of the ideal anatomy by patients' neglect of their physical conditioning and the development of overlying layers of adipose tissue. If every MPS patient had the body of a competitive body builder, with well-defined musculature, the anatomic challenge would be less onerous. Some muscles are particularly difficult to evaluate because they are under other muscles (e.g., piriformis deep to the gluteal muscles of the buttocks). The muscles in the lower extremities seem to be more problematic in this regard than those in the trunk and upper extremities.

A study design, patterned after that used to develop research classification criteria for the fibromyalgia syndrome,[12] has been proposed to validate diagnostic criteria for the MPS involving muscles of the upper torso.[13] Application of this protocol by teams of experts (a Delphi and a blinded examiner) at two centers in different countries confirmed the historically observed outcome that there was poor agreement ($\kappa = 0.21-0.35$) on the diagnosis between pairs of examiners based on the standard examination approaches.[14] The main reason for this situation was that examination of the healthy normal controls by the blinded examiner disclosed a very high proportion that exhibited a taut band, an area of tenderness, a local twitch response, a jump sign, and even referral of pain. The best examination discriminators of MPS patients from healthy normal controls were painfully restricted range of motion, muscle strength limited by pain, skin rolling test, and pressure pain threshold according to algometry. A second component of the study involved use of validated questionnaire instruments that examined subjective pain, dysfunctional sleep, physical function, anxiety, and depression. The questionnaire instruments were more consistently effective in distinguishing MPS from healthy normal control (HNC) than were the examination measures. Of particular interest were the findings of sleep dysfunction, anxiety, and depression in MPS patients. Further analyses of these data will probably result in recommendation of a combined diagnostic profile for MPS that involves elements from the medical history, validated questionnaire instruments, and musculoskeletal examination.

Although there are certainly critics of the Simons and Travell clinical criteria for the diagnosis of the MPS, there is general agreement among physicians treating patients with musculoskeletal pain that such a condition does exist. A national survey of 1663 American Pain Society members[15] resulted in 403 completed surveys being returned. The participants responded to questions about the legitimacy of the MPS as a unique condition, whether or not they considered it to be distinct from the FMS, and which signs or symptoms were important to its diagnosis. Of the respondents, 88% indicated that MPS is a legitimate diagnosis and 81% believed that it is distinct from the FMS. When examined by specialty, the perception of legitimacy ranged from 50% to 100%, with osteopaths and orthopedists (poorly sampled at only 0.5% and 1.2% of the respondents, respectively) reporting the lowest legitimacy (50% to 60%, respectively), and anesthetists and physiatrists, composing 67% of the respondents, indicated over 90% legitimacy for the MPS. The latter groups were generally (83%) convinced that MPS is distinct from FMS. When asked about which findings were essential to the diagnosis of MPS, the respondents showed strong support for regional pain, the presence of TrPs, a normal neurologic examination, and pain that decreases with local injection. The respondents considered irrelevant, or placed much less importance on finding, palpable nodules, a local twitch response, and a decreased range of muscle motion.

As the advocates of the MPS construct strive for uniformity in their approach to diagnosis, there is also value in striving for uniform and logical terminology. If the essence of the condition is conceptualized, it is the TrP. Many authors have referred to this construct as a "myofascial TrP," as if there were some type of TrP. It has been suggested that the term used be simply *TrP*, because the term *myofascial* adds nothing of significance. This has already become the editorial policy of the *Journal of Musculoskeletal Pain*.

Prevalence Estimates

The prevalence of MPS in the general population is uncertain. That information is difficult to obtain because there are, as yet, no validated diagnostic criteria for the condition. Thus, it has not been possible to confidently seek out the disorder on a large scale using screening survey instruments.

In a study designed to examine the prevalence of the FMS in a Midwestern community, Wolfe and associates[16] have found that about 60% of the general population in their study did not currently have pain. About 30% of the general population had acute or regional pain (the latter would include MPS), and about 10% had chronic widespread pain (the category for FMS). Follow-up examination revealed that about 2% of the general population (all within the 10% with chronic widespread pain subgroup) met criteria for the classification of the FMS, but the patients who reported having regional pain were not examined to confirm the presence of MPS (Fig. 23–1A).

In a study designed to document the prevalence of MPS in a general internal medicine practice, Skootsky and coworkers[17] screened 201 patients and more thoroughly evaluated 172, who presented to an academic health care center for various reasons; 54 patients, whose presenting complaints included musculoskeletal pain, were retained for additional testing. The approach was first to eliminate those who had pain conditions clearly unrelated to the MPS. The remainder were given a detailed TrP examination, guided by body pain diagrams that had been completed by the patients. When a muscle was found to contain a TrP, it was digitally compressed for 5 to 20 seconds to see whether that maneuver would intensify the pain. The diagnosis of MPS was made when the patient exhibited regional pain intensified by digital pressure, and the referral pattern corresponded with established referral maps. It was discovered that 16 patients (30% of 54, 8% of 201) in an academic general internal medicine practice satisfied criteria for the diagnosis

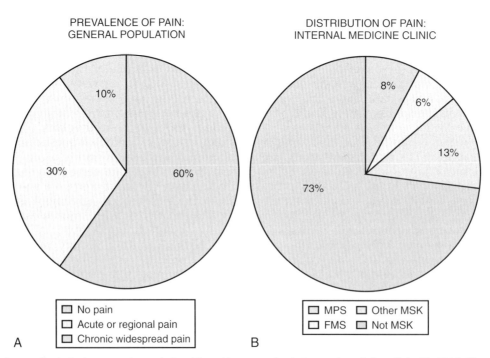

Figure 23–1. Prevalence of pain in the general population **(A)** and in an academic internal medicine clinic **(B)**. FMS, fibromyalgia syndrome; MPS, myopathic pain syndrome; MSK, musculoskeletal.

of MPS. As shown in Figure 23–1B, this would be slightly higher than the reported prevalence of the FMS (about 6%) in an academic internal medicine practice.[18]

Related Syndromes

Two areas of the body that deserve special attention regarding MPS are the muscles of mastication[19] and the muscles of the pelvis.[20-22]

Dentists typically diagnose and manage the temporomandibular syndrome, now referred to as myofascial pain dysfunction (MPD) syndrome. A classic study[19] of MPD, from the University of Minnesota School of Dentistry, identified 164 patients with this condition from among 296 patients presenting with pain in the head and neck. In the patients with MPD, there was tenderness in at least one muscle of mastication, referral of the pain to an expected zone of reference, and frequent comorbid conditions, such as postural or emotive factors. In most cases (66%), the symptoms emerged gradually, but in others there was a history of antecedent dental work or motor vehicle accident.

The muscles of the pelvis can contribute to pain that can be confused with low back pain or with female organ pathology in which urethral pain, vulvodynia, or dyspareunia can be manifest.[20-23] Pelvic area muscles with MPS (e.g., piriformis, iliopsoas, obturator internus) can refer pain to pelvic structures, causing the dysfunction, or they can compress nerves (sciatic nerve, pudendal nerve), which are then responsible for the symptoms. The interested reader is referred to the original publications for help with anatomic perspective, examination methods, and management.

Proposed Pathogenesis

Several authors have published theories about the predisposing factors and initiating events that may be responsible for the onset of the MPS.[4,5,24-26] Briefly, it has been suggested that predisposing factors, such as body asymmetry and poor posture, can conspire with mechanical stressors, radiculopathy,[27,28] nutritional inadequacies, endocrine dysfunctions, or anger or other psychological factors to initiate the symptoms of the MPS.

Exploration of the TrP using needle electromyography (EMG) in a rabbit model of MPS[29] and in symptomatic humans[30] has led to the finding of spontaneous electrical activity (SEA).[31] In a controlled research study, an electromyographer found this SEA phenomenon significantly more often when probing with an electromyographic needle in the location of a human TrP site than in the location of a control site.[32] Because local infusion of phentolamine eliminated this SEA phenomenon and the pain, it was speculated that the trigger point has the characteristic adrenergic dependency of the muscle spindle.[31,33,34] Others have argued that the TrP is anatomically located at a neuromuscular junction.[26,32,34] The evidence seems to support a spinal reflex that could involve the spindle and neuromuscular junction within the muscle, spinal cord, and radicular nerves that connect the muscle to the cord.

The most dramatic demonstration of objective abnormalities in MPS has come from microanalysis of interstitial fluid samples obtained from human skeletal muscle TrPs.[35,36] The concentrations of proteins, bradykinin, calcitonin gene-related peptide, substance P, tumor necrosis factor α, interleukin-1β, serotonin, and norepinephrine were found to be significantly higher in this fluid. Local ischemia is suggested by a lower than normal pH in the region of the TrP ($P < 0.01$).

Management Approaches

Most authors have advised the use of a systematic, comprehensive, multidisciplinary approach to the treatment of MPS.[4,5,24,37] It has been emphasized that important components of such a program should include the services of an empathetic provider, who is well informed about this condition, has made an accurate diagnosis, has identified predisposing and perpetuating factors, and makes strategic use of both physical modalities and medications of proven efficacy. These appear to be surprisingly confident interventions for a condition whose very diagnosis is plagued by uncertainty.

A simple physical intervention, which is often at least temporarily effective, involves repeatedly applying a cold spray over the TrP in line with the involved muscle fibers, followed by gentle massage of the TrP, with stretching of the affected muscle.[4,5] Observing a dramatic therapeutic success with this procedure has the effect of generating belief in the MPS concept on a broader scale. It also represents a teachable moment for patient education, because the patient can learn to abort progression of future attacks at an early stage by applying his or her own local stretch and massage. On the other hand, it is acknowledged that this approach is more readily applied to a superficial muscle, such as the trapezius fibers around the neck, than for a more deeply positioned muscle, such as the piriformis or iliopsoas muscles of the pelvis.

The skills of an experienced physical therapist can be used to teach better posture, body mechanics, and relaxation techniques and to provide TrP massage, postisometric relaxation, reciprocal inhibition, and other manual modalities.[4,5]

A more invasive approach to therapy is local injection or dry needling of the TrP.[4,5,38] Whereas the pain of MPS in a given muscle can be eliminated by local anesthesia of the relevant sensory and motor nerves, that approach provides only temporary relief. The more lasting approach is referred to as TrP injection. After the symptomatic (active) TrP has been identified, small amounts of a local anesthetic can be injected into the muscle using short jabs of the needle into the location of the TrP.

It is believed that local anesthetic offers no long-term benefit but does make the procedure less uncomfortable. Many practitioners argue in favor of dry needling because the overall results are similar and the patient is not placed at risk of being sensitized to an adverse reaction from the anesthetic.[39] The effectiveness of the needling procedure is explained by local structural damage to the TrP caused by repeated passes of the needle. It is less clear whether scar tissue formation in the area represents an impediment to recurrence or a nidus favoring it. Typically, several local needlings over a period of weeks or months are required to achieve a cure. The required course is recognized to be substantially longer when MPS is complicated by the comorbidity of FMS.[40] Some have found additional usefulness in the injection of botulinum toxin,[41] but others have failed to demonstrate a significant effect in controlled clinical trials.[42] Based on clinical observations by Hubbard,[43] it would seem reasonable to consider a trial of phenoxybenzamine in MPS to inhibit function of the muscle spindle.

Therefore, it seems likely that the MPS is a legitimate clinical construct that has not yet achieved the recognition it deserves, partly because the MPS is challenging to diagnose, but more importantly because diagnostic criteria have not yet been validated. This is not likely to change until experts in the field feel the need for validated criteria and put their collective efforts to the task so that the results will be more universally accepted. Until that is accomplished, the MPS will remain in a form of clinical and scientific limbo. When it does happen, the next steps would be possible—to conduct believable epidemiologic, pathologic, and therapeutic studies. The outcomes of such studies would substantially advance the field, both scientifically and in the arena of public opinion.

FIBROMYALGIA SYNDROME

Diagnostic Criteria

Before 1990, there were no widely accepted criteria for the diagnosis of FMS, so the situation with that condition was comparable to that of the MPS today. The results of a multicenter research study, sanctioned by the American College of Rheumatology (ACR),[12] have led to the development of research criteria for the classification of FMS (Table 23–1). Almost immediately, these criteria were widely accepted. Epidemiologic, biologic, and therapeutic studies were undertaken with greater confidence; reports about FMS increased from about 15 to over 100 annually. These criteria required only two simple components—a history of widespread pain for at least 3 months and allodynia to digital pressure at 11 or more of 18 anatomically defined tender points[12] (TePs; Table 23–2). They exhibited moderately high sensitivity (88.4%) and specificity (81.1%) for FMS against controls (pain-free normals and patients with other painful conditions).

The TeP of FMS is conceptually and physiologically different from the TrP of MPS in that TePs are symmetrically widespread in the body, not necessarily

Table 23–1. American College of Rheumatology (ACR) Criteria for Research Classification of Fibromyalgia Syndrome (FMS)

CRITERION	DESCRIPTION
1. History	Chronic, widespread (four quadrants) soft tissue pain for 3 mo
2. Examination	Pain (1+ or greater severity) induced by 4 kg of digital palpation pressure at 11 of 18 anatomically defined tender points (TePs; see Table 23–2)
3. 1 and 2 are true	When 1 and 2 are true, sensitivity and specificity for FMS > 80%

Adapted from Wolfe F, Smythe HA, Yunus MB, et al: The American College of Rheumatology 1990 Criteria for the Classification of Fibromyalgia. R eport of the Multicenter Criteria Committee. Arthritis Rheum 1990;33:160-172.

Table 23–2. Eighteen Anatomically Defined Tender Points in Fibromyalgia Syndrome

NUMBER	OFFICIAL AMERICAN COLLEGE OF RHEUMATOLOGY BILATERAL TENDER POINT SITES
1, 2	Occiput—suboccipital muscle insertions.
3, 4	Low cervical—anterior aspects of C5-7 intertransverse spaces
5, 6	Trapezius—midpoint of upper border
7, 8	Supraspinatus—origins above scapula spine, near medial border
9, 10	Second rib—upper lateral surface of second costochondral joint
11, 12	Lateral epicondyle—2 cm distal to epicondyles
13, 14	Gluteal—upper outer buttock, anterior fold of muscle
15, 16	Greater trochanter—posterior to trochanteric prominence
17, 18	Knees—medial fat pad, just proximal to medial condyle

Adapted from Wolfe F, Smythe HA, Yunus MB, et al: The American College of Rheumatology 1990 Criteria for the Classification of Fibromyalgia. Report of the Multicenter Criteria Committee. Arthritis Rheum 1990;33:160-172.

located in muscles, and do not refer pain. The anatomic location of the tenderness at FMS TePs is deep to the skin in various soft tissue structures, such as skeletal muscles, ligaments, and bursae, but there has never been convincing evidence that the painful tissues are histologically abnormal. The amount of pressure to use for this examination can be standardized against an algometer, but a reasonably accurate estimate of the correct amount of pressure (4 kg) can be obtained by pressing the examining thumb against a surface until the blood flow to the distal one fourth of the thumb nail blanches. The amount of perceived discomfort can be accentuated and prolonged by applying the stimulus repetitively to induce wind-up.[44]

Three clinical measures have been useful in globally assessing the severity of pain in a given FMS patient. These are the total tender point count (TTP), tender point index (TPI, also known as the myalgic score) and the average pain threshold (APT). The TTP is the number of TePs (range, 0 to 18) that are reported by the patient to be painful with 4 kg of digital palpation pressure. Although a TTP value of 11 is critical in classifying FMS, that measure lacks sensitivity to change as a research outcome. Because the TPI and APT are severity scales, they are more sensitive to changes in pain severity with time. The TPI is influenced more by the affective status of the patient than is the APT. The TPI is obtained by summing the severity of tenderness to 4 kg of digital pressure at all 18 TePs, using the following scale: nontender, 0; tender without physical response, 1; tender plus wince or withdrawal; 2, tender plus exaggerated withdrawal, 3; and too painful to examine, 4 (range, 0 to 72). The APT is calculated as the average algometric pressure required to induce the transition from the sensation of pressure to the perception of pain at all 18 TePs.

Many criticisms have been leveled against the ACR criteria for the diagnosis of FMS. One relates to the fact that the criteria are largely subjective and were not specifically validated for use in community practice, where most clinical diagnoses are made. Although this criticism is legitimate, the same type of concern is conspicuously absent regarding the ACR-endorsed classification criteria developed in a similar manner for other rheumatic diseases.

Another criticism of the ACR criteria, without any objective data to support it, has been that making the diagnosis of FMS might somehow be detrimental to the FMS patient's illness, actually having the effect of making the patient worse. This argument however, was repudiated by the study of White and colleagues.[45]

A third criticism of the ACR criteria has been that the diagnosis requires 11 TePs; however, some clinic patients, with a history of widespread pain, exhibit fewer than 11 TePs. As a result, the physician is uncertain about what to call the patient's illness, but there can be several responses. It is known that 10% of those in the general population experience chronic widespread pain, whereas only 2% meet criteria for FMS.[16] It was reasoned at the time that when research on this 2% (with FMS, the most severe of those with widespread STP) discovers effective therapies, they could be applied to the remaining 8%, with reasonable hope of benefit. If pathologic mechanisms were found in the 2%, they could later be more efficiently sought in the 8%. Perhaps the real concern is the lack of a name for those in the 8% subgroup. It is curious that the same critics who object to giving people with widespread allodynia the diagnosis of FMS are troubled by not having a name for the excluded 8%.

This issue was indirectly addressed by the results of a study[46] in which the investigator proposed to compare, in a single practice, FMS diagnoses made by three different approaches: (1) ACR criteria for FMS carefully applied by a nurse; (2) a diagnosis of FMS defined by specific threshold scores on two self-report questionnaires; and (3) a diagnosis of FMS based on the clinician's personal opinion about who

should be included. The patients were to be evaluated by all three criteria so that the denominator would be the same. Of the 120 patients who were diagnosed with FMS by at least one of these three methods, only 50% met the ACR criteria, 69% met the dual-questionnaire criteria, and 84% were identified by the clinician. The composition of each diagnosis group was different, although there was overlap. The implication is that if ACR criteria are not used for community diagnosis of FMS, those diagnosed will be different from the current definition of FMS. If this is true, the established clinical, epidemiologic, pathologic, and therapeutic information in the FMS database would no longer be directly relevant and would have to be reassessed. Even as it is, the FMS population is composed of subgroups. It now seems best to keep FMS criteria the same and call the 8% something else, even if they prove to benefit from FMS therapy. This would remain until an entirely new basis can be agreed on for conceptualizing this multimodal condition.

Finally, it has been argued, especially in Europe, that the gatekeepers of medicine will not examine patients to document TePs, so the criteria will prove to be impractical in the clinic. Clearly, the primary care physician (PCP) does have limited time with the patient and may only be able to serve as a triage officer. Considering that possibility, a four-phase program has been envisioned to facilitate the efficient screening, referral, and management of those with FMS (Box 23–4). The plan begins in phase 1, with a simple screening questionnaire (Fig. 23–2) given to all patients entering the PCP's waiting room. The objective is to identify people who have chronic widespread pain (WSP), according to the body pain diagram. In phase 2, persons with WSP would be evaluated for TePs by the PCP or, more likely, by the secondary care physician, to make the FMS diagnosis. At that level, the patient would be screened for comorbidities, perhaps with a small strategic battery of validated questionnaires. In phase 3, the patient with a serious or recalcitrant comorbid condition may be referred to a tertiary specialist for management of that specific problem. Phase 4 provides for adjustment of therapeutic interventions based on the results of serial outcome assessment.

Prevalence Estimates

The FMS has been found in all ethnic groups studied to date; it is not limited to affluent or industrialized nations. With prevalence estimates ranging from 2% to almost 12% in the general population, it must be viewed as a common medical condition.[16] Its prevalence increases with age, most dramatically in women, with a peak in the fifth to seventh decade (7.4%-10%). Middle-aged women are four to seven times more likely to be affected than men of similar age. By contrast, the gender distribution of childhood FMS is almost equal and many children outgrow their symptoms.[47] About 15% of patients seen in rheumatology clinics are classified as having FMS,

---

**BOX 23–4. PROPOSED PLAN FOR SCREENING AND COMPREHENSIVE CARE OF
FIBROMYALGIA SYNDROME (FMS)**

Phase 1: Pain Screening and Primary Care
A simple screening questionnaire that the receptionist for a primary care health professional (primary care physician [PCP], chiropractors, nurse practitioner, physician assistant, general practitioner, general internists) would give to every patient entering the waiting room until all the primary care professional's regular patients had been assessed. Thereafter, it may be given only to new patients. When the PCP reviews the form of a patient with pain (question 1 answered "yes"), a decision about the symptom's distribution would be made (localized pain, regional pain, widespread pain). A second decision would be whether to initiate care for the patient's symptoms or refer the patient for further care of this problem.

**Phase 2: Comorbidity Screening and
Secondary Care**
Based on the findings on the screening materials, the patient identified as having widespread pain would be examined by the PCP or referral physician to make the diagnosis (FMS, if that applies). The next stage would be a screening for comorbid conditions by a well-informed and willing PCP or consultant (rheumatologist, neurologist, pain specialist, internist, physiatrist). The patient would begin an exercise program and counseling with a professional specifically trained to provide

advanced care for FMS. Problems found in counseling (e.g., marital, financial, psychiatric) would spin off to an experienced specialist (e.g., counselor, psychologist, psychiatrist, disability advisor, financial counseling).

Phase 3: Comorbidity Screening and Tertiary Care
Based on second-line screening for comorbidities, care would begin for those additional diagnoses. This phase may invoke referral to tertiary subspecialty care (e.g., cardiologist, gastroenterologist, neurologist, neurosurgeon, physical therapist, psychiatrist, physiatrist, obstetrician-gynecologist, urologist). This care would be integrated with follow-up by the primary care resource.

**Phase 4: Long-term Primary Care and
Follow-up Assessment**
The primary or secondary care health professional would continue to follow the patient over time, assessing the status of care for pain and comorbidities. There would be monitoring for side effects to medications and for new problems intruding on the continuity of the fibromyalgia that might or might not be related to it. In this phase, it is important not to assume that every new symptom presenting in an FMS patient is a component of the FMS. Health care providers will need to know what is and is not expected with FMS.

---

whereas the prevalence of FMS is about 6% in other practice settings. In 1997, the annual direct cost of care for the average FMS patient in the United States was estimated to be more than $2000.[48] Multiplied by the 6 million U.S. patients with FMS, that figure predicts an annual direct cost of more than $12 billion (Fig. 23–3).

Little is known about the incidence of FMS but risk factors for its development may include physical trauma, a febrile illness, or a family history of FMS, but these may not be mutually exclusive. A study conducted in Israel[49] has shown that automobile accidents with whiplash neck injury are more likely to result in symptomatic FMS than industrial accidents that cause a bony fracture of a lower extremity (22% vs. 2% for all subjects, more than 30% for female accident victims). A narrowed cervical canal may be an important risk factor for the development of chronic pain following a whiplash injury.[50]

Clinical Presentation

The clinical manifestations of FMS are usually more complex than body pain alone. Associated symptoms (comorbidities) often require further investigation and specific management. For example, patients describe disordered sleep, obstructive sleep apnea,

fatigue, cognitive dysfunction, dizziness, headaches, psychological distress, depression, anxiety, chest pains, dysesthesia in the hands, cold intolerance, restless legs, and irritable bowel or irritable bladder syndrome. These comorbid symptoms clearly contribute to the suffering experienced by FMS patients. As a result, affected individuals tend to leave their jobs and otherwise restrict social interactions until they feel isolated, alone, and out of touch with others.

Cognitive Dysfunction

People with FMS frequently complain about diminished cognitive function. This ranges from difficulty concentrating when reading a book to short-term memory deficits. Research has suggested that FMS patients perform poorly on a range of cognitive tasks,[51] exhibiting premature cognitive aging, with the main evidence of abnormality coming from distraction or multitasking experiments.

Affective Distress

Before FMS was better understood as a condition of central sensitization, patients with this condition

Phase 1: Screening Questionnaire

Instructions: Answer Yes or No to each of the following questions. If you answer "No to question 1, you are done. You do not need to read any of the other questions. When you are done, please return the completed questionnaire to the office clerk.

Yes No

☐ ☐ 1. Have you had body pain for at least three months?

☐ ☐ 2. Was your body pain one of your reasons for coming to the doctor today?

Instructions: If you answered Yes to question 1, mark a slanted line across the line below to indicate how severe your pain has been over the past two weeks.

| No pain | | Severe pain |

Instructions: If you answered Yes to question 1, use a pencil or pen, to <u>mark darkly</u> on the body diagrams the locations of your pain during the last week.

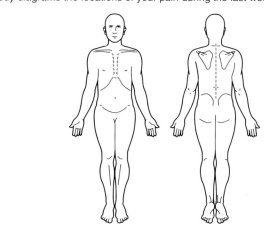

Figure 23–2. Screening questionnaire for chronic widespread pain as seen in the fibromyalgia syndrome. The findings supportive of the fibromyalgia syndrome would be chronic pain from question 1, the relative severity of the pain from question 3, and widespread pain from question 4. Each question could also be applied to other categories of soft tissue pain and patients with localized or regional musculoskeletal pain, if present, would be identified by the body pain diagram. APT, average pain threshold; TPI, tender point index.

Below this line is for office use only. Please do not mark below this line.

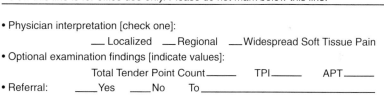

- Physician interpretation [check one]:
        __ Localized   __ Regional   __ Widespread Soft Tissue Pain
- Optional examination findings [indicate values]:
        Total Tender Point Count_____   TPI_____   APT_____
- Referral: ____Yes   ____No   To_____

were often suspected of having a psychiatric disorder. Indeed, the frequencies of depression and anxiety in FMS were each found to be about 40% at the time of the FMS diagnosis,[52] but that left 60% who were not actively depressed or anxious. Depression also occurs with rheumatoid arthritis (RA; 20% to 30%), cancer, and other chronic conditions (14% to 33%). In these settings, the psychological comorbidities are believed to result from the pain and physical limitation imposed by the disease. The same could be true for FMS. Sexual abuse in childhood is no longer a viable hypothesis for the cause of FMS.[53]

Insomnia

Most FMS patients experience chronic insomnia. Some have difficulty falling asleep (initial insomnia),

but most awaken feeling distressingly alert after only a few hours of sleep (midinsomnia) and are then unable to sleep soundly again until it is almost morning (terminal insomnia). People with FMS typically awaken in the morning feeling painfully stiff, cognitively sluggish, and unrefreshed by their sleep. It is surprising that these chronically sleep-deprived individuals have difficulty napping during the day.

Stiffness

The morning stiffness experienced by most FMS patients is remarkable because it lasts so long and is so severe. The typical stiffness of osteoarthritis (OA) is usually 5 to 15 minutes, whereas that of inflammatory RA patients is 30 minutes to 2 hours. By comparison, the stiffness of FMS patients is typically 45

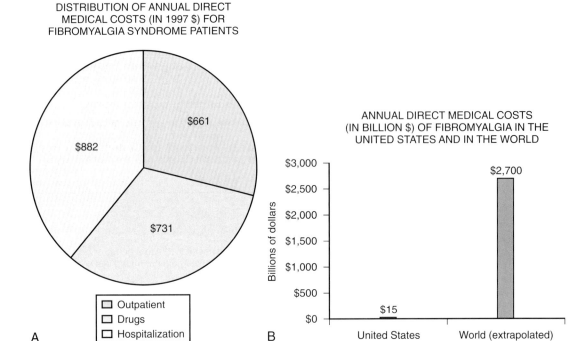

DISTRIBUTION OF ANNUAL DIRECT
MEDICAL COSTS (IN 1997 $) FOR
FIBROMYALGIA SYNDROME PATIENTS

$661

$882

$731

☐ Outpatient
☐ Drugs
☐ Hospitalization

A

ANNUAL DIRECT MEDICAL COSTS
(IN BILLION $) OF FIBROMYALGIA IN THE
UNITED STATES AND IN THE WORLD

$2,700

$15

United States   World (extrapolated)

B

Figure 23–3. Direct medical costs associated with the fibromyalgia syndrome. **A,** Distribution of average, annual direct medical costs (in 1997 dollars) for individual fibromyalgia syndrome patients. The total is $2,274 in 1997 dollars, which would need to be adjusted for inflation since that time. This amount does not include the cost of assistance in the home, cost of work income lost, or toll on the family resulting from an affected individual. **B,** Annual direct medical costs (in billions of 1997 dollars) for the fibromyalgia syndrome in the United States and extrapolated for the world. In this representation, the costs in the United States appear trivial next to costs worldwide. The extrapolation is relatively accurate in terms of numbers of affected individuals, but probably fails because the level of care provided and the cost of that care may be radically different among countries.

minutes to 4 hours. The best clinical correlate with morning stiffness in FMS is pain, so patients may not be clearly distinguishing these seemingly different symptoms.

Fatigue

About 80% of FMS patients complain of fatigue and a small subgroup meet the new criteria for CFS. The fatigue of CFS (a feeling of weakness) is qualitatively and quantitatively different from that of FMS (a feeling of tiredness). The differential diagnosis of fatigue is difficult because it must include various sleep disorders, chronic infections, autoimmune disorders, psychiatric comorbidities, and neoplasia. Fatigue may also result from residual levels of sedating medication, such as tricyclic antidepressant drugs, or other sedatives often used to treat the insomnia of FMS.

Irritable Bowel Syndrome and Dyspepsia

Irritable bowel syndrome (IBS) and benign dyspepsia are common gastrointestinal conditions, occurring in 30% to 50% of FMS patients. A feature common

to both FMS and IBS may be central sensitization. These may be synergistic in regard to the patient's perception of his or her illness and have a modulating effect on the clinical outcome. A common differential diagnosis is lactose intolerance, which can cause intermittent cramping, diarrhea, and flatulence. A simple litmus test of the feces will show acidic pH when lactose intolerance is the cause of diarrhea.

Irritable Bladder (Urethral) Syndrome

About 60% of FMS patients experience urinary urgency and nocturia on a regular basis. Up to 12% of FMS patients fulfill the diagnostic criteria for the female urethral syndrome.[54] This is defined as the presence of urinary frequency, dysuria, suprapubic discomfort, and urethral pain, despite sterile urine. Many patients report having been treated with antibiotics frequently for culture-negative urinary tract infections. Intensive investigations often fail to disclose a specific cause. Eliminating coffee from the patient's diet may be therapeutic. A new self-report questionnaire instrument has been developed to facilitate screening for this condition in FMS patients.[55]

Related Syndromes

It is currently believed that when the 1990 ACR classification criteria are met, it is appropriate to classify the affected patient as having FMS irrespective of, or in addition to, any other legitimate medical diagnoses. Conversely, patients with other chronic diseases can develop FMS at any time in the course of their symptoms. For want of better terminology, in the setting of another painful condition or inflammatory disorder, the FMS condition has been referred to as secondary FMS. That terminology is not intended to imply that the FMS is caused by the other condition, but the terminology is entrenched and serves a purpose. Secondary FMS may not be clinically distinguishable from that of primary FMS[12] but, increasingly, there are laboratory findings that distinguish these FMS subgroups.[56]

As examples of a secondary FMS, almost 30% of patients with RA, 40% of systemic lupus erythematosus patients, and 50% of Sjögren's syndrome patients have concomitant FMS. Patients with a rheumatic disease and FMS seem to experience articular pain disproportionate to their synovitis. This must be considered when treating the rheumatic condition because increasing the dosage of antirheumatic medications in the absence of active inflammation may have little effect on the pain amplified by FMS. The best results are obtained by treating each condition separately.

Rheumatic disease patients with concomitant FMS should be warned that a transient increase in FMS symptoms may occur with each decrease in glucocorticoid dosage (steroid withdrawal FMS), so the usual FMS therapy may need to be increased transiently. This is a surprising phenomenon, because glucocorticoid is not helpful in treating primary FMS. To avoid interference with a steroid taper by emergent FMS, it is best to decrease the dosage of glucocorticoid used to treat the rheumatic disease in graduated steps at about 2-week intervals. The rate of the taper depends on the current dosage—for prednisone equivalent to 60 mg/day, step down directly to 30 mg/day; then, by 5-mg/dose steps, from 30 to 15 mg/day, then, by 2.5-mg/dose steps to 5 mg/day, and then, by 1-mg/dose steps, until the lowest effective dosage has been achieved.

Infectious and inflammatory conditions that seem to be associated with FMS include hepatitis C, tuberculosis, syphilis, and Lyme disease. The prevalence of overlap may depend on the community prevalence of the infectious disease. An academic practice in a Lyme-endemic area evaluated 788 patients with apparent infection for a mean of 2.5 years.[57] Of those with Lyme disease, 20% met criteria for FMS. The symptoms of FMS developed 1 to 4 months after infection, often in association with Lyme arthritis. The signs of Lyme disease generally resolved with antibiotic therapy, but the FMS symptoms often persisted. The largest subgroup of the 788 patients did not have Lyme disease but did meet criteria for FMS or chronic fatigue syndrome.

An association between subacute bacterial endocarditis and FMS has not been formally explored, but the characteristic somatic symptoms with endocarditis (arthralgias, myalgias) suggest that diagnostic confusion could occur.

Pathogenesis

The cause of FMS is still unknown. Theories regarding its cause have undergone a gradual transition from a psychiatric process, as some still view it, to a muscle disorder, as currently classified in the Medline Index, to a genetically determined central nervous system disorder of chronic widespread allodynia, neuroendocrine function, and cytokine participation, as it should now be considered.

The situation with FMS has changed dramatically in just a few years of concentrated research. In contrast with just 2 decades ago, when FMS patients were often viewed as healthy complainers without any real abnormalities, there are now classification criteria to aid in making the diagnosis. Whereas patients were once considered to be depressed somatizers, the psychiatric model is no longer adequate. The pathogenesis was once diligently sought in "painful muscles," but symptoms now appear to have better fit with a central sensitization model. Although it was stated that there are no abnormal test findings in FMS, abnormalities in neurochemical mediators of central nervous system nociceptive function are clearly present in ways consistent with the patterns of symptoms.

The roles of neurochemicals as neurotransmitters and modulators of the nociceptive process have been studied extensively in animals[58]; the findings are now at least theoretically relevant to human FMS with allodynia.[59] It is believed that these agents participate in descending inhibition of nociception. This line of reasoning has led to the measurement of neurotransmitter levels in biologic fluids obtained from FMS patients. Several major classes of biochemical participants in the nociceptive process are the biogenic amines (e.g., serotonin, norepinephrine, dopamine), excitatory amino acids (e.g., glutamic acid, glutamine, aspartic acid, asparagine, glycine, arginine), neurokinins (e.g., substance P, calcitonin gene-related protein, arginine vasopressin, neuropeptide Y), nerve growth factor, and probably nitric oxide. The biogenic amines are generally considered to be antinociceptive whereas the excitatory amino acids, substance P, nerve growth factor, and perhaps even nitric oxide would more likely be pronociceptive. Animal and human data are available; most human data come directly from studies of FMS patients.

Moldofsky and Walsh[60] were the first to suggest that serotonin (5-hydroxytryptamine, 5-HT) might be involved in the pathogenesis of FMS, both in failing to attenuate persistent pain and to correct the chronic deficiency in slow-wave sleep. They found a clinical correlate between FMS pain and the plasma concentration of tryptophan (TRP). More recently, the serum and cerebrospinal fluid (CSF) of FMS patients were found to exhibit low concentrations of TRP.[61,62] Early findings of a low serum concentration of 5-HT[63] have been supported by other investigators.[64] The levels of 5-HT have not yet been reported in the CSF of FMS patients but the levels of its immediate precursor, 5-hydroxytryptophan (5-HTP) and its metabolic product, 5-hydroxyindole acetic acid (5-HIAA) have been studied. In FMS, both were found to exhibit lower than normal CSF concentrations relative to the CSF of HNC.[62,65] In addition, 5-HIAA was measured in 24-hour urine samples of patients with FMS and compared with the results from HNC.[66] The rate of 5-HIAA excretion was significantly lower in FMS than in the HNC, lower in female than in male FMS patients, and lower in female FMS than in female HNC patients.[66] Even the numbers of active FMS TePs correlated with the concentration of 5-HT in FMS sera.[67]

The role of α-adrenergic agonists such as norepinephrine (NE) in the antinociception system of FMS patients may be similar to that of 5-HT, but a number of unique features of this biogenic amine have attracted attention.[68] The concentration of methoxy-hydroxyphenylglycol (MHPG), the inactive metabolite of NE, is significantly lower than normal in FMS CSF.[65] Considering the possibility that the elevated CSF substance P (SP) level might be lowered by an α2-adrenergic agonist, the effects of tizanidine were studied in those with FMS before drug administration and after 2 months of therapy while still taking the drug.[69] The result was a significant lowering of the CSF SP level, although not to normal levels, and simultaneous improvement in clinical symptoms. Unfortunately, the two changes did not correlate significantly.

The concentration of homovanillic acid, the inactive metabolite of dopamine, was found to be significantly lower than normal in FMS CSF.[65] This finding, which would imply low CNS levels of dopamine in FMS, was complemented by a study of the role of dopamine receptors in the function of the hypothalamus and pituitary in FMS.[70]

The neuropeptide, SP, is an 11–amino acid peptide that has several important roles in the process of nociception. Activated, small, thinly myelinated A-delta and C-fiber afferent neurons respond to noxious peripheral stimuli by releasing SP into laminae I and V (A-delta) and lamina II (C-fiber) of the spinal cord dorsal horn. With random interstitial diffusion, SP or its C-terminal peptide fragment makes contact with its neurokinin-1 (NK1) effector receptor. The mechanism of SP action in the dorsal horn of the spinal cord is not entirely clear but it appears not to be a signal transporter, as is glutamic acid. Rather, SP apparently facilitates nociception by arming or alerting spinal cord neurons to incoming nociceptive signals from the periphery.

Vaeroy and associates,[71] working in Norway, were the first to recognize that the concentration of SP was elevated (average threefold increase) in the CSF of FMS patients compared with HNC subjects. Their findings have now been reproduced in three other clinical studies.[72-74] The biologic relevance of substance P in CSF to the pain of primary FMS is still uncertain. An important question is whether an elevated CSF SP level is unique to FMS. An earlier report[75] has indicated that CSF SP concentrations are lower than normal in various chronic painful conditions. For example, CSF SP levels were found to be lower than normal in diabetic neuropathy[76] and chronic low back pain.[77] By contrast, elevated levels of CSF SP have been found in patients with painful rheumatic diseases, whether or not they have concomitant FMS.[78] In painful osteoarthritis of the hip, the elevated CSF SP level prior to surgical treatment returned to normal after successful total hip arthroplasty (complete replacement of the hip joint with mechanical components), which left the patients almost free from hip pain.[79]

The elevated CSF SP level in FMS has prompted much speculation about the cause. Nerve growth factor was known to stimulate the production of substance P in small, afferent, unmyelinated neurons. It was therefore an exciting development to have found elevated levels of nerve growth factor (NGF) in the CSF of primary FMS patients, but not in FMS with an associated painful inflammatory condition (secondary FMS).[80] This suggests that there may be different mechanisms for the elevated SP level in primary FMS and FMS associated with inflammatory diseases.[12] In primary FMS, the elevated CSF SP level seems to be induced by nerve growth factor, whereas in secondary FMS the cause may be inflammation in the periphery.

Another approach for understanding the cause of FMS has been through genetic studies. About one third of FMS patients have reported that another family member, usually a female, has a similar, chronic pain condition or has already been given the diagnosis of FMS.[81] Published studies have documented familial patterns. Some have predicted an autosomal dominant mode of inheritance for FMS[82,83] and evidence for this has increased.[84] In a study by Yunus and coworkers,[85] a linkage of FMS with the histocompatibility locus was examined by the sibship method. A complete genome scan of families with two or more FMS-affected members has been undertaken[86] using samples of deoxyribonucleic acid (DNA) from a large number of FMS multicase families for comparison with clinical and laboratory genotypic features. Meanwhile, several candidate genes have been proposed to directly explain specific metabolic abnormalities that have been consistently observed in FMS. A study of 80 multicase FMS families has already examined markers spanning the genomic regions for the following: the serotonin transporter (HTTLPR, three regional markers) on chromosome 17; the serotonin receptor 2A (HTR2A, three regional markers) on chromosome 13; and the histocompatibility locus antigen (HLA, two regional markers) region of chromosome 6.[87] No evidence for linkage was found in the HTTLPR region. Fami-lies with an older age of onset were linked to the HLA region (logarithm of the odds [LOD] = 3.02,

$P = 0.00057$), suggesting an immune-mediated pathogenesis. In the HTR2A region, the results indicated a moderately strong linkage to families with a younger age of onset, less severe pain, lower levels of depression, and absence of the irritable bowel syndrome (LOD = 5.56, $P = 0.000057$). The HTR2A genome is polymorphically imprinted, so the issue of parent of origin will need to be considered in future studies. Bioinformatics mining and further sequencing of genes in the HTR2A region will help identify specific polymorphisms for further clinical association testing.

Another appealing gene candidate as a causative factor in FMS would be the catechol-O-methyltransferase (COMT) enzyme, which physiologically inactivates catecholamines such as dopamine, norepinephrine, endorphins, and catecholamine-containing drugs. Polymorphism (actually dimorphism) in the gene encodes for variations in COMT enzyme activity. The COMT gene exists in two forms, L and H, which make copies differing by a single amino acid (either valine or methionine) at the variable site. This small variation has a large effect on the activity of COMT. Subjects with the LL phenotype, who have two copies of the methionine version, make three- to fourfold less COMT than the HH variants, which contain valine at the variable site. The significance of COMT polymorphism (LL, LH, or HH) in FMS was assessed by Gursoy and colleagues.[88] Sixty-one patients with FMS and 61 demographically matched HNCs were included in the study. Although no significant difference was found between LL and LH separately, the LL and LH genotypes together were more highly represented in FMS than in the HNC groups ($P = 0.024$). In addition, HH genotypes in FMS were significantly lower than in the HNC groups ($P = 0.04$).

The much higher prevalence of FMS in women has led to speculation regarding gender-specific causes. For example, in an epidemiologic study of a Midwestern community,[89] the curves representing pain thresholds (sensitivity to a pressure stimulus) in men and women consistently showed lower values for women. Because the examination component of the ACR criteria for FMS involves the response to a fixed pressure stimulus of 4 kg, it is not surprising that these criteria have identified more women than men with FMS. Understanding the mechanisms responsible for this gender-related difference in pain thresholds is incomplete. Measurements of female hormones have not been very fruitful. One possible explanation is that men normally make substantially more 5-HT in their brains than women.[90]

Many symptoms of FMS resemble those observed in patients with hormone deficiencies. This observation has led to the study of neuroendocrine function in FMS.[91] Subsets of those with FMS exhibit functional abnormalities in the hypothalamic-pituitary-adrenal (HPA) axis, sympathoadrenal (autonomic nervous) system, hypothalamic-pituitary-thyroid (HPT) axis, hypothalamic-pituitary-gonadal (HPG) axis, or hypothalamic–pituitary–growth hormone (HGH) axis.[92] In FMS patients, the HPA axis exhibits an exaggerated adrenocorticotropic hormone (ACTH) response to insulin-induced hypoglycemia or stressful exercise. Despite this dramatic rise in serum ACTH level in FMS, the level of cortisol did not rise commensurately. Mediators that regulate the HPA include corticotropin-releasing factor, serotonin, norepinephrine, substance P, and interleukin-6 (IL-6).[93,94]

Growth hormone was studied because it was known to be produced during delta wave sleep (stages 3 and 4, non–random eye movement), which many FMS patients fail to achieve normally. An alternative means of monitoring growth hormone production has been to measure the plasma levels of insulin-like growth factor-1 (IGF-1, previously known as somatomedin C) which has a long half-life. An age-adjusted deficiency of IGF-1 has been documented in FMS.[95] In addition, administration of human growth hormone to FMS patients was effective in reducing the severity of FMS symptoms.[96]

The reasons why these endocrinopathies would be associated with a chronic pain syndrome are not entirely clear. It may be that central nervous system abnormalities in the availability of biogenic amines such as serotonin, norepinephrine, or dopamine are responsible for the abnormal regulation of the neuroendocrine system.[65] These systems interact and are interdependent, so in susceptible individuals, a partial failure of one system may lead to subtle malfunctions of others.

A comprehensive review of immune function abnormalities has been published,[97] but more current information is available. An early epidemiologic search for serum antinuclear antibodies (ANAs) disclosed that almost one third of FMS patients exhibit low titers of these autoantibodies,[98] but more recent reports have reduced that to 14%,[99] or as low as 8.8% in FMS compared with 8.9% in patients with osteoarthritis.[100] There have been intermittent reports of lymphocyte immune abnormalities in people with FMS but the outcomes of those studies were variable and hard to interpret in light of the clinical picture.[97] More recently, two studies have critically evaluated the possible role of cytokines in patients with FMS.[101,102] Serum IL-8 and IL-6 from in vitro–stimulated peripheral blood mononuclear cell (PBMC) cultures were significantly higher for the FMS subjects. The serum IL-8 level was most dramatically elevated in FMS patients who were also depressed, but it also correlated with pain intensity and the duration of FMS symptoms. Its production in vitro is stimulated by substance P, which may help explain the elevation of both these cytokines, even in different fluid compartments of FMS patients. It is therefore of interest that IL-6 has been successfully administered to people with FMS, with the finding that it substantially modulated the severity of FMS-related symptoms.[93]

To summarize FMS pathogenesis, the recognition of allodynia as a manifestation of abnormal central nociceptive processing has changed the collective view of FMS. It has led research on this condition in a new direction, toward the study of central sensitization.

Some abnormalities found in FMS—namely, the low 5-HT and elevated SP levels—are logically consistent with a pain amplification syndrome. The extent to which these mechanisms are unique to FMS will be critical in determining the direction of future research. Certainly, a better understanding of the cause of FMS will help develop more effective therapy.

Management Approaches

The objectives of FMS treatment are to reduce pain, improve sleep, restore physical function, maintain social interaction, and reestablish emotional balance. A reasonable community objective might be to reduce the need for expensive health care resources. To achieve these goals, patients will need a combination of social support, education, physical modalities, and medication.[103,104]

ADEPT

It is reasonable to view treatment approaches in categories and sometimes an acronym can help the physician remember them. For that purpose, a six-step outline of therapy has been developed; ADEPT living stands for *a*ttitude, *d*iagnosis, *e*ducation, *p*hysical modalities, *t*reatment with medication, and *l*iving.[105]

Attitude
Attitude refers to the preparation, or frame of mind, that each participant brings to the therapeutic interaction. Clinicians must be prepared to accept FMS as a real condition that exerts a tremendous impact on the patient's life. Empathy will be more therapeutic than baseless recriminations. For the patient's part, it will be important to realize that FMS is just one of thousands of conditions of concern to the health care provider, the presenting symptoms for different medical conditions can be very similar, therapy for FMS is still experimental, and the physician's time with each patient is necessarily limited. The attitudes of family members, employers, policy makers, and politicians all have a important impact on the patient's condition.

Diagnosis
The correct diagnosis should be made, not only to identify the FMS, but also to disclose any comorbid medical conditions. If the patient has concomitant hypothyroidism, diabetes mellitus, or renal insufficiency, the approach to management will also need to accommodate these other conditions. For example, when rheumatoid arthritis and FMS are evident in the same patient, treatment is more successful when both conditions are treated as if the other were not present.

Education
Education is crucial to the management of the FMS. Understanding is power when it comes to main-taining a proper attitude, adapting to limitations, and taking an active role in the therapeutic program. Several studies have examined the effects of cognitive-behavioral therapies on outcome in FMS and have demonstrated positive effects on pain scores, pain coping, pain behavior, depression, and physical functioning.[106] Such gains are often maintained for several months after completion of the therapy and periodic booster sessions may prolong the benefits. Support groups have been viewed negatively by some clinicians, regarded as an environment for learning discontent. On the other hand, joining a resource-oriented support group can help FMS patients come to terms with a complicated illness.

Physical Modalities
A variety of physical modalities have been proposed as interventions for the FMS that can be logically segregated into two categories—those that patients can accomplish for themselves and those that require active participation by a trained therapist. At home, the patient can pace usual activities by setting a clock to time necessary work activity and then balance the work time with an equal period of rest. Progressive exercise, heat applied as a shower or bath, and Jacobson relaxation techniques can all be self-directed therapies, with minimal cost.[106]

Aerobic exercise was among the first nonpharmacologic strategies advocated for FMS patients, with convincing evidence for benefit.[106] Its goals are to maintain function for everyday activities and to prolong life through cardiovascular fitness. If carried out at low impact, with an intensity sufficient to challenge aerobic capacity, exercise can also reduce pain, improve sleep, balance mood, improve stamina, instill new perspectives, restore cognition, and facilitate a sense of well-being.[107] Patients who can exercise sustain less negative impact of FMS in their lives.

On the other hand, it is recognized that imprudent levels of exertion can temporarily worsen pain. When the diagnosis of FMS is first made, the patient usually is deconditioned and has already learned to fear the pain induced by exercise. When prescribing exercise for FMS patients, the clinician should begin with low-intensity exercise, such as walking in place in a swimming pool, and minimize eccentric muscle contractions.[108] Continuation of the exercise program will be facilitated by a gradual reduction of pain. A potential role for pyridostigmine in this process has been proposed.[109]

Most patients report benefit from heat in the form of a hot bath, hot water bottle, electric heat pad, or sauna. Many find that a hot bath or shower can be more effective than analgesic medication for headache, body pain, and stiffness. The application of heat can relax muscles, facilitate exercise, and improve a sense of well-being. Cold applications are preferred by some. Light massage that gradually progresses to deep sedative palpation of large body surfaces can reduce muscle tension, but its influence on the body pain usually lasts only 1 or 2 days.

Treatments

In the ADEPT acronym, treatments refer to therapies advised and/or performed by health care professionals. Surgery will be addressed first because there is no surgical therapy specific for FMS. Many patients with FMS have unnecessary or marginally beneficial surgical procedures (e.g., carpal tunnel release[110]) because they have pain and are insistent that something be done, and there are surgeons who are so poorly informed about FMS that they carry out procedures without researching the FMS further. This is not to say that surgery should not be performed on patients with FMS if it is clearly indicated. The danger is primarily in performing a surgical procedure to manage pain.

The most exciting new developments regarding FMS therapy relate to new medications being developed and tested specifically for this condition. The theoretical background relating these agents to FMS has been based on various biochemical or physiological abnormalities found in FMS[42,111,112] and known to be important contributors to pain pathogenesis. One way of viewing the therapeutic goals of pharmaceutical therapy would be to say that FMS has three main domains (or symptoms) that represent targets for therapeutic intervention (see Fig. 23–4A), such as pain, insomnia, and depression, but others could be substituted. The dramatic rate of progress can be attributed directly to the efforts of pharmaceutical companies. Some newer agents are already available on the market for other indications (but off-label for FMS). Others are approaching release, and others are in various stages of development. The following discussion is intended to illustrate the direction of medication therapy for this condition.

It seems logical that analgesics should be an important component of a multimodal treatment program for a painful condition such as FMS, but nonsteroidal anti-inflammatory drugs have not been effective as monotherapy. Perhaps the more important role of such agents is to contribute synergy with other medications. For example, there is evidence that acetaminophen enhances the benefit achieved from tramadol (Ultram) therapy[113]—hence, the development of Ultracet.

The use of opioids in FMS patients is controversial, but clinical experience would indicate that they are *not* effective in this condition. The bias of most authors is that opioids should not be used in FMS patients until well-designed, controlled, clinical studies have shown unequivocal benefit. Thus, the risk of habituation is not justified. When patients are taking an opioid, it is recommended that proactive treatment be undertaken to manage anticipated side effects, such as constipation and pruritus. The aim of opioids in severe cases should not be merely pain relief but rather to clearly demonstrate improvement in physical function. If improvement in function is not achieved, side effects are difficult to control, or maladaptive behavior ensues, these agents should be discontinued and not restarted.

The in vivo synthesis of 5-HT can be augmented by the administration of 5-HTP, which benefits from one-way kinetics in conversion to 5-HT. It is effective in the treatment of FMS at a dosage of 100 mg three times daily,[114] and it is available over the counter in the United States.

Tricyclic antidepressant drugs are effective in low dosage, improving sleep and enhancing the effects of analgesics. The largest experience is available for amitriptyline in low doses (10 to 25 mg) given at night to improve sleep. Cyclobenzaprine is a comparable drug, with a bedtime dose of 5 to 10 mg. A combination of fluoxetine and amitriptyline was found to be more effective than either agent alone.[115]

Tramadol was a drug designer's improvement on the tricyclic drugs. Reuptake inhibition of serotonin and norepinephrine is combined with weak μ-opioid agonism. It reduces the impact of pain on FMS patients.[116] As monotherapy, it significantly reduces the severity of experienced pain but is not helpful with insomnia or depression. In combination with acetaminophen, a substantial synergy has been noted.[113] Nausea and dizziness can be limiting at first, in about 20% of patients, but initiating therapy with just one tablet at bedtime for 1 to 2 weeks can reduce the frequency of that adverse effect and allow progressive increase of the dosage by about one tablet every 4 days to full therapeutic levels. A typical maintenance dosage for FMS is 300 to 400 mg/day in three to four divided doses, concomitant with acetaminophen at 2 to 3 g/day in divided doses.

Selective serotonin reuptake inhibitor (SSRI) drugs were developed for the treatment of depression. In usual antidepressant dosages, these agents are effective as monotherapy for depression when present in FMS but not for FMS body pain. In very high dosages (fluoxetine, 80 mg/day), they may exhibit analgesic effects but it is unlikely that the drug is still selective.[117]

The analgesic effects of the tricyclic drugs, not apparent with normal dosages of SSRIs, have suggested that the small contribution from inhibition of the norepinephrine transporter might be critical to their pain-relieving effect. In the tricyclics, there is a large—up to 900-fold—difference between the serotonin reuptake inhibition activity and that of norepinephrine.

Two new variants on the SSRI concept have been developed to achieve better balance between reuptake inhibition of serotonin and norepinephrine. One class (exemplified by duloxetine) exhibits almost equivalent serotonin and norepinephrine reuptake inhibition activity (SNRI), whereas the other class (norepinephrine selective reuptake inhibitor [NSRI], exemplified by milnacipran) has norepinephrine reuptake inhibition that is even more potent than 5-HT.

Duloxetine has antidepressant activity, which may be an important reason for choosing it to treat FMS patients who are depressed (about 40% of FMS patients are depressed). In dosages of 60 to 120 mg once daily in the morning, duloxetine can be effective in controlling FMS body pain, whether or not the patient is depressed.[118,119] It is well tolerated by most FMS patients. Nausea, dry mouth, constipation, diarrhea, and anorexia are reported more frequently with active drug than with placebo. Duloxetine has now been released in the United States for neuropathic pain and depression, but is in line for the FMS indication as well. To some extent, the adverse effects can be averted by starting the drug in a low dosage (30 mg in the morning) and gradually building on that as tolerated, perhaps increasing the morning dosage by 30 mg every week.

Milnacipran is available in Europe but is still under investigation. It is not yet available in the United States.

Tropisetron is a 5-HT$_3$ antagonist that has been subjected to controlled study in Europe for the treatment of FMS.[120] A responder group, exhibiting a rapid and steady decrease in pain intensity, has been distinguished from a nonresponder group, which showed almost no response. There seems to be a bell-shaped dose-response curve; the best effects are seen in patients receiving 5 mg tropisetron (39% responder rate) but that effect is lost at higher dosages. Treatment with tropisetron is well tolerated, limited mainly by gastrointestinal side effects.

Because the substance P level is markedly elevated in the spinal fluid of FMS patients, it was assumed that it is important to the pathogenesis of FMS. The discovery and characterization of the substance P receptor (neurokinin-1 [NK-1] receptor) gave rise to hopes that developing potent NK-1 receptor blockade drugs would provide new treatment options. Unfortunately, the potent NK-1 antagonists that were developed failed to exhibit much analgesic activity in FMS.[121] On the other hand, blocking that receptor resulted in antidepressant activity; one could wonder whether some of the antidepressant effect of duloxetine relates to its ability to inhibit the production of substance P. If that is the case, why is pregabalin not more effective as an antidepressant?

The pain amplification of central sensitization can be inhibited or attenuated by *N*-methyl-D-aspartate (NMDA) receptor antagonists. Two NMDA receptor antagonists, ketamine and dextromethorphan, have been studied in FMS and were both found to exhibit beneficial effects on spontaneous pain and allodynia.[122] In the case of ketamine, about 50% of FMS patients benefited. The concept of FMS subgroups was advanced by these findings because ketamine clearly identified responsive and unresponsive subjects from among otherwise comparable FMS patients. Ketamine's usefulness as a therapeutic agent in FMS has been further limited by frequent adverse effects, such as psychological disturbances (e.g., feelings of unreality, altered body image perception, modulation of hearing and vision), dizziness, anxiety, aggression, and nausea.

Drugs with anticonvulsant activity have the potential to raise the threshold for pain fiber depolarization, as they do for central neurons to reduce seizure activity. Pregabalin is a ligand for the rather recently discovered α_2-δ subunit of voltage-gated calcium channels.[123,124] It has analgesic, anxiolytic, and anticonvulsant activity in animal models. It reduces the release of several neurochemicals, including glutamate, norepinephrine, and substance P. It was found to be effective in reducing the severity of body pain, improving quality of sleep, and reducing fatigue in FMS.[125] Pregabalin is now available in the United States but is scheduled because of its mild antianxiolytic activity. In therapeutic dosages (300 to 600 mg/day in two or three divided doses), it is generally well tolerated. Adverse effects can include dose-related dizziness and somnolence that resolve despite continuous therapy with the drug. This observation suggests that it is helpful to start at a low dosage and increase it gradually (perhaps weekly) to help the patient adapt.[†] One approach is to start with 100 to 150 mg at bedtime and increase the nighttime dosage weekly to 300 to 450 mg before adding a smaller morning dosage to achieve 450 to 600 mg/day. Weight gain (about 6 lb) and peripheral edema occur in 6% to 12% of patients, without evidence for an effect on the heart or kidneys.

Sodium oxybate, a metabolite of gamma-aminobutyric acid (GABA), exhibits sedative hypnotic activity. It influences both pre- and postsynaptic GABA-B receptors.[126] This scheduled drug is already approved by the U.S. Food and Drug Administration (FDA) for the treatment of narcolepsy with cataplexy and excessive daytime sleepiness. It is available from only one pharmacy in the United States, which delivers the properly prescribed medication directly to the home of the patient. It was predicted that sodium oxybate would be beneficial in the management of the insomnia of FMS, but it is also effective in reducing the pain of FMS.[127] In a small, randomized, placebo-controlled clinical trial with FMS patients,[128] oxybate was shown to significantly increase the total sleep time, enhance slow-wave sleep, reduce alpha intrusion into slow-wave sleep, decrease nighttime awakenings, reduce daytime fatigue, and increase production of growth hormone. It also was observed to decrease the severity of the perceived pain significantly and reduce the tender point index. A more recent study has supported these findings.[129] In therapeutic dosages (3 to 6 g/day, in two divided doses at night), oxybate was well tolerated, as illustrated by the high rate of study completion. Nausea (15%) and dizziness (7%) were the most common oxybate dose-related adverse events, but these generally resolved with continued therapy.

Study Considerations: Number Needed to Treat

The term *number needed to treat* (NNT) refers to the number of patients with a given condition that would

---

[†] The FDA-approved dosage is 300 mg (150 mg twice daily) or 450 mg (225 mg twice daily), but physicians experienced with the care of FMS have preferred to emphasize nighttime dosing.

need to be treated with a specific intervention to achieve a specified outcome for one hypothetical patient. This is a useful measure because it directly compares the efficacy of different interventions and is easily explained to patients. For example, the clinician could learn that for every four patients treated with medicine X, one of those patients will achieve a 50% improvement in body pain. The problem from the standpoint of FMS is that only the more recent FMS therapeutic trials have provided responder data in the format required to calculate NNT. The information needed from a placebo-controlled trial includes the total numbers of subjects in each treatment group (active and placebo) and the numbers in each group who achieved the specified outcome. The placebo-controlled trial must be blinded and parallel in design. Although the NNT is probably a feature of the drug in such a trial, there may be other methodologic variables that could influence its magnitude. For example, a trial that incorporates a placebo run-in, with exclusion of placebo responders, could artificially increase the effect size and lower the NNT, whereas studies of different durations, populations, or dosages may improperly favor one agent over another. Based on calculations by the UBC calculator[130] and realizing that early studies may not feature the ideal regimen for a given drug, and may involve different durations of study, NNT values for 50% improvement in perceived (self-report visual analogue scale) pain (95% confidence intervals) for several new medications used to treat FMS include the following: duloxetine (Cymbalta), NNT = 6 (range, 3 to 16), pregabalin (Lyrica), NNT = 6 (range, 4 to 17), sodium oxybate (Xyrem), NNT = 7 (range, 3 to 222).[119,129,131] Table 23–3 compares these values with NNT values for clinical regimens used to manage other medical conditions.

A range of comparison NNT values for interventions used to treat common clinical situations can be found on the Bandolier NNT website[132]: celecoxib, 200 mg, for postoperative dental pain to achieve at least 50% relief over 4 to 6 hours, NNT = 4 (range, 2.9 to 4.9); bypass graft of a stenotic lesion in the left main coronary artery to prevent one death over a 2-year period, NNT = 6; simvastatin to prevent one major coronary event over a period of 6 years, NNT = 15; treating hypertension in persons older than 60 years to prevent one coronary event, NNT = 18; prophylactic use of low-dose aspirin in unstable angina to prevent one myocardial infarction or death in 1 year, NNT = 25; prophylactic use of low-dose aspirin in healthy U.S. physicians to prevent one myocardial infarction or death in 1 year, NNT = 500.

Strategic Polypharmacy and Newer Therapeutic Agents

The use of specific combinations of the newer therapeutic agents, strategic polypharmacy, in the management of FMS has been proposed.[105] It should be pointed out, however, that there are no published

Table 23–3. Number Needed to Treat (NNT): Comparisons of Values for Drug Treatment of Fibromyalgia Syndrome (FMS) with Management of Other Common Medical Conditions

CONDITION	NNT VALUE*
FMS: 50% Improvement in Perceived Self-Report Visual Analogue Scale for Pain	
Duloxetine (Cymbalta)[114]	6 (3-16)[†]
Pregabalin (Lyrica)[124]	6 (4-17)[†]
Sodium oxybate (Xyrem)[125]	7 (3-222)[†]
Other Conditions	
Celecoxib, 200 mg, for postoperative dental pain to achieve at least 50% relief over 4-6 hr	4 (2.9-4.9)
Bypass graft of stenotic lesion in left main coronary artery to prevent one death over 2-yr period[‡]	6
Simvastatin to prevent one major coronary event over a period of 6 yr[‡]	15
Treating hypertension in persons >60 yr to prevent one coronary event[‡]	18
Prophylactic use of low-dose aspirin in unstable angina to prevent one myocardial infarction or death in 1 yr[‡]	25
Prophylactic use of low-dose aspirin in healthy U.S. physicians to prevent one myocardial infarction or death in 1 yr[‡]	500

*NNT, 95% confidence intervals.
[†]Calculations made by using the UBC calculator (www.healthcare.ubc.ca/calc/clinsig.html).
[‡]Bandolier NNT website (www.jr2.ox.ac.uk/bandolier/index.html).

data on the consequences of combining drugs that are effective in monotherapy. Will the resultant benefit be additive, synergistic, or combative for people with FMS? If synergistic, will dual therapy allow the effective use of lower dosages of those drugs to avoid the emergence of adverse effects? The critical principles of this concept for FMS are that complementary medications should be from different drug classes, have different mechanisms of action, and not be synergistic for any serious adverse effect. For example, tramadol therapy may help control pain, whereas a sleep aid might be added for insomnia (see Fig. 23–4B). An SSRI for depression would not be added for the same patient because the biogenic amine transporter inhibition mechanism is the same for tramadol and the SSRI. Combining them would increase the risk of the patient developing the hyperserotonin syndrome.

For an FMS patient whose two most prominent symptoms are pain and depression, the use of duloxetine would be logical, and it might be chosen as first-line monotherapy. Duloxetine could be used to treat the pain in an FMS patient even if depression were not present, because it has been found to be equally effective for pain whether or not depression is present.[119] In an FMS patient with pain and insomnia, the use of pregabalin or oxybate would be logical. Obviously, either of these drugs could be used to treat the pain, even if insomnia were not present. In an FMS patient with three prominent symptoms (e.g., pain, insomnia, depression), the use of either

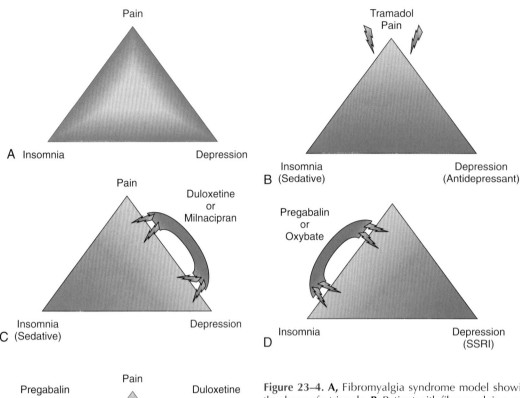

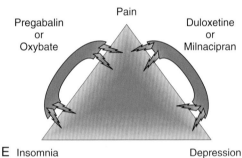

Figure 23–4. A, Fibromyalgia syndrome model showing three important domains in the shape of a triangle. **B,** Patient with fibromyalgia syndrome whose most troublesome manifestation is widespread body pain **C,** Patient with fibromyalgia syndrome who has moderate widespread body pain and depression, which are compromising her quality of life. This is a good setting for monotherapy with duloxetine or milnacipran. Pregabalin and oxybate would not be useful for the depression but duloxetine is therapeutic for both depression and pain. **D,** Patient with fibromyalgia syndrome who has moderate widespread body pain and insomnia, which leave her uncomfortable, fatigued, and cognitively impaired. **E,** Patient with fibromyalgia syndrome who has an impaired quality of life because, in addition to the severe widespread allodynia, she sleeps very poorly and is currently depressed. See text for details.

pregabalin or oxybate in combination with duloxetine would be logical and safe because their mechanisms of action and elimination are different. Because there is little published research experience with such a regimen, it must be considered clinically experimental, tailored to the individual patient, and carefully monitored for safety.

Figure 23–4 provides an exercise in understanding the potential role of newer medications in the management of patients with FMS who exhibit different patterns of actively symptomatic domains. In Figure 23–4A, three important fibromyalgia syndrome symptom domains are shown in the shape of a triangle. Widespread body pain is critical to the construct but a large majority of patients (more than 80%) experience moderately severe insomnia and about one third are depressed at any point in time.

Figure 23–4B illustrates a patient with fibromyalgia syndrome whose most troublesome manifestation is widespread body pain. She believes that she sleeps

well and exhibits no evidence to suggest current depression. It seems clear that the domain of widespread allodynia should be the focus of therapy. The analgesic tramadol is being used to treat the pain. Pregabalin, duloxetine, or oxybate could also be used as monotherapy for the pain but tramadol may be adequate at 100 mg three or four times daily. If an element of depression were to present in such a patient, it would be wise to treat that interactively or with a medication that has a mechanism other than inhibition of a biogenic amine reuptake, because that is tramadol's mechanism of action. If an occasional sleepless night is reported, instruction about sleep hygiene habits should be reviewed and a mild sedative could be prescribed.

In Figure 23–4C, the FMS patient has both moderately widespread body pain and depression. Together, they are compromising her quality of life. This is a good setting for monotherapy with duloxetine or milnacipran. Pregabalin and oxybate would not be useful with the depression, but duloxetine is therapeutic for both depression and pain independently.

In Figure 23–4D, the FMS patient has moderate widespread body pain and insomnia that leave her uncomfortable, fatigued, and cognitively impaired. This is a good setting for monotherapy with pregabalin or sodium oxybate. Duloxetine may be helpful for the fatigue and dyscognition but is not useful as a treatment for insomnia.

In Figure 23–4E, the FMS patient has an impaired quality of life. In addition to the severe widespread allodynia, she sleeps poorly and is currently depressed. She cannot get comfortable in any position, asleep or awake. She is nearly always on the verge of tears and is irritable. Her behavior alienates her from those she loves when she most needs their support. This is a setting for treating the symptoms aggressively. The patient needs help with her mood and her sleep. This situation should invoke the use of strategic polypharmacy with duloxetine or milnacipran and pregabalin or oxybate. If the use of two drugs seems inappropriate, consider how many patients with chronic diseases (e.g., hypertension, diabetes, hyperlipidemia, cancer, congestive heart disease, rheumatoid arthritis) are successfully managed with a single drug. It certainly is the exception rather than the rule.

It still may be wise to adapt the patient to one drug at a time, so that it would be easier to identify the cause of an adverse effect. In that setting, duloxetine might be the first-line drug, with gradual dosage escalation to full therapeutic dosage of 90 to 120 mg in the morning. Then, pregabalin could be initiated at nighttime, with weekly increases in dosage, again striving for full therapeutic dosage (450 to 600 mg/day), mainly given at night (300 to 450 mg at night and 75 to 150 mg in the morning). If pregabalin were not tolerated, then oxybate could take its place as the sedating analgesic agent.

Other Comorbidities

Management of other specific symptomatic domains in FMS deserves separate attention.

Dysfunctional Sleep

Since the original description of dysfunctional sleep in people with FMS, it has been clear that this symptom should be a focus of therapy. Despite that, management of insomnia in FMS remains nonspecific and empirical. The sedating tricyclic biogenic amine reuptake drugs, such as amitriptyline and cyclobenzaprine, have been the most commonly prescribed medications for FMS insomnia. These are not ideal for this role because they cause a number of adverse effects and are subject to tachyphylaxis, but a 1-month holiday from all biogenic amine reuptake transporters can restore effectiveness.[133] SSRIs are so stimulatory that they can interfere with sleep, so they should be taken in the morning, never at bedtime. Benzodiazepines, such as alprazolam and clonazepam, reduce anxiety and allow less troubled sleep

induction in FMS. Clonazepam can also help control nocturnal myoclonus and bruxism when these conditions are comorbid with FMS. Newer hypnotic drugs, such as zopiclone and zolpidem, improve sleep without correcting the disturbed sleep pattern seen on the electroencephalogram and without any measurable influence on FMS pain.[134] Rebound (withdrawal insomnia) with zolpidem is problematic but can be avoided if patients use the drug no more than three times weekly (alternate days). Two medications more recently used in the FMS setting—pregabalin and oxybate—will likely meet the needs for this indication, because they are effective for both pain and sleep.[125,128,129] In addition, both actually correct the non–rapid eye movement sleep pattern abnormalities seen with FMS.

Fatigue and Daytime Tiredness

Fatigue in FMS is probably the direct result of chronic insomnia. In addition, a small subpopulation of FMS patients is sufficiently depressed to make usual activities of daily life seem overwhelming. Overlap of FMS with medical conditions such as sleep apnea, hypothyroidism, diabetes, chronic infection, or anemia can also drain energy, so they should be included in the differential diagnosis. Mild exercise can reduce fatigue in FMS. For the patient who wears out before the end of the day, pacing of the day's duties, interspersed with mandatory rest periods, can conserve energy. The pharmacologic therapy of fatigue in FMS will increasingly rely on the improved rest that can be achieved with pregabalin or oxybate.[125,128,129] Duloxetine therapy has also relieved fatigue in FMS patients with only marginal improvement in sleep.[119] When tricyclic biogenic amine reuptake inhibitors such as amitriptyline or cyclobenzaprine are used for insomnia, the beneficial effect on sleep can be offset by daytime sedation and impaired cognition. These effects can sometimes be ameliorated by adding a low dose of an SSRI, such as fluoxetine, in the morning.[115] It seems unwise to treat the daytime fatigue of FMS with stimulants such as caffeine or ephedrine derivatives, because the exhausted brain will eventually require restorative rest.

Dysautonomia

Orthostatic hypotension may respond to liberal intake of water, increased dietary salt, the use of compressive stocking hose, or a combination of these, but occasionally will require the addition of a mineralocorticoid.[135] Patients may benefit from avoiding the effects of caffeine and nicotine. Mild cardiac rhythm dysautonomia may be viewed more as a marker of FMS than as a comorbid condition requiring intervention.

Irritable Bowel Syndrome

The treatment of IBS in FMS relies on general measures that include dietary adaptations such as avoiding caffeine, alcohol, fat, or specific foods that can be identified as worsening symptoms. Depending on the predominant form of IBS (constipation-predominant, diarrhea-predominant, or combination of constipation and diarrhea) experienced by the patient, somewhat selective symptomatic medications can be used. Pain can be treated with antispasmodic agents and tricyclics. For the diarrhea-predominant form, classic antidiarrheal agents such as loperamide and diphenoxylate can be used. In refractory cases, cholestyramine or antibiotics can be considered. Alosetron (Lotronex) is indicated for severe cases of diarrhea-predominant IBS but there is a black box warning regarding the use of this potent serotonin-3 receptor antagonist. It can cause ischemic colitis and serious complications of constipation, such as hospitalization, blood transfusion, surgery, and death. Distribution of this drug is restricted to prescription by physicians who have been specifically trained in its use. For the constipation-predominant form of IBS, a diet high in fiber and osmotic laxatives such as lactulose, psyllium (Metamucil), and sorbitol or magnesium preparations can be helpful. Sometimes four prunes per day will facilitate a more normal stool consistency. Tegaserod maleate (Zelnorm) had been used for this purpose for some time but it has been withdrawn from the market because of liver toxicity.

Irritable Bladder or Urethral Syndrome

The treatment of the irritable bladder or urethral syndrome in FMS includes general measures and medication. It is important to maintain high fluid intake, avoid foods that irritate the bladder (fruits, fruit juices, coffee), and perform pelvic floor exercises regularly. Medications that can be helpful include antispasmodics, muscle relaxants, urinary anesthetics, and tricyclic agents. Interstitial cystitis may or may not relate to the FMS. It is generally best managed by an interested and empathetic urologist.

CONCLUSION

To summarize, FMS is a criteria-based diagnosis that can identify a moderately severe chronic pain condition affecting women more often than men. It is not a diagnosis of exclusion. The current research classification of FMS depends on a history of widespread pain and prominent tenderness to palpation at 11 or more 18 anatomically defined tender points. Research is being undertaken to develop clinical case criteria for FMS that can be validated for use in community practice. Other manifestations of FMS can include severe insomnia, body stiffness, affective symptoms, irritable bowel, and urethral syndrome. The therapy of FMS is still multidimensional but dramatic improvements have occurred, particularly in regard to medications that target two or more symptomatic domains of the disorder. A simple acronym—ADEPT living—can help the clinician recall the elements of effective therapy (see earlier discussion).

SUMMARY

- The general term for the conditions discussed in this chapter should be *soft tissue pain* (STP) disorders. This avoids the pitfalls of other current terms and enables use of a classification system that facilitates many related diagnoses.
- The term *localized STP* encompasses episodic bursitis, tendinitis, or epicondylitis when one of these conditions occurs in a single location of the body. These conditions can benefit from rest, a change in regular use patterns, and brief use of anti-inflammatory medications.
- Myofascial pain syndrome (MPS) is a regional STP disorder characterized by spontaneous regional pain, tenderness in a skeletal muscle trigger point (TrP), and referral of pain when the TrP is activated by digital pressure or needle penetration.
- MPS exhibits physiologic features of a spinal reflex. It responds to improved posture, cold spray with stretching, dry needling, local anesthesia of the radicular nerve, local phentolamine injection, or local injection of botulinum toxoid.
- Fibromyalgia syndrome (FMS) is a generalized STP disorder characterized by chronic widespread pain and tenderness in many symmetrically distributed, anatomically characterized sites in the body.
- FMS is a central neuropathic disorder that exhibits many objective abnormalities in the central nervous system. There are a number of important comorbidities; these may include MPS, severe insomnia, and reactive depression. An intensive search for effective therapies has produced many gratifying successes.

References

1. Russell IJ: A new journal. J Musculoskel Pain 1993;1:1-7.
2. Travell J: Identification of myofascial trigger point syndromes: A case of atypical facial neuralgia. Arch Phys Med Rehabil 1981;62:100-106.
3. Kellgren JH: Observations on referred pain arising from muscle. Clin Sci 1939;3:175-190.
4. Simons DG, Travell JG, Simons LS: Myofascial Pain and Dysfunction: The Trigger Point Manual, 2nd ed, vol 1: Upper Half of Body. Baltimore, Williams & Wilkins, 1999.
5. Travell JG, Simons DG: Myofascial Pain and Dysfunction: The Trigger Point Manual, vol 2: Lower Half of Body. Baltimore, Williams & Wilkins;1992.
6. Hsieh C-YJ, Hong C-Z, Adams AH, et al: Interexaminer reliability of the palpation of trigger points in the trunk and lower limb muscles. Arch Phys Med Rehabil 2000;81:258-264.
7. Delaney GA, McKee AC: Inter- and intra-rater reliability of the pressure threshold meter in measurement of myofascial trigger point sensitivity. Am J Phys Med Rehabil 1993;72:136-139.
8. Gerwin R, Shannon S, Hong C-Z, et al: Interrater reliability in myofascial trigger point examination. Pain 1997;69:65-73.
9. Nice DA, Riddle DL, Lamb RL, et al: Intertester reliability of judgements of the presence of trigger points in patients with low back pain. Arch Phys Med Rehabil 1992;73:893-898.
10. Wolfe F, Simons DG, Fricton J, et al: The fibromyalgia and myofascial pain syndromes: A preliminary study of tender points and trigger points in persons with fibromyalgia, myo-

fascial pain syndrome and no disease. J Rheumatol 1992;19: 944-951.

11. Gerwin RD, Shannon S, Hong CZ, et al: Interrater reliability in myofascial trigger point examination. Pain 1997;69:65-73.

12. Wolfe F, Smythe HA, Yunus MB, et al: The American College of Rheumatology 1990 Criteria for the Classification of Fibromyalgia. Report of the Multicenter Criteria Committee. Arthritis Rheum 1990;33:160-172.

13. Russell IJ: Reliability of clinical assessment measures for the classification of myofascial pain syndrome. J Musculoskel Pain 1999;7:309-324.

14. Staffel K, del Moral OM, Lacomba MT, et al: Factors that influence the reliability of clinical assessment for the classification of the myofascial pain syndrome (MPS). J Musculoskel Pain 2007;15:36.

15. Harden RN, Bruehl SP, Gass S, et al: Signs and symptoms of the myofascial pain syndrome: A national survey of pain management providers. Clin J Pain 2000;16:64-72.

16. Wolfe F, Ross K, Anderson J, et al: The prevalence and characteristics of fibromyalgia in the general population. Arthritis Rheum 1995;38:19-28.

17. Skootsky SA, Jaeger B, Oye RK: Prevalence of myofascial pain in general internal medicine practice. West J Med 1989;151: 157-160.

18. Campbell SM, Clark S, Tindall EA, et al: Clinical characteristics of fibrositis. I. A "blinded," controlled study of symptoms and tender points. Arthritis Rheum 1983;26:817-824.

19. Fricton JR, Kroening R, Haley D, et.al. Myofascial pain syndrome of the head and neck: A review of clinical characteristics of 164 patients. Oral Surg Oral Med Oral Pathol 1985;60:615-623.

20. FitzGerald MP, Kotarinos R: Rehabilitation of the short pelvic floor. II: Treatment of the patient with the short pelvic floor. Int Urogynecology J 2003;14:269-275.

21. FitzGerald MP, Kotarinos R: Rehabilitation of the short pelvic floor. I: Background and patient evaluation. Int Urogynecology J 2003;14:261-268.

22. Prendergast SA, Weiss JM: Screening for musculoskeletal causes of pelvic pain. Clin Obstet Gynecol 2003;46: 773-782.

23. Siocumb JC: Neurological factors in chronic pelvic pain: Trigger points and the abdominal pelvic pain syndrome. Am J Obstet Gynecol 1984;149:536-543.

24. Borg-Stein J: Treatment of fibromyalgia, myofascial pain, and related disorders. Phys Med Rehabil Clin North Am 2006; 17:491-510.

25. Simons DG: Myofascial pain syndrome: One term but two concepts: A new understanding. J Musculoskel Pain 1995;3: 7-13.

26. Simons DG: Myofascial trigger paints: The critical experiment. J Musculoskel Pain 1997;5:113-118.

27. Samuel AS, Peter AA, Ramanathan K: The association of active trigger points with lumbar disc lesions. J Musculoskel Pain 2007;15:11-18.

28. Gunn CC: Radiculopathic pain: Diagnosis and treatment of segmental irritation or sensitization. J Musculoskel Pain 1997;5:119-134.

29. Hong C-Z, Torigoe Y: Electromyographic characteristics of localized twitch responses in responsive taut bands of rabbit skeletal muscle. J Musculoskel Pain 1994;2:17-43.

30. Donaldson CCS, Skubick D, Clasby R, et al: The evaluation of trigger-point activity using dynamic EMG techniques. Am J Pain Manage 1994;4:118-122.

31. Hubbard DR, Berkoff GM: Myofascial trigger points show spontaneous needle EMG activity. Spine 1993;18:1803-1807.

32. Couppé C, Midttun A, Hilden J, et al: Spontaneous needle EMG activity in myofascial trigger points in the infraspinatus muscle: A blinded assessment. J Musculoskel Pain 2001;9: 7-16.

33. Donaldson CCS, Nelson DV, Schulz R: Disinhibition in the gamma motoneuron circuitry: A neglected mechanism for understanding myofascial pain syndromes? Appl Psychophys Biofeedback 1998;23:43-57.

34. Rivner MH: The neurophysiology of myofascial pain syndrome. Curr Pain Headache Rep 2001;5:432-440.

35. Shah JP, Phillips TM, Danoff JV, et al: An in vivo microanalytical technique for measuring the local biochemical milieu of human skeletal muscle. J Appl Physiol 99:1977-84, 2005.

36. Gerwin RD, Dommerholt J, Shah JP: An expansion of Simons' integrated hypothesis of trigger point formation. Curr Pain Headache Rep 2004;8:468-75.

37. Criscuolo CM: Interventional approaches to the management of myofascial pain syndrome. Curr Pain Headache Rep 2001;5(5):407-411.

38. Borg-Stein J, Stein J: Trigger points and tender points: One and the same? Does injection treatment help? Rheum Dis Clin North Am 1996;22:305-322.

39. Baldry P: Superficial dry needling at myofascial trigger point sites. J Musculoskel Pain 1995;3:117-126.

40. Hong CZ, Hsueh TC: Difference in pain relief after trigger point injections in myofascial pain patients with and without fibromyalgia (comment). Arch Phys Med Rehabil 1996;77: 1161-1166.

41. Porta M: A comparative trial of botulinum toxin type A and methylprednisolone for the treatment of myofascial pain syndrome and pain from chronic muscle spasm. Pain 2000;85:101-105.

42. Wheeler AH, Goolkasian P, Gretz SS: A randomized, double-blind, prospective pilot study of botulinum toxin injection for refractory, unilateral, cervicothoracic, paraspinal, myofascial pain syndrome. Spine 1998;23:1662-1666.

43. Hubbard DR: Personal communication. March 2000, Phoenix, Ariz.

44. Staud R, Vierck CJ, Cannon RL, et al: Abnormal sensitization and temporal summation of second pain (wind-up) in patients with fibromyalgia syndrome. Pain 2001;91:165-175.

45. White KP, Nielson WR, Harth M, et al: Does the label "fibromyalgia" alter health status, function, and health service utilization? A prospective, within-group comparison in a community cohort of adults with chronic widespread pain. Arthritis Rheum 2002;47:260-265.

46. Katz RS, Wolfe F, Michaud K: Fibromyalgia diagnosis: A comparison of clinical, survey, and American College of Rheumatology criteria. Arthritis Rheum 2006;54:169-176.

47. Buskila D: Fibromyalgia in children—lessons from assessing nonarticular tenderness (editorial). J Rheumatol 1996;23: 2017-2019.

48. Wolfe F, Anderson J, Harkness D, et al: A prospective, longitudinal, multicenter study of service utilization and costs in fibromyalgia. Arthritis Rheum 1997;40:1560-1570.

49. Buskila D, Neumann L, Vaisberg G, et al: Increased rates of fibromyalgia following cervical spine injury: A controlled study of 161 cases of traumatic injury. Arthritis Rheum 1997;40:446-452.

50. Pettersson K, Karrholm J, Toolanen G, et al: Decreased width of the spinal canal in patients with chronic symptoms after whiplash injury. Spine 1995;20:1664-1667.

51. Park DC, Glass JM, Minear M, et al: Cognitive function in fibromyalgia patients. Arthritis Rheum 2001;44:2125-2133.

52. Ahles TA, Khan SA, Yunus MB, et al: Psychiatric status of patients with primary fibromyalgia, patients with rheumatoid arthritis, and subjects without pain: A blind comparison of DSM-III diagnoses. Am J Psychiat 1991;148:1721-1726.

53. Raphael KG, Widom CS, Lange G: Childhood victimization and pain in adulthood: A prospective investigation. Pain 2001;92:283-293.

54. Wallace DJ: Genitourinary manifestations of fibrositis: An increased association with the female urethral syndrome. J Rheumatol 1990;17:238-239.

55. Brand K, Kristjanson L, Wisniewski S, et al: Development of the fibromyalgia bladder index (abstract). J Musculoskel Pain 2004;13(Suppl):46.

56. Giovengo SL, Russell IJ, Larson AA: Increased concentrations of nerve growth factor (NGF) in cerebrospinal fluid of patients with fibromyalgia. J Rheumatol 1999;26:1564-1569.

57. Steere A, Taylor E, McHugh GL, et al: The overdiagnosis of Lyme disease. JAMA 1993;269:1812-1816.

58. Malmberg AB, Yaksh TL: Hyperalgesia mediated by spinal glutamate or substance P receptor blocked by spinal cyclo-oxygenase inhibition. Science 1992;257:1276-1279.

59. Russell IJ: Neurochemical pathogenesis of fibromyalgia syndrome. J Musculoskel Pain 1996;1&2:61-92.

60. Moldofsky H, Warsh JJ: Plasma tryptophan and musculoskeletal pain in nonarticular rheumatism ("fibrositis syndrome"). Pain 1978;5:65-71.

61. Russell IJ, Michalek JE, Vipraio GA, et al: Serum amino acids in fibrositis/fibromyalgia syndrome. J Rheumatol 1989; 19(Suppl):158-163.

62. Russell IJ, Vipraio GA, Acworth I: Abnormalities in the central nervous system (CNS) metabolism of tryptophan (TRY) to 3-hydroxykynurenine (OHKY) in fibromyalgia syndrome (FS). Arthritis Rheum 1993;36:S222.

63. Russell IJ, Michalek JE, Vipraio GA, et al: Platelet 3H-imipramine uptake receptor density and serum serotonin levels in patients with fibromyalgia/fibrositis syndrome. J Rheumatol 1992;19:104-109.

64. Hrycaj P, Stratz T, Müller W: Platelet 3H-imipramine uptake receptor density and serum serotonin levels in patients with fibromyalgia/fibrositis syndrome (comment). J Rheumatol 1993;20:1986-1987.

65. Russell IJ, Vaeroy H, Javors M, et al: Cerebrospinal fluid biogenic amine metabolites in fibromyalgia/fibrositis syndrome and rheumatoid arthritis. Arthritis Rheum 1992;35:550-556.

66. Kang Y-K, Russell IJ, Vipraio GA, et al: Low urinary 5-hydroxy-indole acetic acid in fibromyalgia syndrome: Evidence in support of a serotonin-deficiency pathogenesis. Myalgia 1998;1:14-21.

67. Wolfe F, Russell IJ, Vipraio G, et al: Serotonin levels, pain threshold, and fibromyalgia symptoms in the general population. J Rheumatol 1997;24:555-559.

68. Bennett RM, Clark SR, Campbell SM, et al: Symptoms of Raynaud's syndrome in patients with fibromyalgia: A study utilizing the Nielsen test, digital photoplethysmography, and measurements of platelet alpha 2-adrenergic receptors. Arthritis Rheum 1991;34:264-269.

69. Russell IJ, Michalek JE, Xiao Y, et al: Therapy with a central alpha-2-agonist (tizanidine) decreases cerebrospinal fluid substance P, and may reduce serum hyaluronic acid as it improves the clinical symptoms of the fibromyalgia syndrome. Arthritis Rheum 2002;46:S614.

70. Malt EA, Olafsson S, Aakvaag A, et al: Altered dopamine D2 receptor function in fibromyalgia patients: A neuroendocrine study with buspirone in women with fibromyalgia compared to female population-based controls. J Affect Disord 2003;75:77-82.

71. Vaeroy H, Helle R, Forre O, et al: Elevated CSF levels of substance P and high incidence of Raynaud's phenomenon in patients with fibromyalgia: New features for diagnosis. Pain 1988;32:21-26.

72. Russell IJ, Orr MD, Littman B, et al: Elevated cerebrospinal levels of substance P patients fibromyalgia syndrome. Arthritis Rheum 1994;37:1593-1601.

73. Welin M, Bragee B, Nyberg F, et al: Elevated substance P levels are contrasted by a decrease in met-enkephalin-arg-phe levels in csf from fibromyalgia patients. J Musculoskel Pain 1995;3(Suppl 1):4.

74. Bradley LA, Alberts KR, Alarcon GS, et al: Abnormal brain regional cerebral blood flow (rCBF) and cerebrospinal fluid (CSF) levels of substance P (SP) in patients and non-patients with fibromyalgia (FM). Arthritis Rheum 1996;39(Suppl): S212.

75. Sjostrom S, Tamsen A, Hartvig P, et al: Cerebrospinal fluid concentrations of substance P and (met)enkephalin-Arg6-Phe7 during surgery and patient-controlled analgesia. Anesth Analg 1988;67:976-981.

76. Tsigos C, Diemel LT, Tomlinson DR, et al: Cerebrospinal fluid levels of substance P and calcitonin-gene-related peptide: Correlation with sural nerve levels and neuropathic signs in sensory diabetic polyneuropathy. Clin Sci 1993;84:305-311.

77. Sjostrom S, Tamsen A, Hartvig P, et al: Cerebrospinal fluid concentrations of substance P and (met)enkephalin-Arg6-Phe7 during surgery and patient-controlled analgesia. Anesth Analg 1988;67:976-981.

78. Russell IJ: Unpublished data, 2002.

79. Nyberg F, Liu Z, Lind C, et al: Enhanced CSF levels of substance P in patients with painful arthrosis but not in patients with pain from herniated lumbar discs. J Musculoskel Pain 1995;3(Suppl 1):2.

80. Giovengo SL, Russell IJ, Larson AA: Increased concentrations of nerve growth factor in cerebrospinal fluid of patients with fibromyalgia. J Rheumatol 1999;26:1564-1569.

81. Russell IJ: Unpublished data, 1994.

82. Buskila D, Neumann L, Hazanov I, et al: Familial aggregation in the fibromyalgia syndrome. Semin Arthritis Rheum 1996;26:605-611.

83. Pellegrino MJ, Waylonis GW, Sommer A: Familial occurrence of primary fibromyalgia. Arch Phys Med Rehabil 1989;70:61-63.

84. Buskila D, Neumann L, Hazanov I, et al: Familial aggregation in the fibromyalgia syndrome. Semin Arthritis Rheum 1996;26:605-611.

85. Yunus MB, Khan MA, Rawlings KK, et al: Genetic linkage analysis of multicase families with fibromyalgia syndrome. J Rheumatol 1999;26:408-412.

86. Dudek DM, Arnold LM, Iyengar SK, et al: Genetic linkage of fibromyalgia to the serotonin receptor 2A region on chromosome 13 and the HLA region on chromosome 6. Am J Hum Genet 2003;72:468.

87. Arnold LM, Hudson JI, Hess EV, et al: Family study of fibromyalgia. Arthritis Rheum 2004;50:944-952.

88. Gursoy S, Erdal E, Herken H, et al: Significance of catechol-O-methyltransferase gene polymorphism in fibromyalgia syndrome. Rheumatol Int 2003;23:104-107.

89. Wolfe F, Ross K, Anderson J, et al: The prevalence and characteristics of fibromyalgia in the general population. Arthritis Rheum 1995;38:19-28.

90. Nishizawa S, Benkelfat C, Young SN, et al: Differences between males and females in rates of serotonin synthesis in human brain. Proc Natl Acad Sci U S A 1997;94:5308-5313.

91. Crofford LJ, Pillemer SR, Kalogeras KT, et al: Hypothalamic-pituitary-adrenal axis perturbations in patients with fibromyalgia. Arthritis Rheum 1994;37:1583-1592.

92. Crofford LJ: Neuroendocrine abnormalities in fibromyalgia and related disorders. Am J Med Sci 1998;315:359-366.

93. Torpy DJ, Papanicolaou DA, Lotsikas AJ, et al: Responses of the sympathetic nervous system and the hypothalamic-pituitary-adrenal axis to interleukin-6: A pilot study in fibromyalgia. Arthritis Rheum 2000;43:872-880.

94. Pillemer SR, Bradley LA, Crofford LJ, et al: The neuroscience and endocrinology of fibromyalgia. Arthritis Rheum 1997;40:1928-1939.

95. Bennett RM, Clark SR, Campbell SM, et al: Low levels of somatomedin C in patients with the fibromyalgia syndrome. A possible link between sleep and muscle pain. Arthritis Rheum 1992;35:1113-1116.

96. Bennett RM, Clark SC, Walczyk J: A randomized, double-blind, placebo-controlled study of growth hormone in the treatment of fibromyalgia. Am J Med 1998;104:227-231.

97. Caro XJ: Is there an immunologic component to the fibrositis syndrome? Rheum Dis Clin North Am 1989;15:169-186.

98. Yunus MB, Hussey FX, Aldag JC: Antinuclear antibodies and connective tissue disease features in fibromyalgia syndrome: A controlled study. J Rheumatol 1993;20:1557-1560.

99. Dinerman H, Goldenberg DL, Felson DT: A prospective evaluation of 118 patients with the fibromyalgia syndrome: Prevalence of Raynaud's phenomenon, sicca symptoms, ANA, low complement, and Ig deposition at the dermal-epidermal junction. J Rheumatol 1986;13:368-373.

100. Al Allaf AW, Ottenwell L, Puller T: The prevalence and significance of positive antinuclear antibodies in patients with fibromyalgia syndrome: 2-4 years' follow-up. Clin Rheumatol 2002;21:472-477.

101. Gur A, Karakoc M, Nas K, et al: Cytokines and depression in cases with fibromyalgia. J Rheumatol 2002;29:358-361.

102. Wallace DJ, Linker-Israeli M, Hallegua D, et al: Cytokines play an aetiopathogenetic role in fibromyalgia: A hypothesis and pilot study. Rheumatol 2001;40:743-749.
103. Russell IJ, Bieber C: Myofascial pain and fibromyalgia syndrome. In McMahon SB, Koltzenburg M (eds): Wall and Melzack's Textbook of Pain, 5th ed. London, Elsevier, 2005, pp 669-681.
104. Russell IJ: Fibromyalgia syndrome: Approaches to management. Bull Rheum Dis 1996;45:1-4.
105. Russell IJ: Fibromyalgia syndrome: Approach to management. Prim Psychiatry 2006;13:76-84.
106. Burckhardt CS: Nonpharmacologic management strategies in fibromyalgia. Rheum Dis Clin North Am 2002;28:291-304.
107. Jones KD, Clark SR: Individualizing the exercise prescription for persons with fibromyalgia. Rheum Dis Clin North Am 2002;28:419-436.
108. Jones KD, Clark SR, Bennett RM: Prescribing exercise for people with fibromyalgia. AACN Clin Issues 2002;13:277-293.
109. Paiva ES, Deodhar A, Jones KD, et al: Impaired growth hormone secretion in fibromyalgia patients: Evidence for augmented hypothalamic somatostatin tone. Arthritis Rheum 2002;46:1344-1350.
110. Meyer HP, Van der Westhuizen FD: Impact of spinal surgery in patients with fibromyalgia syndrome and back pain. J Musculoskel Pain 2004;12(Suppl 9):61.
111. Staud R: Evidence of involvement of central neural mechanisms in generating fibromyalgia pain. Curr Rheumatol Rep 2002;4:299-305.
112. Russell IJ: Advances in fibromyalgia: Possible role for central neurochemicals. Am J Med Sci 1998;315:377-384.
113. Bennett RM, Kamin M, Karim R, et al: Tramadol and acetaminophen combination tablets in the treatment of fibromyalgia pain: A double-blind, randomized, placebo-controlled study. Am J Med 2003;114:537-545.
114. Caruso I, Sarzi Puttini P, Cazzola M, et al: Double-blind study of 5-hydroxytryptophan versus placebo in the treatment of primary fibromyalgia syndrome. J Int Med Res 1990;18:201-209.
115. Goldenberg D, Mayskiy M, Mossey C, et al: A randomized, double-blind crossover trial of fluoxetine and amitriptyline in the treatment of fibromyalgia. Arthritis Rheum 1996;39:1852-1859.
116. Russell IJ, Kamin M, Bennett RM, et al: Efficacy of tramadol in treatment of pain in fibromyalgia. J Clin Rheumatol 2000;6:250-257.
117. Arnold LM, Hess EV, Hudson JI, et al: A randomized, placebo-controlled, double-blind, flexible-dose study of fluoxetine in the treatment of women with fibromyalgia. Am J Med 2002;112:191-197.
118. Arnold LM, Lu Y, Crofford LJ, et al: A double-blind, multicenter trial comparing duloxetine with placebo in the treatment of fibromyalgia patients with or without major depressive disorder. Arthritis Rheum 2004;50:2974-2984.
119. Arnold LM, Rosen A, Pritchett YL, et al: A randomized, double-blind, placebo-controlled trial of duloxetine in the treatment of women with fibromyalgia with or without major depressive disorder. Pain 2005;119:5-15.
120. Stratz T, Farber L, Varga B, et al: Fibromyalgia treatment with intravenous tropisetron administration. Drug Exp Clin Res 2001;27:113-118.
121. Russell IJ: The promise of substance P inhibitors in fibromyalgia. Rheum Dis Clin of North Am 2002;28:329-342.
122. Henriksson KG, Sorensen J: The promise of N-methyl-D-aspartate receptor antagonists in fibromyalgia. Rheum Dis Clin North Am 2002;28:343-351.
123. Dooley DJ, Donovan CM, Meder WP, et al: Preferential action of gabapentin and pregabalin at P/Q-type voltage-sensitive calcium channels: Inhibition of K^+-evoked (3H)-norepinephrine release from rat neocortical slices. Synapse 2002;45:171-190.
124. Taylor CP: Meeting report: The biology and pharmacology of calcium channel proteins Presented at the Pfizer Satellite Symposium at the 2003 Society for Neuroscience Meeting. CNS Drug Rev 2004;10:159-164.
125. Crofford LJ, Rowbotham MC, Mease PJ, et al: Pregabalin for the treatment of fibromyalgia syndrome: Results of a randomized, double-blind, placebo-controlled trial. Arthritis Rheum 2006;52:1264-1273.
126. Carter LP, Flores LR, Wu H, et al: The role of GABA-B receptors in the discriminative stimulus effects of gamma-hydroxybutyrate in rats: Time course and antagonism studies. J Pharmacol Exp Ther 2003;305:668-674.
127. Scharf MB, Hauck M, Stover R, et al: Effect of gamma-hydroxybutyrate on pain, fatigue, and the alpha sleep anomaly in patients with fibromyalgia. Preliminary report. J Rheumatol 1998;25:1986-1990.
128. Scharf MB, Baumann M, Berkowitz DV: The effects of sodium oxybate on clinical symptoms and sleep patterns in patients with fibromyalgia. J Rheumatol 2003;30:1070-1074.
129. Russell IJ, Perkins AT, Michalek JE; Oxybate for FMS Study Group: Sodium oxybate relieves pain and improves sleep in fibromyalgia syndrome (FMS): A randomized, double-blind, placebo-controlled, multi-center clinical trial. Arthritis Rheum 2007 (submitted).
130. UBC clinical significance calculator: Available at www.healthcare.ubc.ca/calc/clinsig.html.
131. Crofford LJ, Rowbotham MC, Mease PJ, et al: Pregabalin for the treatment of fibromyalgia syndrome: Results of a randomized, double-blind, placebo-controlled trial. Arthritis Rheum 52:1264-73, 2005.
132. Bandolier: Evidence-based health care. Available at www.jr2.ox.ac.uk/bandolier/ index.html.
133. Carette S, Bell JJ, Reynolds WJ, et al: Comparison of amitriptyline, cyclobenzaprine, and placebo in the treatment of fibromyalgia: A randomized, double-blind clinical trial. Arthritis Rheum 1994;37:30-40.
134. Moldofsky H, Lue FA, Mously C, et al: The effect of zolpidem in patients with fibromyalgia: A dose-ranging, double-blind, placebo-controlled, modified crossover study. J Rheumatol 1996;23:529-533.
135. Borg-Stein J: Management of peripheral pain generators in fibromyalgia. Rheum Dis Clin North Am 2002;28:305-317.

24 Headache Disorders

David M. Biondi

Headache is a common medical condition that has high prevalence in the general population.[1,2] In the United States, headache accounts for several million outpatient medical visits each year and more than a million patient-days bedridden each month.[3] Migraine alone, recognized by the World Health Organization as a highly disabling condition,[4] has an annual prevalence of 12% to 13% (18.2% for women and 6.5% for men), therefore affecting more than 30 million people in the United States alone.[5] Migraine is a public health concern in the United States that has been associated with annual socioeconomic losses in the billions of dollars from missed workdays, reduced work productivity, and direct medical costs.[3,6] The magnitudes of worldwide prevalence and socioeconomic burden of migraine are similar.[2,7,8] Chronic daily headache, a condition defined as 15 or more headache days per month, is estimated to affect 3% to 5% of the world population[9-12] and is associated with an unknown but predictably large socioeconomic burden.

There are hundreds of potential causes for head and face pain. Pain-sensitive structures of the head include the scalp, peripheral nerves, muscles, periosteum, dural linings of the brain, and both intracranial and extracranial blood vessels. The brain parenchyma itself is insensate. Primary headache disorders are those that are not attributable to an identifiable structural or disease-related etiology and include the major diagnostic categories of tension-type, migraine, and cluster headache. Primary headaches are classified by their presenting signs and symptoms. In the general population, the most prevalent primary headache disorder is tension-type headache, but migraine is the most prevalent disabling primary headache disorder. Arguably due to its symptom intensity and associated disability, migraine is the most common primary headache disorder among clinic patients who present with a chief complaint of headache or admit to experiencing significant headaches when questioned.[13]

The treatment of primary headache disorders, especially migraine, has vastly improved over the last two decades as preclinical and clinical research better defines the pathogenesis and identifies specific treatment targets for each headache type. In contrast, secondary headache disorders are those that are attributed to another condition, an underlying structural abnormality, or a disease process and include a broad range of conditions such as headaches associated with intracranial tumor, blood vessel abnormalities, hemorrhage, infection, trauma, medication, metabolic disorder, or other systemic medical conditions. Secondary headaches are defined by their etiologic cause and treatments are specifically targeted to address that cause as well as to provide palliative pain relief.

HEADACHE CLASSIFICATION AND DIAGNOSIS

Before 1988, there were no systematic or internationally recognized criteria for the evaluation and diagnosis of headaches. The Headache Classification Subcommittee of the International Headache Society published the first International Classification of Headache Disorders (ICHD) in 1988.[14] The second edition of the ICHD (ICHD-2) was published in early 2004.[15] The diagnostic criteria and headache classifications are based on clinical and epidemiologic research as well as expert consensus. The ICHD-2 has been recognized by the WHO and is used as a basis for headache diagnoses included in the International Classification of Diseases (ICD-10). The ICHD-2 uses a hierarchical system that is divided into three parts (Table 24–1). The first part has four major categories of primary headache disorders subclassified into a total of 57 subtypes and subforms. The second part has eight major categories of secondary headache disorders subclassified into a total of 152 subtypes and subforms. The third part defines cranial neuralgias, facial pain, and other headaches yet to be defined. Although all classification systems have limitations when applied to clinical practice, the ICHD-2 provides a tool by which headaches can be diagnosed and studied in a consistent manner throughout the international research and academic community. It also provides a thoughtfully devised framework for headache diagnosis in the medical office or clinic settings. With an improved understanding of characteristics specific to a headache type, arriving at an accurate headache diagnosis can and has substantially improved treatment outcomes through mechanism-based and evidence-based treatment strategies.

Table 24–1. Headache Classification Categories

1. Migraine
   1.1 Migraine without aura (previously used term: common migraine)
   1.2 Migraine with aura (previously used term: classic migraine)
2. Tension-type headache
   2.1 Infrequent episodic tension-type headache
   2.2 Frequent episodic tension-type headache
   2.3 Chronic tension-type headache
3. Cluster headache and other trigeminal autonomic cephalalgias
   3.1 Cluster
       3.1.1 Episodic cluster headache
       3.1.2 Chronic cluster headache
4. Other Primary Headaches
5. Headache attributed to head and/or neck trauma
6. Headache attributed to cranial or cervical vascular disorder
7. Headache attributed to nonvascular intracranial disorder
   7.1 Headache attributed to high cerebrospinal fluid pressure
   7.2 Headache attributed to low cerebrospinal fluid pressure
   7.3 Headache attributed to noninfectious inflammatory disease
   7.4 Headache attributed to intracranial neoplasm
8. Headache attributed to a substance or its withdrawal
   8.1 Headache induced by acute substance use or exposure
   8.2 Medication overuse headache (MOH)
9. Headache attributed to infection
10. Headache attributed to disorder of homeostasis
11. Headache or facial pain attributed to disorder of the cranium, neck, eyes, ears, nose, sinuses, teeth, mouth, or other facial or cranial structures
12. Headache attributed to psychiatric disorder
13. Cranial neuralgias and central causes of facial pain
14. Other headache, cranial neuralgia, central or primary facial pain

Adapted from Headache Classification of the International Headache Society: The International Classification of Headache Disorders, 2nd edition. Cephalalgia 2004;24(Suppl 1):1-160 (not inclusive of all subtypes and subforms).

THE HEADACHE EVALUATION

Headache History

Although secondary headache disorders account for only a small proportion of headache presentations in the outpatient setting,[2] the medical evaluation must first exclude these potentially serious or life-threatening conditions. A thorough understanding of the patient's headache history, current pain characteristics, and all associated symptoms are the first step toward making a headache diagnosis. Comprehensive physical and neurologic examinations are necessary to determine an accurate headache diagnosis. Diagnostic tests are sometimes necessary to confirm clinical impressions if the headache history, headache characteristics, or physical examinations are inconsistent with or atypical for primary headache disorders. Because attack frequency, temporal attack profiles, and associated symptoms define the various headache disorders, a detailed headache history is invaluable. A headache history may be modeled after information needed to establish a headache diagnosis based on ICHD-2 diagnostic criteria (Table 24–2). A headache questionnaire com-

Table 24–2. Headache History

1. Initial Headache Presentation and Progression
   a. Acute, fulminant, or cataclysmic
   b. Subacute or gradual
   c. Chronic or protracted
   d. Paroxysmal
   e. Cyclic
   f. Prodromal symptoms or neurologic aura
   g. Any precipitating event, illness, or activity
2. Pain Location
   a. Generalized, holocephalic
   b. Unilateral with or without side shift
   c. Focal or discretely localized
   d. Bilateral or bandlike
3. Pain Expression
   a. Intermittent
      (1) Frequency
      (2) Duration
   b. Constant
   c. Intensity (mild, moderate, severe)
   d. Level of disability
4. Pain Quality
   a. Throbbing, pounding
   b. Squeezing, viselike, tightening, pressure
   c. Boring, drilling, knifelike
   d. Stabbing, jolting, shocklike, shooting
   e. Burning, searing
5. Associated Signs and Symptoms
   a. Nausea, vomiting, diarrhea
   b. Photophobia, phonophobia, osmophobia
   c. Paresthesia, numbness
   d. Scalp sensitivity
   e. Muscle weakness
      (1) Focal
      (2) Generalized
   f. Dizziness, vertigo, dysequilibrium
   g. Blurred vision, visual scotoma, diplopia, visual field cuts
   h. Cognitive dysfunction, language disturbances, confusion, altered consciousness
   i. Autonomic signs
      (1) Lacrimation, rhinorrhea nasal congestion, miosis, mydriasis, flushing, diaphoresis, blood pressure alterations, syncope
6. Diurnal, Weekly, Monthly, or Annual Headache Cycles or Patterns
7. Headache Triggers, Exacerbating Factors, and Ameliorating Factors
8. Family Headache History

pleted by the patient before the physician visit can save time during a patient encounter but direct questioning of the patient is more likely to uncover small nuances and unusual features of the headache presentation that may be missed on a structured form alone. Headache-associated symptoms and signs that are not typical of ICHD-defined primary headache disorders and progressive worsening of headache attacks or attack patterns over time are features that can imply a secondary headache disorder. If these features are present, a secondary headache disorder will need to be ruled out through appropriate diagnostic investigation. It is not unusual for a patient to experience more than one type of primary headache disorder such as a combination of tension-type and migraine headaches. The initial evaluation and treatment course will often focus on the headache that is most concerning or disabling for the patient but all headache presentations merit further evaluation. A patient's detailed headache diary can be a helpful tool for confirming a provisional or uncertain headache diagnosis.

Initial Headache Presentation and Headache Progression

Factors initiating or inciting recurrent headaches, the temporal pattern of individual attacks, and progression of attack patterns over time can provide essential information regarding a headache's etiology. Episodic or chronic headaches beginning for the first time in patients 50 years of age or older hold greater risk of being attributed to an underlying condition such as tumor, temporal arteritis, or other systemic disorder; therefore patients in this age group usually require more intense medical attention and diagnostic evaluation. Headaches that begin suddenly during or after physical exertion, Valsalva, sexual activity, or head injury might be associated with intracranial hemorrhage or related to an abnormality at the craniocervical junction such as a Chiari malformation. A headache that has a sudden onset and is immediately at maximal pain intensity is concerning for the possibility of intracranial hemorrhage from a ruptured aneurysm or arteriovenous malformation (AVM). Headache associated with apoplexy of the pituitary can also have a cataclysmic onset. Rare cases of referred head pain associated with myocardial ischemia have been reported.[16] Physical exertion can also incite primary headaches such as migraine or benign exertional headache and because of this association, a purely history-based diagnosis can sometimes be difficult. Severe headaches that begin during pregnancy and postpartum might be related to intracranial venous thrombosis, which can be accompanied by altered consciousness or focal neurologic signs but alternatively might be related to the exacerbating effect of rapidly changing hormonal levels on a primary headache disorder such as migraine. Head pain referred from the neck (cervicogenic headache) can begin after neck injury associated with sports, motor vehicle accidents, or accidental falls. Subacute or gradual headache progression over hours to weeks might be indicative of a subdural hematoma, infection, or vasculitis. A chronic progressive or protracted headache course might suggest an intracranial tumor or metabolic disorder. The chronic progressive pattern can also indicate transformation of episodic migraine to chronic migraine as a consequence of medication overuse. Paroxysmal headache attacks can describe several primary headache disorders such as migraine or cluster but might also be associated with cerebral ischemia or epilepsy. A predictable monthly headache pattern can describe hormonally related migraine attacks while a predicable diurnal headache pattern can describe cluster or migraine headaches. Headaches that occur during sleep can be suggestive of an intracranial tumor or sleep disorder such as apnea or excessive snoring but this can also be a pattern observed in cases of cluster and migraine.

Head Pain Location

Alternating hemicrania or side shift during a headache attack is typical of migraine but migraine pain can also have holocephalic or occipital localization. Neck pain is reported during a majority of migraine attacks and may be the first symptom of a migraine attack.[17] Cluster headache is invariably unilateral without side shift and is typically located around the orbit or temple. Focal or discretely localized pain without change in its location might be indicative of a fixed intracranial lesion or peripheral nerve injury in the scalp or upper neck. Side locked head pain with predominant neck pain is suggestive of cervicogenic headache. Bilateral pressure or bandlike headache is a common presentation for tension-type headache but if it is persistent or progressive, it might be indicative of an abnormal elevation of cerebrospinal fluid pressure or an intracranial mass.

Pain Duration and Attack Frequency

Tension-type headache attack duration can range from 30 minutes to 7 days. Episodic migraine attacks typically last from 4 to 72 hours. Cluster attacks last from 15 to 180 minutes and may occur several times every day including during sleep. Paroxysmal hemicranial attacks last 2 to 30 minutes and occur more than five times per day. The SUNCT syndrome (short-lasting, unilateral, neuralgiform headache with conjunctival injection and tearing) is defined by attacks lasting between 5 and 240 seconds that can occur from 3 to 200 times per day. In general it is not possible to classify secondary headache disorders based on time course, diurnal frequency, or clinical symptoms owing to the wide variety of etiologies and pathogenic mechanisms as well as lack of stereotypic characteristics.

Pain Quality

Tension-type headache has a mild to moderate pain intensity and is described as squeezing, bandlike, or viselike. Migraine pain is typically moderate to severe in intensity and is described as throbbing, pounding, or jabbing. Migraine might also be described as a constant, intense pressure—"like my head is going to explode." Cluster headache pain is often described with terms such as *drilling*, *boring*, and *piercing*. Many patients describe cluster pain as a feeling perceived as analogous to "a hot poker jammed into my eye." Burning, jabbing, or shooting are terms sometimes used to describe cluster or well-established migraine attacks but are more commonly descriptors for cranial neuralgia. Pain associated with secondary headache disorders such as intracranial tumor, infection, or psychiatric conditions is most often holocephalic or well-circumscribed in location, constant in duration, variable in pain intensity, and progressive in its course.

Symptoms Associated with Headache

Obtaining a complete list of headache-associated symptoms is an essential component of the headache history because headache accompaniments are criteria used to classify primary headache disorders, but they also can be key indicators that raise suspicion for underlying pathology. Fixed or long-lasting (more than 1 hour) neurologic deficits, hemiplegia, confusion, diplopia, alterations of consciousness, and seizures are rare accompaniments of primary headache disorders and suggest a secondary headache disorder. Episodic nausea, vomiting, and hypersensitivity to sensory stimuli such as light, sound, or odors are common accompaniments of migraine. Protracted and projectile vomiting suggests intracranial pathology and elevated intracranial pressure. High blood pressure, slow pulse rate, and altered consciousness also might indicate elevated intracranial pressure due to an intracranial mass lesion or an obstruction to cerebrospinal fluid flow. Headache exacerbated by the supine position, Valsalva, and physical exertion might indicate an elevated CSF pressure syndrome such as idiopathic intracranial hypertension, also known as pseudotumor cerebri. Headache that is most severe when the patient is sitting or standing but dramatically improves when supine suggests a low cerebrospinal fluid pressure syndrome. Cluster and other trigeminal autonomic cephalalgias (TACs), such as benign paroxysmal hemicrania and SUNCT, are associated with cranial parasympathetic symptoms such as lacrimation, nasal congestion, rhinorrhea, and face sweating that occur ipsilateral to the head pain.

Other Information from the Headache History

In cases of migraine, a family history of severe headache or migraine is very common and can be a reassuring aspect of the headache history, especially when evaluating children who are experiencing intense headache or adults experiencing migraine-like headaches for the first time. Migraine patients are consistently recognized to have attack triggers such as emotional or physical stress, missed meals, alterations in usual sleep patterns, weather changes, humidity, and strong sensory stimuli including bright light, glare, noise, or perfume scents. Menstrually related and pharmacologically induced hormonal changes are well known migraine triggers. Consuming alcohol during an active cluster cycle invariably triggers cluster attacks but also can incite migraine attacks in susceptible individuals. In cases of chronic or treatment refractory headache, special attention is given to the medication history. New medications, both prescribed and over the counter (OTC), taken by the patient for a coexisting condition can cause headache as a side effect or due to interference with other headache treatments. Headaches might occur after taking certain prescribed medications such as nitrates, calcium channel blockers, antidepressants, or insulin, among others. Caffeine overuse (more than 200 mg per day) is suspected to be an important dietary factor contributing to the transformation of intermittent to chronic migraine in some individuals.[18] A complete medication history is particularly important in patients with migraine because the frequent use of acute migraine medications such as 5-HT$_{1B/D}$ agonists (triptans), ergot derivatives, and

analgesics (non-opioid or opioid, OTC or prescribed) even if taken for another painful condition might cause a progressive worsening of headache intensity and frequency in some patients, a condition commonly known as "analgesic rebound headaches" and classified in the ICHD-2 as medication overuse headache (MOH).[19-22] The frequent use of prescription medications such as opioid analgesics and combination analgesics, especially those containing caffeine, are recognized headache triggers and catalysts for migraine transformation.[21]

PHYSICAL EXAMINATION, LABORATORY TESTING, AND NEUROIMAGING

Detailed general physical and neurologic examinations are needed to confirm the provisional headache diagnosis. A comprehensive examination of all body systems is recommended, but there are some key aspects of the physical examination that are particularly important in the evaluation of headache patients (Table 24–3). There are findings from the history and physical examinations that warrant urgent or more aggressive medical attention (Table 24–4). Diagnostic testing is necessary if the clinical history and examination suggest an underlying structural abnormality or disease process.[23] There are no laboratory or imaging tests specific for or diagnostic of primary headache disorders. Although there are no universally accepted evidence-based guidelines for the use of neuroimaging in the evaluation of patients with headache, clinical guidance may be gained from the medical literature, expert consensus, and general standard of care amongst headache specialists in the United States (Table 24–5).[23] Although there is insufficient evidence to guide the selection of a specific neuroimaging test for all headache presentations, an evidence-based guideline for neuroimaging of non-acute headache in the primary care setting has been developed (Table 24–6).[23] Electroencephalography has not been found helpful in the routine evaluation of headache.[24]

Table 24–3. Key Aspects of the Physical Examination in a Headache Evaluation

1. Vital signs, heart and carotid artery auscultation
2. Clinical observations
   a. Mental status and general functioning
   b. Speech content and fluency
   c. Facial expression and physical body gestures
   d. Gait equilibrium and coordination
3. Optic funduscopic examination
4. Neurologic functions
   a. Cranial nerves evaluation with special attention to eye movements, face strength, and symmetry
   b. Pronator drift, fine motor control of the fingers, somatic muscle strength, and symmetry
   c. Deep tendon reflexes and Babinski's responses
5. Musculoskeletal evaluation
   a. Neck range of movement and suppleness
   b. Myofascial tender or trigger points
   c. Temporomandibular joint problems

Table 24–4. Ominous Findings in the History and Physical Examination of Headache Patients

1. Sudden onset of headache (thunderclap headache)
2. Fever, rash, and/or stiff neck (meningismus) associated with the headache
3. Papilledema (optic nerve head swelling)
4. Dizziness, unsteadiness, dysarthria, weakness, or changes in sensation (numbness or tingling) especially if profound, static, and occurring for the first time
5. Migraine auras or other previously experienced neurologic migraine accompaniments lasting longer than 1 hour
6. Presence of confusion, drowsiness, or loss of consciousness
7. Headache is triggered by exertion, coughing, bending, or sexual activity
8. Headache is progressively worsening and/or resistant to treatment
9. Previously experienced headache characteristics or accompaniments have substantially changed
10. Persistent or severe vomiting accompanies the headache
11. Headaches beginning after age of 50 are associated with a higher risk of arteritis or intracranial tumors. Specifically ask about unexplained weight loss, sweats, fevers, myalgia, arthralgia, and jaw claudication, which are typical accompaniments of giant cell (temporal) arteritis
12. Headache occurring in a patient with human immunodeficiency virus or cancer
13. Frequent emergency department or acute care use
14. Daily or near-daily use of pain relievers or the need to take more than the recommended dosage of pain relievers to control headache symptoms

Table 24–5. Neuroimaging in the Evaluation of Headache

1. Urgent Neuroimaging Recommended
   a. Thunderclap or abrupt onset headache with abnormal neurologic examination
   b. Headache associated with seizure or altered consciousness
   c. Prior to lumbar puncture in situations where headache is accompanied by
      (1) Signs of increased intracranial pressure
      (2) Fever and nuchal rigidity
      (3) Localizing neurologic signs
2. Routine Neuroimaging Recommended
   a. Isolated or first time "thunderclap" headache without focal neurologic examination
   b. Significant change in previous headache characteristics or progressive worsening of headache pattern over hours, days, or weeks
   c. Predominant occipitonuchal headache
   d. New onset of or change in previous headache characteristics in an older individual
   e. Headache accompanied by abnormal neurologic examination, including papilledema, unilateral loss of sensation, weakness, hyperreflexia, or dysequilibrium.
   f. New onset headache in patient who
      (1) Is HIV positive or immunocompromised
      (2) Has a prior diagnosis of cancer
      (3) Is in a population at high risk for intracranial disease
3. Neuroimaging Generally Not Required
   a. Migraine with normal neurologic examination
   b. Recurrent migraine attacks with stable and stereotypical presentations
   c. Tension type headache with normal neurologic examination
   d. Other headaches with normal neurologic examination

Table 24–6. Guidance for the Selection of Diagnostic Neuroimaging

Non–Contrast-Computed Tomography
Recommended when urgent neuroimaging is necessary in cases of:
- Suspected intracranial hemorrhage
- Suspected elevated intracranial pressure or focal neurologic deficit prior to lumbar puncture
- Headache associated with neurologic changes
- Headache presenting with a substantial change in previously experienced headache characteristics

Contrast-Enhanced Computed Tomography
Recommended if abnormality is found on non–contrast CT, or a vascular abnormality or tumor is suspected and an urgent evaluation is necessary.

Magnetic Resonance Imaging
1. Recommended as an initial or urgent diagnostic examination if there is suspicion of venous sinus thrombosis or vasculitis
2. Recommended when an abnormality is suspected in the posterior cranial fossa or at the craniocervical junction
3. Recommended when an aneurysm or vascular malformation is suspected; evaluated with magnetic resonance angiography (MRA)
4. If an abnormality is detected on CT, MRI may further define the abnormality

COMMON PRIMARY HEADACHE DISORDERS

Tension-Type Headache

Episodic tension-type headache (TTH) is the most prevalent primary headache disorder in the general population.[25] Despite its high prevalence, episodic TTH is the least studied of the primary headache disorders[15] and is not often brought to the attention of medical practitioners. In contradistinction to episodic TTH, frequent and chronic TTH can be associated with a high level of personal disability. Although chronic TTH would undoubtedly result in substantial personal and socioeconomic burden, episodic TTH is also associated with a large socioeconomic impact due to its high prevalence.[25] Infrequent TTH (Box 24–1) is defined by its headache frequency of less than 1 headache day per month on average. The pain is generally characterized by bilateral, nonpulsating, squeezing pain having a mild to moderate intensity that is not aggravated by routine physical activity. TTH attacks last from 30 minutes to 7 days in duration. Nausea and vomiting are absent in episodic TTH. Symptoms associated with TTH can include photophobia or phonophobia but not both. Frequent TTH is defined by headache episodes with the clinical features of infrequent TTH but a frequency of more than 1 but less than 15 headache days per month. Chronic TTH is characterized by a frequency of 15 or more headache days per month. Chronic TTH has the clinical features of infrequent TTH but mild nausea may be present.

MIGRAINE

Migraine without aura is a highly prevalent, neurologic disorder most commonly characterized by

BOX 24–1. TENSION-TYPE HEADACHE

2.1 Infrequent Episodic Tension-type Headache
Diagnostic criteria
A. At least 10 episodes occurring on <1 day per month on average (<12 days per year) and fulfilling criteria B-D
B. Headache lasting from 30 minutes to 7 days
C. Headache has at least two of the following characteristics:
   1. bilateral location
   2. pressing/tightening (non-pulsating) quality
   3. mild or moderate intensity
   4. not aggravated by routine physical activity such as walking or climbing stairs
D. Both of the following:
   1. no nausea or vomiting (anorexia may occur)
   2. no more than one of photophobia or phonophobia
E. Not attributed to another disorder

From Headache Classification of the International Headache Society: The International Classification of Headache Disorders, 2nd edition. Cephalalgia 2004;24(Suppl 1):1-160.

BOX 24–2. MIGRAINE

1.1 Migraine without Aura
Diagnostic criteria
A. At least 5 attacks fulfilling criteria B-D
B. Headache attacks lasting 4-72 hours (untreated or unsuccessfully treated)
C. Headache has at least two of the following characteristics:
   1. unilateral location
   2. pulsating quality
   3. moderate or severe pain intensity
   4. aggravation by or causing avoidance of routine physical activity (e.g., walking or climbing stairs)
D. During headache at least one of the following:
   1. nausea and/or vomiting
   2. photophobia and phonophobia
E. Not attributed to another disorder

1.2.1 Typical Aura with Migraine Headache
Diagnostic criteria
A. At least 2 attacks fulfilling criteria B-D
B. Aura consisting of at least one of the following but no motor weakness:
   1. fully reversible visual symptoms including positive features (e.g., flickering lights, spots or lines) and/or negative features (i.e., loss of vision)
   2. fully reversible sensory symptoms including positive features (i.e., pins and needles) and/or negative features (i.e., numbness)
   3. fully reversible dysphasic speech disturbances
C. At least two of the following:
   1. homonymous visual symptoms and/or unilateral sensory symptoms
   2. at least one aura symptom develops gradually over greater than or equal to 5 minutes and/or different aura symptoms occur in succession over greater than or equal to 5 minutes
   3. each symptom lasts greater than or equal to 5 minutes and less than or equal to 60 minutes
D. Headache fulfilling criteria B-D for migraine without aura begins during the aura or follows aura within 60 minutes
E. Not attributed to another disorder

From Headache Classification of the International Headache Society: The International Classification of Headache Disorders, 2nd edition. Cephalalgia 2004;24(Suppl 1):1-160.

attacks and other neurologic accompaniments of intense head pain lasting 4 to 72 hours in duration.[5,15] Migraine is three times more prevalent in women. The headache of migraine is classically unilateral, frontotemporal in location, throbbing in quality, and moderate to severe in intensity. The pain is aggravated by routine physical activity and can alternate from one side of the head to the other both during and between attacks. Migraine is also defined by common associated features, which include sensitivity to environmental stimuli (i.e., light, sound, smell, motion), nausea and vomiting (Box 24–2). Migraine with aura differs only by the presence of fully reversible focal neurologic symptoms that usually develop gradually over 5 to 20 minutes and resolve within 60 minutes. The aura can precede the onset of headache by as much as 60 minutes or occur concurrently with headache onset. Aura can occasionally occur after the migraine headache is well established. Typical aura is characterized by visual, sensory, and speech symptoms alone or in combination. The aura of migraine is usually a mix of "positive" and "negative" neurologic phenomena such as visual scintillation followed by visual scotoma or sensory paresthesia followed by numbness. Migraine aura is a gradually progressive event classically typified by a visual hallucination moving from central to peripheral across the visual field or a "march" of sensory paresthesia up an arm to the face that progressively and completely resolves in reverse order from the region first affected.

Aura-like symptoms can be caused by secondary conditions such as vascular malformations, tumors, ischemia, and epilepsy but these events are often defined by a very short or long duration (less than 5 minutes or more than 1 hour), lack of the characteristic progression or "march" of symptoms, dense neurologic deficits, altered levels of consciousness, and demonstrable neurologic examination abnormalities. Status migrainosis is a migraine attack that lasts longer than 72 hours and is associated with intense pain and disability. The migraine attack is often refractory to usual outpatient treatments but is otherwise typical of the episodic migraine attacks previously experienced by the patient. Chronic migraine is defined by 15 or more headache days per month, of which eight or more headaches are migraine for at least 3 months in the absence of medication overuse or other underlying condition. In a majority of cases, chronic migraine transforms from episodic migraine over a period of months to years; some are associated with medication overuse while others are not.[10,26] In general, the clinical presentation of chronic migraine is similar to chronic TTH but the frequent or daily TTH is punctuated by intermittent migraine or migraine-like attacks. Chronic migraine is covered in more detail later in this chapter.

Personal and Socioeconomic Burden Associated with Migraine

High health care utilization and disability have been associated with migraine. Hu and colleagues estimated that more than 93% of the economic burden of migraine, estimated to be $13 billion in 1999, was due to absenteeism and reduced productivity.[3] Disability in migraine is a result of increased absence from usual occupational and social roles, development of coexisting behavioral and psychological conditions, and disease-related morbidities such as treatment side effects. Severely disabled patients (i.e., those having chronic daily headache) account for a disproportionate amount of the economic and health care burden of migraine. The most disabled half of migraine patients are responsible for roughly 90% of lost work time attributable to migraine,[27] a higher proportion of direct costs associated with treatment and medical utilization,[28] and higher proportion of indirect costs in the way of absenteeism and reduced productivity.[29] Others have reported that 20% of a population-based sample of migraine patients accounted for 77% of absenteeism and 40% accounted for 75% of lost productivity.[29]

Migraine Comorbidity

Sleep disturbance, depression, anxiety, panic disorder, bipolar disorder, epilepsy, obsessive-compulsive behavior, fibromyalgia, and cognitive impairment are more prevalent in chronic headache and migraine populations. Breslau reported that migraine patients were three times more likely to develop depression than those without migraine, six times more likely to have panic disorder, and five times more likely to have generalized anxiety disorder.[30] A positive correlation was also found for the association of migraine with obsessive-compulsive and bipolar disorders. Hamilton rating scores for anxiety and depression were found to be higher in headache patients.[31] The recognition of comorbid medical conditions not only provides therapeutic opportunities by revealing potential pharmacologic treatments that are common to the coexisting disorders but it also assists in avoiding or minimizing an iatrogenic worsening of one

Table 24–7. Potential Therapeutic Opportunities and Limitations for Migraine Preventive Treatment Based on Comorbid Conditions

Potential Therapeutic Opportunities	
COMORBID/COEXISTING DISORDER	**PROPHYLACTIC MEDICATIONS TO CONSIDER**
Depression	TCA, SNRI, SSRI, MAOI
Anxiety	TCA, β-adrenergic blockers, SSRI, MAOI
Bipolar disorder	AED
Epilepsy	AED
Sleep disturbance	TCA
Fibromyalgia	TCA, SNRI
Stroke	Aspirin

Potential Therapeutic Limitations	
COMORBID/COEXISTING DISORDER	**PROPHYLACTIC MEDICATIONS TO AVOID**
Depression	β-adrenergic blockers
Bipolar disorder	TCA, MAOI, SNRI, SSRI
Epilepsy	TCA, MAOI, SNRI, SSRI
Stroke	Ergot derivatives, beta-adrenergic blockers

AED, antiepileptic drug; MAOI, monoamine oxidase inhibitor; SNRI, serotonin norepinephrine reuptake inhibitor; TCA, tricyclic antidepressant; SSRI, selective serotonin reuptake inhibitor.

condition by treatments prescribed for another (Table 24–7).

CLUSTER

Cluster is much less prevalent than migraine (0.1% to 0.4% in the United States) but is associated with a high level of disability due to multiple daily attacks of severe pain, many of which abruptly interrupt sleep (Box 24–3).[32,33] Men are affected approximately four times more commonly than women. Episodic cluster occurs in recurrent cycles of attacks that last from 2 weeks to 3 months in duration. When a cluster cycle is active, attacks can occur from once every other day up to eight attacks per day. The attacks of cluster are characterized by severe or extremely severe pain occurring unilaterally in the orbital or temporal regions. The pain is strictly unilateral during an attack and may rarely shift sides from cycle to cycle. Attacks tend to "cluster" at predictable times during the day. Many attacks classically occur within 60 to 120 minutes of initiating sleep, during the rapid eye movement (REM) sleep phase.[34] Individual attacks last from 15 to 180 minutes in duration. A hallmark of cluster is the association of prominent cranial parasympathetic autonomic features that include lacrimation, conjunctival injection, nasal congestion, rhinorrhea, eyelid swelling, facial sweating, miosis, and ptosis ipsilateral to the pain. Because of this association, cluster and clinically related headache syndromes are sometimes called *trigeminal autonomic cephalalgias* (TACs). During the attack, the patient is restless and agitated, which

BOX 24–3. CLUSTER HEADACHE

3.1 Cluster Headache
Diagnostic criteria
A. At least 5 attacks fulfilling criteria B-D
B. Severe or very severe unilateral orbital, supra-orbital and/or temporal pain lasting 15-180 minutes if untreated
C. Headache is accompanied by at least one of the following:
   1. ipsilateral conjunctival injection and/or lacrimation
   2. ipsilateral nasal congestion and/or rhinor-rhea
   3. ipsilateral eyelid edema
   4. ipsilateral forehead and facial sweating
   5. ipsilateral miosis and/or ptosis
   6. a sense of restlessness or agitation
D. Attacks have a frequency from one every other day to 8 per day
E. Not attributed to another disorder

3.1.1 Episodic Cluster Headache
Diagnostic criteria
A. Attacks fulfilling criteria A-E for 3.1 Cluster headache
B. At least two cluster periods lasting 3-365 days and separated by pain-free remission periods of greater than or equal to 1 month

3.1.2 Chronic Cluster Headache
Diagnostic criteria
A. Attacks fulfilling criteria A-E for 3.1 Cluster headache
B. Attacks recur over >1 year without remission periods or with remission periods lasting <1 month

From Headache Classification of the International Headache Society: The International Classification of Headache Disorders, 2nd edition. Cephalalgia 2004;24(Suppl 1):1-160.

is in contradistinction to the migraine patient who prefers to be calm and motionless.

The characteristics of migraine, tension-type headache, and cluster headache are summarized in Table 24–8.

CERVICOGENIC HEADACHE

Neck pain and cervical muscle tenderness are common and prominent symptoms of primary headache disorders.[35] Conversely, head pain can be referred from bony structures or soft tissues of the neck, a condition commonly called *cervicogenic headache*.[36] The prevalence of cervicogenic headache in the general population is estimated to be 0.4% to 2.5%, but may be as high as 20% in patients with chronic headache.[37] The mean age of patients with this condition is 42.9 years, and it is four times more prevalent in women than in men.

Cervicogenic headache is characterized by unilateral head pain of fluctuating intensity that is increased by movement of the head and radiates from occipital to frontal regions (Box 24–4).[36,38-40] Neck movement or sustained awkward head positioning precipitates the headache. The headache does not shift from side to side. The pain is typically nonthrobbing, non-lancinating, of moderate to severe intensity, and of variable attack duration. Patients with cervicogenic headache may have restricted neck range of motion, and may have ipsilateral neck, shoulder, or arm pain. One problem with this definition is that the proposed clinical features of cervicogenic headache may mimic those commonly associated with primary headache disorders, such as tension-type headache, migraine without aura, or hemicrania continua. Cervicogenic headache may be associated with certain symptoms typical of migraine, including nausea, phonophobia and photophobia, dizziness, and

Table 24–8. Characteristics of the Common Primary Headache Disorders

MIGRAINE WITHOUT AURA	MIGRAINE WITH AURA	TENSION-TYPE HEADACHE	CLUSTER HEADACHE
Recurrent headache attacks lasting 4 to 72 hours and having: At least 2 of the following: • Unilateral location • Pulsating quality • Moderate or severe intensity • Aggravation by routine physical activity And at least 1 of the following: • Nausea and/or vomiting • Photophobia and phonophobia Can evolve to a very frequent (chronic) migraine condition with or without acute or analgesic medication overuse.	Recurrent disorder manifesting in attacks of reversible focal neurologic symptoms that usually develop gradually over 5 to 20 minutes and last for less than 60 minutes. Typical aura consists of visual and/or sensory and/or speech symptoms. Headache with the features of migraine without aura usually follows the aura symptoms. Less commonly, headache lacks migrainous features or is completely absent.	Episodic headache attacks lasting 30 minutes to 7 days and having: At least 2 of the following: • Bilateral location • Pressing/tightening (nonpulsating) quality • Mild or moderate intensity • Not aggravated by routine physical activity And both of the following: • No nausea or vomiting • No more than one of photophobia or phonophobia Can evolve to frequent or chronic tension-type headache.	Episodic attacks of severe, strictly unilateral, orbital, supraorbital, and/or temporal pain lasting 15 to 180 minutes if untreated. At least 1 of the following is present ipsilateral to the pain: • Conjunctival injection and/or lacrimation • Nasal congestion and/or rhinorrhea • Eyelid edema • Forehead and facial sweating • Miosis and/or ptosis Attacks have a frequency from once every other day to 8 times a day. Most patients are restless or agitated during an attack.

BOX 24–4. CERVICOGENIC HEADACHE

11.2.1 Cervicogenic Headache
Diagnostic criteria:
A. Pain, referred from a source in the neck and perceived in one or more regions of the head and/or face, fulfilling criteria C and D
B. Clinical, laboratory and/or imaging evidence of a disorder or lesion within the cervical spine or soft tissues of the neck known to be, or generally accepted as, a valid cause of headache[1]
C. Evidence that the pain can be attributed to the neck disorder or lesion based on at least one of the following:
   1. Demonstration of clinical signs that implicate a source of pain in the neck[2]
   2. Abolition of headache following diagnostic blockade of a cervical structure or its nerve supply using placebo or other adequate controls[3]
D. Pain resolves within 3 months after successful treatment of the causative disorder or lesion

Notes
[1] Tumors, fractures, infections, and rheumatoid arthritis of the upper cervical spine have not been validated formally as causes of headache, but are n-3evertheless accepted as valid causes when demonstrated to be so in individual cases. Cervical spondylosis and osteochondritis are not accepted as valid causes fulfilling criterion B. When myofascial trigger points are the cause, the headache should be coded under 2. Tension-type headache.
[2] Clinical signs acceptable for criterion C1 must have demonstrated reliability and validity. The future task is the identification of such reliable and valid operational tests. Clinical features such as neck pain, focal neck tenderness, history of neck trauma, mechanical exacerbation of pain, unilaterality, coexisting shoulder pain, reduced range of motion in the neck, nuchal onset, nausea, vomiting, photophobia, and so on, are not unique to cervicogenic headache. These may be features of cervicogenic headache, but they do not define the relationship between the disorder and the source of the headache.
[3] Abolition of headache means complete relief of headache, indicated by a score of zero on a visual analogue scale (VAS). Nevertheless, acceptable as fulfilling criterion C2 is ≥ 90% reduction in pain to a level of <5 on a 100-point VAS.
From Headache Classification of the International Headache Society: the International Classification of Headache Disorders, 2nd edition. Cephalalgia 2004;24(Suppl 1):1-160.

ipsilateral blurred vision.[37] As a result, distinguishing cervicogenic headache from other headache types can be difficult.

The best-described subtypes of cervicogenic headache are C2 neuralgia and third occipital headache. C2 neuralgia headache can result from lesions or injury affecting the C2 spinal nerve. C2 neuralgia is typically described as a deep or dull pain that radiates from the occipital to parietal, temporal, frontal, and periorbital regions. A paroxysmal sharp or shocklike pain centered in the occipital region is often superimposed over the constant pain. Ipsilateral eye lacrimation and conjunctival injection are common associated signs. Arterial or venous compression of the C2 spinal nerve or its dorsal root ganglion has

been implicated as a cause for C2 neuralgia in some cases.[41-44] Third occipital headache involves the third occipital nerve (dorsal ramus C3), which innervates the C2-3 zygapophyseal joint. The C2-3 zygapophyseal joint and the third occipital nerve appear most vulnerable to trauma from acceleration-deceleration ("whiplash") injuries of the neck.[45] Pain from the C2-3 zygapophyseal joint is referred to the occipital region of the head but is also referred to the frontotemporal and periorbital regions. Third occipital headache appears to be a common cause of cervicogenic headache. In a study of 100 patients who had whiplash, the prevalence of third occipital headache was 27%.[46] The majority of cervicogenic headaches occurring after whiplash will resolve within a year of the trauma.[47]

Anatomy

The first three cervical spinal nerves and their rami are the primary peripheral nerve structures that can refer pain to the head.[48] The anatomic locus for cervicogenic headache is the trigeminocervical nucleus in the upper cervical spinal cord, where sensory nerve fibers in the descending tract of the trigeminal nerve (trigeminal nucleus caudalis) are believed to interact with sensory fibers from the upper cervical roots. This functional intersection of upper cervical and trigeminal sensory pathways is believed to allow the bidirectional transmission of pain signals between the neck and the trigeminal sensory receptive fields of the face and head.[49]

Diagnostic Criteria and Testing

In addition to the ICHD-2 diagnostic criteria, the Cervicogenic Headache International Study Group (CHISG) has proposed another set of diagnostic criteria for cervicogenic headache[38] (Table 24–9). These criteria have an obligatory requirement for symptoms or signs of neck involvement that may be fulfilled if head pain is precipitated by neck movement, sustained awkward head positioning, or by external pressure over the upper cervical or occipital region on the symptomatic side. These criteria may also be fulfilled by the combination of both restricted neck range of motion and ipsilateral neck, shoulder, or arm pain that is vague and nonradicular or radicular in nature. The CHISG criteria also require confirmatory evidence by anesthetic blocks, but this requirement is only obligatory for scientific studies, not clinical diagnosis.

Anesthetic blockade of the zygapophyseal joint, cervical nerve, or medial branch is used to confirm the diagnosis of cervicogenic headache and possibly predict the treatment modalities that will most likely provide the greatest efficacy. Fluoroscopic or interventional magnetic resonance imaging (iMRI) guided blockade may be necessary to assure accurate and specific localization of the pain source.[50-52] The diagnosis of cervicogenic headache can be made in certain

Table 24–9. The Cervicogenic Headache International Study Group Criteria

Major Criteria of Cervicogenic Headache
(I) Symptoms and signs of neck involvement:
  (a) precipitation of head pain, similar to the usually occurring one:
    (1) by neck movement and/or sustained awkward head positioning, and/or:
    (2) by external pressure over the upper cervical or occipital region on the symptomatic side
  (b) restriction of the range of motion (ROM) in the neck
  (c) ipsilateral neck, shoulder, or arm pain of a rather vague nonradicular nature or, occasionally, arm pain of a radicular nature.
Points (I) (a through c) are set forth in a surmised sequence of importance. It is obligatory that one or more of the phenomena in point (I) are present. Point (a) suffices as the sole criterion for positivity within group (I); points (b) or (c) do not. Provisionally, the combination of (I) (b and c) has been set forth as a satisfactory combination within (I). The presence of all three points (a, b, and c) fortifies the diagnosis (but still point [II] is an additional obligatory point for scientific work).
(II) Confirmatory evidence by diagnostic anesthetic blockades
Point (II) is an obligatory point in scientific works
(III) Unilaterality of the head pain, without sideshift
For scientific work, point (III) should preferably be adhered to
Head Pain Characteristics
(IV) (a) moderate-severe, nonthrobbing, and nonlancinating pain, usually starting in the neck
  (b) episodes of varying duration, or
  (c) fluctuating, continuous pain
Other Characteristics of Some Importance
(V) (a) only marginal effect or lack of effect of indomethacin
  (b) only marginal effect or lack of effect of ergotamine and sumatriptan
  (c) female sex
  (d) not infrequent occurrence of head or indirect neck trauma by history, usually of more than only medium severity
None of the single points under (IV) and (V) are obligatory.
Other Features of Lesser Importance
(VI) Various attack-related phenomena, only occasionally present:
  (a) nausea
  (b) phonophobia and photophobia
  (c) dizziness
  (d) ipsilateral "blurred vision"
  (e) difficulties on swallowing
  (f) ipsilateral edema, mostly in the periocular area

cases without doing an anesthetic procedure, if the diagnosis is based on a careful history, physical examination, and a complete neurologic assessment. However, it has been argued that cervicogenic headache cannot be diagnosed on clinical grounds alone because the definitive criterion is complete relief of pain after controlled anesthetic blocks of cervical structures or their nerve supply.[48] In support of the latter viewpoint, a study that evaluated 71 patients with chronic neck pain and headache found no distinguishing features on history or examination that confirmed a definitive diagnosis of third occipital headache before nerve blocks.[46] Diagnostic imaging such as plain films, cervical spine magnetic resonance imaging (MRI), and computed tomography (CT)

myelography cannot confirm the diagnosis of cervicogenic headache but can lend support to its diagnosis.[53] Imaging is primarily used to search for secondary causes of pain that may require surgery or other, more aggressive forms of treatment.[54]

Treatment of Cervicogenic Headache

There is no proven effective treatment for cervicogenic headache. However, a number of different treatment modalities are available. A comprehensive, multidisciplinary pain treatment program provides the best opportunity for success and can significantly decrease the protracted course of costly treatment and disability that is often associated with this challenging pain disorder.

Physical therapy may provide long-term improvement for cervicogenic headache. In a randomized controlled trial with unblinded treatment and blinded assessment of 200 patients with cervicogenic headache, those assigned to 6 weeks of treatment with either manipulative therapy, exercise therapy, or a combination of both therapies had a significant reduction in headache frequency at 12 months, the primary outcome measure, compared with controls who received no treatment.[55] Combined treatment was not significantly better than either treatment alone. The intensity of headache may initially worsen during or after physical therapy, especially if it is vigorously applied. Physical treatment is better tolerated when initiated with gentle muscle stretching and manual cervical traction. Therapy can be slowly advanced as tolerated to include strengthening and aerobic conditioning. Using anesthetic blockade for temporary pain relief may enhance patient tolerance of physical therapy.

Although the concept has not been adequately confirmed in clinical trials, complete relief of pain by diagnostic blockade of the cervical spinal nerve, medial branch, or zygapophyseal joint is likely to predict response to radiofrequency neurotomy.[56] Percutaneous radiofrequency neurotomy can be considered for cervicogenic headache if diagnostic anesthetic blockade of cervical nerve, medial branch, or zygapophyseal joint blockade is temporarily successful in providing complete pain relief.[56-58] However, the benefit of this procedure for cervicogenic headache is not established by adequate randomized controlled trials. In the setting of neck pain, radiofrequency neurotomy appears to be beneficial in patients selected on the basis of complete pain relief with diagnostic blockade. This point is illustrated by a randomized controlled trial involving 24 patients with chronic cervical zygapophyseal joint pain (but *not* cervicogenic headache) confirmed with double-blind, placebo-controlled local anesthesia.[58] Patients assigned to active treatment (n = 12) had a significantly longer pain relief compared with those assigned to controls. In contrast, radiofrequency neurotomy compared with sham treatment was not beneficial in patients with cervicogenic headache selected on the basis of purely clinical criteria, as shown in a randomized controlled trial of 12 patients.[59] A major limitation of this study is that all included patients had an incomplete response to diagnostic anesthetic blockade and thus might not be expected to respond to radiofrequency denervation.[60] For patients with third occipital headache selected on the basis of controlled diagnostic blocks of the third occipital nerve, one series of 49 patients reported that treatment with radiofrequency neurotomy was successful with complete relief of pain in 43 patients (88%).[61] The median duration of relief was 297 days. After recurrence, headache relief could be reestablished by repeating the procedure. Side effects of the procedure were consistent with denervation of the third occipital nerve and included mild ataxia, numbness, and temporary dysesthesia; none of these side effects required intervention. Small uncontrolled retrospective studies suggest that some patients may obtain relief from intra-articular steroid injections at the C2-3 zygapophyseal joint.[62] Cervical epidural steroid injections may give short-term pain relief in cases of multilevel disk or spine degeneration.[63]

Pharmacologic treatments for chronic cervicogenic headache include medications that are used for the preventive or palliative management of neuropathic pain, such as tricyclic antidepressants, anticonvulsants, and others. However, these medications have not been evaluated in controlled clinical trials for the treatment of cervicogenic headache. Available evidence suggests that pharmacologic therapy does not provided substantial pain relief for cervicogenic headache in most cases.[37] In addition, patients with chronic cervicogenic headache may overuse or become dependent on analgesics. Despite these observations, the judicious short-term use of analgesic medication may provide enough pain relief to allow greater patient participation in a physical therapy and rehabilitation program.

A variety of surgical interventions, such as neurectomy, dorsal rhizotomy, and microvascular decompression of nerve roots or peripheral nerves, have been performed for presumed cases of cervicogenic headache. However, the available data are limited to small observational studies, and these have generally reported that surgery is associated with only incomplete or temporary benefit for pain relief.[43,44,64,65] Intensification of pain or anesthesia dolorosa are potential adverse outcomes that must be considered when contemplating the use of surgical interventions. Surgical interventions are not recommended unless the pain is refractory to all reasonable nonsurgical treatments and there is compelling radiologic evidence of a surgically correctable lesion.

CHRONIC DAILY HEADACHE

Chronic daily headache (CDH) refers to a group of complex and disabling headache disorders estimated to affect more than 4% of the general population in the United States. The estimated prevalence of chronic migraine (CM) alone is 1.3%.[10] Patients with CDH account for most of the referrals to headache

specialty practices[66] but chronic migraine is overrepresented in this population because it is associated with greater disability than chronic tension-type headache. Among patients with CDH, many are overusing prescribed or over-the-counter medications. In migraine patients, the frequent use of analgesics and acute migraine medications can act as a catalyst for the transformation of episodic to CM, a condition subclassified as medication overuse headache (MOH) in the ICHD-2 and commonly known as "rebound headache." Some of the common issues confounding management of patients who experience CM are medication overuse, psychiatric comorbidity, refractoriness to pharmacologic treatments, and disability. Despite aggressive treatment, most patients continue to experience frequent or episodic migraine attacks.[21,22,67]

Classification of Chronic Daily Headache

CDH is clinically defined by a frequency of 15 or more headache days per month. Primary CDH are those headache conditions not associated with a structural or systemic pathology (i.e., chronic tension-type or chronic migraine headache). Secondary forms of CDH include those caused by cranial tumors, cerebrovascular disorders or malformations, intracranial or pericranial infection, disorders of cerebrospinal fluid pressure, medication side effects, cervicogenic headache, pericranial or facial muscular disorders, and head or neck trauma.

In practice, primary CDH has a broad range of clinical presentations.[68,69] When categorizing CDH by attack duration, chronic cluster, chronic paroxysmal hemicrania, and hypnic headache have frequent attacks that generally last less than 4 hours while chronic migraine, chronic tension-type headache, and hemicrania continua last longer than 4 hours or, more commonly, present with constant daily pain. Most cases of CDH in the general population are chronic tension-type headache while most cases evaluated in specialty headache clinics evolve from a pattern of episodic migraine attacks to become chronic migraine[15] or sometimes called "transformed" migraine. The ICHD-2 defines CM as migraine headache occurring on 15 or more days per month for more than 3 months in the absence of medication overuse and not attributed to another disorder.[15] Epidemiologic studies have suggested that this definition will not accurately identify a large proportion of patients who actually have clinically apparent CM. Revised criteria have defined CM as a disorder with 15 or more headache days per month, of which eight or more headache episodes meet ICHD-2 diagnostic criteria for migraine. New daily persistent headache (NDPH) is a headache disorder that is characterized by a daily headache pattern from onset.

Approximately 75% of patients with chronic migraine had originally experienced episodic migraine without aura.[70] As chronic migraine develops, the headache tends to lose its frequent episodic presentation and evolves to a constant headache pattern having clinical characteristics of chronic tension-type headache. Superimposed on the constant head pain are intermittent, but usually frequent, intense headache episodes that have typical features of migraine.[15,68] Patients with CM are often sensitive to a variety of sensory stimuli such as light, sound, smell, and touch even between migraine attacks.[71] Other symptoms of CM include chronic nausea, diminished appetite, poor sleep, dizziness, dysequilibrium, fatigue, cognitive inefficiency, and behavioral and mood changes. There are many "intrinsic" and "extrinsic" stimuli that can exacerbate the intensity of pain and migraine-associated symptoms. These stimuli include hormonal cycles, emotional stress, hunger, physical exertion, illness, exposure to bright light or loud noise, strong odors, and dramatic variation of ambient temperature or weather change. In general, patients with CM appear to be "hypersensitive" and "hyperresponsive" to sensory or physical stimuli.

MEDICATION OVERUSE HEADACHE

Chronic headache associated with medication overuse has been identified as a common problem in general medical practice.[19] Despite general acceptance of the medication overuse headache (MOH) diagnosis, controversy and debate still surround the true nature of this condition.[72] MOH is described in clinical terms as a chronic headache syndrome associated with frequent use of acute migraine or analgesic medication that is characterized by an insidious increase of headache frequency and intensity, poor response to alternative acute medications, reduced efficacy of preventive medications, predictable early morning awakenings because of headache, cyclic onset or exacerbation of headache intensity following the last dose of medication or prior to the next scheduled dose, and development of drug dependency or addiction. The ICHD-2 defines specific subclassifications of MOH based on the medication that is overused, frequency of medication ingestion, and improvement in the chronic headache pattern after withdrawal of the overused medication.[15] The ICHD-2 has divided MOH into specific subcategories related to overuse of ergot derivatives, triptans, simple analgesics, opioid analgesics, and combination medications such as those containing various combinations of simple analgesics, butalbital, and caffeine. In general, MOH is defined by a frequency of 15 or more headache days per month induced by frequent or daily use of a medication for greater than 3 months. In addition, the headache resolves or reverts to its previous pattern within 2 months after discontinuation of the overused medication. The quantification of "overuse" in terms of treatment days per month varies from one medication to another. MOH has been primarily studied in the migraine population and indeed migraine patients may be the primary headache population at greatest risk for developing this syndrome.[73-76] The differential risk of migraine patients to develop transformation to a chronic pain disorder is based on clinical long-term observations

and expert consensus. Medication-induced chronic headache has been observed to occur in migraine patients but not others who were taking opioid analgesics for conditions other than headache, for example, arthritis or bowel hypermotility.[73-76] In a study that retrospectively analyzed the medical records of more than 32,000 patients with various pain disorders over a period of 11 years, the use of daily or weekly analgesics at the time of initial medical evaluation increased the risk of developing chronic pain years later.[73] Although the risk of developing chronic pain was observed in patients with all of the targeted pain disorders (neck pain, low back pain, migraine and nonmigraine headache), the greatest risk was for patients with migraine (RR 13.3; 95% CI 2 to 2.8) when compared to those with nonmigraine headache (RR 6.2; 95% CI 5 to 7.7), neck pain (RR 2.4; 95% CI 2 to 2.8), and low back pain (RR 2.3; 95% CI 2 to 2.8). This study appears to support the long-held belief that patients with migraine are more vulnerable to escalation in the frequency of painful events and amplification of pain intensity as a consequence of frequent analgesic use.

Up to 80% of patients presenting to U.S. headache specialty clinics with a chief complaint of CDH use analgesics on a daily or near-daily basis.[77,78] In contrast, population-based studies and surveys of headache specialty or general medical practices in Europe and Asia report medication overuse in 1% to 30% of patients presenting with CDH.[11,12,79,80] These reports suggest that most patients who experience CDH in the general population worldwide do so independent of medication overuse. Because of contrasting reports, headache specialists have debated whether analgesic overuse is a cause or consequence of CM.[72] Fueling this debate are the observations that many patients continue to experience frequent headache after the withdrawal of overused medications.[21,22,67] The pathogenic basis for migraine transformation is unknown. Perhaps migraine has a continuum of clinical expression that progresses or transforms to a chronic pain disorder as a consequence of neural plasticity, toxicity, or dysregulation. Whether the neuroadaptive changes associated with chronic migraine can reach a state of irreversibility is unknown. Clinical studies that have identified longer lifetime duration of migraine and longer duration of medication overuse are negative predictors for CDH treatment outcomes after the withdrawal of overused medications[20,81,82] lend support to the concern that recovery from the neuroadaptive changes associated with CM and MOH may be incomplete.

PATHOGENESIS OF MIGRAINE, CHRONIC MIGRAINE, AND CHRONIC DAILY HEADACHE

Migraine is a heritable disorder.[83] Genetic studies have suggested a heterogeneous genotype for the most common forms of migraine thereby giving rise to the numerous phenotypic expressions of migraine encountered in clinical practice. The risk of developing CDH and CM also seems to be linked to genetics.[84] The relative risk of developing CDH is 2.1 to 3.9 times greater in first-degree relatives compared to the general population. Although phenotypically dissimilar, some researchers hypothesize that migraine and tension-type headache share a similar pathogenic basis.[85]

Knowledge of migraine pathophysiology has evolved from a belief that migraine is a vascular condition to recognition that migraine is a complex neurovascular disorder. Headache is just one of many neurologic and systemic symptoms associated with migraine. Although one of the most common symptoms of migraine attacks, headache may not occur in all attacks.[15] Although far from fully understood, several lines of evidence suggest that migraine is associated with cortical hyperexcitability, prolonged recovery of cortical neurons after depolarization, secondary changes in brain perfusion, altered trigeminal nociceptor function, trigeminal-mediated neurogenic inflammation in the meninges and around cranial blood vessels, dysmodulation of central pain processing, and sensitization of both peripheral and central pain pathways originating from the head and neck regions.[86-88] Although the presence of scalp sensitivity during a migraine attack has been long observed in clinical practice, the recognition that this clinical feature of migraine represents allodynia[89,90] has opened new opportunities for preclinical investigation, identification of novel treatment targets, and improving clinical management strategies for migraine.

Scientific evidence supports the concept that central sensitization occurs during migraine attacks.[91] Sensitization of central trigeminal sensory pathways during migraine is characterized by spontaneous pain that is independent of peripheral sensory input, allodynia, hyperalgesia, and expansion of nociceptive sensory fields, which emulate the clinical characteristics of neuropathic pain disorders. Prolonged sensitization of peripheral and central trigeminal nociceptive pathways has been proposed as a mechanism for both chronic migraine and chronic tension-type headache.[92,93]

Plasticity of serotonin (5HT) receptors and the 5HT neurotransmitter system in the brain after chronic analgesic exposure has been demonstrated in animal models.[94] This change was associated with a loss of analgesic efficacy and facilitation of pain transmission. A hypothesis that similar effects underlie the development of chronic daily headache after analgesic overuse in humans has been presented. Other research using animal models has identified neurons that facilitate pain transmission, called "on-cells," which display increased firing patterns during opiate withdrawal thereby resulting in hyperalgesia and enhanced nociception.[95]

Repeated episodes of headache may be associated with changes in central nervous system structure or function. Specialized brain imaging techniques have demonstrated abnormal nonheme iron deposition in the region of the periaqueductal gray matter of the rostral brainstem in migraine patients but not in nonmigraine control subjects.[96] The amount of iron deposition had a positive association with the subjects' lifetime duration of migraine. This change was hypothesized to be a consequence of iron-catalyzed free radical cell damage "accentuated by repeated episodes of hyperoxia" during migraine attacks, thereby suggesting that repeated attacks of migraine over time results in structural injury to antinociceptive systems of the brainstem and ultimately impaired pain modulation.

There is further evidence to support the theory that migraine causes structural injury to neurologic systems. Impaired visual function in migraine patients was hypothesized to be the result of changes in the primary visual cortex as a consequence of cerebral ischemia occurring during attacks of migraine with aura.[97] Similarly, dysfunction of visual systems has been linked with visual cortex injury from repeated migraine auras possibly through the effects of NMDA-associated neurotoxicity, repeated transient hypoxia, or cortical ischemia.[98] High migraine frequency, especially in cases of migraine with aura, has been linked to deep white matter lesions in the cerebral hemispheres and subclinical strokes in the cerebellum.[98,99] It is unknown whether the white matter lesions are consequences of ischemic or metabolic (i.e., glutamate or nitric oxide–related) injury. Further evidence suggesting migraine-associated neuroplasticity or neuronal injury includes interictal abnormalities in cognitive function,[100] subclinical cerebellar dysfunction,[101] and abnormalities at the neuromuscular junction[102] in migraine patients.

Several hypotheses may explain the pathophysiologic basis of CM, including possible associations with low central neuronal serotonin, dysregulation of neuronal 5-HT receptors, hyperexcitability of central pain pathways, low central beta-endorphin levels, dysfunction of NMDA receptors,[103] and others.[104,105] The mechanisms of chronic tension-type headache are even more obscure. Tenderness of pericranial muscles, increased pericranial muscle stiffness, and increased surface electromyographic activity have been observed.[106]

EPIDEMIOLOGY AND DEMOGRAPHICS OF CHRONIC DAILY HEADACHE

An epidemiologic study has estimated that the 1-year prevalence of CDH in the United States is 4.1%.[10] Categorized into specific primary headache disorders, the 1-year prevalence was 2.2% for chronic tension-type headache, 1.3% for CM, and 0.6% for other chronic headache types. Women were twice as likely to have CDH. The prevalence of CDH was found to be similar in selected European and Asian populations.[11,80] Approximately 75% of all patients with CM report that their chronic headache condition had transformed from episodic migraine and many cases were associated with medication overuse.[19] Although the true prevalence is not known, MOH appears to be a greater problem in the United States when compared to other populations around the world. It was estimated that 10% of patients evaluated at headache centers in Europe have MOH but up to 80% of patients presenting to U.S. headache clinics have MOH.[107] For the most part, caffeine intake was not systematically assessed in the global population studies; therefore its effect on migraine transformation cannot be determined. Some risk factors for the development of chronic migraine include analgesic and ergot overuse, depression, sleep disturbances, head injury, and life stressors.[108-112] Depression was reported to be present in 80% of patients with CDH presenting to headache specialty practices.[9] Another study found psychiatric comorbidity was reported to affect 90% of patients with primary CDH. In this study, 69% had generalized anxiety and 25% had major depression.[113] It has been observed that depression improves in parallel with improvement of the daily headache pattern and withdrawal of overused medications. Psychiatric comorbidity likely contributes to the intractability of headache and level of headache-related disability. Other factors associated with headache progression or poor treatment responses have been identified, such as headache frequency, body mass index, and highest education level achieved[114] (Table 24-10).

PROGNOSIS FOR CHRONIC DAILY HEADACHE AND MEDICATION OVERUSE HEADACHE

Long-term outcomes have generally been favorable for a majority of CDH patients who successfully complete inpatient, multidisciplinary headache management programs that combine pharmacologic and behavioral interventions.[115-118] In an evaluation of 50 hospitalized patients who became headache-free after treatment with repeated dosing of intravenous dihydroergotamine, 72% demonstrated improvement in headache activity at 3 months and 87% showed improvement after 2 years.[115] A synopsis of 22 reports published between 1975 and 1991 revealed that the success rate for management of MOH after withdrawal of overused medications ranged between 48% and 91%. Almost half of these studies reported success rates of 77% or greater.

Table 24-10. Some Factors Associated with Headache Progression

Risk Factors
Female gender
Caucasian race
Analgesic overuse
Analgesic use with all attacks
Earlier age of headache onset
High frequency of attacks at baseline
Head trauma
Oral contraceptive use
Previous ineffective prophylaxis
Occurrence of vomiting
Attack onset upon awakening
Family history of coronary artery disease
Obesity (body mass index 30 or greater)

Yet the long-term benefits of medication withdrawal for CDH has been variable. Two studies found that 35% to 43% of patients with CDH continued to experience CDH at 1 and 2 years after treatment. Even among those who improved, a return to the "baseline" (i.e., before development of CDH) headache pattern was rare.[119,120] Another study found that 60% of migraine patients receiving treatment in a primary care setting continued to experience disability at 1 year and 20% continued to experience significant pain and disability at 2 years.[29] Patients with CDH generally respond poorly to traditional migraine treatments, develop occupational and social impairment, and experience treatment-related complications or side effects. When psychological disorders and behavioral conditions co-occur with CDH, clinical manifestations of the disorder and treatment strategies become increasingly more complex.[9]

A meta-analysis of 29 studies involving 2612 patients with chronic headache associated with medication overuse revealed that the original primary headache was migraine in 65% and tension-type headache in 27%.[121] The mean lifetime durations of the original primary headache disorder and CDH were 20.4 years and 5.9 years, respectively. The mean duration of frequent drug use was 10.3 years. In the 17 studies that provided outcomes after medication withdrawal, 72.4% of patients reported either no headache or a greater than 50% improvement in the number of headache days experienced within 1 to 6 months after withdrawing the overused medication. In the three studies that provided outcomes for greater than 9 months (9 to 35 months) after medication withdrawal, at least 50% improvement was maintained in 60%, 70%, and 73%.[20,81,82] Another review analyzing published studies reported a 1-year relapse rate of 60% after medication withdrawal.[122] Factors that improved positive treatment outcomes included lifetime headache duration of less than 10 years, medication overuse less than 5 years, migraine as the primary headache disorder, regular use of appropriate prophylactic medications, history of ergotamine overuse, and maintenance of complete abstinence from the overused medication.

GENERAL TREATMENT STRATEGIES FOR HEADACHE, MIGRAINE, AND CHRONIC DAILY HEADACHE

The management of headache disorders is generally more successful when individualized and multidisciplinary treatment strategies are used. Educating patients about pathogenesis and treatment of their headache disorder has great importance for improving treatment compliance. Realistic goals and expectations for treatment outcome should be discussed early in the course of treatment. Realistic expectations include an understanding that treatment will not be a cure but is expected to result in a reduction of headache frequency, duration, and severity. Gathering an inventory of all over-the-counter and prescribed medications previously and currently used by the patient is needed to assess the possibility of medication overuse headache (MOH). Although patients with MOH often find the concepts of headache transformation and MOH difficult to understand, educating them about the consequences of frequent medication use and the reasons for limiting or withdrawing overused medications is essential to improve the likelihood of treatment success. Patients with MOH must be prepared for the high probability that their headaches will worsen before any improvement is achieved. It is also important to recognize that the benefit of medication withdrawal and time required to gain meaningful migraine control can be delayed weeks or months, especially if abortive or analgesic medications had been overused for an extended period of time.[123] A discussion of "bridge treatment," a treatment strategy used to reduce the inevitable increase in headache intensity during withdrawal, will help reassure the patient that a pain management plan is available and lessen the anxiety associated with their beliefs and misconceptions of medication withdrawal. Identification and treatment of anxiety and depression are essential because these conditions may contribute to poor coping skills, catastrophizing behaviors, and continued disability. Stress reduction, relaxation exercises, and biofeedback are excellent adjuncts to pharmacologic treatments and are highly recommended.[124,125] Psychological or psychiatric treatment interventions are sometimes needed. Close follow-up and frequent emotional support are necessary for most patients.

NONPHARMACOLOGIC MANAGEMENT OF HEADACHE

Nonpharmacologic treatment strategies are essential components of a successful headache management program (Table 24–11). Presumably as a consequence

Table 24–11. Nonpharmacologic Options for Migraine Treatment and Prevention

1. Lifestyle adjustments and trigger avoidance
   a. Maintain a regular meal schedule: avoid missing meals and fasting
   b. Maintain a regular sleep and wake schedule
      (1) Reduce fatigue
      (2) Avoid oversleeping
      (3) Remain as consistent as possible
         (a) Weekends
         (b) Holidays
         (c) Vacations
   c. Dietary restrictions
      (1) Reduce caffeine consumption
      (2) Avoid excessive consumption of sugar or carbohydrates
      (3) Avoid or limit alcohol consumption
   d. Avoid tobacco products
   e. Maintain a regular exercise schedule: aerobic exercise and cardiovascular conditioning
2. Coping and relaxation strategies
   a. Stress management
   b. Relaxation training
   c. Biofeedback training

of neuronal hypersensitivity and hyperreactivity, patients with migraine and CDH do not adapt well to changes or inconsistencies in their environment or physiology. Genuine attempts to identify, reduce, and withdraw headache triggers are recommended. Improvement of sleep patterns, developing daily routines, getting regular exercise, and eating a well-balanced, healthy diet are essential for successful treatment outcomes. Although food triggers may be important for some migraine patients, they are difficult to identify in most. Typical food triggers include chocolate, aged cheeses (cheddar, brie, gruyere), beer, wine (especially red and rosé), sherry, champagne, buttermilk, processed meats (bacon, hot dogs, cold cuts, canned ham), sour cream, nuts, seeds, and peanut butter. Headache patients who have identified an association between their headache attacks and reactive hypoglycemia might do better on a diet that reduces carbohydrate load or follows a schedule of several small meals throughout the day. Missed meals and hunger are notorious headache triggers. Excessive caffeine use (more than 500 mg/day) can trigger or worsen headaches while smaller doses may be helpful as an adjunct to acute treatment. One or two small servings of caffeinated drinks each day might be permissible for some patients while others cannot tolerate even small caffeine doses.

Regular participation in physical therapy can reduce disability and behaviors related to disability through physical and aerobic reconditioning, exercise, muscle stretching, and improvement of posture.[125] To be effective, exercise must be practiced regularly because infrequent physical exertion by a deconditioned headache patient is more likely to trigger acute headache than help. Occupational therapy can provide helpful training in the use of thermal modalities or other nonpharmacologic pain management techniques, proper pacing of daily activities, and vocational counseling.

The contribution of cognitive, emotional, and behavioral factors to headache-related disability is often underestimated.[126] Functional imaging studies of the brain show that anticipation of pain produces cerebral activation patterns similar to those seen during actual painful experiences.[127] These results suggest that maladaptive neuronal consequences associated with the expectation of pain or constant attention to pain may contribute to worsening of the pain condition. Psychological and behavioral treatments that address emotional or psychological aspects of headache are therefore valuable components of a pain management program. Cognitive-behavioral strategies and behavior modification techniques are used to reduce illness behavior and increase self-efficacy by providing an "internal locus of control" rather than complete reliance on medication. Behavioral techniques are also important for their medication-sparing or medication-augmenting effects. Many of these treatments, such as biofeedback, have demonstrated efficacy in reducing the frequency and severity of migraine attacks, as well as associated disability.[128]

PHARMACOLOGIC MANAGEMENT OF HEADACHE

The pharmacologic management of migraine and other headaches involves acute treatment of episodic headache events and preventive treatment to reduce headache frequency (Tables 24–12 and 24–13). Pharmacologic treatments for the acute and preventive management of cluster headache are somewhat different than those used for migraine (Tables 24–14 and 24–15). For management of CDH, strong emphasis is placed on preventive management and limiting the use of acute or abortive medications. Rational combinations of multiple, synergistic medications for headache prevention is often needed in cases of very frequent or chronic headache.

In most cases of MOH, the overused medication must be tapered or withdrawn before substantial headache control can be achieved. Medication-induced toxicity may be encountered when a patient

Table 24–12. Selected Headache and Migraine Acute Pain Medications

DRUG CLASS	COMMENTS/PROPOSED MOA*	DOSAGE RANGE†
Simple analgesics		
Acetaminophen	Inhibition of prostaglandin synthesis; enhanced serotonin release	650-3000 mg/day
Nonsteroidal anti-inflammatory drugs (NSAIDs)		
Aspirin	Inhibition of prostaglandin synthesis; enhanced serotonin release	650-3000 mg/day
Naproxen		500-1500 mg/day
Ibuprofen		600-2400 mg/day
Ketoprofen		75-225 mg/day
Flurbiprofen		100-300 mg/day
Ketorolac		10-30 mg mg/day (PO) or
Others		30-60 mg/day (IM)
Analgesic Combinations		
Aspirin, acetaminophen, and caffeine	**Analgesics**: Inhibition of prostaglandin synthesis and enhanced serotonin release	Various dosage combinations for oral administration
Butalbital, acetaminophen or aspirin, and caffeine	**Butalbital**: Inhibition of pain transmission in central pain pathways; sedation	
Isometheptene, acetaminophen, and dichloralphenazone	**Caffeine**: adenosine receptor agonist; inhibition of pain transmission in the CNS; enhances GI absorption of simple analgesics.	
Opioid analgesics		
Codeine	Agonists at endorphin receptors: inhibit release of various chemical mediators of pain in the peripheral and central nervous systems	Various dosages and routes of administration (oral, rectal suppository, injectable, transdermal)
Hydrocodone		
Oxycodone		
Morphine		
Meperidine		
Others		
Ergot derivatives		
Ergotamine tartrate	Agonists at serotonin, adrenergic, and dopamine receptors; multiple other actions; inhibits pain transmission and blocks release of inflammatory neuropeptides	Oral 1-2 mg (6 mg daily maximum)
Dihydroergotamine		Rectal suppository 1-2 mg (4 mg daily maximum)
		Injectable 0.5-1 mg (SC, IM, IV)
		Nasal spray 2 mg/day
5-HT$_{1B/D}$ agonists (Triptans)		Injectable
Sumatriptan	Agonists at serotonin receptors; inhibits pain transmission and blocks release of inflammatory neuropeptides	— Suma 6 mg
Zolmitriptan		Nasal spray
Rizatriptan		— Suma 5, 20 mg
Naratriptan		— Zolmi 5 mg
Almotriptan		Orally dissolvable tablet
Frovatriptan		— Zolmi 2.5, 5 mg
Eletriptan		— Riza 5, 10 mg
		Oral tablet
		— Suma 25, 50, 100 mg
		— Zolmi 2.5, 5 mg
		— Riza 5, 10 mg
		— Nara 1, 2.5 mg
		— Almo 6.25, 12.5 mg
		— Frova 2.5 mg
		— Ele 20, 40 mg

*The precise MOA for most acute headache and migraine drugs is not known.
†Refer to the package insert for specific dosing instructions, interactions and adverse effects.
CNS, central nervous system; 5-HT, serotonin; GI, gastrointestinal; MOA, mechanism of action.

Table 24–13. Selected Migraine Preventive Medications

DRUG CLASS	COMMENTS/PROPOSED MOA*	DOSAGE RANGE (MG/DAY)[†]
β-Adrenergic blockers		
Atenolol	β-Adrenergic and 5-HT$_{2B/2C}$ receptor antagonist; inhibits	50-200
Metoprolol	sensitization or facilitation of pain transmission	50-200
Nadolol		20-240
Propranolol[‡]		60-320
Timolol[‡]		20-30
TCAs		
Amitriptyline	a) Down-regulation of 5-HT$_2$ receptors	25-150
Desipramine	b) Inhibition of pain transmission in central	25-150
Doxepin	nociceptive pathways by enhancing effect of	25-200
Nortriptyline	serotonin and norepinephrine in the CNS	25-150
Protriptyline	c) Modulate neuronal sensitivity to GABA, substance P,	10-40
	and endogenous opioids	
Other antidepressants		
Venlafaxine (SNRI)	Enhances neuronal concentrations of monoaminergic	75-225
Duloxetine (SNRI)	neurotransmitters	40-60
Fluoxetine (SSRI)		20-60
Antiepileptic drugs		
Divalproex sodium[‡]	Generally ↑ GABA activity in brain and stabilize nerve	500-1500
Topiramate[‡]	membrane activation thresholds	50-200
Zonisamide		300-600
Gabapentin		1200-3600
Others		
CCBs		
Diltiazem HCl	a) Prevent vasoconstriction	240-360
Verapamil	b) Increase cerebral blood flow	90-360
	c) Interfere with calcium-dependent enzyme activation	
	that leads to sensitization of central pain pathways	
Serotonin antagonists		
Ergot derivatives		
Methylergonovine	5-HT$_{2B/2C}$ receptor antagonists	0.6-2.0
Methysergide[‡§]	Methysergide—weak 5-HT$_{1B/D}$ receptor agonist	4-10
Non-ergot drugs		
Cyproheptadine	Cyproheptadine—histamine receptor antagonist	4-12
MAOIs		
Phenelzine	Inhibition of monoamine oxidase, increasing available	30-90
Tranylcypromine	5-HT and NE	30-60
Other Treatments		
Botulinum toxin A	Contraindicated in patients with neuromuscular	25-200 units injected/treatment
	disease.	
Riboflavin (vitamin B$_2$)	Efficacy after 3-4 months of treatment.	400
Magnesium	Efficacy after 3-4 months of treatment.	400-600
Coenzyme Q10	Efficacy after 3-4 months of treatment.	150-300

CCB, calcium channel blocker; CNS, central nervous system; 5-HT, serotonin; MAOI, monoamine oxidase inhibitor; MOA, mechanism of action; NE, norepinephrine; SNRI, serotonin norepinephrine reuptake inhibitor; SSRI, selective serotonin reuptake inhibitor; TCA, tricyclic antidepressant;
*The MOA for most of the prophylactic drugs is not known. Their prophylactic effects were discovered by chance when they were used for other purposes. However, based on the presumed pathophysiology of migraine, a rationale for their use in migraine prophylaxis has been hypothesized.
[†]Refer to the package insert for specific dosing instructions, interactions, and adverse effects.
[‡]FDA approved for migraine prophylaxis in adults.
[§]No longer commercially available in the United States.

is overusing acute medications or aggressive multiple drug treatment protocols are being prescribed. Ergotism, serotonin syndrome, anticholinergic toxicity, and neuroleptic malignant syndrome are potentially dangerous consequences of medication toxicity that require prompt identification and initiation of rescue and palliative treatments (Table 24–16). In addition, patients who are overusing abortive medications will often require treatment for one or more abstinence syndromes (Table 24–17). Treatments for abstinence can be initiated in an outpatient setting but some cases having greater medical acuity or complexity may require inpatient management for close monitoring and emotional support.

Medication withdrawal or detoxification may be attempted as an outpatient with patients who are motivated, reliable, and compliant. Most patients will require some type of palliative treatment to reduce the peak intensity of withdrawal pain. Some overused medications such as simple analgesics, caffeine, ergotamines, and triptans can usually be withdrawn without taper. Patients taking large daily dosages of opioid analgesics, butalbital compounds, or benzodiazepines will usually require a slow scheduled taper of the overused medication or replacement with another medication that will protect against potentially serious consequences of abstinence such as seizure, delirium, or psychiatric mani-

Table 24–14. Selected Cluster Acute Pain Medications

DRUG CLASS	COMMENTS/PROPOSED MOA*	DOSAGE†
Oxygen		
100% O$_2$ via face mask	Unknown	7-10 liters/minute for 15-20 minutes
5-HT$_{1B/D}$ agonists (Triptans)		
Sumatriptan	Agonists at serotonin receptors; inhibits pain	Injectable
Zolmitriptan	transmission and blocks release of	— Suma 6 mg‡
	inflammatory neuropeptides	Nasal spray
		— Suma 5, 20 mg
		— Zolmi 5 mg
Ergot derivatives		
Ergotamine tartrate	Agonists at serotonin, adrenergic, and dopamine	Rectal suppository 1-2 mg (4 mg daily
	receptors; multiple other actions; inhibits pain	maximum)
Dihydroergotamine	transmission and blocks release of	Injectable 0.5-1 mg (SC, IM, IV)
	inflammatory neuropeptides	Nasal spray 2 mg/day
Opioid analgesics		
Morphine	Agonists at endorphin receptors	Various dosages by rectal suppository
Dihydromorphone		Nasal Spray
Butorphanol		

*The MOA for these drugs in cluster is not known.
†Refer to the package insert for specific dosing instructions, interactions, and adverse effects.
‡FDA approved for acute treatment of cluster headaches in adults.

Table 24–15. Selected Cluster Preventive Medications

DRUG CLASS	COMMENTS/PROPOSED MOA*	DOSAGE RANGE (mg/day)†
CCB	a) Prevent vasoconstriction	
Verapamil	b) Increase cerebral blood flow	120-480
	c) Interfere with calcium-dependent enzyme activation that leads to sensitization of central pain pathways	
Antiepileptic drugs		
Divalproex sodium	Generally ↑ GABA activity in brain and	500-1500
Topiramate	stabilize nerve membrane activation	50-200
Zonisamide	thresholds	300-600
Serotonin antagonists		
Ergot derivatives		
Methylergonovine	5-HT$_{2B/2C}$ receptor antagonists	0.6-2.0
Methysergide‡	Methysergide—weak 5-HT$_{1B/D}$ receptor	4-10
Non-ergot drugs	agonist	
Cyproheptadine	Cyproheptadine—histamine receptor antagonist	4-12
Others		
Lithium carbonate	Unknown	450-900
Melatonin	Unknown	10 mg (at bedtime)
Bridge treatments§	Administered immediately after initiation of a cluster cycle to provide quick relief while titrating preventive medications	
Prednisone	Unknown	60 (after 3 days start tapering over 2 weeks)

CCB, calcium channel blocker; MOA, mechanism of action; 5-HT, serotonin.
*The MOA for prophylactic drugs used for cluster is not known. Their prophylactic effects were discovered by chance when they were used for other purposes.
†Refer to the package insert for specific dosing instructions, interactions, and adverse effects.
‡No longer commercially available in the United States.
§None of the listed medications are FDA approved for this use.

festations. Butalbital compounds have historically been one of the most commonly overused drugs in cases of MOH at specialty headache centers in the United States.[129] Because of its long serum half-life, phenobarbital loading and tapered withdrawal has been used for the management of butalbital withdrawal in cases of overuse.[130] A conversion ratio of 30 mg phenobarbital for each 100 mg of butalbital has been used in clinical practice.[131] Many of the combination analgesics with butalbital contain caffeine, which may also require tapering in order to ease the substantial effects of caffeine withdrawal, including headache exacerbation and irritability. Instructing the patient to temporarily increase dietary sources of caffeine and tapering back over time is effective in most cases. If the overused agents are short-acting opioid analgesics, replacement and tapering with equianalgesic dosages of long acting

Table 24–16. Medication Toxicity Syndromes

Ergotism (Ergotamine Toxicity)
1. Clinical features of ergotism
   a. Acute ergot toxicity—vomiting, diarrhea, thirst, burning paresthesias, rapid and weak pulse, mental confusion, hallucinations, seizures, unconsciousness
   b. Chronic ergot toxicity—gangrene, myalgias, nausea, vomiting, diarrhea, dizziness, confusion, hallucinations, depression, paranoid ideation, hemiplegia
2. Treatment is generally supportive after medication is withdrawn
Serotonin Syndrome
1. Clinical features of the serotonin syndrome
   a. Hyperthermia, rigidity, restlessness, hyperreflexia, tremor, myoclonus, dramatic alteration in mental status, convulsions, and extreme fluctuations in vital signs
   b. This condition can (rarely) be fatal
2. Treatment is generally supportive after medications are withdrawn; cyproheptadine, a serotonin antagonist may be helpful in management of this syndrome; antiepileptic medications and benzodiazepines may also be helpful.
Tricyclic Antidepressant Toxicity
1. Clinical features of tricyclic antidepressant toxicity
   a. Cardiovascular—dysrhythmia, conduction block, asystole, hypotension, hypertension
   b. Central nervous system—agitation, delirium, hallucinations, dystonia, myoclonus, seizures
   c. Anticholinergic—anhydrosis, flushed skin, hyperthermia, urinary bladder retention, mydriasis, hypomotility of the gut
   d. This condition can be fatal if untreated
2. Treatment is generally supportive including cardiovascular and respiratory resuscitation, alkalinization of the blood, acetylcholinesterase inhibitors, parasympathomimetic drugs, and treatment of seizures with benzodiazepines.
Neuroleptic Malignant Syndrome (NMS)
1. Clinical features of NMS
   a. Hyperthermia/fever, muscle rigidity, diaphoresis, dysphagia, tremor, incontinence, tachycardia, altered blood pressure control, increased serum CPK, and altered states of consciousness
   b. This condition can rarely be fatal due to respiratory and renal failure.
2. Treatment is generally supportive including cardiovascular and respiratory resuscitation, cooling blankets, hydration, and sedation with benzodiazepines. Medications potentially effective for reducing symptoms of NMS include dantrolene, bromocriptine, and amantadine.

Table 24–17. Treatment of Medication Withdrawal Syndromes

Opiate/Narcotic Withdrawal
1. Clonidine (Catapres) PO, TD
2. Tizanidine (Zanaflex) PO
3. Opiate taper
   a. Long-acting opiates, PO
      (1) MSContin (morphine sulfate), OxyContin (oxycodone), or methadone
Barbiturate Withdrawal
1. Phenobarbital substitution and protracted taper
2. Benzodiazepine substitution and protracted taper
3. Protracted taper of the offending barbiturate
4. Carbamazepine substitution and taper
Benzodiazepine Withdrawal
1. Protracted benzodiazepine taper using the offending benzodiazepine or a substituted medication having longer serum half-lives such as diazepam, lorazepam, or clonazepam
2. Carbamazepine, divalproex sodium, or clonidine may be helpful as adjunct treatments
Ergotamine Tartrate Withdrawal
1. Dihydroergotamine (DHE) IV protocol
2. No triptans for at least 24 hours after the last ergotamine dose
Triptan Withdrawal
1. No DHE or ergotamines for at least 24 hours after last triptan dose
Caffeine Withdrawal
1. Sudden caffeine withdrawal can cause headache (52%), fatigue, and depression
2. Treat by tapering caffeine consumption

IV, intravenous; PO, oral tablet; TD, transdermal patch.

opioids such as methadone or sustained-release morphine can reduce the potential for intense rebound headache pain and opioid withdrawal symptoms. Clonidine delivered by transdermal patch or tablet can used for further control of the clinical manifestations of opioid withdrawal and abstinence.

Temporary palliation of pain during the withdrawal of overused medications in cases of MOH, may be accomplished with several different analgesic strategies that are commonly called "bridge treatments." These treatment strategies generally provide marginal pain relief but the relief is usually substantial enough to allow patient compliance with the medication withdrawal process. Some of the outpatient bridge treatment strategies include a short course of steroids,[132] a scheduled course of a long-acting nonsteroidal anti-inflammatory analgesic such as naproxen or ketoprofen, a 3-day course of self-administered subcutaneous or intramuscular dihydroergotamine, a 3-day course of intranasal dihydroergotamine, or a brief course of a scheduled triptan.[133] None of these treatments have been proven effective in rigorously conducted scientific trials nor has any one approach demonstrated superiority. Even so, general consensus appears to favor the use of one or more bridge treatment strategies in the management of drug withdrawal for cases of MOH.

Migraine prevention may work best if initiated before the development of daily headache patterns.[134] General guidelines for determining the need for migraine preventive treatment include experiencing more than two migraine attacks per month, headache-related disability occurring three or more days per month, symptomatic medications are ineffective or contraindicated, abortive medications or analgesics are likely to be used more than two days per week, or the occurrence of profound migraine-associated disability, prolonged migraine auras, or migraine-associated stroke. Because of the daily or very frequent occurrence of headache and consequent disability, most patients with CDH will require prophylaxis unless contraindicated. In cases of MOH, prophylaxis can be initiated simultaneously with the discontinuation or tapering of the overused medication. Sequential trials of prophylactic medications, singly or in combination, are sometimes required. Repeat trials of medications that had previously failed while the patient was overusing abortive medications are reasonable. Selection of the best prophylactic medication for an individual patient can be based on comorbid or coexisting medical and psychiatric conditions (see Table 24–7), but optimal treatment for all coexisting conditions is imperative. Preventive treatment may fail when used in an inadequate dosage or for an inadequate duration. Each new preventive medication or dosage change may require 8 weeks or more before optimum efficacy is attained. Medication noncompliance is another common cause of treatment failure. To improve compliance, patients should be given a good understanding of their medications, dosing schedules, treatment goals, and realistic expectations for treatment outcomes. Written instructions or preprinted information sheets can be helpful to address these issues. Many patients with migraine and CDH are overly sensitive to medication side effects, especially those related to the central nervous system; therefore treatment is usually initiated with a low dose followed by a slow incremental titration of the medication dosage to achieve a predetermined target dosage, desirable therapeutic effect, or, intolerable side effects. Other causes for failure of preventive treatment include ongoing analgesic, ergotamine, or triptan overuse; incorrect headache diagnosis; development of a new headache disorder, concurrent medical condition that has headache as a clinical feature; or significant psychiatric comorbidity. Asking the patient to maintain a headache diary can help determine treatment efficacy and guide adjustments of treatment.

Combination Drug Therapy

Clinical experience suggests that the rational use of more than one prophylactic medication is more effective than monotherapy in many cases of frequent migraine and CDH (Table 24–18). Most clinical drug trials are aimed at establishing the safety and efficacy of a single drug compared with placebo in the preventive management of migraine or CDH, rather than establishing the efficacy of combination therapy. However, patients who do not respond to an effectively dosed headache preventive drug might obtain greater benefit from combining preventive medications. The rationale for this treatment strategy is based on the assumption that medications with different but complementary pharmacologic mecha-

Table 24–18. Preventive Medication Combinations (Rational Multiple Drug Therapy) for Migraine and Chronic Daily Headache

1. Beta-blocker and a tricyclic or selective serotonin reuptake inhibitor
   a. Fluoxetine may increase cardiovascular activities of propranolol and metoprolol; therefore use together with caution
2. Calcium channel blocker and a tricyclic or selective serotonin reuptake inhibitor antidepressant
3. Tricyclic antidepressant and a selective serotonin reuptake inhibitor
   a. Watch blood levels of the tricyclic antidepressant (TCA) especially when combined with fluoxetine
   b. Be aware of the serotonin syndrome (see Table 24–16)
4. Divalproex sodium or other antiepileptic and a tricyclic antidepressant
   a. Watch blood levels of the TCA when combined with divalproex sodium
5. Ergot derivative and β-blocker, calcium channel blocker, or tricyclic antidepressant
6. Monoamine oxidase inhibitor and a tricyclic antidepressant
   a. TCAs that may be used include nortriptyline, amitriptyline, or doxepin
   b. Monoamine oxidase inhibitor (MAOI) and TCA are started at the same time or MAOI is added to established TCA treatment
   c. Do not add TCA to established MAOI treatment

nisms of action will have additive or synergistic effects. Clinical experience suggests that rational multiple drug treatment improves efficacy and reduces the development of tolerance and treatment failure over time.[135] Despite these observations, systematic trials are still needed to clearly assess the effects, potential advantages, and disadvantages of combination drug therapy.

Scheduled Opioid Treatment

Although opioid analgesics have demonstrated efficacy in the acute treatment of episodic migraine in some reports,[136] other medications such as dihydroergotamine and ketorolac have been at least equally effective but with fewer side effects.[137,138] In other studies, morphine has generally demonstrated low efficacy in the acute treatment of migraine.[139,140] Furthermore, scientific study has linked opioid tolerance and elevated pain sensitivity, a condition commonly called "opioid-induced hyperalgesia";[141] this phenomenon may be similar, if not identical, to the consequences of frequent medication use in cases of MOH or "analgesic rebound" in the migraine population.

There is little evidence in the medical literature that will help determine the efficacy of opioid analgesics for the preventive management of CDH. A 5-year study at a large headache specialty clinic enrolled 385 patients who received scheduled opioid analgesics for the management of chronic intractable headache.[142] Approximately half of the patients were in the study between 3 and 5 years when the report was written. Analyses of this group demonstrated that

26% reported significant improvement, which was defined as a subjective improvement in headache intensity of at least 50%. Despite reporting improvement in pain intensity, many of these patients did not return to work nor did they demonstrate improvement in various parameters of disability. The majority of patients who reported significant pain relief were not able or were not willing to give up other analgesic medications so as to rely primarily on opioid analgesics alone. Approximately 50% of all patients in the study for longer than 3 years voluntarily discontinued use of the opioid analgesics because of side effects or failure to experience substantial pain relief.

Another study of scheduled opioid analgesics for the management of CDH conducted at a university-based headache clinic reported similar results.[143] Over 7 years, 70 patients with chronic daily or near daily headaches were treated with scheduled, long-acting opioid analgesics. A positive treatment response, defined as 50% or better reduction in headache days per month, was reported by 34% of patients but only 26% had a sustained response over a mean of 2 years. Approximately 10% of patients indicated that they were "much better" but their headache diaries did not demonstrate an objective measure of improvement. Of the treatment nonresponders, roughly 22% could not tolerate opioid-induced side effects. Opioid tolerance was observed in four treatment responders. In all patients, attempts were made to taper the opioid analgesics but headache characteristics or attack patterns worsened almost immediately in every case.

Because the frequent or chronic use of opioid analgesics by migraine patients is recognized to incite the transformation of episodic migraine to chronic migraine, a phenomenon that appears similar to opioid-induced hyperalgesia affecting other chronic noncancer pain syndromes,[144] the use of opioid analgesics for the acute management of frequent migraine or preventive management of chronic migraine is not generally recommended. Referral to a headache specialty program is recommended if the use of frequent or scheduled opioid analgesics is being considered.

Outpatient Infusion Therapy

Short courses of parenteral medications may be required for patients experiencing status migrainosus (refractory acute migraine) or patients who are unable to tolerate the exacerbation of pain intensity associated with the withdrawal of overused medications (Table 24–19). This treatment strategy may be initiated under close medical supervision for patients who are unable or unwilling to receive inpatient hospital treatment. Reliable and cooperative patients who are medically stable and have a social support system are good candidates.

Hospitalization

Patients with CDH will sometimes require hospitalization for comfort, close observation, and protection

Table 24–19. Parenteral Treatment Protocols for the Management of Chronic Daily Headache*

1. Dihydroergotamine (DHE) IV, IM; 0.5-1 mg every 8 hours for 9 doses
   a. Premedicate with an antiemetic especially when DHE is given IV
2. Phenothiazines (Compazine, Thorazine) IV, IM; i.e., chlorpromazine 10-20 mg IV or prochlorperazine 5-10 mg IV every 8 hours for 6 to 9 doses
   a. Analgesic, antiemetic, and sedative
   b. Premedicate with diphenhydramine 25-50 mg IV to reduce likelihood of akathisias or dystonic reactions
3. Droperidol (Inapsine) IV, IM; 0.625-2.5 mg IV every 8 hours for 6 to 9 doses
   a. Analgesic, antiemetic, and sedative
   b. Parenteral diphenhydramine as needed for akathisias and dystonic reactions
   c. Rule out QT prolongation on EKG prior to use
4. Ketorolac (Toradol) IV, IM; 30 mg IV every 8 hours for 3 days
   a. Dosage adjustment required for patient with renal failure or renal disease
5. Magnesium sulfate IV; 1000 mg IV two times a day (4 hours apart) for 2 to 3 days
6. Diphenhydramine (Benadryl) IV; 50-100 mg IV every 8 hours for 3 days
7. Valproate sodium (Depacon) IV; 500-1000 mg IV every 12 hours for 2 to 3 days
   a. Monitor serum valproic acid levels
8. Corticosteroids IV; various formulations
9. Intravenous fluid hydration and replenishment

Note: Avoid use of opioid analgesics because they may perpetuate head pain through mechanisms associated with opioid-induced hyperalgesia (rebound headache syndrome).
*Refer to the package insert for specific dosing instructions, interactions and adverse effects.

Table 24–20. Guidance for Hospital Admission of Patients with Chronic Daily Headache

1. Narcotic addiction/dependency
2. Butalbital/barbiturate addiction/dependency
3. Benzodiazepine addiction/dependency
4. Ergotamine tartrate dependency
5. Inability or unwillingness of the patient to discontinue analgesic medications due to rebound pain, dependency, addiction or withdrawal symptoms
6. Intractable headache not responding to appropriate, aggressive outpatient or emergency department interventions
7. Poor psychosocial situations or lack of emotional support structure at home.
8. Coexisting medical condition(s) would make outpatient medication withdrawal risky; unstable vitals
9. Patient has persistent nausea, vomiting, and diarrhea, which have caused dehydration, electrolyte imbalance, and prostration requiring IV fluids and intensive monitoring of vital signs.
10. Severe coexisting psychiatric disease

from toxic side effects of medication, consequences of medication withdrawal, and suicidal ideation. Hospitalization guidelines will be different for individual headache centers, geographic regions, and insurance providers (Table 24–20). Many hospitalized patients have failed outpatient attempts to withdraw overused medications. Most patients require intense monitoring of their cardiovascular or neurologic status. In addition, many patients are safer under close observation and supportive care of trained medical personnel especially when faced with disabling pain, delirium, suicidal ideation, risk of seizures, dehydration, or other conditions of medical instability associated with medication toxicity or withdrawal. A patient's psychological status and toleration for the intense symptoms associated with medication withdrawal need individual consideration when evaluating the need for hospitalization. Hospitalization allows for intensive acute pain management, concerted patient education, supervised practice of coping strategies, and creation of a plan for management of future headache episodes. Owing to the availability of close medical supervision and emergency resuscitation equipment or teams, hospitalization also allows for greater treatment efficiency and safety when making rapid medication transitions or titration. Medication adjustments can be made on a day-to-day or sometimes hour-to-hour basis depending on the patient's response to treatment and tolerance for side effects.

The goals of hospitalization can vary depending upon the purpose of the admission or the manner in which the headache management program is designed. A short (1 to 3 day) length of stay might be primarily used to "break" a headache pattern by delivering one or more parenteral treatment protocols and to initiate withdrawal of overused medication when required (see Table 24–19). The most widely recognized parenteral treatment protocol is intravenous dihydroergotamine (DHE) and metoclopramide administered every 8 hours for nine doses.[145] Other parenteral treatment protocols include chlorpromazine or prochlorperazine, droperidol, ketorolac, magnesium, valproic acid, or diphenhydramine administered alone or in various combinations. Treatment protocols designed to attenuate the clinical consequences of the abstinence syndromes associated with withdrawal of medications such as opioid analgesics, barbiturates, and benzodiazepines are often required (see Table 24–17). A longer length of stay (1 to 4 weeks) may be needed for patients who have experienced significant disability, medication toxicity, drug dependency, and psychiatric morbidity. This type of program takes an integrated, multidisciplinary approach that often follows a rehabilitation model of care. Components of the rehabilitation approach often include the services of psychology, physical therapy, occupational therapy, skilled nursing staff, pharmacy staff, and social work. Other services that may be used based upon each patient's need include psychiatry, chemical dependency, dietary, clergy, and vocational rehabilitation specialists. Employing an integrated, multidisciplinary model of pain management and rehabilitation has demonstrated greater therapeutic gain in outcome studies measured at the time of or subsequent to hospital discharge.[146-148]

CONCLUSION

Episodic migraine, chronic migraine, and other forms of chronic daily headache are common neurologic disorders that can be associated with vast personal and socioeconomic burdens. There is evidence to suggest that the incidence of migraine and possibly other primary headache disorders are determined by a combination of genetic, physiological, and environmental influences. High headache attack frequency and frequent use of analgesic medications are two modifiable risk factors that have been associated with the transformation of episodic to chronic migraine. The best way to manage chronic daily headache especially in the case of migraine is to prevent its occurrence a priori through timely establishment of a headache diagnosis, early use of prophylaxis (nonpharmacologic and pharmacologic), and aggressive attack management.

For patients who have MOH, successful management is best achieved after all overused acute medications are withdrawn. Developing a comprehensive headache management strategy before initiating a medication withdrawal schedule will ease patient anxiety and potentially enhance compliance. One or more "bridge treatments" are available to palliate the acute exacerbation of head pain intensity that frequently occurs as overused medications are withdrawn. Hospitalization for intensive pain management, close observation, and patient safety is required in some cases. Scientific evidence is needed to determine the relative efficacy and safety of the various parenteral treatment protocols used for bridge treatment. The utility, safety, and value of rational drug combinations for headache prophylaxis also need validation. Until clinical trials establish uniform, evidence-based, treatment guidelines, expert consensus and current standards of practice support the use of these yet unproven treatments for the management of chronic headache.

Preclinical, clinical, and longitudinal, epidemiologic studies are crucial to address the current hypothesis that neuroplasticity and neuronal injury might underlie the transformation of episodic to chronic headache and whether these functional or structural neuronal consequences are reversible once established. Improved understanding of these processes and of pain mechanisms in general will help to establish the importance of appropriate and aggressive headache treatment as well as the potential role for neuroprotection and disease modification in the lifelong management of migraine and other headache disorders.

References

1. Rasmussen BK: Epidemiology of headache. Cephalalgia 2001;21(7):774-777.
2. Rasmussen BK, Jensen R, Schroll M, et al: Epidemiology of headache in a general population—a prevalence study. J Clin Epidemiol 1991;44:1147-1157.

3. Hu XH, Markson Le, Lipton RB et al: Burden of migraine in the United States: Disability and economic costs. Arch Intern Med 1999;159:813-818.
4. Menken M, Munsat TL, Toole JF: The global burden of disease study. Arch Neurol 2000;57:418-420.
5. Lipton RB, Stewart WF, Diamond S, et al: Prevalence and burden of migraine in the United States: Data from the American Migraine Study II. Headache 2001;41(7):646-657.
6. Osterhaus JT, Gutterman DL, Plachetka JR: Healthcare resource and lost labor costs of migraine headache in the US. Pharmacoeconomics 1992;2:67-76.
7. Edmeads J, Mackell JA: The economic impact of migraine: An analysis of direct and indirect costs. Headache 2002;42(6):501-509.
8. Gerth WC, Carides GW, Dasbach EJ, et al: The multinational impact of migraine symptoms on healthcare utilization and work loss. Pharmacoeconomics 2001;19(2):197-206.
9. Scher AI, Lipton RB: The frequent headache epidemiology (FrHE) study. Pain 2003;16:81-89.
10. Scher AI, Stewart WF, Liberman J, et al: Prevalence of frequent headache in a population sample. Headache 1998;38:497-506.
11. Castillo J, Munoz P, Guitera V, et al: Epidemiology of chronic daily headache in the general population. Headache 1999;39:190-196.
12. Ravishankar K: Headache pattern in India-a headache clinic analysis of 1000 patients. Cephalalgia 1997;17:316-317.
13. Dowson A: Landmark study. Cephalalgia 2002;22:590.
14. Headache Classification of the International Headache Society: Classification and diagnostic criteria for headache disorders, cranial neuralgias and facial pain. Cephalalgia 1988;8(Suppl 7):1-96.
15. Headache Classification of the International Headache Society: The International Classification of Headache Disorders, 2nd edition. Cephalalgia 2004;24(Suppl 1):1-160.
16. Lipton RB, Lowenkopf T, Bajwa, ZH, et al: Cardiac cephalgia: A treatable form of exertional headache. Neurology 1997;49(3):813-816.
17. Kaniecki RG: Migraine and tension-type headache: An assessment of challenges in diagnosis. Neurology 2002;58:S15.
18. Bigal ME, Sheftell FD, Rapoport AM, et al: Chronic daily headache: Identification of factors associated with induction and transformation. Headache 2002;42:575-581.
19. Rapoport AM, Stang P, Gutterman DL, et al: Analgesic rebound headache in clinical practice: Data from a physician survey. Headache 1996;36:14-19.
20. Schneider P, Aull S, Baumgartner C, et al: Long-term outcome of patients with headache and drug abuse after inpatient withdrawal: Five-year follow-up. Cephalalgia 1996;16:481-485.
21. Fritsche G, Eberl A, Katasarava Z, et al: Drug-induced headache: Long-term follow-up of withdrawal therapy and persistence of drug misuse. Eur Neurol 2001;45:229-235.
22. Pini LA, Cicero AF, Sandrini M: Long-term follow-up of patients treated for chronic headache with analgesic overuse. Cephalalgia 2001;21:878-883.
23. Frishberg B, Rosenberg JH, Matchar DB, et al: Evidence-based guidelines in the primary care setting: Neuroimaging in patients with nonacute headache. Available at www.aan.com/go/practice/guidelines.
24. American Academy of Neurology Practice Parameter: The electroencephalogram in the evaluation of headache. Neurology 1995;45:1411-1413.
25. Schwartz BS, Stewart WF, Simon D, et al: Epidemiology of tension-type headache. JAMA 1998;279:381-383.
26. Diener HC, Dahlof CGH: Headache associated with chronic use of substances. In Olesen J, Tfelt-Hansen P, Welsh KMA (eds): The Headaches (ed 2). Philadelphia, Lippincott Williams & Wilkins, 2000, pp 871-878.
27. Lipton RB, Stewart WF, Simon D: Work-related disability: Results from the American Migraine Study. Cephalalgia 1996;16:231-238.
28. Clouse JC, Osterhaus JT: Healthcare resource use and costs associated with migraine in a managed healthcare setting. Pharmacoeconomics 1994;28:659-664.
29. VonKorff M, Stewart WF, Simon DJ, et al: Migraine and reduced work performance: A population based diary study. Neurology 1998;50:1741-1745.
30. Breslau N: Psychiatric comorbidity in migraine. Cephalalgia 1998;18(Suppl 22):56-61.
31. Mitsikostas DD, Thomas AM: Comorbidity of migraine and depressive disorders. Cephalalgia 1999;19:211-217.
32. Swanson JW, Yanagihara T, Stang PE, et al: Incidence of cluster headaches: A population-based study in Olmstead County, Minnesota. Neurology 1994;44:433-437.
33. Finkel AG: Epidemiology of cluster headache. Curr Pain Headache Rep 2003;7:144-149.
34. Biondi DM: Headaches and their relationship to sleep. Dent Clin North Am 2001;45:685-700.
35. Blau, JN, MacGregor EA: Migraine and the neck. Headache 1994;34:88.
36. Sjaastad O, Saunte C, Hovdahl H, et al: "Cervicogenic" headache. An hypothesis. Cephalalgia 1983;3:249.
37. Haldeman S, Dagenais S: Cervicogenic headaches: A critical review. Spine J 2001;1:31.
38. Sjaastad O, Fredriksen TA, Pfaffenrath V: Cervicogenic headache: Diagnostic criteria. The Cervicogenic Headache International Study Group. Headache 1998;38:442.
39. Pollmann W, Keidel M, Pfaffenrath V: Headache and the cervical spine: A critical review. Cephalalgia 1997; 17:801.
40. Sjaastad O, Fredriksen TA, Pfaffenrath V: Cervicogenic headache: Diagnostic criteria. Headache 1990;30:725.
41. Jansen J, Bardosi A, Hildebrandt J, et al: Cervicogenic, hemicranial attacks associated with vascular irritation or compression of the cervical nerve root C2. Clinical manifestations and morphological findings. Pain 1989;39:203.
42. Sharma RR, Parekh HC, Prabhu S, et al: Compression of the C-2 root by a rare anomalous ectatic vertebral artery. Case report. J Neurosurg 1993;78:669.
43. Pikus HJ, Phillips JM: Characteristics of patients successfully treated for cervicogenic headache by surgical decompression of the second cervical root. Headache 1995;35:621.
44. Pikus HJ, Phillips JM: Outcome of surgical decompression of the second cervical root for cervicogenic headache. Neurosurgery 1996;39:63.
45. Lord SM, Barnsley L, Wallis BJ, et al: Chronic cervical zygapophyseal joint pain after whiplash: A placebo-controlled prevalence study. Spine 1996;21:1737.
46. Lord SM, Barnsley L, Wallis BJ, et al: Third occipital nerve headache: A prevalence study. J Neurol Neurosurg Psychiatry 1994;57:1187.
47. Drottning M, Staff PH, Sjaastad O: Cervicogenic headache (CEH) after whiplash injury. Cephalalgia 2002;22:165.
48. Bogduk N: The neck and headaches. Neurol Clin 2004;22:151.
49. Bogduk N: The anatomical basis for cervicogenic headache. J Manipulative Physiol Ther 1992;15:67.
50. Stolker RJ, Vervest AC, Groen GJ: The management of chronic spinal pain by blockades: A review. Pain 1994;58:1.
51. Schellhas KP: Facet nerve blockade and radiofrequency neurotomy. Neuroimaging Clin N Am 2000;10:493.
52. Bovim G, Berg R, Dale LG: Cervicogenic headache: Anesthetic blockades of cervical nerves (C2-C5) and facet joint (C2/C3). Pain 1992;49:315-320.
53. Fredriksen TA, Fougner R, Tangerud A, et al: Cervicogenic headache: Radiological investigations concerning head/neck. Cephalalgia 1989;9:139.
54. Delfini R, Salvati M, Passacantilli E, et al: Symptomatic cervicogenic headache. Clin Exp Rheumatol 2000;18:S29.
55. Jull G, Trott P, Potter H, et al: A randomized controlled trial of exercise and manipulative therapy for cervicogenic headache. Spine 2002;27:1835.
56. Blume HG: Cervicogenic headaches: Radiofrequency neurotomy and the cervical disc and fusion. Clin Exp Rheumatol 2000;18:S53.
57. McDonald GJ, Lord SM, Bogduk N: Long-term follow-up of patients treated with cervical radiofrequency neurotomy for chronic neck pain. Neurosurgery 1999;45:61.

58. Lord SM, Barnsley L, Wallis BJ, et al: Percutaneous radio-frequency neurotomy for chronic cervical zygapophyseal-joint pain. N Engl J Med 1996;335:1721.

59. Stovner LJ, Kolstad F, Helde G: Radiofrequency denervation of facet joints C2-C6 in cervicogenic headache: A random-ized, double-blind, sham-controlled study. Cephalalgia 2004; 24:821.

60. Bogduk N: Cervicogenic headache. Cephalalgia 2004;24: 819.

61. Govind J, King W, Bailey B, et al: Radiofrequency neurotomy for the treatment of third occipital headache. J Neurol Neu-rosurg Psychiatry 2003;74:88.

62. Slipman CW, Lipetz JS, Plastaras CT, et al: Therapeutic zyg-apophyseal joint injections for headaches emanating from the C2-3 joint. Am J Phys Med Rehabil 2001;80:182.

63. Reale C, Turkiewicz AM, Reale CA, et al: Epidural steroids as a pharmacological approach. Clin Exp Rheumatol 2000;18: S65.

64. Bovim G, Fredriksen TA, Stolt-Nielsen A, et al: Neurolysis of the greater occipital nerve in cervicogenic headache. A follow up study. Headache 1992;32:175.

65. Poletti CE, Sweet WH: Entrapment of the C2 root and gan-glion by the atlanto-epistrophic ligament: Clinical syndrome and surgical anatomy. Neurosurgery 1990;27:288.

66. Silberstein SD, Lipton RB: Overview of diagnosis and treat-ment of migraine. Neurology 1994;44:6-16.

67. Linton-Dahlof P, Linde M, Dahlof C: Withdrawal therapy improves chronic daily headache associated with long-term misuse of headache medication: A retrospective study. Ceph-alalgia 2000;20:658-662.

68. Silberstein SD, Lipton RB, Sliwinski M: Classification of daily and near-daily headaches: Field trial of revised IHS criteria. Neurology 1996;47:871-875.

69. Silberstein SD, Lipton RB, Solomon S, et al: Classification of daily and near-daily headaches: Proposed revisions to the IHS criteria. Headache 1994;34:1-7.

70. Moschiano F, D'Amico D, Schieroni F, et al: Neurobiology of chronic migraine. Neurol Sci 2003;24(Suppl 2):S94-S96.

71. Vingen JV, Sand T, Stover LJ: Sensitivity to various stimuli in primary headaches: A questionnaire study. Headache 1999; 39:552-558.

72. Tepper SJ, Dodick DW: Debate: Analgesic overuse is a cause, not consequence of chronic daily headache. Headache 2002; 42:543-554.

73. Zwart JA, Dyb G, Hagen K, et al: Analgesic use: A predictor of chronic pain and medication overuse headache. The Head-HUNT Study. Neurology 2003;61:160-164.

74. Bahra A, Walsh M, Menon S, et al: Does chronic daily head-ache arise de novo in association with regular analgesic use? (Abstract). Cephalalgia 2000;20:294.

75. Lance F, Parkes C, Wilkinson M: Does analgesic abuse cause headache de novo? Headache 1988;38:61-62.

76. Wilkinson SM, Becker WJ, Heine JA: Opiate use to control bowel motility may induce chronic headache in patients with migraine. Headache 2001;41:303-309.

77. Rapoport AM: Analgesic rebound headache. Headache 1988; 28:662-665.

78. Solomon S, Lipton RB, Newman LC: Clinical features of chronic daily headache. Headache 1992;32:325-329.

79. Granella F, Farina S, Malferrani G, et al: Drug abuse in chronic headache: A clinico-epidemiologic study. Cephalalgia 1987; 7:15-19.

80. Wang SJ, Fuh JL, Lu SR, et al: Chronic daily headache in Chinese elderly: Prevalence risk factors and biannual follow-up. Neurology 2000;54:314-319.

81. Diener HC, Dichgans J, Scholz E, et al: Analgesic-induced chronic headache: Long-term results of withdrawal therapy. J Neurol 1989;236:9-14.

82. Baumgartner C, Wessely P, Bingol C, et al: Long-term prog-nosis of analgesic withdrawal in patients with drug-induced headache. Headache 1989;29:510-514.

83. Gardner KL: Genetics of migraine: An update. Headache 2006;46(Suppl 1):S19-S24.

84. Montagna P, Cevoli S, Marzocchi N, et al: The genetics of chronic headaches. Neurol Sci 2003;24(Suppl 2): S51-S56.

85. Silberstein SD: Tension-type headache and chronic daily headache. Neurology 1993;43:1644-1649.

86. Williamson DJ, Hargreaves RJ: Neurogenic inflammation in the context of migraine. Microsc Res Tech 2001;53: 167-178.

87. Aurora SK: Pathophysiology of migraine headache. Curr Pain Headache Rep 2001;5:179-182.

88. Edvisson L: Pathophysiology of primary headaches. Curr Pain Headache Rep 2001;5:71-78.

89. Burstein R, Yarnitsky D, Goor-Aryeh I, et al.: An association between migraine and cutaneous allodynia. Ann Neurol 2000;47:614-624.

90. Burstein R, Cutrer FM, Yarnitsky D: The development of cutaneous allodynia during a migraine attack: Clinical evi-dence for sequential recruitment of spinal and supraspinal nociceptive neurons in migraine. Brain 2000;123:1703-1709.

91. Strassman AM, Raymond SA, Burstein R: Sensitization of meningeal sensory neurons and the origin of headaches. Nature 1996;384:560-564.

92. Jensen R, Olesen J: Initiating mechanisms of experimentally induced tension-type headache. Cephalalgia 1996;16:175-182.

93. Bendtsen L, Ashina M: Sensitization of myofascial pain path-ways in tension-type headache. In Oleson J, Tfelt-Hansen P, Welch KMA (eds): The Headaches, ed 2. Philadelphia, Lip-pincott Williams & Wilkins, 2000, pp 573-577.

94. Srikiatkhachorn A, Tarasub N, Govitrapong P: Effect of chronic analgesic exposure on the central serotonin system: A possible mechanism of analgesic abuse headache. Head-ache 2000;40:343-350.

95. Fields HL, Heinricher MM, Mason P: Neurotransmitters as nociceptive modulatory circuits. Ann Rev Neurosci 1991;14: 219-245.

96. Welch KMA, Nagesh V, Aurora SK, et al: Periaqueductal gray matter dysfunction in migraine: Cause or the burden of illness? Headache 2001;41:629-637.

97. Chronicle E, Mulleners W: Might migraine damage the brain? Cephalalgia 1994;14:415-418.

98. Wong TY, Klein R, Sharrett AR, et al: Cerebral white matter lesions, retinopathy, and incident clinical stroke. JAMA 2002; 288:67-74.

99. Kruit MC, van Buchem MA, Hofman PAM, et al: Migraine as a risk factor for subclinical brain lesions. JAMA 2004;291: 427-434.

100. Mulder EJCM, Linssen WHJP, Passchier J, et al: Interictal and postictal cognitive changes in migraine. Cephalalgia 1999:19: 557-565.

101. Sandor PS, Mascia A, Seidel L, et al: Subclinical cerebellar impairment in the common types of migraine: A three-dimensional analysis of reaching movements. Ann Neurol 2001;49:668-672.

102. Jacome DE: Neuromuscular transmission in migraine: A single-fiber EMG study in clinical subgroups. Neurology 2002;58:1316-1367.

103. Welsh KMA, Goadsby PJ: Chronic daily headache. Curr Opin Neurol 2002;15:287-295.

104. Srikiatkhachorn A, Anthony M: Platelet serotonin in patients with analgesic induced headache. Cephalalgia 1996;16:423-426.

105. Srikiatkhachorn A, Manseesri S, Govitrapong P, et al: Derange-ment of serotonin system in migraine patients with analgesic abuse headache: Clues from the platelets. Headache 1998; 38:43-49.

106. Sandrini G, Antonaci F, Pucci E: Comparative study with EMG, pressure algometry, and manual palpation in tension-type headache and migraine. Cephalalgia 1994;14:451-457.

107. Gladstone J, Eross E, Dodick D: Chronic daily headache: A rational approach to a challenging problem. Semin Neurol 2003;23:265-276.

108. Sandrini G, Manzoni GC, Zanferrari C, et al: An epidemio-logical approach to the nosology of chronic daily headache. Cephalalgia 1993;3(Suppl 12):72-77.

109. Granella F, Cavallini A, Sandrini G, et al: Long-term outcome of migraine. Cephalalgia 1998;18(Suppl 2):30-33.

110. Hernandez-Latorre MA, Roig M: Natural history of migraine in childhood. Cephalalgia 2000;20:573-579.
111. Katsarava Z, Schneeweiss S, Kurth T, et al: Incidence and predictors for chronicity of headache in patients with episodic migraine. Neurology 2004;62:788-790.
112. Cologno D, Torelli P, Manzoni GC: Possible predictive factors in the prognosis of migraine with aura. Cephalalgia 1999;19:824-830.
113. Verri AP, Cecchini P, Galli C, et al: Psychiatric comorbidity in chronic daily headache. Cephalalgia 1998;18:45-49.
114. Scher AI, Stewart WF, Ricci JA, et al: Factors associated with the onset and remission of chronic daily headache in a population-based study. Pain 2003;106:81-89.
115. Silberstein SD, Silberstein JR: Chronic daily headache: Prognosis following inpatient treatment with repetitive IV DHE. Headache 1992;32:439-445.
116. Hoodin F, Brines BJ, Lake III AE, et al: Behavioral self-management in an inpatient headache treatment unit: Increasing adherence and relationship to changes in affective distress. Headache 2000;40:377-387.
117. Grazzi L, Andrasik F, D'Amico D, et al: Behavioural approach in the treatment of chronic daily headache with drug overuse: A 3-year follow-up study. Cephalalgia 2000;20:300.
118. Wall DJ, Haugh MJ: Biofeedback as an adjunct to repetitive intravenous dihydroergotamine in the treatment of refractory headache. Headache 1993;33:285.
119. Scher AI, Lipton RB, Stewart WF: Natural history and prognostic factors for chronic daily headache: Results from the Frequent Headache Epidemiology Study. Neurology 2002;58(Suppl 3):A171.
120. Lu SR, Fuh JL, Chen WT, et al: Chronic daily headache in Taipei, Taiwan: Prevalence, follow-up and outcome predictors. Cephalalgia 2001;20:900-906.
121. Diener HC, Dahlof CGH: Headache associated with chronic use of substances. In Olesen J, Tfelt-Hansen P, Welch KMA (eds): The Headaches, ed 2. Philadelphia, Lippincott Williams & Wilkins; 2000, pp 871-878.
122. Zed PJ, Loewen PS, Robinson G: Medication-induced headache: Overview and systematic review of therapeutic approaches. Ann Pharmacother 1999,33:61-72.
123. Mathew NT, Kurman R, Perez F: Drug induced refractory headache-clinical features and management. Headache 1990;30:634-638.
124. Campbell JK, Penzien DB, Wall EM: Evidence-based guidelines for migraine headache: Behavioral and physical treatments. U.S. Headache Consortium 2000. Available at www.aan.com/go/practice/guidelines.
125. Biondi DM: Physical treatments for headache: A structured review. Headache 2005;45:738-746.
126. Rome HP, Rome JD: Limbically augmented pain syndrome (LAPS): Kindling, corticolimbic, sensitization, and the conversions of affective and sensory symptoms in chronic pain disorders. Pain Med 2000;1:7-23.
127. Ploghaus A, Tracey I, Gati JS, et al: Dissociating pain from its anticipation in the human brain. Science 1999;284:1979-1981.
128. Goslin RE, Gray RN, McCrory DC, et al: Behavioral and physical treatments for migraine headache. Technical Review 2.2, February 1999. Prepared for the Agency for Health Care Policy and Research. Available from the national Technical Information Service; NTIS Accession No. 127946.
129. Meskunas CA, Tepper SJ, Rapoport AM, et al: Medications associated with probable medication overuse headache reported in a tertiary care headache center over a 15-year period. Headache 2006;46:766-772.
130. Loder E, Biondi D: Oral Phenobarbital loading: A safe and effective method of withdrawing patients with headache from butalbital compounds. Headache 2003;43:904-909.
131. Hayner G, Galloway G, Wiehl WO: Haight Ashbury free clinics' drug detoxification protocols: Part 3: Benzodiazepines and other sedative hypnotics. J Psychoactive Drugs 1993;25:331-335.
132. Krymchantowski AV, Barbosa JS: Prednisone as initial treatment of analgesic-induced daily headache. Cephalalgia 2000;20:107-113.
133. Sheftell FD, Rapoport AM, Coddon DR: Naratriptan in the prophylaxis of transformed migraine. Headache 1999;39:506-510.
134. Rothrock JF, Kelly NM, Brody ML, et al: A differential response to treatment with divalproex sodium in patients with intractable headache. Cephalalgia 1994;14:241-244.
135. Loder E, Biondi D: General principles of migraine management: The changing role of prevention. Headache 2005;45(Suppl 1):S33-S47.
136. Silberstein SD: Practice parameter: Evidence-based guidelines for migraine headache (an evidence-based review). Report of the Quality Standards Subcommittee of the American Academy of Neurology. Neurology 2000;55:754-762.
137. Carleton SC, Shesser RF, Pietrzak MP, et al: Double-blind, multicenter trial to compare the efficacy of intramuscular dihydroergotamine plus hydroxyzine versus intramuscular meperidine plus hydroxyzine for the emergency department treatment of acute migraine headache. Ann Emerg Med 1998;32:129-138.
138. Larkin GL, Prescott JE: A randomized, double-blind comparative study of the efficacy of ketorolac tromethanine versus meperidine in the treatment of severe migraine. Ann Emerg Med 1992;21:919-924.
139. Sicuteri F: Opioid receptor impairment underlying mechanism in "pain diseases?" Cephalalgia 1981;1:77-82.
140. Panconesi A, Anselmi B, Franchi G: Increased adverse effects of opiates in migraine patients. Cephalalgia 1995;15:159-160.
141. Meng ID, Porreca F: Basic Science: Mechanisms of medication overuse headache. Headache Curr 2004;1:47-54.
142. Saper JR, Lake AE III, Hamel RL, et al: Daily scheduled opioids for intractable head pain: Long-term observations of a treatment program. Neurology 2004;62:1687-1694.
143. Rothrock J: From the role of chronic opioid therapy in managing chronic daily headache: A roundtable discussion. Presented at the Annual Scientific Meeting of the American Headache Society. Seattle, WA, 2002.
144. Biondi DM: Opioid resistance in chronic daily headache: A synthesis of ideas from the bench and bedside. Curr Pain Headache Rep 2003;7:67-75.
145. Raskin NH: Repetitive intravenous dihydroergotamine as therapy for intractable migraine. Neurology 1986;36:995-997.
146. Freitag FG, Lake AE III, Lipton R, et al: Inpatient treatment of headache: An evidence-based assessment. Headache 2004;44:342-360.
147. Lake AE III, Saper JR, Madden SF, et al: Comprehensive inpatient treatment for intractable migraine: A prospective long-term outcome study. Headache 1993;33:55-62.
148. Saper JR, Lake AE III, Madden SF, et al: Comprehensive/tertiary care for headache: A 6-month outcome study. Headache 1999;39:249-263.

CHAPTER
25 Dental and Facial Pain

Noshir R. Mehta, Steven J. Scrivani, and Raymond Maciewicz

Craniofacial pain disorders deserve special consideration, given the complex anatomy and specialized sensory innervation of the head and neck. Many craniofacial syndromes also are unique, and represent a clinical diagnostic challenge. This chapter presents an introduction to practical issues regarding assessment and treatment of common craniofacial pain disorders, using the International Headache Society's diagnostic classification scheme[1] (Boxes 25–1 to 25–3).

PAIN CAUSED BY PATHOLOGY OF THE HEAD, FACE, AND ORAL CAVITY

The specialized structures of the head and face have a rich, sensory innervation supplied by the trigeminal system, lower cranial nerves, and upper cervical roots. As such, pain is one of the most prominent symptoms of disease in this area. In most cases, the acute pain symptoms closely correlate with other signs and symptoms of disease. However, correlation between pain and symptoms may not be evident in a number of more complex, chronic pain problems, particularly those involving the masticatory system.[2]

Dental Pain

Tooth pulp has a specialized and possibly exclusively nociceptive innervation.[3] In contrast, periodontal tissues are innervated by a wide variety of sensory afferents. Dental pain is usually well localized and the quality of pain can range from a dull ache to severe electric shocks, depending on the specific etiology and extent of disease (Box 25–4). Dental pain is typically provoked by thermal or mechanical stimulation of the damaged tooth. Clinical and radiographic findings of dental decay, tooth fracture, or abscess drainage may confirm the source of dental pain.

BOX 25–1. INTERNATIONAL HEADACHE SOCIETY, INTERNATIONAL CLASSIFICATION OF HEADACHE DISORDERS II

14 Categories
- The primary headaches: 1-4
- The secondary headaches: 5-12
- Cranial neuralgias, central and primary facial pain, and other headache disorders: 13-14

BOX 25–2. HEADACHE OR FACIAL PAIN ATTRIBUTED TO DISORDERS OF CRANIUM, NECK, EYES, EARS, NOSE, SINUSES, TEETH, MOUTH, OR OTHER FACIAL OR CRANIAL STRUCTURES (11.1-8)

11.2—Neck
Cervicogenic headache
11.3—Eyes
Acute glaucoma
Latent or manifest squint
Ocular inflammatory disorders
11.5—Sinus disorders ("sinus headache")
11.6—Teeth, jaws, or related structures
11.7—Temporomandibular joint disorders (TMDs)

BOX 25–3. CRANIAL NEURALGIAS, CENTRAL AND PRIMARY FACIAL PAIN, AND OTHER HEADACHES (13.1-19)

13.1—Trigeminal neuralgia
13.2—Glossopharyngeal neuralgia
13.8—Occipital neuralgia
13.12—Constant pain caused by compression, irritation, or distortion of cranial nerves or upper cervical roots by structural lesions
13.15—Head or facial pain attributed to herpes zoster
Postherpetic neuralgia
13.18—Central causes of facial pain
Anesthesia dolorosa
Central post-stroke pain
Facial pain attributed to multiple sclerosis
Persistent idiopathic facial pain
Burning mouth syndrome

Acute dental pain typically responds to local treatments (e.g., ice packs and reduced mechanical stimulation), or systemic, nonsteroidal anti-inflammatory drugs (NSAIDs). Opioid analgesics also are occasionally indicated, depending on the extent of objective pathology. Opioids should only be used short term, and in combination with NSAIDs. In many cases, treatment with antibiotic agents is appropriate and palliative until a definitive dental intervention is performed.

Disorders of the Periodontium (Periodontal Disease)

Chronic periodontal disease is an immune-mediated inflammatory process initiated by pathogenic oral microorganisms[4] and resulting in either focal or generalized areas of destruction of the tooth-supporting structures and surrounding bone. Chronic periodon-

---

BOX 25–4. DENTAL AND ORAL SURGICAL CONDITIONS

- Dentoalveolar pathology
  - Pulpal
  - Periodontal
- Odontogenic and nonodontogenic pathology
- Trigeminal neuralgia and "equivalents"
- Headache and neck pain
- Temporomandibular disorders
- Oral mucous membrane disease
- Oral manifestations of systemic disease
- Neuropathic pain (persistent idiopathic facial pain)

---

titis is generally not a chronically painful disorder. Typically, patients may notice gingival sensitivity and tenderness, or gingival enlargement caused by inflammation and bleeding with brushing or probing examination. There is loss of gingival attachment around the necks of and soft tissue pocketing around the roots of the tooth with loss of bone support, which may result in tooth sensitivity, tenderness, and mobility. In the presence of an acute infection in the periodontal tissues, tenderness to the touch, erythema, and bleeding may be evident. An acute periodontal abscess may cause swelling and purulence (Table 25–1). When inflammation or infection (i.e., acute pericoronitis) occurs in the soft tissue or bone around an erupting or partially erupted tooth (particularly third molars, otherwise known as "wisdom teeth"), similar signs and symptoms may be seen with pain as a primary complaint.

The pain of periodontal disorders is also generally responsive to NSAIDs, opioid analgesic agents, or combination analgesic agents. An acute abscess also may have to be locally incised and drained. Areas of generalized periodontitis may be treated with tooth scaling and curettage of the gingival pocketing and possibly local or systemic antibiotic therapy.

Oral Mucous Membrane Disorders

Diseases of the oral mucosa are numerous and caused by a variety of local and systemic etiologies. Typically these diseases produce pain and oral mucosal lesions including vesicles, bullae, erosions, erythema, or red and white patches (Table 25–2). Pain may be a symptom of the primary disease process, secondary to an associated process (i.e., infection), or related to

---

Table 25–1. Odontogenic Pain

DIAGNOSIS	PULPITIS	PERIODONTAL	CRACKED TOOTH	DENTINAL
Diagnostic features	Spontaneous or evoked deep/diffuse pain in compromised dental pulp. Pain may be sharp, throbbing, or dull.	Localized deep continuous pain in compromised periodontium (e.g., gingiva, periodontal ligament) exacerbated by biting or chewing.	Spontaneous or evokes brief sharp pain in a tooth with history of trauma or restorative work (e.g., crown, root canal).	Brief, sharp pain evoked by different kinds of stimulus to the dentin (e.g., hot or cold drinks).
Diagnostic evaluation	Look for deep caries and recent or extensive dental work. Pain provoked or exacerbated by percussion, thermal, or electrical stimulation of affected tooth. Dental x-rays helpful (periapical).	Tooth percussion over compromised periodontium provokes pain. Look for inflammation or abscess (e.g., periodontitis, apical dental x-rays helpful (bitewings, periapical).	Presence of tooth fracture may be detectable by x-ray. Percussion should elicit pain. Dental x-rays are helpful (periapical taken from different angles).	Exposed dentin or cementum as a result of recession of periodontium. Possible erosion of dentinal structure. Cold stimulation reproduces pain.
Treatment	Medication: nonsteroidal anti-inflammatory drugs (NSAIDs), non-opiate analgesics. Dentistry: remove carious lesion, tooth restoration, endodontic treatment or tooth extraction.	Medication: NSAIDs, non-opiate analgesics, antibiotics, mouthwashes. Dentistry: drainage and debridement of periodontal pocket, scaling and root planing, periodontal surgery, endodontic treatment or tooth extraction.	Medication: NSAIDs, non-opiate analgesics. Dentistry: depends on level of the tooth fracture—restoration, treatment, or extraction of the tooth.	Medication: mouthwash (fluoride), desensitizing toothpaste. Dentistry: fluoride or potassium salts, tooth restoration, endodontic treatment. Patient education, diet, toothbrushing force and frequency, proper toothpaste.

Table 25–2. Common Painful Mucosal Conditions

Infections	Herpetic stomatitis
	Varicella zoster
	Candidiasis
	Acute necrotizing gingivostomatitis
Immune/Autoimmune	Allergic reactions (toothpaste, mouthwashes, topical medications)
	Erosive lichen planus
	Benign mucous membrane pemphigoid
	Aphthous stomatitis and aphthous lesions
	Erythema multiforme
	Graft-versus-host disease
Traumatic and Iatrogenic Injuries	Factitial, accidental (burns: chemical, solar, thermal)
	Self-destructive (rituals, obsessive behaviors)
	Iatrogenic (chemotherapy, radiation)
Neoplasia	Squamous cell carcinoma
	Mucoepidermoid carcinoma
	Adenocystic carcinoma
	Brain tumors
Neurologic	Burning mouth syndrome and glossodynia
	Neuralgias
	Postviral neuralgias
	Post-traumatic neuropathies
	Dyskinesias and dystonias
Nutritional and Metabolic	Vitamin deficiencies (B_{12}, folate)
	Mineral deficiencies (iron)
	Diabetic neuropathy
	Malabsorption syndromes
Miscellaneous	Xerostomia, secondary to intrinsic or extrinsic conditions
	Referred pain from esophageal or oropharyngeal malignancy
	Mucositis secondary to esophageal reflux
	Angioedema

damaged oral mucosa (i.e., mouth movements, chewing foods, thermal, chemical). The pain is often treated with systemic and local analgesic agents.

Disorders of the Maxilla and Mandible

Numerous disorders of the bony substrate of the jaws can produce pain. These disorders are generally classified as being of odontogenic or nonodontogenic origin, cystic, cystic-like or tumor, or benign or malignant (either primary or metastatic disease). Often additional historical or examination findings warrant further evaluation (i.e., swelling, mass, discoloration, numbness, weakness, bleeding, drainage, tooth loss or mobility). Pain complaint can be treated symptomatically until a definitive diagnosis is established and definitive therapy is initiated (Table 25–3).

Salivary Gland Disorders

Disorders of the three major pairs of salivary glands (parotid, submandibular, and sublingual) and many hundreds of minor salivary glands within the oral cavity also may produce pain as a primary or associated complaint. These disorders often are accompanied by other signs and symptoms (including swelling, drainage, cervical adenopathy, or generalized symptoms of systemic infection) depending on the etiology of the disorder. Disorders of the parotid gland can locally extend to produce otologic symptoms, or cranial nerve (V, VII, or IX) involvement. Disorders of the submandibular gland may result in symptoms of impaired swallowing or impairment of cranial nerves V, IX, or XII (Box 25–5).

Burning Mouth/Tongue Disorder (Oral Burning)

Burning mouth/tongue disorder (BMD) is an idiopathic pain condition of the oral mucous membranes. It can be focal (inside the lips, tongue) or generalized and is typically described as a constant, bilateral burning painful sensation. BMD generally affects middle-aged or older females and has been attributed to numerous oral disorders (i.e., mucous membrane disease, Sjögren's syndrome/dry mouth, fungal infections) and systemic diseases (i.e., vitamin deficiencies, diabetes mellitus, immune connective tissue disorders, vasculitides). More recent evidence suggests that BMD is more likely a neuropathic pain disorder of either peripheral or central origin. Some recent taste-testing data and functional brain imaging studies seem to support this hypothesis[5-10] (Table 25–4). The current treatments for BMD focus on this hypothesis and use both topical (oral mucosa) and systemic antineuropathic pain medications (see Chapters 21, 33, and 34); however, there is little evidence such treatments are effective in BMD.

Sinus Disorders

Patients frequently describe their facial pain problem as a "sinus headache." However, sinus disorders do not cause chronic headaches, and the clinician should look for a more specific etiology for pain symptoms in such cases.[11] Diseases of the nose and paranasal sinuses typically cause acute pain associated with multiple other symptoms that are generally related to the specific nasal or sinus disease (i.e., allergic,

---

BOX 25–5. SALIVARY GLAND DISEASE

- Inflammatory
- Noninflammatory
- Infectious
- Obstructive
- Immunologic (Sjögren's syndrome)
- Tumors
- Others (red herrings)

Table 25–3. Temporomandibular Disorders

DIAGNOSIS	TMJ ARTICULAR DISORDERS	MUSCLE DISORDERS	MYOFASCIAL DISORDERS
Diagnostic features	Pain localized in the preauricular area during jaw function. Usually presence of painful click or crepitus during mouth opening. Limited opening (<35 mm), deviated or painful jaw movements.	Tenderness of the masticatory muscles. Dull, aching pain exacerbated by jaw function or palpation	Diffused dull or aching pain affecting multiple groups of muscles of the head and neck region, as well as other parts of the body
Diagnostic evaluation	Internal derangement of the TMJ with abnormal function of the disk-condyle complex, or degeneration of the joint surface. Palpation is painful. Possible joint swelling in acute phases. MRI, CT, of the joint may rule out tumors and advanced degenerative stages.	Tenderness during palpation of the masticatory muscles and tendons. Possible limited range of jaw movement and during passive stretching examination. Can be associated with a parafunctional habit (bruxism or early morning pain).	Presence of trigger or tender points in one or more groups of muscles. Pain can radiate to distant areas with stimulation of the trigger points. Rule out presence of lupus erythematosus.
Treatment	Patient education and self-care. Medication: NSAIDs, non-opiate analgesics. Physical therapy: exercise program. Occlusal splints. Oral maxillofacial surgery: arthrocentesis, arthroscopic surgery, open surgery.	Patient education and self-care. Medication: topical and systemic NSAIDs., non-opiate analgesics, muscle relaxants, antidepressants, (usually TCAs), anxiolytics, anticonvulsants, BTX, trigger point injections and vapocoolant spray. Physical therapy: TENS, massage, exercise program. Occlusal splints Cognitive-behavior: biofeedback, relaxation, coping skills.	Same as muscle disorders.

BTX, botulinum toxin; CT, computed tomography; MRI, magnetic resonance imaging; NSAIDs, nonsteroidal anti-inflammatory drugs; TCAs, tricyclic antidepressants; TENS, transcutaneous electrical nerve stimulation; TMJ, temporomandibular joint.

Table 25–4. Trigeminal Neuropathic Pain Disorders

DIAGNOSIS	TRIGEMINAL NEURALGIA	DEAFFERENTION PAIN	ACUTE AND POST-HERPETIC NEURALGIA	BURNING MOUTH SYNDROME
Diagnostic features	Brief severe lancinating pain evoked by mechanical stimulation of trigger zone (pain-free between attacks). Usually unilateral, affects the V2/V3 areas (rarely V1). Possible pain remission periods (for months/years)	Spontaneous or evoked pain with prolonged after-sensation after tactile stimulation. Trigger zone as a result of surgery (tooth extraction) or trauma. Positive and negative descriptors (e.g., burning, nagging, boring).	Pain associated with herpetic lesions, usually in the V1 dermatoma. Spontaneous pain (burning and tingling), but may present as dull and aching. Occasional lancinating evoked pain.	Constant burning pain of the mucous membranes of the tongue, mouth. Hard or soft palate, or lips. Usually affects women >50 years of age.
Diagnostic evaluation	MRI for evidence of tumor or vasocompression of the trigeminal tract or root (cerebellopontine angle). Rule out MS, especially in young adults.	Etiologic factors such as trauma or surgery in the painful area. Order MRI if the area is intact to rule out peripheral or central lesions.	Small cutaneous vesicles (AHN) or scarring (PHN), usually affecting V1. Loss of normal skin color. Corneal ulceration can occur. Sensory changes in affected area (e.g., hyperesthesia, dysesthesia).	Rule out salivary gland dysfunction (xerostomia) or tumor, Sjögren's syndrome, candidiasis, geographic or fissured tongue, and chemical or mechanical irritations. Nutrition and menopause.
Treatment	Medication: anticonvulsants (e.g., carbamazepine, gabapentin); antidepressants (e.g., amitriptyline, nortriptyline, desipramine); non-opiate analgesics, BTX. Combination of baclofen and anticonvulsants can produce good results. Surgery: microvascular decompression of trigeminal root, ablative surgeries (e.g., rhizotomy, gamma knife).	Medication: anticonvulsants (e.g., carbamazepine, gabapentin); antidepressants; non-opiate analgesics; topical agents (e.g., lidocaine 5% patches). Surgery: ablative surgeries (e.g., rhizotomy, gamma knife).	Medication: acyclovir (acute phase) anticonvulsants, antidepressants; non-opiate analgesics; topical agents (e.g., lidocaine 5% patches). Surgery: ablative surgeries (e.g., rhizotomy, gamma knife).	Medication: anticonvulsants, benzodiazepines, antidepressants; non-opiate analgesics; topical agents (e.g., lidocaine, mouthwashes). Cognitive-behavioral: biofeedback, relaxation, coping skills.

AHN, acute herpetic neuralgia; BTX, botulinum toxin; MRI, magnetic resonance imaging; MS, multiple sclerosis; PHN, post-herpetic neuralgia.

Table 25–5. Paranasal, Periocular, Periauricular, and Head and Neck Cancer Pain

DIAGNOSIS	PARANASAL SINUS PAIN	PERIOCULAR PAIN	PERIAURICULAR PAIN	HEAD AND NECK CANCER
Diagnostic features	Bilateral or unilateral throbbing or pressure frontal area pain, exacerbated by leaning forward or palpitation over the sinus.	Pain or tenderness with or without eye movements, deep orbital pain, and referred pain.	Diffuse aching or sudden pain with or without aural discharge (e.g., otitis media).	Variety of symptoms. Pain may be caused by tumor, nerve compression, secondary infection, second myofascial pain, deafferentation, radiotherapy, chemotherapy.
Diagnostic evaluation	History of chronic allergies, frequent URIs, sinusitis, headaches of various types, sinus surgery. Refer to ENT specialist for endoscopic and/or CT study (e.g., sinus opacification).	Examine eyelids, lacrimal function, conjunctiva, sclera. Ophthalmoscopy and ophthalmology referral. Rule out primary headache, temporal arteritis, orbital pseudotumor.	The area is innervated by multiple cranial and cervical nerves so complete functional and structural examiantion necessary (e.g., inspect tympanic membrane, TMJ and myofascia). CT and MRI invaluable for mastoiditis and cholesteatoma.	Complete evaluation by multidisciplinary team, CT, MRI, endoscopy, biopsy, and surveillance. Treatment coordination by oncologist.
Treatment	ENT evaluation/treatment Medication: sinusitis— topical decongestants; systemic antibiotics. Chronic sinus pain— NSAIDs; non-opiate analgesics; topical agents (lidocaine spray); anticonvulsants, antidepressants; BTX. Surgery	Proper ophthalmologic evaluation and treatment. Medication: NSAIDs; non-opiate analgesics; systemic antibiotics, topical corticosteroids, BTX across forehead and glabellar areas in selected cases. Surgery	Proper ENT evaluation and treatment. Medication: NSAIDs; non-opiate analgesics; systemic antibiotics, topical corticosteroids, BTX in selected cases. Surgery	Oncologist evaluation and treatment. Medication: anticonvulsants, antidepressants, opiate or non-opiate analgesics, topical agents, muscle relaxants. Surgery: ablative surgeries.

BTX, botulinum toxin; CT, computed tomography; ENT, ear, nose, and throat; MRI, magnetic resonance imaging; NSAIDs, nonsteroidal anti-inflammatory drugs; TMJ, temporomandibular joint; URIs, upper respiratory infections.

inflammatory, infections) (Table 25–5). Acute dento-alveolar pathology of the maxillary posterior teeth often has signs and symptoms consistent with sinus disease. In addition, acute dentoalveolar inflammatory or infections (dental abscess) can cause secondary maxillary sinus inflammation or infection. These are typically acute in nature, but can become chronic. This condition is often confused with other facial pain and headache disorders.

Disorders of the Eye and Ear

Numerous disorders can exhibit pain in and around the eye and ear and as such need to be evaluated for any primary ophthalmologic or otologic disease. Very often pain in and around these structures is also associated with a variety of other craniofacial and headache syndromes (Boxes 25–6 to 25–8).

Tumors

Numerous intra- and extracranial tumors can cause oral cavity, oropharyngeal, facial, and head pain as a primary symptom. Cancers of the upper aerodigestive tract, jaws, base of skull, and neck may demonstrate pain along with other associated signs and symptoms. In addition, numerous intracranial tumors and lesions (i.e., vascular malformations) can exhibit facial pain and headache. These are primarily tumors

BOX 25–6. HEADACHE AND FACIAL PAIN SYNDROMES WITH EYE PAIN

- Cluster headache and cluster-tic syndrome
- Paroxysmal hemicrania
- SUNCT syndrome
- Trigeminal neuralgia
- Sphenopalatine neuralgia (Sluder's neuralgia)
- Icepick headache
- Ice cream headache
- Hypnic headache
- Eye pain, headache, and lung cancer
- Nonorganic pain and headache (psychosomatic and psychiatric disorders)

SUNCT, short-lasting, unilateral, neuralgiform headache attacks, conjunctival injection, tearing.

of the cerebellopontine angle (CPA); however, various primary brain neoplasms and metastatic disease have been associated with facial pain and headache. Headache and facial pain of unknown origin should warrant a careful evaluation for an underlying occult tumor[12-14] (see Boxes 25–6 and 25–7).

Patients presenting with facial pain or headache should undergo a comprehensive medical history and careful physical examination with particular attention to the cranial neurologic examination.

Consideration should be given to obtaining appropriate imaging studies including computed tomography (CT), magnetic resonance imaging (MRI), and magnetic resonance angiography (MRA).

Temporomandibular Joint Disorders

Myofascial disorders are an extremely common cause of chronic head and neck pain. In fact, myofascial factors are important contributors to symptoms in almost half of all chronic pain patients that seek medical assistance.[15,16] In the craniocervical region these conditions frequently involve the masticatory and craniocervical postural muscles. The conditions are grouped together under the heading "temporomandibular joint/myofascial pain dysfunction" (TMD) syndrome,[17] in order to emphasize common diagnostic features. TMD is most common in young adults, and women are affected far more often than men.

Muscle pain and tenderness is a prominent feature of TMD. It is usually accompanied by restriction of functional movement ("dysfunction"). Patients often present with reduced jaw opening, as well as impaired cervical and upper extremity range of motion.

In addition to pain, TMD may include additional complaints including the following[18-20]: headache, face pain, eye pain, ear symptoms, temporomandibular joint symptoms, neck pain, and arm and back symptoms.

Headache

Symptoms of bilateral head and face pain involve multiple postural muscles or the muscles of mastication. The pain is dull and aching, with a chronic or persistent temporal pattern.[21-25] Pain is typically moderate in intensity, and patients often exhibit daily symptoms that can wax and wane in severity. Pain exacerbations are often provoked by functional use of the affected muscles. Morning headaches may be related to nocturnal bruxism and or sleep disorders.[26] Increasing pain during the day may be related to muscle use or maintenance of head posture.[17]

Face Pain

Pain in the sides of the mandible or pain described by the patient as "sinus" pain in the zygomatic or orbital area may have a musculoskeletal origin.[27] Daytime clenching and acute or chronic stress, combined with a reduction of dental vertical dimension (height) related to loss of posterior teeth can create muscle trigger points or muscle fatigue. This is particularly noticed by the patient after meals and reported as "a heavy and tired feeling" in the jaw muscles. Face pain related to sinuses and other pathologies is discussed later in the chapter.

Eye Pain

TMD complaints frequently include pain symptoms that involve the eye and periorbital region.[27-31] The pain is typically referred from other muscular sites, including the suboccipital region. Orbital pain symptoms are often described as unilateral, constant, and "boring." This is frequently seen in patients with a history of trauma or chronic upper cervical vertebral subluxations or nerve root impingements related to the occiput and the atlantoaxial region. In addition, entrapment of the greater occipital nerve at the occiput level can produce this type of pain often diagnosed as occipital neuralgia. This can be frequently amenable to physical medicine along with changes in head posture and mandibular position.

Ear Symptoms

Pain, stuffiness, and tinnitus may have a musculoskeletal etiology.[32,33] Mandibular posture related to the maxilla affects the masticatory elevator muscles. The medial pterygoids are intimately related in the left-to-right balance of the mandible on tooth closure.

The tensor tympani and tensor palati are actually one muscle with a raphe that wraps around the hamulus notch of the maxilla. Improper growth of the maxilla during development may affect eustachian tube function and may contribute to middle ear infections in children and stuffiness and changes in pressure in the ear in adults.

Tinnitus and other types of sounds may also have a musculoskeletal etiology. Specifically, cervical factors and mandibular postural factors have been seen in subjects with tinnitus. A combination of physical medicine and dental mouth guard therapy has been effective in some cases in which there has been a history of trauma or childhood growth affecting the proper expansion of the maxilla. Ear pain that is sharp and jabbing on movement of the mandible is frequently seen in patients who have an internal derangement of the temporomandibular joint. This type of pain usually is unilateral and ipsilateral to the joint in question. Ear pain and symptoms such as stuffiness in the absence of positive otologic findings are among the most common reasons for evaluation of dental and maxillomandibular-related imbalance. Treatment can often alleviate the symptoms completely or reduce the effect on the patient in conjunction with standard medical intervention.[34-39]

Temporomandibular Joint (TMJ) Symptoms

Pain and sounds are very common with TMJ disorders.[40,41] Pain is usually unilateral and may be related to trauma or bruxism in the presence of missing posterior teeth resulting in injury or anterior disk displacement without reduction and subsequent "locking" of the TMJ. Treatment often includes a combination of dental, medical, and physical medicine, mouth guard therapy,[42] and stress management through biofeedback relaxation.[17,26]

Neck Pain

Neck stiffness and pain are commonly part of the umbrella of TMD.[43,44] Trauma, habitual posturing, and musculoskeletal tension chronically affect the cervical area, creating pain, stiffness, and trigger points in the muscles of the head and neck. It is well documented that the trigeminal and cervical nerve systems are interactive in the maintenance of head, neck, and jaw posture.[45] Examination of dental factors in patients with chronic neck pain is important[46] because studies examining the relationships within the maxillomandibular position and cervical spine have shown that loss of vertical dimension of the teeth and a deep bite can adversely affect cervical muscle function, leading to chronic stiffness, pain, and reduction of range of motion.[47]

Arm and Back Symptoms

Patients presenting with TMJ disorders often also have other musculoskeletal findings including shoul-

der pain and pain radiating down the arm that may or may not be accompanied by tingling and or numbness. Physical examination may reveal positive signs for thoracic outlet syndrome, costoclavicular syndrome, vertebral subluxations or nerve impingement of the brachial plexus of nerves, and even previously undiagnosed rotator cuff injuries.[48] The treatment requires a thoughtful multimodal approach for the various areas affected.

Internal Derangements of the Temporomandibular Joints

The TMJ is a synovial diarthrodial joint that forms the articulation between the temporal bone and the condylar head of the mandible (Fig. 25–1). The joint allows for sliding as well as hinge movement of the mandible during functional mastication. The condyles are not perfectly round but are wider mediolaterally than anteroposteriorly (Fig. 25–2). Individual variations in form are thought to follow functional loads and depend on the thickness of connective tissue layer that covers the articulating surfaces.[49,50] The condyles travel within their respective mandibular fossae. Each mandibular fossa or glenoid fossa

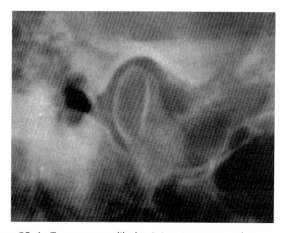

Figure 25–1. Temporomandibular joint. Note space between the head of the condyle and the bony confines of the articular fossa for allowance of movement.

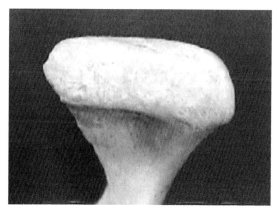

Figure 25–2. Condylar head. Space is not round but wider mediolaterally than anteroposteriorly.

forms the temporal component of the TMJ. It is a concave area on the inferior border of the squamous part of the temporal bone that is also referred to as the articular fossa.[51]

Between the bones that form the TMJ lie interposing disks or articular cartilages[52] (Fig. 25–3). Each articular disk is the structure of dense fibrous connective tissue and divides the joint cavity into two separate compartments, the upper diskotemporal space, and lower diskomandibular space. Both compartments are lubricated by synovial fluid, a plasma-like fluid secreted by the synovial membrane.[53] The inferior surface of the disk is concave to match the articular surface of the condyle, whereas the superior surface of the disk is convex to adapt to the concave surface of the articular fossa (Fig. 25–4). The articular disk is firmly attached to the medial and lateral poles

of the condyle. The lateral ligamentous attachments are relatively thin and weak compared with the medial pole attachments and tend to tear more frequently than the medial ligamentous attachments.

Viewed sagittally the articular disk is divided into three parts: a thicker anterior section called the anterior band, a middle thinner intermediary zone, and a broader posterior band, which is the thickest of the three (see Fig. 25–3). The thinner intermediary zone, along with the two broader anterior and posterior zones, gives the articular cartilage its classic bowtie appearance seen in magnetic resonance images.

In the adult, the central part of the articular disk is avascular and lacks innervations, which allows for changes in the central thin part of the disk to occur without pain. The articular disk has a random arrangement of type I collagen fibers, elastic fibers, and glycosaminoglycans composed of chondroitin sulfate, dermatan sulfate, and hyaluronic acid. The disks allow for movement of rotation in the upper joint compartment and translation in the lower joint compartment.[54] This functionally correlates to rotation being the first 22.5 mm of mouth opening and translation from that point to full-mouth opening ranging from 45 to 55 mm between the front teeth. In each joint complex (Fig. 25–5) the anterior part of the articular cartilage attaches to the superior head of the lateral pterygoid muscle, whereas the inferior head of the lateral pterygoid muscle attaches into the fovea of the condyle. This attachment of the superior head of the lateral pterygoid is variable in human beings and studies have shown the superior head of the lateral pterygoid muscle attachment to range from 40% to 60% of insertion into the articular disk.[55] The posterior part of the articular cartilage blends into loose retrodiskal tissue. This retrodiskal tissue, which consists of blood vessels, loose connective tissue and nerves, is one of the main reasons that mandibular motion is allowed. On full mouth closure the retrodiskal tissue is squeezed like a sponge and allows for full seating of the condyle in its fossa (see

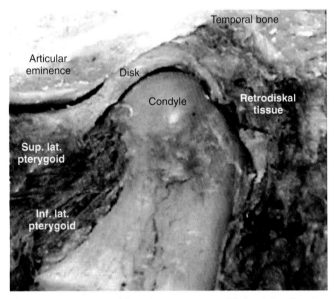

Figure 25–3. Dissected human temporomandibular joint showing the articular disk lying interposed between the condyle and the fossa of the temporal bone. Note the two heads of the lateral pterygoid muscle anterior to the condyle and the retrodiskal tissue posteriorly.

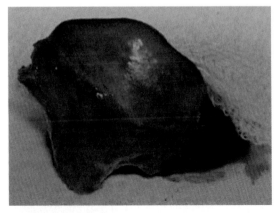

Figure 25–4. Articular disk seen from above. Smooth fibrocartilage disk has taken the shape of the condyle on which it sat. Also note the color of the surrounding tissue with nerves and blood supply.

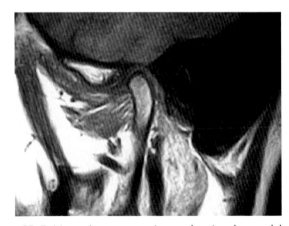

Figure 25–5. Magnetic resonance image showing the condyle and fossa with interposing disk. Note the superior head of the lateral pterygoid attaching to the disk and the condylar head and the inferior head attaching to the fovea of the condyle.

Fig. 25–3). As the mouth is opened and the condyles move forward in their respective fossa the blood vessels in the retrodiskal tissues expand to fill the void left by the translating condyles and their interposing articular cartilages. This act, similar to a sponge being squeezed and then being filled, is repeated during jaw function. It is also the region that is injured if a sudden opening and closing of the mandible happens as a result of a blow or injury to the mandible. This leads to bleeding in the joint space followed by pain and limitation of movement.

Disorders of the Temporomandibular Joint

Temporomandibular disorders fall in the 11th major category of the International Headache Society's (IHS) Classification and Diagnostic Criteria for Headache Disorders, Cranial Neuralgias, and Facial Pain[1] (see Box 25–2). According to IHS, temporomandibular articular disorders (IHS Classification 11.7) are broadly divided into congenital or developmental disorders and inflammatory disorders.

Congenital or developmental disorders such as aplasia, hypoplasia, hyperplasia, and neoplasia can be odontogenic or nonodontogenic and primarily are esthetic and functional problems. Neoplastic lesions of the bone produce pain in more advanced stages.[56] Neoplastic lesions can be primary (e.g., osteoma, osteoblastoma, chondroblastoma, and benign giant cell tumors) or metastatic (e.g., squamous cell carcinoma, nasopharyngeal tumors, and parotid gland adenoid cystic carcinomas) tumors.[57]

Disk derangement disorders or articular disk displacements are by far the most common TMJ articular disorders and characterized by abnormal position of the articular disk to the head of the condyle or temporal fossa. Disk displacement usually starts with the presence of a "clicking" or "popping" sound in the TMJ on opening and closing the mouth. Pain is typically a symptom as long as there is full function. Disk displacements are usually anterior or anteromedial in nature although posterior and lateral displacements have been described in the literature (see Fig. 25–3). This may be related in part to the thinnest diskal attachments being on the lateral pole of the condyle as well as the medial direction of pull by the lateral pterygoid and inward direction of condylar movement during mouth opening.[58] Disk displacement therefore clinically suggests torn or stretched collateral diskal ligaments that bind the disk to the condyle.

In **disk displacement with reduction,** a clicking sound on mouth opening and closing may be present. The term *reduction* is used to describe the misaligned disk temporarily coming back (or slipping back) to its proper interposition between the condyle and fossa during full opening (Figs. 25–6 and 25–7). On closing the mouth, the disk again displaces as the teeth come closer together. This repetitive ongoing displacement on opening and closing produces a reciprocal noise (clicks) and is hence termed *reciprocal*

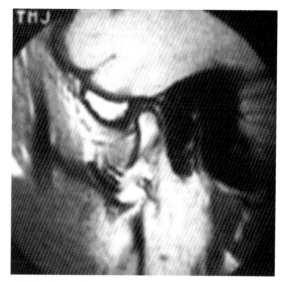

Figure 25–6. Magnetic resonance image of an anteriorly displaced disk that lies at the 10 o'clock position to the head of the condyle with the teeth together.

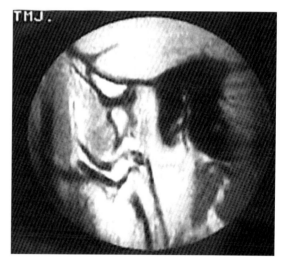

Figure 25–7. Opening movement with a clinical "click" sound allows the disk and condyle from image in Figure 25–6 to assume a normal open position.

clicking. This stage may actually represent a physiologic accommodative stage without need for therapy other than discussion regarding its anatomic significance. With progression to the next stage, intermittent "locking" as a result of the momentary impedance of the disk to the travel path of the condyle happens as a sequela of a chronic clicking condition in subjects who tend to clench and grind their teeth at night (nocturnal parafunction) and have missing posterior teeth with subsequent overclosure of the bite. The teeth act as the doorstop for the TMJs and support the ultimate position of the TMJ on full closure. Good dental vertical dimension without shift on closure is essential in reducing the risk factors for progression (Fig. 25–8). Bite appliance therapy has been shown to be effective in muscular[59-61] and disk displacement problems.[42]

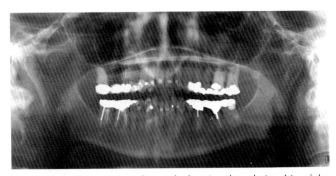

Figure 25–8. Panoramic radiograph showing the relationship of the teeth, dental occlusion, and the temporomandibular joints. The height of the teeth acts as a doorstop for the positioning of the condyles in their respective fossae.

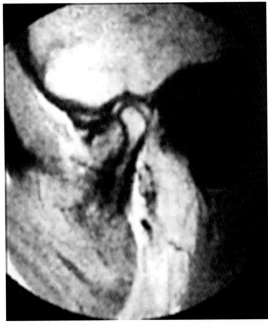

Figure 25–9. Anterior disk displacement without reduction. The disk is folded in front of the head of the condyle, thus preventing full opening of the mandible.

Disk displacement without reduction is sometimes referred to as a "closed lock." This suggests that the disk has been permanently displaced and the disk's shape has been permanently changed such that it physically prevents the condyle of the mandible from translating to a full open position (Fig. 25–9). There is a limitation of jaw opening to 22 to 25 mm with pain and a deviation of the mandible to the side of the lock. As a result, there is reduction in the chewing capability due to pain, inflammation at the affected joint, and possible changes in the normal occlusion or "bite." An MRI of the TMJ is the gold standard to assess soft tissue details of the articular cartilage and its displacement whereas hard-tissue CT scans are generally performed to assess chronic osteoarthritic or bony changes.[62,63]

TMJ dislocation is also known as open lock or condylar subluxation in which the condyle translates

beyond the anterior eminence of the articular fossa with subsequent trapping in this open-mouth position. Chronic hypertranslation can usually be managed by the subject's physically manipulating the jaw. If the condition is chronic the subject knows to relax the jaw-closing muscles and slip the condyle back into position. The most common subluxation occurs during yawning or opening the mouth widely. If the problem is related to trauma or to a sudden acute translation, then the subluxation is considered to be an acute dislocation and requires medial intervention in which the muscles are relaxed by anesthesia or analgesics followed by manual manipulation of the joint with a downward and backward motion. Follow-up with anti-inflammatory medication, ice and rest, or a dental appliance may be necessary until the acute stage subsides.[64]

Inflammatory disorders including capsulitis and synovitis are relatively common in the TMJ secondary to macro- or microtrauma, irritation, or infections. These disorders may exhibit pain on function and inflammation with extreme tenderness on palpation of the TMJ. MRI imaging may show effusions in the T2-weighted signal and the inability to completely bring the teeth together accompanied by pain in the ear. Joint inflammation also may be a result of polyarthritis of systemic origin, which generally is seen secondarily to connective tissue diseases.

Osteoarthritis (noninflammatory): Primary osteoarthritis is a degenerative condition of the joints characterized by hard tissue abrasion and degradation of the articular surface of the condyle related to overload. This is frequently seen in subjects with a long history of missing teeth or maloccluded dentures. This process is generally slow, not associated with symptoms of pain during the early stages, and may remain relatively benign over the life of the subject. Primary osteoarthritis is usually identified by a hard-tissue radiograph screening (e.g., dental panoramic image), a tomograph or dental CT scan, or presence of grating (crepitus) noises in the joint during movement (Fig. 25–10).

Secondary osteoarthritis is usually identified by a single prior event such as trauma or infection, or may result from rheumatoid arthritis. An idiopathic degenerative condition primarily affecting adolescent females is termed condylysis. It is seen as a sudden lysis of the condyle creating a rapid change in the bite of the individual with shift of the jaw and resultant open bite, which is notable by the subject. The etiology of condylysis is not clear but has been known to be associated in young females with rheumatoid arthritis.[65]

Ankylosis is usually related to trauma to the joint with subsequent bleeding and restricted mandibular movement; ankylosis may be fibrous or bony in nature. Fibrous ankylosis usually is seen in the upper joint compartment as a result of adhesions forming after a joint bleed and prolonged immobility. Limited jaw opening (usually one or two fingers placed horizontally between the central incisors) is typically present. Bony ankylosis has no movement associated

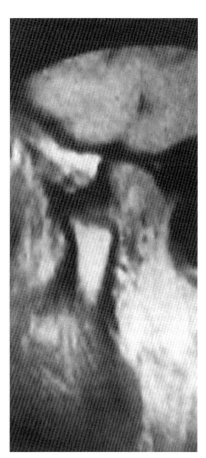

Figure 25–10. Magnetic resonance image of a degenerative joint. The disk is folded in front of the head of the condyle, thus preventing full opening of the mandible.

with it. Both conditions may require surgical release followed by postsurgical mobilization techniques.[64]

Fracture, caused by trauma to any part of the face, may result in bony fractures of the condylar neck, condylar head, body of the mandible, and maxilla and temporal fossa and may result in reduction in opening, pain, and fibrosis of bony ankylosis if untreated. Uncomplicated (nondisplaced) fractures require no immediate treatment as long as function is not compromised.[64]

MUSCULAR DISORDERS OF THE CRANIOFACIAL COMPLEX

Muscular pain and dysfunction are the most common symptoms in patients with temporomandibular disorders. The masticatory muscles are affected in a fashion similar to other striated skeletal muscles of the body. Because the ligaments, nerves, and muscles function as a complex unit to stabilize the head, maintain functional airway space, and allow for three-dimensional movement of the mandible (i.e., craniocervical-mandibular or the stomatognathic system), breakdown of this complex and finely tuned system may commonly result in muscular disorders leading to pain in the head, face, and neck. For consistency this section also follows the International Headache Society's Classification and Diagnostic Criteria for Headache Disorders, Cranial Neuralgias, and Facial Pain[1] (see Box 25–2), which addresses the issue of muscle pain under the following headings: (1) myalgia caused by trauma, (2) myalgia secondary to parafunction, (3) myalgia secondary to postural hypertonicity, (4) myofascial pain, (5) reflex splinting/trismus, (6) spasm (sustained), (7) myositis, and (8) contracture (fibrosis).

Myalgia as a Result of Trauma

Tissue injury initiates an inflammatory reaction that induces pain.[39] The exact nature of the pain depends on the location, severity, and type of injury. Injury in a muscle that does not have constant use allows for resolution of the inflammatory process. For masticatory muscles, it is difficult to completely eliminate movement because of the need for speech, swallowing, and chewing, which may contribute to a prolonged healing process.

Masticatory muscle injury can occur from acute muscle strain or direct trauma. Soft-tissue injury results in bleeding, inflammation, and swelling causing myalgia, muscle spasm, muscle splinting, or myositis.[66] Myofascial trigger points may occur in many locations within the muscle and are considered[67] the primary source of muscular pain.

Injury results in a deep sharp ache on contraction of the muscle. Depending on the area of injury, the pain may emanate from the tendon attachments (tendinitis), fascial component (myofascitis), or body of the muscle (myospasm and myositis). The temporalis tendon attachment to the coronoid process is the most frequent site of masticatory tendinitis. In the presence of acute or chronic internal derangement of the TMJ complex, the muscles that support and move the joints can be secondarily affected. Protective muscle splinting prevents further injury to the joint. Immobilization of the injured joint is frequently seen with anterior disk displacement without reduction (closed lock). Splinting of the masticatory elevator muscles is maintained until the joint is healed.

The presence of elevator spasm may cause a health care provider who is unfamiliar with TMD to prescribe muscle relaxants; however, these agents may lead to more injury, whereas proper treatment of the joint's internal derangement would result in cessation of the muscle splinting. If the internal derangement is not adequately treated, the muscles remain chronically shortened and may eventually undergo contracture.[68] A patient with acute closed lock often presents with a history of clicking and may not be able to pinpoint an eliciting event. The patient may awaken with the jaw locked, whereas at other times, it may occur during mastication. Typically, the patient will have loss of posterior support through tooth wear, tooth breakdown, or missing or poorly restored posterior teeth.[68] Treatment may require dental surgery under general endotracheal anesthesia to allow the joints to relocate back because the normal protection afforded by the muscles is missing.

Closed lock may be accompanied by a change in occlusion resulting from disk displacement or spasm of the lateral pterygoid. There may be a shift of the occlusion to the contralateral side with a corresponding posterior open bite developing on the ipsilateral side. The patient may attempt to position the posterior teeth into contact but is hampered by joint pain and the lateral pterygoid, pulling the mandible in the opposite side.[69-72]

In acute trauma, the occlusion settles back to its preinjured state once the TMJ inflammation has subsided. However, the joint will continue to be loaded and healing will be delayed if the patient has a parafunctional habit or a decreased vertical dimension.[68] In such cases, the joint may become chronically inflamed and the muscles of mastication may continue to be in a state of protective splinting or spasm.

If a patient has a combination of acute trauma, loss of posterior teeth, and moderate to severe parafunction, anterior disk displacement with intermittent locking of the TMJ will likely occur. Patients often report a history of trauma followed by a variable period of clicking, progressively increasing in frequency and culminating in abrupt disappearance of sound and inability to open the mouth. The differential of sound diagnosis of a patient who has limited opening must include internal derangement and muscle trismus.

Myalgia secondary to injury of the cervical spine can affect the masticatory muscles and result in headaches and facial pain. Once the masticatory muscles are secondarily affected they in turn affect the mandibular position. Mandibular dysfunction results from masticatory muscle involvement and in tightening up the muscles of the cervical spine, thereby perpetuating the cycle. As such, a significant proportion of TMD patients also present with a history of cervical injury, thus treatment of this craniofacial and cervical syndrome requires that both the jaw and neck be treated in a multidisciplinary manner.[73]

Muscle disorders may occur secondarily to rotations, fixations, fusions, or injury, or locking of the facets of the cervical, thoracic, lumbar, and sacral vertebrae. The history, physical examination, and radiographic evaluation will elucidate the acuteness and severity of the vertebral problem. Disk herniations can secondarily affect the cervical muscles through protective splinting, which can eventually lead to chronic postural changes. Nerve impingement and nerve root injuries also can affect muscle function. Cervical problems are frequently comorbid conditions seen in TMD patients[73,74] (Fig. 25–11). A reduction in the space between the posterior spine of the atlas and base of the occiput[75] may cause pain by compression of the suboccipital tissues. The pain will be perceived as a headache starting from the back of the head.[76]

Acute or long-standing trauma can cause a shift in the occiput/atlas relationship and may lead to chronic tension in the suboccipital muscles with resulting fixation and nerve irritation of the C1 and C2 nerves.

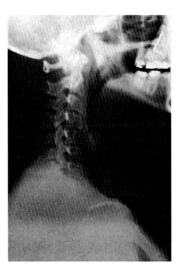

Figure 25–11. Cervical radiograph of patient with whiplash injury. Note the loss of normal curve, especially at C4-C6; also note the reduction of the suboccipital space between occiput and atlas. (From Kaplan AS, Assael LA: Temporomandibular Disorders: Diagnosis and Treatment. Philadelphia, Saunders, 1991.)

The pain will be referred from the back of the head to the eye, side of the head, skin over the TMJ, and angle of the mandible, radiating into the neck. Rotation of the atlas is commonly seen in patients with TMD and may be linked to changes in occlusal contact patterns and instability of mandibular position.[77] Osteoarthritic degeneration and ligament and muscle injury also occur at this level in acceleration-deceleration injuries. A disruption of the CI-C2 articulation also may result in excessive stretching or kinking of the vertebral artery, which may lead to temporary vertebrobasilar syndrome with symptoms of vertigo, nausea, tinnitus, and visual disturbances.[78]

The patient with a combined craniofacial cervical syndrome will have a history of direct or indirect injury to the head and neck. The injury is usually a low-grade impact to the body that causes a sudden twist or flexion extension of the neck. Symptoms may include headaches, nausea, visual disturbances, neck weakness, pain, and stiffness accompanied by noises on rotation, flexion, and extension of the head. Depending on the level of the initial injury, branches of the cervical and brachial plexus also may be affected. Secondary muscles affected can cause superimposed acute or chronic pain. Occlusal appliances may be worn to reduce muscle tension.[79]

Myalgia Secondary to Parafunction

Oral parafunction includes bruxism, clenching, lip biting, thumb sucking, and any other oral habit not associated with mastication, deglutition, and speech. Bruxism and clenching are the most common of the parafunctional activities with a prevalence of up to 90% in the general population.[80,81] In most patients, parafunction occurs in a milder intermittent form and does not require treatment. Moderate or severe bruxism and clenching can damage oral structures causing wear of the teeth, breakdown of the periodontium in the presence of inflammation, and internal derangement and muscular dysfunction.[82]

Studies on bruxism and clenching have reported excessive force occurring for extended periods (normal tooth contact during a 24-hour period is about 20 minutes, occurring during chewing and swallowing).[83] Parafunctional forces exceed normal masticatory forces with the resultant force vector primarily horizontal. Under such conditions, damage is likely to occur to the teeth and periodontium. Ironically, most treatments are designed to protect the occlusion in function rather than in parafunction. The detrimental effects of parafunction will cause breakdown in the weakest structure, which may include teeth, periodontium, TMJ, or muscles. The patient can therefore present with both tooth and joint pathology.[82]

Bruxism and clenching have been explained historically by theories of occlusion, but to date have yet to be substantiated by research. Nocturnal bruxism is currently classified as a sleep disorder, the duration and intensity of which vary nightly based on the emotional stress and before-sleep activities of the individual. Sleep studies have shown that bruxism occurs during body movement and the rapid eye movement (REM) stage of sleep and during the transition from a deeper to a lighter stage of sleep.[84]

Numerous studies have been done on the personality characteristics of "bruxers."[85-88] People who clench and grind their teeth have been shown to exhibit higher degrees of anxiety, aggressiveness, and hostility. The conclusions of these and other studies have confirmed an emotional etiology of diurnal (daytime) parafunction,[89-91] which includes lip biting, nailbiting, thumb sucking, clenching, and habitual bruxism. The pathologic effects are the same as those for nocturnal parafunction.

Associated internal derangement of the TMJ can occur in the presence of myalgia of the elevator or lateral pterygoid muscles. Excessive contraction of the elevator muscles will load the TMJ if posterior tooth support has been compromised. Chronic contraction of the lateral pterygoid muscle from parafunction may predispose a patient to internal derangement if there is attachment to the articular disk. Excessive muscle tension generated during sleep may cause muscle tears and myositis with swelling. Patients may present with pain in the cervical muscles due to chronic bruxism and clenching. Electromyographic studies have shown an interrelationship of cervical muscle activity and occlusal contact. The patient may report restless sleep, waking up with limited mandibular range of motion and headache, facial pain, and neck pain. The pain and stiffness usually improve as the day progresses; thus if a patient complains of stiffness and pain increasing as the day progresses, diurnal activity should be suspected. The patient may report high levels of stress and depression. Palpable muscle soreness primarily affects the elevators and the lateral pterygoid. Increased pain

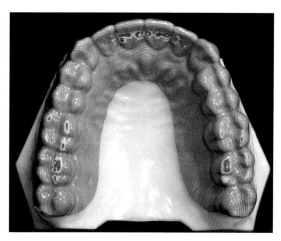

Figure 25–12. Bruxcore device for monitoring tooth grinding or clenching. The multiple layers allow for quantifying by surface microdots missing and depth by color change.

will be noted if the patient is asked to clench on the wear facets by moving the mandible laterally—a provocation test.

A testing device known as a Bruxcore has been used as a means of quantifying nocturnal activity[92] (Fig. 25–12). A portable electromyographic biofeedback instrument also has been used to monitor bruxism.[93] A tape recorder can monitor bruxing noises but is not very reliable because clenching does not produce significant noise. Repeated monitoring on different nights at a sleep laboratory will give the most accurate monitoring; however, this is rarely necessary. Electromyographic analysis may show a higher resting tension level than normal but is dependent on the specific type of muscle disorder and the specific muscle being analyzed.

The treatment of parafunctional activity includes therapeutic modalities for stress management including biofeedback, medication, and psychological counseling. The goal is to decrease parafunction to within the adaptive capacity of the individual. Protective treatment of the oral structures is best accomplished with occlusal appliances, worn at night, during the day, or both, that reduce loading on the TMJ, stress on the dentition and periodontium, and muscle activity[94] (Figs. 25–13 and 25–14).

Myalgia Secondary to Postural Hypertonicity

A healthy craniocervical complex maintains a stable head position through a series of learned complex antagonistic muscle interactions. Studies on different head postures have shown that forward head posture (FHP) leads to shortening and greater tension of the posterior cervical muscles.[78] The trapezius, sternocleidomastoid, and deeper muscles contract to prevent the head from tipping forward, leading to muscle hyperactivity and chronic tension.

Often the patient develops a level of tension that leads to pain. Over time, shortened muscles tend to develop trigger points that may result in a loss of

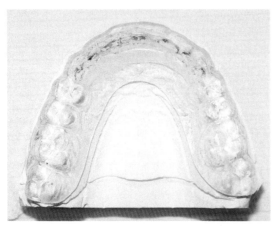

Figure 25–13. A maxillary dental night guard with anterior contact to reduce bruxism forces helps unload teeth and allows muscles and nerves to relax. The guard is usually made of dental acrylic.

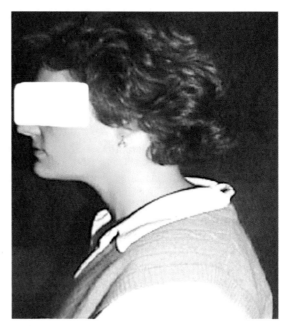

Figure 25–15. Patient with a forward head posture and rounded shoulders due to adaptive work position.

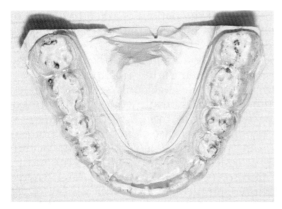

Figure 25–14. Lower hard full-coverage bite plate usually worn during the day, for patients with maxillomandibular dysfunction. Contact is usually bilateral and equal.

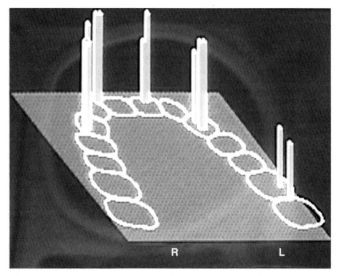

Figure 25–16. T-Scan electronic bite assessment of the patient in Figure 25–15 with head in forward position as in previous figure.

normal cervical lordosis.[78] The body adapts to FHP by rounding of the shoulders, leading to chronic shortening of the pectoral muscles, which further maintains FHP. Pectoral muscle tension along with FHP leads to upper thoracic breathing and tighter intercostal muscles. The anterior and middle scalenes may entrap the brachial plexus at the thoracic outlet, or the first rib can be pulled up to the clavicle resulting in costoclavicular entrapment.[78]

Mehta and Forgione[95] have discussed the effect of chronic forward head posture and the relative position of the occiput, atlas, and axis with respect to each other and the craniomandibular complex. FHP and cervical muscle tension can lead to changes in occlusal contacts. Analyzing occlusal contact in maximum intercuspation with the patient in a supine position will not allow an accurate evaluation of occlusion in function. Likewise, posture and stability of the cervical region should be considered before definitive occlusal therapy is instituted (Figs. 25–15 to 25–17).

Proper positioning during sleep is important for resting the postural muscles. A patient who habitually sleeps on his or her stomach and twists the neck at 90 degrees experiences the same effects as the individual who keeps the head turned to one side all day long. People who sleep on their sides with the arms outstretched under the pillow and head may have a tendency to entrap the brachial plexus at the costoclavicular level. This side position can be abusive to the cervical muscles and can result in acute torticollis of the sternocleidomastoid muscle. Neck stiffness and trigger points are observed in patients with sleep habits that involve strained head positions.

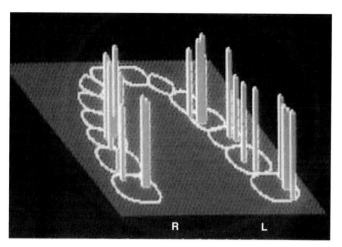

Figure 25–17. Same patient's bite with head in a more upright posture and shoulders straight. Note the shift of the bite to the posterior even position.

Standing posture may be affected by leg length discrepancies, hip rotation, and flat feet, all of which may contribute to cervical and low back symptoms. Shoes that are uneven or have extremely high heels tend to cause a secondary protective adjustment of the postural muscles that may result in chronic muscular shortening, trigger points, and spasm. Shifts in body posture and compensatory cervical changes affect mandibular position and tooth contact patterns.[27] Clinically the patient reports pain and stiffness related to sleep or daily activity accompanied by chronic aching in the postural cervical muscles especially evident in the trapezius and sternocleidomastoid. The patient may report a feeling of the head being too heavy on the neck and pain and burning at the root of the neck. Other presenting signs include pain on palpation including trigger points and acute spasm, limited active range of motion with pain, and FHP. Cervical and spinal plain films, CT, or MRI scans may be needed to evaluate spinal curvature and to rule out other pathology. The treatment of the affected muscle groups and correction of the posture include short-term exercise to increase range of motion and improve postural position, muscle re-education to strengthen the muscles in the therapeutic postural position, and maintenance of muscle flexibility with a home exercise program to maintain the therapeutic postural position.[66]

Myofascial Pain and Trigger Points

A myofascial trigger point is defined as a hyperirritable locus within a taut band of skeletal muscle that is located in muscular tissue or in its associated fascia or tendon. The spot is painful on compression and can evoke characteristic referred pain and autonomic phenomena.[67] Active trigger points may cause pain spontaneously or during movement. Latent trigger points, which affect almost half of the population by

early adulthood,[93] are usually not painful but create weakness and restriction of movement in a muscle. These trigger points can be activated by sudden overloading contraction, viral infection, cold temperature, fatigue, and increased emotional stress. Because of the complex nature of the myofascial trigger points and their common presence in acute and chronic muscle dysfunction, an understanding of their clinical features is necessary. According to Travell and Simons,[96] there are seven clinical features:

- Local tenderness over the trigger point
- Referred pain, tenderness, and autonomic phenomena
- Palpable taut band associated with the trigger points
- A local twitch response of a trigger point is usually present in a palpable taut band
- Perpetuation of trigger points
- A therapeutic effect when stretching a muscle with trigger points
- Weakness and fatigability of muscles afflicted with trigger points

Myofascial pain often refers pain to the head and neck, which is considered by some to constitute tension-type headaches. Myofascial pain and trigger points of the masticatory muscles can send pain to the eyes, ears, TMJ, and the teeth depending on the specific muscles. The pain is usually a dull or intense ache that varies but is strongly related to posture or muscle activity and can usually be localized by the patient on a diagrammatic representation of the body. The muscles of posture and mastication are commonly affected by trigger points. The pain may occur in the same dermatome, myotome, or sclerotome. Satellite trigger points may occur within the pain reference zone. Clinically there is a restricted movement with pain on passive stretching, and strong contraction dramatically increases pain. Resistive testing reveals weakness caused by protective splinting.

Trigger points are palpated by rubbing the fingertip lightly along the long axis of the muscle. If present, a taut band is located first, then the more sensitive trigger point. Applying pressure on a trigger point elicits a grimace or an involuntary sound from the patient called the "jump sign." Snapping palpation of the taut band produces a local twitch response (LTR), confirming the presence of the trigger point. Final confirmation comes on reproduction of the patient's pain by digital pressure.[96]

Pressure algometers quantify the amount of pressure applied to the trigger point, which allows the clinician to document the severity of the trigger point and may be used to objectively record the efficacy of treatment (Fig. 25–18).

Thermography may help visualize "hot spots" that are 5 to 10 cm in diameter, although it is not clear if the thermographic presentation reflects the trigger point itself or zone of referred pain. As such, thermography has little application in differentiating a trigger point from a referred pain zone.

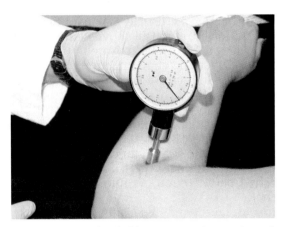

Figure 25–18. Pressure threshold meter to test for muscle tenderness or trigger points.

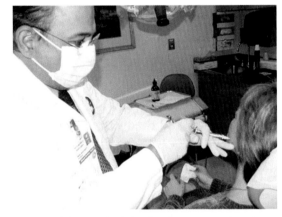

Figure 25–19. Trigger point injection for trigger point of masseter.

The treatment of myofascial trigger points includes spraying the involved muscle with ethyl chloride or fluoromethane followed by stretching, hot compresses, and range-of-motion exercises. Trigger point injections of procaine (0.5% solution in saline) or lidocaine (2% without epinephrine) have also been commonly used (Fig. 25–19) along with botulinum toxin (Botox) more recently. Other techniques involve ischemic compression for 30 to 60 seconds and acupressure. Pharmacologic treatments include analgesics, muscle relaxants, antidepressants, and NSAIDs. Physical therapy modalities such as myofascial release and craniosacral technique including postural correction and exercise have been effective in managing myofascial trigger points. Stress and nutritional and hormonal factors also should be addressed.[94] With the masticatory muscles, occlusal appliances may be used.[42,79] Dental guards or appliances have been found to be effective in reducing muscle symptoms and trigger points in mandibular elevators (see Figs. 25–13 and 25–16).

Muscle Splinting

Muscle splinting[78] is a reflex mechanism in which skeletal muscles stabilize an injured area and protect it from further injury. The involved muscles become hypertonic and painful. An associated feeling of weakness, although alarming to the patient, is a normal body defense to reduce function of the affected part. Muscle splinting often is a sequela to muscle injury and follows myositis. If splinting remains over a protracted period, muscle spasm may follow, leading to a chronic cycle of myofascial pain and dysfunction.[76]

In the masticatory system, splinting of the elevator muscles may affect dental occlusal contact patterns. Because of the accompanying weakness, occlusal forces and chewing are affected. Pain limits jaw activity, mimicking trismus or an anteriorly displaced disk without reduction (closed lock). Injury to the cervical muscles causes protective splinting and decreased mobility of the head and neck. The accompanying weakness is frightening to patients, who report that they cannot keep their head upright for any appreciable period of time. Pain in the cervical muscles is present with reduced movement of the head and neck.

Pain is elicited on palpation and stretching of the masticatory muscle. Muscle tightness and muscle weakness may be noticed during evaluation of range of motion and muscle palpation. Electromyographic changes are not seen during rest. Electromyographic activity of the masticatory muscles is normal as activity is increased until pain is experienced, at which point the activity is decreased in response to the splinting action. Thermography does not show any change unless myositis is present.

Initially, therapy should consist of restriction of movement of the affected area, although if there is a noticeable shift of the mandible, the patient may complain of difficulty in keeping the mandible in a relaxed position. An intraoral splint during this acute phase allows for occlusal stability. As healing progresses, the dental splint may need to be adjusted or withdrawn to permit return to normal occlusion.[78] In the presence of pain that results from an inability of the muscles to maintain a stable head posture, a reverse soft cervical collar may be prescribed until initial healing occurs. This modification prevents the mandible from being displaced by the collar thereby secondarily affecting the TMJ. Once the muscles are capable of normal control, the collar should not be worn. Injections initially are not indicated. Ice, rest, and relaxation form the basis of acute therapy. Stretching, ultrasound, or light massage can be used in the initial stages. Once the muscles have started to heal, splinting decreases. At this stage, muscle therapy can begin with an aim to regain mobility. Mobilization techniques, gentle stretching, and range-of-motion exercises are required to prevent ongoing myospasm, contracture, and atrophy.

Muscle Spasm (Sustained)

A muscle spasm is defined as the painful contraction of a striated muscle caused by trauma, tension, or disease.[64,66] The spasm manifests as pain and interference in function. Muscular fiber contractions occur in response to increased excitability of alpha motoneurons. The maintenance of a muscle spasm is thought to be caused by the ischemia induced in a skeletal muscle by its continued contraction. With muscle fatigue, lactic acid accumulates, leading to the release of bradykinin and pain. In the masticatory musculature, a spasm of the masseter or temporalis muscle results in limited range of motion, which in turn causes a deflection to the ipsilateral side on opening. If a spasm is isometric, the muscle is rigid and resistant to stretch. Condylar position can be affected in true spasm of the elevator muscles and may predispose a patient to internal derangement. In a true spasm of the elevator muscles, the patient presents with an inability to separate the upper and lower teeth. In the cervical area, a muscle spasm can create severe pain and rigidity of the neck, secondary vertebral shifts and locking, entrapment of nerves with pain radiating to the innervated area, and forced adaptation to a new postural position, eventually affecting the middle and low back muscles. In addition to severe headaches and dysfunction, cervical immobility has been known to affect the maxillomandibular relationship, resulting in a malocclusion.

Spastic muscles must be differentiated from the painful soft muscle of myositis, relatively normal albeit painful muscle splinting, and localized taut bands and areas of myofascial trigger points. A muscle in spasm has a stiff hard surface that is painfully resistant to stretch. Electromyographic recordings show a high degree of standing tension but a decrease in electromyographic activity in contrast to the contralateral side. Pressure threshold meters and tissue compliance measurements may be useful for identification of the particular muscles in spasm. Thermography is also being investigated for routine diagnostic use.[97-99]

Initial treatment should be directed toward eliminating the cycling spasm. The patient should be restricted to movement within painless limits, but some function is necessary to regain a normal stretch reflex, which helps relax the muscle. In spasm of a masticatory muscle a stabilization (flat plane) appliance can be used to disengage the teeth if there is sufficient opening to be able to make a temporary emergency splint. Splints are thought to work by shutting off proprioceptive input from the teeth, which may play a role in the maintenance of spastic activity. Muscle relaxants administered judiciously can help reduce dysfunction and spasm and act as adjuncts to other therapy such as injections, spray and stretch techniques using vapocoolants (ethyl chloride or fluoromethane spray), and massage and acupressure techniques.[78,100] As the muscle starts to respond to treatment, stretching and range-of-motion exercises can be instituted to prevent contractures and bring the muscle into full function.[55] The use of passive jaw motion exercises is suggested for ongoing range-of-motion therapy. Structural factors such as the bite should be corrected only after the muscle is pain-free and fully functional.[78]

Myositis

Injury caused by a direct blow to a muscle can trigger a localized inflammatory response accompanied by swelling, pain, and immobilization of the part.[78] Pain is described generally as dull, deep, boring, and constant. Episodes of sharp pain related to movement of the affected area also may be reported. Injury to the head and neck muscles results in an accompanying reduction in neck movement along with changes in shoulder height and head posture as a means of protecting against further trauma. The pain may be perceived by the patient as a headache. An accompanying feeling of weakness in the neck will be experienced.

Patients with myositis of the masticatory musculature may complain of pain in the face or jaw accompanied by a change in the bite with inability to chew, swallow, and speak comfortably. Locally, the area may appear swollen and discolored because of extravasation of inflammatory products. An inflamed muscle on palpation is evident as a soft painful mass. Pain is associated with active as well as passive movement of the affected part. The skin surface may be warm to touch. The patient may present with low-grade fever if there is secondary infection. Surface electromyographic evaluation shows a low resting tension and an inability of the muscle to function fully as a result of protective splinting, evidenced by low electromyographic readings. Pressure threshold measurements, using a threshold meter, show a reduction from the baseline threshold of force that induces discomfort. Thermography demonstrates increased temperature over the site of injury. Proximal to the injury may be a cold spot showing vasoconstriction, which may affect healing.

The initial therapy of the acute symptoms of myositis includes the immediate application of ice to the affected part to reduce swelling. Mouth opening should be restricted, a dental intraoral bite guard is used to control closure, and an NSAID is typically prescribed. A methylprednisolone (Medrol) dose pack can be ordered to control the swelling and an antibiotic added if there is secondary infection. After the acute symptoms have subsided, treatment includes heat and mobilization of the affected area and institution of an exercise program to regain full range of motion followed by a muscle-strengthening program.

Fibrosis and Contracture

Myotatic contracture occurs in muscles that are not allowed to function within their full range of motion. The muscle tends to lose its stretch reflex capabilities, and a gradual shortening of the muscle occurs. Pain or immobilization of a part for a prolonged period leads to myotatic contracture.[64]

In the masticatory musculature, this problem occurs secondary to the inability of patients to open their mouths fully. Patients frequently report avoiding opening wide for fear of hearing clicking or crepitus, whereas others may not open wide because of pain. Over time, this practice leads to the development of a habituated protective pattern causing myotatic contracture. Likewise, restricted movement of the cervical region results in myotatic contracture. This condition is alleviated with treatment.

Myofibrotic contracture often occurs as a result of an inflammatory process leading to fibrous changes in the muscle or its sheath. Trauma to a muscle and the resultant inflammation and muscle splinting may lead to irreversible fibrosis. Radiation therapy, incision through a muscle with fibrotic healing, and disuse for long periods (>6 weeks) also can result in myofibrotic contracture. In patients with masticatory muscle involvement, myotatic or myofibrotic contracture appears with limited interincisal opening. If the elevator muscles are involved, there is deviation on opening but not on protrusion, and lateral movement is normal.

Pain is not present unless there is sudden and forceful stretching or biting. Usually a history of injury or long-term immobility of the mandible exists. Acute or chronic malocclusion does not occur as a result of contracture. Palpation generally does not elicit pain, especially with a myofibrotic type of contracture.

Decreased electromyographic activity is seen when the muscle is contracted. Pressure and pain tolerance meters show lower thresholds. Plain radiography, CT scan, arthrography, or MRI scan of the TMJ can be done to rule out internal derangement.

The treatment for myotatic contracture is gradual stretching of the involved muscle with ultrasound used as adjunct therapy. Massage and myofascial release along with daily stretching and exercise bring the muscle slowly back to function. Myofibrotic contracture is irreversible and requires surgical intervention for a patient whose function is severely impaired.

GENERAL MANAGEMENT OF TEMPORO-MANDIBULAR DISORDER PATIENTS

The overall management goals mimic those of other orthopedic or rheumatologic disorders. In the craniofacial and cervical patients, the reduction of occlusal loading, stabilization of the TMJ, and relaxation of muscles allow for easier function of the joint. Because the majority of patients with temporomandibular disorders present with a chronic pain history of the head and neck, multidisciplinary management tends to be more successful than individual treatments. Conservative management techniques aimed at behavioral modification, supportive medication, physical medicine, and intraoral occlusal guards tend to be successful in 85% to 90% of patients. The key to successful management is accurate diagnosis of the precipitating and perpetuating factors in the individual.

It is well documented that chronic pain and disability have a strong psychological component and most patients require some form of treatment ranging from simple home health tips on time management and cognitive behavioral intervention to structured psychological and psychiatric intervention, which may include a comprehensive stress management program (sleep management, electromyography [EMG] biofeedback, and progressive relaxation) and lifestyle changes. Physical medicine treatments address the structural aspects of temporomandibular and craniocervical disorders and may include myofascial and craniosacral physical therapy, orthopedic correction for the cervical spine, muscle education, and TMJ pain relief therapies (ultrasound, pulsed radiofrequency energy, transcutaneous electrical nerve stimulation [TENS]). Medications for pain or sleep and specific psychiatric and nerve-related issues should be instituted during the course of other treatments. Modification of the patient's nutritional factors, daily activities, and posture is important to the overall effectiveness of the treatment program.

Patients who present with craniocervical and mandibular dysfunctions and a history of trauma often have chronic headaches and neck pain in addition to the specific TMD. In these patients it is beneficial to add orthopedic intraoral appliances, referred to as night guards, bite plates, bite splints, or bruxism guards, which are effective in relaxing jaw muscles, relieving jaw and joint pain, and stabilizing the maxillomandibular bite relationship. These appliances should be used as a short-term treatment until symptoms subside. In some cases in which the patient needs to wear the guard for longer periods, an upper nighttime guard and lower daytime guard may be given to protect against developing dental decay or periodontal breakdown. Dental corrections of the bite should not be attempted until the pain and dysfunction have subsided. Surgery of the TMJ is usually not initially recommended unless there is an acute injury or a specific joint-related problem that has not been resolved with nonsurgical management.

Neuropathic Pain Syndromes

Neuropathic pain syndromes result from pathology in the peripheral or central nervous system. These disorders are particularly common in the head and neck, probably a result of the dense and specialized sensory innervation of this region. For practical purposes, craniocervical neuropathic pain disorders can be divided into two main groups: (1) trigeminal neuralgia (TN) and (2) a more heterogeneous group of neuralgic disorders termed "painful post-traumatic trigeminal neuropathy" (PTN) (see Box 25–3).

Trigeminal Neuralgia

TN is a well-recognized disorder characterized by brief paroxysms of severe, unilateral, electric pain in the trigeminal region. TN has an incidence of 4 per 100,000 people.[101,102] The condition is most common in adults older than age 50, and women are affected only slightly more often than men[103]; however, TN has no geographic or ethnic preference. The pain in TN typically consists of "lightning bolts" of momentary pain that radiate within the second or third trigeminal divisions. In individual patients, the attacks are stereotyped, typically recurring with the same intensity and in the same distribution. Despite the severity of TN pain, however, most patients are symptom-free between attacks and exhibit a normal clinical sensory examination between pain episodes.[104-108] Many TN patients demonstrate a discrete (<10 mm) sensory "trigger zone" in the oral mucosa or perioral skin; light touch or thermal stimulation within the trigger zone evokes a TN pain attack. Although a trigger zone is not a requirement for TN, the presence of a trigger zone is pathognomonic for the TN diagnosis. White and Sweet[109] emphasized that TN has five major clinical features:

- The pain is paroxysmal.
- The pain is confined to the trigeminal distribution.
- The pain is unilateral.
- The bedside clinical sensory examination is normal.
- The pain may be provoked by light touch to the face (trigger zones).

These criteria were incorporated, largely unchanged, into the official research diagnostic criteria published by the International Association for the Study of Pain[110] and the International Headache Society[1] (see Box 25–3). TN appears to result from a chronic, partial injury to the trigeminal sensory nerve root as it enters the brainstem.[105-108,111-114] Consistent with this view is the presence of a separate disease process affecting the trigeminal nerve roots in 5% to 10% of patients with TN symptoms. This is usually multiple sclerosis (MS) or a benign tumor (schwannoma, meningioma) in the cerebellopontine angle (CPA). These cases are usually termed *symptomatic trigeminal neuralgia*. In the remaining majority of TN cases, imaging studies and laboratory tests are negative. These cases are usually termed *idiopathic trigeminal neuralgia*. Despite the idiopathic label, increasing evidence documents that subtle forms of chronic nerve root injury (such as compression by a vascular loop) produce trigeminal root irritation in these cases.

In summary, the diagnosis of TN is based on a clinical history consistent with widely accepted, specific diagnostic criteria. For patients that meet the criteria, a careful physical examination and cranial imaging studies are essential to differentiate primary from symptomatic TN.

Clinical Management

Medical as well as surgical treatments are available to manage the severe pain attacks of TN. The present authors use a diagnostic and management algorithm for TN. The patients should initially receive a trial of medical therapy with an antiepileptic drug (AED) (Boxes 25–9 and 25–10). A series of clinical trials during the past 50 years demonstrate that oral AEDs

---

BOX 25–9. ANTICONVULSANTS

- Phenytoin (Dilantin)
- Carbamazepine (Tegretol)
- Baclofen (Lioresal)*
- Clonazepam (Klonopin)
- Gabapentin (Neurontin)
- Lamotrigine (Lamictal)
- Topiramate (Topamax)
- Oxcarbazepine (Trileptal)
- Tiagabine (Gabitril)
- Levetiracetam (Keppra)
- Zonisamide (Zonegran)
- Pregabalin (Lyrica)
  - Lidocaine
  - Mexiletine (Mexitil)

*Baclofen is a muscle relaxant with CNS effects and is effective in treating TN as part of a combined therapy.

BOX 25–10. PHARMACOLOGIC EFFECT AND MECHANISM OF PAIN RELIEF

- CBZ   Na channel
- OXC
- CLO   GABA
- BAC   GABA-B
- GBP   Na, Ca channel
- LTG   Na channel, inh GLU
- TOP   Na channel, GABA, AMPA
- TGB   GABA RI
- Suppress spontaneous ectopic neuronal activity
- Reduce neuronal hypersensitivity
- Segmental inhibition of signaling

AMPA, alpha amino-3-hydroxy-5-methylisoxazole-4-propionic acid; BAC, baclofen; CBZ, carbamazepine; CLO, clonazepam; GABA, gamma-aminobutyric acid; GBP, gabapentin; GLU, glutamate; LTG, lamotrigine; Na, sodium; OXC, oxcarbazepine; TGB, tiagabine; TOP, topiramate.

---

are effective in TN with gabapentin or carbamazepine as the initial drugs of choice, with baclofen as part of a combined therapy. The AED dosage should be progressively increased to therapeutic "anticonvulsant" levels. Single-drug AED therapy provides substantial relief from the recurrent attacks of facial pain in the large majority of TN patients. If a patient does not respond to single AED therapy, adding a second AED may increase the chance of a therapeutic response. The lack of response of the patient to the AEDs warrants a search for other causes of the patient's pain.

Surgical options are also available for patients in a variety of clinical situations. Three procedures are commonly recommended:

- Percutaneous retrogasserian radiofrequency lesion[115-117]

- Posterior fossa microvascular decompression[118-120]
- Gamma knife radiotherapy[121,122]

These procedures substantially reduce or eliminate pain attacks in as many as 90% of TN patients.

Atypical Trigeminal Neuralgia

Many authors use the diagnosis "atypical TN"[123-125] to describe cases in which the clinical findings do not fully meet the standard diagnostic criteria for TN. However, there is general agreement that atypical TN patients are less responsive to anticonvulsants and surgical intervention than patients with "standard" TN.[125-131] It is reasonable to assume that the TN is probably neither homogeneous nor unique; however, the general diagnosis of atypical TN seems misleading because the term does not identify a meaningful subset of TN patients that could be examined more closely. Nonetheless, the clinical problem of atypical TN is a real one because patients suffering from complex facial pain disorders often present with a spectrum of symptoms, some of which may be quite similar to the TN criteria.

PAINFUL POST-TRAUMATIC TRIGEMINAL NEUROPATHY

A significant number of patients develop chronic facial pain following trauma to sensory nerves in the craniocervical region.[132,133] These cases are distinct from TN, and usually grouped according to the nature and location of the painful nerve damage (neuralgia). We usually classify this group under the heading "painful post-traumatic trigeminal neuropathy" (PTN). Patients with PTN exhibit chronic or recurrent pain in the area of the previous nerve injury, numbness, dysesthesias, and chronic burning sensations. Diagnostic evaluations rule out any other cause of pain. Most craniocervical neuralgias meet these general PTN criteria although individual clinical features vary depending on the specific syndrome. Common examples of craniocervical neuralgias include postherpetic neuralgia, inferior alveolar neuralgia following mandibular third molar extraction, and infraorbital neuralgia following maxillary trauma.

Patients with PTN represent a significant clinical challenge because the symptoms of PTN respond poorly, if at all, to AED or surgical therapies commonly used in TN. The general approach to clinical management in PTN is similar to that for other forms of neuropathic pain and discussed in Chapter 21.

CONCLUSION

Craniocervical pain is a common clinical complaint and often a diagnostic challenge. Given the complex anatomy of the region and the numerous discrete syndromes, a multidisciplinary approach is frequently indicated for the evaluation of difficult or refractory cases.

SUMMARY

- Pain syndromes that involve the face, head, and neck are very common in clinical practice. These syndromes are often unique, and deserving of special attention.
- The common descriptive terms for cranial pain complaints are frequently misleading. To avoid confusion, pain clinicians should be familiar with the International Headache Society's Classification and Diagnostic Criteria for Headache Disorders, Cranial Neuralgias, and Facial Pain. Clinicians should be comfortable distinguishing painful conditions that arise from structural pathology, headache syndromes, myofascial pain disorders, and primary neuralgias.
- Clinicians should be familiar with the clinically relevant features of craniocervical anatomy and distinctive neurobiology of pain transmission in this region.
- Chronic/recurrent pain syndromes are extremely common in the head and neck, and myofascial pain disorders are among the most common causes of pain and dysfunction in this group. Myofascial syndromes overlap several common diagnoses, including TMJ myofascial pain dysfunction syndrome, tension headache, and most cases of occipital neuralgia. Pain clinicians should be aware of the diagnostic features, potential causes, and exacerbating factors for such disorders. Pain clinicians should also understand how these factors are associated with the various multidisciplinary options currently recommended for treatment.
- Pain clinicians should be aware of the unique anatomy and physiology of the TMJ, and how jaw position and dental occlusion can contribute to myofascial pain symptoms.
- Bruxism and sleep disorders are common contributors to craniocervical pain that occurs in the morning.
- Bite appliances in conjunction with stress management and physical therapy may be a viable treatment option for patients with craniofacial and myofascial pain.
- Trigeminal neuralgia (TN) is a unique neurogenic disorder. Patients who meet the clinical TN diagnostic criteria may benefit substantially from anticonvulsant drugs or surgical therapy. Patients with other forms of neurogenic facial pain have a poorer prognosis.

References

1. The International Classification of Headache Disorders, 2nd ed. Cephalalgia 2004;24(Suppl 1):9-160.
2. Cohen S, Hargreaves KM: Pathways of the Pulp, 9th ed. Philadelphia, Mosby, 2002.
3. Mason P, Strassman A, Maciewicz R: Is the jaw-opening reflex a valid model of pain? Brain Res 1985;357:137-146.
4. Offenbacher S: Periodontal diseases: Pathogenesis. Ann Periodontol 1996;1:821-878.
5. Bartoshuk LM, Duffy VB, Reed D, Williams A: Supertasting, earaches and head injury: Genetics and pathology alter our taste worlds. Neurosci Biobehav Rev 1996;20:79-87.
6. Grushka M, Sessle BJ: Burning mouth syndrome. Dent Clin North Am 1991;35:171-184.
7. Mott AE, Grushka M, Sessle BJ: Diagnosis and management of taste disorders and burning mouth syndrome. Dent Clin North Am 1993;37:33-71.
8. Ship JA, Grushka M, Lipton JA, et al: Burning mouth syndrome: An update. J Am Dent Assoc 1995;126:842-853.
9. Forssell H, Jaaskelainen S, Tenovuo O, Hinkka S: Sensory dysfunction in burning mouth syndrome. Pain 2002;99:41-47.

10. Eliav E, Gracely RH, Nahlieli O, Benoliel R: Quantitative sensory testing in trigeminal nerve damage assessment. J Orofac Pain 2004;18:339-344.
11. Tepper SJ: New thoughts on sinus headache. Allergy Asthma Proc 2004;25:95-96.
12. Nguyen M, Maciewicz R, Bouckoms A, et al: Facial pain in patients with cerebellopontine angle meningiomas. Clin J Pain 1986;2:3-9.
13. Cheng TM, Cascino TL, Onofrio BM: Comprehensive study of diagnosis and treatment of trigeminal neuralgia secondary to tumors. Neurology 1993;43:2298-2302.
14. Mathews ES, Scrivani SJ: Percutaneous stereotactic radiofrequency thermal rhizotomy for the treatment of trigeminal neuralgia. Mt Sinai J Med 2000;67:288-299.
15. Gelb H: Present-day concepts in diagnosis and treatment of craniomandibular disorders. N Y State Dent J 1985;51:266-271.
16. Gelb H: Clinical Management of Head, Neck and TMJ Pain and Dysfunction, 2nd ed. Philadelphia, Saunders, 1985.
17. Johansson A, Unell L, Carlsson GE, et al: Gender difference in symptoms related to temporomandibular disorders in a population of 50-year-old subjects. J Orofac Pain 2003;17:29-35.
18. Magnusson T, Egermark I, Carlsson GE: A longitudinal epidemiologic study of signs and symptoms of temporomandibular disorders from 15 to 35 years of age. J Orofac Pain 2000;14:310-319.
19. Carlsson GE, Egermark I, Magnusson T: Predictors of signs and symptoms of temporomandibular disorders: A 20-year follow-up study from childhood to adulthood. Acta Odontol Scand 2002;60:180-185.
20. Alghamdi N, Mehta N: The effectiveness of multifaceted treatment of TMDS: 500 patients drawn from a pool of 5000. J Dent Res 2001;80:86.
21. Bonjardim LR, Gaviao MB, Pereira LJ, et al: Signs and symptoms of temporomandibular disorders in adolescents. Pesqui Odontol Bras 2005;19:93-98.
22. Kapur N, Kamel IR, Herlich A: Oral and craniofacial pain: Diagnosis, pathophysiology, and treatment. Int Anesthesiol Clin 2003;41:115-150.
23. Egermark I, Magnusson T, Carlsson GE: A 20-year follow-up of signs and symptoms of temporomandibular disorders and malocclusions in subjects with and without orthodontic treatment in childhood. Angle Orthod 2003;73:109-115.
24. Sipila K, Zitting P, Siira P, et al: Temporomandibular disorders, occlusion, and neck pain in subjects with facial pain: A case-control study. Cranio 2002;20:158-164.
25. Nassif NJ, Talic YF: Classic symptoms in temporomandibular disorder patients: A comparative study. Cranio 2001;19:33-41.
26. Macfarlane TV, Blinkhorn AS, Davies RM, et al: Oro-facial pain in the community: Prevalence and associated impact. Community Dent Oral Epidemiol 2002;30:52-60.
27. Mehta NR, Forgione AG, Rosenbaum RS, Holmberg R: "TMJ" triad of dysfunctions: A biologic basis of diagnosis and treatment. J Mass Dent Soc 1984;33:173.
28. Hijzen TH, Slangen JL: Myofascial pain-dysfunction: Subjective signs and symptoms. J Prosthet Dent 1985;54:705-711.
29. Rasmussen P: Facial pain. IV. A prospective study of 1052 patients with a view of precipitating factors, associated symptoms, objective psychiatric and neurological symptoms. Acta Neurochir (Wien) 1991;108:100-109.
30. de las Penas CF, Cuadrado ML, Gerwin RD, Pareja JA: Referred pain from the trochlear region in tension-type headache: A myofascial trigger point from the superior oblique muscle. Headache 2005;45:731-737.
31. Kalina R, Orcutt J: Ocular and periocular pain. In Bonica JJ (ed): The Management of Pain. Philadelphia, Lea & Febiger, 1990, pp 759-768.
32. Curtis AW: Myofascial pain-dysfunction syndrome: The role of nonmasticatory muscles in 91 patients. Otolaryngol Head Neck Surg 1980;88:361-367.
33. Alvarez DJ, Rockwell PG: Trigger points: Diagnosis and management. Am Fam Physician 2002;65:653-660.
34. Kuttila S, Kuttila M, Le BY, et al: Characteristics of subjects with secondary otalgia. J Orofac Pain 2004;18:226-234.
35. Kuttila M, Le BY, Savolainen-Niemi E, et al: Efficiency of occlusal appliance therapy in secondary otalgia and temporomandibular disorders. Acta Odontol Scand 2002;60:248-254.
36. Kuttila SJ, Kuttila MH, Niemi PM, et al: Secondary otalgia in an adult population. Arch Otolaryngol Head Neck Surg 2001;127:401-405.
37. Wright EF, Syms CA, III, Bifano SL: Tinnitus, dizziness, and nonotologic otalgia improvement through temporomandibular disorder therapy. Mil Med 2000;165:733-736.
38. Bush FM, Harkins SW, Harrington WG: Otalgia and aversive symptoms in temporomandibular disorders. Ann Otol Rhinol Laryngol 1999;108:884-892.
39. Wazen JJ: Referred otalgia. Otolaryngol Clin North Am 1989;1205-1215.
40. Egermark I, Carlsson GE, Magnusson T: A 20-year longitudinal study of subjective symptoms of temporomandibular disorders from childhood to adulthood. Acta Odontol Scand 2001;59:40-48.
41. Matsumoto MA, Matsumoto W, Bolognese AM: Study of the signs and symptoms of temporomandibular dysfunction in individuals with normal occlusion and malocclusion. Cranio 2002;20:274-281.
42. Simmons HC, III, Gibbs SJ: Anterior repositioning appliance therapy for TMJ disorders: Specific symptoms relieved and relationship to disk status on MRI. Cranio 2005;23:89-99.
43. Fink M, Wahling K, Stiesch-Scholz M, Tschernitschek H: The functional relationship between the craniomandibular system, cervical spine, and the sacroiliac joint: A preliminary investigation. Cranio 2003;21:202-208.
44. Ciancaglini R, Testa M, Radaelli G: Association of neck pain with symptoms of temporomandibular dysfunction in the general adult population. Scand J Rehabil Med 1999;31:17-22.
45. Svensson P, Wang K, Sessle BJ, Rendt-Nielsen L: Associations between pain and neuromuscular activity in the human jaw and neck muscles. Pain 2004;109:225-232.
46. Kushida CA, Morgenthaler TI, Littner MR, et al: Practice parameters for the treatment of snoring and obstructive sleep apnea with oral appliances: An update for 2005. Sleep 2006;29:240-243.
47. Chakfa AM, Mehta NR, Forgione AG, et al: The effect of stepwise increases in vertical dimension of occlusion on isometric strength of cervical flexors and deltoid muscles in nonsymptomatic females. Cranio 2002;20:264-273.
48. Abduljabbar T, Mehta NR, Forgione AG, et al: Effect of increased maxillo-mandibular relationship on isometric strength in TMD patients with loss of vertical dimension of occlusion. Cranio 1997;15:57-67.
49. Dibbets JM, van der Weele LT: Prevalence of structural bony change in the mandibular condyle. J Craniomandib Disord 1992;6:254-259.
50. Buchbinder D, Kaplan A: Biolog. In Kaplan AS, Assael LA (eds): Temporomandibular Disorders: Diagnosis and Treatment. Philadelphia, Saunders, 1991.
51. Pullinger AG, Bibb CA, Ding X, Baldioceda F: Contour mapping of the TMJ temporal component and the relationship to articular soft tissue thickness and disk displacement. Oral Surg Oral Med Oral Pathol 1993;76:636-646.
52. Pullinger AG, Bibb CA, Ding X, Baldioceda F: Relationship of articular soft tissue contour and shape to the underlying eminence and slope profile in young adult temporomandibular joints. Oral Surg Oral Med Oral Pathol 1993;76:647-654.
53. Ward DM, Behrents RG, Goldberg JS: Temporomandibular synovial fluid pressure response to altered mandibular positions. Am J Orthod Dentofacial Orthop 1990;98:22-28.
54. Axelsson S, Holmlund A, Hjerpe A: Glycosaminoglycans in normal and osteoarthrotic human temporomandibular joint disks. Acta Odontol Scand 1992;50:113-119.
55. Wongwatana S, Kronman JH, Clark RE, et al: Anatomic basis for disk displacement in temporomandibular joint (TMJ) dysfunction. Am J Orthod Dentofacial Orthop 1994;105:257-264.

56. Brecht K, Johnson CM, III: Complete mandibular agenesis: Report of a case. Arch Otolaryngol 1985;111:132-134.
57. Warner BF, Luna MA, Robert NT: Temporomandibular joint neoplasms and pseudotumors. Adv Anat Pathol 2000;7:365-381.
58. Elfving L, Helkimo M, Magnusson T: Prevalence of different temporomandibular joint sounds, with emphasis on disc-displacement, in patients with temporomandibular disorders and controls. Swed Dent J 2002;26:9-19.
59. Wright EF, Clark EG, Paunovich ED, Hart RG: Headache improvement through TMD stabilization appliance and self-management therapies. Cranio 2006;24:104-111.
60. Al-Ani Z, Gray RJ, Davies SJ, et al: Stabilization splint therapy for the treatment of temporomandibular myofascial pain: A systematic review. J Dent Educ 2005;69:1242-1250.
61. Castroflorio T, Talpone F, Deregibus A, et al: Effects of a functional appliance on masticatory muscles of young adults suffering from muscle-related temporomandibular disorders. J Oral Rehabil 2004;31:524-529.
62. Miller VJ, Karic VV, Myers SL, Exner HV: The temporomandibular opening index (TOI) in patients with closed lock and a control group with no temporomandibular disorders (TMD): An initial study. J Oral Rehabil 2000;27:815-816.
63. Placios E, Volvasoni G, Shannon M, Reed C: Magnetic Resonance of the Temporomandibular Joint: Clinical Consideration Radiography Management. New York, Thieme, 1990.
64. Okeson J: Orofacial pain: Guidelines for assessment diagnosis and management. The American Academy of Orofacial Pain. Lombard, Ill, Quintessence, 1996.
65. Stegenga B, de Bont LG, Boering G, Van Willigen JD: Tissue responses to degenerative changes in the temporomandibular joint: A review. J Oral Maxillofac Surg 1991;49:1079-1088.
66. Kraus H: Diagnosis and treatment of muscle pain. Lombard, IL, Quintessence, 1988.
67. Travell J, Rinzler SH: The myofascial genesis of pain. Postgrad Med 1952;11:425-434.
68. Bell D: Clinical Management of Temporomandibular Disorders. Chicago, Year Book, 1982, pp 55-58.
69. De Boever JA, Carlsson GE, Klineberg IJ: Need for occlusal therapy and prosthodontic treatment in the management of temporomandibular disorders. Part II: Tooth loss and prosthodontic treatment. J Oral Rehabil 2000;27:647-659.
70. De Boever JA, Carlsson GE, Klineberg IJ: Need for occlusal therapy and prosthodontic treatment in the management of temporomandibular disorders. Part I. Occlusal interferences and occlusal adjustment. J Oral Rehabil 2000;27:367-379.
71. Karlsson S, Cho SA, Carlsson GE: Changes in mandibular masticatory movements after insertion of nonworking-side interference. J Craniomandib Disord 1992;6:177-183.
72. Wenneberg B, Nystrom T, Carlsson GE: Occlusal equilibration and other stomatognathic treatment in patients with mandibular dysfunction and headache. J Prosthet Dent 1988;59:478-483.
73. Padamsee M, Mehta N, Forgione A, Bansal S: Incidence of cervical disorders in a TMD population. J Dent Res 1994;74.
74. Fitz-Ritzon D: Neuroanatomy and neurophysiology of the upper cervical spine. In Vernon H (ed): Upper Cervical Spine. Baltimore, Williams & Wilkins,
75. Rocabado M: Biomechanical relationship of the cranial, cervical, and hyoid regions. J Craniomandibr Pract 1983;1:61-66.
76. Rocabado M: Biomechanical relationship of the cranial, cervical, and hyoid regions. J Craniomandib Pract 1983;1:61-66.
77. Grace A: Pathomechanics of the upper cervical spine. In Vernone H (ed): Upper Cervical Syndrome. Baltimore, Williams & Wilkins, 1988.
78. Mehta N: Muscular disorders. In Kaplan AS, Assael LA (eds): Temporomandibular Disorder: Diagnosis and Treatment. Philadelphia, Saunders, 1991, pp 118-141.
79. Gelb H, Tarte J: A two-year clinical dental evaluation of 200 cases of chronic headache: The craniocervical-mandibular syndrome. J Am Dent Assoc 1975;91:1230-1236.
80. Wruble MK, Lumley MA, McGlynn FD: Sleep-related bruxism and sleep variables: A critical review. J Craniomandib Disord 1989;3:152-158.
81. Glaros AG, Rao SM: Bruxism: A critical review. Psychol Bull 1977;84:767-781.
82. Mehta NR, Forgione AG, Maloney G, Greene R: Different effects of nocturnal parafunction on the masticatory system: The weak link theory. Cranio 2000;18:280-286.
83. Graf H: Bruxism. Dent Clin North Am 1969;13:659-665.
84. Reding GR, Rubright WC, Zimmerman SO: Incidence of bruxism. J Dent Res 1966;45:1198-1204.
85. Jorgic-Srdjak K, Ivezic S, Cekic-Arambasin A, Bosnjak A: Bruxism and psychobiological model of personality. Coll Antropol 1998;22(Suppl):205-212.
86. Marbach JJ: Is there a myofascial, temporomandibular disorder personality? J Mass Dent Soc 1995;44:12-17.
87. Pierce CJ, Chrisman K, Bennett ME, Close JM: Stress, anticipatory stress, and psychologic measures related to sleep bruxism. J Orofac Pain 1995;9:51-56.
88. Fischer WF, O'Toole ET: Personality characteristics of chronic bruxers. Behav Med 1993;19:82-86.
89. Glickman I, Haddad AW, Martignoni M, et al: Telemetric comparison of centric relation and centric occlusion reconstructions. J Prosthet Dent 1974;31:527-536.
90. Mehta NR, Roeber FW, Haddad AW, Glickman I: Photoelastic model for occlusal force analysis. J Dent Res 1975;54:1243.
91. Mehta NR, Roeber FW, Haddad AW, et al: Stresses created by occlusal prematurities in a new photoelastic model system. J Am Dent Assoc 1976;93:334-341.
92. Forgione A: A simple but effective method quantifying bruxism behavior. J Restorative Dent 1974;53:127.
93. Mejias JE, Mehta NR: Subjective and objective evaluation of bruxing patients undergoing short-term splint therapy. J Oral Rehabil 1982;9:279-289.
94. Rugh J: Behavioral therapy. In Mohl G, Zarb G, Carlsson G, Rugh J (eds): A Textbook of Occlusion. Lombard, Ill, Quintessence, 1988, pp 329-337.
95. Mehta N, Forgione A: The effect of macroposture and body mechanics on dental occlusion. In Gelb H (ed): New Concepts in Craniomandibular and Chronic Pain Management. St. Louis, Mosby-Year Book, 1994, p 35.
96. Travell JG, Simons DG: Myofascial Pain and Dysfunction: The Trigger Point Manual: The Upper Extremities, Vol. 1. Baltimore, Williams & Wilkins, 1983, pp 29-30.
97. Fikackova H, Ekberg E: Can infrared thermography be a diagnostic tool for arthralgia of the temporomandibular joint? Oral Surg Oral Med Oral Pathol Oral Radiol Endod 2004;98:643-650.
98. McBeth SB, Gratt BM: Thermographic assessment of temporomandibular disorders symptomology during orthodontic treatment. Am J Orthod Dentofacial Orthop 1996;109:481-488.
99. Lund JP, Widmer CG, Feine JS: Validity of diagnostic and monitoring tests used for temporomandibular disorders. J Dent Res 1995;74:1133-1143.
100. Rocabado M: Biomechanical relationship of the cranial, cervical, and hyoid regions. J Craniomandibular Pract 1983;1:61-66.
101. Zakrzewska JM: Trigeminal neuralgia. Prim Dent Care 1997;4:17-19.
102. Ransohoff J: Surgical treatment of trigeminal neuralgia current status (in memory of Byron Stookey, M.D.). Headache 1969;9:20-26.
103. Fothergill J: Of a Painful Affection of the Face. London, Medical Society of London, 1776. 104. Amols W: Differential diagnosis of trigeminal neuralgia and treatment. Headache 1969;9:50-53.
105. Bayer DB, Stenger TG: Trigeminal neuralgia: An overview. Oral Surg Oral Med Oral Pathol 1979;48:393-399.
106. Bowsher D: Trigeminal neuralgia: An anatomically oriented review. Clin Anat 1997;10:409-415.
107. Canavero S, Bonicalzi V, Pagni CA: The riddle of trigeminal neuralgia. Pain 1995;60:229-231.
108. Carney LR: Considerations on the cause and treatment of trigeminal neuralgia. Neurology 1967;17:1143-1151.

109. White JC, Sweet WH: Pain and the Neurosurgeon, 2nd ed. Springfield Ill, Charles C Thomas, 1969.
110. Merskey H, Bogduk N: Classification of Chronic Pain: Descriptions of Chronic Pain Syndromes and Definitions of Pain Term, 2nd ed. Seattle, Wash., IASP Press, 1994.
111. Etiology of trigeminal neuralgia: (Editorial). JAMA 1965; 194:553.
112. Adams CB: Trigeminal neuralgia: Pathogenesis and treatment. Br J Neurosurg 1997;11:493-495.
113. Anastasiades P: [Idiopathic neuralgia of the trigeminal nerve]. Stomatologia (Athenai) 1980;37:233-242.
114. Brachmann F: [The etiology and pathogenesis of trigeminal neuralgia]. Zahnarztl Prax 1966;17:112-114.
115. Scrivani SJ, Keith DA, Mathews ES, Kaban LB: Percutaneous stereotactic differential radiofrequency thermal rhizotomy for the treatment of trigeminal neuralgia. J Oral Maxillofac Surg 1999;57:104-111.
116. Sweet WH: Controlled thermocoagulation of trigeminal ganglion and rootlets for differential destruction of pain fibers: Facial pain other than trigeminal neuralgia. Clin Neurosurg 1976;23:96-102.
117. Taha JM, Tew JM, Jr: Treatment of trigeminal neuralgia by percutaneous radiofrequency rhizotomy. Neurosurg Clin North Am 1997;8:31-39.
118. Adams CB, Kaye AH, Teddy PJ: The treatment of trigeminal neuralgia by posterior fossa microsurgery. J Neurol Neurosurg Psychiatry 1982;45:1020-1026.
119. Burchiel KJ, Clarke H, Haglund M, Loeser JD: Long-term efficacy of microvascular decompression in trigeminal neuralgia. J Neurosurg 1988;69:35-38.
120. Campbell RL, Trentacosti CD, Eschenroeder TA, Harkins SW: An evaluation of sensory changes and pain relief in trigeminal neuralgia following intracranial microvascular decompression and/or trigeminal glycerol rhizotomy. J Oral Maxillofac Surg 1990;48:1057-1062.
121. Alberico RA, Fenstermaker RA, Lobel J: Focal enhancement of cranial nerve V after radiosurgery with the Leksell gamma knife: Experience in 15 patients with medically refractory trigeminal neuralgia. AJNR 2001;22:1944-1948.
122. Young RF, Vermulen S, Posewitz A: Gamma knife radiosurgery for the treatment of trigeminal neuralgia. Stereotact Funct Neurosurg 1998;70(Suppl 1):192-199.
123. Cusick JF: Atypical trigeminal neuralgia. JAMA 1981;245: 2328-2329.
124. Shankland WE: Trigeminal neuralgia: Typical or atypical? Cranio 1993;11:108-112.
125. Tyler-Kabara EC, Kassam AB, Horowitz MH, et al: Predictors of outcome in surgically managed patients with typical and atypical trigeminal neuralgia: Comparison of results following microvascular decompression. J Neurosurg 2002;96:527-531.
126. Brown CR, Shankland W: Atypical trigeminal neuralgia. Pract Periodontics Aesthet Dent 1996;8:285.
127. Dworkin SF: Benign chronic orofacial pain: Clinical criteria and therapeutic approaches. Postgrad Med 1983;74:239-8.
128. Frediani F: Typical and atypical facial pain. Ital J Neurol Sci 1999;20:S46-S48.
129. Greenberg MS: Trigeminal neuralgia or atypical facial pain. Oral Surg Oral Med Oral Pathol Oral Radiol Endod 1996;82:361-362.
130. Tancioni F, Gaetani P, Villani L, et al: Neurinoma of the trigeminal root and atypical trigeminal neuralgia: Case report and review of the literature. Surg Neurol 1995;44:36-42.
131. Turp JC, Gobetti JP: Trigeminal neuralgia versus atypical facial pain: A review of the literature and case report. Oral Surg Oral Med Oral Pathol Oral Radiol Endod 1996;81: 424-432.
132. McFarland HR: Chronic traumatic trigeminal neuralgia. South Med J 1982;75:814-816.
133. Sweet WH: Deafferentation pain after posterior rhizotomy, trauma to a limb, and herpes zoster. Neurosurgery 1984;15: 928-932.

CHAPTER
26 Visceral Pain

Klaus Bielefeldt and G. F. Gebhart

Chronic visceral pain is very common. Abdominal pain is among the main reasons for physician visits with more than 12 million consultations each year in the United States.[1] Patients with visceral pain present unique challenges to the treating physician. Pain is generally poorly localized, typically associated with strong autonomic reactions and changes in visceral function. Pain management, in turn, may further alter visceral function, with opioid effects on the gastrointestinal tract providing a good example. Potential treatment effects on visceral function, such as slowed intestinal transit, can exacerbate the pain or lead to additional discomfort, thus showing that rational and effective pain management needs to be based on an understanding of the anatomic and physiologic basis of visceral function *and* pain.

PHYSIOLOGIC BASIS OF VISCERAL SENSATION AND PAIN

Anatomy and Physiology of Visceral Afferent Pathways

Many viscera, such as the gastrointestinal tract, arise from midline structures. As a result, they receive a bilateral innervation. Equally, appropriate visceral stimuli activate both hemispheres of the brain, with a predominance of the left side in most right-handed individuals.[2,3] In addition, organs in the chest cavity and most viscera within the abdomen receive a dual afferent innervation with vagal and spinal nerves conveying sensory input to the central nervous system (Fig. 26–1). Even though vagal fibers do not reach pelvic organs, the distal colon, bladder, prostate, and uterus also have a complex sensory innervation with afferents projecting through the thoracolumbar (hypogastric) and lumbosacral (pelvic) nerve to the spinal cord.

The vagus nerve is predominantly comprised of afferent fibers (80% or more), which project via the nodose and jugular ganglia to the nucleus of the solitary tract in the brainstem. Spinal afferents pass through prevertebral (sympathetic) ganglia to the dorsal root ganglia and send their endings to the dorsal horn and central gray of the spinal cord. Information about noxious stimuli is relayed rostrally through the spinothalamic tract. In addition, post-synaptic dorsal horn neurons within the central gray send their central processes through the medial aspect of the dorsal columns, a pathway that has only recently been recognized as uniquely important in visceral pain.[4] Thus two ascending fiber tracts convey sensory input about noxious events in the viscera to the brain: the spinothalamic tract and the dorsal column.

Most physiologic studies characterizing the properties of visceral sensory pathways rely on responses to defined mechanical stimuli. Vagal afferents form a relatively homogeneous group that is activated by low-intensity mechanical stimuli and encodes stimulus intensity over a wide range. The low threshold of activation is consistent with the presumed primary role of these sensory pathways, namely regulation of physiologic processes. In contrast, two classes of mechanosensitive spinal afferents can be distinguished based on their response characteristics: low threshold fibers are similarly activated by low-intensity stimuli and continue to encode stimulus intensity over a wide range, whereas high-threshold fibers are activated by intense, potentially noxious intensities of mechanical stimuli. Thus spinal high-threshold fibers resemble specialized nociceptors that have been described and characterized best in skin, suggesting that they play a primary role in visceral nociception.[5,6] However, because mechanosensitive visceral afferents encode stimulus intensity over a wide range and because they also exhibit the property of sensitization after visceral insult, it is reasonable to consider that both low- and high-threshold mechanosensitive afferents can contribute to visceral pain conditions. Moreover, independent of their threshold to mechanical stimuli, most visceral sensory neurons are polymodal, meaning they respond to multiple stimulus modalities, including endogenous and exogenous chemicals contained in luminal contents, temperatures (heat or cold), and stretch.

Mucosal Signaling and Visceral Sensation

In the airways, gastrointestinal tract, and urinary bladder, nerve fibers are found in close proximity to epithelial cells, which often exhibit specializations with secretory vesicles on the basal surface.[7-9] This structural organization suggests that visceral epithelial cells function as an interface between a chemical

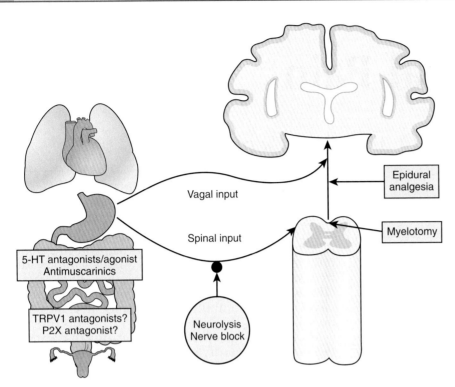

Figure 26–1. Schematic description of visceral innervation and potential targets for analgesic therapy. As indicated by the arrows, most viscera receive a dual sensory innervation with vagal and spinal afferents. Current symptomatic treatment of peripheral targets relies largely on agents interfering with intestinal contractility. However, the capsaicin receptor (TRPV1) and purinergic P2X receptors constitute promising targets for the treatment of visceral pain. Neurolytic block, myelotomy, and epidural analgesia all target spinal afferent pathways involved in relaying visceral pain.

or mechanical stimulus and the nervous system. Functional studies support this interpretation and reveal an important role of epithelial elements in visceral sensation and nociception. The best described example is serotonin released from enteroendocrine cells in the gastrointestinal tract. The gut is the major source of this signaling molecule and contains 95% of the body's serotonin. Much of this serotonin is stored in specialized enteroendocrine (enterochromaffin) cells and can be released by chemical or mechanical stimuli, activating intrinsic and extrinsic neurons.[7] Within the urinary tract, epithelial cells release adenosine triphosphate (ATP), which acts on purinergic receptors (P2X receptors) and is involved in normal micturition as well as bladder pain.[10] Finally, bladder epithelial cells also express the capsaicin receptor TRPV1, an ion channel that is activated by acid, temperature, endogenous lipid mediators, and the pungent substance (capsaicin) contained in hot pepper. Animals with a targeted deletion of this channel display altered micturition behavior, again pointing to the importance of epithelial cells in visceral sensation.[11]

Sensitization of Visceral Afferent Pathways

Visceral afferents can sensitize in response to inflammation or injury. The release of mediators, such as prostaglandins or bradykinin, rapidly alters the properties of ion channels, leading to an increase in neuron excitability. In addition, cytokines and growth factors may trigger transcriptional changes, affecting the properties of sensory neurons through changes in gene expression. The increased peripheral input (*peripheral sensitization*) may secondarily alter

sensory processing in the central nervous system (*central sensitization*), with both contributing to visceral pain syndromes. One easily recognized consequence of sensitization of visceral afferent pathways is increased tenderness to palpation over a larger area than normal.[12] Both peripheral and central mechanisms contribute to the increased sensitivity and expanded areas of referral, both of which are common in patients with irritable bowel, dyspepsia, and interstitial cystitis.

Central Processing of Visceral Sensation and Pain

Vagal afferents project to the nucleus of the solitary tract, and from there via the parabrachial nucleus and ventromedial thalamus to the insular cortex.[13] They form many connections with the hypothalamus, supraoptic nucleus, anterior cingulated cortex, and amygdala, which are essential for autonomic and emotional responses to visceral stimulation.[14,15] Spinal afferents also project to the thalamus, but are preferentially found in the ventral posterolateral nucleus, which is connected to cortical areas, including the insula. The lateral components primarily serve discriminative functions associated with pain perception (e.g., location and intensity), while the medial thalamic nuclei, the main target of vagal input, is more closely linked to emotional and autonomic responses triggered by pain. Consistent with the bilateral innervation of organs originating from midline structures, most visceral stimuli activate both cerebral hemispheres, albeit with a preferential activation of one—mostly the left—side.[2,16,17] Studies using functional brain imaging have not demonstrated striking differences in the processing of visceral and nonvisceral pain. However, visceral pain preferentially activates the perigenual portion of the anterior cingulate cortex, whereas nonvisceral pain is primarily represented in the mid cingulate cortex. The physical proximity or even overlap between processing of visceral pain and emotion in the perigenual portion of the anterior cingulate cortex provides a potential explanation for the stronger emotional response to painful visceral stimuli compared to nonvisceral stimuli.[18-20] The representation of vagal *and* spinal afferent inputs to cortical structures, most notably the insula and anterior cingulated cortex, also support a role for both sensory pathways in the complex experience of pain.

Visceral Pain Stimuli

Visceral events that can produce conscious sensation or acute pain in humans include traction of the mesentery, distention of hollow organs, strong contractions of muscle layers surrounding such hollow organs, ischemia, and chemical irritants.[12,21] As routine endoscopic interventions have established, cutting or burning—two clearly noxious stimuli when applied to skin—are not perceived when applied in the viscera, thus setting visceral apart from nonvisceral sensation. Because of its sensitizing influences on sensory pathways, visceral inflammation can trigger pain or increase excitability of visceral afferent pathways (e.g., enhancing low-threshold input into a noxious range), which can become chronic (e.g., chronic pancreatitis). Finally, while not studied in as much detail, malignancies can trigger chronic pain due to direct effects of the tumor on afferent nerves (e.g., nerve compression, release of chemicals) or due to indirect effects, such as distention of a hollow organ.[22]

Clinical Implications

Current evidence suggests that spinal afferents primarily serve the discriminatory function of nociception, encoding location and intensity of visceral pain. Thus treatment strategies, such as regional block or surgical dissection, generally target spinal afferent pathways.

Unilateral nerve blocks or neurolysis are often ineffective, which is partly due to the fact that most viscera receive bilateral innervation and are innervated by two sets of nerves.

Visceral pain is a complex experience associated with strong emotional and autonomic reactions. The emotive component of visceral pain is at least in part due to the central projections of spinal *and* vagal sensory pathways, both of which can activate the perigenual area of the anterior cingulate cortex, an area closely associated with emotional processing. Considering the complex innervation of most viscera by spinal and vagal afferent pathways, these neuroanatomic findings provide an explanation for why regional blocks or nerve dissections often result in only partial or temporary effects.

Impaired function of viscera, such as decreased transit of material in the gut, may significantly contribute to pain due to distention or strong contractions of visceral muscles or the composition of luminal contents. Thus, effective pain management needs to combine analgesic therapies with treatment strategies targeting specific visceral function.

REGIONAL BLOCK AND NEURAL ABLATION

Surgical and nonoperative approaches have been developed to perform transient nerve blocks or more permanently destroy sensory pathways involved in visceral pain. Whereas pain is a common symptom of many disorders involving different viscera, malignancies are the primary cause of severe pain syndromes, prompting consideration of ablative or neurolytic procedures. In view of the often transient nature of pain relief after ablative therapies, most studies targeting visceral sensory pathways have involved patients with inoperable cancers and relatively short life expectancy. Because these patients typically present in advanced stages of their disease, surgical denervation plays only a minor role in the treatment. Chemical neurolysis, generally using high concentrations of ethanol, can achieve comparable results without subjecting patients to the risk of an operation. Since the first description by Kappis nearly 100 years ago,[23] several techniques have been developed to optimize the targeted delivery of neurolytic agents and/or minimize the likelihood of adverse effects. Most of these approaches use imaging methods, such as fluoroscopy, ultrasound, or computerized tomography. Despite the wealth of literature, though, few systematic studies have addressed the efficacy, outcomes, or adverse effects of these interventions. Problems assessing the effects of visceral pain management with peripheral blocks are further confounded by differences in type, concentration, and amount of the neurolytic agent, primarily ethanol, in both definition and measurement end points and in follow-up time. Only four randomized controlled trials have been published comparing ablative therapies with conventional pharmacologic pain management.[24-27] All of them showed at least transiently improved pain levels and a concomitant decrease in opioid use, thus supporting the utility of nerve blocks in appropriately selected patients.

Celiac Plexus and Splanchnic Nerve Block

Spinal afferents innervating organs in the upper abdomen traverse the celiac plexus with two distinct ganglia located caudal to origin of the celiac artery. The afferents travel centrally behind the crural diaphragm in the splanchnic nerves. The traditional dorsal approach uses the twelfth rib and spinal process of the first lumbar vertebra as landmarks.[28,29] With the patient in the prone position, a needle is advanced about 7 cm lateral of the midline at a 30- to 45-degree angle and tilted slightly cranially to reach the lateral wall of the body of the first lumbar vertebra. The needle is then moved anteriorly by about 2 cm. If aspiration does not yield blood return, water-soluble contrast (3 to 5 mL), often mixed with a local anesthetic, is injected under fluoroscopic control. To more directly target the celiac plexus, the needle can be placed about 2 cm more anterior, which requires piercing the diaphragmatic crura and positions the needle close to the anterolateral aspect of the aorta. Severely ill patients with respiratory compromise and patients with significant ascites or recent abdominal surgery often poorly tolerate being in the prone position for the time required to complete this procedure. Therefore an anterior approach has been developed with advancement of the needle from the epigastric area toward the body of the first lumbar vertebra. If the appropriate position is confirmed, the neurolytic agent, generally phenol or ethanol, is given. Current approaches mostly rely on the tissue destructive properties of ethanol, which is used in concentrations between 50% and 99% and volumes between 10 and 50 mL per injection. Injections are generally performed bilaterally to effectively destroy afferent pathways. A recent report suggested that radiofrequency ablation may provide an alternative to chemical neurolysis.[30] Additional studies are needed before allowing conclusions about efficacy and safety of this approach.

Various imaging techniques have been used to improve the efficacy of neurolysis and to decrease the potential of adverse effects. The celiac ganglia are too small to allow direct visualization with CT scanning or transabdominal ultrasound. Using endoscopic ultrasonography, the scanner can be brought into close proximity of the plexus. However, the ganglia do not differ in echogenicity from surrounding structures, thus again not allowing direct imaging of the target structure. Therefore, all of these approaches rely on identifying the celiac artery as the main landmark. Computed tomography (CT) allows guidance of the needle to the target area and a three-dimensional reconstruction of the area affected by the neurolytic agent, based on the spread of radio-opaque contrast.[31] Repeated imaging with radiation exposure of patient and staff is required during the procedure. Whereas ultrasound allows real-time guidance without radiation exposure, air in the overlying structures often interferes with sound penetration and imaging, thus limiting its utility for patients undergoing celiac plexus block.[32] Endoscopic ultrasound with the use of an endoscopically advanced needle has been successfully used. Ethanol injection alters the echogenicity of the affected tissue, thus allowing direct visualization of the spread of the neurolytic agent.[33] Despite the theoretical advantages, published studies have not yet demonstrated the superiority of one of these approaches.

Surgical Nerve Ablation

One randomized controlled trial and several small case series have used surgical approaches to ablate the celiac ganglia or splanchnic nerves. The direct visualization during a surgical exploration allows targeted injection of neurolytic agents into the celiac plexus, if a curative resection cannot be performed.[34] Due to advances in preoperative imaging, fewer patients currently undergo exploratory laparotomies, thus limiting the number of patients who might undergo an intraoperative celiac plexus block. With the advent of minimally invasive surgery, thoracoscopic resection of splanchnic nerves has been reported. As is true for the less invasive procedures, approaches have not been standardized with unilateral and bilateral resection with or without vagotomy being performed to achieve pain control in these patients.[35-37]

Efficacy of Neural Block and Ablation

Differences in patient selection, techniques, and outcome measures complicate a comparison of published results (Table 26–1). A meta-analysis published in 1995 concluded that nearly 90% of patients with various malignancies experienced good pain relief for about 3 months after the procedure.[29] Even though most case series report similar results, it is important to determine whether ablative therapy actually improves pain control or quality of life in comparison to conventional treatment involving the systemic use of analgesic substances. A small randomized controlled trial demonstrated similar pain control, but lower adverse effects due to opioid consumption in patients treated with neurolytic block.[24] Subsequent studies point at a slight advantage of ablative treatment over pharmacotherapy. Intraoperative celiac plexus block with 50% ethanol led to stable pain levels in patients with inoperable pancreatic cancer, while patients receiving saline injection as control experienced a significant increase in pain scores during follow-up. This improvement in pain control was associated with a significantly lower use of opioids.[34] In a post-hoc analysis, patients with significant pain who underwent celiac plexus block lived longer compared to control subjects. However, there was no overall survival benefit when the comparison was made using the original study design as a template for the analysis. Importantly, most patients had low pain intensities at the beginning of the trial with average pain levels of approximately 2 on a visual analogue scale of 0 to 10. Three subsequent trials comparing neurolytic celiac plexus block to analgesic therapy confirmed better pain relief after ablative therapy. In two studies, the improvement was transient with progressive recurrence of pain after about 1 to 2 months.[25,26] Most patients still required opioids, albeit at lower dosages compared to control subjects in the two smaller studies.[25,26] A recent study by Wong and colleagues did not confirm this decrease in opioid consumption. Consistent with results shown by Kawamata and colleagues,[26] their results also demonstrated that appropriate dosing of opioids achieves good pain control and a comparable quality of life that does not differ between treatment groups.[27] None of these investigations demonstrated

Table 26–1. Published Trials of Regional Blocks for Chronic Visceral Pain

TRIAL DESIGN	DISEASES	TREATMENT	PATIENTS	FOLLOW-UP	OUTCOME MEASURE	IMPROVEMENT	REFERENCE
Randomized controlled trial	Pancreatic cancer	Neurolytic CPB	65	6 months	VAS pain score	Stable score (2.3) compared to increase in controls (3.5)	12
Randomized controlled trial	Pancreatic cancer	Neurolytic CPB	12	15 weeks	Complete pain relief (VAS pain score)	1 (8%) 10 when combined with analgesics	19
Randomized controlled trial	Pancreatic cancer	Neurolytic CPB	10	10 weeks	VAS pain score	Decrease from 5.5 to 3	9
Randomized controlled trial	Pancreatic cancer	Neurolytic CPB	50	1 year	VAS pain score ≤5	86%	24
Case series	Pancreatic cancer	Neurolytic CPB	11	1-18 weeks	≥75 % pain relief	5 (55%)	21
Case series	Pancreatic cancer	Neurolytic CPB	12	54 days	Duration of pain relief (days) by VAS	25 ± 23 days	23
Case series	Various malignancies	Neurolytic CPB	34	4 weeks	≥75% pain relief	18 (53%)	13
Case series	Pancreatic cancer	Neurolytic CPB	50	3 months	VAS pain score ≤3	37 (74%)	20
Case series	Pancreatic cancer	Neurolytic CPB	22	8 weeks	VAS pain score	Decrease from 6.59 to 3.13	14
Case series	Pancreatic cancer	Neurolytic CPB	35	8 weeks	Opioid consumption	Decrease from 94.3 ± 9.3 to 45.6 ± 7.6 mg/day	22
Case series	Pancreatic cancer	Intraoperative neurolytic CPB	15	30 weeks	Complete pain relief without opioids	10 (97%)	18
Case series	Various malignancies	Neurolytic CPB	53	30 days	Pain relief	23 (43%)	2
Case series	Pancreatic cancer	Neurolytic CPB	58	6 months	Decrease in pain score >2 points	31 (54%)	8
Case series	Various disorders	Neurolytic CPB	10	Up to 2 years	Pain relief	6 (60%)	4
Case series	Various malignancies	Neurolytic sympathetic block	25	8 weeks	VAS pain score	Significant reduction	3
Case series	Refractory cardiac ischemia	SGB	46	Not given	Pain relief	31 (67%)	16
Case series	Refractory cardiac ischemia	PVB	21	Not given	Pain relief	11 (52%)	16
Prospective trial	Pancreatitis	Neurolytic CPB	18	8 weeks	Improved pain score	6 (33%)	7
Case series	Pancreatitis	Neurolytic CPB and drainage operation	18	36 months	Complete pain relief	17 (94%)	1
Case series	Pancreatitis	CBP with bupivacaine and triamcinolone	90	Up to 52 weeks	Improved pain score	50 (55%)	6
Case series	Pancreatitis	Splanchnic RFA	12	18 months	VAS pain score	Improvement in 10 (83 %)	5
Case series	Pancreatic cancer	SX	24	8 weeks	Opioid consumption	Decrease from 90.1 ± 7.7 to 41.5 ± 5.2 mg/day	22
Case series	Pancreatic cancer	SX ± vagotomy	20	Up to 12 months	Pain relief	16 (80%)	11
Case series	Pancreatitis	SX	8	>3 months	Pain relief and 50% decrease in opioid use	3 (38%) 5 after repeat SX	17
Case series	Pancreatitis	SX	17	12 months	VAS pain score	Decrease 8.2 to 2.1	15
Case series	Refractory cardiac ischemia	SX	10	11.5 months	Angina severity score	Decrease from 10 to 2.1	10

CPB, celiac plexus block; PVB, paravertebral block; RFA, radiofrequency ablation; SGB, stellate ganglion block; SX, splanchnicectomy; VAS, visual analogue scale.

a significant effect of neurolytic plexus block on patient survival.

Because progressive worsening during the development of a pain syndrome may affect the efficacy of ablative procedures, one small study randomly enrolled patients to perform early and late neurolytic blocks, defined by the use of low or high dosages of opioids, respectively.[38] Even though both groups reported better pain control than medically treated controls, there were no significant differences between the groups. Similarly, the limited information about the various approaches with or without direct imaging or even direct surgical destruction of peripheral afferent pathways remains inconclusive.

A randomized controlled trial reported improved pain control after bilateral splanchnic nerve blockade compared to a celiac plexus block.[39] This assessment was based on a more significant decrease in pain intensity from baseline scores rather than a difference in the primary end point pain measured by visual analogue scale. Thus confirmatory studies are needed to establish whether splanchnic nerve destruction is indeed superior to neurolysis of the celiac plexus. De Cicco and colleagues examined the spread of contrast injected before the neurolytic agent using CT scanning.[31] In their retrospective study, the pattern was a good predictor of pain control with optimal results obtained in patients in whom contrast spread bilaterally above and below the origin of the celiac artery. However, case series using CT guidance do not report better response rates compared to the conventional approach.[31,32,40] The more recently introduced endoscopic ultrasound allows visualization of the area of interest during the injection of the neurolytic agent. Only one small and underpowered study compared this approach with CT guidance, reporting better results with endoscopic ultrasonography.[41] However, published case series reveal results that fall within the range achieved with other techniques.[33,42]

Similarly, the results of surgical interventions with neurolytic or neuroablative therapy remain inconclusive. Whereas the only randomized controlled trial demonstrated good pain relief and a decrease in opioid consumption,[34] a case series evaluating different palliative operations for pancreatic cancer did not confirm the decrease in opioid use after celiac plexus block.[43] Smaller case series report improved pain control in about 60% to 80% of patients after thoracoscopic splanchnicectomy done unilaterally or bilaterally with or without a vagotomy.[35-37,44-48] Poor definition of end points, limited assessment of analgesic effects, the lack of appropriate control groups, and the fact that comparable results were obtained using a variety of often quite different approaches clearly demonstrate the need for appropriately designed studies. Only two observational studies compared surgical approaches to conventional management strategies. Splanchnicectomy reduces opioid requirements compared to systemic pharmacotherapy, but not compared to celiac plexus block.[37,48] Overall, the current data do not support the superiority of one approach over another. Thus the choice that patients and physicians face should primarily focus on the available expertise, favoring one technique over other techniques.

Nerve Block or Ablative Therapy in Benign Disorders

As described, pain relief after neurolytic block is often transient, thus decreasing the enthusiasm to use such approaches in patients with benign disorders and long life expectancies. Therefore less information is available about the efficacy of nerve blocks in such patients. Several case series combining about 150 patients with chronic pancreatitis have been published, making this the largest patient group with benign diseases. Initial response rates vary between 50% and 90% with limited follow-up in the majority of cases.[30,36,41,47,49,50] Due to concerns about the use of neurolytic agents, the largest series combined bupivacaine with triamcinolone.[50] Although about half of the patients reported an initial benefit, sustained responses after 24 weeks were seen in only 10% of cases. The different techniques do not permit comparisons with results obtained in patients with pancreatic cancer. However, the apparently lower response rates are consistent with a complex etiology of chronic pain syndromes in patients with benign disorders. Using differential neuraxial blockade, Conwell and colleagues determined that primarily visceral pain was present only in about one fifth of patients with chronic pancreatitis, with the majority experiencing "central pain," defined by persistent pain despite surgical anesthesia through epidural administration of lidocaine.[51] Moore and associates reported results of stellate ganglion and paravertebral blocks with bupivacaine in 59 patients with refractory angina due to coronary artery disease.[52] About 60% of the patients experienced pain relief for more than 2 weeks. However, the benefit was transient and most patients required multiple interventions to maintain some benefit. Taken together, current data do not support the routine use of ablative therapies in patients with chronic pancreatitis, with limited data suggesting some benefit of transient nerve blocks in patients with ischemic heart disease.

Adverse Effects of Neurolytic Block

Transient pain is the most common side effect reported with ethanol as the neurolytic agent. Whereas the use of local anesthetic before the ethanol injection decreases the incidence of this adverse effect, at least 10% to 30% of patients experience significant pain during and within the first hours after the procedure.[32,40,42,53] The destruction of sympathetic efferent pathways causes vasodilation of splanchnic vessels, resulting in hypotension in up to 20% of patients.[25,40,42] Similarly, the unopposed parasympathetic drive can lead to diarrhea, which again is reported by about one fifth of patients.[24,25,42,53] All of these problems can generally be managed medically by appropriate premedication, hydration, postprocedural observation, and appropriate symptomatic therapy. More significant adverse effects are rare, but have been reported for all different approaches.

The posterior approach may traverse the kidney as well as the pleural space, potentially leading to hematuria or pneumothorax.[28,29,53] The anterior approach requires advancing the needle through liver, stomach, and colon. Although this is largely inconsequential, clinically relevant perforations can occur and may be difficult to diagnose due to the neurolytic block and often concomitantly administered analgesia.[54] Therefore all patients should be well hydrated, receive an intravenous fluid bolus before the nerve block is performed, and remain under observation for at least 2 to 4 hours after the procedure. The delivery of neurolytic agents in close proximity to major vessels is another potential source of complications. When performed under fluoroscopic control, contrast administration should confirm extraluminal positioning of the needle. In all cases, aspiration should assure that the needle is not inside a vessel before the neurolytic agent is injected. However, indirect effects, such as mesenteric venous thrombosis, may rarely occur despite these precautions.[55] Spread of the neurolytic agent within the retroperitoneal space with injury of lumbar nerves has been reported in some cases.[29] Paraparesis is the most feared and mostly irreversible complication, which is thought to be caused by injury to the nutrient vessels supplying the spinal cord.[28,29] Even though sufficiently powered studies addressing the likelihood of these adverse effects are not available, current evidence suggests that the incidence does not differ between the different approaches.[33,42,48]

Clinical Implications

Neurolytic celiac or splanchnic nerve block is a moderately effective method to decrease pain in patients with intra-abdominal malignancies, and has been best studied in patients with pancreatic cancer. The benefit is often transient, and may decrease the need for opioids, but does not affect life expectancy or quality of life compared to conventional pain management. Adverse effects occur in about 20% of patients, are largely minor and transient, and can be managed by appropriate medical therapy. Approaches using different imaging techniques or even direct operative visualization does not affect outcome or the incidence of side effects.

SPINAL TREATMENT TARGETS FOR VISCERAL PAIN

Epidural block or pharmacotherapy and surgical myelotomy can be performed to treat chronic visceral pain syndromes. Two aspects unique to visceral pain syndromes warrant some specific discussion of spinal treatment targets. First, preliminary studies suggest that patients with ischemic heart disease may derive significant benefit from epidural blocks.

Second, unlike nonvisceral pain, which is primarily relayed to supraspinal sites via the spinothalamic tract, functional and neuroanatomic studies have convincingly demonstrated that a dorsal column ascending pathway plays an important role in visceral pain.[56,57] Only few studies have systematically evaluated the clinical efficacy of these approaches over long time periods, thus limiting the ability to fully assess their therapeutic value at this point.

Epidural Analgesia and Visceral Pain

Spinal drug delivery through epidural catheters allows the delivery of opioids and other agents without a significant risk of systemic adverse effects. Acute or chronic epidural drug delivery alleviates visceral pain in patients with malignant and some patients with benign disorders.[51,58] Interestingly, high thoracic epidural anesthesia significantly improved angina in patients with refractory pain due to coronary artery disease and decreased documented episodes of cardiac ischemia as judged by ST depressions.[59,60] A recent study provided further insights into the underlying mechanism by demonstrating improved cardiac perfusion during high epidural analgesia, likely due to a concomitant block of sympathetic pathways.[61] Considering the limited information about the use of epidural analgesia in visceral pain, safety issues remain largely unaddressed. However, it is likely that incidence and nature of adverse effects will be similar to the previously reported complication rate of epidural drug delivery, which is addressed in more detail in Chapter 51 and 69.[62-64]

Even though systematic studies have not specifically addressed the efficacy of epidural drug delivery in patients with chronic visceral pain syndromes, currently available data support its use in patients with refractory pain due to ischemic heart disease.

Myelotomy and Visceral Pain

Since its introduction about 20 years ago, midline myelotomy has been used to treat patients with refractory pain due to visceral malignancies.[65] The nature of this intervention as a "rescue" treatment in patients who failed other therapies limits the ability to judge its clinical efficacy. No randomized controlled trials have determined its efficacy or adverse effects compared with optimized standard treatment. Case series report improved pain control in about 60% of patients, with symptoms reoccurring in up to half of the patients.[66-68]

Clinical Implications

As is true for all ablative therapies, midline myelotomy appears to provide only partial and transient pain relief. In the absence of more conclusive studies, myelotomies should be reserved for patients with intractable pain due to terminal disease.

MECHANISM-ORIENTED PHARMACOTHERAPY OF VISCERAL PAIN

Visceral pain is often associated with abnormalities of organ function, such as constipation, nausea, cardiac failure, or dysuria. These abnormalities may be due to the same underlying problem, caused by the pain syndrome or its treatment, or even cause the pain. Thus evaluation of patients with visceral pain syndromes should always go hand in hand with appropriate functional evaluation of the affected organ system.

Serotonin and Gastrointestinal Pain Management

As described above, the gastrointestinal tract contains 95% of the body's serotonin (5-HT), where it is involved in many different functions. Different serotonin receptors are found on neurons, smooth muscle, and epithelial cells. The ligand-gated 5-HT$_3$ receptor has been found on vagal and spinal afferents and is involved in visceral sensation, including the perception of nausea.[69,70] Metabotropic 5-HT receptors exert more complex effects on gut function as they act on multiple targets, including muscle and nerve cells, with limited studies suggesting that 5-HT$_4$ agonists and 5-HT$_1$ antagonists may decrease visceral sensation in experimental animals and healthy volunteers.[71-73] Currently, selective 5-HT$_3$ receptor antagonists and 5-HT$_4$ receptor agonists are available for clinical use in the United States. Even though there is some experience with other serotonin receptor blockers, this experience is limited, mostly demonstrating physiologic changes in healthy controls or short-term effects in patients with mild abdominal discomfort.

Clinical Efficacy of Serotonin Agonists and Antagonists

The 5-HT$_3$ antagonist alosetron has been successfully used in patients with functional bowel disease, characterized by abdominal pain and diarrhea. Whereas initial reports only demonstrated improved symptoms in women, a recent study suggests that it may be similarly efficacious in men.[74-77] Only one study followed up patients for more than 4 months and demonstrated that efficacy remains unchanged for nearly 1 year.[77] However, the effect is relatively modest with a recent meta-analysis showing a small odds ratio (1.8) favoring the active agent over placebo, translating into a number needed to treat of about 7.[78] Other 5-HT$_3$ receptor antagonists, such as ondansetron, play an important role in the treatment of severe nausea and vomiting but do not affect visceral pain.[69]

Tegaserod, a 5-HT$_4$ agonist, has been tested in patients with abdominal pain or discomfort associated with constipation. Tegaserod significantly accelerates gastrointestinal transit and alleviates symptoms of constipation, including associated discomfort and pain.[79,80] Using global improvement scores, currently available data suggest a relatively low odds ratio (2.0) favoring tegaserod over placebo with a number needed to treat of about 7.[81]

Adverse Effects of Serotonin Agonists and Antagonists

The most common side effect of alosetron and related agents is constipation, which is reported by 20% to 40% of patients.[81] Alosetron has been linked to ischemic colitis, a potentially fatal disease, which led to a temporary withdrawal from the market.[78] It is currently only available under a restricted access program with stringent monitoring. Tegaserod generally triggers mild side effects with diarrhea being the most commonly cited adverse event with an incidence of about 7% to 9%.[81]

Smooth Muscle Relaxants and Visceral Pain

Stretch and tension are adequate stimuli for visceral sensation, corresponding to distention of a hollow viscus or contraction of the tunica muscularis.[21] Visceral muscle is morphologically and functionally distinct from striated muscle, thus potentially allowing the use of pharmacologic interventions that may not significantly affect striated muscle. Several strategies emerged or are currently under investigation. Most rely on the block of muscarinic receptors, the main excitatory signaling mechanism between parasympathetic neurons and visceral smooth muscle. Less commonly used strategies employ agonists for α-adrenergic receptors or L type calcium channel blockers to affect the contractility of visceral smooth muscle. The latter two approaches have largely been used in healthy volunteers, showed only limited efficacy in small studies involving patients with different painful disorders, and carry a significant risk of adverse effects, primarily symptomatic hypotension.[82-87] Therefore, the discussion of spasmolytic agents focuses on muscarinic receptor antagonists, with the best evidence emerging from studies performed in patients with functional diseases of the gastrointestinal tract.

Clinical Efficacy of Smooth Muscle Relaxants

Two recently published meta-analyses concluded that compared to placebo, patients receiving anticholinergic drugs are twice as likely to report an overall benefit, which includes pain relief.[88,89] However, many of the patients experienced relatively mild pain at baseline with only moderate pain relief compared to placebo.[90,91]

Adverse Effects of Smooth Muscle Relaxants

About 10% of patients experience largely minor adverse effects, mostly due to effects on mucous membranes, the urinary tract and eye, with dry mouth, urinary retention, and problems with accommodation. Based on the mechanisms of action, anticholinergic drugs are contraindicated in patients with known glaucoma and should be avoided in patients with micturition problems.

Botulinum Toxin and Visceral Pain

The clinical use of botulinum toxin has expanded significantly beyond the initial target, spastic motor disorders of skeletal muscles.[92] More than 10 years ago, it was shown to affect smooth muscle as well, leading to symptomatic improvement in patients with achalasia.[93] As anecdotal evidence suggested a decrease in pain independent of its effect on muscle activity, botulinum toxin has been increasingly used to treat various pain syndromes, presumably by directly altering peripheral transmitter release from nociceptive afferent nerve terminals.[94] Essentially all the studies focusing on patients with visceral pain are case series. Often, patients present with associated impairment of visceral function, such as dysphagia, gastroparesis, or voiding dysfunction. Botulinum toxin is mostly injected into target areas under direct visualization with endoscopy, using total dosages of 100 to 200 U of the toxin.

Clinical Efficacy of Botulinum Toxin

Few studies have focused on pain and systematically examined changes in pain intensity after treatment with botulinum toxin. In patients with various esophageal motility disorders characterized by pain, injection of botulinum toxin into the distal esophagus significantly improved the pain score from severe to mild in about two thirds of patients for a mean time of 5 months.[95] In a smaller case series of patients suffering from diffuse esophageal spasm with severe chest pain, endoscopically guided injection of botulinum toxin along the tubular esophagus resulted in nearly complete alleviation of pain for 6 months.[96] There are limited results about the effects of this neurotoxin in other areas of the gastrointestinal tract, suggesting potential benefit in disorders associated with pain.[97] In the urinary tract, botulinum toxin has been successfully used to treat voiding disorders. A recently published case series suggests some effect in interstitial cystitis, an idiopathic disorder characterized by pelvic pain, urinary urgency, and increased frequency of micturitions.[98]

Adverse Effects of Botulinum Toxin

The generally low dosages of locally injected botulinum toxin do not cause systemic side effects. Adverse effects are largely limited to transient pain or infectious complications at the injection site. Injection in close proximity to striated muscle, most notably sphincteric muscle for bladder or rectum, may lead to transient incontinence.

κ-Opioids and Visceral Pain

Opioids are potent analgesics for nonvisceral as well as visceral pain. However, the use of opioids, most of which are agonists at the mu (μ) opioid receptor, for visceral pain is confounded by the high incidence of gastrointestinal side effects such as nausea, vomiting, and constipation. Especially in patients with gastrointestinal disorders, these unwanted effects may become dose-limiting. As peripheral visceral afferents express κ-opioid receptors, κ-agonists were developed to take advantage of their analgesic properties and the lower likelihood of adverse effects.[99] Animal and acute studies in human volunteers demonstrated increased thresholds to painful visceral stimuli, consistent with a potential analgesic effect.[100] However, central effects with significant dysphoria limit the use of κ-agonists to peripherally acting agents.

Clinical Efficacy of κ-Opioid Agonists

A single small study reported κ-agonist–induced pain relief in patients with chronic pancreatitis who were refractory to μ-opioid agonists. However, patients were only studied acutely after a single administration of the agonist.[101] Several randomized controlled trials examined the effects of fedotozine, a κ-opioid agonist, in patients with chronic abdominal pain due to functional disorders over a period of at least 6 weeks. While they reported an overall benefit, the effect was rather small compared to placebo.[102-104]

Adverse Effects Due to κ-Opioid Agonists

Randomized controlled trials did not report a significantly higher incidence of adverse effects after administration of peripherally acting κ-opioid agonists compared to placebo.[81]

Clinical Implications

The improved understanding of normal visceral function and sensation has led to the development of new therapeutic strategies. In the gastrointestinal tract, muscarinic receptor antagonists and serotonin receptor agonists and antagonists alter function and may improve discomfort associated with functional disorders. Similar targeted treatments are currently under development using drugs that interact with purinergic receptors and the heat- and acid-sensitive ion channel TRPV1 (capsaicin receptor).

In a small number of patients with associated changes in visceral function, localized injection of botulinum toxin A under endoscopic guidance may transiently alleviate symptoms including pain.

References

1. Russo MW, Wei JT, Thiny MT, et al: Digestive and liver diseases statistics, 2004. Gastroenterology 2004;126:1448-1453.
2. Aziz Q, Anderson LC, Valind S, et al: Identification of human brain loci processing esophageal sensation using positron emission tomography. Gastroenterology 1997;113:50-59.
3. Kern M, Hofmann C, Hyde J, et al: Characterization of the cerebral cortical representation of heartburn in GERD patients. Am J Physiol Gastrointest Liver Physiol 2004;286: G174-181.

4. Willis WD: Dorsal root potentials and dorsal root reflexes: A double-edged sword. Exp Brain Res 1999;124:395-421.
5. Bielefeldt K, Christianson JA, Davis BM: Basic and clinical aspects of visceral sensation: Transmission to the CNS. Neurogastroenterol Motil 2005;17:488-499.
6. Cervero F: Visceral pain: Mechanisms of peripheral and central sensitization. Ann Med 1995;27:235-239.
7. Gershon MD: Review article: Roles played by 5-hydroxytryptamine in the physiology of the bowel. Aliment Pharmacol Ther 1999;13(suppl 2):15-30.
8. Adriaensen D, Timmermans JP, Brouns I, et al: Pulmonary intraepithelial vagal nodose afferent nerve terminals are confined to neuroepithelial bodies: An anterograde tracing and confocal microscopy study in adult rats. Cell Tissue Res 1998;293:395-405.
9. Birder LA: More than just a barrier: Urothelium as a drug target for urinary bladder pain. Am J Physiol Renal Physiol 2005;289:F489-F495.
10. Cockayne DA, Hamilton SG, Zhu QM, et al: Urinary bladder hyporeflexia and reduced pain-related behaviour in p2x3-deficient mice. Nature 2000;407:1011-1015.
11. Birder LA, Kanai AJ, De Groat WC, et al: Vanilloid receptor expression suggests a sensory role for urinary bladder epithelial cells. Proc Natl Acad Sci U S A 2001;98:13396-13401.
12. Mayer EA, Gebhart GF: Basic and clinical aspects of visceral hyperalgesia. Gastroenterology 1994;107:271-293.
13. Saper CB: The central autonomic nervous system: Conscious visceral perception and autonomic pattern generation. Annu Rev Neurosci 2002;25:433-469.
14. Zagon A: Does the vagus nerve mediate the sixth sense? Trends Neurosci 2001;24:671-673.
15. Michl T, Jocic M, Heinemann A, et al: Vagal afferent signaling of a gastric mucosal acid insult to medullary, pontine, thalamic, hypothalamic and limbic, but not cortical, nuclei of the rat brain. Pain 2001;92:19-27.
16. Silverman DH, Munakata JA, Ennes H, et al: Regional cerebral activity in normal and pathological perception of visceral pain. Gastroenterology 1997;112:64-72.
17. Derbyshire SWG: A systematic review of neuroimaging data during visceral stimulation. Am J Gastroenterol 2003;98:12-20.
18. Vogt BA: Pain and emotion: Interactions in subregions of the cingulate gyrus. Nat Rev Neurosci 2005;6:533-544.
19. Strigo IA, Bushnell MC, Boivin M, et al: Psychophysical analysis of visceral and cutaneous pain in human subjects. Pain 2002;97:235-246.
20. Strigo IA, Duncan GH, Boivin M, et al: Differentiation of visceral and cutaneous pain in the human brain. J Neurophysiol 2003;89:3294-3303.
21. Corsetti M, Gevers AM, Caenepeel P, et al: The role of tension receptors in colonic mechanosensitivity in humans. Gut 2004;53:1787-1793.
22. Kocoglu H, Pirbudak L, Pence S, et al: Cancer pain, pathophysiology, characteristics and syndromes. Eur J Gynaecol Oncol 2002;23:527-232.
23. Kappis M: Sensibilität und lokale anästhesie im chirurgischen gebiet der bauchhöhle mit besonderer berücksichtigung der splanchnicusanästhesie. Beitr Klin Chir 1919;115:161-175.
24. Mercadante S: Celiac plexus block versus analgesics in pancreatic cancer pain. Pain 1993;52:187-192.
25. Polati E, Finco G, Gottin L, et al: Prospective randomized double-blind trial of neurolytic coeliac plexus block in patients with pancreatic cancer. Br J Surg 1998;85:199-201.
26. Kawamata M, Ishitani K, Ishikawa K, et al: Comparison between celiac plexus block and morphine treatment on quality of life in patients with pancreatic cancer pain. Pain 1996;64:597-602.
27. Wong GY, Schroeder DR, Carns PE, et al: Effect of neurolytic celiac plexus block on pain relief, quality of life, and survival in patients with unresectable pancreatic cancer: A randomized controlled trial. JAMA 2004;291:1092-1099.
28. Mercadante S, Nicosia F: Celiac plexus block: A reappraisal. Reg Anesth Pain Med 1998;23:37-48.
29. Eisenberg E, Carr DB, Chalmers TC: Neurolytic celiac plexus block for treatment of cancer pain: A meta-analysis. Anesth Analg 1995;80:290-295.
30. Garcea G, Thomasset S, Berry DP, et al: Percutaneous splanchnic nerve radiofrequency ablation for chronic abdominal pain. A N Z J Surg 2005;75:640-644.
31. De Cicco M, Matovic M, Balestreri L, et al: Single-needle celiac plexus block: Is needle tip position critical in patients with no regional anatomic distortions? Anesthesiology 1997;87:1301-1308.
32. Marcy PY, Magne N, Descamps B: Coeliac plexus block: Utility of the anterior approach and the real time colour ultrasound guidance in cancer patient. Eur J Surg Oncol 2001;27:746-749.
33. Levy MJ, Wiersema MJ: EUS-guided celiac plexus neurolysis and celiac plexus block. Gastrointest Endosc 2003;57:923-930.
34. Lillemoe KD, Cameron JL, Kaufman HS, et al: Chemical splanchnicectomy in patients with unresectable pancreatic cancer. A prospective randomized trial. Ann Surg 1993;217:447-455.
35. Le Pimpec Barthes F, Chapuis O, Riquet M, et al: Thoracoscopic splanchnicectomy for control of intractable pain in pancreatic cancer. Ann Thorac Surg 1998;65:810-813.
36. Moodley J, Singh B, Shaik AS, et al: Thoracoscopic splanchnicectomy: Pilot evaluation of a simple alternative for chronic pancreatic pain control. World J Surg 1999;23:688-692.
37. Stefaniak T, Basinski A, Vingerhoets A, et al: A comparison of two invasive techniques in the management of intractable pain due to inoperable pancreatic cancer: Neurolytic celiac plexus block and videothoracoscopic splanchnicectomy. Eur J Surg Oncol 2005;31:768-773.
38. De Oliveira R, Dos Reis MP, Prado WA: The effects of early or late neurolytic sympathetic plexus block on the management of abdominal or pelvic cancer pain. Pain 2004;110:400-408.
39. Suleyman Ozyalcin N, Talu GK, Camlica H, et al: Efficacy of coeliac plexus and splanchnic nerve blockades in body and tail located pancreatic cancer pain. Eur J Pain 2004;8:539-545.
40. Fields S: Retrocrural splanchnic nerve alcohol neurolysis with a CT-guided anterior transaortic approach. J Comput Assist Tomogr 1996;20:157-160.
41. Gress F, Schmitt C, Sherman S, et al: A prospective randomized comparison of endoscopic ultrasound- and computed tomography-guided celiac plexus block for managing chronic pancreatitis pain. Am J Gastroenterol 1999;94:900-905.
42. Gunaratnam NT, Sarma AV, Norton ID, et al: A prospective study of EUS-guided celiac plexus neurolysis for pancreatic cancer pain. Gastrointest Endosc 2001;54:316-324.
43. Van Geenen RC, Keyzer-Dekker CM, van Tienhoven G, et al: Pain management of patients with unresectable peripancreatic carcinoma. World J Surg 2002;26:715-720.
44. Buscher HCJL, Jansen JBMJ, Van Dongen R, et al: Long-term results of bilateral thoracoscopic splanchnicectomy in patients with chronic pancreatitis. Br J Surg 2002;89:158-162.
45. Hammond B, Vitale GC, Rangnekar N, et al: Bilateral thoracoscopic splanchnicectomy for pain control in chronic pancreatitis. Am Surg 2004;70:546-549.
46. Krishna S, Chang VT, Shoukas JA, et al: Video-assisted thoracoscopic sympathectomy-splanchnicectomy for pancreatic cancer pain. J Pain Symptom Manage 2001;22:610-616.
47. Noppen M, Meysman M, D'haese J, et al: Thoracoscopic splanchnicolysis for the relief of chronic pancreatitis pain: Experience of a group of pneumologists. Chest 1998;113:528-531.
48. Okuyama M, Shibata T, Morita T, et al: A comparison of intraoperative celiac plexus block with pharmacological therapy as a treatment for pain of unresectable pancreatic cancer. J Hepato-Biliary-Pancreatic Surg 2002;9:372-375.
49. Chan C, Vilatoba M, Bartolucci A, et al: Improved reduction in pain in chronic pancreatitis with combined intraoperative celiac axis plexus block and lateral pancreaticojejunostomy. Curr Surg 2001;58:220-222.

50. Gress F, Schmitt C, Sherman S, et al: Endoscopic ultrasound-guided celiac plexus block for managing abdominal pain associated with chronic pancreatitis: A prospective single center experience. Am J Gastroenterol 2001;96:409-416.

51. Conwell DL, Vargo JJ, Zuccaro G, et al: Role of differential neuroaxial blockade in the evaluation and management of pain in chronic pancreatitis. Am J Gastroenterol 2001;96:431-436.

52. Moore R, Groves D, Hammond C, et al: Temporary sympathectomy in the treatment of chronic refractory angina. J Pain Symptom Manage 2005;30:183-191.

53. Rykowski JJ, Hilgier M: Efficacy of neurolytic celiac plexus block in varying locations of pancreatic cancer: Influence on pain relief. Anesthesiology 2000;92:347-354.

54. Takahashi M, Yoshida A, Ohara T, et al: Silent gastric perforation in a pancreatic cancer patient treated with neurolytic celiac plexus block. J Anesth 2003;17:196-198.

55. Fitzgibbon DR, Schmiedl UP, Sinanan MN: Computed tomography-guided neurolytic celiac plexus block with alcohol complicated by superior mesenteric venous thrombosis. Pain 2001;92:307-310.

56. Al-Chaer ED, Lawand NB, Westlund KN, et al: Visceral nociceptive input into the ventral posterolateral nucleus of the thalamus: A new function for the dorsal column pathway. J Neurophysiol 1996;76:2661-2674.

57. Willis WD, Al-Chaer ED, Quast MJ, et al: A visceral pain pathway in the dorsal column of the spinal cord. PNAS 1999;96:7675-7679.

58. Gilmer-Hill HS, Boggan JE, Smith KA, et al: Intrathecal morphine delivered via subcutaneous pump for intractable pain in pancreatic cancer. Surg Neurol 1999;51:6-11.

59. Gramling-Babb P, Miller MJ, Reeves ST, et al: Treatment of medically and surgically refractory angina pectoris with high thoracic epidural analgesia: Initial clinical experience. Am Heart J 1997;133:648-655.

60. Olausson K, Magnusdottir H, Lurje L, et al: Anti-ischemic and anti-anginal effects of thoracic epidural anesthesia versus those of conventional medical therapy in the treatment of severe refractory unstable angina pectoris. Circulation 1997;96:2178-2182.

61. Nygard E, Kofoed KF, Freiberg J, et al: Effects of high thoracic epidural analgesia on myocardial blood flow in patients with ischemic heart disease. Circulation 2005;111:2165-2170.

62. Rice I, Wee MYK, Thomson K: Obstetric epidurals and chronic adhesive arachnoiditis. Br J Anaesth 2004;92:109-120.

63. Aldrete JA, Williams SK: Infections from extended epidural catheterization in ambulatory patients. Reg Anesth Pain Med 1998;23:491-495.

64. Anderson VC, Burchiel KJ: A prospective study of long-term intrathecal morphine in the management of chronic non-malignant pain. Neurosurgery 1999;44:289-300.

65. Gildenberg PL: Myelotomy through the years. Stereotact Funct Neurosurg 2001;77:169-171.

66. Hwang S-L, Lin C-L, Lieu A-S, et al: Punctate midline myelotomy for intractable visceral pain caused by hepatobiliary or pancreatic cancer. J Pain Symptom Manage 2004;27:79-84.

67. Kim YS, Kwon SJ: High thoracic midline dorsal column myelotomy for severe visceral pain due to advanced stomach cancer. Neurosurgery 2000;46:85-90.

68. Nauta HJ, Wehman JC, Koliatsos VE, et al: Intraventricular infusion of nerve growth factor as the cause of sympathetic fiber sprouting in sensory ganglia. J Neurosurg 1999;91:447-453.

69. Camilleri M: Serotonergic modulation of visceral sensation: Lower gut. Gut 2002;51(suppl 1):i81-i86.

70. Tack J, Sarnelli G: Serotonergic modulation of visceral sensation: Upper gastrointestinal tract. Gut 2002;51(suppl 1):i77-i80.

71. Coffin B, Farmachidi JP, Rueegg P, et al: Tegaserod, a 5-HT$_4$ receptor partial agonist, decreases sensitivity to rectal distension in healthy subjects. Aliment Pharmacol Ther 2003;17:577-585.

72. Schikowski A, Thewissen M, Mathis C, et al: Serotonin type-4 receptors modulate the sensitivity of intramural mechano-receptive afferents of the cat rectum. Neurogastroenterol Motil 2002;14:221-227.

73. Tack J, Coulie B, Wilmer A, et al: Influence of sumatriptan on gastric fundus tone and on the perception of gastric distension in man. Gut 2000;46:468-473.

74. Camilleri M, Chey WY, Mayer EA, et al: A randomized controlled clinical trial of the serotonin type 3 receptor antagonist alosetron in women with diarrhea-predominant irritable bowel syndrome. Arch Intern Med 2001;161:1733-1740.

75. Camilleri M, Mayer EA, Drossman DA, et al: Improvement in pain and bowel function in female irritable bowel patients with alosetron, a 5-HT$_3$ receptor antagonist. Aliment Pharmacol Ther 1999;13:1149-1159.

76. Chang L, Ameen VZ, Dukes GE, et al: A dose-ranging, phase II study of the efficacy and safety of alosetron in men with diarrhea-predominant IBS. Am J Gastroenterol 2005;100:115-123.

77. Chey WD, Chey WY, Heath AT, et al: Long-term safety and efficacy of alosetron in women with severe diarrhea-predominant irritable bowel syndrome. Am J Gastroenterol 2004;99:2195-2203.

78. Cremonini F, Delgado-Aros S, Camilleri M: Efficacy of alosetron in irritable bowel syndrome: A meta-analysis of randomized controlled trials. Neurogastroenterol Motil 2003;15:79-86.

79. Camilleri M: Treating irritable bowel syndrome: Overview, perspective and future therapies. Br J Pharmacol 2004;141:1237-1248.

80. Kamm MA, Muller-Lissner S, Talley NJ, et al: Tegaserod for the treatment of chronic constipation: A randomized, double-blind, placebo-controlled multinational study. Am J Gastroenterol 2005;100:362-372.

81. Kuiken SD, Tytgat GN, Boeckxstaens GE: Review article: Drugs interfering with visceral sensitivity for the treatment of functional gastrointestinal disorders—The clinical evidence. Aliment Pharmacol Therapeut 2005;21:633-651.

82. Richter JE, Dalton CB, Bradley LA, et al: Oral nifedipine in the treatment of noncardiac chest pain in patients with the nutcracker esophagus. Gastroenterology 1987;93:21-28.

83. Bharucha AE, Camilleri M, Zinsmeister AR, et al: Adrenergic modulation of human colonic motor and sensory function. Am J Physiol Gastrointest Liver Physiol 1997;273:G997-1006.

84. Tack J, Caenepeel P, Corsetti M, et al: Role of tension receptors in dyspeptic patients with hypersensitivity to gastric distention. Gastroenterology 2004;127:1058-1066.

85. Thumshirn M, Camilleri M, Choi MG, et al: Modulation of gastric sensory and motor functions by nitrergic and alpha(2)-adrenergic agents in humans. Gastroenterology 1999;116:573-585.

86. Viramontes BE, Malcolm A, Camilleri M, et al: Effects of an alpha 2-adrenergic agonist on gastrointestinal transit, colonic motility, and sensation in humans. Am J Physiol Gastrointest Liver Physiol 2001;281:G1468-1459.

87. Davenport K, Timoney AG, Keeley FX: Conventional and alternative methods for providing analgesia in renal colic. BJU Int 2005;95:297-300.

88. Poynard T, Regimbeau C, Benhamou Y: Meta-analysis of smooth muscle relaxants in the treatment of irritable bowel syndrome. Aliment Pharmacol Therapeut 2001;15:355-361.

89. Quartero AO, Meineche-Schmidt V, Muris J, et al: Bulking agents, antispasmodic and antidepressant medication for the treatment of irritable bowel syndrome. Cochrane Database System Rev 2005;CD003460.

90. Jones RH, Holtmann G, Rodrigo L, et al: Alosetron relieves pain and improves bowel function compared with mebeverine in female nonconstipated irritable bowel syndrome patients. Aliment Pharmacol Ther 1999;13:1419-1427.

91. Battaglia G, Morselli-Labate AM, Camarri E, et al: Otilonium bromide in irritable bowel syndrome: A double-blind, placebo-controlled, 15-week study. Aliment Pharmacol Therapeut 1998;12:1003-1010.

92. Bhidayasiri R, Truong DD: Expanding use of botulinum toxin. J Neurolog Sci 2005;235:1-9.

93. Pasricha PJ, Ravich WJ, Kalloo AN: Botulinum toxin for achalasia. Lancet 1993;341:244-245.

94. Mense S: Neurobiological basis for the use of botulinum toxin in pain therapy. J Neurol Neurosurg Psychiatry 2004; 251(suppl 1): 1-7.

95. Miller LS, Pullela SV, Parkman HP, et al: Treatment of chest pain in patients with noncardiac, nonreflux, nonachalasia spastic esophageal motor disorders using botulinum toxin injection into the gastroesophageal junction. Am J Gastroenterol 2002;97:1640-1646.

96. Storr M, Thammer J, Dunkel R, et al: Modulatory effect of adenosine receptors on the ascending and descending neural reflex responses of rat ileum. BMC Neurosci 2002;3:21.

97. Bromer MQ, Friedenberg F, Miller LS, et al: Endoscopic pyloric injection of botulinum toxin a for the treatment of refractory gastroparesis. Gastrointest Endosc 2005;61: 833-839.

98. Smith CP, Radziszewski P, Borkowski A, et al: Botulinum toxin a has antinociceptive effects in treating interstitial cystitis. Urology 2004;64:871-875.

99. Riviere PJ: Peripheral kappa-opioid agonists for visceral pain. Br J Pharmacol 2004;141:1331-1334.

100. De Schepper HU, Cremonini F, Park M-I, et al: Opioids and the gut: Pharmacology and current clinical experience. Neurogastroenterol Motil 2004;16:383-394.

101. Eisenach JC, Carpenter R, Curry R: Analgesia from a peripherally active [kappa]-opioid receptor agonist in patients with chronic pancreatitis. Pain 2003;101:89-95.

102. Dapoigny M, Abitbol JL, Fraitag B: Efficacy of peripheral kappa agonist fedotozine versus placebo in treatment of irritable bowel syndrome. A multicenter dose-response study. Dig Dis Sci 1995;40:2244-2249.

103. Delvaux M, Louvel D, Lagier E, et al: The agonist fedotozine relieves hypersensitivity to colonic distention in patients with irritable bowel syndrome. Gastroenterology 1999;116: 38-45.

104. Read NW, Abitbol JL, Bardhan KD, et al: Efficacy and safety of the peripheral kappa agonist fedotozine versus placebo in the treatment of functional dyspepsia. Gut 1997;41:664-668.

27 Acute Pain Management in Children

Santhanam Suresh and Sally Tarbell

The study of pain management in infants, children, and adolescents has seen a resurgence in the last decade. Data emphasizing the efficacy of adequate pain control and decreases in adverse neurohormonal changes have led to better care of infants and children.[1] Despite adequate pain control, there may be changes in biobehavioral factors when there is exposure to pain during the neonatal period.[2] Although the management of pain in infants and children has improved, there is still a need for further improvement. As we enter an era in which pain has been identified as a major part of patient well-being, we have no choice but to improve pain control in children.

DEVELOPMENTAL NEUROBIOLOGY OF PAIN

The study of pain in neonates has been a major focus for many neuroscientists. Even at birth, nociceptive pathways are well developed. A recent study of brain perfusion in response to pain has demonstrated significant changes in perfusion to noxious stimuli compared with non-noxious stimuli.[3] Newborn rats seem to have intense proliferation of A- and C-fibers at the site exposed to pain; a pattern of hyperalgesia appears to develop in these animals.[4] Human neonates exposed to repeated heel sticks may have cutaneous hyperalgesia, which can be reversed with topical local anesthesia.[5] More studies in the area of pain and neonates have been published in the last decade, signifying the interest in the neurobiology of pain as well as the importance of pain management in infants and children.[6]

CLINICAL MEASUREMENT OF PEDIATRIC ACUTE PAIN

Measures of acute pain in infants and young children, particularly the younger ones, rely on observer reports. These instruments gather information about one or more of the following: pain-related behaviors such as facial expression, body movements, and vocalizations, physiologic changes such as heart rate and oxygen saturation, and the child's behavioral state. These measures have usually been developed to assess either procedural pain (e.g., Premature Infant Pain Profile, PIPP[7]; Neonatal Facial Coding System, NFCS[8,9]) or postoperative pain (e.g., Children's Hospital of Eastern Ontario Pain Scale, CHEOPS[10]; Toddler-Preschooler Postoperative Pain Scale, TPPPS[11]). There is no one scale that is the gold standard for pain assessment in infants and preverbal children, and therefore the specific scale chosen will depend on the young child's characteristics (e.g., whether or not the child is neurologically impaired) and the type of pain being assessed.[12] Although these scales have been shown to have construct validity and internal and inter-rater reliability, there are intrinsic limits to their specificity for pain. For example, physiologic parameters can vary because of other conditions not associated with pain (Table 27–1).[13-25]

Children 5 years and older can typically provide self-reports on one of several validated visual analogues (e.g., Coloured Analogue Scale, CAS[20]) or faces scales (e.g., Faces Pain Scale—Revised, FPS-R[14,22]; Oucher[16]). McGrath and Hillier[26] have developed a separate Facial Affective Scale (FAS) designed to measure pain affect, as distinct from pain intensity. It is noteworthy that faces scales anchored with a smiling face produce higher pain ratings than those anchored with a neutral face.[27] The well-documented discordance between observer's ratings of a child's pain and the child's self-report[28-31] allows the clinician to consider the child's self-report as the gold standard whenever this can be obtained reliably, usually in children 5 years of age and older. There is preliminary evidence that children with developmental delay who are verbal can use self-rating methods such as a visual analogue scale (VAS) to assess their pain.[25] However, for those children with significant developmental delay who are nonverbal, Chambers and colleagues[28] have developed scales that rely on caregiver observations that identify core pain cues in this vulnerable group of children, such as the Non-Communicating Children's Pain Checklist—Revised (NCCPC-R)[23] and a version of the NCCPC for postoperative pain (NCCPC-PV).[24] The core pain cues include crying (with or without tears), screaming or yelling, inability to be comforted, face

Table 27–1. Clinical Measurement of Pediatric Acute Pain

AGE GROUP	MEASURE	TYPE OF MEASUREMENT	TYPE OF PAIN
Neonates and infants	Premature Infant Pain Profile, PIPP (preterm and full-term neonates)[7]	Behavioral, physiologic; gestational age	Procedural
	Neonatal Facial Coding System, NFCS (preterm and full-term neonates, infants ≤ 18 mo)[8,9]	Facial expression	Procedural, postoperative
	COMFORT scale (0-3yr)[13]	Behavioral, physiologic	Procedural, postoperative
Toddlers and preschoolers	Faces scales[14,15]	Self-report	Procedural, postoperative
	Oucher (≥3 yr)[16]	Self-report	Procedural
	Poker chip tool (4-8 yr)[17]	Self-report	Procedural
	Toddler-Preschooler Postoperative Pain Scale, TPPPS (1-5 yr)[11]	Behavioral	Postoperative
	Children's Hospital of Eastern Ontario Pain Scale, CHEOPS (1-7 yr)[18]	Behavioral	Postoperative
	Children's and Infants' Postoperative Pain Scale, CHIPPS (0-4 yr)[19]	Behavioral, physiologic; alertness, calmness	Postoperative
School-age children and adolescents	Coloured Analog Scale, CAS (≥5 yr)[20]	Self-report	Procedural, recurrent, chronic
	Visual Analogue Scale, VAS (≥5 yr)[20,21]	Self-report	Procedural, recurrent, chronic
	Faces scales[14,22]	Self-report	Procedural, recurrent, chronic
Noncommunicating children, children with cognitive impairment	Non-Communicating Children's Pain Checklist-Postoperative Version (NCCPC-PV), Non-Communicating Children's Pain Checklist-R (NCCPC-R)[23,24]	Behavioral	Procedural, postoperative, injury, pain related to chronic medical condition
	VAS[25]	Self-report	Procedural

contorted or looking distressed, flinching from contact, and appearing tense or stiff.[32] Terstegen and colleagues[33] have studied children with profound cognitive impairment and found 23 observable behaviors that were sensitive to postsurgical pain. Another recent pain assessment tool that can be used in all ages, including mentally challenged children, is the FLACC scale (**f**aces, **l**egs, **a**ctivity, **c**ry, **c**onsolability)[34] Each category is scored on a 0 to 2 scale, which results in a total score of 0 to 10 (0 = relaxed and comfortable; 1 to 3 = mild discomfort; 4 to 6 = moderate pain; 7 to 10 = severe discomfort).

Most measures developed so far have focused on acute, procedure-related pain. Changes in the behavioral and sensory aspects of pain that could habituate when pain becomes chronic may not be captured by these scales.[28] The systematic evaluation of chronic pain in children, which includes but moves beyond the sensory aspects of the pain, is described in Chapter 8. For further information on the measurement of acute pediatric pain, see reviews by Franck and associates (2000),[12] Johnston and colleagues (2003),[35] and Gaffney and coworkers (2003).[36]

NONMEDICAL MANAGEMENT OF ACUTE PAIN IN CHILDREN

Management of pain through nonmedical techniques, including environmental and behavioral strategies, has been found to be effective in modulating pain, both independently and in conjunction with pharmacologic interventions in children.[37-40] Nonmedical pain management strategies vary across developmental stages, and there are now empirically supported strategies for children of all ages (Table 27-2).[41-68] A number of mechanisms have been proposed to account for the effectiveness of specific nonpharmacologic pain management strategies, including activation of pain inhibitory pathways that descend to the dorsal horn of the spinal cord,[69-71] modulation of affective states, such as anxiety and negative affect, known to amplify the perception of pain,[36,72] lessening the association of painful procedures with distress and pain by attentional diversion,[47,73] altering or reinterpreting the sensation of pain (e.g., hypnotic suggestions for numbness),[74,75] and directing attention away from a painful stimulus.[66,69,73] Cognitive-behavioral therapy (e.g., relaxation, problem solving, cognitive coping skills) and distraction techniques such as deep breathing, cartoon videos, party blowers, and hypnosis have strong empirical support for their efficacy in children undergoing painful procedures (see Table 27-2). Distraction methods are hypothesized to work by engaging and absorbing the child's attention away from the pain,[52,76,77] thereby reducing perceived pain intensity, as well as inhibiting neural activity that underlies pain perception.[69] It has further been hypothesized that the extent to which children can redirect their attention away from pain and

Table 27–2. Nonmedical Methods of Pediatric Acute Pain Management

AGE OF CHILD	METHOD	EXAMPLES OF USES
Neonates, infants (<1 yr)	Swaddling[41]	Heel lance
	Positioning, skin-to skin contact; "kangaroo care"[35]	Heel lance
	Pacifier[42,43]	Immunization, heel lance
	Sucrose[44]	Injection, heel lance
	Breast-feeding[45,46]	Immunization, heel lance
	Toys, videos, distraction[47]	Immunization
Toddlers, preschoolers, early school age (2-6 yr)	Distraction, bubble blowing,[48] party blower[49,50]	Injection
	Video[51,52]	Immunization
	Interactive toys[53,54]	Injection
	Music[55]	VCUG, injections, chemotherapy administration by subcutaneous port, IM
	Nonprocedural talk[56]	Injection
	Breathing techniques[58]	Injection
	Imaginative Involvement[59]	BMA
	Hypnosis, hypnoanalgesia[59,60]	VCUG, venipuncture, LP, BMA
	Procedural Preparation: modeling, provision of procedural & sensory information, coaching[54,62-64]	LP, BMA, VCUG, Surgery, Immunization
School age (7-11 yr)	Distraction[64]	Immunization
	Hypnosis, hypnoanalgesia[59,60]	BMA, LP, IV insertion, VCUG
	Cognitive-behavioral therapy (CBT); includes relaxation techniques, imagery, cognitive coping skills, filmed modeling, reinforcement and incentives, behavioral rehearsal, coaching by parent or staff[63]	Burn wound care, venipuncture, LP, BMA, chemotherapy administration
	Procedural preparation—modeling, provision of procedural and sensory information[54,63,65]	VCUG, BMA, LP, EGD
Adolescent (≥12 yr)	Distraction, including virtual reality[67]	Burn wound care
	Hypnosis, hypnoanalgesia[59,67,68]	BMA, LP, surgery, VCUG
	Cognitive-behavioral therapy (CBT); includes relaxation techniques, imagery, cognitive coping skills, filmed modeling, reinforcement and incentives, behavioral rehearsal, coaching by parent or staff[63]	BMA, LP, venipuncture, chemotherapy administration
	Procedural preparation—modeling, provision of procedural and sensory information[63,66]	BMA, LP, EGD

BMA, bone marrow aspiration; EGD, esophagogastroduodenoscopy; LP, lumbar puncture; VCUG, voiding cystourethography.

pain-related concerns will determine the effectiveness of the psychological pain management techniques,[77] although this later hypothesis requires further empiric validation.

There is evidence that optimal pain coping strategies will vary according to the phase of a procedure; for example, while preparing for a procedure, the child may benefit from non–procedure-related conversation, whereas during the procedure, engaging in deep breathing may be most helpful.[49,78] There is also strong support for the influence of interactions of medical staff and parental caregivers on improving or exacerbating the child's pain and distress during painful procedures; for example, reassurance, apologies, empathy, criticism from caregivers, and giving control to the child tend to increase the child's distress behaviors, whereas distraction techniques such as directing the child to use a coping strategy such as deep breathing serve to reduce the child's distress.[50,79-81] Although it is typical for younger children to evidence more behavioral distress with painful procedures,[40,82] they are still capable of learning and being coached in pain management strategies that can help reduce their pain and behavioral distress.

Typically, children 7 years old or younger require parental or staff coaching to use self-management strategies such as deep breathing or positive self-talk.[47] Advances are being made in the management of procedural distress for children subjected to repeated painful procedures, such as those undergoing cancer treatment. One study has found that the child's negative exaggeration of a past lumbar puncture (LP) resulted in higher distress at subsequent LPs.[83] A cognitive intervention designed to modify these negative perceptions was found to be effective in reducing distress at subsequent procedures.[83] Chen and colleagues have also presented preliminary data suggesting that the few children who received midazolam for their procedure remembered many details from their prior procedure, which may account for the continued anticipatory anxiety that children display at subsequent procedures, in spite of being administered a medication with amnestic effects.[63] For additional reviews regarding nonmedical methods for acute pain management in children, see Blount and associates(2006),[84] Chen and coworkers (2000),[63] Powers (1999),[56] Kazak and Kunin-Batson (2001),[85] and Stevens (2001).[86]

PAIN TREATMENT MODALITIES

Depending on pain secondary to the surgical incision or a medical condition, it can be treated using various analgesics. The use of multimodal analgesia is beneficial for the management of pain. The ultimate goal of analgesia is to provide a consistent approach to pain, with minimal adverse effects. A pain treatment plan developed prior to the patient's surgery, based on the potential tissue insult from surgery, will help achieve more comprehensive management of pain. An organizational chart based on the multimodal management of pain could alter the approach to pain control.

Mild Analgesics

Sucrose

Opioid peptides in the ventral striatum and cingulate gyrus may play a role in regulating positive responses to energy-rich food such as fat and sugar. Hence, the administration of oral doses of glucose and sucrose can provide mild analgesia. A Cochran database review has suggested that the sucrose may be effective in reducing procedural pain in neonates.[87] Although an optimal dose has not been determined, doses in the range of 0.01 to 0.1 g have been shown to reduce procedural pain. This very innocuous technique can be used for most procedural pain in infants younger than 6 months of age.

Acetaminophen

This is a commonly used analgesic therapy for most common medical and surgical conditions. A higher dose of oral or rectal acetaminophen may be needed to obtain therapeutic levels. Generally, an initial rectal dose of 30 mg/kg is recommended, followed by subsequent doses of 20 mg/kg at 4- to 6-hour intervals. This produces therapeutic plasma levels that may be adequate for managing pain.[88,89] Although intravenous acetaminophen is available in Europe and has been used extensively in pediatric patients, it is not yet available in the United States. The daily dosage of acetaminophen must be limited to 100 mg/kg in children, 75 mg/kg in infants, and 60 mg/kg for neonates.[90] Although rare, the incidence of hepatic toxicity with high doses of acetaminophen should always be presented cautiously to parents, so that injudicious use of the medication is avoided.[91] Acetaminophen may not be an effective analgesic as an adjuvant for major surgical procedures in infants, and hence other classes of analgesics, including non-steroidal anti-inflammatory drugs (NSAIDs) or N-methyl-D-aspartic acid (NMDA) receptor antagonists may have to be considered.[92] A newer nitric oxide–releasing version of acetaminophen with analgesic and anti-inflammatory properties has been shown to have significant opioid-sparing effects in experimental models. This may offer a tremendous advantage over the current preparations of acetaminophen[93] (Table 27–3).

Nonsteroidal Anti-inflammatory Drugs

Aspirin has been avoided in children because of its association with Reye's syndrome. It still has a role in certain painful pediatric diseases, including Kawasaki's disease.[94] The more common NSAIDs in pediatric use are ibuprofen and diclofenac, mainly in Europe.[95-97] The intravenous preparation is available for use in children. Neonatal clearance of NSAIDs improves with age. Ibuprofen is metabolized by cytochrome P-450 (CYP) 2C9 and 2C8 subgroups.[98] In neonates, CYP 2C9 activity is low and improves after birth in the first 3 months. The two isomers, R-ibuprofen and S-ibuprofen, have different half-lives (10 and 25.5 hours, respectively). Assays producing pharmacokinetic data in neonates could therefore be skewed. Single-isomer NSAIDs are now emerging, with a better analgesic profile and fewer side effects.[99] Although there are conflicting views about the use of intravenous ketorolac following orthopedic surgery in animal experiments, a short duration of therapy does not seem to affect bone healing.[100] NSAIDs are excellent adjuvants to opioids for pain relief. In certain surgeries that could lead to postoperative bleeding, it may be wise to avoid using ketorolac.[101] The recommended dose for intravenous ketorolac is 0.5 mg/kg, with a maximum 30 mg/dose. The oral dose of ibuprofen is 10 to 15 mg/kg. Newer cyclooxygenase-2 (COX-2) inhibitors that have been intro-

Table 27–3. Oral Dosage Guidelines for Non-Opioid Analgesics

DRUG	DOSE (MG/KG)*	TOTAL DOSE (MG)†	RECOMMENDED INTERVAL (HR)	MAXIMUM DAILY DOSE (MG/KG)*	MAXIMUM TOTAL DAILY DOSE (MG)†
Acetaminophen	10-15‡	650-1000	4	100	4000
Ibuprofen	6-10§	400-600	4-6	40	2400
Naproxen	5-6	250-375	12	24	1000

*Weight < 60 kg.
†Weight > 60 kg.
‡See text for detailed explanation about dosing in neonates and infants.
§See text for pharmacogenetic variability.
Adapted from Berde CB, Sethna NF: Analgesics for the treatment of pain in children. N Engl J Med 2002;347:1094-1103.

duced to clinical practice are used rarely in children except in certain chronic painful conditions, including rheumatoid arthritis.[102] Adult studies have shown that COX-2 inhibitors can be effectively and safely used following spinal fusion surgery.[103] The risk of atherothrombosis has to be weighed heavily when choosing COX-2 inhibitors for pain relief in chronic pain states.

N-Methyl-D-Aspartate Receptor Antagonists

The N-methyl-D-aspartate (NMDA) class of drugs is more commonly used in the pediatric population than in their adult counterparts. Ketamine is the most commonly used NMDA receptor antagonist in pediatric patients. The S enantiomer has four times the potency of the R enantiomer.[104] Although not used independently for providing pain relief, ketamine is used as an adjuvant to other analgesics and has an opioid-sparing effect in postoperative pain control.[104] We use ketamine as an adjuvant in patients who seem to exhibit signs of opioid tolerance. Doses of 0.05 to 0.1 mg/kg/hr are normally provided as a continuous infusion. We have recently used other NMDA receptor antagonists, including dextromethorphan[105] and magnesium,[106] as adjuvants to pain management.

Tramadol

This is being used increasingly for pain control in children.[107,108] The absence of respiratory depression, along with the decrease in postoperative nausea and vomiting, makes it an attractive alternative to conventional opioids.[109] It is metabolized to o-desmethyl tramadol by cytochrome P2D6 (CYP2D6).[110] The clearance of tramadol reaches 84% in full-term neonates.[98] The recommended dose for tramadol is 1 mg/kg orally every 6 hours. In children who may have significant obstructive apnea, tramadol offers an attractive alternative over intravenous morphine with regard to respiratory embarrassment.[111]

Opioids

Opioids form the mainstay of analgesic management, particularly in the acute postoperative setting. They are also used extensively in the management of pain in chronic painful conditions, including sickle cell disease and cystic fibrosis,[112] and for the management of pain in cancer patients. A detailed description of opioids and their mechanism of action is found in Chapters 31 and 32.

Pharmacokinetics of Opioids

Opioids have lower clearance in neonates and infants and reach the normal mature values in the first 6 months of life.[113] The active metabolites of morphine are excreted by the kidneys; these can accumulate in children with compromised renal function and in neonates because of their decreased renal clearance. Opioid-induced respiratory depression can be accentuated in neonates and infants whose respiratory reflex responses to airway obstruction and hypoxemia are immature at birth but mature during the first year of life.[90] A brief description of commonly used opioids in pediatric practice for acute pain control will be presented here. Adverse effects of opioids, including respiratory depression, nausea and vomiting, pruritus, and itching, can be effectively managed and can result in a positive postoperative outcome (Table 27–4).

Codeine

Codeine is perhaps the most commonly used opioid in children. It is usually prescribed for most postoperative pediatric patients in combination with acetaminophen. Codeine is converted to morphine by cytochrome P-450 2D6. Many children younger than 12 years lack CYP2D6 maturity and cannot convert codeine to morphine.[114] Consequently, although they exhibit the adverse effects of codeine, such as nausea and vomiting, they do not experience any analgesic effects. Codeine is associated with significant nausea and vomiting and may lead to a worse postoperative outcome compared with other available opioids. The recommended dosage is 0.5 to 1 mg/kg.

Oxycodone

Oxycodone is a fairly powerful analgesic that can provide excellent analgesia without the adverse effects associated with oral codeine. It is metabolized in the liver by cytochrome P-450 rather than by hepatic glucuronidation. It has higher oral bioavailability than morphine and has a slightly longer half-life. It has a better profile than other oral opioids for postoperative pain control. A dose of 0.1 to 0.2 mg/kg is generally used every 4 to 6 hours for pain control.[90] It is available in combination with oral acetaminophen for pain control in children.

Table 27–4. Management of Adverse Effects of Opioids

ADVERSE EFFECT	INITIAL MANAGEMENT	SECONDARY MANAGEMENT
Pruritus	Benadryl, hydroxyzine	IV low-dose naloxone
Nausea, vomiting	Phenergan	Ondansetron, IV naloxone
Urinary retention	Decrease opioid dose	Urinary catheterization
Respiratory depression	Decrease opioid dose	IV naloxone

Hydrocodone

This is a commonly used analgesic in postsurgical patients. It has the advantage of providing powerful analgesia with minimal adverse effects. The dose of hydrocodone is 0.15 mg/kg every 6 hours. It is available as an elixir. The total dosage should be restricted to a maximum of 15 mg/day.

Morphine

Morphine still remains the mainstay for managing acute pain in children. It is mainly metabolized by the hepatic enzyme uridine 5-diphosphate glucuronosyltransferase-2B7 (UGT2B7) into morphine-3-glucuronide (M3G) and morphine-6-glucuronide (M6G). A single nucleotide polymorphism, A118G of the μ-opioid receptor gene, may lead to decreased potency of morphine and M6G,[115] which may explain the ineffectiveness of morphine in certain populations. The recommended oral dose is 0.5 to 1 mg/kg every 3 to 4 hours. When given intravenously, a dose of 0.1 mg/kg administered every 2 to 4 hours will provide adequate analgesia. Associated adverse effects of morphine include respiratory depression, itching, and potential for nausea and vomiting and urinary retention. In children undergoing major surgical procedures, a patient-controlled analgesia system may provide sustained adequate analgesia (see later). There have been recent reports of morphine-induced hyperalgesia, particularly when patients have been on long-term opioids.[116]

Fentanyl

Although fentanyl was originally studied in neonates because of its immense cardiovascular stability, it has found a place in daily analgesia management, particularly in the operating room for immediate control of pain in the intraoperative and immediate postoperative periods. The dose of fentanyl is 0.5 to 1 μg/kg, given every 1 to 2 hours. Fentanyl has significant hemodynamic stability and may be useful, particularly in children who have cardiovascular instability. There are other forms of fentanyl available, including transmucosal fentanyl and transdermal fentanyl, both of which have no indication for use in an acute pain setting,

Hydromorphone

This is a potent opioid that can be used in a postoperative setting for pain control. Intravenous doses of 0.02 mg/kg every 2 to 4 hours provide analgesia during surgical procedures. Oral hydromorphone, 0.04 to 0.08 mg/kg every 3 to 4 hours, can provide adequate analgesia. Hydromorphone has a similar risk profile to morphine in terms of respiratory depression.

Methadone

Methadone has seen a resurgence in use for acute postoperative pain control. We routinely use methadone as a single dose prior to removal of epidural catheters or in conjunction with other oral opioids, especially oxycodone, in children who have undergone major surgery and are being converted to oral medication. The half-life of methadone in children is longer than in adults.[117] We administer 200 μg/kg, followed by a dose of 25 to 75 μg/kg every 8 to 12 hours, based on the surgical procedure and the potential for severe pain. The oral bioavailability of the drug is good, making it a potentially viable alternative to other oral opioids when parenteral opioids are discontinued.

Patient-Controlled Analgesia

Patient-controlled analgesia (PCA) has revolutionized the management of pain in children and adolescents. Most children who undergo major surgery are given an option to use PCA in the postoperative period. There are many controlled trials that have supported the safety and efficacy of PCA in children older than 6 years.[118] Although the use of nurse-controlled or parent-controlled analgesia[119] has been controversial because of the safety profile, the judicious use of PCA, whether it is nurse- or parent-controlled, can provide excellent pain relief in the postoperative period for the cognitively impaired child or for infants. We prefer the use of morphine and hydromorphone in older children and adolescents and fentanyl in infants because of its greater titratability. A possible reason for the greater efficacy of PCA in comparison with conventional methods is because of its on-demand availability to patients at all times. A low-dose basal infusion seems to be appropriate for children and has not been associated with any adverse outcomes. In children who may experience greater pain in the postoperative period, such as after spinal fusion, may need additional continuous infusions of adjuvant medications, including NMDA receptor antagonists such as ketamine, for additional pain control. Provided is a sample form for managing patient-controlled analgesia in children (Appendix 27–1). A simple conversion sheet to convert patients from one opioid to another is shown in Figure 27–1. Recently, we have added continuous epidural analgesia in addition to PCA for patients undergoing spinal fusion (see Appendix 27–2).

Regional Anesthesia

There has been greater enthusiasm among health care personnel who take care of children to use regional anesthesia for pain management. Although there is controversy regarding the use of regional anesthesia in children under general anesthesia, there is consensus among pediatric anesthesiologists about the use of safely providing a regional anesthetic technique under general anesthesia.[120] It is important to follow safety guidelines for dosage of local anesthetics in children (Table 27–5). Techniques regarding the use of regional anesthesia are described in detail in Chapters 46 to 50.

Caudal Analgesia

The most commonly used regional technique in children is a caudal block, which is used for most analgesia for surgery performed below the umbilicus. The technique is simple and requires a basic understanding of the anatomy of the space. A blunt styletted needle is passed through the sacrococcygeal ligament into the caudal space. A "pop" is felt when the caudal space is accessed. Newer techniques, including the use of nerve stimulation[121] and ultrasonography,[122] can be used to localize the caudal space. Local anesthetics include bupivacaine, 0.125% or 0.25%, with 1:200,000 epinephrine at a dose of 1 mL/kg (maximum dosage, 30 mL).

Spinal Anesthesia

This has been advised especially for former preterm infants who are undergoing hernia repair as a method

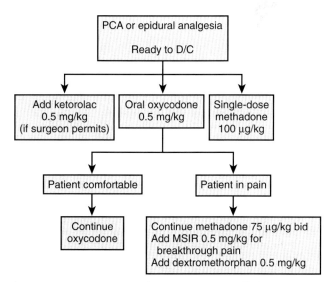

Figure 27–1. Conversion from patient-controlled or epidural analgesia to oral analgesics. D/C, discontinue; MSIR, morphine sulfate immediate release..

to avoid apnea and bradycardia.[123] The procedure is performed in infants awake, without the use of general anesthesia. Although a good technique, it has its limitations because of the lack of adequate training to perform this block on a routine basis.[124]

Epidural Analgesia

With improved techniques and increasing needle and catheter availability for children, the use of central neuraxial blocks, particularly epidural analgesia, has been increasing. Epidural analgesia combined with general anesthesia has been the most commonly used modality in children. It is imperative to use standardized dosing parameters for a single injection as well as for continuous infusion in neonates, infants, and children to avoid local anesthetic toxicity[125] (see Table 27–5). There are a few caveats for use in children, including the following:

1. Use of saline for testing loss of resistance, particularly in the neonate and infant, because of the potential risk of air embolism.[126]
2. Caution while accessing the epidural space. Depth varies in children and the distance from skin to the epidural space could be as little as 1 to 2 cm. Formulas are available for determining epidural depth space, but this is not always predictable.[127]
3. Test dose with epinephrine-containing solution. Intravenous injection may not always lead to an increase in heart rate or blood pressure. A more predictable measure is a change in T waves on an electrocardiographic rhythm monitor.[128] This is our primary measure for potential intravenous injection.

Epidural catheter insertions have to be carried out using sterile techniques. Our preference is to leave the catheter in for approximately 72 hours. Catheter placement can be facilitated using a stimulating technique or ultrasonography.[122,129] A dedicated pain treatment service can facilitate the use of epidural analgesia. We have also reported the use of patient-controlled epidural analgesia (PCEA), which can be very effective in adolescents and children who may experience greater pain, particularly while ambulating after extensive surgery.[130] An epidural analgesia order sheet is provided for reference (Appendix 27–2).

Table 27–5. Local Anesthetic Solution Dosing Guidelines*

DRUG	ROUTE OF ADMINISTRATION	Age Group		
		NEONATES	CHILDREN	ADOLESCENTS
Bupivacaine	Bolus	2	3	4
Bupivacaine	Continuous infusion	0.2	0.3	0.4
Ropivacaine	Bolus dose	2	3	4
Ropivacaine	Continuous infusion	0.2	0.3	0.4
Levobupivacaine		2	2	3

*In mg/kg.

Adjuvants to Epidural Analgesia

Common adjuvants to epidural analgesia in children include fentanyl (2 to 5 µg/mL), hydromorphone (0.2 µg/kg/hr to 0.4 µg/kg/hr), or clonidine (1 µg/mL) to prolong or provide better analgesia. A study conducted in our institution has shown that the use of freshly added epinephrine (1:200,000) provides an equivalent degree of analgesia compared with clonidine, 2 µg/mL.[131]

Further Considerations

Adverse Effects of Opioids

Although the use of patient-controlled analgesia and epidural analgesia has improved the quality of pain control in children, they are also associated with adverse effects, including nausea, vomiting, constipation, respiratory depression, and pruritus. Although respiratory depression is a major complication associated with opioids, the other adverse effects are more common and can cause a significant degree of discomfort to the patient. Opioid-induced bowel distention, particularly in the child who is on large doses of opioids or following bowel resection, is a common adverse effect. If oral medication can be tolerated, we administer oral naloxone, 20 µg/kg every 4 to 6 hours, with excellent relief.[132] Alternatively, a small dose of intravenous naloxone may be helpful in decreasing minor adverse effects, including urinary retention, pruritus, and nausea and vomiting[133] (see Table 27–4).

Peripheral Nerve Blocks

Techniques for performing nerve blocks are explained in detail elsewhere in this text. Local anesthetic doses for peripheral nerve blocks in children are based on weight, and large doses are generally avoided. Using ultrasonography, a new pharmacodynamic model has been created to decrease the total dose of local anesthetic solution needed for pain relief following peripheral nerve blocks.[134] Commonly used peripheral nerve blocks in children, with their indications, are shown in Box 27–1.[135-146]

CONCLUSION

Acute pain management in children has seen a tremendous transformation in the last few years. The addition of safer medications, with a better safety profile, has clearly advanced the field of pain management in neonates, infants, and children. With greater emphasis by the U.S. Food and Drug Administration to recognize the unique needs of pediatric patients, we have a mandate to study and continue further research in infants and children.

> **BOX 27–1. COMMONLY USED PERIPHERAL NERVE BLOCKS IN CHILDREN**
>
> **Head and Neck**
> Trigeminal branches(V1, V2, V3) for scalp surgery,[135] cleft lip, cleft palate, nasal surgery,[136] mandibular surgery, craniotomy[137]
> Cervical plexus for mastoid surgery,[138] thyroid surgery[139]
>
> **Upper Extremity**
> Brachial plexus,[140] commonly axillary or infraclavicular
> Digital blocks for common plastic surgery procedures[141]
>
> **Lower Extremity**
> Femoral nerve for fractures[142]
> Lateral femoral cutaneous nerve for graft excision from lateral thigh[143]
> Sciatic nerve block (infragluteal or popliteal fossa)[144]
> Ankle block
> Trunk block
> Intercostal blocks for rib fractures, excisions
> Ilioinguinal nerve blocks for hernia repair[134]
> Penile blocks for circumcision, penile surgery[145]
> Rectus sheath blocks for umbilical hernia repair[146]

References

1. Anand KJ: Neonatal stress responses to anesthesia and surgery. Clin Perinatol 1990;17:207-214.
2. Taddio A, Katz J, Ilersich AL, et al: Effect of neonatal circumcision on pain response during subsequent routine vaccination. Lancet 1997;349:599-603.
3. Slater R, Cantarella A, Gallella S, et al: Cortical pain responses in human infants. J Neurosci 2006;26:3662-3666.
4. Reynolds ML, Fitzgerald M: Long-term sensory hyperinnervation following neonatal skin wounds. J Comp Neurol 1995; 358:487-498.
5. Fitzgerald M, Woolf CJ, Shortland P: Collateral sprouting of the central terminals of cutaneous primary afferent neurons in the rat spinal cord: Pattern, morphology, and influence of targets. J Comp Neurol 1990300:370-385.
6. Carbajal R, Lenclen R, Jugie M, et al: Morphine does not provide adequate analgesia for acute procedural pain among preterm neonates. Pediatrics 2005;115:1494-1500.
7. Stevens B: Pain management in newborns: How far have we progressed in research and practice? Birth 1996;23:229-235.
8. Grunau RE, Oberlander T, Holsti L, et al: Bedside application of the Neonatal Facial Coding System in pain assessment in neonates. Pain 1998;76:277-286.
9. Peters JW, Koot HM, Grunau RE, et al: Neonatal Facial Coding System for assessing postoperative pain in infants: Item reduction is valid and feasible. Clin J Pain 2003;19: 353-363.
10. McGrath PJ, Johnson G, Goodman JT: CHEOPS: A Behavioral Scale for Rating Postoperative Pain in Children. In Fields HL, Dubner R, Cervero F (eds): Advances in Pain Research and Therapy. New York, Raven Press, 1985, pp 395-402.
11. Tarbell SE, Cohen IT, Marsh J: The Toddler-Preschooler Postoperative Pain Scale: An observational scale for measuring postoperative pain in children aged 1-5. Preliminary report. Pain 1992;50:273-280.

12. Franck LS, Greenberg CS, Stevens B: Pain assessment in infants and children. Pediatr Clin North Am 2000;47:487-512.

13. van Dijk M, de Boer JB, Koot HM, et al: The reliability and validity of the COMFORT scale as a postoperative pain instrument in 0 to 3-year old infants. Pain 2000;84:367-377.

14. Champion GD, Goodenough B, von Baeyer CL, et al: Measurement of pain by self-report. In Finley G, McGrath P (eds): Measurement of Pain in Infants and Children. Seattle, IASP Press, 1998, pp 123-160.

15. Hicks CL, von Baeyer CL, Spafford PA, et al: The Faces Pain Scale—Revised: Toward a common metric in pediatric pain measurement. Pain 2001;93:173-183.

16. Beyer JE, Denyes MJ, Villarruel AM: The creation, validation, and continuing development of the Oucher: A measure of pain intensity in children. J Pediatr Nurs 1992;7:335-346.

17. Hester NO, Foster RL, Kristensen K: Measurement of pain in children: Generalizability and validity of the pain ladder and poker chip tool. In Tyler DC, Krane EJ (eds): Pediatric Pain. New York, Raven Press, 1990, pp 79-84.

18. McGrath PA, deVeber LL, Hearn MT: Multidimensional pain assessment in children. In Fields HL, Dubner R, Cervero F (eds): Advances in Pain Research and Therapy. New York, Raven Press, 1985, pp 387-393.

19. Buttner W, Finke W: Analysis of behavioural and physiological parameters for the assessment of postoperative analgesic demand in newborns, infants and young children: A comprehensive report on seven consecutive studies. Paediatr Anaesth 2000;10:303-318.

20. McGrath PA, Seifert CE, Speechley KN, et al: A new analogue scale for assessing children's pain: An initial validation study. Pain 1996;64:435-443.

21. Varni JW, Thompson KL, Hanson V: The Varni/Thompson Pediatric Pain Questionnaire. I. Chronic musculoskeletal pain in juvenile rheumatoid arthritis. Pain 1987;28:27-38.

22. Good M, Stanton-Hicks M, Grass JA, et al: Relaxation and music to reduce postsurgical pain. J Adv Nurs 2001;33:208-215.

23. Breau LM, McGrath PJ, Camfield C, et al: Psychometric properties of the non-communicating children's pain checklist—revised. Pain 2002;99:349-357.

24. Breau LM, Finley GA, McGrath PJ, et al: Validation of the non-communicating children's pain checklist-postoperative version. Anesthesiology 2002;96:528-535.

25. Benini F, Trapanotto M, Gobber D, et al: Evaluating pain induced by venipuncture in pediatric patients with developmental delay. Clin J Pain 2004;20:156-163.

26. McGrath PA, Hillier LM: Controlling children's pain. In Gatchel RJ, Turk DC (eds): Psychological Approaches to Pain Management. New York, Guilford, 1996, pp 331-370.

27. Chambers CT, Hardial J, Craig KD, et al: Faces scales for the measurement of postoperative pain intensity in children following minor surgery. Clin J Pain 2005;21:277-285.

28. Chambers CT, Reid GJ, Craig KD, et al: Agreement between child and parent reports of pain. Clin J Pain 1998;14:336-342.

29. Bhat R, Abu-Harb M, Chari G, et al: Morphine metabolism in acutely ill preterm newborn infants. J Pediatr 1992 May;120(5):795-9 1998:795-799.

30. Maciocia PM, Strachan EM, Akram AR, et al: Pain assessment in the paediatric Emergency Department: Whose view counts? Eur J Emerg Med 2003;10:264-267.

31. Cohen LL, Blount RL, Cohen RJ, et al: Dimensions of pediatric procedural distress: Children's anxiety and pain during immunizations. J Clin Psychol Med Settings 2004;11:41-47.

32. Stallard P, Williams L, Velleman R, et al: Brief report: Behaviors identified by caregivers to detect pain in noncommunicating children. J Pediatric Psychol 2002;27:209-214.

33. Terstegen C, Koot HM, de Boer JB, et al: Measuring pain in children with cognitive impairment: Pain response to surgical procedures. Pain 2003;103:187-198.

34. Voepel-Lewis T, Merkel S, Tait AR, et al: The reliability and validity of the Face, Legs, Activity, Cry, Consolability observational tool as a measure of pain in children with cognitive impairment. Anesth Analg 2002;95:1224-1229.

35. Johnston CC, Stevens B, Pinelli J, et al: Kangaroo care is effective in diminishing pain response in preterm neonates. Arch Pediatr Adolesc Med 2003;157:1084-1088.

36. Gaffney A, McGrath PJ, Dick B: Measuring pain in children: Developmental and instrument issues. In Schecter NL, Berde CB, Yaster M (eds): Pain in Infants, Children and Adolescents, 2nd ed. Baltimore, Lippincott Williams & Wilkins, 2003, pp 128-141.

37. Jay SM, Elliot CH, Woody PD, et al: An investigation of cognitive-behavior therapy combined with oral valium for children undergoing painful medical procedures. Health Psychol 1991;10:317-322.

38. Kashikar-Zuck S, Swain NF, Jones BA, et al: Efficacy of cognitive-behavioral intervention for juvenile primary fibromyalgia syndrome. J Rheumatol 2005;32:1594-1602.

39. Robins PM, Smith SM, Glutting JJ, et al: A randomized controlled trial of a cognitive-behavioral family intervention for pediatric recurrent abdominal pain. J Pediatr Psychol 2005;30:397-408.

40. Kazak AE, Biancamaria P, Boyer BA, et al: A randomized controlled prospective outcome study of a psychological and pharmacological intervention protocol for procedural distress in pediatric leukemia. J Pediatr Psychol 1996;21:615-631.

41. Fearon I, Kisilevsky BS, Hains SM, et al: Swaddling after heel lance: Age-specific effects on behavioral recovery in preterm infants. J Dev Behav Pediatr 1997;18:222-232.

42. Reis EC, Roth EK, Syphan JL, et al: Effective pain reduction for multiple immunization injections in young infants. Arch Pediatr Adolesc Med 2003;157:1115-1120.

43. Field T, Goldson E: Pacifying effects of non-nutritive sucking on term and pre-term neonates during heelstick procedures. Pediatrics 1984;74:1012-1015.

44. Stevens BJ, Yamada J, Ohlsson A: Sucrose for analgesia in newborn infants undergoing painful procedures. Cochrane Database System Rev 2004;(3):CD001069.

45. Shah PS, Aliwalas LL, Shah V: Breastfeeding or breast milk for procedural pain in neonates. Cochrane Database System Rev 2006;(3):CD004950.

46. Rostami S, Nikrooz L, Alijani H, et al: Comparison of efficacy of breast-feeding with oral glucose on infant vaccination pain. Pain Res Management 2006;11:72b.

47. Cohen LL: Reducing infant immunization distress through distraction. Health Psychol 2002;21:207-211.

48. Sparks L: Taking the "ouch" out of injections for children: Using distraction to decrease pain. MCN Am J Matern Child Nurs 2001;26:72-78.

49. Blount RL, Bachanas PJ, Powers SW, et al: Training children to cope and parents to coach them during routine immunizations: Effects on child, parent, and staff behaviors. Behav Ther 1992;23:689-705.

50. Manimala M, Blount RL, Cohen LL: The influence of parental reassurance and distraction on children's reactions to an aversive medical procedure. Child Health Care 2000;29:161-177.

51. Cohen LL, Blount RL, Panopoulos G: Nurse coaching and cartoon distraction: An effective and practical intervention to reduce child, parent, and nurse distress during immunizations. J Pediatr Psychol 1997;22:355-370.

52. McLaren JE, Cohen LL: A comparison of distraction strategies for venipuncture distress in children. J Pediatr Psychol 2005;30:387-396.

53. Dahlquist LM, Pendley JS, Landthrip DS, et al: Distractions interventions for preschoolers undergoing intramuscular injections and subcutaneous port access. Health Psychol 2002;21:94-99.

54. Salmon K, McGuigan F, Pereira JK: Brief report: Optimizing children's memory and management of an invasive medical procedure: The influence of procedural narration and distraction. J Pediatr Psychol 2006;31:522-527.

55. Fowler-Kerry S, Lander JR: Management of injection pain in children. Pain 1987;30:169-175.

56. Powers SW: Empirically supported treatments in pediatric psychology: Procedure-related pain. J Pediatr Psychol 1999;24:131-145.

57. Gonzalez JC, Routh DK, Armstrong FD: Effects of maternal distraction versus reassurance on children's reactions to injections. J Pediatr Psychol 1993;18:593-604.

58. French GM, Painter EC, Coury DL: Blowing away shot pain: A technique for pain management during immunization. Pediatrics 1994;93:384-388.

59. Kuttner L, Solomon R: Hypnotherapy and imagery for managing children's pain. In Schecter NL, Berde CB, Yaster M (eds): Pain in Infants, Children and Adolescents, 2nd ed. Baltimore, Lippincott Williams & Wilkins, 2003, pp 317-328.

60. Butler LD, Symons BK, Henderson SL, et al: Hypnosis reduces distress and duration of an invasive medical procedure for children. Pediatrics 2005;115:77-85.

61. Smith GM, Hale J, Pasnikowski EM, et al: Astrocytes infected with replication-defective adenovirus containing a secreted form of CNTF or NT3 show enhanced support of neuronal populations in vitro. Exp Neurol 1996;139:156-166.

62. Christiano B, Tarbell SE: Brief report: Behavioral correlates of postoperative pain in toddlers and preschoolers. J Pediatr Psychol 1998;149-154.

63. Chen E, Joseph MH, Zeltzer LK: Behavioral and cognitive interventions in the treatment of pain in children. Pediatr Clin North Am 2000;47:513-525.

64. Cohen LL, Blount RL, Cohen RJ, et al: Comparative study of distraction versus topical anesthesia for pediatric pain management during immunizations. Health Psychol 1999;18:591-598.

65. Claar RL, Walker LS, Smith CA: The influence of appraisals in understanding children's experiences with medical procedures. J Pediatr Psychol 2002;27:553-563.

66. Hoffman HG, Doctor JN, Patterson DR, et al: Virtual reality as an adjunctive pain control during burn wound care in adolescent patients. Pain 2000;85:305-309.

67. Liossi C, Hatira P: Clinical hypnosis versus cognitive behavioral training for pain management with pediatric cancer patients undergoing bone marrow aspirations. Int J Clin Exp Hypn 1999;47:104-116.

68. Jones CWE: Hypnosis and spinal fusion by Harrington rod instrumentation. Am J Clin Hypnosis 1997;19:155-157.

69. Bushnell MC, Villemure C, Duncan GH: Psychophysiological and neurophysiological studies of pain modulation by attention. In Price DD, Bushnell MC (eds): Psychological Methods of Pain Control: Basic Science and Clinical Perspectives. Seattle, IASP Press, 2003, pp 99-116.

70. Melzack R, Wall PD: Pain mechanisms: A new theory. Science 1965;150:971-979.

71. Holliday MA, Pinckert TL, Kiernan SC, et al: Dorsal penile nerve block vs topical placebo for circumcision in low-birth-weight neonates. Arch Pediatr Adolesc Med. 1999;153:476-480.

72. Rhudy JL, Meagher MW: Fear and anxiety: Divergent effects on human pain thresholds. Pain 2000;84:65-75.

73. DeMore M, Cohen LL: Distraction for pediatric immunization pain: A critical review. J Clin Psychol Med Settings 2005;12:281-291.

74. Haythornwhite JA, Lawrence J, Fauerbach J: Brief cognitive interventions for burn pain. Ann Behav Med 2001;23:42-49.

75. Rainville P, Price DD: The neurophenomenology of hypnosis and hypnoanalgesia. In Price DD, Bushnell MC (eds): Psychological Methods of Pain Control: Basic Science and Clinical Perspectives. Seattle, IASP Press, 2004, pp 235-267.

76. Harrison A: Comparing nurses' and patients' pain evaluations: A study of hospitalized patients in Kuwait. Soc Sci Med 1993;36:683-692.

77. Zeltzer LK, Bush JP, Chen E, et al: A psychobiologic approach to pediatric pain: Part II. Prevention and treatment. Curr Prob Pediatr 1997;27:264-284.

78. Blount RL, Powers SW, Cotter MC, et al: Making the system work: Training pediatric oncology patients to cope and their parents to coach them during BMA/LP procedures. Behav Modif 1994;18:6-31.

79. Blount RL, Schaen ER, Cohen LL: Commentary: Current status and future directions in acute pediatric pain assessment and treatment. J Pediatr Psychol 1999;24:150-152.

80. Blount RL, Corbin SM, Sturges JW, et al: The relationship between adult's behavior and child coping and distress during BMA/LP procedures: A sequential analysis. Behav Ther 1989;20:585-601.

81. Bouwmeester J, Gonzalez Candel A: [Special forms of analgesia: Patient-controlled analgesia]. Tijdschrift Kindergeneeskde 1993;61:52-54.

82. Task Force on Pain Management, Catholic Health Association: Pain management. Theological and ethical principles governing the use of pain relief for dying patients. Health Prog 1993;74:30-39, 65.

83. Chen E, Zeltzer LK, Craske MG, et al: Alteration of memory in the reduction of children's distress during repeated aversive medical procedures. J Consult Clin Psychol 1999;67:481-490.

84. Blount RL, Piira T, Cohen LL, et al: Pediatric procedural pain. Behav Modif 2006;30:24-49.

85. Kazak AE, Kunin-Batson A: Psychological and integrative interventions in pediatric procedure pain. In Finley GA, McGrath PJ (eds): Acute and Procedure Pain in Infants and Children. Seattle, IASP Press, 2001, pp 77-100.

86. Stevens B: Acute pain management in infants in the neonatal intensive care unit. In Finley GA, McGrath PJ (eds): Acute and Procedure Pain in Infants and Children. Seattle, IASP Press, 2001, pp 101-128.

87. Stevens B, Yamada J, Ohlsson A: Sucrose for analgesia in newborn infants undergoing painful procedures. Cochrane Database Syst Rev 2004;(3):CD001069.

88. Birmingham PK, Tobin MJ, Henthorn TK, et al: Twenty-four-hour pharmacokinetics of rectal acetaminophen in children: An old drug with new recommendations. Anesthesiology 1997;87:244-252.

89. Birmingham PK, Tobin MJ, Fisher DM, et al: Initial and subsequent dosing of rectal acetaminophen in children: A 24-hour pharmacokinetic study of new dose recommendations. Anesthesiology 2001;94:385-389.

90. Berde CB, Sethna NF: Analgesics for the treatment of pain in children. N Engl J Med 2002;347:1094-1103.

91. Mohler CR, Nordt SP, Williams SR, et al: Prospective evaluation of mild to moderate pediatric acetaminophen exposures. Ann Emerg Med 2000;35:239-244.

92. van der Marel CD, Peters JW, Bouwmeester NJ, et al: Rectal acetaminophen does not reduce morphine consumption after major surgery in young infants. Br J Anaesth 2007;98:372-379.

93. Gaitan G, Ahuir FJ, Herrero JF: Enhancement of fentanyl antinociception by subeffective doses of nitroparacetamol (NCX-701) in acute nociception and in carrageenan-induced monoarthritis. Life Sci 2005;77:85-95.

94. Baumer JH, Love SJ, Gupta A, et al: Salicylate for the treatment of Kawasaki disease in children. Cochrane Database Syst Rev 2006;(4):CD004175.

95. Bruce E, Franck L, Howard RF: The efficacy of morphine and Entonox analgesia during chest drain removal in children. Paediatr Anaesth 2006;16:302-308.

96. Lesko SM, Mitchell AA: An assessment of the safety of pediatric ibuprofen. A practitioner-based randomized clinical trial. JAMA 1995;273:929-933.

97. St. Charles CS, Matt BH, Hamilton MM, et al: A comparison of ibuprofen versus acetaminophen with codeine in the young tonsillectomy patient. Otolaryngol Head Neck Surg 1997;117:76-82.

98. Anderson BJ, Palmer GM: Recent pharmacological advances in paediatric analgesics. Biomed Pharmacother 2006;60:303-309.

99. Jackson ID, Heidemann BH, Wilson J, et al: Double-blind, randomized, placebo-controlled trial comparing rofecoxib with dexketoprofen trometamol in surgical dentistry. Br J Anaesth 2004;92:675-680.

100. Reuben SS: Effect of nonsteroidal anti-inflammatory drugs on osteogenesis and spinal fusion. Reg Anesth Pain Med 2001;26:590-591.

101. Rusy LM, Houck CS, Sullivan LJ, et al: A double-blind evaluation of ketorolac tromethamine versus acetaminophen in pediatric tonsillectomy: Analgesia and bleeding. Anesth Analg 1995;80:226-229.

102. Brunner HI, Kim KN, Ballinger SH, et al: Current medication choices in juvenile rheumatoid arthritis. II, Update of a survey performed in 1993. J Clin Rheumatol 2001;7: 295-300.
103. Reuben SS: A new class of COX-2 inhibitors offer an alternative to NSAIDs in pain management after spinal surgery. Spine 2001;26:1505-1506.
104. Subramaniam K, Subramaniam B, Steinbrook RA: Ketamine as adjuvant analgesic to opioids: A quantitative and qualitative systematic review. Anesth Analg 2004;99:482-495.
105. Hasan RA, Kartush JM, Thomas JD, et al: Oral dextromethorphan reduces perioperative analgesic administration in children undergoing tympanomastoid surgery. Otolaryngol Head Neck Surg 2004;131:711-716.
106. Suresh S, Lozono S, Hall SC: Large-dose intravenous methotrexate-induced cutaneous toxicity: Can oral magnesium oxide reduce pain? Anesth Analg 2003;96:1413-1414.
107. Antila H, Manner T, Kuurila K, et al: Ketoprofen and tramadol for analgesia during early recovery after tonsillectomy in children. Paediatr Anaesth 2006;16:548-553.
108. Khosravi MB, Khezri S, Azemati S: Tramadol for pain relief in children undergoing herniotomy: A comparison with ilioinguinal and iliohypogastric blocks. Paediatr Anaesth 2006; 16:54-58.
109. Bozkurt P: Use of tramadol in children. Paediatr Anaesth 2005;15:1041-1047.
110. Allegaert K, Anderson BJ, Verbesselt R, et al: Tramadol disposition in the very young: An attempt to assess in vivo cytochrome P-450 2D6 activity. Br J Anaesth 2005;95:231-239.
111. Hullett BJ, Chambers NA, et al: Tramadol vs morphine during adenotonsillectomy for obstructive sleep apnea in children. Paediatr Anaesth 2006;16:648-653
112. Ravilly S, Robinson W, Suresh S, et al: Chronic pain in cystic fibrosis. Pediatrics 1996;98(4 Pt 1):741-747.
113. Chay PC, Duffy BJ, Walker JS: Pharmacokinetic-pharmacodynamic relationships of morphine in neonates. Clin Pharmacol Ther 1992;51:334-342.
114. Williams DG, Patel A, Howard RF: Pharmacogenetics of codeine metabolism in an urban population of children and its implications for analgesic reliability. Br J Anaesth 2002;89:839-845.
115. Lotsch J, Skarke C, Liefhold J, et al: Genetic predictors of the clinical response to opioid analgesics: Clinical utility and future perspectives. Clin Pharmacokinet 2004;43:983-1013.
116. Chu LF, Clark DJ, Angst MS: Opioid tolerance and hyperalgesia in chronic pain patients after one month of oral morphine therapy: A preliminary prospective study. J Pain 2006;7:43-48.
117. Berde CB, Sethna NF, Holzman RS: Pharmacokinetics of methadone in children and adolescents in the perioperative period. Anesthesiology 1987;67:A519.
118. Berde CB, Lehn BM, Yee JD, et al: Patient-controlled analgesia in children and adolescents: A randomized, prospective comparison with intramuscular administration of morphine for postoperative analgesia. J Pediatr 1991;118:460-466.
119. Malviya S, Voepel-Lewis T, Tait AR, et al: Pain management in children with and without cognitive impairment following spine fusion surgery. Paediatr Anaesth 2001;11:453-458.
120. Krane EJ, Dalens BJ, Murat I, et al: The safety of epidurals placed during general anesthesia. Reg Anesth Pain Med 1998;23:433-438.
121. Tsui BC, Tarkkila P, Gupta S, et al: Confirmation of caudal needle placement using nerve stimulation. Anesthesiology 1900;91:374-378.
122. Rapp HJ, Folger A, Grau T: Ultrasound-guided epidural catheter insertion in children. Anesth Analg 2005;101:333-339.
123. Cote CJ, Zaslavsky A, Downes JJ, et al: Postoperative apnea in former preterm infants after inguinal herniorrhaphy. A combined analysis. Anesthesiology 1995;82:809-822.
124. Suresh S, Hall SC: Spinal anesthesia in infants: Is the impractical practical? Anesth Analg 2006;102:65-66.
125. Berde C: Epidural analgesia in children. Can J Anaesth 1994;41:555-560.
126. Sethna NF, Berde CB: Venous air embolism during identification of the epidural space in children. Anesth Analg 1993;76:925-927.
127. Suresh S, Wheeler M: Practical pediatric regional anesthesia. Anesthesiol Clin North Am 2002;20:83-113.
128. Freid EB, Bailey AG, Valley RD: Electrocardiographic and hemodynamic changes associated with unintentional intravascular injection of bupivacaine with epinephrine in infants. Anesthesiology 1993;79:394-398.
129. Tsui BC, Guenther C, Emery D, et al: Determining epidural catheter location using nerve stimulation with radiological confirmation. Reg Anesth Pain Med 2000;25: 306-309.
130. Birmingham PK, Wheeler M, Suresh S, et al: Patient-controlled epidural analgesia in children: Can they do it? Anesth Analg 2003;96:686-691.
131. Wheeler M, Patel A, Suresh S, Roth et al: The addition of clonidine 2 microg.kg-1 does not enhance the postoperative analgesia of a caudal block using 0.125% bupivacaine and epinephrine 1:200,000 in children: A prospective, double-blind, randomized study. Paediatr Anaesth 2005;15: 476-483
132. Culpepper-Morgan JA, Inturrisi CE, Portenoy RK, et al: Treatment of opioid-induced constipation with oral naloxone: A pilot study. Clin Pharmacol Ther 1992;52:90-95.
133. Maxwell LG, Kaufmann SC, Bitzer S, et al: The effects of a small-dose naloxone infusion on opioid-induced side effects and analgesia in children and adolescents treated with intravenous patient-controlled analgesia: A double-blind, prospective, randomized, controlled study. Anesth Analg 2005; 100:953-958.
134. Willschke H, Bosenberg A, Marhofer P, et al: Ultrasonographic-guided ilioinguinal/iliohypogastric nerve block in pediatric anesthesia: What is the optimal volume? Anesth Analg 2006;102:1680-1684.
135. Suresh S, Wagner AM: Scalp excisions: Getting "ahead" of pain. Pediatr Dermatol 2001;18:74-76.
136. Molliex S, Navez M, Baylot D, et al: Regional anesthesia for outpatient nasal surgery. Br J Anaesth 1996;76:151-153.
137. Suresh S, Bellig G: Regional anesthesia in a very low-birth-weight neonate for a neurosurgical procedure. Reg Anesth Pain Med. 2004;29:58-59.
138. Suresh S, Barcelona SL, Young NM, et al: Postoperative pain relief in children undergoing tympanomastoid surgery: Is a regional block better than opioids? Anesth Analg 2002;94:859-862.
139. Aunac S, Carlier M, Singelyn F, et al: The analgesic efficacy of bilateral combined superficial and deep cervical plexus block administered before thyroid surgery under general anesthesia. Anesth Analg 2002;95:746-750.
140. Tobias JD: Brachial plexus anaesthesia in children. Paediatr Anaesth 2001;11:265-275.
141. Wagner AM, Suresh S: Peripheral nerve blocks for warts: Taking the cry out of cryotherapy and laser. Pediatr Dermatol 1998;15:238-241.
142. Tobias JD: Continuous femoral nerve block to provide analgesia following femur fracture in a paediatric ICU population. Anaesth Intens Care 1994;22:616-618.
143. Khan ML, Hossain MM, Chowdhury AY, et al: Lateral femoral cutaneous nerve block for split skin grafting. Bangladesh Med Res Council Bull 1998;24:32-34.
144. Konrad C, Johr M: Blockade of the sciatic nerve in the popliteal fossa: A system for standardization in children. Anesth Analg 1998;87:1256-1258.
145. Broadman LM: Blocks and other techniques pediatric surgeons can employ to reduce postoperative pain in pediatric patients. Semin Pediatr Surg 1999;8:30-33.
146. de Jose Maria B, Gotzens V, Mabrok M: Ultrasound-guided umbilical nerve block in children: A brief description of a new approach. Paediatr Anaesth 2007;17:44-50.

APPENDIX

27–1 Sample Patient-Controlled Analgesia Order Sheet

CHECK (✓) OFF EACH ORDER AS TRAN-SCRIBED			Patient label
	DATE	TIME ANESTHESIA: PCA ORDER SHEET - MORPHINE ORDERED Page 1 of 1	
		ANESTHESIA PCA ORDERS – MORPHINE	
		Inpatient and Emergency Department Orders	
		1. NO ADDITIONAL SEDATIVES / OPIOIDS to be given during PCA unless discussed with Anesthesia Service.	
		2. Patient weight = _____ kg	
		3. Allergies _____	
		Type of Reaction: _____	
		4. Morphine Sulfate = 1 mg/ml	
		5. Mode: ☐ PCA ☐ Continuous ☐ PCA + Continuous	DO NOT WRITE IN THIS SPACE
		6. Continuous Infusion = _____ mg/hr (0.01 – 0.02 mg/kg/hr)	
		7. PCA Bolus Dose = _____ mg (0.01 – 0.02 mg/kg)	
		8. Lockout = _____ minutes (5 – 15 minutes)	
		9. One hour limit = _____ mg (0.2 mg/kg)	
		10. PCA Operator: (CIRCLE ALL THAT APPLY) Patient Parent Nurse	
		11. Give PCA operation instructions to patient/parent	
		12. Cardiorespiratory monitor: ☐ Yes ☐ No	
		13. Continuous pulse oximetry	

Physician's Orders

NURSE'S SIGNATURE   DOCTOR'S SIGNATURE

FORM—(Rev. 9/03)   ☐ CHECK HERE IF FORMULARY LISTED GENERIC EQUIVALENT IS UNACCEPTABLE

	CHECK (✓) OFF EACH ORDER AS TRAN-SCRIBED	
Physician's Orders		DATE TIME ANESTHESIA: PCA ORDER SHEET - MORPHINE ORDERED Page 2 of 2
		14. Assess pain relief, level of consciousness, and vital signs per PCA Nursing Protocol.
		15. If respiratory rate < 12, $SpO_2 \leq 92\%$, patient is cyanotic and/or the patient is unarousable, **stop PCA, apply supplemental O_2, and STAT page Anesthesia Service**
		16. For itching, administer diphenhydramine 0.1 – 0.5 mg/kg = _____ mg (maximum 25 mg) IV over 20 minutes q 4 hours prn. Hold if patient is somnolent.
		17. For nausea/vomiting, administer ondansetron 0.1 mg/kg = _____ mg (maximum 4 mg) IV over 5 minutes q 6 hours prn.
		18. Contact Anesthesia Pain Service APN or Anesthesia Resident for inadequate analgesia, side effect management, other questions, and to evaluate for PCA discontinuation.

NURSE'S SIGNATURE	DOCTOR'S SIGNATURE

FORM—(Rev. 5/05)

☐ CHECK HERE IF FORMULARY LISTED GENERIC EQUIVALENT IS UNACCEPTABLE

27–2 Sample Patient-Controlled Analgesia Conversions: Dosing Parameters

CHECK (✓) OFF EACH ORDER AS TRAN-SCRIBED		
	DATE TIME ANESTHESIA: ORDER SHEET - EPIDURAL ANALGESIA ORDERED Page 1 of 2	Patient label

Physician's Orders

ANESTHESIA ORDERS – EPIDURAL ANALGESIA

1. NO ADDITIONAL SEDATIVES / OPIOIDS to be given during Epidural infusion unless discussed with Anesthesia Service.

2. Maintain IV access during epidural infusion.

3. Patient weight = _____ kg

4. Allergies _____

   Type of Reaction: _____

5. Solution: _____% (0 – 0.125%) bupivacaine with fentanyl _____ mcg/ml (0 – 10 mcg/ml)
   Other Solution: _____

6. Mode: ☐ Continuous infusion ☐ Patient Controlled Epidural Analgesia - PCEA
   ☐ PCEA + Continuous

7. Administer above epidural solution via a well-labeled pump into epidural catheter at _____ ml per hour.

8. PCEA Bolus Dose = _____ mg (0.5 – 3 ml)

9. Lockout = _____ minutes (15 – 30 minutes)

10. One hour limit = _____ ml - Bupivacaine dose (infusion + demand) ≤ 0.4 mg/kg/hr. for patients > 3 mo., ≤ 0.2 mg/kg for patients < 3 mo., < 0.3 mg/kg for thoracic catheters

11. PCEA Operator: (CIRCLE ALL THAT APPLY)   Patient   Parent   Nurse

12. Give PCEA operation instructions to patient/parent

13. Cardiorespiratory monitor: ☐ Yes   ☐ No
    alarm limits: respiratory rate less than _____, heart rate less than _____

14. Continuous pulse oximetry.

15. Assess pain relief, level of consciousness, and vital signs per Epidural Nursing Protocol.

16. If respiratory rate < 12, SpO_2 ≤ 92%, patient is cyanotic and/or the patient is unarousable, **stop infusion, apply supplemental O_2, and STAT page Anesthesia Service**

DO NOT WRITE IN THIS SPACE

NURSE'S SIGNATURE

DOCTOR'S SIGNATURE

FORM—(Rev. 5/05)   ☐ CHECK HERE IF FORMULARY LISTED GENERIC EQUIVALENT IS UNACCEPTABLE

	CHECK (✓) OFF EACH ORDER AS TRAN-SCRIBED	DATE TIME ANESTHESIA: ORDER SHEET - EPIDURAL ANALGESIA ORDERED Page 2 of 2	
Physician's Orders		17. If patient is allowed to ambulate per surgeon's order, ambulate with assistance. Monitors may be disconnected while patient ambulates.	
		18. Assess dependent skin areas for pressure sores q shift. Notify Anesthesia if sores are present.	
		19. For itching, administer diphenhydramine 0.1 – 0.5 mg/kg = _____ mg (maximum 25 mg) IV over 20 minutes q 4 hours prn. Hold if patient is somnolent.	
		20. For nausea/vomiting, administer ondansetron 0.1 mg/kg = _____ mg (maximum 4 mg) IV over 5 minutes q 6 hours prn.	
		21. Diazepam, starting dose 0.02 – 0.04 mg/kg= _____ mg IV PRN q 6 hours for muscle spasm or anxiety	
		22. If no urine output after 8 hrs. call surgical service to evaluate patient for urinary retention.	
		23. Assess catheter dressing for signs of infection, soiling, or catheter displacement (fluid leaking into dressing) every shift. If any of these occur stop infusion and notify Anesthesia.	
		24. Stop infusion and page Anesthesia if: a. systolic blood pressure is < 60 mm Hg in a patient < 1 yr. old or < 70 mm Hg in a patient > 1 yr. old b. the patient or nurse notes increased leg weakness or numbness or signs of local anesthetic toxicity such as ringing in ears, metallic taste in mouth, lip numbness, slurred speech.	
		25. Contact Anesthesia Pain Service APN or Resident for inadequate analgesia, side effect management, other questions, and to evaluate for epidural discontinuation.	
NURSE'S SIGNATURE		DOCTOR'S SIGNATURE	

FORM—(Rev. 5/05)   ☐ CHECK HERE IF FORMULARY LISTED GENERIC EQUIVALENT IS UNACCEPTABLE

Copyright: Children's Memorial Hospital, Chicago, IL.

28 Assessment of Pain in Older Patients

Susan L. Charette and Bruce A. Ferrell

Pain is a common yet frequently overlooked complaint among older patients. Population-based studies have estimated that the prevalence of pain may be as high as 25% to 50% in community-dwelling older persons and 45% to 80% in nursing home residents.[1-5] Unfortunately, many physicians and patients incorrectly view pain as an expected part of aging. Older patients frequently have multiple comorbid conditions, and their medical care is typically directed toward the management of the underlying disease processes. Little attention may be paid to the alleviation of associated symptoms such as pain. As a result, pain is a significant problem that frequently goes unrecognized and undertreated.[5,6]

Pain must be accepted as a real and important issue for older patients. It can have multiple causes, variable presentations, and numerous meanings. Uncontrolled pain can negatively affect functional status, psychosocial well-being, and quality of life. The consequences of pain include impaired mobility, decreased socialization, depression, sleep disturbances, and increased health use and costs.[2,7,8] Pain may also negatively affect common geriatric conditions, including gait impairment, falls, polypharmacy, cognitive dysfunction, and malnutrition.[4] Given this potential for negative consequences, it is recommended that older persons be assessed for pain on their initial presentation to any health care provider.[1]

Effective pain management requires an accurate pain assessment. After a thorough initial assessment, ongoing reassessment is needed to ensure adequacy of the therapeutic plan, evaluate for new sources of pain, and monitor for side effects from the current treatment regimen. This chapter reviews potential challenges and important pearls for the assessment of chronic pain in older patients.

DEFINITIONS AND DESCRIPTIONS OF PAIN

Before discussing assessment, a review of the common definitions and descriptions of pain is useful. Pain may be defined as an unpleasant sensory and emotional experience associated with actual or potential tissue damage, or described in terms of such damage.[9]

Although pain often results from a physical insult, there are no reliable biologic markers for the presence or intensity of pain.[10] Ultimately, it is the patient's self-report that provides the most accurate and reliable evidence for the existence of pain.[1,10-12]

Acute pain typically has a distinct onset, an obvious source, and a relatively short duration.[10] Acute pain may be self-limited or signify a serious condition that needs urgent attention. Patients may present with an acute physical response, including signs such as an elevated heart rate, elevated blood pressure, diaphoresis, and mild increase in temperature. The intensity of acute pain usually correlates to the level of tissue damage, and typically disappears after the underlying cause has been treated.

Chronic pain is more difficult to define. It is characterized by a longer duration and is usually associated with chronic medical conditions. Although chronic pain may lack distinct physiologic signs similar to those of acute pain, it is often associated with long-term changes in functional status and psychosocial well-being. Chronic pain is often defined arbitrarily as pain lasting longer than 3 to 6 months or beyond the time frame expected for healing.[10] For other conditions, the underlying disease and the associated chronic pain are synonymous with one another.[10] Common examples include fibromyalgia and osteoarthritis. Chronic pain may also present as recurrent attacks of acute pain, such as intermittent headaches and recurring mechanical low back pain. Given the range of processes that can produce chronic pain, it is essential to carefully diagnose the cause and review the natural history of the associated pain syndrome with the patient.

Chronic pain may result from one or more physiologic mechanisms that perpetuate pain. Treatment plans specifically targeting the underlying pathophysiology are more likely to be effective. Chronic pain is typically generated by a nociceptive or neuropathic mechanism. Nociceptive pain is the result of inflammation, traumatic injury, tissue destruction, or mechanical deformation that serves as a stimulus to a primary afferent sensory neuron.[10] Nociceptive pain can be visceral, derived from internal organs and viscera, or somatic, relating to muscle, soft tissue (ligaments, tendons), bones, joints, or skin.[13] This type of pain is often described as a deep aching, throbbing, gnawing, or sore sensation; examples include rheumatoid arthritis and polymyalgia rheumatica. Neuropathic pain results from nerve damage in the central or peripheral nervous system.[14] It is commonly experienced as burning, severe shooting pains, or persistent numbness or tingling. The diagnosis of neuropathic pain is often made by the presence of hyperalgesia (a stimulus that was previously only noxious now results in intense pain, such as a pinprick) or allodynia (stimulus that was typically not painful is now painful, such as light touch). Common examples include postherpetic neuralgia and poststroke central pain. Usually, nociceptive pain responds well to analgesics, whereas neuropathic pain may respond to nonanalgesic drugs such as antidepressants, anticonvulsants, or local anesthetics.[10] In addition to the pain descriptions provided by patients, the response to treatment or lack thereof may be useful in determining the underlying type of pain.

Research over the last 2 decades has suggested that chronic pain, whether nociceptive or neuropathic, can be perpetuated by remodeling within the spinal cord and brain. That is, after an event such as peripheral tissue injury or nerve injury, changes can occur in the central nervous system at the level of the spinal cord and thalamus via physiologic, biochemical, cellular, and molecular mechanisms.[15] This neural plasticity, or ability for prolonged stimuli to induce changes in the central nervous system, is considered to be an important factor in the development of persistent pain after correction of the underlying pathology, and may lead to the development of hyperalgesia, allodynia, and the spread of pain to areas other than those involved with the initial pathology.[16] Animal studies have suggested that prolonged pain from a visceral source may also induce changes at the level of the dorsal column and thalamus, and that this neural plasticity may be a primary factor in chronic visceral pain.[17] Such changes in humans may help explain the persistence and intensity of pain observed with chronic conditions such as phantom limb pain, complex regional pain syndrome, and other neuropathic pain problems.

ASSESSMENT

Barriers to Effective Pain Assessment in Older Patients

The assessment of pain in older patients can be challenging. Social, cultural, and professional barriers have been documented that affect how patients, health care providers, and society perceive pain and the disabilities associated with it (Box 28-1). Misconceptions of the meaning, prevalence, and importance of pain are commonplace. Identifying the barriers that exist at the patient and health provider levels is an essential component of pain assessment and management.

BOX 28-1. BARRIERS TO PAIN ASSESSMENT AND MANAGEMENT

Patient-related Barriers
Cognitive impairment
Sensory impairment—vision and hearing
Ageist attitudes
Fear of the meaning of pain
Fear of pain medication side effects
Implications of tests and interventions
Language issues
Cultural background

Social and Institutional Barriers
Stigma of chronic pain and physical disability
Fear of addiction to pain medications
Controlled substances laws
Poor reimbursement

Health Professional Barriers
Misconceptions and prejudice regarding pain
Lack of adequate education in pain management

There are a variety of patient-related barriers that make pain assessment difficult. Cognitive impairment is a common problem among older patients and can impede the assessment of pain. Cognitively impaired older people who retain communication skills are usually able to report experienced pain when asked; however, as their cognitive impairment advances, self-reports of pain decrease.[18] Other methods of pain assessment can be used in the cognitively impaired patient (see discussion in a later section). Another common obstacle is sensory impairment. In particular, most older patients experience some degree of vision and hearing impairment. These deficits may interfere with their ability to receive and provide information during a pain assessment.[3]

Unfortunately, ageist attitudes about pain are held by many older patients. The misconception that pain is a normal and expected part of aging is counterproductive to the evaluation and management of pain.[5] Additional patient-centered barriers include fears about the meaning of pain as well as the implications of tests and interventions. Some patients may fear that their pain represents a serious, underlying medical problem, and worry that divulging their pain to their physician will lead to tests, more pain, and an unfavorable diagnosis. Others may be concerned about the potential for drug interactions with their current medications and possible side effects. Often, older patients have concerns about the cost of medications, including those for pain control. Other patients, however, do not want to bother their health care provider or the staff at their residence, sometimes out of fear of reprisal.[5,19]

Finally, language and cultural issues may present barriers to effective pain assessment. The language or wording used by physicians may differ from that used by their older patients. Thus, older adults may deny "pain" but admit to having "discomfort" when questioned.[11] Cultural background can influence a patient's pain experience and his or her description of the pain, and these factors should be considered during the assessment.[11]

Social and institutional factors also pose significant barriers to effective pain assessment. Patients frequently voice their unease about the potential for addiction to pain medications, and the media magnifies these concerns with stories of misuse and abuse among celebrities, for example. Other patients may choose not to report their pain because of fears about the implication of chronic pain and the potential stigma associated with the diagnosis of a disabling medical condition. In addition, the process of prescribing pain medications can be inconvenient because of restricted formularies by insurance companies, the need for special prescriptions for narcotic pain relievers, and constraints in pharmacy service availability, especially in the long-term care setting. Finally, labor-intensive pain assessment and management services receive poor reimbursement compared with other diagnoses; this lack of adequate compensation may dissuade physicians and other health care professionals from addressing this common patient issue.

Barriers to the effective assessment of pain are common among the health care professionals who care for older patients. Physicians and nurses may have misconceptions about pain, similar to their patients. Research has shown that physicians underestimate pain in patients, whether they are cognitively intact or impaired, and older patients often receive inadequate analgesia.[20,21] Second, historically, physicians and nurses have received inadequate training in pain assessment and management. These health professionals typically lack an adequate background to perform an effective pain assessment; one study has shown that over 25% of senior internal medicine residents felt inadequately prepared to manage pain.[22] Finally, patient care is often focused on active medical issues, and pain frequently falls to the bottom of the problem list. Multiple medical conditions may detract from the treatment of pain and often leave health care providers with inadequate time to address this symptom.

Recognizing these challenges is an important first step in the assessment and management of pain. Patients should be asked routinely about pain and reassured that their concerns are important and valid. Their questions about the meaning of pain, necessary tests, and side effects of medications need to be answered. For those who are unable to communicate or have significant cognitive impairment, the patient's family or primary decision maker should be included in the assessment and plan. Education and training of nurses and physicians in the evaluation of pain, particularly as it relates to older adults, are crucial. The next section will address effective means for pain assessment in older patients and how to overcome these barriers in clinical practice.

Assessment of Chronic Pain

Accurate pain assessment is the most critical component of effective pain management.[10] Initial assessment is essential to identify the underlying cause(s), understand what modalities and medications have helped and those that have not or that have caused complications or side effects, and make optimal recommendations for an effective treatment plan.[1] In addition, the pain assessment should include an evaluation for acute pain that might indicate a new concurrent illness rather than an exacerbation of a chronic pain condition.[1] Reassessment after therapy has been initiated is essential to reevaluate the response to treatment, monitor for side effects, and determine whether other sources of pain have developed. The pain assessment should uncover the sequence of events that led to the persistent pain complaint, and ultimately will establish the diagnosis, plan of care, and likely prognosis.[1] This section will review the basics of pain assessment and other related issues, including functional status, psychological and social factors, assessment tools, and evaluation in the cognitively impaired.

History

The assessment of pain should begin with a thorough account of the patient's pain history and medical problems. Given that chronic pain is typically associated with an ongoing medical diagnosis, accurate history taking provides the necessary background to identify the probable source. Past medical and surgical history, including reports of prior trauma or injury, are especially valuable. An evaluation of the medication list and a review of systems provide important details that may be helpful in determining the diagnosis and developing a treatment plan. In addition, a psychosocial history, including alcohol consumption and illicit drug use, should be obtained, because these factors may complicate the patient's pain experience and its management.

The pain history provides insight into the patient's pain experience. First, an evaluation of the pain characteristics should be pursued, including features such as intensity, character, frequency (or pattern, or both) location, duration, and precipitating and relieving factors.[1] Second, the patient should be asked about any recent event or activity that may be the source of the pain or have prompted an exacerbation or flare. Third, the patient should be asked questions about her or his use of analgesics and other therapies for the pain. This history should include current and previously used prescription medications, over-the-counter medications, and complementary or alternative remedies, as well as their effectiveness and any side effects experienced.[1] In addition, inquiry regarding the use and helpfulness of other types of treatments such as physical therapy, chiropractic manipulation, massage, and acupuncture should be obtained. Finally, it is important to inquire about the patient's knowledge, attitudes, and beliefs regarding pain and its management.[1] In particular, pain may have different meanings for different people; some may view their pain as an "atonement for their sins" or "God's will," and others may believe that their symptoms are a sign that the end of life is near. An awareness of the patient's thoughts and ideas about pain is important, and may affect the expression of pain as well as treatment options and their effectiveness.

Most patients can report pain; all you have to do is ask them. This self-report provides the most accurate and reliable evidence for the existence of pain and its intensity.[1,10-12] It is imperative that physicians, nurses, and other health care providers, as well as family and caregivers, listen to patient's complaints of pain and take them seriously.[1] Even those with mild to moderate cognitive impairment can answer simple questions about pain, and this information may be helpful in completing the assessment and developing a management plan.[7] Older patients often use words other than "pain" to describe what they are feeling.[10] Many patients may not admit to having pain; however, they may use words such as "hurting," "aching," "soreness," or "discomfort" to characterize the sensation.[1,21] These words should be kept in mind and used when asking about pain. The history directs the physical examination and lays the groundwork for the management plan. Box 28-2 outlines some useful questions that may be incorporated into a pain interview to help characterize a patient's pain and its impact on his or her life.

Physical Examination

The physical examination is an integral component of the pain assessment. It builds on the history, and should especially focus on potential pain sources and areas of concern identified during the history taking. The examination should include a careful evaluation of the location of reported pain and common sites for pain referral.[1] In particular, the musculoskeletal and nervous systems should receive special attention, because they are the most frequent sources of pain.[1] The musculoskeletal examination should include an evaluation for trigger points of myofascial pain, tender points of fibromyalgia, inflammation, muscle spasm, deformities such as scoliosis and kyphosis, joint alignment, fracture, and gait disturbances.[1,10] In addition, joint range of motion and reproduction of aggravating movements may be useful to identify underlying physical impairment associated with pain and the need for rehabilitation.[10] Gait should be formally evaluated to see whether it contributes to or is affected by the pain process; the timed "get-up and go" test is an effective performance-based measure of functional status and gait.[23] The nervous system evaluation should search for evidence of weakness, hyperalgesia, hyperpathia, allodynia, numbness, paresthesia, and signs of autonomic neuropathies.[1,10,11] The physical examination may also provide information on the status and contribution of other medical

---

BOX 28–2. SAMPLE QUESTIONS IN A PAIN INTERVIEW

1. How strong is your pain right now? What was the worst or average pain over the past week?
2. How many days over the past week have you been unable to do what you would like to do because of your pain?
3. Over the past week, how often has pain interfered with your ability of take care of yourself—for example, with bathing, eating, dressing, and going to the toilet?
4. Over the past week, how often has pain interfered with your ability to take care of your home-related chores, such as going grocery shopping, preparing meals, paying bills, and driving?
5. How often do you participate in pleasurable activities such as hobbies, socializing with friends, and travel? Over the past week, how often has pain interfered with these activities?
6. How often do you do some type of exercise? Over the past week, how often has pain interfered with your ability to exercise?
7. How often does pain interfere with your ability to think clearly?
8. How often does pain interfere with your appetite? Have you lost weight?
9. How often does pain interfere with your sleep? How often over the past week?
10. Has pain interfered with your energy, mood, personality, or relationships with other people?
11. Over the past week, how often have you taken pain medication?
12. How would you rate your health at the present time?

From AGS Panel on Persistent Pain in Older Persons: The management of persistent pain in older persons. J Am Geriatr Soc 2002;50:S205-S224. With permission.

---

problems to the patient's pain. Health care providers who specialize in the evaluation and treatment of these systems, including physical therapists, physiatrists, rheumatologists, and neurologists, may be able to provide additional assistance with the physical diagnosis of the pain source and the treatment plan, and should be considered for consultation.[1]

Functional Status

A patient's functional status may be adversely affected by pain, and the resulting functional losses may significantly affect quality of life and general well-being. Both the history and physical examination should address functional status to identify activity limitations and physical deficits caused by the underlying pain.[5] Impairments in functional status may range from difficulties in performing instrumental activities of daily living, such as driving and house cleaning, to an inability to perform basic activities of daily living, such as bathing, transfers, or toileting. Although many questions asked during the assessment may provide much of this information, validated functional status scales such as the Lawton Instrumental Activities of Daily Living Scale and the Katz Activities of Daily Living Scale may be incorporated into the assessment to address specific activities in an organized format.[24,25] Another way to elicit information about the impact of pain on a patient's function and behaviors is to ask the patient about his or her participation in activities such as hobbies, physical exercise, and socialization with family and friends.[11] One way to address these issues is to ask a question that addresses the global impact of the pain on one's life, such as "How many days over the past 6 months have you been unable to do what you would like to do because of your pain"?[26] The information on functional status obtained during the pain assessment should be incorporated into the goals of the treatment plan, and these should aim to maximize the patient's independence and enhance quality of life.[10]

Psychological and Social Assessment

Although pain can have a significant impact on physical function, its potential effect on the psychosocial well-being of older patients should not be overlooked. Depression is a common problem among older persons. Research has supported an association between pain and depressed mood in this patient population.[8] Many patients with chronic pain will experience concomitant depressive symptoms or anxiety.[4] The initial pain assessment should include an evaluation of psychological function, including mood, self-efficacy, pain coping skills, helplessness, and pain-related fears.[1] The Geriatric Depression Scale is a useful screening tool for depression and may be a useful adjunct during a comprehensive pain assessment.[27] Other validated instruments for the assessment of depression include the Hamilton Depression Rating Scale and the Cornell Scale for Depression in Dementia.[28,29] Counseling, supportive group therapy, biofeedback, or psychoactive medications may be indicated for patients with an underlying mood disorder, and they should be referred to these services.[10]

An evaluation of the patient's social situation should be included as part of the initial pain assessment. Important issues include the patient's social support system, presence of caregivers, family relationships, work history, living arrangements, cultural environment, spirituality, and health care accessibility.[1] Cultural and social factors may influence a patient's experience with and expression of pain, as well as his or her pain management choices and likelihood of compliance. Awareness of this background information during the initial assessment will be extremely useful for the development of the pain management plan and for reassessment.

Measurement of Pain Intensity and Pain Assessment Scales

Various pain assessment scales have been designed for research and to assist health care practitioners in the evaluation of pain. There are multidimensional and unidimensional instruments for the assessment of pain. Multidimensional instruments have been developed to evaluate patients for multiple pain-related factors. These instruments typically ask questions from a number of domains, including pain intensity, location, temporal effects, affective aspects, and functional status. The McGill Pain Questionnaire (MPQ), the Brief Pain Inventory (BPI), and the Geriatric Pain Measure are three validated multidimensional tools for the assessment of pain.[30-32] Although these instruments and others collect numerous important data points relevant to a person's pain experience, they are often long, time-consuming, and difficult to score at the bedside, and it can be a challenge to implement such tools in the clinical setting.[10]

Unidimensional instruments typically focus on one domain of the pain experience, such as pain intensity. These tools take less time to administer and are more practical for use in various clinical settings.[10] Pain intensity may be a primary factor that determines the impact of pain on a person's overall functioning and well-being, and may be a useful end point for monitoring disease progression and the effectiveness of intervention strategies.[11] Many unidimensional pain intensity scales have been created to help quantify pain severity. Numeric rating scales have patients rate the intensity of their pain, typically on a scale from 0 to 10. For example, the verbal 0 to 10 scale has patients rate their current pain on a scale from 0, no pain, to 10, the worst pain imaginable.[33,34] Verbal descriptor scales (VDS) have patients identify the phrase or adjective that best quantifies the intensity of their pain such as no pain, mild pain, moderate pain, severe pain, extreme pain, and the most intense pain imaginable.[7,34] A variation of the VDS is the pain thermometer that lists adjectives of pain vertically, from the bottom of the thermometer or no pain to the top of the thermometer or pain as bad as it could be.[1,19] Facial pain scales shows a series of progressively distressed facial expressions along a continuum and patients are asked to choose the face that reflects the intensity of their current pain.[35] The Visual Analogue Scale consists of a 10-cm line denoted by no pain on the left end of the line and most pain imaginable on the right end of the line; patients are asked to mark the intensity of their pain on the line.[7,34]

Although the literature demonstrates fair to good reliability and validity for these instruments in the geriatric population, there are potential limitations to their use in patients with lower levels of education, deficits in vision and hearing, and moderate to advanced cognitive impairment.[11] The pain reports of older patients, especially those with cognitive impairment, are influenced by pain at the moment, so rather than using these scales to ask about recent

Table 28–1. Pain Assessment Instruments

INSTRUMENT	VALIDITY*	RELIABILITY*	SUBSCALES	EASE OF USE†
Multidimensional				
McGill Pain Questionnaire[30]	+ + + +	+ + +	5	+ + +
Brief Pain Inventory[31]	+ + + +	+ + +	2	+
Geriatric Pain Measure[32]	+ + + +	+ + +	5+	
Unidimensional				
Verbal 0-10 Scale[33]	+ + + +	+ +	N/A	+
Visual Analogue Scale[34]	+ + + +	+ +	N/A	+ + +
Faces Pain Scale[35]	+ + + +	+ +	N/A	+ +
Present pain intensity[30]	+ + + +	+ + +	N/A	+ +

*Relative strength of tool (in our opinion): +, weak; + + + +, strong.
†Relative ease of use (in our opinion): +, easy; + + + +, difficult.

or past pain experience, it is best to use them to evaluate current pain.[10] Table 28–1 outlines examples of common multidimensional and unidimensional assessment tools.

Pain Assessment in the Cognitively Impaired

Cognitive impairment is an important consideration in the assessment of pain in older patients. Although a potential barrier, research has suggested that the self-report of pain from patients with mild to moderate cognitive impairment is reliable and valid.[18,33] Thus, the assessment of pain in those with early cognitive impairment should begin with the patient's self-report and a thorough history, as described earlier. Of the available pain intensity scales, the Pain Thermometer and the VDS are generally recommended for use in patients with mild to moderate cognitive impairment.[11,34]

The evaluation of pain is more challenging in patients with severe cognitive impairment. Some individuals may be able to convey their needs through "yes" and "no" answers to simple questions.[10] However, for patients who are unable to make their needs known, the best method of pain assessment remains a subject of great debate. One area of research has focused on observational indicators of pain.[11] This type of assessment focuses on the behavioral manifestation of pain; potential indicators include nonverbal cues and behaviors, vocalizations, facial expressions, and changes in unusual behaviors (Box 28–3). The most reliable behavior may relate to guarding during examination or routine activities such as walking, morning care, and transfers.[1] In addition, an atypical behavior in a patient with severe dementia should trigger assessment for pain as a possible cause.[1] Family members, caregivers, and others who know the patient well may provide useful qualitative information about the patient's pain and changes in behavior; however, their quantitative assessment is often less reliable.[10]

BOX 28–3. BEHAVIORAL MANIFESTATIONS OF PAIN IN THE COGNITIVELY IMPAIRED

Facial Expressions
Slight frown; sad, frightened face
Grimacing, wrinkled forehead, closed or tightened eyes
Any distorted expression
Rapid blinking

Verbalizations, Vocalizations
Sighing, moaning, groaning
Grunting, chanting, calling out
Noisy breathing
Asking for help
Verbally abusive

Body Movements
Rigid, tense body posture, guarding
Fidgeting
Increased pacing, rocking
Restricted movement
Gait or mobility changes

Changes in Interpersonal Interactions
Aggressive, combative, resisting care
Decreased social interactions
Socially inappropriate, disruptive
Withdrawn

Changes in Activity Patterns or Routines
Refusing food, appetite change
Increase in rest periods
Sleep, rest pattern changes
Sudden cessation of common routines
Increased wandering

Mental Status Changes
Crying or tears
Increased confusion
Irritability or distress

From AGS Panel on Persistent Pain in Older Persons: The management of persistent pain in older persons. J Am Geriatr Soc 2002; 50:S205-S224. With permission.

CONCLUSION

Pain is a unique experience for every person. An effective pain assessment sets the groundwork for optimal pain management. An understanding of the patient's personal pain history is essential, and should include detailed information on the pain complaint, prior treatments and their efficacy, functional status, and psychosocial well-being. Barriers exist at multiple levels and present considerable challenges to pain assessment in older patients. A multifaceted approach that targets education, research, and public policy is needed if we are to break down these barriers. The training of physicians, nurses, and other health care professionals must include curricula on pain assessment and management in older patients. Continued research into the optimal tools and approaches to the evaluation and treatment of chronic pain is critical. In particular, further understanding of the role of neural plasticity in chronic pain and the development of interventions to reduce or block the maladaptive response of the brain and spinal cord to injury are needed. Finally, it is imperative that our leaders in medicine, social institutions, and government recognize the prevalence and impact of chronic pain in older adults. With the aging of the population, the importance and relevance of these issues will continue to grow in the future. Public policy must address the need for improvements in the evaluation and management of chronic pain in older patients.

Acknowledgment

This chapter originally appeared in *Clinics in Geriatric Medicine*[36] and is reprinted with permission from Elsevier.

References

1. AGS Panel on Persistent Pain in Older Persons: The management of persistent pain in older persons. J Am Geriatr Soc 2002;50:S205-S224.
2. Helme RD, Gibson SJ: Pain in older people. In Crombie IK, Croft PR, Linton SJ, et al (eds): Epidemiology of Pain. Seattle, IASP Press, 1999, pp 103-112.
3. Ferrell BA: Pain evaluation and management in the nursing home. Ann Intern Med 1995;123:681-687.
4. Ferrell BA: Pain management in elderly people. J Am Geriatr Soc 1991;39:64-73.
5. Ferrell BA, Ferrell BR, Osterweil D: Pain in the nursing home. J Am Geriatr Soc 1990;38:409-414.
6. Bernabei R, Gambassi G, Lapane K, et al: Management of pain in elderly patients with cancer. SAGE Study Group. Systematic evaluation of geriatric drug use via epidemiology. JAMA 1998;279:1877-1882.
7. Ferrell BA, Ferrell BR, Rivera L: Pain in cognitively impaired nursing home patients. J Pain Symptom Manage 1995;10:591-598.
8. Parmelee PA, Katz IR, Lawton MP: The relation of pain to depression among institutionalized aged. J Gerontol 1991;46:P15-P21.
9. Merskey H, Lindblom V, Mumford JM, et al: Part III. Pain terms—a current list with definitions and notes on usage. In Merskey H, Bogduk N (eds): Classification of Chronic Pain, 2nd ed. Seattle, IASP Press, 1994, pp 207-213.
10. Ferrell BA: Pain. In Osterweil D, Brummel-Smith K, Beck JC, (eds): Comprehensive Geriatric Assessment. New York, McGraw-Hill, 2000, pp 381-397.
11. Herr KA, Garand L: Assessment and measurement of pain in older adults. Clin Geriatr Med 2001;17:457-478.
12. Turk DC, Melzack R: The measurement of pain and the assessment of people experiencing pain. In Turk DC, Melzack R (eds): Handbook of Pain Assessment. New York, Guilford Press, 1992, pp 3-12.
13. Myer RA, Campbell JN, Raja SN: Peripheral and neural mechanisms of nociception. In Wall PD, Melzack R (eds): Textbook of Pain, 3rd ed. New York, Churchill Livingstone, 1994, pp 13-44.
14. Bennett GF: Neuropathic pain. In Wall PD, Melzack R (eds): Textbook of Pain, 3rd ed. New York, Churchill Livingstone, 1994, pp 201-224.
15. Coderre TJ, Katz J, Vaccarino AL, et al: Contribution of central neuroplasticity to pathological pain: Review of clinical and experimental evidence. Pain 1993;52:259-285.
16. Marcus DA: Treatment of nonmalignant chronic pain. Am Fam Physician 2000;61:1331-1338.
17. Saab CY, Park YC, Al-Chaer ED: Thalamic modulation of visceral nociceptive processing in adult rats with neonatal colon irritation. Brain Res 2004;1008:186-192.
18. Parmelee PA, Smith B, Katz IR: Pain complaints and cognitive status among elderly institution residents. J Am Geriatr Soc 1993;41:517-522.
19. Herr KA, Mobily PR: Complexities of pain assessment in the elderly: Clinical considerations. J Gerontol Nurs 1991;17:12-19.
20. Morrison RS, Siu AL: A comparison of pain and its treatment in advanced dementia and cognitively intact patients with hip fracture. J Pain Symptom Manage 2000;19:240-248.
21. Sengstaken EA, King SA: The problems of pain and its detection among geriatric nursing home residents. J Am Geriatr Soc 1993;41:541-544.
22. Blumenthal D, Gokhale M, Campbell EG, et al: Preparedness for clinical practice: Reports of graduating residents at academic health centers. JAMA 2001;286:1027-1034.
23. Mathias S, Nayak US, Isaacs B: Balance in elderly patients: The "get-up and go" test. Arch Phys Med Rehabil 1986;67:387-389.
24. Katz S, Ford AB, Moskowitz RW, et al: Studies of illness in the aged. The index of activities of daily living: A standardized measure of biological and psychological function. JAMA 1963;85:914-919.
25. Lawton MP, Brody EM: Assessment of older people: Self-maintaining and instrumental activities of daily living. Gerontologist 1969;9:179-186.
26. Von Korff M, Dworkin SF, Le Resche L, et al: An epidemiologic comparison of pain complaints. Pain 1988;32:173-183.
27. Yesavage JA, Brink TL, Rose TL, et al: Development and validation of a geriatric depression screening scale: A preliminary report. J Psychiatr Res 1983;17:37-49.
28. Hamilton M: A rating scale for depression. J Neurol Neursurg Psychiatry 1960;23:56-62.
29. Alexopoulos GS, Abrams RC, Young RC, et al: Cornell scale for depression in dementia. Biol Psychiatry 1988;23:271-284.
30. Melzack R: The McGill Pain Questionnaire: Major properties and scoring methods. Pain 1975;1:277-299.
31. Daut RL, Cleeland CS, Flanery RC: Development of the Wisconsin Brief Pain Questionnaire to assess pain in cancer and other diseases. Pain 1983;17:197-210.
32. Ferrell BA, Stein WM, Beck JC: The Geriatric Pain Measure: Validity, reliability and factor analysis. J Am Geriatr Soc 2000;48:1669-1673.
33. Ferrell BA: Pain in cognitively impaired nursing home residents. J Pain Symptom Manage 1995;10:591-598.
34. Herr KA, Mobily PR: Comparison of selected pain assessment tools for use with the elderly. Appl Nurs Res 1993;6:39-46.
35. Herr KA, Mobily PR, Kohout FJ, et al: Evaluation of the Faces Pain Scale for the use with the elderly. Clin J Pain 1998;14:29-38.
36. Charette SL, Ferrell BA: Rheumatic diseases in the elderly: Assessing chronic pain. Clin Geriatr Med 2005;21:563-576.

CHAPTER

29 Managing Pain during Pregnancy and Lactation

James P. Rathmell, Christopher M. Viscomi, and Marjorie Meyer

Pain occurs during pregnancy in almost all women. Even during the course of an otherwise uncomplicated pregnancy, common musculoskeletal conditions can cause severe pain. Less commonly, patients who have had long-standing painful disorders will enter pregnancy and present management challenges. This chapter will review the most current safety data regarding maternal use of common pain medications during pregnancy and in the breastfeeding mother. Along with an overview of common painful musculoskeletal conditions of pregnancy, an approach to the management of chronic pain during pregnancy is given.

USE OF MEDICATIONS DURING PREGNANCY

Medical management of the pregnant patient should begin with attempts to minimize the use of all medications and use nonpharmacologic therapies whenever possible. When opting for drug therapy, the clinician must consider any potential for harm to the mother, the fetus, and the course of pregnancy. The degree of protein binding and lipid solubility of the medication, speed of maternal metabolism, and molecular weight all affect placental transfer of medications from mother to fetus. With the exception of large polar molecules (such as heparin and insulin), almost all medications will reach the fetus to some degree.

Approximately 3% of newborns will have a significant congenital malformation.[1] Only 25% of fetal malformations have a known genetic cause, and only 2% to 3% have a clear environmental link, such as maternal medication exposure during organogenesis.[2] One of the major limitations in evaluating any medication's potential for causing harm to a developing human fetus is the degree of species specificity for congenital defects. A classic example of this specificity is the drug thalidomide; nonprimate studies have revealed no teratogenic effects, but severe limb deformities occurred in human offspring when thalidomide was prescribed during pregnancy.[3]

The most critical period for minimizing maternal drug exposure is during early development, from conception through the tenth menstrual week of pregnancy (the tenth week following start of the last menstrual cycle). Drug exposure prior to organogenesis (prior to the fourth menstrual week) usually causes an all-or-none effect—the embryo either does not survive or develops without abnormalities.[4] Drug effects later in pregnancy typically lead to single- or multiple-organ involvement, developmental syndromes, or intrauterine growth retardation.[2] Certain medications may not influence fetal organ development directly, but have the potential to influence the physiology of pregnancy adversely. For example, nonsteroidal anti-inflammatory drugs (NSAIDs) may delay the onset of labor, decrease amniotic fluid volume, or place a newborn at risk for pulmonary hypertension or renal injury.

The U.S. Food and Drug Administration (FDA) has developed a five-category labeling system for all approved drugs in the United States (Table 29–1). This labeling system rates the potential risk for teratogenic or embryotoxic effects based on available scientific and clinical evidence. It is important to note that the FDA classification system has been revised to address neonatal influences other than teratogenicity. For example, ibuprofen is associated with decreased amniotic fluid and constriction of the ductus arteriosus, with a special class B_m designation. Because few medications have undergone large-scale testing during human pregnancy, most medications are category C, indicating incomplete knowledge and potential for benefit and harm with drug therapy. More specifically, our present knowledge about the adverse effects of uncontrolled pain, as well as the risks of administering medications during pregnancy, remain incomplete and the physician will be left to weigh the risks against the benefits of instituting pharmacologic therapy for each individual.

Table 29–1. FDA Pregnancy Risk Classification for Pain Management Medications

FDA CLASSIFICATION	DEFINITION	EXAMPLES
Category A	Controlled human studies have indicated no apparent risk to fetus. The possibility of harm to the fetus seems remote.	Multivitamins
Category B	Animal studies have not not indicated a fetal risk or animal studies have indicated a teratogenic risk, but well-controlled human studies have failed to demonstrate a risk.	Acetaminophen Butorphanol, nalbuphine* Caffeine Fentanyl, hydrocodone, methadone, meperidine, morphine, oxycodone, oxymorphone* Ibuprofen, naproxen, indomethacin Metoprolol Paroxetine, fluoxetine Prednisolone, prednisone
Category C	Studies have indicated teratogenic or embryocidal risk in animals, but no controlled studies have been done in women; there have been no controlled studies in animals or humans.	Aspirin, ketorolac Codeine, propoxyphene* Gabapentin, pregabalin Lidocaine, mexiletine Nifedipine Propranolol Sumatriptan
Category D	There has been positive evidence of human fetal risk but, in certain cases, the benefits of the drug may outweigh the risks involved.	Amitriptyline, imipramine Diazepam Phenobarbital Phenytoin Valproic acid
Category X	There has been positive evidence of significant fetal risk, and the risk clearly outweighs any possible benefit.	Ergotamine

*All opioid analgesics are FDA risk category D if used for prolonged periods or in large doses near term.
FDA, U.S. Food and Drug Administration.
Adapted from Fed Reg 1980;44:37434-37467.

USE OF MEDICATIONS IN THE BREAST-FEEDING MOTHER

The same physicochemical properties that facilitate transplacental drug transfer affect drug accumulation in breast milk. High lipid solubility, low molecular weight, minimal protein binding, and the un-ionized state all facilitate excretion of medications into breast milk. The neonatal dose of most medications obtained through breast-feeding is 1% to 2% of the maternal dose.[5] Even with minimal exposure via breast milk, neonatal drug allergy and slower infant drug metabolism must be considered.[6] Only small amounts of colostrum are excreted during the first few postpartum days; thus, early breast-feeding poses little risk to the infant whose mother received medications during delivery.[7]

Most breast milk is synthesized and excreted during and immediately following breast-feeding. Taking medications after breast-feeding or when the infant has the longest interval between feedings and avoidance of long-acting medications will minimize drug transfer via breast milk.[8] However, effective treatment of chronic pain often necessitates the use of long-acting medications, particularly long-acting opioids. To aid physicians in drug selection and to provide advice to lactating mothers, the American Academy of Pediatrics has categorized medications in relation to the safety of maternal ingestion by breast-feeding mothers[9] (Table 29–2).

MEDICATIONS COMMONLY USED IN PAIN MANAGEMENT

Nonsteroidal Anti-inflammatory Drugs (NSAIDs)

Although the exact mechanism of action is uncertain, NSAIDs decrease pain by inhibiting prostaglandin synthesis. During pregnancy, prostaglandins modulate many key processes, including stimulation of uterine activity, maintaining patency of the fetal ductus arteriosus (essential for adequate in utero blood flow), and promoting fetal urine production (which contributes to the level of amniotic fluid in the second and third trimesters). As expected, alteration of prostaglandin metabolism then has varied effects on the pregnancy, depending on the timing and duration of use. For example, short-term use of indomethacin in the second trimester is effective for the treatment of pain caused by degenerating fibroids; use for long periods of time (more than 48 hours) in the third trimester has been associated with narrowing of the ductus arteriosus[10,11] and oligohydramnios.[12] To complicate this picture further, aspirin, the prototypical NSAID, is used in a therapeutic manner in low doses (80 to 160 mg/day) to decrease the incidence of pregnancy complications in certain high-risk groups but is associated with premature narrowing of the ductus arteriosus at higher doses.[13] Therefore, NSAID use in pregnancy must be carefully planned to achieve the proposed benefit and avoid fetal risk.

Table 29–2. Classification of Maternal Medication Use during Pregnancy

CLASSIFICATION	DEFINITION	EXAMPLES
Category 1	These medications should not be consumed during lactation. Strong evidence exists that serious adverse effects on the infant are likely with maternal ingestion of these medications during lactation.	Ergotamine
Category 2	The effects on human infants are unknown, but caution is urged.	Amitriptyline, desipramine, doxepin, fluoxetine, imipramine, trazadone Diazepam, lorazepam, midazolam
Category 3	These medications are compatible with breast-feeding.	Carbamazepine, phenytoin, valproate Atenolol, propranolol, diltiazem Codeine, fentanyl, methadone, morphine, propoxyphene Butorphanol Lidocaine, mexiletine Acetaminophen Ibuprofen, indomethacin, ketorolac, naproxen Caffeine

Adapted from American Academy of Pediatrics Committee on Drugs: Transfer of drugs and other chemicals into human milk. Pediatrics 2001;108: 776-789.

In general, if NSAID use is indicated, the duration should be short (less than 48 hours) in the absence of monitoring fetal ductus flow and amniotic fluid volume. All NSAID use for pain should be discontinued by 34 weeks' gestation to prevent pulmonary hypertension in the newborn.[14]

There is no role for routine use of NSAIDs for pain other than that related to rheumatologic disease or uterine fibroids. In the largest published series of NSAID use during pregnancy to date, Ostensen and Ostensen[15] have detailed a series of 88 women with rheumatic disease, comparing outcome in 45 who received NSAID therapy during pregnancy with 43 who were not treated during pregnancy. The most common agents used were naproxen (23/45) and ibuprofen (8/45). NSAIDs were most frequently used during the first and second trimesters because many patients stopped therapy once pregnancy was recognized; many of the rheumatic conditions remitted later in pregnancy. They found no significant differences in pregnancy outcome (duration of pregnancy and labor, vaginal delivery rate, maternal bleeding requiring transfusion, or incidence of congenital anomalies) or the health status of offspring at long-term follow-up (ranging from 6 months to 14 years). The authors concluded that NSAID therapy limited to periods of active rheumatic disease until weeks 34 to 36 did not adversely effect the neonate.[15] It is of note, however, that women with rheumatic disease have poor pregnancy outcome in general, so these outcome data should not be applied to the general obstetric population. Uterine fibroids grow during pregnancy, with peak growth and highest incidence of fibroid degeneration in the second trimester. Short courses of indomethacin (usually 48 hours) have been beneficial in reducing pain related to degenerating fibroids.

Despite the physiologic effects of NSAIDs, the results of the Collaborative Perinatal Project have suggested that first-trimester exposure to aspirin does not pose appreciable teratogenic risk,[16] nor does ibuprofen or naproxen, the most commonly used NSAIDs. Patients who conceive while taking NSAIDs can be reassured that this will not impair pregnancy outcome.

Aspirin has well-known platelet-inhibiting properties and, theoretically, may increase the risk of peripartum hemorrhage. Neonatal platelet function is inhibited for up to 5 days after delivery in aspirin-treated mothers.[17] Although low-dose aspirin therapy (60 to 80 mg/day) has not been associated with maternal or neonatal complications, higher doses appear to increase the risk of intracranial hemorrhage in neonates born prior to 35 weeks' gestation.[12]

Ketorolac is an NSAID available for oral and parenteral administration. According to the manufacturer's prescribing information,[18] ketorolac did not cause birth defects in the offspring of pregnant rabbits. However, ketorolac administration during labor did lead to dystocia in rodents. Ketorolac shares the platelet-inhibiting properties of other NSAIDs.[19] Although ketorolac has not undergone evaluation for its effects on the fetal ductus arteriosus or renal vasculature, it is likely to have effects similar to those of other NSAIDs. Until more information is available, it may be prudent to choose more extensively studied NSAIDs for use during pregnancy.

Based on our clinical experience and a review of the available literature, we have formulated guidelines for the use of NSAIDs during pregnancy (Box 29–1). Because of the antiplatelet properties of NSAIDs, many anesthesiologists are concerned about the risk of epidural hematoma formation as a result of epidural catheter placement. To date, there are no outcome studies on which to base recommendations. There is no evidence that low-dose aspirin therapy or use of other NSAIDs increases the risk of epidural hematoma formation following spinal or epidural placement.[20] As part of our routine history and physical examination of the parturient, we screen for any

BOX 29–1. GUIDELINES FOR USE OF NSAIDS DURING PREGNANCY

- Consider nonpharmacologic management or acetaminophen use first.
- Consider use of a mild opioid or opioid-acetaminophen combination analgesic.
- Continue aspirin or other NSAID if the symptoms cannot be controlled nonpharmacologically or with acetaminophen alone.
- Institute close fetal monitoring during the second trimester. If high doses of NSAIDs are required, periodic fetal ultrasound, including fetal echocardiography, should be used to monitor amniotic fluid volume and patency of the ductus arteriosus.
- Discontinue NSAID use after weeks 34 to 36 to reduce the risks of peripartum bleeding, neonatal hemorrhage, and persistent fetal circulation.

evidence of bleeding diathesis or easy bruising and, in their absence, proceed with epidural placement without further laboratory testing. This practice is consistent with the practice guidelines published by the American Society of Regional Anesthesia.[21]

In breast-feeding women, salicylate transport into breast milk is limited by its highly ionized state and high degree of protein binding. Caution should still be exercised if more than occasional or short-term aspirin use is contemplated during lactation, because neonates have very slow elimination of salicylates.[22] Both ibuprofen and naproxen are also minimally transported into breast milk and are considered compatible with breast-feeding[9]; these agents are generally better tolerated than indomethacin.[23] Little information is available on the safety of maternal ketorolac use during lactation. One study has found that ketorolac concentrations ranged from 1% to 4% of maternal serum levels in breast milk.[24] Taking into account the bioavailability of ketorolac after oral administration, this would likely result in neonatal blood levels between 0.16% and 0.40% of the maternal dose. The American Academy of Pediatrics considers ketorolac to be compatible with breast feeding.[9]

Acetaminophen provides similar analgesia without the anti-inflammatory effects seen with NSAIDs. Acetaminophen has no known teratogenic properties, does not inhibit prostaglandin synthesis or platelet function, and is hepatotoxic only in extreme overdosage.[12,25] If persistent pain demands use of a mild analgesic during pregnancy, acetaminophen appears to be a safe and effective first-choice agent. Acetaminophen does enter breast milk, although maximal neonatal ingestion would be less than 2% of a maternal dose.[26] Acetaminophen is considered compatible with breast-feeding.[9]

Opioid Analgesics

Much of our present knowledge about the effects of chronic opioid exposure during pregnancy is derived from the study of opioid-abusing patients.[27-29] Chronic opioid use in pregnancy is associated with low birth weight and decreased head circumference, although the contribution of comorbidities, including polysubstance abuse and smoking, is not clear. Enrollment and compliance with methadone therapy for opioid dependence improves birth weight and prolongs gestation, supporting the role of therapy during gestation.

There is no evidence to suggest a relationship between exposure to any of the opioid agonists or agonist-antagonists during pregnancy and large categories of major or minor malformations. The Collaborative Perinatal Project monitored 50,282 mother-child pairs and included exposures to codeine, propoxyphene, hydrocodone, meperidine, methadone, morphine, or oxycodone.[16] Only codeine was found to have an association with malformation (respiratory), but this has not been confirmed by other studies. No evidence was found for either agent to suggest a relationship to large categories of major or minor malformations. Overall, opioid analgesics are a reasonable choice for pain control in early pregnancy, with teratogenic risk category B for all except codeine and propoxyphene, which are risk category C when medication is used for a short time.

It is important to note that all opioid medications are risk category D when used for long periods during pregnancy. This increased risk warning is caused by the potential for neonatal opioid dependence when mothers are treated with opioid medications for prolonged periods during pregnancy. Abrupt cessation of opioids in the opioid-dependent patient late in pregnancy can precipitate fetal withdrawal in utero, characterized by fetal tachycardia and fetal death.[30] Therefore, pregnant women who are opioid-dependent, regardless of whether use is prescription or illicit, should not undergo acute withdrawal late in pregnancy without careful fetal monitoring. The general recommendation is to offer continuation of narcotic medication (for prescription use) or opioid substitution therapy such as methadone for women using illicit drugs, with entry into treatment programs.[31] Additional benefits of treatment programs include improved prenatal care, higher birth weight, and reduction of infectious risk to the neonate.

Neonates exposed to opioid medications in utero can develop dependence and manifest withdrawal symptoms in the first few days of life. Characterized in mild cases by irritability and increased tone, severe neonatal withdrawal is associated with poor feeding and seizures.[32] Neonatal abstinence syndrome occurs in from 30% to 90% of infants exposed to heroin or methadone in utero[28,29,33] when mothers are treated for illicit opioid use. Patients requiring methadone for the treatment of chronic pain tend to require lower doses of methadone and their infants have a lower incidence of neonatal abstinence syndrome, approximately 11%.[34] Most infants who have narcotic withdrawal are symptomatic by 48 hours postpartum, but there are reports of withdrawal symptoms beginning 7 to 14 days postpartum.[28] Neonates with prenatal exposure to opiates for long periods may require very slow weaning (as slow as a 10% reduction every third day) to prevent withdrawal symptoms.[35] The American Academy of Pediatrics considers methadone to be compatible with breast-feeding.[9]

Recognition of infants at risk for neonatal abstinence syndrome and institution of appropriate supportive and medical therapy typically results in little short-term consequence to the infant.[36,37] The long-term effects of in utero opioid exposure are unknown. Chasnoff has considered environmental and socioeconomic factors that influence child development and concluded that no definite data exist to demonstrate long-term developmental sequelae from in utero opioid exposure.[38]

Fentanyl is one of the most common parenteral opioid analgesics administered during the perioperative period. As with all opioid analgesics, administration of fentanyl to the mother immediately prior to delivery may lead to respiratory depression in the newborn.[39] Maternal administration of fentanyl or other opioids may also cause loss of the normal variability in fetal heart rate. Loss of fetal heart rate variability can signal fetal hypoxemia, so administration of opioids during labor may deprive obstetric caregivers of a useful tool for assessing fetal well-being.[40]

Meperidine undergoes extensive hepatic metabolism to normeperidine, which has a long elimination half-life (18 hours). Repeated dosing can lead to accumulation, especially in patients with renal insufficiency.[41] Normeperidine causes excitation of the central nervous system that manifest as tremors, myoclonus, and generalized seizures.[42] Significant accumulation of normeperidine is unlikely in the parturient who receives single or infrequent doses; however, meperidine offers no advantages over other parenteral opioids.

Although mixed agonist-antagonist opioid analgesic agents are widely used to provide analgesia during labor, they do not appear to offer any advantage over pure opioid agonists. In a blinded randomized comparison of meperidine and nalbuphine during labor, the two agents appeared to provide comparable analgesic effects as well as similar neonatal Apgar and neurobehavioral scores.[43] Use of nalbuphine[44] or pentazocine[45] during pregnancy can lead to neonatal abstinence syndrome. Nalbuphine may also cause a sinusoidal fetal heart rate pattern after maternal administration, thereby complicating fetal assessment.[46]

Low-affinity opioid agonists, such as tramadol (Ultram), are being used with increasing frequency, in part because of a perceived lessening of the abuse and addiction potential. There is no evidence that acute use of tramadol for labor analgesia has any advantages over more traditional opioids. The intramuscular application of tramadol in mothers in labor reaches the neonate almost freely, confirming a high degree of placental permeability. The neonate already possesses the complete hepatic capacity for the metabolism of tramadol into its active metabolite.[47] However, the renal elimination of the active tramadol metabolite M1 is delayed, in line with the slow maturation process of renal function in neonates. Neonates born to women who are chronically receiving tramadol during pregnancy carry a risk of withdrawal. There are no studies on the relative rates of neonatal abstinence syndrome comparing tramadol with other opioid analgesics. Breast-feeding is of unknown risk when the mother is receiving tramadol.

Postoperative analgesia for most pregnant women undergoing nonobstetric surgery can be readily provided using narcotic analgesics (Tables 29–3 and 29–4). Fentanyl, morphine, and hydromorphone are all safe and effective alternatives when a potent opioid is needed for parenteral administration. There are a range of safe and effective oral analgesics—for mild pain, acetaminophen alone or in combination with hydrocodone is a good alternative; for moderate pain, oxycodone alone or in combination with acetaminophen is effective; more severe pain may require

Table 29–3. Oral Analgesics for Treating Pain during Pregnancy*

DRUG	EQUIANALGESIC ORAL DOSE (mg)	HOW SUPPLIED	FDA RISK CATEGORY
Acetaminophen	—	325-, 500-, 625-mg tabs; 500 mg/15 mL elixir	B
Codeine	60	15-, 30-, 60-mg tabs; 15 mg/5 mL elixir	C[†]
Acetaminophen with codeine	—	300 · 15-,300 · 30-, 300 · 60-mg tabs; 120 · 12/5 mL elixir	C[†]
Hydrocodone	60	—[‡]	B[†]
Acetaminophen with hydrocodone	—	500 · 2.5, 500 · 5, 500 · 7.5, 660 · 10 mg tabs; 500 · 7.5/15 mL elixir	C[†]
Oxycodone	10	5-mg tabs; 5 mg/5 mL elixir	B[†]
Acetaminophen with oxycodone	—	325 · 5-, 500 · 5-mg tabs; 325 · 5/5 mL elixir	C[†]
Morphine	20	15-, 30-mg tabs; 10-, 20-mg/5 mL elixir	B[†]
Hydromorphone	2	2-, 4-, 8-mg tabs; 5 mg/5 mL elixir	B[†]

*There is wide variability in the duration of analgesic action from patient to patient. All the oral agents listed are generally started with dosing every 4 to 6 hours. The dosing interval can then be adjusted as needed to maintain adequate analgesia.
[†]All opioid analgesics are FDA risk category D if used for prolonged periods or in large doses near term.
[‡]There is no oral formulation of hydrocodone alone available in the United States.

Table 29–4. Analgesics for Moderate to Severe Pain During Pregnancy*

DRUG	EQUIANALGESIC PARENTERAL DOSE	EQUIANALGESIC ORAL DOSE
Fentanyl	50 μg	—
Hydromorphone	1 mg	2-4 mg
Morphine	5 mg	30-60 mg
Meperidine	50 mg	150-300 mg

*There is wide variability in the duration of analgesic action from patient to patient. All the parenteral agents listed are generally started with parenteral dosing every 3 to 4 hours and the oral agents every 4 to 6 hours. The dosing interval can then be adjusted as needed to maintain adequate analgesia.

morphine or hydromorphone, both of which are available for oral administration.

Narcotic analgesics can also be administered into the intrathecal or epidural compartments to provide postoperative analgesia. Such neuraxial administration of hydrophilic agents (e.g., morphine) greatly reduces total postoperative opioid requirements while providing excellent analgesia.[48] Spinal or epidural delivery of opioids can be used to minimize maternal plasma concentrations, thereby reducing placental transfer to the fetus or exposure of the breast-feeding infant.

Buprenorphine is an opioid agonist-antagonist currently used for office-based treatment of opioid dependence but is increasing in use for the treatment of chronic pain. Obstetricians and anesthesiologists will therefore encounter patients treated with buprenorphine with increasing frequency. The pharmacologic action provides a ceiling effect (at approximately 24 mg/day) and antagonism of the μ-opioid receptor when given with pure μ agonists, characteristics that lessen the abuse potential and allow for office-based therapy. The μ agonist effects in opioid-naïve individuals, combined with κ-receptor actions, has made buprenorphine a potential treatment option for chronic pain.[49] In the buprenor-phine-maintained patient, however, acute pain can be difficult to treat because of the partial antagonist activity at the μ receptor. Whereas treatment of opioid dependence requires only once-daily dosing, opioid-dependent patients receiving buprenorphine with mild pain may receive analgesia simply by splitting the same daily dose into dosing intervals every 6 hours.[50]

Opioids are excreted into breast milk. Pharmacokinetic analysis has demonstrated that breast milk concentrations of codeine and morphine are equal to or somewhat higher than maternal plasma concentrations.[51] Meperidine use in breast-feeding mothers via patient-controlled analgesia (PCA) has resulted in significantly greater neurobehavioral depression of the breast-feeding newborn than equianalgesic doses of morphine.[52] After absorption from the infant's gastrointestinal tract, opioids contained in ingested breast milk undergo significant first-pass hepatic metabolism. Morphine undergoes glucuronidation to inactive metabolites.[51] Meperidine undergoes N-demethylation to the active metabolite normeperidine.[53] Normeperidine's half-life is markedly prolonged in the newborn,[54] so that regular breast-feeding leads to accumulation and the resultant risks of neurobehavioral depression and seizures. The American Academy of Pediatrics considers the use of many opioid analgesics, including codeine, fentanyl, methadone, morphine, and propoxyphene, to be compatible with breast-feeding.[9] There are insufficient data to determine the safety of buprenorphine with breast-feeding; however, the excretion of buprenorphine into breast milk is minimal.[55]

Local Anesthetics

Few studies have focused on the potential teratogenicity of local anesthetics. Lidocaine and bupivacaine do not appear to pose significant developmental risk to the fetus. In the Collaborative Perinatal Project,[16] only mepivacaine had any suggestion of teratogenicity; however, the number of patient exposures was inadequate to draw conclusions. Animal studies have found that continuous exposure to lidocaine throughout pregnancy does not cause congenital anomalies, but may decrease neonatal birth weight.[56] Continuous exposure to local anesthetics is unusual, but might be seen with the frequent use of local anesthetic patches or creams, which are used for postherpetic neuralgia and other neuropathic pain states.

Neither lidocaine nor bupivacaine appear in measurable quantities in breast milk after epidural local anesthetic administration during labor.[7] Intravenous infusion of high doses (2 to 4 mg/min) of lidocaine for suppression of cardiac arrhythmias has led to minimal levels in breast milk.[57] Based on these observations, continuous epidural infusion of dilute local anesthetic solutions for postoperative analgesia should result in only small quantities of drug actually reaching the fetus. The American Academy of Pediatrics considers local anesthetics to be safe for use in the nursing mother.[9]

Mexiletine is an orally active antiarrhythmic agent with structural and pharmacologic properties similar to those of lidocaine. This agent has shown promise in the treatment of neuropathic pain. Mexiletine is lipid-soluble and freely crosses the placenta. There are no controlled studies in humans of mexiletine use during pregnancy. However, studies in rats, mice, and rabbits using doses up to four times the maximum daily dose in humans have demonstrated an increased risk of fetal resorption but not teratogenicity.[58] Mexiletine appears to be concentrated in breast milk; however, based on expected breast milk concentrations and average daily intake of breast milk, the infant would receive only a small fraction of the usual pediatric maintenance dose of mexiletene.[59] Mexiletine is rated risk category C by the FDA and its use should be undertaken cautiously during pregnancy. The American Academy of Pediatrics considers mexiletine use to be compatible with breast-feeding.[9]

Steroids

Most corticosteroids cross the placenta, although prednisone and prednisolone are inactivated by the placenta.[2] Fetal serum concentrations of prednisone are less than 10% of maternal levels. Among 145 patients exposed to corticosteroids during their first trimester of pregnancy, no increase in malformations was seen.[16] The use of corticosteroids during a limited trial of epidural steroid therapy in the pregnant patient probably poses minimal fetal risk (see further discussion later in this chapter).

In the mother who is breast-feeding, less than 1% of a maternal prednisone dose appears in the nursing infant over the next 3 days.[60] This amount of steroid exposure is unlikely to affect infant endogenous cortisol secretion.[60]

Benzodiazepines

Benzodiazepines are among the most frequently prescribed of all drugs and are often used as anxiolytic agents, to treat insomnia, and as skeletal muscle relaxants in patients with chronic pain.[61] First-trimester exposure to benzodiazepines may be associated with an increased risk of congenital malformations. Diazepam may be associated with cleft lip or cleft palate,[62] as well as with congenital inguinal hernia.[63] However, epidemiologic evidence has not confirmed the association of diazepam with cleft abnormalities; the incidence of cleft lip and palate remained stable after the introduction and widespread use of diazepam.[64] Epidemiologic studies have confirmed the association of diazepam use during pregnancy with congenital inguinal hernia.[64] Benzodiazepine use immediately before delivery also increases the risk of fetal hypothermia, hyperbilirubinemia, and respiratory depression.[65]

Two other benzodiazepines have been evaluated for teratogenicity. Chlordiazepoxide has been reported to produce a fourfold increase in congenital anomalies, including spastic diplegia, duodenal atresia, and congenital heart disease.[66,67] However, a study of over 200,000 Michigan Medicaid recipients did not support these earlier findings.[68] Instead, this study found a high coprevalence of alcohol and illicit drug use in patients receiving benzodiazepines. Benzodiazepine use alone did not appear to be a risk factor for congenital anomalies. Oxazepam use during pregnancy has also been associated with congenital anomalies, including a syndrome of dysmorphic facial features and central nervous system defects.[69] In addition to the risks of teratogenesis, neonates who are exposed to benzodiazepines in utero may experience withdrawal symptoms immediately after birth.[70]

In the breast-feeding mother, diazepam and its metabolite desmethyldiazepam can be detected in the infant's serum for up to 10 days after a single maternal dose. This is caused by the slower metabolism in neonates compared with adults.[71] Clinically, infants who are nursing from mothers receiving diazepam may show sedation and poor feeding.[71] It appears most prudent to avoid any use of benzodiazepines during organogenesis, near the time of delivery, and during lactation.

Antidepressants

Antidepressants are often used in the management of migraine headaches, as well as for analgesic and antidepressant purposes in chronic pain states. Selective serotonin reuptake inhibitors (SSRIs) have become the mainstay for treatment of depression and are widely prescribed. As with most medications, increased use has been associated with increased reports of adverse effects in pregnancy and the neonate. Although initially thought to be safe in early pregnancy, unpublished epidemiologic reports from GlaxoSmithKline have raised concern that paroxetine, one of the most widely prescribed antidepressants, may be associated with an increase in malformations when used in the first trimester, particularly cardiovascular malformations.[72] This recent retrospective epidemiologic study of 3581 pregnant women exposed to paroxetine or other antidepressants during the first trimester has suggested an increased risk of overall major congenital malformations for paroxetine compared with other antidepressants (odds ratio, [OR], 2.20; 95% confidence interval [CI], 1.34 to 3.63). There was also an increased risk for cardiovascular malformations with the use of paroxetine compared with other antidepressants (OR, 2.08; 95% CI, 1.03 to 4.23); 10 out of 14 infants with cardiovascular malformations had ventricular septal defects. Use late in pregnancy has also recently become a concern, with reports of a neonatal abstinence syndrome, including jitteriness or seizures,[73] and pulmonary hypertension in the newborn.[74] These data have initiated a reevaluation regarding the risks and benefits of SSRIs during pregnancy and have raised the FDA risk category from B to C. It is important to note that although the relative risk of adverse outcomes has increased, the incidence of malformations (1% to 3%) and pulmonary hypertension (0.5% to 1%) remain low, whereas the presence of severe depression in pregnant women is high (15%). As with all medications, the risk of no medication must be carefully weighed against the risk of treatment; there are many women who will need to remain on their antidepressant throughout pregnancy, and the low incidence of adverse outcomes remains reassuring.

Although tricyclic antidepressants have had a more limited role in the treatment of depression, they can be of benefit in patients with chronic pain. Amitriptyline, nortriptyline, and imipramine are all rated risk category D by the FDA. Desipramine and all other conventional antidepressant medications are category C.[75] Amitriptyline is teratogenic in hamsters (encephaloceles) and rats (skeletal defects).[12] Imipramine has been associated with several congenital defects in rabbits, but not in rats, mice, or monkeys.[76] Although there have been case reports of human neonatal limb deformities after maternal amitriptyline and imipramine use, large human population studies have not revealed association with any congenital malformation, with the possible exception of cardiovascular defects after maternal imipramine use.[12] There have been no reports linking maternal desipramine use with congenital defects. Withdrawal syndromes have been reported in neonates born to mothers using nortriptyline, imipramine, and desipramine, with symptoms including irritability, colic, tachypnea, and urinary retention.[12]

Amitriptyline, nortriptyline and desipramine are all excreted into human milk. Pharmacokinetic modeling has suggested that infants are exposed to about 1% of the maternal dose.[77] In a critical review of the literature regarding use of antidepressants during breast-feeding, Wisner and colleagues have concluded that amitriptyline, nortriptyline, desipramine, clomipramine, and sertraline are not found in quantifiable amounts in nurslings and reported no adverse effects; they have recommended use of these agents as the antidepressants of choice for breast-feeding women.[77] Fluoxetine is also excreted into human milk and has a milk-to-plasma ratio of about 0.3. No controlled studies are available to guide fluoxetine therapy during lactation[12]; however, colic and high infant serum levels have been reported.[78] Maternal doxepin use has also been associated with elevated plasma levels of the metabolite *N*-desmethyldoxepin and respiratory depression in a nursing infant.[79] The American Academy of Pediatrics considers all antidepressants to have unknown risk during lactation.[9]

Duloxetine, a selective norepinephrine reuptake inhibitor (SNRI), is representative of a new class of drug that combines inhibition of serotonin and norepinephrine reuptake. Duloxetine is efficacious for depression and neuropathic pain, and may have particular efficacy in diabetic neuropathy. Duloxetine is FDA pregnancy category C, indicating potential risks and benefits. Neonates born to mothers receiving SSRI or SNRI drugs may have a withdrawal reaction, as discussed earlier. Although the relative risks and benefits of breast-feeding when a woman is receiving duloxetine have not been fully evaluated, the manufacturer advises against its use during breast-feeding.

Anticonvulsants

A number of anticonvulsant medications are used in pain management. However, most data regarding the fetal risk of major malformation in women taking anticonvulsants are derived from the treatment of epilepsy. Among one group of epileptic women receiving phenytoin, carbamazepine, or valproic acid, the risk of a congenital defect was approximately 5%,[80] or twice that of the general population. Neural tube defects and, to a lesser extent, cardiac abnormalities predominate in the offspring of women taking carbamazepine and valproic acid[81] and can be detected during routine prenatal screening (elevated alpha-fetoprotein level). Inadequate maternal folate absorption associated with anticonvulsant use during pregnancy may contribute to neural tube defects.[81] The fetal hydantoin syndrome has been associated with phenytoin, carbamazepine, and valproate use during pregnancy; the syndrome consists of variable dysmorphic features, including microcephaly, mental deficiency, and craniofacial abnormalities.[81] The appearance of this syndrome may be predicted by fetal genetic screening[82] or by measuring amniocyte levels of the enzyme responsible for phenytoin metabolism.[83] Whereas anticonvulsants have teratogenic risk, epilepsy itself may be partially responsible for fetal malformations.[81] It is possible that pregnant women taking anticonvulsants for chronic pain may have a lower risk of fetal malformations than those taking the same medications for seizure control.

Patients contemplating childbearing who are receiving anticonvulsants should have their pharmacologic therapy critically evaluated. Those taking anticonvulsants for neuropathic pain should strongly consider discontinuation during pregnancy, particularly during the first trimester. Consultation with a perinatologist is recommended if continued use of anticonvulsants during pregnancy is being considered. Frequent monitoring of serum anticonvulsant levels and folate supplementation should be initiated, and maternal alpha-fetoprotein screening may be considered to detect fetal neural tube defects.

Gabapentin is a newer anticonvulsant that is being used for the treatment of neuropathic pain syndromes. Little information exists about the safety of gabapentin in pregnant women. In their prescribing information, the manufacturer[84] has reported a series of nine women who received gabapentin during their pregnancies. Four women elected pregnancy termination, four had normal outcomes, and one neonate had pyloric stenosis and an inguinal hernia. Insufficient data exist to counsel patients regarding the fetal risk of gabapentin use during pregnancy.

A new drug similar to gabapentin is pregabalin, which combines anticonvulsant activity and affinity to the gamma aminobutyric acid receptor. The main applications of pregabalin are for the treatment of pain associated with diabetic neuropathy and postherpetic neuralgia. Pregabalin is listed as FDA pregnancy risk category C, but the risks during breast-feeding are unknown.

The use of anticonvulsants during lactation does not seem to be harmful to infants. Phenytoin, carbamazepine, and valproic acid appear in small amounts in breast milk, but no adverse effects have been noted.[12] No data exist on gabapentin use during lactation.

Ergot Alkaloids

Ergotamine can have significant therapeutic efficacy for the episodic treatment of migraine headaches. However, even low doses of ergotamine are associated with significant teratogenic risk, and higher doses have caused uterine contractions and spontaneous abortion.[75] During lactation, ergot alkaloids are associated with neonatal convulsions and severe gastrointestinal disturbances.[12] Occasionally, methylergonovine is systemically administered to treat uterine atony and maternal hemorrhage immediately after delivery. This brief exposure does not contraindicate breast-feeding.[85]

Caffeine

Caffeine is often used in combination analgesics for the management of vascular headaches. Early studies of caffeine ingestion during pregnancy have suggested an increased risk of intrauterine growth retardation, fetal demise, and premature labor.[86] However, these early studies did not control for concomitant alcohol and tobacco use. Subsequent research, which controlled for these confounding factors, has found no added risks with moderate caffeine ingestion, but ingestion of more than 300 mg/day was associated with decreased birth weight.[87] Caffeine ingestion combined with tobacco use increases the risk of delivering a low-birth-weight infant.[88] Ingestion of modest doses of caffeine (100 mg/m², a dose similar to that found in two cups of brewed coffee) in caffeine-naïve subjects produces modest cardiovascular changes in mother and fetus, including increased maternal heart rate and mean arterial pressure, increased peak aortic flow velocities, and decreased fetal heart rate.[89] The modest decrease in fetal heart rate and increased frequency of fetal heart rate accelerations may confound interpretation of fetal heart tracings. Caffeine ingestion is also associated with an increased incidence of tachyarrhythmia in the newborn, including supraventricular tachyarrhythmias, atrial flutter, and premature atrial contractions.[90] Many over-the-counter analgesic formulations contain caffeine (typically in amounts from 30 to 65 mg/dose), and use of these preparations must be considered when determining total caffeine exposure.

Moderate ingestion of caffeine during lactation (up to two cups of coffee/day) does not appear to affect the infant. Breast milk usually contains less than 1% of the maternal dose of caffeine, with peak breast milk levels appearing 1 hour after maternal ingestion. Excessive caffeine use may cause increased wakefulness and irritability in the infant.[91]

Sumatriptan

Sumatriptan is a selective serotonin agonist that has achieved widespread use because of its efficacy in the treatment of migraine headaches. It has been associated with fetal malformations in rabbits, but not in rats.[92] Limited data in humans have not demonstrated any strong teratogenic effects.[75,93] Sumatriptan does not share uterine contractile properties with ergotamine, and would not likely have abortifacient effects.[94] Beginning in January 1996, Glaxo Welcome established a registry to evaluate the risk of sumatriptan use during pregnancy prospectively.[95] At the time of this writing, 124 pregnancies had early exposure to sumatriptan, with a 4% birth defect rate. This rate is close to the expected rate in the general population and no particular clustering of defects has been noted. Sumatriptan is labeled risk category C by the FDA.

The use of sumatriptan during lactation has not been well studied. One study of a single 6-mg dose of subcutaneous sumatriptan given to lactating women found total breast milk sumatriptan to be only 0.24% of the maternal dose. Because sumatriptan is poorly absorbed from the infant GI tract, only 14% of the drug ingested by the fetus would be bioavailable. Even this minor exposure could be largely avoided by expressing and discarding all milk for 8 hours after injection.[96]

Beta Blockers

Propranolol and other beta blockers are used for chronic prophylaxis against migraine and non-migraine vascular headaches. There is no evidence that propranolol is teratogenic. Fetal effects noted with maternal consumption of propranolol include decreased weight, potentially because of a modest decrease in maternal cardiac output, with consequent diminished placental perfusion.[97] Cox and associates[98] have presented an in-depth review of the use of beta blockers, calcium channel blockers, and other antiarrhythmic agents during pregnancy.

In the lactating mother, propranolol doses of up to 240 mg/day appear to have minimal neonatal effects. The average neonatal exposure at this maternal dose is less than 1% of the therapeutic dose.[99] Atenolol is concentrated in breast milk, but still results in subtherapeutic levels in the infant.[100]

EVALUATION AND TREATMENT OF PAIN DURING PREGNANCY

We have been asked to consult on numerous patients with uncontrolled pain during the course of pregnancy. Often, severe pain was arising from an extreme form of one of the more common musculoskeletal pain syndromes of pregnancy. Thus, a working knowledge of the painful musculoskeletal conditions that occur during pregnancy is essential. We also discuss evaluation of back pain and migraine headaches during pregnancy, because these are among the most common problems encountered in practice. Although sickle cell pain crisis is less common, it provides a good example of the approach to managing chronic recurrent pain during the course of pregnancy.

Musculoskeletal Considerations in Pregnancy

Abdominal Wall and Ligamentous Pain

Abdominal wall pain during pregnancy typically results in prompt evaluation by an obstetrician. One of the most common causes of abdominal pain early in pregnancy is miscarriage, which presents with

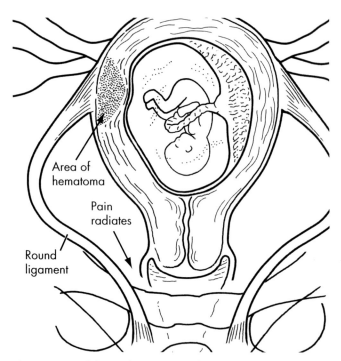

Figure 29–1. Abdominal pain arising from stretch and hematoma formation in the round ligament usually presents between 16 and 20 weeks' gestation, with pain and tenderness over the round ligament, which radiates to the pubic symphysis. (Adapted with permission from Chamberlain G: ABC of antenatal care. Abdominal pain in pregnancy. Br Med J 1991;302:1390-1394.)

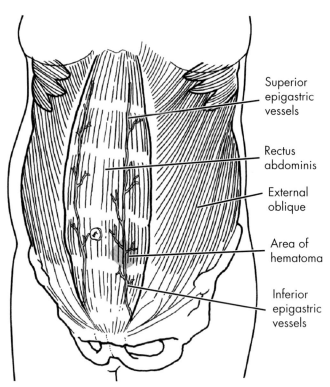

Figure 29–2. Stretch of the abdominal wall in pregnancy can lead to tearing of the rectus abdominis muscle or inferior epigastric veins and formation of a painful hematoma within the rectus sheath. Pain is well localized and can be severe, often starting after a bout of coughing or sneezing. (Adapted with permission from Chamberlain G: ABC of antenatal care. Abdominal pain in pregnancy. Br Med J 1991;302:1390-1394.)

abdominal pain and vaginal bleeding. Unruptured ectopic pregnancy and ovarian torsion may present with vague hypogastric pain and suprapubic tenderness. Once these conditions requiring the immediate attention of an obstetrician have been ruled out, myofascial causes of abdominal pain should be considered.

The round ligaments stretch as the uterus rises in the abdomen. If the pull is too rapid, small hematomas may develop in the ligaments (Fig. 29–1). This usually begins at 16 to 20 weeks' gestation, with pain and tenderness localized over the round ligament which radiates to the pubic tubercle.[101] Treatment is bed rest and local warmth, along with oral analgesics in more severe cases.

Less common is abdominal pain arising from hematoma formation within the sheath of the rectus abdominis muscle (Fig. 29–2). As the uterus expands, the muscles of the abdominal wall become greatly overstretched. Rarely, the rectus muscle may dehisce or the inferior epigastric veins rupture behind the muscle. Severe pain localized to a single segment of the muscle often follows a bout of sneezing. Diagnosis of rectus hematoma is made when localized pain is exacerbated by tightening the abdominal muscles (raising the head in the supine position). Ultrasonography can be helpful in confirming the

diagnosis. Conservative management with bed rest, local heat, and mild analgesics is often all that is needed.

Hip Pain

Two relatively rare conditions, osteonecrosis and transient osteoporosis of the hip, both occur with somewhat greater frequency during pregnancy.[102] Although the exact cause is not known, high levels of estrogen and progesterone in the maternal circulation and increased interosseous pressure may contribute to the development of osteonecrosis.[103] Transient osteoporosis of the hip is a rare disorder characterized by pain and limitation of motion of the hip and osteopenia of the femoral head.[104] Both conditions present with hip pain during the third trimester, which may be sudden or gradual in onset. Osteoporosis is easily identified, with plain radiography demonstrating osteopenia of the femoral head and preservation of the joint space. Osteonecrosis is best evaluated with magnetic resonance imaging (MRI), which will demonstrate changes before they appear on plain radiographs. Both conditions are managed symptomatically during pregnancy. Limited weight bearing is essential in transient osteoporosis of the hip to avoid fracture of the femoral neck.[104]

Posterior Pelvic Pain

Causative Factors

The hormonal changes that occur during pregnancy lead to widening and increased mobility of the sacroiliac synchondroses and the symphysis pubis as early as the 10th to 12th week of pregnancy. Sacroiliac pain is described by many pregnant women, located in the posterior part of the pelvis distal and lateral to the lumbosacral junction.[105] Many terms have been used in the literature to describe this type of pain, including *sacroiliac dysfunction, pelvic girdle relaxation,* and even *sacroiliac joint pain.*[105]

Clinical Presentation

The pain radiates to the posterior part of the thigh and may extend below the knee, leading to misinterpretation as sciatica. The pain is less specific than sciatica in distribution and does not extend to the ankle or foot. Differentiating between back and posterior pelvic problems is a challenge; Ostgaard and coworkers have attempted to separate the two entities by defining the syndrome of "posterior pelvic pain" (Box 29–2).

Back Pain

Causative Factors

Back pain occurs at some time during pregnancy in about 50% of women[106-108] and is so common that it is often regarded as a normal part of pregnancy. The lumbar lordosis becomes markedly accentuated during pregnancy and may contribute to the development of low back pain.[109] Endocrine changes

during pregnancy may also play a role in the development of back pain. Relaxin, a polypeptide secreted by the corpus luteum, softens the ligaments around the pelvic joints and cervix, allowing accommodation of the developing fetus and facilitating vaginal delivery. This laxity may cause pain by an exaggerated range of motion.[110]

Clinical Presentation

Although radicular symptoms often accompany low back pain during pregnancy, herniated nucleus pulposus (HNP) has an incidence of only 1:10,000.[111] The prevalence of lumbar intervertebral disk bulge and herniation was determined by MRI in 45 pregnant women and 41 asymptomatic nonpregnant women of childbearing age. Fifty-three percent of pregnant and 54% of nonpregnant women had disk abnormalities at one or more levels.[112] The authors concluded that pregnant women do not have an increased prevalence of lumbar intervertebral disk abnormalities. Direct pressure of the fetus on the lumbosacral nerves or lumbar plexus has been postulated as the cause of radicular symptoms.[107]

One group investigated patient characteristics associated with back pain during pregnancy. Of note, maternal age, weight gain during pregnancy, the baby's weight, number of previous pregnancies, and number of prior children[107] were all unassociated with increased likelihood of back pain. A subsequent study reported that back problems before pregnancy increased the risk of back pain, as did young age and multiparity.[108]

Ostgaard and associates[108] prospectively followed 855 pregnant women from the 12th week of gestation until childbirth. Back pain occurred in 49% of women at some point during the average 28 weeks of observation. The authors classified back pain into three groups (Fig. 29–3)—in one group, pain was localized to the sacroiliac area and increased as pregnancy progressed (see earlier discussion of posterior pelvic pain); in the other two groups, pain was localized to the mid thoracic area (high back) or the lumbar area (low back) and decreased or did not change during the course of pregnancy. True sciatica with a dermatomal distribution occurred in only 10 women (1%).

Evaluation of the Patient with Back and Posterior Pelvic Pain

Evaluation begins with a thorough history, which will often point the clinician to other causes.[113] Patients with both preterm labor and premature rupture of membranes may present with low back pain[114,115] accompanied by uterine contractions and changes in the cervical os. Urologic disorders, including hydronephrosis, pyelonephritis, and renal calculi, may also present with low back discomfort.[116] Major morphologic changes occur in the collecting system

---

BOX 29–2. SIGNS AND SYMPTOMS OF THE SYNDROME OF "POSTERIOR PELVIC PAIN"

- A history of time- and weight-bearing–related pain in the posterior pelvis, deep to the gluteal area
- A positive "posterior pelvic provocation test" (see Fig. 29–5)
- A pain drawing with well-defined markings of stabbing pain in the buttocks distal and lateral to the L5-S1 area, with or without radiation to the posterior thigh or knee, but not into the foot (see Fig. 29–6)
- Free movements in the hips and spine and no nerve root symptoms
- Pain when turning in bed

Adapted with permission from Ostgaard HC, Zetherstrom G, Roos-Hanson E, et al: Reduction of back and posterior pelvic pain in pregnancy, Spine 1994;19:894-900.

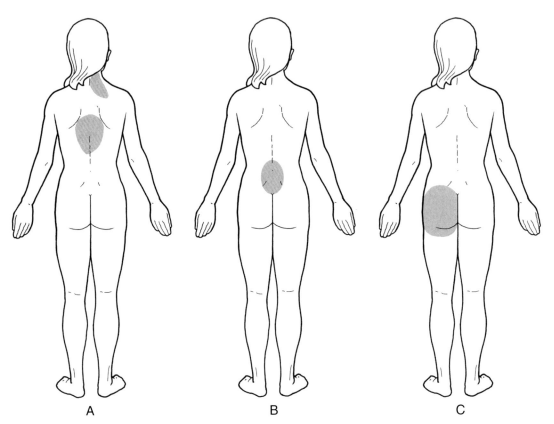

Figure 29–3. Three types of pain were reported by a group of 855 women studied between 12 menstrual weeks of pregnancy and delivery. Back pain was reported by 49% of the women at some point during pregnancy. **A,** High back pain (10%). **B,** Low back pain (40%). **C,** Sacroiliac pain (50%). (Adapted with permission from Ostgaard HC, Andersson GBJ, Karlsson K: Prevalence of back pain in pregnancy. Spine 1991;16:549-552.)

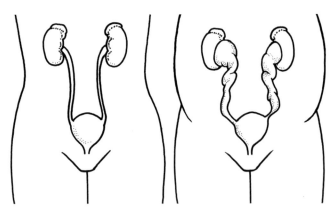

Figure 29–4. Elevated progesterone levels and pressure from the expanding uterus lead to dilation of the ureters in pregnancy. Stasis in the urinary tract can lead to pyelonephritis. (Adapted with permission from Chamberlain G: ABC of antenatal care. Abdominal pain in pregnancy. Br Med J 1991;302:1390-1394.)

of pregnant women including dilation of the calices, renal pelvis, and ureters[117] (Fig. 29–4). The physical examination should include complete back and neurologic evaluations. Particular attention should be directed toward the pelvis and sacroiliac joints during the examination. Posterior pelvic pain (sacroiliac dysfunction) can often be distinguished from other causes of low back pain based on physical examination (Figs. 29–5 and 29–6; Table 29–5; see Box 29–2). Positive straight leg raise (typical low back pain with or without radiation to the ipsilateral lower extremity) during physical examination is consistent with sacroiliac subluxation or herniated nucleus pulposus. Unilateral loss of knee or ankle reflex or the presence of a sensory or motor deficit is suggestive of lumbar nerve root compression.

Pregnancy is not an absolute contraindication to radiographic evaluation. Radiation exposure during pregnancy leads to concerns about resultant congenital anomalies, mental retardation, and increased risk of subsequent cancers.[118] No detectable growth or mental abnormalities have been associated with fetal exposure to less than 10 rad; the dose received during a typical three-view spinal series typically does not exceed 1.5 rad.[119] Plain radiographs will contribute vital information primarily when fracture, dislocation, and destructive lesions of the bone are suspected.

MRI has revolutionized diagnostic imaging during pregnancy, proving effective and reliable in the diagnosis of many structural abnormalities.[120] Although MRI appears to be safe during pregnancy, there are no long-term studies examining the safety of fetal exposure to intense magnetic fields during gestation.[121] Schwartz[119] has presented a thorough and

Table 29–5. Sacroiliac Subluxation: Criteria for Diagnosis and Common Confirmatory Signs

CRITERION OR SIGN	DESCRIPTION
Diagnostic Criterion	
Sacral pain	The pain is usually unilateral and, in some cases, radiates to the buttock, lower abdomen, anterior medial thigh, groin, or posterior thigh.
Positive Piedallu's sign	Forward flexion of the lower back results in asymmetrical movement of the posterior superior iliac spines (PSISs), with one PSIS becoming higher than the other.
Positive pelvic compression	Pain in the sacral area is provoked by direct bilateral downward pressure on the anterior superior iliac spines (ASISs).
Asymmetry of the ASIS	The ASISs should be examined with the patient in the supine position to eliminate the effect of leg length discrepancy; in sacroiliac subluxation, one ASIS will be higher than the other.
Confirmatory Sign	
Straight leg raise	Passive raising of the patient's leg, with the knee extended and the patient in the supine position, causes pain, usually at the end range.
Flexion block	With the patient in the supine position, the knee is flexed at 90 degrees and then passively pressed toward the chest; flexion is blocked to half the expected range on the painful side.
Positive Patrick's test	Placing one heel on the opposite knee, in the recumbent position, and simultaneously rotating the leg outward provokes pain,
Pain at Baer's point	A point of acute tenderness is found just to the side and below the umbilicus on the painful side, which is about one third of the way between the umbilicus and ASIS.

Adapted with permission from Daly JM, Frame PS, Rapoza PA: Sacroiliac subluxation: A common, treatable cause of low back pain in pregnancy, Fam Pract Res J 1991;11:149-159.

insightful review of neurodiagnostic imaging of the pregnant patient. Practical guidelines for the use of radiographic studies in the evaluation of pregnant patients are given in Box 29–3.

Electromyography and nerve conduction studies (collectively referred to as EMG) serve as good screening tests in the patient with new onset of low back pain accompanied by sensory or motor symptoms. When the clinical presentation is confusing, EMG can aid in differentiating peripheral nerve lesions, polyneuropathies, and plexopathies from single radiculopathies. However, false-negative EMG results are common, especially in the case of a herniated nucleus pulposus causing compression of a single nerve root.[122]

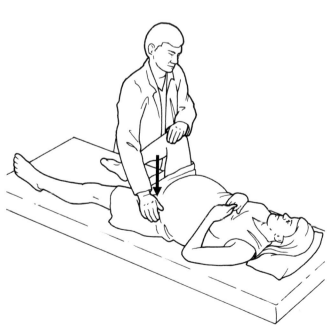

Figure 29–5. The posterior pelvic provocation test. (Adapted with permission from Ostgaard HC, Zetherstrom G, Roos-Hanson E, et al: Reduction of back and posterior pelvic pain in pregnancy. Spine 1994;19:894-900.)

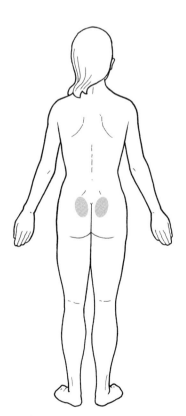

Figure 29–6. Areas where pain is felt when the posterior provocation test is performed in women with posterior pelvic pain. (Adapted with permission from Ostgaard HC, Zetherstrom G, Roos-Hanson E, et al: Reduction of back and posterior pelvic pain in pregnancy. Spine 1994;19:894-900.)

**BOX 29–3. GUIDELINES FOR USE OF
NEURODIAGNOSTIC IMAGING IN
THE PREGNANT PATIENT**

- Determine the necessity of a radiologic examination and the risks involved.
- If possible, perform the examination only during the first 10 postmenses days; if the patient is pregnant, delay the examination until the third trimester, or preferably postpartum.
- Determine the most efficacious use of radiation for the problem.
- Use magnetic resonance imaging if possible.
- Avoid direct exposure to the abdomen and pelvis.
- Avoid contrast agents.
- Do not avoid radiologic testing purely for the sake of pregnancy. Remember, you are responsible for providing the best possible care for the patient. The risk to the pregnant patient of not having an indicated radiologic examination is also an indirect risk to the fetus.
- If significant exposure is incurred by a pregnant patient, have a radiation biologist (usually stationed in the radiology department) review the radiology examination history carefully so that an accurate dose estimate can be ascertained.
- The decision to terminate pregnancy because of excessive radiation exposure is an extremely complex issue. Because any increased risk of malformations is considered to be negligible unless radiation doses exceed 0.1 to 0.15 Gy (10 to 15 rad), the amount of exposure that an embryo or fetus would likely receive from diagnostic procedures is well below the level for which a therapeutic abortion should be considered.
- Consent forms are neither required nor recommended. The patient should be informed verbally that any radiologic examinations ordered during pregnancy are considered necessary for her medical care. She should also be informed that the risks to the fetus from computed tomography or plain film radiography are very low and that there are no known risks to humans of magnetic resonance imaging. Having the patient sign a consent increases the perceived risks and adds needlessly to her concerns during and after the examination.

Adapted with permission from Schwartz RB: Neurodiagnostic imaging of the pregnant patient. In Devinsky O, Feldmann E, Mainline B (eds): Neurologic Complications of Pregnancy. New York, Raven Press, 1994, pp 243-248.

Prevention and Treatment

Few of the commonly used strategies to prevent low back pain during pregnancy are universally effective. Patients who were instructed in basic lifting techniques experienced significantly less backache than a control group who did not receive similar instruction.[94] Aerobic exercise can be prescribed safely throughout pregnancy[123]; however, maintenance of good physical conditioning may not alter the incidence of back pain during pregnancy.[124] Nonetheless, the American College of Obstetricians and Gynecologists recommends specific muscular conditioning exercises to promote good posture and prevent low back pain during pregnancy.[125]

Treatment begins with counseling the patient about the common causes of back pain during pregnancy. Reassurance and simple changes in the patient's activity level will often suffice to reduce symptoms to a tolerable level. If pain remains poorly controlled, referral to a physical therapist for evaluation and instruction in body mechanics and low back exercises may be beneficial.[126] Acupuncture also reduces pain, and may be more efficacious compared with group physiotherapy. Aquatic exercise programs can be particularly helpful to the parturient and offer the added benefit of reducing the effects of gravity on the mother's musculoskeletal system. Water gymnastics appear to decrease the number of workdays missed for pregnancy-associated back pain. Massage and the surface application of heat or ice may also be useful.[127] Although rigorous clinical trials are lacking, transcutaneous electrical nerve stimulation (TENS) appears to produce clinically meaningful pain relief for various painful disorders in which pain has a limited distribution.[128,129] The safety of TENS use during pregnancy has not been closely examined; however, the stimulation parameters used in conventional TENS units are likely to produce only localized currents in biologic tissues.[128] Limited data suggest that TENS is safe for use during pregnancy[130] and may be useful in patients with pain in a limited distribution.

For posterior pelvic pain of sacroiliac origin, Daly and colleagues[110] have described successful treatment of in 10 of 11 women (91%) using rotational manipulation of the sacroiliac joint. In a similar group of women with posterior pelvic pain, Ostgaard and coworkers[105] have demonstrated a reduction in pain and sick leave using periodic classes during pregnancy in which a physiotherapist described simple anatomy, posture physiology, lifting and working techniques, muscle training, and relaxation training. Some pain relief was reported by the majority of women with posterior pelvic pain who used a nonelastic trochanteric belt in the same study[105] (Fig. 29–7). For women who suffer primarily with back pain at night, Thomas and associates[131] have reported relief of symptoms and improved sleep in 57 of 92 women using a wedge-shaped pillow designed to support the abdomen of a pregnant woman lying on her side.

Although the incidence of herniated nucleus pulposus during pregnancy is low, radicular symptoms are common and often accompany sacroiliac subluxation and myofascial pain syndromes. Use of epidural steroids outside of pregnancy remains controversial.[132] The strongest evidence for efficacy of epidural steroids appears to be in patients with

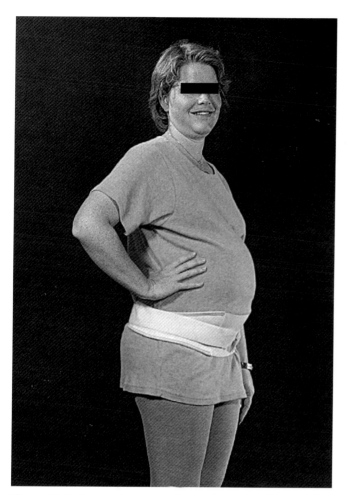

Figure 29–7. Proper placement of a trochanteric belt to stabilize painful pelvic joints and decrease back pain.

symptoms attributable to acute disk pathology.[133] Whereas the risk to the fetus following a single dose of an epidural corticosteroid appears to be low, it is our opinion that epidural steroids should be reserved for the parturient with the new onset of signs (e.g., unilateral loss of deep tendon reflex, sensorimotor change in a dermatomal distribution) and symptoms consistent with lumbar nerve root compression. In such patients, we believe that it is reasonable to proceed with epidural steroid placement prior to obtaining imaging studies. Resolution of the radicular symptoms after epidural steroid treatment may well obviate the need for imaging studies.

Acetaminophen is the first analgesic to consider for management of minor back pain. While NSAIDs are the cornerstone of the pharmacologic management of back pain in nonpregnant individuals, their use during pregnancy remains controversial. Short-term use of ibuprofen or naproxen appears to be safe during the first and second trimesters.[12] Severe back pain may require treatment with narcotics and necessitate hospital admission for parenteral administration of opioid analgesics (see Tables 29–3 and 29–4). Progressive ambulation over several days using the assistance and instruction of a skilled physical therapist is usually successful. Short courses of oral or parenteral opioids appear to add little risk to the fetus.

Migraine Headache during Pregnancy

Causative Factors and Clinical Presentation

Almost 25% of women suffer from migraine headaches,[134] with the peak incidence during childbearing years. Migraines occur more often during menstruation, which has been attributed to a sudden decline in estrogen levels.[135] During pregnancy, a sustained 50- to 100-fold increase in estradiol occurs. Indeed, 70% of women have reported improvement or remission of migraines during pregnancy.[75]

Migraine headaches rarely begin during pregnancy. Many clinicians believe that initial presentation of headaches during pregnancy should initiate a thorough search for potentially serious causes.[75,136] One report of nine women presenting with migraine-like headaches during pregnancy found that four were severely thrombocytopenic, two met criteria for preeclampsia, and one had a threatened abortion.[136] The literature is replete with reports of intracranial pathology that mimicked migraines during pregnancy, including strokes, pseudotumor cerebri, tumors, aneurysms, arteriovenous malformations, and cerebral venous thrombosis.[75] Metabolic causes of headache during pregnancy include illicit drug use (most notably, cocaine[137]), anti-phospholipid antibody syndrome, and choriocarcinoma.[138]

Evaluation

Patients who present with their first severe headache during pregnancy should receive a complete neurologic examination and be strongly considered for MRI, toxicology screening, and serum coagulation profiles. In the patient who presents with sudden onset of the "worst headache of my life," a subarachnoid hemorrhage should be ruled out.[75] Progressively worsening headaches in the setting of sudden weight gain should suggest preeclampsia or pseudotumor cerebri. The triad of elevated blood pressure, proteinuria, and peripheral edema points toward preeclampsia; hyperreflexia and an elevated serum uric acid level are also found in patients with preeclampsia.

Treatment and Prevention

For pregnant women with a history of migraines prior to pregnancy and a normal neurologic examination, the therapeutic challenge is to achieve control of the headaches while minimizing risk to the fetus. Nonpharmacologic techniques, including relaxation, biofeedback, and elimination of certain foods, often suffice for treatment. Marcus and colleagues[139] have demonstrated significant reduction in headache that continued throughout pregnancy and at the 1-year follow-up using a combination of relaxation training, thermal biofeedback, and physical therapy exercises.

If pharmacologic therapy appears warranted, acetaminophen with or without caffeine is safe and effective.[140] Ibuprofen and naproxen both appear to be safe for use during the first two trimesters.[12] The short-term use of mild opioid analgesics such as hydrocodone, alone or in combination with acetaminophen, also appears to carry little risk (see Table 29–3). When oral analgesics prove ineffective, hospital admission and administration of parenteral opioids may be required (see Table 29–4).

Until more information is available on the safety of sumatriptan during pregnancy, it should be used only after other strategies have failed. Ergot preparations should be avoided during pregnancy and lactation.

A history of three to four incapacitating headaches per month warrants consideration of prophylactic therapy.[140] Daily oral propranolol or atenolol are reasonable choices, although patients should understand that their use is associated with small for gestational age infants. Longer acting agents should lead to less fluctuation in maternal and fetal blood concentrations, and perhaps less fluctuation in the drug effects on fetal heart rate. Based on this theoretical advantage, we prefer to use long-acting agents (e.g., atenolol or sustained-release propranolol).

Although antidepressants are effective for prophylactic therapy in nonpregnant patients, the most commonly used medications of this class (imipramine, amitriptyline, and nortriptyline) are all FDA category D. Limited anecdotal experience with calcium channel blockers (verapamil, nifedipine, and diltiazem are all FDA class C) or minidose aspirin (80 mg/day) suggests that they may be effective prophylactic agents during pregnancy.[75,140]

Pain in the Pregnant Patient with Sickle Cell Disease

Causative Factors and Clinical Presentation

Sickle cell disease is an inherited multisystem disorder. The presence of abnormal hemoglobin in red blood cells leads to the cardinal features of the disease, chronic hemolytic anemia and recurrent painful episodes. Vaso-occlusive crisis is the most common maternal complication noted in parturients with sickle cell hemoglobinopathies.[141] Vaso-occlusive crises follow a characteristic pattern of recurrent sudden attacks of pain, usually involving the abdomen, chest, vertebrae, and extremities. One prospective study has demonstrated that the clinical course of women with sickle cell disease is not adversely affected by their pregnancy, as measured by the rate of painful episodes over a 100-day period.[142] The rate was constant before, during, and after the first pregnancy and subsequent pregnancies. Painful episodes occurred at some time during the course of 50% of pregnancies.

Most crises during pregnancy are vaso-occlusive and are often precipitated by urinary tract infection, preeclampsia or eclampsia, thrombophlebitis, or pneumonia. Clinically, the individual will describe pain in the bones or joints but may also perceive the soft tissues as being affected. Visceral pain is also common and may be related to events in the liver or spleen. Painful episodes can be variable in severity and duration, with most episodes lasting from 3 to 5 days.[143]

Evaluation

Because laboratory evaluation is nonspecific, diagnosis of vaso-occlusive crisis begins with excluding other causes for the painful episode, particularly occult infection.[141] Complete assessment and the acute management of sickle cell crisis in pregnancy has been reviewed by Martin and coworkers.[144]

Treatment

Management of vaso-occlusive crisis during pregnancy is primarily supportive and symptomatic. General management begins with aggressive hydration to increase intravascular volume and decrease blood viscosity.[144] Supplemental oxygen is essential in those patients with hypoxemia. Partial exchange transfusions to reduce polymerized hemoglobin S remain an integral part of the management of sickle cell disease[145]; prophylactic transfusion may reduce the incidence of severe sickling complications during pregnancy.[146]

Education about how pregnancy interacts with sickle cell disease can help reduce depression or anxiety, often decreasing the pain that the patient is experiencing. Biofeedback has been shown to reduce the pain of sickle cell crises and the number of days that analgesics were taken.[147] Physical therapy techniques (e.g., exercise, splinting, local application of heat) can also be helpful.[148] TENS may be helpful when pain is isolated to a limited region.[149]

The severity of pain dictates the pharmacologic approach to managing sickle cell pain. Although nonopioid analgesics may suffice, oral or parenteral opioids are often required (see Tables 29–3 and 29–4). Acetaminophen remains the nonopioid analgesic of choice during pregnancy. Although NSAIDs can be useful adjuncts, particularly for controlling bone pain, they should be used cautiously during pregnancy. Oral analgesic combinations containing acetaminophen and hydrocodone or another weak to moderate potency opioid can be added for more severe pain.

For the hospitalized patient with severe sickle cell pain, potent opioid analgesics administered intravenously may be necessary to control pain adequately (see Table 29–4). Morphine sulfate is well tolerated and effective for control of severe sickle cell pain[150]; fentanyl and hydromorphone provide reasonable alternatives for patients who cannot tolerate morphine. Administration of morphine via a patient-controlled analgesia (PCA) device allows patients a sense of control over their illness. Weisman and

Schecter[151] have noted that significantly higher doses of opioids may be necessary for the control of vaso-occlusive crisis pain as compared with postoperative pain. In our practice, we aggressively treat individuals with severe sickle cell pain with potent opioids administered via PCA (most often using morphine). As the pain of vaso-occlusive crisis begins to resolve, patients are transitioned to a long-acting oral opioid (such as sustained-release morphine). This approach allows earlier ambulation and hospital discharge. All opioids are then tapered over the following 7 to 10 days.

The use of regional anesthesia has not been formally studied in sickle cell disease. Continuous epidural analgesia of a low-dose local anesthetic offers the theoretic advantage of increased microvascular blood flow while providing pain relief without opioids. Finer and associates[152] have reported the successful management of a pregnant woman in the midst of a pain crisis using a continuous epidural infusion. In parturients who have pain localized to the trunk or lower extremities and who are intolerant of opioids, continuous epidural analgesia may be a reasonable alternative.

Acute Pain in the Opioid-dependent Patient

Acute pain in the pregnant patient is most often encountered during labor and delivery. Both pain control and withdrawal symptoms are mediated through the μ-opioid receptor. Therefore, narcotic pain medication requires availability of the μ-opioid receptor, which in opioid-dependent patients is also occupied by opioid agonist therapy for dependence. No randomized or controlled studies are available to determine whether anesthetic needs differ in opioid-dependent patients compared with control patients. One descriptive study has found that 24% of opioid-dependent women had difficulty with labor analgesia and 74% had difficulty with postcesarean analgesia.[153] These statistics may overestimate the difficulty in pain control, because it was not clear that treatment of opioid dependence was adequate prior to treatment for acute pain. When opioid dependence is untreated and combined with acute pain, opioid needs reflect the combined therapies rather than treatment for pain alone. Although no randomized clinical trials have been performed, we have found that epidural analgesia with a standard dose of local anesthetic and low-dose opioid (e.g., $^1/_{16}$% bupivacaine with fentanyl, 2 μg/mL) provides adequate intrapartum analgesia.

Intrathecal or epidural analgesia using only opioids may not be effective in reducing the need for systemic narcotics. Sustained administration of μ-opioid agonists by any route can induce both opioid tolerance and abnormal pain that is similar to neuropathic pain.[154] Although previously attributed to pharmacologic tolerance, patients maintained on methadone may experience opioid-induced hyperalgesia, a paradoxical effect mediated in part by the neurotransmitter N-methyl-D-aspartate (NMDA) and possibly by the novel neuropeptide dynorphin.[155] Interestingly, dynorphin may be an important mediator of chronic neuropathic pain, a common complaint among opioid-dependent patients.

There are no trials that investigate opioid use and pain control after vaginal or abdominal delivery in opioid-tolerant patients. Recently published guidelines for the treatment of acute pain in patients maintained on methadone or buprenorphine provide a reasonable approach until more data are available.[50] Patients maintained on methadone for opioid dependence should have their methadone continued at the same dose in addition to standard-dose opiates as needed for acute pain. Use of nonopioid analgesics should be included, but additional opioid medication should not be withheld. This additional short-acting opioid medication can be gradually discontinued as clinically indicated. If patients are unable to tolerate oral medication, methadone can be administered intramuscularly or subcutaneously in two to four divided doses.

Patients maintained on buprenorphine pose a more difficult dilemma in the postoperative period. As a combined opioid agonist-antagonist, continued administration of buprenorphine can block the μ-mediated analgesic effect of additional short-acting opioids.[156] It is of note that although nonpregnant patients receive a combination of buprenorphine and naloxone, monotherapy is prescribed during pregnancy with buprenorphine to avoid naloxone exposure by the neonate.[157] Pain control options, in addition to nonopioid analgesics, include the following[50]: (1) adding short-acting opioids with the realization that larger doses may be needed; (2) dividing the daily dose of buprenorphine into 6-hour intervals, which can take advantage of the short-term analgesic effect of buprenorphine; and (3) discontinuing buprenorphine and initiating methadone at 30 mg/day, with increasing titration in 5- to 10-mg intervals daily to alleviate withdrawal symptoms. In this way, short-acting opioids can be used for pain and methadone can be used to prevent withdrawal, with less direct antagonism at the μ-opioid receptor. This approach is best attempted with the help of an addiction specialist, because restarting the buprenorphine after the acute pain has been resolved can precipitate withdrawal if not carefully managed. In general, buprenorphine should be restarted only when patients have mild withdrawal symptoms (not before) to prevent antagonistic effects at the μ-opioid receptor.

CONCLUSION

Many physicians find themselves apprehensive about treating pain in pregnant patients. Evaluation and treatment are limited by the relative contraindication of radiography in the workup and the risks associated with pharmacologic therapy during pregnancy. Nonetheless, familiarity with common pain problems, as well as the maternal and fetal risks of pain medications, can allow the pain physician to help women achieve a more comfortable pregnancy. A single health care provider should be designated to coordinate specialist evaluations and integrate their suggestions into a single integrated plan of care.

References

1. Klingberg MA, Weatherall JA: Epidemiologic Methods for Detection of Teratogens, New York, 1990, S Karger, pp 203-211.
2. Niebyl JR: Nonanesthetic drugs during pregnancy and lactation. In Chestnut DH (ed): Obstetric Anesthesia: Principles and Practice. St. Louis, Mosby, 1994, pp 229-240.
3. Blake DA, Niebyl JR: Requirements and limitations in reproductive and teratogenic risk assessment. In Niebyl JR (ed): Drug Use in Pregnancy. Philadelphia, Lea and Febiger, 1988, pp 1-9.
4. Rice SA: Anaesthesia in pregnancy and the fetus: Toxicology aspects. In Reynolds F (ed): Effects on the baby of maternal analgesia and anaesthesia. London, WB Saunders, 1993, pp 88-89.
5. American Academy of Pediatrics Committee on Drugs: Transfer of drugs and other chemicals into human milk. Pediatrics 1989;84:924-936.
6. Berlin CM: Pharmacologic considerations of drug use in the lactating mother. Obstet Gynecol 1981;58:175-235.
7. Dailland P: Analgesia and anaesthesia and breast feeding. In Reynolds F (ed): Effects on the Baby of Maternal Analgesia and Anaesthesia. London, WB Saunders, 1993, pp 268-296.
8. Vorherr H: Drug excretion in breast milk. Postgrad Med 1974;56:97-104.
9. American Academy of Pediatrics Committee on Drugs: Transfer of drugs and other chemicals into human milk. Pediatrics 2001;108:776-789.
10. Moise KJ, Huhta JC, Sharif DS, et al: Indomethacin in the treatment of premature labor: Effects on the fetal ductus arteriosus. N Engl J Med 1988;319:327-331.
11. Leal SD, Cavalle-Garrido T, Ryan G, et al: Isolated ductal closure in utero diagnosed by fetal echocardiography. Am J Perinatol 1997;14:205-210.
12. Briggs GG, Freeman RK, Yaffe SJ: Drugs in Pregnancy and Lactation. Baltimore, Williams & Wilkins, 1990.
13. Coomarasamy A, Honest H, Papaioannou S, et al: Aspirin for prevention of preeclampsia in women with historical risk factors: A systematic review. Obstet Gynecol 2003;101:1319-1332.
14. Alano MA, Ngougmna E, Ostrea EM Jr, et al: Analysis of nonsteroidal antiinflammatory drugs in meconium and its relation to persistent pulmonary hypertension of the newborn. Pediatrics 2001;107:519-523.
15. Ostensen M, Ostensen H: Safety of nonsteroidal antiinflammatory drugs in pregnant patients with rheumatic disease. J Rheumatol 1995;23:1045-1049.
16. Slone D, Heinonen OP, Kaufman DW, et al. Aspirin and congenital malformations. Lancet 1976;1:1373-1375.
17. Stuart JJ, Gross SJ, Elrad H, et al: Effects of acetylsalicylic acid ingestion on maternal and neonatal hemostasis. N Engl J Med 1982;307:909-912.
18. Ketorolac prescribing information. Palo Alto, Cal, Syntex Laboratories, 1997.
19. Dordoni PL, Della Ventura M, Stefanelli A, et al: Effect of ketorolac, ketoprofen, and nefopam on platelet function. Anaesthesia 1994;49:1046-1049.
20. Sage DJ: Epidurals, spinals and bleeding disorders in pregnancy: A review. Anaesth Intens Care 1990;18:319-326.
21. American Society of Regional Anesthesia: Practice guidelines, 2006. Available at http://www.asra.com/Consensus Statements.
22. Levy G, Garrettson JK: Kinetics of salicylate elimination by newborn infants of mothers who ingested aspirin before delivery. Pediatrics 1974;62:201-220.
23. Skeith KJ, Wright M, Davis P: Differences in NSAID tolerability profiles. Fact or fiction? Drug Safety 1994;10:183-195.
24. Wischnik A: The excretion of ketorolac tromethamine into breast milk after multiple oral dosing. Eur J Clin Pharmacol 1989;36:521-524.
25. Paracetamol: International Agency for Research on Cancer Monogr Eval Carcinog Risks Hum 1990;50:307-332.
26. Notorianni LJ, Oldham HG: Passage of paracetamol into human milk. Br J Clin Pharmacol 1987;24:63-67.
27. MacGregor SN: Drug addiction and pregnancy. In Dilts PV, Sciarra JJ (eds): Gynecology and Obstetrics Philadelphia, JB Lippincott, 1976, pp 1-18.
28. Zelson M, Lee SJ, Casalino M: Neonatal narcotic addiction. N Engl J Med 1973;289:1216-1220.
29. Strauss ME, Andresko M, Stryker JC, et al: Methadone maintenance during pregnancy: Pregnancy, birth and neonate characteristics. Am J Obstet Gynecol 1974;120:895-900.
30. Rementeria JL, Nunaq NN: Narcotic withdrawal in pregnancy: Stillbirth incidence with a case report. Am J Obstet Gynecol 1973;116:1153-1156.
31. Rayburn WF, Bogenschutz MP: Pharmacotherapy for pregnant women with addictions. Am J Obstet Gynecol 2004;191:1885-1897.
32. Osborn DA, Jeffery HE, Cole M: Opioid treatment for opioid withdrawal in newborn infants. Cochrane Database Syst Rev.(3):2005:CD002059
33. Ostrea EM, Chavez CJ, Strauss ME: A study of factors that influence the severity of neonatal narcotic withdrawal. J Pediatr 1976;88:642-645.
34. Sharpe C, Kuschel C: Outcomes of infants born to mothers receiving methadone for pain management in pregnancy. Arch Dis Child Fetal Neonatal Ed 2004;89:F33-F36.
35. Franck LS, Gregory GA: Clinical evaluation and treatment of infant pain in the neonatal intensive care unit. In Schecter NL, Berde CB, Yaster M (eds): Pain in Infants, Children, and Adolescents. Baltimore, Williams & Wilkins, 1993, pp 527-528.
36. Finnegan LP, Connaughton JF, Kron RE, et al: Neonatal abstinence syndrome: Assessment and management. Addict Dis 1975;2:141-158.
37. Levy M, Spino M: Neonatal withdrawal syndrome: Associated drugs and pharmacologic management, Pharmacotherapy 1993;13:202-211.
38. Chasnoff IJ: Effects of maternal narcotic versus nonnarcotic addiction on neonatal neurobehaviour and infant development. In Pinkert TM (ed): Consequences of Maternal Drug Abuse. Washington DC, National Institute on Drug Abuse, 1985, pp 84-85.
39. Carrie LES, O'Sullivan CM, Seegobin R: Epidural fentanyl in labour. Anaesthesia 1981;36:965-969.
40. Rayburn W, Rathke A, Leuschen MP, et al: Fentanyl citrate analgesia during labor. Am J Obstet Gynecol 1989;161:202-206.
41. Hagmeyer KO, Mauro LS, Mauro VF: Meperidine-related seizures associated with patient-controlled analgesia pumps. Ann Pharmacother 1993;27:29-32.
42. Tang R, Shimomura S, Rotblatt M: Meperidine-induced seizures in sickle-cell patients. Hosp Formulary 1980;76:764-772.
43. Frank M, McAteer EJ, Cattermole R, et al: Nalbuphine for obstetric analgesia. Anaesthesia 1987;42:697-703.
44. Sgro C, Escousse A, Tennebaum D, et al: Perinatal adverse effects of nalbuphine. Lancet 1990;336:1070-1076.
45. Scanlon JW: Pentazocine and neonatal withdrawal symptoms [letter]. J Pediatr 1974;85:735-736.
46. Feinstein SJ, Lediero, JG, Vintzileos AM, et al: Sinusoidal fetal heart rate pattern after administration of nalbuphine. Am J Obstet Gynecol 1986;154:159-160.
47. Claahsen-van der Grinten HL, Verbruggen I, van den Berg PP, et al: Different pharmacokinetics of tramadol in mothers treated for labour pain and in their neonates. Eur J Clin Pharmacol 2005;61:523-529.
48. Eisenach JC, Grice SC, Dewan DW: Patient-controlled analgesia following cesarean delivery: A comparison with epidural and intramuscular narcotics, Anesthesiology 1988;68:444-448.
49. Johnson RE, Fudala PJ, Payne R: Buprenorphine: Considerations for pain management. J Pain Symptom Manage 2005;29:297-326.
50. Alford DP, Compton P, Samet JH: Acute pain management for patients receiving maintenance methadone or buprenorphine therapy. Ann Intern Med. 2006;144:127-134.

51. Findlay JWA, DeAngelis RL, Kearney MF, et al: Analgesic drugs in breast milk and plasma. Clin Pharmacol Ther 1981;29:625-633.
52. Wittels B, Scott DT, Sinatra RS: Exogenous opioids in human breast milk and acute neonatal neurobehaviour: A preliminary study. Anesthesiology 1990;73:864-869.
53. O'Donoghue SEF: Distribution of pethidine and chlorpromazine in maternal, fetal and neonatal biologic fluids. Nature 1971;229:124-125.
54. Kuhnert BR, Kuhnert PA, Philipson EH, et al: Disposition of meperidine and normeperidine following multiple doses in labor. Am J Obstet Gynecol 1985;151:410-415.
55. Marque P, Chevrel J, Lavignasse P, et al: Buprenorphine withdrawal syndrome in a newborn. Clin Pharmacol Ther 1997;62:569-571.
56. Fujinaga M, Mazze RI: Reproductive and teratogenic effects of lidocaine in Sprague-Dawley rats, Anesthesiology 1986;65:626-632.
57. Zeisler JA, Gardner TD, DeMesquita SA: Lidocaine excretion in breast milk. Drug Intell Clin Pharm 1986;20:691-693.
58. United States Pharmacopeial Convention: Drug Information for the Health Care Professional, 12th ed. Rockville, Md, United States Pharmacopeia Dispensing Information, 1992.
59. Lewis AM, Johnston A, Patel L, et al: Mexilitene in human blood and breast milk. Postgrad Med J 1981;57:546-547.
60. Katz FH, Duncan BR: Entry of prednisone into human milk. N Engl J Med 1975;293:1154-1158.
61. Dellemijn PLI, Fields H: Do benzodiazepines have a role in chronic pain management? Pain 1994;57:137-152.
62. Safra MJ, Oakley GP Jr: Association between cleft lip with and without cleft palate and prenatal exposure to diazepam. Lancet 1975;2:47-80.
63. Laegreid L, Olegard R, Wahlstrom J, et al: Abnormalities in children exposed to benzodiazepines in utero. Lancet 1987;1:108-109.
64. Rosenberg L, Mitchell AA, Parsells JA, et al: Lack of relation of oral clefts to diazepam use during pregnancy. N Engl J Med 1983;309:1282-1285.
65. Scanlon JW: Effects of benzodiazepines on the neonate. N Engl J Med 1975;292:649-650.
66. Milkovich L, Van den Berg BJ: Effects of prenatal meprobamate and chlodiazepoxide on human embryogenic and fetal development. N Engl J Med 1974;291:1268-1271.
67. Rothman KJ, Flyer DC: Exogenous hormones and other drug exposures in children with congenital heart disease. Am J Epidemiol 1979;109:433-439.
68. Bergman U, Rosa F, Baum C: Effects of exposure to benzodiazepines during fetal life. Lancet 1992;340:694-696.
69. Laegreid L, Olegard R: Teratogenic effects of benzodiazepine use during pregnancy. J Pediatr 1989;114:126-131.
70. Athinarayanan P, Pierog SH, Nigm SK, et al: Chlordiazepoxide withdrawal in the neonate. Am J Obstet Gynecol 1976;124:212-213.
71. Erkolla R, Kanto J: Diazepam and breast feeding. Lancet 1972;1:1235-1236.
72. Williams M, Wooltorton E: Paroxetine (Paxil) and congenital malformations. CMAJ 2005;173:1320-1321.
73. Moses-Kolko EL, Bogen D, Perel J, et al: Neonatal signs after late in utero exposure to serotonin reuptake inhibitors: Literature review and implications for clinical applications. JAMA. 2005;293:2372-2383.
74. Chambers CD, Hernandez-Diaz S, Van Marter LJ, et al: Selective serotonin-reuptake inhibitors and risk of persistent pulmonary hypertension of the newborn. N Eng J Med 2006;354:579-587.
75. Hainline B: Neurologic complications of pregnancy: Headache. Neurol Clin 1994;12:443-460.
76. Shepard TH: Catalog of Teratogenic Agents. Baltimore, Johns Hopkins University Press, 1989, pp 345.
77. Wisner KL, Perel JM, Findling RL: Antidepressant treatment during breast-feeding. Am J Psychiatry 1996;153:1132-1137.
78. Lester BM, Cucca J, Andreozzi L, et al: Possible association between fluoxetine hydrochloride and colic in an infant. J Am Acad Chil Adolesc Psychiatry 1993;32:1253-1255.
79. Matheson I, Pande H, Alertsen AR: Respiratory depression caused by N-desmethyldoxepin in breast milk [letter]. Lancet 1985;2:1124.
80. Spiedel BD, Meadow SR: Maternal epilepsy and abnormalities of the fetus and newborn. Lancet 1972;2:839-843.
81. Yerby MS: Pregnancy, teratogenesis, and epilepsy. Neurol Clin 1994;12:749-771.
82. Strickler SM, Miller MA, Andermann E: Genetic predisposition to phenytoin-induced birth defects. Lancet 1985; 2:746-749.
83. Buehler BA, Delimont D, Van Waes M, et al: Prenatal prediction of the risk of the fetal hydantoin syndrome. N Engl J Med 1990;322:1567-1572.
84. Gabapentin prescribing information. New York, Pfizer, 1996.
85. Del Pozo E, Brun Del Re R, Hindselmann M: Lack of effects of methergonavine on postpartum breast lactation. Am J Obstet Gynecol 1975;123:845-846.
86. Van Den Berg BJ: Epidemiologic observations of prematurity: Effects of tobacco, coffee, and alcohol. In Reed DM, Stanley FJ (ed): The Epidemiology of Prematurity, Baltimore, Urban and Schwarzenberg, 1977, pp 157-176.
87. Martin TR, Bracken MB: The association between low birth weight and caffeine consumption during pregnancy. Am J Epidemiol 1987;126:813-821.
88. Beaulac-Baillargeon L, Desrosiers C: Caffeine-cigarette interaction on fetal growth. Am J Obstet Gynecol 1987; 157:1236-1240.
89. Miller RC, Watson WJ, Hackney AC, Seeds JW: Acute maternal and fetal cardiovascular effects of caffeine ingestion. Am J Perinatol 1994;11:132-136.
90. Hadeed A, Siegel S: Newborn cardiac arrhythmias associated with maternal caffeine use during pregnancy, Clin Pediatr 1993;32:45-47.
91. Findlay JWA, Deangelis RL, Kearney MF, et al: Analgesic drugs in breast milk and plasma. Clin Pharmacol Ther 1981;29:625-633.
92. Ezaki H, Utusumi M, Tokado H: Reproductive study on sumatriptan succinate in rats by oral route. Yakuri Chiryo 1993;21:2071-2091.
93. Humphrey PPA, Feniuk W, Marriott AS: Pre-clinical studies on the anti-migraine drug, sumatriptan. Eur Neurol 1991;31:282-290.
94. Feniuk W, Humphrey PP, Perren MJ: GR43175 does not share the complex pharmacology of the ergots. Cephalgia 1989;9:35-39.
95. Eldridge R: Personal communication. June 1997.
96. Wojnar-Horton RE, Hackett LP, Yapp P, et al: Distribution and excretion of sumatriptan in human milk. Br J Clin Pharmacol 1996;41:217-221.
97. Pruyn SC, Phelan JP, Buchanan GC: Long-term propranolol therapy in pregnancy: Maternal and fetal outcome. Am J Obstet Gynecol 1979;135:485-489.
98. Cox JL, Gardner MJ: Treatment of cardiac arrythmias during pregnancy. Prog Cardiovasc Dis 1993;36:137-178.
99. Bauer JH, Pape B, Zajicek J, et al: Propranolol in human plasma and breast milk. Am J Cardiol 1979;63:860-862.
100. White WB, Andreoli JW, Wong SH, et al: Atenolol in human plasma and breast milk. Obstet Gynecol 1984;63:42-44.
101. Chamberlain G: ABC of antenatal care: Abdominal pain in pregnancy. Br Med J 1991;302:1390-1394.
102. Heckma JD, Sassard R: Musculoskeletal considerations in pregnancy. J Bone Joint Surg 1994;76A: 1720-1730.
103. Hungerford DS, Lennox DW: The importance of increased interosseous pressure in the development of osteonecrosis of the femoral head: Implications for treatment. Orthop Clin North Am 1985;16:635-654.
104. Bruinsma BJ, LaBan MM: The ghost joint: Transient osteoporosis of the hip. Arch Phys Med Rehabil 1990;71:295-298.
105. Ostgaard HC, Zetherstrom G, Roos-Hansson E, Svanberg B: Reduction of back and posterior pelvic pain in pregnancy. Spine 1994;19:894-900.
106. Mantle MJ, Holmes J, Currey HLF: Backache in pregnancy II: Prophylactic influence of back care classes. Rheum Rehabil 1981;20:227-232.

107. Fast A, Shapiro D, Ducommun EJ, et al: Low back pain in pregnancy. Spine 1987;12:368-371.

108. Ostgaard HC, Andersson GBJ, Karlsson K: Prevalence of back pain in pregnancy. Spine 1991;16:549-552.

109. MacEvilly M, Buggy D: Back pain and pregnancy: A review. Pain 1996;64:405-414.

110. Daly JM, Frame PS, Rapoza PA: Sacroiliac subluxation: A common, treatable cause of low back pain in pregnancy. Fam Pract Res J 1991;11:149-159.

111. LaBan MM, Perrin JCS, Latimer FR: Pregnancy and the herniated lumbar disc. Arch Phys Med Rehabil 1983;64:319-321.

112. Weinreb JC, Wolbarsht LB, Cohen JM, et al: Prevalence of lumbosacral intervertebral disc abnormalities in MR images of pregnant and asymptomatic nonpregnant women. Radiology 1989;170:125-128.

113. Rungee JL: Low back pain during pregnancy. Orthopedics 1993;16:1339-1344.

114. Iams JD, Stilson R, Mohnson RF, et al: Symptoms that precede preterm labor and preterm premature rupture of the membranes. Am J Obstet Gynecol 1990;62:486-490.

115. Katz M, Goodyear K, Creasy RK: Early signs and symptoms of preterm labor. Am J Obstet Gynecol 1990;162:1150-1153.

116. Roy C, Sussine C, LeBras Y, et al: Assessment of painful ureterohydronephrosis during pregnancy by MR urography. Eur Radiol 1996l6:334-338.

117. Waltzer WC: The urinary tract in pregnancy. J Urology 1981;125:271-276.

118. Little JB: Biologic effects of low-level radiation exposure. In Taveras JM (ed): Radiology: Diagnosis, Imaging, Intervention. Philadelphia, JB Lippincott, 1994, pp 3-6.

119. Schwartz RB: Neurodiagnostic imaging of the pregnant patient. In Devinsky O, Feldmann E, Mainline B (eds): Neurological Complications of Pregnancy. New York, Raven Press, 1994, pp 243-248.

120. Mattison DR, Angtuaco T, Miller FC, Quick GJ: Magnetic resonance imaging in maternal and fetal medicine. J Perinatol 1989;9:411-419.

121. Kanal E: Pregnancy and the safety of magnetic resonance imaging. Magn Reson Imaging Clin North Am 1994;2:309-317.

122. Wilbourn AJ, Aminoff MJ: Electrodiagnosis. In Rothman RH, Simeone FA (eds): The Spine. Philadelphia, WB Saunders, 1992, pp 163-171.

123. Wolfe LA, Hall P, Goodman L, et al: Prescription of aerobic exercise during pregnancy. Sports Med 1989;8:273-301.

124. Berg G, Hammar M, Moller-Nielsen J, et al: Low back pain during pregnancy. Obstet Gynecol 1988;71:71-75.

125 American College of Obstetricians and Gynecologists: Planning for Pregnancy, Birth and Beyond. New York, Dutton, 1996, pp 92-95.

126. Gleeson PB, Pauls JA: Obstetrical physical therapy. Phys Therapy 1988;68:1699-1702.

127. Pauls JA: Therapeutic Approaches to Women's Health: A Program of Exercise and Education. Gaithersburg, Md, Aspen, 1995.

128. Robinson AJ: Transcutaneous electrical nerve stimulation for control of pain in musculoskeletal disorders. J Orthop Sports Phys Ther 1996;24:208-227.

129. Reeve J, Menon D, Corabian P: Transcutaneous electrical nerve stimulation. TENS: A technology assessment. J Technol Assess Health Care 1996;12:299-324.

130. Evans AT, Samuels SN, Marshall C, et al: Suppression of pregnancy-induced nausea and vomiting with sensory afferent stimulation. J Reprod Med 1993;38:603-606.

131. Thomas IL, Nicklin J, Pollock H, et al: Evaluation of a maternity cushion (Ozzlo Pillow) for backache and insomnia in late pregnancy. Aust N Z J Obstet Gynaecol 1989;29:133-138.

132. Koes BW, Scholten RJPM, Mens JMA, et al: Efficacy of epidural steroid injections for low back pain and sciatica: A systematic review of randomized clinical trials. 1995; Pain 63:279-288.

133. Benzon HT: Epidural steroid injections for low back pain and lumbosacral radiculopathy. Pain 1986;24:277-295.

134. Rasmussen BK, Rigmor J, Schroll M: Epidemiology of headache in a general population: A prevalence study. J Clin Epidemiol 1991;44:1147-1157.

135. Sommerville BW: The role of estradiol withdrawal in the etiology of menstrual migraine. Neurology 1972;22:355-365.

136. Chanceller MD, Wroe SJ: Migraine occuring for the first time during pregnancy. Headache 1990;30:224-227.

137. Levine SR, Brust CJM, Futrell M, et al: Cerebrovascular complications of the use of the crack form of alkaloidal cocaine. N Engl J Med 1990;323:699-704.

138. Donaldson JO: Thrombophillic coagulopathies and pregnancy-associated cerebrovascular disease. Current Obstet Gynaecol 1991;1:186-192.

139. Marcus DA, Scharff L, Turk D: Nonpharmacological management of headaches during pregnancy. Psychosom Med 1995;7:527-535.

140. Silverstein SD: Headaches and women: Treatment of the pregnant and lactating migraineur. Headache 1993;33:533-540.

141. Powars DR, Sandhu M, Niland-Weiss J, et al: Pregnancy in sickle cell disease. Obstet Gynecol 1986;67:217-228.

142. Smith JA, Espeland M, Bellevue R, et al: Pregnancy in sickle cell disease: Experience of the cooperative study of sickle cell disease. Obstet Gynecol 1996;87:199-204.

143. Shapiro BS: The management of pain in sickle cell disease. Pediatr Clin North Am 1989;36:1029-1045.

144. Martin JN, Martin RW, Morrison JC: Acute management of sickle cell crisis in pregnancy. Clin Perinatol 1986;13:853-868.

145. Wayne AS, Kevy SV, Nathan DG: Transfusion management of sickle cell disease. Blood 1993;81:1109-1123.

146. Howard RJ, Tuck SM, Pearson TC: Pregnancy in sickle cell disease in the UK: Results of a multicentre survey of the effect of prophylactic blood transfusion on maternal and fetal outcome. Br J Obstet Gynaecol 1995;102:947-951.

147. Cozzi L, Tyron WW, Sedlaceck K: The effectiveness of biofeedback-assisted relaxation in modifying sickle cell crisis. Biofeedback Self Regul 1987;12:51-61.

148. Alcorn R, Bowser B, Henley EJ, et al: Fluidotherapy and exercise in the management of sickle cell anemia. Phys Ther 1984;64:1520-1522.

149. Wang WC, George SL, Wilimas JA: Transcutaneous nerve stimulation treatment of sickle cell pain. Acta Haematol 1988;80:99-102.

150. Chamberlain G: Medical problems in pregnancy, II. BMJ 1991;302:1327-30.

151. Weisman SJ, Schechter NL: Sickle cell anemia: Pain management. In Sinatra RS, Hord AH, Ginsberg B, et al (eds): Acute Pain: Mechanisms and Management. St. Louis, Mosby Year Book, 1992, pp 508-516.

152. Finer P, Blair J, Rowe P: Epidural analgesia in the management of labor pain and sickle cell crisis: A case report. Anesthesiology 1988;68:799-800.

153. Cassidy B, Cyna AM: Challenges that opioid-dependent women present to the obstetric anaesthetist. Anaesth Intens Care 2004;32:494-501.

154. Dovertya M, Whitea JM, Somogyia AA, et al: Hyperalgesic responses in methadone maintenance patients. Pain 2001;90:91-96.

155. Vanderah T, Gardell LR, Burgess SE, et al: Dynorphin promotes abnormal pain and spinal opioid antinociceptive tolerance. J Neurosci 2000;20:7074-7079.

156. Fudala PJ, Bridge P, Herbert S, et al: Office-based treatment of opioid addiction with a sublingual-tablet formulation of buprenorphine and naloxone. N Engl J Med 2003;349:949-958.

157. U.S. Department of Health and Human Services: Clinical Guidelines for the Use of Buprenorphine in the Treatment of Opioid Addiction (Publ. No. 04-3939, Treatment Improvement Protocol 40). Rockville, Md, U.S. Department of Health and Human Services, 2004, pp 67-69.

CHAPTER

30 Pain in Selected Neurologic Disorders

Randall P. Brewer

Chronic pain is an accompaniment of many neurologic disorders. Although chronic pain may be the defining feature in certain neurologic disorders, neurologists and primary care practitioners often focus primarily on treatments aimed to address the primary neurologic condition (disease-based treatments). Thus, it is important for the pain specialist to acquire a pathophysiologic understanding of the specifics of the pain that accompanies these conditions and embark on treatment strategies to complement disease-based treatments and improve the quality of life in affected individuals. Common neuropathic pain disorders will be given specific attention in the chapter on neuropathic pain syndromes (see Chapter 21), which includes discussions of complex regional pain syndrome, postherpetic neuralgia, and diabetic peripheral neuropathy. Another neuropathic pain syndrome, phantom pain, is specifically addressed in Chapter 22. The neuroanatomic basis and pathophysiology underlying the pain associated with these disorders have been detailed in Chapters 7 through 9.

The symptoms of pain accompanying neurologic disorders are remarkably similar, despite the varied causes of neurologic conditions. The details of advanced therapeutic strategies will be covered in the chapters describing classes of pharmacologic and interventional management techniques. The discussion here will focus on the prevalence, symptoms, and characteristics of a selection of neurologic disorders characterized by or having symptomatic pain as a dominant feature during the course of the illness. Although it is not possible to include every disorder in which pain is a feature, this chapter includes those that the pain specialist is likely to encounter at some frequency during the course of his or her practice in the management of chronic pain. Because of the success that leaders in the field of pain medicine have achieved in the recognition of pain, information regarding the pain associated with each disorder discussed in this chapter may be worthy of a more detailed dissertation (see the reference list for detailed reviews in the literature of each disorder, when available).

Pain associated with neurologic disorders may be broadly characterized as occurring in two basic forms:

(1) neuropathic pain resulting from a pathologic entity or lesion(s) within the central or peripheral nervous system; and (2) pain occurring as a secondary feature of the neurologic disorder as a result of nervous system dysfunction. The former category is widely accepted as neuropathic pain, as defined by the International Association for the Study of Pain in 1994.[1] Lesions associated with the development of chronic neuropathic pain typically involve damage or dysfunction along the small-fiber peripheral nervous system, spinothalamic pathways within the spinal cord, medial lemniscus and trigeminal pathways in the brainstem, and thalamocortical pathways to the parietal cerebral cortex of the brain. Thus, the location of the neuropathic pain in a given disorder typically follows the neuroanatomic substrate as defined by the location of the lesion(s) affected by the condition. The pain complaints are characterized by numerous pain descriptors, such as burning, shooting, stabbing, aching, and shocklike, with accompanying sensory phenomena such as numbness and tingling. The pain accompanying these disorders is often a combination of constant and intermittent pain experiences. Additionally, the pain typically has components of stimulus-dependent and stimulus-independent pains. As defined in Chapter 21, stimulus-dependent phenomena include allodynia, hyperalgesia, and hyperpathia. Attention to the dominant pain description, type, and nature of evoked (stimulus-dependent) pain subtypes allows the clinician to adjust treatment strategies accordingly.

Secondary pain syndromes that arise from nervous system dysfunction may include components of neuropathic or nociceptive pain. Examples of secondary pain syndromes include myofascial pains secondary to spasticity, muscle cramps, and regional myofascial dysfunction. Musculoskeletal pain may stem from bone and joint disorders precipitated or aggravated by paralysis, falls, generalized immobility, and spasticity. Immobility predisposes to decubitus ulcers, disordered intestinal motility, osteoporosis (vertebral compression fractures), and focal peripheral nerve entrapments. During the clinical evaluation of the neurologic patient with chronic pain, it is important

Table 30–1. Pain Syndromes in Neurologic Disorders

PRIMARY DISORDER	PAIN LOCATION(S)	PAIN DESCRIPTORS	EXAMPLES OF SECONDARY PAIN TYPES
Peripheral neuropathy	Stocking-glove	Burning, tingling, stabbing, dysesthesias	Ischemia (diabetes, vasculitis), musculoskeletal, visceral (autonomic neuropathy)
Spinal cord disorders	Radicular, transitional zone pain, deafferentation pain	Constant burning, tingling, aching, evoked shooting pain	Decubitus ulcers, musculoskeletal (spine, osteoporosis), spasticity-related, visceral (dysautonomia), secondary neuropathic
Brain and brainstem lesions	Contralateral extremities, ipsilateral face (brainstem)	Aching, burning, dysesthesias, sharp	Musculoskeletal (frozen shoulder), decubitus ulcers, spasticity-related secondary neuropathic
Basal ganglia disorders	Trunk, extremities	Aching, squeezing, gnawing	Musculoskeletal, secondary neuropathic

Table 30–2. Painful Peripheral Neuropathies

CLASSIFICATION BY CAUSE	EXAMPLES
Metabolic disorders	Diabetes mellitus, vitamin deficiency (thiamine, vitamin B_{12}), uremia
Toxins	Ethanol, heavy metals (arsenic, lead), industrial solvents
Drug-induced	Chemotherapy, isoniazid, antiretroviral therapy
Trauma	Complex regional pain syndrome type II, neuromas, postamputation pain, peripheral nerve trauma
Entrapments	Peroneal, ulnar, median (carpal tunnel syndrome), posterior tibial (tarsal tunnel syndrome)
Autoimmune	Connective tissue disorders, vasculitis, paraneoplastic disorders, Guillain-Barré syndrome, chronic inflammatory demyelinating polyneuropathy
Infectious	Lyme disease, spirochetal infection, herpes zoster, cytomegalovirus infection
Hereditary	Familial amyloid polyneuropathy, Fabry's disease

to distinguish pain that is a direct result of the neurologic disorder from pain that may be secondary to the accompanying disability or primary disease process. Prevention and treatment of secondary sources of pain requires constant diligence and periodic reassessment by the treating pain specialist. Table 30–1 summarizes the types of pain syndromes common in neurologic disorders.

PERIPHERAL NERVOUS SYSTEM DISORDERS

The peripheral nervous system is comprised of motor and sensory axons of the anterior horn cells (motor fibers) and dorsal root ganglia (sensory fibers), peripheral autonomic ganglia and their axons, and peripheral ganglia of the gastrointestinal tract. Pain is frequently a dominant symptom in the course of the development of peripheral nervous system disorders, especially those that affect the "small fibers" of the sensory peripheral nervous system. These fiber types (A-delta and C fibers) are characterized by slower axonal conduction and conveyance of the sensory modalities of pain, warmth, and cold. Injuries to spinal nerve roots, dorsal root ganglia, and peripheral nerves are characterized by sensory and motor dysfunction according to the site(s) of pathologic involvement. The symptoms of peripheral nervous systems disorders are thus characterized by neuropathic pain described as numbness, tingling, and shooting or stabbing pain. Of the most common peripheral nervous system disorders, pain from peripheral neuropathies is commonly encountered in the clinical practice of pain medicine. The most common peripheral neuropathy, diabetic peripheral neuropathy, is delineated in Chapter 21. Table 30–2 includes a general classification of painful neuropathies; a few specific examples are discussed in the following sections.

Autoimmune Peripheral Nervous System Disorders

Autoimmune peripheral nervous system disorders include the neuropathies caused by connective tissue diseases, systemic vasculitis, and autoimmune disorders of peripheral myelin. Neuropathic pain may precede the diagnosis of systemic or focal vasculitis or occur during the course of established disease. When neuropathy precedes the diagnosis of vasculitis, the absence of more severe systemic symptoms may delay the diagnosis.[2] Inflammation leading to ischemia of focal peripheral nerves may lead to the clinical syndrome of mononeuropathy multiplex. This syndrome is characterized by pain, numbness, and weakness in the distribution of multiple peripheral nerves. The peripheral nerves most commonly affected include the ulnar nerves, median nerves, and the peroneal nerves. Dysfunction in the territories of these nerves typically will occur at sites of peripheral nerve entrapment and at sites distal from locations usually associated with peripheral entrapments. A distal symmetrical polyneuropathy may also occur in the setting of vasculitis and connective tissue disease. This syndrome is characterized by numbness, tingling and pain in a characteristic symmetric stocking-glove distribution. Symptoms typically begin in the feet, with burning, aching and dysesthesias. Not uncommonly, asymmetry of the progression of the neuropathy leads to the consideration of autoimmune vasculitis and may assist in the clinical diagnosis.

Acute inflammatory demyelinating polyneuropathy, known as Guillain-Barré syndrome, occurs at an annual incidence of approximately 1 per 100,000.[3] Paresthesias or dysesthesias typically precede the development of weakness, which proceeds in an ascending pattern. Contemporary treatment strategies have limited the disability associated with the disorder, but a small proportion of patients may have resulting disability and chronic pain. During the acute phase of the illness, pain is often a prominent symptom. A review of pain in the Guillain-Barré syndrome has highlighted the importance of recognizing the primary components of pain and secondary pain syndromes.[4] Deep aching, throbbing pain in the low back associated with radiation into the lower extremities is typically the most excruciating and disabling pain during the acute episode. A positive straight leg raise may accompany the acute pain. Accompanying the low back and radicular pain, myofascial pain may coincide with the development of muscle spasm, cramping, and muscular tenderness. Stabbing, shocklike or electric pain may be present in the extremities and face. Ectopic impulses caused by acute nerve root inflammation may be the pathologic mechanism associated with the acute neuropathic pain component in Guillain-Barré syndrome. Chronic neuropathic pain may actually persist beyond treatment and recovery of the paralytic disorder in a small proportion of patients.[4] Finally, the autonomic nervous system dysfunction present in Guillain-Barré syndrome may lead to the development of visceral pain secondary to ileus and urinary retention, headaches, and cardiovascular instability.

The treatment of primary neuropathic pain in the Guillain-Barré syndrome includes the use of antineuropathic agents in addition to the immune-based therapy of the primary disease. Antineuropathic agents commonly used include tricyclic antidepressants, anticonvulsants, and opioids (oral and parenteral, when necessary). In severe cases, epidural local anesthetics or opioids may be of benefit in the acute stage. Treatments beneficial for secondary pain syndromes include muscle relaxants (e.g., baclofen, tizanidine) for acute myofascial pain and supportive measures for the acute dysautonomia (e.g., intravenous fluid administration, stool softeners, urinary drainage).

Human Immunodeficiency Virus–Related Neuropathies

Nervous system complications of human immunodeficiency virus (HIV) type 1 infection have been reviewed by Price.[5] Peripheral neuropathic pain is recognized as a common accompaniment to HIV infection. Neuropathic pain may complicate any stage of the infection, resulting in disordered sleep and ambulation, disability, and psychosocial distress. Whereas symptomatic neuropathic pain is estimated

to occur at a prevalence of 10% to 15%, pathologic evidence of peripheral nerve degeneration is universally present following death from HIV infection.[6] The peripheral neuropathic pain syndromes characteristic of HIV infection are summarized in Table 30–3.

During the acute course of seroconversion, acute inflammatory demyelinating polyneuropathy may present with numbness, weakness, and peripheral neuropathic pain. The disorder may be the initial manifestation of HIV seroconversion. The course may present similar to that of Guillain-Barré syndrome, although with a higher incidence of more severe weakness, atrophy, and profound sensory loss. The treatment of moderate to severe cases uses the standard strategies for the treatment of Guillain-Barré syndrome (e.g., immunotherapy, antineuropathic agents, epidural infusions). The acute polyneuropathy associated with seroconversion typically resolves with mild, if any, residual sequelae of neuropathic pain. The chronic form of the disorder, chronic inflammatory polyneuropathy, manifests in the intermediate to late stages of the disease. It manifests as neuropathic pain associated with more severe sensory loss, weakness, and gait disturbance.

With the advent of successful antiretroviral therapy, long-term survival rates for those with HIV infection have increased and, as a result, there has been an associated increase in the incidence of chronic neuropathic pain attributable to the treated disease as well as the treatments. In addition to the neuropathies associated with primary HIV infection, antiretroviral agents may be neurotoxic. In particular, the dideoxynucleoside family of nucleoside analogue reverse transcriptase inhibitors have been shown to have specific peripheral neurotoxic effects.[7] Antiretroviral induced neuropathies are manifested by distal dysesthesias, burning, tingling, and shooting pains. Allodynia may be experienced during ambulation and can be debilitating. Difficulty with sleep is a common accompaniment secondary to allodynia and spontaneous dysesthesias.

Table 30–3. Peripheral Nervous System Pain in Human Immunodeficiency Virus (HIV) Infection

STAGE OF DISEASE	PAIN SYNDROME
Early	Acute inflammatory demyelinating polyneuropathy
Intermediate	Antiretroviral neurotoxicity
	Chronic inflammatory demyelinating polyneuropathy
	Autoimmune vasculitic mononeuropathy multiplex
	HIV-induced sensory axonal polyneuropathy
Late	Antiretroviral neurotoxicity
	HIV-induced sensory axonal polyneuropathy
	Cytomegalovirus polyradiculopathy
	Cytomegalovirus mononeuropathy multiplex
	Neurosyphilis

A distal symmetric HIV-induced sensory axonal polyneuropathy may occur in the intermediate or late stages of infection. The polyneuropathy manifests as burning pain, numbness, and evoked dysesthesias beginning in the lower extremities, with variable progression to upper extremity involvement. Similar to the antiretroviral neuropathies, allodynia may impair sleep and ambulation. Another intermediate stage phenomenon, vasculitic mononeuropathy multiplex, may coexist with other peripheral nervous system symptoms of HIV infection. Symptoms of vasculitic neuropathy are similar to those that characterize the connective tissue disorders. Pain, numbness, dysesthesias, and motor symptoms are multifocal and asymmetric. These often persist, despite treatment of the primary disease.

During the course of the illness, especially if untreated or refractory to treatment, opportunistic infections may contribute to the neurologic symptoms. Cytomegalovirus infection may give rise to a progressive polyradiculopathy or mononeuropathy multiplex, or both. The polyradiculopathy presents with the development of pelvic and lower extremity radicular pain and urinary retention and may progress to cauda equina syndrome. Rapid progression, with ascending paralysis, central nervous system involvement, and death, occurs in untreated cases.[8] Reactivation of other latent nervous system infections such as neurosyphilis, herpes simplex virus, and toxoplasmosis have been well characterized in advanced HIV, and may lead to neuropathic peripheral or central pain syndromes.

The treatment of HIV-related peripheral neuropathy and neuropathic pain follows the usual course of management of neuropathic pain syndromes in general. However, in comparison with other neuropathic syndromes, such as postherpetic neuralgia and diabetic peripheral neuropathy, the neuropathic pain associated with HIV and HIV-related neuropathies has proven difficult to treat. In particular, the antiepileptic drug, lamotrigine, has been shown to be of benefit in refractory cases.[9]

Idiopathic Sensory Polyneuropathy

A significant number of patients will exhibit symptoms of peripheral neuropathic pain in a characteristic stocking-glove distribution without a definable causative agent. The disorder is estimated to occur in approximately 25% of those 65 years of age and older and in as many as 50% of those 85 and older. In many cases, the disorder is characterized by loss of peripheral pain and temperature sensation. However, in a significant proportion of cases, complaints of burning, tingling, and symptoms of restless legs syndrome may predominate. This syndrome may be associated with difficulties with ambulation, falls, and a reduction in the quality of life.[10] It is hypothesized that age-related changes to the peripheral nervous system may contribute to the development of age-related idiopathic sensory neuropathy. As is

true for other sensory neuropathies, symptoms are typically worse at night. This may lead to disrupted sleep and failed attempts at restoring sleep, with therapy aimed toward minimizing insomnia. In most cases, the physical examination reveals evidence of loss of pain and temperature sensation distally in the lower extremities. In more severe cases, there may be loss of large fiber sensation, with deficits in vibration and joint position sense. It is imperative to exclude vitamin deficiencies, insulin resistance, and incipient diabetes mellitus in the evaluation of these patients. Therapy is aimed toward achieving restorative sleep and minimizing awakenings secondary to pain. An antineuropathic agent, such as a tricyclic antidepressant or anticonvulsant given at bedtime, represents common first-line therapy. An open-label study using topical lidocaine 5% has demonstrated improvement in symptoms over baseline, without significant adverse effects.[11]

Subacute Sensory Neuronopathy

Sensory neuronopathy is a rare disorder characterized as an autoimmune response to antigens found on cells in the dorsal root ganglia. The disorder may also result from the effects of drugs or neurotoxins (cisplatin or pyridoxine). It is characterized by ataxia and sensory loss, frequently with painful dysesthesias beginning in the lower extremities and rarely in the upper extremities, trunk, or facial region. This disorder is slowly progressive and may not improve following immunotherapy aimed at removal of paraneoplastic or autoimmune antibodies. This disorder has been most commonly associated with small cell cancer of the lung, Sjögren's syndrome, and the presence of anti-Hu antibodies. In addition to immunotherapy aimed at treatment of the primary disorder or tumor resection (if relevant), symptomatic therapy is aimed at reduction of the neuropathic pain components and prevention of a secondary pain syndrome through limb protection and ambulatory assistive devices. When the disorder is associated with toxin or drug exposure, treatment is typically limited to supportive measures and treatment of any neuropathic pain components.[12]

Tabes Dorsalis

Perhaps once the most commonly encountered chronic neuropathic pain condition, neurosyphilitic involvement of the dorsal root entry zone represents a classic neurologic pain disorder. The disorder is characterized by "lightning pains" involving the lower extremities. Similar pains may occur in the trunk, thorax, and abdomen. Tabetic pain may occur for brief periods (seconds or minutes) or last for several days. Occasionally, visceral involvement predominates, known as "visceral crises." These are characterized by attacks of epigastric or pelvic pain accompanied by nausea and vomiting. The physical examination is remarkable for loss of sensory modalities distally in the lower extremities. There may also be significant ataxia, hypotonia, and dysautonomia. The neuropathologic hallmark of tabes dorsalis is inflammatory infiltrates along the dorsal roots, with degeneration of the posterior columns. Therapy involves standard antibiotic therapy to eradicate the *Treponema pallidum* organism. Antineuropathic agents such as anticonvulsants and tricyclic antidepressants are used for symptomatic therapy. Argyll Robertson pupils (miotic pupils that are unresponsive to light but react with accommodation) are usually present. Although characteristic of the disorder, the classic finding of Charcot joints is the result of deep anesthesia caused by the disorder. Although an important secondary complication of the neurologic syndrome, once the disorder has reached the stage of profound joint hypalgesia, the protective mechanism of pain (and therefore the need for aggressive therapy) has been severely attenuated.

PAIN ASSOCIATED WITH SPINAL DISORDERS

Disorders of the spinal cord are commonly associated with pain. The causes and locations of the spinal cord disorders typically determine the need for surgical or medical management of the primary condition. Pain may be a prominent element in the presentation of certain spinal cord disorders (e.g., acute spinal cord injury) or occur as a late effect of the disease or therapy (e.g., radiation treatment, tumor resection). The characteristics of the pain experience, variable presentations, and secondary pain generators are common to all disorders of the spinal cord. In an effort to highlight the aspects of the pain associated with disorders of the spinal cord, a few selected examples are discussed in the following sections. Table 30–4 summarizes the pain syndromes associated with spinal cord disorders.

Spinal Cord Injury

New cases of traumatic spinal cord injury are estimated to number approximately 11,000 new cases/

Table 30–4. Pain in Spinal Cord Disorders

TYPE OF PAIN	SYNDROME
Neuropathic	Transitional ("end zone") pain
	Deafferentation pain
	Radicular pain
	Cauda equina
	Syringomyelia (may include facial pain)
	Peripheral entrapments (ulnar, peroneal, median)
Nociceptive	Traumatic spinal instability
	Spondylotic arthropathy (facet syndrome)
	Osteoporosis (compression fractures), aseptic necrosis
	Musculoskeletal overuse (rotator cuff syndrome, joint pain), pressure sores, decubitus ulcers
Visceral	Autonomic dysreflexia, bladder atony, intestinal inertia

year.[13] Longitudinal studies of patients with spinal cord injury have noted that 23% of persons with spinal cord injury report pain at 6 weeks; the proportion of patients with pain increases to 41% the year following the injury.[14] Following the acute injury, pain is commonly located at the site of spinal trauma. During the weeks to months in recovery, several patterns of pain may emerge. The pattern of pain is somewhat dependent on the extent of spinal cord injury, as well as details regarding any concomitant nerve root injuries that may have occurred as a result of the initial injury. Typically, patients with partial spinal cord lesions associated with moderate or mild neurologic deficits may have severe, debilitating neuropathic pain as major sequelae. Plexus and nerve root avulsions associated with the initial injury often give rise to a distinct focus of neuropathic pain, which must be independently assessed and treated.

The most dominant pain type following spinal cord injury is that of central neuropathic pain. The neuropathic pain emanates from the area of injury and extends variably into areas of sensory loss. The pain may be more intense from the transition of complete sensory loss to normal sensation. This is known as "end zone pain" or "transitional pain" and may be associated with severe allodynia, hyperalgesia, and spontaneous attacks of intense lancinating pain. Commonly, the pain follows a single or multiple root distributions. In the areas with sensory loss, there may be deafferentation pain characterized by constant burning and aching. With lesions above the midthoracic level, the presence of pain caused by spasticity in the upper or lower extremities may predominate. Intense muscular spasms, jerks, and hypertonicity will commonly be associated with neuropathic pain complaints. Usually, the patient may have numerous musculoskeletal regions of ongoing pain, which may be the result of the initial traumatic episode or aggravated by chronic disability.

The pain associated with spinal cord injury impairs the quality of life in these individuals. It is significantly associated with disordered sleep, exercise, work, and activities of daily living. It may impair the patient's ability to engage in social, recreational, and self-care activities. The treatment of pain following spinal cord injury tends to be directed toward the type of pain experience and the tolerability of the agent relative to the patient's confounding medical history. Antineuropathic drugs such as gabapentin and other antiepileptics, tricyclic antidepressants, and topical local anesthetics may be of assistance in amelioration of the symptoms of neuropathic pain. Pain related to spasticity and myofascial pain is usually treated with oral muscle relaxants such as baclofen. In patients intolerant or resistant to oral baclofen, intrathecal baclofen has been proven efficacious in the control of chronic lower extremity spasticity. Musculoskeletal pain associated with the initial trauma, or emerging disorders, may respond to local anesthetic or corticosteroid injections, nonsteroidal anti-inflammatory drugs, and opioids.

Syringomyelia

Syringomyelia involves cavitation in the central canal of the spinal cord. Syringomyelia may have a post-traumatic (especially following hematomyelia), congenital (associated with Arnold Chiari malformation), or postinfectious (associated with arachnoiditis) cause, or may be associated with intramedullary spinal cord tumors. Post-traumatic syringomyelia involves the presence of new neurologic deficits above a previous level of paraplegia or quadriplegia. Increased levels of sensory loss, spasticity, and progressive atrophy may accompany increasing levels of neuropathic pain. Dissociated sensory loss describes the loss of pain and temperature sensation resulting from involvement of the crossing of the spinothalamic second-order neurons, with sparing of dorsal column function. Worsening spasticity is attributable to increasing involvement of the descending corticospinal tracts. Atrophy and fasciculations indicate involvement of the anterior horn cell columns by the syrinx.

The pain associated with syringomyelia is generally neuropathic in nature. Patients with a cervical syrinx will present with pain and numbness along multiple cervical root distributions (arm pain and dysesthesia) and often describe burning that may be associated with significant allodynia and hyperalgesia. Pain and temperature sensory loss may be associated with unrecognized trauma. Extension of the syrinx into the upper cervical region may be associated with ipsilateral facial pain caused by the involvement of the descending trigeminal tract and nucleus. Thoracic syringomyelia will present with neuropathic pain in a trunk or abdominal distribution, dissociated distal sensory loss, spasticity, and urinary retention. Lower thoracic syringomyelia will exhibit symptoms of dysfunction of the conus medullaris, with prominent sacral neuropathic pain and urinary retention.

Treatment of syringomyelia may involve neurosurgical drainage of the syrinx or surgical resection of a spinal cord tumor (when present), or both. Syrinx drainage is primarily performed to limit neurologic progression; however, alleviation of central pain following syrinx drainage is not common.[15] Medical treatment of the central neuropathic pain associated with syringomyelia is often associated with only partial efficacy and a high frequency of treatment refractoriness. Treatment modalities include anti-convulsants, antidepressants, local anesthetics, spinal cord stimulation, and intrathecal drug administration.[16]

MULTIPLE SCLEROSIS

Multiple sclerosis is a relapsing, remitting, and chronic progressive disorder of central myelin. The disease is characterized by acute exacerbations of neurologic deficits. These exacerbations are associated with acute inflammation of central myelin. Areas of prominent involvement include the optic

---

BOX 30–1. PAIN CONDITIONS ASSOCIATED WITH MULTIPLE SCLEROSIS

Neuropathic Pain
　Acute transverse myelitis
　Acute radicular pain
　Chronic myelopathy (deafferentation pain, transitional pain, radicular pain)
　Focal peripheral neuropathies (secondary to disability)

Myofascial Pain
　Spasticity secondary to myelopathy
　Regional myofascial pain (overuse syndromes, posture and gait disorders)
　Diffuse myofascial pain (chronic fatigue, sleep deprivation)

Musculoskeletal Pain
　Overuse syndromes (wheelchair-bound patients)
　Accelerated osteoporosis because of immobility

Headaches

---

nerves, periventricular white matter, brainstem, and spinal cord. Estimates have suggested that over 50% of patients who have the chronic form of multiple sclerosis also experience chronic pain.[17] Because of the chronic nature of the disorder and the multiple sites of neurologic involvement, a multidisciplinary approach is recommended for optimizing outcomes.[18] Box 30–1 summarizes the pain conditions associated with multiple sclerosis.

Trigeminal neuralgia has a well-known association with brainstem demyelination in those with multiple sclerosis. Sharp, lancinating facial pain may occur spontaneously or may be evoked by tactile stimulation. An uncommon finding in the idiopathic disorder, trigeminal sensory loss is more common in patients with multiple sclerosis. During acute exacerbations of multiple sclerosis, patients may have significant axial spine pain or radicular pain caused by demyelination along the dorsal root entry zones. Cervical demyelination may be associated with acute neck pain and electric shock–like pain along the axial spine (Lhermitte's phenomenon). Following an acute exacerbation, patients typically may be left with a neurologic deficit that may include spasticity, ataxia, and sensory loss. Following acute transverse myelitis, patients with persistent neurologic deficits often have lingering central neuropathic pain. The pattern of the neuropathic pain is similar to that described for spinal cord injury. Elements of deafferentation pain, end zone pain, and chronic radicular pain may be present concomitantly or individually in a patient with multiple sclerosis.

The types of secondary pain experienced by patients with multiple sclerosis include chronic myofascial pain related to spasticity and sleep deprivation, chronic headaches, and musculoskeletal pain related to disability. With the increasing burden of disease, it is likely that the intensity, locations, and complexity of the pain in multiple sclerosis progress, along with the neurologic disorder. The pain has significant impact on psychosocial functioning, daily activities, mood, and sleep.[19]

The treatment of chronic pain in multiple sclerosis involves alleviation of primary neuropathic pain with a contemporary pharmacologic regimen and referral for specific immunotherapy during periods of acute exacerbation. Concomitant myofascial pain may be effectively treated with oral muscle relaxants such as baclofen and tizanidine. Intrathecal baclofen used for chronic lower extremity spasticity is recognized as an effective therapy in patients with an incomplete response to oral therapy. In ambulatory patients, a regular exercise regimen may be of benefit in alleviating diffuse myofascial pain symptoms. Concomitant sleep disorders and depression should be addressed and treated with nonpharmacologic means (e.g., sleep hygiene measures, cognitive-behavioral therapy if required) and pharmacologic modalities when appropriate.

PAIN IN NEUROMUSCULAR DISORDER

Neuromuscular disorders describe a heterogeneous group of neurologic conditions associated with diseases of the peripheral motor nerves, neuromuscular junction, muscles (muscular dystrophies, myopathies), and anterior horn cells. In a large series of patients with postpolio syndrome, a large proportion of patients (80%) reported muscular and joint pains.[20] The common feature in these conditions is the notable loss of muscular power, tone, and muscular atrophy. Syndromes with slow progression over time are characterized by disorders of ambulation, which may lead to chronic disability and incapacitation. With the progression of disease, there may be concomitant musculoskeletal pain associated with the loss of neuromuscular support of the axial spine and pelvic and shoulder girdles. As is common in other chronic pain syndromes, the pain may be associated with significant psychosocial distress and mood and sleep disorders. In patients with neuromuscular disorders, muscle and joint pains predominate. Patients with mixed peripheral nervous system disorders may also have a component of neuropathic pain. Neuropathic pain may also be incited by peripheral nerve entrapments, which may be considered to be a secondary pain disorder caused by chronic disability and loss of muscular protection over sites of neural compression.

BRAIN CENTRAL PAIN SYNDROMES

In addition to lesions of the spinal cord, lesions of the brain or brainstem may lead to neuropathic central pain. Tumors, vascular malformations, inflammatory diseases (postinfectious encephalomyelitis, meningitis abscess), intracerebral hemorrhages, and stroke may be associated with the development of chronic pain, which therefore depends chiefly on the site of the lesion in the central nervous system, not the size of the lesion nor the specific pathology. The neuroanatomic substrate for brain central neuropathic pain involves a lesion along the somatosensory pathways in the brainstem trigeminothalamic pathways, medial lemniscus, thalamus, thalamocortical projections, and somatosensory cerebral cortex. The classic and most characteristic neuropathic central pain condition is that of central poststroke pain.

Central poststroke pain is estimated to occur in approximately 10% of individuals after the first year following a stroke. Poststroke pain was characterized by Dejerine and Roussy (in 1906) following lesions of the somatosensory thalamus.[21] Poststroke pain typically coexists with a concomitant contralateral sensory deficit. The pain may emerge weeks or even months following the initial vascular event. The pain may be described as diffuse burning or aching, interspersed with episodes of spontaneous lancinating or sharp pains. Remarkably, there may be a very mild motor deficit in comparison with the significant pain and hemihypesthesia. Patients with brainstem infarctions, particularly lateral medullary infarcts (Wallenberg's syndrome), may also be affected with central neuropathic pain. Ipsilateral neuropathic facial pain may coexist with contralateral sensory deficits and central neuropathic pain.[22]

The recognition of central neuropathic pain following a lesion of the central nervous system is important to minimize the disability and quality of life disruption that may accompany a chronic, yet static, neurologic disorder. Attention to secondary pain disorders such as a frozen shoulder following stroke, decubitus ulcers, and muscular spasticity is important in the assessment of the pain. Pharmacologic management of central poststroke pain often provides incomplete or partial results. Antidepressants may be indicated for the treatment of the neuropathic pain in addition to a concomitant mood disorder. Antiepileptics and tricyclic antidepressants may be of benefit for the relief of lancinating sharp pains and constant burning pain. Centrally acting muscle relaxants such as baclofen or tizanidine are important adjuvant therapies when a concomitant pain syndrome is produced by muscular spasticity. The pharmacologic management of central poststroke pain has been recently reviewed.[23]

PAIN IN MOVEMENT DISORDERS

Movement disorders are characterized as slowly progressive disorders of the motor system that have the primary component of dysfunction in the execution of normal motor function—hence, the term *movement disorders*. Clinical symptoms of movement disorders involve abnormalities of gait, coordination, fine motor control, and muscular tone. Movement disorders may be the result of dysfunction in numerous deep brain regions known as the basal ganglia. These regions include the globus pallidus, putamen, caudate nucleus, substantia nigra, subthalamic nucleus, and motor nuclei of the thalamus. Certain movement disorders are characterized by dysfunction secondary to neuronal loss in specific brain regions, such as the loss of dopamine-producing cells in the substantia nigra in patients with idiopathic Parkinson's disease. Loss of important components of motor system control in the movement disorders may lead to secondary dysfunction in other deep brain nuclei because of the loss of specific inhibitory or facilitory neural input. The causes of movement disorders include genetic syndromes, toxin- and drug-induced disorders, post-traumatic states, and poststroke syndromes. However, the causes of most movement disorders remain elusive, but improved understanding of acquired genetic factors coupled with environmental influences has enhanced our understanding of the pathogenesis of many of the movement disorders.

Parkinson's Disease

First described by James Parkinson in 1817, Parkinson's disease is a slowly progressive movement disorder characterized by resting tremor, rigidity, and bradykinesia. The incidence of idiopathic Parkinson's disease ranges from 5 to 20 per 100,000 persons/year. It typically occurs in older individuals with a variable pattern of progression. It may progress over a decade and result in rigid immobility or assume a more indolent course of slow progressive loss of motor control over several decades. The symptoms of Parkinson's disease have been ameliorated by the advent of dopaminergic agents, which significantly improve the symptoms of bradykinesia and rigidity.

With progression of the disease, patients typically have significant motor fluctuations with "on" periods of relative ease of movement interspersed with "off" periods of rigidity, bradykinesia, and tremor. It is during the off periods when many patients with Parkinson's disease experience pain. The pain may be described as muscular tightness and cramping. Accompanying pain symptoms may also take the form of restless legs syndrome and peripheral dysesthesias. It is estimated that pain occurs in over 50% of patients with Parkinson's disease.[24] The treatment of the underlying pain involves obtaining a careful history of the motor fluctuations and accompanying sensory phenomena. Motor symptoms are best treated with dopaminergic agents, whereas the sensory manifestations may require treatment with antineuropathic agents, such as anticonvulsants or tricyclic antidepressants.[25] Secondary pain complaints may be proactively managed by symptomatic treatment of arthralgias, management of concomitant osteoarthritis, and prevention of falls.

Dystonia

Dystonia describes a heterogeneous group of movement disorders characterized by disordered control of muscle groups. It is typically related to the simultaneous contractions of agonist and antagonist muscle groups. The dystonias are classified according to the extent of neuromuscular involvement—focal, segmental, multifocal, or generalized. The causes of dystonia include several hereditary syndromes, postinfectious, post-traumatic (usually following peripheral nerve trauma), and idiopathic forms. Clinical examples of syndromes of dystonia include those characterized by abnormal posturing of the trunk (torsion dystonia) or head and neck (cervical dystonia). Pain is a prominent feature of the dystonias, occurring as a result of sustained muscle contraction (intracellular acidosis). In most cases, the treatment of dystonia includes dopaminergic agents, anticholinergic agents, muscle relaxants (e.g., baclofen), and benzodiazepines. In the focal dystonias, especially idiopathic cervical dystonia, the use of locally injected botulinum toxin has resulted in significant symptomatic benefit.[26]

References

1. Mersky H, Bogduk N: Classification of chronic pain. Seattle, IASP Press, 1994, pp 1-222.
2. Davies L, Spies JM, Pollard JD, et al: Vasculitis confined to the peripheral nerves. Brain 1996;119:1441-1448.
3. Hughes RA: Epidemiology of peripheral neuropathy. Curr Opin Neurol 1995;8:335-338.
4. Petland B, Donald SM: Pain in the Guillain-Barré syndrome: A clinical review. Pain 1994;59:159-164.
5. Price RW: Neurologic complications of HIV infections. Lancet 1996;348:445-452.
6. Verma A: Epidemiology and clinical features of HIV-1 associated neuropathies. J Periph Nerv Syst 2001;6:8-13.
7. Simpson DM: Selected peripheral neuropathies associated with human immunodeficiency virus infection and antiretroviral Therapy. J Neurovirol 2002;8(Suppl 2):33-41.
8. Anders HJ. Goebel FD: Neurologic manifestations of cytomegalovirus infection in the acquired immunodeficiency syndrome. Int J STD AIDS 1999;10:151-159.
9. Simpson DM, McArthur JC, Olney R, et al: Lamotrigine for HIV-associated painful sensory neuropathies, a placebo-controlled trial. Neurology 2003;60:1508-1514.
10. Mold JW, Vesely SK, Keyl BA, et al: The prevalence, predictors, and consequences of peripheral sensory neuropathy in older patients. J Am Board Fam Pract 2004;17:309-318.
11. Herrmann DN, Barbano RL, Hart-Gouleaus, et al: An open-label study of the lidocaine patch 5% in painful idiopathic sensory polyneuropathy. Pain Med 2005;6:379-384.
12. Kuntzer T, Antoine JC, Steck AJ: Clinical features and pathophysiological basis of sensory neuronopathies (ganglionopathies). Muscle Nerve 2004;30: 255-268.
13. Go BK, DeVivo MJ, Richards JS: The epidemiology of spinal cord injury. In Stover SL, DeLisa JA, Whiteneck GG (eds):. Spinal Cord Injury. Gaithersburg, Md, Aspen, 1995, pp 170-184.
14. Kennedy P, Frankel H, Gardner B, et al: Factors associated with acute and chronic pain following traumatic spinal cord injuries. Spinal Cord 1997;35:814-817.
15. Milhorat TH, Kotzen RM, Mu HTM, et al: Dysesthetic pain in patients with syringomyelia. Neurosurgery 1996;38:940-947.
16. Todor DR, Mu HT, Milhorat TH: Pain and syringomyelia: A review. Neurosurg Focus 2000;8:E11.
17. Kassirer MR, Osterberg DH: Pain and chronic multiple sclerosis. J Pain Sympt Manage 1987;2:95-97.
18. Crayton HJ, Rossman HS: Managing the symptoms of multiple sclerosis: A multimodal approach. Clin Ther 2006;28: 445-460.
19. Schapiro RT: Management of spasticity, pain, and paroxysmal phenomena in multiple sclerosis. Curr Neurol Neurosci Rep 2001;1:299-302.

20. Halstead LS, Rossi CD: New problems in old polio patients: Results of a survey of 539 polio survivors Orthopedics 1985;8:845-850.
21. Dejerine J, Roussy G: La syndrome thalamique. Revue Neurologique, Paris. 1906;14:521-532.
22. MacGowan DJL, Janal MN, Clark WC, et al: Central post-stroke pain in Wallenberg's lateral medullary infarction: Frequency, character and determinants in 63 Patients. Neurology 1997;49:120-125.
23. Frese A, Husstedt IW, Rangelstein EB, et al: Pharmacologic treatment of central post-stroke pain. Clin J Pain 2006;22: 252-260.
24. Goetz CG, Tanner CM, Levy M, et al: Pain in idiopathic Parkinson's disease. Mov Disord 1986,1:45-50.
25. Drake DF, Harkins S, Qutubuddin A: Pain in Parkinson's disease: Pathology to treatment, medication to deep brain stimulation. Neurorehabilitation 2005;20:335-341.
26. Bhidayasiri R, Tarsy D: Treatment of dystonia. Exp Rev Neurother 2006;6:863-886.

31 Major Opioids and Chronic Opioid Therapy

Megan H. Cortazzo and Scott M. Fishman

Derivatives from the opium plant have been described as analgesics and used for pain control since 3500 BC. It was not until 1806 that a pure opioid substance was isolated. This substance was called "morphine," named after the Greek god Morpheus.[1] Since that time, the opium plant has yielded other derivatives and synthetic analogues of morphine have been produced for medicinal use.

Despite development of many novel classes of analgesics, opioids remain the gold standard in the treatment of malignant and nonmalignant nociceptive pain. Although they have been proven to produce analgesia for a wide array of pain states, they are neither without side effects nor controversy. The goal of this chapter is to review clinically relevant aspects of selected opioids, including side effects and pharmacology, and review current consensus on rational opioid prescribing.

GENERAL CONSIDERATIONS OF OPIOID ADMINISTRATION

Opioid Receptors

Multiple systems are involved in the modulation of pain perception, including the endogenous opioid system. The natural endogenous opioids include the endogenous peptides—β-endorphins, enkephalins, and dynorphins. Since the 1973 discovery of opioid receptors in the central nervous system (CNS), the body of literature describing their function and location has grown immensely.[2,3] Opioid receptors have integral roles in the endogenous antinociceptive system and, as such, are located throughout the central and peripheral nervous system. The best described opioid receptors are labeled mu (μ), kappa (κ), and delta (δ) and are prominently located in the CNS, particularly in the dorsal horn of the spinal cord,[4] as well as on dorsal root ganglia and peripheral nerves.[5,6] The three identified opioid receptors, μ, κ, and δ, belong to a superfamily of guanine (G) protein–coupled receptors located at presynaptic and post-synaptic sites in the CNS and in peripheral tissues.[7]

The μ-opioid receptor modulates input from mechanical, chemical, and thermal stimuli at the supraspinal level. The κ receptor is similar to the μ receptor in that it influences thermal nociception but, in addition, it also modulates chemical visceral pain. The δ receptors influence mechanical and inflammatory pain.[8] An opioid agonist such as morphine binds with an opioid receptor to produce analgesia as well as undesired side effects, such as respiratory depression and constipation, largely via interaction with the μ receptor. In a study using knockout mice that lacked the μ receptor, it was found that they have no response to morphine with respect to analgesia, respiratory depression, constipation, or physical dependence.[9]

Distribution, Metabolism, and Excretion

The amount of opioid required to produce analgesia has significant interindividual variability. Factors responsible for this include opioid receptor individuality as well as variations in opioid absorption and clearance. Such individual variability requires careful titration of an opioid to the desired response. The onset, duration, and intensity of analgesia will depend on the delivery of drug to the target and on the length of time that the receptor is occupied. The number of receptors occupied and length of time that the opioid activates its target receptor depends on the perfusion, plasma concentration, pH, and permeability coefficient of the drug.[10]

The metabolic pathway for each opioid is based on molecular variables of the specific opioid. Opioids with hydroxyl groups, such as morphine and hydromorphone, undergo hepatic metabolism via uridine diphosphate glucuronosyl transferase (UGT) enzymes. UGT adds a glucuronic acid moiety, forming glucuronide metabolites (hydromorphone 3-glucuronide, morphine 6-glucuronide, and morphine 3-glucuronide.) These metabolites are then excreted through the kidney. Patients with renal impairment are particularly prone to deleterious effects from metabolite accumulation.[11]

The cytochrome P-450 (CYP) system contains two polymorphic isoforms that metabolize certain opioids. The first CYP isoform, responsible for the biotransformation of codeine, oxycodone, and hydrocodone, is 2D6. It is estimated that up to 10% of whites lack this enzyme, making them "poor metabolizers" of certain opioids and thus providing another cause of the high interindividual variability seen in patients treated with opioids.[11] The 3A4 isoform of the CYP system is involved in the biotransformation of fentanyl and methadone to their inactive forms.[12] Because there are other drugs that interact with 3A4 isoenzymes, the metabolism of methadone and fentanyl can be problematically decelerated or accelerated. For example, macrolide antibiotics inhibit the enzyme, which decreases clearance of methadone and fentanyl, whereas anticonvulsants such as phenytoin induce the activation of this enzyme system and increase methadone and fentanyl clearance.[13,14] Excretion of most opioid metabolites is via the kidneys, but some of the glucuronide conjugates are excreted in bile and methadone is primarily excreted in the feces.[11]

Administration

Multiple routes of administration is one of the many clinically useful characteristics of opioids. Administration can range from intrathecal, intravenous, or oral to rectal, sublingual, buccal, intranasal, or transdermal. Depending on the clinical situation, one route may be more advantageous over another. For example, a patient who requires continuous opioid delivery but is unable to take medications orally may benefit from a transdermal delivery system, such as is currently available in a transdermal patch containing fentanyl. Fentanyl is also available as a rapid-onset transmucosal delivery product. Neuraxial routes of opioid delivery are widely used in peri- and postoperative care, as well as for terminally ill patients.

The goal of effective opioid therapy in chronic pain is to provide sustained analgesia over regular intervals.[15] This requires consideration of a number of factors, including knowledge of equianalgesic dosages between opioids and pharmacologic properties and side effects of specific opioid agents. Pain in the opioid-tolerant patient is particularly challenging, because typical dosages for the opioid-naïve patient do not apply and exact opioid requirements may require careful titration.

Whether fixed dosing is better than PRN is controversial, with each method having advantages for particular situations. With fixed dosing, there is a consistent opioid delivery, theoretically reaching steady state.[16] Presumably, this avoids the peak and trough effect that can be associated with on-demand dosing, and may prevent delays in delivery that can occur in on-demand schedules. One problem for opioid-naïve patients who receive fixed doses of opioids that have longer half-lives is that they may experience excessive side effects or toxicity because of the difficulty in predicting exact opioid requirement and potential accumulation. For example, morphine may take less than 24 hours to reach steady state levels, whereas methadone can take up to 1 week. When there is a need to assess a patient's analgesia threshold, PRN dosing of an opioid with a short half-life may be used or conservative fixed dosing may be applied for opioids that have a short half-life, supplemented with PRN "rescue" dosing.

Analgesic therapy with long-acting opioids (LAOs) offers convenient dose intervals that can attain safe, effective, steady-state levels. Several controlled-release opioids are available, including morphine (MS Contin, Oramorph SR, Kadian), oxycodone (OxyContin), and fentanyl (Duragesic patch). Oxymorphone has recently received U.S. Food and Drug Administration (FDA) approval for use in an oral controlled-released formulation. Methadone can be used as an LAO, but it poses specific issues and concerns for clinicians distinct from those of other opioids (see later discussion). Methadone has a faster onset and longer analgesic effect than many other opioids and may be ideal in some situations. However, these effects may also limit its use. Methadone is not specifically formulated for sustained release like other LAOs, which essentially release a short-acting opioid (SAO) throughout the drug's passage through the GI tract. Methadone simply has an intrinsically longer plasma half-life than other typical opioids such as hydromorphone (Dilaudid) or morphine and therefore can be advantageous in patients with GI motility issues, such as short gut syndrome.

Although sustained- and immediate-release opioid preparations have made the oral route a practical option, some cancer patients are unable to tolerate oral delivery.[17] In those cases, transdermal, buccal, rectal, intravenous, or subcutaneous infusions are often a practical alternative option. With infusion, the first-pass effect is eliminated, potentially offering some advantages. Compared with the oral route, there may be faster onset of analgesia, with uncomplicated access. Compared with the intramuscular route, administration is often less painful and may be safer in patients with bleeding disorders or reduced muscle mass.

Adverse Effects

The most commonly encountered side effects associated with opioids include constipation, nausea, vomiting, sedation, urinary retention, pruritus, and respiratory depression. Any of these side effects can significantly limit therapy, but tolerance to them usually ensues shortly after initiation of opioids. However, constipation is a major exception because it does not resolve with the prolonged use of opioids. Particular attention should be given to older adults and patients with hepatic or renal insufficiency. Tolerance and physical dependency are also commonly associated with opioid therapy. These are pharmacologic properties related to opioids that are frequently misinterpreted as indicators of addiction. Addiction is also a potential risk associated with opioid use (see later discussion). Physicians should anticipate any or all of these adverse effects, remain vigilant through-out therapy, and follow patients closely, particularly when initiating therapy and when escalating opioid doses.

Constipation

The most common side effect of opioid administration is constipation, and unfortunately, tolerance to it usually does not develop. Constipation can cause significant discomfort, nausea, and emesis. The underlying mechanism of opioid-induced constipation is thought to be decreased gastric motility related to opioid binding to highly concentrated opioid receptors located in the antrum of the stomach and the proximal small bowel.[18,19] There is limited evidence that certain opioids at equianalgesic doses produce more or less constipation than others. Because the transdermal route bypasses initial exposure to the GI tract, transdermal fentanyl has been postulated to produce less constipation than orally administration opioids.[20-22] However, current data are not convincing, particularly because transdermal opioids are well known to result in significant constipation that requires aggressive laxative therapy, irrespective of whether they produce less constipation than oral agents.

When initiating any opioid, it is important to prescribe medications to maintain regular bowel motility concomitantly. Treatment for opioid-induced constipation should include an active laxative, such as senna, lactulose, or bisacodyl; passive agents such as stool softeners or fiber-based bulking agents may be ineffective because they rely on triggering gastric motility, which in the case of opioids is usually inhibited. Alternatively, use of an adjunctive agent with a side effect profile that includes diarrhea, such as misoprostol, can coexist well with constipating opioids. However, misoprostol should be used with caution in females of childbearing age because it can initiate uterine contractions and miscarriage.[23,24]

Nausea and Emesis

Nausea and vomiting are often seen in patients who take opioids, but it is usually a transient side effect that often only lasts 2 to 3 days. The underlying mechanism of nausea and vomiting appears to be related to several causative factors. One of these is activation of receptors in the brainstem site that produces afferent input into the medullary chemoreceptor trigger zone, which is responsible for afferent input to the emetic center of the brain. These areas are dense in neurotransmitter receptors that correspond to the antiemetic agents used clinically. Other potential causes of nausea are stimulation of receptors in the vestibular apparatus or constipation.[25,26] Another underappreciated cause of opioid-related nausea is constipation, which will often respond to treatments that increase motility.

In evaluating a patient who reports nausea and vomiting while taking opioids, one should determine important history-related factors to the nausea, such as when the patient last moved his or her bowels, whether it worsens with movement, or whether there is a temporal relationship between opioid ingestion and onset of nausea. The choice of antiemetic agent depends on the historical aspects surrounding the reported side effect. Patients who experience nausea when they are more ambulatory may be more likely to have vestibule-related nausea. In such cases, drugs such as meclizine, promethazine, or scopolamine may be useful for relieving this type of induced nausea. Droperidol, prochlorperazine, ondansetron, or hydroxyzine may have greater benefit for nausea that is not associated with movement, a type of nausea thought to be related to chemoreceptor trigger zone–associated activation.[27,28] One should also ensure that reversible metabolic causes, intracranial pathology, or other factors such as medications are not the origin of nausea or emesis before it is solely attributed to opioids.

There are several approaches in treating opioid-induced nausea and vomiting. An antiemetic may be added, often choosing an agent that offers secondary benefits such as promotility, sedative, antipruritic, anxiolytic, or antipsychotic effects, depending on the needs of the individual patient. Another option is to decrease the opioid dose to the minimum acceptable dose for adequate analgesia that can reduce side effects. Based on the observation that tolerance to opioid-induced nausea accrues rapidly, the dose that had previously been reduced may be titrated slowly upward with increasing analgesia and without nausea. If nausea is protracted, one may consider changing to a different opioid. The emetogenic response to opioids is idiosyncratic and a different opioid may not produce nausea.[29]

Pruritus

Opioid-induced pruritus occurs more frequently with opioids delivered by the intravenous or neuraxial route compared with oral administration. Tolerance to pruritus usually develops fairly quickly, but in rare cases can be more persistent. The underlying mechanism of pruritus appears to be related to histamine release, which activates C-fiber itch receptors on C-fibers that are distinct from pain-transmitting C-fibers. Clinically, pruritus is often limited to the face and perineum, but can become generalized and severe. Treatment includes antihistamines, but the therapeutic effect may be related to sedation more than a direct antihistaminergic effect.[29] In patients receiving intrathecal or intravenous morphine who have significant pruritus that is unresponsive to antihistamines, low dosages of nalbuphine, a μ-receptor antagonist and κ-receptor agonist, may effectively reduce pruritus without reversing analgesia.[30,31]

Sedation

Opioid-naïve patients or patients on chronic opioids who are undergoing a dose escalation often experience sedation and drowsiness. Sedation is usually temporary as patients accommodate to the new medication or new dose, and it has been demonstrated that patients who are on a stable dose of opioids for 7 days rarely have psychomotor impairment.[32-34] The importance of this fact cannot be overemphasized because patients are increasingly being prescribed opioids for cancer- and non–cancer-related pain. Patients and others may question whether it is safe to operate a motor vehicle while taking opioids. This is a controversial issue and strong arguments may be made on both sides. Some physicians may recommend taking no precautions whereas others may counsel their patients never to drive while on opioids. Emerging evidence is not completely clear on this issue, but some studies have suggested that patients on long-term opioid therapy may be alert enough to drive safely.[35,36] However, it seems prudent to restrict driving, at least for 1 week or longer at onset or on dose escalation of an opioid regimen.

Sedation that persists despite an adequate adjustment period to the opioid dose can become as problematic as the pain itself. In such cases, lowering the dose of opioid to the minimal acceptable analgesic level, increasing (widening) the dosing interval, or changing to another opioid that may not be as sedating may be considered.[29] It is important to consider other causes of sedation such as other medications (e.g., benzodiazepines, antiemetics, tricyclics, muscle relaxants), renal or hepatic dysfunction leading to accumulation, or progression of the patient's primary disease state itself. If sedation is thought to be secondary to accumulating levels of the drug or its metabolites, changing to a different agent that is not as dependent on renal clearance or does not have active metabolites, such as fentanyl, may reduce sedation. For continued unremitting sedation, and after limiting CNS depressants, attempting opioid dose reduction, and attention being given to all other underlying causes, psychostimulants may be useful (e.g., amphetamines, modafinil).

Respiratory Depression

One of the most serious concerns and feared complications of opioid prescribing is the risk of respiratory depression. The underlying mechanism of respiratory depression is μ-receptor–induced depression of brainstem centers that subserve respiratory drive.[37] It has long been recognized that in patients who have combined intrathecal-epidural and oral or intravenous opioids, depressed respiratory drive may occur more rapidly. Although there is minimal evidence to support this claim, recognizing that this as a possible risk often supports an acceptable risk management–oriented approach to opioid administration. In addition, combining opioids with other sedating drugs can hasten respiratory depression. Clinically, the patient manifests sedation as the first sign of respiratory depression, which can pose a problem in detection during the evening hours when the patient is sleeping. Because respiratory depression can be seen after administration of epidural and intrathecal opioids, often delayed and not appearing until approximately 12 hours after injection, the signs of sedation may be lost during sleep. Therefore, it is advisable to use alarmed pulse oximetry in patients in whom clinical suspicion is warranted.[29]

Pain is a powerful physiologic stimulant of respiratory drive and opposes the respiratory depressant effects of opioids. In patients in whom pain relief is anticipated from a non-opioid analgesic treatment (e.g., neurolytic procedure, radiation therapy, adjuvant analgesics, surgery), reduction in opioid dose may be required.[37]

If a patient is nonarousable and opioid-induced respiratory depression is suspected, the specific opioid receptor antagonist naloxone should be administered. Care must be taken when giving naloxone to patients who have been on opioids for longer than 1 week or older adult patients, because severe withdrawal symptoms, seizures, and severe pain can be induced and can be deleterious. Naloxone administration has also induced congestive heart failure in susceptible patients. Naloxone often is packaged in an ampule containing 0.4 mg, which can then be diluted in 10 mL normal saline and 0.5-mL boluses (0.02 mg/0.5 mL) given every 2 minutes.[37]

Opioid Tolerance and Physical Dependence

There are substantial differences that distinguish tolerance, dependence, and addiction from each other. Unfortunately, these concepts are frequently misunderstood and can lead to the undertreatment of pain. In 2001, the American Pain Society (APS), American Academy of Pain Medicine (AAPM), and American Society of Addiction Medicine (ASAM) approved definitions of addiction, physical dependence, and tolerance with the hope of reducing misguided treatment of patients who require opioids for pain treatment. In a patient who is chronically administered opioids, it should be anticipated that she or he will develop physical dependence and tolerance, but the maladaptive behavior changes witnessed in patients with addiction (see later discussion) should not necessarily follow.[38]

Tolerance

The term *opioid tolerance* is often used to describe the phenomenon that occurs when a fixed dose of an opioid results in decreasing analgesia, thus requiring higher doses of medication to achieve the same or less effect over time.[29] The mechanisms responsible for this phenomenon are not entirely understood, but the N-methyl-D-aspartate (NMDA) receptor has been demonstrated to be involved.[39,40] The clinical usefulness of the NMDA receptor involvement has yet to be determined fully, but nonhuman studies have continued to promulgate the potential for using NMDA receptor antagonists in conjunction with opioids to attenuate tolerance and physical dependence.[41,42] A subpopulation of dorsal horn neurons expressing NMDA receptors treated with high-dose morphine have been shown to have enhanced NMDA receptor–mediated activity.[41] Furthermore, μ-receptor antagonists and NMDA receptor antagonist treatment of this subpopulation has attenuated the increased activity.[41] Another study has demonstrated that "morphine-tolerant" rats treated with an NMDA receptor antagonist reversed morphine-induced tolerance.[42] The relevance of these findings at the bedside have, to date, not been clear.

Human studies on the NMDA effect on tolerance have been less promising. There has been great hope that NMDA receptor antagonists such as ketamine or dextromethorphan might potentiate the analgesic effect of opioids, but there has not been much convincing evidence from replicated trials.[43,44] In a double-blind controlled clinical trial comparing morphine and a combination of morphine and dextromethorphan, statistical differences in analgesia or dose were not seen between groups.[45] Nonetheless, basic concepts continue to support the understanding that the NMDA receptor is a key component in the development of opioid-induced tolerance. In particular, ketamine continues to be a drug of major interest because of its potential to improve opioid performance through preventing tolerance and enhancing opioid-induced analgesia.[46-48]

When it is suspected that a patient has become tolerant to one medication, the cause may be opioid tolerance but it may also relate to increased pain that requires dosing adjustment. The need for dose escalation in a patient treated with chronic opioids should always stimulate consideration that the underlying disease may be progressing. When opioid-induced tolerance is present, an opioid rotation can be performed. This is based on the clinical observation that patients often have intraindividual analgesic responses to different opioids, and improved analgesia with less side effects may occur when a different opioid is used.[49] Although the full mechanism of this phenomenon is not completely understood, it is usually thought to occur because of incomplete tolerance, possibly relating to differing μ-opioid and other opioid receptor affinities of one opioid versus another. When an opioid rotation is performed in an opioid tolerant patient as opposed to an opioid-naïve patient, equal analgesic doses may not be necessary. The patient may respond with analgesia to half of the equianalgesic dose and, if not, may be titrated to an adequate analgesic effect that is less than would be expected by calculation of equianalgesic conversion from standard formulas. This is a potentially useful phenomenon whereby the overall opioid requirement of the patient may be reduced, achieving an opioid-sparing effect.

Physical Dependence and Withdrawal

Physical dependence is a physiologic state that manifests when a medication is abruptly stopped, resulting in a withdrawal syndrome. It is *not* synonymous with addiction. This separation of physical dependence and addiction is supported by evidence of two distinct anatomic areas within the central nervous system that are involved in physical dependence versus addiction. Noradrenergic neurons within the locus coeruleus are implicated in the maintenance of dependence and development of withdrawal, whereas the ventral tegmental dopaminergic area and orbitofrontal glutamatergic projections to the nucleus accumbens are particularly thought to subserve addiction.[46,50] It has been shown that drugs of abuse such as heroin, cocaine, nicotine, alcohol, phencyclidine, and cannabis initiate their habit-forming actions by activating a common reward pathway in the brain.[51] There is also evidence for the involvement of noradrenergic neurons in the development of withdrawal. Not only do norepinephrine levels change in the brain following opioid dependence, but the administration of an α₂ agonist such as clonidine or a β antagonist such as propranolol attenuates many of the symptoms of opioid withdrawal but does not reverse addiction.[52]

The clinical presentation of opioid withdrawal usually begins with irritability, anxiety, insomnia, diaphoresis, yawning, rhinorrhea, and lacrimation. If it progresses without intervention, a flulike condition develops, with chills, myalgias, fever, abdominal cramping, nausea, diarrhea, tachycardia, and other features of a heightened adrenergic state. Although uncomfortable for the patient, it is self-limiting and lasts approximately 3 to 7 days. Opioid withdrawal may be seen in patients who abruptly discontinue opioids or who have relative discontinuation because of taking SAOs after accommodating to the longer plasma half-life of LAOs.[29]

It is usually possible to taper patients from opioids and to prevent withdrawal symptoms. Although faster tapering can be accomplished without the advent of withdrawal symptoms, if time allows, few patients will be symptomatic with decreasing the dose by 10% to 20% every 48 to 72 hours over a prolonged period (usually 2 to 3 weeks, depending on the dose).[53] If, however, a patient develops symptoms of withdrawal during discontinuation or taper, clonidine 0.2 to 0.4 mg/day may be used to decrease discomfort.[54] Clonidine is often maintained for 4 days during a short-acting opioid taper and 14 days during a long-acting opioid taper. Once opioids have been discontinued, clonidine can be tapered over approximately 1 week.[29]

Addiction

Opioid addiction is a disorder characterized by opioid use resulting in physical, psychological, or social dysfunction (or a combination of these) and continued use of the opioid, despite the dysfunction. Neurobiologic evidence has suggested that this phenomenon may be subserved by positive reinforcement and sensitization of the dopaminergic system in the brain, which may explain the continued seeking of a substance destructive to the patient's life.[55] Patients who are receiving an inadequate dose of opioid medication often engage in drug-seeking behavior to obtain more pain medications for pain relief, which is often mistaken for the true drug-seeking behavior of addiction. Physicians are often challenged to distinguish true addiction from pseudoaddiction because, on the surface, pseudoaddiction may appear similar to addiction, with features such as drug seeking and self-escalation. However, unlike addiction, with increased doses of opioids, the pseudoaddicted patient notes pain relief and improved function. Other common signs of pseudoaddiction and inadequate analgesia may include the following:

- Requesting analgesics by name
- Demanding, manipulative behavior
- Clock watching
- Taking opioid drugs for an extended period
- Obtaining opiate drugs from more than one physician

Whereas pseudoaddiction resolves when the patient obtains adequate analgesia, true addictive behavior does not. Addiction exists in direct contradistinction to what is seen in a patient with pseudoaddiction who goes through dose escalation. In opioid addiction, aberrant behavior not only continues despite opioid increase, but is usually further stimulated and promoted by increased exposure to the addicting drug. Addiction is a difficult diagnosis to make on the basis of a single visit, and there is no one single behavior or diagnostic test that can confirm the diagnosis. The Committee on Pain of the American Society of Addiction Medicine has defined addiction in the context of pain treatment with opioids as a persistent pattern of dysfunctional opioid use.[56] Patient behaviors may be used cumulatively to support the diagnosis of addiction, but absolute conclusions cannot always be made, particularly without longitudinal information over extended periods. Many behaviors may indicate the possibility of addiction to some degree (Table 31–1).

Nonadherence to opioids may be related to many possibilities, including adverse effects, forgetfulness, incompatibility with lifestyle, and confusion about the drug regimen. It may rarely be related to aberrant behaviors such as diversion or drug abuse, and the astute physician will maintain a position of vigilance without feeling compelled to reach immediate conclusions. If a physician chooses to pursue pain treatment with an abusable drug in a patient at risk for addiction, collaborating with an addiction specialist or psychiatrist may be well advised to ensure that the necessary resources to support an appropriate risk management program are available. As always, high vigilance and tempered judgment are required.

The prevalence of addiction, abuse, or dependence in patients with chronic pain is not known exactly, but is estimated to range from 3% to 19%.[57] Treating chronic pain in a person with a history of addiction is challenging, but is not an absolute contraindication. Even when there is no history of addiction in a patient with chronic pain, the fear of the potential of addiction frequently impedes the appropriate management of the patient's analgesic requirements. Although a low percentage of the population with chronic pain appears to have an addiction problem, the remainder of the population has been shown to receive suboptimal analgesia because of the prescriber's fears of patient misuse of the opioid.[58]

Table 31–1. Aberrant Behaviors Indicative of Addiction

BEHAVIORS *LESS* INDICATIVE OF ADDICTION	BEHAVIORS *MORE* INDICATIVE OF ADDICTION
Expresses anxiety or desperation over recurrent symptoms	Buys pain medications from a street dealer
Hoards medications	Steals money to obtain drugs
Takes someone else's pain medications	Tries to get opioids from more than one source
Aggressively complains to physician for more drugs	Performs sex for drugs
Requests a specific drug or medication	Sees two physicians at once without them knowing
Uses more opioids than recommended	Performs sex for money to buy drugs
Drinks more alcohol when in pain	Steals drugs from others
Expresses worry over changing to a new drug, even if it offers potentially fewer side effects	Prostitutes others for money to obtain drugs
Takes (with permission) someone else's prescription opioids	Prostitutes others for drugs
Raises dose of opioids on own	Forges prescriptions
Expresses concern to physician or family members that pain might lead to use of street drugs	Sells prescription drugs
Asks for second opinion about pain medications	
Smokes cigarettes to relieve pain	
Has used opioids to treat other symptoms	

From Passik SD, Kirsh KL, Donaghy KB, et al: Pain and aberrant drug-related behaviors in medically ill patients with and without histories of substance abuse. Clin J Pain 2006;22:173-181.

SELECTED OPIOIDS

Although therapeutic options to provide analgesia continue to emerge, opioids remain the gold standard of currently available analgesics. Despite the widespread use of opioids for the treatment of acute and chronic pain, controversy exists over whether opioids should be used in the treatment of chronic nonmalignant pain. There are proponents on each side of the controversy, and part of the fear of prescribing opioids stems from an inaccurate understanding of appropriate outcomes for prescribing opioids and risks of abuse or side effects. Although opioids can be a useful tool to provide adequate analgesia for patients, fear of patients developing addiction, dependence, or untoward side effects often precludes physicians from prescribing opioids.[59] If it is decided to initiate opioid therapy in patients with chronic nonmalignant pain, the decision should be based on a well thought-out rationale for treatment, with clear end points in mind.

SAOs are generally used for acute pain, whereas LAOs are prescribed for patients with chronic pain syndromes. Because SAOs have relatively brief peak serum blood levels of active analgesic metabolites, using them to treat persistent baseline chronic pain will require frequent dosing. This roller coaster effect is thought to promote nonoptimal pain-related behaviors, which is why LAOs are considered to be more useful in such cases.

SAOs are often combined with other analgesics such as acetaminophen, nonsteroidal anti-inflammatory drugs (NSAIDs), or aspirin which may offer drug-sparing effects because less medication may be used. Although combination opioids may help reduce potential opioid-related side effects and toxicity, there is the potential of harm to major organs from the nonopioid components (e.g., acetaminophen, NSAIDs, aspirin). When using combination opioids, physicians must be aware of renal and liver function problems, as well as the potential harm that could occur to the GI system. Patients must be educated about the risks of taking other analgesics such as acetaminophen, NSAIDs, and aspirin in conjunction with the combination opioids. Moreover, physicians must also consider that the compounded non-opioid drug is likely to have a ceiling effect beyond which it is no longer efficacious. Because opioids induce tolerance and have no ceiling effect, the pharmacologically appropriate need for increased opioid may inadvertently push the dose of a combination drug to appropriate levels for the opioid component but to toxic levels for the nonopioid agent. Although reviewing all available opioids is beyond the scope of this chapter, we will review the most commonly used opioids for pain management. Minor opioids such as hydrocodone are discussed in Chapter 32.

Codeine

Codeine is an alkaloid found in very low concentrations in opium; it is now derived from morphine. It is frequently administered in combination with acetaminophen, butalbital, and caffeine.[54] It has been shown to be an effective analgesic in chronic non-malignant pain, but with limitations.[60] It is a weak μ-opioid agonist and has a half-life of 2.5 to 3 hours. The major metabolic pathway leads to glucuronidation of codeine to codeine 6-glucuronide (C6G), with a minor metabolic pathway catalyzed by the polymorphically expressed enzyme CYP2D6 through N-demethylation of codeine to norcodeine and O-demethylation of codeine to morphine.[10] Evidence has suggested that the analgesic effects of codeine rely on its conversion to morphine and patients with genetic variations in the enzymes needed to make this conversion may find codeine to be less effective.[61] The genetic polymorphism of CYP2D6 is responsible for the variable response to the medication. Patients with the genotype CYP2D6 PM (poor metabolizers) do not achieve adequate analgesia with codeine. In addition, certain medications that inhibit CYP2D6, such as quinidine, paroxetine, fluoxetine, and bupropion, can alter the phenotype of normal patients with normal genetics, thus decreasing the therapeutic analgesic effect of codeine.[62] Urinary excretion products of codeine include codeine (70%), norcodeine (10%), morphine (10%), normorphine (4%), and hydrocodone (1%).[54] This may be important to remember when interpreting urine toxicology screens of patients taking codeine.

Morphine

Morphine, a hydrophilic phenanthrene derivative, is the prototypical opioid against which all other opioids are compared for equianalgesic potency. Because of its hydrophilic nature, it has a delayed transport across the blood–brain barrier, thus delaying its onset of action. Conversely, it has a longer duration of action, 4 to 5 hours, when compared with its plasma half-life of 2 to 3 hours.[24] Metabolism of morphine to its two major metabolites, morphine 6-glucuronide (M6G) and morphine 3-glucuronide (M3G), occurs mainly in the liver (see Table 31–2). Although the parent compound produces analgesia and side effects, M6G may also produce some analgesia along with some adverse effects. M6G accounts for 5% to 15% of morphine's metabolites and is a μ and δ agonist, accounting for its analgesic effects. It has been demonstrated that M6G does not exert antinociceptive effects in knockout mice lacking the μ receptor.[63]

M3G, which accounts for 50% of morphine's metabolites, does not appear to possess opioid agonism, but may produce effects that oppose morphine's analgesic actions, such as allodynia, hyperalgesia, myoclonus, and seizures.[10] Oral administration of morphine has been shown to result in higher levels of M3G and M6G compared with the intravenous, intramuscular, or rectal routes, which bypass hepatic metabolism.[64] Chronic administration of morphine ultimately results in higher circulating levels of M3G and M6G metabolites than the parent compound.[65] It has been found that patients receiving chronically high morphine doses metabolize morphine to hydromorphone and test positive for hydromorphone on urine toxicology screens.[66] This is of critical importance in patients using morphine for chronic pain who undergo urine drug screening.

Although extrahepatic metabolism of morphine has been shown to occur in gastric and intestinal epithelia, morphine should be used with caution in patients with decreased hepatic function, such as those with cirrhosis.[10] In addition, glucuronides have been shown to undergo deconjugation back to the parent compound by colonic flora and reabsorbed as morphine.[10] Morphine metabolites are excreted by the kidney, so caution should also be taken when prescribing morphine to patients with renal impairment because accumulation of M6G and M3G can be toxic. Currently available forms of morphine include short- and long-acting preparations. Short-acting agents may be compounded for almost any route of administration and long-acting preparations generally use specialized sustained-release matrix technology, such as that found in MS Contin, Kadian, Oramorph SR, and Avinza.

Oxycodone

Oxycodone is a semisynthetic opioid that is closely related to morphine. It has been available for analgesia since 1917, when it was introduced into clinical practice in Germany.[67] It is processed from thebaine, an organic compound found in opium. Like morphine, currently available forms of oxycodone include short- and long- acting preparations. Short-acting oxycodone may be used alone (e.g., Roxicodone) or may be compounded with acetaminophen (e.g., Percocet, Roxicet, Endocet) or aspirin e.g., Percodan). Long-acting oxycodone preparations are designed for oral administration, using specialized sustained-release technology (e.g., OxyContin and similar generics).

Oxycodone has a high bioavailability, 60%, when compared with morphine, which has a bioavailability of 33%, making it almost twice as potent as morphine.[54] Oxycodone is a prodrug that undergoes hepatic metabolism via the CYP2D6 isoenzyme, whereby it is converted into its active metabolite, oxymorphone, a μ-opioid agonist, and its inactive metabolite, noroxycodone. Oxymorphone is reportedly often undetectable and is 14 times more potent than the parent compound.

Similar to codeine, there is genetic polymorphism in 10% of the population, which accounts for significant variations in the metabolism of oxycodone. This variation accounts for the fact that some patients require higher than usual doses of oxycodone to achieve analgesia. Another factor to be considered when prescribing oxycodone is whether other potential competitors of the CYP2D6 isoenzyme are being prescribed. Such interacting medications include neuroleptics, tricyclic antidepressants, and

selective serotonin reuptake inhibitors (SSRIs). Cases of serotonin syndrome have been described in the liter-ature when SSRIs and oxycodone were used concomitantly.[67,68]

Meperidine

The use of meperidine for analgesia has been declining recently because of its potential for neurotoxicity. It is a weaker μ-opioid agonist than morphine with 10% its potency, more rapid onset, and shorter duration of action.[65] The half-life of meperidine is 3 hours and it is hepatically demethylated to its neurotoxic metabolite, normeperidine, which has a half-life of 12 to 16 hours. Normeperidine has been well documented to cause CNS hyperactivity and seizures.[24] Excretion of normeperidine is via the kidneys; therefore, caution should be taken when administering meperidine to patients with renal impairment or those prone to CNS hyperactivity. Initially, toxic effects may be seen as subtle mood changes that can progress to naloxone-irreversible tremors, myoclonus, and seizures. Chronic administration of meperidine in patients with normal renal function and administration of meperidine in conjunction with SSRIs, monoamine oxidase (MAO) inhibitors, tramadol, and methadone can also result in neurotoxic side effects.[65]

Hydromorphone

Hydromorphone has a strong affinity for the μ receptor. It is a hydrogenated ketone analogue of morphine and can be formed by N-demethylation of hydrocodone.[69] Hydromorphone is similar to morphine in that it is hydrophilic and has a similar duration of analgesia, but differs with respect to side effects and potency. Pruritus, sedation, nausea, and vomiting occur less frequently. Further, hydromorphone is five times more potent than morphine when administered orally (see Table 31–3), and seven times more potent when administered parenterally. Although essentially hydrophilic, it is 10 times more lipophilic than morphine. This lipophilicity may be an advantage when treating patients who are unable to take oral medications and cannot maintain IV access, such as is in hospice environments. It can be given subcutaneously at 10 or 20 mg/mL; this route delivers approximately 80% of the dose absorbed through IV delivery.[69] Onset of analgesia occurs in 30 minutes after oral administration and 5 minutes after intra-venous administration, with peak analgesic effects occurring within 8 to 20 minutes.[70]

Hydromorphone is metabolized in the liver to hydromorphone 3-glucuronide (H3G) and, like its parent compound, is excreted renally. Similar to M3G, H3G lacks analgesic effect but may be an active metabolite that potentiates neurotoxic effects such as allodynia, myoclonus, and seizures.[10] Production of H3G is relatively low so the risk of neurotoxic side effects is relatively low, except in patients with renal insufficiency, in whom H3G may accumulate.[65]

Fentanyl

Fentanyl is a highly lipophilic agent with a high affinity for the μ-opioid receptor. It is 75 to 125 times more potent and has a faster onset of action than morphine.[65] Because of its higher potency, smaller quantities of the medication can be delivered to the patient compared with other opioids. Although fentanyl is considered to be a short-acting medication, its lipophilic nature allows for long-acting transdermal and very rapid-onset transmucosal administration for the treatment of chronic and acute pain, respectively.[65] Although there are other minor pathways, fentanyl undergoes hepatic biotransformation via CYP3A4 N-dealkylation to norfentanyl. Its half-life and onset of action vary greatly by route of administration. (Transmucosal fentanyl undergoes first-pass metabolism and has an onset of action within 5 to 10 minutes.)

The transdermal fentanyl patch is used for some patients with chronic pain or pain related to cancer. Transdermal fentanyl has been used for acute postoperative pain but may be associated with hypoventilation.[71] Transdermal patches are typically placed on a hairless part of the body that is flat and free of any defects that could interfere with adherence of the patch. Patients should be advised to avoid submerging the patch in hot water or placing a heating pad over the area, because this influences absorption. Patients report local skin erythema or irritation as the most common side effect.[72]

Transdermal fentanyl is an alternative choice for patients who have significant GI issues, such as persistent emesis, chronic nausea, "short gut" syndrome, or believed to be at risk of diverting oral medications. The patch offers the opportunity to have the patient return the used patches for inspection at the time of prescription refill. Theoretically, transdermal delivery may induce less constipation than oral opioids because it avoids direct exposure to the GI tract, but this is questionable in light of the common finding of significant constipation for almost all who use transdermal opioids.

Unlike other LAOs, transdermal fentanyl may be challenging to titrate because of variation in individual patient characteristics such as skin perspiration, skin temperature, fat stores, and muscle bulk.[10] The rate of achieving therapeutic serum levels can be variable, ranging from 1 to 30 hours (mean, 13 hours). Because of the wide variation of reaching therapeutic levels, a short-acting oral analgesic or IV patient-controlled analgesia (PCA) may be necessary to address breakthrough pain while the transdermal opioid effect is ramping up or to prevent withdrawal symptoms if rotation is from another opioid. Achieving steady-state levels may require up to 6 days and the amount of SAO required after steady state is achieved will help determine whether the dose of fentanyl must be increased.[10] If the patch is removed, however, it may take up to 16 hours for serum fentanyl concentrations to drop by 50%.

Oral transmucosal fentanyl has a more rapid onset of analgesia than other SAOs and offers some special advantages. Because it is transmucosal, it avoids the GI tract and first-pass hepatic metabolism and has a rapid onset of action, within 10 to 15 minutes. One study has compared IV morphine with transmucosal fentanyl in an acute postoperative setting and demonstrated similar onset of analgesia.[73] Transmucosal fentanyl can be beneficial for patients with acute breakthrough pain. To date, a major limitation for using this route has been cost.

Methadone

Methadone is an attractive choice for analgesia because of several of its unique properties, but it also has many features that distinguish it from other opioids that have raised its potential for adverse outcomes. Its attributes include no known neurotoxic or active metabolites, high absorption and bioavailability, and multiple receptor activities, including μ- and δ-opioid agonism, NMDA antagonism, and serotonin reuptake blockade. Methadone has been shown to have approximately a threefold bioavailability compared with morphine.[74,75] In patients who require high-dose LAOs, methadone appears to be a theoretical second-line choice because of the lack of accumulation of neurotoxic metabolites that induce myoclonus, hallucinations, seizures, sedation, and confusion. Unfortunately, it is methadone's unique pharmacokinetics and pharmacodynamics that render its effects somewhat unpredictable.

Methadone is structurally unrelated to other opioid-derived alkaloids. It is a racemic mixture of two enantiomers, the D isomer (S-methadone) and L isomer (R-methadone). R-Methadone accounts for its opioid receptor affinity and thus its opioid effect. Animal studies have demonstrated that methadone has a lower affinity for the μ receptor than morphine.[76] This may explain why methadone may have fewer μ-opioid–related side effects than morphine. Methadone, however, has a higher affinity for the δ receptor than morphine.[77]

Methadone has a slow but variable elimination half-life, averaging approximately 27 hours, which may be related to its lipophilicity and extensive tissue distribution.[75] The delayed clearance of methadone is the basis for its use in maintenance therapy because it can prevent the onset of withdrawal symptoms for 24 hours or longer. Surprisingly, although methadone may be efficacious for purposes of opioid maintenance therapy, potentially preventing withdrawal symptoms for 24 hours or longer, its analgesic half-life is shorter than 24 hours, usually found to range from 6 to 8 hours. This discrepancy is related to its biphasic elimination. The alpha elimination phase lasts 8 to 12 hours and correlates with the period of analgesia that lasts approximately 6 to 8 hours. The beta elimination phase ranges from 30 to 60 hours and is responsible for preventing withdrawal symptoms; this is exploited in maintenance therapy.[65]

Methadone has multiple drug interactions related to inducers or inhibitors of the CYP system, particularly the 3A4 subtype.[78] Because these interactions are not commonly seen with other opioids, drug interactions with methadone may not be as readily anticipated or detected. In addition to interacting with drugs, 3A4 is an autoinducible enzyme, which accounts for the fact that methadone can bring about its metabolism and increase its clearance with prolonged use.[76]

Other issues affecting methadone absorption and accumulation are gastric and urinary pH. Decreased gastric pH, such as in patients taking proton pump inhibitors, results in increased rates of methadone absorption. Renal failure and hemodialysis do not alter the excretion of methadone; however, as urinary pH increases, methadone clearance in the urine decreases. Urine pH higher than 6 can reduce methadone clearance from 30% to almost 0%, resulting in increased circulating levels.[76] Most methadone is eliminated via the feces.[10] Another source of methadone's potential metabolic instability relates to it avid protein binding. Acute changes in protein binding may lead to sudden increases or decreases in circulating methadone levels.[76]

The difference between methadone and other LAOs is that methadone's duration of effect is intrinsically long-acting, whereas most other LAOs are sustained-released forms, based on compounding technology. It is beneficial in patients with impaired GI absorption. In addition, methadone is available as a powder, which allows it to be formulated for almost any route of administration. Methadone pills can be broken and cut in half and it is also available as a liquid elixir (1 or 10 mg/mL). This avoids having to crush pills, offering a potential advantage in patients with gastrostomy tubes. In addition, because methadone elixir has a low-concentration formulation, a careful and precise titration of methadone can be performed to achieve adequate analgesia.[76]

One of the most disturbing aspects of methadone use in the United States has been the reported increase in methadone-related deaths.[79,80] Although the mechanism for these deaths is not exactly clear, many appear to be related to overdose and drug interactions. In some cases, overdose may be related to the misunderstanding of standard conversion rates for methadone from other opioids. Contrary to conventional wisdom, methadone appears to be more potent (milligram for milligram) in patients who are being switched to methadone from high doses of other opioids. Whereas standard conversion tables may suggest that the ratio of conversion from morphine to methadone may be from 1:1 to 1:3, these ratios were taken from studies on acute pain or normal controls. Many of these conversion tables were developed more than 20 years ago, far before recent increases in methadone use as a chronic analgesic. In cases in which much higher preswitch dosages are converted to methadone, the appropriate morphine-to-methadone ratio may range from 1:5 to 1:20 or higher. Obviously, such a counterintuitive dosing phenomenon leads to the potential for overdose.

Another possible source of methadone-related mortality includes torsade de pointes arrhythmias, which have been reported in some patients.[81] Although a prospective study has demonstrated an increase in the QT interval of patients taking methadone, it was also concluded that the magnitude of the increase is less than with other antiarrhythmic drugs and is not higher than QT interval widening with other drugs, such as tricyclic antidepressant therapy.[82] Use of methadone requires awareness of possible QT prolongation and the possible additive effect that other QT prolonging agents may have when combined with methadone.

Table 31–2 shows the oral bioavailability, half-lives, duration of action, and metabolites of selected opioids. Table 31–3 shows the equianalgesic doses of different opioids.

RATIONAL OPIOID PRESCRIBING

Patients with moderate to severe chronic pain who have been treated with non-opioid therapies and have not improved may benefit from opioid analgesics. Even though the selection of a short- or long-acting

Table 31–3. Equianalgesic Doses of Opioids

OPIOID	ORAL EQUIANALGESIC DOSE (mg)
Morphine	10
Meperidine	100
Oxycodone	7
Hydromorphone	2
Methadone	10-20
Oxymorphone	1.5
Butorphanol	2
Buprenorphine	0.3
Hydrocodone	10
Codeine	80
Tramadol	40
Propoxyphene	43-45

Table 31–2. Selected Opioids: Oral Bioavailability, Half-lives, Duration of Action, and Metabolites

OPIOID	AVAILABILITY (%)	HALF-LIFE (HR)	DURATION OF ACTION (HR)	METABOLITES
Morphine	10-45	2-3	4-5	M6G, M3G
Oxycodone (OxyContin)	60-80	4.5	12	Oxymorphone, noroxycodone
Methadone	60-95	8-80 (average, 27)	6-8	—
Hydromorphone	24	2.3	3-4	H3G
Oxymorphone (Opana ER)	10	9 ± 3	12	O3G, 6-hydroxyoxymorphone

H3G, hydromorphone 3-glucuronide; M3G, morphine 3-glucuronide; M6G, morphine 6-glucuronide; O3G: oxymorphone 3-glucuronide.

opioid appears to be empiric, a rational approach to opioid choice can be aided by a thorough review of the patient's medical history, especially paying close attention to hepatic and renal function, previous experiences with opioids, and other medical and psychiatric factors. If the patient is opioid-naïve, low-dose SAOs such as propoxyphene, hydrocodone, or oxycodone may be initiated and carefully titrated to establish an opioid requirement. Because of the rapid clearance and brief half-life of SAOs, toxic accumulation of the medications are far lower than with LAOs. The severity and duration of the patient's pain should help guide whether PRN or fixed dosing is required. In patients with acute pain secondary to an injury or surgery for which rapid healing is expected, PRN dosing is reasonable. However, in patients with the expectation of prolonged recovery or chronic pain with significant baseline or persistent pain, opioids may be administered in fixed-dosing intervals as well as in PRN intervals for breakthrough pain. Scheduled dosing decreases clock-watching anxiety and reinforcement of pain behaviors. If a patient is able to tolerate an SAO and its side effects, consolidation of the daily opioid requirement into an equianalgesic LAO regimen may be an appropriate next step.

Opioids can produce reliable analgesia and, although their use is not without potential adverse effects, these can be anticipated and often preempted or otherwise mitigated. In managing chronic pain with a multidisciplinary approach, opioid therapy can become an integral portion of the treatment plan. However, it is not uncommon to combine opioid treatment with other modalities, including psychological treatment and physical rehabilitation. Simultaneously, interventional pain procedures and adjunctive analgesics may be useful as well.

Although opioids may be excellent analgesics, they are often used as a second-line treatment for chronic pain, mainly because chronic pain may respond to non-opioid treatments that might carry fewer risks. When other pharmacologic, rehabilitative, or interventional procedures are not appropriate or are unsuccessful, chronic opioid therapy should be considered.

The effectiveness of opioid therapy for certain types of chronic pain, such as neuropathic pain, remains controversial. Because antidepressants and anticonvulsants have been shown to provide less than 50% pain relief, on average, opioids have been used in the treatment of chronic neuropathic pain, despite their narrow therapeutic window.[83] When treating neuropathic pain, it has been shown that opioid potency may be relatively lower than for other conditions. The basis of this seems to be secondary to changes that occur in the endogenous opioid system after nerve injury. It appears that endogenous peptide levels and opioid receptor density decrease in nociceptive pathways.[84] It also appears that γ-aminobutyric acid (GABA)–ergic tone decreases after nerve injury and that the inhibitory effect of morphine on dorsal horn neuron projections after nerve injury is reduced compared with noninjured nerves.[85]

Despite these findings, there is compelling evidence in the literature showing efficacy of opioids for neuropathic pain; a recent trial demonstrated that combining gabapentin and morphine for the treatment of neuropathic pain was superior to either alone.[86]

In forms of chronic pain unrelated to nerve injury that have not responded well to other treatments, opioid therapy has been shown to be more effective in reducing pain than placebo or anti-inflammatory medications alone. However, studies have struggled to show substantial improvements in overall functioning with opioid therapy. In a meta-analysis comparing analgesia and function in subjects taking opioids, NSAIDs, or placebo, there was no statistical difference among groups with regard to improved function. It should be noted, however, that this study did not use adjunctive medications or physical therapy.[87] This emphasizes the point that although opioids may be effective, if used as the sole agent for changing all the primary and secondary effects of chronic pain, they may not be effective enough. The importance of a multidisciplinary approach to the treatment of chronic pain syndromes cannot be overstated.

The use of opioids requires a comprehensive strategy, including consideration of other potentially effective therapies that have less risk and end points of treatment. Rational prescribing also requires consideration of all potential risks associated with the treatment and should include a plan to avoid or deal with these risks.

Considerations for Opioid Prescribers

Because opioids are controlled substances with potential for abuse, they are regulated by the Drug Enforcement Administration (DEA) and other state agencies. A surging public health crisis of prescription drug abuse has led to increasing concern over the potential for prescription opioids to be diverted and abused. To address this issue, the APS, AAPM, and ASAM have advanced a joint statement on pain and addiction to assist prescribers in developing rational approaches to prescribing.[88] In 2004, the Federation of State Medical Boards of the United States revised its 1998 model policy for the use of controlled substances in the treatment of pain,[89] which offers clear practice expectations for state medical boards to adopt for reviewing physician practices. The model policy emphasizes the importance of a history and physical examination; informed consent for treatment; frequent monitoring to evaluate therapeutic effectiveness, including the patient's functional status; referral to a specialist if the patient presents with a complex history or is not responding to treatment as expected; and transparent documentation.[89]

Treatment End Points

Because pain is a subjective experience, using "pain relief" as a treatment end point is a subjective and nontestable marker of therapeutic success or failure.

One of the most feared consequences of chronic opioid therapy is drug addiction, which, as discussed earlier, presents as compulsive use of the opioid that causes dysfunction and the continued use of the opioid, despite the dysfunction (i.e., negative impact or harm to the patient's life). Because effective analgesia should improve function, and because of fear of the side effect of addiction, which hinges on dysfunction, a major focus of chronic opioid therapy should be functional improvement as an objective end point. It is expected that patients who are treated carefully and judiciously with opioids and achieve analgesia should have some functional gains. This is in contradistinction to the addict who becomes impaired by substance abuse, manifest by dysfunction. The challenge for physicians treating chronic pain with opioids is to devise a system of objective markers that distinguish function from dysfunction and that emphasize a wide spectrum of therapeutic goals.

There are several markers of functional improvement that can be used in patients treated with chronic opioids. Several standardized functional measurements (e.g., Short Form 36 [SF-36], Oswestry Disability Index [ODI]) can be used to measure subjective pain reduction with supportive and objective evidence of improvement of functional status and effect on quality of life. However, psychological and social factors, as well as the status of coexistent disease, may influence perception of pain, suffering, and entitlement, and can alter the overall assessment.[90-92] Unfortunately, not all these parameters will improve concomitantly or proportionally following the initiation of opioid therapy. If factors related to psychological and physical reconditioning have not been addressed, pain perception and the reduction of pain after an opioid trial may be less than optimal.

Determining effective treatment end points during an opioid trial may require flexibility in considering the many possible variations in efficacy and functional gain. A central question that may be useful at the beginning of an opioid trial is, "What do you need to do with this medicine that you cannot do now?" What follows should be the creation of a list of reasonably attainable functional goals that cover multiple domains of the patient's life. Equally important in documenting this list is the process by which the goals will be attained and how the patient plans to document progress of each functional goal for the clinician on every subsequent follow-up visit. Each goal is followed regularly and adjusted, based on progress. Expectations may need to be reduced if goals are not being met or may be advanced as the patient improves.

One approach to determining whether a patient is benefiting from opioid therapy is to gather collateral information from others involved in the patient's care and life. Input from physical and occupational therapists, psychologists, family members, and caregivers may prove to be invaluable. Evidence of improved function may include gains in employment, increased activities of daily living, and socializing with family and friends. On the contrary, if a patient becomes dysfunctional in employment, social, or private life, concerns about possible medication-related deterioration should be raised, including addiction. However, decreased function is not pathognomonic of addiction. It may be related to other factors beyond a patient's control such as sedation, cognitive impairment, or other external causes. If these or other external problems are not the cause of a patient's deteriorating mental or physical health, it may be helpful to consider seeking additional support in the form of a multidisciplinary program or referral to other specialty providers, such as psychologists, social workers, psychiatrists, or addiction specialists.

It remains controversial as to whether subjective relief without objective evidence of improved quality of life is sufficient to justify chronic use of opioids. Pain reduction is a subjective variable. Its use as an assessment tool for therapeutic success only represents a single aspect of adequate chronic opioid therapy. For example, consider the patient with significant disability related to pain that is rated 6 on a pain severity scale of 1 to 10. Although opioid therapy may not be successful in significantly reducing subjective pain scores, this does not signify treatment failure. In fact, despite no reported reduction in pain scores, objective signs of return to work and increased physical activity clearly demonstrate that treatment has improved the patient's quality of life. Conversely, if an opioid trial is characterized by subjective reports of marked pain relief, but there are no observable functional gains and possibly even signs of persistent sedation with decreased physical activity, voluntary unemployment, dysfunctional interpersonal relationships, or diminished physical activity, the physician must consider why the patient would regard this as a positive outcome and attempt to resolve any underlying conditions or misunderstandings.

As noted by the Federation of State Medical Boards, a critical aspect of safe opioid management is documentation of a patient's care, including current functional status on initial evaluation and throughout follow-up.[87] Documentation not only requires clarity of events but should offer transparency about the physician's decision process, particularly in regard to risk-benefit considerations, choices, and plans for risk management. Vigilance for decreased function is important; this may help reveal problems such as addiction, progressive disease, or pain unresponsive to opioids.

Another critical issue to consider during the course of treatment is when to discontinue opioid therapy if the treatment is deemed to be ineffective. Many factors must be considered before a treatment is considered to be a failure, including inadequate dosing, inappropriate dosing schedule, improper drug delivery route, opioid-insensitive pain, side effects limiting dose escalation, and social and psychological issues.

Appropriate durations of effective opioid therapy remain controversial. There are currently no clear guidelines and consensus regarding this issue. With opioid use, tolerance can develop and may require an increase in dose or an opioid rotation to maintain sufficient therapeutic effect. Periodic opioid dose escalation or opioid rotation may be necessary for patients who are achieving analgesia and functional gains from therapy. In such cases, functional decline might be consistent with pseudoaddiction because of inadequate treatment. Full consideration of treatment efficacy related to adverse effects and to the progression of underlying disease must be made when formulating decisions regarding length of treatment; these must be reconsidered on a regular basis. Once opioid therapy has been initiated, it may be difficult to know whether pain would be present without opioid therapy unless opioids are tapered.

References

1. Maher TJ, Pasarapa C: Opioids (bench). In Smith HS (ed): Drugs for Pain. Philadelphia, Hanley & Belfus, 2003, pp 83-96.
2. Pert CB, Snyder SH: Opiate receptor: Demonstration in nervous tissue. Science 1973;179:1011-1014.
3. Simon EJ, Hiller JM, Edelman I: Stereospecific binding of the potent narcotic analgesic [^{3}H]-etorphine to rat-brain homogenate. Proc Natl Acad Sci U S A 1973;70:1947-1949.
4. Besse D, Lombard MC, Zajac JM, et al: Pre- and post-synaptic distribution of mu, delta and kappa opioid receptors in the superficial layers of the cervical dorsal horn of the rat spinal cord. Brain Res 1990;521:15-22.
5. Hassan AHS, Ableitner A, Stein C, et al: Inflammation of the rat paw enhances axonal transport of opioid receptors in the sciatic nerve and increases their density in the inflamed tissue. Neuroscience 1993;55:185-195.
6. Stein C, Pfluger M, Yassouridis A, et al: No tolerance to peripheral morphine analgesia in presence of opioid expression in inflamed synovia. J Clin Invest 1996;98:793-799.
7. Stoelting RK, Hillier S: Opioid agonists and antagonists. In Stoelting RK, Hillier SC: Handbook of Pharmacology and Physiology in Anesthetic Practice, 2nd ed. Philadelphia, Lippincott Williams & Wilkins, 2006, pp 78-117.
8. Martin M, Matifas A, Maldonado R, et al: Acute antinociceptive responses in single and combinatorial opioid receptor knockout mice: Distinct mu, delta and kappa tones. Eur J Neurosci 2003;24:198-205.
9. Keiffer BL: Opioids: First lessons from knockout mice. Trends Pharmacol Sci 1999;20:19-26.
10. Janicki PK, Parris WC: Clinical pharmacology of opioids. In Smith HS (ed): Drugs for Pain. Philadelphia, Hanley & Belfus, 2003, pp 97-118.
11. Mervyn D: Opioids in renal failure and dialysis patients. J Pain Symptom Manage 2004;28:497-504.
12. Labroo RB, Paine MF, Thummel KE, et al: Fentanyl metabolism by human hepatic and intestinal cytochrome P4503A4: Implications for interindividual variability in disposition, efficacy, and drug interactions. Drug Metab Dispos 1997; 25:1072-1080.
13. Davis MP, Walsh D: Methadone for relief of cancer pain: A review of pharmokinetics, pharmacodynamics, drug interactions and protocols of administration. Support Care Cancer 2001;9:73-83.
14. Tempelhoff R, Modica PA, Spitznagel EL: Anticonvulsant therapy increases fentanyl requirements during anaesthesia for craniotomy. Can J Anaesth 1990;37:327-332.
15. Portenoy RK: Current pharmacotherapy of chronic pain. J Pain Symptom Manage 2000; 19(Suppl 1):S16-S20.
16. Reder RF: Opioid formulations: Tailoring to the needs in chronic pain. J Pain Symptom Manage 2001;5(Suppl A): 109-111.
17. Mercadante S, Fulfaro F: Alternatives to oral opioids for cancer pain. Oncology (Williston Park) 1999;13:215-220.
18. Polack JM, Bloom SR: Neuropeptides of the gut: A newly discovered control mechanism. World J Surg 1979;3:393-405.
19. DeLuca A, Coupar IM: Insights into opioid action in the intestinal tract. Pharmacol Ther 1996;69:103-115.
20. Choi YS, Billings JA: Opioid antagonists: A review of their role in palliative care, focusing on use in opioid-related constipation. J Pain Symptom Manage 2002;24:71-79.
21. Radbruch L, Sabotowski R, Loick G, et al: Constipation and the use of laxatives: A comparison between transdermal fentanyl and oral morphine. Pall Med 2000;14:111-119.
22. Ahmedzai S, Brooks D: Transdermal fentanyl versus sustained-release oral morphine in cancer pain: Preference, efficacy, and quality of life. J Pain Symptom Manage 1997;13:254-261.
23. Agra Y, Sacristan A, Gonzalez M, et al: Efficacy of senna versus lactulose in terminal cancer patients treated with opioids. J Pain Symptom Manage 1998;15:1-7.
24. Inturrisi CE: Clinical pharmacology of opioids for pain. Clin J Pain 2002;18:S3-S13.
25. Simoneau II, Hamza MS, Mata HP, et al: The cannabinoid agonist WIN55,212-2 suppresses opioid-induced emesis in ferrets. Anesthesiology 2001;94:882-887.
26. Foss JF, Bass AS, Goldberg LI: Dose-related antagonism of the emetic effect of morphine by methylnaltrexone in dogs. J Clin Pharmacol 1993;33:747-751.
27. Frederich ME: Nonpain symptom management. Prim Care 2001;28:299-316.
28. Cherny NI, Portenoy RK: The management of cancer pain. CA Cancer J Clin 1994;44:262-303.
29. Wilsey BL, Mahajan GM, Fishman: Opioid therapy in chronic non-malignant pain. In Smith HS (ed): Drugs for Pain. Philadelphia, Hanley & Belfus, 2003, pp 119-131.
30. Charuluxanan S, Kyokong O, Somboonviboon W, et al: Nalbuphine versus propofol for treatment of intrathecal morphine-induced pruritus after cesarean delivery. Anesth Analg 2001;93:162-165.
31. Charuluxanan S, Kyokong O, Somboonviboon W, et al: Nalbuphine versus ondansetron for prevention of intrathecal morphine-induced pruritus after cesarean delivery. Anesth Analg 2003; 96:1789-793.
32. Zacny JP: Should people taking opoids for medical reasons be allowed to work and drive? Addiction 1996;91:1581-1584.
33. Zacny JP: A review of the effects of opiates on psychomotor and cognitive functioning in humans. Exp Clin Psychopharmacol 1995;3:432-466.
34. Bruera E, Macmillan K, Hanson J, et al: The cognitive effects of the administration of narcotic analgesics in patients with cancer pain. Pain 1989;39:13-16.
35. Sabotowski R, Schwalen S, Rettig K, et al: Driving ability under long-term treatment with transdermal fentanyl. J Pain Symptom Manage 2003;25:38-47.
36. Fishbain DA, Cutlet RB, Rosomoff HL, et al: Are opioid dependent/tolerant patients impaired in driving-related skills? A structured evidence-based review. J Pain Symptom Manage 2003;25:38-47.
37. Holtzman M, Fishman SM: Opioid receptors. In Benzon HT, Raja SN, Molloy RE, et al (eds): Essentials of Pain and Regional Anesthesia. Philadelphia, Elsevier Churchill Livingstone, 2005, pp 87-93.
38. American Academy of Pain Medicine, the American Pain Society and the American Society of Addiction Medicine: Definitions related to the use of opioids for the treatment of pain. A consensus document from the American Academy of Pain Medicine, the American Pain Society and the American Society of Addiction Medicine, 2001. Available at http://www.ampainsoc.org/advocacy/opioids2.htm.
39. Price DD, Mayer DJ, Mao J, et al: NMDA-receptor antagonists and opioid receptor interactions as related to analgesia and tolerance. J Pain Symptom Manage 2000;19(Suppl 1) S7-S11.
40. Bespalov AY, Zvartau EE, Beardsley PM: Opioid-NMDA receptor interactions may clarify conditioned (associative) components of opioid analgesic tolerance. Neurosci Biobehav Rev 2001;25:343-353.
41. Zhao M, Joo DT: Subpopulation of dorsal horn neurons displays enhanced N-methyl-D-aspartate receptor function after chronic morphine exposure. Anesthesiol 2006;104:815-825.

42. Adam F, Bonnet F, Le Bars D: Tolerance to morphine analgesia: Evidence for stimulus intensity as a key factor and complete reversal by a glycine site-specific NMDA antagonist. Neuropharmacology 2006;51:191-202.

43. Tucker A, Kim Y, Nadeson R, et al: Investigation of the potentiation of the analgesic effect by ketamine in humans: A double-blinded randomised controlled, crossover study of experimental pain. BMC Anesthesiol 2005;5:2.

44. Schmid RL, Sandler AN, Katz J: Use and efficacy of low-dose ketamine in the management of acute postoperative pain: A review of current techniques and outcomes. Pain 1999;82: 111-125.

45. Galer BS, Lee D, Ma T, et al: MorphiDex (morphine sulfate/dextromethorphan hydrobromide combination) in the treatment of chronic pain: Three multicenter, randomized, double-blind, controlled clinical trials fail to demonstrate enhanced opioid analgesia or reduction in tolerance. Pain 2005; 115:284-295.

46. Kalivas PW, Volkow ND: The neural basis of addiction: A pathology of motivation and choice. Am J Psychiatry 2005;162:1403-1413.

47. Lossignol DA, Obiols-Portis M, Body JJ: Successful use of ketamine for intractable cancer pain. Support Care Cancer 200513:188-193.

48. Subramaniam K, Subramaniam B, Steinbrook RA: Ketamine as adjuvant analgesic to opioids: A quantitative and qualitative systematic review. Anesth Analg 2004;99:482-895.

49. Indelicato R, Portenoy RK: The art of oncology: When the tumor is not the target. Opioid rotation in the management of refractory cancer pain. J Clin Oncol 2002;20:348-352.

50. Bozarth MA, Wise RA: Neural substrates of opiate reinforcement. Prog Neuropsychopharmacol Biol Psychiatry 1983; 7:569-575.

51. Wise RA: Neurobiology of addiction. Curr Opin Neurobiol 1996;6:243-251.

52. Maldonado R: Participation of noradrenergic pathways in the expression of opiate withdrawal: Biochemical and pharmacological evidence. Neurosci Biobehav Rev 1997;21:91-104.

53. Pappagallo M: Aggressive pharmacologic treatment of pain. Rheum Dis Clin North Am 1999;25:193-213.

54. Wilsey BL, Fishman SM: Minor and short-acting opioids. In Benzon HT, Raja SN, Molloy RE (eds): Essentials of Pain and Regional Anesthesia. Philadelphia, Elsevier Churchill Livingstone, 2005, pp 107-112.

55. Lyvers M: Drug addiction as a physical disease: The role of physical dependence and other chronic drug-induced neurophysiological changes in compulsive drug self-administration. Exp Clin Psychopharmacol 1998;6:107-125.

56. American Society of Addiction Medicine: Public policy statement on definitions related to the use of opioids in pain treatment. J Addict Dis 1998;17:129-133.

57. Fishbain DA, Rosomoff HL, Rosomoff RS: Drug abuse, dependence and addiction in chronic pain patients. Clin J Pain 1992;8:77-85.

58. Passik SD: Responding rationally to recent report of abuse/diversion of Oxycontin. J Pain Symptom Manage 2001; 21:359.

59. Potter M, Schafer S, Gonzalez-Mendez F, et al: Opioids for chronic nonmalignant pain. Attitudes and practices of primary care physicians in the UCSF/Stanford Collaborative Research Network. University of California, San Francisco. J Fam Pract 2001;50:145-151.

60. Arkinstall W, Sandler A, Goughnour B, et al: Efficacy of controlled-release codeine in chronic non-malignant pain: A randomized, placebo-controlled clinical trial. Pain 1995;62: 169-178.

61. Eckhardt K, Li S, Ammon S, et al: Same incidence of adverse drug events after codeine administration irrespective of the genetically determined differences in morphine formation. Pain 1998;76:27-33.

62. Susce MT, Carmichael-Murray E, deLeon J: Response to hydrocodone, codeine and oxycodone in a CYP2D6 poor metabolizer. Prog Neuropsychopharmacol Biol Psychiatry 2006; 30:1356-1358.

63. Loh H, Hiu HC, Cavalli A, et al: Mu Opioid receptor knockout mice: Effects on ligand-induced analgesia and morphine lethality. Brain Res Mol Brain Res 1998;54:321-326.

64. Peterson GM, Randall CT, Paterson J: Plasma levels of morphine and morphine glucuronides in the treatment of cancer pain: Relationship to renal function and route of administration. Eur J Pharmacol 1990;38:121-124.

65. Mahajan G, Fishman SM: Major opioids in pain management. In Benzon HT, Raja SN, Molloy RE et al (eds): Essentials of Pain and Regional Anesthesia. Philadelphia, Elsevier Churchill Livingstone, 2005, pp 94-105.

66. Cone EJ, Heit H, Caplan YH, et al: Evidence of morphine metabolism to hydromorphone in pain patients chronically treated with morphine. J Analyt Toxicol 2006;30:1-5.

67. Kalso E: Oxycodone. J Pain Symptom Manage 2005;29: S47-S56.

68. Karunatilake H, Buckly NA: Serotonin syndrome induced by fluvoxamine and oxycodone. Ann Pharmacol 2006; 40:155-157.

69. Sarhill N, Declan W, Nelson KA: Hydromorphone: Pharmacology and clinical applications in cancer patients. Support Care Cancer 2001;9:84-96.

70. Coda B, Tanaka A, Jacobson RC, et al: Hydromorphone analgesia after intravenous bolus administration. Pain 1997; 71:41-48.

71. Sandler A: Transdermal fentanyl: Acute analgesic clinical studies. J Symptom Manage 1992; 7:S27-S35.

72. Gourlay GK: Treatment of cancer pain with transdermal fentanyl. Lancet Oncol 2001;2:165-172.

73. Lichtor JL, Sevarino FB, Joshi GP, et al: The relative potency of oral transmucosal fentanyl of moderate to severe postoperative pain. Anesth Analg 1999;89:732-738.

74. Kristensen K, Blemmer T, Angelo HR, et al: Stereoselective pharmacokinetics of methadone in chronic pain patients. Ther Drug Monit 1996;18:221-227.

75. Rostami-Hodjegan A, Wolff K, Hay AW, et al: Population pharmacokinetics of methadone in opioid users: Characterization of time-dependent changes. Br J Clin Pharmacol 1999;48: 43-52.

76. Fishman SM, Wilsey B, Mahajan G, et al: Methadone reincarnated: Novel clinical applications with related concerns. Pain Med 2002;3:339-348.

77. Davis MP, Walsh D: Methadone for relief of cancer pain: A review of pharmacokinetics, pharmacodynamics, drug interactions, and protocols of administration. Support Care Cancer 2001;9:73-83.

78. Garrido MJ,Troconiz IF: Methadone: A review of its pharmacokinetic/pharmacodynamic properties. J Pharmacol Toxicol Methods 1999;42:61-66.

79. Ballesteros MF, Budnitz DS, Sanford CP, et al: Increase in deaths because of methadone in North Carolina [letter]. JAMA 2003;290:40.

80. Walker PW, Klein D, Kasza L: High-dose methadone and ventricular arrhythmias: A report of three cases. Pain 2003;103:321-324.

81. Krantz Mj, Lewkowiez L, Hayes H, et al: Torsades de pointes associated with very high dose methadone. Ann Intern Med 2002;137:501-504.

82. Gil M, Sala M, Anguera I, et al: QT prolongation and torsades de pointes in patients infected with human immunodeficiency virus and treated with methadone. Am J Cardiol 2003; 92:995-997.

83. McQuay H, Moore R: An Evidence-based Resource for Pain Relief. Oxford, Oxford University Press, 1999.

84. Przewlocki R, Przewlocka B: Opioids in neuropathic pain. Curr Pharm Des 2005;11:3013-3025.

85. Chen YP, Chen SR, Pan HC: Effect of morphine on deep dorsal horn projection neurons depends on spinal GABAergic and glycinergic tone: Implications for reduced opioid effect in neuropathic pain. J Pharmacol Exp Ther 2005;315: 696-703.

86. Gilron I, Bailey JM, Tu D, et al: Morphine, gabapentin, or their combination for neuropathic pain. N Engl J Med 2005; 352:1324-1334.

87. Furlan AD, Sandoval JA, Mailis-Gagnon A: Opioids for chronic noncancer pain: A meta-analysis of effectiveness and side effects. CMAJ 2006;174:1589-1594.

88. American Academy of Pain Medicine and the American Pain Society: The use of opioids for the treatment of chronic pain: A consensus statement from the American Academy of Pain Medicine and the American Pain Society, 1996. Available at www.ampainsoc.org/advocacy/opoids.htm.

89. Federation of State Medical Boards of the United States: Model Policy for the Use of Controlled Substances for the Treatment of Pain, 2004. Available at www.fsmb.org/pdf/2004_grpol_Controlled_Substances.pdf.

90. Working RH, Hazel RD, Banks SM: Toward a model of the pathogenesis of chronic pain. Semin Clin Neuropsychiatry 1999;4:176-185.

91. Vlaeyen JW, Crombez G: Fear of movement/(re) injury, avoidance and pain disability in chronic low back pain patients. Manual Ther 1999;4:187-195.

92. Feldman SI, Downey G, Schaffer-Nets R: Pain, negative mood, and perceived support in chronic pain patients: A daily diary study people with reflex sympathetic dystrophy syndrome. J Consult Clin Psychol 1999;67:776-785.

CHAPTER

32 Minor and Short-Acting Analgesics, Including Opioid Combination Products

Steven P. Stanos and Mark D. Tyburski

The use of naturally occurring plant materials for the relief of pain dates back to early times. Advances in antipyretic and analgesic medicines began in the late 1800s with the development of salicylic acid, antipyrine, phenacetin, and acetaminophen.[1] These basic medicines are still used today to various degrees in both over-the-counter (OTC) and prescription preparations—the minor analgesics salicylic acid and acetaminophen are widely marketed and heavily consumed. Minor analgesics for acute and chronic pain include a number of prescription and OTC agents, which may be useful in isolation or as adjuvants in a more comprehensive multimodal pharmacologic approach. Adjuvants refer to agents that enhance the effect of other medications but may not be fully effective when used alone. A population survey has reported that the use of OTC medications, many of which include minor analgesics, account for the most common method of relieving pain (53%). This is closely followed by physical exercise (52%) and prescription medications (35%).[2]

The minor analgesics reviewed in this chapter include oral acetaminophen, opioid combination preparations, tramadol, steroids, and caffeine, as well as topical compounds and delivery systems (Box 32–1). See the chapters in this text that discuss opioids, anticonvulsants, antidepressants, and NSAIDs for complete information on those topics (Chapters 31, 33, 34, and 35). Additional combination OTC forms using minor analgesics include convenience combinations—those that contain aspirin, acetaminophen, or ibuprofen plus other remedies such as nasal decongestants, antihistamines, cough suppressants, or antacids. These are useful for treating the sequelae of a primary illness (e.g., cold and flu symptoms, insomnia, cough) and any pain symptoms that may coexist.[3]

Prescribing habits regarding the use of analgesics for the treatment of various musculoskeletal conditions continues to evolve. Caudill-Slosberg and colleagues[4] have compared prescribing habits between 1980 and 1981 to those between 1999 and 2000, and demonstrated a significant increase in those patients receiving a prescription for acute and chronic musculoskeletal pain. Increases were seen with nonselective nonsteroidal anti-inflammatory drugs (NSAIDs) and cyclooxygenase-2 (COX-2) agents, as well as more potent opioids, including combination opioid preparations containing acetaminophen and NSAIDs.

Minor analgesics are widely used, with reported prevalence rates of twice-weekly use of approximately 8.7% for prescription drugs and 8.8% for OTC analgesics. Analgesic use has constituted the largest selling group of OTC medications in a number of population studies.[5] Daily use was more common for prescribed analgesics, whereas OTC analgesics were used a few times per week.[6,7] Among prescription and OTC medications, acetaminophen, ibuprofen, and aspirin were the most commonly used, by 17% to 23% of the population.[8] Use of analgesics, many of which include minor agents, accounts for a significant cost of health care dollars. In a recent population study, analgesic costs ranked second behind diagnostic imaging in expenditures for the treatment of acute low back pain.[7] Chronic use of prescription and OTC analgesics (i.e., aspirin, nonaspirin NSAIDs, and acetaminophen) may continue for longer than 1 year. In the same survey, approximately 2.3 million adults reported using nonaspirin NSAIDs and 2.6 million used acetaminophen on a frequent basis for longer than 5 years.[9] This widespread use occurs despite a general knowledge of the increased risks of gastrointestinal (GI), renal, and/or cardiac toxicity with short-

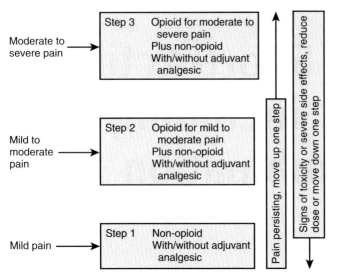

Figure 32–1. The World Health Organization (WHO) analgesic ladder. (Adapted from World Health Organization: Cancer Pain Relief. Geneva, World Health Organization, 1990.)

BOX 32–1. MINOR ANALGESICS

Minor opioids and combination products
Acetaminophen
Tramadol
Oral steroids
Caffeine and combination products
Topical medications (analgesics, rubefacients, local anesthetics, cooling agents, heating agents)
Over-the-counter convenience products

---

term and chronic use. Unfortunately perceptions remain that as a class of medications, OTC and prescription NSAIDs are relatively safe. This misbelief leads to frequent inappropriate use and the potential for serious adverse events.[10] The increased availability and marketing of OTC agents has likely contributed to patient misuse, with consumers still unaware of the potential catastrophic risks associated with their use—60% of people cannot identify the active ingredient in their analgesics and 40% of Americans believe that OTC drugs are too weak to cause significant harm.[11]

The use of OTC and prescription analgesics is not only confined to the outpatient setting. Significant use of these agents in nursing home facilities was reported in a group of Medicare beneficiaries during 2001. Patients averaged 8.8 unique medications per month, including 2.9 OTC medications. Of these subjects, 70% used non-opioid OTC analgesics and 19.0% used non-opioid prescription analgesics.[12]

SPECIFIC DRUGS

Minor Opioids

In this chapter, minor opioids are defined as analgesic combination products with codeine, propoxy-

phene, hydrocodone, or oxycodone. These products continue to account for a large percentage of prescriptions written for chronic nonmalignant pain. Combination opioid analgesics—compounds containing acetaminophen or anti-inflammatory medications—make up a significant amount of opioids prescribed by primary care physicians[13] and pain specialists. Combination analgesics are advocated in several treatment guidelines, including the three-step analgesic ladder of the World Health Organization[14,15] (Fig. 32–1). Since the 1990s, the use of minor analgesic combinations containing oxycodone and hydrocodone has continued to increase, whereas the use of those containing propoxyphene and codeine has declined. Clinic type (e.g., primary care, spine center, pain center), geographic, and socioeconomic variables may also affect prescribing practices.[16]

Opioid analgesics as a class, can be categorized into three chemical groups: (1) synthetic phenlypiperidines (e.g., meperidine, fentanyl); (2) synthetic pseudopiperidines (e.g., methadone, propoxyphene); and (3) naturally occurring alkaloids derived directly from the poppy seed (e.g., heroin, morphine, codeine) and their semisynthetic derivatives (e.g., hydromorphone, oxycodone, oxymorphone).[17] This chapter will review codeine, propoxyphene, oxycodone, hydrocodone, and tramadol, all natural or synthetic opioids used in isolation or in combination forms for the treatment of mild to moderate pain (Tables 32–1 and 32–2).

Pharmacokinetics and Pharmacodynamics

An understanding of pharmacokinetics and pharmacodynamics is essential for appropriately prescribing minor opioid analgesics, interpreting related toxicology screens, and appreciating potential mechanisms for adverse side effects. In general, medications are primarily metabolized by the cytochrome P-450 (CYP) and glucuronidation pathways. Opioid analgesics, like any medication, may be metabolized by the CYP drug-metabolizing enzyme system 2D6. Genetic polymorphism of CYP2D6 may lead to variability in enzyme breakdown and clinical effectiveness of the medication. Deficiency of CYP2D6 may be seen in whites (7%) and those of Asian descent (1%).[18] These enzyme systems can be induced (activated) or inhibited by various agents, including drugs, alcohol, and cigarette smoke, as well as endogenous substances. Inducers are agents that activate the CYP enzyme system, leading to increased metabolism and reduced drug effect. Inhibitors may impair the CYP enzyme system, limiting metabolism of the drug, and thus increasing drug effect. Although pharmacokinetic drug-drug interactions may affect serum levels of a drug, this may be subclinical in most patients, with significant interactions occurring rarely in vivo, in only 10% to 15% of patients.[19] Patient response to individual opioids may vary markedly. Recent evidence has supported more than one mechanism for μ-opioid analgesic reaction, which may be related to receptor polymorphism.[20]

Table 32–1. Minor and Short-Acting Opioids

CLASS	NAME	ADULT DOSE	HALF-LIFE (ONSET)	MECHANISM OF ACTION	OTHER
Natural opium alkaloids	Codeine with acetaminophen or acetylsalicylic acid (ASA) (Tylenol No. 2, No. 3, No. 4, Empirin No. 3, No. 4, Capital with Codeine, Aceta, Fioricet with Codeine, Fiorinal with Codeine	PO: 15-60 mg q4h (max daily acetaminophen (APAP)-ASA dose, 4 g)	2.5-3.5 hr PO (30-60 min)	Opioid agonist activity at multiple receptors—μ (supraspinal analgesia and euphoria), κ (spinal analgesia and sedation), δ (dysphoria, psychotomimetic effects)	Compared with morphine—decreased analgesia, constipation, respiratory distress, sedation, emesis, and physical dependence; increased antitussive effects
Phenanthrene derivatives	Hydrocodone plus ASA or acetaminophen (Lortab, Lortab ASA, Vicodin, Norco, Vicoprofen, ZTuss, P-V-Tussin, Tussafed HC)	PO: 5-10 mg q4-6h (max daily APAP/ASA dose, 4 g)	3.8 hr (10-30 min)	Opioid agonist activity at multiple receptors—μ (supraspinal analgesia and euphoria), κ (spinal analgesia and sedation), δ (dysphoria, psychotomimetic effects)	Compared with morphine—equivalent analgesia, respiratory depression, and physical dependency; equivalent antitussive effects
	Oxycodone (with or without acetaminophen or ASA) (OxyIR, Roxicodone) Oxycodone plus ASA (Percodan, Endodan, Roxiprin) Oxycodone plus acetaminophen (Percocet, Endocet, Tylox, Roxicet, Roxilox)	PO: 5-30 mg q4-6h (4 g max dose of ASA/APAP); sustained-release: 10/10-160 mg q12h	2-5 hr (10-15 min)	Opioid agonist activity at multiple receptors: μ (supraspinal analgesia and euphoria), κ (spinal analgesia and sedation), δ (dysphoria, psychotomimetic effects)	Compared with morphine—more potent analgesia, constipation, antitussive effects, respiratory depression, sedation, emesis, and physical dependence
Diphenylheptane derivative	Propoxyphene, with or without acetaminophen (Darvon, Darvon-N) Propoxyphene plus acetaminophen (Darvocet A500, Propacet 100)	PO: 65 mg q4h (max, 390 mg/day); napsylate, 100 mg q4h (max, 600 mg/day)	6-12 hr (15-60 min)	Opioid agonist activity at multiple receptors: μ (supraspinal analgesia and euphoria), κ (spinal analgesia and sedation), δ (dysphoria, psychotomimetic effects)	Compared with morphine—less analgesia, sedation, emesis, respiratory depression, and physical dependence

Table 32–2. Opioid Combination Products

DRUG CLASS	DRUG NAME	TRADE NAME	AVAILABLE DOSE	TYPICAL DOSE	COMMENTS	HALF-LIFE
Para-aminophenol derivatives/natural opium alkaloids	Acetaminophen (APAP)/codeine phosphate	Tylenol with Codeine elixir, Tylenol with codeine No. 2, No. 3, No. 4	(120/12 mg/5 mL liquid; 300/15 mg, 300/30 mg, 300/60 mg (tablets)	Elixir—children <3 yr, safe dosage not established; 3-6 yr, 5 mL (1 tsp) 3-4 times daily; 7-12 yr, 10 mL 3-4 times daily: adults, 15 mL q4h; tablets and capsules, 15-60 mg codeine q4-6h	Codeine phosphate, max, 360 mg daily; acetaminophen, max, 4000 mg daily	Acetaminophen, 1-4 hr; codeine, 2.5-3 hr
			650/30 mg (tablets)	30-60 mg codeine q4-6h	Codeine phosphate, max, 360 mg daily; acetaminophen, max, 4000 mg daily	Acetaminophen, 1-4 hr; codeine, 2.5-3 hr
Acetylsalicylic acid/natural opium alkaloids	Aspirin/codeine phosphate	Empirin with Codeine No. 3, No. 4	325/30 mg, 325/60 mg (tablets)	1-2 tablets q4h	Codeine phosphate, max, 360 mg daily	Aspirin, 2.5-3.5 hr; codeine, 2.5-3 hr
Para-aminophenol derivatives/phenanthrene derivatives	Hydrocodone bitartrate/acetaminophen	Vicodin, Lorcet-HD, Lortab, Norco, Maxidone, Anexsia	2.5/500 mg, 5/500 mg, 7.5/325 mg, 7.5/500 mg, 7.5/650 mg, 7.5/750 mg, 10/325 mg, 10/500 mg, 10/650 mg, 10/660 mg, 10/750 mg (tablets)	1-2 tablets q4-6h	Dosage typically limited by acetaminophen, max, 4000 mg daily	Hydrocodone, 3.5-4.1 hr
	Oxycodone/acetaminophen	Percocet, Endocet, Tylox, Roxicet, Roxilox	5/325 mg, 7.5/325 mg, 5/500 mg (Tylox), 7.5/500 mg, 10/325 mg, 10/650 mg (tablets); Roxicet; 5/325 mg)/5 mL (solution) (Roxicet)	1-2 tablets q4-6h	Acetaminophen, max, 4000 mg daily	Acetaminophen, 1-4 hr; oxycodone, 3.1-3.7 hr
Acetylsalicylic acid/phenanthrene derivatives	Oxycodone/aspirin	Percodan, Endodan, Roxiprin	4.8/325 mg tablet	1 tablet q4-6h	Aspirin, max, 4000 mg daily	Aspirin, 2.5-3.5 hr; oxycodone, 3.1-3.7 hr
Propionic acid/phenanthrene derivatives	Hydrocodone bitartrate/ibuprofen	Vicoprofen	7.5/200 mg (tablets)	1 tablet q4-6h	Marketed for short-term management of acute pain; NSAIDs may increase risk of serious cardiovascular thrombotic events, myocardial infarction, stroke	Hydrocodone, 3.5-4.1 hr; ibuprofen, 4-6 hr
	Oxycodone/ibuprofen	Combunox	5/400 mg (tablets)	1-2 tablets q4-6h	Max dosage ibuprofen, 2400-3200 mg daily	Oxycodone, 3.1-3.7 hr; ibuprofen, 1.8-2.6 hr
Diphenylheptane derivatives	Propxyphene HCl/APAP		65/650 mg (tablets)	1 tablet q4-6h	Structurally related to methadone; propoxyphene HCl, max, 390 mg daily	Propoxyphene, 6-12 hr; norpropoxyphene, 30-36 hr; acetaminophen, 1-4 hr
	Propxyphene HCl/aspirin/caffeine	Darvon Compound 65	65/389/32.4 mg (tablets)	1-2 tablets q4-6h	Structurally related to methadone; propoxyphene HCl, max, 390 mg daily	Propoxyphene, 6-12 hr; norpropoxyphene, 30-36 hr; aspirin, 2.5-3.5 hr; caffeine, 3-6 hr
	Propoxyphene napsylate/APAP	Darvocet-N 50, Darvocet-N 100, Darvocet A500, Propacet 100	50/325 mg (N 50), 100/650 mg (N 100), 100/500 mg (A500) (tablets)	1-2 tablets q4-6h	Structurally related to methadone; propoxyphene napsylate, max, 600 mg daily	Propoxyphene, 6-12 hr; norpropoxyphene, 30-36 hr; acetaminophen, 1-4 hr

Table 32–3. Combination Analgesics for Mild to Moderate Pain

AGENT	ONSET (min)	DURATION OF ACTION (hr)	EQUIANALGESIC ORAL DOSE (mg)*	DEA SCHEDULE
Oxycodone combinations	10-15	4-6	30[†]	II
Hydrocodone combinations	30-60	4-6	30	III
Codeine combinations	30-60	4-6	130	III
Propoxyphene combinations	15-60	4-6	130	IV
Tramadol combinations	60	6-7	100	Not scheduled

DEA, U.S. Drug Enforcement Agency.
*Doses reflect opioid component only and are equianalgesic to 30 mg morphine.
[†]Doses for moderate to severe pain not necessarily equivalent to 30 mg morphine
From Gutstein HB, Akil H: Opioid analgesics. In Hardman JG, Limbird LE, Gilman AG (eds): Goodman and Gilman's The Pharmacological Basis of Therapeutics, 10th ed. New York: McGraw Hill, 2001, pp 569-619.

Morphine, hydromorphone, and oxymorphone are not metabolized by CYP but are metabolized by uridine diphosphate glucuronosyltransferase (UGT) enzymes. Except for morphine and codeine, UGT enzymes metabolize medications primarily to inactive metabolites. Morphine is converted to large quantities of relatively inactive morphine-3-glucuronide (M3G) and smaller quantities of the active metabolite, morphine-6-glucuronide (M6G). M6G is 50 times more potent than morphine. M3G may account for central nervous system (CNS) toxicity, including lowering of seizure thresholds.[21] Equianalgesic oral doses of the various minor opioid combination products compared with those of morphine are listed in Table 32–3.

Codeine

Along with morphine and thebaine, codeine (methylmorphine) is a naturally occurring opium alkaloid derivative. Codeine, a weak analgesic, is similar in structure to morphine, but with an affinity to the μ-opioid receptor that is 300 times lower. Classically, codeine is thought to be metabolized by O-demethylation to its primary active metabolite, morphine, by CYP2D6 enzyme.[22] Studies have demonstrated that only a small percentage of the total dose (3%)[23] is converted by CYP2D6 to morphine. Approximately 80% is directly glucuronidated by UGT2B7 to codeine-6-glucuronide (C6G), an additional active metabolite. The remaining inactive metabolites are primarily norcodeine (2%) and normorphine (2.4%).[24] Nonfunctional CYP2D6 renders codeine ineffective, perhaps because of genetic mutations or deletions[25] or pharmacologic inhibition.[26] Codeine effects not related to morphine formation include cognitive impairment,[27] sedation, dizziness, euphoria and dysphoria, headache, blurred vision,[28] and prolongation of gastrointestinal transit time.[29] The average half-life of codeine is 2.5 hours.

Efficacy
When used alone, codeine is typically prescribed in doses of 30 to 60 mg every 4 to 6 hours, with an onset of analgesia at 30 to 60 minutes and a duration of effect lasting 4 to 6 hours.

Codeine has been shown to be an effective cough suppressant (10 to 120 mg/day) and is present in a number of OTC cold and cough convenience preparations.[30] However, codeine's potential opioid analgesic effect has long been questioned. Houde's classic study in the 1960s reported the analgesic effects of codeine (32 mg) to be no more than 650 mg of aspirin, although both were more than placebo.[31] The NNT (number needed to treat—the number of patients needed to receive the medication to achieve at least 50% pain relief) of 60 mg codeine has been reported as 16.7,[32] leading to its widespread use as a combination analgesic.

Codeine (10 to 60 mg) is more commonly prescribed in combination with acetaminophen (APAP; 400 to 1000 mg), aspirin, or NSAIDs such as ibuprofen (400 mg). A systematic review of codeine and acetaminophen trials for acute noncancer pain concluded that the benefit over codeine alone is only modest (5%).[33] A systematic review of trials of APAP alone or in combination with codeine noted efficacy with patients prescribed APAP plus 60 mg codeine as compared with APAP alone. At doses more than 60 mg, there was diminishing incremental analgesia with increasing dose and a higher incidence of side effects (e.g., constipation, nausea, and sedation).[34] A head-to-head study of codeine (30 mg)-acetaminophen (300 mg) and hydrocodone (7.5 mg)-acetaminophen (500 mg) showed significant relief of moderate to severe acute (6 hours) postoperative pain compared with placebo, but the analgesia was no greater than that achieved with hydrocodone-acetaminophen.[35]

Propoxyphene (Dextropropoxyphene)

Propoxyphene (dextropropoxyphene) is a mild synthetic opioid originally synthesized in the 1950s and primarily marketed in its hydrochloride form as Darvon (65 mg; maximum, 400 mg/day), propoxyphene napsylate (Darvocet-N 50, Darvocet-N 100), and in Europe as co-proxamol (32.5 mg dextropropoxyphene plus 325 mg of paracetamol). By the late

1960s, propoxyphene was the most widely prescribed analgesic in the United States.[36] Reports of propoxyphene overdoses led to warnings by the U.S. Food and Drug Administration (FDA) in 1978 and a subsequent reduction in use.[37] Propoxyphene use continues, however, primarily for older adults, because of its perceived safety profile.[38] However, Smith[39] has suggested that its analgesic activity is lower than that of aspirin. Because of the increasing number of fatal overdoses of co-proxamol and limited evidence supporting its efficacy versus acetaminophen for acute and chronic pain, the British government announced the gradual withdrawal of co-praxamol from British markets in January 2005.[40]

Propoxyphene has a half-life of approximately 6 hours. Its major active metabolite, norpropoxyphene, has a variable half-life (30 to 36 hours), leading to accumulation with repeated dosing and possibly contributing to cardiac and central nervous system toxicity. Norpropoxyphene has fewer central nervous system effects than propoxyphene but accumulates in cardiac tissue, leading to a local anesthetic effect and prolongation of action potentials, in some cases fatal torsade de pointes.[41] A meta-analysis has concluded there is little evidence to support the use of a propoxyphene-acetaminophen combination as compared with acetaminophen alone for cases of moderate short-term pain.[42]

Oxycodone

Oxycodone is a semisynthetic opioid analgesic derived from the opium alkaloid thebaine. Human studies have demonstrated it to have an analgesic potency 1.5 times that of morphine after oral administration.[43] A number of active metabolites have been proposed as contributing to the clinical pharmacokinetics of oxycodone. One theory supports 3-O-demethylation by CYP2D6 to oxymorphone. Oxymorphone is a potent μ-opioid ligand, with two to five times higher receptor affinity compared with morphine. Although potent, oxymorphone accounts for only 10% of oxycodone metabolites. Oxymorphone has been available for a number of years for parenteral and rectal use, and was more recently reformulated and released in an immediate-release and extended-release scheduled II formulation. In vitro studies have shown that O-demethylation of oxycodone accounts for 13% of oxidative metabolism. Oxidation of oxycodone primarily occurs via N-demethylation by CYP3A4/5 to noroxycodone, representing the most abundant circulating metabolite in human studies. Unfortunately, noroxycodone has weak affinity for μ-opioid receptors.[44]

In vivo, oxycodone has potent μ-opioid receptor effects, but data suggest that the intrinsic antinociceptive effects may be additionally mediated by κ-opioid receptors.[45] This has led some to consider oxycodone as an ideal medication for opioid rotation in patients not responsive to morphine, a classic μ-opioid receptor agonist.[46,47] Recent studies have proposed non-CYP2D6 metabolites (noroxycodone, noroxymorphone, noroxycodols, oxycodols) as additional substances responsible for μ-opioid receptor binding and analgesic effects.[48] Animal studies have recently demonstrated conflicting gender-related differences in female versus male rats when examining the antinociceptive effects of oxycodone.[49]

Hydrocodone

Hydrocodone is similar in structure to codeine but is six to eight times more potent.[50] Hydrocodone is a prodrug and undergoes CYP2D6 metabolism to hydromorphone and CYP3A4 metabolism to noroxycodone. Hydrocodone is less potent than morphine by receptor affinity and demonstrates a relative analgesic potency of 0.59 compared with morphine. The discrepancy between hydrocodone's binding affinity and potency compared with that of morphine is possibly the result of active hydrocodone metabolites or intrinsic efficacy of receptor activation, which is more efficient for hydrocodone compared with morphine.[51] Hydrocodone is marketed as a combination product with APAP, ibuprofen, and aspirin.

Efficacy

The hydrocodone-ibuprofen combination product was introduced in the United States in 1997 as a fixed dose of hydrocodone (7.5 mg) and ibuprofen (200 mg), and has demonstrated efficacy for acute postoperative pain.[52] Neither hydrocodone (7.5 mg) nor ibuprofen (200 mg) given alone was superior to placebo, supporting the concept of analgesic synergy with the two agents. Similar findings were demonstrated in acute low back pain[53] and postoperative obstetric and gynecologic pain.[54] Hydrocodone-APAP (7.5, 200 mg), one and two tablets, was compared with a fixed-dose combination of codeine (30 mg) and APAP (300 mg). The two-tablet dose of combination hydrocodone-APAP was more effective than the one-tablet dose and one or two tablets of the fixed codeine-APAP combination.[55]

Acetaminophen

Acetaminophen (APAP, paracetamol) and acetaminophen combination products (i.e., containing opioids) are commonly prescribed as a minor analgesic for acute and chronic pain (see Table 32–2). The American College of Rheumatology and similar European professional colleges have recommended it as a first-line pharmacologic therapy for the treatment of osteoarthritis (OA).[56,57] Prescription APAP is available as an opioid-containing combination product (e.g., codeine, hydrocodone, oxycodone), whereas OTC preparations may be combined with pseudoephedrine or dextromethorphan as convenience drugs.

Mechanism of Action and Description

Acetaminophen (paracetamol) is a *p*-aminophenol analgesic introduced in the late 1800s in Germany, a product of the rapidly developing chemical industry. Newly synthesized compounds included synthetic antipyretics and analgesics such as aceto-phenetidin (phenacetin), antipyrine (phenazone), and acetylsalicylic acid (ASA; aspirin).[58] Paracetamol, the active metabolite of phenacetin, was found to demonstrate less intense GI side effects, leading to its use as an analgesic. Paracetamol was formerly introduced in the United States in the 1950s and, although was found in the 1960s to have hepatotoxic effects with unintentional misuse and overdose, it became one of the most widely used OTC and combination prescription analgesics worldwide.

Although acetaminophen has been in use since the 1890s, its pharmacologic mechanism of action remains unclear. Generally, it has known analgesic and antipyretic activity, with no known peripheral anti-inflammatory or platelet effects. Its antipyretic activity may be secondary to the blockade of prostaglandin (PG) production and inhibition of prostaglandin endoperoxide H_2 synthase (PGHS) and COX centrally. Acetaminophen may block COX activity by reducing the active form of COX to an inactive form but with only limited effects in the GI tract and peripherally at sites of inflammation, thus contributing to a lower GI side effect profile as compared with NSAIDs.[59] Also, recent studies have suggested central analgesic qualities may be related to decreasing the activation of a subtype of endogenous opioid peptide, β-endorphin.[60]

APAP is available in oral and rectal formulations and is rapidly absorbed from the GI tract, mainly the small intestine.[61] APAP has a $t_{1/2}$ of between 1.25 and 3 hours and serum therapeutic levels of 10 to 30 µg/mL. Twenty-five percent of the dose undergoes first-pass metabolism in the liver. Up to 90% of APAP is metabolized in the liver via glucuronidation and sulfate conjugation, forming nontoxic metabolites. The remaining 10% undergoes oxidative metabolism

via the CYP system (CYP2E1 and CYP1A2), which is responsible for the formation of the potentially hepatotoxic and nephrotoxic metabolite N-acetyl-p-benzoquinoneimine (NAPQI; Fig. 32–2). This minor pathway becomes more critical when the enzyme system responsible for sulfonation and glucuronidation becomes saturated with doses greater than 150 mg/kg, increasing the total fraction of NAPQI. Approximately 85% of the dose is excreted in the urine within 24 hours of oral dosing. NAPQI is itself detoxified by conjugation with glutathione.[62] Case reports have suggested that clinical situations of low glutathione levels (e.g., chronic hepatitis C, malnourishment, HIV infection, cirrhosis) may place these patients at greater risk for adverse events from acetaminophen. However, one study has found no significant evidence that these populations are at higher risk for acetaminophen toxicity.[63] There are few clinically significant pharmacokinetic interactions with therapeutic doses of APAP. Although case reports have attributed an elevated international normalized ratio (INR) to APAP and oral anticoagulant drug interactions,[64] randomized controlled studies have found no evidence of clinically significant INR changes.[65] Although studies have demonstrated an association, there is no clear evidence of cause and effect.[66]

Risks and Precautions

Acetaminophen-induced toxicity is often associated with liver and renal dysfunction. Acetaminophen

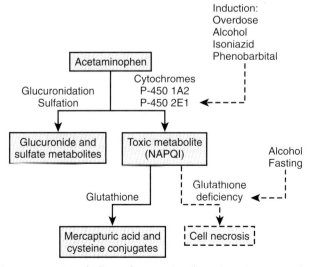

Figure 32–2. Metabolism of acetaminophen. NAPQI, N-acetyl-p-benzoquinoneimine. (From Barkin RL: Acetaminophen, aspirin, or ibuprofen in combination analgesic products. Am J Ther 2001;8: 433-442.)

BOX 32–2. ACETAMINOPHEN DOSING CONSIDERATIONS

Dosing for Mild Pain
- 325-1000 mg PO, per rectum, q4-6h
- Maximum dose: 1 g/dose; 4 g/24 hr
- American Liver Foundation: Patients should not exceed 3 g/day for any prolonged period.*

Renal Impairment
- Adjust dose frequency.
- CrCl = 10-50 mL/min, q6h; CrCl < 10 mL/min, q8h

Hepatic Impairment
- Use with caution.
- Consider decreasing dose; monitor liver function; avoid chronic use.

Counseling Patients
Acetaminophen (APAP) in over-the-counter products:
- Regular-strength APAP products commonly contain 325 mg/tablet.
- Extra-strength APAP products commonly contain 500 mg/tablet.

*Based on recent study by Watkins and Seeff.[68]

hypersensitivity reactions are rare, but severe reactions are possible. In general, chronic administration of acetaminophen may cause depletion of glutathione stores, leading to a greater production of the hepatoxic and nephrotoxic metabolite, NAPQI. Current recommendations for a maximum daily dosage of APAP are approximately 4 g/day for adults and 75 mg/kg/day for infants or children[67] (Box 32–2). Unintentional liver injury, such as hepatic necrosis or acute liver failure (ALF) from self-medication with OTC and prescription acetaminophen products, can develop with dosages exceeding 4 g/day.

The serum alanine aminotransferase (ALT) level may be elevated with acute use of recommended doses of acetaminophen. Watkins and Seeff[68] studied healthy adults given 4 g of acetaminophen for 14 days. They found that 31% to 44% of the study subjects, which included patients on acetaminophen and various opioid-acetaminophen combination products, demonstrated elevations at three times the upper limit of normal (typically considered clinically significant). Opioids were found to have no additional effect on ALT levels. Elevation of liver function is not routinely seen with chronic use and is thought to occur because of cellular adaptation.[68] This acetaminophen tolerance may be characterized by possible downregulation of CYP bioactivation and increases in glutathione production by liver hepatocytes.[69]

The concomitant use of alcohol and APAP resulting in increased risk, lower threshold for hepatic and renal toxicity, or both remains controversial, and has been primarily reported in retrospective reviews and case reports.[70] Acute and chronic alcohol use contributes to drug-induced hepatotoxicity via induction of CYP2E1 and NAPQI formation.[71] Enhanced ethanol-related toxicity was demonstrated only in patients at high risk with APAP levels above 300 mg/mL, a level far above the package insert recommendation of no more than three alcoholic beverages daily.[72] Ethanol may block the formation of NAPQI when consumed with APAP.[73] Other inducers of hepatic isoenzymes CYP2E1 and CYP1A2 commonly used for pain management include carbamazepine, oxcarbazepine, barbiturates, and phenytoin[74] (Table 32–4). Most importantly, the risk of acetaminophen-induced hepatotoxicity may be increased in patients with alcoholic hepatic disease, viral hepatitis, or alcoholism because of a reduction in glucuronide conjugation and subsequent depletion of glutathione reserves.

Chronic acetaminophen prescribing should be avoided in patients with renal disease, although the exact mechanism of injury is unknown and may be relevant only for patients with preexisting renal compromise or systemic disease.[75] Patients with a history of salicylate hypersensitivity characterized by drug-induced urticaria have demonstrated an 11% cross-reactivity to acetaminophen.[76] Acetaminophen use has been shown to be associated with hypertension in two large prospective studies in women.[77,78] Similar studies in healthy men failed to show an association with acetaminophen use and hypertension.[79] Analgesics, in general, may modestly affect blood pressure via a number of mechanisms—primarily through kidney or systemic COX-2 inhibition of prostaglandins—leading to an imbalance between vasodilators PGI_2 and PGE_2 and vasoconstrictors $PGF_{2\alpha}$ and thromboxane A_2. These effects on PG synthesis are greater with NSAIDs compared with acetaminophen.[80]

Clinical Use

Although a number of guidelines have recommended APAP as a first-line agent, advantages over NSAIDs in managing OA-related pain remain controversial. A double-blinded trial of paracetamol, 4 g/day, for 1 month was as effective as both analgesic and anti-inflammatory doses of ibuprofen in patients with knee OA.[81] More recent studies have demonstrated the efficacy of both a traditional NSAID (diclofenac)[82] and a COX-2 inhibitor (celecoxib)[83] versus APAP in hip and knee osteoarthritis cohorts. A Cochrane Database review of acetaminophen for the chronic pain of osteoarthritis found the drug to be less effective than NSAIDs in pain reduction scores, although the superiority of NSAIDs over acetaminophen appeared to be more evident in OA patients with more severe pain. Both NSAID and acetaminophen groups had similar efficacy with regard to functional status.[84] Recent evidence has suggested that acetaminophen may retain anti-inflammatory action comparable to that of NSAIDs in patients with knee osteoarthritis. Brandt and associates[85] performed a pilot study of 30 subjects diagnosed with osteoarthritis of the knee and showed that treatment with acetaminophen results in similar significant decreases in mean total knee effusion volume (measured by magnetic resonance imaging, MRI) as those treated with NSAIDs.

Tramadol

Tramadol, (±)cis-2-[(dimethylamino)methyl]-1-(3-methoxyphenyl)-cyclohexanol hydrochloride, is a syn-

Table 32–4. Agents that Increase Risk of Acetaminophen Hepatotoxicity through Cytochrome P-450 (CYP) Induction

CYP1A2	CYP2E1
Barbiturates	Ethanol
Bupropion (possible)	Isoniazid
Caffeine	
Carbamazepine	
Charcoal-broiled food	
Cruciferous vegetable	
Dihydralazine	
Isoniazid	
Phenytoin	
Primidone	
Rifampin	
Ritonavir	
Sulfinpyrazone	

Adapted from Barkin RL: Acetaminophen, aspirin, or ibuprofen in combination analgesic products. Am J Ther 2001;8:433-442.

thetic racemic mixture typically used for its centrally acting analgesic properties. However, clinical and basic science studies have described numerous mechanisms of action at central and peripheral sites. Tramadol is classified as a weak synthetic opioid, with mild serotonin and norepinephrine reuptake-inhibiting effects.[86,87]

Mechanism of Action and Description

The most well-studied mechanism of action for tramadol is its weak affinity for opioid receptors, the most significant of which is at the μ receptor. However, tramadol-induced analgesia is only partially inhibited by the opiate antagonist naloxone, suggesting additional non-opioid analgesic mechanisms.[88] Tramadol also displays an inhibitory effect on central neuronal norepinephrine (NE) and serotonin (5-HT) reuptake systems. More recently, noted actions include a local anesthetic effect, anti-inflammatory effects in rat experimental models, and reduction of substance P levels in human synovial fluid.[89,90] Although α_2 agonist activity has also been reported, concentrations in the range of 10 to 100 μmol/L do not bind significantly to α_2- adrenergic receptors.

Opioid Receptors

Tramadol's affinity for the μ receptor appears to be approximately 10 times weaker than codeine, 60 times weaker than dextropropoxyphene, and 6000 times weaker than morphine.[88] (Table 32-5). The active O-demethylated metabolite M1 has a 300 times higher affinity for the μ receptor than the parent compound and is up to six times more potent in producing analgesia.[91]

Central Neuronal Actions

Multiple actions affecting descending inhibitory pain pathways have been reported.[92,93] The first system involves neurons originating in the periaqueductal gray matter (PAG) in the midbrain that synapse at the nucleus raphe magnus (RM), from where fibers then project to the spinal cord. Reuptake inhibition

of 5-HT may contribute to pain inhibition. Another pathway originates at the locus coeruleus (LC) in the pons, projecting fibers to the spinal cord. Norepinephrine released from this pathway inhibits pain responses at the spinal cord by an α-adrenergic mechanism.

Activation of these descending pain inhibition pathways stimulates interneurons that inhibit transmission of painful stimuli in the dorsal horn by the action of endogenous opioids. Opioid receptor activity has been proposed to be mediated by the dextrorotatory (+) enantiomer as compared with the levorotary (−) enantiomer.[94] The (−) enantiomer is approximately 10 times more potent than its (+) counterpart in the inhibition of NE uptake, and the (+) enantiomer is approximately 4 times more potent than the (−) enantiomer in the inhibition of 5-HT uptake. M1 retains higher affinity for the μ-opioid receptor (300 to 400 times) and possesses greater analgesic activity than the parent compound. The M1 (+) enantiomer acts at the μ receptor, whereas the M1 (−) enantiomer mainly inhibits NE reuptake[92,93] (Table 32–6).

Formulations include immediate- and sustained-release (SR) oral forms (SR, every 12-hour dosing; extended-release [ER] form, every 24-hour dosing), injectable solutions for subcutaneous, intravenous, spinal, or intramuscular administration, and a rectal formulation. SR formulations are available in a number of countries worldwide, but only the ER formulation is currently available in the United States. In addition, an orally disintegrating tablet version of tramadol (Ralivia FlashDose) for the treatment of moderate to moderately severe pain is under development.[95] Tramadol is currently recommended for the treatment of moderate to moderately severe pain in patients unresponsive to previous oral therapies or who have a contraindication to COX-2 selective or nonselective NSAIDs.[9]

History

Tramadol has been available in Germany since 1977, where it remains one of the most widely prescribed analgesics. Prior to its U.S. release in 1995, clinical[96] and epidemiologic studies[97] suggested that tramadol demonstrates a low abuse potential, leading the Drug

Table 32–5. Affinity of Tramadol and Selected Compounds for Opioid Receptors

| DRUG | K_i Values (μmol/L)* | | |
	μ RECEPTOR	δ RECEPTOR	κ RECEPTOR
Morphine	0.00034	0.092	0.66
Dextropropoxyphene	0.034	0.38	1.22
Codeine	0.2	5.1	6.0
Tramadol	2.1	57.6	42.7
Imipramine	3.7	12.7	1.8

K_i, constant of inhibition.
*Lower K_i = higher binding affinity.
From Hennies HH, Friderichs E, Schneider J: Receptor binding, analgesic and antitussive potency of tramadol and other selected opioids. Arzneimittelforschung 1988;38:877-880.

Abuse Advisory Committee (DAAC) to recommend FDA approval of tramadol as a nonscheduled analgesic.[98] Current studies continue to support the low abuse potential of tramadol. A postmarketing survey has demonstrated limited evidence of tramadol use–related dependence, withdrawal, and abuse.[99] Another study assessing the prevalence of abuse compared tramadol with NSAIDs and hydrocodone-containing analgesics in patients with chronic noncancer pain.[100] This study used an abuse index that identified subjects according to the following behaviors: (1) increased dose without physician approval; (2) used for purposes other than intended; (3) demonstrated an inability to stop use; and (4) experienced withdrawal. The percentage of subjects who scored positive (at least one behavior) during a 12-month period was 2.5% for NSAIDs, 2.7% for tramadol, and 4.9% for hydrocodone.

Formulations

Currently available oral formulations of tramadol include 50-mg scored immediate-release (IR) tablets, SR tablets and capsules (every 12-hour dosing available worldwide, but not in the United States), ER once-daily tablets, and combination tablets consisting of tramadol, 37.5 mg, plus acetaminophen, 325 mg.[101] The SR preparations are available in strengths of 50, 100, 150, and 200 mg dosed on a twice-daily schedule. The recently approved ER tramadol hydrochloride tablets (Ultram ER) are available in 100-, 200-, and 300-mg strengths dosed on a once-daily basis. The bioavailability of Ultram ER 200 mg relative to 50 mg tramadol IR every 6 hours is approximately 85% to 90%. Steady-state plasma

concentrations of tramadol and M1 are achieved within 4 days of once-daily dosing. Important pharmacokinetic parameters of the 200-mg ER formulation include time of maximum concentration (T_{max}) of 12 hours and 15 hours for tramadol and the M1 metabolite, respectively, as compared with tramadol, 50 mg IR (tramadol, 1.5 hours; M1, 1.9 hours)[101] (Table 32–7).

Once-daily Ultram ER was formulated to counter the need to dose IR tramadol hydrochloride (Ultram) every 6 hours, improve compliance, and decrease sleep interruptions because of more stable serum concentrations. The bioavailability of ER tramadol is comparable with that of IR tramadol and demonstrates steady-state bioequivalence (AUC [area under the plasma drug concentration versus time curve] and maximum concentration [C_{max}] values) as compared with IR tramadol administered four times daily.[101] Tramadol ER (200 mg) has a longer T_{max} (tramadol, 12 hours; M1 metabolite, 15 hours) as compared with IR tramadol (tramadol, 1.5 hours; M1 metabolite, 1.9 hours) but reaches steady-state plasma concentrations (tramadol and M1) within 4 days with once-daily dosing.

Tramadol ER (100, 200, 300 mg) was found to be superior to placebo in average change from baseline pain, from 1 through 12 weeks, in a randomized trial of osteoarthritis of the knee. The average tramadol ER dose was 276 mg/day.[102]

Pharmacokinetics

Maximal serum concentration of oral tramadol is reached in approximately 2 hours.[103] The mean bioavailability after a single dose is 68%,[104] and this

Table 32–6. Affinity between Tramadol, Two Enantiomers, and Its Active Metabolite M1, Opioid Receptors, and Inhibition of Serotonin and Norepinephrine Reuptake

	Affinity for Opioid Receptors (K_i, μmol/L)			Reuptake Inhibition	
PRODUCT	**μ**	**δ**	**κ**	**NOREPINEPHRINE**	**SEROTONIN**
(±) Tramadol	2.1	57.6	42.7	0.78	0.9
(+) Tramadol	1.3	62.4	54.0	2.51	0.53
(−) Tramadol	24.8	213	53.5	0.43	2.35
(+) M1	0.0034				
Morphine	0.00034	0.092	0.57	Inactive	Inactive
Imipramine	3.7	12.7	1.8	0.0066	0.021

K_i, constant of inhibition.
Modified from Grond S, Sablotzki A:. Clinical pharmacology of tramadol. Clin Pharmacokinet 2004;43:879-923; and Mattia C, Coluzzi F: Tramadol. Focus on musculoskeletal and neuropathic pain. Minerva Anestesiol 2005;71:565-584.

Table 32–7. Pharmacokinetic Properties of Immediate- and Extended-Release Tramadol and Its M1 Metabolite

	Tramadol		M1 Metabolite	
PHARMACOKINETIC PARAMETER	**ULTRAM ER**	**ULTRAM IR**	**ULTRAM ER**	**ULTRAM IR**
C_{max} (μg/L)	335	383	95	104
C_{min} ((μg/L)	187	228	69	82
T_{max} (hr)	12	1.5	15	1.9

Table 32–8. Primary Kinetic Parameters of Tramadol*

| PARAMETER | Young Healthy Volunteers | | Older Healthy Volunteers | | PATIENTS WITH RENAL FAILURE (IV, $n = 10$) | PATIENTS WITH HEPATIC FAILURE (PO, $n = 12$) |
	IV ($n = 10$)	PO ($n = 10$)	PO ($n = 12$; AGE = 65-75 yr)	PO ($n = 8$; AGE >75 yr)		
T_{max} (hr)	—	1.9	2.0	2.1	—	1.9
C_{max} (µg/L)	409	290	324	415	894	433
AUC (µ/L × hr)	3709	2488	2508	3854	7832	7848
$t_{1/2\beta}$ (hr)	5.2	5.1	6.1	7.0	10.8	13.3
TC (L/hr)	28.8	42.6	47.6	29.5	16.8	16.3

*Depending on patient's age and hepatic and renal failure.
AUC, area under the plasma drug concentration versus time curve; TC, total clearance; C_{max}, maximum plasma concentration; $t_{1/2\beta}$, elimination half-life; T_{max}, time necessary to reach the maximum plasma concentration.
From Mattia C, Coluzzi F:. Tramadol. Focus on musculoskeletal and neuropathic pain. Minerva Anestesiol 2005;71:565-584.

increases to 90% to 100% after multiple doses. The mean bioavailability after IM administration is 100%, and after rectal administration is 78%. Tramadol is 20% bound to plasma proteins and crosses the placenta.[105] Metabolism is primarily hepatic via the CYP enzyme system. Tramadol is excreted by the kidneys (90%) and feces (10%). Biotransformation in the liver creates 23 metabolites; the primary metabolite is O-desmethyltramadol (M1).[106] Polymorphism of the CYP2D6 isoenzyme in the liver (present in approximately 7% to 10% of whites) may cause attenuation of analgesia in poor metabolizers. These patients may require higher loading doses and more rescue analgesia.[107] The elimination half-life of tramadol is 5 to 6 hours and of M1 is approximately 8 hours. Adjustments in dosage are required for patients with hepatic and renal failure and in geriatric patients (Table 32–8).[108] Bioequivalence has been demonstrated between IR and SR-ER formulations[91] (see Table 32–7).

Management Considerations

For improved tolerability of tramadol, various titration regimens have been proposed (Table 32–9). An alternate example of a titration schedule for patients with moderate to moderately severe chronic pain using the IR 50-mg tablets is as follows:
1. Start at 25 mg/day and titrate in 25-mg increments as separate doses every 3 days to reach 100 mg/day (25 mg four times daily).
2. Increase total daily dose by 50 mg as tolerated every 3 days to reach 200 mg/day (50 mg four times daily).
3. After titration, tramadol, 50 to 100 mg, can be administered as needed for pain relief every 4 to 6 hours, not to exceed 400 mg/day.

Patients with moderately severe pain needing more immediate pain control may benefit from a more aggressive dosing schedule. In this case, the increased risk of adverse events associated with higher initial doses must be clearly discussed and acceptable. In this subset of patients, tramadol, 50 to 100 mg, may be administered as needed every 4 to 6 hours, not to exceed 400 mg total per 24-hour period.

Table 32–9. Sample Tramadol Dosing Schedules

TRAMADOL DOSE (mg)	DAY
Chronic Pain	
25 qAM	1
25 bid	2
25 tid	3
25 qid	4
50 qAM, 25 noon, 25 afternoon, 50 qhs	5-7
50 qid	8-10
50-100 qid	11-X
Acute or Subacute Pain	
50 q6h	1-3
100 q6h	4-X

The initial recommended dose of tramadol SR formulations is 50 to 100 mg twice daily. Titration to doses of 150 to 200 mg twice daily pending side effect tolerability and efficacy of pain relief as needed may be carried out. Tramadol ER dosage recommendations include an initial dose of 100 mg daily, titrating up by 100 mg every 5 days, to a maximum daily dosage of 300 mg.

Risks and Precautions

Compared with traditional opioid analgesics, tramadol retains a more favorable side effect profile and may present a lower risk of addiction with chronic usage.[109]

Common Side Effects
The most common reported side effects include nausea, vomiting, dizziness, fatigue, sweating, dry mouth, drowsiness, sedation, and orthostatic hypotension. The incidence of side effects has been reported to be as high as 16.8% in patients with chronic pain complaints. Controlled-release formulations may produce a lower incidence of side effects (6.5%).[110]

Despite its improved side effect profile and early consideration as an alternative to pure µ-opioid receptor agonist medications, reports of overdose and fatality have led to a change in the package insert information, which includes a contraindication for use in patients with past or present histories of addiction or dependence on opioids.[97] Other more severe side effects include angioedema,[111] bleeding complications because of the increased effects of oral anticoagulants,[112] and serotonin toxicity.[113-115]

Tramadol and Serotonin Toxicity (Serotonin Syndrome)

Concomitant use of tramadol with other serotonergic medications (e.g., selective serotonin receptor inhibitors [SSRIs], monoamine oxidase inhibitors [MAOIs], and serotonin norepinephrine reuptake inhibitors [SNRIs]; Box 32–3) has been associated with case reports of serotonin toxicity.[116] Given the fact that a number of medication classes commonly used in pain management may predispose patients to mild to severe symptoms of serotonin toxicity, a review to gain a more clear understanding of serotonin toxicity and serotonin syndrome is in order.

Definition. Serotonin toxicity is an iatrogenic drug-induced toxidrome, a group of signs and symptoms presenting together with a particular type of chemical poisoning. Life-threatening serotonin toxicity, although rare, is usually precipitated by ingestion of MAOIs and SSRIs leading, in some cases, to hyperpyrexia and death.[117,118] The pathophysiology remains unclear but may involve overstimulation of $5-HT_{1A}$ and $5-HT_2$ receptors in the brain. Serotonin toxicity has been described by Gillman and Whyte as a triad

---

Table 32–10. Clinical Triad of Serotonin Toxicity (ST)

PARAMETER	MANIFESTATIONS
Neuromuscular hyperactivity	Tremor, clonus, myoclonus, hyperreflexia
Autonomic hyperactivity	Diaphoresis, fever, tachycardia, tachypnea, mydriasis
Altered mental status	Agitation, excitement, confusion

---

involving neuromuscular hyperactivity, autonomic hyperactivity, and altered mental status (Table 32–10).[115]

Sternbach proposed criteria for serotonin syndrome in one of the earlier published comprehensive reviews of serotonin syndrome.[113] In 2000, Radomski and associates[114] published an updated review of the subject, with revised diagnostic criteria (Table 32–11).

Mechanisms of Serotonin Toxicity. Serotonin toxicity may be related to mechanisms and potency of drugs. Tricyclic antidepressants (TCAs) exhibit a 100-fold variability in affinity for the serotonin transporter in humans. Overdose of amitriptyline alone does not precipitate serotonin toxicity.[119] More potent TCAs, such as clomipramine, may actually have more potent serotonergic effects clinically and in overdose. In overdoses of SSRIs or SNRIs such as venlafaxine alone, 15% exhibit moderate serotonin toxicity without life-threatening symptomatology or pyrexia.[120] Although venlafaxine has less potency than amitriptyline at the receptor level, it precipitates serotonin toxicity more frequently than SSRIs (30% vs. 15%). This may be related to mechanisms other than serotonin reuptake inhibition.[121] Trazodone and nefazodone differ compared with TCAs and SSRIs in that they are primarily $5-HT_{2A}$ antagonists. Neither exhibit serotonergic side effects nor induce signs of serotonin toxicity in overdose.[118]

A number of other pharmacologic agents, including illicit substances, enhance 5-HT activity and must be considered in the workup for possible serotonin toxicity (e.g., buspirone, ergot alkaloids, amphetamine, cocaine, TCAs, MAOIs[122]; see Box 32–3).

Clinical Use of Tramadol Formulations

Earlier reports evaluating the effectiveness of tramadol in varied painful conditions yielded conflicting results. In comparative studies of acute pain, oral tramadol was found to have efficacy similar to propoxyphene in a postoperative pain study and comparable efficacy to codeine for pain related to dental surgery.[123] However, tramadol hydrochloride, 50 and 100 mg, was found to have efficacy similar to placebo for pain after total hip arthroplasty,[124] but provided

---

BOX 32–3. SEROTONERGIC DRUGS

Serotonin (5-HT) Reuptake Inhibitors
Paroxetine, sertraline, fluoxetine, fluvoxamine, citalopram
Venlafaxine, milnacipran, duloxetine
Clomipramine, imipramine
Tramadol, meperidine, fentanil, methadone, dextromethorphan, dextropropoxyphene

Serotonin Precursors
5-Hydroxytryptophan, L-tryptophan

$5-HT_{1A}$ Antagonists
LSD, dihydroergotamine, bromocriptine, buspirone

Serotonin Releasers
Amphetamine, MDMA ("ecstasy")

Monoamine Oxidase Inhibitors
Tranylcypromine, phenelzine, nialamide, isoniazid, iproniazid, isocarbozaxid
Pargyline, selegiline, procarbazine
Moclobemide

Adapted from Gillman PK: A review of serotonin toxicity data: Implications for the mechanisms of antidepressant drug action. Biol Psychiatry 2006;59:1046-1051.

Table 32–11. Spectrum of Serotonin Syndrome

MILD STATE OF SEROTONIN-RELATED SYMPTOMS	SEROTONIN SYNDROME (FULL-BLOWN FORM)		TOXIC STATES
Single symptom may predominate	At least four major or three major and two minor of the following:		Coma
Most Common Are:	*Major*	*Minor*	Generalized tonic-clonic seizures
Tremor	Mental Symptoms		Fever (may exceed 40° C)
Myoclonus	Impaired consciousness	Restlessness	Disseminated intravascular coagulation and renal failure
Diaphoresis and shivering	Elevated mood	Insomnia	
	Neurologic Symptoms		
	Myoclonus	Uncoordination	
	Tremor	Dilated pupils	
	Shivering	Akathesia	
	Rigidity		
	Hyperflexia		
	Vegetative Symptoms		
	Fever	Tachycardia	
	Sweating	Tachypnea, dyspnea	
		Diarrhea	
		Hypertension, hypotension	

Coincidence with the addition or increase of a known serotonergic agent. Clinical features were not an integral part of the underlying psychiatric disorder prior to commencing the serotonergic agent. Other causes (e.g., infectious, metabolic or endocrine, substance abuse or withdrawal) have been ruled out. A neuroleptic drug has not been started or increased in dosage prior to the onset of the signs and symptoms listed above.
From Gnanadesigan N, Espinoza RT, Smith R, et al: Interaction of serotonergic antidepressants and opioid analgesics: Is serotonin syndrome going undetected? J Am Med Dir Assoc 2005;6:265-269.

inferior analgesia to hydrocodone-acetaminophen in an emergency room acute musculoskeletal pain cohort consisting of fracture, sprain-strain, and contusion.[125]

More recent clinical and evidence-based practice has found tramadol to be useful in a wide range of painful conditions, including osteoarthritis,[126] post-amputation phantom limb and residual limb pain,[127] postoperative pain reduction after arthroscopic knee surgery,[128] and cancer-related pain.[129] Guidelines for the pharmacologic management of OA have recommended tramadol for those patients who fail to achieve analgesia with acetaminophen, COX-2 inhibitors, or NSAIDs.[56,130]

The 2004 Cochrane Collaboration review of tramadol for neuropathic pain identified a number of eligible trials, including two trials comparing tramadol with placebo,[131,132] one comparing tramadol with clomipramine,[133] and one comparing tramadol with morphine for cancer pain.[134] Tramadol was found to be effective for the treatment of neuropathic pain based on this limited number of short-term studies (4 to 6 weeks). The NNT for tramadol in neuropathic pain states (3.5) was similar to that for other commonly used medications—2.4 for TCAs, 2.5 for carbamazepine, and 3.7 for gabapentin.

Tramadol-Acetaminophen

A number of different strengths of combination tramadol and acetaminophen compounds are available in the United States and Europe. The combination takes advantage of potential synergy between the two compounds demonstrated in animal and human models, suggesting an initial onset of analgesia of acetaminophen (20 minutes) followed by tramadol (approximately 50 minutes).[135] A meta-analysis of dental pain has demonstrated that the combination of acetaminophen plus tramadol has a similar rapid onset of efficacy as paracetamol alone, but levels of analgesia are maintained for a longer period as compared with tramadol alone.[136] Tramadol-acetaminophen combination products contain less tramadol by dose (in the United States, 37.5 vs. 50 mg) and relatively less acetaminophen (325 mg as compared with 500 mg [extra strength acetaminophen]) and thus may lower the potential incidence of organ toxicity (liver) when taken within the range of recommended doses.[91] Tramadol-acetaminophen combination products have demonstrated efficacy for acute and chronic pain conditions.[137] Combination tramadol, 37.5 mg, plus APAP, 325 mg, may provide analgesia equivalent to codeine and APAP in patients with chronic osteoarthritis, but with greater tolerability.[138] The most common treatment-related adverse event includes somnolence, nausea, and constipation with a mean dosage of 4.1 tablets daily.[139] Figure 32–3 illustrates NNT data from a meta-analysis evaluating the efficacy of tramadol-acetaminophen combination for moderate to severe postoperative pain.[140]

Oral Steroids

The first glucocorticoid was isolated in 1935. This naturally occurring corticosteroid, cortisone, was later laboratory synthesized in 1944. Four years later, Hench and colleagues at the Mayo Clinic were able

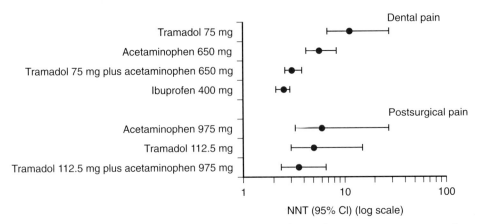

Figure 32–3. Meta-analysis evaluating tramadol-acetaminophen combination for moderate to severe postoperative pain. CI, confidence interval; NNT, number needed to treat. (From Edwards JE, McQuay HJ, Moore RA: Combination analgesic efficacy: Individual patient data meta-analysis of single-dose oral tramadol plus acetaminophen in acute postoperative pain. J Pain Symptom Manage 2002;23:121-130.)

to obtain a portion of the total 9 g of synthetic cortisone available from Merck for clinical trial use. They injected this "compound E" (cortisone) into patients with rheumatoid arthritis. Accounts describe the treatment of multiple patients with 100-mg injections, with astonishing results—patients experienced dramatic pain reduction and remarkable improvement in their functional mobility. Reports have noted that one of their formerly totally bedridden patients was able to get out of bed and tried to dance. However, when the supplies ran out just 1 week later, all the treated patients went into remission.[141] This report led not only to the widespread use of cortisone in the treatment of rheumatologic conditions, but also earned Hench the joint award (along with Kendall and Reichstein) of the Nobel Prize in Medicine and Physiology in 1950. As oral steroid preparations evolved, their use increased in addition to injection therapy as a method of producing systemic levels for chronic treatment regimens. Pulsed dosing schedules are now routinely used for disease management and episodic flares of a wide range of disorders, including rheumatic, pulmonary, dermatologic, neurologic, ophthalmologic, hematologic, and endocrine disorders. Exogenous glucocorticoid administration has been to shown to have a suppressive effect on the hypothalamic-pituitary-adrenal (HPA) axis. Some believe that this can occur in as little as 5 days of using high supraphysiologic doses, whereas at physiologic doses this may not occur for 3 to 4 weeks. Thus, a tapered dosing schedule is typically recommended when treatment exceeds 2 to 3 weeks.[142] The use of steroids in the treatment of painful conditions is largely based on the premise that there is an inflammatory role in the mediation of pain.[143] Chronic use of oral steroids occurs in the treatment of rheumatologic inflammatory conditions (e.g., rheumatoid arthritis, polymyalgia rheumatica, Crohn's disease), as well as cancer pain. In addition, oral steroids are commonly used for short-term or pulsed dosing schedules for conditions such as complex regional pain syndrome (CRPS), RA flares, gouty or osteoar-

thritis flares, painful radiculopathy, bursitis, carpal tunnel syndrome, and other acute or chronic musculoskeletal conditions.[144-146]

Mechanism of Action and Description

Adrenocortical steroids such as prednisone, methylprednisolone, and dexamethasone act by inhibiting multiple cellular mechanisms, including the accumulation of inflammatory cells at sites of inflammation, macrophage phagocytosis, lysosomal enzyme release and synthesis, and release of mediators of inflammation. In regard to their ability to attenuate pain responses, this action is likely related to their strong anti-inflammatory action. Steroids suppress or prevent cell-mediated immune responses, and decrease or prevent tissue response to the inflammatory process. The mechanisms for reduction of cancer pain are thought to be secondary to inhibition of prostaglandin synthesis and reduction in peritumor and perineural edema by decreasing capillary permeability.[143]

Oral prednisone is readily absorbed in the GI tract. It is highly protein-bound (up to 70% to 90%) and distributes widely into a variety of tissues. The plasma half-life ($t_{1/2}$) of prednisone is 3.4 to 4 hours, with a biologic $t_{1/2}$ of 18 to 36 hours. It is metabolized in the liver to its active metabolite prednisolone, which is further metabolized to inactive compounds. The active metabolite and inactive compounds are excreted in the urine and the drug is not removed by hemodialysis.[147] The pharmacodynamics of commonly used glucocorticoids are presented in Table 32–12.

Prednisone tablets are available in multiple dosage forms, ranging from 2.5- to 50-mg tablets. Other glucocorticoids commonly prescribed for painful conditions include methylprednisolone (Medrol Dosepak) and dexamethasone (Table 32–13). The Medrol Dosepak consists of 21 4-mg tablets, taken in a tapering fashion (one tablet daily), from six tablets on day

Table 32–12. Pharmacodynamics of Common Glucocorticoids

AGENT	EQUIVALENT GLUCOCORTICOID DOSE (mg)	RELATIVE GLUCOCORTICOID ACTIVITY	RELATIVE MINERALOCORTICOID ACTIVITY*	HALF-LIFE IN PLASMA (hr)	BIOLOGIC HALF-LIFE (hr)
Cortisone	25	0.8	0.8	0.5	8-12
Cortisol	20	1	1	1.5-2	8-12
Methylprednisolone	4	5	0.5	>3.5	18-36
Prednisolone	5	4	0.6	2.1-3.5	18-36
Prednisone	5	4	0.6	3.4-3.8	18-36
Triamcinolone	4	5	0	2->5	18-36
Dexamethasone	0.75	20-30	0	3-4.5	36-54
Betamethasone	0.6	20-30	0	3-5	36-54

*Clinically—sodium and water retention, potassium depletion.
Adapted from Jacobs JWD, Bijlsma JWJ: Glucocorticoid therapy. In Kelly W, Harris E, Ruddy S, et al (eds): Kelly's Textbook of Rheumatology, 7th ed. Philadelphia, WB Saunders, 2005, Table 57–1.

Table 32–13. Commonly Prescribed Oral Glucocorticoids

AGENT	TRADE NAME	AVAILABLE DOSE FORM
Methylprednisolone	Medrol	2-, 4-, 8-, 16-, 24-, 32-mg tablets
Prednisone	Deltasone, Sterapred	2.5-, 5-, 10-, 20-, 50-mg tablets
	Prednisone Intensol (oral concentrate)	5 mg/mL
Dexamethasone	Decadron	0.25-, 0.5-, 0.75-, 1.5-, 4-, 8-mg tablets
	Decadron elixir (oral concentrate)	0.5 mg/5 mL

BOX 32–4. COMMON GLUCOCORTICOID DOSING SCHEDULES

Prednisone taper—prednisone, 10-mg tablets
   3 tablets PO bid × 4 days, 2 tablets PO bid × 3 days, 1 tablet PO bid × 3 days.
Medrol Dosepak—methylprednisolone, 4-mg tablets
   Day 1: 2 tablets before breakfast, 1 tablet after lunch and dinner, and 2 tablets at bedtime. (total = 6 tablets). If given later in the day, may take all 6 tablets at once or in divided doses.
   Day 2: 1 tablet before breakfast, 1 tablet after lunch and dinner, and 2 tablets at bedtime.
   Day 3: Same as day 2, except 1 tablet at bedtime.
   Day 4: 1 tablet before breakfast, after lunch, and at bedtime.
   Day 5: 1 tablet after breakfast and at bedtime.
   Day 6: 1 tablet after breakfast.
Dexamethasone taper—dexamethasone, 8-mg tablets
   Tapering schedule over 7 days: 64, 32, 24, 16, 8, 8, 8 mg

---

1 to one tablet on day 6. See Box 32–4 for common glucocorticoid dosing schedules.

Risks and Precautions

In general, long-term administration at physiologic replacement doses do not lead to adverse effects. Similarly, short-term dosing at supraphysiologic levels typically does not cause adverse effects. Many have recommended a tapering dose schedule to avoid glucocorticoid withdrawal, which can occur in as little as 5 days at high supraphysiologic doses or 3 to 4 weeks at physiologic doses.[142] Suppression of the HPA axis can persist for up to 12 months after cessation of prolonged corticosteroid therapy, and supplementation may be required during periods of physiologic stress such as surgery, acute blood loss, or infection. Because of the depression and prevention of cell-mediated immune responses, oral corticosteroids are not well tolerated by patients with immunocompromised states, whether acute or chronic. However, they do play an adjuvant role in the management of cancer pain.[148] In these cases, new pain complaints in cancer patients or palliative care patients must be vigilantly monitored because, in the presence of opioid analgesics and corticosteroid therapy, symptoms may be less severe and related to a new diagnosis, such as appendicitis.[149]

A population-based study examining over 2400 patients on long-term oral glucocorticoid therapy found that side effects are associated with cumulative and average dose in a dose-dependent fashion. The study allowed for the use of varied glucocorticoid preparations and converted them into a prednisone-equivalent dose. The most common side effects, with approximate prevalence, included weight gain (70%), skin bruising (53%), sleep disturbance (45%), mood symptoms (42%), cataracts (15%), acne (15%), and fractures (12%). Increasing daily dosage was more significantly associated with fractures and sleep disturbance than increased duration of use.[150]

Prednisone use during pregnancy is schedule D during the first trimester and schedule C for the

Table 32–14. FDA* Pregnancy Categories for Drugs

CATEGORY	DESCRIPTION
A	No fetal risk in controlled studies
B	No risk to human fetus despite possible animal risk, or no risks in animal studies but human studies lacking
C	Human risk cannot be ruled out. Animal studies may or may not show risk
D	Evidence of risk to human fetus

*FDA, U.S. Food and Drug Administration.

second and third trimesters (Table 32–14). First-trimester exposure to systemic corticosteroids (category C) has been associated with intrauterine growth retardation and increased incidence of cleft lip, with or without cleft palate. If necessary, the maternal benefits of short courses of oral corticosteroids may outweigh the fetal risks when given beyond the first trimester.[151]

Clinical Use

Oral corticosteroids have a limited role in the treatment of painful conditions. They may be useful in the treatment of acute painful inflammatory conditions, including complex regional pain syndrome (CRPS), carpal tunnel syndrome, rotator cuff arthropathy–adhesive capsulitis, and painful cervical or lumbar radiculopathy. Steroids have been and continue to be administered by multiple routes for CRPS therapy. After early reports of success with systemic steroids,[152] Christensen and coworkers[146] studied 23 patients and reported that 30 mg/day of oral prednisone is significantly better than placebo based on their stated clinical outcome measures. Braus and colleagues[153] studied the effects of methylprednisolone, 32 mg/day for 2 weeks, followed by a taper over 2 weeks for the treatment of CRPS in poststroke patients. This randomized study showed a significant clinical improvement in steroid-treated patients at 4 weeks. A recent investigation into the effects of chronic methylprednisolone treatment on the rat CRPS type I model (tibia fracture) has revealed that glucocorticoids reverse hindpaw edema and warmth after fracture, with persistent effects after discontinuation of treatment. However, glucocorticoid treatment has no effect on the allodynia, hindpaw unweighting, or periarticular bone loss observed after tibia fracture.[154]

The use of minor analgesics for the cancer pain population is common. The most commonly used opioid coanalgesics are NSAIDs and acetaminophen, but up to 39% of cancer patients take various types of corticosteroids, with dexamethasone being the most common formulation. These patients have a wide range of diagnoses, with breast, lung, and colorectal cancers topping the list. This cross-sectional study did not specifically determine whether each adjuvant medication was given specifically for pain control as opposed to other diseases, but other studies

have documented the usefulness of corticosteroids for the rational polypharmacy of cancer pain management.[148,155,156] Efficacy has been demonstrated for neuropathic pain because of tumor compression (malignant compression of the spinal cord, brachial, or lumbosacral plexus), tumor-induced bone pain, and hepatic capsule distention secondary to liver metastases.[143,157] In addition to NSAIDs and disease-modifying antirheumatic drugs (DMARDs), low-dose oral corticosteroids may also be helpful in managing joint symptoms caused by chemotherapy-induced arthropathy.[158]

Despite the lack of many directed controlled clinical trials, corticosteroids are frequently prescribed in an adjunctive role for palliation and control of side effects of chemotherapy; therefore, these agents may play a dual role in selected patients. Many consider that corticosteroids may help with prevention of chemotherapy-induced nausea and emesis and hypersensitivity reactions. In addition, they may also help with asthenic symptoms and fatigue, as well as appetite stimulation.[145,159]

The use of oral glucocorticoids in the form of methylprednisolone, or prednisone burst or taper, is common practice in the acute treatment of disk herniation with radicular pain complaints. Although there has been a significant increase in studies evaluating the efficacy of fluoroscopically guided epidural steroid injections,[160] there is a paucity of reports of the usefulness of oral or systemic corticosteroids for this pain population. In the only prospective, double-blind, randomized controlled trial evaluating the use of oral corticosteroids in the treatment of radicular pain, a tapering dose of dexamethasone over 7 days was not superior to placebo for early or long-term relief of lumbosacral radicular pain. Dexamethasone, however, was superior to placebo for reducing stretch-invoked pain during straight-leg raising. This study did allow the concurrent use of meperidine, oxycodone, and acetaminophen for analgesia.[161] Systemic dexamethasone taper via the intramuscular route has been studied to a limited degree, with conflicting results.[162,163] The rationale for the use of oral corticosteroids is based on the observance that proinflammatory mediators and neurosensitizing chemicals are released from the damaged intervertebral disk.[164,165] One study has suggested that epidurally administered glucocorticoids do not appear to have a negative effect on the spontaneous resorption of disk herniations.[166]

In most musculoskeletal injuries, there is a close relationship between injury and pain. Therefore, individual treatments in a comprehensive management program may serve dual purposes—reducing inflammation to control local damage and concurrently reducing pain. Although there are few trials that evaluate the efficacy of oral corticosteroids in musculoskeletal injuries, clinical practice reveals that their use is widespread. A questionnaire-based study involving 99 physicians at a national sports medicine conference found that 59% of physicians prescribe oral corticosteroids for musculoskeletal injuries, with prednisone being the most commonly used.[167] The study did not differentiate whether the medication was being prescribed specifically for pain or for its anti-inflammatory properties, but prescriptions were written for acute and chronic conditions equally.

Although the mainstays of treatment for carpal tunnel syndrome include neutral wrist splints, ergonomic evaluation and modification of biomechanics, oral NSAIDs, steroid injection, and surgical release of the transverse carpal ligament, there is evidence to suggest that oral corticosteroids may play a role in the short-term management of symptoms in patients with mild to moderate symptoms and in those not interested in or awaiting surgical release of the transverse carpal ligament. Studies have examined varied dosing and duration of treatment regimens with prednisolone (10 days to 3 weeks, with dosing of up to 25 mg daily); results suggest that regardless of dosing, the global symptom score (GSS) is improved in patients treated with oral corticosteroid versus placebo.[144]

Short-term dosing of oral prednisolone, at variable doses, has been studied in adhesive capsulitis. Binder and associates[168] used 10 mg daily for 4 weeks, followed by 5 mg daily for 2 weeks. Night pain was significantly lower in the treatment group at 8 weeks. However, by 5 months, this difference had resolved. Over the total 8-month period, no difference was found in pain at rest or with movement, range of motion, or cumulative recovery curve between the oral steroid group and the control group that received no specific therapy. Other studies have evaluated a 3-week course of 30 mg prednisolone daily that resulted in a significant reduction in pain and disability, improved active range of motion, and improved participant-rated improvement at 3 weeks. By 6 weeks, the improvements were still noted, but none of the values were statistically significant; at 12 weeks, the placebo group was favored.[145]

The use of oral corticosteroids for the treatment of rheumatoid arthritis has been studied since 1949, when Hench and coworkers[169] showed treatment efficacy in an uncontrolled trial. Although oral corticosteroids may show beneficial effects in regard to radiologic progress of the disease,[170] they are more commonly used during episodes of symptomatic flares to control pain or during bridge therapy of slower acting agents.[171,172] A meta-analysis evaluating the effectiveness of low-dose prednisolone versus placebo and NSAIDs found that low-dose prednisolone (less than 15 mg daily) shows greater effect over placebo and NSAIDs for joint tenderness and pain.[172]

Caffeine

Caffeine is an important adjuvant compound used in combination with OTC and prescription analgesics. Caffeine exhibits antinociceptive effects and analgesic properties when used in combination with opioid analgesics.[173] Caffeine combination products have been studied in a number of pain conditions, including headache,[174] oral surgery,[175] low back pain,[176] and postpartum-related pain.[177] Caffeine (65 to 130 mg) was shown to increase the potency of other analgesics by 40%.[178] OTC headache medications typically include 65 or 32.5 mg of caffeine combined with acetaminophen, 250 to 500 mg, and/or ASA, 250 to 520 mg (Table 32-15).

Mechanism of Action and Description

Caffeine, a methylxanthine, is a nonselective adenosine receptor antagonist that blocks multiple adenosine receptors (A1,A2A, A2B, and A3) in peripheral tissues and the central nervous system.[179,180] Centrally, caffeine may increase dopamine and norepinephrine as well as act as a vasoconstrictor of vessels, contributing to its analgesic effect in certain headache conditions.[181] A recent animal study using a fixed dose of aspirin, acetaminophen (paracetamol), and caffeine demonstrated increased secretion of norepinephrine and reduction in dopamine in rat striatal tissue.[182]

Clinical Use

Studies examining the relationship between dietary caffeine intake and chronic low back pain have yielded conflicting results.[183,184] One review, including over 10,000 patients in 30 trials, found that caffeine is successful as an adjuvant for analgesia. Without the combination of caffeine, 40% higher doses of aspirin, acetaminophen, or salicylamide would have been required to achieve equivalent analgesia. When used for the treatment of nonmigrainous headaches, 65 mg of caffeine was found to be as effective as 648 mg of acetaminophen.

Topical Medications

Topical medications for pain include topical analgesics, counterirritants, heat and cold preparations, and patches. Topical analgesics constitute a growing area of development in pain management, a growing

Table 32-15. Components of Caffeine-Containing Over-the-Counter Medications

NAME	CAFFEINE (mg)	ACETAMINOPHEN (mg)	NSAID (mg)
Excedrin Tension Headache	65	500	N/A
Excedrin Migraine	65	250	250 ASA
Goody's Extra Strength Headache Powder	32.5	260	520 ASA

ASA, acetylsalicylic acid; NSAID, nonsteroidal anti-inflammatory drug.

section of the OTC analgesic market, and a smaller evolving niche market of compounding pharmacies in the United States and Europe. Compounding pharmacies can serve a unique service in providing customized compounding of various creams and gels for topical use. Commonly used medications include ketamine, gabapentin, cyclobenzaprine, and various NSAIDs.[185]

The use of OTC and prescription topical analgesics continues to grow. Use of topical analgesics may represent a viable option for patients because of the safety concerns of NSAIDs in the popular media and scientific literature.[186] The FDA's black box warnings of prescription and OTC NSAIDs, including COX-2 inhibitors,[187] may have led to renewed interest in safer pharmacologic alternatives to oral medications. In general, topical preparations have considerably less potential for systemic adverse effects and organ toxicity. Interestingly, a recent meta-analysis of randomized placebo controlled trials for osteoarthritis found topical NSAIDs to be more effective than oral nonselective NSAIDs and COX-2 inhibitors and second to intra-articular steroid injections, as measured by patient-perceived improvement during the first 2 to 3 weeks following treatment.[188] Topical analgesics comprise approximately 6% of the U.S. OTC analgesic market.[189] Commonly prescribed topical medications include the following: lidocaine 5% patches, indicated for postherpetic neuralgia (PHN)[190]; topical TCAs, including doxepin and amitriptyline, for neuropathic pain states[191,192]; and counterirritants and vanilloid receptor agonists, such as capsaicin, for neuropathic pain.[193] This section will review various prescription strength and OTC topical medication classes, including analgesics, anesthetics, counterirritants, and hot or cold products used commonly for the treatment of acute and chronic pain conditions (Table 32–16).

Topical Preparations

Topical agents may potentially achieve a similar level of efficacy compared with oral formulations without the associated systemic side effects. Some evidence has shown that topically delivered agents can accumulate to therapeutic concentrations within the local tissues to which they have been applied while maintaining low serum levels and subsequently resulting in less organ toxicity. Table 32–17 lists the benefits and limitations of dermal and transdermal delivery systems.[194-215]

Delivery of topical agents can be by passive and active methods. Passive methods involve application of drugs to the skin (e.g., by ointments, creams, gels, patches) and may include modified systems that enhance the driving force through the skin. These include thermodynamic and permeability enhancers, such as penetration enhancers, prodrugs, and liposomes. Passive methods currently on the market are usually well tolerated but are limited by skin irritation, poor adhesion, and limitation in size because of practical cosmetic issues.[194]

"Topical" versus "Transdermal"

"Topical" and "transdermal" are distinct modes of medication delivery to the skin. Both delivery methods must transverse the stratum corneum, the major barrier to delivering treatment. Transdermal methods deliver medication through percutaneous absorption, with the goal of achieving similar therapeutic systemic levels as active oral preparations.

Table 32–16. Topical Medications

CLASS	INGREDIENTS
Counterirritants (rubefacients)	Capsaicin, 0.025%, 0.075%, 0.1%; camphor; salicylic acid; trolamine salicylate; poison ivy, marsh tea; benzyl nicotinate
Local anesthetics	Benzocaine; lidocaine 5% patch, ointment; EMLA—lidocaine 2.5%/prilocaine 2.5%
Cooling agents	Menthol; peppermint oil
Heating agents	Iron, charcoal, table salt, water (ThermaCare heat wrap)

Table 32–17. Benefits and Limitations of Analgesia by Cutaneous Delivery

BENEFITS	LIMITATIONS
First-pass metabolism, other variables associated with gastrointestinal tract (e.g., pH, gastric emptying time) avoided[195-197]	Diffusion across stratum corneum only occurs for molecules <500 Da[199]
Reduced side effects, minimization of drug concentration peaks and troughs in blood[197,198]	Topical agents must have both aqueous, lipid solubility[200]
Ease of dose termination in case of untoward side effects	Both intra- and interindividual variability in skin permeability, as well as between healthy/diseased skin, causes variable efficacy[201,202]
Delivery can be sustained, controlled over prolonged period[203,204]	
Direct access to target site[205]	Skin enzymes can cause metabolism before cutaneous absorption, reducing drug potency[211]
Convenient, painless administration[195,196]	
Improved patient acceptance, adherence to therapy[206-208]	Localized skin irritation (e.g., erythema, edema) can be common reactions[212-215]
Ease of use—may reduce overall health treatment costs[209,210]	
Provides viable solution for treatment when oral dosing not feasible (e.g., in unconscious or nauseated patients)[197]	

Da, dalton.
From Brown MB, Martin GP, Jones SA, et al: Dermal and transdermal drug delivery systems: Current and future prospects. Drug Deliv 2006;13:175-187.

Transdermal pharmacotherapies can be administered distal to the site of injury (e.g., SR nicotine and clonidine patches, long-acting fentanyl delivery systems). In contrast, topical agents use cutaneous delivery to target the site of application specifically. The sites of action for topical agents are the soft tissues and peripheral nerves underlying the site of application.[216] Serum levels generally remain relatively low and systemic side effects or drug-drug interactions are consequently more unlikely.[216]

The vehicle in which the active ingredient(s) are delivered can affect the skin penetration depth and absorption rate into the epidermis.[216] Primarily, the penetration of topical modalities is limited by the relatively dense stratum corneum, a layer of flattened dead cells or keratinocytes covering the live epidermis.[217,218] Once past this relatively impermeable barrier, analgesics may access cutaneous nociceptors, including the unmyelinated C-fibers of the epidermal layer. Below the epidermis, the dermal layer also contains nociceptive fibers, along with fibroblasts, connective tissue, blood vessels, hair follicles, and glands.[218]

Animal models have suggested that the variability in transcutaneous absorption rates between topical agents is likely derived from their ability to negotiate the superficial skin.[219] Ideally, the most effective topical agent will have a low molecular weight (less than 500 Da),[217] and both hydrophobic features to transverse the stratum corneum and hydrophilic components to penetrate the predominantly aqueous epidermis.[219,220] Occlusive dressings and specialized delivery agents may also help improve penetration.[220] Lecithin organogels (LOs) are biocompatible jelly-like phases, composed primarily of hydrated phospholipids and organic liquid.[221] Poloxamer-lecithin organogel (PLO) is a commonly used vehicle that includes a viscosity-enhancing agent that facilitates oil-in-water preparations and is used by a number of compounding pharmacies.[222] PLO also includes lecithin and propylene glycol, which help disperse the drug more uniformly. Additionally, polyethylene glycol and limonene[223] have been used as topical penetration enhancers, increasing the absorption rate of NSAIDs by up to 75-fold.[220]

Modalities

Active delivery of medication may be enhanced by the use of physical modalities, including iontophoresis and phonophoresis.[224] Iontophoresis is the migration of charged particles across biologic membranes under an electric field, usually applied transcutaneously.[225] This method, generally under the direction of a physical therapist or other health care professional, uses low-level current to enhance the permeability of the topically applied agent (e.g., corticosteroid, NSAID). Phonophoresis involves the migration of drug through the skin via an ultrasound (US) transducer. Phonophoresis is commonly used in the treatment of musculoskeletal conditions to enhance the delivery of topical NSAIDs to inflamed tissues.[226]

Topical Treatment Options: Clinical Trial Evidence

Nonsteroidal Anti-inflammatory Drugs

Topical NSAIDs are more widely used and studied in Europe as compared with the United States. Several proposed peripheral mechanisms of their analgesic activity include the inhibition of PGE synthesis, the lipoxygenase pathway, and excitatory amino acids, as well as modulation of G protein–mediated signal transduction.[216] A large variety of topical NSAID formulations is available commercially (Table 32–18).

Pharmacokinetic data suggest that topically applied NSAIDs can result in enhanced local concentrations, without significant toxic systemic levels. Heyneman and colleagues[220] reviewed single- and multiple-dose NSAID absorption studies. Collectively, these indicated that following topical administration of NSAIDs, peak plasma levels are less than 10% of the concentrations obtained from oral dosing (range, 0.2% to 8.0%), with total systemic absorption from topical application only 3% to 5% of the oral route. The time to achieve C_{max} following topical application ranged from 2.2 to 23 hours, approximately 10 times longer than the time required for the equivalent oral dose. Topical NSAIDs generally achieve steady-state concentration within 2 to 5 days of repeated application.[220]

Furthermore, penetration studies indicate that topically applied NSAIDs reach therapeutic concentrations below the site of application.[220] A two-way crossover design assessed the levels of subcutaneous and muscle absorption of 800 mg of oral ibuprofen compared with 16 g of 5% ibuprofen gel administered to the thigh.[227] Microdialysis probes inserted 25 to 30 mm into the muscle found average values of 63.5 ± 90.3 and 213.4 ± 117 ng/hr/mL of ibuprofen for the oral and topical routes, respectively. The ibuprofen concentrations in the dermis were 22.5-fold greater when delivered topically; the mean values of ibuprofen in the subcutaneous tissue were 731.2 ± 605.0 and 176.6 ± 122.9 ng/hr/mL for the topical and oral routes, respectively.[227] Another study of 100 patients who underwent knee arthroscopy evaluated ketoprofen concentrations in intra-articular tissues following a single application of a 30-mg plaster, multiple applications of plasters over a 5-day period, or a 50-mg oral dose.[228] The median C_{max} levels in the cartilage for topical and oral administration were 568.9 and 85.7 ng/g, respectively (a 6.8-fold difference). In contrast, the plasma values were 18.7 ng/mL for topically administered ketoprofen and 2595.3 ng/mL for the oral route. Overall, when administered by a topical route, the ketoprofen levels were 30-fold greater in cartilage than in plasma.[228]

Relative to all other topically administered drugs, NSAIDs have accumulated the largest amount of clinical evidence for their use.[216] A meta-analysis by Moore and associates[229] considered 86 randomized

Table 32–18. Topical Nonsteroidal Anti-inflammatory Drugs

FORMULATION	ACTIVE INGREDIENT	BRAND	STRENGTH
Ointment	Indomethacin		10%
Solution (lotion)	Diclofenac	Pennsaid	1.5%
Cream	Diclofenac	Voltaren Emulgel	1%
	Ibuprofen	Dolgit (5%)	5%, 10%, 15%
	Benzydamine	Difflam	3%
	Salicylic acid	Fostex	2%
Spray	Indomethacin		1%, 4%
Patch/plaster	Diclofenac/diclofenac epolamine (DHEP)		65- to 180-mg plaster, 1% patch
	Flurbiprofen	TransAct	40-mg patch
Gel	Piroxicam	Feldene	0.5%
	Diclofenac	DDA Emulgel	1% / 1.16%
	Felbinac	Traxam	3%
	Eltenac		0.1%, 0.3%, 1%
	Ketoprofen	Powergel, Tiloket gel	2.5% / 5%
	Indomethacin		1%
	Naproxen sodium	Naprosyn gel	10%
	Ibuprofen		1%
	Salicylic acid	Keralyt gel	3%
Drops	Ketorolac	Acular	0.2%
	Flurbiprofen	Ocufen	0.03%
	Suprofen	Profenal	1%
	Diclofenac	Voltaren	0.1%
Foam	Ketoprofen		15%
	Felbinac	Traxan	3%

Adapted from Vaile JH, Davis P: Topical NSAIDs for musculoskeletal conditions. A review of the literature. Drugs 1998;56:783-799.

controlled trials of NSAIDs for the treatment of pain conditions. This review included a total of 10,160 patients. Following 1 to 2 weeks of topical application, placebo-controlled trials demonstrated the benefit of NSAIDs for the treatment of acute pain conditions, such as soft tissue trauma, sprains, and strains, as well as chronic pain conditions, such as osteoarthritis and tendonitis. Overall, the NNT was 3.9 for acute pain conditions—more specifically, 2.6 for ketoprofen, 3.5 for ibuprofen, and 4.2 for piroxicam. For chronic pain conditions, the NNT was 3.1 (range, 2.7 to 3.8). Side effects encountered for all pain conditions studied were minimal; topical NSAIDs rarely induced local skin reactions (3.6%) or adverse systemic effects (less than 0.5%).[229] Similarly, a smaller meta-analysis of 26 double-blinded, placebo-controlled trials by Mason and coworkers[230] found that topical NSAID treatment is safe and effective for acute pain following 1 week of application.

A meta-analysis of randomized controlled trials has assessed the efficacy of topical NSAIDs relative to placebo or oral formulations for the treatment of osteoarthritis.[231] Compared with placebo, a positive treatment effect was observed for topical NSAIDs during weeks 1 and 2 of treatment only, with effect sizes of 0.41 (95% confidence interval [CI], 0.16 to 0.66) and 0.40 (95% CI, 0.15 to 0.65), respectively. In contrast, even during the first week, topical NSAIDs were found to provide inferior analgesia compared with oral versions, and topical agents induced more local side effects. The authors concluded that no trial evidence has supported the benefit of NSAIDs over placebo for treating osteoarthritis after 2 weeks of application, and even suggested that current practice guidelines on osteoarthritis that advocate the use of

topical NSAIDs[56,232,233] be revised.[231] However, two recent randomized, controlled trials of topical diclofenac solution for the treatment of pain secondary to knee osteoarthritis reported benefit at 4 and 12 weeks of application.[234,235] Measured by Western Ontario and McMaster Universities (WOMAC) osteoarthritis index scores, relative to baseline, the study group had a 42.9% decrease in pain at 4 weeks and a 45.7% decrease after 12 weeks, compared with 26.9% and 33.3% decrease in pain for the vehicle control groups, respectively. Measurements of physical function, stiffness, and pain on walking indicated similar benefit of the topical diclofenac over placebo in both studies. Probably because of the skin penetration enhancer dimethyl sulfoxide (DMSO), 30 of 84 patients in the 4-week study group and 68 of 164 patients in the 12-week study group reported skin irritation (typically dryness), leading to discontinuation by 5 patients in each of the treatment groups, respectively.[234,235]

Various novel NSAID patches and plasters have been developed, conferring a more constant, continuous delivery of a standardized dose of analgesic, although individual skin variability affects the actual amount absorbed. Galer and colleagues[236] used a multicenter, randomized, parallel design trial to assess the efficacy of a topical diclofenac patch for treatment of pain from sports-related soft tissue injuries, such as sprains, strains, or contusions. A diclofenac epolamine 1.3% or placebo patch was applied twice daily on 222 patients for 2 weeks. The study group achieved statistically significant pain intensity differences from placebo on clinic visits at day 3 ($P = 0.036$) and day 14 ($P = 0.044$) following treatment initiation, but not on day 7. Forty percent of participants given the placebo reported adverse events, whereas 34% of study group patients reported side effects.[236] A similar study comparing a diclofenac patch (140 mg diclofenac sodium) and placebo applied within 3 hours of blunt, soft tissue trauma-type injury found statistically significant analgesic effect over placebo ($P < 0.0001$) as measured by tenderness produced by pressure and time required to reach pain resolution at the site of injury ($P < 0.0001$). Adverse events, most commonly local cutaneous reactions, were experienced in a similar frequency by both groups.[237]

Topical diclofenac 1.5% solution (Pennsaid) is presently approved in Canada and Europe for the treatment of osteoarthritis. Topical diclofenac 1.5% in a carrier containing DMSO solution applied three times daily demonstrated efficacy when compared with vehicle-controlled solution and placebo in osteoarthritis of the knee. Adverse effects included skin irritation (36%), most commonly skin dryness, leading to discontinuation in only 6% of cases.[234] A similar study of knee OA found that diclofenac 1.5% solution (40 drops, four times daily) demonstrated improvements in pain, physical function, patient global assessment, stiffness, and pain on walking.[235]

Topical ketoprofen has been suggested to demonstrate more favorable physicochemical properties compared with other available NSAIDs, including greater lipophilicity and more rapid absorption.[238] Some studies have demonstrated plasma ketoprofen levels to correlate with measures of efficacy in a postoperative orthopedic cohort for up to 12 hours of oral dosing. Another study found variability in serum levels of topical ketoprofen (20%) in a PLO-based formulation after a single application, with a low rate and extent of systemic absorption (approximately 0.5%).[239] A placebo-controlled study of patients with pain from ankle sprain assessed the analgesia achieved over a 2-week period by the application of a 100-mg topical ketoprofen patch.[240] There was significantly less spontaneous pain observed for the study group compared with the control group during all visits (days 3 to 4, 7 ± 1, and 14 ± 2). Most notably, there was a 49.9- $\pm$ 20.2-mm (−73%) decrease in pain from baseline at day 7 ± 1 for patients given the ketoprofen patch, compared with a 37.6- $\pm$ 24.3-mm (−57%) decrease among the patients given a placebo patch. The intergroup difference in pain relief was significant ($P = 0.0007$), but the difference in adverse events (AEs) was not. Thirty-one percent of the study group and 24% of the control group experienced AEs.[240] A similar study with a topical ketoprofen patch, 100 mg, demonstrated efficacy in symptomatic tendinitis, finding a reduction in pain after 1 week in the treatment group (−38.4 $\pm$ 25.6 mm) compared with placebo (−25.8 $\pm$ 24.5 mm).[241]

Ketoprofen, an arylpropionic acid derivative, has been associated with an increasing number of case reports describing contact allergic and photosensitization skin reactions in Europe and Asia.[242,243] The unique photoallergy may be related to ketoprofen's benzophenone structure.[244] Caution or avoidance of use may be necessary during periods of significant skin exposure to sun.

Topical Counterirritants and Hot or Cold Preparations

An increased understanding of nociceptor physiology, including a greater understanding of thermosensation, has been spurred by identification of proteins called vanilloid receptors, detectors of noxious heat, and subsequent identification of a new family of thermosensation receptors, the transient receptor protein channel (TRPV) family.[245] The vanilloid receptor (TRPV1) is a nonselective cation receptor activated by capsaicin, the pungent agent found in chili peppers. TRPV1 is also activated by heat (higher than 43° C) and decreased pH, and enhanced by bradykinin and nerve growth factor.[246] The TRPV2 receptor, which is 50% identical to TRPV1, may mediate high-threshold noxious heat (higher than 52° C). TRPV3 is activated by increased temperature (higher than 31° C) and is expressed in the skin, tongue, and nervous system, where it may act as a "warm sensitive neuron."[246] Another TRPV receptor, the cold- and menthol-sensitive receptor (CMRI), has been identified and may help us better understand cold thermosensation and the development of targeted cold-producing analgesics. Pharmacologic studies of menthol have suggested possible κ-opioid receptor effects, contributing additional analgesic properties to the substance.[247]

Review and Physiology

Counterirritants such as capsaicin, camphor, menthol, and garlic represent a category of analgesics that excite and subsequently desensitize nociceptive sensory neurons[248] (Table 32–19). Although many of the group's members have had a long history of common medical use, it was not until recently that their molecular mechanisms of action were elucidated. All these pungent plant derivatives act on the TRPV superfamily, a group of structurally similar, thermosensitive ion channels. As noted earlier, members include TRPV1 (also called vanilloid receptor subtype 1 [VR1]), TRPV3, TRPM8, and TRPA1,[249] which are activated by capsaicin, camphor, menthol, and garlic, respectively[248] (Fig. 32–4). These thermosensitive receptors detect a wide range of temperatures, ranging from noxious heat to extreme cold, as well as other stimuli, including heat, protons, lipids, changes in extracellular osmolarity and/or pressure, and depletion of intracellular Ca^{2+} stores.[250] These proteins are expressed in primary sensory neurons as well as other tissues. On the activation of TRP receptors, the release of CGRP, substance P, and other inflammatory neurotransmitters is induced, producing local irritation and inflammation.[251] This can lead to two types of desensitization, acute or "pharmacologic" desensitization characterized by a diminished response during a constant agonist application, and a longer period of tachyphylaxis, or "functional" desensitization, characterized by desensitization to

Table 32–19. Topical Counterirritants and Hot and Cold Preparations

PRODUCT	Ingredients (%)				
	METHYL SALICYLATE	MENTHOL	CAMPHOR	CAPSAICIN	OTHER
Icy Hot balm	29	7.6			
Ben-Gay Ultra Strength	30	10	4		
Ben-Gay patch		1.4			
Salon Patch				0.025	
Mineral Ice		2			
Capzasin-HP				0.1	
Flexall Ultra Plus	10	16	3.1		
Aspercreme					Trolamine salicylate, 10

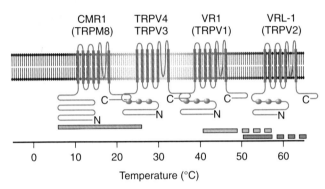

Figure 32–4. Transient receptor protein (TRP) family receptors and their thermosensitivity. (From Tominaga M, Caterina MJ: Thermosensation and pain. J Neurobiol 2004;61:3-12. With permission.)

other stimuli such as chemicals, pressure, or temperature.[248]

Capsaicin

As early as the 19th century, the selective effects of capsaicin on sensory nerve fibers were recognized.[218] The spicy ingredient in chili peppers has been used to relieve neuropathic pain, uremic pruritus, and bladder overactivity, as well as to provide analgesia.[252] Capsaicin has been recommended in a number of treatment guidelines for the treatment of osteo-arthritis.[233] Currently, nonprescription creams, lotions, and patches containing 0.025% to 0.075% capsaicin by weight are available for the treatment of musculoskeletal and neuropathic pain.[253] The mechanism of capsaicin is characterized by a paradoxic biphasic pharmacologic action on sensory neurons. An initial excitatory phase (pain and inflammation), mediated by activation of the TRPV1 receptor, is followed by the secondary analgesic phase that has been attributed to long-term desensitization of nociceptors and depletion of substance P.[254] A systematic review of topical capsaicin for the relief of musculoskeletal pain pooled the results of three double-blind, placebo-controlled trials of a total of 368 patients.[255] After 4 weeks of treatment with capsaicin 0.025% or plaster, the mean response rate (percentage of patients with at least 50% pain relief) was 38% (range, 34% to 42%), and the placebo response rate was 25% (range, 17% to 37%). The NNT was 8.1 and approxi-

mately one third of patients experienced local, treatment-related adverse events.[255] An older meta-analysis reported that capsaicin cream provides better pain relief for osteoarthritis than placebo (odds ratio, 4.36; 95% CI, 2.77 to 6.88).[256] However, products with low concentrations of capsaicin require multiple applications to provoke the desensitization of nerves,[252] and may be problematic for daily use because of potential adverse application effects such as burning or irritation of the eyes or other mucous membranes if not adequately removed from the hands after application.[218] Additionally, burning and pain on application reduce patient adherence and may adversely limit efficacy.[218,252] The combination of topical capsaicin (0.025%) with 3.3% doxepin provided more rapid analgesia when compared with treatment with either of these two agents independently.[257]

Camphor

Camphor is derived from the wood of the camphor laurel tree (*Cinnamomum camphora*). Historically, the sweet-smelling compound has had many medicinal uses, including as a decongestant, cough suppressant, and antipruritic agent.[248] OTC camphor-containing balms have also been used to provide analgesia. Recent studies have implicated three receptors in camphor's mechanism of action: TRPV3, the capsaicin receptor TRPV1, and the garlic receptor TRPA1.[248]

Menthol

In contrast, menthol—the component that confers mint smell and flavor to the *Mentha* species—is often included in eutectic formulations of local anesthetic agents.[247] Anecdotally, menthol induces tingling and cooling sensations when applied topically. Menthol confers analgesia through its Ca^{2+} channel–blocking actions. In addition to binding TRPM8,[249,253] menthol binds κ-opioid receptors and may also confer an additional opioid analgesic effect.[247] Furthermore, similar to other terpenes, menthol is an effective topical permeation enhancer for water-soluble drugs, such as the TCA imipramine.[258]

Salicylates

Topical rubefacients containing salicylates, another type of counterirritant, have an unidentified mechanism of action.[259] It is thought that analgesia is conferred by a mode different than that of NSAIDs, yet salicylates are often found in many topical preparations. Further randomized, clinical trial evidence of salicylates has been systematically reviewed by Mason and coworkers.[259] Three double-blind, placebo-controlled trials examined topical salicylates for the treatment of acute musculoskeletal pain. The study groups exhibited significantly better pain reductions than placebo (relative benefit, 3.6; 95% CI, 2.4 to 5.6; NNT, 2.1; range, 1.7 to 2.8). The long-term efficacy data and adverse events reported were poor for chronic musculoskeletal pain, but information from six double-blind, placebo-controlled trials indicated a relative benefit versus control of 1.5 (range, 1.3 to 1.9; NNT, 5.3; range, 3.6 to 10.2).

CONCLUSION

Analgesics play an important role in the treatment of many acute and chronic pain conditions. They represent the first line of agents in the World Health Organization's analgesic ladder, and range from OTC convenience medications to adjuvants in the treatment of musculoskeletal, arthritis, spine-related, and cancer pain conditions. Although considered relatively safe compared with many other prescription-strength medications, minor analgesics must be used with caution. Side effects and adverse events related to common use and misuse of these medications include liver toxicity (acetaminophen), gastrointestinal, renal, and cardiac toxicity (NSAIDs and COX-2 inhibitors), and physiologic dependence, tolerance, and addiction (combination opioid analgesics and tramadol products).

Topical analgesics (e.g., patches, creams, solutions) represent a growing area of development in pain management because of the relative ease of application, potential for reduced systemic side effects, and lowered risk of end-organ damage. Advancements in pharmaceutical delivery systems may also aid in the development and more widespread use of various OTC and prescription-strength topical compounds. The pain clinician should be cognizant of the vast array of ingredients found in various OTC topical analgesics and counterirritants, including capsaicin, menthol, camphor, and methylsalicylates.

SUMMARY

- Regular use of OTC analgesic medications is a common method used by patients for relieving various pain-related conditions.
- Minor opioid analgesics include propoxyphene, hydrocodone, oxycodone, and tramadol individual and combination products.
- Patient responses to individual opioids and opioid combination products may vary significantly. This is likely explained by opioid receptor polymorphisms and differences in pharmacokinetics and genetic variation related to enzymatic breakdown by hepatic metabolic systems.

- True serotonin toxicity and serotonin syndrome are rare but potentially deadly conditions seen in the field of pain management characterized clinically by changes in mental status and autonomic and neuromuscular hyperactivity.
- The use of OTC and prescription-strength topical preparations represents a growing area of development in pain medicine, with significantly less potential for systemic adverse effects and organ toxicity than oral formulations.
- Compared with other topically administered medications, topical NSAIDs have accumulated the largest amount of clinical evidence for their use in acute versus chronic musculoskeletal conditions.

References

1. Haas H: History of antipyretic analgesic therapy. Am J Med 1983;75:1-3.
2. Turunen JH, Mantyselka PT, Kumpusalo EA, et al: How do people ease their pain? A population-based study. J Pain 2004;5:498-504.
3. Hersh EV, Moore PA, Ross G: Over-the-counter analgesics and antipyretics: A critical assessment. Clin Ther. 2000;20:500-548.
4. Caudill-Slosberg MA, Schwartz LM, Woloshin S: Office visits and analgesic prescriptions for musculoskeletal pain in US: 1980 vs. 2000. Pain 2004;109:514-519.
5. Finnish Statistics on Medicines. Helsinki, Finland, National Agency for Medicines and Social Insurance Institution, 2003.
6. Turunen JH, Mantyselka PT, Kumpusalo EA, et al: Frequent analgesic use at population level: Prevalence and patterns of use. Pain 2005;115:374-381.
7. Vogt MT, Kwoh CK, Cope DK, et al: Analgesic usage for low back pain: Impact on health care costs and service use. Spine 2005;30:1075-1081.
8. Kaufman DW, Kelly JP, Rosenberg L, et al: Recent patterns of medication use in the ambulatory adult population of the United States: The Slone survey. JAMA 2002;287:337-344.
9. Paulose-Ram R, Hirsch R, Dillon C, et al: Frequent monthly use of selected non-prescription and prescription non-narcotic analgesics among U.S. adults. Pharmacoepidemiol Drug Saf 2005;14:257-266.
10. Wilcox CM, Cryer B, Triadafilopoulos G: Patterns of use and public perception of over-the-counter pain relievers: Focus on nonsteroidal anti-inflammatory drugs. J Rheumatol 2005;32:2218-2224.
11. Roumie CL, Griffin MR: Over-the-counter analgesics in older adults: A call for improved labelling and consumer education. Drugs Aging 2004;21:485-498.
12. Simoni-Wastila L, Stuart BC, Shaffer T: Over-the-counter drug use by Medicare beneficiaries in nursing homes: Implications for practice and policy. J Am Geriatr Soc 2006;54:1543-1549.
13. Adams NJ, Plane MB, Fleming MF, et al: Opioids and the treatment of chronic pain in a primary care sample. J Pain Symptom Manage 2001;22:791-796.
14. American Pain Society: Principles of Analgesic Use in the Treatment of Acute and Cancer Pain, 4th ed. Glenview, Ill, American Pain Society, 1999.
15. World Health Organization: Cancer Pain Relief. Geneva, World Health Organization, 1990.
16. Luo X, Pietrobon R, Sun SX, et al: Estimates and patterns of direct health care expenditures among individuals with back pain in the United States. Spine. 2004;29:79-86.
17. Armstrong SC, Cozza KL: Pharmacokinetic drug interactions of morphine, codeine, and their derivatives: Theory and clinical reality, Part I. Psychosomatics 2003;44:167-171.
18. Bertilsson L, Dahl ML, Dalen, et al: Molecular genetics of CYP2D6: Clinical relevance with focus on psychotropic drugs. Br J Clin Pharmacol 2002;53:111-122.

19. Lin JH, Lu AY: Inhibition and induction of cytochrome P450 and the clinical implications. Clin Pharmacokinet 1998;35:361-390.

20. Pasternak GW: Molecular biology of opioid analgesia. J Pain Symptom Manage 2005;29(Suppl 5):S2-S9.

21. Lotsch J: Opioid metabolites. J Pain Symptom Manage 2005;29(Suppl 5):S10-24.

22. Sindrup SH, Prosen K, Bjerring P, et al: Codeine increases pain thresholds to copper vapour laser stimuli in extensive but not in poor metabolisers of sparteine. Clin Pharmacol Ther 1990;48:686-693.

23. Quiding H, Lundqvust G, Boreus LO, et al: Analgesic effect and plasma concentrations of codeine and morphine after two dose levels of codeine following oral surgery. Eur J Clin Pharmacol 1993;44:319-323.

24. Vree T, Versy-Van WC: Pharmacokinetics and metabolism of codeine in humans. Biopharm Drug Dispos 1992;13:445-460.

25. Caraco Y, Sheller J, Wood AJ: Pharmacogenetic determination of the effects of codeine and prediction of drug interactions. J Pharmacol Exp Ther 1996;278:1165-1174.

26. Desmeules J, Gascon MP, Dayer P, et al: Impact of environmental and genetic factors on codeine analgesia. Eur J Clin Pharmacol 1991;41:23-26.

27. Bachs L, Skurtveit S, Morland J: Codeine and clinical impairments in samples in which morphine is not detected. Eur J Clin Pharmacol 2003;58:785-789.

28. Eckhardt K, Li S, A mmon S, et al: Same incidence of adverse drug events after codeine administration irrespective of the genetically determined differences in morphine formation. Pain 1998;76:27-33.

29. Hasselstrom J, Yue QY, Sawa J: The effect of codeine on gastrointestinal transit in extensive and poor metabolisers of debrisoquine. Eur J Clin Pharmacol 1997;53:145-148.

30. Homsi J, Walsh D, Nelson K: Important drugs for cough in advanced cancer. Support Care Cancer 2001;9:565-574.

31. Houde R, Wallenstein S, Beaver W: Evaluation of analgesics in patients with cancer pain. In Lasagna L (ed): Clinical Pharmacology: International Encyclopaedia of Pharmacology and Therapeutics. Oxford, Pergamon Press, 1966.

32. McQuay H, Moore R: An Evidence-based Resource for Pain Relief. Oxford, Oxford University Press, 1988.

33. De Craen AJ, Giulio G, Lampe-Schoenmaeckers, et al: Analgesic efficacy and safety of paracetamol-codeine combinations versus paracetamol alone: A systemic review. BMJ 1996;313:321-325.

34. Moore A, Collins S, Carroll D, et al: Paracetamol with and without codeine in acute pain: A quantitative systematic review. Pain 1997;70:193-201.

35. Forbes JA, Bates JA, Edquist IA, et al: Evaluation of two opioid-acetaminophen combinations and placebo in postoperative oral surgery pain. Pharmacotherapy 1994;14:139-146.

36. Young RJ: Dextropropoxyphene overdosage. Pharmacological considerations and clinical management. Drugs 1983;26:70-79.

37. Litman RE, Diller J, Nelson F: Deaths related to propoxyphene or codeine or both. J Forensic Sci 1983;28:128-38.

38. Kamal-Bahl S, Stuart BC, Beers MH: National trends in and predictors of propoxyphene use in community-dwelling older adults. Am J Geriatr Pharmacother 2005;3:186-195.

39. Smith R: Federal government faces painful decision on Darvon. Science 1971;203:857-58.

40. Duff G: Withdrawal of co-proxamol products and interim updated prescribing information. Letter to healthcare professionals, January 31, 2005. Available at www.mhra.gov.uk/CEM/CMO/2005/2.

41. Ulens C, Daenens P, Tytgat J: Norpropoxyphene-induced cardiotoxicity is associated with changes in ion selectivity and gating of HERG currents. Cardiovasc Res 1999;44:568-78.

42. Li Wan Po A, Zhang WY: Systematic overview of co-proxamol to assess analgesic effects of addition of dextropropoxyphene to paracetamol. BMJ 1997;315:1565-1571.

43. Kalso E, Vainio A, Mattila MJ, et al: Morphine and oxycodone in the management of cancer pain: Plasma levels determined by chemical and radioreceptor assays. Pharmacol Toxicol 1990;67:322-328.

44. Heiskanen T, Olkkola KT, Kalso E: Effects of blocking CYP2D6 on the pharmacokinetics and pharmacodynamics of oxycodone. Clin Pharmacol Ther 1998;64:603-611.

45. Nozaki C, Saitoh A, Kamei J: Characterization of the antinociceptive effects of oxycodone in diabetic mice. Eur J Pharmacol 2006;535:141-151.

46. Ross FB, Mith MT: The intrinsic antinociceptive effects of oxycodone appear to be kappa-opioid receptor mediated. Pain 1997;73:151-157.

47. Riley J, Ross JR, Rutter D, et al: No pain relief from morphine? Individual varation in sensitivity to morphine and the need to switch to an alternative opioid in cancer patients. Support Care Cancer 2006;14:56-64.

48. Lalovic B, Kharasch E, Hoffer C, et al: Pharmacokinetics and pharmacodynamics of oral oxycodone in healthy human subjects: Role of circulating active metabolites. Clin Pharmacol Ther 2006;79:461-79.

49. Holman JR, Wala EP: Characterization of the antinociceptive effect of oxycodone in male and female rats. Pharmacol Biochem Behavior 2006;83:100-108.

50. Beaver WT: Analgesic Efficacy of Hydrocodone and its Combinations: A Review. Spring House, Pa, Smith Simon, 1988.

51. Hardy JR: Opioids in cancer pain. In Davis M, Glare P, Hardy J (eds): Hydrocodone. Oxford, Oxford University Press, 2005, pp 59-67.

52. Wideman GL, Keffer M, Morris E, et al: Analgesic efficacy of a combination of hydrocodone with ibuprofen in postoperative pain. Clin Pharmacol Ther 1999;65:66-76.

53. Palangio M, Morris E, Doyle RT, et al: Combination hydrocodone and ibuprofen versus combination oxycodone and acetaminophen in the treatment of moderate or severe acute low back pain. Clin Ther 2002;24:87-99.

54. Palangio M, Wideman GL, Keffer M, et al: Combination hydrocodone and ibuprofen versus combination oxycodone and acetaminophen in the treatment of postoperative obstetric or gynecologic pain. Clin Ther 2000;22:600-612.

55. Palangio M, Damask MJ, Morris E, et al: Combination hydrocodone and ibuprofen versus combination codeine and acetaminophen for the treatment of chronic pain. Clin Ther 2000;22:879-892.

56. American College of Rheumatology Subcommittee on Osteoarthritis Guidelines: Recommendations for the medical management of osteoarthritis of the hip and knee: 2000 Update. Arthritis Rheum 2000;43:1905-1915.

57. Pendleton A, Arden N, Dougados M, et al: EULAR recommendations for the management of knee osteoarthritis: Report of a task force of the Standing Committee for International Clinical Studies Including Therapeutic Trials (ESCISIT). Ann Rheum Dis 2000;59:936-944.

58. Prescott LF: Paracetamol (Acetaminophen): A Critical Bibliographic Review, 2nd ed. Florence, Ky, Routledge, 2001.

59. Lucas R, Warner TD, Vojnovic I, et al: Cellular mechanisms of acetaminophen: Role of cyclo-oxygenase. FASEB J 2005;19:635-637.

60. Shen H, Sprott H, Aeschlimann A, et al: Analgesic action of acetaminophen in symptomatic osteoarthritis of the knee. Rheumatology 2006;45:765-770.

61. Heading RC, Ni mmo J, Prescott LF, et al: The dependence of paracetamol absorption on the rate of gastric emptying. Br J Pharmacol 1973;47:415-421.

62. Toes MJ, Jones AL, Prescott L: Drug interactions with paracetamol. Am J Ther 2005;12:56-66.

63. Lauterburg BH: Analgesics and glutathione. Am J Ther 2002;9:225-233.

64. Gebauer MG, Nyfort-Hansen K, Henschke PJ, et al: Warfarin and acetaminophen interaction. Pharmacotherapy 2003;23:109-112.

65. Gadisseur AP, Van Der Meer FJ, Rosendaal FR: Sustained intake of paracetamol (acetaminophen) during oral anticoagulant therapy with coumarins does not cause clinically

important INR changes: A randomized double-blind clinical trial. J Thromb Haemost 2003;1:714-717.

66. Hylek EM, Heiman H, Skates SJ, et al: Acetaminophen and other risk factors for excessive warfarin anticoagulation. JAMA 1998;279:657-662.

67. Kurtovic J, Riordan SM: Paracetamol-induced hepatotoxicity at recommended dosage. J Intern Med 2003;253:240-243.

68. Watkins PB, Seeff LB: Drug-induced liver injury. Hepatology 2006;43:618-631.

69. Shayiq RM, Roberts DW, Rothstein K, et al: Repeat exposure to incremental doses of acetaminophen provides protection against acetaminophen-induced lethality in mice: An explanation for high acetaminophen dosage in humans without hepatic injury. Hepatology 1999;29:451-463.

70. Rumack BH: Acetaminophen misconceptions. Hepatology 2004;40:10-15.

71. Whitcomb DC, Block GD: Association of acetaminophen hepatotoxicity with fasting and ethanol use. JAMA 1994; 272:1845-1850.

72. Smilkstein MJ, Rumack BH: Chronic ethanol use and acute acetaminophen overdose toxicity [abstract]. Clin Toxicol 1998;36:476.

73. Thummel KE, Slattery JT, Ro H, et al: Ethanol and production of the hepatotoxic metabolite of acetaminophen in healthy adults. Clin Pharmacol Ther 2000;67:591-599.

74. Hansten PD, Horn JR: Cytochrome P450 enzymes and drug interactions. In Top 100 Drug Interactions—A Guide to Patient Management. Edmonds, Wash, H&H Publications, 2005, pp 157-170.

75. Fored CM, Ejerblad E, Lindblad P, et al: Acetaminophen, aspirin, and chronic renal failure. N Engl J Med 2001;345: 1801-1808.

76. Asero R: Risk factors for acetaminophen and nimesulide intolerance in patients with NSAID-induced skin disorders. Ann Allergy Asthma Immunol 1999;82:554-558.

77. Curhan GC, Willett WC, Rosner B, et al: Frequency of analgesic use and risk of hypertension in younger women. Arch Intern Med 2002;162:2204-2208.

78. Dedier J, Stampfer MJ, Hankinson SE, et al: Non-narcotic analgesic use and the risk of hypertension in U.S. women. Hypertension 2002;40:604-608.

79. Kurth T, Hennekens CH, Sturmer T, et al: Analgesic use and risk of subsequent hypertension in apparently healthy men. Arch Intern Med 2005;165:1903-1909.

80. Seppala E, Laitinen O, Vapaatalo H: Comparative study on the effects of acetylsalicylic acid, indomethacin and paracetamol on metabolites of arachidonic acid in plasma, serum and urine in man. Int J Clin Pharmacol Res 1983;3:265-269.

81. Bradley JD, Brandt KD, Katz BP, et al: Comparison of an anti-inflammatory dose of ibuprofen, an analgesic dose of ibuprofen, and acetaminophen in the treatment of patients with osteoarthritis of the knee. N Engl J Med 1991;325:87-91.

82. Case JP, Baliunas AJ, Block JA: Lack of efficacy of acetaminophen in treating symptomatic knee osteoarthritis: A randomized, double-blind, placebo-controlled comparison trial with diclofenac sodium. Arch Intern Med 2003;163:169-178.

83. Pincus T, Koch G, Lei H, et al: Patient preference for placebo, acetaminophen (paracetamol) or Celecoxib Efficacy Studies (PACES): Two randomised, double blind, placebo controlled, crossover clinical trials in patients with knee or hip osteoarthritis. Ann Rheum Dis 2004;63:931-939.

84. Towheed TE, Judd MJ, Hochberg MC, et al: Acetaminophen for osteoarthritis. Cochrane Database Syst Rev 2003;(2): CD004257.

85. Brandt KD, Mazzuca SA, Buckwalter KA: Acetaminophen, like conventional NSAIDs, may reduce synovitis in osteoarthritic knees. Rheumatology (Oxford) 2006;45:1389-1394.

86. Gutstein HB, Akil H: Opioid analgesics. In Hardman JG, Limbird LE, Gilman AG (eds): Goodman & Gilman's The Pharmacological Basis of Therapeutics, 10th ed. New York, McGraw Hill, 2001, pp 569-619.

87. Roth SH: Efficacy and safety of tramadol HCl in breakthrough musculoskeletal pain attributed to osteoarthritis. J Rheumatol 1998;25:1358-1363.

88. Hennies HH, Friderichs E, Schneider J: Receptor binding, analgesic and antitussive potency of tramadol and other selected opioids. Arzneimittelforschung 1988;38:877-880.

89. Bianchi M, Rossoni G, Sacerdote P, et al: Effects of tramadol on experimental inflammation. Fundam Clin Pharmacol 1999;13:220-225.

90. Bianchi M, Broggini M, Balzarini P, et al: Effects of tramadol on synovial fluid concentrations of substance P and interleukin-6 in patients with knee osteoarthritis: Comparison with paracetamol. Int I mmunopharmacol 2003;3:1901-1908.

91. Grond S, Sablotzki A: Clinical pharmacology of tramadol. Clin Pharmacokinet 2004;43:879-923.

92. Gillen C, Haurand M, Kobelt DJ, et al: Affinity, potency and efficacy of tramadol and its metabolites at the cloned human mu-opioid receptor. Naunyn Schmiedeberg Arch Pharmacol 2000;362:116-121.

93. Valle M, Garrido MJ, Pavon JM, et al: Pharmacokinetic-pharmacodynamic modeling of the antinociceptive effects of main active metabolites of tramadol, (+)-O-desmethyltramadol and (–)-O-desmethyltramadol in rats. J Pharmacol Exp Ther 2000;293:646-653.

94. Raffa RB, Nayak RK, Liao S, et al: The mechanism of action and pharmacokinetics of tramadol hydrochloride. Rev Cont Pharmacol 1995;6:485-498.

95. Tramadol—Biovail Corporation. Drugs R D 2004;5:182-183.

96. Yanagita T: Drug dependence potential of 1-(m-methoxy-phenyl)-2-dimethylaminomethyl)-cyclohexan-1-ol hydrochloride (tramadol) tested in monkeys. Arzneimittelforschung 1978;28:158-163.

97. Preston KL, Jasinski DR, Testa M: Abuse potential and pharmacological comparison of tramadol and morphine. Drug Alcohol Depend. 1991;27:7-17.

98. U.S. Food and Drug Administration: Minutes of the FDA Drug Abuse Advisory Committee #27, 1994.

99. Cicero TJ, Adams EH, Geller A, et al: A postmarketing surveillance program to monitor Ultram (tramadol hydrochloride) abuse in the United States. Drug Alcohol Depend 1999;57: 7-22.

100. Adams EH, Breiner S, Cicero TJ, et al: A comparison of the abuse liability of tramadol, NSAIDs, and hydrocodone in patients with chronic pain. J Pain Symptom Manage 2006; 31:465-476.

101. Ultram prescribing information. Raritan, NJ, Ortho-McNeil, 2004.

102. Babul N, Noveck R, Chipman H, et al: Efficacy and safety of extended-release, once-daily tramadol in chronic pain: A randomized 12-week clinical trial in osteoarthritis of the knee. J Pain Symptom Manage 2004;28:59-71.

103. Liao S, Hill JF, Nayak RK: Pharmacokinetics of tramadol following single and multiple oral doses in man [abstract]. Pharm Res 1992;9(Suppl):308.

104. Lintz W, Barth H, Osterloh G, et al: Bioavailability of enteral tramadol formulations. 1st communication: Capsules. Arzneimittelforschung 1986;36:1278-1283.

105. Lee CR, McTavish D, Sorkin EM: Tramadol: A preliminary review of its pharmacodynamic and pharmacokinetic properties, and therapeutic potential in acute and chronic pain states. Drugs 1993;46:313-340.

106. Wu WN, McKown LA, Liao S: Metabolism of the analgesic drug Ultram (tramadol hydrochloride) in humans: API-MS and MS/MS characterization of metabolites. Xenobiotica 2002;32:411-425.

107. Stamer UM, Lehnen K, Hothker F, et al: Impact of CYP2D6 genotype on postoperative tramadol analgesia. Pain 2003;105: 231-238.

108. Mattia C, Coluzzi F: Tramadol: Focus on musculoskeletal and neuropathic pain. Minerva Anestesiol 2005;71:565-584.

109. Desmeules JA: The tramadol option. Eur J Pain 2000;4(Suppl A):15-21.

110. Nossol S, Schwarzbold M, Stadler T: Treatment of pain with sustained-release tramadol 100, 150, 200 mg: Results of a post-marketing surveillance study. Int J Clin Pract 1998;52: 115-121.

111. Hallberg P, Brenning G: Angioedema induced by tramadol—a potentially life-threatening condition. Eur J Clin Pharmacol 2005;60:901-903.

112. Hedenmalm K, Lindh JD, Sawe J, et al: Increased liability of tramadol-warfarin interaction in individuals with mutations in the cytochrome P450 2D6 gene. Eur J Clin Pharmacol 2004;60:369-372.

113. Sternbach H: The serotonin syndrome. Am J Psychiatry 1991;148:705-713.

114. Radomski JW, Dursun SM, Reveley MA, et al: An exploratory approach to the serotonin syndrome: An update of clinical phenomenology and revised diagnostic criteria. Med Hypotheses 2000;55:218-224.

115. Gillman PK, Whyte IM: Serotonin syndrome. In Haddad P, Dursun S, Deakin B (eds): Adverse Syndromes and Psychiatric Drugs. Oxford, Oxford University Press, 2004, pp 37-49.

116. Gillman PK: Monoamine oxidase inhibitors, opioid analgesics and serotonin toxicity. Br J Anaesth 2005;95:434-441.

117. Dunkley EJ, Isbister GK, Sibbritt D, et al: The Hunter Serotonin Toxicity Criteria: Simple and accurate diagnostic decision rules for serotonin toxicity. QJM 2003;96:635-642.

118. Isbister GK, Hackett LP: Nefazodone poisoning: Toxicokinetics and toxicodynamics using continuous data collection. J Toxicol Clin Toxicol 2003;41:167-173.

119. Dawson AH: Cyclic antidepressant drugs. In Dart RC (ed): Medical Toxicology, 3rd ed, vol 1. Baltimore, Lippincott Williams & Wilkins, 2004, pp 834-843.

120. Whyte IM, Dawson AH, Buckley NA: Relative toxicity of venlafaxine and selective serotonin reuptake inhibitors in overdose compared to tricyclic antidepressants. QJM 2003;96:369-374.

121. Bamigbade TA, Davidson C, Langord RM, et al: Actions of tramadol, its enantiomers and principal metabolite, O-desmethyltramadol, on serotonin (5-HT) efflux and uptake in the rat dorsal raphe nucleus. Br J Anaesth 1997;79:352-356.

122. Gillman PK: A review of serotonin toxicity data: Implications for the mechanisms of antidepressant drug action. Biol Psychiatry 2006;59:1046-1051.

123. Sunshine A: New clinical experience with tramadol. Drugs 1994;47(Suppl 1):8-18.

124. Stubhaug A, Grimstad J, Breivik H: Lack of analgesic effect of 50 and 100 mg oral tramadol after orthopedic surgery: A randomized, double-blind, placebo and standard active drug comparison. Pain 1995;62:111-118.

125. Turturro MA, Paris PM, Larkin GL: Tramadol versus hydrocodone-acetaminophen in acute musculoskeletal pain: A randomized double-blind clinical trial. Ann Emerg Med 1998;32:139-143.

126. Babul N, Noveck R, Chipman H, et al: Efficacy and safety of extended-release, once-daily tramadol in chronic pain: A randomized 12-week clinical trial in osteoarthritis of the knee. J Pain Sym Management 2004;28:59-71.

127. Wilder-Smith CH, Hill LT, Laurent S: Postamputation pain and sensory changes in treatment-naïve patients: Characteristics and responses to treatment with tramadol, amitriptyline, and placebo. Anesthesiology 2005;103:619-628.

128. Akinci SB, Saricaoglu F, Atay OA, et al: Analgesic effect of intra-articular tramadol compared with morphine after arthroscopic knee surgery. Arthroscopy 2005;21:1060-1065.

129. Leppert W, Luczak J: The role of tramadol in cancer pain treatment—a review. Support Care Cancer 2005;13:5-17.

130. Simon L, Lipman AG, Jacox A, et al: Guidelines for the Management of Osteoarthritis, Rheumatoid Arthritis and Juvenile Chronic Arthritis Pain. Glenview Ill, American Pain Society, 2002.

131. Harati Y, Gooch C, Swenson M, et al: Double-blind randomized trial of tramadol for the treatment of the pain of diabetic neuropathy. Neurology 1998;50:1842-1846.

132. Sindrup SH, Andersen G, Madsen C, et al: Tramadol relieves pain and allodynia in polyneuropathy: A randomised, double-blind, controlled trial. Pain 1999;83:85-90.

133. Gobel H, Stadler TH: Treatment of pain because of postherpetic neuralgia with tramadol: Results of an open, parallel pilot study vs. clomipramine with and without levomepromazine. Clin Drug Invest 1995;10:208-214.

134. Leppert W: Analgesic efficacy and side effects of oral tramadol and morphine administered orally in the treatment of cancer pain. Nowotwory 2001;51:257-266.

135. Tallarida RJ, Raffa RB: Testing for synergism over a range of fixed ratio drug combinations: Replacing the isobologram. Life Sci 1996;58:PL23-PL28.

136. Medve RA, Wang J, Karim R: Tramadol and acetaminophen tablets for dental pain. Anesth Prog 2001;48:79-81.

137. Schug SA: Combination analgesia in 2005—a rational approach: Focus on paracetamol-tramadol. Clin Rheumatol 2006;25(Suppl 1):S16-S21.

138. Cicero TJ, Inciardi JA, Adams EH, et al: Rates of abuse of tramadol remain unchanged with the introduction of new branded and generic products: Results of an abuse-monitoring system, 1994-2004. Pharmacoepidemiol Drug Saf 2005;14:851-859.

139. Emkey R, Rosenthal N, Wu SC, et al: CAPSS-114 Study Group. Efficacy and safety of tramadol/acetaminophen tablets (Ultracet) as add-on therapy for osteoarthritis pain in subjects receiving a COX-2 nonsteroidal antiinfla mmatory drug: A multicenter, randomized, double-blind, placebo-controlled trial. J Rheumatol 2004;31:5-7.

140. Edwards JE, McQuay HJ, Moore RA: Combination analgesic efficacy: Individual patient data meta-analysis of single-dose oral tramadol plus acetaminophen in acute postoperative pain. J Pain Symptom Manage 2002;23:121-130.

141. Glyn J: The discovery and early use of cortisone. J R Soc Med 1998;91:513-517.

142. Hopkins RL, Leinung MC: Exogenous Cushing's syndrome and glucocorticoid withdrawal. Endocrinol Metab Clin North Am 2005;34:371-384

143. Rousseau P: The palliative use of high-dose corticosteroids in three terminally ill patients with pain. Am J Hosp Palliat Care 2001;18:343-6.

144. Chang MH, Ger LP, Hsieh PF, et al: A randomised clinical trial of oral steroids in the treatment of carpal tunnel syndrome: A long term follow up. J Neurol Neurosurg Psychiatry 2002;73:710-714.

145. Buchbinder R, Hoving JL, Green S, et al: Short course prednisolone for adhesive capsulitis (frozen shoulder or stiff painful shoulder): A randomised, double-blind, placebo-controlled trial. Ann Rheum Dis 2004;63:1460-1469.

146. Christensen K, Jensen EM, Noer I: The reflex dystrophy syndrome response to treatment with systemic corticosteroids. Acta Chir Scand 1982;148:653-655.

147. Deltasone prescribing information. Kalamazoo, Mich, Pharmacia & Upjohn, 2002.

148. Lussier D, Huskey AG, Portenoy RK: Adjuvant analgesics in cancer pain management. Oncologist 2004;9:571-591.

149. Amigo P, Mazuryk ME, Watanabe S, et al: Recent onset of abdominal pain in a patient with advanced breast cancer. J Pain Symptom Manage 2000;20:77-80.

150. Curtis JR, Westfall AO, Allison J, et al: Population-based assessment of adverse events associated with long-term glucocorticoid use. Arthritis Rheum 2006;55:420-426.

151. Carmichael SL, Shaw GM: Maternal corticosteroid use and risk of selected congenital anomalies. Am J Med Genet 1999;86:242-4.

152. Kozin F, McCarty DJ, Sims J, et al: The reflex sympathetic dystrophy syndrome. I. Clinical and histologic studies: Evidence for bilaterality, response to corticosteroids and articular involvement. Am J Med 1976;60:321-331.

153. Braus DF, Krauss JK, Strobel J: The shoulder-hand syndrome after stroke: A prospective clinical trial. Ann Neurol 1994;36:728-733.

154. Guo TZ, Wei T, Kingery WS: Glucocorticoid inhibition of vascular abnormalities in a tibia fracture rat model of complex regional pain syndrome type I. Pain 2006;121:158-167.

155. Greenberg HS, Kim JH, Posner JB: Epidural spinal cord compression from metastatic tumor: Results with a new treatment protocol. Ann Neurol 1980;8:361-366.

156. Watanabe S, Bruera E: Corticosteroids as adjuvant analgesics. J Pain Symptom Manage 1994;9:442-445.

157. Weissman DE: Glucocorticoid treatment for brain metastases and epidural spinal cord compression: A review. J Clin Oncol 1988;6:543-551.
158. Kim MJ, Ye YM, Park HS, et al: Chemotherapy-related arthropathy. J Rheumatol 2006;33:1364-1368.
159. Wooldridge JE, Anderson CM, Perry MC: Corticosteroids in advanced cancer. Oncology (Williston Park) 2001;15: 225-234.
160. DePalma MJ, Bhargava A, Slipman CW: A critical appraisal of the evidence for selective nerve root injection in the treatment of lumbosacral radiculopathy. Arch Phys Med Rehabil 2005;86:1477-1483.
161. Haimovic IC, Beresford HR: Dexamethasone is not superior to placebo for treating lumbosacral radicular pain. Neurology 1986;36:1593-1594.
162. Green LN: Dexamethasone in the management of symptoms because of herniated lumbar disc. J Neurol Neurosurg Psychiatry 1975;38:1211-1217.
163. Hedeboe J, Buhl M, Ramsing P: Effects of using dexamethasone and placebo in the treatment of prolapsed lumbar disc. Acta Neurol Scand 1982;65:6-10.
164. Saal JS, Franson RC, Dobrow R, et al: High levels of inflammatory phospholipase A_2 activity in lumbar disc herniations. Spine 1990;15:674-678.
165. McLain RF, Kapural L, Mekhail NA: Epidural steroid therapy for back and leg pain: Mechanisms of action and efficacy. Spine J 2005;5:191-201.
166. Autio RA, Karppinen J, Kurunlahti M, et al: Effect of periradicular methylprednisolone on spontaneous resorption of intervertebral disc herniations. Spine 2004;29:1601-1607.
167. Harmon KG, Hawley C: Physician prescribing patterns of oral corticosteroids for musculoskeletal injuries. J Am Board Fam Pract 2003;16:209-212.
168. Binder A, Hazleman BL, Parr G, et al: A controlled study of oral prednisolone in frozen shoulder. Br J Rheumatol 1986;25:288-292.
169. Hench PS, Kendall EC, Slocumb CH, et al: The effect of a hormone of the adrenal cortex (17-hydroxy-11-dehydrocorticosterone: compound E) and of pituitary adrenocorticotropic hormone on rheumatoid arthritis. Proc Staff Meet Mayo Clin 1949;24:181-197.
170. Kirwan JR: The effect of glucocorticoids on joint destruction in rheumatoid arthritis. The Arthritis and Rheumatism Council Low-Dose Glucocorticoid Study Group. N Engl J Med 1995;333:142-146.
171. Harris ED, Emkey RD, Nicols JE, et al: Low-dose prednisone therapy in rheumatoid arthritis: A double-blind study. J Rheumatol 1983;10:713-721.
172. Gotzsche PC, Johansen HK: Meta-analysis of short-term low dose prednisolone versus placebo and non-steroidal anti-inflammatory drugs in rheumatoid arthritis. BMJ 1998;316: 811-818.
173. Saynok J, Yaksh TL: Caffeine as an analgesic adjuvant: A review of pharmacology and mechanisms of action. Pharmacol Rev 1993;45:43-85.
174. Mighardi JR, Armellmo JJ, Friedman M, et al: Caffeine as an analgesic adjuvant in tension headache. Clin Pharmacol Ther 2004;56:576-586.
175. Forbes JA, Beaver WT, Jones KF, et al: Effects of caffeine on ibuprofen analgesia in postoperative oral surgery pain. Clin Pharmaol Ther 1991;49:674-684.
176. Kuntz D, Brossel R: [Analgesic effect and clinical tolerability of the combination of paracetamol 500 mg and caffeine 50 mg versus paracetamol 400 mg and dextropropoxyphene 30 mg in back pain.] Presse Med 1996;25:1171-1174.
177. Laska EM, Sunshine A, Zigelbom I, et al: Effect of caffeine on acetaminophen analgesia. Clin Pharmacol Ther 1983;33: 498-509.
178. Laska EM, Sunhine A, Mueller F, et al: Caffeine as an analgesic adjuvant. JAMA 1984;21:1711-1718.
179. Godfrey L, Yan L, Clarke G, et al: Modulation of paracetamol antinociception by caffeine and by selective adenosine A2 receptor antagonists in mice. Eur J Pharmacol 2006;531: 80-86.
180. Abo-Salem OM, Hayallah AM, Bilkei-Gorzo A: Antinociceptive effects of novel A2B adenosine antagonists. J Pharm Exp Therapeutics 2004;308:358-366.
181. Sawnok J, Yaksh TL: Caffeine as an analgesic adjuvant: A review of pharmacology and mechanisms of action. Pharmacol Rev 1993;45:43-85.
182. Fiebich BL, Candelario-Jalil E, Mantovani M, et al: Modulation of catecholamine release from rat striatal slices by the fixed combination of aspirin, paracetamol and caffeine. Pharmacol Res 2006;53:391-396.
183. Currie SR, Wilson KG, Gauthier ST: Caffeine and chronic low back pain. Clin J Pain 1995;11:214-219.
184. McPartland JM, Mitchell JA: Caffeine and chronic back pain. Arch Phys Med Rehabil 1997;78:61-63.
185. Jones M: Chronic neuropathic pain: Pharmacological interventions in the new millennium. Int J Pharm Compound 2000;4:6-15.
186. Grosser T, Fries S, FitzGerald GA: Biological basis for the cardiovascular consequences of COX-2 inhibition: Therapeutic challenges and opportunities. J Clin Invest 2006;116: 4-15.
187. U.S. Food and Drug Administration: Alert for healthcare professionals: Prescription non-steroidal anti-inflammatory drugs (NSAIDs), 2005. Available at www.fda.gov/cder/drug/Info Sheets/HCP/NS_NSAIDsHCP.pdf.
188. Bjordal JM, Klovning A, Elisabeth LA, et al: Short-term efficacy of pharmacotherapeutic interventions in osteoarthritic knee pain: A meta-analysis of randomized placebo-controlled trials. Eur J Pain 2007;11:125-38.
189. Unites States Analgesics. Industry Profile, Reference Code: 72-751. www.Datamonitor.com.
190. Rowbotham MC, Davies PS, Verkempinck C, et al: Lidocaine patch: Double-blind controlled study of a new treatment method for post-herpetic neuralgia. Pain 1996;65:39-44.
191. McCleane G: Topical application of doxepin hydrochloride, capsaicin and a combination of both produces analgesia in chronic human neuropathic pain: A randomized, double-blind, placebo-controlled study. Br J Clin Pharmacol 2000; 49:574-579.
192. Gerner P, Kao G, Srinivasa V, et al: Topical amitriptyline in healthy volunteers. Reg Anesth Pain Med 2003;28: 289-293.
193. Capsaicin Study Group: Treatment of painful diabetic peripheral neuropathy with topical capsaicin: A multicenter, double-blind, vehicle-controlled study. Arch Intern Med 1991;151:2225-2229.
194. Brown MB, Martin GP, Jones SA, et al: Dermal and transdermal drug delivery systems: Current and future prospects. Drug Deliv 2006;13:175-187.
195. Cleary GW: Transdermal delivery systems; a medical rationale. In Shah VP, Maibach HI (eds): Topical Drug Bioavailability, Bioequivalence, and Penetration. New York, Plenum Press, 1993, pp 17-68.
196. Henzl MR, Loomba PK: Transdermal delivery of sex steroids for hormone replacement therapy and contraception: A review of principles and practice. J Reprod Med 2003; 48:525-540.
197. Kornick CA, Santiago-Palma J, Moryl N, et al: Benefit-risk assessment of transdermal fentanyl for the treatment of chronic pain. Drug Saf. 2003;26:951-973.
198. Cramer MP, Saks SR: Translating safety, efficacy and compliance into economic value for controlled release dosage forms. Pharmacoeconomics 1994;5:482-504.
199. Bos JD, Meinardi MM: The 500 Dalton rule for the skin penetration of chemical compounds and drugs. Exp Dermatol 2000;9:165-169.
200. Yano T, Nakagawa A, Tsuji M, et al: Skin permeability of various non-steroidal anti-inflammatory drugs in man. Life Sci 1986;39:1043-1050.
201. Southwell D, Barry BW, Woodford R: Variations in permeability of human skin within and between specimens. Int J Pharm 1984;18:299-309.
202. Larsen RH, Nielsen F, Sorensen JA, et al: Dermal penetration of fentanyl: Inter- and intraindividual variations. Pharmacol Toxicol 2003;93:244-248.

203. Varvel JR, Shafer SL, Hwang SS, et al: Absorption characteristics of transdermally administered fentanyl. Anesthesiology 1989;70:928-934.
204. Yang SI, Park HY, Lee SH, et al: Transdermal eperisone elicits more potent and longer-lasting muscle relaxation than oral eperisone. Pharmacology 2004;71:150-156.
205. Long CC: Common skin disorders and their topical treatment. In Walters KA (ed): Dermatological and Transdermal Formulations. New York, Marcel Dekker, 2002, pp 41-60.
206. Payne R, Mathias SD, Pasta DJ, et al: Quality of life and cancer pain: Satisfaction and side effects with transdermal fentanyl versus oral morphine. J Clin Oncol 1998;16:1588-1593.
207. Jarupanich T, Lamlertkittikul S, Chandeying V: Efficacy, safety and acceptability of a seven-day, transdermal estradiol patch for estrogen replacement therapy. J Med Assoc Thai 2003;86:836-845.
208. Archer DF, Cullins V, Creasy GW, et al: The impact of improved compliance with a weekly contraceptive transdermal system (Ortho Evra) on contraceptive efficacy. Contraception 2004;69:189-195.
209. Whittington R, Faulds D: Hormone replacement therapy: I. A pharmacoeconomic appraisal of its therapeutic use in menopausal symptoms and urogenital estrogen deficiency. Pharmacoeconomics 1994;5:419-445.
210. Frei A, Andersen S, Hole P, et al: A one-year health economic model comparing transdermal fentanyl with sustained-release morphine in the treatment of chronic noncancer pain. J Pain Palliat Care Pharmacother 2003;17:5-26.
211. Steinstrasser I, Merkle HP: Dermal metabolism of topically applied drugs: Pathways and models reconsidered. Pharm Acta Helv Apr 1995;70:3-24.
212. Hogan DJ, Maibach HI: Adverse dermatologic reactions to transdermal drug delivery systems. J Am Acad Dermatol 1990;22(5 Pt 1):811-814.
213. Carmichael AJ: Skin sensitivity and transdermal drug delivery: A review of the problem. Drug Saf 1994;10:151-159.
214. Toole J, Silagy S, Maric A, et al: Evaluation of irritation and sensitisation of two 50 microg/day oestrogen patches. Maturitas 2002;43:257-263.
215. Murphy M, Carmichael AJ:. Transdermal drug delivery systems and skin sensitivity reactions: Incidence and management. Am J Clin Dermatol 2000;1:361-368.
216. Galer BS: Topical Medications. In Loeser JD, Butler SH, Chapman CR, et al (eds): Bonica's Management of Pain, 3rd ed. Philadelphia, Lippincott Williams & Wilkins, 2001, pp 1736-1742.
217. Brown MB, Martin GP, Jones SA, et al: Dermal and transdermal drug delivery systems: Current and future prospects. Drug Deliv 2006;13:175-187.
218. Bley KR: Recent developments in transient receptor potential vanilloid receptor 1 agonist-based therapies. Expert Opin Investig Drugs 2004;13:1445-1456.
219. Vaile JH, Davis P: Topical NSAIDs for musculoskeletal conditions. A review of the literature. Drugs 1998;56:783-799.
220. Heyneman CA, Lawless-Liday C, Wall GC: Oral versus topical NSAIDs in rheumatic diseases: A comparison. Drugs 2000;60:555-574.
221. Kumar R, Katare OP: Lecithin organogels as a potential phospholipid-structured system for topical drug delivery: A review. AAPS PharmSciTech 2005;6:E298-E310.
222. Franckum J, Ramsay D, Das NG, et al: Pluronic lecithin organogel for local delivery of anti-inflammatory drugs. Int J Pharm Compounding 2004;8:101-105.
223. Yamane MA, Williams AC, Barry BW: Terpene penetration enhancers in propylene glycol/water co-solvent systems: Effectiveness and mechanism of action. J Pharm Pharmacol 1995;47:978-989.
224. Weber DC, Hoppe KM: Physical agent modalities. In Braddom RL (ed): Physical Medicine and Rehabilitation, 3rd ed. Philadelphia, WB Saunders, 2006, pp 459-477.
225. Lekas MD: Iontophoresis treatment. Otolaryngol Head Neck Surg 1979;878:292-298.
226. Klaiman MD, Shrader JA, Danoff JV, et al: Phonophoresis versus ultrasound in the treatment of co mmon musculoskeletal condtions. Med Sci Sports Exerc 1998;30:1349-1355.

227. Tegeder I, Muth-Selbach U, Lotsch J, et al: Application of microdialysis for the determination of muscle and subcutaneous tissue concentrations after oral and topical ibuprofen administration. Clin Pharmacol Ther 1999;65:357-368.
228. Rolf C, Engstrom B, Beauchard C, et al: Intra-articular absorption and distribution of ketoprofen after topical plaster application and oral intake in 100 patients undergoing knee arthroscopy. Rheumatology (Oxford) 1999;38:564-567.
229. Moore RA, Tramer MR, Carroll D, et al: Quantitative systematic review of topically applied non-steroidal anti-inflammatory drugs. BMJ 1998;316:333-338.
230. Mason L, Moore RA, Edwards JE, et al: Topical NSAIDs for acute pain: A meta-analysis. BMC Musculoskelet Disord 2004;5:10.
231. Lin J, Zhang W, Jones A, et al: Efficacy of topical non-steroidal anti-inflammatory drugs in the treatment of osteoarthritis: Meta-analysis of randomised controlled trials. BMJ 2004;329:324.
232. Scott DL, Shipley M, Dawson A, et al: The clinical management of rheumatoid arthritis and osteoarthritis: Strategies for improving clinical effectiveness. Br J Rheumatol 1998;37:546-554.
233. Jordan KM, Arden NK, Doherty M, et al: EULAR Recommendations 2003: An evidence based approach to the management of knee osteoarthritis: Report of a Task Force of the Standing Committee for International Clinical Studies Including Therapeutic Trials (ESCISIT). Ann Rheum Dis Dec 2003;62:1145-1155.
234. Bookman AA, Williams KS, Shainhouse JZ: Effect of a topical diclofenac solution for relieving symptoms of primary osteoarthritis of the knee: A randomized controlled trial. CMAJ 2004;171:333-338.
235. Roth SH, Shainhouse JZ: Efficacy and safety of a topical diclofenac solution (pennsaid) in the treatment of primary osteoarthritis of the knee: A randomized, double-blind, vehicle-controlled clinical trial. Arch Intern Med 2004;164:2017-2023.
236. Galer BS, Rowbotham M, Perander J, et al: Topical diclofenac patch relieves minor sports injury pain: Results of a multicenter controlled clinical trial. J Pain Symptom Manage 2000;19:287-294.
237. Predel HG, Koll R, Pabst H, et al: Diclofenac patch for topical treatment of acute impact injuries: A randomised, double blind, placebo controlled, multicentre study. Br J Sports Med 2004;38:318-323.
238. Beetge E, du Plessis J, Muller DG, et al: The influence of the physicochemical characteristics and pharmacokinetic properties of selected NSAIDs on their transdermal absorption. Int J Pharm 2000;193:261-264.
239. Dowling TC, Arjomand M, Lin ET, et al: Relative bioavailability of ketoprofen 20% in a poloxamer-lecithin organogel. Am J Health Syst Pharm 2004;61:2541-2544.
240. Mazieres B, Rouanet S, Velicy J, et al: Topical ketoprofen patch (100 mg) for the treatment of ankle sprain: A randomized, double-blind, placebo-controlled study. Am J Sports Med 2005;33:515-523.
241. Mazieres B, Bouanet S, Guillon Y, et al: Topical ketoprofen in the treatment of tendonitis: A randomized, double-blind, placebo-controlled study. J Rheumatol 2005;32:1563-1570.
242. Matthieu L, Meuleman L, Van Hecke E, et al: Contact and photocontact allergy to ketoprofen: The Belgian experience. Contact Dermatitis 2004;50:238-241.
243. Sugiura M, Hayakawa R, Kato Y, et al: Cases of photocontact dermatitis because of ketoprofen. Contact Dermatitis 2000;43:16-19.
244. Durbize E, Vigan M, Puzenat E, et al: Spectrum of cross-photosensitization in 18 consecutive patients with contact photoallergy to ketoprofen: Associated photoallergies to non-benzophenone-containing molecules. Contact Dermatitis 2003;48:144-149.
245. Julius D: The molecular biology of thermosensation. In Dostrovsky JO, Carr DB, Koltzenburg M (eds): Proceedings of the Tenth World Congress on Pain. Progress In Pain Research And Management, vol 24. Seattle, IASP Press, 2003, pp 63-70.

246. Clapham DE: TRP channels as cellular sensors. Nature 2003;426:517-524.
247. Galeotti N, Di Cesare Mannelli L, Mazzanti G, et al: Menthol: A natural analgesic compound. Neurosci Lett 2002;322(3): 145-148.
248. Xu H, Blair NT, Clapham DE: Camphor activates and strongly desensitizes the transient receptor potential vanilloid subtype 1 channel in a vanilloid-independent mechanism. J Neurosci 2005;25:8924-8937.
249. Tominaga M, Caterina MJ: Thermosensation and pain. J Neurobiol 2004;61:3-12.
250. Gunthorpe MJ, Benham CD, Randall A, et al: The diversity in the vanilloid (TRPV) receptor family of ion channels. Trends Pharmacol Sci 2002;23:183-191.
251. Bautista DM, Movahed P, Hinman A, et al: Pungent products from garlic activate the sensory ion channel TRPA1. Proc Natl Acad Sci U S A 2005;102:12248-12252.
252. Szallasi A: Vanilloid (capsaicin) receptors in health and disease. Am J Clin Pathol 2002;118:110-121.
253. McKemy DD, Neuhausser WM, Julius D: Identification of a cold receptor reveals a general role for TRP channels in thermosensation. Nature 2002;416:52-58.
254. Szallasi A, Blumberg PM: Vanilloid (capsaicin) receptors and mechanisms. Pharmacol Rev 1999;51:159-212.
255. Mason L, Moore RA, Derry S, et al: Systematic review of topical capsaicin for the treatment of chronic pain. BMJ 2004;328:991.
256. Zhang WY, Li Wan Po A: The effectiveness of topically applied capsaicin: A meta-analysis. Eur J Clin Pharmacol 1994;46:517-522.
257. McLean G: Topical application of doxepin hydrochloride, capsaicin and a combination of both produces analgesia in chronic human neuropathic pain: A randomized, double-blind, placebo-controlled study. Br J Clin Pharmacol 2000; 49:574-579.
258. Jain AK, Thomas NS, Panchagnula R: Transdermal drug delivery of imipramine hydrochloride. I. Effect of terpenes. J Control Release 2002;79:93-101.
259. Mason L, Moore RA, Edwards JE, et al: Systematic review of efficacy of topical rubefacients containing salicylates for the treatment of acute and chronic pain. BMJ 2004;328: 995.

CHAPTER
33 Antidepressants as Analgesics

Gary McCleane

The second half of the twentieth century saw the introduction of a range of therapeutic agents that were shown to have an antidepressant effect. Among these agents were those with a tricyclic chemical structure that led to their classification as tricyclic antidepressants (TCAs). Even before their introduction into clinical practice, the concept of a link between depression and pain was obvious and the possibility that this link was causal encouraged the use of antidepressants for those patients who exhibited the features of both pain and depression.

In 1962, Kuipers reported a case series in which the TCA imipramine was used in patients with "non-articular rheumatism" and in whom 60% to 70% experienced pain relief.[1] Similarly, Scott reported his double-blind trial in patients with rheumatoid arthritis, osteoarthritis, and ankylosing spondylitis in whom imipramine provided significantly more pain relief than placebo.[2] In both these reports, it was postulated that the pain relief produced is secondary to mood elevation, rather than an intrinsic analgesic effect of the antidepressant. It is now recognized that the pain relief apparent with the use of antidepressants can be independent of any alteration in mood caused by the drug,[3] although it has been noted with, for example, doxepin treatment that pain reduction is intimately associated with reduction in depression.[4]

Therefore, the focus of this chapter is on the potential pain-reducing potential of drugs otherwise associated with the treatment of depression. However, pain rarely exists in isolation and any muscle relaxation, mood enhancement, or improvement in the quality and duration of sleep, all of which are potential effects of antidepressant use, are often welcome accompaniments of any pain relief that is produced.

CLASSIFICATION OF ANTIDEPRESSANTS

Antidepressants are currently classified partly on the basis of their chemical structure and partly on their primary in vivo effects (Box 33–1).

Tricyclic Antidepressants

The structures of some TCAs are shown in Figure 33–1.

Analgesic Mechanism of Action

It is now clear that the tricyclic antidepressants have a number of diverse effects that contribute to their analgesic effect (Table 33–1). The extent to which each individual TCA exerts these effects differs, which may account for differences in the effectiveness and propensity to cause side effects in patients when members of this class of drugs are used. As will be noted later in this chapter, not all the proposed modes of action of TCAs are the result of central effects, with a number of possible peripheral actions now becoming apparent.

Serotonergic Effect
The presence of a descending bulbospinal inhibitory influence on spinal neural activity is now well defined. When 5-hydroxytryptamine (5-HT) antagonists are administered, the antinociceptive effect of the TCAs are inhibited.[5] Similarly, when central 5-HT systems are depleted using p-chlorophenylalanine, the antinociceptive effects of TCAs are again reduced.[6-9]

Some tricyclics interfere with serotonin reuptake into nerve terminals.[10-12] In addition, some TCAs alter serotonin binding to receptors on neural tissue.[13,14]

Noradrenergic Effect
In a similar fashion to the serotonergic effect of TCAs, the descending bulbospinal noradrenergic inhibitory influence is thought to be important in their analgesic effect. Depletion of central norepinephrine systems with α-methyl p-tyrosine inhibits the antinociceptive actions of the antidepressants[6-9] and α-adrenoreceptor antagonists also have the same effect.[15-17] Specifically, when phentolamine, a nonspecific α_1- and α_2-adrenoreceptor antagonist, is given with a TCA, antinociception is inhibited.[18] However, when the α_1-adrenoreceptor antagonist prazosin is coadministered with the TCA amitriptyline in

BOX 33–1. CLASSIFICATION OF ANTIDEPRESSANTS

Monoamine Oxidase Inhibitors
- Harmaline
- Iproclozide
- Iproniazid
- Isocarboxazid
- Moclobemide
- Nialamide
- Selegiline
- Toloxatone
- Tranylcypromine

Dopamine Reuptake Inhibitors
- Amineptine
- Bupropion

Serotonin-Norepinephrine Reuptake Inhibitors (SNRIs)
- Desipramine
- Duloxetine
- Milnacipran
- Nefazodone
- Venlafaxine

Selective Serotonin Reuptake Inhibitors (SSRIs)
- Alaproclate
- Citalopram
- Escitalopram
- Etoperidone
- Fluoxetine
- Fluvoxamine
- Paroxetine
- Sertraline
- Zimeldine

Selective Serotonin Reuptake Enhancer
- Tianeptine

Tricyclic Antidepressants (TCAs)
- Amitriptyline
- Clomipramine
- Desipramine
- Dothiepin
- Doxepin
- Imipramine
- Lofepramine
- Nortriptyline
- Protriptyline
- Trimipramine
- Iprindole
- Opipramol

Tetracyclic Antidepressants
- Amoxapine
- Maprotiline
- Mianserin
- Mirtazapine

mice, antinociception is observed. Conversely, when amitriptyline is coadministered with the α_2-adrenoreceptor antagonist RX821002, antinociception is observed,[16] suggesting that TCAs derive at least part of their antinociceptive effect by interacting with α_2 adrenoreceptors rather than the α_1 receptors.

Opioidergic Effect
Although the serotonergic and noradrenergic effects of TCAs were originally thought to be the primary mechanism of action of this drug class, it is now clear that other actions may also be important. When clomipramine is administered to rats in the formalin test, the opioid antagonist naloxone can completely antagonize the antinociceptive effect of that TCA.[18] Similarly, administration of the delta (δ)-opioid antagonist naltrindole with antidepressants displaces their antinociceptive dose-response curves to the right, whereas administration of the enkephalin catabolism inhibitor acetorphan with the antidepressants dothiepin, amitriptyline, or sibutramine enhances their antinociceptive effects.[19] Chronic antidepressant administration can modify opioid receptor densities[20] and increase opioid levels in certain brain regions.[21,22]

N-Methyl-D-Aspartate Receptor Effect
Reynolds and Miller have observed that desmethylimipramine and imipramine both prevent Ca^{2+} influx into cultured cortical neurons of the rat produced by N-methyl-D-aspartate (NMDA). They also noted that other TCAs had a similar but less intense effect.[23] Others have observed that antidepressants bind to the NMDA receptor complex[23,24] and that chronic administration of antidepressants alters NMDA binding characteristics.[25] There is some debate as to the importance of a NMDA effect in regard to the analgesic effect of antidepressants.[26]

Adenosine Receptor Effect
Adenosine is known to produce analgesia,[27] and antidepressants inhibit the uptake of adenosine into neuronal preparations.[28] The antinociceptive effect of the antidepressants is inhibited by adenosine receptor antagonists.[29-31] Adenosine receptors have both peripheral and central representation (see later discussion).

Sodium Channel Effect
Anecdotal evidence has long been present for a sodium channel–blocking or local anesthetic–type effect with TCAs. Individual patients have reported that holding a TCA tablet over a sore tooth causes pain reduction and localized numbness.

A number of other therapeutic agents used in pain management are known to have a sodium channel blocking effect. These include the local anesthetics and certain antiepileptic drugs. Results of animal studies have confirmed that TCAs have sodium channel–blocking effects[32-37] and it is therefore likely that this effect has at least some involvement in their analgesic actions.

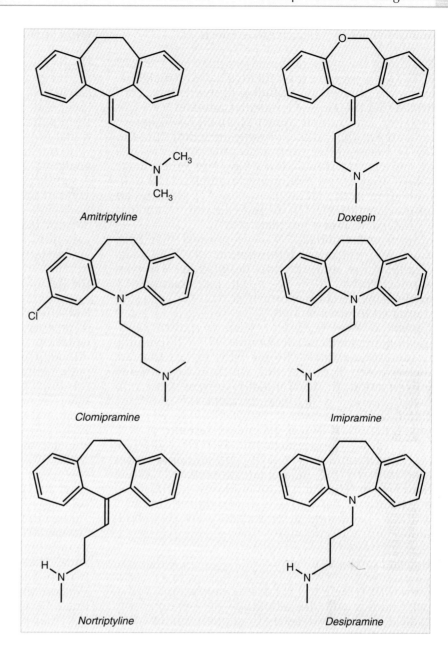

Figure 33–1. Tricyclic antidepressants.

Table 33–1. Mode of Action of Tricyclic Antidepressants

EFFECT	MODE OF ACTION
Serotonergic	Interferes with serotonin reuptake
	Alters serotonin binding to receptors
Noradrenergic	Interacts with α_2 adrenoreceptors
Opioidergic	Modifies opioid receptor densities
	Increases opioid levels in some brain areas
N-Methyl-D-aspartate (NMDA) receptor	Binds to NMDA receptor complex
	Alters NMDA binding characteristics
Adenosine receptor	Inhibits adenosine uptake
Sodium channel	Blocks sodium channels
Calcium channel	Increases densities of L-type calcium channels
Other receptors	Inhibits histaminic, cholinergic, muscarinic, and nicotinic receptors

Calcium Channel Effect

Although acute treatment with an antidepressant has no observable effect on calcium channels, chronic treatment with citalopram and chlorprothixene (but not imipramine) increases the density of L-type calcium channels. It also has an antinociceptive effect, with this effect being nullified by nifedipine administration.[38]

Other Effects

Antidepressants also interact with histaminic, cholinergic muscarinic, and cholinergic nicotinic receptors in an inhibitory manner.[26] These interactions may contribute to the side effects of the antidepressants (e.g., dry mouth, sedation, urinary retention).

Animal Studies of Antinociceptive Effects

Because of the many proposed pharmacologic effects of TCAs, one would expect them to have an analgesic-antinociceptive effect. A number of studies have confirmed that this class of antidepressant does have this property. For example, Abdel-Salam and colleagues[39] have shown that antidepressants, including those in the TCA class, display antinociceptive properties in a rat tail electric stimulation assay, and others have shown that chronic administration decreases self-mutilation in the rat autotomy test,[40,41] produces an antinociceptive effect in the formalin test,[42,43] and has a similar action in a hot plate test.[44]

Ardid and Guilbaud[45] have confirmed that both acute and chronic administration of TCAs (e.g., clomipramine, amitriptyline, desipramine) have an antinociceptive effect in a rat mononeuropathy model. This effect on neuropathic pain has been substantiated in other studies.[46,47]

Some of the TCAs also seem to possess anti-inflammatory effects. For example, when imipramine is administered on a chronic basis to rats that are then exposed to carrageenin, which induces intense inflammation, the local inflammatory response normally observed is significantly reduced.[48] Similarly, clomipramine reduces carrageenin-induced skin inflammation in a dose-dependent fashion, as well as decreasing the prostaglandin E_2 (PGE_2)–like biologic and immunologic activity and substance P concentration in the inflammatory exudate.[49] When both amitriptyline and imipramine are administered on a chronic basis to rats with adjuvant-induced arthritis, behavioral tests suggest that they both induce antinociception.[50]

Human Experimental Pain

Even with a single 100-mg dose of imipramine, verbal pain ratings and the amplitude of somatosensory evoked cerebral potentials to suprathreshold intradermal electric stimuli are reduced significantly, more than in subjects taking placebo.[51] Similarly, a single oral dose of desipramine has been shown to increase subjective pain thresholds and the nociceptive withdrawal reflex threshold to percutaneous electrical stimulation of the sural nerve.[52] Poulsen and associates[53] have examined the effect of a single oral dose of 100 mg of imipramine on pain detection and tolerance thresholds to heat and pressure, thresholds of quadriceps femoris muscle withdrawal reflex to single and repeated electrical stimulation of the sural nerve, and continuous pain ratings during the cold pressor test in 12 healthy volunteers. They found that imipramine significantly increases pain thresholds to heat and pressure, as well as the pain tolerance threshold and reflex threshold to single electrical stimulation. Pain ratings during the cold pressor test and pain detection thresholds to heat and pressure were unaltered.[53] These studies have suggested that TCAs can have a differential hypoanalgesic effect in different human experimental pain tests.

Tricyclic Antidepressants in Clinical Pain Management

Historically, TCAs were used in human pain management before their modes of action as analgesics were elucidated. The fact that they can reduce pain and independently elevate mood, as well as normalize sleep patterns and cause muscle relaxation, are additional potential benefits of their use.

In no human field of use is the evidence of an analgesic effect greater than that of neuropathic pain. A significant body of evidence underpins the use of TCAs in a number of specific neuropathic pain conditions and, because the features of neuropathic pain are not dependent on the causal disease or neural irritation, it is widely accepted that the evidence of analgesia with specific conditions is strong enough to allow uniform use for any condition manifesting the symptoms of neuropathic pain.

Postherpetic Neuralgia

A prototypic neuropathic pain condition, neural irritation, and destruction make this a particularly difficult condition to treat. With established postherpetic neuralgia (PHN), palliation rather than cure is the only prospect. Perhaps in no other condition have TCAs made such an impact. Evidence has suggested that amitriptyline,[54-57] nortriptyline,[58] and desipramine[59] are among the TCAs that can usefully alleviate the suffering associated with this condition. As an example of potential efficacy, Watson and coworkers have reported "good to excellent" pain relief in 16 of 24 patients studied,[54] and Max and colleagues[57] have reported that 47% of 58 patients studied in their randomized controlled trial obtained "moderate or greater" pain relief with amitriptyline. Interestingly, in a study comparing amitriptyline with the tetracyclic antidepressant maprotiline (which has a predominantly noradrenergic effect) Watson and associates[55] have noted that "amitriptyline relieves some patients with postherpetic neuralgia. Many patients suffer side effects and better therapies are necessary." Incidentally, the pain relief produced by amitriptyline was greater than that apparent after maprotiline use.

Watson and coworkers[58] have compared the effect of nortriptyline and amitriptyline and found both to have an analgesic effect, but that nortriptyline has fewer side effects. Kishore-Kumar and colleagues[59] have examined the effect of desipramine on PHN and confirmed an analgesic effect. They stated that "other antidepressants—notably amitriptyline—are known to ameliorate postherpetic neuralgia, but those agents are often toxic." Almost 2 decades after this study, amitriptyline is still considered a front-line agent, and arguably the preferential first therapeutic agent for the treatment of PHN.

Painful Diabetic Neuropathy

Again, strong evidence exists for pain relief produced by TCAs in patients with painful diabetic neuropathy (PDN). Amitriptyline,[3,60] desipramine,[60-62] clomipramine,[62] imipramine,[63-65] and nortriptyline[66] have all been shown to have an analgesic effect in this condition.

In terms of comparative efficacy, Max and associates[60] found that desipramine is of equal efficacy to amitriptyline, whereas Sindrup and coworkers[62] found that clomipramine tends to produce better pain relief than desipramine. When dose-response is considered, Sindrup and colleagues[65] found that when imipramine is used, a dose-response relationship does exist. Although a dose-response relationship is also noted when clomipramine is used, this does not seem to be the case with desipramine treatment.[62]

Painful Mononeuropathy and Polyneuropathy

Some evidence exists for an analgesic effect when clomipramine is used in the treatment of painful mononeuropathy and polyneuropathy pain. Langohr and associates[67] have compared treatment with clomipramine and acetylsalicylic acid in a blinded crossover study and were able to show a greater analgesic effect during the clomipramine treatment phase.

Pain Associated with Spinal Cord Injury

Not all studies examining the effect of TCAs on neuropathic pain have produced a positive result. Cardenas and coworkers[68] studied 84 patients with spinal cord injury (SCI) pain who were randomized to receive amitriptyline or an active placebo, benztropine mesylate. No significant differences in measured pain parameters were found between the treatment groups or when comparing pretreatment and treatment periods. This evidence is in contrast to that presented by others who have suggested a beneficial effect of TCAs in SCI pain, although their evidence is based on case reports rather than blinded, placebo-controlled trials.[69,70] In contrast to the negative response in studies of SCI pain, Leijon and Boivie[71] have reported a useful analgesic effect when amitriptyline is used in patients with central post-stroke pain.

Fibromyalgia

Although the use of TCAs in patients with fibromyalgia is widespread, consideration of the evidence supporting their use is difficult. This is largely because fibromyalgia is a complex disorder that manifests itself in a spectrum of symptoms and signs. From a broad perspective, there can be little doubt that antidepressants do improve the symptoms of fibromyalgia in a some patients.[72] O'Malley and colleagues[73] have undertaken a meta-analysis of studies that examine the effect of antidepressants in patients with fibromyalgia. They have calculated that the odds ratio for improvement with antidepressant therapy is 4.2 (95% confidence interval, 2.6 to 6.8). They concluded that antidepressant therapy has a positive effect on sleep, fatigue, pain, and well-being, but not on trigger points. They also found that in only one of the five studies that measured depression scores was there a correlation between symptom improvement and depression scores.[72] When TCAs are specifically considered, Arnold and associates[74] have concluded from their meta-analysis that TCAs produce the largest improvement in sleep quality, with modest improvement found in measures of stiffness and tenderness.

In terms of the number of patients who can improve with antidepressant treatment, Carette and coworkers[75] found that after 1 month of treatment for fibromyalgia, 21% were improved (as opposed to 0% on placebo) and after 6 months of treatment, these had increased to 36% and 19%, respectively.

Osteoarthritis

Historically, an analgesic effect of TCAs was first noted in patients with joint pain.[1] Limited evidence has suggested that TCAs can reduce joint pain caused by osteoarthritis.[50]

Low Back Pain

Although a diagnosis of low back pain is extremely wide and nonspecific and encompasses a wide range of differing problems, it does represent a significant clinical problem for many practitioners. A single report of a randomized, controlled trial of the use of doxepin in patients with low back pain has suggested that it can reduce pain and decrease indices of depression.[76]

Cancer-related Neuropathic Pain

TCAs seem to exert an analgesic effect in a range of pain conditions, but Mercadante and colleagues[77] have reported that amitriptyline failed to produce any pain relief in 16 patients with advanced cancer who had features of neuropathic pain. However, their study numbers were small, the neuropathic pain may not have been present in isolation given the cancer diagnosis, and any neuropathic pain arising in association with cancer could have been emanating from a diverse number of neural structures irritated by tumor deposits.

Human Immunodeficiency Virus
Sensory Neuropathy

TCAs do not seem to be effective in this condition.[78]

Comparative Studies

Morello and associates[79] have studied 28 patients with painful diabetic neuropathy in a crossover study comparing the effect of amitriptyline and gabapentin. They found that the pain relief produced by the TCA is of similar magnitude and quality to that obtained with gabapentin.

Overall Effectiveness

One way of displaying the potential efficacy of any agent is to consider the numbers needed to treat (NNT; Table 33–2). In terms of analgesic medication, this represents the number of patients needing to take the treatment to obtain a 50% or more reduction in their pain.

Selective Serotonin Reuptake Inhibitors

TCAs have analgesic potential for various pain conditions and have a diverse range of pharmacologic

Table 33–2. Numbers Needed to Treat (NNT) Using Tricyclic Antidepressants for Pain

CONDITION	NNT
Painful diabetic neuropathy	3.0
	3.4
	1.3
Postherpetic neuralgia	2.3
	2.1
	2.2
Atypical facial pain	2.8
Central pain	1.7

Data from McQuay HJ, Tramer M, Nye BA, et al: A systematic review of antidepressants in neuropathic pain. Pain 1996;68:217-227; Collins SL, Moore R, McQuay HJ, et al: Antidepressants and anticonvulsants for diabetic neuropathy and postherpetic neuralgia: A quantitative systematic review. J Pain Symptom Manage 2000;20:449-458; and McQuay HJ, Moore RA: Antidepressants and chronic pain. BMJ 1997;314:763-764.

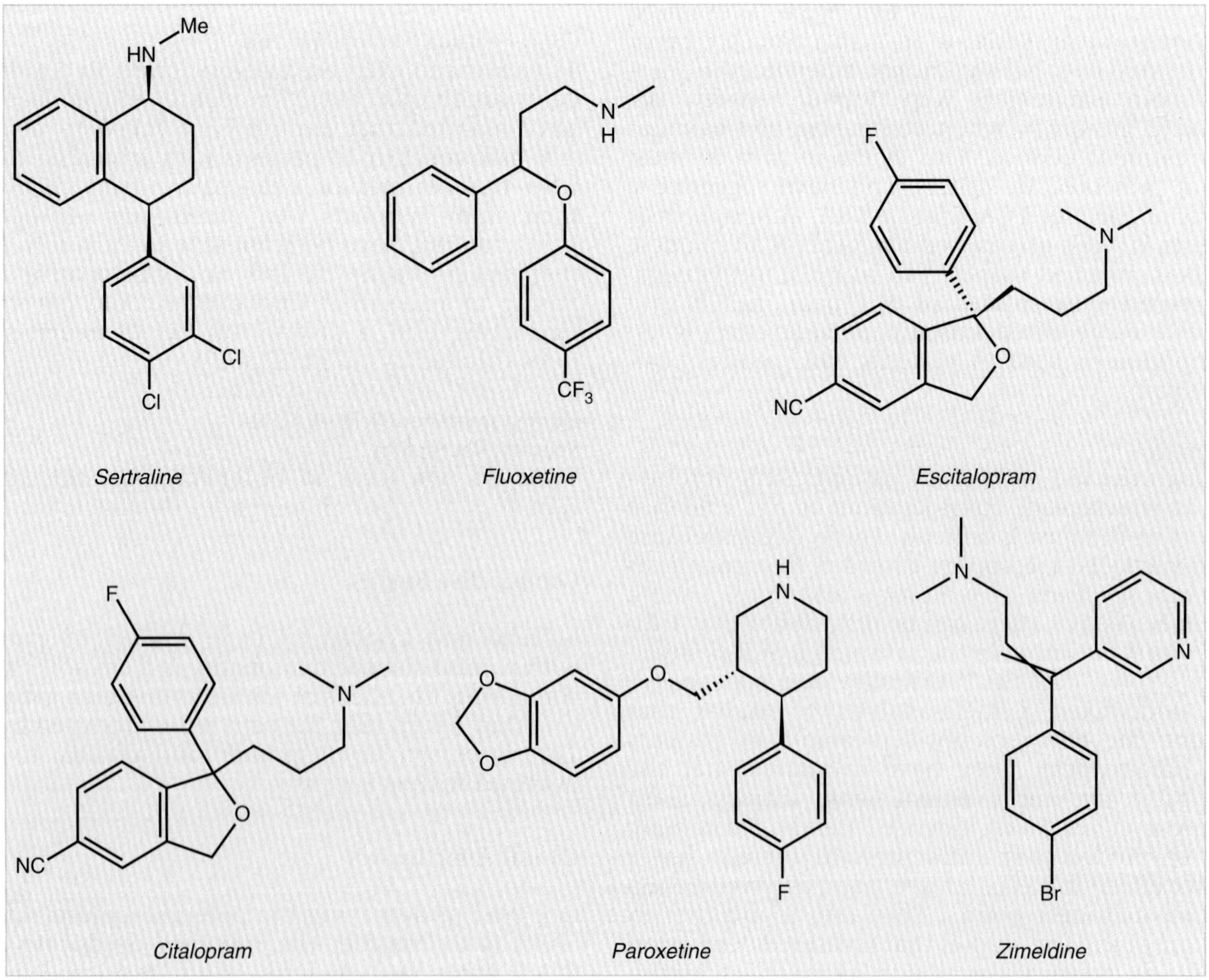

actions, but these actions can also increase their propensity to cause side effects. It was hoped that with the advent of antidepressants with more specific modes of action, analgesia would still be associated with their use and the potential to produce side effects would be reduced.

When the antinociceptive effect of the selective serotonin reuptake inhibitors (SSRIs; Fig. 33–2) were examined in a mouse hot plate pain test, fluvoxamine induced a dose-dependent antinociceptive effect, whereas fluoxetine and citalopram induced only a weak antinociceptive effect.[80] Escitalopram failed to elicit any antinociceptive effect. The antinociceptive effect of these three SSRIs was not blocked by the opioid antagonist naloxone. In contrast, again using a mouse hot plate test, paroxetine produced an antinociceptive effect that was inhibited by naloxone, suggesting that this SSRI may act not only because of its serotonergic effect, but also because of an interaction with the opioidergic system.[81] In the same study, paroxetine-induced antinociception was inhibited by the 5-hydroxytryptamine (5-HT; serotonin) 5-HT$_3$ antagonist ondansetron, but not by the 5-HT$_2$ receptor antagonist ketanserin.

Figure 33–2. Selective serotonin reuptake inhibitors (SSRIs).

When considering the overall results from studies, it has been calculated that the NNT for one patient to get 50% pain reduction is 5 for paroxetine and 15.3 for fluoxetine.[82] This leads to the conclusion that evidence for the effectiveness of SSRIs in pain management is limited, at best.[83,84]

SSRIs and Human Pain

Painful Diabetic Neuropathy

A number of studies have examined the effect of SSRIs on PDN. Sindrup and colleagues[85] have compared the effects of paroxetine with imipramine. Paroxetine did produce pain relief, but less than that obtained with imipramine. On the other hand, use of paroxetine was associated with fewer side effects than imipramine.[85] Max and colleagues[60] have compared the effect of amitriptyline, desipramine, fluoxetine, and placebo in patients with PDN. When subjects were considered in terms of percentage of those who derived moderate or greater pain relief, the results were 74% of those receiving amitriptyline, whereas for desipramine, fluoxetine, and placebo the results were 61%, 48%, and 41% respectively. Citalopram has also been studied and found to be relatively effective, with few side effects.[86]

Fibromyalgia

A number of studies have suggested that SSRIs have little effect on fibromyalgia (FM) pain. In one, Norregaard and associates[87] studied 22 patients with FM and compared the effect of citalopram with placebo. After 8 weeks of treatment (4 weeks on placebo, 4 weeks on citalopram), no changes were observed in any pain parameter measured, nor in depression scores. Similarly, Anderberg and coworkers[88] have found no difference with citalopram treatment when results were analyzed on an intent to treat basis, although there were reductions in pain and well-being scores in those completing the study.

Serotonin-Norepinephrine Reuptake Inhibitors

Serotonin-norepinephrine reuptake inhibitors (SNRIs; Fig. 33–3) selectively block the reuptake of norepinephrine and serotonin, 5-HT. Milnacipran blocks 5-HT and norepinephrine reuptake with equal affinity, whereas duloxetine has a 10-fold selectivity for 5-HT and venlafaxine a 30-fold selectivity for 5-HT.[89]

SNRIs and Animal Pain Studies

The likely effects of drugs on humans can often be predicted by testing that uses specific animal pain models. However, there may be species differences in response; in human clinical practice, mixed pain states are common, whereas animal models are based on specific pain types.

When formalin is applied to animal paws, a two-stage response is observed, which can be measured electrophysiologically or by behavioral observation. Both duloxetine (an SNRI) and citalopram (an SSRI) attenuate the second phase of the formalin response.[90] When compared with venlafaxine and milnacipran, duloxetine attenuates the second phase of this test more significantly.[91]

In the tail flick test (a test of acute nociception), duloxetine has minimal effect,[90-92] whereas in the hot plate test, some antinociceptive response with duloxetine is also observed.[90,92] In the chronic nerve constriction injury model of neuropathic pain, venlafaxine[93] and duloxetine[90] both have a significant antinociceptive effect.

SNRIs in Clinical Pain Management

Duloxetine is the first antidepressant to have a specific pain indication in the United States, the treatment of painful diabetic neuropathy (diabetic peripheral neuropathic pain).[94] SNRIs may also be useful for other conditions.

Painful Diabetic Neuropathy

It is well established that duloxetine reduces the pain associated with diabetic neuropathy.[95-97] Bearing in mind the relatively high risk of side effects when TCAs are used in treatment of this condition, dropout rates from studies are as low as 12% with duloxetine use[95] and long-term studies examining the use of this drug for up to 52 weeks have shown that it has a favorable safety profile when used over this prolonged period.[96] Duloxetine treatment has been associated with modest adverse changes in glycemia in patients with diabetic peripheral neuropathic pain, which does not impact on the significant improvement in pain observed with duloxetine treatment.[98]

Fibromyalgia

Traditionally, TCAs have been used in the treatment of FM. However, their side effect profiles often reduce compliance. Conversely the SSRIs have a more acceptable side effect profile but are relatively ineffective. The SNRIs, however, combine a relatively low risk of side effects with a relatively high chance of alleviating symptoms.

In a number of large studies, duloxetine has been found to be efficacious, not only in terms of pain reduction, but also in many of the other problematical complaints associated with this condition.[97,99] For example, in a study of 207 subjects, Arnold and colleagues[99] have found that duloxetine significantly reduces pain, number of tender points, and stiffness scores while significantly increasing the tender point pain threshold when compared with placebo. Furthermore, measures of quality of life were improved by active treatment. In an even larger study of 354 patients with FM, Arnold and associates[100] have confirmed their previous findings and have also shown that the beneficial effects of duloxetine therapy are independent of its effect on mood.

These positive effects with duloxetine therapy seem to be reproduced by other SNRIs, with milnacipran[101,102] and venlafaxine[103] also having been shown to have a positive effect. In Vitton and coworkers'[101]

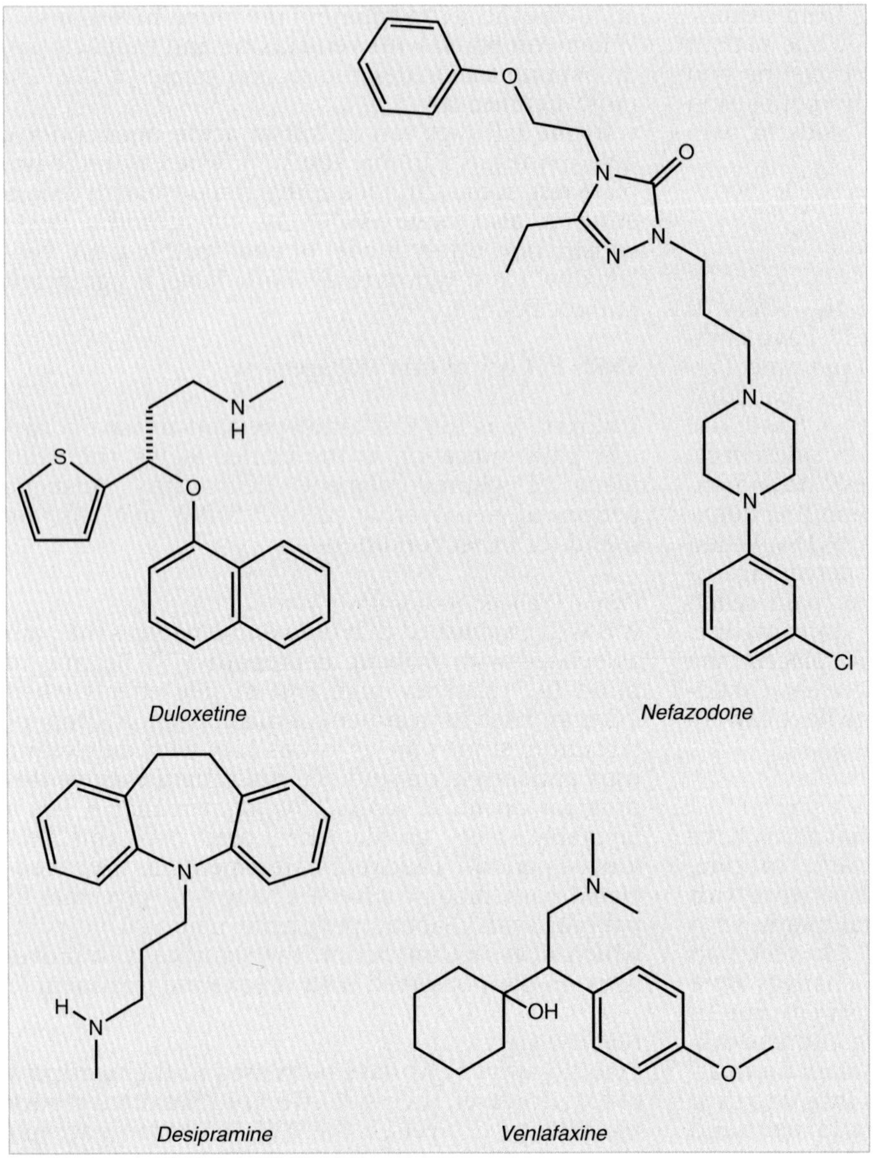

Duloxetine

Nefazodone

Desipramine

Venlafaxine

Figure 33–3. Serotonin-norepinephrine reuptake inhibitors (SNRIs).

study of the use of milnacipran in subjects with FM, of the 125 subjects enrolled in the study, 37% reported at least a 50% reduction in pain intensity (as opposed to 14% in the placebo group).

Tetracyclic Antidepressants

Limited evidence for an analgesic effect with tetracyclic antidepressants (Fig. 33–4) exists. When amitriptyline is compared with the tetracyclic antidepressant maprotiline in patients with postherpetic neuralgia, even though maprotiline displays analgesic properties, those of amitriptyline are more pronounced.[65] In animal nociceptive models, mirtazapine displays antinociceptive properties with evidence of antinociceptive effect in the hot plate chronic nerve constriction model of neuropathic pain and in the second phase of the formalin response.[90]

Monoamine Oxidase Inhibitors

Renowned for their multiple side effects, drug interactions, and necessity for a tyramine-free diet when they are used, monoamine oxidase inhibitors (MAOIs; Fig. 33–5) have no place in pain management. Little evidence exists for any analgesic effect.[104]

Dopamine Reuptake Inhibitors

Although classified as a dopamine reuptake inhibitor (Fig. 33–6), bupropion also has noradrenergic activity. Evidence of an analgesic effect is limited, although Semenchuk and colleagues[105] have found that 73% of subjects studied in their placebo-controlled trial with neuropathic pain obtain pain relief with bupropion treatment.

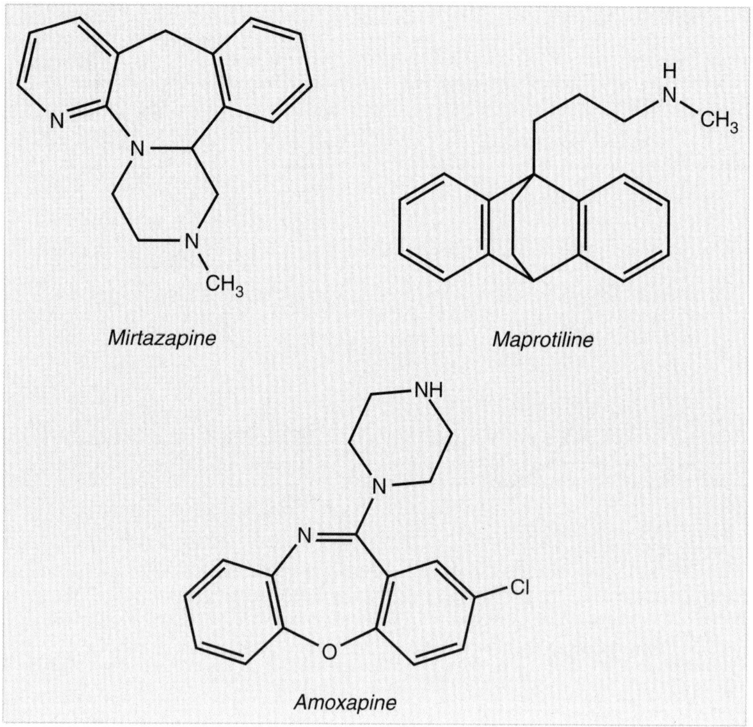

Figure 33–4. Tetracyclic antidepressants.

ANTIDEPRESSANTS: SAFETY AND SIDE EFFECTS

The safety of the antidepressants can be considered both from the perspective of normal usage and in overdose. Buckley and colleagues[106] have provided an interesting insight into the potential dangers of antidepressants when taken in overdose. They calculated the number of deaths per million prescriptions (Table 33–3).

The implications for use of these drugs are obvious. Careful consideration needs to be given to the use of desipramine if there is any danger that the drug may be taken in overdose. The data in the study cited[106] are from the United Kingdom, but a similar picture is likely elsewhere. In one study in Virginia, TCAs were found to be the most common antidepressants used in suicide attempts.[107]

In terms of overall comparative tolerability, one would expect that the newer antidepressants would be better tolerated than the TCAs. In a meta-analysis reviewing the tolerability of TCAs and SSRIs (when used for the treatment of depression), Arroll and colleagues[108] have found that the numbers needed to harm (NNH)—in this case the numbers of subjects receiving the treatment—for one to need to drop out because of side effects was calculated as 5 to 11 for the TCAs and 21 to 94 for the SSRIs. In sharp contrast, Wilson and Mottram[109] have studied the use of antidepressants in older depressed patients and concluded that ". . . TCA-related drugs are comparable to SSRIs in terms of tolerability" but did note that the use of TCAs is associated with an increased risk of dry mouth, drowsiness, dizziness, and lethargy when compared with SSRIs.

Among the SSRIs, it seems that fluoxetine has a greater chance of causing adverse gastrointestinal effects than other SSRIs.[110]

Effect of Antidepressants on Weight

Weight gain is common with antidepressant use. When they are used for the treatment of depression, mood alteration may have an effect on appetite and well-being. TCAs are more likely to cause weight gain (which may interfere with compliance) than the SSRIs.[111]

Cholinergic-Type Side Effects

Cholinergic-type side effects may also complicate TCA use. These include dry mouth, sedation, and urinary retention.

Risk of Falls

In a study of U.S. veterans, French and colleagues[112] have shown that of 2212 hip fracture patients, 70% had taken medication prior to the fracture, which may have contributed to their fall. Patients were twice as likely to have taken a TCA or SSRI as a matched control.

Use of Antidepressants in Pregnancy

Concern always exists when medication is taken during pregnancy. It seems that neither TCA nor SSRI use during pregnancy is associated with an increased risk of major fetal malformation, but poor neonatal adaptation has been reported.[113]

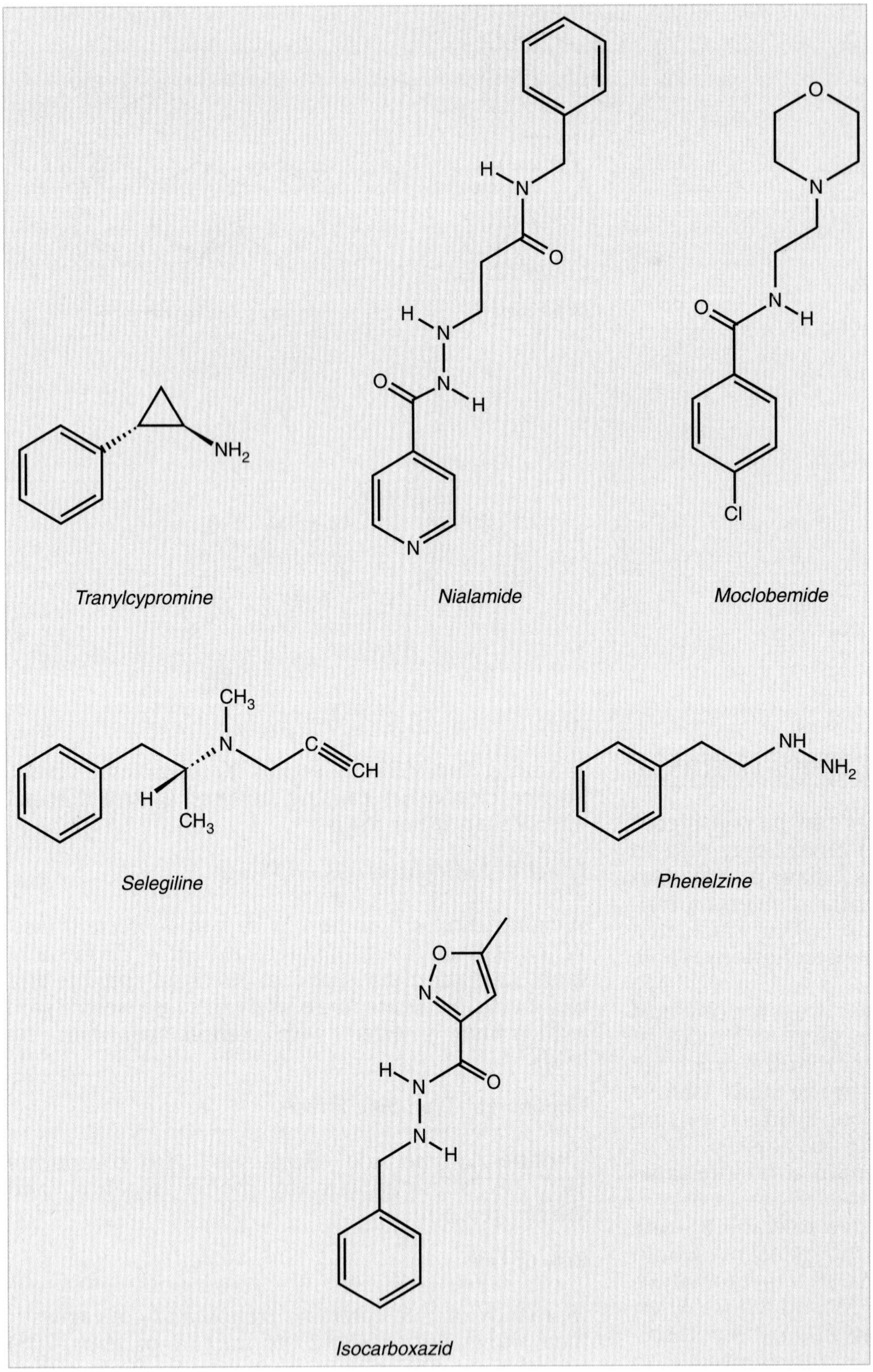

Tranylcypromine

Nialamide

Moclobemide

Selegiline

Phenelzine

Isocarboxazid

Figure 33–5. Monoamine oxidase inhibitors (MAOIs).

Automobile Driving

Use of any potentially sedative medication leads to concerns about its use while driving. Ramaekers[114] has concluded that after acute dosing of sedating antidepressants (e.g., amitriptyline, imipramine, doxepin, mianserin), a measure of driving ability gave comparable results to individuals whose blood alcohol concentration was 0.8 mg/mL. When treatment was continued for 1 week, driving performance returned to that of the placebo group, except for those taking mianserin where impairment continued. It was also noted that concomitant use of a benzodiazepine with the antidepressant makes driving impairment significant. When SSRIs are considered, no impairment of driving ability has been noted.[115] Consequently, when a TCA is given, the patient should be warned to avoid driving until he or she stabilizes on a fixed dose of

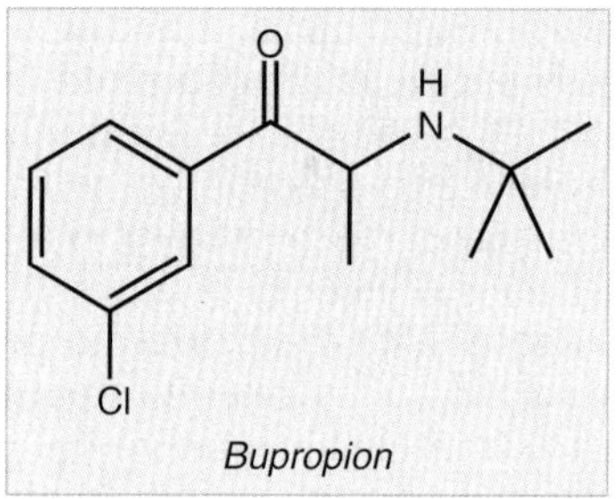

Figure 33–6. Dopamine reuptake inhibitor.

Table 33–3. Numbers of Deaths per Million Prescriptions of Antidepressants

CLASS OF ANTIDEPRESSANT	ANTIDEPRESSANT	DEATHS PER MILLION PRESCRIPTIONS
Tricyclic antidepressants (TCAs)	Desipramine	200.9
	Dothiepin	53.3
	Amitriptyline	38.0
	Imipramine	32.8
	Clomipramine	12.5
	Nortriptyline	5.5
Selective serotonin reuptake inhibitors (SSRIs)	Fluvoxamine	3.0
	Citalopram	1.9
	Fluoxetine	0.9
	Paroxetine	0.7
Serotonin-norepinephrine reuptake inhibitors (SNRIs)	Venlafaxine	13.2
	Nefazodone	0

Data from Buckley NA, McManus PR: Fatal toxicity of serotonergic and other antidepressant drugs: Analysis of United Kingdom mortality data. BMJ 2002;325:1332-1333.

the TCA. Also, the patient should be warned of the potential for driving ability to be influenced over the longer term when the TCA is taken with other sedative medication.

SSRIs and Nonsteroidal Anti-inflammatory Drugs

De Jong and colleagues[116] have studied 15,445 new users of antidepressants with or without nonsteroidal anti-inflammatory drug (NSAID) use. They counted the number of first prescriptions of peptic ulcer drugs, with or without an NSAID, from day 2 after starting until 10 days after antidepressant commencement. In the 691 individuals given TCAs and who were not on NSAIDs, the incidence of peptic ulcer drug request was 0.051. In the SSRI-only group (1181 subjects), the incidence was 1.2. When a SSRI was taken with an NSAID (86 subjects), the incidence of peptic ulcer drug request was 12.4% as opposed to 2.5% in the TCA-NSAID cohort. This would suggest that some caution needs to be taken when SSRIs are given to patients taking NSAIDs.

Paradoxical Pain

We have seen that strong evidence exists for TCAs having a useful analgesic effect. However, two studies have provided interesting and thought-provoking insights into the possibility that perhaps TCAs can produce pain symptoms as well as relieve them. In the first study, Esser and Sawynok[46] studied rats with a chronic constriction injury to lumbar nerve roots that produced features of neuropathic pain. When amitriptyline was systemically administered, thermal hyperalgesia was completely reversed in the injured paw. It also produced an antihyperalgesic effect on that side but had no effect on mechanical allodynia. However, and of more importance, the systemic administration of amitriptyline produced hyperesthesia on the contralateral (uninjured) side. In the second study, Esser and coworkers[47] again looked at a rat neuropathic pain model and found that amitriptyline reduces thermal hyperalgesia on the injured side but has no effect on allodynia. They again noted contralateral hyperesthesia with amitriptyline use. The significance of these results for human use of TCAs is not known, but warrants investigation.

Possible Analgesic Effect When Applied Topically

Peripheral Mode of Action

So far, this discussion has revolved around the use of antidepressants by the oral route of administration. Unfortunately, such systemic use also produces systemic side effects, which, particularly with the TCAs, may reduce patient compliance.

We have earlier reviewed the potential modes of action of TCAs when given as oral analgesics. These include effects on the serotonergic and noradrenergic pathways, sodium and potassium channels, and adenosine, NMDA, and opioid receptors. Not all these potential pharmacologic targets, however, have exclusively central representation.

Adenosine Receptors

At peripheral nerve terminals in rodents, adenosine α_1 receptor activation produces antinociception by decreasing cyclic adenosine monophosphate (cAMP) levels, whereas adenosine α_2 receptor activation produces pronociception by increasing cAMP levels in the sensory nerve terminals. Adenosine α_3 receptor activation produces pain behaviors as a result of the release of histamine and 5-HT from mast cells and subsequent actions of the sensory nerve terminal.[117] Caffeine acts as a nonspecific adenosine receptor antagonist. When systemic caffeine is administered with systemic amitriptyline, the normal effect on thermal hyperalgesia is blocked. When amitriptyline is administered into a neuropathic pain site, an antihyperalgesic effect is recorded, but not when it is given into the contralateral paw. This antihyperalgesic effect is blocked by caffeine,[118] suggesting that at least part of the effect of peripherally applied amitriptyline is mediated through peripheral adenosine receptors.

Sodium Channels

Sudoh and colleagues[119] administered various TCAs by a single injection into rat sciatic notches. They measured the duration of complete sciatic nerve blockade and compared this with that of bupivacaine. They found that amitriptyline, doxepin, and imipramine produce a longer complete sciatic nerve block than bupivacaine, whereas trimipramine and desipramine produce a shorter block. Nortriptyline and maprotiline failed to produce any block. When the effect of topical application of amitriptyline is compared with that of lidocaine, amitriptyline is seen to produce longer cutaneous analgesia than lidocaine.[120] These studies suggest, therefore, that from a mode of action perspective, TCAs could well have an analgesic effect when applied peripherally.

Animal Evidence of Antinociceptive Effects

Neuropathic Pain

When amitriptyline is applied to rodent paws made neuropathic by a chronic nerve constriction injury, an antinociceptive effect is observed. When amitriptyline is applied to the contralateral paw, no antinociceptive effect is observed in the paw on the injured side.[46,47,118] When desipramine and the SSRI fluoxetine are considered, desipramine has a similar antinociceptive effect when applied topically, whereas fluoxetine does not.[121]

Formalin Test

It seems that when amitriptyline[122,123] and desipramine[121] are coadministered peripherally with formalin, both the first- and second-phase responses are reduced. When amitriptyline is administered peripherally along with formalin, Fos immunoreactivity in the dorsal region of the spinal cord is significantly lower than in animals in which formalin is administered alone.[124]

Visceral Pain

Using a noxious colorectal distention model in the rat, Su and Gebhart[125] have shown that the antidepressants imipramine, desipramine, and clomipramine reduce the response to noxious colorectal distention by 20%, 22%, and 46%, respectively, when compared with control-treated animals.

Thermal Injury

Thermal hyperalgesia is produced by exposing a rodent hind paw to 52° C for 45 seconds. Locally applied amitriptyline at the time of thermal injury produces antihyperalgesic and analgesic effects, depending on the concentration used. When amitriptyline is applied after the injury, the analgesic but not the antihyperalgesic effect is retained.[126]

Human Pain

Human evidence of an analgesic effect with the topical application of TCAs is limited. A small randomized, placebo-controlled trial (RCT) of 40 subjects with neuropathic pain of mixed cause showed a reduction of 1.18 on a 0 to 10 linear visual analogue score (LVAS) relative to placebo use with the application of doxepin 5% cream. Minor side effects were seen in only three subjects.[127] A larger RCT involving 200 subjects, again with neuropathic pain of mixed cause, suggested that 5% doxepin cream reduces the LVAS by approximately 1 relative to placebo, and that time to effect is about 2 weeks. Again, side effects were minor and infrequent.[128] A pilot study examining the effect of topical amitriptyline application failed to produce any pain relief, but the maximum therapy duration was 7 days,[129] and therefore the study may have been terminated before the time to maximal effect had been reached. Case studies of a useful reduction in pain when 5% doxepin cream is applied topically in subjects with complex regional pain syndrome type I (CRPS)[130] and when doxepin is used as an oral rinse in patients with oral pain as a result of cancer or cancer therapy[131] have been reported.

Although the results of studies in humans of an analgesic effect with topical doxepin are interesting, more research is needed to verify this and other effects of TCAs when administered by this method. The evidence would suggest that topically applied doxepin has a local effect and that the consequences of systemic administration and systemic side effects can be substantially reduced.

CONCLUSION

There is compelling evidence of an antinociceptive effect when TCAs are used in animal pain models. This is substantiated by the recognition that TCAs have a number of effects, including serotonergic and noradrenergic effects, and actions on opioid, NMDA, and adenosine receptors and on sodium and potassium channels, which could account for their antinociceptive properties. The results of animal studies, a large number of human clinical studies, as well as extensive and long-term use of TCAs in clinical practice, suggest that these agents have a pain-reducing potential for various pain conditions, including neuropathic pain and pain associated with fibromyalgia.

The analgesic effect seen when TCAs are used is only present to a slight degree with SSRIs, although their side effect potential is substantially less. The more recently introduced SNRIs appear to have a more favorable side effect profile than TCAs, with many of their analgesic effects. It could be argued, therefore, that SNRIs should be the first choice when an antidepressant is chosen to treat pain, and that TCAs should be reserved for use when there is therapeutic failure with an SNRI.

The potential for a peripheral mode of action of the TCAs may allow them to be used as topical analgesics, with the reassurance that at least some of their effects are local. Thus, it is possible that systemic side effects can be avoided.

References

1. Kuipers RK: Imipramine in the treatment of rheumatic pain. Acta Rheum Scand 1962;8:45-51.

2. Scott WA: The relief of pain with an antidepressant in arthritis. Practitioner 1969;202:802-807.

3. Max MB, Schafer SC, Gracely RH, et al: Amitriptyline relieves diabetic neuropathy pain in patients with normal or depressed mood. Neurology 1987;37:589-596.

4. Ward NG, Bloom VL, Friedel RO: The effectiveness of tricyclic antidepressants in the treatment of coexisting pain and depression. Pain 1979;7:331-341.

5. Ardid D, Guilbaud G: Antinociceptive effects of acute and "chronic" injections of tricyclic antidepressant drugs in a new model of mononeuropathy in rats. Pain 1992;49: 279-287.

6. Sierralta F, Pinardi G, Miranda HF: Effect of p-chlorophenylalanine and alpha-methyltyrosine on the antinociceptive effect of antidepressant drugs. Pharmacol Toxicol 1995;77: 276-280.

7. Valverde O, Mico JA, Maldonado R, et al: Participation of opioid and monoaminergic mechanisms on the antinociceptive effect induced by tricyclic antidepressants in two behavioural pain tests in mice. Prog Neuropsychopharmacol Biol Psychiatry 1994;18:1073-1092.

8. Tura B, Tura SM: The analgesic effect of tricyclic antidepressants. Brain Res 1990;518:19-22.

9. Botney M, Fields HL: Amitriptyline potentiates morphine analgesia by a direct action on the central nervous system. Ann Neurol 1983;13:160-164.

10. Langer SZ, Moret C, Raisman R, et al: High-affinity ^{3}H-imipramine binding in rat hypothalamus: Association with uptake of serotonin but not norepinephrine. Science 1980;210:1133-1135.

11. Ross SB, Renyi AL: Tricyclic antidepressant agents. II. Effect of oral administration on the uptake of ^{3}H-noradrenaline and ^{14}C-5-hydroxytryptamine in slices of the midbrain-hypothalamus regions of the cat. Acta Pharmacol Toxicol 1975;36:395-408.

12. Segawa T, Kuruma I: Influences of drugs on the uptake of 5-hydroxytryptamine by nerve-ending particles of rabbit brain stem. J Pharm Pharmacol 1968;20:320-322.

13. Fillion G, Fillion MP: Modulation of affinity of post-synaptic receptors by antidepressant drugs. Nature 1981;292:349-351.

14. Segawa T, Mizuta T, Nomura Y: Modification of central 5-hydroxytryptamine binding sites in synaptic membranes from rat brain after long-term administration of tricyclic antidepressants. Eur J Pharmacol 1979;58:75-83.

15. Mico JA, Gibert-Rahola J, Casas J, et al: Implication of α_1- and α_2-adrenergic receptors in the antinociceptive effect of tricyclic antidepressants. Eur Neuropsychopharmacol 1997;7: 139-145.

16. Gray AM, Pache DM, Sewell RD: Do α_2-adrenoreceptors play a role in the antinociceptive mechanism of action of antidepressant compounds? Eur J Pharmacol 1999;378:161-168.

17. Schreiber S, Backer MM, Pick GG: The antinociceptive effect of venlafaxine in mice is mediated through opioid and adrenergic mechanisms. Neurosci Lett 1999;273:85-8.

18. Ansuategui M, Naharro L, Feria M: Noradrenergic and opioidergic influences on the antinociceptive effect of clomipramine in the formalin test in rats. Psychopharmacology 1989;98:93-96.

19. Gray AM, Spencer PS, Sewell RD: The involvement of the opioidergic system in the antinociceptive mechanism of action of antidepressant compounds. Br J Pharmacol 1998;124:669-674.

20. Hamon M, Gozlan H, Bourgoin S, et al: Opioid receptors and neuropeptides in the CNS in rats treated chronically with amoxapine or amitriptyline. Neuropharmacology 1987;26: 531-539.

21. DeFelipe MC, De Ceballos ML, Gil C, et al: Chronic antidepressant treatment increases enkephalin levels in n. accumbens and striatum of the rat. Eur J Pharmacol 1985;112:119-122.

22. Sacerdote P, Brinzi A, Mantegazza P, et al: A role for serotonin and beta-endorphin in the analgesia induced by some tricyclic antidepressant drugs. Pharmacol Biochem Behav 1987;26:153-158.

23. Reynolds IJ, Miller RJ: Tricyclic antidepressants block N-methyl-D-aspartate receptors: Similarities to the action of zinc. Br J Pharmacol 1988;95:95-102.

24. Kitamura Y, Zhao XH, Takei M, et al: Effects of antidepressants on the glutamergic systems in mouse brain. Neurochem Int 1991;19:257-263.

25. Skolnick P, Layer RT, Popik P, et al: Adoption of N-methyl-D-aspartate (NMDA) receptors following antidepressant treatment: Implications for the pharmacotherapy of depression. Pharmacopsychiatry 1996;29:23-26.

26. Sawynok J, Esser MJ, Reid AR: Antidepressants as analgesics: An overview of central and peripheral mechanisms of action. J Psychiatr Neurosci 2001;26:21-29.

27. Sawynok J: Adenosine receptor activation and nociception. Eur J Pharmacol 1998;347:1-11.

28. Phillis JW, Wu PH: The effect of various centrally active drugs on adenosine uptake by the central nervous system. Comp Biochem Physiol 1982;72C:179-187.

29. Pareek SS, Chopde CT, Thahus Desai PA: Adenosine enhances analgesic effect of tricyclic antidepressants. Ind J Pharmacol 1994;26:159-161.

30. Sierralta F, Pinardi G, Mednez M, et al: Interaction of opioids with antidepressant-induced antinociception. Psychopharmacol 1995;122:347-348.

31. Esser MJ, Sawynok J: Caffeine blockade of the thermal antihyperalgesic effect of acute amitriptyline in a rat model of neuropathic pain. Eur J Pharmacol 2000;399:131-139.

32. Barber MJ, Starmer CF, Grant AO: Blockade of cardiac sodium channels by amitriptyline and diphenylhydantoin. Circ Res 1991;69:677-696.

33. Habuchi Y, Furukawa T, Tanaka H, et al: Blockade of Na$^+$ channels by imipramine in guinea-pig cardiac ventricular cells. J Pharmacol Exp Ther 1991;256:1072-1081.

34. Bou-Abboud E, Nattel S: Molecular mechanisms of the reversal of imipramine-induced sodium channel blockade by alkalinization in human cardiac myocytes. Cardiovasc Res 1998;38:395-404.

35. Deffois A, Fage D, Carter C: Inhibition of synaptosomal veratridine-induced sodium influx by antidepressants and neuroleptics used in chronic pain. Neurosci Lett 1996;220: 117-120.

36. Pancrazio JJ, Kamatchi GL, Roscoe AK, et al: Inhibition of neuronal Na$^+$ channels by antidepressant drugs. J Pharmacol Exp Ther 1998;284:208-214.

37. Song J-H, Ham S-S, Shin Y-K, et al: Amitriptyline modulation of Na$^+$ channels in rat dorsal root ganglion neurons. Eur J Pharmacol 2000;401:297-305.

38. Antkiewicz-Michaluk L, Romanska I, Michaluk J, et al: Role of calcium channels in effects of antidepressant drugs on responsiveness to pain. Psychopharmacol (Berl) 1991;105:269-274.

39. Abdel-Salam OM, Nofal SM, El-Shenawy SM: Evaluation of the anti-inflammatory and anti-nociceptive effects of different antidepressants in the rat. Pharmacol Res 2003;48:157-165.

40. Abad F, Manuel F, Boada J: Chronic amitriptyline decreases autotomy following dorsal rhizotomy in rats. Neurosci Lett 1989;99:187-190.

41. Seltzer Z, Tal M, Sharav Y: Autotomy behaviour in rats following peripheral deafferentation is suppressed by daily injections of amitriptyline, diazepam and saline. Pain 1989;37:245-250.

42. Acton J, McKenna JE, Melzack R: Amitriptyline produces analgesia in the formalin pain test. Exp Neurol 1992; 117:94-96.

43. Lund A, Mjellem-Joly N, Hole K: Chronic administration of desipramine and zimelidine changes the behavioural response in the formalin test in rats. Neuropharmacology 1991; 30:481-487.

44. Otsuka N, Kiuchi Y, Yokogawa F, et al: Antinociceptive efficacy of antidepressants: Assessment of five antidepressants

and four monoamine receptors in rats. J Anesth 2001;
15:154-158.

45. Ardid D, Guilbaud G: Antinociceptive effects of acute and "chronic" injections of tricyclic antidepressant drugs in a new model of mononeuropathy in rats. Pain 1992;49:279-287.

46. Esser MJ, Sawynok J: Acute amitriptyline in a rat model of neuropathic pain: Differential symptom and route effects. Pain 1999;80:643-653.

47. Esser MJ, Chase T, Allen GV, et al: Chronic administration of amitriptyline and caffeine in a rat model of neuropathic pain: Multiple interactions. Eur J Pharmacol 2001;430: 211-218.

48. Michelson D, Misiewicz-Poltorak B, Raybourne RB, et al: Imipramine reduces the local inflammatory response to carrageenin. Agents Actions 1994;42:25-28.

49. Bianchi M, Rossoni G, Sacerdote P, et al: Effects of clomipramine and fluoxetine on subcutaneous carrageenin-induced inflammation in the rat. Inflamm Res 1995;466-469.

50. Butler SH, Weil-Fugazza J, Godefroy F, et al: Reduction of arthritis and pain behaviour following chronic administration of amitriptyline or imipramine in rats with adjuvant-induced arthritis. Pain 1985;23:159-175.

51. Bromm B, Meier W, Scharein E: Imipramine reduces experimental pain. Pain 1986;25:245-257.

52. Coquoz D, Porchet HC, Dayer P: Central analgesic effects of antidepressant drugs with various mechanisms of action: Desipramine, fluvoxamine and moclobemide. Schweiz Med Wochenschr 1991;121:1843-1845.

53. Poulsen L, Arendt-Nielsen L, Brosen K, et al: The hypoalgesic effect of imipramine in different human experimental pain models. Pain 1995;60:287-293.

54. Watson CP, Evans RJ, Reed K, et al: Amitriptyline versus placebo in postherpetic neuralgia. Neurology 1982;32:671-673.

55. Watson CP, Chipman M, Reed K, et al: Amitriptyline versus maprotiline in postherpetic neuralgia: A randomized, double-blind, crossover trial. Pain 1992;48:29-36.

56. Watson CP, Evans RJ: A comparative trial of amitriptyline and zimelidine in post-herpetic neuralgia. Pain 1985;23: 387-394.

57. Max MB, Schafer SC, Culnane M, et al: Amitriptyline, but not lorazepam, relieves postherpetic neuralgia. Neurology 1988;38:1427-1432.

58. Watson CP, Vernich L, Chipman M, et al: Nortriptyline versus amitriptyline in postherpetic neuralgia: A randomized trial. Neurology 1998;51:1166-1171.

59. Kishore-Kumar R, Max MB, Schafer SC, et al: Desipramine relieves postherpetic neuralgia. Clin Pharmacol Ther 1990;47: 305-312.

60. Max MB, Lynch SA, Muir J, et al: Effects of desipramine, amitriptyline and fluoxetine on pain in diabetic neuropathy. N Eng J Med 1992;326:1250-1256.

61. Max MB, Kishore-Kumar R, Schafer SC, et al: Efficacy of desipramine in painful diabetic neuropathy: A placebo-controlled trial. Pain 1991;45:3-9.

62. Sindrup S, Gram LF, Skjold T, et al: Clomipramine vs desipramine vs placebo in the treatment of diabetic neuropathy symptoms. A double-blind cross-over study. Br J Clin Pharmacol 1990;30:683-691.

63. Kvinesdal B, Molin J, Froland A, et al: Imipramine treatment of painful neuropathy. JAMA 1984;251:1727-1730.

64. Sindrup SH, Ejlertsen B, Froland A, et al: Imipramine treatment in diabetic neuropathy: Relief of subjective symptoms without changes in peripheral and autonomic nerve function. Eur J Clin Pharmacol 1989;37:151-153.

65. Sindrup S, Gram LF, Skjold T, et al: Concentration-response relationship in imipramine treatment of diabetic neuropathy symptoms. Clin Pharmacol Ther 1990;47:509-515.

66. Gomez-Perez FJ, Rull JA, Dies H, et al: Nortriptyline and fluphenazine in the symptomatic treatment of diabetic neuropathy: A double-blind cross-over study. Pain 1985;23: 395-400.

67. Langohr HD, Stohr M, Petruch F: An open and double-blind cross-over study on the efficacy of clomipramine (Anafranil) in patients with painful mono- and polyneuropathies. Eur Neurol 1982;21:309-317.

68. Cardenas DD, Warms CA, Turner JA, et al: Efficacy of amitriptyline for relief of pain in spinal cord injury: Results of a randomized controlled trial. Pain 2002;96:365-673.

69. Donovan WH, Dimitrijevic MR, Dahm L, et al: Neurophysiological approaches to chronic pain following spinal cord injury. Paraplegia 1982;20:135-146.

70. Frakash AE, Portenoy RK: The pharmacological management of chronic pain in the paraplegic patient. J Am Paraplegia Soc 1986;9:41-50.

71. Leijon G, Boivie J: Central post-stroke pain—a controlled trial of amitriptyline and carbamazepine. Pain 1989;36:27-36.

72. Rossy LA, Buckelew SP, Dorr N, et al: A meta-analysis of fibromyalgia treatment interventions. Ann Behav Med 1999; 21:180-191.

73. O'Malley PG, Balden E, Tomkins G, et al: Treatment of fibromyalgia with antidepressants: A meta-analysis. J Gen Intern Med 2000;15:659-666.

74. Arnold LM, Keck PE, Welge JA: Antidepressant treatment of fibromyalgia. A meta-analysis and review. Psychosomatics 2000;41:104-13.

75. Carette S, Bell MJ, Reynolds WJ, et al: Comparison of amitriptyline, cyclobenzaprine, and placebo in the treatment of fibromyalgia. A randomized, double-blind clinical trial. Arthritis Rheum 1994;37:32-40.

76. Hameroff SR, Cork RC, Scherer K, et al: Doxepin effects on chronic pain, depression and plasma opioids. J Clin Psychiatry 1982;43:22-27.

77. Mercadante S, Arcuri E, Tirelli W, et al: Amitriptyline in neuropathic cancer pain in patients on morphine therapy: A randomized placebo-controlled, double-blind crossover study. Tumori 2002;88:239-242.

78. Kieburtz K, Simpson D, Yiannoutsos C, et al: A randomized trial of amitriptyline and mexiletine for painful neuropathy in HIV infection. Neurology 1998;51:1682-1688.

79. Morello CM, Leckband SG, Stoner CP, et al: Randomized double-blind study comparing the efficacy of gabapentin with amitriptyline on diabetic peripheral neuropathy pain. Arch Intern Med 1999;159:1931-1937.

80. Schreiber S, Pick CG: From selective to highly selective SSRIs: A comparison of the antinociceptive properties of fluoxetine, fluvoxamine, citalopram and escitalopram. Eur Neuropsychopharmacol 2006;16:464-468.

81. Duman EN, Kesim M, Kadioglu M, et al: Possible involvement of opioidergic and serotinergic mechanisms in antinociceptive effect of paroxetine in acute pain. J Pharmacol Sci 2004;94:161-165.

82. McQuay HJ, Moore RA: Antidepressants and chronic pain. BMJ 1997;314:763-764.

83. Saarto T, Wiffen PJ: Antidepressants for neuropathic pain. Cochrane Database Syst Rev 2005;(3):CD005454.

84. Staiger TO, Gaster B, Sullivan MD, et al: Systematic review of antidepressants in the treatment of chronic low back pain. Spine 2003;28:2450-2455.

85. Sindrup SH, Gram LF, Brosen K, et al: The selective serotonin reuptake inhibitor paroxetine is effective in the treatment of diabetic neuropathy symptoms. Pain 1990;42:135-144.

86. Sindrup SH, Bjerre U, Dejgaard A, et al: The selective serotonin reuptake inhibitor citalopram relieves the symptoms of diabetic neuropathy. Clin Pharmacol Ther 1992;52: 547-552.

87. Norregaard J, Volkmann H, Danneskiold-Samsoe B: A randomized controlled trial of citalopram in the treatment of fibromyalgia. Pain 1995;61:445-449.

88. Anderberg UM, Marteinsdottir I, von Knorring L: Citalopram in patients with fibromyalgia—a randomized, double-blind, placebo-controlled study. Eur J Pain 2000;4:27-35.

89. Stahl SM, Grady MM, Moret C, et al: SNRIs: Their pharmacology, clinical efficacy, and tolerability in comparison with other classes of antidepressants. CNS Spectr 2005;10:732-747.

90. Bomholt SF, Mikkelsen JD, Blackburn-Munro G: Antinociceptive effects of the antidepressants amitriptyline, dulox-

etine, mirtazapine and citalopram in animal models of acute, persistent and neuropathic pain. Neuropharmacology 2005; 48:252-263.

91. Ivengar S, Webster AA, Hemrick-Luecke SK, et al: Efficacy of duloxetine, a potent and balanced serotonin-norepinephrine reuptake inhibitor, in persistent pain models in rats. J Pharmacol Exp Ther 2004;311:576-584.

92. Jones CK, Peters SC, Shannon HE: Efficacy of duloxetine, a potent and balanced serotinergic and noradrenergic reuptake inhibitor, in inflammatory and acute pain models in rodents. J Pharmacol Exp Ther 2005;312:726-732.

93. Mochizucki D: Serotonin and noradrenaline reuptake inhibitors in animal models of pain. Hum Psychopharmacol 2004;19S:S15-S9.

94. Smith TR: Duloxetine in diabetic neuropathy. Expert Opin Pharmacother 2006;7:215-223.

95. Rashkin J, Pritchett YL, Wang F, et al: A double-blind, randomized multicenter trial comparing duloxetine with placebo in the management of diabetic peripheral neuropathic pain. Pain Med 2005;6:346-356.

96. Rashkin J, Smith TR, Wong K, et al: Duloxetine versus routine care in the long-term management of diabetic peripheral neuropathic pain. J Palliat Med 2006;9:29-40.

97. Goldstein DJ, Lu Y, Detke MJ, et al: Duloxetine vs. placebo in patients with painful diabetic neuropathy. Pain 2005;116: 109-118.

98. Hardy T, Sachson R, Shen S, et al: Does treatment with duloxetine for neuropathic pain impact glycemic control? Diabetes Care 2007;30:21-26.

99. Arnold LM, Lu Y, Crofford LJ, et al: A double-blind, multicenter trial comparing duloxetine with placebo in the treatment of fibromyalgia patients with or without major depressive disorder. Arthritis Rheum 2004;50:2974-2984.

100. Arnold LM, Rosen A, Pritchett YL, et al: A randomized, double-blind, placebo-controlled trial of duloxetine in the treatment of women with fibromyalgia with or without major depressive disorder. Pain 2005;119:5-15.

101. Vitton O, Gendreau M, Gendreau J, et al: A double-blind placebo-controlled trial of milnacipran in the treatment of fibromyalgia. Hum Psychopharmacol 2004;19:S27-S35.

102. Gendreau RM, Thorn MD, Gendreau JF, et al: Efficacy of milnacipran in patients with fibromyalgia. J Rheumatol 2005;32:1975-1985.

103. Sayar K, Aksu G, Ak I, et al: Venlafaxine treatment of fibromyalgia. Ann Pharmacother 2003;37:1561-1565.

104. Hannonen P, Malminiemi K, Yli-Kerttula U, et al: A randomized, double-blind, placebo-controlled study of moclobemide and amitriptyline in the treatment of fibromyalgia in females without psychiatric disorder. Br J Rheumatol 1998;37:1279-1286.

105. Semenchuk MR, Sherman S, Davis B: Double-blind, randomized trial of bupropion SR for the treatment of neuropathic pain. Neurology 2001;57:1583-1588.

106. Buckley NA, McManus PR: Fatal toxicity of serotinergic and other antidepressant drugs: Analysis of United Kingdom mortality data. BMJ 2002;325:1332-1333.

107. Vieweg WV, Linker JA, Anum ES, et al: Child and adolescent suicides in Virginia: 1987-2003. J Child Adolesc Psychopharmacol 2005;15:6556-6563.

108. Arroll B, Macgillivray S, Ogston S, et al: Efficacy and tolerability of tricyclic antidepressants and SSRIs compared with placebo for treatment of depression in primary care: A meta-analysis. Ann Fam Med 2005;3:449-456.

109. Wilson K, Mottram P: A comparison of side effects of serotonin reuptake inhibitors and tricyclic antidepressants in older depressed patients: A meta-analysis. Int J Geriatr Psychiatry 2004;19:754-762.

110. Brambilla P, Cipriana A, Hotopf M, et al: Side-effect profile of fluoxetine in comparison with other SSRIs, tricyclic and

newer antidepressants: A meta-analysis of clinical trial data. Pharmacopsychiatry 2005;38:69-77.

111. Fava M: Weight gain and antidepressants. J Clin Psychiatry 2006;11:S37-S41.

112. French DD, Campbell R, Spehar A, et al: Outpatient medications and hip fractures in the US: A national veterans study. Drugs Aging 2005;22:877-885.

113. Eberhard-Gran M, Eskild A, Opjordsmoen S: Treating mood disorders during pregnancy: Safety considerations. Drug Saf 2005;28:695-706.

114. Ramaekers JG: Antidepressants and driver impairment: Empirical evidence from a standard on-the-road test. J Clin Psychiatry 2003;64:20-29.

115. Ridout F, Meadows R, Johnsen S, et al: A placebo-controlled investigation into the effects of paroxetine and mirtazapine on measures related to car driving performance. Hum Psychopharmacol 2003;18:261-269.

116. De Jong JC, Van den Berg PB, Tobi H, et al: Combined use of SSRIs and NSAIDs increases the risk of gastrointestinal adverse effects. Br J Clin Pharmacol 2003;55:591-595.

117. Sawynok J: Adenosine receptor activation and nociception. Eur J Pharmacol 1998;317:1-11.

118. Esser MJ, Sawynok MJ: Caffeine blockade of the thermal antihyperalgesic effect of acute amitriptyline in a rat model of neuropathic pain. Eur J Pharmacol 2000;399:131-139.

119. Sudoh Y, Cahoon EE, Gerner P, et al: Tricyclic antidepressant as long-acting local anesthetics. Pain 2003;103:49-55.

120. Haderer A, Gerner P, Kao G, et al: Cutaneous analgesia after transdermal application of amitriptyline versus lidocaine in rats. Anesth Analg 2003;96:1707-1710.

121. Sawynok J, Esser MJ, Reid AR: Peripheral antinociceptive actions of desipramine and fluoxetine in an inflammatory and neuropathic pain test in the rat. Pain 1999;82: 149-158.

122. Sawynok J, Reid AR, Esser MJ: Peripheral antinociceptive action of amitriptyline in the rat formalin test: Involvement of adenosine. Pain 1999;80:45-55.

123. Sawynok J, Reid A: Peripheral interactions between dextromethorphan, ketamine and amitriptyline on formalin-evoked behaviours and paw edema in rats. Pain 2003;102: 179-186.

124. Heughan CE, Allen GV, Chase TD, et al: Peripheral amitriptyline suppresses formalin-induced Fos expression in the rat spinal cord. Anesth Analg 2002;94:427-431.

125. Su X, Gebhart GF: Effects of tricyclic antidepressants on mechanosensitive pelvic nerve afferent fibers innervating the rat colon. Pain 1998;76:105-114.

126. Oatway M, Reid A, Sawynok J: Peripheral antihyperalgesic and analgesic actions of ketamine and amitriptyline in a model of mild thermal injury in the rat. Anesth Analg 2003;97:168-173.

127. McCleane GJ: Topical doxepin hydrochloride reduces neuropathic pain: A randomized, double-blind, placebo controlled study. Pain Clinic 1999;12:47-50.

128. McCleane GJ: Topical application of doxepin hydrochloride, capsaicin and a combination of both produces analgesia in chronic human neuropathic pain: A randomized, double-blind, placebo-controlled study. Br J Clin Pharmacol 2000;49: 574-579.

129. Lynch ME, Clarke AJ, Sawynok J: A pilot study examining topical amitriptyline, ketamine, and a combination of both in the treatment of neuropathic pain. Clin J Pain 2003;19: 323-328.

130. McCleane GJ: Topical application of doxepin hydrochloride can reduce the symptoms of complex regional pain syndrome: A case report. Injury 2002;33:88-89.

131. Epstein JB, Truelove EL, Oien H, et al: Oral topical doxepin rinse: Analgesic effect in patients with oral mucosal pain due to cancer or cancer therapy. Oral Oncology 2001;37:632-637.

CHAPTER
34 Anticonvulsants

Timothy L. Lacy, Stelian Serban, Brian McGeeney, Sudhir Rao, and Marco Pappagallo

Since 1993, there have been eight novel anticonvulsants (antiepileptic drugs [AEDs]) approved by the U.S. Food and Drug Administration (FDA) and two newer intravenous preparations of anticonvulsant drugs (valproic acid, fosphenytoin).[1] These exciting additions have some advantages over the older agents—phenytoin, carbamazepine, valproate, primidone, and ethosuximide. Both newer and older AEDs have great usefulness in a range of disorders beyond their anticonvulsant efficacy. The newer agents generally have a better side effect profile, fewer drug-drug interactions, less enzyme induction, new mechanisms of action, and a broader spectrum of activity than the older agents.

Blood levels of AEDs, used in the past as a guide to treatment, are not required for the newer agents and are therefore used less commonly. Guidelines for the use of the newer drugs for the management of epilepsy have been developed in the United States and United Kingdom.[2-5] Although there are similarities between these guidelines, there are also differences in the suggested treatment regimens. The British guidelines are more conservative by recommending the use of the new medications as a first choice only for specific clinical conditions, such as contraindications to or lack of efficacy of older drugs. The long-term outcome and cost-effectiveness of the newer agents has been studied in a randomized controlled trial.[4] Approximately 150,000 people in the United States are diagnosed with epilepsy every year and most are well controlled by a single drug. As many as 35% of the remaining patients have continued seizures, however, and the newer agents allow greater options for monotherapy or adjunctive treatment. Although initially developed as AEDs, these have also been frequently used for the treatment of neuropathic pain, migraine prophylaxis, and treatment of bipolar disorder, among other conditions. One agent, carbamazepine, was originally approved by the FDA not for epilepsy but for trigeminal neuralgia. The field of pain management, in particular, has seen large increases in the use of AEDs as adjuvant analgesics, particularly for neuropathic pain.[6] In the United States, five AEDs have FDA approval for pain syndromes (Table 34–1)—carbamazepine for trigeminal neuralgia, gabapentin and pregabalin for postherpetic neuralgia and neuropathic pain associated with diabetic polyneuropathy,

and divalproex and topiramate for migraine prophylaxis. There have been great advances in understanding how these agents work and how to use them most effectively, but much has yet to be learned. All AEDs modify the excitability of neurons and act on diverse molecular targets. Once a target is identified, its contribution to the effect of interest has to be elucidated.

The use of anticonvulsants is associated with adverse effects, such as rash, which can occur in up to 10% of those taking phenytoin, carbamazepine, or lamotrigine. Other AEDs, such as valproate and carbamazepine, are known for their propensity to cause weight gain. Generally, lamotrigine, levetiracetam, and phenytoin are weight-neutral and topiramate, zonisamide, and felbamate are associated with weight loss.[3-7]

MECHANISMS OF ACTION

The main actions of AEDs (Table 34–2) can be summarized as modulation of voltage-gated calcium or sodium channels, glutamate antagonism, enhancing the gamma-aminobutyric acid(GABA) inhibitory system, or a combination of these effects.

Voltage-Gated Calcium Channels

Modulation of voltage-gated calcium channels is a major mechanism of action of some AEDs.[7] The intracellular free Ca^{2+} concentration is only 1 in 10,000 that of the extracellular environment, and the influx of calcium through calcium channels has important effects on neurons. Voltage-gated calcium channels can be divided into high-voltage activated (HVA) and low-voltage activated (T type). Hagiwara and colleagues[8] first suggested the existence of different calcium channels, each with different kinetics for opening and closing. Electrophysiologic characteristics allow a division into high-voltage activated and low-voltage activated channels, depending on the threshold of activation. The HVA group is further divided into types L, P/Q, N, and R.[9] These require a large membrane depolarization and are mainly responsible for calcium entry and neurotransmitter release from presynaptic nerve terminals. Low-voltage

Table 34–1. FDA-Approved Pain Indications for Anticonvulsants

AGENT	INDICATION
Carbamazepine	Trigeminal neuralgia
Gabapentin	Post-herpetic neuralgia (PHN)
Pregabalin	Post-herpetic neuralgia
	Neuropathic pain associated with diabetic fibromyalgia polyneuropathy
Divalproex	Migraine prophylaxis
Topiramate	Migraine prophylaxis

Table 34–2. Mechanism of Action of Anticonvulsants

MECHANISM OF ACTION	AGENTS
Modulation of voltage-gated calcium channels	Phenobarbital, lamotrigine, zonisamide, valproic acid, gabapentin, pregabalin, ethosuximide
Modulation of voltage-gated sodium channels	Phenytoin, lamotrigine, carbamazepine, oxcarbazepine, zonisamide
Modulation of gamma-aminobutyric acid	Benzodiazepine, valproic acid, gabapentin, topiramate, felbamate, barbiturates, tiagabine, vigabatrin
Modulation of glutamate	Ketamine, felbamate, memantine—NMDA receptors; topiramate-kainate antagonist, AMPA antagonist

AMPA, α-amino-3-hydroxy-5-methyl-4-isoxazolepropionic acid; NMDA, N-methyl-D-aspartate.

channels regulate firing by participating in bursting and intrinsic oscillations. The spike and wave discharges from the thalamus in absence seizures are dependent on T-type calcium channels; these discharges are inhibited by valproic acid or ethosuximide. The N-type HVA calcium channels are thought to be largely responsible for neurotransmitter release at synaptic junctions and inactivate rather quickly. The P/Q-type calcium channel is so named because it was first described in the Purkinje cells of the cerebellum in 1989. The T-type channel, named after the transient currents elicited, starts to open with weak depolarization, near resting potential. L-type channels are found in high concentration in skeletal muscle and in many other tissues, such as neuronal and smooth muscle, where it has been most studied. The voltage-gated calcium channel is composed of five polypeptide subunits and is the target of many drugs. Calcium channels consist of an alpha protein, along with several auxiliary subunits; the alpha protein forms the channel pore.

Pregabalin and gabapentin are amino acid derivatives of GABA and have been demonstrated to have antiseizure activity and analgesic activity in neuropathic and other chronic pain states.[6] Both agents reduce nociceptive behavior in animal models of neuropathic pain or inflammation in addition to the anti-seizure effect. They bind to the alpha$_2$-delta (α_2-δ) subunit of voltage-gated calcium channels with high affinity.[7] The binding of gabapentin or pregaba-

lin to the α_2-δ subunit results in inhibition of calcium influx at presynaptic voltage-gated calcium channels. This binding affinity correlates with their antinociceptive and anticonvulsant potencies. Animal models have demonstrated increased expression of the α_2-δ subunit of the calcium channel in the dorsal root ganglion secondary to peripheral nerve injury.[10] This subunit is not upregulated in all models of hyperalgesia. The increased expression may explain the relative selectivity of these agents for neuropathic or inflammatory pain. In addition to these actions, gabapentin has also been demonstrated to elevate GABA levels in the brain.[11] Other anticonvulsants can act on HVA calcium channels, including phenobarbital, lamotrigine, and possibly levetiracetam, although they are likely to have more important effects on other channels.

The T-type low-voltage activated calcium channels are also involved in the transmission of neuropathic pain from the periphery and in the spinal cord. Both ethosuximide and zonisamide inhibit these channels. However, this channel is involved in thalamocortical bursting, and it has been suggested that this has an inhibitory role on the transmission of pain centrally; therefore, the use of these medications may be of limited value as antinociceptive agents.

Voltage-Gated Sodium Channels

When neurons are depolarized and approaching an action potential, the voltage-gated sodium channels quickly change conformation in response and permit flow of sodium ions. Activation of sodium channels (and other voltage-gated ion channels) derives from the outward movement of charged residues because of an altered electrical field across the membrane. Sodium channels play an essential role in the action potential of neurons and other electrically excitable cells, such as myocytes. The flow of sodium ions is terminated by channel inactivation in a few milliseconds (fast inactivation). Sodium channels can cycle open and closed rapidly, which may result in seizures, neuropathic pain, or paresthesias. The structure of the channel is essentially a rectangular tube, with its four walls formed from four subunits, the four domains of a single polypeptide. A region near the N-terminus protrudes into the cytosol and forms an inactivating particle. It has been demonstrated that a short loop of amino acid residues acting as a flap or hinge blocks the inner mouth of the sodium channel, resulting in fast inactivation.[12] The highly conserved intracellular loop is the inactivating gate that binds to the intracellular pore and inactivates it within milliseconds. Site-directed antibody studies against this intracellular loop have prevented this fast inactivation. Phenytoin does not appear to act directly through this mechanism. Unlike local anesthetics, the binding and unbinding of phenytoin are slow.[13]

The voltage-gated sodium channel can be divided into an α subunit and one or more auxiliary β subunits. At least nine α subunits have been functionally characterized—Nav 1.1 through Nav 1.9.[14] The sodium channels 1.2, 1.8, and 1.9 are preferentially expressed on peripheral sensory neurons, where they are important in nociception and may be a future target for channel-specific analgesics.[15] Seven of the nine sodium channel subtypes have been identified in sensory ganglia, such as the dorsal root ganglia and trigeminal ganglia. The sodium channel 1.7 is also present in large amounts in the peripheral nervous system. Sodium channel 1.2 is expressed in unmyelinated neurons and Nav 1.4 and Nav 1.5 are muscle sodium channels. Sodium channel mutations have been described that cause well-recognized syndromes. A mutation of sodium channel 1.4 is responsible for hyperkalemic periodic paralysis and an inherited long QT syndrome can be caused by mutation of Nav 1.5. A mutation of Nav 1.1 has been shown to be responsible for a syndrome of generalized epilepsy.[16,17]

Increased expression of sodium channels has been demonstrated in peripheral and central sensory neurons in neuropathic pain; it is one mechanism for the observed hyperexcitability of pain pathways.[18] Anticonvulsants modulating the gating of sodium channels are phenytoin, lamotrigine, carbamazepine, oxcarbazepine, and zonisamide, with some evidence for topiramate and valproic acid. It is important to note that at clinical concentrations, the sodium channel is only weakly blocked when hyperpolarized. When the neuronal membrane is depolarized, there is a much greater inhibition in the channel.[7] Binding of the channel by anticonvulsants is slow compared with local anesthetics. The slow binding of AEDs ensures that the kinetic properties of the normal action potentials are not altered. Generally, AEDs have no role in the treatment of acute pain, although they have demonstrated efficacy for chronic pain conditions. Interestingly, the local application of phenytoin and carbamazepine has an antinociceptive effect that is more potent than lidocaine.[19] It has been demonstrated that phenytoin, carbamazepine, and lamotrigine bind to a common recognition site on sodium channels and is likely the result of their two phenol groups, which act as binding elements.[20] At normal resting potentials, AEDs have little effect on action potentials. In addition to the fast current of the open channel, there is also a persistent sodium current. This current, carried by persistent openings, is a small fraction of the fast current but may have an important role in regulating excitability. There is evidence that a numbers of AEDs, such as phenytoin, valproate, and topiramate, also act by blocking the persistent sodium current, which is separate from the fast sodium current.

Gamma-Aminobutyric Acid Modulation

GABA is the main inhibitory neurotransmitter in the central nervous system (CNS) and acts through ligand-gated ion channels. The potentiation of GABA inhibitory transmission is an important mechanism of action of certain AEDs.[7] There is also evidence that GABA acts as a trophic factor during brain development.[21] GABA is synthesized from glutamate by two isoforms of glutamic acid decarboxylase enzymes, GAD65 and GAD67. GABA activity is rapidly terminated at the synapse by reuptake into nerve terminals and is metabolized by a reaction catalyzed by GABA transaminase (GABA-T). Tiagabine is an AED that acts by inhibiting the GABA transporters that remove GABA from the synaptic cleft, thus prolonging the effect of GABA. The AED vigabatrin, currently unavailable in the United States, is a GABA analogue that acts as an irreversible inhibitor of GABA-T, resulting in markedly elevated brain GABA levels. GABA acts through fast chloride-permeable ionotropic (intrinsic channel pore) GABA-A receptors and through slower metabotropic (G protein–coupled) GABA-B receptors. Bicuculline is an antagonist of GABA-A, but not GABA-B. An ionotropic GABA-C receptor has been described, also with an intrinsic chloride-sensitive channel but insensitive to the antagonist bicuculline.

A number of AEDs act on the GABA system by direct action on the GABA-A receptor (benzodiazepines) or by indirect pathways (e.g., valproate, gabapentin) that increase GABA synthesis and turnover. Topiramate and felbamate also modulate the GABA-A receptor. Mice lacking functional GABA-B receptors have been shown to exhibit seizures and hyperalgesia.[22]

Mutation of GABA receptor genes can cause epilepsy, such as a mutation of the α subunit (GABRA1) of the GABA-A receptor described in a French-Canadian family with juvenile myoclonic epilepsy.[23] Bromides, first introduced by English physician Charles Locock in the 1850s, are now thought to act by enhancing GABA-A receptor affinity for GABA and increasing the ion current. Drugs that enhance GABA activity generally have a broad spectrum of activity against seizure disorders, although they are not effective against absence seizures. Generally, GABA-A receptors are composed of α, β, and δ_2 subunits, with each containing a large N-terminal portion, four transmembrane regions, and a short C-terminal extracellular portion. Phenobarbital and other barbiturates act on sodium, calcium, and GABA-linked ion channels but their most important action is on the GABA-A receptor, with a different mechanism than that of those in the benzodiazepine family. Barbiturates prolong openings of the channel, leading to more passage of ion. Topiramate and felbamate appear to act in part through action at the GABA-A receptor also. Benzodiazepines bind to the GABA-A receptor, where the δ_2 subunit is necessary for their action. The action of benzodiazepines is conferred by the γ_2 subunit and adjacent α_1, α_2, α_3, or α_5 subunits.

Glutamate Modulation

Glutamate is the main excitatory neurotransmitter in the CNS and most of its actions are mediated through ionotropic (ligand-gated) receptors. There are also metabotropic (G protein–coupled) receptors. The ionotropic glutamate receptors are the *N*-methyl-D-aspartate (NMDA), α-amino-3-hydroxy-5-methyl-4-isoxazolepropionic acid (AMPA), and kainate receptor subtypes, which have numerous differences. The AMPA receptors show fast gating and desensitize strongly, whereas NMDA receptors gate more slowly, only weakly desensitize, and are blocked by magnesium in a strongly voltage-dependent manner. Efficient agonist action at NMDA receptors also requires the coagonist glycine. The glutamate receptor ion channel has similarities with the K$^+$ channel. Ketamine is an NMDA antagonist used to treat refractory status epilepticus and is also an anesthetic agent. In analgesic clinical trials, antagonists of glutamate have been disappointing. Felbamate is also an NMDA antagonist. Lower affinity antagonists of NMDA include memantine and ketamine. The potential side effects of felbamate, aplastic anemia and liver failure, would make the use of this drug unlikely at this time. Topiramate selectively inhibits kainate receptors and, to a lesser extent, AMPA receptors. AMPA receptors are the primary mediators of fast excitatory transmission under basal signaling conditions.

SPECIFIC ANTICONVULSANT DRUGS

The remainder of this chapter discusses different anticonvulsant drugs and their specific properties. Starting and maintenance dosing regimens are shown in Table 34–3.

Phenytoin and Fosphenytoin

Merrit and Putnam[24] first described the usefulness of phenytoin for treating seizures when they described its ability to suppress electric shock–induced seizures in animals. Phenytoin was able to control seizures without producing sedation. More recently, Mattson and colleagues[25] have performed a large blinded study of phenytoin, phenobarbital, primidone, and carbamazepine in 622 patients with new-onset partial and secondarily generalized tonic-clonic seizures.

Phenytoin and carbamazepine were the most efficacious and least toxic. Intravenous phenytoin is often used to treat status epilepticus; it acts quickly and is suitable for a loading dose. In addition to widespread use for seizures, phenytoin was the first AED to be used for neuropathic pain, with a 1942 report on its use in trigeminal neuralgia. Subsequent controlled trials investigating its analgesic potential have been unimpressive. Phenytoin is known for nonlinear metabolism, which is manifest as marked increases in plasma level with small dose increases after saturation of metabolism. Around 95% of a phenytoin dose is excreted as metabolites from the cytochrome P-450 system. The half-life varies by dose; it is between 12 and 36 hours, which allows for once-daily administration. More frequent administration can reduce peak dose symptoms and a steady state concentration is not reached for at least 2 or 3 of days because of long half-life.

Phenytoin is still extensively used in the United States for the management of partial and generalized seizures but has a number of drawbacks.[26] It is highly protein bound, has multiple drug-drug interactions, and the intravenous formulation has disadvantages. Parenteral phenytoin is dissolved in 40% propylene glycol and 10% ethanol with a pH of 12 and intravenous administration can easily cause hypotension. The drug is administered at up to 50 mg/min. Extravasation may cause a severe tissue reaction. The parenteral form cannot be given by the intramuscular route, unlike fosphenytoin. It should be diluted with saline, not dextrose. Parenteral phenytoin crystallizes into insoluble phenytoin when admixed with solutions of 5% dextrose in water. Phenytoin exhibits nonlinear elimination at therapeutic concentrations. The therapeutic range is 10 to 20 μg/mL, with a free level of 1 to 2 μg/mL. Only the free drug concentration is biologically active. Side effects (Table 34–4) include rash in 5% to 10% of patients. Phenytoin may cause a hypersensitivity syndrome manifesting as fever, rash, and lymphadenopathy. An association between erythema multiforme in patients on phenytoin undergoing whole brain radiation has been

Table 34–3. Starting and Maintenance Dosing Regimens for Anticonvulsants

ANTICONVULSANT	REGIMEN
Phenytoin	Loading, 20 mg/kg; maintain at 5-8 mg/kg, often 300 mg daily; bid or daily regimen orally; IV formulation infusion, maximum, 50 mg/min
Fosphenytoin	Loading, 20 mg/kg; up to 150 mg/min IV; full loading by IM route possible; large-volume IM tolerated well
Carbamazepine	200 mg daily; maintain 600-1200 mg daily, lower in older adults; tid regimen; slow-release forms (Tegretol XR, Carbatrol) given bid
Oxcarbazepine	300 mg bid; maintain 1200 mg/day; up to 2400 mg/daily
Gabapentin	300 mg daily; maintain 900-3600 mg/day
Pregabalin	150 mg daily; maintain 300-600 mg/day; tid or bid regimen
Phenobarbital	Loading, 20 mg/kg, divided into two doses; start orally at 60-90 mg daily; maintain 90-120 mg daily
Levetiracetam	500 mg bid; maintain 1000-3000 mg daily
Topiramate	25 mg daily; maintain 200-400 mg/day bid regimen; for migraine, usually 50-100 mg
Valproic acid	250 mg daily; Depakene, tid; Depakote, bid; Depacon, IV formulation, 100 mg/mL, requires dilution, slow infusion twice daily
Zonisamide	100 mg once daily, then bid with higher doses; increase by 100 mg/wk; maximum, 400 mg daily
Lamotrigine	50 mg daily (25 mg if taking valproic acid); increase slowly over 4-6 wk to maintenance of 300-500 mg/day, bid
Clonazepam	0.5 mg tid; maintain 2-6 mg/day

Table 34–4. Major Side Effects of Anticonvulsants

ANTICONVULSANT	SIDE EFFECTS
Phenytoin	Hypotension, extravasation may cause severe tissue reaction, hypersensitivity syndrome (fever, rash, lymphadenopathy), nystagmus, ataxia, encephalopathy, seizures, fetal hydantoin syndrome, osteoporosis
Carbamazepine	Rash, neurotoxicity, diplopia, hyponatremia, agranulocytosis
Oxcarbazepine	Rash, hyponatremia, low serum thyroid concentrations
Phenobarbital	Cognitive dysfunction, hyperactivity in children
Gabapentin, pregabalin	Dizziness, fatigue, somnolence, weight gain, peripheral edema
Topiramate	Parasthesias, drowsiness, fatigue, cognitive effects, dysgeusia, nephrolithiasis, weight loss
Levetiracetam	Somnolence, headache, anxiety
Valproate	Drowsiness, tremor, nausea, weight gain, hepatotoxicity, pancreatitis, encephalopathy, increased risk of spina bifida
Lamotrigine	Rash, Stevens-Johnson syndrome
Zonisamide	Hyperthermia, oligohidrosis, weight loss
Benzodiazepine	Drowsiness, ataxia

described and it would be prudent to avoid phenytoin in such circumstances.[27] Nystagmus occurs early in toxicity, followed by ataxia progressing to encephalopathy. Phenytoin toxicity is rarely reported to exacerbate seizures. The drug may result in birth defects, referred to as the fetal hydantoin syndrome. Phenytoin use is a risk factor for osteoporosis because of multiple effects on calcium metabolism; supplemental vitamin D and calcium is often recommended.[28] One study of 75 cancer patients with various pain syndromes looked at the use of phenytoin, buprenorphine, or both for the relief of cancer pain; there was a mild effect in favor of phenytoin.[29]

Fosphenytoin is a phosphate ester prodrug and is entirely metabolized to phenytoin, with a bioavailability of phenytoin at around 100%.[30] Fosphenytoin has certain advantages over phenytoin, such as the ability for rapid IV infusion and availability for intramuscular injection. Disadvantages include cost when compared with generic phenytoin.

Carbamazepine

Carbamazepine has been used in the United States since the 1980s to treat partial and generalized tonic-clonic seizures. Carbamazepine was first approved by the FDA for the treatment of trigeminal neuralgia, not for epilepsy. In addition to its anticonvulsant and trigeminal neuralgia indications, it is used frequently for bipolar disorder. It was one of the first AEDs studied for the relief of neuropathic pain. The analgesic properties of carbamazepine were first reported in 1962.[31] It is chemically related to the tricyclic antidepressants; reports have included studies of its use for postherpetic neuralgia, painful diabetic neuropathy, poststroke pain, and pain in Guillain-Barré syndrome. Newer generation AEDs are often compared with carbamazepine for efficacy and side effects. A major clinical trial compared carbamazepine, phenytoin, phenobarbital, and primidone for the treatment of partial and secondarily generalized tonic-clonic seizures.[25] Treatment success was highest with carbamazepine and phenytoin, intermediate with phenobarbital, and least favorable for primi-

done. Carbamazepine exhibits nonlinear time-dependent kinetics because of autoinduction.

Metabolism involves oxidation to a 10,11-epoxide, which is further hydrolyzed. Both steps become more efficient over time and the patient often needs an increase in dose after a few weeks of treatment. The half-life can shorten considerably. The autoinduction of enzymes is quickly reversed with discontinuation, so caution is advised when restarting after a few days of absence.[32] Generally, the dose does not correlate well with blood levels and older adults require a smaller dose for adequate levels. The therapeutic range is 4 to 12 mg/dL; the elimination half-life varies from 38 hours after a single dose to 12 hours after chronic monotherapy. The starting dosage of carbamazepine is 100 or 200 mg/day; it is available in an oral suspension as well as a tablet formulation. Carbamazepine is typically given twice daily. Enzyme-inducing drugs shorten the half-life of carbamazepine. The drug does not have the cosmetic side effects of phenytoin (see Table 34–4). Slow-release formulations are available, reducing the serum fluctuations that may reduce peak dose side effects. The development of rash, generally within the first few weeks, occurs in up to 10% of patients. It has been suggested that a slow introduction reduces the chance of this side effect, which warrants discontinuation. Neurotoxicity generally occurs above 12 mg/dL and often includes diplopia. The carbamazepine 10,11-epoxide is the major metabolite of carbamazepine and is responsible for many of the side effects. Hyponatremia is not uncommon with carbamazepine, although only a minority of patients will be symptomatic. The exact mechanism for hyponatremia is unclear but it appears to be an effect on the renal tubules not attributable to the syndrome of inappropriate antidiuretic hormone (SIADH).

Oxcarbazepine

Oxcarbazepine is an anticonvulsant drug with a chemical structure similar to carbamazepine but with a different metabolism.[33] Oxcarbazepine was developed as a structural variation of carbamazepine to avoid the production of the epoxide metabolite, implicated in many of the side effects. Oxcarbazepine does have other differences that separate it from carbamazepine. Clinical trials for the antiseizure effect have used dosages from 600 to 2400 mg/day.[34] Rash occurs in about 3% of patients taking oxcarbazepine and cross-reactions with carbamazepine have been reported (see Table 34–4). Hyponatremia also occurs with oxcarbazepine, more so in older patients, and it may be more frequent in those taking oxcarbazepine than carbamazepine. In a postmarketing survey of 947 patients, 23% had a serum sodium level lower than 135 mEq/L and 1% required discontinuation of the medication.[35] Compared with carbamazepine, fewer patients will develop rash or hypersensitivity to oxcarbazepine. Oxcarbazepine is not associated with idiosyncratic hepatic or hematologic effects. Low serum thyroid hormone concentrations have been reported in patients on long-term treatment of oxcarbazepine for epilepsy.

The mechanism of action of oxcarbazepine mainly involves blockade of sodium currents but differs from carbamazepine by modulating different types of calcium channels. Oxcarbazepine and carbamazepine block sodium currents (see earlier), but oxcarbazepine does this at low concentrations. Oxcarbazepine is metabolized by reduction and glucuronidation, resulting in a monohydroxy derivative (MHD). The plasma terminal half-life of oxcarbazepine is between 1 and 2.5 hours, whereas the plasma MHD terminal half-life averages 9.3 ± 1.8 hours after administration of a single dose. Oxcarbazepine metabolism is not induced or inhibited by the cytochrome P-450 (CYP450) system and its metabolites are passed in the urine. High-dose oxcarbazepine can cause some inhibition of CYP450 enzymes. When switching patients from carbamazepine to oxcarbazepine, the physician should be aware of the effect of loss of enzyme induction on the metabolism of concurrent medications. Involvement of hepatic CYP450-dependent enzymes in the metabolism of the drug is minimal. This allows for better combining of oxcarbazepine with other AEDs such as valproate.[33] The bioavailability of the oral form is high (more than 95%).

There is limited but increasing evidence of the experimental use of oxcarbazepine for pain. One study has reported the antinociceptive effects of carbamazepine and oxcarbazepine in an inflammatory paw pressure test in rats.[36] The study demonstrated significant dose- and time-dependent reduction in nociception with both agents individually. Furthermore, the challenge of caffeine, which is a competitive antagonist at both adenosine α_1- and α_2-receptors, or a selective adenosine α_1-receptor antagonist, to the model significantly reduced the antinociceptive effect of carbamazepine and oxcarbazepine. This is further evidence for the important role of adenosine receptors in the actions of carbamazepine and oxcarbazepine.

Several multicenter double-blind randomized trials have suggested that oxcarbazepine has substantial efficacy in alleviating the pain associated with trigeminal neuralgia, with relatively few clinically significant adverse events (e.g., vertigo, dizziness, ataxia, fatigue)[37,38] In most cases, pain relief was noted within 24 to 48 hours of receiving oxcarbazepine treatment. In addition, some patients obtained pain relief with oxcarbazepine despite having previously responded poorly to carbamazepine in terms of efficacy or tolerability. These trials reported a comparable analgesic effect between oxcarbazepine and carbamazepine, leading to the conclusion that oxcarbazepine offers an alternative to carbamazepine for the treatment of newly diagnosed or refractory trigeminal neuralgia.[39,40]

Evidence that oxcarbazepine may also be effective in treating painful diabetic neuropathy is accumulating. This suggests that oxcarbazepine may significantly improve pain scores in patients with painful diabetic neuropathy.[41]

Phenobarbital

Phenobarbital has an FDA indication for the treatment of partial and generalized tonic-clonic seizures. A parenteral form is available and is often used to control status epilepticus. It is one of the oldest AEDs and is not currently used often as much for monotherapy, having been replaced by newer agents. It still retains an important place in the management of neonatal seizures because of its predictable pharmacokinetics and efficacy. It induces hepatic enzymes and is approximately 50% protein-bound. Its half-life is 4 days and its blood level may be increased with the addition of valproate or tricyclic antidepressants. A concern in the use of phenobarbital is its effect on cognition and behavior; it has been associated with hyperactivity in children (see Table 34–4).

Pregabalin

Pregabalin has been demonstrated to have anticonvulsant, analgesic, and anxiolytic activity in animal models and in clinical trials.[42,43] As noted earlier, the presumed mechanism of action is similar to that of gabapentin—binding to the α_2-δ subunit of voltage-gated calcium channels, resulting in inhibition of calcium influx. The pharmacokinetics are predictable, in contrast to those of gabapentin. The drug has high bioavailability and an elimination half-life of 6.3 hours. It does not bind to plasma proteins, undergo hepatic metabolism, or have any effect on the CYP450 system. Ninety percent is excreted unchanged in the urine. The dosage needs to be adjusted in patients with renal impairment. The antiseizure activity of pregabalin has been studied at dosages from 300 to 600 mg.[44-46]

Three randomized double-blind trials of 5 to 8 weeks' duration have been conducted using pregabalin for painful diabetic neuropathy.[42,43] Dosages ranged from 300 to 600 mg, given in divided doses three times daily. There were significant improvements in pain and sleep scores from week 1 on. Pregabalin was studied in four randomized, double-blind, placebo-controlled trials as adjunctive treatment for partial seizures.[46,48] Dosages ranged from 50 to 600 mg daily; statistically significant reductions in seizure frequency were noted.

Pregabalin has also been shown to be effective in the treatment of post-herpetic neuralgia (PHN), fibromyalgia, and generalized anxiety disorder.[50-55] In a multicenter, double-blind, placebo-controlled randomized clinical trial studying PHN, pregabalin-treated patients had greater decreases in pain than patients treated with placebo.[49] Secondary outcome measures, including sleep, were also studied, and patients treated with pregabalin in this setting appeared to experience sleep improvement compared with placebo-treated patients.

Gabapentin

Gabapentin is used as an adjunctive medication for partial seizures and generalized tonic-clonic seizures, but most of its use in the United States is for neuropathic pain.[56,57] In addition to binding to calcium channels, other proposed mechanisms include reducing the release of monoamines.[58] Previously proposed mechanisms of analgesic action included sodium channel modulation of action potentials and augmentation of inhibitory pathways by increasing GABAergic transmission.[59] It is available in oral formulations and is absorbed by both diffusion and facilitated transport via an amino acid transport mechanism. The facilitated transport is saturable, leading to nonlinear kinetics and bioavailability somewhat related to dose. The drug is not metabolized and is eliminated unchanged in the kidneys. The half-life is roughly 6 hours. Those with renal impairment may need a smaller dose and patients on dialysis need a maintenance dose because gabapentin is removed during dialysis. Gabapentin does not induce enzymes and is known for its lack of drug interactions and low protein binding. The most common side effects are somnolence, dizziness, and fatigue, and it can cause weight gain. It is thought to be relatively safe, even in overdose. It is generally given three times daily to control seizures, and can be started at 300 mg at night and increased briskly. Liquid formulations are available. Gabapentin has been studied in a wide range of pain syndromes, including multiple sclerosis–related central pain and spasms, complex regional pain syndrome, migraine, trigeminal neuralgia, HIV-related neuropathy, spinal cord injury pain, cluster headache, diabetic painful peripheral neuropathy, and PHN, for which it has an FDA indication.[6,56-60]

A randomized, double-blind, active placebo-controlled crossover trial in patients with painful diabetic neuropathy or PHN received lorazepam (active placebo), controlled-release morphine, gabapentin, and a combination of gabapentin and morphine. Each was given orally for 5 weeks. The study results indicated that the best analgesia is obtained from the gabapentin-morphine combination, with each medication given at a lower dose than when given as a single agent.[60] Other studies have demonstrated that the concomitant administration of gabapentin reduces opioid requirements postoperatively.[61,62] Some putative mechanisms for synergy include morphine increasing gabapentin levels and a combined inhibitory action in the brain, spinal cord, and periphery.[63,64]

Topiramate

Topiramate is a sulfamate-substituted derivative of D-fructose.[65] It has multiple mechanisms of action and has broad use in seizure disorders. Topiramate blocks voltage-sensitive sodium channels, limits sustained repetitive firing, and binds to GABA-A receptors to enhance GABA activity through nonbenzodiazepine and nonbarbiturate mechanisms. It increases the opening frequency of chloride ion channels in GABA-A receptors and can block AMPA-kainate glutamate receptors, acting as a negative modulator of glutamate at this receptor. Topiramate reduces the activity of L-type calcium channels and is a carbonic anhydrase inhibitor. Topiramate exhibits linear pharmacokinetics over its dose range and has a half-life of 19 to 25 hours. The oral bioavailability is about 85% and is not affected by food. It is a mild enzyme inducer and increases the clearance of ethinylestradiol at dosages higher than 200 mg/day. Enzyme-inducing drugs may reduce the serum level of topiramate. Common side effects (see Table 34–4) include paresthesias because of carbonic anhydrase inhibition, drowsiness, fatigue, and cognitive complaints. It also commonly causes dysgeusia. The incidence of nephrolithiasis was 1.5% in clinical trials and mild weight loss is often noted. The propensity to reduce weight in some patients has led to investigation of its potential as a weight-reducing agent.[66] Two large trials on migraine prophylaxis with topiramate were published in 2004 and topiramate received FDA approval for this indication.[67,68]

The particular mechanisms of action responsible for its efficacy for the relief of migraine are unknown. A study by Storer and Goadsby[69] has demonstrated the inhibition of trigeminocervical neurons by topiramate consistent with its clinical effect. Anesthetized cats were studied with a microelectrode in the trigeminal nucleus and trigeminal activation by electrical stimulation of the superior sagittal sinus. Three placebo-controlled studies on the use of topiramate for painful diabetic neuropathy did not demonstrate a significant pain-relieving effect.[70]

Levetiracetam

Levetiracetam is a newer AED, approved in 1999 as adjunctive therapy for partial seizures in adults. The drug has a number of favorable characteristics and is being investigated for adjuvant use in areas such as pain.[71] It has linear kinetics, is not significantly bound to plasma proteins (10%), has no important drug interactions, demonstrates high oral bioavailability, and is eliminated partly unchanged (66%) by the kidneys. It has a half-life of 6 to 8 hours. Hence, it has favorable pharmacokinetic characteristics. It appears that inhibition of voltage-gated sodium channels or T-type calcium channels is not involved in the anticonvulsant effects of levetiracetam, which does not appear to have direct GABA-A receptor effects. The mechanism of action of levetiracetam thus does not involve modulation of the four main systems. Evidence has suggested that levetiracetam reduces the inhibitory action of zinc and other negative allosteric modulators (beta-carbolines) on GABA- and glycine-gated currents.[72] It has been shown that levetiracetam binds to SV2A, a synaptic vesicle protein; this is thought to be involved in its anticonvulsant action. The protein SV2A interacts with the presynaptic protein synaptotagmin, considered the primary calcium sensor for regulating calcium-dependent exocytosis of synaptic vesicles.[73] The most common side effects include somnolence and headache, and it can cause anxiety (see Table 34–4). Levetiracetam is not metabolized by the liver. There is no significant interaction with other AEDs or oral contraceptives. Because of the scarcity of data to support its use as an analgesic, studies confirming its analgesic effect would be required prior to integration into an analgesic regimen.

Valproate

First synthesized in 1882, valproate became available in the 1960s as an antiepileptic agent and received FDA approval in 1978 as an immediate-release formulation.[74] The drug has a broad spectrum of use in seizure disorders, including absence seizures, and is now also used extensively by psychiatrists for mood disorders. An enteric-coated formulation of divalproex sodium became available in 1983; this is sodium valproate and valproic acid in a 1:1 ratio. Valproic acid, but not divalproex, is available in generic form. Divalproex has FDA approval for monotherapy and adjunctive therapy for partial seizures, manic episodes associated with bipolar disorder, and migraine prophylaxis. Evidence for its use as an acute treatment for migraine is lacking but some experts will attest to its benefits at a dose of 1000 mg IV, and it is used off-label for other psychiatric problems.

The exact molecular mechanisms responsible for its clinical effects are unknown. The catabolism of GABA is inhibited and the synaptic release of GABA is increased. Valproate is highly bound to plasma proteins, although somewhat less in older adults and those with liver or kidney disease. It has a half-life of 16 hours. Valproate is extensively metabolized—the most significant pathway is conjugation with glucuronic acid, and this pathway can be saturated within the therapeutic range. The general therapeutic range is 50 to 100 µg/mL. Valproate has complex interactions with other anticonvulsants but should not alter the metabolism of steroid contraceptives because it does not induce enzymes. Levels higher than 125 µg/mL often have adverse effects on the CNS, including drowsiness and tremors. Valproate may alter the pharmacokinetics of other drugs. Both carbamazepine and phenobarbital can reduce the level of valproate by 30% to 40%. Valproate can displace phenytoin from its protein-binding sites, increasing the free fraction of phenytoin. The most frequent side effects include nausea, vomiting, tremor, and weight gain (see Table 34–4). Most GI disturbances are not long-lasting. Other side effects such as alopecia, dizziness, emotional lability, and peripheral edema have been reported. Valproate is known for idiosyncratic reactions, unlike most other AEDs. Hepatotoxicity and pancreatitis may occur, with the hepatic effects seen more frequently in those younger than 2 years.[75] Ammonia levels may increase; if severe, this can cause encephalopathy. Valproate is a known teratogen, increasing especially the risk of spina bifida in 2% of infants born to mothers taking valproic acid.

Lamotrigine

Lamotrigine received FDA approval in 1994; it is used as an adjunctive agent for partial seizures and as monotherapy for partial and generalized seizures.[76,77] It also received FDA approval in 2003 for use as a treatment for bipolar disorder. Compared with phenytoin and carbamazepine, patients treated with lamotrigine were less likely to experience adverse events such as dizziness, somnolence, and cognitive impairment.[75] There is little dose-dependent toxicity, so monitoring laboratory values is not necessary. The most concerning side effect is rash, known to occur more often with rapid titration; it can present as Stevens-Johnson syndrome[78] (see Table 34–4). The risk of rash is similar to that with phenytoin or carbamazepine, from 5% to 10%; the risk of Stevens-Johnson syndrome is increased in those taking valproate. Enzyme-inducing drugs reduce the serum level of lamotrigine. Lamotrigine has no effect on liver enzymes, is metabolized via glucuronidation, and is 55% protein-bound, with a half-life of 30 hours. It needs a slow titration, at least 4 to 6 weeks. The coadministration of valproate leads to higher levels of lamotrigine. Lamotrigine has been reported useful for the neuropathic pain of sciatica.[79] Controlled trials have been conducted on the analgesic effects of lamotrigine on HIV-associated painful neuropathy, spinal cord injury pain, and central post-stroke pain.[80,82] In patients with incomplete spinal cord injury (SCI), lamotrigine significantly reduces pain at or below the SCI level. Patients with brush-evoked allodynia and wind-up–like pain in the area of maximal pain are more likely to have a positive effect from lamotrigine than patients without these evoked pains (7 of 7 vs. 1 of 14). Although this trial showed no significant effect on spontaneous and evoked pain in complete and incomplete spinal cord injury, lamotrigine has reduced spontaneous pain in patients with incomplete SCI and evoked pain in the area of spontaneous pain.[81]

Pain following a stroke, previously known as the thalamic pain syndrome, is a common severe central pain condition. In a community-based study of stroke, the prevalence of poststroke pain was found to be 8%, and 5% of patients developed moderate to severe pain. In patients older than 80 years, 11% developed central pain after a stroke.[82] Central poststroke pain (CPSP) is characterized by pain in those body areas that have lost part of their sensory innervation because of the stroke. Although the exact mechanisms underlying CPSP are unknown, it has been suggested that disruption of the spinothalamic tract or its cortical projection is a necessary requirement for the occurrence of central pain. Loss of such nervous activity to the thalamus is assumed to create a neuronal hyperactivity in the thalamus or other brain structures, similar to that seen in other neuropathic pain conditions.[82] Oral lamotrigine, 200 mg daily, is a well-tolerated and moderately effective treatment for central poststroke pain. Lamotrigine may be an alternative to tricyclic antidepressants for the treatment of CPSP.[82]

Approximately one third of patients with AIDS have distal sensory polyneuropathy (DSP) characterized by pain, numbness, and burning, primarily in the soles and dorsum of the feet.[80] Progressive and painful, DSP may significantly impair a patient's quality of life. It reduces functional ability by rendering walking difficult. DSP is a toxic effect of dideoxynucleoside analogue antiretroviral therapy (ART) that limits a patient's ability to remain on an antiviral regimen containing these compounds. HIV-associated DSP and antiretroviral toxic neuropathy are clinically indistinguishable and many patients have an overlap syndrome, with contributions from both disorders. The cause of DSP associated with AIDS or ART is unknown.[80] Lamotrigine was found to be effective in relieving pain in patients with HIV-associated peripheral neuropathy who were receiving neurotoxic ART.

Tiagabine

Tiagabine became available in the United States in 1997 for partial seizures in those older than 12 years.[83] The drug blocks the uptake of GABA, prolonging its effect. It does not affect liver enzymes and is metabolized by the CYP450 system. Its half-life of approximately 8 hours is reduced considerably in the presence of enzyme-inducing medications. It has not been studied extensively for the relief of pain. In the animal tail flick model, it does have an antinociceptive effect, and it was reported useful in a pilot study to treat tonic spasms in multiple sclerosis.[84,85] Postmarketing reports have shown that tiagabine use is associated with new-onset seizures and status epilepticus in patients without epilepsy. Dose may be an important predisposing factor in the development of seizures, although seizures have been reported in patients taking as little as 4 mg/day. In most cases, patients were using concomitant medications (e.g., antidepressants, antipsychotics, stimulants, narcotics) that are thought to lower the seizure threshold. Some seizures occurred near the time of a dose increase, even after periods of prior stable dosing.

Zonisamide

Zonisamide is indicated for adjunctive therapy in the treatment of partial seizures in adults and became available in the United States in 2000.[86] It blocks repetitive firing of voltage-sensitive sodium channels and reduces voltage-sensitive T-type calcium currents. It has a long half-life, approximately 65 hours, and it is completely absorbed. It may be administered once or twice daily. Zonisamide is metabolized by the CYP450 system but does not induce enzymes. The most common side effects in trials were dizziness, ataxia, and anorexia (see Table 34–4). Zonisamide is contraindicated in those with sulfonamide allergy because it is a sulfonamide derivative, and the drug is approximately 40% bound to plasma proteins. Uncommon side effects include hyperthermia and oligohidrosis. There have been case reports on usefulness for poststroke pain and headache.

A randomized, double-blind, placebo-controlled pilot study of the efficacy of zonisamide in the treatment of painful diabetic neuropathy has revealed that pain scores on the visual analogue scale and Likert (psychometric response) scales decrease more for the zonisamide group compared with the placebo group, but these differences did not reach statistical significance.[87] A larger randomized controlled trial is needed to establish the efficacy and tolerability of zonisamide for painful diabetic neuropathy. A 16-week randomized, double-blind, placebo-controlled trial with an optional single-blind extension of the same treatment for another 16 weeks has revealed that zonisamide and a hypocaloric diet result in more weight loss than placebo and a hypocaloric diet in the treatment of obesity.[88]

Benzodiazepines

As described earlier, benzodiazepines facilitate the actions of GABA in the CNS as a result of their binding to the GABA-A receptor. Clonazepam and clobazam (clobazam is not available in the United States) are useful as adjunctive treatment for refractory epilepsies.[89] Clonazepam is 47% protein-bound and is extensively metabolized. Diazepam and lorazepam have extensive use in the emergency management of seizures and status epilepticus. The side effects of drowsiness, ataxia, and the development of tolerance to the antiseizure effect (see Table 34–4) limit the usefulness of clonazepam and other benzodiazepines for chronic use. Diazepam is available as a rectal gel for quick onset in the acute management of seizures. Clonazepam is also used for chronic facial pain and has had some success in small clinical trials.[90] The only randomized double-blind trial of a benzodiazepine for pain was lorazepam when it was compared with amitriptyline for PHN, but it was found to be less effective.[91]

Vigabatrin

Vigabatrin is an irreversible inhibitor of GABA transaminase and is used as adjunctive therapy in those with partial seizures.[26] It is not currently available in the United States. It is also useful in infantile spasms and is the drug of choice for children with infantile spasms secondary to tuberous sclerosis. It is more effective for partial seizures than generalized seizures. Headache and drowsiness are the most prevalent side effects (see Table 34–4). Visual field defects and adverse psychiatric reactions have been reported. The drug is rapidly and completely absorbed after oral administration and does not exhibit significant protein binding. It is eliminated unchanged in the urine, with minimal metabolism. The elimination half-life is 5-7 hours but the pharmacodynamic half-life is considerably longer, enabling a once- or twice-daily dosing schedule. The role of vigabatrin in pain management is unknown.

References

1. LaRoche SM, Helmers S: The new antiepileptic drugs. JAMA 2004;291:605-614.
2. French JA, Kanner AM, Bautista J, et al: Efficacy and tolerability of the new antiepileptic drugs. 1. Treatment of new onset epilepsy. Neurology 2004;62:1252-1260.
3. French JA, Kanner AM, Bautista J, et al: Efficacy and tolerability of the new antiepileptic drugs. II. Treatment of refractory epilepsy. Neurology 2004;62:1261-1273.
4. National Institute for Clinical Excellence: Newer drugs for epilepsy in adults, 2004. Available at www.nice.org.uk/Docref.asp?d=110081.
5. National Institute for Clinical Excellence: Newer drugs for epilepsy in children, 2004. Available at www.nice.org.uk/Docref.asp?d=113359.
6. Tremont-Lukats IW, Megeff C, Backonja MM: Anticonvulsants for neuropathic pain syndromes: Mechanisms of action and place in therapy. Drugs 2000;601029-1052.
7. Rogawski M, Loscher W: The neurobiology of antiepileptic drugs. Nat Rev Neurosci 2004;10:685-692.
8. Hagiwara S, Ozawa S, Sand O: Voltage clamp analysis of two inward current mechanisms in the egg cell membrane of a starfish. J Gen Physiol 1975;65:617-644.
9. Yamakage M, Namiki A: Calcium channels—basic aspects of their structure, function and gene encoding; anesthetic action on the channels—a review. Can J Anesth 2002;49:151-164.
10. Luo ZD, Chaplan SR, Higuera ES, et al: Upregulation of dorsal root ganglion (alpha)2(delta) calcium channel subunit and its correlation with allodynia in spinal nerve-injured rats. J Neurosci 2001;21:1868-1875.
11. Errante LD, Williamson A, Spencer, D et al: Gabapentin and vigabatrin increase GABA in the human neocortical slice. Epilepsy Res 2002;49:203-210.
12. Golden AL: Mechanisms of sodium channel inactivation. Curr Opin Neurobiol 2003;13:284-290.
13. Kuo CC, Bean BP: Slow binding of phenytoin to inactivated sodium channels in rat hippocampal neurons. Mol Pharmacol 1994;46:716-725.
14. Yu F, Catterall W: Overview of the voltage-gated sodium channel family. Genome Biol 2003;4:207.
15. Priestley T: Voltage-gated sodium channels and pain. Curr Drug Targets CNS Neurol Disord 2004;3:441-456.
16. Lossin C, Wang DW, Rhodes TH, et al: Molecular basis of an inherited epilepsy. Neuron 2002;34:877-884.
17. Spampanato J, Kearney JA, de Haan G, et al: A novel epilepsy mutation in the sodium channel SCN1A identifies a cytoplasmic domain for beta subunit interaction. J Neurosci 2004;3;24:10022-10044.
18. Gold MS, Weinreich D, Kim CS, et al: Redistribution of Na(V) 1.8 in uninjured axons enables neuropathic pain. J Neurosci 2003;23:158-166.
19. Todorovic SM, Rastogi AJ, Jevtovic-Todorvic V: Potent analgesic effects of anticonvulsants on peripheral thermal nociception in rats. Br J Pharmacol 2003;140:255-260.
20. Kuo C: A common anticonvulsant binding site for phenytoin, carbamazepine, and lamotrigine in neuronal Na⁺ channels. Mol Pharmacol 1998;54:712-721.
21. Owens DF, Kriegstein AR: Is there more to GABA than synaptic inhibition? Nat Rev Neurosci 2002;3:715-727.
22. Schuler V, Lüscher C, Blanchet C, et al: Epilepsy, hyperalgesia, impaired memory, and loss of pre- and postsynaptic GABA(B) responses in mice lacking GABA(B(1)). Neuron 2001;31:47-58.
23. Cossette P, Lortie A, Vanasse M, et al: Autosomal dominant juvenile myoclonic epilepsy and GABRA1. Adv Neurol 2005;95:255-263.
24. Merrit HH, Putnam TJ: A new series of anti-convulsant drugs tested by experiments on animals. Arch Neurol Psychiatry 1938;39:1003-1015.
25. Mattson RH, Cramer JA, Collins JF, et al: Comparison of carbamazepine, phenobarbital, phenytoin, and primidone in partial and secondarily generalized tonic-clonic seizures. N Engl J Med 1985;313:145-151.
26. Browne TR, Holmes GL: Handbook of Epilepsy, 3rd ed. Philadelphia, Lippincott Williams & Wilkins, 2004.
27. Ahmed I, Reichenberg J, Lucas A, et al: Erythema multiforme associated with phenytoin and cranial radiation therapy: A report of three patients and review of the literature. Int J Dermatol 2004;43:67-73.
28. Orwoll ES, Klein RF: Osteoporosis in men. Endocr Rev 1995;16:87-116.
29. Yajnik S, Singh GP, Singh G, et al: Phenytoin as a coanalgesic in cancer pain. J Pain Symptom Manage 1992;7:209-213.
30. Fischer JH, Patel TV, Fischer PA: Fosphenytoin: Clinical pharmacokinetics and comparative advantages in the acute treatment of seizures. Clin Pharmacokinet 2003;42:33-58.
31. Blom S: Trigeminal neuralgia: Its treatment with a new anticonvulsant drug. Lancet 1962:1:839-840.
32. Schaffler L, Bourgeois BF, Lunders HO: Rapid reversibility of autoinduction of carbamazepine metabolism after temporary discontinuation. Epilepsia 1994;35:195-198.
33. Kalis MM, Huff NA: Oxcarbazepine, an antiepileptic agent. Clin Ther 2001;23:680-700.
34. Barcs G, Walker EB, Elger CE, et al: Oxcarbazepine placebo-controlled, dose-ranging trial in refractory partial epilepsy. Epilepsia 2000;41:1597-1607.
35. Friis ML, Kristensen O, Boas J, et al: Therapeutic experiences with 947 epileptic out-patients in oxcarbazepine treatment. Acta Neurol Scand 1993;87:224-227.
36. Tomic MA, Vuckovic SM, Stepanovic-Petrovic RM, et al: The anti-hyperalgesic effects of carbamazepine and oxcarbazepine are attenuated by the treatment with adenosine receptor antagonists. Pain 2004;111:253-260.
37. Zakrzewska JM, and Patsalos PN: Oxcarbazepine: A new drug in the management of intractable trigeminal neuralgia. J Neurol Neurosurg Psychiatry 1989;52:472-476.
38. Farago F: Trigeminal neuralgia: Its treatment with two new carbamazepine analogues. Eur Neurol 1987;26:73-83.
39. Lindstrom P: The analgesic effect of carbamazepine in trigeminal neuralgia. Pain 1987;4:S85.
40. Beydoun A: Neuropathic pain: From mechanisms to treatment strategies. J Pain Symptom Manage 2003;25:S1-S3.
41. Carranza E, Mikoshiba I: Rationale and evidence for the use of oxcarbazepine in neuropathic pain. J Pain Symptom Manage 2003;25:S31-S35.
42. Lesser H, Sharma U, LaMoreaux L, et al: Pregabalin relieves symptoms of painful diabetic neuropathy: A randomized controlled trial. Neurology 2004;63:2104-2110.
43. Rosenstock J, Tuchman M, LaMoreaux L, et al: Pregabalin for the treatment of painful diabetic peripheral neuropathy: A double-blind, placebo-controlled trial. Pain 2004;110:628-638.
44. Sabatowski R, Galvez R, Cherry DA, et al: Pregabalin reduces pain and improves sleep and mood disturbances in patients

with post-herpetic neuralgia: Results of a randomized, placebo-controlled trial. Pain 2004;109:26-35.

45. Pary R: High-dose pregabalin is effective for the treatment of generalized anxiety disorder. Evid Based Ment Health. 2004 Feb;7(1):17.

46. Arroyo S, Anhut H, Kugler AR, et al: Pregabalin add-on treatment: A randomized, double-blind, placebo-controlled, dose-response study in adults with partial seizures.Epilepsia 2004;45:20-27.

47. Beydoun AA, Uthman BM, Ramsay RE, et al: Pregabalin add-on trial: Double-blind multi-center study in patients with partial epilepsy [abstract]. Epilepsia 2000;41(Suppl 7):253-254.

48. French JA, Kugler AR, Robbins JL, et al: Dose-response trial of pregabalin adjunctive therapy in patients with partial seizures. Neurology 2003;60:1631-1637.

49. Dworkin RH, Corbin AE, Young Jr JP, et al: Pregabalin for the treatment of postherpetic neuralgia: A randomized, placebo-controlled trial. Neurology 2003;60:1274-1283.

50. Sabatowski R, Galvez R, Cherry DA, et al: Pregabalin reduces pain and improves sleep and mood disturbances in patients with postherpetic neuralgia: Results of randomized, placebo-controlled clinical trial. Pain 2004;109:26-35.

51. Van Seventer R, Bladin C, Hoggart B, et al: Pregabalin dosed twice a day (BID) efficaciously and safely treats neuropathic pain associated with postherpetic neuralgia [abstract]. J Pain 2004;5(Suppl 1):58.

52. Van Seventer R, Baldin C, Hogart B, et al: Pregabalin dosed BID efficacious for improving sleep interference in patients suffering from postherpetic neuralgia: Results of a large, randomized, placebo-controlled trial [abstract]. J Pain 2004;5 (Suppl 1):60.

53. Frampton J, Foster R: Pregabalin in the treatment of postherpetic neuralgia. Drugs 2005;65:111-118.

54. Crofford LJ, Rowbotham MC, Mease PJ, et al: Pregabalin for the treatment of fibromyalgia syndrome: Results of a randomized, double-blind, placebo-controlled trial. Arthritis Rheum 2005;52:1264-1273.

55. Tarride J, Gordon A, Montserrat V, et al: Cost-effectivenes of pregabalin for the management of neuropathic pain associated with diabetic peripheral neuropathy and postherpetic neuralgia: A Canadian perspective. Clin Ther 2006;28:1922-1934.

56. Chadwick DW, Anhut H, Greiner MJ, et al: A double-blind trial of gabapentin monotherapy for newly diagnosed partial seizures. International Gabapentin Monotherapy Study Group 945-77. Neurology 1998;51:1282-1288.

57. Rowbotham M, Harden N, Stacey B, et al: Gabapentin for the treatment of postherpetic neuralgia: A randomized controlled trial. JAMA 1998;280:1837-1842.

58. Schlicker E, Reimann W, Göthert M: Gabapentin decreases monoamine release without affecting acetylcholine release in the brain. Arzneimittelforschung 1985;35:1347-1349.

59. Wail AW, McLean MJ: Limitation by gabapentin of high-frequency action potential firing by mouse central neurons in cell culture. Epilepsy Res 1994;17:1-11.

60. Stillman M: Clinical approach to patients with neuropathic pain.Cleve Clin J Med 2006;73:726-739.

61. Gilron I, Bailey JM, Tu D, et al: Morphine, gabapentin, or their combination for neuropathic pain. N Engl J Med 2005;352:1324-1334.

62. Eckhardt K, Ammon S, Hofmann U, et al: Gabapentin enhances the analgesic effect of morphine in healthy volunteers. Anesth Analg 2000;91:185-191.

63. Turan A, Karamanlioglu B, Memis D, et al: Analgesic effects of gabapentin after spinal surgery. Anesthesiology 2004;100:935-938.

64. Singh L, Field MJ, Ferris P, et al: The antiepileptic agent gabapentin (Neurontin) possesses anxiolytic-like and antinociceptive actions that are reversed by D-serine. Psychopharmacology (Berl) 1996;127:1-9.

65. Glauser T: Topiramate. Epilepsia 1999;4 (Suppl 5):S71-S80.

66. Astrup A, Caterson I, Zelissen P: Topiramate: Long-term maintenance of weight loss by a low-calorie diet in obese subjects. Obes Res 200412:1658-1669.

67. Silberstein SD, Neto W, Schmitt J, et al; MIGR-001 Study Group: Topiramate in migraine prevention: Results of a large controlled trial. Arch Neurol 2004;61:490-495.

68. Brandes JL, Saper JR, Diamond M, et al: Topiramate for migraine prevention: A randomized controlled trial. JAMA 2004;291:965-973.

69. Storer RJ, Goadsby PJ: Topiramate inhibits trigeminovascular neurons in the cat. Cephalalgia 2004;24:1049-1056.

70. Thienel U, Neto W, Schwabe SK, et al; Topiramate Diabetic Neuropathic Pain Study Group: Topiramate in painful diabetic polyneuropathy: Findings from three double-blind placebo-controlled trials. Acta Neurol Scand 2004;110:221-231.

71. Price MJ: Levetiracetam in the treatment of neuropathic pain: Three case studies. Clin J Pain 2004;20:33-36.

72. Rigo JM, Hans G, Nguyen L, et al: The anti-epileptic drug levetiracetam reverses the inhibition by negative allosteric modulators of neuronal GABA- and glycine-gated currents. Br J Pharmacol 2002;136:659-672.

73. Lynch BA, Lambeng N, Nocka K, et al: The synaptic vesicle protein SV2A is the binding site for the antiepileptic drug levetiracetam. Proc Natl Acad Sci USA. 2004;101:9861-9866.

74. DeVane LC: Pharmacokinetics, drug interactions, and tolerability of valproate. Psychopharmacol Bull 2003;37(Suppl 2):25-42.

75. Eadie MJ, Hooper WD, Dickinson RG: Valproate-associated hepatotoxicity and its biochemical mechanisms. Med Toxicol 1988;3:85-106.

76. Brodie MJ, Richens A, Yuen AWC, et al: Double-blind comparison of lamotrigine and carbamazepine in newly diagnosed epilepsy. Lancet 1995;345:476-479.

77. Steiner TJ, Dellaportas CI, Findley LJ: Lamotrigine monotherapy in newly diagnosed untreated epilepsy: A double-blind comparison with phenytoin. Epilepsia 1999;40:601-607.

78. Roujeau JC, Stern RS: Severe adverse cutaneous reactions to drugs. N Eng J Med 1994;331:1272-1285.

79. Eisenberg E, Damunni G, Hoffer E, et al: Lamotrigine for intractactable sciatica: Correlation between dose, plasma concentration and analgesia. Eur J Pain 2003;7:485-491.

80. Simpson DM, McArthur JC, Olney R, et al: Lamotrigine for HIV-associated painful sensory neuropathies: A placebo-controlled trial. Neurology 2003;60:1508-1414.

81. Finnerup NB, Sindrup SH, Bach FW, et al: Lamotrigine in spinal cord injury pain: A randomized controlled trial. Pain 2002;96:375-383.

82. Vestergaard K, Anderson G, Gottrup H, et al: Lamotrigine for central poststroke pain: A randomized controlled trial. Neurology 2001;56:184-190.

83. Leach JP, Brodie MJ: Tiagabine. Lancet 1998:351:203-207.

84. Giardina WJ, Decker MW, Porsolt, et al: An evaluation of the GABA uptake blocker tiagabine in animal models of neuropathic and nociceptive pain. Drug Dev Res 1998:44:106-113.

85. Solaro C, Tanganelli P: Tiagabine for treating painful tonic spasms in multiple sclerosis: A pilot study. J Neurol Neurosurg Psychiatry 2004;75:341.

86. Sackellares JC, Ramsey RE, Wilder BJ, et al: Randomized, controlled clinical trial of zonisamide as adjunctive treatment for refractory partial seizures. Epilepsia 2004;45:610-617.

87. Alti A, Dogra S: Zonisamide in the treatment of painful diabetic neuropathy: A randomized, double-blind, placebo-controlled pilot study. Pain Med 2005;6:225-234.

88. Gadde KM, Franciscy DM, Wagner HR, et al: Zonisamide for weight loss in obese adults: A randomized, controlled trial. JAMA 2003;289:1820-1825.

89. Levy RH, Mattson RH, Meldrum BS, et al: Antiepileptic Drugs, 5th ed. Philadelphia, Lippincott Williams & Wilkins, 2002.

90. Smirne S, Scarlato G: Clonazepam in cranial neuralgias. Med J Aust 1977;1:93-94.

91. Max MB, Schafer SC, Culnane M, et al: Amitriptyline, but not lorazepam, relieves postherpetic neuralgia. Neurology 1988:38:1427-1432.

CHAPTER

35 Nonsteroidal Anti-inflammatory Drugs, Acetaminophen, and COX-2 Inhibitors

Asokumar Buvanendran and Scott S. Reuben

Nonsteroidal anti-inflammatory drugs (NSAIDs) are a diverse group of chemically unrelated compounds that are classified together based on their therapeutic property of possessing an anti-inflammatory action (Fig. 35–1).[1] NSAIDs are the most widely prescribed drugs for the treatment of acute and chronic pain with sales in millions of dollars in the United States and account for about 6 to 7 billion dollars in sales worldwide.

Extracts from the bark and leaves of willow, myrtle, and other plants have therapeutic effects based on the presence of salicylic acid, which was first used for the treatment of fever in 1763 by Edward Stone. In 1829, Henri Leroux, in France, obtained a compound of salicylic acid (known as salicin) in crystalline form and succeeded in splitting it to obtain the acid in its pure state. Professor Hermann Koble, in Germany, discovered the compound's chemical structure and succeeded in synthesizing it in 1859. Sodium salicylate was first used for the treatment of rheumatic fever in 1875. Bayer Pharmaceutical started manufacturing aspirin (acetylsalicylic acid) by 1914 and currently sells about 11 billion tablets annually. Shortly after aspirin was first manufactured, other drugs with diverse chemical structures but similar antipyretic, anti-inflammatory, and analgesic properties were discovered; these were grouped together as NSAIDs. John R. Vane elucidated the mechanism of NSAIDs in 1971 and shared the Nobel Prize in Physiology and Medicine with Sune Bergstrom and Bengt Samuelson in 1982.

MECHANISM OF ACTION

Prostaglandin Synthesis and Pharmacology

Von Euler[2] coined the term *prostaglandin* (PG) to describe an extract from semen that contracted

uterine smooth muscle. Although PGs are derived from arachidonic acid and other polyunsaturated fatty acids, the 20-carbon polyunsaturated essential fatty acid (arachidonic acid) is the major source in mammalian tissues. PGs derived from arachidonic acid contain two double bonds (prostaglandin E_2 [PGE_2], thromboxane and prostacyclin). Analogous compounds synthesized from eicosatrienoic (linoleic) and eiocosapentaenoic acids contain one less or more double bond in the side chains (PGE_1, PGE_3, respectively).[3] The various groups of PGs, thromboxanes, hydroxy acids, and leukotrienes, which retain the 20-carbon unsaturated fatty acid structure, are collectively known as eicosanoids. The three fatty acid precursors (eicosapentaenoic acid) are derived directly or indirectly from dietary fat and are esterified into cell membranes.[4] Their release, usually as a result of trauma, is the major stimulus for eicosanoid production, because PGs cannot be stored and are released as soon they are synthesized.[5] Cell membrane disruption leads to the release of phospholipid, which is converted to arachidonic acid by the action of phospholipase A_2. Arachidonic acid in turn acts as a substrate for cyclooxygenase (COX). COX-catalyzed peroxidation of arachidonic acid results in a cyclic structure, whereas peroxidation catalyzed by lipo-oxygenase produces straight-chain hydroxy-peroxy acids, which can then be converted to hydroxy acids (Fig. 35–2).

Prostaglandins are also involved in the pyretic response. After injection of pyrogens, there is a rise in PG levels in the cerebrospinal fluid (CSF) that is prevented by pretreatment with aspirin.[6] It is of interest that acetaminophen, which is antipyretic but not anti-inflammatory, blocks brain PG synthetase. Prostanoids do not generally activate nociceptors directly, but sensitize them to mechanical stimuli and chemical mediators of nociception, such as bradykinin.[7]

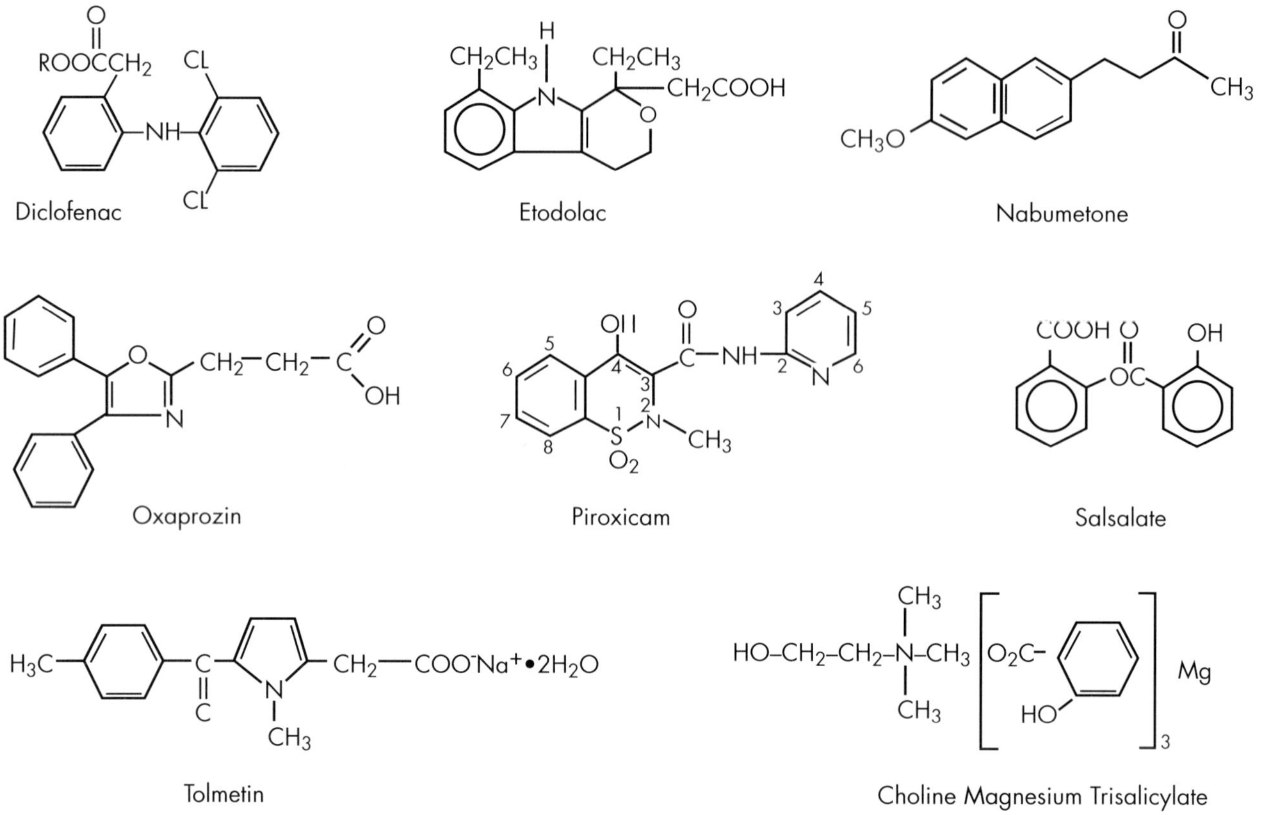

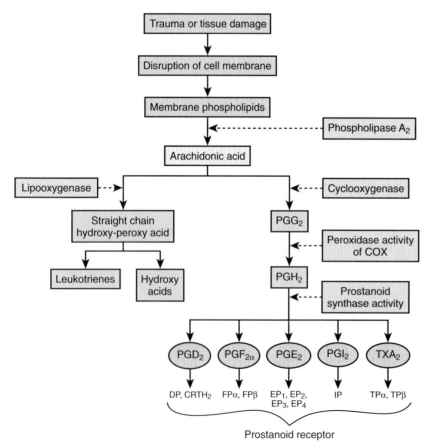

Figure 35–1. Structures of several different NSAIDs, revealing the wide variation in chemical structures of the compounds that are grouped into this one therapeutic class.

Figure 35–2. Pathway for the formation of prostaglandins. COX, cyclooxygenase; CRTH₂, chemoattractant receptor-homologous molecule; DP, PGD receptor; EP₁, EP₂, EP₃, EP₄, PGE receptors; FPα, PGF receptor α; FPβ, PGF receptor β; IP, PGI receptor; PG, prostaglandin; TPα, TXA₂ receptor α; TPβ, TXA₂ receptor β; TXA₂, thromboxane A₂.

PGE_2 is the predominant eicosanoid released from endothelial cells of small blood vessels[8] and is a key mediator of both peripheral and central pain sensitization.[4] As the prostanoid most associated with inflammatory responses, the formation of PGE_2 at inflammatory sites is often considered an indicator of local COX activity, and suppression of PGE_2 is an indicator of a decreased inflammatory process.[9] The production of PGE_2 is slow in onset and of long duration in response to inflammation.[10] It is currently recognized that COX is encoded by two genes.[11] Although the isomerization of PGH_2 into PGE_2 has been well characterized biochemically and pharmacologically, the enzyme responsible, PGE synthase, has been only purified and cloned rather recently.[12] This enzyme is one of the membrane-associated proteins in the eicosanoid and glutathione metabolism superfamily, which consists of six proteins with divergent functions.[13]

COX-1 and COX-2 Selectivity

The existence of a COX isoform that is positively and negatively regulated by cytokines and glucocorticoids, respectively, was long suspected, but it was only in the early 1990s that an inducible COX isoenzyme (COX-2) was successfully cloned.[14] The identification of two COX isoforms, COX-1 and COX-2, has generated intense efforts to characterize the relative contribution of each isoform to prostanoid production in specific situations. The development of isoform-specific antagonists has been extremely useful, first as experimental tools and, more recently, for clinical therapy.

COX-1 and COX-2 are membrane-associated enzymes with a 60% amino acid sequence homology.[15] The major sequence differences occur in the membrane-binding domains. Structural and functional studies of the COX isoforms have revealed a homodimer profile. Both isoenzymes are composed of three independent folding units: (1) an epidermal growth factor–like domain; (2) a membrane-binding moiety; and (3) an active enzymatic domain that consists of a long hydrophobic channel.[16] In spite of their remarkable structural similarity, the two COX isoforms have different gene expression profiles, distinct kinetic properties, and different interactions with phospholipase A_2 and synthases.[15] The genes for COX-1 and COX-2 are located on human chromosomes 9 and 1, respectively.[17] Whereas COX-1 represents a housekeeping gene that lacks a TATA box, the promoter of the immediate-early gene COX-2 contains a TATA box and binding sites for several transcription factors, including nuclear factor kappa B (NF-κB), the nuclear factor for interleukin-6 (IL-6) expression (NF IL-6), and the cyclic AMP (cAMP) response element-binding protein.[18]

COX-1 is expressed constitutively and produces prostanoids that fine-tune physiologic processes requiring instantaneous or continuous regulation (e.g., hemostasis).[15] COX-2 expression is usually low but can be induced by numerous factors, including neurotransmitters, growth factors, proinflammatory cytokines, lipopolysaccharide, calcium, phorbol esters, and small-peptide hormones.[19] However, there are exceptions to the original constitutive versus inducible theory of COX expression. COX-1 expression can be induced in some stress conditions, such as nerve injury, and many tissues, including the central nervous system (CNS) and the kidney, constitutively express COX-2.[19] In the spinal cord, there are detectable basal levels of both COX-1 and COX-2, which might enable immediate reactions to transmitter release that result in prostanoid production.[20]

It has been suggested that there is another COX enzyme formed as a splice variant of COX-1, known as COX-3.[21] Canine COX-3 expressed by transfected insect cells can be inhibited by therapeutic concentrations of analgesic or antipyretic drugs, or both, such as acetaminophen, phenacetin, antipyrine, and dipyrone. However, it has been reported that this COX-1 variant (COX-3) is not expressed in humans,[22] rats, or mice, because the corresponding additional intron 1 sequence in the mRNA transcript spans 94 (human) or 98 (rat and mouse) nucleotides, thus shifting the coding sequence out of frame.[23,24]

Peripheral and Central Induction of COX-2

The original hypothesis formulated by Vane in his Nobel Prize–winning work on the mechanism of action of NSAIDs was that these compounds inhibit prostanoid production in the periphery, preventing a sensitizing action of PGE_2 on the peripheral terminals of sensory fibers.[25] More recently, peripheral inflammation has also been shown to induce a widespread increase in COX-2[26] and PGE synthase (PGES) expression in the CNS. The proinflammatory cytokine interleukin-1β (IL-1β) is upregulated at the site of inflammation and plays a major role in inducing COX-2 in local inflammatory cells by activating the transcription factor NF-κB.[27] IL-1β is also responsible for the induction of COX-2 in the CNS in response to peripheral inflammation, but this is not the result of neural activity arising from the sensory fibers innervating the inflamed tissue or of systemic IL-1β in the plasma. Instead, peripheral inflammation produces some other signal molecule that enters the circulation, crosses the blood-brain barrier, and acts to elevate IL-1β levels, leading to COX-2 expression in neurons and non-neuronal cells in many different areas of the spinal cord.[4,28] An elevation of COX-2 also occurs at many levels in the brain and spinal cord, mainly in the endothelial cells of the brain vasculature.[29]

Thus, there appear to be two forms of input from peripheral inflamed tissue to the CNS. The first is mediated by electrical activity in sensitized nerve fibers innervating the inflamed area, which signals the location of the inflamed tissue as well as the onset, duration, and nature of any stimuli applied to this tissue.[25] This input is sensitive to peripherally acting COX-2 inhibitors and to neural blockade with local anesthetics, as with epidural anesthesia.[30] The second is a humoral signal originating from the inflamed tissue, which acts to produce a widespread induction of COX-2 in the CNS. This input is not affected by regional anesthesia[28,31] and will only be blocked by centrally acting COX-2 inhibitors.[28,30,32] This implies that patients who receive neuraxial anesthesia for surgery might also need a centrally acting COX-2 inhibitor for optimal reduction of postoperative pain and the postoperative stress response.[30,32]

Therefore, the permeability of the blood-brain barrier to currently used NSAIDs and COX-2 inhibitors becomes important.[33,34] Inhibitors of COX-2 that penetrate the blood-brain barrier more effectively might represent more efficient pain killers and could also act to reduce many of the more diffuse aspects of inflammatory pain, such as generalized aches and pains, depression, and loss of appetite, which are key aspects in determining the quality-of-life response to treatment.[35] The main process whereby a drug passes from the bloodstream to the CNS is passive diffusion, for which lipophilicity and ionization are critical determinants of transfer.[36] The CSF represents a convenient sampling point for drugs that enter the central nervous system; however, there are very few NSAIDs for which CSF pharmacokinetics have been defined. For example, the CSF-to-plasma concentration ratio of oxyphenbutazone has been determined to be 0.0074 (0.7%). This ratio is close to the free fraction of oxyphenbutazone in plasma, which is about 0.5%.[37] The high lipid solubility of indomethacin allows it to cross into the CSF rapidly and equilibrate with the free plasma concentration.[38] Similar results have been noted with ketoprofen.[39]

Prostanoid Receptors: Expression, Regulation, and Function

The first prostanoid receptor to be isolated and cloned was the thromboxane A_2 (TXA_2) receptor,[40] a guanine (G) protein–coupled receptor with seven transmembrane domains. Homology screening of complementary DNA (cDNA) libraries has resulted in the isolation and identification of seven other prostanoid receptors that had been predicted pharmacologically: the PGD receptor (DP), four PGE receptors (EP_1, EP_2, EP_3, and EP_4), the PGF receptor (FP), and the PGI receptor (IP). Prostanoid receptors are expressed in many tissues and cell types. Among the EP receptors, EP_3 and EP_4 are the most widely distributed, whereas EP_1 and EP_2 distribution is restricted to the kidney, stomach, and uterus, as well as to neuronal and nonneuronal cells in the nervous system.[41] EP_1, EP_3, and EP_4 mRNAs are expressed in primary sensory neurons in the dorsal root and trigeminal ganglia,[42] suggesting involvement in PGE_2-mediated peripheral sensitization. Inflammation affects the expression levels of many prostanoid receptor subtypes. Further studies are needed to determine which of the EP receptors are involved with analgesia and appropriate antagonists.

The inhibition of prostaglandin biosynthesis may only partly explain the therapeutic effects of NSAIDs.[43] Another postulated mechanism includes interactions with the adenylate cyclase system. Indomethacin and some other NSAIDs inhibit phosphodiesterase, thereby elevating the intracellular concentration of cyclic AMP.[44]

PHARMACOKINETICS

NSAIDs are weak acids with pK_a values typically lower than 5. Because weak acids will be 99% ionized 2 pH units above their pK_a, these anti-inflammatory agents will be present in the body mostly in the ionized form.

General Factors Affecting NSAID Pharmacokinetics

Although NSAIDs differ in their individual pharmacokinetic properties, some general factors affecting NSAID pharmacokinetics can enable clinicians to select among the different agents available.

Absorption

Most NSAIDs are rapidly absorbed following oral administration, with peak plasma concentrations generally reached within 2 to 3 hours after administration. Slow-release dosage forms have been developed to maintain active plasma levels for prolonged time periods. Factors affecting gastric emptying may have a profound effect on the time course of the clinical effect of the NSAID administered. The extent of drug absorption from the gastrointestinal (GI) tract is more important than the rate.[45] The rectal route of administration has been used to minimize the GI side effects that are a common feature of these agents. In general, the rate and extent of NSAID absorption is comparable for the rectal and oral routes.[46]

Distribution

All NSAIDs are lipid-soluble, weakly acidic, and highly bound to plasma proteins, with the exception of aspirin. In most cases, less than 1% of the total plasma concentration is in the unbound form. Albumin is the major binding protein for NSAIDs. Disease conditions that cause hypoalbuminemia will result in an increased free fraction of NSAID in plasma, thus affecting the distribution and elimination of these agents.[47] Most NSAIDs have distribution volumes between 0.1 and 0.15 L/kg.

In inflammatory joint diseases, the effect of an NSAID is related to levels in the affected synovial fluid. These levels correlate closely with the drug concentration at the active site, because there is simple transport of drugs across the synovial membrane.[48,49] The amount of drug in synovial fluid is dependent on the level of albumin in the joint, which is lower than in plasma.[50]

Elimination

Hepatic biotransformation is the main elimination pathway of most of the NSAIDs.[51] Most are metabolized by cytochrome P-450–mediated oxidation, glucuronide conjugation, or both. Renal excretion of nonmetabolized drug is a minor elimination pathway for most NSAIDs, accounting for less than 10% of the administered dose. Some NSAID metabolites are also excreted to a significant extent via the bile.

Pathophysiologic Conditions Affecting NSAID Kinetics

Renal failure and hepatic disease are common disorders that affect the kinetics of NSAIDs.

Renal Failure

Renal failure has a variety of influences on drug kinetics, not only reducing the renal excretion of drugs and metabolites normally excreted in urine, but also affecting the absorption, distribution, and biotransformation of drugs.

Absorption and Distribution

The absorption of NSAIDs is not impaired in renal failure patients. However, the plasma protein binding of many acidic compounds such as the NSAIDs is impaired in renal failure patients.[52] The result is an increase in the volume of distribution of the unbound fraction of the drug in plasma.

Elimination

An increase in the unbound fraction of the drug in plasma may lead to an increase in total plasma clearance of the NSAID. The clearance of those NSAIDs for which formation of acyl glucuronides is a major elimination pathway is significantly reduced in patients with renal failure.[53] Of the acyl glucuronides, NSAIDs (e.g., diflunisal, ketoprofen, naproxen, indoprofen, benoxaprofen, tiaprofenic acid) are usually excreted rapidly in urine, but accumulate in the plasma of patients with renal failure. The effect of renal failure on the oral clearance of several NSAIDs (e.g., ibuprofen, fenbufen, isoxicam, piroxicam) is small.[54] Most of these compounds are metabolized by oxidative pathways. All NSAIDs are highly bound to plasma proteins and hemodialysis will not likely result in increased elimination of these agents. No dosage adjustments are therefore necessary for patients being administered NSAIDs who are undergoing hemodialysis.[53]

Hepatic Disease

Impaired liver function can affect the disposition of NSAIDs.

Absorption and Distribution

Most NSAIDs are low-clearance drugs and liver disease should theoretically not be expected to interfere with the oral bioavailability of these agents. Because the liver is the major organ for the synthesis of albumin, the major binding protein for NSAID in plasma, it would be expected that hepatic dysfunction could lead to alterations in the unbound drug fraction present in plasma.

Elimination

Because most NSAIDs have a small total intrinsic clearance (oral clearance) relative to blood flow, hepatic clearance is essentially independent of flow and reflects drug-metabolizing capacity. The elimination of ibuprofen does not seem to be affected in patients with liver disease.[55]

SPECIFIC DRUGS

Generic and trade names of NSAIDs are given in Table 35–1.

Salicylates

The major salicylates currently used are aspirin, diflunisal, choline magnesium trisalicylate, and salsalate.

Aspirin

Aspirin is the most studied and commonly used NSAID. Aspirin has an elimination half-life that increases from 2.5 hours at low doses to 19 hours at

Table 35–1.   Generic and Trade Names of Nonsteroidal Anti-inflammatory Drugs

GENERIC NAME	TRADE NAMES
Aspirin	
Diflunisal	Dolobid
Diclofenac	Voltaren, Cataflam, Arthrotec (combination with misoprostol)
Indomethacin	Indocin
Sulindac	Clinoril
Tolmetin	Tolectin
Ketorolac	Toradol
Etodolac	Lodine, Lodine XL
Ibuprofen	Motrin, Advil, Vicoprofen (combination with hydrocodone), Combunox (combination with oxycodone)
Flurbiprofen	Ansaid
Naproxen	Naproxen, Aleve
Ketoprofen	Orudis
Fenoprofen	Nalfon, Nalfon 200
Oxaprozin	Daypro
Mefenamic	Ponstel
Meclofenamic	Meclomen
Phenylbutazone	Butazolidin
Piroxicam	Feldene
Nabumetone	Relafen
Acetaminophen	Tylenol
Celecoxib	Celebrex
Rofecoxib	
Valdecoxib	
Meloxicam	Mobic

high doses. It is well absorbed in the stomach and small intestine, with a peak blood level achieved 1 hour after an oral dose. There is then rapid conversion of aspirin to salicylates from a high first-pass effect, which occurs in the wall of the small intestine and the liver. The metabolic pathways follow first-order and zero-order kinetics.[56]

Aspirin inhibits the biosynthesis of prostaglandins by irreversible acetylation and consequent inactivation of COX. This is in contrast to the action of newer NSAIDs, which are reversible inhibitors of the COX enzyme.[57] Although most cells can synthesize new cyclooxygenase, platelets cannot; thus, the acetylation of their microsomal enzyme lasts for the life of the platelet (10 to 14 days). The ability of aspirin to acetylate proteins may be one reason for its superiority as an anti-inflammatory agent as compared with other salicylate derivatives. Of all the NSAIDs, only aspirin has been associated with Reye's syndrome, a combination of seizures, coma, and sometimes death related to the use of aspirin during a viral illness in children.[58]

Diflunisal

Diflunisal is potentially better tolerated in the GI system because it is not metabolized to salicylic acid in plasma, based on a study comparing diflunisal, 250 and 500 mg twice daily, versus aspirin, 600 mg four times daily.[59] It has a short half-life relative to aspirin and less inhibition of platelets compared with aspirin.[60]

Choline Magnesium Trisalicylate and Salsalate

Both are nonacetylated salicylates that have a minimal effect on platelet function and less effect on GI mucosa than their acetylated counterparts. They produce similar analgesia and blood levels of salicylate as those of the acetylated class.[61]

Acetaminophen

Acetaminophen is a *p*-aminophenol derivative with analgesic and antipyretic properties similar to those of aspirin. Antipyresis probably occurs because of direct action on the hypothalamic heat-regulating centers via the inhibiting action of endogenous pyrogen.[62] Recently, it has been hypothesized that acetaminophen may be acting via the serotonergic pathway to provide analgesia.[63] Although equipotent to aspirin in inhibiting central PG synthesis, acetaminophen has no significant peripheral PG synthetase inhibition. Doses of 650 mg have been shown to be more effective than doses of 300 mg, but little additional benefit is seen at doses above 1000 mg, indicating a possible ceiling effect.[64]

Acetaminophen has few side effects in the usual dosage range; no significant GI toxicity or platelet functional changes occur. It is almost entirely metabolized in the liver, and the minor metabolites are responsible for the hepatotoxicity seen in overdose.[65] Inducers of the cytochrome P-450 enzyme system in the liver (e.g., alcohol) increase the formation of metabolites and therefore increase hepatotoxicity. In certain patients (chronic ethanol users, patients suffering from malnutrition, and fasting patients), repeating therapeutic or slightly excessive doses may precipitate hepatotoxicity. A dosage of 2600 to 3200 mg/day may represent a safer chronic daily dosage and dosing should not exceed 4 g/day.[66] Toxic doses may be a function of baseline glutathione levels and other dose-related factors. Acetaminophen is completely and rapidly absorbed following the oral route. Peak serum concentrations are achieved within 2 hours of a therapeutic dose and therapeutic serum concentrations are 10 to 20 μg/mL.[67] About 90% of acetaminophen is hepatically metabolized to sulfate and glucuronide conjugates for renal excretion, with a small amount secreted unchanged in the urine.[68]

The bioavailability of rectally administered acetaminophen is variable. It is approximately 80% of that of tablets and the rate of absorption is slower, with maximum plasma concentration achieved about 2 to 3 hours after administration.[69] Doses of 40 to 60 mg/kg of rectal acetaminophen have been shown to have an opioid-sparing effect in postoperative pain models.[70] Propacetamol, an injectable prodrug of paracetamol, is completely hydrolyzed within 6 minutes of administration and 1 g of propacetamol yields 0.5 g of paracetamol. Injectable paracetamol has been shown to reduce opioid consumption by about 35% to 45%[71] in postoperative pain studies.[72] There is widespread use of paracetamol (IV acetaminophen), except in the United States. In a study examining the analgesic serum concentrations of paracetamol, it has been demonstrated that a ceiling effect of paracetamol may be present at intravenous doses of 5 mg/kg, which corresponds to a serum concentration of 14 mg/mL.[73]

Recent data have demonstrated that acetaminophen can deplete pulmonary antioxidant levels, leading to an increased risk of newly diagnosed asthma.[74] Previous research has demonstrated that acetaminophen may be associated with an increased risk of newly diagnosed asthma if used for 14 days or more per month. Increasing use of acetaminophen may be associated with increased prevalence of asthma and chronic obstructive pulmonary disease (COPD).

Acetic Acid Derivatives

This group of NSAIDs contains two subclasses, pyroleacetic acids (indomethacin, sulindac, tolmetin, ketorolac, etodolac) and phenylacetic acids (diclofenac, bromfenac).

Indomethacin

Indomethacin has good oral and rectal absorption, although the extent of absorption varies widely among patients. There is also a large interpatient variability in elimination half-life, caused by extensive enterohepatic recirculation of the drug. It is highly bound to albumin. Metabolism involves demethylation and deacetylation in the liver, with subsequent excretion of inactive metabolites and unchanged drug in the bile and urine.[75] Its clinical application is somewhat limited by a relatively high incidence of side effects (primary gastritis and renal dysfunction), but it is used in patients with acute gouty arthritis and osteoarthritis.

Sulindac

Sulindac was developed as the result of a search for a drug similar to indomethacin but with lower toxicity. The lower GI toxicity with sulindac may occur because sulindac is an inactive prodrug that is converted after absorption by liver microsomal enzymes to sulindac disulfide, which appears to be the active metabolite.[76] It is eliminated from the plasma, predominantly by excretion in the bile, but is subject to enterohepatic circulation. Peak plasma levels of 0.1 to 0.2 mg/100 mL occur 2 to 3 hours after an oral dose of 200 mg. Steady-state plasma levels of the sulfide are reached after 4 to 5 days of therapy with 200 mg twice daily by mouth. It is available in 150- and 200-mg tablets and is administered twice daily for the treatment of gouty arthritis, osteoarthritis, and various inflammatory diseases.[77]

Huskisson and Franchimont[77] have reported that only 25% of patients have GI problems; constipation is predominant. As mentioned earlier, sulindac was considered in early studies to be the least nephrotoxic of the NSAIDs, but more recent studies have failed to support this contention.[78] Sulindac seems to have less effect on the CNS than indomethacin, possibly because it has an indene rather than indole nucleus, present in both indomethacin and serotonin, an important mediator in the CNS.

Tolmetin and Etodolac

Both these drugs have fewer side effects than other NSAIDs. Tolmetin is available in 100- and 200-mg tablets and has a half-life of 60 minutes. It is excreted in the urine partly unchanged, partly conjugated, and as an inactive dicarboxylic acid metabolite.[79] Tolmetin can cause edema because of sodium retention and abnormal liver function, both of which are reversible on discontinuation of this NSAID.

Etodolac is an acidic compound with a pK_a of 4.65. It is manufactured as tablets and capsules, with a normal dosage ranging from to 1 to 1.2 g daily. Clinical doses of 200 to 300 mg twice daily for the relief of low back or shoulder pain has been equated to analgesia with naproxen, 500 mg twice daily.[80] From large clinical trials, it has been found that the incidence of abdominal pain and dyspepsia is similar to that with several other NSAIDs, and gastrointestinal

ulceration occurs in less than 0.3% of patients.[81] Dyspepsia occurs with etodolac in 10% of patients, with a somewhat lower incidence of abdominal pain.

Ketorolac

Ketorolac is currently the only parenteral NSAID for clinical analgesic use in the United States. Although indomethacin has been available as an injectable form for years, it was used only in low dosages for the treatment of patent ductus arteriosus. Ketorolac is almost entirely bound to plasma proteins (more than 99%), which results in a small apparent volume of distribution, with extensive metabolism by conjugation and excretion via the kidney.[82] The analgesic effect occurs within 30 minutes, with maximum effect between 1 to 2 hours and duration of 4 to 6 hours.[83] Ketorolac demonstrates analgesia well beyond its anti-inflammatory properties, which are between those of indomethacin and naproxen, but ketorolac can provide analgesia 50 times that of naproxen. It has an antipyretic effect 20 times that of aspirin and thus can mask a febrile response when given routinely to patients postoperatively. Several studies have demonstrated efficacy comparable to or exceeding that of morphine for treatment of moderate postoperative pain treatment, but with fewer side effects.[84] Although ketorolac prolongs bleeding time, it does not do so excessively; however, postoperative bleeding associated with intraoperative ketorolac use has been reported.[85] There is evidence that ketorolac may be acting at the CNS in addition to its peripheral mode of action.[32,38] Dental surgery studies with ketorolac have also indicated that ketorolac acts centrally,[86] but measurements of drug levels in CSF have demonstrated poor penetration of the compound from plasma.[87]

Oral ketorolac was approved for use in the United States approximately 3 years after the parenteral form and has an efficacy similar to that of naproxen and ibuprofen.[88] However, the parenteral form can be administered at single doses of 30 to 60 mg or as 30 mg IM or IV every 6 hours, whereas the oral dose is limited to 10 to 20 mg for no more than 5 days because of GI toxicity. However, the appropriate analgesic dose of ketorolac is controversial. Since ketorolac has been marketed, there have been reports of death caused by GI and operative site bleeding.[89] As a consequence, the drug's license was suspended in Germany and France. In a response to these adverse events, the drug's manufacturer has recommended reducing the dose of ketorolac from 150 to 120 mg/day.[83] The European Committee for Proprietary Medicinal Products has recommended a further maximal daily dose reduction to 60 mg for older patients and to 90 mg for younger adults.[90] Currently, there is consensus that the dose should be as low as 7.5 to 10 mg every 6 hours.[91,92] Although ketorolac has been available in an injectable formulation, studies are underway to determine the efficacy of this drug when administered intranasally.[93] The intranasal route of administration may offer the added advantage of better brain penetration via the olfactory route and provide higher levels of the drug in the CNS and CSF,[94] with minimal GI side effects.

Diclofenac

Oral diclofenac is a carboxylic acid functional group with rapid and complete absorption. Diclofenac binds extensively to plasma albumin. Substantial concentrations of drug are attained in synovial fluid, which may be one of the sites of action of diclofenac.[95] Concentration-effect relationships have been established for total bound, unbound, and synovial fluid diclofenac concentrations.[96] Diclofenac is eliminated following biotransformation to glucuroconjugated and sulfate metabolites that are excreted in urine, with very little drug eliminated unchanged. The metabolism of diclofenac in humans is partitioned between acyl glucuronidation and phenyl hydroxylation; the former reaction is catalyzed primarily by uridine 5′-diphosphoglucuronosyl transferase 2B7, whereas the latter is catalyzed by cytochrome P-450 (CYP) 2C9 and 3A4.[97]

Diclofenac differs from the other NSAIDs by having a high first-pass effect and hence lower oral bioavailability. Diclofenac may also have a significantly higher incidence of hepatotoxicity than other NSAIDs. The excretion of conjugates may be related to renal function. Conjugate accumulation occurs in end-stage renal disease; however, no accumulation is apparent on comparison of younger and older adults.[98] Dosage adjustments for older adults, children, or patients with various disease states (e.g., hepatic disease, rheumatoid arthritis) may not be required. Significant drug-drug interactions have been demonstrated with aspirin, lithium, digoxin, methotrexate, cyclosporine, cholestyramine, and colestipol.[99]

A parenteral form has been used in Europe, with one study showing it to be effective in reducing opioid requirements and reducing pain after thoracotomies.[100] Diclofenac sodium has also been tested in clinical trials in a gel form for pain relief of superficial burns, with good success.[101]

Propionic Acid Derivatives

This class of compounds includes ibuprofen, fenoprofen, ketoprofen, flurbiprofen, and naproxen. A newer drug in this class is oxaprozin, which has received attention because it has a once-daily dosage regimen, but it has no distinct advantage over other NSAIDs.[102]

Ibuprofen

Ibuprofen is well absorbed, and peak plasma levels of 15 to 20 μg/mL are achieved about 1 to 2 hours after a single dose. The half-life is about 3.5 hours. The drug is mostly metabolized in the liver, with less than 10% excreted unchanged in the urine and bile.[103] Ibuprofen at a dose of 1200 mg/day has a predominately analgesic effect in arthritis patients. At the high end of the recommended dosage, 2400 mg/day, it produces GI side effects, of which nausea and dyspepsia are predominant. Renal side effects of ibuprofen appear to be dose-dependent, and have not been reported at the recommended over-the-counter drug dosage (0.2 to 0.8 g/day). Even at anti-inflammatory doses (more than 1.6 g/day), renal side effects are almost exclusively encountered in patients with low intravascular volume and low cardiac output, particularly in older adults.[104] The concomitant administration of ibuprofen antagonizes the irreversible platelet inhibition induced by aspirin. Therefore, treatment with ibuprofen in patients with increased cardiovascular risk may limit the cardioprotective effects of aspirin.[105]

Ketoprofen

The drug is available in oral form and reaches its peak plasma level in 0.5 to 2 hours. The half-life is 2.4 hours, with an analgesic duration of 4 to 6 hours.[106] The maximum recommended dosage is 300 mg/day. Ketoprofen, 100 mg, has been tried as a patch that directly delivers the compound to the site of injury. Pharmacokinetic data indicate that the plasma levels of ketoprofen, 100 mg administered orally, are higher than when applied via a patch. Because the patch facilitates ketoprofen delivery over a 24-hour period, the drug remains continually present in the tissue adjacent to the site of application. High tissue but low plasma ketoprofen concentrations mean that although tissue concentrations are high enough to exert a therapeutic effect, plasma concentrations remain low enough to minimize systemic adverse events.[107]

Fenoprofen

The calcium derivative of fenoprofen is more common; it is well absorbed, and achieves a peak plasma level of 20 to 30 μg/mL 2 hours after a single oral dose, with a plasma half-life of 2 to 3 hours.[108] The drug is available as 300-mg capsules and the recommended dosage is 2.4 g/day. Steady-state plasma levels are reached within the first 24 hours of therapy. Fenoprofen is well tolerated compared with aspirin and causes minimal occult GI bleeding; nevertheless, dyspepsia remains the most common side effect. Most of the drug is excreted as glucuronide in the urine.

Naproxen

Naproxen is well absorbed in the upper GI tract and is highly bound to plasma albumin. Because of its long half-life of 13 hours, it is suitable for twice-daily administration.[109] It takes about 3 days for equilibrium to be reached. Excretion is almost entirely in the urine, mainly as an inactive glucuronide metabolite.

Naproxen is available as 250-, 375-, and 500-mg tablets and has been used for the treatment of arthritis and other inflammatory diseases, with efficacy superior to aspirin.[110] It causes less GI irritation than aspirin. Naproxen increases bleeding time by inhibiting platelet aggregation. When given during pregnancy, it can cross the placenta in 20 minutes and cause neonatal jaundice.

Oxaprozin

Oxaprozin is effective in the management of adult rheumatoid arthritis, osteoarthritis, ankylosing spondylitis, soft tissue disorders, and postoperative dental pain. Oxaprozin has a high oral bioavailability (95%), with peak plasma concentrations at 3 to 5 hours after dosing.[111] It is metabolized in the liver by oxidative and conjugative pathways and readily eliminated by the renal and fecal routes. Oxaprozin's strong analgesic qualities are particularly useful in painful musculoskeletal conditions because, for example, it inhibits COX-1 and COX-2 isoenzymes, inhibits nuclear translocation of NF-κB and of metalloproteinases, and modulates the endogenous cannabinoid system.[112] In a randomized study of patients with refractory shoulder pain, oxaprozin, 1200 mg once daily, was superior to three doses/day of diclofenac (50 mg) in reducing pain and improving quality of life.[113]

Oxaprozin can diffuse easily into inflamed synovial tissues after oral administration.[114] Although discovered more than 20 years ago, it is now under intensive investigation because of its unusual pharmacodynamic properties. Other than being a nonselective COX inhibitor, the drug is capable of inhibiting both anandamide hydrolase in neurons, with consequent potent analgesic activity, and NF-κB activation in inflammatory cells.[112] Moreover, oxaprozin induces apoptosis of activated monocytes in a dose-dependent manner. Because monocyte, macrophage, and NF-κB pathways are crucial for the synthesis of proinflammatory and histotoxic mediators in inflamed joints, oxaprozin appears to have pharmacodynamic properties exceeding those presently assumed as markers of classic NSAIDs.[115]

Oxicam Derivatives

The only NSAID in this class in clinical use is piroxicam. Unlike other NSAIDs, peak serum concentration following oral dosing is attained more slowly, with a duration of 5.5 hours. It is notable for its long elimination half-life of 48.5 hours, so it may take up to 1 week to achieve steady-state blood concentrations, although it does also allow for once-daily dosing.[116]

Pyrazolone Derivatives

The only drug in clinical use in this class is phenylbutazone. Although phenylbutazone is a very effective anti-inflammatory and analgesic, it has been associated with aplastic anemia and agranulocytosis; therefore, it cannot be recommended for long-term use.[117] Thus, it is not often clinically used.

Anthranilic Acid Derivatives

These NSAIDs are unique because they block prostaglandin synthesis and the tissue response to prostaglandins. Mefenamic acid has been associated with severe pancytopenia and many other side effects. Therefore, it cannot be used longer than 1 week.[118] Meclofenamate has a high incidence of GI toxicity and is also not a first-line drug. It is well absorbed orally; peak plasma levels are reached after 2 hours, with a half-life of about 4 to 6 hours.

Naphthylalkanones

This newer class of NSAIDs is most noted for its non-acidic chemical structure, similar to naproxen but unlike that of other clinically used NSAIDs. The only clinically available NSAID in this class is nabumetone. Studies have shown that its use results in fewer gastric lesions than aspirin, naproxen, or ibuprofen.[119] Also, dosages of 1 g/day for 7 days in volunteers resulted in no changes in bleeding time. Only 35% of the drug is converted to its active form after oral administration. None of the parent drug can be measured in plasma after oral administration because of the rapid biotransformation that occurs during the first-pass effect, which makes nabumetone a prodrug.[120]

Meloxicam

Meloxicam is a relatively new NSAID approved for the treatment of osteoarthritis in the United States. It has also been evaluated for the treatment of rheumatoid arthritis, ankylosing spondylitis, and acute rheumatic pain.[121] Meloxicam has been shown to be COX-2–preferential, particularly at its lowest therapeutic dose, and is anti-inflammatory by inhibiting prostanoid synthesis in inflammatory cells. Because it is COX-2–preferential, it would be expected to have less GI toxicity than nonselective NSAIDs. In clinical trials of meloxicam in osteoarthritis, it was found to be as effective as piroxicam, diclofenac, and naproxen, with fewer GI symptoms and a lower incidence of perforations, obstructions, and bleeds.[122]

Meloxicam has a plasma half-life of approximately 20 hours and is convenient for once-daily administration in 7.5- and 15-mg tablets.[123] Neither moderate renal nor hepatic insufficiency significantly alters the pharmacokinetics of meloxicam in short-term studies; however, it should not be used in patients with renal failure. Furthermore, dose adjustment is not required in older adults. Drug-drug interaction studies have demonstrated that meloxicam interacts with some medications, including cholestyramine, lithium, and some inhibitors of cytochrome P-450 2C9 and 3A4. Consequently, increased clinical vigilance should be maintained when co-prescribing some medications with meloxicam. No interactions have been observed following the concomitant administration of food, cimetidine, antacid, aspirin, β-acetyldigoxin, methotrexate, warfarin, or furosemide.

Concentration-dependent therapeutic and toxicologic effects have yet to be extensively elucidated for meloxicam.[123] Its pharmacokinetic profile is characterized by a prolonged, almost complete, absorption and the drug is more than 99.5% bound to plasma proteins. Meloxicam is metabolized to four biologically inactive main metabolites, which are excreted in urine and feces. Steady-state plasma concentrations are achieved within 3 to 5 days. The pharmacokinetic parameters of meloxicam are linear over the dose range 7.5 to 30 mg and bioequivalence has been shown for a number of different formulations.

COX-2 Inhibitors

COX-2 specific inhibitors were developed with the aim of reducing the incidence of serious GI adverse effects associated with the administration of traditional NSAIDs on the assumption that these side effects were mediated by COX-1. The assessment of COX-1 and COX-2 selectivity in vitro using whole-blood assays (Table 35–2) of the cellular capacity to produce prostanoids has shown that selectivity is a continuous variable of COX inhibitors.

The initial COX-2 inhibitors approved by the U.S. Food and Drug Administration (FDA) were celecoxib and rofecoxib. Overall, a meta-analysis of clinical studies evaluating COX-2 inhibitors compared with traditional NSAIDs for postoperative pain has shown that the analgesic efficacy of COX-2 inhibitors 0 to 6 hours postoperatively is similar to or better than that of ibuprofen.[124] Initial clinical trials using COX-2 inhibitors for the management of pain have evaluated efficacy in the immediate postoperative period and have demonstrated a reduction in postoperative opioid consumption.[125] A meta-analysis has examined whether there is any advantage of multimodal analgesia with acetaminophen, NSAIDs, or COX-2 inhibitors when added to patient-controlled analgesia of morphine.[126] The results suggested that all the analgesic agents provide an opioid-sparing effect (25% to 55%). The use of NSAIDs was associated with a decrease in the incidence of postoperative nausea and vomiting and sedation. In addition, the use of COX-2 inhibitors or acetaminophen did not decrease the incidence of opioid-related adverse events when compared with placebo. Clinical trials of COX-2 inhibitors used during the preoperative period and into the postoperative period (2 weeks) for patients undergoing both major surgery[127] and minimally invasive surgery[128] have demonstrated improved clinical outcomes. It is also possible that early and aggressive sustained treatment with COX-2 inhibitors might ameliorate the longer lasting elements of postoperative pain and prevent the transformation of acute into chronic pain.[129]

It has recently been demonstrated that the preoperative administration of oral COX-2 inhibitors can reduce CSF PGE_2 levels in humans during the perioperative period, resulting in improved outcomes following hip replacement surgery.[30] In addition to reducing CSF PGE_2 levels, the COX-2 inhibitors[30,32] were able to modulate the level of CSF IL-6. The exact mechanism responsible for the reduction in the interleukin level has yet to be determined, but is probably related to the PGE_2 pathway.[30]

Celecoxib

Celecoxib was the first COX-2 inhibitor approved by the FDA, in December 1998. It now has been approved for the relief of pain from osteoarthritis, rheumatoid arthritis, acute pain, dysmenorrhea, and familial adenomatous polyposis. It has good selectivity for the COX-2 enzyme (see Table 35–2). It is available in 100-, 200-, and 400-mg capsules, with a maximum recommended dosage of 400 mg/day for chronic pain. The recommended dose for the management of acute pain is 400 mg followed by 200 mg within the first 24 hours. If celecoxib is administered with aluminum- or magnesium-containing antacids, plasma levels of celecoxib are reduced. Peak plasma levels occur 3 hours after oral administration, and the drug crosses into the CSF.[33] Celecoxib is 97% protein-bound, with an apparent volume of distribution of 400 L. It is metabolized via cytochrome P-450 2C9 and eliminated predominantly by the liver. It is not indicated for pediatric use and is a category C drug for pregnancy. Celecoxib can increase lithium levels in the plasma, whereas concomitant fluconazole (Diflucan) administration can increase the levels of celecoxib. The drug has a half-life of about 11 hours.[130] Adverse events noted in the various clinical trials include headache, edema, dyspepsia, diarrhea, nausea, and sinusitis. It is contraindicated in patients who have a sulfonamide allergy or a known hypersensitivity to aspirin or other NSAIDs. Because celecoxib does

Table 35–2. IC_{50} Ratios for Inhibition of COX-1 and COX-2 in Human Whole Blood*

DRUG	IC_{50} RATIO
Lumiracoxib	700
Etoricoxib	344
Rofecoxib	272
Valdecoxib	61
Celecoxib	30
Meloxicam	18
Naproxen	0.7
Ibuprofen	1.5
Indomethacin	0.02
Aspirin	0.007

*Higher ratio indicates greater COX-2 selectivity.
IC_{50}, concentration needed to inhibit 50% of COX-1 and COX-2.

not interfere with platelet function,[131] it can be administered perioperatively as a multimodal analgesic without the increased risk of bleeding.[125]

Recently, the efficacy and upper GI safety of celecoxib, compared with nonspecific NSAIDs, was evaluated in 13,274 patients with osteoarthritis (SUCCESS-I study).[132] Patients were randomly assigned to either celecoxib 100 or 200 mg twice daily or nonselective NSAID therapy (diclofenac 50 mg twice daily or naproxen 500 mg twice daily) for 12 weeks. This study revealed that both dosages of celecoxib are as effective as the nonselective NSAIDs in treating osteoarthritis. Furthermore, significantly more gastric ulcer–related complications occurred within the nonselective NSAID group of patients (0.8/100 patient-years) compared with the celecoxib group (0.1/100 patient-years) (odds ratio, 7.02; $P = .008$). The number of cardiovascular thromboembolic events was low and similar between the groups. The results of the SUCCESS-I study are different from those of the CLASS trial,[133] which did not demonstrate an advantage of celecoxib in reducing the incidence of upper GI ulcer complications; this was attributed by the SUCCESS-I study authors to the low dropout rate and design of the newer study.

Rofecoxib

Rofecoxib is a selective COX-2 inhibitor indicated for use in osteoarthritis, rheumatoid arthritis, dysmenorrhea, and acute pain. The drug is administered orally, with a bioavailability of 93%, and 87% of the absorbed dose is bound to plasma proteins.[134] The metabolism of rofecoxib in the liver (via cytosolic reduction) yields metabolites that have no COX-1 or COX-2 activity. Although metabolized via the liver, dosage adjustment for patients with liver disease is not necessary. In addition, the metabolites are predominately eliminated from the body in the urine. Analgesic efficacy occurs 0.7 to 1.5 hours after oral dosing and continues for more than 24 hours.[135] Steady-state plasma concentrations of rofecoxib are achieved after 4 days, a function of its 17-hour half-life. It is supplied in 12.5-, 25-, and 50-mg tablets including a suspension (5 mL contains 12.5 mg or 25 mg). Although not approved by the FDA, rofecoxib suspension has been commonly used for the management of acute pain in pediatric patients. The maximum daily recommended dosage for acute pain is 50 mg/day for 5 days.

Rofecoxib has less effect on the GI mucosa and therefore less likelihood of GI complications compared with other NSAIDs; adverse events reported with rofecoxib include dyspepsia, peripheral edema, and hypertension.[136] Because rofecoxib has no effect on platelet aggregation[137] and has minimal interaction with warfarin,[138] it has been used extensively in the perioperative arena as a preemptive analgesic for various types of surgeries.[30,127,138,139] Larger clinical trials and long-term follow-up studies undertaken to demonstrate the efficacy of this compound in the

prevention of cancer have demonstrated an increased incidence of cardiovascular events[140] and prompted the voluntary withdrawal of rofecoxib by the manufacturer in 2004 (see more detailed discussion later).

Valdecoxib and Parecoxib

Valdecoxib is a derivative of isoxazole and binds noncovalently to COX-2, forming a tight and relatively stable enzyme-inhibitor complex. It is a potent inhibitor of PGE_2 production in humans.[141] The primary hydroxylated metabolite of valdecoxib, SC-66905, which accounts for 10% to 15% of the parent compound in human plasma, has lower COX-2 inhibitory activity than that of valdecoxib and does not contribute significantly to the clinical effects of valdecoxib. Valdecoxib and its metabolite SC-66905 are also the active moieties of a parenteral COX-2 inhibitor, parecoxib sodium.[142]

Valdecoxib has good oral bioavailability (83%) and a minimal first-pass effect. It achieves maximal plasma concentration in 3 hours, with an elimination half-life of about 8 to 11 hours.[143] It is metabolized by the liver via the cytochrome P450 3A4 isoenzyme. About 70% of the dose is excreted in the urine as metabolites. Valdecoxib has been approved for use in osteoarthritis (10 mg), rheumatoid arthritis (10 mg),[144] and acute pain (up to 40 mg). Several clinical studies have demonstrated the efficacy of valdecoxib in patients undergoing oral surgery[145,146] and major orthopedic surgery at doses of 40 mg.[147] Common adverse events reported include GI[148] and renal events.[149] Clinical studies in high-risk cardiac patients that demonstrated a significant increased incidence of major cardiovascular adverse events and the identification of increased risk for serious skin reactions (e.g., toxic epidermal necrolysis, Stevens-Johnson syndrome, erythema multiforme) led to the withdrawal of this COX-2 inhibitor from the U.S. market in 2005.

CONTROVERSIES ABOUT NSAIDS

Several controversial issues exist regarding the routine perioperative administration of NSAIDs. These include a possible deleterious effect on fracture and tendon healing, an increased risk of perioperative bleeding, and concerns regarding cardiovascular safety. NSAIDs are currently recommended in a multimodal analgesic approach for the management of perioperative pain.[150] Practice guidelines for acute pain management in the perioperative setting have specifically stated that "unless contraindicated, all patients should receive an around-the-clock regimen of NSAIDs, COX-2 inhibitors, or acetaminophen."[151]

Concerns About Increased Risk of Bleeding

The routine perioperative use of NSAIDs may predispose patients to an increased risk of bleeding.[152,153] In contrast, the COX-2 selective inhibitors can be administered preemptively to surgical patients without the added risk of increased perioperative bleeding reported with conventional NSAIDs.[154-156] Therefore, we believe that COX-2 inhibitors offer a significant advantage compared with nonspecific NSAIDs for a variety of orthopedic surgical procedures (e.g., total joint arthroplasty, anterior cruciate ligament [ACL] reconstruction, spinal fusion surgery) and for pediatric patients undergoing tonsillectomy.[156] Prior to the introduction of COX-2 inhibitors, patients undergoing elective total joint arthroplasty were instructed to discontinue their use of NSAIDs 7 to 10 days prior to surgery because of the concern of a twofold increase in the incidence of perioperative bleeding, resulting in higher transfusion requirements.[155] We have observed that discontinuing NSAIDs before total joint arthroplasty results in an arthritic flare, not only in the operative joint, but also in other arthritic joints, leading to increased perioperative pain. Increased pain before total joint arthroplasty is one of the causes for increased postoperative pain, prolonged hospital admission, and impaired rehabilitation.[157] The perioperative administration of COX-2 inhibitors for total joint arthroplasty has been shown to result in a reduction in perioperative pain and improvement in outcomes without an added risk of increased perioperative bleeding.[127,158]

Bone Healing

Another concern regarding the perioperative use of NSAIDs is the possible deleterious effect on osteogenesis and spinal fusion.[159-162] Prostaglandins have been known for many years to have potent effects on bone metabolism, including osteoblastic and osteoclastic activity, as well as being essential for bone repair.[163] The exact mechanism by which NSAIDs impair spinal fusion has not yet been elucidated. It has been hypothesized that the effect may be mediated by an inhibition of the inflammatory process, with a concomitant reduction in blood flow in the early period of osteogenesis, decreased mesenchymal cell proliferation, or inhibition of calcification of the bone matrix.[159-161] Many investigators have recommended that NSAIDs not be used in the multimodal management of acute pain for patients undergoing spinal fusion surgery.[159-162] Although the data are conflicting, a large body of literature derived from laboratory animal studies has suggested that COX-2 inhibitors delay or inhibit bone healing.[159-161] However, in these studies, COX-2 inhibitors were administered over several weeks to months at doses higher than those approved for acute pain.

Recently, it has been suggested that the deleterious effects of COX-2 inhibitors on fracture healing may be avoidable with short-term treatment.[164] In addition to limiting NSAIDs to short-term use, physicians should prescribe the lowest effective dose for bone surgeries. In a retrospective study of 434 consecutive patients undergoing elective decompressive posterior lumbar laminectomy with instrumented spinal fusion, the short-term perioperative administration of celecoxib, rofecoxib, or low-dose ketorolac (110 mg/day) had no significant deleterious effect on nonunion.[165] In contrast, higher doses of ketorolac (120 to 240 mg/day), even when administered for less than 1 week, resulted in a significant increase in the incidence of nonunion following spinal fusion surgery. Further evidence for the safety of COX-2 inhibitors following spinal fusion surgery has been demonstrated in a recent prospective, double-blind, randomized study in humans.[166] This was the first prospective study demonstrating that the perioperative administration of celecoxib for 5 consecutive days following spinal fusion surgery results in no increased incidence of nonunion at 1 year follow-up compared with placebo. In addition, we have reported that patients who are given celecoxib report a significantly lower incidence of chronic donor site pain (4/40, 10%) compared with placebo (12/40, 30%) at 1 year following surgery.[166]

Cardiovascular Effects

Another concern about the perioperative administration of NSAIDs and COX-2 inhibitors for short-term use is their possible role in increasing cardiovascular morbidity.[167] Theoretical concerns concerning this risk were based on a fivefold increase in the incidence of myocardial infarction noted in the Vioxx Gastrointestinal Outcome Research (VIGOR) study.[136] This study used rofecoxib, 50 mg daily, for a median of 9 months in a high-risk rheumatoid arthritis patient population in which the use of aspirin was precluded. It was argued at the time that the findings did not represent an increased cardiovascular risk because of rofecoxib but rather a protective effect of naproxen in the control population, as well as precluding the use of aspirin. Other clinicians attributed the increased adverse cardiovascular events to a prothrombotic state caused by selective COX-2 inhibitors.[168] COX-1 mediates the production of thromboxane A_2 in platelets, leading to platelet aggregation and vasoconstriction. In contrast, COX-2 catalyzes endothelial prostacyclin synthesis, which counteracts thromboxane A_2, leading to vasodilation and inhibition of platelet aggregation. Because selective COX-2 inhibitors decrease prostacyclin formation, these NSAIDs may potentially disrupt homeostasis and create a prothrombotic effect (see full discussion later, "Adverse Events").[169]

Epidemiologic database studies, which reflected actual drug use and included higher risk patients, also found a correlation between normal- or high-dose rofecoxib use and adverse cardiovascular outcomes.[140,170] The drug manufacturer voluntarily withdrew rofecoxib from the world market on September 30, 2004 after examining the interim results from the Adenomatous Polyp Prevention on Vioxx (APPROVe) study.[140] This long-term, randomized, prospective, placebo-controlled study was designed to investigate the effects of 3 years of treatment with rofecoxib, 25 mg daily, on the risk of recurrent neo-plastic polyps of the large bowel in patients with a history of colorectal adenomas. The study revealed a 1.7-fold increased risk of myocardial infarction or cerebrovascular accident with rofecoxib compared with placebo, which became apparent after 18 months of treatment. During the first 18 months, the event rates were similar in both groups.

Subsequently, on December 17, 2004, the Adenoma Prevention with Celecoxib (APC) trial was halted because of an increased occurrence of cardiovascular events. The APC trial examined the efficacy of cele-coxib (200 or 400 mg twice daily) with placebo for 33 months for the prevention of colorectal adenoma.[170] Celecoxib was associated with a dose-related 2.3- to 3.4-fold increase in serious adverse cardiovascular events. Similar to the APPROVE study,[140] the increased risk did not become apparent until after 12 months of treatment. It was argued that these results were not consistent with an extensive database or with two other large long-term placebo-controlled studies; the Prevention of Spontaneous Adenomatous Polyps (PreSAP) trial[171] included patients taking 400 mg of celecoxib daily or placebo for an average of 32 months and the Alzheimer's Disease Anti-Inflammatory Pre-vention Trial (ADAPT).[172] The latter study found no increased risk with celecoxib, 200 mg daily, but noted a statistically significant increase in cardiovascular risk with naproxen. This study is of significant clini-cal importance because previous prospective, long-term COX-2 inhibitor studies have used placebo for comparison, whereas this was the first trial to compare its use with a nonspecific NSAID.[173]

Valdecoxib and the parenteral prodrug parecoxib have also been associated with the potential risk of adverse postoperative cardiovascular events, includ-ing an increase in cerebrovascular events (2.9% vs. 0.7%) and myocardial infarctions (1.6% vs. 0.7%) after administration of a supramaximal dose (40 mg twice daily) for 14 days following coronary artery bypass grafting (CABG) surgery.[174] However, no increases in cardiovascular events were observed with a therapeutic dosing of parecoxib followed by valde-coxib for general and orthopedic surgeries.[144,146,147]

We are now left to determine whether the increased cardiac risk associated with COX-2 inhibition is unique to this subclass of drugs or whether it is char-acteristic of all NSAIDs. A joint meeting of the FDA's Arthritis Advisory Committee and the Drug Safety and Risk Management Advisory Committee con-vened in February 2005 to discuss the safety of COX-2 inhibitors and nonspecific NSAIDs. These committees jointly reaffirmed that COX-2 inhibitors are important treatment options for pain manage-ment and that the preponderance of data have dem-onstrated that the cardiovascular risk associated with celecoxib is similar to that associated with commonly used older nonspecific NSAIDs.[175] The rationale behind this conclusion was that COX-2 inhibitors collectively increase cardiovascular risk compared with placebo but not when compared with nonselec-tive NSAIDs. It was noted that short-term use of

NSAIDs does not appear to increase cardiovascular risk and that rigorous scientific studies are needed to characterize the longer term cardiovascular risks of these analgesics.

Subsequently, on April 7, 2005, the FDA announced a series of changes applicable to the entire class of NSAIDs. These included a FDA boxed warning for the potential increased risk of cardiovascular events and GI bleeding associated with all prescription NSAIDs, including celecoxib. The manufacturers were asked to revise their labeling to include a medication guide for patients to help make them aware of the potential for cardiovascular and GI adverse events. In addition, the FDA has requested that the manufacturers of all over-the-counter NSAIDs revise their labels to include more specific information about the potential cardio-vascular and GI risks, and include information to assist consumers in the safe use of these drugs. Finally, the FDA concluded that the overall risk-benefit profile of valdecoxib is unfavorable, and requested that the manufacturer voluntarily withdraw valdecoxib from the market because of the following:

1. The lack of adequate data on the cardiovascular safety of long-term use of valdecoxib, along with the increased risk of adverse cardiovascular events when used in short-term CABG trials[174] that the FDA believes may be relevant to chronic use.
2. Reports of serious and potentially life-threatening skin reactions, including deaths, in patients taking valdecoxib. The risk of these reactions in individual patients is unpredictable, because they occur in patients with and without a prior history of sulfa allergy, and after both short- and long-term use.
3. Lack of demonstrated advantages for valdecoxib compared with other NSAIDs.

The manufacturer agreed to suspend sales and marketing of valdecoxib pending further discussions with the FDA. The FDA noted that all NSAIDs can lead to the onset of new hypertension or worsening of preexisting disease; either may contribute to an increased incidence of cardiovascular events. Because patient response to thiazides or loop diuretics may be impaired, close monitoring of blood pressure is recommended. Fluid retention and edema have also been observed in some patients taking NSAIDs; caution should therefore be exercised in patients with fluid retention, hypertension, or heart failure.

CANCER PREVENTION WITH NSAIDS AND COX-2 INHIBITORS

Although COX-2 inhibitors such as rofecoxib and celecoxib have been blamed for increasing the risk of adverse cardiac events, researchers in the oncology community have been pointing to the potential of these drugs as anticancer agents. NSAIDs appear to reduce the risk of developing cancer and may hold promise as anticancer drugs.[176] Because COX-2 is overexpressed in various cancer tissues and is respon-sible for cell proliferation and apoptosis, NSAIDs may be a potential molecular target for chemoprevention strategies.[177]

Recent studies have demonstrated that high levels of COX-2 expression are associated with a significantly greater likelihood of subsequent breast cancer in women with atypical hyperplasia; a fourfold increase in breast cancer was documented in one study.[178] Because COX-2 may be important for the development of some types of breast cancer, it may be a good target for treatment strategies. Because of its greater long-term tolerability, COX-2 inhibitors may have greater potential for chemoprevention compared with nonspecific NSAIDs such as aspirin. If further studies support the association of COX-2 inhibitors and reduced breast cancer risk, then the drug's potential benefits will need to be weighed against its cardiovascular risks.

Interest in COX-2 as a therapeutic target for colorectal cancer derives from epidemiologic studies that have consistently shown a 40% to 50% reduction in colorectal incidence among chronic users of NSAIDs.[179] COX-2 proteins are overexpressed in approximately 80% of human colorectal cancers and in 40% of colorectal adenomas relative to normal mucosa.[180] From pooled randomized trials, there is evidence that NSAIDs significantly reduce the recurrence of sporadic adenomatous polyps, regression, and possibly prevention of colorectal adenomas and cancers.[181] This increased interest in COX-2 inhibitors for colorectal cancer has led to large trials of COX-2 inhibitors, which led to the secondary results of increased cardiovascular effects and the termination of these oncology trials.[140,171]

ADVERSE EVENTS

Allergy and Hypersensitivity

All NSAIDs, including acetylsalicylic acid, may induce hypersensitivity reactions, which are of two general types. Both may be related to the inhibition of PG synthesis. They are (1) the syndrome of asthmatic attacks in patients with vasomotor rhinitis, nasal polyposis, and bronchial asthma and (2) the syndrome of urticaria and angioedema. Prostaglandin E_2 is a bronchodilator. It stabilizes histamine stores in mastocytes and thus helps inhibit the inflammatory response.[182] In a susceptible person, the result of the inhibition of PG biosynthesis may be spontaneous degranulation of mastocytes, with release of histamine in the respiratory tract and skin, leading to bronchoconstriction and asthma as well as urticaria.

Gastrointestinal Effects

The first evidence that aspirin could damage the stomach was reported in 1938 based on gastroscopic observations.[183] In the 1950s and 1960s, case control studies appeared, indicating that melena is associated with NSAID use. NSAIDs cause hemorrhagic gastric erosions in the corpus and antrum of the stomach. The mortality rate attributed to NSAID-related GI toxic effects is 0.22%/year, with an annual relative

risk of 4.21. It has been estimated that 16,500 NSAID-related deaths occur because of gastric complications, similar to the number of deaths annually from acquired immunodeficiency syndrome (16,685) and higher than the deaths caused by multiple myeloma and asthma. Some risk factors identified for the development of NSAID-induced ulcers include advanced age; history of ulcer; concomitant use of corticosteroids; higher doses of NSAIDs, including the use of more than one NSAID; concomitant administration of anticoagulation; serious systemic disorder; cigarette smoking; consumption of alcohol; and concomitant infection with *Helicobacter pylori*.

The mechanisms by which NSAIDs cause ulceration in the stomach are their topical irritant effect on the epithelium and their ability to suppress PG synthesis.[184] The ability of NSAIDs to cause gastric damage correlates with the time and dose dependency for PG suppression in the stomach.[185] Inhibition of PG synthesis leads to a reduction in the ability of the gastric mucosa to defend itself against luminal irritants; bicarbonate secretions, blood flow, and epithelial cell turnover are influenced by PGs. Another feature of NSAIDs that likely contributes to gastric bleeding from preexisting ulcers is their effect on platelet aggregation through the suppression of thromboxane synthesis.[186] Mediators in the pathway whereby decreased PG levels cause gastric irritation and damage have been extensively studied. These mediators include leukotrienes,[187] tumor necrosis factor α,[188] and neutrophil adherence substances.[189]

NSAID-induced enteropathy has been documented in the small intestine and colon, although the exact mechanism is not fully understood. Various preventive strategies have been developed to reduce NSAID gastroenteropathy.[190] Enteric-coated and slow-release formulations of NSAIDs have been ineffective in preventing the gastric side effects seen with NSAID consumption. Other agents used for the prevention of ulcer formation with NSAIDs include sucralfate (controversy exists about its efficacy), histamine 2 (H_2) receptor antagonists (famotidine), proton pump inhibitors (omeprazole), and prostaglandins (misoprostol).

NSAID gastric-induced complications led to the development of COX-2 inhibitors. Preferential use of COX-2 inhibitors,[191] because of their gastric enteropathy safety properties, has led to the increased incidence of cardiovascular effects noted after they were introduced, which finally led to the withdrawal of some COX-2 inhibitors from the market. Because of the post–COX-2 inhibitor withdrawal period, guidelines for gastric protection when NSAIDs are needed have been suggested.[190] For patients with no cardiovascular risk factors that require aspirin prophylaxis and who are at low or no risk for GI complications, monotherapy with one of the traditional nonselective NSAIDs can be prescribed. For patients who do not require aspirin prophylaxis and who are at risk for NSAID-induced GI complications, an initial approach would be to prescribe a COX-2 inhibitor or a traditional NSAID and proton pump inhibitor. On the other hand, for patients with cardiovascular risk who require aspirin prophylaxis, COX-2 inhibitors should be avoided; for patients with no GI risk factors, traditional NSAIDs can be used and, if they are at risk for GI complications, a proton pump inhibitor must also be prescribed.[192]

Hematologic and Cardiovascular Effects

All NSAIDs, including COX-2 inhibitors, may cause an increased risk of serious cardiovascular thrombotic events, myocardial infarction, and stroke. Arachidonic acid is converted into prostaglandin endoperoxides PGG_2 and PGH_2 by the action of cyclooxygenase (see Fig. 35–2). These are in turn converted to TXA_2 in platelets by the action of TXA_2 synthase, but in vascular endothelium they are converted to PGI_2 by the action of PGI_2 synthase. TXA_2 functions as a platelet activator and vasoconstrictor, whereas PGI_2 is a platelet inhibitor and vasodilator. Furthermore, activated platelets divert some of their endoperoxides to vascular cells ("endoperoxide steal") to provide more substrate for PGI_2 formation.[193] Platelet activity, therefore, is the result of a constant balance between the effects of PGI_2 in the endothelium and TXA_2 in the platelets. Platelets are especially vulnerable to COX inhibition because, unlike most other cells, they cannot regenerate this enzyme. Presumably, this reflects the inability of platelets to synthesize proteins independently. This means that aspirin, which irreversibly acetylates the COX enzyme, causes inhibition of platelet aggregation for the life span of the platelet, which is 7 to 10 days.[193] In contrast, nonselective NSAIDs reversibly inhibit the COX enzyme, causing a transient reduction in the formation of TXA_2 and inhibition of platelet activation, which resolves after most of the drug is eliminated.[193] A single dose of 300 to 900 mg of ibuprofen can inhibit platelet aggregation for 2 hours after administration, but the effect is largely dissipated by 24 hours.[194] Similarly, both sulindac and diclofenac also cause a short-term (less than 24 hours) reduction in platelet aggregation. Antiplatelet effects of long-acting NSAIDs such as piroxicam, however, can last for several days after the drug is discontinued.[195] Overall, nonaspirin NSAIDs cause "transient, dose-dependent, and modest bleeding time abnormalities,"[193] which often do not exceed normal limits.

Although in vitro studies examining the effect of NSAIDs on platelet function have provided much information, it is ultimately the clinical effect in patients that is of greatest interest. The test most commonly used to assess clinical platelet function has been the bleeding time. Unfortunately, this test is highly operator-dependent and is subject to much technical artifact. In addition, its clinical use as a preoperative tool for predicting intraoperative bleeding remains controversial. There is also uncertainty as to whether bleeding time assessed on the forearm correlates with prolonged bleeding in other areas of the body.[194,195] Therefore, bleeding time is no longer used as a preoperative tool for assessing the risk of perioperative bleeding.

Studies have shown variable clinical effects of NSAIDs on bleeding. In one study of patients undergoing total hip replacement surgery, 140 patients had more intraoperative and postoperative blood loss when using NSAIDs than those who did not.[196] Other studies have confirmed that finding and noted more complications in patients using NSAIDs with half-lives longer than 6 hours.[152] On the other hand, no difference was found in clinical blood loss during total hip replacement or transurethral resection of the prostate in patients taking diclofenac compared with those taking a placebo preoperatively in other studies.[197,198]

In addition to a potential increase in perioperative bleeding, NSAIDs and COX-2 inhibitors may cause an increased incidence of serious cardiovascular thrombotic events, myocardial infarction, and stroke (as noted earlier in "Controversies About NSAIDs").[175] An unbalanced biosynthesis of PGI_2 and TXA_2 seems to play a role in atherogenesis and thrombosis. It is postulated that prolonged administration of COX-2 inhibitors, which inhibit PGI_2, may lead to several adverse effects. These include a rise in blood pressure, initiation and early development of atherosclerosis, and architectural and functional responses of blood vessels to such stress. These changes may predispose individuals to an exaggerated thrombotic response on rupture of an atherosclerotic plaque.[199] Aspirin and traditional NSAIDs suppress the activities of COX-1 and COX-2 and therefore reduce both thromboxane A_2, and PGI_2 levels. In contrast, COX-2 inhibitors suppress the production of PGI_2 without affecting thromboxane A_2 synthesis.[200] These mechanisms may be responsible for the increased incidence of acute myocardial infarctions observed with prolonged use of COX-2 inhibitors.

Finally, most NSAIDs potentiate the anticoagulant activity of warfarin by displacing the protein-bound drug or by inhibiting the metabolism by hepatic microsomal enzymes.[193] Thus, they should be used with caution in patients taking oral anticoagulants, especially older patients, who undergo a significant increase in bleeding and hospitalizations when the two are used in combination.[201]

Renal Toxicity

Aspirin as well as other NSAIDs cause a transient decrease in renal function. This effect may occur more often in patients with underlying renal disease.[202] The postulated mechanism is the inhibition of the renal synthesis of PG, which may be important in the autoregulation of renal blood flow. Aspirin may also block the diuretic effect of spironolactone by inhibiting its binding to the tubular cell receptor.

The renal profile of traditional NSAIDs and COX-2 inhibitors may be described by the following: sodium retention is COX-2 inhibition–mediated and glomerular filtration rate (GFR) changes are caused by inhibition of COX-1 and COX-2. All NSAIDs, including COX-2 inhibitors, are associated with hypertension and edema. Most of these events are of minor clinical significance, with discontinuation rates caused by hypertension and edema when used over the short term.[203] Most cases resolve with continuation of therapy, which is generally seen over 1 to 8 weeks. The risk factors for NSAID-induced renal toxicity include chronic NSAID use, multiple NSAID use, dehydration, volume depletion, congestive heart failure, vascular disease, hyperreninemia, shock, sepsis, systemic lupus erythematosus, hepatic disease, sodium depletion, nephrotic syndrome, diuresis, concomitant drug therapy (e.g., diuretics, angiotensin-converting enzyme [ACE] inhibitors, beta blockers, potassium supplements), and patient age 60 years or older.[202]

Hepatic Toxicity

Aspirin is clearly hepatotoxic in certain situations, and this effect is non–dose-dependent. However, the effect is reversible when the drug is discontinued.[204]

Central Nervous System Effects

Direct toxic reactions are of several types. Symptoms of the ear in the form of tinnitus or deafness are usually an early warning of toxicity. Toxic manifestations are directly related to free drug levels, which vary inversely with albumin levels; the adverse event is typically reversed when the dose is reduced or discontinued. The most frequently implicated class of drugs in hypersensitivity-induced aseptic meningitis is the NSAIDs. Four NSAIDs—ibuprofen, sulindac, tolmetin, and naproxen—have all been implicated as causing drug-induced aseptic meningitis. Patients typically complain of fever, headache, and stiff neck, which generally commence within weeks of beginning therapy.[205]

USE IN SPECIFIC POPULATIONS

Pregnant and Lactating Women

When administered to pregnant women, salicylates may reach substantial levels in the fetus. Birth defects have not been reported to occur in regular users; however, there is experimental evidence to show that it is teratogenic in monkeys.[206] Aspirin taken at term may delay the onset of labor for 3 to 10 days, and it has been associated with increased bruising of the newborn child, particularly when instrumentation was necessary. The administration of aspirin or indomethacin at term to delay the onset of labor has been reported to cause serious pulmonary vascular disease in the newborn infant.

Pediatric Use

NSAIDs are often used "off-label" in pediatric populations.[207] In the United States and Canada, NSAIDs approved for children include ibuprofen, naproxen, tolmetin, aspirin, and choline magnesium salicylate. In the United Kingdom, diclofenac, indomethacin, piroxicam, and mefenamic acid are also approved for use in children. Review of available pharmacokinetic data prior to use of any NSAID not approved for pediatric populations is suggested to minimize adverse effects and maximize efficacy.[208] The GI toxicity from NSAIDs in children does exist, but frequency estimates vary. In a large retrospective study of 702 children examined for gastropathy, only 5 patients (10 events) were documented with gastric ulcers or gastritis.[209] Other toxicities related to NSAID use in children are renal (rare) and skin reactions, which are all reversible.[210]

Oral administration of ibuprofen or acetaminophen (15 mg/kg) every 4 to 6 hours on a fixed dose and the option of using opioid as an adjustable dose could be beneficial for the relief of pain in pediatric patients. When oral administration is not possible, rectal ibuprofen (40 mg/kg/day) or indomethacin is useful. When oral or rectal routes are not optimal, the only intravenous NSAID is ketorolac, 0.8 mg/kg, to a maximum of 60 mg/day.[211] Ketorolac can be of great benefit in pediatric patients with sickle cell crisis, but renal function in these patients needs to be closely monitored.

Older Adults

The absorption of NSAIDs is not affected by the diminished active transport systems in the GI tract seen in older adult patients, because most of the absorption of these compounds occurs via passive diffusion.[212] Changes in body composition, such as decrease in albumin levels in older adult patients might be expected to increase toxicity of highly protein-bound compounds; however, these seldom produce clinically important effects if hepatic and renal function are normal.[213]

Piroxicam and ibuprofen have been shown to have longer plasma half-lives in older women and men, respectively.[214,215] These drugs also undergo biotransformation largely by oxidation. There is evidence that drugs undergoing biotransformation by phase II reactions are more slowly eliminated, as may be the case with naproxen and ketoprofen.[216,217] Acute renal failure may occur, especially in older adult patients, when the renin-angiotensin system is activated and a PG inhibitor is prescribed.[217]

Older patients are subject to a number of diseases, for which they receive multiple medications. Drug-drug interaction is therefore a serious issue. Some important examples include the interaction of NSAIDs such as phenylbutazone or azapropazone with warfarin, leading to an enhanced anticoagulation effect.[218] Indomethacin nullifies the hypotensive effects of atenolol, propranolol, prazosin, captopril, and thiazide diuretics. It also blunts the diuretic response of furosemide, triamterene, and spironolactone. Phenylbutazone and oxyphenbutazone increase the rate of synthesis of the cytochrome P-450 enzyme, reducing the hydroxylation activity of tolbutamide; thus, the plasma half-life of this agent is prolonged, resulting in hypoglycemia. Azapropazone also enhances the hypoglycemic action of tolbutamide. Salicylate in therapeutic doses has been shown to enhance the effects of oral hypoglycemic agents, especially chlorpropamide.

COMBINATION DRUGS

To enhance the efficacy and safety of NSAID analgesia, other drugs have been formulated in combination with NSAIDs. Formulations of ibuprofen containing hydrocodone are available, and diclofenac has also been formulated in combination with misoprostol. Although such combinations are more convenient, there is no evidence that they are any more effective or safer than when administered as separate drugs. Caffeine, long sold in combination with acetaminophen and aspirin in over-the-counter analgesia preparations, has also been studied in combination with ibuprofen.[219,220] The effect of the added analgesia from the caffeine is measurable but not substantial. The enhanced NSAID analgesia seen in combination with caffeine probably does not result from alterations in absorption or distribution of the NSAID.[221]

An oxycodone-ibuprofen combination, 5 mg/400 mg, is manufactured as Combunox. It is an oral fixed-dose combination tablet with analgesic, anti-inflammatory, and antipyretic properties. It is approved in the United States for short-term use (up to 7 days) for management of acute, moderate, and severe pain and is the first and only fixed-dose combination of ibuprofen and oxycodone.[222] A single dose of oxycodone-ibuprofen (5 mg /400 mg) provided better analgesia than low-dose oxycodone or ibuprofen administered alone in most trials. It is generally well tolerated after single or multiple doses and short-term use is not expected to produce any of the serious adverse effects typically associated with the long-term use of opioids or NSAIDs.

NEW DRUGS IN DEVELOPMENT

There are some new drugs in clinical use in Europe; however, these have not yet been approved by the FDA.

Etoricoxib

Etoricoxib (MK-663) is a dipyridinyl derivative that contains a phenyl group attached to the central ring. Etoricoxib is highly selective for COX-2 (IC_{50} ratio, 344; see Table 35–2), with substantial distribution into tissue and 92% bound to plasma.[223] It distributes rapidly, reaching peak concentration within 1 to 2 hours and has an elimination half-life of approximately 22 hours.[224] Etoricoxib is metabolized via cytochrome P-450–dependent oxidation, which results in prolonged elimination in patients with

liver disease. The highest recommended daily dosage for chronic use is 60 to 90 mg; for acute pain, the dose is 120 mg.[225]

Clinical trials of etoricoxib have had demonstrated analgesic efficacy with various types of arthritis,[226] acute dental pain,[227] dysmenorrhea, and chronic pain conditions, such as back pain. Adverse effects include GI, renal, and cardiovascular manifestations. There is a 40% relative risk reduction in GI side effects with etoricoxib compared with those of other NSAIDs. To date, available data on the cardiovascular safety in 6700 patients, with 6500 patient-years of follow-up, have demonstrated a relative risk of 1.1 for etoricoxib compared with placebo. There is currently a 30,000-patient study being undertaken to evaluate the cardiovascular risk of this drug.

Lumiracoxib

Lumiracoxib is structurally distinct from other COX-2 inhibitors; it is a phenylacetic acid derivative with a short mean plasma half-life of 4 hours, but it provides analgesic efficacy for 24 hours with a single dose.[228] Lumiracoxib has been found to bind and interact with the COX-2 enzyme via a mechanism different from that of other COX-2 selective inhibitors and carboxylate-containing nonselective COX inhibitors. The carboxylate group of lumiracoxib forms hydrogen bonds with the catalytic Tyr 385 and with Ser 530 on COX-2, rather than with the larger hydrophobic side pocket or with Arg 120.[229] Lumiracoxib is highly selective for COX-2 (see Table 35–2). It has been shown clinically to provide analgesia for the treatment of knee osteoarthritis,[230] acute pain after dental surgery,[231] and pain after major joint replacement surgery.[232] Like other COX-2 inhibitors, lumiracoxib has been shown to have a reduced incidence of GI side effects. In a large controlled study (TARGET study) of 18,325 patients, lumiracoxib, 400 mg daily, was shown to cause fewer gastric ulcers compared with patients taking NSAIDs.[233] It is being investigated for the treatment of pain from various types of arthritis and dysmenorrhea. It is 99% protein-bound, with a volume of distribution of 13 L and bioavailability of 74% after oral administration.

References

1. Flowers R, Moncada S, Vane J: Analgesic, anti-pyretics and anti-inflammatory agents: Drugs employed in the treatment of gout. In Gilman A, Goodman L, Rall T, et al (eds): The Pharmacological Basis of Therapeutics, 7th ed. New York, Macmillan, 1985, pp 674-715.
2. Von Euler US: On the specific vasodilating and plain muscle stimulating substance from accessory genital glands in man and certain animals (prostaglandin and vestiglandin). J Physiol 1937;88:213-234.
3. Park JY, Pillinger MH, Abramson SB: Prostaglandin E_2 synthesis and secretion: The role of PGE_2 synthases. Clin Immunol 2006;119:229-240.
4. Samad TA, Sapirstein A, Woolf CJ: Prostanoids and pain: Unraveling mechanisms and revealing therapeutic targets. Trends Mol Med 2002;8:390-396.

5. Cashman J, McAnulty G: Nonsteroidal anti-inflammatory drugs in perisurgical pain management: Mechanisms of action and rationale for optimum use. Drugs 1995;49:51-70.

6. Ferreira SH, Vane JR: New aspects of the mode of action of non-steroidal anti-inflammatory drugs. Annu Rev Pharmacol 1974;14:57-73.

7. Ferreira SH: Prostaglandins, aspirin-like drugs and analgesia. Nature 1972;240:200-203.

8. Gerritsen ME, Cheli CD: Arachidonic acid and prostaglandin endoperoxide metabolism in isolated rabbit and coronary microvessels and isolated and cultivated coronary microvessel endothelial cells. J Clin Invest 1983;72:1658-1671.

9. Giuliano F, Warner TD: Origins of prostaglandins E₂: Involvement of cyclooxygenase (COX)-1 and COX-2 in human and rat systems. J Pharmacol Therp 2002;102:1001-1006.

10. Higgs GA: Arachidonic acid metabolism, pain and hyperalgesia: The mode of action of non-steroid mild analgesics. Br J Pharmacol 1980;10:233-235S.

11. Dray A, Bevan S: Inflammation and hyperalgesia: The team effort. Trends Pharm Sci 1993;14:287-62.

12. Mancini JA, Blood K, Guay J, et al: Cloning, expression, and up-regulation of inducible rat prostaglandin E synthase during lipopolysaccharide-induced pyresis and adjuvant-induced arthritis. J Biol Chem 2001;276:4469-4475.

13. Jakobsson PJ, Morgenstern R, Mancini J, et al: Common structural features of MAPEG—a widespread superfamily of membrane-associated proteins with highly divergent functions in eicosanoid and glutathione metabolism. Protein Sci 1999;8:689-692.

14. O'Banion MK, Sadowski HB, Winn V, et al: A serum and glucocorticoid-regulated 4-kilobase mRNA encodes a cyclooxygenase-related protein J Biol Chem 1991;266:23261-23267.

15. Smith WL, DeWitt DL, Garavito RM, et al: Cyclooxygenases: Structural, cellular biology. Annu Rev Biochem 2000;69:145-182.

16. Everts B, Wahrborg P, Hedner T, et al: COX-2 specific inhibitors—the emergence of a new class of analgesic and anti-inflammatory drugs. Clin Rheumatol 2000;19:331-343.

17. Kraemer SA, Meade EA, DeWitte DL: Prostaglandin endoperoxide synthase gene structure: Identification of the transcriptional start site and 5′ flanking regulatory sequences. Arch Biochem Biophys 1992;293:391-400.

18. Chun KS, Surh YJ: Signal transduction pathways regulating cyclooxygenase-2 expression: Potential molecular targets for chemoprevention. Biochem Pharmacol 2004;68:1089-1100.

19. O'Banion MK: Cyclooxygenase-2: Molecular biology, pharmacology and neurobiology. Crit Rev Neurobiol 1999;13:45-82.

20. Yaksh TL, Dirig DM, Conway CM, et al: The acute antihyperalgesic action of nonsteroidal, anti-inflammatory drugs and release of spinal prostaglandin E₂ is mediated by the inhibition of constitutive spinal cyclooxygenase-2 (COX-2) but not COX-1. J Neurosci 2001;21:5847-5853.

21. Chandrasekharan NV, Dai H, Roos KL, et al: COX-3, a cyclooxygenase-1 variant inhibited by acetaminophen and other analgesic/antipyretic drugs: Cloning, structure and expression. Proc Natl Acad Sci U S A 2002;99:13926-13931.

22. Qin N, Zhang SP, Reitz TL, et al: Cloning, expression and functional characterization of human cyclooxygenase-1 splicing variants: Evidence for intron 1 retention. J Pharmacol Exp Ther 2005;315:1298-305.

23. Dinchuk JE, Liu RQ, Trzaskos JM: COX-3: In the wrong frame in mind. Immunol Lett 2003;86:121.

24. Cui JG, Kuroda H, Chandrasekharan NV, et al: Cyclooxygenase-3 gene expression in Alzheimer hippocampus and in stressed human neural cells. Neurochem Res 2004;29:1731-1737.

25. Vane JR: The mode of action of aspirin and similar compounds. J Allergy Clin Immunol 1976;58:691-712.

26. Kroin JS, Buvanendran A, McCarthy RJ, et al: Cyclooxygenase-2 (COX-2) inhibitor potentiates morphine antinociception at the spinal level in a post-operative pain model. Reg Anesth Pain Med 2002;27:451-455.

27. Dai YQ, Jin DZ, Zhu XZ, et al: Triptolide inhibits COX-2 expression via NF-kappa B pathway in astrocytes. Neurosci 2006;55:154-160.

28. Samad TA, Moore KA, Sapirstein A, et al: Interleukin-1 beta–mediated induction of COX-2 in the CNS contributes inflammatory pain hypersensitivity. Nature 2001;410:471-475.

29. Laflamme N, Lacroix S, Rivest S: An essential role of interleukin-1 beta in mediating NF-kappa B activity and COX-2 transcription in cells of the blood-brain barrier in response to a systemic and localized inflammation but not during endotoxemia. J Neurosci 1999;9:10923-10930.

30. Buvanendran A, Kroin JS, Berger RA, et al: Up-regulation of prostaglandin E₂ and interleukins in the central nervous system and peripheral tissue during and after surgery in humans. Anesthesiology 2006;104:403-410.

31. Kroin JS, Ling ZD, Buvanendran A, et al: Upregulation of spinal cyclooxygenase-2 in rats after surgical incision. Anesthesiology 2004;100:364-369.

32. Reuben SS, Buvanendran A, Kroin JS, et al: Postoperative modulation of central nervous system prostaglandins E₂ by cyclooxygenase inhibitors after vascular surgery. Anesthesiology 2006;104:411-416.

33. Dembo G, Park SB, Kharasch ED: Central nervous system concentration of cyclooxygenase-2 inhibitors in humans. Anesthesiology 2005;102:409-415.

34. Buvanendran A, Kroin JS, Tuman KJ, et al: Cerebrospinal fluid and plasma pharmacokinetics of the cyclooxygenase 2 inhibitor rofecoxib in humans: Single and multiple oral drug administration. Anesth Analg 2005;100:1320-1324.

35. Bartfai T: Immunology telling the brain about pain. Nature 2001;410:425-427.

36. Bonati M, Kanto J, Tognoni G: Clinical pharmacokinetics of cerebrospinal fluid. Clin Pharmacokinet 1982;7:312-325.

37. Gaucher A, Netter P, Faure G, et al: Diffusion of oxyphenbutazone into synovial fluid, synovial tissue, joint cartilage and cerebrospinal fluid. J Clin Pharmacol 1982;25:107-112.

38. Bannwarth B, Netter P, Pourel J, et al: Clinical pharmacokinetics of nonsteroidal anti-inflammatory drugs in the cerebrospinal fluid. Biomed Pharmacother 1989;43:121-126.

39. Netter P, Lapicque F, Bannwarth B, et al: Diffusion of intramuscular ketoprofen into the cerebrospinal fluid. Eur J Clin Pharmacol 1985;29:319-321.

40. Ushikubi F, Nakajima M, Hirata M, et al: Purification of the thromboxane A2/prostaglandin H2 receptor from human blood platelets. J Biol Chem 1989;264:16496-16501.

41. Sugimoto Y, Narumiya S, Ichikawa A, et al: Distribution and function of prostanoid receptors: Studies from knockout mice. Prog Lipid Res 2000;39: 289-314.

42. Oida H, Namba T, Sugimoto Y, et al: In situ hybridization studies of prostacyclin receptor mRNA expression in various mouse organs. Br J Pharmacol 1995;116:2828-2837.

43. Smith MJH: Aspirin and prostaglandins; some recent developments. Agents Actions 1978;8:427-429.

44. Saini SS, Gessell-Lee DL, Peterson JW: The COX-2 specific inhibitor celecoxib inhibits adenylyl cyclase. Inflammation 2003;27:79-88.

45. Cooke AR, Hunt JN: Relationship between pH and absorption of acetylsalicylic acid from the stomach. Gut 1969;10:77-78.

46. Eller MG, Wright C 3rd, Della-Coletta AA: Absorption kinetics of rectally and orally administered ibuprofen. Biopharm Drug Dispos 1989;10:269-278.

47. Evans AM, Hussein Z, Rowland M: Influence of albumin on the distribution and elimination kinetics of diclofenac in the isolated perfused rat liver: Analysis by the impulse-response technique and the dispersion model. J Pharm Sci 1993;82: 421-428.

48. Soren A: Kinetics of salicylates in blood and joint fluid. J Clin Pharmacol 1957;15:173-177.

49. Makela AL, Lempiainen M, Ylijoki H: Ibuprofen levels in serum and synovial fluid. Scand J Rheumatol Suppl 1981;39:15-17.

50. Fowler PD, Shadforth MF, Crook PR, et al: Plasma and synovial fluid concentrations of diclofenac sodium and its major hydroxylated metabolites during long-term treatment

of rheumatoid arthritis. Eur J Clin Pharmacol 1983;25:389-394.

51. Davies NM, Skjodt NM: Choosing the right nonsteroidal anti-inflammatory drug for the right patient: A pharmacokinetic approach. Clin Pharmacokinet 2000;38:377-392.
52. Gibaldi M: Drug distribution in renal failure. Am J Med 1977;62:471-474.
53. Verbeeck RK: Pathophysiologic factors affecting the pharmacokinetics of nonsteroidal antiinflammatory drugs. J Rheumatol Suppl 1988;17:44-57.
54. Cook ME, Wallin JD, Thakur VD: Comparative effects of nabumetone, sulindac, and ibuprofen on renal function. J Rheumatol 1997;24:1137-1144.
55. Menkes CJ: Renal and hepatic effects of NSAIDs in the elderly. Scand J Rheumatol Suppl 1989;83:11-13.
56. Levy G: Clinical pharmacokinetics of aspirin. Pediatrics 1978;62:867-872.
57. Flower RJ: Drugs which inhibit prostaglandin biosynthesis. Pharmacol Rev 1974;26:33-67.
58. Farrell G: Liver disease produced by nonsteroidal anti-inflammatory drugs. In Farrell G (ed): Drug-Induced Liver Disease. Edinburgh, Churchill Livingstone, 1994, p 371.
59. Huskisson EC, Williams TN, Shaw LD, et al: Diflunisal in general practice. Curr Med Res Opin 1978;5:589-592.
60. Green D, Davis RO, Holmes GI, et al: Effects of diflunisal on platelet function and fecal blood loss. Clin Pharmacol Ther 1981;30:378-384.
61. Levitt MJ, Kann J: Choline magnesium trisalicylate: Comparative pharmacokinetic study of once-daily and twice-daily dosages. J Pharm Sci 1984;73:977-979.
62. Lipton JM, Rosenstein J: Thermoregulatory disorders after removal of a craniopharyngioma from the third cerebral ventricle. Brain Res Bull 1981;7:369-673.
63. Pickering G, Loriot MA, Libert F, et al: Analgesic effect of acetaminophen in humans: First evidence of central serotonergic mechanism. Clin Pharmacol Ther 2006;79:371-378.
64. Skoglund LA, Skjelbred P, Fyllingen G: Analgesic efficacy of acetaminophen 1000 mg, acetaminophen 2000 mg, and the combination of acetaminophen 1000 mg and codeine phosphate 60 mg versus placebo in acute postoperative pain. Pharmacotherapy 1991;11:364-369.
65. Stewart DM, Dillman RO, Kim HS, et al: Acetaminophen overdose: A growing health care hazard. Clin Toxicol 1979;14:507-513.
66. Bertin P, Keddad K, Jolivet-Landreau I: Acetaminophen as symptomatic treatment of pain from osteoarthritis. Joint Bone Spine 2004;71:266-274.
67. Douglas DR, Sholar JB, Smilkstein MJ: A pharmacokinetic comparison of acetaminophen products (Tylenol Extended Relief vs regular Tylenol). Acad Emerg Med 1996;3:740-744.
68. Steventon GB, Mitchell SC, Waring RH: Human metabolism of paracetamol (acetaminophen) at different dose levels. Drug Metabol Drug Interact 1996;13:111-117.
69. Blume H, Ali SL, Elze M, et al: [Relative bioavailability of paracetamol in suppositories preparations in comparison to tablets.] Arzneimittelforschung 1994;44:1333-1338.
70. Cobby TF, Crighton IM, Kyriakides K, et al: Rectal paracetamol has a significant morphine-sparing effect after hysterectomy. Br J Anaesth 1999;83:253-256.
71. Peduto VA, Ballabio M, Stefanini S: Efficacy of propacetamol in the treatment of postoperative pain. Morphine-sparing effect in orthopedic surgery. Acta Anaesthesiol Scand 1998;42:293-298.
72. Delbos A, Boccard E: The morphine-sparing effect of propacetamol in orthopedic postoperative pain. J Pain Symptom Manage 1995;10:279-286.
73. Hahn TW, Mogensen T, Lund C, et al: Analgesic effect of i.v. paracetamol: Possible ceiling effect of paracetamol in postoperative pain: Acta Anaesthesiol Scand 2003;47:138-145.
74. Eneli I, Sadri K, Camargo C Jr, et al: Acetaminophen and the risk of asthma: The epidemiologic and pathophysiologic evidence. Chest 2005;127:604-612.
75. Duggan DE, Hogans AF, Kwan KC, et al: The metabolism of indomethacin in man. J Pharmacol Exp Ther 1972;181:563-575.
76. Wood LJ, Mundo F, Searle J, et al: Sulindac hepatotoxicity: Effects of acute and chronic exposure. Aust N Z J Med 1985;15:397-401.
77. Huskisson EC, Scott J: Sulindac: Trials of a new anti-inflammatory drug. Ann Rheum Dis 1978;37:89-92.
78. Quintero E, Gines P, Arroyo V, et al: Sulindac reduces the urinary excretion of prostaglandins and impairs renal function in cirrhosis with ascites. Nephron 1986;42:298-303.
79. Grindel JM, Migdalof BH, Plostnieks J: Absorption and excretion of tolmetin in arthritic patient. Clin Pharmacol Ther 1979;26:122-128.
80. Pena M: Etodolac analgesic effects in musculoskeletal and postoperative pain. Rheumatol Int 1990;10:9-16.
81. Schattenkirchner M: An updated safety profile of etodolac in several thousand patients. Eur J Rheumatol Inflamm 1990;10:56-65.
82. Gills JC, Brogden RN: Ketorolac: A reappraisal of its pharmacodynamics and pharmacokinetic properties and therapeutic use in pain management. Drugs 1997;53:139-188.
83. Toradol IV/IM prescribing information (discontinued 2006). Nutley, NJ, Roche Laboratories, 1994.
84. Stouten E, Armbruster S, Houmes RJ, et al: Comparison of ketorolac and morphine for postoperative pain after major surgery. Acta Anaesthesiol Scand 1992;36:716-721.
85. Greer I: Effects of ketorolac tromethamine on hemostasis. Pharmacotherapy 1990;10:71S-76S.
86. Gordon SM, Brahim JS, Rowan J, et al: Peripheral prostanoid levels and nonsteroidal anti-inflammatory drug analgesia: Replicate clinical trials in a tissue injury model. Clin Pharmacol Ther 2002;72:175-183.
87. Rice ASC, Lloyd J, Bullingham RES, et al: Ketorolac penetration into the cerebrospinal fluid of humans. J Clin Anesth 1993;5:459-462.
88. Forbes JA, Kehm CJ, Grodin CD, et al: Evaluation of ketorolac, ibuprofen, acetaminophen, and an acetaminophen-codeine combination in postoperative oral surgery pain. Pharmacotherapy 1990;10:94S-105S.
89. Strom BL, Berlin JA, Kinman JL, et al: Parenteral ketorolac and risk of gastrointestinal and operating site bleeding. A postmarketing surveillance study. JAMA 1996;275:376-382.
90. Choo V, Lewis S: Ketorolac doses reduced. Lancet 1993;10:109.
91. Sevarino FB, Sinatra RS, Paige D, et al: The efficacy of intramuscular ketorolac in combination with intravenous PCA morphine for postoperative pain relief. J Clin Anesth 1992;4:285-288.
92. Reuben SS, Connelly NR, Lurie S, et al: Dose-response of ketorolac as an adjunct to patient-controlled analgesia morphine in patients after spinal fusion surgery. Anesth Analg 1998;93:98-102.
93. Vyas TK, Shahiwala A, Marathe S, et al: Intranasal drug delivery for brain targeting. Curr Drug Deliv 2005;2:165-175.
94. Quadir M, Zia H, Needham TE: Development and evaluation of nasal formulation of ketorolac. Drug Deliv 2000;7:223-229.
95. Elmquist WF, Chan KK, Sawchuk RJ: Transsynovial drug distribution: Synovial mean transit time of diclofenac and other nonsteroidal antiinflammatory drugs. Pharm Res 1994;11:1689-1697.
96. Chan KK, Vyas KH, Brandt KD: In vitro protein binding of diclofenac sodium in plasma and synovial fluid. J Pharm Sci 1987;76:105-108.
97. Tang W: The metabolism of diclofenac—enzymology and toxicology perspectives. Curr Drug Metab 2003;4:319-329.
98. Morgan GJ, Poland M, DeLapp RE: Efficacy and safety of nabumetone versus diclofenac, naproxen, ibuprofen, and piroxicam in the elderly. Am J Med 1993;9:19S-27S.
99. Davies NM: Anderson KE: Clinical pharmacokinetics of diclofenac: Therapeutic insights and pitfalls. Clin Pharmacokinet 1997;33:184-213.
100. Rhodes M: Nonsteroidal anti-inflammatory drugs for post-thoracotomy pain. J Thorac Cardiovasc Surg 1992;103:17-20.
101. Magnette J, Kienzler JL, Alexkandrova I, et al: The efficacy and safety of low-dose diclofenac sodium 0.1% gel for the

symptomatic relief of pain and erythema associated with superficial natural sunburn. Eur J Dermatol 2004;14:48-46.

102. Miller L: Oxaprozin: A once-daily nonsteroidal anti-inflammatory drug. Clin Pharm 1992;11:591-603.

103. Brooks CD, Schlagel CA, Sekhar NC, et al: Tolerance and pharmacology of ibuprofen. Curr Ther Res 1973;15:180-181.

104. Mann JF, Goerig M, Brune K, et al: Ibuprofen as an over-the-counter drug: Is there a risk for renal injury? Clin Nephrol 1993;39:1-6.

105. Catella-Lawson F, Reilly MP, Kapoor SC, et al: Cyclooxygenase inhibitors and the antiplatelet effect of aspirin. N Engl J Med 2001;345:1809-1817

106. Geisslinger G, Menzel S, Wissel K, et al: Pharmacokinetics of ketoprofen enantiomers after different doses of the racemate. Br. J Clin Pharmacol 1995;40: 73-75.

107. Mazieres B: Topical ketoprofen patch. Drugs 2005;6:337-344.

108. Gruber CM Jr: Clinical pharmacology of fenoprofen: A review. J Rheumatol 1976;2(Suppl 3):8-17.

109. Ryley NJ, Lingam G: A pharmacokinetic comparison of controlled-release and standard naproxen tablets. Curr Med Res Opin 1988;11:10-15.

110. Sevelius H, Segre E, Bursick K: Comparative analgesic effects of naproxen sodium, aspirin, and placebo. J Clin Pharmacol 1980;20:480-485.

111. Davis NM: Clinical pharmacokinetics of oxaprozin. Clin Pharmacokinet 1998;35:425-436.

112. Kean WF: Oxaprozin: Kinetic and dynamic profile in the treatment of pain. Curr Med Res Opin 2004;20:1275-1277.

113. Heller B, Tarricone R: Oxaprozin versus diclofenac in NSAID-refractory periarthritis of the shoulder. Curr Med Res Opin 2004;20:1279-1287.

114. Kurowski M, Thabe H: The transsynovial distribution of oxaprozin. Agents Actions 1989;27:458-460.

115. Dallegri F, Bertolotto M, Ottonello L, et al: A review of the emerging profile of the anti-inflammatory drug oxaprozin. Expert Opin Pharmacother 2005;6:777-785.

116. Caldwell JR: Comparison of the efficacy, safety, and pharmacokinetic profiles of extended-release ketoprofen and piroxicam in patients with rheumatoid arthritis. Clin Ther 1994;16:222-235.

117. Bottiger LE: Phenylbutazone, oxyphenbutazone and aplastic anaemia. Br Med J 1977;23:265.

118. Grant DJ, MacConnachie AM: Nonsteroidal anti-inflammatory drugs in elderly people. Mefenamic acid is more dangerous than most. BMJ 1995;311:392.

119. Porro GB, Montrone F, Petrillo M, et al: Gastroduodenal tolerability of nabumetone versus naproxen in the treatment of rheumatic patients. Am J Gastroenterol 1995;90:1485-1488.

120. Dahl S: Nabumetone A: A "nonacidic" nonsteroidal anti-inflammatory drugs. Ann Pharmacother 1993;27:456-463.

121. Fleischmann R, Iqbal I, Slobodin G: Meloxicam. Expert Opin Pharmacother 2003;3:1501-1512.

122. Vidal L, Kneer W, Baturone M, et al: Meloxicam in acute episodes of soft tissue rheumatism of the shoulder. Inflamm Res 2001;50:S24-S29.

123. Gates BJ, Nguyen TT, Setter SM, et al: Meloxicam: A reappraisal of pharmacokinetics, efficacy and safety. Expert Opin Pharmacother 2005;6:2117-2140.

124. Romsing J, Moniche S: A systemic review of COX-2 inhibitors compared with traditional NSAIDs, or different COX-2 inhibitors for postoperative pain. Acta Anaesthesiol Scand 2004;48:525-546.

125. Reuben SS, Connelly NR: Postoperative analgesic effects of celecoxib or rofecox after spinal fusion surgery. Anesth Analg 2000;91:1221-1225.

126. Elia N, Lysakowski C, Tramer M: Does multimodal analgesia with acetaminophen, nonsteroidal antiinflammatory drugs, or selective cyclooxygenase-2 inhibitors and patient-controlled analgesia morphine offer advantages over morphine alone? Anesthesiology 2005;103:1296-1304.

127. Buvenandran A, Kroin JS, Tuman KJ, et al. Effects of perioperative administration of a selective cyclooxygenase 2 inhibitor on pain management and recovery of function after knee replacement. JAMA 2003;290:2411-2418.

128. Buvanendran A, Tuman KJ, McCoy DD, et al: Anesthetic techniques for minimally invasive total knee arthroplasty. J Knee Surg 2006;19:133-136.

129. Reuben SS, Gutta SB, Maciolek H, et al: Effect of initiating a multimodal analgesic regimen upon patient outcomes after anterior cruciate ligament reconstruction for same-day surgery: A 1200-patient case series. Acute Pain 2004;6:87-93.

130. Kessenich C: Cyclooxygenase 2 inhibitors: An important new drug classification. Pain Manage Nurs 2001;2:13-18.

131. Leese PT, Hubbard RC, Karim A, et al: Effects of celecoxib, a novel cyclooxygenase-2 inhibitor, on platelet function in healthy adults: A randomized, controlled trial. J Clin Pharmacol 2000;40:124-132.

132. Singh G, Fort JG, Goldstein JL, et al: Celecoxib versus naproxen and diclofenac in osteoarthritis patients: SUCCESS-I study. Am J Med 2006;119:255-266.

133. Silverstein FE, Faich G, Goldstein JL, et al: Gastrointestinal toxicity with celecoxib vs nonsteroidal anti-inflammatory drugs for osteoarthritis and rheumatoid arthritis: The CLASS study: A randomized controlled trial. Celecoxib Long-term Arthritis Safety Study. JAMA 2000;284:1247-1255.

134. Weaver A: Rofecoxib: Clinical pharmacology and clinical experience. Clin Ther 2001;23:1323-1338.

135. Depre M, Ehrich E, Van Hecken A, et al: Pharmacokinetics of COX-2 specificity and tolerability of supratherapeutic doses of rofecoxib in humans. Eur J Clin Pharmacol 2000;56:167-174.

136. Bombardier C, Laine L, Reicin A, et al : Comparison of upper gastrointestinal toxicity of rofecoxib and naproxen in patients with rheumatoid arthritis. N Engl J Med 2000;343:1520-1528.

137. Silverman DG, Halaszynski T, Sinatra R, et al: Rofecoxib does not compromise platelet aggregation during anesthesia and surgery. Can J Anaesth 2003;50:1004-1008.

138. Sinatra RS, Shen QJ, Halaszynski T, et al: Preoperative rofecoxib oral suspension as an analgesic adjunct after lower abdominal surgery: The effects on effort-dependent pain and pulmonary function. Anesth Analg 2004;98:135-140.

139. Horattas MC, Evans S, Sloan-Stakleff KD, et al: Does preoperative rofecoxib (Vioxx) decrease postoperative pain with laparoscopic cholecystectomy? Am J Surg 2004;188:271-276.

140. Bresalier RS, Sandler RS, Quan H, et al; Adenomatous Polyp Prevention on Vioxx (APPROVe) Trial Investigators: Cardiovascular events associated with rofecoxib in a colorectal adenoma chemoprevention trial. N Engl J Med 2005; 352:1092-1102.

141. Alsalameh S, Burian M, Mahr G, et al: The pharmacological properties and clinical use of valdecoxib, a new cyclooxygenase-2 selective inhibitor. Aliment Pharmacol Ther 2003;17:489-501.

142. Jain KK: Evaluation of intravenous parecoxib for the relief of acute post-surgical pain. Expert Opin Invest Drugs 2000;9:2717-2723.

143. Yuan JJ, Yang DC, Zhang JY, et al: Disposition of a specific cyclooxygenase-2 inhibitor, valdecoxib, in humans. Drug Metab Dispos 2002;30:1013-1021.

144. Fenton C, Keating GM, Wagstaff AJ, et al: Valdecoxib: A review of its use in the management of osteoarthritis, rheumatoid arthritis, dysmenorrhoea and acute pain. Drugs 2004;64:1231-1261.

145. Daniels SE, Desjardins PJ, Talwalker S, et al: The analgesic efficacy of valdecoxib vs oxycodone/acetaminophen after oral surgery. J Am Dent Assoc 2002;133:611-621.

146. Fricke J, Varkalis I, Zwillich S, et al: Valdecoxib is more efficacious than rofecoxib in relieving pain associated with oral surgery. Am J Ther 2002;9:89-97.

147. Camu F, Beecher T, Recker DP, et al: Valdecoxib, a COX-2 specific inhibitor, is an efficacious opioid-sparing analgesic in patients undergoing hip arthroplasty. Am J Ther 2002;9: 43-51.

148. McAdam BF, Catella-Lawson, Mardini IA, et al: Systemic biosynthesis of prostacyclin by cyclooxygenase COX-2: The

human pharmacology of a selective inhibitor of COX-2. Proc Natl Acad Sci 1999;96:272-277.

149. Goldstein JL, Eisen GM, Agrawal N, et al: Reduced incidence of upper gastrointestinal ulcer complications with the COX-2 selective inhibitor, valdecoxib. Aliment Pharmacol Ther 2004;20:527-538.

150. U.S. Department of Health and Human Services, Acute Pain Management Guideline Panel: Acute pain management: Operative or medical procedures and trauma—clinical practice guideline (AHCPR Publication No. 92-0032). Rockville, Md, Agency for Health Care Policy and Research, U.S. Department of Health and Human Services, 1992, pp 15-26.

151. Ashburn MA, Caplan RA, Carr DB, et al. Practice guidelines for acute pain management in the perioperative setting. An updated report by the American Society of Anesthesiologists task force on acute pain management. Anesthesiology 2004;100:1573-1581.

152. Connelly C, Panush R: Should nonsteroidal anti-inflammatory drugs be stopped before elective surgery? Arch Intern Med 1991;151:1963-1966.

153. Marret, Flahault A, Samama CM, et al: Effects of postoperative, nonsteroidal, antiinflammatory drugs on bleeding risk after tonsillectomy: Meta-analysis of randomized controlled trials. Anesthesiology 2003;98:1497-1502.

154. Souter AJ, Fredman B, White PF: Controversies in the perioperative use of nonsteroidal anti-inflammatory drugs. Anesth Analg 1994;79:1178-1190.

155. Reuben SS, Fingeroth R, Krushell R, et al: Evaluation of the safety and efficacy of the perioperative administration of rofecoxib for total knee arthroplasty. J Arthroplasty 2002;17:26-31.

156. Joshi W, Connelly NR, Reuben SS, et al: An evaluation of the safety and efficacy of administering rofecoxib for postoperative pain management. Anesth Analg 2003;97:35-38.

157. Gajraj NM: The effect of cyclooxygenase-2 inhibitors on bone healing. Reg Anesth Pain Med 2003;28:456-465.

158. Dumont AS, Verma S, Dumont RJ, et al: Nonsteroidal anti-inflammatory drugs on bone metabolism in spinal fusion surgery. A pharmacological quandary. J Pharmacol Toxicol Methods 2000;43:31-39.

159. Maxy RJ, Glassman SD: The effect of non-steroidal anti-inflammatory drugs on osteogenesis and spinal fusion. Reg Anesth Pain Med 2001;26:156-158.

160. Wedel DJ, Berry D: He said, she said, NSAIDs. Reg Anesth Pain Med 2003;28:372-375.

161. Kawaguchi H, Pilbeam CC, Harrison JR, et al: The role of prostaglandins in the regulation of bone metabolism. Clin Orthop 1995;313:36-46.

162. Gerstenfeld LC, Thiede M, Seibert K, et al: Differential inhibition of fracture healing by non-selective and cyclooxygenase-2 selective non-steroidal anti-inflammatory drugs. J Orthop Res 2003;21:670-675.

163. Gerstenfeld LC, Einhorn TA: COX inhibitors and their effects on bone healing. Expert Opin Drug Saf 2004;3:131-136.

164. Reuben SS, Ablett D, Kaye R: High-dose nonsteroidal anti-inflammatory drugs compromise spinal fusion. Can J Anaesth 2005;52:506-512.

165. Reuben SS, Kuppinger J, Ekman EF: The effect of perioperative celecoxib administration on acute and chronic donor site pain following spinal fusion surgery. Anesth Analg 2005;100:S-298.

166. Reuben SS, Ekman EF, Raghunathan K, et al: The effect of cyclooxygenase-2 inhibition on acute and chronic donor-site pain after spinal-fusion surgery. Reg Anesth Pain Med 2006;31:6-13.

167. Bhattacharyya T, Smith RM: Cardiovascular risks of coxibs: The orthopaedic perspective. J Bone Joint Surg Am 2005;87:245-246.

168. Levesque LE, Brophy JM, Zhang B: The risk of myocardial infarction with cyclooxygenase-2 inhibitors: A population study of elderly adults. Ann Intern Med 2005;142:481-489.

169. Solomon DH, Schneeweiss S, Glynn R, et al: Relationship between selective cyclooxygenase-2 inhibitors and acute myocardial infarction in older adults. Circulation 2004;109:2068-2073.

170. Solomon SD, McMurray JV, Pfeffer MA, et al; Adenoma Prevention with Celecoxib (APC) Study Investigators: Cardiovascular risk associated with celecoxib in a clinical trial for colorectal adenoma prevention. N Engl J Med 2005;352:1071-1080.

171. Levin B: Overview of colorectal chemoprevention trials, 2002. Available at http://www.fda.gov/ohrms/dockets/ac/05/slides/2005-4090s1_9_FDA-Levin.ppt.

172. National Institutes of Health: Use of non-steroidal anti-inflammatory drugs suspended in large Alzheimer's disease prevention trial, 2004. Available at http://www.nia.nih.gov/Alzheimers/ResearchInformation/NewsReleases/PR20061117 ADAPTstatement.htm.

173. Couzin J: Clinical trials. Halt of Celebrex study threatens drug's future and other trials. Science 2004;306:2170.

174. Ott E, Nussmeier NA, Duke PC, et al: Efficacy and safety of the cyclooxygenase 2 inhibitors parecoxib and valdecoxib in patients undergoing coronary artery bypass surgery. J Thorac Cardiovasc Surg. 2003;125:1481-1492.

175. U.S. Food and Drug Administration Memorandum: Analysis and recommendations for agency action regarding nonsteroidal anti-inflammatory drugs and cardiovascular risk, 2005. Available at http://www.fda.gov/cder/drug/infopage/COX2/NSAIDdecisionMemo.pdf.

176. Thun MJ, Henley SJ, Partrono C: Nonsteroidal anti-inflammatory drugs as anticancer agents: Mechanistic, pharmacologic and clinical issues. J Natl Cancer Inst 2002;94:252-266.

177. Hampton T: Breast cancer prevention strategies explored. JAMA 2006;295:2128-2130.

178. Hartmann LC, Sellers TA, Frost MH, et al: Benign breast disease and the risk of breast cancer. N Engl J Med 2005;353:229-237.

179. Giovannucci E, Egan KM, Hunter DJ, et al: Aspirin and the risk of colorectal cancer in women. N Engl J Med 1995;333:609-614.

180. Sinicrope FA, Lemoine M, Xi L et al: Reduced expression of cyclooxygenase 2 proteins in hereditary nonpolyposis colorectal cancers relative to sporadic cancers. Gastroenterology 1999;117:350-358.

181. Asano TK, McLeod RS: Nonsteroidal anti-inflammatory drugs (NSAID) and aspirin for preventing colorectal adenomas and carcinomas. Cochrane Database Syst Rev 2004;(2):CD004079.

182. Szczklik A, Gryglewski RJ, Czerniawska-Mysik G: Clinical patterns of hypersensitivity to nonsteroidal anti-inflammatory drugs and their pathogenesis. J Allergy Clin Immunol 1977;60:276-284.

183. Douthwaite AH, Lintott SAM: Gastroscopic observation of the effect of aspirin and certain other substances on the stomach. Lancet 1938;2:1222-1225.

184. Wallace JL, McCafferty DM, Carter L, et al: Tissue-selective inhibition of prostaglandin synthesis in rat by tepoxalin: Anti-inflammatory without gastropathy. Gastrenterology 1993;105:1630-1636.

185. Lanza FL: A review of gastric ulcer and gastroduodenal injury in normal volunteers receiving aspirin and other nonsteroidal anti-inflammatory drugs. Scand J Gastroenterol 1989;24:24-31.

186. Hawkey CJ, Hawthrone AB, Hudson N, et al: Separation of the impairment of hemostasis by aspirin from mucosal injury in the human stomach. Clin Sci 1991;81:565-573.

187. Vaananen PM, Keenan CM, Grisham MB, et al: A pharmacological investigation of the role of leukotrienes in the pathogenesis of experimental NSAID gastropathy. Inflammation 1992;16:227-240.

188. Santucci L, Fiorucci S, Giansanti M, et al: Pentoxifylline prevents indomethacin-induced acute gastric mucosal damage in rats: Role of tumour necrosis factor alpha. Gut 1994;35:909-915.

189. Wallace JL, Granger DN: The pathogenesis of NSAID-gastropathy—are neutrophils the culprits? Trends Pharmacol Sci 1992;13:129-131.

190. Wallace JL: Nonsteroidal anti-inflammatory drugs and gastroenteropathy: The second hundred years. Gastroenterology 1997;112:1000-1016.

191. De Smet B, Fendrick AM, Stevenson JG, et al: Over and underutilization of cyclooxygenase-2 selective inhibitors by primary care physicians and specialists. J Gen Intern Med 2006;21:694-697.

192. Fendrick AM: COX-2 inhibitor use after Vioxx: Careful balance or end of the rope? Am J Manag Care 2004;10:740-741.

193. Schafer A: Effects of nonsteroidal anti-inflammatory drugs on platelet function and systemic hemostasis. J Clin Pharmacol 1995;35:209-219.

194. Lind S: The bleeding time does not predict surgical bleeding. Blood 1991;77:2547-2552.

195. Weintraub M, Case K, Kroening B: Effects of piroxicam on platelet aggregation. Clin Pharmacol Ther 1978;23:134-135.

196. An H, Mikhail W, Jackson W, et al: Effects of hypotensive anesthesia, nonsteroidal anti-inflammatory drugs, and polymethylmethacrylate on bleeding in total hip arthroplasty patients. J Arthroplasty 1991;6:245-250.

197. Lindgren U, Djupsjo H: Diclofenac for pain after hip surgery. Acta Anaesthesiol Scand 1985;56:28-31.

198. Bricker S, Savage M, Hanning C: Perioperative blood loss and nonsteroidal anti-inflammatory drugs: An investigation using diclofenac in patients undergoing transurethral resection of the prostate. Eur J Anaesthesiol 1987;4:429-434.

199. Egan KM, Wang M, Fries S, et al: Cyclooxygenases, thromboxane, and atherosclerosis: Plaque destabilization by cyclooxygenase-2 inhibition combined with thromboxane receptor antagonism. Circulation 2005;111:334-342.

200. Borer JS, Simon LS: Cardiovascular and gastrointestinal effects of COX-2 inhibitors and NSAIDs: Achieving balance. Arthr Res Ther 2005;7:S14-22.

201. Shorr R, Ra W, Daugherty J, Griffin M: Concurrent use of nonsteroidal anti-inflammatory drugs and oral anticoagulants places elderly persons at high risk for hemorrhagic peptic ulcer disease. Arch Intern Med 1993;153:1665-1670.

202. Taber SS, Mueller BA: Drug-associated renal dysfunction. Crit Care Clin 2006;22:357-374.

203. Barkin RL, Buvanendran A: Focus on the COX-1 and COX-2 agents: Renal events of nonsteroidal and anti-inflammatory drugs–NSAIDs. Am J Ther 2004;11:124-129.

204. O'Connor N, Dargan PI, Jones AL: Hepatocellular damage from non-steroidal anti-inflammatory drugs. QJM 2003;96:787-791.

205. Marinac J: Drug and chemical-induced aseptic meningitis: A review of the literature. Ann Pharmacother 1992;26:813-822.

206. Wilson JG: Factor determining the teratogenicity of drugs. Annu Rev Toxicol 1974;14:205-217.

207. Fahey SM, Silver RM: Use of NSAIDs and COX-2 inhibitors in children with musculoskeletal disorders. Curr Issues 2003;23:794-799.

208. Keenan GF, Giannini EH, Athreya BH. Clinically significant gastropathy associated with nonsteroidal anti-inflammatory drug use in children with juvenile rheumatic arthritis. J Rheumatol 1995;22:1149-1151.

209. Levy ML, Barron KS, Eichemfield A, et al: Naproxen-induced pseudoporphyria: A distinctive photodermatis. J Pediatr 1990;117:660-664.

210. Watcha MF, Jones MB, Lagueruela R, et al: Comparison of ketorolac and morphine as adjuvants during pediatric surgery. Anesthesiology 1992;76:368-372.

211. Kean WF, Buchanan WW: Variables affecting the absorption of non-steroidal anti-inflammatory drugs from the gastrointestinal tract. Jpn J Rheumatol 1987;1:159-170.

212. Buchanan WW: Implications of NSAID therapy in elderly patients. J Rheumatol 1990;17:29-32.

213. Richardson CJ, Blocka KLN, Ross SG, et al: Effects of age and sex on piroxicam disposition. Clin Pharmacol Ther 1985;37:13-18.

214. Greenblatt DJ, Abernethy DR, Matlis R, et al: Absorption and disposition of ibuprofen in the elderly. Arthritis Rheum 1984;27:1066-1069.

215. Upton RA, Williams RL, Kelly J, et al: Naproxen pharmacokinetics in the elderly. Br J Clin Pharmacol 1984;18:207-214.

216. Advenier C, Roux A, Gobert C, et al: Pharmacokinetics of ketoprofen in the elderly. Br J Clin Pharmacol 1983;16:65-70.

217. Blackshear JL, Davidman M, Stillman MT: Identification of risk factors for renal insufficiency from non-steroidal anti-inflammatory drugs. Arch Intern Med 1983;143:1130-1134.

218. Koopmans PP, Thien TH, Gribnau FWJ: Influence of non-steroidal anti-inflammatory drugs on diuretic treatment of mild to moderate essential hypertension. Br Med J 1984;289:1492-1494.

219. Forbes J, Beaver W, Jones K, et al: Evaluation of caffeine on ibuprofen analgesia in postoperative oral surgery pain. Clin Pharmacol Ther 1991;49:674-684.

220. McQuay H, Angell K, Carroll D, et al: Ibuprofen compared with ibuprofen plus caffeine after third molar surgery. Pain 1996;66:247-251.

221. Castaneda-Hernandez G, Castillo-Mendez M, Lopez-Munoz F, et al: Potentiation by caffeine of the analgesic effect of aspirin in the pain-induced function impairment model in the rat. Can J Physiol Pharmacol 1994;72:1127-1131.

222. Oldfield V, Perry CM: Oxycodone/ibuprofen combination tablet: A review of its use in the management of acute pain. Drugs 2005;65:2337-2354.

223. Cochrane DJ, Jarvis B, Keating GM: Etoricoxib. Drugs 2002;62:2637-2651.

224. Agrawal NG, Rose MJ, Matthews CZ, et al: Pharmacokinetics of etoricoxib in patients with hepatic impairment. J Clin Pharmacol 2003;43:1136-1148.

225. Matsumoto AK, Cavanaugh PF: Etorocoxib. Drugs Today 2004;40:395-414.

226. Leung AT, Malmstrom K, Gallacher AE, et al: Efficacy and tolerability profile of etoricoxib in patients with osteoarthritis: A randomized, double-blind, placebo and active-comparator controlled 12-week efficacy trial. Curr Med Res Opin 2002;18:49-58.

227. Chang DJ, Chang DJ, Desjardins PJ, King TR, et al: The analgesic efficacy of etoricoxib compared with oxycodone/acetaminophen in an acute postoperative pain model: A randomized, double-blind clinical trial. Anesth Analg 2004;99:807-815.

228. Mangold KB, Gu H, Rodriguez LC, et al: Pharmacokinetics and metabolism of lumiracoxib in healthy male subjects. Drug Metab Dispos 2004;32:566-571.

229. Esser R 2005, Bery C, Du Z, et al: Preclinical pharmacology of luxiracoxib: A novel selective inhibitor of cyclooxygenase-2. Br J Pharmacol 2005;144:538-550.

230. Lehmann R, Brzosko M, Kopsa P, et al: Efficacy and tolerability of lumiracoxib 100 mg once daily in knee osteoarthritis: A 13-week, randomized, double blind study vs placebo and celecoxib. Curr Med Res Opin 2005;21:517-526.

231. Zelenakas K, Fricke JR Jr, Jayawardene S, et al: Analgesic efficacy of single oral doses of lumiracoxib and ibuprofen in patients with postoperative dental pain. Int J Clin Pract 2004;58:251-256.

232. Chan VW, Clark AJ, Davis JC, et al: The post-operative analgesic efficacy and tolerability of lumiracoxib compared with placebo and naproxen after total knee or hip arthroplasty. Acta Anaesthesiol Scand 2005;49:1491-1500.

233. Schnitzer TJ, Beier J, Geusens P, et al: Efficacy and safety of four doses of lumiracoxib versus diclofenac in patients with knee or hip primary osteoarthritis: A phase II, four-week, multicenter, randomized, double-blind, placebo-controlled trial. Arthritis Rheum 2004;51:549-557.

CHAPTER
36 Skeletal Muscle Relaxants

Kenneth C. Jackson II and Charles E. Argoff

The term *skeletal muscle relaxant* is often used to describe a diverse group of medications commonly used in the treatment of back pain (Table 36–1).[1-4] Medications commonly referred to as skeletal muscle relaxants include carisoprodol, chlorzoxazone, cyclobenzaprine, metaxalone, methocarbamol, and orphenadrine.[5] All these agents are labeled by the U.S. Food and Drug Administration (FDA) with an indication for the relief of discomfort associated with an acute, painful, musculoskeletal condition. Oral baclofen and tizanidine are also commonly used to treat acute musculoskeletal conditions and are considered by many clinicians as muscle relaxants, despite the lack of an indication in this regard. Baclofen and tizanidine do have FDA indications for the treatment of spasticity caused by multiple sclerosis, spinal cord disease, or injury. Benzodiazepines, principally diazepam, are also commonly used and indicated for adjunctive relief of skeletal muscle spasm and are often considered in discussions regarding skeletal muscle relaxants.

In discussing this broad class of medications, it becomes difficult to cull out the actual intended therapeutic outcomes. These agents are typically prescribed during the initial presentation of an acute low back pain problem, often the result of a soft tissue mechanical injury. The injury normally occurs in the muscles, ligaments, and/or tendons, structures around the lumbar spine. The presentations may include local pain and tenderness, muscle spasm, and limited range of motion. Muscle spasm is often the most difficult to define and is the subject of controversy among some clinicians.[6] Muscle spasm can be described as a vicious pain-spasm-pain cycle that provides protection to compromised tissues and structures. Following the interpretation of pain impulses, an involuntary reflex muscle contraction at the site of injury can occur and can lead to local ischemic injury. This can further facilitate the pain-spasm-pain paradigm. Muscle spasm phenomena may be considered a variation of a myofascial pain presentation.[7]

MECHANISM OF ACTION

In considering the above discussion of muscle spasm pathophysiology, one begins to discern the problem with defining the activity of the skeletal muscle relaxants. In specific terms, the exact mechanism of action for these various agents has not been fully elucidated.

It is generally accepted that skeletal muscle relaxants have the ability to depress polysynaptic reflexes within the dorsal horn via a variety of mechanisms (Box 36–1), which in turn may produce relaxation of skeletal muscle tissue in an indirect manner.[1-3] In animal studies, these agents exert their muscle-relaxing effects by inhibiting interneuronal activity and blocking polysynaptic neurons in the spinal cord and descending reticular formation in the brain.[1] It is interesting to note that other sedating agents also depress polysynaptic reflexes, making it difficult to determine whether skeletal muscle relaxants produce their clinical activity via sedation or a change in the pain-spasm-pain cycle.

INDICATIONS FOR USE

Despite the common use of skeletal muscle relaxants, relatively little data exist to elucidate their role in the treatment of back pain, especially chronic back pain.[8,9] None of the agents discussed in this chapter have an indication for use in the setting of chronic back pain, but in one survey of the use of skeletal muscle relaxant use in the United States, muscle relaxants, although indicated for short-term treatment, are most often prescribed on a long-term basis.[10] In general, skeletal muscle relaxants, excluding baclofen and tizanidine, maintain FDA labeling as adjuncts for treatment of short-term acute low back pain (LBP) and are commonly used to treat muscle spasms and associated pain for periods of 1 to 3 weeks. This time frame coincides with how long many patients may expect it will take to recover from an initial acute low back insult. In this context, it may be difficult to discern the role of these agents, other than the palliative analgesic quality that they may provide for patients. Skeletal muscle relaxant selection is dependent on an evaluation of adverse effects, contraindications, patient tolerability, and clinical experience. This discussion will also include a brief review of the clinical use of botulinum toxin as a treatment for musculoskeletal pain.

SPECIFIC DRUGS

Carisoprodol (Soma)

Carisoprodol is available as a 350-mg tablet and in combination with aspirin (Soma Compound) and

Table 36–1.　Skeletal Muscle Relaxant Profiles

DRUG	ONSET OF ACTION	DURATION (hr)	SIDE EFFECTS	IMPORTANT DRUG INTERACTIONS
Carisoprodol	30 min	4-6	Drowsiness, N/V, dizziness, ataxia; withdrawal potential	Additive effects with alcohol and other CNS depressants
Chlorzoxazone	~1 hr	3-4	N/V, headache, drowsiness, dizziness	Additive effects when taken with alcohol or other CNS depressants
Cyclobenzaprine	~1 hr	12-24	Drowsiness, dizziness, dry mouth	Additive effects with barbiturates, alcohol, other CNS depressants; seizures with tramadol and MAOIs; additive effects with TCAs
Metaxalone	1 hr	4-6	Dizziness, headache, drowsiness, N/V, rash	Additive effects when taken with alcohol or other CNS depressants
Methocarbamol	30 min (PO)	N/A	Dizziness, blurred vision, drowsiness	Additive effects when taken with alcohol or other CNS depressants
Orphenadrine	1 hr (PO)	4-6	Tachycardia, lightheadedness, N/V, dry mouth	Propoxyphene (confusion, anxiety, tremors)
Diazepam	30 min (PO)	Variable, depending on elimination	Sedation, fatigue, hypotension, ataxia, respiratory depression	Potentiation of effects when taken with phenothiazines, opioids, barbiturates, MAOIs
Baclofen	3-4 days (PO) 30 min (IT)	Variable (PO); 4-6 hr (IT)	Drowsiness, slurred speech, hypotension, constipation, urinary retention	Antidepressants (short-term memory loss); additive effects with imipramine
Tizanidine	2 weeks	Variable	Drowsiness, dry mouth, dizziness, hypotension, increased spasm, or muscle tone	Additive effects with alcohol and other CNS depressants; reduced clearance with oral contraceptives

CNS, central nervous system; IT, intrathecal; N/V, nausea and vomiting; TCA, tricyclic antidepressant.

BOX 36–1. CLASSIFICATION OF AGENTS BY PROPOSED MECHANISM OF ACTION

CNS Depressants
Antihistamine—orphenadrine
Sedatives—carisoprodol, chlorzoxazone, metaxalone, methocarbamol
TCA-like—cyclobenzaprine

Central α_2 Agonists
Tizanidine

GABA Agonists
Baclofen, benzodiazepines

CNS, central nervous system; GABA, gamma-aminobutyric acid; TCA, tricyclic antidepressant.

Table 36–2.　Comparative Dosing of Commonly Used Muscle Relaxants

AGENT	DOSAGE
Baclofen	Initially, 5-10 mg PO qid
Carisoprodol	350 mg PO qid
Chlorzoxazone	250-750 mg PO qid
Cyclobenzaprine	5-10 PO tid
Diazepam	2-10 mg PO qid
Metaxalone	800 mg PO qid
Methocarbamol	750-1500 mg PO qid
Orphenadrine	100 mg PO bid
Tizanidine	4-8 mg PO qid

with aspirin and codeine (Soma Compound with Codeine). Carisoprodol dosing should not exceed four doses in a 24-hour period (Table 36–2). Similar to other muscle relaxants, carisoprodol has additive effects when taken with alcohol or other central nervous system (CNS) depressants.

Carisoprodol is converted in the liver to meprobamate (Miltown), a schedule intravenous (IV) controlled substance. Meprobamate is well known to produce phenomena that result in physical and psychological dependence.[11-16] Substance abuse appears to be problematic with carisoprodol, probably as a consequence of meprobamate formation. In recent years, several states have begun listing carisoprodol

as a controlled substance in their state formularies. However, carisoprodol is not considered a controlled substance at the federal level. Because of the dependence potential, carisoprodol should be cautiously tapered as opposed to immediately discontinued following long-term use.

Chlorzoxazone (Paraflex, Parafon Forte DSC)

Chlorzoxazone is available as 250- and 500-mg tablets, taken up to four times daily. It has been suggested that chlorzoxazone may be less effective than the other skeletal muscle relaxants.[8] It does not have any significant drug-drug interactions, but does have a significant adverse effect profile that includes a rare idiosyncratic hepatocellular reaction.[17] The role of this agent is unclear, considering the potential lack of efficacy and significant toxicity profile.[18]

Cyclobenzaprine (Flexeril)

Cyclobenzaprine is available as 5- and 10-mg tablets, with recommended dosing of up to three times daily. Cyclobenzaprine is more structurally and pharmacologically related to the tricyclic antidepressants than to the CNS depressant skeletal muscle relaxants. As with other skeletal muscle relaxants, cyclobenzaprine does not have activity directly on muscle tissue, with animal data suggesting that this agent acts primarily in the brainstem. The net result of this action is a reduction in tonic somatic motor activity.[19] Although no human evidence exists to support this mechanism, it is interesting to note that the newer 5-mg dose has yielded similar clinical efficacy with less sedation than the more sedating 10-mg dose.[20] In the future, this may prove to be an important distinction with the CNS depressant agents. In an open-label study of patients with acute neck or low back pain associated with muscle spasm who were randomized to be treated for 7 days with cyclobenzaprine 5 mg PO three times daily alone or cyclobenzaprine 5 mg PO three times daily in combination with ibuprofen, at doses of 400 mg PO three times daily or 800 mg three times daily, no significant treatment differences were found among these groups.[21]

Because of the structural relationship to tricyclic antidepressants (TCAs), clinicians must be cognizant of the anticholinergic side effects, such as dry mouth, urinary retention, and constipation, seen with cyclobenzaprine. Use of cyclobenzaprine is contraindicated in the setting of arrhythmias, congestive heart failure, hyperthyroidism, or during the acute recovery phase of a myocardial infarction. A recent report has suggested that coadministration with proserotonergic agents such as selective serotonin reuptake inhibitors (SSRIs) may predispose patients to life-threatening serotonin syndrome.[22]

Cyclobenzaprine labeling suggests that concomitant use with tramadol may place patients at higher risk for developing seizures.[19] Concomitant use of cyclobenzaprine with monoamine oxidase inhibitors or use within 14 days after their discontinuation is contraindicated. It can enhance the effects of agents with CNS depressant activity. Older adults appear to have a higher risk for CNS-related adverse reactions, such as hallucinations and confusion, when using cyclobenzaprine. Withdrawal symptoms have been noted with the discontinuation of chronic cyclobenzaprine use. Use of a medication taper may be warranted for patients with chronic use.

Metaxalone (Skelaxin)

Metaxalone is available as a 400- and 800-mg tablet and has a recommended dose of 800 mg three or four times daily. Metaxalone does not have any significant drug-drug interactions and appears to have a fairly benign side effect profile, although fatalities attributed to the use of metaxalone have been reported..[23,24] Hemolytic anemia and impaired liver function have been seen with the use of metaxalone,

but both are uncommon. Metaxalone is contraindicated in patients who have severe renal or hepatic impairment. It is known to cause an elevation in the cephalin flocculation test, necessitating serial liver function assessments. Metaxalone can also produce a false-positive result for Benedict's test. In this scenario, alternatives to urine glucose testing may be necessary.[25] Although FDA-approved over 30 years ago, there are few published placebo-controlled studies comparing metaxalone with placebo for the treatment of musculoskeletal pain.[26]

Methocarbamol (Robaxin, Robaxisal)

Methocarbamol is available in oral and parenteral forms for IV or intramuscular use. However, many complications have arisen with the injectable form, including pain, sloughing of the skin, and thrombophlebitis. The oral dosage form of the medication is marketed as a 500- and 750-mg tablet, with a recommended daily dosage range of 4000 to 4500 mg as three or four divided doses daily. For difficult situations, the dose for the first 24 to 48 hours can be up to 6 to 8 g/day. Methocarbamol is also combined with aspirin and marketed as Robaxisal. Similar to metaxalone, although FDA-approved over 30 years ago, there are few published placebo-controlled studies comparing methocarbamol with placebo for the treatment of musculoskeletal pain.[27]

Orphenadrine Citrate (Norflex, Norgesic, Norgesic Forte)

Orphenadrine is a direct descendant of diphenhydramine, and thus exhibits antihistaminic and anticholinergic properties. Like methocarbamol, orphenadrine is available in a parenteral dosage formulation. There have been reports of severe adverse reactions with parenteral use (e.g., anaphylactoid reaction), making this formulation difficult to use. Orphenadrine is available as a 100-mg tablet (Norflex) and in combination with aspirin (Norgesic) and caffeine (Norgesic Forte).

Orphenadrine use with propoxyphene may cause confusion, anxiety, and tremors, perhaps because of additive effects. Orphenadrine's anticholinergic actions have been noted to produce significant adverse effects at high dosages, such as tachycardia, palpitations, urinary retention, and blurred vision.[28]

Diazepam (Valium)

This is the most commonly prescribed and referenced benzodiazepine for the treatment of muscle spasms.[29] Diazepam demonstrates hypnotic, anxiolytic, antiepileptic, and antispasmodic properties. With respect to muscle relaxation, gamma-aminobutyric acid (GABA)–mediated presynaptic inhibition at the spinal level is thought to be the main mechanism of action for diazepam. Sedation and abuse potential are the main concerns with this agent and class. It is important to taper this agent slowly after long-term use, as opposed to abrupt removal, to avoid any withdrawal symptoms. Diazepam is available in a wide range of dosages and each patient should be treated on an individual basis. The recommended dosage range for musculoskeletal pain is 2 to 10 mg four times daily.

Baclofen (Lioresal)

Baclofen is chemically related to GABA, and produces its effects by inhibiting monosynaptic and polysynaptic transmission along the spinal cord. This drug is mainly used for spasticity associated with CNS disorders (multiple sclerosis [MS], spinal cord lesions). Studies have shown baclofen to be superior with respect to efficacy when compared with diazepam.[2] Baclofen is unique in that it can be administered intrathecally in cases of severe spasticity and for patients who do not tolerate or have failed oral therapy. It has also found a niche in the treatment of trigeminal neuralgia because of a more favorable side effect profile. Baclofen is available in 10- and 20-mg tablets, with a therapeutic range of 40 to 80 mg daily. However, the dose should be started at 5 mg three times daily and tapered up to a therapeutic level of 5 mg every 3 to 5 days. It should be tapered slowly after long-term use to avoid a withdrawal reaction and rebound phenomena, and should be used with caution in older patients and patients with renal impairment.

Tizanidine (Zanaflex)

Tizanidine (Zanaflex) is a short-acting inhibitor of excitatory (presynaptic) motor neurons at the spinal and supraspinal levels, producing agonistic activity at the noradrenergic α_2 receptors. This activity results in the inhibition of neurotransmitter release from spinal interneurons and the concomitant inhibition of facilitatory spinal pathways that enhance muscle movement. Tizanidine is related chemically to clonidine, but has significantly lower antihypertensive effects.[30] The main adverse effect for most patients is profound sedation.[31] Currently, tizanidine is FDA-approved for the management of increased muscle tone associated with spasticity resulting from CNS disorders, such as multiple sclerosis or spinal cord injury. There are currently two published studies on the use of tizanidine in the setting of back pain or muscle spasm, either alone or in combination with ibuprofen, as well as one report of effective use for myofascial pain.[32-34] In a multicenter placebo-controlled study evaluating the efficacy and safety of tizanidine for the treatment of low back pain, tizanidine was found to provide more pain relief and less restriction of movement compared with placebo. Drowsiness was the most common side effect but, as the authors pointed out, for patients with acute low back pain, especially at night, this adverse effect may actually be desired.[32] In a separate study, 105 patients with acute low back pain were given tizanidine 4 mg PO three times daily in conjunction with ibuprofen

400 mg PO three times daily, or ibuprofen 400 mg PO three times daily with placebo. The study results suggested that the tizanidine-ibuprofen combination is more effective for the treatment of moderate or severe acute low back pain than ibuprofen only.[33] Tizanidine is available as 2- and 4-mg tablets; treatment should be instituted with a 4-mg single dose, increasing by 2- to 40-mg increments up to a therapeutic dose. The maximum daily dose should not exceed 36 mg.

Tizanidine should be used with caution in the setting of renal impairment. Tizanidine clearance is decreased by 50% in patients with creatinine clearance lower than 25 mL/min. Coadministration with alcohol can increase the area under the curve (AUC) of tizanidine by approximately 20% and increase the maximum concentration (C_{max}) by approximately 15%. Use with oral contraceptives can decrease the clearance of tizanidine and place patients at higher risk for sedating adverse effects.

Botulinum Toxin (Botox, Myobloc)

Botulinum toxin is a potent neurotoxin produced by the gram-positive anaerobic bacterium *Clostridium botulinum*. Of the seven known immunologically distinct serotypes of botulinum toxin (A to G), only types A and B have been developed for routine commercial use. Historically, the toxin's primary mechanism of action has been linked to its ability to inhibit the release of acetylcholine from cholinergic nerve terminals. However, it is now appreciated that these neurotoxins may also inhibit the release of glutamate, substance P, and calcitonin gene-related peptide. These effects may strongly contribute to the analgesic effects of these toxins.[35-37] Botulinum toxin has been studied in a number of chronic pain conditions associated with painful muscle spasm, including cervicogenic headache, temporomandibular joint disorders, craniocervical dystonia syndromes, chronic myofascial pain, and chronic low back pain.

The potential benefit of the use of botulinum toxin for the treatment of cervicogenic headache associated with "whiplash" injuries has been studied over the last decade. In 1997, Hobson and Gladish[38] reported that botulinum toxin type A injections could be effective in reducing cervicogenic headache resulting from cervical whiplash type injuries. In a randomized, double-blind, placebo-controlled study, Freund and Schwartz[39] have found that the botulinum toxin type A–treated patients demonstrate significant greater improvement from baseline with respect to pain reduction and cervical range of motion. Mixed results have been observed in evaluating the effect of botulinum toxin injection on temporomandibular joint and other orofacial-related pain. In an open-label study completed by Freund and Schwartz,[40] patients with temporomandibular joint dysfunction believed to be related to myofascial dysfunction were treated with a total of 200 units of botulinum toxin A (masseter and temporalis muscles injected), with most patients experiencing pain reduction as well as improvements in jaw function. Von Lindern and colleagues'[41] study of patients with chronic facial pain associated with muscular hyperactivity also demonstrated improvement in botulinum toxin type A–treated patients. However, in a placebo-controlled crossover trial evaluating botulinum toxin type A inpatients with chronic moderate to severe orofacial pain of muscular origin, no statistically significant differences were seen between placebo and active treatment.[42]

There have been several published evaluations of the use of botulinum toxin for the treatment of myofascial pain in the cervicothoracic regions. In a small crossover trial ($N = 6$), patients whose cervical myofascial trigger points were injected with botulinum toxin type A had an average of 30% pain reduction.[43] In a separate study, Wheeler and associates[44] completed a randomized, double-blind, prospective, placebo-controlled study in 33 patients with chronic cervical myofascial pain who were injected with either 50 or 100 units of botulinum toxin type A or normal saline. No clear benefit was found in the botulinum toxin–treated patients. Porta,[45] in a single-blinded study, evaluated the potential difference between "conventional" lidocaine-methylprednisolone trigger point injections and botulinum toxin type A injections for myofascial pain treatment and concluded that although each group received benefit, the duration of benefit was longer in the botulinum toxin–treated group.

Botulinum toxin injections have also been studied in the treatment of chronic low back pain. In one study, 31 patients with chronic low back pain were randomized to be treated with 200 units of botulinum toxin A into five sites (L1-5 or L2-S1, 40 units/site) or placebo injections. Pain and disability were measured at 3 and 8 weeks following injection using the visual analogue scale and the Oswestry Low Back Pain and Disability Questionnaire. At 3 and 8 weeks, the pain reduction experienced by the botulinum toxin–treated group was greater than that experienced by the placebo group and, at 8 weeks, there was less disability in the botulinum toxin–treated group compared with placebo.[46] The precise role of botulinum toxin injection therapy in the management of conditions associated with chronic muscle spasm remains to be determined.

CONCLUSION

Available clinical data indicate that skeletal muscle relaxants are more effective than placebo with respect to relieving acute low back pain.[8] Most of this information is dated, however, with study designs and analyses that would not be acceptable if this research were conducted today. In general terms, no data support any one agent being more efficacious than another. Some reports have suggested that chlorzoxazone may be less effective than other agents, which puts into question the viability of using this agent.[8,47]

Most clinical guidelines list skeletal muscle relaxants as optional agents for use individually or in combination with an NSAID. The Agency for Health Care Policy and Research (AHCPR) guidelines, published in 1995, specifically noted that skeletal muscle relaxants alone or in combination with an NSAID are no more effective than using an NSAID alone.[48] This conclusion has been supported in systematic reviews by van Tulder and colleagues.[8,47] Skeletal muscle relaxants have been shown to more effective than placebo for patients with acute LBP with respect to outcomes such as short-term pain relief, global efficacy, and improvement of physical outcomes,[49-52] but there remains no quality evidence that allows for a direct comparison of skeletal muscle relaxants with NSAIDs. Most clinicians and researchers agree that skeletal muscle relaxants may be of benefit to patients with acute low back pain by reducing the duration of their discomfort and accelerating recovery. A meta-analysis of cyclobenzaprine use in acute low back pain by Browning and associates[53] has concluded that despite limitations in the available evidence, the combination of an NSAID with cyclobenzaprine appears to be warranted. It is probably best to consider the use of skeletal muscle relaxants as an adjunct or alternative to NSAIDs, especially in cases in which NSAID toxicity is a concern or when NSAID monotherapy proves suboptimal.

Skeletal muscle relaxants have CNS depressant effects and should be used with caution, particularly for patients with concomitant use of alcohol, anxiolytics, opioid analgesics, or other sedating medications. There is strong evidence that skeletal muscle relaxants are associated with higher risks for total adverse effects, especially those related to the central nervous system.[8,9,47] The most common and consistent adverse effects noted with the central nervous system were drowsiness and dizziness.[25]

Thus, skeletal muscle relaxants remain an enigmatic collection of agents with an ill-defined role in the treatment of acute and chronic back pain. This is partly because of the nature of their discovery and early clinical applications that predate more modern research approaches. Considering the many issues currently facing clinicians (e.g., adverse effects of NSAIDs), it will become necessary to reevaluate the role and use of skeletal muscle relaxants in the future.

References

1. Elenbaas JK: Centrally acting oral skeletal muscle relaxants. Am J Hosp Pharm 1980;37:1313-1323.
2. Waldman HJ: Centrally acting skeletal muscle relaxants and associated drugs. J Pain Symptom Manage 1980;9:434-441.
3. Balano KB: Anti-inflammatory drugs and myorelaxants: Pharmacology and clinical use in musculoskeletal disease. Prim Care 1996;23:329-334.
4. Patel AT, Ogle AA: Diagnosis and management of acute low back pain. Am Fam Physician 2000;61:1779-1786, 1789-1790.
5. Jackson KC: Evaluation of skeletal muscle relaxant use for acute musculoskeletal pain and injury in ambulatory care. J Pain 2003;4(Suppl 1):84.

6. Johnson EW: The myth of skeletal muscle spasm. Am J Phys Med Rehabil 1989;68:1.

7. Rivner MH: The neurophysiology of myofascial pain syndrome. Curr Pain Headache Rep 2001;5:432-440.

8. van Tulder MW, Touray T, Furlan AD, et al: Muscle relaxants for non-specific low back pain. Cochrane Database Syst Rev 2003(3):CD004252.

9. Chou R, Peterson K, Helfand M: Comparative efficacy and safety of skeletal muscle relaxants for spasticity and musculoskeletal conditions: A systematic review. J Pain Symptom Manage 2004;28:140-175.

10. Dillon C, Paulose-Ram R, Hirsch R, et al: Skeletal muscle relaxant use in the United States: Data from the Third National Health and Nutrition Examination Survey (NHANES III). Spine 2004;29:892-896.

11. Littrell RA, Hayes LR, Stillner V: Carisoprodol (Soma): A new and cautious perspective on an old agent. South Med J 1993;86:753-756.

12. Bailey DN, Briggs JR: Carisoprodol: An unrecognized drug of abuse. Am J Clin Pathol 2002;117:396-400.

13. Reeves RR, Carter OS, Pinkofsky HB, et al: Carisoprodol (soma): Abuse potential and physician unawareness. J Addict Dis 1999;18:51-56.

14. Reeves RR, Carter OS, Pinkofsky HB: Use of carisoprodol by substance abusers to modify the effects of illicit drugs. South Med J 1999;92:441.

15. Rust GS, Hatch R, Gums JG: Carisoprodol as a drug of abuse. Arch Fam Med 1993;2:429-432.

16. Elder NC: Abuse of skeletal muscle relaxants. Am Fam Physician 1991;44:1223-1226.

17. Powers BJ, Cattau EL Jr, Zimmerman HJ: Chlorzoxazone hepatotoxic reactions: An analysis of 21 identified or presumed cases. Arch Intern Med 1986;146:1183-1186.

18. Jackson KC: Low back pain pharmacotherapy. Drugs Today (Barc) 2004;40:765-772.

19. Flexeril prescribing information. Fort Washington, Pa, McNeil Consumer & Specialty Pharmaceuticals, April 2003.

20. Borenstein DG, Korn S: Efficacy of a low-dose regimen of cyclobenzaprine hydrochloride in acute skeletal muscle spasm: Results of two placebo-controlled trials. Clin Ther 2003;25:1056-1073.

21. Childers MK, Borenstein D, Brown RL, et al: Low-dose cyclobenzaprine versus combination therapy with ibuprofen for acute neck or back pain with muscle spasm: A randomized trial. Curr Med Res Opin 2005;21:1485-1493.

22. Keegan MT, Brown DR, Rabinstein AA: Serotonin syndrome from the interaction of cyclobenzaprine with other serotoninergic drugs. Anesth Analg 2006;103:1466-1468.

23. Moore KA, Levine B, Fowler D: A fatality involving metaxalone. Forens Sci Int 2005;149:49-51.

24. Poklis JL, Ropero Miller JD, Garside D, et al: Metaxalone (Skelaxin)-related death. J Anal Toxicol 2004;28:537-541.

25. Toth PP, Urtis J: Commonly used muscle relaxant therapies for acute low back pain: A review of carisoprodol, cyclobenzaprine hydrochloride, and metaxalone. Clin Ther 2004;26:1355-67.

26. Dent RW, Ervin DK: A study of metaxalone (Skelaxin) vs. placebo in acute musculoskeletal disorders: A cooperative study. Curr Ther Res Clin Exp 1975;18:433-440.

27. Tisdale SA, Ervin DK: A controlled study of methocarbamol (Robaxin) in acute painful musculoskeletal conditions. Curr Ther Res Clin Exp 1975;17:525-530.

28. Gareri P, De Fazio P, Cotroneo A, et al: Anticholinergic drug-induced delirium in an elderly Alzheimer's dementia patient. Arch Gerontol Geriatr 2007;44(Suppl 1):199-206.

29. Cherkin DC, Wheeler KJ, Barlow W, et al: Medication use for low back pain in primary care. Spine 1998;23:607-614.

30. Coward DM: Tizanidine: Neuropharmacology and mechanism of action. Neurology 1994;44(Suppl 9):S6-S10.

31. Smith HS, Barton AE: Tizanidine in the management of spasticity and musculoskeletal complaints in the palliative care population. Am J Hospice Palliat Care 2000;17:50-58.

32. Berry H, Hutchinson DR: A multicentre placebo-controlled study in general practice to evaluate the efficacy and safety of tizanidine in acute low back pain. J Int Med Res 1988;16:75-82.

33. Berry H, Hutchinson DR: Tizanidine and ibuprofen in acute low back pain: Results of a double-blind multicentre study in general practice. J Int Med Res 1988;16:83-91.

34. Malanga GA, Gwynn MW, Smith R, et al: Tizanidine is effective in the treatment of myofascial pain syndrome. Pain Physician 2002;5:422-432.

35. Guyer BM: Mechanism of botulinum toxin in the relief of chronic pain. Curr Rev Pain 1999;3:427-431.

36. Gobel H, Heinze A, Heinze-Kuhn K, et al: Botulinum toxin A in the treatment of headache syndromes and pericranial pain syndromes. Pain 2001;91:195-199.

37. Hallet M: How does botulinum toxin work? Ann Neurol 2000; 48:7-8.

38. Hobson DE, Gladish DF: Botulinum toxin injection for cervicogenic headache. Headache 1997;37:253-255.

39. Freund BJ, Schwartz M: Treatment of chronic cervical-associated headache with botulinum toxin A: A pilot study. Headache 2000;40:231-236.

40. Freund B, Schwartz M, Symington J: Botulinum toxin: New treatment for temporomandibular disorders. Br J Oral Maxillofac Surg 2000;38:466-471.

41. von Lindern JJ, Niederhagen B, Berge S, et al: Type A botulinum toxin in the treatment of chronic facial pain after neck dissection. Head Neck 2004;26:39-45.

42. Nixdorf DR, Heo G, Major PW: Randomized controlled trial of botulinum toxin A for chronic myogenous orofacial pain. Pain 2002;99:465-473.

43. Cheshire WP, Abashian SW, Mann JD: Botulinum toxin in the treatment of myofascial pain syndrome. Pain 1994;59:65-69.

44. Wheeler AH, Goolkasian P, Gretz SS: A randomized, double-blind, prospective pilot study of botulinum toxin for refractory, unilateral, cervicothoracic, paraspinal, myofascial pain syndrome. Spine 1998;23:1662-1666.

45. Porta M: A comparative trial of botulinum toxin type A and methylprednisolone for the treatment of myofascial pain syndrome and pain from chronic muscle spasm. Pain 2000;67:101-105.

46. Foster L, Clapp L, Erickson M, et al: Botulinum toxin and chronic low back pain: A randomized, double-blind study. Neurology 2001;56:1290-1293.

47. van Tulder MW, Koes BW, Bouter LM: Conservative treatment of acute and chronic nonspecific low back pain: A systematic review of randomized controlled trials of the most common interventions. Spine 1997;22:2128-2156.

48. Bigos SJ, Bowyer OR, Braen GR, et al: Clinical Practice Guideline No. 14: Acute Low Back Problems in Adults (Publ. No. 95-0642). Rockville, Md, U.S. Department of Health and Human Services, Agency for Health Care Policy and Research, 1994.

49. Barrata R: A double-blind study of cyclobenzaprine and placebo in the treatment of acute musculoskeletal conditions of the low back. Curr Ther Res 1982;32:646-652.

50. Berry H, Hutchinson D: A multicentre placebo-controlled study in general practice to evaluate the efficacy and safety of tizanidine in acute low-back pain. J Int Med Res 1988;16:75-82.

51. Lepisto P: A comparative trial of dS 103-282 and placebo in the treatment of acute skeletal muscle spasms caused by disorders of the back. Ther Res 1979;26:454-459.

52. Gold R: Orphenadrine citrate: Sedative or muscle relaxant? Clin Ther 1978;1:451-453.

53. Browning R, Jackson JL, O'Malley PG: Cyclobenzaprine and back pain: A meta-analysis. Arch Intern Med 2001;161:1613-1620.

CHAPTER
37 Neuraxial Agents

Robert W. Hurley and Steven P. Cohen

Medication delivery to the spinal cord or the dorsal nerve roots via the intrathecal or epidural route exploits the endogenous pharmacology of the neuraxis to produce pain relief in patients. These methods of delivery require a certain degree of expertise, and are commonly used by anesthesiologists and interventional pain management specialists. The first neuraxial administration of a medication was described by Leonard Corning in 1885, first in a dog and then in a man suffering from "seminal incontinence."[1] Fourteen years later, Augustus Bier reported the first case whereby cocaine was administered intrathecally to provide surgical anesthesia.[2] The first use of a neuraxial technique to treat chronic pain was in 1901, when Sicard administered local anesthetic epidurally via the caudal route.[3] Another significant breakthrough occurred in 1942, when Manalan used a catheter to administer medication continuously for labor analgesia.[4] The epidural injection of steroids for the treatment of sciatica was first described in 1953.[5] Several years after the discovery of the endogenous opioid receptors and their respective agonists, Wang and colleagues[6] reported treating cancer pain with intrathecal morphine.

This chapter will focus on current and potential pharmacologic agents administered into the epidural or intrathecal space to produce antinociception in animals or analgesia in humans (Table 37–1). The outcomes of neuraxial anesthesia and analgesia on postsurgical morbidity, as well as on long-term neuraxial analgesia, either by intrathecal pump or a tunneled epidural catheter, is covered elsewhere in this text and hence are not addressed here.

PERIPHERAL NERVE NEUROTRANSMITTERS AND THE SPINAL CORD

A variety of mechanical, thermal, or chemical stimuli can result in the sensation of pain. Information about these painful or noxious stimuli is carried to higher brain centers by receptors and neurons distinct from those that carry innocuous somatic sensory information. Small-diameter A-delta and C-fibers primarily transmit nociceptive information. Neurotransmission by A-delta and C-fibers is accomplished via the release of numerous peptides, including substance P, calcitonin gene-related peptide, galanin, vasoactive intestinal peptide and somatostatin into the spinal cord. The excitatory amino acid glutamate is also present within small-diameter primary afferents and can be released by noxious stimulation, resulting in the activation of second-order neurons in the dorsal horn of the spinal cord.[7] The presynaptic nerve terminal of the primary afferent in the spinal cord is a potential therapeutic target. It possesses many receptor systems that can enhance transmission by increasing the release of excitatory amino acids and other transmitters, activating voltage-gated calcium channels and purinergic receptors, and inhibiting pathways involved in the modulation of pain such as α_2-adrenergic, cholinergic, serotonergic, and opioid receptors and gamma-aminobutyric acid (GABA) systems.[8-10]

Primary afferent neurons release neurotransmitters that activate postsynaptic receptors on second-order projection neurons in the spinal cord. Second-order neurons in the dorsal horn possess a wide variety of neurotransmitter receptors. A subset of these receptors results in depolarization of the neuron, leading to increased nociceptive transmission. These include the excitatory amino acid, N-methyl-D-aspartate (NMDA), DL-α-amino-3-hydroxy-5-methylisoxazole propionic acid (AMPA)–kainate, metabotropic glutamatergic (mGlu), and substance P receptors. Activation of other receptors results in hyperpolarization of postsynaptic neurons, thereby inhibiting transmission of noxious stimuli. These include the opioid, GABA$_A$, and serotonin receptors. Neurotransmission by second-order neurons on bulbar or thalamic targets is primarily through glutamate, resulting in depolarization of postsynaptic AMPA and NMDA receptor–containing neurons.[11]

NEURAXIAL AGENTS

Local Anesthetics

The most widely used drugs for neuraxial analgesia are local anesthetics, which most commonly are used to provide surgical anesthesia, postoperative pain relief, and relief of cancer pain. An extensive discussion of these agents is given in Chapter 44 and therefore the discussion of local anesthetic agents will be brief. The propagation of nerve impulses in the form of an action potential to carry sensory or motor information requires ion flux through specific channels

Table 37–1. Neuraxial Pharmacotherapy Agents

CLASSIFICATION	DRUG	CONDITIONS STUDIED	DOSE	CLINICAL EVIDENCE FOR EFFICACY
Adrenergic	Clonidine	CBP, LP, MP, PP, CP	Single dose (30-450 µg intrathecal; 100-900 µg epidural) Infusion (150-1200 µg/day intrathecal)	Moderate evidence for postoperative pain Strong evidence for cancer pain Moderate evidence for neuropathic pain Moderate evidence for labor pain Weak evidence for central pain
Cholinergic	Neostigmine	PP, LP, MP	Single dose (10-750 µg intrathecal; 75-300 µg epidural)	Moderate evidence for intrathecal administration for postoperative pain (however, significantly limited by side effects, primarily nausea) Moderate evidence for epidural administration for postoperative pain Weak evidence for epidural administration in labor pain Weak evidence for epidural administration in malignant pain
GABAergic	Midazolam	PP, LP, CBP	Single dose (1-2 mg intrathecal; 2-5 mg epidural) Infusion (500-1500 µg/day intrathecal)	Moderate evidence for postoperative pain Moderate evidence for labor pain Weak/mixed evidence for chronic back pain
	Baclofen	CP, NP, CBP	Infusion (50-500 µg/day intrathecal)	Strong evidence for central pain Moderate evidence for neuropathic pain Weak evidence for chronic back pain
Glutamatergic	Ketamine	NP, MP, PP	Single dose (25-50 mg intrathecal; 20-50 mg epidural) Infusion (2-50 mg/day intrathecal)	Weak/mixed evidence for postoperative pain; intrathecal administration associated with dysphoria Weak evidence for malignant pain Weak evidence for neuropathic pain
	CPP	NP		No evidence for neuropathic pain
Calcium channel blocker	Ziconotide	PP, MP, NP	Infusion (0.24-170 µg/day intrathecal)	Moderate evidence for neuropathic and malignant pain
	Verapamil	PP	Single dose (5 mg epidural)	Weak evidence for postoperative pain
	Nimodipine	CP	Infusion (48 mg/day epidural)	Weak evidence for postoperative pain
Adenosine	Adenosine	AP, PP, LP, NP	Single dose (500-2000 µg intrathecal)	No evidence for cancer pain Weak/mixed evidence for acute pain No evidence for postoperative pain No evidence for labor pain Weak evidence for neuropathic pain
	R-PIA	NP	Single dose (50 nmol intrathecal)	Weak evidence for neuropathic pain
Cyclooxygenase	Ketorolac	AP	Single dose (0.25-2.0 mg intrathecal)	No evidence for acute pain
	Acetylsalicylic acid	MP	Single dose (120-720 mg intrathecal)	Weak evidence for malignant pain
Somatostatin	Somatostatin	PP, MP	Single dose (250 µg epidural) Infusion (250-3000 µg/day epidural)	Weak/mixed evidence for postoperative pain Weak evidence for malignant pain
	Octreotide	CP	Infusion (480-700 µg/day intrathecal)	Weak evidence for central pain
Dopamine	Droperidol	MP, PP	Single dose (2.5 mg epidural) Infusion (1.25-5.0 mg/day)	Weak/mixed evidence for postoperative pain Weak evidence for malignant pain

AC, acute pain; CBP, chronic back pain; CP, central pain; LP, labor pain; MP, malignant (cancer) pain; NP, neuropathic pain; PP, postoperative pain.
Evidence of efficacy: strong, one or more placebo-controlled trials coupled with evidence from other studies; moderate, one placebo-controlled study with moderate support from comparative or open-label studies; weak, one controlled trial with no other supporting studies; weak/mixed, mixed evidence from placebo-controlled studies or other supporting studies; no evidence, the evidence against outweighs the evidence supporting efficacy.

in the nerve membrane. When resting membrane potential depolarizes to threshold levels, an influx of sodium ions through voltage-gated ion channels occurs, resulting in an action potential. Local anesthetic agents bind to these channels reversibly and block the conductance of sodium ions through the channels, thereby inhibiting nerve conduction.[12] Sodium channels are complex three-dimensional structures that are integral membrane proteins in the lipid bilayer of cells. Local anesthetics gain access to the sodium channel from the plasma or cytoplasmic side of the channel protein and bind within the pore of the channel.[12] The binding of sodium channels by local anesthetics is state-dependent. The local anesthetic can bind to the channel when it is open (active), closed (inactivated) or in resting states. Specifically, the receptor has the highest affinity when the channel is open or closed and the lowest affinity in the resting state.[13] These processes are not sensory-specific; thus, local anesthetics are capable of blocking the transmission of all nerve fibers, not just A-delta and C fibers. As such, a major limiting factor in the use of local anesthetics in ambulatory patients is motor blockade.

Opioids

Opioid analgesics exert their actions through inhibition of target cell activity. The existence of multiple types of opioid receptors was originally proposed by Martin and associates.[14] Subsequent in vitro and in vivo pharmacologic studies, using alkaloid-derived and synthetic compounds, have provided support for the existence of multiple opioid receptor subtypes including mu (μ), delta (δ), and kappa (κ) receptors.[15,16] Molecular cloning techniques have thus far identified three gene families that encode for these receptors.[17,18] In addition, an "orphan" opioid receptor (ORL1), which shares substantial sequence homology but does not bind prototypic opioid receptor agonists with high affinity, has also been identified.[19] All the opioid receptors belong to the guanosine triphosphate (GTP)–binding protein superfamily of metabotropic receptors. Agonist binding to opioid receptors results in activation of inwardly rectifying potassium channels, inhibition of the N-type and L-type calcium channels, inhibition of adenylate cyclase activity, or a combination of these, all processes whereby neuronal excitability can be suppressed.

Although peripherally located opioid receptors have been identified, the predominant analgesic sites are believed to reside in the central nervous system. In the brain, these receptor sites include the brainstem, thalamus, forebrain, and mesencephalon. In the spinal cord, they include postsynaptic receptors located on cells originating in the dorsal horn, as well as presynaptic receptors found on the spinal terminals of primary afferent fibers.[8]

The effects of opioids are determined not only by their affinity for endogenous receptors, but by their ability to reach those receptors. The onset of analgesia is similar for intrathecal and epidural narcotics, suggesting that the penetration of neural tissue and not the meninges is the rate-limiting step. Intrathecal opioids exert their analgesic properties by presynaptically inhibiting the release of glutamate, substance P, and calcitonin gene-related peptide, molecules believed to be responsible for transmitting nociceptive signals across synapses. Epidurally administered narcotics may work by an additional mechanism. The systemic absorption of an epidural bolus of lipophilic opioids (e.g., fentanyl and sufentanil) is similar to that which follows an intramuscular injection, and may play a role in the analgesic effects.[20,21] The conflicting results as to how epidural lipophilic opioids exert their pain-relieving properties may be explained by differing modes of administration. For example, a bolus of epidural fentanyl appears to produce analgesia mostly via spinal mechanisms, whereas uptake into the systemic circulation plays a major role in the analgesic effects produced by continuous epidural infusion. In contrast, hydrophilic opioids such as morphine are more likely to diffuse across dural membranes, where their primary analgesic effect is through receptors in the dorsal horn.[22]

Lipid solubility determines in part several other important characteristics of intrathecal opioids, including the spread of analgesia and side effects. Highly water-soluble opioids such as morphine exhibit a greater degree of rostral spread when injected into the subarachnoid or epidural space than lipid-soluble compounds, so that in pain conditions requiring higher spinal levels or more extensive coverage, the may confer a higher degree of analgesia. Conversely, because many adverse effects of intrathecally administered opioids, such as nausea and vomiting and delayed respiratory depression, are the result of interaction with opioid receptors in the brain, the more water-soluble compounds are associated with a higher incidence of these problems.

Whereas the earliest studies on the chronic use of intrathecal opioids were conducted in patients suffering from cancer pain, more recent studies have found intrathecal and epidural narcotics to be effective for nonmalignant pain as well.[23,24] These conditions include not only nociceptive pain but also neuropathic pain—a heterogeneous group of disorders originally believed to be resistant to narcotics. Certain aspects of neuropathic pain, such as tactile allodynia, may be less responsive to the effects of intrathecally administered opiates. Many neuropathic conditions therefore require adding nonopioid adjuvants to intrathecally administered opioids for successful pain relief.[25,26]

When opioids are administered directly into the cerebrospinal fluid (CSF), only a fraction of the systemic dose is required because there are no anatomic barriers to be crossed, and vascular reuptake is slow. Not all side effects of intrathecal opioids are dose-related, but in many cases the drastic reduction in dosage translates into reduced side effects. One of the primary indications for a trial with intrathecal or epidural narcotics is a good analgesic response to systemic opioids coupled with intractable side effects. Among the adverse opioid effects reduced by switching from oral formulations to intrathecal administration are sedation and constipation. Those that may be increased include pruritus, urinary retention, and edema. The mechanisms contributing to the various adverse effects of opioids are incompletely understood, but are probably multifactorial. These include those that are mediated via interaction with specific opioid receptors and those that are not. Undesirable effects not mediated by opioid receptors, such as CNS excitation and hyperalgesia, cannot be reversed with naloxone. The incidence of the various opioid-induced side effects depends on different factors, including the opioid infused, route of administration and dosage, extent of disease, concurrent drug use (including oral narcotics), age, concomitant medical problems, and prior exposure to opioids. The most frequent side effects of intrathecal morphine are constipation, urinary retention, nausea and vomiting, and libido disturbances.[27]

Adrenergic Agonists

α-Adrenergic receptors are widely distributed throughout the body. α_1-Adrenergic receptors play an essential role in the regulation of systemic vascular resistance (SVR), but have no known significant role in analgesia. Their α_2 counterparts are present throughout the peripheral and central nervous system and play a substantial role in modulating pain signals. It is thought that agonist binding to these receptors produces activation of a G protein–modulated second messenger system. However, depending on the particular α subunit—α_{2a}, α_{2b}, or α_{2c}—different physiologic consequences may occur, and the neuronal responses can be inhibitory or excitatory.[28] The α_{2b} subtype produces hemodynamic responses (primarily hypotension), whereas the α_{2a} receptor is responsible for analgesia and sedation.[28,29] The mechanism of action of neuraxial α_2 agonists is similar to that of opioids. Presynaptically, they bind to α_2 receptors on small primary afferent neurons, resulting in hyperpolarization and diminished release of neurotransmitters involved in pain transmission. On postsynaptic neurons, α_2 agonists hyperpolarize the cell by increasing potassium conductance through G_i-coupled potassium channels. Clonidine is the prototypic nonselective α_2 agonist used to produce antinociception, although it has substantial hemodynamic side effects because of its nonselectivity. A newer agent, dexmedetomidine, is a selective α_{2a} receptor agonist that contains analgesic and sedative properties, with fewer cardiovascular effects.[30] α-Adrenergic agonists have also been shown to activate spinal cholinergic neurons, which may contribute to their analgesic effects. In addition to their antinociceptive properties, α_2 agonists produce dose-dependent sedation, presumably by inhibitory mechanisms involving the brainstem.

The antihypertensive medication clonidine is the most studied α_2 agonist for neuraxial use; α_2 agonists have been administered intrathecally in humans since 1985. Although clonidine is U.S. Food and Drug Administration (FDA)–approved for epidural use only in cancer pain, clinical reports have shown it to be effective intrathecally and epidurally for nonmalignant pain as well.[31,32] Studies have shown that clonidine may prolong and enhance the effects of intrathecal and epidural anesthesia when coadministered with local anesthetics, and that adding it to opioids can extend the duration of pain relief for labor analgesia and postoperative pain.[33-35] However, for acute pain, the evidence that adding clonidine to an epidural or intrathecal opioid is more effective than either analgesic alone is weak and inconsistent.[36] Neuraxial clonidine has shown efficacy in treating central pain and spasticity after spinal cord injury.[37] α_2-Receptor agonists may also be suitable for patients suffering from neuropathic pain. In a randomized, placebo-controlled study evaluating epidural clonidine in refractory reflex sympathetic dystrophy, Rauck and coworkers[38] found that 300 µg of clonidine is equally effective but associated with less side effects than 700 µg.

Wu and colleagues[39] have compared the effects of preoperative epidural clonidine followed by patient-controlled epidural analgesia (PCEA) with clonidine, morphine, and ropivacaine with a control group that received preoperative epidural saline followed by PCEA with morphine and ropivacaine in 40 patients scheduled for elective colorectal surgery. Patients in the clonidine group exhibited longer PCEA trigger times, lower pain scores at rest and while coughing, less morphine consumption, and a faster return of bowel function throughout the 72-hour postoperative period compared with patients in the control group. Interestingly, the concentrations of certain proinflammatory cytokines were also decreased in the clonidine group 12 and 24 hours following surgery. The most common side effects of neuraxial clonidine are sedation, hypotension, and bradycardia. Hypotension and bradycardia are likely the result of α_2 effects on preganglionic fibers in the thoracic spinal cord. Sedation results from actions at supraspinal sites.

Clonidine has undergone extensive neurotoxicity testing in animals. The continuous intrathecal infusion of clonidine alone (2 mg/mL at 100 µL/h) and clonidine combined with morphine in dogs was not associated with any spinal neurotoxicity, and was reported to decrease the magnitude of inflammation associated with intrathecal morphine administration.[40] Clonidine is currently considered to be a second-line drug for neuraxial use in patients with chronic pain.[26]

Cholinergic Agonists

Cholinergic receptors are divided into the G protein–coupled (metabotropic) receptors (the muscarinic subtype) and ion channel (ionotropic) receptors (the nicotinic subtype). Pharmacologic molecular cloning studies have led to the classification of muscarinic acetylcholine receptors (mAChRs) in central and peripheral tissues into five distinct muscarinic receptor subtypes—M1, M2, M3, M4, and M5. Studies of radioligand binding and analysis of the mRNA of muscarinic receptors have demonstrated the existence of M1, M2, M3, and M4 receptors in the spinal cord. Neuronal nicotinic acetylcholine receptors (nAChRs) are pentameric ligand-gated ion channels, and molecular cloning has identified nine α and three β subunits. These subunits assemble to form functional receptors in heteromeric combinations or as homopentamers. Receptor subunit composition underlies the differences in functional properties, and there is considerable variation in subunit expression throughout the spinal cord.

In animal models, the intrathecal administration of muscarinic cholinergic agonists results in antinociception, an effect that is reversed by muscarinic antagonists.[41] In contrast, the intrathecal administration of nicotinic agonists results in a decrease in nociceptive threshold (hyperalgesia), an increase in spontaneous pain behaviors,[42] or both in most studies, but antinociception in others.[43] The increase in pain-related behaviors after the intrathecal administration of nicotinic agonists may be the result of an associated increase in excitatory transmitter release. This hyperalgesia is reversed by administration of intrathecal nicotinic or glutamate receptor antagonists.[44,45] The diversity of nAChR subunits probably contributes to the seemingly paradoxical analgesic and hyperalgesic effects of nicotinic agonists. However, the predominant analgesic effects of neuraxial cholinergic drugs are thought to be mediated by muscarinic M1 and M3 receptors found in dorsal root ganglia and superficial laminae of the dorsal horn, with a more modest contribution by nicotinic receptors.[46] The cholinesterase inhibitors, including neostigmine and physostigmine, increase the amount of available acetylcholine by inhibiting its metabolism. These drugs have been found in numerous animal studies to produce antinociception, anti-allodynia, and antihyperalgesia after neuraxial administration.[47,48]

Because of the lack of available selective muscarinic agonists and the paradoxical and unpredictable effects of neuraxially administered nicotinic agonists, human research has focused on the administration of cholinesterase inhibitors, primarily neostigmine. Despite promising data from animal studies, the administration of intrathecal neostigmine by itself to humans has been somewhat disappointing. After preclinical toxicity screening, neostigmine was introduced into clinical trials for intrathecal administration. Intrathecal administration was found to produce analgesia to experimental pain stimuli in naïve volunteers and patients suffering from cancer and postoperative pain.[49-51] Unfortunately, the pain relief was accompanied by severe and debilitating nausea; therefore, the use of intrathecal neostigmine as a sole analgesic is not currently recommended. However, the addition of neostigmine to intrathecal opioids and local anesthetics has been found to prolong and enhance analgesia, with only a modest increase in the incidence of nausea and vomiting. In a study examining the postoperative analgesic effects of intrathecal bupivacaine with various combinations of fentanyl and neostigmine after abdominal hysterectomy, intrathecal neostigmine reduced postoperative pain scores and opioid requirements to a similar degree as fentanyl, with the greatest effect observed in patients receiving the high dose (25 µg) neostigmine-fentanyl combination.[52]

In a clinical study comparing different combinations of neuraxial analgesics for labor analgesia in healthy parturients, patients receiving the four-drug combination of bupivacaine, fentanyl, clonidine, and neostigmine had significantly longer analgesia than those receiving bupivacaine and fentanyl or bupivacaine, fentanyl, and clonidine.[53] This enhanced analgesia of neuraxial neostigmine with local anesthetics was confirmed in a randomized, double-blind study by Kumar and colleagues[54] assessing the addition of neostigmine, ketamine, and midazolam to bupivacaine in 80 children administered a single-shot caudal injection for inguinal hernia repair. The duration of complete analgesia was significantly longer in the neostigmine-bupivacaine group than in patients who received midazolam-bupivacaine, ketamine-bupivacaine, or bupivacaine alone. In addition to enhancing sensory blockade, combining neostigmine with an assortment of other intrathecal medications may also prolong muscle weakness and increase sedation.[55] The most commonly encountered side effects of intrathecal neostigmine are nausea, vomiting, and at doses exceeding 150 µg, sedation and leg weakness. At low doses, neostigmine is devoid of significant hemodynamic effects. However, at higher doses (750 µg), increases in blood pressure, heart rate, respiratory rate, and anxiety may occur.

Epidural administration of neostigmine alone or in combination with local anesthetics or opioids has been found to decrease postoperative pain effectively. Omais and associates[56] examined postoperative analgesia following the epidural administration of neostigmine and the intrathecal administration of morphine and bupivacaine in patients undergoing orthopedic surgery. The addition of 60 µg of epidural neostigmine resulted in decreased consumption of adjuvant analgesics and a prolonged time to first request for additional analgesia, with a small increase in nausea. Most clinical studies evaluating epidural neostigmine have been performed in the area of obstetric anesthesia. Roelants and coworkers[57] conducted a prospective, randomized trial assessing the value of combining epidural neostigmine with sufentanil for pain relief in the first stage of labor. The authors concluded that adding 500 µg of neostigmine to 10 µg of sufentanil produced comparable analgesia to 20 µg of sufentanil, with no additional side effects. In a randomized controlled study evaluating various doses of epidural neostigmine in parturients undergoing elective cesarean sections with bupivacaine-fentanyl intrathecal anesthesia, Kaya and colleagues[58] found that the addition of epidural neostigmine to an intrathecal anesthetic confers moderate analgesic benefits compared with saline over the first 24 hours. No dose-response relationship was found between the lowest (75 µg) and highest (300 µg) doses, although patients in the 300-µg neostigmine group experienced more intraoperative shivering and sedation. Thirty-five percent of patients who received 300 µg of neostigmine experienced nausea up to 4 hours postoperatively, although this trend was not quite statistically significant.

Unfortunately, there are few studies evaluating the long-term use of neuraxial neostigmine for chronic pain. Lauretti and associates[59] found that the epidural administration of a low dose of neostigmine (100 µg) in combination with morphine is associated with improved analgesia when compared with opioid treatment alone in terminal cancer patients followed for 20 days. This improvement was not associated with an increased incidence of adverse effects. Neostigmine is currently considered a fifth-line drug for long-term intrathecal use in chronic pain patients.[26]

Gamma-Aminobutyric Acid Agonists

Three types of GABA receptor are currently recognized—$GABA_A$, $GABA_B$, and $GABA_C$. Only $GABA_A$ and $GABA_B$ receptors are present in significant quantities within the CNS. The $GABA_A$ receptor is a ligand-gated ion channel. Activation of this receptor by GABA results in an influx of chloride ions and stabilization of the membrane potential, which decreases neuronal excitability. The receptor possesses two binding sites for GABA, as well as sites at which barbiturates, inhalational anesthetics, neurosteroids, and benzodiazepines bind to modulate the action of GABA. The receptor itself is a pentameric arrangement of different subunits. In contrast, the $GABA_B$ receptor is a metabotropic receptor. Activation of the $GABA_B$ receptor by GABA results in activation of inwardly rectifying potassium channels, inhibition of calcium channels, inhibition of adenylate cyclase activity, or a combination of these effects, all of which serve to suppress neuronal excitability.

In laboratory animals, $GABA_A$ agonists including muscimol, isoguvacine, and midazolam have antiallodynic and antihyperalgesic effects in chronic pain models, whereas the $GABA_A$ antagonists bicuculline and picrotoxin induce allodynia and hyperalgesia in naïve rats. However, $GABA_A$ receptors are also closely linked to large-diameter afferents, and therefore are likely involved in modulating innocuous sensation as well. Similar to $GABA_A$ receptors, $GABA_B$ receptors are found in greatest abundance in the superficial dorsal horn of the spinal cord. Within the GABAergic system, nociceptive transmission is primarily thought to be regulated by $GABA_B$ receptor activity. The $GABA_B$ receptor agonist baclofen blocks the activity of peripheral C and A-delta nociceptive fibers. Furthermore, in the spinal cord, $GABA_B$ receptors are found on interneurons as well as on terminals from primary afferent neurons. $GABA_B$ receptor agonists administered via the intrathecal or epidural route

produce pre- and postsynaptic inhibition and therefore block the release of glutamate, substance P, and calcitonin gene-related peptide (CGRP) from primary afferents, and GABA from interneurons.

In naïve animals, intrathecal administration of antagonists to either receptor results in increased pain behaviors, suggesting that tonic release of GABA in the spinal cord prevents innocuous stimuli from being perceived as noxious. In animal models of acute and persistent nociception, $GABA_B$ agonists such as baclofen produce antinociception and antiallodynia, respectively, at doses at which no motor impairment is observed.[60,61] In contrast, the highly selective $GABA_A$ agonist muscimol was found to be effective only in animal models of persistent nociception.[62] In the same study, midazolam, which is the only $GABA_A$ agonist currently available for human use, was ineffective in acute or persistent pain models at doses that do not produce substantial motor impairment. In summary, the results from animal studies suggest that both $GABA_A$ and $GABA_B$ receptor agonists could be used to treat chronic pain.

In human studies, both $GABA_A$ and $GABA_B$ agonists have been shown to contain analgesic effects when injected into the intrathecal or epidural space. The literature has indicated that the neuraxial administration of $GABA_A$ agonists in combination with local anesthetics increases the duration of motor and sensory block, increases the time to first analgesic request, and decreases postoperative analgesic requirements. The administration of the $GABA_A$ agonist midazolam via the intrathecal or epidural route in combination with a mixture of other analgesics, including local anesthetics and opioids, was found to reduce opioid requirements and enhance postoperative analgesia for different surgical procedures.[63-66] Sajedi and Islami[67] have found that the addition of 5 mg of midazolam to epidural lidocaine results in the faster onset of sensory loss and longer durations for motor and sensory blockade than patients who received 3 mg of midazolam or placebo during elective lower limb surgery. In a double-blind study evaluating the effects of adding intrathecal midazolam to bupivacaine in patients undergoing hemorrhoidectomy, the addition of midazolam was found to expedite the onset of intrathecal analgesia in a dose-dependent manner.[68] In a pediatric population, the combination of bupivacaine and midazolam delivered via a caudal injection delayed the child's first request for adjuvant analgesics when compared with bupivacaine alone.[54] Other studies have found intrathecal midazolam to be effective in treating chronic mechanical low back pain, musculoskeletal pain, and neurogenic pain.[69] The administration of subarachnoid midazolam was not shown to be effective in treating pain associated with peripheral vascular disease and malignancy.[69]

The safety of the neuraxial administration of midazolam is controversial. Numerous animal studies have shown evidence of neurotoxicity with intrathecal midazolam. Svensson and coworkers[70] found histologic evidence of neuronal death in the spinal cords of rats after 20 consecutive days of 100 mcg intrathecal injections of midazolam. Unfortunately, the relative doses and concentrations of midazolam used in these animal studies were many times higher than those used in human studies. Malinovsky and colleagues[71] reported that midazolam (1 mg/mL) produces histologic pathology greater than that of lidocaine or saline controls. Similar results were obtained by Erdine and associates,[72] who found that rabbits infused with both preservative-containing and preservative-free intrathecal midazolam (300 µg daily, 1 mg/mL) over 5 days displayed vascular and other histologic spinal cord lesions on microscopic examination.

Part of the controversy revolves around the pH of the medications administered. In an attempt to resolve this Bozkurt and colleagues[73] administered normal saline, midazolam, and a saline vehicle control with the same acidic pH as midazolam epidurally in newborn rabbits. During electron microscopy examination on days 2 and 7, both the acidic midazolam and saline groups displayed significant pathologic spinal cord changes, such as the degeneration of vacuoles, cytoplasm, and neurofilaments, disruption of myelin sheaths, lysis of cell membranes, perivascular edema, and pyknosis of nuclei. In contrast, the normal pH saline group displayed normal histology on spinal cord sectioning. More recent studies using multiple doses of commercially available concentrations of midazolam in two animal species have found no histopathologic or behavior differences compared with saline controls.[74]

Currently, the use of midazolam as an intrathecal analgesic is not FDA-approved because of safety concerns. However, in clinical studies, there have been no reported adverse cardiovascular (hypotension or bradycardia), urologic (urinary hesitance or incontinence), or gastrointestinal (nausea or vomiting) side effects when compared with local anesthetic alone. In one human study involving 1100 patients who were administered intrathecal local anesthetic or local anesthetic and midazolam, 2 mg, for surgery, the authors reported no increased incidence of postoperative neurologic signs or symptoms or any other complications between the two groups.[75] Midazolam is currently considered a fourth-line neuraxial treatment for chronic pain.[26]

Numerous studies support the use of neuraxial baclofen for spasticity in humans. Multiple clinical trials have shown intrathecal baclofen to be effective for a variety of central pain conditions as well, including stroke, spinal cord injury, cerebral palsy, and multiple sclerosis.[76-79] Intrathecal baclofen has also been found to be an effective treatment for noncentral neuropathic pain conditions such as phantom pain and complex regional pain syndrome.[80-82] In a small study by Lind and associates,[83] it was found that the addition of intrathecal baclofen in patients being treated with spinal cord stimulation for neuropathic improves pain scores to a greater degree than concomitant treatment with oral baclofen. The beneficial effect of intrathecal baclofen is dose-

dependent, peaking at 50 µg. Neuraxial baclofen has also been found to be a benefit in the treatment of musculoskeletal pain. Loubser and Akman[84] found that intrathecal baclofen reduced musculoskeletal but not neurogenic pain in 12 patients with chronic spinal cord injury–related pain. Based on the results of this study and the temporal disparity regarding its analgesic effects on central pain and muscle spasm, it is likely that different pain-relieving mechanisms exist for these two conditions.

At therapeutic doses, baclofen is associated with numerous adverse effects, including drowsiness, flaccidity, headache, confusion, hypotension, weight gain, constipation, nausea, urinary frequency, and sexual dysfunction.[85] Intrathecal baclofen overdose can lead to respiratory depression, seizures, obtundation and, if not adequately treated, death. Withdrawal from abrupt cessation of intrathecal baclofen treatment can also be life-threatening, and there is some evidence to suggest that replacement with oral baclofen may not always be adequate to control the symptoms.[86] Baclofen is currently considered a fourth-line treatment for chronic pain.[26]

Glutamatergic Receptor Antagonists

Similar to GABAergic and cholinergic receptors, glutamatergic receptors are divided into the G protein–coupled (metabotropic) receptors (mGluRs), and ion channel (ionotropic) receptors, which include NMDA, AMPA, and kainate receptors. NMDA receptors contain ion channels permeable to calcium, sodium, and potassium. The NMDA ion channel is somewhat unique in that ambient concentrations of magnesium block NMDA responses in a use- and voltage-dependent manner.[87] In addition to the glutamate binding site, the NMDA receptor has binding sites for glycine, which functions as an obligatory coagonist, phencyclidine-like compounds, and endogenous protons and polyamines. Endogenous protons inhibit NMDA receptors via their interactions with an extracellular proton sensor on one of the receptor subunits. Endogenous polyamines such as spermine and spermidine bind at a separate site but shield this proton receptor, thereby potentiating NMDA receptor actions.[87] AMPA and kainate receptors function as ion channels permeable to sodium and potassium. Activation of the ionotropic receptors results in depolarization and neuronal excitation. Metabotropic glutamate receptors are divided into three groups. Group I receptors are positively coupled to phosphatidylinositol hydrolysis, and activation of these receptors ultimately results in increases in intracellular calcium levels. The second and third groups of mGluRs are similar to opioid receptors in that they are negatively coupled to adenylate cyclase; hence, activation of these receptors results in neuronal inhibition.

In animal studies, selective agonists at the NMDA, AMPA, kainate, and group I mGlu receptors applied intrathecally produce spontaneous pain behavior in naïve animals and result in allodynia and hyperalgesia in neuropathic and inflammatory models of persistent pain. Antagonists to these receptors reverse these nociceptive responses.

In humans, there are no AMPA, kainate, or mGluR agonists or antagonists available for clinical use. As such, the most widely researched glutamate modulators are the NMDA receptor antagonists. Perhaps the most studied NMDA antagonist for neuraxial use is ketamine, a noncompetitive NMDA antagonist that has been administered both epidurally and intrathecally in humans for acute and chronic pain relief. Following tissue injury, the activation of spinal NMDA receptors induces a state of facilitated processing from repetitive small afferent fiber stimulation, leading to an increased response to high- and low-threshold stimulation and enhanced receptor field size. This process, considered to abolish "wind-up pain" is thought to be responsible for phenomena such as allodynia and hyperalgesia. In a case report by Kristensen and colleagues,[88] the intrathecal administration of CPP (3-[2-carboxypoperazin-4-yl] propyl-1-phosphonic acid), a competitive NMDA antagonist, was noted to suppress "wind-up" but not spontaneous pain or allodynia in a patient with a peripheral nerve injury. Four hours after the last injection of CPP, psychomimetic side effects developed that were attributed to the rostral spread of medication. In combination with intrathecal morphine alone or with other agents in patients suffering from cancer pain, the addition of intrathecal ketamine was shown to enhance the analgesic effects of opioids and other drugs while reducing the development of tolerance.[89]

Bion[90] has reported that hyperbaric intrathecal ketamine mixed with epinephrine provides adequate short-term anesthesia in young soldiers undergoing field surgery. However, a more recent open-label study by Hawksworth and Serpell[91] of 10 male patients undergoing prostate surgery found that the high frequency of psychomimetic disturbances, the short duration of action, and the high incidence of incomplete anesthesia preclude its use as a sole anesthetic agent. Similar findings were reported by Kathirvel and associates[92] in a prospective study involving 30 healthy women undergoing brachytherapy application for cervical cancer. The authors found that although the addition of 25 mg of ketamine had local anesthetic-sparing effects, it neither extended postoperative analgesia nor reduced postoperative analgesic requirements. Compared with patients who received bupivacaine alone, those who received bupivacaine and ketamine experienced an increased incidence of nausea, vomiting, sedation, dizziness, and "strange feelings." In an interesting case report, the long-term intrathecal administration of the S(+)- ketamine enantiomer was found to be effective in a patient with severe neuropathic cancer pain refractory to conventional therapy.[93] This study reported no adverse side effects and found low plasma concentrations of ketamine after the third week of treatment.

Epidurally administered ketamine has been found to be a clinically more viable treatment than intrathecal delivery, with a lower incidence of dysphoric and other adverse effects. In a randomized, double-blind study by Choe and coworkers,[94] epidurally administered ketamine was found to prolong the duration of analgesia and decrease the number of patients requiring supplemental injections when combined with epidural morphine for upper abdominal surgery. In a study involving patients undergoing hepatic resection, the combination of epidural ketamine and morphine was found to provide superior pain relief to morphine alone. In older patients, the epidural ketamine dose was reduced by 33% (20 vs. 30 mg).[95] There were no reports of psychomimetic effects, neurologic findings, or any other complications in this study. In a study by Himmelseher and colleagues[96] assessing the impact of adding S(+)-ketamine to epidural anesthesia with ropivacaine in patients undergoing knee arthroplasty, the combination group experienced significantly longer pain relief than patients receiving local anesthetic alone.

Not all studies have found epidural ketamine to be beneficial. Lauretti and associates[97] found no benefit to adding epidural ketamine to clonidine in 56 patients undergoing orthopedic surgical procedures. The 24-hour postoperative pain scores, time to first rescue medication, and quality of analgesia were similar in the clonidine, ketamine, and clonidine-ketamine combination groups. Weir and Fee,[98] in a double-blind study, found that adding ketamine to epidural bupivacaine for knee replacement surgery failed to prolong postoperative analgesia or reduce analgesic requirements, but did result in significantly more side effects. Most of the existing literature has demonstrated that epidural ketamine in doses ranging from 0.5 to 1 mg/kg is well tolerated in patients of all age groups and is most effective when combined with opioids or local anesthetics.

The potential neurotoxicity of intrathecal ketamine remains a subject of controversy. In most countries, racemic formulations (50% S(+)- and 50% R(−)-ketamine) are available either preservative-free or with preservatives such as benzethonium chloride and chlorobutanol. Karpinski and coworkers[99] reported a terminal cancer patient who received a 3-week intrathecal infusion of racemic ketamine and was found to have subpial vacuolar myelopathy on autopsy. Stotz and colleagues[100] reported a similar finding. On postmortem examination of a terminal cancer patient who received a 7-day trial of intrathecal ketamine, focal lymphocytic vasculitis close to the catheter injection site was found. Although no human studies of preservative-free racemic or pure S(+)-ketamine have been performed to examine the histopathologic effects in humans, preservative-free racemic ketamine has been shown to be without apparent neurotoxic effects after repeated administration in animals.[101] Ketamine is not currently FDA-approved for neuraxial use in the United States and is considered a sixth-line medication for the treatment of chronic pain.[26]

Calcium Channel Antagonists

Voltage-dependent calcium channel (VDCC) conduction plays an integral role in pain transmission. Diversity among these voltage-gated calcium channels was originally described through differences in the biophysical properties of calcium currents recorded from individual neurons. Multiple distinct voltage-gated calcium currents were observed, including the L-type responsive to dihydropyridines, the T-type response to ethosuximide, and the N-type and P/Q-type responsive to conotoxins. Molecular cloning has led to the identification of multiple genes encoding calcium channels corresponding to the biophysical and pharmacologic profiles of the receptor subtypes. VDCCs are found in the plasma membrane of all excitable cells, including neurons of the peripheral and central nervous systems. These calcium channels are found in high concentrations in the dorsal horn of the spinal cord and dorsal root ganglia.

Neuraxial administration of some VDCC modulators has been shown to produce antinociception, antiallodynia, and antihyperalgesia in animals. High-threshold VDCCs, including N and P/Q channels, are primarily found at synaptic sites involved in the release of transmitters; L-type channels are mainly observed at cell bodies and dendrites.[102] Several VDCCs have been found to colocalize in the same neuron; therefore, antagonists to a given channel type usually block only a fraction of the VDCCs present and hence may have additive effects when combined. Finally, the relative importance of the various channel types depends on the functional status of the neuron. For instance, in acute models of nociception in uninjured naïve animals, there is a large body of evidence for N-types, limited evidence for L-types, and no evidence that P/Q types produce antinociception. However, under conditions of persistent nociception induced in animals by chemical, inflammatory, or neuropathic stimuli, all three of these subtypes have been found to have antiallodynic or antihyperalgesic properties.[103] Although the physiologic and pharmacologic properties of VDCCs are largely determined by the molecular identity of the α_1 subunit, the auxiliary subunits, including $\alpha_2\delta_1$, also play a substantial role in receptors' characteristics. Gabapentin and pregabalin are two medications originally designed as structural analogues of GABA. However, neither drug is an agonist at $GABA_A$ or $GABA_B$ receptors, and neither drug acutely alters GABA uptake. It is likely that their analgesic effects are mediated at the $\alpha_2\delta_1$ subunits of VDCCs, for which both have substantial affinity.[104] Intrathecal gabapentin has no effect on an animal's nociceptive threshold in the uninjured state, but has antihyperalgesic and antiallodynic properties in animal models of chronic pain.[105] A substantial portion of the effects of gabapentin are mediated by the N-type VDCC.[105]

Ziconotide, an N-type calcium channel blocker, is a synthetic form of the peptide ω-conotoxin MVIIA isolated from the venom of the marine cone snail *Conus magus*. It potently blocks N-type VDCCs in vitro and inhibits wind-up. In a double-blind study in humans examining the effects of a continuous intrathecal infusion of ziconotide started prior to surgical incision and continued for 48 to 72 hours postoperatively, patients in the treatment group had lower pain scores and decreased postoperative patient-controlled analgesia (PCA) morphine requirements compared with those receiving a placebo infusion. Patients who received both high- and low-dose ziconotide infusions reported lower pain scores and had reduced postoperative opioid requirements compared with those receiving a placebo infusion.[106] However, in four of the six patients receiving high-dose ziconotide (7 vs. 0.7 μg/hr), adverse effects such as blurred vision, nystagmus, dizziness, and sedation necessitated discontinuing the infusion. In a multicenter, double-blind, placebo-controlled study evaluating intrathecal ziconotide for the treatment of refractory pain in 111 patients with cancer and AIDS, Staats and coworkers[107] found that the treatment group obtained significantly better pain relief than control patients (53% vs. 18% improvement). The observation that there was no loss of efficacy for ziconotide in the maintenance phase is consistent with animal studies showing the absence of tolerance with calcium channel blockers. The most common side effects noted in this study were confusion, somnolence, and urinary retention. All side effects were reversible, with their incidence decreasing after the initial dosing period. Currently, ziconotide is considered to be a fourth-line treatment.[26]

Epidural administration of VDCC modulators has also been performed. In a double-blind study conducted in healthier cohorts, adding a low dose of the L-type calcium channel blocker verapamil (5 mg) to epidural bupivacaine both pre- and post-surgical incision was found to reduce postoperative analgesic requirements in patients undergoing abdominal surgery.[108] In a case report, Filos and colleagues[109] have described modest and short-lived analgesic benefit of epidural nimodipine in two terminal cancer patients. The authors reported significant discomfort on administration, but no increased incidence of sedation, mood disturbances, or hypotension was noted in the treatment group.

Adenosine Agonists

Extracellular adenosine and adenosine triphosphate (ATP) have been proposed as neurotransmitters. Adenosine is believed to modulate the transmission of nociceptive information by its action at peripheral, spinal, and supraspinal receptor sites. These receptors are divided into two groups, purinergic 1 (P_1) and purinergic 2 (P_2) receptors, at which adenosine and ATP act, respectively. These receptors can be further subdivided into adenosine A_1, A_{2a}, A_{2b}, and A_3 receptors, all of which are metabotropic, and ATP P_{2X} and

P_{2Y} receptors, which are ionotropic and metabotropic, respectively.

Numerous studies in animals have demonstrated that intrathecal or systemic administration of adenosine and adenosine analogues inhibit pain behavior in response to noxious stimuli in acute and chronic models of nociception. Neuraxially administered A_1 receptor agonists produce antinociceptive properties in a number of acute, inflammatory, and neuropathic pain models.[110] In contrast, the intrathecal administration of ATP results in pronociceptive behaviors and a decrease in nociceptive thresholds[111] through the activation of the P_{2X} receptor. Activation of spinal P_{2Y} receptors results in antinociception[112] but this effect is subordinate to the pronociceptive properties of the P_{2X} receptor.

In a phase I clinical safety study published in 1998 by Rane and associates,[113] the intrathecal injection of adenosine in 12 healthy volunteers reduced areas of secondary allodynia after skin inflammation and decreased forearm ischemic tourniquet pain, but had no effect on the cold pressor test. No adverse side effects were noted, although one patient who received a 2000-µg injection (ranges tested were from 500 to 2000 µg) experienced transient low back pain. In a case report on a patient with neuropathic leg pain and tactile-allodynia, a single intrathecal injection of the A_1 agonist R-phenylisopropyl adenosine (R-PIA) provided relief of the patient's stimulus-dependent pain.[114] However, 1000 µg of intrathecal adenosine produced no significant impact on postoperative analgesic requirements or Visual Analogue Scale (VAS) pain scores in women undergoing hysterectomies compared with placebo.[115]

In a randomized double-blind study conducted in 25 health parturients, Rane and coworkers[116] found no clinically or statistically significant benefit when a one-time dose of adenosine, 500 µg, was added to intrathecal sufentanil for labor pain. In a study of a different formulation of adenosine marketed in the United States, Eisenach and colleagues[117] found that intrathecal adenosine reduces hyperalgesia and allodynia associated with intradermal capsaicin injection, but has no effect on acute noxious chemical or thermal stimulation. A follow-up study by the same group of investigators showed that intrathecal adenosine reduces areas of allodynia by 25% in volunteers given subdermal capsaicin.[118] These findings are consistent with those of Rane and associates[116] and indicate that adenosine may be more effective for neuropathic pain than for acute pain. The only side effects noted in the initial safety studies were headache and back pain.

There are no published studies investigating the long-term infusion of intrathecal adenosine in patients with chronic pain. To date, all human studies assessing neuraxial adenosine have been in either the perioperative setting or experimental pain models. Although adenosine shows promise as a treatment for chronic pain, it is premature to comment on its safety or efficacy. Currently, adenosine is considered a fifth-line treatment for chronic pain.[26]

Cyclooxygenase Inhibitors

There is a growing body of research that implicates the cyclooxygenase (COX) isoenzymes COX-1 and COX-2 as playing a role in the development and maintenance of spinal neuropathic pain.[119] In the spinal cord, prostaglandin E_2 (PGE_2) acts presynaptically to increase the release of glutamate from primary afferent C fibers and postsynaptically to excite dorsal horn neurons directly by activation of nonselective cation currents.[120-122] Both effects promote the development and maintenance of central sensitization and enhanced pain states. Intrathecal administration of nonsteroidal anti-inflammatory drugs (NSAIDs) prevents the development of hyperalgesia and inhibits the release of PGE_2.[123,124] In an animal experiment using a peripheral nerve injury model, the COX-1–selective NSAID ketorolac provided significantly longer antinociception than the COX-2–selective NSAID NS-398 (6 days vs. 2 hours).[125] These findings are consistent with experiments showing potent antinociceptive effects without neurotoxicity following intrathecal ketorolac administration.[126] In a study by Parris and coworkers[127] investigating intrathecal ketorolac and morphine in an animal model of neuropathic pain, it was demonstrated that both drugs possess antinociceptive properties, with morphine being more potent than ketorolac for all outcome measures except cold allodynia, in which the effects of the two drugs were found to be similar.

In humans, there have been several studies examining the analgesic effects of intrathecal aspirin in patients with chronic refractory pain.[128,129] In a large study conducted in 60 cancer patients with intractable pain, a single intrathecal dose of isobaric lysine acetylsalicylate (doses ranged from 120 to 720 mg) resulted in excellent relief in 78% of cases, with the duration of analgesia lasting from 3 weeks to 1 month on average. The only significant side effect was fatigability. An open-label, dose-escalating, phase I safety study assessing preservative-free intrathecal ketorolac in young healthy volunteers demonstrated no adverse side effects other than a dose-dependent decrease in heart rate lasting 1 hour after injection. Of note, the threshold to heat in these volunteers was unaffected by any dose of neuraxial ketorolac.[130] In a report by Lauretti and colleagues,[131] inadvertent epidural diclofenac injection by family members in two terminal cancer patients was reported to provide pain relief ranging from several hours to 2 days after several previously unsuccessful epidural trials. Although the intrathecal use of nonselective COX-1 inhibitors appears to hold promise in the treatment of neuropathic pain, long-term efficacy and safety studies are lacking. Ketorolac is currently considered a fifth-line treatment of chronic pain.[26]

Other Neuraxial Agents

Somatostatin Agonists

There is extensive literature on the use of neuraxial somatostatin for pain relief. To date, at least six somatostatin receptors have been identified, dispersed throughout the periaqueductal gray, ventral horn, primary afferent neurons, and substantia gelatinosa. The antinociceptive effects of somatostatin result from presynaptic inhibition. Stimulation of somatostatin receptors results in hyperpolarization of the cell via a G protein–coupled inwardly rectifying potassium current. This serves to block coupled calcium channels, reduce transmitter release, and decrease the synthesis of cAMP.

Epidural somatostatin has been demonstrated in several studies to provide postoperative pain relief for patients undergoing major surgical procedures.[132,133] In an open-label study assessing the effect of 250 µg of epidural somatostatin on postoperative pain after abdominal surgery, complete pain relief (no other analgesics required) was obtained in all eight patients.[133] In two patients, an epidural somatostatin infusion also provided adequate intraoperative analgesia. There were no reported side effects in this pilot study.

There are also reports of intrathecal and epidural somatostatin being used for the relief of cancer pain. In a study performed by Mollenholt and associates[134] examining the efficacy of continuous intrathecal and epidural infusions of somatostatin in eight patients with intractable cancer pain unresponsive to opioids, demyelination of spinal nerve roots and dorsal columns were noted in two of the eight patients at autopsy. None demonstrated any clinical signs of neurologic deficits during treatment. Because the patients were receiving other treatments for cancer, including chemotherapy and radiation treatment, the pathologic changes could not definitively be attributed to somatostatin. All patients in this investigation required rapid dose escalation over a relatively short period, perhaps indicating the development of tolerance. Analgesia was rated as either "good" or "excellent" in six of the eight patients. One patient experienced nausea, headache, and vertigo during the last 5 days of somatostatin treatment, and another became agitated and tremulous during the first night of therapy.

In another report, intrathecal octreotide, a synthetic analogue of somatostatin with a longer half-life, was noted to provide long-term pain relief in two patients, one of whom was suffering from refractory central pain secondary to multiple sclerosis.[135] In this patient, a double-blind case report with saline resulted in a sharp increase in pain during the 2-week placebo period, necessitating an increase in supplemental opioids. The patient continued on the intrathecal somatostatin therapy for 5 years, with no adverse side effects. The increase in somatostatin required during this period was modest, from 20 to 29 µg/hr.

Not all studies examining intrathecally administered somatostatin for pain relief have found the drug to be of benefit. In a randomized controlled trial assessing epidural diamorphine and somatostatin in 24 patients undergoing cholecystectomy, only the patients who received intraoperative diamorphine required less postoperative analgesics.[136] The neurax-

ial use of somatostatin was associated with minimal side effects. However, neuraxial somatostatin and its analogues have been reported to produce substantial neurotoxicity in animals,[137,138] and there have been no recent clinical trials assessing neuraxial somatostatin as an analgesic. Octreotide is currently considered a sixth-line treatment of chronic pain.[26]

Dopamine Agonists

The mechanism by which neuraxial droperidol exerts its antinociceptive effects has not been fully delineated, but may involve D_1 and D_2 receptors in descending dopaminergic tracts in the dorsal horn of the spinal cord.[139] When administered parenterally, neuroleptic drugs have been demonstrated to have analgesic as well as sedative and antiemetic effects in humans. In several clinical studies including two randomized controlled trials, the butyrophenone droperidol was shown to potentiate epidural analgesia with opioids.[140-142] In a double-blind, placebo-controlled study, Wilder-Smith and associates[143] demonstrated that the combination of epidural droperidol and intravenous sufentanil significantly reduces both the duration of analgesia and adverse effects compared with IV sufentanil alone. Less nausea, vomiting, and pruritus were reported in the group receiving combination therapy. A more recent randomized, controlled study by Gurses and coworkers[144] showed that a one-time bolus of epidural droperidol in combination with epidural tramadol increased the quality and duration of analgesia over tramadol alone in the immediate postoperative period in 90 patients who underwent abdominal surgery. Finally, Bach and colleagues[142] conducted a retrospective study assessing the effect of adding epidural droperidol to epidural opioids in 20 patients with chronic pain, 17 of who suffered from malignancy. It was found that the addition of droperidol to epidural morphine results in significantly reduced opioid requirements and improved pain relief (80% of patients reported decreased pain), with 7 patients reporting reversible side effects.

The potential benefits of combining epidural droperidol with opioids include a reduction in opioid-related side effects, including nausea, vomiting, pruritus, urinary retention, and hypotension. Side effects of epidural droperidol include sedation, respiratory depression, and parkinsonian effects.

There are no studies to date on the long-term intrathecal use of neuroleptics. The literature that does exist on neuraxial neuroleptics primarily deals with the intrathecal effects of droperidol in animals or epidural droperidol in the perioperative setting.

CONCLUSION

The use of neuraxial analgesics to modulate pain has generated intense interest in recent years. Compared with oral and intravenous routes of administration, the intrathecal and epidural administration of analgesics is associated with a reduced incidence of most, but not all, side effects. To date, most of the literature regarding intrathecal analgesics has been conducted in surgical and cancer patients, in whom the development of cumulative side effects, tolerance, and system malfunction is less of a concern than for chronic, nonmalignant pain patients. In these patients, treatment with neuraxial analgesics is more controversial, with long-term safety and efficacy studies surprisingly scarce. One area that demonstrates particular promise is combining various neuraxial analgesics to enhance efficacy and reduce side effects and tolerance. In addition to the agents mentioned in this chapter, other substances that show promise for future study include nitric oxide inhibitors, dynorphins, calcitonin, neurotensin, antidepressants, beta blockers, and cannabinoids. Clearly, more research is needed to determine the best candidates for neuraxial therapy and which drug combinations have the best efficacy and side effect profiles.

References

1. Corning JL: Spinal anesthesia and local medication of the cord. N Y Med J 1885;42:483-485.
2. Bier A: Versuche über Cocainisirung des Ruckenmarkes. Dtsch Z Chir 1899;51:361-369.
3. Sicard A: Les injection medicamenteuses extra-durales par voie sacrococcygienne. Cr Soc Biol Paris 1901;53:396-398.
4. Manalan SA: Caudal block anesthesia in obstetrics. J Indiana Med Assoc 1942;35:564-565.
5. Lievre J-A, Bloch-Michel H, Pean G, et al: L'hydrocortisone en injection locale. Rev Rhumat Mal Osteo-Articul 1953;4: 310-311.
6. Wang JK, Nauss LA, Thomas JE: Pain relief by intrathecally applied morphine in man. Anesthesiology 1979;50: 149-151.
7. Aanonsen LM, Lei S, Wilcox GL: Excitatory amino acid receptors and nociceptive neurotransmission in rat spinal cord. Pain 1990;41:309-321.
8. Glaum SR, Miller RJ, Hammond DL: Inhibitory actions of mu- and delta-opioid receptor agonists on excitatory transmission in lamina II neurons of adult rat spinal cord. J Neurosci 1994;14:4965-4971.
9. Hammond DL: J.J. Bonica Lecture—2001: Role of spinal GABA in acute and persistent nociception. Reg Anesth Pain Med 2001;26:551-557.
10. Stone LS, Broberger C, Vulchanova L, et al: Differential distribution of alpha$_{2A}$ and alpha$_{2C}$ adrenergic receptor immunoreactivity in the rat spinal cord. J Neurosci 1998;18: 5928-5937.
11. Blomqvist A, Ericson AC, Craig AD, et al: Evidence for glutamate as a neurotransmitter in spinothalamic tract terminals in the posterior region of owl monkeys. Exp Brain Res 1996;108:33-44.
12. Ragsdale DS, McPhee JC, Scheuer T, et al: Molecular determinants of state-dependent block of Na$^+$ channels by local anesthetics. Science 1994;265:1724-1728.
13. Butterworth JFt, Strichartz GR: Molecular mechanisms of local anesthesia: A review. Anesthesiology 1990;72:711-734.
14. Martin WR, Eades CG, Thompson JA, et al: The effects of morphine- and nalorphine- like drugs in the nondependent and morphine-dependent chronic spinal dog. J Pharmacol Exp Ther 1976;197:517-532.
15. Lord JA, Waterfield AA, Hughes J, et al: Endogenous opioid peptides: Multiple agonists and receptors. Nature 1977; 267:495-499.
16. Martin WR, Eades CG, Thompson WO, et al: Morphine physical dependence in the dog. J Pharmacol Exp Ther 1974;189: 759-771.
17. Chen Y, Mestek A, Liu J, et al: Molecular cloning and functional expression of a mu-opioid receptor from rat brain. Mol Pharmacol 1993;44:8-12.
18. Kieffer BL, Befort K, Gaveriaux-Ruff C, et al: The delta-opioid receptor: Isolation of a cDNA by expression cloning and pharmacological characterization. Proc Natl Acad Sci U S A 1992;89:12048-12052.
19. Mollereau C, Parmentier M, Mailleux P, et al: ORL1, a novel member of the opioid receptor family: Cloning, functional expression and localization. FEBS Lett 1994;341:33-38.
20. Nordberg G: Pharmacokinetic aspects of spinal morphine analgesia. Acta Anaesthesiol Scand Suppl 1984;79:1-38.
21. Guinard JP, Mavrocordatos P, Chiolero R, et al: A randomized comparison of intravenous versus lumbar and thoracic epidural fentanyl for analgesia after thoracotomy. Anesthesiology 1992;77:1108-1115.
22. Bernards CM, Shen DD, Sterling ES, et al: Epidural, cerebrospinal fluid, and plasma pharmacokinetics of epidural opioids (part 1): Differences among opioids. Anesthesiology 2003;99: 455-465.
23. Paice JA, Winkelmuller W, Burchiel K, et al: Clinical realities and economic considerations: Efficacy of intrathecal pain therapy. J Pain Symptom Manage 1997;14:S14-S26.
24. Yue SK, St Marie B, Henrickson K: Initial clinical experience with the SKY epidural catheter. J Pain Symptom Manage 1991;6:107-114.
25. Bennett G, Burchiel K, Buchser E, et al: Clinical guidelines for intraspinal infusion: Report of an expert panel. Polyanalgesic Consensus Conference 2000. J Pain Symptom Manage 2000;20:S37-43.
26. Hassenbusch SJ, Portenoy RK, Cousins M, et al: Polyanalgesic Consensus Conference 2003: An update on the management of pain by intraspinal drug delivery—report of an expert panel. J Pain Symptom Manage 2004;27:540-563.
27. Winkelmuller M, Winkelmuller W: Long-term effects of continuous intrathecal opioid treatment in chronic pain of nonmalignant etiology. J Neurosurg 1996;85:458-467.
28. Kamibayashi T, Maze M: Clinical uses of alpha$_2$-adrenergic agonists. Anesthesiology 2000;93:1345-1349.
29. Stone LS, MacMillan LB, Kitto KF, et al: The α_{2a} adrenergic receptor subtype mediates spinal analgesia evoked by α_2 agonists and is necessary for spinal adrenergic-opioid synergy. J Neurosci 1997;17:7157-7165.
30. Hall JE, Uhrich TD, Barney JA, et al: Sedative, amnestic, and analgesic properties of small-dose dexmedetomidine infusions. Anesth Analg 2000;90:699-705.
31. Ackerman LL, Follett KA, Rosenquist RW: Long-term outcomes during treatment of chronic pain with intrathecal clonidine or clonidine/opioid combinations. J Pain Symptom Manage 2003;26:668-677.
32. Rainov NG, Heidecke V, Burkert W: Long-term intrathecal infusion of drug combinations for chronic back and leg pain. J Pain Symptom Manage 2001;22:862-871.
33. Dobrydnjov I, Samarutel J: Enhancement of intrathecal lidocaine by addition of local and systemic clonidine. Acta Anaesthesiol Scand 1999;43:556-562.
34. Gautier PE, De Kock M, Fanard L, et al: Intrathecal clonidine combined with sufentanil for labor analgesia. Anesthesiology 1998;88:651-656.
35. Roelants F, Lavand'homme PM, Mercier-Fuzier V: Epidural administration of neostigmine and clonidine to induce labor analgesia: Evaluation of efficacy and local anesthetic-sparing effect. Anesthesiology 2005;102:1205-1210.
36. Walker SM, Goudas LC, Cousins MJ, et al: Combination spinal analgesic chemotherapy: A systematic review. Anesth Analg 2002;95:674-715.
37. Middleton JW, Siddall PJ, Walker S, et al: Intrathecal clonidine and baclofen in the management of spasticity and neuropathic pain following spinal cord injury: A case study. Arch Phys Med Rehabil 1996;77:824-826.
38. Rauck RL, Eisenach JC, Jackson K, et al: Epidural clonidine treatment for refractory reflex sympathetic dystrophy. Anesthesiology 1993;79:1163-1169.
39. Wu CT, Jao SW, Borel CO, et al: The effect of epidural clonidine on perioperative cytokine response, postoperative pain,

and bowel function in patients undergoing colorectal surgery. Anesth Analg 2004;99:502-509.

40. Yaksh TL, Horais KA, Tozier NA, et al: Chronically infused intrathecal morphine in dogs. Anesthesiology 2003;99:174-187.

41. Naguib M, Yaksh TL: Characterization of muscarinic receptor subtypes that mediate antinociception in the rat spinal cord. Anesth Analg 1997;85:847-853.

42. Rueter LE, Meyer MD, Decker MW: Spinal mechanisms underlying A-85380-induced effects on acute thermal pain. Brain Res 2000;872:93-101.

43. Damaj MI, Patrick GS, Creasy KR, et al: Pharmacology of lobeline, a nicotinic receptor ligand. J Pharmacol Exp Ther 1997;282:410-419.

44. Khan IM, Marsala M, Printz MP, et al: Intrathecal nicotinic agonist-elicited release of excitatory amino acids as measured by in vivo spinal microdialysis in rats. J Pharmacol Exp Ther 1996;278:97-106.

45. Khan IM, Taylor P, Yaksh TL: Stimulatory pathways and sites of action of intrathecally administered nicotinic agents. J Pharmacol Exp Ther 1994;271:1550-1557.

46. Yoon MH, Choi JI, Jeong SW: Antinociception of intrathecal cholinesterase inhibitors and cholinergic receptors in rats. Acta Anaesthesiol Scand 2003;47:1079-1084.

47. Hwang JH, Hwang KS, Leem JK, et al: The antiallodynic effects of intrathecal cholinesterase inhibitors in a rat model of neuropathic pain. Anesthesiology 1999;90:492-499.

48. Buvanendran A, Kroin JS, Kerns JM, et al: Characterization of a new animal model for evaluation of persistent postthoracotomy pain. Anesth Analg 2004;99:1453-1460.

49. Hood DD, Eisenach JC, Tuttle R: Phase I safety assessment of intrathecal neostigmine methylsulfate in humans. Anesthesiology 1995;82:331 343.

50. Klamt JG, Dos Reis MP, Barbieri Neto J, et al: Analgesic effect of subarachnoid neostigmine in two patients with cancer pain. Pain 1996;66:389-391.

51. Lauretti GR, Reis MP, Prado WA, et al: Dose-response study of intrathecal morphine versus intrathecal neostigmine, their combination, or placebo for postoperative analgesia in patients undergoing anterior and posterior vaginoplasty. Anesth Analg 1996;82:1182-1187.

52. Lauretti GR, Mattos AL, Reis MP, et al: Combined intrathecal fentanyl and neostigmine: Therapy for postoperative abdominal hysterectomy pain relief. J Clin Anesth 1998;10:291-296.

53. Owen MD, Ozsarac O, Sahin S, et al: Low-dose clonidine and neostigmine prolong the duration of intrathecal bupivacaine-fentanyl for labor analgesia. Anesthesiology 2000;92:361-366.

54. Kumar P, Rudra A, Pan AK, et al: Caudal additives in pediatrics: A comparison among midazolam, ketamine, and neostigmine coadministered with bupivacaine. Anesth Analg 2005;101:69-73.

55. Tan PH, Chia YY, Lo Y, et al: Intrathecal bupivacaine with morphine or neostigmine for postoperative analgesia after total knee replacement surgery. Can J Anaesth 2001;48:551-556.

56. Omais M, Lauretti GR, Paccola CA: Epidural morphine and neostigmine for postoperative analgesia after orthopedic surgery. Anesth Analg 2002;95:1698-1701.

57. Roelants F, Lavand'homme PM: Epidural neostigmine combined with sufentanil provides balanced and selective analgesia in early labor. Anesthesiology 2004;101:439-444.

58. Kaya FN, Sahin S, Owen MD, et al: Epidural neostigmine produces analgesia but also sedation in women after cesarean delivery. Anesthesiology 2004;100:381-385.

59. Lauretti GR, Gomes JM, Reis MP, et al: Low doses of epidural ketamine or neostigmine, but not midazolam, improve morphine analgesia in epidural terminal cancer pain therapy. J Clin Anesth 1999;11:663-668.

60. Hammond DL, Drower EJ: Effects of intrathecally administered THIP, baclofen and muscimol on nociceptive threshold. Eur J Pharmacol 1984;103:121-125.

61. Hwang JH, Yaksh TL: The effect of spinal GABA receptor agonists on tactile allodynia in a surgically-induced neuropathic pain model in the rat. Pain 1997;70:15-22.

62. Dirig DM, Yaksh TL: Intrathecal baclofen and muscimol, but not midazolam, are antinociceptive using the rat-formalin model. J Pharmacol Exp Ther 1995;275:219-227.

63. Nishiyama T, Gyermek L, Lee C, et al: Analgesic interaction between intrathecal midazolam and glutamate receptor antagonists on thermal-induced pain in rats. Anesthesiology 1999;91:531-537.

64. Valentine JM, Lyons G, Bellamy MC: The effect of intrathecal midazolam on post-operative pain. Eur J Anaesthesiol 1996;13:589-593.

65. Wu YW, Shiau JM, Hong CC, et al: Intrathecal midazolam combined with low-dose bupivacaine improves postoperative recovery in diabetic mellitus patients undergoing foot debridement. Acta Anaesthesiol Taiwan 2005;43:129-134.

66. Yegin A, Sanli S, Dosemeci L, et al: The analgesic and sedative effects of intrathecal midazolam in perianal surgery. Eur J Anaesthesiol 2004;21:658-662.

67. Sajedi P, Islami M: Supplementing epidural lidocaine with midazolam: Effect on sensory/motor block level. Acta Anaesthesiol Taiwan 2004;42:153-157.

68. Kim MH, Lee YM: Intrathecal midazolam increases the analgesic effects of spinal blockade with bupivacaine in patients undergoing haemorrhoidectomy. Br J Anaesth 2001;86:77-79.

69. Borg PA, Krijnen HJ: Long-term intrathecal administration of midazolam and clonidine. Clin J Pain 1996;12:63-68.

70. Svensson BA, Welin M, Gordh T Jr, et al: Chronic subarachnoid midazolam (Dormicum) in the rat. Morphologic evidence of spinal cord neurotoxicity. Reg Anesth 1995;20:426-434.

71. Malinovsky JM, Cozian A, Lepage JY, et al: Ketamine and midazolam neurotoxicity in the rabbit. Anesthesiology 1991;75:91-97.

72. Erdine S, Yucel A, Ozyalcin S, et al: Neurotoxicity of midazolam in the rabbit. Pain 1999;80:419-423.

73. Bozkurt P, Tunali Y, Kaya G, et al: Histological changes following epidural injection of midazolam in the neonatal rabbit. Paediatr Anaesth 1997;7:385-389.

74. Johansen MJ, Gradert TL, Satterfield WC, et al: Safety of continuous intrathecal midazolam infusion in the sheep model. Anesth Analg 2004;98:1528-1535.

75. Tucker AP, Mezzatesta J, Nadeson R, et al: Intrathecal midazolam II: Combination with intrathecal fentanyl for labor pain. Anesth Analg 2004;98:1521-1527.

76. Van Schaeybroeck P, Nuttin B, Lagae L, et al: Intrathecal baclofen for intractable cerebral spasticity: A prospective placebo-controlled, double-blind study. Neurosurgery 2000;46:603-609.

77. Taira T, Kawamura H, Tanikawa T, et al: A new approach to control central deafferentation pain: Spinal intrathecal baclofen. Stereotact Funct Neurosurg 1995;65:101-105.

78. Dario A, Scamoni C, Bono G, et al: Functional improvement in patients with severe spinal spasticity treated with chronic intrathecal baclofen infusion. Funct Neurol 2001;16:311-315.

79. Guillaume D, Van Havenbergh A, Vloeberghs M, et al: A clinical study of intrathecal baclofen using a programmable pump for intractable spasticity. Arch Phys Med Rehabil 2005;86:2165-2171.

80. Zuniga RE, Perera S, Abram SE: Intrathecal baclofen: A useful agent in the treatment of well-established complex regional pain syndrome. Reg Anesth Pain Med 2002;27:90-93.

81. Zuniga RE, Schlicht CR, Abram SE: Intrathecal baclofen is analgesic in patients with chronic pain. Anesthesiology 2000;92:876-880.

82. van Hilten BJ, van de Beek WJ, Hoff JI, et al: Intrathecal baclofen for the treatment of dystonia in patients with reflex sympathetic dystrophy. N Engl J Med 2000;343:625-630.

83. Lind G, Meyerson BA, Winter J, et al: Intrathecal baclofen as adjuvant therapy to enhance the effect of spinal cord stimulation in neuropathic pain: A pilot study. Eur J Pain 2004;8:377-383.

84. Loubser PG, Akman NM: Effects of intrathecal baclofen on chronic spinal cord injury pain. J Pain Symptom Manage 1996;12:241-247.

85. Denys P, Mane M, Azouvi P, et al: Side effects of chronic intrathecal baclofen on erection and ejaculation in patients with spinal cord lesions. Arch Phys Med Rehabil 1998;79: 494-496.

86. Douglas AF, Weiner HL, Schwartz DR: Prolonged intrathecal baclofen withdrawal syndrome. Case report and discussion of current therapeutic management. J Neurosurg 2005;102: 1133-1136.

87. Chizh BA, Headley PM: NMDA antagonists and neuropathic pain—multiple drug targets and multiple uses. Curr Pharm Des 2005;11:2977-2994.

88. Kristensen JD, Svensson B, Gordh T, Jr.: The NMDA-receptor antagonist CPP abolishes neurogenic "wind-up pain" after intrathecal administration in humans. Pain 1992;51:249-253.

89. Muller A, Lemos D: [Cancer pain: Beneficial effect of ketamine addition to spinal administration of morphine-clonidine-lidocaine mixture]. Ann Fr Anesth Reanim 1996;15: 271-276.

90. Bion JF: Intrathecal ketamine for war surgery. A preliminary study under field conditions. Anaesthesia 1984;39:1023-1028.

91. Hawksworth C, Serpell M: Intrathecal anesthesia with ketamine. Reg Anesth Pain Med 1998;23:283-288.

92. Kathirvel S, Sadhasivam S, Saxena A, et al: Effects of intrathecal ketamine added to bupivacaine for spinal anaesthesia. Anaesthesia 2000;55:899-904.

93. Benrath J, Scharbert G, Gustorff B, et al: Long-term intrathecal S(+)-ketamine in a patient with cancer-related neuropathic pain. Br J Anaesth 2005;95:247-249.

94. Choe H, Choi YS, Kim YH, et al: Epidural morphine plus ketamine for upper abdominal surgery: Improved analgesia from preincisional versus postincisional administration. Anesth Analg 1997;84:560-563.

95. Taura P, Fuster J, Blasi A, et al: Postoperative pain relief after hepatic resection in cirrhotic patients: The efficacy of a single small dose of ketamine plus morphine epidurally. Anesth Analg 2003;96:475-480.

96. Himmelseher S, Ziegler-Pithamitsis D, Argiriadou H, et al: Small-dose S(+)-ketamine reduces postoperative pain when applied with ropivacaine in epidural anesthesia for total knee arthroplasty. Anesth Analg 2001;92:1290-1295.

97. Lauretti GR, Rodrigues AM, Paccola CA, et al: The combination of epidural clonidine and S(+)-ketamine did not enhance analgesic efficacy beyond that for each individual drug in adult orthopedic surgery. J Clin Anesth 2005; 17:79-84.

98. Weir PS, Fee JP: Double-blind comparison of extradural block with three bupivacaine-ketamine mixtures in knee arthroplasty. Br J Anaesth 1998;80:299-301.

99. Karpinski N, Dunn J, Hansen L, et al: Subpial vacuolar myelopathy after intrathecal ketamine: Report of a case. Pain 1997;73:103-105.

100. Stotz M, Oehen HP, Gerber H: Histological findings after long-term infusion of intrathecal ketamine for chronic pain: A case report. J Pain Symptom Manage 1999;18:223-228.

101. Errando CL, Sifre C, Moliner S, et al: Subarachnoid ketamine in swine—pathological findings after repeated doses: Acute toxicity study. Reg Anesth Pain Med 1999;24:146-152.

102. Dunlap K, Luebke JI, Turner TJ: Exocytotic Ca^{2+} channels in mammalian central neurons. Trends Neurosci 1995;18: 89-98.

103. Vanegas H, Schaible H: Effects of antagonists to high-threshold calcium channels upon spinal mechanisms of pain, hyperalgesia and allodynia. Pain 2000;85:9-18.

104. Gee NS, Brown JP, Dissanayake VU, et al: The novel anticonvulsant drug, gabapentin (Neurontin), binds to the alpha-2delta subunit of a calcium channel. J Biol Chem 1996; 271:5768-5776.

105. Altier C, Zamponi GW: Targeting Ca^{2+} channels to treat pain: T-type versus N-type. Trends Pharmacol Sci 2004;25:465-470.

106. Atanassoff PG, Hartmannsgruber MW, Thrasher J, et al: Ziconotide, a new N-type calcium channel blocker, administered intrathecally for acute postoperative pain. Reg Anesth Pain Med 2000;25:274-278.

107. Staats PS, Yearwood T, Charapata SG, et al: Intrathecal ziconotide in the treatment of refractory pain in patients with cancer or AIDS: A randomized controlled trial. JAMA 2004;291:63-70.

108. Choe H, Kim JS, Ko SH, et al: Epidural verapamil reduces analgesic consumption after lower abdominal surgery. Anesth Analg 1998;86:786-790.

109. Filos KS, Goudas LC, Patroni O, et al: Analgesia with epidural nimodipine. Lancet 1993;342:1047.

110. Sawynok J: Adenosine receptor activation and nociception. Eur J Pharmacol 1998;347:1-11.

111. Jarvis MF: Contributions of P2X3 homomeric and heteromeric channels to acute and chronic pain. Expert Opin Ther Targets 2003;7:513-522.

112. Okada M, Nakagawa T, Minami M, et al: Analgesic effects of intrathecal administration of P2Y nucleotide receptor agonists UTP and UDP in normal and neuropathic pain model rats. J Pharmacol Exp Ther 2002;303:66-73.

113. Rane K, Segerdahl M, Goiny M, et al: Intrathecal adenosine administration: A phase 1 clinical safety study in healthy volunteers, with additional evaluation of its influence on sensory thresholds and experimental pain. Anesthesiology 1998;89:1108-1115.

114. Karlsten R, Gordh T, Jr.: An A1-selective adenosine agonist abolishes allodynia elicited by vibration and touch after intrathecal injection. Anesth Analg 1995;80:844-847.

115. Sharma M, Mohta M, Chawla R: Efficacy of intrathecal adenosine for postoperative pain relief. Eur J Anaesthesiol 2006;23:449-453.

116. Rane K, Sollevi A, Segerdahl M: A randomised double-blind evaluation of adenosine as adjunct to sufentanil in spinal labour analgesia. Acta Anaesthesiol Scand 2003;47:601-603.

117. Eisenach JC, Hood DD, Curry R: Preliminary efficacy assessment of intrathecal injection of an American formulation of adenosine in humans. Anesthesiology 2002;96:29-34.

118. Eisenach JC, Rauck RL, Curry R: Intrathecal, but not intravenous adenosine reduces allodynia in patients with neuropathic pain. Pain 2003;105:65-70.

119. Lashbrook JM, Ossipov MH, Hunter JC, et al: Synergistic antiallodynic effects of spinal morphine with ketorolac and selective COX1- and COX2-inhibitors in nerve-injured rats. Pain 1999;82:65-72.

120. Malmberg AB, Hamberger A, Hedner T: Effects of prostaglandin E2 and capsaicin on behavior and cerebrospinal fluid amino acid concentrations of unanesthetized rats: A microdialysis study. J Neurochem 1995;65:2185-2193.

121. Ferreira SH, Lorenzetti BB: Intrathecal administration of prostaglandin E2 causes sensitization of the primary afferent neuron via the spinal release of glutamate. Inflamm Res 1996;45:499-502.

122. Baba H, Kohno T, Moore KA, et al: Direct activation of rat spinal dorsal horn neurons by prostaglandin E2. J Neurosci 2001;21:1750-1756.

123. Malmberg AB, Yaksh TL: Hyperalgesia mediated by spinal glutamate or substance P receptor blocked by spinal cyclooxygenase inhibition. Science 1992;257:1276-1279.

124. Malmberg AB, Yaksh TL: Cyclooxygenase inhibition and the spinal release of prostaglandin E2 and amino acids evoked by paw formalin injection: A microdialysis study in unanesthetized rats. J Neurosci 1995;15:2768-2776.

125. Ma W, Du W, Eisenach JC: Role for both spinal cord COX-1 and COX-2 in maintenance of mechanical hypersensitivity following peripheral nerve injury. Brain Res 2002;937:94-99.

126. Korkmaz HA, Maltepe F, Erbayraktar S, et al: Antinociceptive and neurotoxicologic screening of chronic intrathecal administration of ketorolac tromethamine in the rat. Anesth Analg 2004;98:148-152.

127. Parris WC, Janicki PK, Johnson B, Jr., et al: Intrathecal ketorolac tromethamine produces analgesia after chronic constriction injury of sciatic nerve in rat. Can J Anaesth 1996; 43:867-870.

128. Pellerin M, Hardy F, Abergel A, et al: [Chronic refractory pain in cancer patients. Value of the spinal injection of lysine acetylsalicylate. 60 cases.] Presse Med 1987;16:1465-1468.

129. Devoghel JC: Small intrathecal doses of lysine-acetylsalicylate relieve intractable pain in man. J Int Med Res 1983;11:90-91.

130. Eisenach JC, Curry R, Hood DD, et al: Phase I safety assessment of intrathecal ketorolac. Pain 2002;99:599-604.

131. Lauretti GR, Reis MP, Mattos AL, et al: Epidural nonsteroidal antiinflammatory drugs for cancer pain. Anesth Analg 1998;86:117-118.

132. Bagarani M, Amodei C, Beltramme P, et al: [Effects of somatostatin peridurally administered in the treatment of postoperative pain.] Minerva Anestesiol 1989;55:513-516.

133. Chrubasik J, Meynadier J, Scherpereel P, et al: The effect of epidural somatostatin on postoperative pain. Anesth Analg 1985;64:1085-1088.

134. Mollenholt P, Rawal N, Gordh T Jr, et al: Intrathecal and epidural somatostatin for patients with cancer: Analgesic effects and postmortem neuropathologic investigations of spinal cord and nerve roots. Anesthesiology 1994;81:534-542.

135. Paice JA, Penn RD, Kroin JS: Intrathecal octreotide for relief of intractable nonmalignant pain: 5-year experience with two cases. Neurosurgery 1996;38:203-207.

136. Desborough JP, Edlin SA, Burrin JM, et al: Hormonal and metabolic responses to cholecystectomy: Comparison of extradural somatostatin and diamorphine. Br J Anaesth 1989;63:508-515.

137. Gaumann DM, Yaksh TL, Post C, et al: Intrathecal somatostatin in cat and mouse studies on pain, motor behavior, and histopathology. Anesth Analg 1989;68:623-632.

138. Gaumann DM, Grabow TS, Yaksh TL, et al: Intrathecal somatostatin, somatostatin analogs, substance P analog and dynorphin A cause comparable neurotoxicity in rats. Neuroscience 1990;39:761-774.

139. Gao X, Zhang Y, Wu G: Effects of dopaminergic agents on carrageenan hyperalgesia after intrathecal administration to rats. Eur J Pharmacol 2001;418:73-77.

140. Bach V, Carl P, Ravlo O, et al: Extradural droperidol potentiates extradural opioids. Br J Anaesth 1985;57:238.

141. Naji P, Farschtschian M, Wilder-Smith OH, et al: Epidural dropcridol and morphine for postoperative pain. Anesth Analg 1990;70:583-588.

142. Bach V, Carl P, Ravlo O, et al: Potentiation of epidural opioids with epidural droperidol: A one-year retrospective study. Anaesthesia 1986;41:1116-1119.

143. Wilder-Smith CH, Wilder-Smith OH, Farschtschian M, et al: Epidural droperidol reduces the side effects and duration of analgesia of epidural sufentanil. Anesth Analg 1994;79:98-104.

144. Gurses E, Sungurtekin H, Tomatir E, et al: The addition of droperidol or clonidine to epidural tramadol shortens onset time and increases duration of postoperative analgesia. Can J Anaesth 2003;50:147-152.

38 Pharmacology for the Interventional Pain Physician

Renata Variakojis and Honorio T. Benzon

The art and science of interventional pain management is based on expert application of diagnostic and therapeutic injections. Expertise in perineural, neuraxial, and intra-articular injection techniques should be matched with a thorough understanding of the pharmacology of the drugs used in these procedures. This chapter reviews the clinical pharmacology, pharmacokinetics, therapeutic mechanisms, and side effects of radiocontrast agents, corticosteroids, and botulinum toxins. Radiocontrast agents are reviewed in greater detail elsewhere in this text. All these drugs have the potential to produce physiologic toxicity and therefore should be administered appropriately and in the smallest dose that will reliably produce the desired effect; an increase in total dose or volume should not be used to compensate for inadequate injection technique. A discussion of the prospective benefits and known risks of these agents may be included in the process of informed consent.

RADIOCONTRAST AGENTS

Radiocontrast agents play an important role in aiding anatomic structure identification and needle localization under x-ray or fluoroscopic guidance. Iodinated compounds attenuate x-rays passing through the body to a greater degree than bony tissue and, as such, decrease the amount of radiation reaching the image intensifier, or detector.[1] Conventional iodinated contrast agents provide radiopacity via a triiodinated benzoate anion. The significant amount of unbound iodine in these standard ionic solutions leads to a high osmolar concentration, up to eight times more than normal physiologic osmolality. Thus, these ionic, high-osmolality contrast agents have the potential to produce physiologic toxicity. This has led to the development of newer nonionic low-osmolality contrast media, which can deliver equivalent amounts of radiopacity to a target area, with a decrease in the toxic effects attributable to charged particles.[2] These agents contain iodine tightly bound to a benzene ring, with a minimal amount of free iodine. The osmolality of the nonionic agents is near physiologic (300 mOsmol/kg water).

Examples of two commonly used radiocontrast agents are iopamidol (Isovue-M) and iohexol (Omnipaque). Each agent is commercially available in preparations of varying ionic concentration and osmolality. Their properties are listed in Table 38–1.

Both iopamidol and iohexol are absorbed rapidly into the bloodstream following intrathecal, epidural, or paraspinal injection.[3] Plasma levels are measurable within 1 hour of injection and almost all the remaining drug reaches systemic circulation within 24 hours. Both agents undergo minimal metabolism, deiodination, or biotransformation, with more than 90% excreted via the kidneys.[3]

Adverse Reactions

As the use of iodinated contrast agents steadily increases, knowledge of their adverse effects, identification of patient risk factors, and studies of potential treatments are rapidly evolving. The risk of adverse reactions is 4% to 12% with ionic contrast materials and 1% to 3% with nonionic contrast materials.[4] The risk for severe adverse reaction is 0.16% with ionic contrast materials and 0.03% with nonionic contrast materials. The death rate is similar for both ionic and nonionic agents, 1 to 3 per 100,000.[4]

Adverse reactions associated with radiocontrast agents may be chemotactic, related to hyperosmolality, or allergic. Examples of chemotactic reactions include thyrotoxicosis and nephrotoxicity. Hyperosmolal reactions include erythrocyte damage, endothelial damage and thrombosis, vasodilation causing warmth and discomfort, hypervolemia, and cardiovascular depression. Allergic reactions range from flushing, urticaria, and hives to bronchospasm, angioedema, hypotension, bradycardia, loss of consciousness, seizures, and cardiac arrest.

Table 38–1. Radiocontrast Agents Used for Spine Injections

AGENT	CONCENTRATION (weight/vol %)	IONIC CONCENTRATION (mg iodine/mL)	OSMOLALITY (mOsm/kg H₂O)
Isovue-M 200	Iopamidol, 41%	200	300
Isovue-M 300	Iopamidol, 61%	300	616
Omnipaque 180	Iohexol, 39%	180	360
Omnipaque 240	Iohexol, 52%	240	510
Omnipaque 300	Iohexol, 65%	300	672

From Sitzman T, Chen Y, Rallo-Clemans R, et al: Drugs for the interventional pain physician. In Benzon HT, Raja S, Molloy RE, et al (eds): Essentials of pain medicine and regional anesthesia. New York, Elsevier-Churchill Livingstone, 2005, pp 166-180. With permission.

Anaphylactoid Reactions

More than 90% of adverse reactions to radiocontrast material are anaphylactoid.[4] Anaphylactoid reactions are characterized by angioedema, urticaria, bronchospasm, and hypotension. Approximately 60% to 70% of severe reactions to contrast agents occur within 5 minutes, and 80% to 90% within 10 minutes from the start of the injection.[5] Therefore, it is imperative to monitor all patients following radiocontrast administration for a minimum of 30 to 60 minutes. When an anaphylactoid reaction is suspected, prompt treatment with current basic and advanced cardiopulmonary resuscitation techniques is used. This includes administration of oxygen, intravenous fluids, antihistamines (histamine 1 [H₁], histamine 2 H₂ blockers), adrenergic drugs (epinephrine), and corticosteroids.

In patients with a known previous allergic reaction or suspected iodinated contrast material allergy, pretreatment with a regimen of antihistamines and corticosteroids is carried out. A randomized study of the protective effects of pretreatment with corticosteroids in 6763 patients receiving intravenous contrast materials has found that two doses of methylprednisolone (32 mg), given 12 and 2 hours prior to contrast exposure, significantly reduce the incidence of adverse reactions as compared to placebo.[2] The two-dose steroid regimen results in a 31% reduction of all adverse events and a 62% reduction in severe reactions. A recommended regimen, beginning 12 hours prior to contrast exposure, is outlined in Table 38–2.

Renal Injury

Contrast-induced nephropathy (CIN) is a common cause of hospital-acquired acute renal failure and is associated with significant morbidity, health care costs, and mortality.[6] Numerous clinical trials have demonstrated that nephrotoxicity is higher with ionic versus nonionic contrast agents.[7] Certain contrast agents, including iohexol, release the renal vasoconstrictor peptide endothelin from vascular endothelium in a way that may contribute to radiocontrast nephropathy.[8] Nonionic low-osmolality agents have been shown to have a reduced propen-

Table 38–2. Pretreatment Regimen for Previous Radiocontrast Allergic Reactions

WHEN GIVEN	COMPONENTS/DOSAGE
12 hr precontrast exposure	Prednisone, 20 to 50 mg PO Ranitidine, 50 mg PO Diphenhydramine, 25 to 50 mg PO
2 hr precontrast exposure	Prednisone, 20 to 50 mg PO Ranitidine, 50 mg PO Diphenhydramine, 25 to 50 mg PO
Immediate preinjection	Diphenhydramine, 25 mg IV

From Sitzman T, Chen Y, Rallo-Clemans R, et al: Drugs for the interventional pain physician. In Benzon HT, Raja S, Molloy RE, et al (eds): Essentials of pain medicine and regional anesthesia. New York, Elsevier-Churchill Livingstone, 2005, pp 166-180. With permission.

sity to stimulate the release of endothelin and produce less renal vasoconstriction in an animal model, and are associated with a largely reduced risk of radiocontrast nephropathy.[8] Results of a pooled analysis of nonionic contrast agents have shown a significantly lower incidence of CIN after iopamidol compared with iohexol.[7] The difference in the incidence of CIN among nonionic contrast agents may be the result of the number of benzene rings (monomer vs. dimer), iodine content, osmolality, and viscosity of the individual agents.

Risk factors for CIN have been identified; these include preexisiting renal insufficiency, diabetes mellitus, dose of radiocontrast used, advanced congestive heart failure, and intravascular volume depletion.[9] Currently, interventions to prevent radiocontrast-induced nephropathy are a subject of great interest. A variety of therapeutic interventions, including saline hydration, diuretics, mannitol, calcium channel antagonists, theophylline, endothelin receptor antagonists, and dopamine have been used to prevent CIN.[6] More recently, N-acetylcysteine, an antioxidant, and fenoldopam, a dopamine-1 receptor agonist, have been evaluated for their effects on ameliorating acute CIN, with N-acetylcysteine demonstrating a small beneficial effect.[9] Proven preventive measures include volume expansion with intravenous normal saline, alkalinization with sodium bicarbonate, and the use of low-osmolar or iso-osmolar contrast media.[9]

CORTICOSTEROIDS

Corticosteroids (CSs) are key mediators in the maintenance of normal physiology and in the complex adaptive mechanisms that protect an organism in the setting of internal or external stressors.[10] CSs maintain the function and integrity of many important physiologic and biochemical processes, including regulation of protein, carbohydrate, and lipid metabolism.[11,12] Naturally occurring corticosteroids are classified into three functional groups, mineralocorticoids, glucocorticoids, and adrenal androgens.[13] Glucocorticoids (GCs) act primarily to enhance the production of high-energy fuel, glucose, and reduce other metabolic activity not involved in that process.[11] During periods of stress, they are highly protective and their deficiency during critical illness is associated with increased morbidity and mortality.[14] Mineralocorticoids maintain normal fluid and electrolyte balance. Corticosteroids are widely prescribed in clinical medicine because of their anti-inflammatory properties. Injections of glucocorticoids for the relief of vertebrogenic, arthritic, and radiculopathic pains are widely accepted.[3] An understanding of the diverse physiologic effects of therapeutic steroid injections is important in the practice of interventional pain management, so that knowledge of their risks can enhance judicious use of these potent anti-inflammatory agents.

Effects

GCs stimulate hepatic gluconeogenesis, increase hepatic glycogen content, and inhibit insulin-mediated peripheral blood glucose uptake.[11] They modulate protein metabolism by decreasing peripheral protein synthesis while stimulating protein catabolism. GCs inhibit amino acid incorporation into protein of peripheral tissues while stimulating protein and enzyme synthesis in the liver. GC catabolic activity mobilizes glycogenic amino acid precursors from peripheral tissues, such as bone, skin, muscle, and connective tissue.[11] After GC administration, alanine is massively released from muscle, providing a substrate for hepatic gluconeogenesis.[12] CSs regulate lipid metabolism largely by potentiating catecholamine-enhanced activation of cellular lipase, resulting in lipolysis.[12] GC actions on protein and lipid tissues vary in different parts of the body. Whereas cortisol can deplete the protein matrix of the vertebral column (trabecular bone), there may be minimal effect on long bones (compact bone).[11] Similarly, for adipose tissue, the subcutaneous lipid cell mass of the arms and legs decreases while that of the abdomen and interscapular area increases.

CSs have important effects on the function of the cardiovascular system. Cortisol maintains vascular responsiveness to circulating vasoconstrictors and, in high doses, may restore circulatory function in shock associated with hemorrhage, endotoxin, anaphylaxis, and trauma. CSs exhibit a positive ionotropic effect on the myocardium, and improve myocardial cell

uptake of fatty acids for energy metabolism. Cortisol maintains the microcirculation in the setting of acute inflammation by reducing capillary endothelial permeability and preventing edema formation. Hemodynamically, GCs modulate β-adrenergic receptor synthesis and cell density,[15] prevent β-adrenergic receptor desensitization and uncoupling,[16] and inhibit nitric oxide synthase.[17]

GCs modulate the immune response at many levels.[11] They cause leukocytosis by enhancing the release of mature leukocytes from the bone marrow as well as inhibiting their egress from the circulation. They inhibit macrophage activity by impairing phagocytosis, intracellular digestion of antigens, and the production of interleukin 1 (IL-1) and IL-6 inflammatory mediators. GCs interfere with T-cell mediated immunity. They inhibit the production of interferon by T lymphocytes, as well as T-cell growth factor (IL-2). GCs are effective in promoting homograft survival after organ transplantation by suppressing the inflammatory response to antigen-antibody union.

Adrenal Gland and Production of Corticosteroids

All CSs are produced in the cortex of the adrenal gland, which is composed of three distinct zones.[13,18] The outer zone, the zona glomerulosa, produces mineralocorticoids, specifically aldosterone, which is synthesized in response to stimulation by the renin-angiotensin-aldosterone system or hyperkalemia. Aldosterone increases sodium reabsorption and stimulates potassium excretion by the kidneys, and thus regulates extracellular fluid and electrolyte balance and maintains intravascular volume. The middle zone, the zona fasciculata, is the thickest zone, comprising more than 70% of the cortex, and is the site of glucocorticoid production. Cortisol is the primary glucocorticoid, and represents about 80% of GC production.[18] The inner zone, the zona reticularis, produces GCs and in some species small amounts of androgens.

Adrenocortical cells contain large stores of lipid used for steroidogenesis. The adrenal gland has a tremendous capacity to react to acute and chronic stress. Adrenocorticotropic hormone (ACTH) induces physiologic, molecular, and morphologic changes in the adrenal cortex.[19,20] In addition to releasing GCs, the adrenal gland undergoes upregulation of steroidogenic cytochrome P-450 mRNAs,[21,22] as well as hypervascularization and cellular hypertrophy and hyperplasia. These morphologic changes are accompanied by intracellular changes, including an increase in the number of mitochondria, an increase in smooth endoplasmic reticulum, and a decrease in liposomes known to store cholesterol, the substrate for GC biosynthesis.[23,24]

Adrenal insufficiency may result from direct destruction of the adrenal glands (primary adrenal insufficiency) or from the loss of hypothalamic-pituitary integrity (secondary adrenal insufficiency). Primary adrenal insufficiency is associated with deficient production of glucocorticoids, mineralocorticoids, sex hormones, and catecholamines. Chronic primary adrenal insufficiency (Addison's disease) is most commonly caused by autoimmune adrenalitis (slow destruction of the adrenal cortex by cytotoxic lymphocytes).[25] Infection and systemic inflammation may also cause progressive onset of primary adrenal insufficiency, whereas adrenal hemorrhage, necrosis, or thrombosis of the adrenal gland will produce abrupt-onset adrenal insufficiency.[25] The adrenal glands have a large reserve, and approximately 90% of glandular tissue may be disrupted before adrenal insufficiency develops.[14] The signs and symptoms of primary and secondary adrenal insufficiency are similar. Cortisol deficiency is characterized by hypotension, orthostasis, weakness, weight loss, anorexia, lethargy, abdominal cramping, nausea, vomiting, diarrhea, and mental depression.[14] Specific clinical features suggesting primary adrenal insufficiency are hyperpigmentation, vitiligo, autoimmune thyroid disease, and salt craving.[25] The most common cause of secondary adrenal insufficiency is GC therapy. Headaches, visual disturbances, and diabetes insipidus suggest the presence of hypothalamic-pituitary disease.[14] Laboratory findings that suggest the diagnosis of adrenal insufficiency include eosinophilia, hyponatremia (related to an increased release of vasopressin), hyperkalemia, and hypoglycemia.

The function of the adrenal gland may be evaluated by a short corticotropin (ACTH) stimulation test (also known as the cosyntropin stimulation test). The traditional approach is to administer a relatively high dose (250 μg) of synthetic corticotropin intravenously and measure serum cortisol levels before and 30 and 60 minutes after corticotropin. Because a normal response to this supraphysiologic dose of corticotropin (over 100 times greater than stress-induced ACTH levels) does not rule out adrenal insufficiency, many clinicians prefer the low-dose (1 to 2 μg) corticotropin stimulation test, which better approximates ACTH levels found in severe stress.[26]

Steroid Biosynthesis

Adrenal steroids share a common carbon skeleton, the cyclopentanoperhydrophenanthrene ring, comprised of three cyclohexane rings and one cyclopentane ring (Fig. 38–1). Variation among naturally occurring steroid compounds is related to the manner in which hydrogen, hydroxyl, and oxygen radicals

and carbon atoms are attached to the basic steroid nucleus.[13] Cortisol and other anti-inflammatory steroids contain a two-carbon chain attached to position 17, and are termed C21 steroids. Certain structural features are essential for the preservation of biologic activity of all glucocorticoid hormones. Even the commonly administered steroid cortisone must be converted in vivo to hydrocortisone (cortisol) by the liver before it is biologically active.

All human steroids are derived from cholesterol, which has the 17-carbon nucleus. Most of the cholesterol for steroid synthesis is provided by circulating plasma lipoproteins. Cholesterol uptake by the adrenal cortex is mediated by the low-density-lipoprotein (LDL) receptor, whose quantities increase with ACTH stimulation. The first and rate-limiting step in steroid biosynthesis is the conversion of cholesterol to pregnenolone under the control of ACTH and by the cytochrome P-450 enzymes in the mitochondria and smooth endoplasmic reticulum.[18] Corticosterone is the immediate precursor to cortisol, and is the principal glucocorticoid in certain animal species.[18] In humans, cortisol is produced in greater amounts than corticosterone, and accounts for 80% of glucocorticoid production.

ACTH (corticotropin) is synthesized as part of a large precursor, pro-opiomelanocortin (POMC), which is processed into several peptides, including corticotropin, β-lipotropin, and β-endorphin, which are secreted together.[27] ACTH is secreted in periodic bursts and therefore ACTH levels vary throughout the day. The major factors controlling ACTH release include corticotropin-releasing hormone (CRH), the free cortisol level, stress, and the sleep-wake cycle.[11] CRH and vasopressin are the principal regulators of anterior pituitary ACTH secretion. ACTH stimulates the zona fasciculata cells of the adrenal cortex to increase steroid synthesis, and stimulates the release of cortisol, aldosterone, and androgens. Following ACTH stimulation, release of cortisol occurs in 1 to 3 minutes.

Regulation of Secretion

Cortisol secretion is under the control of the hypothalamic-pituitary-adrenal (HPA) axis. Cortisol synthesis depends on three factors—negative feedback by serum cortisol levels, normal circadian cycle, and

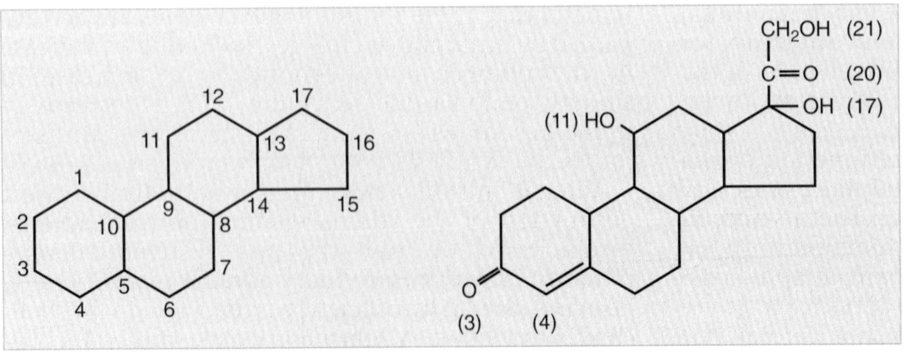

Figure 38–1. Structure of cortisol.

responses to CNS activation by physical and emotional stress. During nonstress periods, cortisol production is under the influence of CNS activation by baroreceptor, chemoreceptor, nociceptor, and emotional afferent signals.

Negative Feedback

Cortisol exerts a negative feedback inhibition of CRH secretion by binding to specific steroid receptors in the CNS.[28] It also inhibits both ACTH secretion and POMC gene transcription. Other inhibitory mechanisms include atrial natriuretic factor and substance P, both of which appear during inflammation. Systemic hypoperfusion, with decreased adrenal blood flow and certain drugs, may also inhibit cortisol synthesis.

Circadian Pattern of Secretion

It is estimated that human cortisol production is approximately 5 to 10 mg/m^2 per day, a value much less than previously reported.[29,30] This amount is the equivalent of about 20 to 30 mg/day of hydrocortisone or 5 to 7 mg/day of oral prednisone.[29] The range of the circadian pattern of cortisol production varies more than threefold. Peak levels of ACTH and cortisol secretion occur between 4 and 8 AM. There is minimal production of cortisol during the evening and the lowest levels are observed between 8 PM and 12 AM.[13] In abnormal sleep-wake cycles, this diurnal pattern will adjust, so that peak cortisol levels occur just prior to awakening.[31] The diurnal variation in adrenal steroidogenesis depends on the integrity of sympathetic innervation. Catecholamines released from the adrenal medulla stimulate adrenocortical steroidogenesis in a direct fashion. Epinephrine and norepinephrine stimulate adrenocortical function by enhancing the transcriptional activity of several steroidogenic factors and enzymes.[22]

CNS Control of Secretion

Baroreceptor and chemoreceptor afferent inputs to the medulla are transmitted via the pons to the hypothalamus. Nociceptive afferent signals activate both the medulla and thalamus, which independently activates the hypothalamus via the paleocortex limbic system.[28] Emotional triggers also activate the hypothalamus through the paleocortex limbic system.[28,32] The arrival of afferent inputs into the hypothalamic paraventricular nucleus stimulates the synthesis of CRH, which is secreted into the hypophyseal portal system to the anterior pituitary, causing ACTH release.[28,32] In addition to neurologic afferent signals, other substances can stimulate the hypothalamus to secrete CRH and cause ACTH release. These include the proinflammatory cytokines IL-1β, IL-6, and tumor necrosis factor α (TNF-α).[28,33] Other substances that influence CRH and ACTH secretion include vasopressin, angiotensin II, norepinephrine (NE), prostaglandin $F_{2\alpha}$ (PGF$_{2\alpha}$), and thromboxane A_2 (TXA$_2$).[32] Cortisol synthesis can increase 5- to 10-fold during severe stress, to a maximal level of approximately 100 mg/m^2 per day.[13,34]

Cortisol in the Circulation

Cortisol circulates in the blood in three forms, free cortisol (5%), protein-bound cortisol, and cortisol metabolites.[11] It is this unbound (free) portion that is the physiologically active hormone. Approximately 90% of cortisol is bound to cortisol-binding globulin (CBG), also known as transcortin, and albumin. CBG has a high affinity for cortisol, but is present in small amounts. The second serum-binding protein, albumin, binds cortisol with less affinity, but is abundantly present. Any disorder that results in decreased albumin levels increases the free fraction of cortisol, thus increasing side effects. During stress, there is a characteristic increase in total cortisol blood levels, including an increase in the unbound percentage.[28] The level of CBG is increased in high-estrogen states, pregnancy, and during administration of contraceptives.[11] Most synthetic glucocorticoids have less affinity for CBG (approximately 70% binding) and this may account for their propensity to produce cushingoid symptoms at low doses. Cortisol primarily is metabolized in the liver, with subsequent renal excretion of the metabolites.

Synthetic Cortisol Analogues

Cortisol has a half-life of 70 to 90 minutes. All synthetic analogues of cortisol have longer half-lives, based on slower rates of metabolism.[12] The half-life does not reflect duration of action, which is best represented by the duration of ACTH suppression. Short-acting GCs include cortisone and hydrocortisone, with durations of action of 8 to 12 hours (Table 38–3). Cortisol (hydrocortisone) is an active agent, whereas the inactive drug, cortisone, must be converted by the liver to cortisol for biologic activity. The intermediate-acting GCs prednisone, prednisolone, methylprednisolone, and triamcinolone have durations of action of 24 to 36 hours. Prednisone is an inactive agent, which is metabolized to the active agent prednisolone by the liver. The longest acting GCs, dexamethasone and betamethasone, have durations of action longer than 48 hours. Short-acting GCs are advantageous when a rapid clinical effect is desired, such as in allergic reactions. Long-acting agents are of interest for their prolonged anti-inflammatory effects, and are well suited for disorders requiring inhibition of ACTH secretion. Because all GCs have some mineralocorticoid effect, their administration can have profound consequences for patients with impaired cardiovascular function. The shorter acting GCs have the highest mineralocorticoid potency, and the long-acting agents have the weakest.

Stress Response

Cortisol levels increase within minutes of stress, whether physical (trauma, surgery, exercise), psycho-

Table 38–3. Properties of Synthetic Cortisol Analogues

DRUG	GLUCOCORTICOID POTENCY (mg)	MINERALOCORTICOID ACTIVITY	DURATION OF ACTION (hr)	PLASMA HALFLIFE (min)
Short-acting				
Cortisone	25	1	8-12	60
Hydrocortisone	20	0.8	8-12	90
Intermediate-acting				
Prednisone	5	0.25	24-36	60
Prednisolone	5	0.25	24-36	200
Methylprednisolone	4	0	24-36	180
Triamcinolone	4	0	24-36	300
Long-acting				
Dexamethasone	0.75	0	36-54	200
Betamethasone	0.6	0	36-54	200

From Nesbitt LT: Minimizing complications from systemic glucocorticosteroid use. Dermatol Clin 1995;13:925-939.

logical (anxiety, depression), or physiologic (hypoglycemia, infection). Pain, fever, and hypovolemia all cause a sustained increase in ACTH and cortisol secretion.[34-36] Surgery is associated with elevations in ACTH and cortisol levels, which usually persist for 24 to 48 hours.[37] The magnitude of the stress response is directly proportional to the extent of surgical trauma. Less extensive procedures such as surgery on the joints, breast, or neck produce a 36% increase in cortisol levels, whereas laparotomy is associated with an 84% increase in the serum cortisol level for 2 days postoperatively.[38] Adult adrenal glands produce about 50 mg of cortisol/24 hours during minor surgery, and 75 to 150 mg/24 hours during major surgery.[39]

Elevated levels of circulating cytokines, which appear within minutes of trauma, stimulate the HPA axis to increase production of cortisol. Increased tissue corticosteroid levels are an important protective and life-sustaining response in these settings. Corticosteroids improve survival in stress by reducing the duration of shock, decreasing the severity of inflammation, improving vessel contractility and hemodynamics, and preventing inflammatory cell recruitment, proliferation, and release of proinflammatory mediators.[40] Corticosteroids also improve outcome by modulating β-receptor responsiveness to catecholamines. GCs both increase the number of β receptors and prevent uncoupling of the β receptor from adenylate cyclase.[15,16] Methylprednisolone acetate administration in critically ill patients receiving catecholamine infusions results in an increase in cardiac index, left ventricular stroke index, and mean arterial pressure.[15]

An intact HPA axis is paramount to survival during periods of major stress and critical illness. Adrenal insufficiency with decreased GC levels is associated with a significantly increased mortality in these settings.[41] The anesthetic drug etomidate, a short-acting hypnotic, was found to account for a dramatic increase in mortality in patients in the ICU of the University Hospital of Glasgow, Scotland. Etomidate was subsequently found to be a selective inhibitor of adrenal 11β-hydroxylase, the enzyme that converts deoxycortisol to cortisol.[41] Adrenal suppression should be suspected in patients receiving corticosteroids, and these patients should receive replacement GCs when facing major surgery or critical illness.

Glucocorticoid Supplementation for Patients Receiving Corticosteroids

Cortisone, a purified glucocorticoid preparation, was introduced into clinical practice in 1949, revolutionizing the treatment of a number of medical diseases and providing physiologic replacement in patients with adrenal insufficiency.[13,42] Shortly thereafter, a number of case reports and studies appeared describing the catastrophic effects of inadequate corticosteroid supplementation in glucocorticoid-treated patients with medical or surgical stresses.[43] Glucocorticoid therapy is the most common cause of secondary adrenal insufficiency.[13] Initially, glucocorticoid administration suppresses CRH and ACTH stimulation. Over time, tertiary iatrogenic adrenal insufficiency develops as the adrenal gland atrophies. Adrenal atrophy may persist for months, following even short courses of corticosteroid therapy.[44]

The dose and duration of corticosteroid administration are only fair predictors of the extent of adrenal suppression, because ACTH and cortisol production vary greatly among individuals. The hypothalamus is the first to be suppressed by steroid dosing, but the first to recover. ACTH levels return to normal after several months. The adrenal glands are the last to be suppressed and the slowest to recover, a process that may take 6 to 12 months. Data regarding corticosteroid-induced adrenal suppression are varied. One study has evaluated the adrenal effects of high-dose, short-term GC therapy with oral prednisone, 25 mg twice daily for 5 days. Five days later, adrenal response to an ACTH challenge remained reduced.[45] It has also been shown that patients treated with 5 mg/day or less of prednisone continue to have an intact HPA axis.[46] The time to recovery from HPA suppression is highly variable, ranging from 2 to 5 days[45] to 9 to 12 months.[47] Suppression of the HPA axis should be anticipated in any patient who has been receiving more than 30 mg/day of hydrocortisone (or 7.5 mg of prednisolone or 0.75 mg of dexamethasone) for more than 3 weeks.[48]

Table 38–4.   Guidelines for Adrenal Supplementation Therapy*

MEDICAL OR SURGICAL STRESS	CORTICOSTEROID DOSAGE
Minor	
Inguinal hernia repair	25 mg of hydrocortisone or 5 mg of methylprednisolone IV on day of procedure only
Colonoscopy	
Mild febrile illness	
Mild-moderate nausea, vomiting	
Gastroenteritis	
Moderate	
Open cholecystectomy	50-75 mg of hydrocortisone or 10-15 mg of methylprednisolone IV on day of procedure;
Hemicolectomy	rapid taper over 1-2 days to usual dose
Significant febrile illness	
Pneumonia	
Severe gastroenteritis	
Severe	
Major cardiothoracic surgery	100-150 mg of hydrocortisone or 20-30 mg of methylprednisolone IV on day of procedure;
Whipple procedure	rapid taper to usual dose over next 1-2 days
Liver resection	
Pancreatitis	
Critically ill	
Sepsis-induced hypotension or shock	50-100 mg of hydrocortisone IV every 6-8 hr or 0.18 mg/kg/hr as a continuous infusion + 50 µg/day of fludrocortisone until shock is resolved; may take several days to a week or more; gradually taper, following vital signs and serum sodium level determination

*Data are based on extrapolation from the literature, expert opinion, and clinical experience. Patients receiving 5 mg/day or less of prednisone should receive their normal daily replacement, but do not require supplementation. Patients who receive more than 5 mg/day of prednisone should receive the above therapy in addition to their maintenance therapy.
From Coursin DB, Wood KE: Corticosteroid supplementation for adrenal insufficiency. JAMA 2002;287:236-240.

Given the large variation in cortisol production in healthy patients, it is difficult to predict the need for GC supplementation during stress. Also, the adrenal response to acute medical illness is variable.[49] Expert recommendations have suggested lower doses and shorter duration of glucocorticoid administration (Table 38–4). Patients undergoing minor procedures such as routine dental work, skin biopsy, inguinal repair, or minor orthopedic surgery only require their normal daily dose of replacement, and not a supplemental dose.[34] Some clinicians have advocated using hydrocortisone continuous infusions to limit the rapid clearance and peaks and nadirs of bolus therapy.[13,34,44] Others have suggested using longer acting glucocorticoid agents, such as methylprednisolone or dexamethasone.[13,34,44]

Therapeutic Effects

Gene Regulation

GCs exert their effects by binding to cytoplasmic GC receptors (GRs) within target cells.[50] GRs are DNA binding proteins, which have a hormone binding site and a DNA binding site. They are expressed in almost every type of cell. The inactive GR is bound to a large protein complex and folded into a conformation that is optimal for binding and prevents the unoccupied receptor from entering the nucleus. Once the GC binds to the GR, the GR complex dissociates and the activated GC translocates to the nucleus and binds to DNA at GC response elements (GREs) in the promoter sequences of target genes.[50] GR expression is regulated by several factors at transcriptional, translational, or post-translational levels.[51] Downregulation of GRs in circulating monocytes and lymphocytes occurs after steroid therapy. A reduction in GR expression by 50% causes various abnormalities, including an increase in circulating cortisol and body fat.[52]

Induction of Transcription

Steroids produce their effects in responsive cells by activating GRs to regulate the transcription of certain target genes.[50] It is estimated that the number of steroid-responsive genes per cell is probably between 10 and 100.[50] When the GR complex binds to the promoter region of target genes, this changes the DNA configuration, exposing previously masked areas. This results in increased binding of other transcription factors to the unmasked areas and the formation of a more stable transcription initiation complex.[50]

Inhibition of Transcription

Steroids inhibit gene transcription by less well understood mechanisms. In some cases, GR binding to negative GC response elements causes steric hindrance to the binding of transcription factors, or the GR may form complexes with these activating transcription factors to inhibit their effect. This mechanism appears to account for the effect of steroids on the transcription of collagenase.[50] Collagenase transcription is induced by tumor necrosis factor α (TNF-α) and phorbol esters, which activate apoprotein-1. The GR complex binds AP-1, forming a protein-protein complex and causing mutual repression of

DNA binding. In another possible mechanism of inhibition of gene transcription, the GR enhances the transcription of specific ribonucleases that break down mRNA.

Anti-inflammatory Actions

GCs are the most potent and effective agents in controlling inflammation through numerous mechanisms, including effects on cytokines, inflammatory mediators, inflammatory cells, nitric oxide synthase, and adhesion molecules.

Effects on Cytokines

Cytokines are important mediators of inflammation and the pattern of their expression largely determines the magnitude and persistence of the inflammatory response.[53] Steroids have potent inhibitory effects on cytokine transcription and synthesis, because they inhibit the transcription of several cytokines relevant in chronic inflammation, including IL-1, IL-3, IL-4, IL-5, IL-6, IL-8, TNF-α, and granulocyte-macrophage colony-stimulating factor (GM-CSF).[54] Steroid-mediated inhibition of cytokine synthesis occurs via three mechanisms—binding of GRs to a negative glucocorticoid response element, inhibiting expression of transcription factors AP-1 and nuclear factor kappa B (NF-κB), and increasing breakdown of mRNA.[50,55,56] Steroids not only block cytokine synthesis, but also interfere with their activity.[50] They inhibit the synthesis of the IL-2 receptor and oppose the AP-1–mediated induction of IL-2 and T-lymphocyte activation and proliferation.

Effects on Inflammatory Mediators

The activation of phospholipase A_2 leads to the hydrolysis of arachidonic acid from membrane phospholipids and the production of arachidonic acid metabolites. Arachidonic acid metabolism via the cyclooxygenase pathway produces prostaglandins and thromboxanes, and the lipooxygenase pathway produces leukotrienes. Steroids increase the synthesis of lipocortin (annexin) 1, a phospholipase A_2 inhibitor, and thus decrease the production of inflammatory mediators such as leukotrienes, prostaglandins, and platelet-activating factor.[50,57] GCs also upregulate the transcription of other anti-inflammatory genes such as neutral endopeptidase and inhibitors of plasminogen activator.[58]

However, the primary anti-inflammatory effect of steroids appears to be the suppression of transcription of genes involved in inflammation.[58] The activated GR binds either to negative GREs or interacts with transcription factors to downregulate gene expression. Additionally, GCs decrease mRNA stability. GC-suppressed genes include those of collagenase, elastase, plasminogen activator, cyclooxygenase (COX)-2, and most chemokines. Steroids directly inhibit the transcription of a cytosolic form of phospholipase A_2 induced by cytokines, and inhibit the gene expression of cytokine-induced COX-2 in monocytes.[59] Cortisol, 6-methylprednisolone, and dexamethasone suppress lipopolysaccharide-induced synthesis of PGE_2 and cyclooxygenase-2 expression and activity in human monocytes.[60]

Steroids affect other inflammatory mediators by effects on their metabolism. Bradykinin is degraded by enzymes such as angiotensin-converting enzyme and neutral endopeptidase (NEP), both of which are induced by steroids. Steroids may also modulate the effects of inflammatory mediators.[50] Thus, although leukotriene B_4 and platelet-activating factor induce *c-fos* and *c-jun* expression in inflammatory cells, steroids inhibit the synthesis of these early genes.[61]

Effects on Inflammatory Cells

GCs interfere with macrophage activity by impairing phagocytosis, intracellular digestion of antigens, and macrophage release of IL-1 and TNF-α.[11] By inhibiting the expression of chemokines, GCs prevent the activation and recruitment of inflammatory cells, including eosinophils, basophils, and lymphocytes.[58] Steroids also markedly decrease the survival of certain inflammatory cells, such as eosinophils. Eosinophil activity is dependent on the presence of cytokines IL-3, IL-5, GM-CSF, and interferon-γ.[62] The presence of these cytokines promotes prolonged eosinophil survival, increased adhesion molecule expression, potentiated eosinophil degranulation, and movement of eosinophils across an endothelial barrier. Steroid administration blocks these cytokine effects, leading to programmed cell death, or apoptosis. GCs cause an expansion in the number of circulating neutrophils secondary to decreased adherence to vascular endothelium (demargination) and stimulation of bone marrow production.[63] GCs interfere with T-cell mediated immunity. They inhibit the production of T lymphocytes by downregulating T-cell growth factors IL-1β and IL-2, and inhibit the release of various T-lymphocyte cytokines.[11]

Effects on Nitric Oxide Synthase

Various cytokines induce nitric oxide synthase (NOS), resulting in increased nitric oxide production. Nitric oxide increases plasma exudation in inflammatory sites. Steroids potently inhibit the inducible form of NOS in macrophages, and steroid pretreatment prevents the induction of NOS expression by endotoxin.[50]

Effects on Adhesion Molecules

Adhesion molecules facilitate the trafficking of inflammatory cells to sites of inflammation. The expression of the adhesion molecules E-selectin, P-selectin, and intracellular adhesion molecule-1 on the surface of endothelial cells is induced by the cytokines IL-1β and TNF-α.[50] These adhesion molecules enable the endothelium to recruit leukocytes actively and nonselectively, including neutrophils, eosinophils, mononuclear cells, and basophils from the circulation.[58] GCs are effective and potent inhibitors of TNF-α and IL-1 release from macrophages, monocytes, and other infiltrating cells. There is a second class of cytokines that selectively activate the endothelium—IL-4 and IL-13, two cytokines associated with allergic diseases. Their release causes the endothelial expression of vascular cell adhesion molecule-1 only. Consequently, only circulating basophils, eosinophils, monocytes, and lymphocytes, but not neutrophils, can bind to the endothelial surface. GCs inhibit cytokine release from lymphocytes and IL-4 release from basophils.[58]

Other Anti-inflammatory Effects

Steroids inhibit plasma exudation from postcapillary venules at inflammatory sites. This effect is delayed, suggesting that gene transcription and protein synthesis are involved.[50] It appears that the antipermeability effect is linked to the synthesis of vasocortin. In addition to nuclear anti-inflammatory effects, GCs also have direct effects on cells and cell membranes. Cortisol stabilizes lysosomal membranes, thus inhibiting lysosomal enzyme release. GCs prevent the sequestration of water intracellularly and the swelling and destruction of cells.[12] GCs inhibit leukocyte accumulation and complement-induced polymorphonuclear neutrophil (PMN) aggregation and decrease PMN chemotaxis, T-cell and B-cell proliferation, and the differentiation and function of macrophages.

Other Mechanisms of Pain Relief

Following peripheral nerve injury, a number of morphologic and biochemical changes occur at the injury site, including the formation of neuromas, which leads to increased electrical excitability. These changes in nerve structure and excitability threshold make the injured nerve abnormally sensitive to physical and chemical stimulation. Ectopic discharge from the injury site leads to a persistent afferent barrage, which maintains neuralgic pains and paresthesias. GCs have been demonstrated to suppress spontaneous ectopic neural discharge originating in experimental neuromas and prevent the later development of ectopic impulse discharge in freshly cut nerves.[64] The effect appears to be mediated by a direct membrane-stabilizing action, rather than an anti-inflammatory action. The topical application of methylprednisolone was noted to block transmission of C-fibers but not the A-beta fibers.[65]

Side Effects

Short courses of GCS therapy (less than 2 to 3 weeks) are usually extremely safe. Side effects from short-term therapy are rare, but may include fluid retention, hyperglycemia, elevated blood pressure, mood changes, menstrual irregularities, gastritis, Cushing's syndrome (Table 38–5), increased appetite, weight gain, increased infections, delayed wound healing, and acneiform eruptions.[31] Long-term GC therapy with near-physiologic GC doses is relatively safe. With long-term supraphysiologic doses of steroids,

Table 38–5. Side Effects of Chronic Glucocorticoid Therapy

SYSTEM AFFECTED	MANIFESTATIONS
Musculoskeletal	Osteoporosis
	Aseptic bone necrosis
	Growth retardation
	Muscle atrophy
	Myopathy
Ophthalmologic	Cataracts
	Glaucoma
	Infection
	Hemorrhage
	Exophthalmos
Gastrointestinal	Nausea, vomiting
	Peptic ulcer disease
	Intestinal perforation
	Pancreatitis
	Esophagitis
Metabolic	Hyperglycemia
	Hyperlipidemia
	Obesity
	Hypocalcemia
	Hypokalemic alkalosis
Cardiovascular	Hypertension
	Edema
	Atherosclerosis
Gynecologic, obstetric	Amenorrhea
	Fetal effects
Hematologic, cellular	Leukocytosis
	Lymphopenia
	Eosinopenia
	Immunosuppression
	Impaired fibroplasias
	Decreased mitotic rate
Nervous	Mood, personality changes
	Psychiatric problems, psychosis
	Seizures
	Pseudotumor cerebri
	Peripheral neuropathy
Cutaneous	Atrophy, striae
	Vascular effects, purpura
	Hair changes
	Pigmentary changes
	Acne, acneiform eruptions
	Infections
HPA axis	Suppression

From: Nesbitt LT: Minimizing complications from systemic glucocorticosteroid use. Dermatol Clin 1995;13:925-939.

more serious side effects may occur[31] (see Table 38–5).

Cushing's Syndrome

Cushing's syndrome is characterized by sudden weight gain, hypertension, glucose intolerance, oligomenorrhea, decreased libido, and spontaneous ecchymoses.[66] The most common presenting sign is centripetal weight gain, involving thickening of the facial fat that rounds the facial contour (moon facies), enlargement of the dorsocervical fat pad (buffalo hump), and truncal obesity. Muscle wasting and weakness are manifested by difficulty climbing stairs and patients are unable to rise from a squatting position without assistance. The development of multiple striae wider than 1 cm on the abdomen or proximal extremities is almost unique to Cushing's syndrome. Mild hirsutism, acne, personality changes, depression, insomnia, and edema also occur. Despite the external signs of excess GC production, patients receiving GCs develop adrenal atrophy and are at risk for adrenal crisis in the setting of stress.[67] Laboratory tests reveal low blood ACTH and cortisol and low urinary cortisol levels.

Skeletal Effects

Osteoporosis, aseptic necrosis, and growth retardation are all potential complications of long-term GC therapy. Osteoporosis occurs in as many as 50% of patients treated with long-term supraphysiologic doses of prednisone.[68] Trabecular bone, found in the axial skeleton (vertebrae and ribs), has a metabolic turnover rate eight times that of cortical bone, and is therefore more susceptible to demineralization.[31,69] Corticosteroid-induced osteoporosis (CIOP) has a multifactorial cause–impaired intestinal absorption of calcium, increased renal excretion of calcium, increased osteoclast activity with resultant bone resorption,[70] inhibition of osteoblast activity with decreased bone synthesis, and secondary hyperparathyroidism. The pathogenesis of corticosteroid-induced osteoporosis differs from postmenopausal osteoporosis in that bone formation appears to be more suppressed compared with bone resorption.[71] The incidence of fractures in patients receiving GCs has been reported to be between 10% and 20%.[72] Patients at greatest risk for corticosteroid-induced osteoporosis are postmenopausal women, children, immobilized patients, and patients with rheumatoid arthritis. Many agents used in postmenopausal osteoporosis, such as activated vitamin D products, hormone replacement therapy, fluoride, calcitonin, and bisphosphonates, have been shown to maintain or improve bone mineral density in corticosteroid-induced osteoporosis.[71]

Aseptic necrosis is a severe musculoskeletal complication of GC therapy. It occurs with greater incidence in patients with systemic lupus erythematosus, alcoholics and other patients with fatty degeneration of the liver, patients with altered lipid metabolism, and renal transplantation patients.[31,73] The mechanism is related to fatty deposits in terminal arterioles of certain sites in bone. The femoral head is the site most commonly affected, although the humeral head or knee may also be involved. Bone pain is almost always the first symptom and precedes radiologic signs of osteonecrosis by up to 6 months.[31] Corticosteroids inhibit both skeletal maturation and linear growth. In children, a compensatory growth spurt may be anticipated when GCs are stopped, with most children reaching their expected height. The greatest danger of therapy is at puberty, when epiphyseal closure occurs.[74] GC inhibition of bone growth is likely related to impaired synthesis of type 1 collagen, with diminished protein matrix for new bone formation, and a decreased effect of growth hormone.

Exogenous growth hormone administration may be considered.

Muscle Effects

The incidence of myopathy secondary to high-dose GC therapy has been reported to vary from 7% to 60%.[75] There is no consistent relationship between the dose and duration of steroid and the occurrence of myopathy. Symptoms include skeletal muscle weakness, tenderness, and pain. Proximal or pelvic muscles are typically affected. Steroid myopathy usually develops from more potent fluorinated steroids, such as triamcinolone, dexamethasone, and betamethasone. Pathologic findings include loss of the thick myofilament, fiber atrophy, and creatinine kinase level elevations. GCs inhibit protein synthesis, primarily in type II muscle fibers, increase cytoplasmic protease activity, leading to myofibrillar destruction, and enhance glutamine synthetase activity in skeletal muscle.[75] Recovery may take months to 1 year; treatment includes a reduction in the GC dose and physical therapy with a rehabilitation exercise program.

Ophthalmologic Effects

Cataracts and glaucoma may occur with chronic GC therapy. Steroid-induced cataracts occur in the posterior subcapsular region of the lens, and may be asymptomatic until well formed.[31] Children are at greatest risk for this complication. Glaucoma is caused by swelling of collagen strands at the angle of the anterior chamber of the eye, with resistance to the outflow of aqueous humor.[31,69] The process is usually reversible after GC therapy is discontinued. Other ophthalmologic complications include an increased risk of ocular infection, most significantly herpes simplex or fungal keratitis, conjunctival or retinal hemorrhage and, in very rare cases, exophthalmos.

Gastrointestinal Effects

Nausea and vomiting are not uncommon with oral steroid therapy. Peptic ulcer disease is slightly increased with GC therapy and is more likely to be gastric than duodenal. GCs cause a decrease in mucus production and mucosal cell renewal. Concomitant use of aspirin and nonsteroidal anti-inflammatory drugs increase this risk and should be avoided, along with tobacco and alcohol, which also are ulcerogenic.[31,76]

Metabolic Effects

Hyperglycemia results from GC effects of increased hepatic glucose synthesis and increased gluconeogenesis. GCs also antagonize peripheral insulin effects, and can occasionally produce insulin resistance. Exacerbation of glucose intolerance is common but the development of new cases of diabetes mellitus is not, and ketoacidosis is rare.[31,69] Weight gain is a common side effect of GC therapy, and may be the result of increased appetite or fluid retention. Increased fat deposits appear centripetally, most commonly on the face, posterior neck, and trunk. Facial edema and fat are estimated to occur in 10% to 25% of patients on steroid therapy for 2 months.

Hyperlipidemia is another metabolic consequence of GC therapy, and is likely secondary to relative insulin resistance. Increased plasma triglyceride levels are more common than increased cholesterol levels.[69] Patients with previous lipid level elevations are at higher risk for this side effect. Electrolyte abnormalities such as hypokalemic alkalosis may also occur, usually with GCs possessing strong mineralocorticoid properties.

Cardiovascular Effects

Hypertension, edema, and atherosclerosis may occur with GC therapy. Elevations in blood pressure occur because of increased sodium retention and vasoconstriction. GCs cause vasoconstriction by potentiating the effect of norepinephrine and opposing the effect of endogenous vasodilators such as histamine. This side effect occurs more frequently in patients with preexisting hypertension, older adults, GCs with high mineralocorticoid potency, and high-dose or prolonged (longer than 2 weeks) glucocorticoid treatment courses. Blood pressure elevations are rare during short-term therapy, but long-term therapy poses the need for sodium restriction and the possible use of a thiazide diuretic. Edema occurs from fluid retention secondary to sodium retention. With initial GC dosing, there is a paradoxical diuresis caused by an early blockade of antidiuretic hormone release.[69] Atherosclerosis may occur at an accelerated rate in certain patients, such as systemic lupus erythematosus (SLE) and renal transplant patients.[77]

Hematologic Effects

Blood cell effects, immunosuppression, and impaired fibroplasia occur with steroid therapy. GCs increase the release of granulocytes from bone marrow, thus increasing the number of circulating leukocytes.[78] Lymphopenia occurs, with predominant depression of T cell production and cytokine release, and minimal effect on B-cell and antibody production.[79] Decreased eosinophil counts and enhanced eosinophil destruction are observed. Erythrocytes demonstrate increased survival, related to decreased autohemolysis and erythrophagocytosis. Immunosuppression is produced by GCs at many levels. Tissue inflammation is reduced by inhibition of cytokine production and by impaired chemotaxis of macrophages, neutrophils, basophils, and eosinophils. There is inhibition of the metabolism of arachidonic acid into prostaglandin and leukotriene mediators, as well as a direct inhibition of COX-2. Steroid therapy increases susceptibility to many bacterial, fungal, viral, and parasitic infections.[80] Wound healing is delayed by GC inhibition of fibroblasts and collagen production. There also is decreased production of ground substance, impaired angiogenesis, and suppression of wound reepithelialization.[81]

Nervous System Effects

Mood changes, nervousness, euphoria, insomnia, and headache are common side effects of GC therapy and are dose-related.[82] Psychosis is an uncommon side effect, and is seen more commonly in patients with previous psychiatric disorders.

Cutaneous Effects

Skin changes typical of the hyperadrenal state may occur; these include purpura, telangiectasia, atrophy, striae, pseudoscars, and facial plethora.[83] The skin becomes thin and fragile. Hair growth changes include transient scalp hair loss and hirsutism on other parts of the body. Hyperpigmentation or hypopigmentation may occur, as well as acneiform eruptions. Steroid acne commonly presents on the back and chest as fine, uniform papulopustules.[31]

Hypothalamic-Pituitary-Adrenal Suppression

HPA axis suppression is related to both dose and duration, and may occur with even short courses of GC therapy. This effect is minimized by single morning doses, and even more so by using an intermediate-acting agent every other morning.[31] The hypothalamus is the first to be suppressed but the quickest to recover after therapy is stopped. The adrenals are the last to be suppressed but the slowest to recover, with recovery taking from 6 to 12 months after long-term GC therapy.[31] To test for HPA axis suppression, a morning serum cortisol level is measured. To test adrenal gland function, the ACTH stimulation test is performed, with measurement of basal and 30- and 60-minute serum cortisol levels in response to an ACTH challenge.

Pregnancy and Lactation

There appears to be no teratogenic contraindication to corticosteroid therapy in pregnancy. However, intrauterine growth retardation has been reported, and steroid use late in pregnancy may cause adrenal suppression in the fetus. Corticosteroids are secreted in small amounts into breast milk, thus exposing the infant to the risk of adrenal suppression.[72]

Complications of Steroid Injections

Epidural steroid injections are used for their anti-inflammatory and membrane-stabilizing effects in the treatment of back pain and radiculopathy arising from nerve root irritation. Although some patients experience no changes in fasting blood glucose or lipid levels after a single epidural injection of dexamethasone,[84] other patients may experience a host of side effects. The depot steroid preparations used for epidural injections may produce ACTH suppression and cushingoid symptoms that can last up to a few weeks.[85] Cushing's syndrome is a reversible metabolic syndrome characterized by obesity, impaired glucose tolerance, hypertension, and gonadal dysfunction. Cushing's syndrome has occurred following a single epidural injection of 60 mg of methylprednisolone[67] or triamcinolone,[86] and has been reported in several patients following repeated epidural steroid injections when 200 mg of methylprednisolone was exceeded.[87]

Steroid myopathy involving the proximal muscles of the lower extremity has been reported following a single epidural triamcinolone injection. The progressive weakness developed over 2 to 4 weeks and did not resolve for 12 to 16 weeks.[86] Lumbar epidural injection of triamcinolone, 80 mg, caused profound HPA axis suppression for 3 weeks, although steroid was undetectable in the plasma during this time. This suggests that GCs act directly on central GC receptors, presumably via CSF absorption.[88] Comparable studies of patients who have received intra-articular steroid injections have shown detectable levels in the circulation and HPA axis suppression for up to 4 weeks.[89]

Epidural injection of triamcinolone, 80 mg, caused a marked reduction in insulin sensitivity in patients with normal glucose tolerance and caused fasting hyperglycemia in patients with a preexisting degree of insulin resistance.[90] In this study, insulin sensitivity and fasting glucose levels were normal 1 week after injection. Because patients with diabetes commonly experience increased insulin requirements for several days following injection, it is suggested that they be given specific advice on the management of their condition following epidural GC injection.

Several other purported adverse reactions have been reported following GC injection. Sterile meningitis and arachnoiditis have been reported following intrathecal injection of methylprednisolone, but may have been related to the polyethylene preservative.[91] Rare anaphylactoid reactions have occurred following intravenous, intramuscular, and soft tissue injections of the succinate salts of methylprednisolone and hydrocortisone.[92-94] Most of these patients were chronically atopic, and in two cases the patients had aspirin sensitivity.[92,95] Signs and symptoms of anaphylaxis reported with the use of various hydrocortisone preparations include bronchospasm, shock, urticaria, and angioedema.[93] Any type of anaphylactic reaction warrants prompt and aggressive life support therapy, including resuscitation of airway, breathing, and circulation, with oxygen support and cardiac life support when indicated.

Coadministration of corticosteroids with preservative-containing local anesthetics (e.g., methylparaben-, propylparaben-, and phenol-containing local anesthetics) may cause precipitation of the steroid. Injection of a steroid precipitate could cause mechanical injury to soft tissue (cartilage, tendon, joint), neural, or vascular structures.

Central Nervous System Events after Transforaminal Epidural Steroid Injections

There have been several reported cases of central nervous system injuries after transforaminal epidural steroid injections (Table 38–6).[96-104] These injuries occurred after injection not only of the steroid but also of the local anesthetic and dye. It has also been reported not only after fluoroscopy but also after computed tomography. These injuries involve the spinal cord in the form of paraplegia or the brain as embolic cerebrovascular accidents. The mechanisms of the spinal cord injuries have been ascribed to injury or spasm of the blood vessels supplying branches to the spinal cord (segmental artery, deep cervical or ascending cervical arteries), proximal intraneural spread of the injectate, or embolization of the particulate steroid through these vessels.[105-107] Injury to these vessels is possible. Huntoon and Martin[102] have shown in cadaver studies that the entry of the ascending cervical and deep cervical vessels in the posterior portion of the cervical intervertebral foramen is within a few millimeters of the path of the needle placed for transforaminal epidural steroid injections, and these findings were confirmed by Hoeft and colleagues.[108] Spasm of the blood vessels occurs after trauma by the needle or after injection of the dye. Another mechanism is embolization of the particulate steroid through these blood vessels, resulting in segmental infarct of the spinal cord or embolization through the vertebral or an end cerebral artery, resulting in cerebral or cerebellar infarct.

Tiso and colleagues[101] and Benzon and associates[107] examined the sizes of the particles in the steroid preparations (Table 38–7). They found that methylprednisolone has a significantly higher percentage of large particles (Fig. 38–2) and that the particles are large enough to occlude the vessels. One type of available betamethasone (Celestone Soluspan) had the smallest particle sizes, followed by triamcinolone acetonide (Figs. 38–3 and 38–4). A compounded form of betamethasone, which can be ordered from compounding companies, does not appear to offer an advantage over triamcinolone, because the sizes of their particles appear to be the same.[107] Whereas Tiso and coworkers[101] noted small particles in dexamethasone and betamethasone sodium phosphate, the short-acting component in the commercial type of betamethasone, Benzon and colleagues[107] noted that the two steroids are pure liquid, with no identifiable

Table 38–6. Adverse Central Nervous System Events after Transforaminal Epidural Steroid Injections

STUDY	SITE	INJECTATE	NEEDLE	EVENT*
Brouwers et al[96]	C6-7	Triamcinolone, 0.5 mL + 0.5% bupivacaine, 0.5 mL	22 G	C3 quadriplegia (spinal cord infarct)
Rozin et al[100]	C7	Methylprednisolone, 80 mg + 0.75% bupivacaine (3 mL total)	25 G, Quincke	Death (brainstem hemorrhage)
Tiso et al[101]	C5-6	Triamcinolone 80 mg + 0.25% bupivacaine, 2 mL	25 G, Quincke	Cerebellar infarct
Karasek and Bogduk[103]	C6-7	Lidocaine 2%, 0.8 mL	? Gauge	Paralysis of all four extremities × 20 min
McMillan[99]	C5-6	Iopamidol, 2 mL	22 G	Cortical blindness × 3 wk (edema of occipital cortex)
Houten and Errico[97]	L3-4, L4-5	Betamethasone, 12 mg + 0.25% bupivacaine (3 mL total)	25 G, spinal	L1 paraplegia (spinal cord edema)
	L3-4	Methylprednisolone, 40 mg + lidocaine, 1%, 1 mL + iodine (Isovue 300), 0.2 mL	20 G, spinal	Low thoracic paraplegia (spinal cord edema)
	S1	Methylprednisolone, 40 mg + 1% lidocaine, 1 mL	22 G, spinal	T10 paraplegia
Huntoon and Martin[102]	L1	Triamcinolone 40 mg + 0.12% bupivacaine, 5 mL	25 G; 22 G, Quincke	T10 paraplegia (spinal cord infarct)
Somayaji et al[104]	L2-L3	Triamcinolone, 40 mg + 0.5% bupivacaine, 1 mL	21 G, spinal	L2 paraplegia (spinal cord infarct)

*The MRI findings in the "Event" column are in parentheses. The cases of Huntoon, Houten, and colleagues had lumbar spine surgeries. The case of Somayaji and associates was performed under computed tomographic guidance.
C, cervical; G, gauge; L, lumbar; S, sacral.
From Benzon HT, Chew TL, McCarthy R, et al: Comparison of the particle sizes of different steroids and the effect of dilution: A review of the relative neurotoxicities of the steroids. Anesthesiology 2007;106:331-338. With permission.

Table 38–7. Percentage Distribution of the Particle Sizes of the Steroids*

SIZE (μm)	MPA 80	MPA 40	TRA	CLTN	BTM REP	BSP	DEX
0-10	60 (49)	53	71 (37)	82 (48)	61	0 (93)	0 (15)
11-20	3 (11)	11	8 (28)	9 (28)	7	0 (6)	0 (15)
21-50	14 (31)	8	9 (31)	6 (23)	10	0 (1)	0 (67)
>50	23 (9)	27	12 (4)	3 (1)	22	0	0 (3)

BTM Rep, betamethasone repository (betamethasone sodium phosphate/betamethasone acetate, compounded betamethasone); BSP, betamethasone sodium phosphate; CLTN, Celestone Soluspan (betamethasone sodium phosphate/betamethasone acetate, commercial betamethasone); DEX, dexamethasone sodium phosphate; MPA 80, methylprednisolone acetate, 80 mg/mL; MPA 40, methylprednisolone acetate, 40 mg/mL; TRA 40, triamcinolone acetonide, 40 mg/mL.
*The results of Tiso and colleagues[101] are in parentheses; they did not state whether the concentration of the methylprednisolone that they examined was 80 mg/mL or 40 mg/mL. They noted particles in betamethasone sodium phosphate and dexamethasone, whereas Benzon and associates[107] did not.
From Benzon HT, Chew TL, McCarthy R, et al: Comparison of the particle sizes of different steroids and the effect of dilution: A review of the relative neurotoxicities of the steroids. Anesthesiology 2007;106:331-338. With permission.

particles. It should be noted that the commercially available betamethasone preparation (Celestone Soluspan) contains 3 mg/mL of betamethasone sodium phosphate and 3 mg/mL of betamethasone acetate. Dexamethasone is long-acting and has minimal or no mineralocorticoid activity, but has increased GC activity, theoretically resulting in a greater elevation of the blood glucose level. One clinical study on dexamethasone has shown it to be slightly less efficacious than triamcinolone.[109] The theoretical disadvantages of dexamethasone are its easy washout from the epidural space and the reports of convulsions after intrathecal injection in animals.[85,107] If transforaminal epidural steroid injections are to be given, then the commercial form of betamethasone is recommended, followed by triamcinolone. The clinician can use dexamethasone if a nonparticulate steroid is preferred; the increased use

of dexamethasone awaits additional studies on its efficacy and neurotoxicity. These events have not been reported after interlaminar injections, so any of the available steroids can be used.

The question of neurotoxicity and possible allergic reactions to steroids arises from the vehicle and preservatives of the commercially available steroids (Table 38–8). Polyethylene glycol, the vehicle used in methylprednisolone and triamcinolone, can decrease the compound action potential of the A, B, and C fibers.[110] However, these changes are reversible, and concentrations above 20% are required for this effect (methylprednisolone and triamcinolone contain only 3% polyethylene glycol). Dexamethasone contains methylparaben and sodium bisulfite, compounds that have been implicated in allergic reactions to local anesthetics.[107] Betamethasone contains benzalkonium chloride, a wetting agent found in

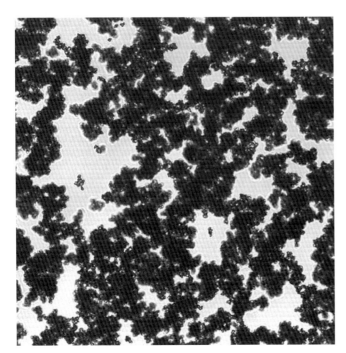

Figure 38–2. Typical microscopic appearance of methylprednisolone 80 mg/mL. The particles are opaque and amorphous in appearance. (From Benzon HT, Chew TL, McCarthy R, et al: Comparison of the particle sizes of different steroids and the effect of dilution: A review of the relative neurotoxicities of the steroids. Anesthesiology 2007;106:331-338. With permission.)

Figure 38–4. Typical microscopic appearance of triamcinolone, 40 mg/mL. Similar to methylprednisolone, the particles are opaque and amorphous in appearance. (From Benzon HT, Chew TL, McCarthy R, et al: Comparison of the particle sizes of different steroids and the effect of dilution: A review of the relative neurotoxicities of the steroids. Anesthesiology 2007;106:331-338. With permission.)

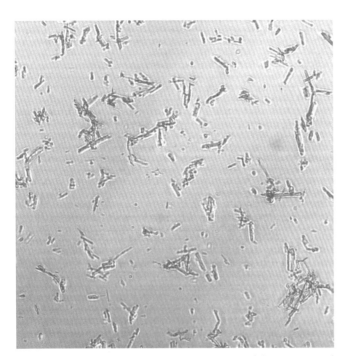

Figure 38–3. Typical microscopic appearances of the commercial form of betamethasone (Celestone Soluspan). The preparation contains 3 mg/mL of betamethasone sodium phosphate and 3 mg/mL of betamethasone acetate. Unlike methylprednisolone and triamcinolone, the particles in Celestone are rodlike and lucent. (From Benzon HT, Chew TL, McCarthy R, et al: Comparison of the particle sizes of different steroids and the effect of dilution: A review of the relative neurotoxicities of the steroids. Anesthesiology 2007;106:331-338. With permission.)

commercial soap preparations, which can cause very rare allergic reactions.

BOTULINUM TOXIN THERAPY

History

Botulinum toxins are produced by the gram-negative anaerobic bacterium *Clostridium botulinum*. They produce flaccid paralysis by preventing the presynaptic release of acetylcholine (Ach) at the neuromuscular junction. There are eight botulinum toxin (BTX) subtypes—A, B, C_1, C_2, D, E, F, and G.[111] Types A, B, E, and F have been described to cause botulism, a syndrome of generalized muscle weakness following the ingestion of botulinum-contaminated food. Botulism affects the extraocular and bulbar muscles early, with visual disturbances often the presenting sign. If muscle weakness progresses to affect the respiratory muscles, respiratory paralysis and death may ensue. BTX was initially used to induce weakness in the lateral rectus muscle of the monkey in a search for a nonsurgical alternative to surgical treatment of strabismus in humans. BTX type A (BTX-A) induced transient weakness in the lateral rectus of the monkey, lasting several months without any significant side effects. BTX-A was used in humans for the treatment of strabismus in 1981. In 1989, the U.S. Food and Drug Administration (FDA) approved the use of BTX-A for the treatment of strabismus, blepharospasm, and hemifacial spasm. In 2000, BTX-B was approved

Table 38–8. Comparison of Steroids in Terms of Component Vehicles and Preservatives

| STEROID | VEHICLE: POLYETHYLENE GLYCOL | Preservatives | | | |
		BENZYL ALCOHOL	METHYLPARABEN	SODIUM BISULFITE	BENZALKONIUM CHLORIDE
Methylprednisolone	+	+	−	−	−
Triamcinolone	±*	+	−	−	−
Betamethasone	−	−	−	−	+
Dexamethasone	−	−	+	+	−

*Triamcinolone acetonide does not contain polyethylene glycol whereas triamcinolone diacetate does; both contain benzyl alcohol. Triamcinolone diacetate was recently discontinued in the United States.
From Benzon HT, Chew TL, McCarthy R, et al: Comparison of the particle sizes of different steroids and the effect of dilution: A review of the relative neurotoxicities of the steroids. Anesthesiology 2007;106:331-338. With permission.

by the FDA for treating cervical dystonia. Since then, the BTXs have been used for the treatment of various medical conditions, including achalasia, anismus, benign prostatic hypertrophy, dysphonia, dystonias, essential tremor, hyperhidrosis, kyphoscoliosis, low back pain, migraine and tension-type headache, myofascial pain, pancreatitis, pelvic floor disorders, rectal fissures, sialorrhea, spasticity, temporomandibular joint syndrome, urinary sphincter dysfunction, and in cosmetic injections for hyperfunctional facial lines.[3]

Pharmacology of Botulinum Toxin

Toxin Structure and Quantification

Botulinum toxin is synthesized as a single-chain polypeptide, consisting of a heavy chain (H chain; molecular weight [MW], 100,000) and a light (L) chain (MW, 50,000). The H chain is responsible for binding to presynaptic cholinergic nerve terminals at the neuromuscular junction, whereas the L chain is the neurotoxic component. The H and L chains are bound together by disulfide bonds, and the toxin is activated by proteolytic enzymes in a cleaving process. BTX is quantified in mouse units (MU); 1 MU is the dose required to kill 50% of a batch of 18- to 20-g female Swiss-Webster mice (LD_{50}). It is estimated that the human lethal dose of BTX-A is about 2800 to 3500 units for a 70-kg adult. The lethal dose of BTX-B in humans is estimated at 144,000 units. However, extrapolations from animal studies are affected by species differences in sensitivity which preclude an accurate determination of the toxic dose in humans. Of all the subtypes, type A appears to be the most potent and has the longest duration of action.

Preparation and Dosing

Two botulinum neurotoxins, types A and B, are used in clinical practice. There are two commercially available type A preparations, Botox and Dysport. Each vial of Botox (Allergan, Inc., Irvine, Cal) contains 100 units of BTX-A, 0.5 mg of human albumin, and 0.9 mg of sodium chloride in a sterile, vacuum-dried form without preservative. Dysport (Ipsen, Ltd., Berkshire, UK) is marketed in other countries in the form of 500-MU vials. Data from patients treated for cervical dystonia suggest that 1 MU of Botox equals 3 to 5 MU of Dysport. There also are two available preparations of the type B toxin (both supplied by Elan Pharmaceuticals, San Diego, Cal); Myobloc is marketed in the United States and Neurobloc is marketed in Europe.

BTX is easily inactivated by heat, shaking, excessive dilution, and surface tension from bubbles during reconstitution. Boiling dissolves the disulfide bonds between the heavy and light chains of BTX, thus rendering the toxin inactive, because neither chain can exert neurotoxicity independently. BTX must be reconstituted with normal saline without a preservative. Dilution of a 100-MU vial may be performed with 1, 2, 5, or 10 mL of 0.9% sodium chloride. This will yield a concentration of 10, 5, 2, or 1 MU/0.1 mL, respectively. The higher concentrations are appropriate for larger muscles—for example, hip flexors or piriformis muscles. Lower concentrations are used for facial injections, such as for the glabella, temporalis, and frontalis muscles. Tuberculin syringes are used to dilute and draw up the toxin. New 30-gauge needles are used to give the injections to reduce discomfort and local trauma and bleeding. BTX should be used within 4 hours of preparation and stored at 2° to 8° C during this time. It has been shown that there is no loss of activity 6 hours after reconstitution at room temperature; however, a 44% loss of activity is observed at 12 hours.[112] Refreezing the toxin after reconstitution causes a 70% reduction in bioactivity at 1 to 2 weeks.

Mechanisms of Action

BTX acts by blocking the presynaptic release of ACh from cholinergic terminals of motor and autonomic nerves. BTX neurotoxicity occurs in three stages–binding, internalization, and proteolysis.[113] Following activation by proteolytic cleavage, the BTX heavy chain binds irreversibly to the presynaptic terminals of cholinergic neurons. The C-terminal region of the heavy chain binds in a serotype-specific manner to receptors on the motor end plates and at autonomic cholinergic ganglia.

Binding induces the formation of an endosome around the toxin molecule. Endocytosis, an energy-dependent process, leads to internalization of the toxin. The newly formed endosome becomes increasingly acidic, and the lowered pH prompts a configurational change in the toxin. This facilitates the formation of a channel through the membrane, which allows for entry of the toxin, specifically the L chain, into the cell. Once inside the cytosol, BTX exerts its proteolytic effect. The L chain acts as a metalloendopeptidase that cleaves different proteins of the protein complex necessary for docking of ACh vesicles to the cell membrane before they can be released. Different BTX subtypes cleave different parts of the SNARE (soluble N-ethylmaleimide-sensitive factor attachment protein receptor) protein complex. BTX types A, E, and C cleave synaptosome-associated protein-25 (SNAP-25). Types B, D, F, and G cleave the synaptic protein synaptobrevin, also known as vesicle-associated membrane protein (VAMP). Type C also cleaves syntaxin. Each of these protein substrates contributes to the formation of the SNARE complex, which is essential for the fusion of ACh-containing vesicles with the presynaptic membrane. SNAREs form coiled bundles that bridge the membrane of the synaptic vesicle with the presynaptic membrane. SNAP-25 interacts with VAMP, located on the vesicle membrane, and VAMP interacts with syntaxin, located on the plasma membrane. Thus, BTX-A cleavage of SNAP-25 prevents the successful docking of ACh vesicles to presynaptic membranes.

Clinical Effects

Botulinum neurotoxins irreversibly inhibit the release of Ach from cholinergic terminals of motor neurons, preganglionic sympathetic fibers, and pre- and post-ganglionic parasympathetic fibers. The BTX molecule cannot cross the blood-brain barrier, and therefore does not have any direct CNS effects.[114] At the neuromuscular junction, BTXs cause a chemical denervation, thereby inhibiting skeletal muscle contraction. Experiments on mouse phrenic nerve have revealed that binding of BTX to nerve terminals takes about 32 to 64 minutes.[115] In humans, clinical effects typically appear after 2 to 3 days, but peak effects are observed at 2 to 6 weeks. The primary muscle relaxant effect is on alpha motor neuron function, but it may also affect the gamma motor neurons in the muscle spindles, resulting in lower muscle resting tone.[116] In both animal and human muscle biopsy studies, muscle atrophy occurs within 2 weeks of injections. Atrophy continues for about 4 weeks and then stabilizes. Muscle mass has been estimated to return to about 70% to 80% of original size after 3 months.[117] Variation in muscle fiber size also occurs.

BTX may also have other mechanisms of analgesia in addition to those related to the relief of muscle spasm. It has been proposed that BTX may have a direct effect on the release of algesic agents from noncholinergic neurons. Specifically, there is evidence to suggest that BTX may block the release of glutamate, substance P, calcitonin g-related peptide, and other substances.[118] The subcutaneous injection of BTX-A into the paws of rats exposed to the formalin experimental pain model, although causing no motor effects, results in reduced pain behaviors, decreased release of glutamate, and inhibition of c-fos expression in the dorsal spinal cord.[119] BTX has affected the release of several neurotransmitters, decreased the release of substance P, and reduced inflammatory pain in an experimental model.[114,119] BTX also appears to have antinociceptive effects that are independent of its effects on muscle activation.

Recovery

BTX-induced chemical denervation is permanent, so skeletal muscle remains paralyzed until new axons and synapses have formed to reestablish the neuromuscular junction. Functional recovery takes place by neurogenesis in the form of axonal sprouting, reinnervation and enlargement of some end plates, and the formation of new smaller end plates.[117] The number of muscle fibers innervated per axon also increases. Sprouting begins within 10 days of BTX exposure.[120] Functional denervation is apparent for 6 weeks up to 6 months following injection, but typically lasts for 3 to 4 months. Recovery is complete after allowing sufficient time for reinnervation and neuromuscular function returns to essentially normal, even after multiple cycles of injection and recovery.

Therapeutic Uses in Pain Management

Cervical Dystonia

The most common form of dystonia is cervical dystonia, characterized by involuntary head and neck movements, either in the form of sustained muscle contraction or intermittent jerking motions. Both types may coexist and cause significant disability. Neck pain with or without headaches is a complaint in 70% of patients. Treatment with oral medications may yield inconsistent and unsatisfactory results. Surgical treatments, including thalamotomy, myelectomy, neurotomy, and selective peripheral denervation of neck muscles may produce limited benefits, but these vary from surgeon to surgeon. The introduction of BTX has revolutionized the treatment of cervical dystonia. It is estimated that treatment with BTX is effective in over 80% of cases, with an average duration of benefit of 3 to 4 months. Controlled clinical trials also have demonstrated a dramatic effect on decreasing the pain component of this syndrome. A survey of 19 studies in which BTX was used for the treatment of cervical dystonia revealed a mean weighted percentage of 76% (range, 50% to 100%) of patients reporting pain relief, from 16 studies that reported pain results.[121] Injections into the superficial neck muscles, such as the sternocleidomastoid, splenius capitis, levator scapulae, and trapezius may be done without electromyelographic guidance. The dose of BTX-A per muscle ranged from 50 to 100 MU. It has been suggested to divide the dose into 25-MU quanta and inject these in an even distribution throughout the length of the muscle. A study of patients with cervical dystonia treated with BTX has revealed that pain relief occurs long before any reduction in muscle spasm can be detected.[122]

Migraine Headache

The finding that BTX may be effective in treating migraine headache occurred in patients who were being treated with pericranial BTX injections for facial wrinkles. This prompted a multicenter, open-label study on the efficacy of BTX for the acute and prophylactic management of migraine.[123] BTX was injected into the glabellar, temporal, frontal, and/or suboccipital muscles of the head and neck. In 77 true migraine patients treated prophylactically with a mean dose of 31 units (range, 5 to 110 units), 51% reported complete response with a mean duration of relief of 4.1 months, and 38% reported a partial response with a mean duration of relief of 2.7 months. In the acute treatment group, 70% of 10 true migraine patients treated with a mean dose of 31 units reported complete response at 1 to 2 hours after treatment. A double-blind, vehicle-controlled study was done on 123 migraineurs in which the patients were randomized to receive the vehicle or BTX-A 25- or BTX-A 75-unit injections at one visit into symmetric points in the frontalis, temporalis, and glabellar muscles.[124] BTX-A, 25 units, was significantly superior to vehicle in reducing migraine frequency and severity, the use of acute migraine medication, and migraine-associated vomiting. The beneficial effects of BTX-A were observed at 2 and 3 months. The 75-unit dose of BTX-A had a higher incidence of side effects, including blepharoptosis, diplopia, and injection site weakness. BTX-B (Myobloc) has been evaluated for treating transformed migraine headaches.[125] Forty-seven patients received injections of 5000 units of BTX-B into three or more muscles. Of these, 64% reported improvement in headache intensity and severity, and all patients experienced a decrease in migraine frequency over 4 weeks.

Tension Headache

Tension-type headache (TH) is characterized as a dull, aching, pressure-like or squeezing feeling; the International Headache Society (IHS) has characterized the pain as pressing or tightening. Because many patients relate their complaints to increased muscle stiffness in the neck and shoulders, a myofascial origin for TH has long been considered. However, the consistent findings of increased scalp tenderness, decreased cephalic pressure pain tolerances, and decreased thermal pain thresholds and tolerances support the presence of hyperalgesia, or dorsal horn sensitization, in chronic TH.[126] A population study of 1000 adult patients has revealed a lifetime prevalence of TH of 78%, with 87% of chronic headache sufferers demonstrating pericranial muscle tenderness and pain threshold abnormalities.[127] BTX has shown efficacy in the treatment of TH. In one retrospective study, 21 patients with chronic TH were injected with BTX-A, 100 units, divided evenly over five injection sites representing the most tender muscle points in the scalp and upper neck.[128] There was a 50% reduction in headache frequency in 18 of the 21 patients and a 50% reduction in tenderness to palpation in 20 patients. In another study, the efficacy of BTX-A was assessed in a randomized, double-blind, placebo-controlled trial in 37 patients.[129] Patients received BTX-A, 100 units, or placebo, divided among six injection sites—two in the temporal muscles and four in the cervical muscles. The actively treated group experienced decreased headache severity and more headache-free days over 3 months following injection. TH is a multifactorial disorder, with peripheral and central pain mechanisms.[129] The efficacy of BTX in this and other headache disorders suggests that BTX may have peripheral and central analgesic effects.

Whiplash Injury

Whiplash injury is sustained by rapid extension followed by flexion of the neck, and often is caused by motor vehicle accidents (MVAs) and sports injuries. Whiplash-associated disorders (WADs) include a number of clinical features, including neck pain, nonspecific headache, and temporomandibular joint pain. Headache occurs in up to 55% of cases, and temporomandibular pain occurs in 35%.[130] Clinical findings in WADs include myofascial tenderness, trigger points in the affected musculature, increased pain with function, and cervical muscle spasm. Up to 87% of patients with WADs have some degree of muscle spasm that contributes to pain and dysfunction.[131] BTX-A has been studied in small trials of WADs and has been found to relieve pain and increase range of motion. A randomized, double-blind, placebo-controlled study has examined the effects of BTX-A in patients with MVA-associated WADs longer than 6 months' duration.[131] Half the patients received BTX-A, 100 units, into five trigger points, and the other 50% received normal saline injections. The muscles treated bilaterally included the splenius capitis, rectus capitis, semispinalis capitis, and trapezius. At 4 weeks postinjection, the BTX-A treatment group demonstrated a significant improvement in range of motion (ROM) and subjective pain. A randomized, placebo-controlled study evaluated the potential benefits of relaxing selected neck muscles with BTX-A.[132] Twenty-eight patients with chronic grade 2 WADs received injections of BTX-A, 100 units, or saline placebo. Each patient received five injections into the five most tender cervical muscular points. At 2 weeks, the BTX-A group showed a trend in improvement in ROM and pain reduction. At 4 weeks postinjection, this group was significantly improved from preinjection levels.

BTX-B has also been studied in WADs. An open-label study evaluated BTX-B for the treatment of 31 patients with chronic headaches following injury.[133] These patients were experiencing headaches radiating from the occipital region to the orbital region for longer than 5 months in addition to restricted neck flexion, rotation, and side bending. BTX-B, 5000 units, was injected in divided doses into the suboccipital muscles (rectus capitis posterior major and minor, obliquus capitis inferior and superior). Of these, 71% experienced a decrease in headache pain and frequency.[133]

Hemifacial Spasm

Hemifacial spasm is usually caused by irritation or compression of the root of the facial nerve by an anomalous blood vessel. This is a slowly progressive syndrome characterized by intermittent tonic or clonic contractions of the muscles supplied by the facial nerve. Treatment with anticonvulsants such as carbamazepine may provide relief initially, but becomes less effective with long-term use. Surgical microvascular decompression of the facial nerve may be highly successful in relieving this condition, but serious potential complications, such as facial paralysis, hearing loss, and stroke, deter many patients from this procedure. BTX injections into the facial muscles have now become the treatment of choice for hemifacial spasm.[134,135] It is recommended that for the first treatment only the orbicularis oculi be injected, with a starting dose of 12.5 units of BTX-A; this initial treatment has led to a decrease in spasms of the lower face.[117] Other commonly injected muscles include the frontalis (5 to 10 MU), risorius (2.5 to 5MU), depressor angulioris (5 MU), platysma (2.5 MU per strand of muscle), and zygomatic major (2.5 MU). The dose for BTX-B is 125 to 250 units per muscle site (total dose, 750 to 5000 units).

Low Back Pain

It is estimated that 80% of adults experience low back pain at some time in their lives. Acute low back pain usually resolves within 6 weeks in 70% to 90% of cases with conservative treatment.[136] Chronic low back pain costs the U.S. economy an estimated 50 billion dollars/year.[137] The efficacy of BTX for the relief of chronic low back pain was investigated in a randomized, double-blind study of 31 patients who had nonradiating back pain for at least 6 months.[138] Fifteen patients received 200 units of BTX-A, 40 units per site at five lumbar paravertebral levels on the side of maximum discomfort, and 16 patients received normal saline. At 3 weeks, 86% of patients in the BTX group and 31% of patients in the saline group reported some degree of pain relief, with 73% in the BTX group reporting more than 50% relief. At 8 weeks, 60% in the BTX group versus 12.5% in the saline group reported pain relief exceeding 50%. BTX was not associated with any increase in low back pain or worsening in functioning.

Myofascial Pain

Myofascial pain syndrome is a regional pain disorder characterized by muscle pain, stiffness, and decreased range of motion. Strain, overload, or trauma are primary causes, whereas coexisting arthropathies, neuropathies, radiculopathies, or visceral disease are potential secondary causes. The classic finding is the "trigger point" described by Travell and Simmons.[139] This is a 3- to 6-mm area of focal tenderness located in a palpable taut band of muscle, which on mechanical stimulation yields both referred pain in a characteristic reference zone and a muscle twitch response. Active trigger points cause myofascial pain, whereas latent trigger points cause restricted range of motion, and may be found in normal individuals. Reactivation of latent trigger points can occur with exposure to cold, emotional or physical stress, trauma, or sleep deprivation. Trigger point injections with local anesthetics and steroids are the treatment of choice and are usually applied in the setting of oral therapy with nonsteroidal anti-inflammatory drugs, muscle relaxants, tricyclic antidepressants, and physical therapy. BTX injections may be used for cases refractory to a series of trigger point injections with local anesthetics and steroids. BTX-A was evaluated for the treatment of chronic myofascial pain in a randomized, double-blind, placebo-controlled study of six patients with myofascial pain involving cervical paraspinal and shoulder girdle muscles.[140] Patients were injected with 50 units of BTX-A or normal saline on two occasions. Four of the 6 patients experienced more than a 30% reduction in pain and muscle spasm following BTX. Onset of the response occurred within the first week, and mean duration of response was 5 to 6 weeks.

Recent studies, however, have shown the lack of efficacy of BTX injections for myofascial pain syndrome. In a randomized, double-blind, crossover study, BTX-A (25 units per trigger point) was found to provide the same degree and duration of pain relief compared with 0.5% bupivacaine.[141] Another study has shown no difference in results between BTX-A, at 5 units per trigger point, and saline.[142] Finally, a study that compared different doses of BTX-A (5, 10, 25, or 50 units per trigger point) with saline showed no differences in the pain scores, pain threshold as measured by pressure algometry, and number of rescue medications.[143] It appears, therefore, that BTX-A does not offer any advantage over bupivacaine or saline, regardless of the dose. It should be noted that doses more than 50 units per muscle may result in weakness of that muscle.

Piriformis Syndrome

Piriformis syndrome affects 5% to 6% of patients referred for low back pain and leg pain treatment.[144] It may occur following trauma to the pelvis, buttock hypertrophy of the piriformis muscle, anatomic abnormalities of the piriformis muscle or sciatic nerve, leg length discrepancy, or piriformis myositis.[145] A history of trauma is present in approximately 50% of cases, but may be as remote as several months, and also may occur following total hip replacement. Parziale and colleagues[144] have characterized the syndrome as having the following features: (1) history of trauma to the sacroiliac or gluteal region; (2) pain in the region of the sacroiliac joint, greater sciatic notch, and piriformis muscle, extending down the leg and causing difficulty walking; (3) acute exacerbation of pain by stooping or lifting that is moderately relieved by traction; (4) palpable, sausage-shaped mass over the piriformis muscle, which is tender to palpation; (5) positive Lasègue sign (pain on voluntary flexion, adduction, and internal rotation of the hip); and (6) possible gluteal atrophy. Additional clinical tests include the Freiberg sign, which is pain on forced internal rotation of the extended thigh, and the Pace sign, which is pain and weakness on resisted abduction of the hip when the patient is seated.[145]

The pain of piriformis syndrome involves the buttock and occasionally the ipsilateral leg, if sciatic nerve irritation is present. There may also be paralumbar pain, or pain radiating to the posterior thigh down to the knee if the posterior cutaneous nerve of the thigh is involved.[145] The pain is exacerbated by prolonged sitting or on rising from a seated position.[146] Initial treatment is conservative and includes physical therapy combined with anti-inflammatory drugs, analgesics, and muscle relaxants to reduce inflammation, spasm, and pain.[145,147] When conservative therapy fails, patients may benefit from local anesthetic, steroid injections, or both into the piriformis muscle, caudal epidural steroid injections,[148] BTX injections, or surgery.[145] A randomized, double-blind study of 72 cases of piriformis syndrome has examined the effect of BTX-A, 200 units, compared with lidocaine and triamcinolone or placebo. BTX-A therapy resulted in 50% pain reduction in 65% of patients as compared with a 32% response in the triamcinolone and lidocaine group and 6% in the placebo group.[149] The techniques of piriformis injection include blind injection of the muscle, nerve stimulator technique to identify the sciatic nerve,[150] fluoroscopy and electromyelographically guided injection,[151] fluoroscopy and nerve stimulator–assisted technique,[145] and computerized tomography to visualize the muscle before injection.[152] In the fluoroscopy and nerve stimulator–assisted technique,[145] the sciatic nerve is identified first with a nerve stimulator, and steroid and saline are injected perisciatically. The needle is then pulled back 0.5 to 1 cm and 1 to 3 mL of dye is injected to outline the piriformis; this is followed by the injection of the steroid and local anesthetic.

Antibody Formation and Adverse Reactions

Repeated injections of BTX-A have been associated with antibody formation, which renders subsequent BTX-A injections ineffective. A study of 32 patients with spasmodic torticollis treated with repeated BTX-A injections has revealed that 4 patients (12.5%) produced antibodies after 2 to 9 months of treatment.[153] The larger doses used in cervical dystonia spasmodic torticollis likely explain this relatively high incidence. The data from numerous studies have suggested that the incidence of antibody formation with BTX-A for the treatment of cervical dystonia is probably less than 5%.[3] Because BTX-A and BTX-B are structurally different, it has long been thought that neutralizing antibodies to BTX-A would not cross-react with BTX-B. It appears that higher toxin doses and frequent injections are the leading factors in the development of neutralizing antibodies.[154] The reported complications of botulinum toxin injection include brachial plexopathy,[155,156] polyradiculoneuritis,[157] and local psoriasiform dermatitis.[158] Muscle weakness occurs if more than 50 units of BTX-A are injected into a muscle.[143]

CONCLUSION

The pain medicine physician should be aware of the pharmacology of the drugs used for interventional pain treatments. These drugs include the radiocontrast agents, steroids, and botulinum toxin. Knowledge of the salient topics related to these drugs will lead to their safer use; these include pretreatment and treatment regimens for patients with a history of allergy to the contrast agents, recommended safeguards to prevent intravascular injection of the steroids during transforaminal injections, and indications for the botulinum toxins. Other drugs used by the interventional physician include local anesthetics and intrathecal agents; these are discussed elsewhere in this text.

SUMMARY

- Nonionic low-osmolality contrast agents have led to the safer use of contrast agents for fluoroscopy. Although allergic reactions are rare, the clinician should be familiar with the pretreatment and treatment regimens recommended for patients with a history of allergy to these agents.
- There are theoretical advantages for the use of the transforaminal technique, but the reports of central nervous system injuries make its continued use in the cervical area inadvisable. These injuries have been described with all the steroids, local anesthetics, and dyes. The use of computed tomography does not prevent the occurrence of these injuries.
- Some recommended precautions in preventing CNS events include aspiration before injection, use of blunt needles, flexible extension tubing, and real-time imaging.

- Steroids with larger particles, such as methylprednisolone, should preferably not be used in transforaminal epidural steroid injections. The commercial form of betamethasone, with its small particles, may be the ideal particulate steroid for transforaminal injections.
- Soluble steroids such as dexamethasone have no particles, are long-acting, and have minimal mineralocorticoid properties (similar to all the other steroids). However, it has increased glucocorticoid activity, similar to betamethasone, and is easily washed out from the epidural space. Definitive prospective, randomized, controlled studies on its efficacy are lacking.
- CNS injuries have not been described with the interlaminar epidural technique. Any of the steroids can be used with this technique.
- Botulinum toxins are effective drugs when used for their FDA-approved indications. Recent studies have shown its lack of efficacy for patients with myofascial pain syndromes.

References

1. Morris TW, Katzberg RW: Intravenous contrast media: Properties and general effects. In Katzberg RW (ed): The Contrast Media Manual. Baltimore, Williams & Wilkins, 1992, pp 1-18.
2. Lasser EC, Berry CC, Talner LB, et al: Pretreatment with corticosteroids to alleviate reactions to intravenous contrast material. N Engl J Med, 1987;317: 845-849.
3. Sitzman T, Chen Y, Rallo-Clemans R, et al: Drugs for the interventional pain physician. In Benzon HT, Raja S, Molloy RE, et al (eds): Essentials of Pain Medicine and Regional Anesthesia. New York, Elsevier Churchill Livingstone, 2005, pp 166-180.
4. Cochran ST: Anaphylactoid reactions to radiocontrast media. Curr Allergy Asthma Rep 2005;5:28-31.
5. Grainger RG: Annotation: Radiological contrast media. Clin Radiol 1987;38:3-5.
6. Asif A, Garces G, Preston RA, et al: Current trials of interventions to prevent radiocontrast-induced nephropathy. Am J Ther 2005;12:127-132.
7. Sharma SK, Kini A: Effect of nonionic radiocontrast agents on the occurrence of contrast-induced nephropathy in patients with mild-moderate chronic renal insufficiency: Analysis of the randomized trials. Cathet Cardiovasc Interv 2005;65:386-393.
8. Heyman SN, Clark BA, Cantley I, et al: Effects of ioversol versus iothalamate on endothelin release and radiocontrast nephropathy. Invest Radiol 1993;28:313-318.
9. Weisbord SD, Palevsky PM: Radiocontrast-induced acute renal failure. J Intens Care Med 2005;20:63-75.
10. Bornstein SR, Chrousos GP: Adrenocorticotropin (ACTH)- and non-ACTH-mediated regulation of the adrenal cortex: Neural and immune inputs. J Clin Endocrinol Metab 1999; 84:1729-1736.
11. Williams GH, Dluhy RG: Disorders of the adrenal cortex. In Braunwald E, Fauci AS, Kasper DL, et al (eds): Harrison's Principles of Internal Medicine. New York, McGraw-Hill, 2001, pp 2084-2105.
12. Melby JC: Clinical pharmacology of systemic corticosteroids. Ann Rev Pharmacol Toxicol 1977;17:511-527.
13. Orth DN, Kovacs WJ: The adrenal cortex. In Wilson JD, Foster DW, Kronenberg HM, et al (eds): Williams Textbook of Endocrinology, 9th ed. Philadelphia, WB Saunders, 1992, pp 517-665.
14. Zaloga GP, Marik P: Endocrine and metabolic dysfunction syndromes in the critically ill. Crit Care Clin 2001; 17:25-41.
15. Saito T, Takanashi M, Gallagher E, et al: Corticosteroid effect on early beta-adrenergic down-regulation during circulatory shock: Hemodynamic study and beta-adrenergic receptor assay. Intens Care Med 1995;21:204-210.
16. Barnes P: Beta-adrenergic receptors and their regulation. Am J Resp Crit Care Med 1995;152: 838-860.
17. Szabo C: Alterations in nitric oxide production in various forms of circulatory shock. New Horiz 1995;3:2-32.
18. Rosol TJ, Yarrington JT, Latendresse J, et al: Adrenal gland: Structure, function, and mechanisms of toxicity. Toxicolo Pathol 2001;29:41-48.
19. Pignatelli D, Magalhaes MM, Magalhaes MC: Direct effects of stress on adrenocortical function. Horm Metab Res 1998;30:464-474.
20. Wolkersdörfer GW, Bornstein SR: Tissue remodeling in the adrenal gland. Biochem Pharmacol 1998;56:163-171.
21. Simpson ER, Waterman MR: Regulation of the synthesis of steroidogenic enzymes in adrenal cortical cells by ACTH. Annu Rev Physiol 1988;50:427-440.
22. Güse-Behling H, Ehrhart-Bornstein M, Bornstein SR, et al: Regulation of adrenal steroidogenesis by adrenaline: Expression of cytochrome P450 genes. J Endocrinol 1992;135: 229-237.
23. Bornstein SR, Ehrhart-Bornstein M, Güse-Behling H, et al: Structure and dynamics of adrenal mitochondria following stimulation with corticotrophin-releasing hormone (CRH). Anat Rec 1992;234:255-262.
24. Nussdorfer GG: Cytophysiology of the adrenal cortex. Int Rev Cytol 1986;98:1-395.
25. Oelkers W: Adrenal insufficiency. N Engl J Med 1996;355: 1206-1211.
26. Richards ML, Caplan RH, Wickus GG, et al: The rapid low-dose (1 μg) cosyntropin test in the immediate postoperative period: Results in elderly subjects after major abdominal surgery. Surgery 1999;125:431-440.
27. Jackson RV, DeCherney GS, DeBold CR, et al: Synthetic ovine corticotrophin-releasing hormone: Simultaneous release of proopiolipomelanocortin peptides in man. J Clin Endocrinol Metab 1984;58:740-743.
28. Burchard K: A review of the adrenal cortex and severe inflammation: Quest of the "eucorticoid" state. J Trauma 2001;51: 800-814.
29. Coursin DB, Wood KE: Corticosteroid supplementation for adrenal insufficiency. JAMA 2002;287:236-240.
30. Esteban NV, Loughlin T, Yergey AL, et al: Daily cortisol production rate in man determined by stable isotope dilution/mass spectrometry. J Clin Endocrinol Metab 1991;72: 39-45.
31. Nesbitt LT: Minimizing complications from systemic glucocorticosteroid use. Curr Ther 1995;13:925-939.
32. Lilly MP, Gann DS: The hypothalamic-pituitary-adrenal-immune axis. Arch Surg 1992;127:1463-1474.
33. Perlstein RS, Whitnall MH, Abrams JS, et al: Synergistic roles of interleukin-6, interleukin-1, and tumor necrosis factor in the adrenocorticotropin response to bacterial lipopolysaccharide in vivo. Endocrinology 1993;132:946-952.
34. Lamberts SWJ, Bruning HA, DeJong FH: Corticosteroid therapy in severe illness. Drug Ther 1997;337:1285-1292.
35. Munck A, Guyre PM, Holbrook JN: Physiological functions of glucocorticoids in stress and their relation to pharmacological actions. Endocrinol Rev 1984;5:25-44.
36. Hiebert JM, Egdhal RH: Cortisol responses to normotensive and hypotensive oligemia in unanesthetized primates. Surg Forum 1972;23:69-77.
37. Cooper CE, Nelson DH: ACTH levels in plasma in preoperative and surgically stressed patients. J Clin Invest 1962; 41;1599-1605.
38. Wade CE, Lindberg JS, Cockrell JL, et al: Upon-admission adrenal steroidogenesis is adapted to the degree of illness in intensive care unit patients. J Clin Endocrinol Metab 1988;67:223-227.
39. Kehlet H, Binder C: Adrenocortical function and clinical course during and after surgery in unsupplemented glucocorticoid-treated patients. Br J Anaesth 1973;45:1043-1048.

40. Annane D, Bellissant E, Bollaert PE, et al: Corticosteroids for severe sepsis and septic shock: A systematic review and meta-analysis. BMJ 2004;329:480.

41. De Jong FH, Mallios C, Jansen C, et al: Etomidate suppresses adrenocortical function by inhibition of 11β-hydroxylation. J Clin Endocrinol Metab 1984;59:1143-1147.

42. Hench PS, Slocumb CH, Polley HF, et al: Effect of cortisone and pituitary adrenocorticotrophic hormone (ACTH) on rheumatic diseases. JAMA 1950;144:1327-1335.

43. Fraser CG, Preuss FS, Bigford WD: Adrenal atrophy and irreversible shock associated with cortisone therapy. JAMA 1952;149:1542-1543.

44. Salem M, Tainsh, RE Jr, Bromberg J, et al: Perioperative glucocorticoid coverage: A reassessment 42 years after emergence of a problem. Ann Surg 1994;219:416-425.

45. Streck WF, Lockwood DH: Pituitary adrenal recovery following short-term suppression with corticosteroids. Am J Med 1979;66:910-914.

46. LaRochelle GE, LaRochelle AG, Ratner RE, et al: Recovery of the hypothalamic-pituitary-adrenal (HPA) axis in patients with rheumatic diseases receiving low-dose prednisone. Am J Med 1993;95:258-264.

47. Graber AL, Ney RL, Nicholson WE, et al: Natural history of pituitary-adrenal recovery following long-term suppression with corticosteroids. J Clin Endocrinol Metab 1965;25:11-16.

48. Cooper MS, Stewart PM: Corticosteroid insufficiency in acutely ill patients. N Engl J Med 2006;348:727-734.

49. Drucker D, Shandling M: Variable adrenocortical function in acute medical illness. Crit Care Med 1985;13:477-479.

50. Barnes PJ, Adcock I: Anti-inflammatory actions of steroids: Molecular mechanisms. Trends in Pharmacol Sci 1993;14:436-441.

51. Burnstein KL, DCidlowski JA: The down side of glucocorticoid receptor regulation. Mol Cell Endocrinol 1992;83:C1-C8.

52. Pepin MC, Pothier F, Barden N: Impaired type II glucocorticoid-receptor function in mice bearing antisense RNA transgene. Nature 1992;355:725-728.

53. Arai K, Lee F, Miyajima A, et al: Cytokines: Coordinators of immune and inflammatory responses Annu Rev Biochem 1990;59:783-836.

54. Guyre PM, Girard MT, Morganelli PM, et al: Glucocorticoid effects on the production and actions of immune cytokines. J Steroid Biochem 1988;30:89-93.

55. Ray A, Laforge, KS, Sehgal PB: On the mechanism for efficient repression of the interleukin-6 promoter by glucocorticoids: Enhancer, TATA box, and RNA start site (Inr motif) occlusion. Mol Cell Biol 1990;10:5736-5746.

56. Kern JA, Lamb RJ, Reed JL, et al: Dexamethasone inhibition of interleukin 1 beta production by human monocytes. Post-transcriptional mechanisms. J Clin Invest 1988;81:237-244.

57. Peers SH, Smillie F, Elderfield AJ, et al: Glucocorticoid and non-glucocorticoid induction of lipocortins (annexins) 1 and 2 in rat peritoneal leukocytes in vivo. Br J Pharmacol 1993;108:66-72.

58. Schwiebert LA, Beck LA, Stellato C, et al: Glucocorticosteroid inhibition of cytokine production: Relevance to antiallergic actions. J Allergy Clin Immunol 1996;97:143-152.

59. O'Banion MK, Winn VD, Young DA: cDNA cloning and functional activity of a glucocorticoid-regulated inflammatory cyclooxygenase. Proc Natl Acad Sci U S A 1992;89:4888-4892.

60. Santini G, Patrignani P, Sciulli MG, et al: The human pharmacology of monocyte cyclooxygenase 2 inhibition by cortisol and synthetic glucocorticoids. Clin Pharmacol Ther 2001;70:475-483.

61. Stankova J, Rola-Pleszcaynski M: Leukotriene B4 stimulates c-fos and c-jun gene transcription and AP-1 binding activity in human monocytes. Biochem J 1992;282:625-629.

62. Sur S, Adolphson CR, Gleich GJ: Eosinophils: Biochemical and cellular aspects. In Middleton E, Reed CE, Ellis EF, et al (eds): Allergy—Principles and Practice, 4th ed. St Louis, Mosby, 1993, p 169.

63. Jantz MA, Sahn SA: Corticosteroids in acute respiratory failure. Am J Respir Crit Care Med 1999;160:1079-1100.

64. Devor M, Govrin-Lippmann R, Raber P: Corticosteroids suppress ectopic neural discharge originating in experimental neuromas. Pain 1985;22:127-137.

65. Johansson A, Hao J, Sjolund B: Local corticosteroid application blocks transmission in normal nociceptive C-fibres. Acta Anaesthesiol Scand 1990;34:3353-3358.

66. Orth DN: Cushing's syndrome. N Engl J Med 1995;332:791-803.

67. Tuel SM, Meythaler JM, Cross LL: Cushing's syndrome from epidural methylprednisolone. Pain 1990;40:81-84.

68. Luckert BP, Raisz LG: Glucocorticoid-induced osteoporosis: Pathogenesis and management. Ann Intern Med 1990;112:352-365.

69. Wolverton SE: Glucocorticosteroids. In Wolverton SE, Wilkin JK (eds): Systemic Drugs for Skin Diseases. Philadelphia, WB Saunders, 1991, pp 87-124.

70. Lester RS: Corticosteroids. Clin Dermatol 1989;7:80-97.

71. Yeap SS, Hosking DJ: Management of corticosteroid-induced osteoporosis. Rheumatology 2002;41:1088-1094.

72. Stanbury RM, Graham E: Systemic corticosteroid therapy—side effects and their management. Br J Ophthalmol 1998;82:704-708.

73. Weiner ES, Abeles M: Aseptic necrosis and glucocorticoids in systemic lupus erythematosus: A reevaluation. J Rheumatol 1989;16:604-608.

74. Wolverton SE: Major adverse effects from systemic drugs: Defining the risks. In Callan J (ed): Current Problems in Dermatology, vol 7. St. Louis, Mosby-Year Book, 1995, pp 1-40.

75. Owczarek J, Jasinska M, Orszulak-Michalak D: Drug-induced myopathies. An overview of the possible mechanisms. Pharmacolog Rep 2005;57:23-34.

76. Piper JM, Ray WA, Daugherty JR, et al: Corticosteroid use and peptic ulcer disease: Role of nonsteroidal anti-inflammatory drugs. Ann Intern Med 1991;114:735-740.

77. Nashel DJ: Is atherosclerosis a complication of long-term corticosteroid treatment? Am J Med 1986;80:925-929.

78. Butterfield JH, Gleich GJ: Anti-inflammatory effects of glucocorticoids on eosinophils and neutrophils. In Schleimer RP, Claman HN, Oronsky A (eds): Anti-inflammatory Steroid Action: Basic and Clinical Aspects. New York, Academic Press, 1989, pp 151-198.

79. Cupps TR: Effects of glucocorticoids on lymphocyte function. In Schleimer RP, Claman HN, Oronsky A (eds): Anti-inflammatory Steroid Action: Basic and Clinical Aspects. New York, Academic Press, 1989, pp 132-150.

80. Truhan AP, Ahmed AR: Corticosteroids: A review with emphasis on complications of prolonged systemic therapy. Ann Allergy 1989;62:375-390.

81. Wahl SM: Glucocorticoids and wound healing. In Schleimer RP, Claman HN, Oronsky A (eds): Anti-inflammatory Steroid Action: Basic and Clinical Aspects. New York, Academic Press, 1989, pp 280-302.

82. Lacomis D, Samuels MA: Adverse neurologic effects of glucocorticosteroids. J Gen Intern Med 1991;6:367-377.

83. Gallant C, Kenny P: Oral glucocorticoids and their complications: A review. J Am Acad Dermatol 1986;14:161-177.

84. Maillefert JF, Aho S, Huguenin MC, et al: Systemic effects of epidural dexamethasone injections. Rev Rhum Engl Ed 1995;62:429-432.

85. Abram SE: Treatment of lumbosacral radiculopathy with epidural steroids. Anesthesiology. 1999;91:1937.

86. Boonen S, Van Distel G, Westhovens R, et al: Steroid myopathy induced by epidural triamcinolone injection. Br J Rheumatol 1995;34:385-386.

87. Knight CL, Burnell JC: Systemic side effects of extradural steroids. Anaesthesia 1980;35:593-594.

88. Jacobs S, Pullan PT, Potter JM, et al: Adrenal suppression following extradural steroids. Anaesthesia 1983;38:953-956.

89. Cook DM, Meikle AW, Bowman R: Systemic absorption of triamcinolone after a single intraarticular injections suppresses the pituitary-adrenal axis [abstract]. Clin Res 1988;36:121A.

90. Ward A, Watson J, Wood P, et al: Glucocorticoid epidural for sciatica: Metabolic and endocrine sequelae. Rheumatology 2002;41:68-71.

91. Nelson DA: Dangers from methylprednisolone acetate therapy by intraspinal injections. Arch Neurol 1988;45:804-806.

92. Goldstein DA, Zimmerman B, Speilberg ST: Anaphylactic response to hydrocortisone in childhood: A case report. Ann Allergy 1985;55:599-600.

93. Peller JS, Bardana EJ Jr: Anaphylactoid reaction to corticosteroid: Case report and review of the literature. Ann Allergy 1985;54:302-305.

94. Freedman MD, Schocket AL, Chapel N, et al: Anaphylaxis after intravenous methylprednisolone administration. JAMA 245: 607-608, 1981.

95. Partridge MR, Gibson GJ: Adverse bronchial reactions to intravenous hydrocortisone in two aspirin-sensitive asthmatic patients. Br Med J 1978;2:1521-1522.

96. Brouwers PJAM, Kottnik EJBL, Simon MAM, et al: A cervical anterior spinal artery syndrome after diagnostic blockade of the right C6 nerve root. Pain 2001;91:397-399.

97. Houten JK, Errico TJ: Paraplegia after lumbosacral nerve root block: Report of three cases. Spine J 2002;2:70-75.

98. Baker R, Dreyfuss P, Mercer S, Bogduk N: Cervical transforaminal injection of corticosteroids into a radicular artery: A possible mechanism for spinal cord injury. Pain 2003;103:211-215.

99. McMillan MR, Crompton C: Cortical blindness and neurological injury complicating cervical transforaminal injection for cervical radiculopathy. Anesthesiology 2003;99:509-511.

100. Rozin L, Rozin R, Koehler SA, et al: Death from transforaminal epidural nerve root block (C7) the result of perforation of the left vertebral artery. Am J Forensic Med Pathol 2003;24:351-355.

101. Tiso RL, Cutler T, Catania JA, et al: Adverse central nervous system sequelae after selective transforaminal block: The role of corticosteroids. Spine J 2004;4:468-474.

102. Huntoon MC, Martin DP: Paralysis after transforaminal epidural injection and previous spinal surgery. Reg Anesth Pain Med 2004;29:494-495.

103. Karasek M, Bogduk N: Temporary neurologic deficit after cervical transforaminal injection of local anesthetic. Pain Med 2004;5:202-205.

104. Somayaji HS, Saifuddin A, Casey ATH, et al: Spinal cord infarction following therapeutic computed tomography-guided left L2 nerve root injection. Spine 2005;30:E106-E108.

105. Rathmell JP, April C, Bogduk N: Cervical transforaminal injection of steroids. Anesthesiology 2004;100:1959-1600.

106. Rathmell JP, Benzon HT. Transforaminal injection of steroid: Should we continue [editorial]? Reg Anesth Pain Med 2004;29:397-399.

107. Benzon HT, Chew TL, McCarthy R, et al: Comparison of the particle sizes of different steroids and the effect of dilution: A review of the relative neurotoxicities of the steroids. Anesthesiology 2007;106:331-338.

108. Hoeft MA, Rathmell JP, Monsey RD, et al: Cervical transforaminal injection and the radicular artery: Variation in anatomical location within the cervical intervertebral foramina. Reg Anesth Pain Med 2006;31:270-274.

109. Dreyfuss P, Baker R, Bogduk N: Comparative effectiveness of cervical epidural steroid injections with particulate and nonparticulate corticosteroid preparations for cervical radicular pain. Pain Med 2006;7:237-242.

110. Benzon HT, Gissen AJ, Strichartz GR, et al: The effect of polyethylene glycol on mammalian nerve impulses. Anesth Analg 1987;66:553-559.

111. Simpson LL: Molecular pharmacology of botulinum toxin and tetanus toxin. Annu Rev Pharmacol Toxicol 1986;26:427-453.

112. Gargland MG, Hoffman HT: Crystalline preparation of botulinum type A (Botox): degradation impotency with storage. Otolaryngol Head Neck Surg 1993;108:135-140.

113. DasGupta BR: Structure and biological activity of botulinum neurotoxin. J Physiol (Paris) 1990;84:220-228.

114. Coffield JA, Considine RV, Simpson LL: The site and mechanism of action of botulinum neurotoxin. In Janckovic J, Hallett, M (eds): Therapy with Botulinum Toxin. New York, Marcel Dekker, 1994, pp 3-13.

115. Yamada S, Kuno Y, Iwanaga H: Effects of aminoglycoside antibiotics on the neuromuscular junction: Part I. Int J Clin Pharmacol Ther Toxicol 1986;24:130-138.

116. Filippi GM, Errico P, Santarelli R, et al: A toxin effects on rat jaw muscle spindles. Acta Otolaryngol (Stockh) 1993;113:400-404.

117. Joseph K, Tsui C: Botulinum toxin as a therapeutic agent. Pharmacol Ther 1996;72:13-24.

118. McMahon HT, Foran P, Dolly JO, et al: Tetanus toxin and botulinum toxins type A and B inhibit glutamate, gamma-aminobutyric acid, aspartate, and met-enkephalin release from synaptosomes. J Biol Chem 1992;267:21338-21343.

119. Cui ML, Khanijou S, Rubino J, et al: Botulinum toxin A inhibits the inflammatory pain in the rat formalin model [abstract]. Soc Neurosci 2000;26:656.

120. Duchen LW: Changes in motor innervation and cholinesterase localization induced by botulinum toxin in skeletal muscle of mouse: Differences between fast and slow muscles. J Neurol Neurosurg Psychiatry 1970;33:40-54.

121. Poewe W, Wissel J: Experience with botulinum toxin in cervical dystonia. In Jankovic J, Hallet M (eds): Therapy with Botulinum Toxin. Marcel Dekker, New York, 1994.

122. Jankovic J, Schwartz K: Botulinum toxin injections for cervical dystonia. Neurology 1990;40:277-280.

123. Binder WJ, Brin MF, Blitzer A, et al: Botulinum toxin type A (Botox) for treatment of migraine headaches: An open-label study. Otolaryngol Head Neck Surg 2000;123:669-676.

124. Silberstein S, Mathew N, Saper J, et al: Botulinum toxin type A as a migraine preventive treatment. Headache 2000;40:445-450.

125. Opida C: Open-label study of Myobloc (botulinum toxin type B) in the treatment of patients with transformed migraine headaches. J Pain 3(Suppl 1):10, 2002.

126. Jensen, R: Pathophysiological mechanisms of tension-type headache: A review of epidemiological and experimental studies. Cephalalgia 1999;19:602-621.

127. Jensen R, Rasmussen BK: Muscular disorders in tension-type headache. Cephalalgia 199616:97-103.

128. Freund BJ, Schwartz M: A focal dystonia model for subsets of chronic tension headache. Cephalalgia 2000;20:433.

129. Smuts JA, Baker MK, Smuts HM, et al: Prophylactic treatment of chronic tension-type headache using botulinum toxin type A. Eur J Neurol 1999;6:S99-S102.

130. Frankell VH: Temporomandibular joint pain syndrome following deceleration injury to the cervical spine. Bull Hosp Joint Dis 1969;26:47-51.

131. Freund BJ, Schwartz M: Treatment of whiplash associated with neck pain with botulinum toxin-A: A pilot study. J Rheumatol 2000;27:481-484.

132. Freund B, Schwartz M: Use of botulinum toxin in chronic whiplash-associated disorder. Clin J Pain 2002;18:S163-S168.

133. Opida CL: Open-label study of Myobloc (botulinum toxin type B) in the treatment of patients with post-whiplash headaches. Poster 204. Presented at the International Conference on Basic and Therapeutic Aspects of Botulinum and Tetanus Toxin, June 2002, Hanover, Germany.

134. O'Day J: Use of botulinum toxin in neuro-ophthalmology. Curr Opin Ophthalmol 2001;12:419-422.

135. Tsui JKC: Botulinum toxin as a therapeutic agent. Pharmacol Ther 1996;72:13-24.

136. Frymoyer JW: Predicting disability from low back pain. Clin Orthop Rel Res 1992;279:101-109.

137. Nachemson A: Newest knowledge of low back pain. Clin Orthop Rel Res 1992;279:8-20.

138. Oster L, Clapp L, Erickson M, et al: Botulinum toxin A and chronic low back pain. Neurology 2001;56:1290-1293.

139. Travell JG, Simons DG: Myofascial Pain and Dysfunction: The Trigger Point Manual, vol 1. Baltimore, Williams & Wilkins, 1983.

140. Cheshire WP, Abashian SW, Mann JD: Botulinum toxin in the treatment of myofascial pain syndrome. Pain 1994;59: 65-69.
141. Graboski CL, Gray DS, Burnham RS: Botulinum toxin A versus bupivacaine trigger point injections for the treatment of myofascial pain syndrome: A randomized double-blind crossover study. Pain 2005;118:170-171.
142. Ojala T, Arokoski JPA, Partanen J: The effect of small doses of botulinum toxin A on neck-shoulder myofascial pain syndrome: A double-blind, randomized, and controlled crossover trial. Clin J Pain 2006;22:90-96.
143. Ferrante FM, Bearn L, Rothrock R, et al: Evidence against trigger point injection technique for the treatment of cervicothoracic myofascial pain with botulinum toxin type A. Anesthesiology 2005;103:377-378.
144. Parziale JR, Hudgins TH, Fishman LM: The piriformis syndrome. Am J Orthop 1996;25:819-823.
145. Benzon HT, Katz JA, Benzon HA, et al: Anatomic considerations, a new injection technique, and a review of the literature. Anesthesiology 2003;98:1442-1448.
146. Barton PM: Piriformis syndrome: A rational approach to management. Pain 1991;47:345-352.
147. Rich B, McKeag D: When sciatica is not disk disease. Phys Sports Med 1992;20:105-115.
148. Mullin V: Caudal steroid injection for treatment of piriformis syndrome. Anesth Analg 1990;71:705-707.
149. Fishman LM, Anderson C, Rosner B: Botox and physical therapy in the treatment of piriformis syndrome. Am J Phys Med Rehabil 2002;81:936-942.
150. Hanania M, Kitain E: Perisciatic injection of steroid for the treatment of sciatica the result of piriformis syndrome. Reg Anesth Pain Med 1998;23:223-228.
151. Fishman SM, Caneris OA, Bandman TB, et al: Injection of the piriformis muscle by fluoroscopic and electromyographic guidance. Reg Anesth Pain Med 1998;23:554-559.
152. Porta M: A comparative trial of botulinum toxin type A and methylprednisolone for the treatment of myofascial pain syndrome and pain from chronic muscle spasm. Pain 2000;85:101-105.
153. Racz GB: Botulinum toxin as a new approach for refractory pain syndromes. Pain Digest 1998;8:353-356.
154. Lang AM: Botulinum toxin for myofascial pain. In Advancements in the Treatment of Neuromuscular Pain. Johns Hopkins University, Office of Continuing Medical Education Syllabus, 1999, pp 23-28.
155. Glanzman RL, Gelb DJ, Drury I, et al: Brachial plexopathy after botulinum toxin injections. Neurology 1990;40: 1143.
156. Sampaio C, Castro-Caldas A, Sales-Luis ML, et al: Brachial plexopathy after botulinum toxin administration for cervical dystonia [letter]. J Neurol Neurosurg Psychiatry 1993; 56:220.
157. Haug BA, Dressler D, Prange HW: Polyradiculoneuritis following botulinum toxin therapy. J Neurol 1990;237: 62-63.
158. Bowden JB, Rapini RP: Psoriasiform eruption following intramuscular botulinum A toxin. Cutis 1992;50:415-416.

CHAPTER
39 Psychological Interventions

Dennis C. Turk and Kimberly S. Swanson

A number of psychological interventions have been developed for patients with chronic pain, with a large body of research supporting their efficacy. Before reviewing the approaches with the greatest empirical support, it is important to consider the plight of the person with chronic pain, the role of psychological factors, and the mechanisms involved in the experience of chronic pain, because these serve as the basis for the development of treatment modalities. We will then outline the various psychological models and conceptualizations of chronic pain and describe the most commonly used treatment interventions.

Note that we will use the terms *patient* and *person* to differentiate the individual who is designated as a patient when he or she is in the health care provider's office, clinic, or hospital from the person with chronic pain when he or she is living outside the constraints of health care facilities. This is an important distinction, because chronic pain is by definition not curable, persisting over extended periods of time for months and even years. Persons with a chronic pain syndrome must learn how to adapt and self-manage their pain, associated symptoms, and lives. Chronic pain might be viewed as analogous to diabetes; in the physician's office, the person with diabetes is a diabetic patient but at all other times is someone who has to learn how to live with diabetes. This involves carrying out all the necessary activities—routinely testing glucose levels (if insulin-dependent), taking medication or injecting with insulin, maintaining an appropriate diet, modulating exercise patterns, and monitoring skin for infections. All these occur outside the formal health care system. Similar behaviors are required of those with various types of chronic pain. In the absence of cure, self-management becomes critical.

PLIGHT OF THE PERSON WITH CHRONIC PAIN

People with chronic and recurrent acute pain (e.g., migraine) often feel rejected by the very elements of society that exist to serve them. They lose faith and may become frustrated and irritated when the health care system that initially might have created expectations for cure turns its back when treatments prove ineffective. They feel victimized and traumatized by repeated and invasive medical procedures; they become disillusioned and feel disbelief when it seems as though medical professionals expect them to find the cause of their pain, and when they have to convince the skeptical provider to take their symptoms seriously.

Although individuals with acute pain can often receive relief from primary health care providers, people with persistent pain become enmeshed in the medical system as they shuttle from physician to laboratory test to imaging procedure in a frustrating search to have their pain diagnosed and successfully treated, if not terminated completely. Thus, at the same time that returning to work and earning an income becomes less possible, medical bills for unsuccessful treatments accumulate. This experience of "medical limbo"—the presence of a painful condition that in the absence of acceptable pathology might have psychiatric causation, suggests malingering, or perhaps even be an undiagnosed but potentially progressive disease—is itself a source of significant and chronic stress that can initiate emotional distress or aggravate a premorbid psychiatric condition.

The person with a chronic pain condition resides in a complex and costly world that is also populated by their significant others, health care providers, employers, and third-party payers. Family members feel increasingly hopeless and distressed as medical costs, disability, and emotional suffering increase while income and available treatment options decline. Health care providers grow increasingly frustrated and feel defeated and ineffective as available treatment options are exhausted while the pain condition remains a mystery and may worsen. Employers, who are already resentful of growing workman's compensation benefits, pay higher costs while productivity suffers, because the employee frequently calls in sick or cannot perform at his or her usual level ("presenteeism"). Third-party payers watch as health care expenditures soar with repeated diagnostic tests, often with inconclusive results. In time, the legitimacy of the individual's report of pain may be questioned, because often a medical reason fails to substantiate the cause of the symptoms.

People with chronic pain may begin to feel that their health care providers, employers, and even family members are blaming them when their condition does not respond to treatment. Some may suggest that the individual is complaining excessively to receive attention, avoid undesirable activities, or be relieved from onerous obligations (e.g., gainful employment, household chores). Others may suggest that the pain is not real, they are feigning or exaggerating their symptoms, and it is all in their head, "psychogenic." Third-party payers may even suggest that the individual is intentionally exaggerating his or her pain to obtain financial gain, whereas others may attribute reported symptoms to the desire to obtain mood-altering medications. In this way they may come to be regarded as wimps, crocks, or fakes.

As a result of these attitudes and the absence of cure or even substantial relief, those with chronic pain may withdraw from society, lose their jobs, alienate family and friends, and become more and more isolated, despondent, depressed, and in general demoralized. Their bodies, the health care system, and their significant other have let them down. They may believe that they have even failed themselves as they relinquish their usual activities and responsibilities, because of symptoms that are intractable but often almost seemingly invisible when not validated by objective pathologic findings. This emotional distress, however, can be exacerbated by other factors, including fear, inadequate or maladaptive support systems, inadequate personal and material coping resources, treatment-induced (iatrogenic) complications, overuse of potent drugs, inability to work, financial difficulties, prolonged litigation, disruption of usual activities, and sleep disturbance.

Fear of pain or movement and (re)injury is an important contributor to disability associated with several chronic pain disorders, including back pain and fibromyalgia syndrome.[1] People with chronic pain often anticipate that certain activities will increase their pain or induce further injury. These fears may contribute to avoidance of activity and subsequently greater physical deconditioning, emotional distress and, ultimately, greater disability. Their failure to engage in activities prevents them from obtaining any corrective feedback about the associations among activity, pain, and injury.

In addition to fear of movement, people with persistent pain may be anxious about the meaning of their symptoms for the future—will their pain increase, will their physical capacity diminish, will they have progressive disability and ultimately end up in a wheelchair or become bedridden? In addition to these anxieties, people in pain may fear that others will not believe that they are suffering or told that they are beyond help and will just have to "learn to live with it." Such fears can contribute to additional emotional distress and increased muscle tension and physiologic arousal that may directly exacerbate and maintain pain. Living with persistent pain conditions requires considerable emotional resilience. It tends to deplete people's emotional reserves, taxing not only the individual but also the capability of family, friends, coworkers, and employers to provide support.

Chronic pain is estimated to be present in up to 20% of the adult U.S. population.[2] If we assume that most people do not live alone but in a social context with significant others, then more than 50% of the population may be affected directly or indirectly. Pain is expensive; health care and indirect costs associated with disability compensation, lost tax revenues, retraining, less than optimal performance on the job, and legal fees exceed $150 billion each year.[3,4] To put it bluntly, pain hurts—it hurts the person with the symptoms, it hurts significant others, and it hurts society.

Despite advances in knowledge of the neurophysiology of pain and the development of new pharmacologic agents with analgesic properties, sophisticated surgical interventions, and advanced technologies (e.g., spinal cord stimulation, implantable drug delivery systems), cure of pain has eluded the best efforts of health care providers. Regardless of the treatment, the amount of pain reduction averages only about 33%; fewer than 50% of persons treated by these interventions obtain even this result, and the extent of improvement in emotional, physical, and social functioning is often below this level.[5]

As noted, chronic pain is by definition incurable. People with chronic pain continually confront noxious sensations and other aversive symptoms that affect every aspect of their lives, social, emotional, interpersonal, and economic, as well as physical. Thus, those with chronic pain are faced with managing their symptoms on their own. Faced with this task, the common response is "How?"

It is well to recall Bonica's[6] comment in the preface to the first edition (1954) of his seminal work, *The Management of Pain* (and repeated in the second edition 36 years later):

The crucial role of psychological and environmental factors in causing pain in a significant number of patients only recently received attention. As a consequence, there has emerged a sketch plan of pain apparatus with its receptors, conducting fibers, and its standard function which [sic] is to be applicable to all circumstances. But . . . in so doing, medicine has overlooked the fact that the activity of this apparatus is subject to a constantly changing influence of the mind.

Based on the overview provided, two conclusions should be obvious: (1) psychological factors play a significant role in the experience, maintenance, and exacerbation, if not the cause, of pain; and (2) because there are no cures for chronic pain and some level of pain will persist in most pain sufferers regardless of treatment, psychological approaches may be useful complements to more traditional medical and surgical approaches.

PSYCHOLOGICAL FORMULATIONS OF CHRONIC PAIN

A number of different psychological perspectives on chronic pain have evolved over time. It is important to consider these initially because psychological treatments are based on different and at times competing psychological principles.

Psychogenic View

As is frequently the case in medicine, when physical explanations seem inadequate or when the results of treatment are inconsistent, reports of pain are attributed to a psychological cause (and thus are "psychogenic"). Although psychogenic views of pain have been discussed since the formulation of psychodynamic theory, a psychodynamic perspective on chronic pain was first described systematically in the 1960s, when people with pain were viewed as having compulsive and masochistic tendencies, inhibited aggressive needs, and feelings of guilt—"pain-prone personalities."[7] It was commonly believed that people with pain had childhood histories fraught with emotional abuse, family dysfunction (e.g., parental quarrels, separation, divorce), illness or death of a parent, early responsibilities, and high motivation toward achievement.[8] Some current research has reported associations between chronic pain and childhood trauma, although the findings are not consistent.[9,10]

Based on the psychogenic perspective, assessment of those with chronic pain is directed toward identifying the psychopathologic tendencies that instigate and maintain pain. Although the evidence to support this model is scarce, the American Psychiatric Association[11] has created a psychiatric diagnosis, somatoform pain disorder. Diagnosis of a pain disorder requires that the person's report of pain must be inconsistent with the anatomic distribution of the nervous system or, if it mimics a known disease entity, cannot be adequately accounted for by organic pathology after extensive diagnostic evaluation. Even in the presence of a medical condition that may cause pain, psychological factors may be implicated and thus the person may receive a psychiatric diagnosis of "pain disorder associated with *both* psychological factors and a general medical condition."[11]

It is assumed that reports of pain will cease once the psychogenic mechanisms have been resolved. Treatment is geared toward helping patients gain insight into the underlying maladaptive psychological contributors.[12,13]

Empiric evidence supporting the psychogenic view is scarce. A number of chronic pain sufferers do not exhibit significant psychopathology. Furthermore, insight-oriented psychotherapy has not been shown to be effective in reducing symptoms for most patients with chronic pain. Studies have suggested that the emotional distress observed in patients with chronic pain more typically occurs in response to the persistence of pain and is not as a causal agent,[14,15] and may resolve once pain is adequately treated.[16] The psychogenic model has thus come under scrutiny, and may be flawed in its view of chronic pain.

Behavioral Formulations

According to the classic or respondent conditioning model, if a painful stimulus is repeatedly paired with a neutral stimulus, the neutral stimulus will come to elicit a pain response. For example, a person who experienced pain after performing a treadmill exercise may become conditioned to experience a negative emotional response to the presence of the treadmill and to any stimulus associated with it (e.g., physical therapist, gym). The negative emotional reaction may instigate muscle tensing, thereby exacerbating pain and further reinforcing the association between the stimulus and pain. Based on this conditioned correlation, people with chronic pain may avoid activities previously associated with pain onset or exacerbation.

In 1976, Fordyce[17] introduced an extension of operant conditioning to chronic pain. This view proposes that acute pain behaviors (e.g., avoidance of activity to protect a painful area from additional pain) may come under the control of external contingencies of reinforcement (responses increase or decrease as a function of their reinforcing consequences) and thus develop into a chronic pain problem. Fordyce underscored the fact that because there is no objective way to measure pain the only way we can know of someone's pain is by their behavior, expressed verbally or nonverbally. Overt pain behaviors include verbal reports, paralinguistic vocalizations (e.g., sighs, moans), motor activity, facial expressions, body postures and gesturing (limping, rubbing a painful body part, grimacing), functional limitations (e.g., reclining for extensive periods of time, inactivity), and behaviors designed to reduce pain (e.g., taking medication, use of the health care system).

The central features of pain behaviors are that they are (1) sources of communication and (2) observable. Observable behaviors are capable of eliciting a response and the consequences of behavior will influence subsequent behavior. Through a learning process, responses that receive positive consequences, especially repeated desirable consequences, will more likely be maintained, whereas behaviors that fail to active positive consequences or that receive negative consequences will be less likely to occur (i.e., extinguished). Pain behaviors may be positively reinforced directly (e.g., attention from a spouse or health care provider, monetary compensation, avoidance of undesirable activity).[18] Pain behaviors may also be maintained by the escape from noxious stimulation through the use of drugs or rest, or the avoidance of undesirable activities such as work. In addition, well behaviors (e.g., activity, working) may not be positively reinforcing and the more rewarding pain behaviors may therefore be maintained.

The operant conditioning model does not concern itself with the initial cause of pain. Rather, it considers pain an internal subjective experience that can be directly assessed and may be maintained even after an initial physical basis of the pain has resolved. The pain behavior originally elicited by organic factors caused by injury or disease may come to occur, totally or in part, in response to reinforcing environmental events.

It is important, however, not to make the mistake of viewing pain behaviors as synonymous with malingering. Malingering involves consciously and purposely faking a symptom such as pain for some gain, usually financial. Contrary to the beliefs of many third-party payers, there is little support for the contention that outright faking of pain for financial gain is prevalent.

The social learning model emphasizes that behavior can be learned not only by actual reinforcement of the individual's behavior but also by observation of what happens to others. This is a particularly powerful way of learning when the others being observed are judged to be similar to the observer. For example, a middle-aged man might learn what to expect by observing how other middle-aged men with similar medical problems are treated. Thus, the development and maintenance of pain behaviors may occur by observational learning and modeling processes. Specifically, people can acquire responses that were not previously in their behavioral repertoire by the observation of others performing these activities. Expectations and actual behavioral responses to nociceptive stimulation are based, at least partially, on prior social leaning history.

Children develop attitudes about health and health care and about the perception and interpretation of symptoms and physiologic processes from their parents and others they confront in their social environment. They learn how others respond to injury and disease and thus may ignore or overrespond to symptoms that they experience based on behaviors modeled in childhood. For example, children of chronic pain patients may exhibit more pain-related responses during stressful times or exhibit more illness behaviors (e.g., complaining, days absent, visit to school nurse) than children of healthy parents based on what they have observed and learned at home.[19]

Expectations and actual behavioral responses to nociceptive stimulation are partially based on prior social learning history. Models can influence the expression, localization, and methods of coping with pain. Even physiologic responses may be conditioned during observation of others in pain.[20]

A central construct of the social learning perspective is that of self-efficacy.[21] This is a personal expectation that is particularly important for patients with chronic pain. A self-efficacy expectation is defined as a personal conviction that a course of action (performing required behaviors) can successfully be executed to produce a desired outcome in a given situation.[21] Given sufficient motivation to engage in a behavior, it is a person's self-efficacy beliefs that determine the choice of activities that he or she will initiate, the amount of effort that will be expended, and how long the individual will persist in the face of obstacles and aversive experiences. In this way, self-efficacy plays an important role in therapeutic change.[22]

Efficacy judgments are based on four sources of information regarding one's capabilities, listed in descending order of effects[17]: (1) one's own past performance at the task or similar tasks; (2) the performance accomplishments of others who are perceived to be similar to oneself; (3) verbal persuasion by others that one is capable; and (4) perception of one's own state of physiologic arousal, which is in turn partly determined by prior efficacy estimation. Performance mastery can then be created by encouraging people to undertake subtasks that are initially attainable but become increasingly difficult, and subsequently approaching the desired level of performance. It is important to remember that coping behaviors are influenced by the person's beliefs that the demands of a situation do not exceed her or his coping resources.

How people interpret, respond to, and cope with illness are determined by cultural norms and perceptions of self-efficacy. These two sets of factors contribute to the marked variability in response to objectively similar degrees of physical pathology noted by health care providers.

Gate-Control Model

Although not a psychological formulation itself, the gate-control model[23] was the first to popularize the importance of central psychological factors in pain perception. Perhaps the most important contribution of the gate-control theory is the way it changed thinking about pain perception. Melzack and Casey[24] have differentiated three systems related to the processing of nociceptive stimulation, all thought to contribute to the subjective experience of pain—sensory-discriminative, motivational-affective, and cognitive-evaluative. Thus, the gate-control theory specifically includes psychological factors as an integral aspect of the pain experience. It emphasizes central nervous system (CNS) mechanisms and provides a physiologic basis for the role of psychological factors in chronic pain.

The gate-control model contradicts the notion that pain is either somatic or psychogenic. Instead, it postulates that both factors have potentiating and moderating effects. According to this model, both the central and peripheral nervous systems interact to contribute to the experience of pain. It is not only these physical factors that guide the brain's interpretation of painful stimuli that are at the center of this model; psychological factors (e.g., thoughts, beliefs, emotions) are also actively involved.

Prior to the Melzack and Wall[23] formulation of the gate-control theory, psychological processes were largely dismissed as reactions to pain. Although the physiologic details of the gate-control model have been challenged,[25] it has had a substantial impact on basic research and can be credited as a source of inspiration for diverse clinical applications to control or manage pain, including neurophysiologically based procedures (e.g., neural stimulation techniques from peripheral nerves and collateral processes in the dorsal columns of the spinal cord), pharmacologic advances, behavioral treatments, and interventions that target modification of attentional and perceptual processes involved in the pain experience.

Cognitive-Behavioral Perspective

The cognitive-behavioral model, perhaps the most commonly accepted model for the psychological treatment of individuals with chronic pain,[26,27] incorporates many of the psychological variables previously described—anticipation, avoidance, and contingencies of reinforcement—but suggests that cognitive factors rather than conditioning factors are of central importance. The model proposes that conditioned reactions are largely self-activated on the basis of learned expectations rather than automatically evoked. The model suggests that behaviors and emotions are influenced by interpretations of events, and emphasis is placed on how people's beliefs and attitudes interact with physical, affective, and behavioral factors. It proposes that conditioned reactions are largely activated by learned expectations rather than being automatically evoked. In other words, it is the individual's information processing that results in anticipatory anxiety and avoidance. The critical factor, therefore, is that people learn to anticipate and predict events and to express appropriate reactions.[28]

From the cognitive-behavioral model, people with pain are viewed as having negative expectations about their own ability to control certain motor skills without pain. Moreover, people with chronic pain tend to believe that they have limited control over their pain. Such negative maladaptive appraisals about the situation and personal efficacy may reinforce the experience of demoralization, inactivity, and overreaction to nociceptive stimulation. These cognitive appraisals and expectations are postulated as having an effect on behavior leading to reduced efforts and activity, which may contribute to increased psychological distress (helplessness) and subsequent physical limitations. If one accepts that pain is a complex subjective phenomenon that is uniquely experienced by each person, then knowledge about idiosyncratic beliefs, appraisals, and coping abilities becomes critical for optimal treatment planning and for evaluating treatment outcome accurately.

Several important factors may facilitate or disrupt people's sense of control: their beliefs and appraisals, their expectations about pain, their ability to cope, their social supports, their disorder, medicolegal and health care systems, and their employers. These factors also influence patients' investment in treatment, acceptance of responsibility, perceptions of disability, adherence to treatment recommendations, support from significant others, expectations for treatment, and acceptance of treatment rationale.

Cognitive interpretations also affect how patients present symptoms to others, including health care providers. Overt communication of pain, suffering, and distress will enlist responses that may reinforce pain behaviors and impressions about the seriousness, severity, and uncontrollability of pain. That is, complaints of pain may induce physicians to prescribe more potent medications, order additional diagnostic tests and, in some cases, perform surgery. Significant others may express sympathy, excuse the person with chronic pain from responsibilities, and encourage passivity, thereby fostering further physical deconditioning.

People with persistent pain often have negative expectations about their own ability and responsibility to exert any control over their pain and often view themselves as helpless. Such negative maladaptive appraisals about their condition, situation, and personal efficacy in controlling their pain and problems associated with pain reinforce their experience of demoralization, inactivity, and overreaction to nociceptive stimulation. These cognitive appraisals are posited as having an effect on behavior, leading to reduced effort, less perseverance in the face of difficulty, lowered activity level, and increased psychological distress. It should be obvious that the cognitive-behavioral perspective integrates the operant conditioning emphasis on external reinforcement and respondent view of conditioned avoidance within the framework of information processing.

The cognitive-behavioral perspective on pain management focuses on providing the patient with techniques to gain a sense of control over the effects of pain on his or her life as well as actually modifying the affective, behavioral, cognitive, and sensory facets of the experience. Behavioral experiences help show pain sufferers that they are capable of more than they assumed, increasing their sense of personal competence. Cognitive techniques (e.g., self-monitoring to identify relationship among thoughts, mood, and behavior, distraction using imagery, and problem solving, described below) help place affective, behavioral, cognitive, and sensory responses under the person's control.

The assumption is that long-term maintenance of behavioral changes will occur only if the person with pain has learned to attribute success to his or her own efforts. It has been suggested that these treatments can result in changes of beliefs about pain, coping style, and reported pain severity, as well as direct behavioral changes. Treatment that results in increases in perceived control over pain and decreased catastrophizing also results in decreases in pain severity and functional disability. When successful rehabilitation occurs, there is a major shift from beliefs about helplessness and passivity to resourcefulness and ability to function regardless of pain, and from an illness conviction to a rehabilitation conviction.

A number of studies have attempted to identify cognitive factors that contribute to pain and disability.[22,29] These studies have consistently demonstrated that a person's attitudes, beliefs, and expectations about their plight, themselves, personal coping strategies, and the health care system affect reports of pain, activity, disability, and response to treatment. For example, people respond to medical conditions in part based on their subjective ideas about their illness and symptoms. When pain is interpreted as signifying ongoing tissue damage or a progressive disease, it is likely to produce considerably more suffering and behavioral dysfunction than if it is viewed as being the result of a stable problem that is expected to improve.

Once beliefs and expectations are formed, they become stable and rigid and relatively impervious to modification. Pain sufferers tend to avoid experiences that could invalidate their beliefs (disconfirmations) and guide their behavior in accordance with these beliefs, even in situations in which these beliefs are no longer valid. It is thus essential for people with chronic pain to develop adaptive beliefs about the relationships among impairment, pain, suffering, and disability, and to deemphasize the role of experienced pain in their regulation of functioning.

Distorted thinking can also contribute to the maintenance and exacerbation of pain. A particularly potent and pernicious thinking style that has been observed in people with chronic pain is catastrophizing—holding negative thoughts about one's situation and interpreting even minor problems as major catastrophes.[30] Research has indicated that people who spontaneously use more catastrophizing thoughts report more pain than those who do not catastrophize.[30]

Coping strategies, or a person's specific ways of adjusting to or minimizing pain and distress, act to alter both the perception of pain intensity and the ability to manage or tolerate pain and continue daily activities. Overt behavioral coping strategies include rest, medication, and use of relaxation. Covert coping strategies include various means of distracting oneself from pain, reassuring oneself that the pain will diminish, seeking information, and problem solving.

Studies have found active coping strategies, such as efforts to function in spite of pain or distracting oneself from pain, to be associated with adaptive functioning, and passive coping strategies, such as depending on others for help with pain control, avoiding activities because of fear of pain or injury, self-medication, and alcohol, to be related to greater pain and depression.[29] Regardless of the type of coping strategy, if people with chronic pain are instructed in the use of adaptive coping strategies, their rating of intensity of pain decreases and tolerance of pain increases.[29] Thus, the perspective on how people function and the emphasis on facilitating self-management are more important than any specific cognitive or behavioral techniques used to bring about changes in thinking and behavior.

Biopsychosocial Model

Although the gate-control theory introduced the role of psychological factors in the maintenance of pain symptoms, it focused primarily on the basic anatomy and neurophysiology of pain. The biopsychosocial model, which expands the cognitive-behavioral model of pain, views illness as a dynamic and reciprocal interaction between biologic, psychological, and sociocultural variables that shape the response to pain.[22,29] What is unique about this model is that it takes into consideration the influence of higher order cognitions, including perception and appraisal. It accepts that people are active processors of information, and that behavior, emotions, and even physiology are influenced by interpretations of events, rather than solely by physiologic factors.[28,29] People with chronic pain may therefore have negative expectations about their own ability and responsibility to exert any control over their pain. Moreover, those with pain behaviors elicit responses from significant others that can reinforce adaptive and maladaptive modes of thinking, feeling, and behaving.

The biopsychosocial model presumes some form of physical pathology or at least physical changes in the muscles, joints, or nerves that generate nociceptive input to the brain. At the periphery, nociceptive fibers transmit sensations that may or may not be interpreted as pain. Such sensation is not pain until subjected to higher order psychological and mental processing that involves perception, appraisal, and behavior. Perception involves the interpretation of nociceptive input and identifies the type of pain (e.g., sharp, burning, punishing). Appraisal involves the meaning attributed to the pain and influences subsequent behaviors. A person may choose to ignore the pain and continue working, walking, socializing, and engaging in previous levels of activity or may choose to leave work, refrain from activities, and assume the sick role. In turn, this interpersonal role is shaped by responses from significant others that may promote the healthy response or the sick role. The biopsychosocial model has been instrumental in the development of cognitive-behavioral treatment approaches for chronic pain, including assessment and intervention (described later in this chapter).[28,29]

Family Systems Perspective

In family systems, and this could be expanded to significant others, not only to traditional concepts of nuclear families, the individual and his or her behavior are placed within a social unit. The family is viewed as an interactional unit, and family members (significant others) have a profound impact on each other's emotions, thoughts, and behaviors. Thus, the functioning of family members is interdependent, and family relationships are important not only for psychological but also physical health.[31,32]

Increasing evidence supports the concept that family members contribute to behavioral risk factors such as smoking, lack of exercise, and poor diet, which can influence the development of numerous chronic illnesses, as well as compliance or noncompliance to treatment regimens.[33] Additionally, families influence the development of chronic pain via operant theory. For example, expressions of acute pain (e.g., reporting pain, grimacing, avoidance of activity, use of pain medication), because they are overt and observable, may be reinforced through expressions of concern from family members. Furthermore, in support of this idea, a number of investigators[34-36] have found that spousal attentiveness to expressions of pain are positively correlated with higher levels of reported pain, pain behavior frequency, and disability.

The experience of chronic stress within the family has also been hypothesized to contribute to the development of chronic illness.[37] Specifically, chronic stress may play an important role in sympathetic nervous system and endocrine dysregulation often found in chronic pain patients.

As noted, pain does not take place in isolation but in a social context. Pain does not occur solely in people's bodies, nor does it occur solely in their brains, but rather it occurs in their lives. The emphasis on the role of significant others is important. It reminds us that treating a chronic pain patient successfully requires that we not only assess and treat the patient but must also target significant others, who can be supportive but can also be impediments to rehabilitation when they are overly punitive or solicitous.[37]

INTERFACES OF PSYCHOLOGY, PHYSIOLOGY, AND NEUROCHEMISTRY

Pain is a biopsychosocial phenomenon, with the implication being that psychological, social, and biologic factors contribute to the experience. Moreover, these factors interact, so that psychological and social factors are reflected in bodily processes and have physiologic consequences, and psychological and social variables are influenced by an individual's unique biology. Advances in research and technology are permitting increased understanding of the intricate associations between biology and behavior.[38]

Psychoneuroendocrinology is a specialized field of research that studies the interactions between behavior and the brain, nervous system, and endocrine system. The primary emphasis of this area is on the hypothalamic-pituitary adrenal (HPA) axis. The HPA axis is believed to be the primary part of the neuroendocrine system that responds to stress.[39-41]

Several investigators have proposed that chronic or extensive activation of the HPA axis can lead to deleterious effects on somatic and psychological well-being.[39-42] Long-term effects of altered secretion of glucocorticoids have adverse effects on various health outcomes, and HPA axis dysregulation has been associated with many chronic pain conditions. There

have been discrepant findings in research regarding enhanced versus attenuated HPA axis activity.[39]

Although the dysregulation cannot be accounted for entirely by psychosocial distress and somatization,[41] the HPA axis release of hormones in the face of psychosocial stress has been established, and HPA axis dysregulation does appear to contribute significantly to the maintenance and severity of chronic pain conditions.[40,42,43]

Psychophysiology is the science of understanding the link between psychology and physiology. Psychophysiology examines how psychological activities (e.g., stressful events or emotions) produce physiologic response. Thus, in chronic pain, psychophysiology examines how exposure to a stressful situation or strong emotions produces a result expressed as the pain experience. Commonly used measures of psychophysiology include measures of brain activity event-related potentials (ERPs), functional magnetic resonance imaging (fMRI), skin temperature, skin conductance (also known as galvanic skin response), cardiac measures (heart rate, heart rhythm, heart rate variability), and muscle responses (electromyogram, muscle tension, and myofascial trigger points).[44,45]

Autonomic dysregulation is the main component of psychophysiology that has been investigated.[45,46] Although autonomic dysregulation as a causative factor in chronic pain has not been confirmed, dysregulation with evidence of sympathetic tone has been demonstrated to be a significant mediator in the long-term maintenance and subjective severity of the pain experience in many chronic pain conditions.[46,47] The results of studies examining psychoneuroimmunology and psychophysiology, along with more recent studies using brain imaging, are not only beginning to confirm the interrelationships between physiologic and psychological factors in chronic pain, they are demonstrating the mechanisms involved in such interactions[38,48] (see Chapter 9).

ASSESSMENT AND EVALUATION

To understand and appropriately treat a person whose primary symptom is pain, one must begin with a comprehensive history and physical examination. Physical examination procedures and sophisticated laboratory and imaging techniques are readily available for use in detecting organic pathology. Physical and laboratory abnormalities, however, correlate poorly with subjective reports of pain, and it is often not possible to make any precise pathologic diagnosis or even to identify an adequate anatomic origin for the pain. Thus, an adequate pain assessment also requires the use of clinical interviews, observation, and assessment tools to help evaluate the myriad psychosocial and behavioral factors that influence the subjective report.

There is no "pain thermometer" that can provide an objective quantification of the amount or severity of pain experienced; it can only be assessed indirectly based on a patient's description, verbally and behaviorally. Patients are usually asked to describe the characteristics (e.g., stabbing, burning), location, and severity of their pain. However, even this can make pain assessment difficult, because pain is a complex, subjective phenomenon comprised of a range of factors and is uniquely experienced by each person. Wide variability in pain severity, quality, and impact may be noted in reports of people with pain as they attempt to describe what appear to be objectively identical phenomena. Their pain descriptions are also colored by cultural and sociologic influences, as well as prior experiences.

Interview

A list of topics that can be covered in an assessment interview is shown in Box 39–1.[49] A functional assessment of the pain can also be used, whereby the person can be asked about the current level of pain or pain over the past week or month, or a diary or journal can be maintained to indicate pain intensity, with ratings recorded several times daily for several days or weeks. Merely inquiring about characteristics of pain, although necessary, is not sufficient. Diaries or journals can provide more information than only the varying pain intensity. A clinician can use information about pain obtained during the interview and from a patient's writings to identify patterns in behavior, including potential antecedents and consequences to pain exacerbation, and treatment decisions can be informed by the availability of such data.

People with pain believe that the cause of their symptoms, trajectory, and beneficial treatments will have important influences on coping with pain and adhering to therapeutic interventions. Thus, when conducting an interview with a person with chronic pain, focus should be on the specific thoughts, behaviors, emotions, and physiologic responses that precede, accompany, and follow pain episodes or exacerbations, including environmental and temporal conditions and consequences associated with the patient's responses (e.g., cognitive, emotional, and behavioral, including frequency, specificity, and generality). It is important to note any patterns of maladaptive thoughts, because these may contribute to a sense of hopelessness, dysphoria, and unwillingness (e.g., fears) about engaging in specific activities.

It is also important to determine expectations and goals for treatment for patients and their significant other(s). For example, an expectation that pain will be eliminated completely may be unrealistic and should be addressed to prevent discouragement if this does not occur. Additionally, formulating treatment goals (e.g., symptom reduction, reduced emotional distress, improved physical, social, and vocational functioning, reduction of inappropriate use of the health care system) is helpful in returning someone to optimal functioning given their age, sex, education, and presence of physical impairments.

Behavioral Observation

A number of different observational procedures have been developed to quantify pain behaviors.[49] Behavioral checklists can identify the frequency and type of pain behaviors exhibited by a person with pain. Such checklists can be self-reports or reports by others—for example, behavioral observation scales can be used by significant others and health care providers can use observational methods to quantify various pain behaviors systematically (e.g., observing the person in the waiting room, while being interviewed, during a structured series of physical tasks, in the presence of a significant other). Noting the type and frequency of pain behaviors can provide detailed information about when someone performs pain behaviors, around whom the behaviors are elicited, and the responses of others to the pain behaviors. It is not surprising to find that people with chronic pain tend to carry out more pain behaviors around others who give them positive reinforcement of the pain behavior (e.g., providing soothing statements, physical intimacy, assistance in performing tasks). Obtaining details about factors that increase and decrease behavior (e.g., patterns) can be used when developing treatment goals.

Self-Report Questionnaires

A number of assessment instruments designed to evaluate a person's attitudes, beliefs, and expectations about themselves, their symptoms, and the health care system have been developed (some common assessment instruments have been described by Melzack and Wall[50]). There are many advantages to the use of standardized instruments—they are easy

---

BOX 39–1. AREAS COVERED IN CLINICAL INTERVIEWS

- Patient's perception about the cause of pain
- Patient's experience of pain (how often and when it occurs) and related symptoms
- Treatments received and currently receiving
- Impact of pain on daily activities
- Impact of pain on interpersonal relationships
- Level and nature of emotional distress
- Current stressors and areas of conflict
- Methods used to cope with symptoms
- Alcohol and substance abuse history and current use
- Behaviors used to let others know pain is present
- Responses by significant others
- Social history
- Education and vocational history
- Receiving or seeking compensation and involvement in litigation
- Concerns and expectations

to administer, require minimal time, assess a wide range of behaviors, and obtain information about behaviors that may be private (sexual relations) or unobservable (thoughts, emotional arousal) and, most importantly, they can be submitted to analyses that permit determination of their reliability and validity. These instruments should not be viewed as alternatives to interviews; rather, they may suggest issues to be addressed in more depth during an interview or investigated with other measures. Additionally, they allow comparison among groups of people with pain and provide valuable information about the functional status of individuals in relation to others with the same condition. Questionnaires have been developed to assess reports of engaging in a range of functional activities, such as the ability to walk up stairs, sit for specific periods of time, lift specific weights, and perform activities of daily living, as well as the severity of the pain experienced when performing these activities.[49,50]

Measures of psychosocial functioning have been developed for use specifically with people with pain to assess psychological distress, impact of pain on their lives, feeling of control, coping behaviors, and attitudes about disease, pain, and health care providers and the person's plight.[49,50] However, these responses to pain may be distorted as a function of the disease or as a result of the medications taken. For example, common measures of depression ask people about their appetites, sleep patterns, and fatigue. Because disease status and medication can affect responses to such questions, scores may be elevated, thus distorting the validity of the responses. Therefore, it is always best to corroborate information gathered from these instruments with other sources, such as personal interview, report by significant other(s), and chart review.

Referral for Psychological Intervention

The health care provider should be alert for red flags that may serve as an impetus for more thorough evaluation by a psychologist who specializes in the treatment of pain. Box 39–2 lists questions worth considering for persons who report persistent or recurring pain. The positive responses to these ques-

---

BOX 39–2. SCREENING QUESTIONS*

1. Has the patient's pain persisted for 3 months or longer, despite appropriate interventions and in the absence of progressive disease? [Yes]
2. Does the patient repeatedly and excessively use the health care system, persist in seeking invasive investigations or treatments after being informed that these are inappropriate, or use opioid or sedative-hypnotic medications or alcohol in a pattern of concern to the patient's physician (e.g., escalating use)? [Yes]
3. Does the patient come in requesting specific opioid medication (e.g., hydromorphone [Dilaudid]; oxycodone [OxyContin])? [Yes]
4. Does the patient have unrealistic expectations of the health care provider or the treatment offered ("total elimination of pain and related symptoms")? [Yes]
5. Does the patient have a history of substance abuse or is he or she currently abusing mind-altering substances? [Yes]
   Patients can be asked, "Have you ever found yourself taking more medication than was prescribed or have you used alcohol because your pain was so bad?" or "Is anyone in your family concerned about the amount of medication you take?" [Yes]
6. Does the patient display a large number of pain behaviors that appear exaggerated (e.g., grimacing, rigid or guarded posture)? [Yes]
7. Does the patient have litigation pending? [Yes]

8. Is the patient seeking or receiving disability compensation? [Yes]
9. Does the patient have any other family members who have had or currently suffer from chronic pain conditions? [Yes]
10. Does the patient demonstrate excessive depression or anxiety? [Yes]
    Straightforward questions such as, "Have you been feeling down?" or "What effect does your pain have on your mood?" can clarify whether this area is in need of more detailed evaluation.
11. Can the patient identify a significant or several stressful life events prior to symptom onset or exacerbation? [Yes]
12. If married or living with a partner, does the patient indicate a high degree of interpersonal conflict? [Yes]
13. Has the patient given up many activities (e.g., recreational, social, familial, in addition to occupational and work activities) because of pain? [Yes]
14. Does the patient have any plans for renewed or increased activities if pain is reduced? [No]
15. Was the patient employed prior to pain onset? [No] If yes, does he or she wish to return to that job or any job? [No]
16. Does the patient believe that he or she will ever be able to resume normal life and normal functioning? [No]

*If there is a combination of more than 6 "yes" answers to questions 1 to 13 and "no" answers to questions 14-16, or if there are general concerns in any one area, consider referral for psychological assessment.

tions should not be viewed as sufficient to make a referral for more extensive evaluation but, when more than six or seven of them are, referral should be considered. These questions need not be regarded as an interview or questionnaire but should be routinely included when interacting with chronic pain patients during the course of the history and physical examination if appropriate. By the end of the evaluation, the health care provider should have elicited enough information to make a decision as to whether a psychological evaluation is warranted.

THERAPEUTIC INTERVENTIONS

There are a number of different clinical approaches to the treatment of chronic pain that have been developed based on the models and variables described, including insight-oriented approaches, behavioral approaches, cognitive-behavioral therapy (CBT), family systems perspective, and biobehavioral interfaces. In addition, there are several specific techniques based on these models that have been used successfully (e.g., motivational interviewing, biofeedback, relaxation, guided imagery, hypnosis, meditation) on their own or as part of more comprehensive treatment regimens. We will briefly describe each of these. Perhaps the most commonly used approach, however, is CBT, which incorporates and integrates many techniques from other approaches.[26,27,51] Thus, we will give more attention to this general approach to patients and treatment.

Insight-oriented therapies

Therapy based on the psychodynamic view and insight-oriented approaches are primarily focused on early relationship experiences that are reconstructed within the context of the therapeutic relationship. The therapeutic relationship is meant to "correct" the person's prior maladaptive experience by reintegrating emotions into symbolic and available mental processes, resulting in improved emotional regulation.[8] It is important for the person with pain and the therapist to have a supportive and trusting relationship. Although insight-oriented psychotherapy may be useful with selected individuals,[13] this approach has rarely been shown to be effective in reducing symptoms for most persons with chronic pain. No randomized controlled trials have been published demonstrating the efficacy of insight-oriented psychotherapy for those with chronic pain problems.

Behavioral Approaches

Respondent Conditioning

If a nociceptive stimulus is repeatedly paired with a neutral stimulus in close temporal proximity, the neutral stimulus will come to elicit a pain response. This is referred to as classic, respondent, or pavlovian conditioning. In chronic pain, many activities that were neutral or even pleasurable may come to elicit or exacerbate pain and are thus experienced as aversive and actively avoided. Over time, a growing number of stimuli (e.g., activities, and exercises) may be expected to elicit or exacerbate pain and will be avoided, a process termed *stimulus generalization*. The anticipatory fear of pain and restriction of activity, and not just the actual nociception, may contribute to disability. Anticipatory fear can also elicit physiologic reactivity that may aggravate pain. Thus, conditioning may directly increase nociceptive stimulation and pain.

As long as activity avoidance succeeds in preventing pain initiation or exacerbation, the conviction of pain sufferers that they remain inactive is difficult to modify. Treatment of pain from the classic conditioning model includes repeatedly engaging in behavior—exposure—that produces progressively less pain than was predicted (corrective feedback), which is then followed by reductions in anticipatory fear and anxiety associated with the activity. Such transformations add support to the importance of quota-based physical exercise programs, with participants progressively increasing their activity levels despite fear of injury and discomfort associated with the use of deconditioned muscles.

Operant Approach

Operant approaches focus on the extinction of pain behaviors by withdrawal of positive attention for pain behaviors and increasing well behaviors by positive reinforcement. The operant learning paradigm does not seek to uncover the cause of pain but focuses primarily on the maintenance of pain behaviors and deficiency in well behaviors. Target pain behaviors are identified, as are their controlling antecedents and consequent reinforcers or punishments,[51] such as overly solicitous, distracting, or ignoring behaviors by a spouse.[34]

Removal of the contingent relationship between overt pain behaviors and its positive or negative consequences, along with positive and negative reinforcement, are used to increase and maintain desired behaviors and decrease pain-compatible behaviors (e.g., with operant behavioral treatment), because patients are expected to be active in setting treatment goals and following through with recommendations.[51] The efficacy of operant treatment has been demonstrated in several studies of those with chronic pain disorders, including low back pain[35] and fibromyalgia syndrome.[52]

Cognitive-Behavioral Therapy

As noted, it is important to make a distinction between the cognitive-behavioral perspective and cognitive and behavioral techniques.[22] Cognitive-behavioral perspective is based on the idea that people believe that they cannot function because of their pain and that they are helpless to improve their

BOX 39–3. ASSUMPTIONS OF THE COGNITIVE-BEHAVIORAL PERSPECTIVE

- People are active processors of information and not passive reactors.
- Thoughts (e.g. appraisals, expectations, beliefs) can elicit and influence mood, affect physiological processes, have social consequences, and also serve as an impetus for behavior; conversely, mood, physiology, environmental factors, and behavior can influence the nature and content of thought processes.
- Behavior is reciprocally determined by individual *and* environmental factors.
- People can learn more adaptive ways of thinking, feeling, and behaving.
- People should be active collaborative agents in changing their thoughts, feelings, behavior, and physiology.

situation (Box 39–3). Treatment goals thus focus on helping patients with pain realize that they can manage problems and on providing skills to respond in more adaptive ways that can be maintained after treatment has ended. These techniques include those described earlier and more specific interventions, as noted here.

The cognitive-behavioral therapy (CBT) approach combines cognitive and behavioral techniques, including assertiveness, stress management, relaxation training, goal setting, guided imagery, and pacing of activities. Biofeedback, meditation, and hypnosis can all be incorporated within the framework of CBT. Therapists assist patients with concerns about the future, returning to work, and physical limitations; they help people build their communication skills, gain a sense of control over their pain, and cope with fear of pain, reinjury, and frustration resulting from the responses of others (e.g., physicians, insurance companies, employers, family, significant others) toward the patient's pain reports or behaviors. Individuals are educated in developing positive coping strategies and are encouraged to increase their activities in a graded fashion. It is expected that they will gain mastery over their pain, which will then result in improved mood.[52]

Four key components of CBT have been described[22]—education, skills acquisition, skills consolidation, and generalization and maintenance. The education component is comprised of helping the patient challenge negative perceptions regarding his or her ability to manage pain through a process termed *cognitive restructuring*, making the person aware of the role of thoughts and emotions in potentiating and maintaining stress and physical symptoms. Steps in cognitive restructuring include identifying maladaptive thoughts during problematic situations (e.g., during pain exacerbations, stressful events), introduction and practice of coping thoughts, shifting from self-defeating to coping thoughts, introduction and practice of positive or reinforcing thoughts, and finally

home practice and follow-up. Using these steps, the therapist encourages patients to test the adaptiveness (not the so-called rationality) of thoughts, beliefs, expectations, and predictions. The crucial element in successful treatment is bringing about a shift from well-established, habitual, and automatic but ineffective responses to systematic problem solving and planning, control of affect, behavioral persistence, and disengagement, when appropriate.[22]

The goal of skills acquisition and consolidation is to help patients learn skills for new pain management behaviors and cognitions, including relaxation, problem-solving, distraction, activity pacing, and communication training. Using role-playing techniques and homework assignments, patients can practice emerging skill sets and evaluate their usefulness for the management of their pain.

Finally, generalization and maintenance are aimed toward solidifying skills and preventing relapse. Problems that arise throughout treatment are viewed as opportunities to assist patients in learning how to handle setbacks and lapses that may occur following treatment. During this phase, they can learn how to anticipate future problems and high-risk situations so they can think about and practice the behavioral responses that may be necessary for successful coping. The goal of this phase is to enable patients to develop a problem-solving perspective, in which they believe that they have the skills and competencies to respond appropriately to problems as they arise. In this manner, attempts are made to help the patient learn to anticipate future difficulties, develop plans for adaptive responding, and adjust behavior accordingly.

The efficacy of CBT has been demonstrated in a large number of studies of chronic pain disorders and has been reviewed extensively.[26,53-55] Evidence suggests that individual and group CBT can help restore function and mood as well as reduce pain and disability-related behaviors.[26,54] Despite the fact that CBT is undoubtedly the intervention used most often for those with chronic pain, there are limitations. For example, although CBT has been found to be helpful for a number of individuals, there are some for whom CBT is not beneficial. Researchers are just beginning to explore different aspects of CBT to answer the question, "What works for whom?"[56-58]

Some specific techniques can be incorporated in CBT when treating chronic pain patients. The specific details involved with these techniques may be less important than the primary objective. Each technique described is designed to help patients feel a sense of control; a common feature is their ability to combat the feelings of helplessness and demoralization experienced by many of those with chronic pain.

Motivational Interviewing

Most people with chronic pain adhere to a biomedical model; for example, the nature of their symptoms is closely aligned with physical pathology. As pain persists, some people may become aware of the role of factors such as emotional stress in their experience of pain. They may begin to consider that they can learn and use self-management techniques to help them adapt to life with a chronic pain condition. Others with chronic pain, however, have difficulty with this expanded perspective. The stage of acceptance of self-management is important, because those who are not ready for the use of psychological techniques will tend to avoid and dismiss such methods. Thus, the clinician needs to be aware of an individual's readiness to accept and undertake the necessary steps to achieve self-management. The assessment process described earlier should help the health care provider determine the patient's readiness for the use of nonphysical approaches.

Motivational interviewing as a treatment intervention was initially developed for those with substance abuse disorders,[52] although it has been increasingly used for chronic pain patients. Specific stages of change have been postulated, and interventional techniques are tailored to each stage.

In the precontemplation stage, patients with chronic pain have not yet begun to consider changing from a purely somatic view of pain, and have adopted a passive role as they wait for the health care provider to identify and provide appropriate treatment. The clinician attempts to assist the person by fostering acknowledgment of risks and problems because of inactivity, such as increased pain and physical deconditioning.[59]

Once patients with chronic pain take responsibility for their prior inactivity, they enter the next of the proposed stages, the contemplation stage. Here, the clinical goal is to encourage the patient to conclude that the risks of inactivity outweigh the perceived benefits. When they are ready to become more active (the preparation stage), the clinician helps outline appropriate structured physical activities in which the patient is willing to participate. Finally, in the action stage, the clinician helps the patient increase the activity level. This is followed by maintenance, geared toward the individual's ongoing motivation and commitment.[59]

It is important for physicians to be tolerant as patients move through these stages. Clinicians can encourage transition to different stages by providing motivational statements, listening with empathy, asking open-ended questions, providing feedback and affirmation, and handling resistance.[52,59] Because motivational interviewing has only been applied to chronic pain rather recently, the efficacy of this intervention with different chronic pain populations is not yet well documented. Motivational interviewing is a general framework for preparing persons for treatment and for adherence to the cognitive-behavioral perspective, and can be readily used with CBT.

Biofeedback

Developed in the 1960s, biofeedback is a self-regulation technique that has been used successfully to treat a number of chronic pain states, such as headache, back pain, chronic myofascial pain, and irritable bowel syndrome.[60,61] The objective of biofeedback is to teach people to exert control over their physiologic processes. During biofeedback, the patient is attached by electrodes to equipment linked to a computer that records physiologic responses. These processes may include skin conductance, respiration, heart rate, heart rate variability, skin temperature, brain wave activity, and muscle tension. The biofeedback equipment converts the readings into visual or auditory signals on a monitor that the patient can observe. In this way, the information recorded is fed back to the person, which helps the individual learn to change physiologic responses by manipulating the auditory or visual signals.

Important forms of biofeedback therapy include electromyographic biofeedback, in which patients (e.g., those with tension headaches), are provided with information fed back to them from the physiologic recordings and taught to manipulate the tension in their frontalis muscle. Patients with migraine are provided with thermal feedback. They are instructed to warm the temperature of their hands using visual or auditory cues. Alternatively, patients may be given biofeedback associated with heart rate variability (HRV), which has been shown to be associated with pain perception.[62,63]

Real-time functional MRI (rtfMRI) has been used as a sophisticated source of biofeedback to help train participants to control activation in the rostral anterior cingulate cortex (rACC) and has shown promising results. This brain region is reputedly involved in pain perception and regulation. When the participants deliberately induced changes in the rACC, there was a corresponding change in their perception of pain.[64]

With practice, most people can learn to control voluntarily important physiologic functions that may be associated directly with pain and stress.[65] Biofeedback generates a state of general relaxation. Typically, patients being treated with biofeedback will be instructed to practice using the methods that have been successful in altering physiologic parameters in the clinic.

The actual mechanisms involved in the success of biofeedback are still unknown. However, the assumption of biofeedback treatment is that the level of pain is maintained or exacerbated by autonomic nervous system dysregulation believed to be associated with the production of nociceptive stimulation (e.g., muscle tension in a person with low back pain). In addition to the physiologic changes accompanying biofeedback, patients are provided with a sense of control over their bodies. Given the high levels of helplessness observed in those with chronic pain problems, the perception of control may be as important as the actual physiologic changes observed. A general sense of relaxation is also an important feature of biofeedback. Again, it is not clear whether the alterations of specific physiologic parameters putatively associated with pain are the most important component of biofeedback compared with the broader relaxation created.

There are many relaxation techniques that have been used in combination with biofeedback and on their own. However, reports are mixed as to whether biofeedback is any more effective than relaxation. The pain condition being treated may differ in regard to the greatest contribution of a possible component (relaxation, sense-of control, general relaxation). Moreover, the components may not be mutually exclusive and may even be synergistic.

Meditation

Meditation is a 2500-year-old practice that has become a popular mental exercise. It is defined as the "intentional self-regulation of attention," a systematic inner focus on particular aspects of inner and outer experience.[66,67] Unlike many approaches in behavioral medicine, such as biofeedback, meditation was developed in a religious or spiritual context. It is regarded as the ultimate goal of spiritual growth, ending suffering, enabling personal transformation, and providing a transcendental experience.[68] However, as a health care intervention, it has been taught effectively, regardless of the individual's cultural or religious background.[69,70]

There are many forms of meditation practice worldwide. Here we will describe two general approaches that have been extensively researched, transcendental meditation and Zen or mindfulness meditation.[71] Transcendental meditation is concentrative in that it involves focus on one of the senses, like a zoom lens focusing on a specific object. For example, the individual repeats a silent word or phrase (mantra) with the goal of transcending the ordinary stream of mental discourse.[68,72] Mindfulness meditation is the opposite of transcendental meditation in that its goal is attempting awareness of the whole perceptual field, like a wide-angle lens. Thus, it incorporates focused attention and whole-field awareness in the present moment. For example, the individual simply observes without judgment, thoughts, emotions, sensations, and perceptions as they arise moment by moment.[69,73] Bonadonna[74] has proposed that those with chronic illness have an altered ability to concentrate; therefore, transcendental meditation may be less useful than mindfulness meditation.

Mindfulness meditation reframes the experience of discomfort in that physical pain, malaise, or suffering becomes the object of meditation. The attention and awareness of discomfort or suffering is another part of human experience; rather than being avoided, which is the most common reaction, it is to be investigated, experienced, and explored.[74] This form of meditation was incorporated into behavioral medicine in the 1980s[69] and has been successfully used as an adjunctive intervention for health conditions such as fibromyalgia syndrome, psoriasis, and cancer pain. Studies have found that mindfulness-based interventions decrease pain symptoms, increase healing speed, improve mood, decrease stress, contain

health care costs, and decrease visits to primary care facilities.[68,75]

Meditation has captured the attention of medicine, behavioral medicine, psychology, and neurocognitive science, partly because experienced meditators demonstrate calmer responses to daily stress and perform better at tasks that require focused attention. Many believe that meditation can confer health benefits.[76,77] Lazar and associates[76] have found that long-term meditation by Western practitioners who were not monks showed increased cortical thickness in areas related to somatosensory, auditory, visual, and interoceptive processing. They found thickening in right Brodmann's areas 9 and 10, which have been shown to be involved in the integration of cognition and emotion. A hypothesis based on this structural change is that by becoming increasingly aware of sensory stimuli during practice, the practitioner is gradually able to use self-awareness to navigate potentially stressful encounters more successfully. This may be useful for those experiencing chronic pain because of the reciprocal relationship between stress and pain symptoms.

Additionally, Lutz and coworkers[77] have observed that Buddhist practitioners at baseline and while in a state of unconditional loving kindness and compassion while meditating have higher self-induced gamma wave synchrony as compared to controls. Gamma wave activity is the synchrony of areas of the brain communicating with each other. This also suggests how meditation may be beneficial for people with chronic pain because of dysregulation within the HPA axis and autonomic nervous system. Furthermore, meditators have demonstrated changes in electroencephalographic activity; specifically, they have higher alpha brain wave activity. This has been found to have beneficial health effects and promote a general sense of well-being.[78-80]

Guided Imagery

Guided imagery can be useful for helping people with pain relax, achieve a sense of control, and distract themselves from pain and accompanying symptoms. This modality involves the generation of mental images by oneself or the practitioner. Thus, it overlaps with available relaxation techniques and hypnosis. Although guided imagery has been advocated as a stand-alone intervention to reduce presurgical anxiety and postsurgical pain and accelerate healing,[81] it is most often used in conjunction with other treatment interventions, such as CBT or relaxation.

With guided imagery, using visualization or imagination, patients are asked to evoke specific images that they find pleasant and engaging. In this way, a detailed representation tailored to the individual can then be created. When the person with chronic pain is feeling pain or is experiencing pain exacerbation, he or she can use imagery to help redirect their attention away from the pain and achieve a psychophysiologic state of relaxation.

Images can be sensory or affective; however, the most successful images tend to be those that involve all the senses (vision, sound, touch, smell, and taste). People with chronic pain are thus encouraged to use images that evoke these senses. Some patients, however, may have difficulty generating a particularly vivid visual image and may find it helpful to listen to a taped description or look at a poster on which they can focus their attention as a way of assisting their imagination.

Hypnosis

Hypnosis has been defined as a "natural state of aroused attentive focal concentration coupled with a relative suspension of peripheral awareness." There are three central components of a hypnotic trance: (1) absorption, or the intense involvement of the central object of concentration; (2) dissociation, in which experiences that would commonly be felt consciously occur outside of conscious awareness; and (3) suggestibility, in which persons are more likely to accept outside input without cognitive censorship or criticism.[82]

Hypnosis has been used as a treatment intervention for pain control at least since the 1850s. It has been shown to be beneficial in relieving pain for people with headache, burn injury, arthritis, cancer, and chronic back pain.[83-85] As with imagery, relaxation, and biofeedback, it is rarely used alone for chronic pain, although it has been used as a psychological model with some success with cancer patients[86]; it is often used concurrently with other treatment interventions. Hypnotic suggestions have been used to instill positive attitudes in people, facilitate compliance with treatment, foster distraction from negative thoughts or stimuli, alleviate anxiety related to medical procedures, reduce reliance on medication, and promote relaxation and rehearsal of adaptive behaviors.[85,87]

A meta-analysis[85] has suggested an overall benefit of the addition of hypnosis to nonhypnotic pain management strategies, although this may be affected by the level of hypnotic suggestibility. Furthermore, there are discrepancies in the literature with regard to the methods used to induce hypnosis, making it difficult to evaluate the efficacy of this intervention accurately.[86] Finally, based on systematic reviews, Patterson and Jensen[83,84] have suggested that hypnosis has more usefulness for the treatment of acute pain than chronic pain. Thus, the degree to which hypnosis is helpful beyond the effectiveness of other interventions and for which populations it is useful remain to be elucidated.

We have only briefly described the range of psychological approaches and techniques that have been used with chronic pain patients. Some illustrative studies have been highlighted and reference made to systematic reviews and meta-analyses; the reader may wish to consult these to learn more about these approaches. These methods can be readily integrated with more comprehensive rehabilitation programs.

They can be useful complements to physical therapy, medication management, and vocational rehabilitation by helping patients become active participants in their own care when pain flares up, as well as being a routine part of a self-management program. Using these techniques, the patient may feel more hopeful, rather than feeling helpless and dependent.

INTERDISCIPLINARY PAIN REHABILITATION PROGRAMS

Psychological approaches and techniques have found strong support in the literature when used on their own. However, interdisciplinary pain rehabilitation programs (IPRPs) are also efficacious, because the cognitive-behavioral perspective and cognitive and behavioral techniques are often important components of these programs[26,54] and have been recommended for use in combination.[55] The premise underlying the development of IPRPs is that patients with complex pain problems are best served by the collaborative efforts of a team of specialists, which often includes physicians, nurses, physical therapists, occupational therapists, vocational counselors, and psychologists. IPRPs operate under the assumption that pain is not just the result of body damage but also has psychological and environmental origins. In other words, IPRPs treat more than pain—they treat the whole person.[88]

The primary goal of IPRPs is to improve physical performance and coping skills and to transfer the responsibility for pain management from the health care provider to the individual. The treatment plan is rehabilitative rather than curative, and encourages people to take a more active role in the management of their pain.

IPRPs adopt the biopsychosocial model of chronic pain, which assumes that all human behavior, including the report of pain, reflects a combination of the events occurring within the person's body, the recognition and appraisal of these events, the affective responses to these events, and the influence of the environment.[88] Comprehensive and concurrent treatment interventions may include drug detoxification, psychological treatment (e.g., relaxation training, problem solving, coping skills training), physical conditioning, acquisition of coping and vocational skills, and education about pain and how the body functions.

Many studies and several meta-analyses have supported the clinical effectiveness of IPRPs.[26,89] In general, compared with pharmacologic, medical, and surgical alternatives, IPRPs appear to be equally effective in reducing pain and significantly more effective in reducing health care consumption, leading to closure of disability claims, increased functional activities, and a higher rate of return to work.[51] Even at long-term follow-up, people who are treated in IPRPs appear to maintain their reductions in pain and emotional distress.[90,91] An additional benefit of IPRPs is that they cost substantially less per person annually than medications and surgeries, rendering treatment more cost-effective.[51]

CONCLUSION

For the person experiencing chronic pain, there is a continuing quest for relief that often remains elusive, leading to feelings of helplessness, hopelessness, demoralization, and outright depression. Emotional distress may be attributed to various factors, including inadequate or maladaptive coping resources, iatrogenic complications, overuse of medication, disability, financial difficulties, litigation, disruption of usual activities, inadequate social support, and sleep disturbances. Thus, chronic pain represents a demoralizing situation; the individual with pain not only faces the stress created by pain but experiences a cascade of ongoing stressors that compromise all aspects of life. Living with chronic pain requires considerable emotional resilience, tends to deplete emotional reserve, and taxes not only the pain sufferer but also the capability of family members and significant others to provide support.

There is a large body of evidence to demonstrate that psychological factors can interfere with or hinder a person's ability to cope with the pain experience. As a result, psychological intervention in the assessment and treatment of chronic pain is becoming standard practice. Psychological treatment can focus on the emotional distress that accompanies chronic pain and provide education and training in the use of cognitive and behavioral techniques, which may reduce perceptions of pain and related disability. Psychologists and psychological principles have played a major role in the understanding and treatment of people with pain, and psychologists have an important function in IPRPs as clinicians and researchers.

None of the treatments described are successful in eliminating pain completely; the same statement can be made in reference to the most commonly used pharmacologic, medical, and surgical interventions.[51] Consequently, most people have to adapt to the presence of chronic pain and learn self-management in the face of persistent pain and accompanying symptoms. The psychological interventions described in this chapter provide a general overview of various treatment strategies. By far, however, treatment with CBT alone or within the context of an IPRP holds the greatest empirical evidence for success. There is a substantial and overwhelming body of research supporting the effectiveness of various psychological approaches. It seems prudent to consider the use of psychological treatment in combination with traditional medical interventions.

Currently, few data are available that consistently identify the characteristics of those who would most likely benefit from the pain treatment methods described in this chapter, although some studies have suggested that individualized treatment is associated with more relief of symptoms than standard treatment.[92-94] Further studies are needed to determine which treatments, and how they should be delivered, are most effective for patients with certain characteristics and result in the fewest iatrogenic complications and adverse events.[55] Positive results will permit more clinically effective and cost-effective ways to treat the difficult population of patients with chronic pain.

Acknowledgments

Support for preparation of this chapter was provided by grants from the National Institutes of Health/ National Institute of Arthritis and Musculoskeletal and Skin Diseases (AR 47298 and AR44724).

References

1. Vlaeyen JWS, Linton SJ: Fear-avoidance and its consequences in chronic musculoskeletal pain: A state of the art. Pain 2000;85:317-322.
2. U.S. Department of Health and Human Services: Prescription Drugs: Abuse and Addiction NIH Publ. No. 01-48881). Rockville, Md, U.S. Department of Health and Human Services, National Institutes of Health, 2001.
3. U.S. Bureau of the Census: Statistical Abstracts of the United States: 1996, 116th ed. Washington, DC, U.S. Bureau of the Census, 1996.
4. National Research Council: Musculoskeletal Disorders and the Workplace. Washington, DC, National Academy Press, 2001.
5. Turk DC: Clinical effectiveness and cost effectiveness of treatments for chronic pain patients. Clin J Pain 2002; 18:355-365.
6. Bonica JJ: History of pain concepts and therapies. In Bonica JJ, Loeser JD, Chapman CR, et al (eds): The Management of Pain, 2nd ed. Philadelphia, Lea & Febiger, 1990, p 12.
7. Engel GL: Psychogenic pain and the pain-prone patient. Am J Med 1959;26:899-918.
8. Frischenschlager O, Pucher I: Psychological management of pain. Disabil Rehabil 2002;24:416-422.
9. Davis DA, Luecken LJ, Zautra AJ: Are reports of childhood abuse related to the experience of chronic pain in adulthood? A meta-analytic review of the literature. Clin J Pain 2005; 21:398-405
10. Raphael K: Childhood abuse and pain in adulthood. More than a modest relationship? Clin J Pain 2005;21:371-373.
11. American Psychiatric Association: Diagnostic and Statistical Manual of Mental Disorders, 4th ed., text rev. Washington, DC, APA Press, 2000.
12. Beutler L, Engle D, Oro'-Beutler M, et al: Inability to express intense affect: A common link between depression and pain? J Consult Clin Psychol, 1986;54:752-759.
13. Basler SC, Grzesiak RC, Dworkin RH: Integrating relational psychodynamic and action-oriented psychotherapies: Treating pain and suffering. In Turk DC, Gatchel RJ (eds): Psychological Approaches to Pain Management: A Practitioner's Handbook, 2nd ed. New York, Guilford Press, 2001, pp 94-127.
14. Okifuji A, Turk DC, Sherman JJ: Evaluation of the relationship between depression and fibromyalgia syndrome: Why aren't all patients depressed? J Rheumatol 2000;27:212-219.
15. Rudy TE, Kerns RD, Turk DC: Chronic pain and depression: Toward a cognitive-behavioral mediational model. Pain 1988;35:129-140.
16. Wallis BJ, Lord S M, Bogduk N: Resolution of psychological distress of whiplash patients following treatment by radiofrequency neurotomy: A randomised, double-blind, placebo-controlled trial. Pain 1997;73:15-22.
17. Fordyce WE: Behavioral Methods for Chronic Pain and Illness. St. Louis, Mosby, 1976.
18. Thieme K, Spies C, Sinha P, et al: Predictors of pain behaviors in fibromyalgia. Arthritis Rheum 2005;53:343-350.

19. Richard, K: The occurrence of maladaptive health-related behaviors and teacher-related conduct problems in children of chronic low back pain patients. J Behav Med 1988;11:107-116.

20. Vaughan KB, Lanzetta JT: Vicarious instigation and conditioning of facial expressive and autonomic responses to a model's expressive display of pain. J Pers Soc Psychol 1980;38:909-923.

21. Bandura A: Self-efficacy: Toward a unifying theory of behavior change. Psychol Rev 1977;84:191-215.

22. Turk DC: Cognitive-behavioral approach to the treatment of chronic pain patients. Reg Anesth Pain Med 2003;6:573-579.

23. Melzack R, Wall PD: Pain mechanisms: A new theory. Science 1965;50:971-979.

24. Melzack R, Casey KL: Sensory, motivational and central control determinants of pain: A new conceptual model. In Kenshalo D (ed); The Skin Senses. Springfield, Ill, Charles C Thomas, 1968, pp 423-443.

25. Dickenson AH: Gate-control theory of pain stands the test of time. Br J Anaesth 2002;88:755-757.

26. Morley S, Eccleston C, Williams A: Systematic review and meta-analysis of randomized controlled trials of cognitive behaviour therapy and behaviour therapy for chronic pain in adults, excluding headache. Pain 1999;80:1-13.

27. Turk DC, Meichenbaum D, Genest M: Pain and Behavioral Medicine: A Cognitive-Behavioral Perspective. New York, Guilford Press, 1983.

28. Turk DC: Understanding pain sufferers: The role of cognitive processes. Spine J 2004;4:1-7.

29. Turk DC, Okifuji A: Psychological factors in chronic pain: Evolution and revolution. J Consult Clin Psychol 2002;70:678-690.

30. Sullivan MJL, Rodgers WM, Kirsch I: Catastrophizing, depression and expectations for pain and emotional distress. Pain 2001;91:147-154.

31. Kerns RD: Family assessment and intervention. In Nicassio PM, Smith TW (eds): Managing Chronic Illness: A Biopsychosocial Perspective. Washington, DC, American Psychological Association, 1995, pp 207-244.

32. Turk DC, Rudy TE, Flor H: Why a family perspective for pain? Int J Family Ther 1985;7:223-234.

33. Schmaling KB, Sher TG (eds): The Psychology of Couples and Illness: Theory, Research, and Practice. Washington, D.C.: APA Press, 2000.

34. Romano JM, Turner JA, Jensen MP, et al: Chronic pain person-spouse behavioral interactions predict person disability. Pain 1995;63:353-360.

35. Turk DC, Kerns RD, Rosenberg R: Effects of marital interaction on chronic pain and disability: Examining the down-side of social support. Rehabil Psychol 1992;37:357-372.

36. Vlaeyen JWS, Haazen IWCJ, Kole-Snijders AMJ, et al: Behavioral rehabilitation of chronic low back pain: Comparison of an operant treatment, an operant-cognitive treatment and an operant-respondent treatment. Br J Clin Psychol 1995;34:95-118.

37. Groth T, Fehm-Wolfsdorf, Hahlweg K: Basic research on the psychobiology of intimate relationships. In Schmaling K, Sher T (eds): The Psychology of Couples and Illness: Theory, Research, and Practice. Washington, DC, APA Press, 2000, pp 13-42.

38. Turk DC, Flor H: Chronic pain: A biobehavioral perspective. In: Gatchel RJ, Turk DC (eds): Psychosocial Factors in Pain: Critical Perspectives. New York, Guilford Press, 1999, pp 18-34.

39. Fries E, Hesse J, Hellhammer J, et al: A new view on hypocortisolism. Psychoneuroendocrinology 2005;30:1010-1016.

40. Gaab J, Baumann S, Budnoik A, et al: Reduced reactivity and enhanced negative feedback sensitivity of the hypothalamus-pituitary-adrenal axis in chronic whiplash-associated disorder. Pain 2005;119:219-224.

41. McBeth J, Chiu YH, Silman AJ, et al: Hypothalamic-pituitary-adrenal stress axis function and the relationship with chronic widespread pain and its antecedents. Arthritis Res Ther 2005;7:R992-R1000.

42. Hammerfald K, Eberle C, Grau M, et al: Persistent effects of cognitive-behavioral stress management on cortisol responses to acute stress in healthy subjects—a randomized controlled trial. Psychoneuroendocrinology 2006;31:333-339.

43. Gaab J, Sonderegger L, Scherrer S, et al: Psychoneuroendocrine effects ofcognitive-behavioral stress management in a naturalistic setting—a randomized controlled trial. Psychoneuroendocrinology 2006;31:428-438.

44. Martinez-Lavin M: Fibromyalgia as a sympathetically maintained pain syndrome. Curr Pain Headache Rep 2004;8:385-389.

45. Martinez-Lavin M, Vidal M, Barbosa RE, et al: Norepinephrine-evoked pain in fibromyalgia. A randomized pilot study [ISRCTN70707830]. BMC Musculoskelet Disord 2002;3:2.

46. Mezzacappa ES, Kelsey RM, Katkin ES, et al: Vagal rebound and recovery from psychological stress. Psychosom Med 2001;63:650-657.

47. Gerwin RD: A review of myofascial pain and fibromyalgia—factors that promote their persistence. Acupunct Med 2005;23:121-134.

48. Rainville P: Brain mechanisms of pain affect, and pain modulation. Curr Opin Neurobiol 2002;12:195-204.

49. Turk DC, Burwinkle TM: Assessment of pain sufferers: Outcomes measures in clinical trials and clinical practice. Rehab Psychol 2005;50:56-64.

50. Turk DC, Melzack R (eds): Handbook of Pain Assessment, 2nd ed. New York, Guilford Press, 2001.

51. Novy DM: Psychological approaches for managing chronic pain. J Psychopathol Behav Assess 2004;26:279-288.

52. Thieme K, Gromnica-Ihle E, Flor H: Operant behavioral treatment of fibromyalgia: A controlled study. Arthritis Rheum 2003;15:314-320.

53. Turner-Stokes L, Erkeller-Yuksel F, Miles A, et al: Outpatient cognitive-behavioral pain management programs: A randomized comparison of a group-based multidisciplinary versus an individual therapy model. Arch Phys Med Rehabil 2003;84:781-788.

54. McCracken LM, Turk DC: Behavioral and cognitive-behavioral treatment for chronic pain: Outcomes, predictors of outcome, and treatment process. Spine 2002;27:2564-2573.

55. Van Tulder MW, Loes B, Seitasal S, et al: Outcome of invasive treatment modalities on back pain and sciatica: An evidence-based review. Eur Spine J 2006;15:S82-S92.

56. Turk DC: Customizing treatment for chronic patients: Who, what, and why. Clin J Pain 1990; 6:255-270.

57. Turk DC: The potential of treatment matching for subgroups of chronic pain patients: Lumping vs. splitting. Clin J Pain 2005;21:44-55.

58. Vlaeyen JWS, Morley S: Cognitive-behavioral treatments for chronic pain: What works for whom? Clin J Pain 2005;21:1-8.

59. Jensen MP, Nielson WR, Kerns RD: Toward the development of a motivational model of pain self-management. J Pain 2003;4:477-492.

60. Astin J A, Shapiro SL, Eisenberg DM, et al: Mind-body medicine: State of the science implications for practice. J Am Board Fam Pract, 2003;16:131-147.

61. Seers K, Carroll D: Relaxation techniques for acute pain management: A systematic review. J Adv Nurs 1998;27:466-475.

62. Rainville P, Bao QV, Chretien P: Pain-related emotions modulate experimental pain perception and autonomic responses. Pain 2005;118:306-318.

63. Storella RJ, Shi Y, O'Connor DM, Pharo GH, et al: Relief of chronic pain may be accompanied by an increase in a measure of heart rate variability. Anesth Analg 1999;89:448-450A.

64. de Charms RC, Maeda F, Glover GH, et al: Control over brain activation and pain learned by using real-time functional MRI. Proc Natl Acad Sci U S A 2005;102:18626-18631.

65. Benson H, Goodale IL: The relaxation response: Your inborn capacity to counteract the harmful effects of stress. J Fla Med Assoc 1981;68:265-267.

66. Goleman DJ, Schwartz GE: Meditation as an intervention in stress reactivity. J Consult Clin Psychol 1976;44:456-466.

67. Shapiro SL, Schwartz GE, Bonner G: Effects of mindfulness-based stress reduction on medical and premedical students. J Behav Med 1998;21:581-599.

68. Astin JA, Shapiro SL, Eisenberg DM, et al: Mind-body medicine: State of the science, implications for practice. J Am Board Fam Pract 2003;16:131-147.

69. Kabat-Zinn J: An outpatient program in behavioral medicine for chronic pain patients based on the practice of mindfulness meditation: Theoretical considerations and preliminary results. Gen Hosp Psychiatry 1982;4:33-47.

70. Kabat-Zinn J, Lipworth L, Burney R: The clinical use of mindfulness meditation for the self-regulation of chronic pain. J Behav Med 1985;8:163-190.

71. Alexander CN, Robinson P, Orme-Johnson DW, et al: The effects of transcendental meditation compared to other methods of relaxation and meditation in reducing risk factors, morbidity, and mortality. Presented at the CIANS-ISBM Satellite Conference Symposium: Lifestyle Changes in the Prevention and Treatment of Disease, Hanover, Germany, 1992.

72. Astin JA: Stress reduction through mindfulness meditation. Effects on psychological symptomatology, sense of control, and spiritual experiences. Psychother Psychosom 1997;66:97-106.

73. Kabat-Zinn J: Full Catastrophe Living. New York, Delacorte Press, 1990.

74. Bonadonna R: Meditation's impact on chronic illness. Holist Nurs Pract 2003;17:309-319.

75. Grossman P, Niemann L, Schmidt S, et al: Mindfulness-based stress reduction and health benefits. A meta-analysis. J Psychosom Res 2004;57:35-43.

76. Lazar SW, Kerr CE, Wasserman RH, et al: Meditation experience is associated with increased cortical thickness. Neuroreport 2005;16:1893-1897.

77. Lutz A, Greischar LL, Rawlings NB, et al: Long-term meditators self-induce high-amplitude gamma synchrony during mental practice. Proc Natl Acad Sci U S A 2004;101:16369-16373.

78. Adelman EM: Mind-body intelligence: A new perspective integrating Eastern and Western healing traditions. Holist Nurs Pract 2006;20:147-151.

79. Cahn BR, Polich J: Meditation states and traits: EEG, ERP, and neuroimaging studies. Psychol Bull 2006;132:180-211.

80. Reed C: Talking up enlightenment. Sci Am 2006;294:23-24.

81. Halpin LS, Speir AM, CapoBianco P, et al: Guided imagery in cardiac surgery. Outcomes Manage 2002;6:132-137.

82. Spiegel D, Moore R: Imagery and hypnosis in the treatment of cancer patients. Oncology 1997;11:1179-1189.

83. Patterson DR, Jensen MP: Hypnosis and clinical pain. Psychol Bull 2003;129:495-521.

84. Jensen M, Patterson DR: Hypnotic treatment of chronic pain. J Behav Med 2006;29:95-124.

85. Montgomery GH, DuHamel KN, Redd WH: A meta-analysis of hypnotically induced analgesia: How effective is hypnosis? Int J Clin Exp Hypn 2000;48:138-153.

86. Syrjala KL, Cummings C, Donaldson GW: Hypnosis or cognitive behavioral training for the reduction of pain and nausea during cancer treatment: A controlled clinical trial. Pain 1992;48:137-146.

87. Pinnell CM, Covino NA: Empirical findings on the use of hypnosis in medicine: A critical review. Int J Clin Exp Hypn 2000;48:170-194.

88. Loeser JD, Turk DC: Multidisciplinary pain management. Semin Neurosurg 2004;15:13-29.

89. Guzman J, Esmail R, Karjalinen K, et al: Multidisciplinary rehabilitation for chronic low back pain: Systematic review. BMJ 2001;322:1511-1516.

90. Olason M: Outcome of an interdisciplinary pain management program in a rehabilitation clinic. Work 2004;22:9-15.

91. Storro S, Moen J, Svebak S: Effects on sick-leave of a multidisciplinary rehabilitation programme for chronic low back, neck, or shoulder pain: Comparison with usual treatment. J Rehabil Med 2004;36:12-16.

92. Bergstrom G, Jensen IB, Bodin L, et al: The impact of psychosocially different patient groups on outcome after a vocational rehabilitation program for long-term spinal pain patients. Pain 2001;93:229-237.

93. Dalton JA, Keefe FJ, Carlson J, et al: Tailoring cognitive behavioral treatment for cancer pain. Pain Manage Nurs 2004;5:3-18.

94. Turk DC, Okifuji A, Sinclair JD, et al: Differential responses by psychosocial subgroups of fibromyalgia syndrome patients to an interdisciplinary treatment. Arthritis Care Res 1998;11:397-404.

40 Physical Medicine Techniques in Pain Management

Martin Grabois, Benoy Benny, and Kwai-Tung Chan

This chapter will focus on physical medicine techniques used to treat patients in pain. At the conclusion of reading this chapter, the reader will have a through understanding of physical medicine techniques and how they fit into the multidisciplinary comprehensive treatment of patients with pain. Although the physical medicine approach can help decrease pain and increase function if combined with medication and behavioral modification, the results can be much more dramatic.

In the previous edition of this text, Linchitz and Sorell[1] defined physical medicine and rehabilitation and the role of the physiatrist. They noted that "Physical medicine and rehabilitation have traditionally been the medical specialty that oversees and prescribes the application of physical modalities to treat disease and disorders, including the rehabilitation of patients with pain. The physiatrist, whose primary perspective is typically one of the functions, is an expert on the musculoskeletal and locomotor systems and is knowledgeable about how to use physical agents and how to coordinate the rehabilitation team. As part of the multidisciplinary medical team, the physiatrist participates in the evaluation and treatment of those with pain."[1]

However, there are not enough physiatrists to treat all patients with pain. Therefore, all physicians need to understand the rationale, indication, counterindications, and prescription of physical medicine techniques and their appropriate use. Many of these techniques can be used for acute, subacute, and chronic pain. However, with the progression to more chronic pain, techniques should be more active and less passive. Although many of these techniques will help decrease pain, the long-term goal should be to increase function in spite of the presence of the pain syndrome.

APPROACH TO TREATMENT

Patients with pain can be evaluated and treated by individual physicians and therapists. This type of approach is more often used and successful in patients with acute or subacute pain. However, as pain becomes more chronic, includes psychosocial vocational issues, or both, a multidisciplinary or interdisciplinary approach is recommended.

Although the terms *multidisciplinary* and *interdisciplinary* are often used interchangeably, multidisciplinary more formally refers to collaboration among members of different disciplines (including various medical specialists and therapists), managed by a leader who directs a range of ancillary services.[2] Interdisciplinary describes a deeper level of consensus-based collaboration in which the entire process (i.e., evaluation, goal setting, and treatment delivery) is orchestrated by the team, facilitated by regular face-to-face meetings, and primarily delivered in a single facility.[2] The interdisciplinary team is commonly led by a pain specialist and includes physical and occupational therapists, pain psychologists, relaxation training experts, vocational, rehabilitation, and therapeutic recreational specialists, social workers, and nurse educators.[3] The role of these team members will be discussed later in this chapter.

It should be noted that comprehensive reviews of the cost-effectiveness and efficacy of interdisciplinary programs have demonstrated significant improvements in return to work, increased function, reduced health care use, and closure of disability claims.[4] These comprehensive programs have also shown clear benefits over conventional management in regard to decreasing pain behavior and improving mood.[4,5] The interdisciplinary model provides ongoing communication for all members of the treatment team, which helps facilitate patients' care while they progress to behavioral, cognitive, and active therapy treatments.[6]

ROLE OF THE THERAPY TEAM

Ideally, a pain program should be comprehensive and interdisciplinary. Typically, the team is led by the physician and consists of physical therapists, occupational therapists, and often recreational therapists, dieticians, and psychologists.[7] The combined assessments by these professionals are used to devise a comprehensive approach to allow the patient to benefit maximally, reintegrate fully into life, and have as few restrictions as possible.

It is important before therapy begins that realistic goals be set. These goals include but should not be limited to decreasing muscle tightness, increasing strength in areas of muscle weakness, increasing general aerobic conditioning, and improving ease in performance of activities of daily living. In general, one wants first to restore flexibility and then increase strength and develop endurance. Completely removing the pain may not be a realistic goal of therapy, but increased function should be. Box 40–1 illustrates the goals of therapy to be accomplished.

Sometimes, the distinction between physical and occupational therapists is lost. Physical therapists focus on the strength, flexibility, and coordination of large muscle groups. They assess and help with strength and flexibility of the legs, pelvic girdle, and trunk and address mobility by ambulation. They also train patients in back and body mechanics.[8] Occupational therapists focus on fine and gross motor strength, flexibility and coordination of the hands, and activities of daily living. For pain patients, they are also good in teaching conservation techniques. They can help patients in their work by instructing them in ergonomics, work simplification, and energy conservation.[9] Another important aspect that they address is proper posture, which can offer significant reduction in pain if put into practice daily. The roles of physical and occupational therapists are presented in Table 40–1.

Recreational therapists help in providing pleasurable outlets to help maintain physical conditioning. Instead of prescribing a boring set of home exercises, incorporating pleasurable activities that are also distracting often increases the patient's interest and cooperation. The psychologist's role is to identify factors that may be complicating the pain experience and help the patient deal with the process in a better way. There are many useful tools and tests to help the psychologist determine other confounding factors so that the patient's functioning can be increased maximally. These include the Minnesota Multiphasic Personality Inventory (MMPI), Beck depression inventory, Oswestry scale, Symptom Checklist 90, and McGill pain questionnaire.[10] The psychologist, working alone or with the team, can encourage pain reduction by teaching the patient stress management and relaxation techniques and patient self-monitoring techniques. Stress reduction can be achieved through cognitive-behavioral therapy.[11]

The physician's role mainly is to lead the team in the complete management of the patient. This includes making sure that there is no disease process that might be causing the pain and, if present, that there is no other treatment or intervention that should be pursued before initiating therapies. It also includes monitoring safe participation in physical rehabilitation while optimizing medication management. If it is thought that the patient could benefit from interventions, it is easier if this is done prior to initiating a comprehensive rehabilitation program.[10]

Physical conditioning programs use a cognitive-behavioral approach plus intensive physical training that includes aerobic capacity, muscle strength and endurance, and coordination. These approaches can be work-related, given and supervised by a physiotherapist or multidisciplinary team, and seem to be effective in reducing the number of sick days for some with chronic back pain when compared with usual care.[12]

BASIC MANAGEMENT CONSIDERATIONS

Clinical Evaluation

Patients with acute or chronic pain may be referred for physical medicine evaluation and treatment as a component of a multidisciplinary management approach or for certain specific treatments. Prior to initiating treatment, it is important to perform a history and physical examination (Chapter 10), review medical records to identify factors contributing to the patient's complaints, and assess the impact of pain on the patient's functioning. Contraindications to physical medicine treatments and/or precautions for treatment should be identified. A careful and thorough history and physical examination also help establish trust between the clinician and patient and facilitate consensus with treatment recommendations.

Table 40–1. Role of Physical Therapists and Occupational Therapists

PHYSICAL THERAPISTS	OCCUPATIONAL THERAPISTS
Loss of flexibility	Joint conservation techniques
Strength and weakness of trunk and limb muscles	Work simplification techniques
Core strengthening	Back conservation
General aerobic conditioning	Posture
Balance and coordination	Energy conservation techniques
Contractures	Activities of daily living and self-care
Assisted mobility	Edema control

BOX 40–1. GOALS OF THERAPY

Restore biomechanical dysfunctions.
Improve strength.
Improve posture.
Improve gait symmetry.
Improve general aerobic conditioning.
Improve efficiency of activities of daily living.
Decrease edema.
Instruct patients to monitor pain response and to pace activity.
Use back or joint conservation techniques.

History

A detailed history is obtained by interviewing the patient and reviewing questionnaires and medical records. It is important to obtain information about the time course, intensity and location of the pain, and relieving and exacerbating factors. The functional state of the patient prior to onset of the problem and the current functional level should be determined to establish a baseline and guide expectations for improvement. The patient's experiences and responses to previous diagnostic and therapeutic interventions should be noted, because they may predict responses to future treatment. Medical conditions that can affect or be affected by physical medicine treatments should be identified. It is also important to obtain information on medications, coexisting psychological and psychiatric disorders, substance abuse or addiction, and involvement in litigation because these can affect the patient's response to treatment.

Physical Examination

A complete physical examination should be done, with a focus on the neurologic and musculoskeletal systems. Active and passive joint range of motion, muscle bulk, strength, and sensation should be assessed and documented. Findings in the involved area should be compared with those on the asymptomatic side, when possible. Patterns of pain and sensory loss can provide clues to the site of nervous system pathology or dysfunction. Signs of vasomotor instability, such as skin temperature and hair, nail, or perspiration changes may indicate autonomic dysfunction. Pain may limit testing of range of motion, strength, and sensation; if this is the case, it should be noted. Reflex testing can be particularly helpful, because it is one of the more objective parts of the examination. Abnormal or asymmetric reflex responses may indicate nervous system dysfunction or pathology. Evidence of prior surgeries or injuries should be noted.

A patient's gait, posture, and movement can provide diagnostic clues to the source and severity of pain. It is helpful to observe the patient and form a general impression prior to carrying out the formal physical examination. Inconsistencies between the patient's complaints and his or her behavior should be noted.

Functional Evaluation

A functional evaluation should be performed on pain patients before, during, and after completion of any treatment or functional restoration program.[7] A functional evaluation may range from direct observation of function by the clinician to formal functional capacity evaluations (FCEs) performed by trained health care personnel.

Functional assessments can provide additional useful information because tests of pain perception, psychological distress, and self-perception of abilities and limitations do not accurately assess a person's physical capacity for work.[13] Physicians and patients often have great difficulty estimating functional limitation and physical ability.[14]

FCEs have existed in one form or another since the 1940s, although their use and application have changed with time. They are primarily used in industrial medicine and legal and disability settings.[15] Reasons for ordering an FCE include the following: making disability determinations, setting goals and planning treatment for industrial rehabilitation, monitoring progress through industrial rehabilitation, determining a person's readiness to return to work after injury, performing pre-employment evaluation, and determining case closure.[16]

Most FCE protocols include some or most of the following components: an interview, record review, self-administered questionnaire, psychological test battery, musculoskeletal evaluation, functional testing, validation of sincerity of effort, and comparisons to specific job requirements.[7,16] Functional testing may include material handling, specific tasks, holding static postures, and repetitive task performance.[7,16] A job analysis should be done prior to administration of an FCE, because measurement of work capacity is specific to the demands posed of a job.[15]

There are scientific and practical limitations associated with FCEs with regard to standardization, validity, and reliability.[15,16] They have not necessarily been shown to predict return to work. However, they may be helpful in charting changes in function, comparing functional disparities to job demands, identifying nonmedical factors influencing ability to work, and used as a tool to guide work restrictions for patients returning to work or for initial therapy prescriptions for patients beginning a rehabilitation program.[7,16]

Psychological Evaluation

A psychological evaluation should be considered when the pain is resulting in significant impairment in psychological, vocational, or social functioning. These evaluations can determine the emotional, cognitive, behavioral, social, or vocational factors that could be affecting the patient's perception of pain.[7]

It is important that the psychological evaluation of a patient in chronic pain be conducted by a clinician who is sensitive to and knowledgeable about the psychological aspects of chronic pain. It should be appreciated that many chronic pain patients may be defensive about a psychological referral and are more likely to be evaluated if they are provided with an appropriate rationale and explanation for the referral. This topic is discussed further in Chapter 13.

Electrodiagnostic Testing

Electrodiagnostic testing encompasses nerve conduction studies (NCS) and electromyography (EMG) which provide information about the peripheral

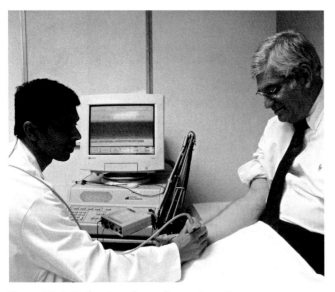

Figure 40–1. Performing electrodiagnostic testing.

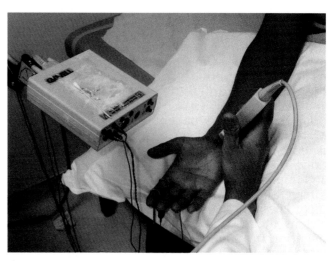

Figure 40–2. Performing nerve conduction studies.

nerves and muscles, and evoked potentials, which is used mainly to asses the central nervous system (Fig. 40–1). Chapter 11 presents a more detailed discussion of the role of electrodiagnostic testing.

Electrodiagnosis can play an important role in identifying an underlying problem in a patient with a pain disorder. Electrodiagnostic testing not only helps in diagnosis but in determining chronicity and severity of the condition, and can even assist in prognosis. Electrodiagnostic testing has another advantage when dealing with the pain patient who is having signs of radiculopathy. Because disk bulges seen by magnetic resonance imaging (MRI) may be found routinely at many levels, EMG testing can help determine whether one of these disk bulges is actually producing nerve damage.[17] This test may also be helpful in those patients who have radiculitis with no structural disk herniation and often a normal MRI scan. EMG has also been shown to help with the diagnosis of spinal stenosis but does not predict future pain.[18] However, a recent report has also shown that EMG does not necessarily correlate with pain severity.[19]

Most physicians will perform NCS and EMG together in the same session. The nerve conduction study usually involves testing of sensory and motor nerves and sometimes reflex studies. The common nerves studied in the lower extremity include the sural, tibial, deep peroneal and, in the upper extremity, the median, ulnar, and radial nerves. The facial and trigeminal nerves are tested less often.

When performing motor NCS, the active electrode is placed over the muscle belly, the reference electrode is placed over the tendon insertion, and the nerve is stimulated at a fixed distance from the muscle. F-wave responses can also be recorded during motor studies; they can indicate the integrity of the entire motor nerve.

When performing sensory NCS (usually done antidromically), the active and reference electrodes are placed over a distal nerve segment and the nerve is stimulated proximally (Fig. 40–2). The EMG study can be done with concentric or monopolar needles. There are two parts of EMG—evaluation of the spontaneous activity and evaluation of the motor unit action potentials (MUAPs). Typically, in neurogenic conditions, the electromyographer will notice fibrillation potentials or positive sharp waves (PSWs) with spontaneous activity that show that the muscle fiber membrane is unstable, enlarged MUAPs, and decreased MUAP recruitment.

Radiculopathy

The sensitivity of EMG in the diagnosis of radiculopathy is lower than MRI, but its specificity is significantly better.[17] EMG not only helps identify which nerve is involved but also the severity and chronicity of the lesion. It is important to remember that in radiculopathy, sensory NCS are normal, because compression of the nerve root usually occurs proximal to the dorsal root ganglion (DRG), which therefore spares it. In S1 radiculopathy, the H reflex is often prolonged.

The diagnosis of radiculopathy relies primarily on the electromyogram. In subacute single nerve root involvement, one should find denervation (fibrillation potentials and/or PSWs) in two or more muscles of that myotome, involvement of the paraspinal muscles at the same level, and no denervation in other myotomes. It usually takes about 3 to 4 weeks for denervation to appear in the extremity muscles, but there may be earlier signs, such as decreased recruitment of motor units in muscles innervated by the involved root or signs of denervation in the paraspinal muscles. A more detailed discussion has been presented in Chapter 11, so Table 40–2 only summarizes abnormalities found by NCS and EMG in some common disorders.

Table 40–2. Summary of Abnormalities on NCS and EMG in Some Common Disorders

DISORDER	MOTOR STUDY	SENSORY STUDY	EMG	F AND H WAVES
Radiculopathy	Usually normal; if severe, may have reduction in amplitude	Normal	Fibs and PSW in muscles supplied by that root	Mild to moderate prolongation of H and F response latencies
Axonal polyneuropathy	Reduced amplitude in distal muscles	Reduced amplitude of distal nerves	Fibs and PSW in distal muscles	Mild to moderate prolongation of H and F response latencies
Demyelinating polyneuropathy	Slowing of conduction velocity (CV); prolongation of distal latency	Reduced amplitude and CV	Fibs, PSW, variable reinnervation; reduced recruitment of motor units	Severe prolongation; absence of F and H
Compression neuropathy	Focal CV slowing across affected segment if mild; reduction in amplitude if severe	Slowing of CV across affected segment; reduction in amplitude if severe	Fibs, PSW in muscles supplied by that nerve	Mild prolongation in F responses
Plexopathy	Reduced amplitude in muscles supplied by affected fibers	Reduced amplitude in sensory nerves traversing affected part of plexus	Fibs and PSW in muscles supplied by affected fibers	Mild to moderate prolongation of F and H latency
Mononeuropathy multiplex	Focal "axonal" lesions of multiple nerves, with markedly decreased amplitude	Reduced or absent responses in affected nerves	Marked abnormalities in muscles supplied by affected nerve	Mild prolongation or absence of H and F responses

CV, conduction velocity; EMG, electromyography; Fibs, fibrillation potential; NCS, nerve conduction studies; PSW, positive sharp waves.

Reflex Sympathetic Dystrophy

Despite the involvement of the sympathetic nerves, electrophysiologic studies do not reveal specific abnormalities unless there is an associated nerve injury. One study has suggested relative reductions in the amplitude of the sympathetic nerve fiber function in the affected area as compared with the affected extremity.[20]

Treatment Goals

The cause of the pain syndrome should be determined from a medical and psychosocial point of view and, if possible, the location of a "pain generator" should be noted.[20] Attempts to decrease or eliminate the pain generator(s) are important and should be carried out first, followed by consideration of other treatment options.[7]

The goals of treatment center on moderating pain, increasing function, decreasing psychosocial issues, and decreasing health care use.[21] These can be achieved by modifying pain medication and pain behavior, decreasing reliance on medical care, and increasing activity through exercise.[6]

The Fordyce model of behavioral modification is useful in the treatment of patients with chronic pain syndromes.[22] The goal in these patients is not to cure the pain but to interrupt the pain behavior reinforcement cycle by rewarding healthy behavior and setting appropriate goals for the patient. These include reduction in the use of medications, modulation of pain response, increased activity, and reduction in pain behaviors.[23]

Role of Medications

Pain commonly limits participation in a physical therapy or rehabilitation program. Adequate pain management is an important component of rehabilitation. Many patients may be pain-free at rest and have incident pain provoked by activity or movement. Analgesic medications that are not timed to the patient's pain may lead to overdosing at rest and underdosing during pain or activity. Simple measures such as taking oral analgesic medications 30 to 60 minutes prior to onset of therapy or other activity that incites pain can provide satisfactory pain relief and increase success of therapy.

In the postoperative setting, patients may benefit from multimodal analgesic techniques; these include use of combinations of analgesic medications and regional-peripheral nerve blocks.[24] Parenterally administered analgesic medications are more effective for treating severe, acute, or rapidly changing pain because of their rapid onset of action and ease of dose titration.[25] Patient-controlled analgesia (PCA) allows self-titration of analgesic medication to an individual's pain and activity level.[26]

Patients with different types of pain—neuropathic, musculoskeletal, inflammatory—will benefit from medications that address the different causes of pain. Some patients have comorbidities that can increase the experience of pain, such as soft tissue inflammation, muscle spasms, or depression.[27] The concurrent use of medications to treat these coexisting symptoms may help reduce the degree of pain experienced.

Role of Physical Modalities

Physical modalities are physical agents and techniques used to produce a therapeutic response. There is a long history of use of physical modalities to treat pain, dating back to ancient human prehistory and civilizations. Physical modalities and techniques commonly used to relieve pain include therapeutic heat and cold, hydrotherapy, ultrasound, electricity, and traction.

It is important to realize that physical modalities do not eliminate pain by themselves and generally should not be prescribed as stand-alone treatments. Rather, they are best used as adjunctive treatments to an active exercise program. Modalities that the patient can safely use at home, such as hot and ice packs and transcutaneous electrical nerve stimulation (TENS), are more useful for chronic pain management. Modalities that require health care personnel to administer are best reserved for those with acute pain syndromes or intermittent exacerbations of chronic pain.

Before prescribing or administering a physical modality, an accurate diagnosis needs to be established and the goals of treatment determined. It is important to be aware of contraindications to the use of a specific modality. Precautions that need to be taken should be specified in the prescription.

PHYSICAL MODALITIES

Therapeutic Heat

Heat is one of the oldest physical modalities used to relieve and reduce pain. In addition to pain relief, heat elicits other physiologic responses in local tissues that may be therapeutic. These include increased blood flow, increased connective tissue extensibility, decreased muscle spasm, decreased joint stiffness, and reduced edema.[28] Heat may also have a modulating effect on pain at spinal and supraspinal levels.[29]

Clinicians considering the use of therapeutic heat should first decide whether superficial or deep heat is required and then choose the appropriate heating modality. Superficial modalities include hot packs, heating pads, heat lamps, paraffin and whirlpool baths, and fluidotherapy. Deep heating agents include ultrasound, short wave, and microwave.

Contraindications to therapeutic heat are listed in Box 40–2. The risk of burns from external heat sources is real and physicians should always write precautions to monitor for burns when heat is prescribed.

Superficial heat is delivered primarily by conduction, convection, and conversion. Modalities that transfer heat by conduction include hot packs (Hydrocollator packs), heating pads, and paraffin baths. These heating modalities generally penetrate to depths of less than 2 cm from the skin. Skin and subcutaneous tissue temperatures are increased by 5° to 6° C after 6 minutes, maintained up to 30 minutes after application.[30]

Heating duration of 15 to 30 minutes may be necessary to increase muscle temperature by 1° C at depths of up to 3 cm.[31] A 1.2°-C increase in knee intra-articular temperature has been demonstrated after superficial heat application.[31]

Hydrocollator packs are hot packs that contain a silicate gel product encased in canvas. These packs are heated and stored in thermostatically controlled water baths. Prior to application, the packs should be wrapped in several layers of towels and excess water allowed to drain off. To minimize risk of burns, hot packs should be placed on the patient rather than under the patient, because body weight and pressure impair circulation and heat dissipation from the heated area.

Heat lamps provide superficial heating through conversion. Heat is generated in tissue through induction of molecular vibration by infrared waves emitted by the lamps. The degree of heating is affected by lamp wattage, angle application, and distance to the body part. Radiant heat from lamps may be preferred when heating of a diffuse area is required or when direct contact of a heating pad with the skin is not desirable.

Paraffin baths are a superficial heat modality commonly used for the treatment of distal extremity pain and stiffness from rheumatoid arthritis, osteoarthritis, and other connective tissue diseases. The two primary methods of application are dip and wrap and dip and immerse.[30] The former is more popular; it consists of dipping and removing the body part from the paraffin bath 8 to 10 times, followed by wrapping to assist in heat retention. The paraffin–mineral oil mixture used should be heated in a bath with a thermostatically controlled heater.

Hydrotherapy is the use of water for medical purposes; it includes treatments as diverse as aquatic therapy and wound care. Patients with painful musculoskeletal conditions can often exercise more easily in water because of reduced weight-bearing and additional support. Warm water also provides heat transferred by convection to immersed body areas. A whirlpool or agitation device can be used to maintain a constant water temperature around the treated areas and provide gentle mechanical stimulation to the immersed body parts.

Fluidotherapy uses glass beads, pulverized corn cobs, or other finely pulverized substances with low heat affinity heated by hot air to form a warm medium, with liquid-like properties. The body part or extremity to be treated is immersed into a cabinet containing this dry and warm medium for treatment.[30] Fluidotherapy is particularly useful for treating limbs affected by complex regional pain syndrome, because it provides gentle tactile desensitization through stimulation of thermoreceptors and mechanoreceptors. Unlike hot packs and paraffin baths, there is no loss of heat over time. Stretching and exercise can also be performed during the heat application.

When deep heating is required, ultrasound, short-wave, and microwave diathermy can be used. These modalities deliver heat to deep tissue via the conversion of physical energy into heat.

Ultrasound uses high-frequency sound waves to deliver energy to the target tissue. The sound waves produce thermal and nonthermal therapeutic effects.[32] Ultrasound waves pass through, are absorbed, or are reflected, depending on the type of tissue encountered. Higher temperatures are generated when ultrasound energy is absorbed. Energy is absorbed more effectively at the muscle-bone interface, resulting in higher tissue temperatures at these areas. Ultrasound is also more effective for heating tendons and ligament compared with muscle, which absorbs ultrasound relatively poorly.

Ultrasound is used clinically to treat subacute and chronic inflammatory soft tissue disorders, such as tendinitis and bursitis. It can also be used for deep heating to facilitate stretching of contractures and shortened soft tissue structures. Low-intensity pulsed ultrasound has been shown to facilitate tissue repair and healing.[32,33] Contraindications to the use of ultrasound are listed in Box 40-3.

Short-wave diathermy uses electromagnetic radiowaves to deliver heat down to 3 to 5 cm below the skin without overheating the skin and subcutaneous tissues. Indications for short-wave diathermy are similar to those for ultrasound. Contraindications include the presence of metal, implanted pacemakers, spinal cord stimulators, surgical implants, and copper-containing intrauterine devices (IUDs) because of the risk of excessive heating.

Microwave diathermy uses electromagnetic radiowaves with frequencies of 915 and 2456 MHz. It is rarely used in current clinical practice. Protective eyewear must be worn during its use to minimize the risk of cataract formation. Because of its more rapid heating of tissues with high water content, it should not be used in patients who have edema, blisters, or hyperhidrosis.

Short-wave and microwave diathermy are not commonly used in clinical practice. This is partly because there are more contraindications (Box 40-4) compared with other heat agents and partly because of the availability and ease of use of other therapeutic heating options.

Therapeutic Cold

Therapeutic cold is another time-tested modality used for pain relief and reduction of edema and muscle spasm. Other effects of cold include reduction in metabolic activity, muscle tone, and spasticity.[30] The rationale for using cold is similar to that of using therapeutic heat—that is, as an adjunctive treatment to physical therapy and exercise.

Therapeutic cold can be delivered by means such as ice packs and slushes, iced whirlpools, ice rubs, chemical ice packs, and evaporative cooling sprays. The same general precautions used for therapeutic heat should be used during therapeutic cold treatments to avoid thermal injury. Contraindications to therapeutic cold are listed in Box 40-5.

Contrast Baths

Contrast baths are a combination of therapeutic heat and cold generally used in the treatment of complex regional pain syndrome and sympathetically mediated pain syndromes. One method is to immerse the limb or body part in a warm bath at a temperature of 38° to 43° C for about 6 minutes, transferring the limb to a cold bath at 13° to 18° C for about 4 minutes, and then followed by a transfer back to the warm bath. This cycle is then repeated several times.[34]

BOX 40-4. CONTRAINDICATIONS TO SHORT-WAVE AND MICROWAVE DIATHERMY

Contraindications to therapeutic heat
Near metallic implants
Over pregnant uterus
Implanted pacemaker

BOX 40-5. CONTRAINDICATIONS TO THERAPEUTIC COLD

Insensate skin
Ischemia
Peripheral vascular diseases
Raynaud phenomenon
Cold insensitivity
Cold urticaria
Cryoglobulinemia
Paroxysmal cold hemoglobinuria

BOX 40-3. CONTRAINDICATIONS TO ULTRASOUND

Contraindications to therapeutic heat
Laminectomy sites
Over pregnant uterus
Over the heart or carotid sinus
Over implanted pacemaker

Transcutaneous Electrical Nerve Stimulation

TENS involves the application of electrical stimulation across the skin to the peripheral nerves. Many acute and chronic pain syndromes have been treated with TENS because of its ease of use and relatively low side effects.[35-37] Based on the gate theory of pain, TENS is thought to block or modulate pain transmission in C fibers through stimulation of the large myelinated A fibers. Research has indicated that there are probably more complex mechanisms to explain its clinical effect.[38]

There are currently many different types of TENS units, which allows for a variety of settings and modes of application. The different TENS modes include conventional narrow pulse duration, high pulse rate, low frequency, burst, modulation, and hyperstimulation.[35] Use of conventional TENS results in a comfortable electrical paresthesia, whereas low-frequency modes result in rhythmic muscle contractions. There are many different protocols for the placement of electrodes and TENS settings. TENS efficacy can be optimized by an individualized approach to parameter settings and electrode placement. When the unit and electrodes are used appropriately, side effects are minimal. Contraindications to the use of TENS are listed in Box 40–6.

Iontophoresis

Iontophoresis is the use of direct electrical current to drive electrically charged molecules actively, such as those in medications, across the skin and into the underlying tissue. It functions more as a drug delivery system rather than as a therapeutic modality. The most popular agents transported are local anesthetics such as lidocaine, steroids, and nonsteroidal anti-inflammatory drugs (NSAIDs). Iontophoresis is generally well tolerated and few complications have been reported.

Traction

Traction is the application of forces in direct opposition to each other to produce a separation of two body parts or stretching of soft tissues. In the area of spine care, traction is commonly used to treat cervical and lumbar pain. Although there is a seemingly endless variety of traction techniques and treatment protocols, most types of traction are applied by a therapist (manual traction), by machine (mechanical traction), or by weight (gravitational traction) in a sustained or intermittent manner.[39]

Traction has been prescribed to treat various spinal disorders, including radiculopathies, disk herniation, disk degeneration, foraminal stenosis, and nonspecific low back pain (Fig. 40–3). Research in this area has been confounded by the multiple types of traction techniques, treatment protocols, and methodologic flaws.[39-44] The benefits of traction for neck and back pain may be mediated through anatomic changes such as diminution of disk protrusion, reduction of disk pressure, widening of disk space and intervertebral foramina, reduction of pressure on exiting nerve roots, stretching or separation of joints and ligaments, and relaxation of muscle spasm.[45]

Contraindications to the use of traction are shown in Box 40–7. Cervical traction should be avoided in patients with rheumatoid arthritis and significant

---

BOX 40–7. CONTRAINDICATIONS TO TRACTION

General Traction
Osteomyelitis or diskitis
Osteoporosis
Spinal cord compression
Malignancy
Unstable fracture
Uncontrolled hypertension
Severe cardiovascular disease

Cervical Traction
Central disk herniation
Hypermobility
Rheumatoid arthritis
Carotid or vertebral artery disease
Temporomandibular joint dysfunction (with chin strap)

Lumbar Traction
Pregnancy
Hemorrhoids and intra-abdominal conditions that may be affected by increased intra-abdominal pressure
Cauda equina syndrome

BOX 40–6. CONTRAINDICATIONS TO TRANSCUTANEOUS ELECTRICAL NERVE STIMULATION

Demand-type cardiac pacemakers
Pregnancy
Over the carotid sinus or eyes
Across the chest

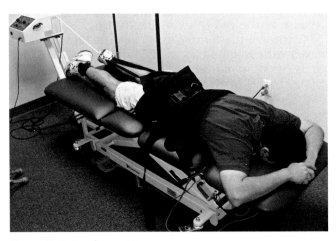

Figure 40–3. Lumbar traction.

vertebral or carotid artery disease. Lumbar traction should be done cautiously, if at all, in patients who are pregnant or who have abdominal conditions that may be worsened by increased intra-abdominal pressure. Inversion lumbar traction can increase systolic and diastolic blood pressures and increase oxygen uptake; it should be avoided in patients with cardiac or pulmonary insufficiency.[46] Despite controversy about to its physical and physiologic effects and benefits, it continues to be part of the treatment armamentarium for spinal pain.

Manual Techniques

Manual medicine refers to hands-on therapy that includes gentle joint stretching or mobilization to improve joint mobility and muscle dysfunctions in the spine or adjacent structures based on the concept that joint restriction contributes to pain.[47] Integral to the skills of ancient surgeons and physicians from Greece to China, manipulation and mobilization are still practiced after thousands of years, not only by chiropractors and medically trained practitioners, but as part of folk practice in many parts of the world. Hippocrates (460-355 BC) was the first in recorded history to describe and illustrate joint manipulation and traction techniques.[48]

There is debate on the long-lasting effects of manual techniques, but few can argue that there is at least subjective short-term relief of neck and low back symptoms. The Agency for Health Care Policy and Research (AHCPR) guidelines include manipulation as an effective strategy for the initial treatment of acute low back pain.[49] Recent studies by Bronfort and Van Tulder and colleagues[50,51] have suggested that manual therapy is effective for the treatment of acute and chronic musculoskeletal pain. A randomized controlled trial comparing spinal manipulative therapy with exercise therapy, in a course of 16 treatments over 2 months, found that spinal manipulation significantly decreases pain and increases functioning and return to work at 12 months compared with exercise therapy.[52] Geisser and associates[53] have shown that patients with chronic low back pain benefit from manual therapy with specific adjuvant exercise.

There are many theories that explain how manual therapy actually reduces pain. Skyba and coworkers[54] have shown that joint manipulation produces a nonopioid form of analgesia mediated by spinal serotonergic and noradrenergic receptors. DiGiovanna[55] theorized that with manual therapy, there is increased circulation via local effects or sympathetic reflex and increased venous and lymphatic drainage that lead to decreased local swelling and edema. Vernon and colleagues[56] have shown that manual therapy causes a change in pain threshold secondary to an increase in serum endorphin levels.

Modern manipulative therapy can range from slow oscillating glides to high-velocity, low-amplitude techniques.[57] It has been shown that spinal manipulative therapy reduces pain over the short term (less than 6 weeks) and long term (more than 6 weeks) compared with sham manipulation, and improves function over the short term.[58]

Types of Manual Therapy

Biomechanical Model (Osteopathic Approach)

This can be used in several ways. Using muscle energy, the manual medicine treatment involves the voluntary contraction of the patient's muscle in a precisely controlled direction against a counterforce applied by the operator.[59] Using strain-counterstrain can help relieve spinal pain by passively putting the joint into its position of greatest comfort.[60]

Manipulation

This is similar to the biomechanical model and is also used by osteopaths and chiropractors. Manipulation refers to a modality in which the practitioner passively, often forcefully, moves (or "thrusts") a bone through its physiologic barrier in an attempt to improve range of motion (ROM) or alignment of a joint. The goal is to improve function and decrease pain. The thrust is a high-velocity, low-amplitude (HVLA) movement. The use of this HVLA is what differentiates manipulation from mobilization.[48] The ROM of a joint during HVLA depends on where the restriction lies in the joint's normal ROM.

When performed appropriately and by a trained person, manipulation can usually result in immediate relief of pain. This is thought to occur because of a decrease in muscle spasm while increasing the ROM and the level of serum endorphins.[55] Contraindications to manipulation include osteoporosis, acute inflammation, infection, vertebral-basilar insufficiency, fracture, or any other cause of structural instability.

Norwegian Approach (Kaltenborn)

The range (hypomobility, hypermobility, or normal mobility) and quality of movement are evaluated using translatoric movement in addition to rotational movements.[61] During treatment, translatoric traction and gliding movements rather than rotational movements are preferred to avoid compressing a joint that is already strained by pathology.[62]

Maitland (Australian) Approach

In this approach, there is continual (ongoing) assessment and reassessment of the patient and consideration of the pathology and anatomy in relation to the signs and symptoms presented by the patient. There is testing of the accessory and physiologic joint movements. Treatment strategies involve use of mobilization, manipulation, adverse neural tissue mobilization, traction, and exercise based on this continual assessment.[45]

McKenzie Approach

This is a popular approach to patients with back pain that uses pain centralization and decentralization

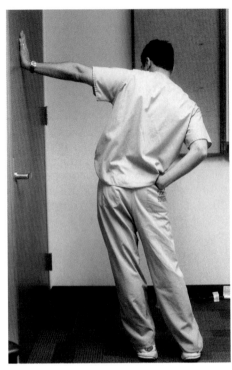

Figure 40–4. McKenzie approach.

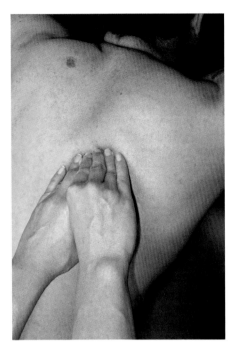

Figure 40–5. Massage.

methods to diagnose and treat spinal pathology. The key concept here is that during movements of the spine, there is a positional change to the nucleus pulposus and that generally a flexed lifestyle leads to a more posterior position of the nucleus. The treatment involves having the patient use repeated movements to treat the spinal pathology (Fig. 40–4).

Myofascial Release
This type of soft tissue treatment stretches the fascial structures of the body along its planes.

Massage

Massage is a general term that refers to application of the hand to soft tissues (e.g., skin, muscles, ligaments, tendons) to produce a therapeutic effect (Fig. 40–5). Massage, even though preferred and appreciated by many, has little objective research to support its long-term benefit.[63] Massage can be subcategorized as classic massage, sports massage, reflexology, shiatsu, and acupuncture. There are many forms of classic massage, including the following:

1. *Stroking or effleurage.* This is light movement, either superficial or deep, over the skin in a slow, rhythmic fashion.[49]
2. *Kneading and pétrissage.* Pétrissage is the application of firm but gentle pressure in a rhythmic fashion while gently grasping the underlying tissues and lifting and squeezing them. Movement is accomplished by gliding of the hands in a centripetal pattern. Kneading lifts, squeezes, and moves larger amounts of tissue than pétrissage.[61]

3. *Friction massage.* This is carried out with the fingers or the ball of the thumb applying pressure in a slow circular pattern. It is used primarily to loosen scars or adhesions.
4. *Tapotement.* This technique involves applying light "chops" or "cups" in series as percussive methods.

Sports massage is massage therapy for athletes that focuses on the muscles. A literature review by Callaghan[63] showed subjective reports of benefit, but little agreement has been documented on the efficacy of massage.

Reflexology is a massage system based on a series of points in the hands and feet that are believed to correspond to a reflex pattern in all areas of the body. Treatment consists of compression of the hands or feet by firm pressure applied by the thumbs of the practitioner.[63]

Shiatsu and acupressure are massage techniques that use pressure applied by the practitioner's fingers over predetermined points. These are the same points and meridians used in acupuncture. Shiatsu, on the other hand, is derived from traditional Japanese massage, called *anma*, and has a more anatomic and physiologic basis.[64]

The indications for massage are muscle cramps, stress and tension, contracture of joints, strains and sprains, tendinitis or tenosynovitis, and edema and lymphedema. Contraindications to massage include local malignancy, local infection, calcification of soft tissues, inflammatory arthritis (gout, infective), bursitis, open wound, bleeding disorder, and entrapment neuropathy.

The theoretic mechanical effects of massage include improved circulation, breakdown of soft tissue adhesions, and activation of the peripheral nervous system. Arterial flow, venous flow, and lymphatic flow are all theoretically improved with massage.[65] Benefits for the peripheral circulation include improvement in local nutrition and removal of waste products.[63] This helps decrease aches in muscles and facilitate healing. Activation of the peripheral nervous system is thought to be beneficial via the gate control theory of Melzak and Wall[66,67] and the inhibition of overactive proprioceptors.

Role of Exercise

In physiology, we learn that regular exercise may increase strength, muscle bulk, and stamina. Physiologically, exercise does not directly reduce pain, although reports have indicated that the performance of exercise modulates pain by a physiologic mechanism that has not yet been fully elucidated.[68] Reports on the efficacy or benefit of therapies is mixed but most physicians agree that being more active rather than less active is more beneficial for most pain patients. A recent Cochrane review has shown that those performing exercises consisting of strengthening, trunk stabilization, and advice to stay active had more beneficial results than those in a placebo group.[69]

Exercise has systemic and local effects on the body. Systemically, it increases blood flow and cardiac output; locally, it helps in increasing flexibility of the muscles and mobilizing joints. In addition, it also strengthens weak muscles, builds endurance and speed, and establishes balance and coordination.[18] Therapeutic exercise should include not only flexibility and strengthening but also exercises for redeveloping the normal patterns of movement of specific muscle groups.[18]

Physical inactivity, if helpful, is only helpful during the acute inflammatory phase of an injury, and activities should be rapidly resumed unless an obvious risk of structural damage is present.[70]

With sprains and strains of joints and ligaments, the acronym RICE is used—**r**est, **i**ce, **c**ompression, and **e**levation. Kellet[71] has explained that the duration of rest and icing should be 48 to 72 hours, so progressive mobilization within the limits of pain is prescribed. Acute soft tissue injury should be rested, supported, and iced, and nonpainful early mobilization is probably beneficial.

Exercise for Patients with Low Back Pain

Regarding low back pain, the benefit of rest is debatable, with a trend to shorter periods of rest or none at all. It was believed 30 years ago that there does need to be a period of rest, ranging from days to longer than 1 month. Deyo and colleagues[70] have noted that there is no advantage in bed rest and that there are fewer missed days and better disability scores in those that do not have complete bed rest. Hagen and associates,[72] in a literature search of musculoskeletal controlled trials, have deduced that "bed rest compared to advice to stay active will, at best, have small effects, and at worst might have harmful effects on acute low back pain."

For patients with back pain, it has been shown that both stretching and strengthening exercises are important. Khalil and colleagues[73] studied patients with myofascial low back pain and have noted that stretching plus a multimodality rehabilitation program compared with only a rehabilitation program improves measures of muscle function and significantly decreases pain in 2 weeks. Takemasa and associates[74] have shown that strengthening exercises not only improve strength but also reduce pain. Several studies have shown that exercises, whether flexion-based (Fig. 40–6) or extension-based (Fig. 40–7), improve back pain over only modality treatment groups.[75,76]

It is important to understand that in chronic pain patients, physical therapy alone will not completely eradicate the pain. Physical therapy and exercise, however, can decrease the musculoskeletal sequelae of chronic pain. Exercise can improve the patient's tolerance of functional activity by increasing flexibility, strengthening weaker muscles, and improving aerobic endurance.

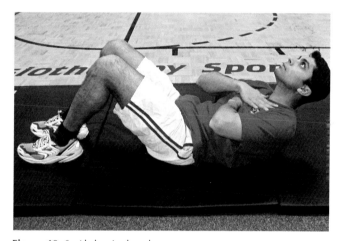

Figure 40–6. Abdominal curls.

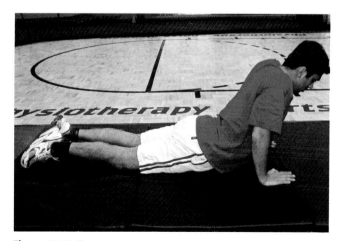

Figure 40–7. Prone press-ups.

Table 40–3. Indications and Precautions for Different Types of Exercise

EXERCISE	INDICATION	PRECAUTIONS
Isometric	Range of motion over joint not desired because of fracture or painful arthritis	Evaluation of blood pressure with sustained contraction; only strengthens muscle at that length
Isotonic	Low weight strengthening; intense weight training for competitive body building	Weak person may incur tendon injury; only to be done with a spotter; may cause severe injury if improperly done
Isokinetic	Strengthening with arc and velocity of motion controlled; more suitable for noncompetitive weight trainer	May raise systolic blood pressure mostly at maximal torque; requires access to facility with machines

Data from Haig AJ, Tong HC, Yamakawa KS, et al: Predictors of pain and function in persons with spinal stenosis, low back pain, and no back pain. Spine 2006;31:2950-2957.

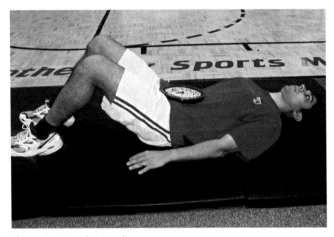

Figure 40–8. Pelvic rock.

Types of Exercises

There are three main types of therapeutic exercises—stretching, strengthening, and endurance activities. Strengthening exercises involve the application of weights or resistance to a muscle group during several repetitions of maximal effort to increase the force of the muscle. Stretching involves the sustained static lengthening of a muscle to increase the flexibility of that specific muscle. Figure 40–8 demonstrates stretching exercises. Endurance exercises involve the application of repeated movements with low resistance to large locomotive muscle groups to increase cardiopulmonary stamina.

There are three types of strengthening exercises. Isometric exercises involve a force being exerted against a fixed object or a muscle contraction that holds an object in one position. Isotonic exercises involve a force being exerted against weight, which moves it through a range of motion (e.g., hand-held weights). Isokinetic exercises occur when a force is exerted against an object that moves it at a fixed velocity. Table 40–3 lists the indications and precautions for these types of exercises.[8] Table 40–4 summarizes some useful exercises and assistive devices for various medical and surgical painful diagnoses.[9]

Table 40–4. Useful Exercises and Assistive Devices in Different Disease Entities

DIAGNOSIS	EXERCISES TO CONSIDER
Reflex sympathetic dystrophy	Edema control
	Gentle desensitization
	Assisted range of motion
	Prevent secondary contracture
Facet arthropathy	Sustained hamstring stretches
	Pelvic tilts (abdominal and gluteal strengthening)
	Lumbar stabilization
	Posture monitoring
	Back conservation techniques
Hip arthritis	Cane to unweight limb
	Hip extension and abduction
Knee arthritis	Cane use
	Joint conservation techniques (e.g., straight-leg raises and short-range quadriceps contractions)
Spondylolisthesis	Core strengthening
	Bracing in flexion
Osteoporosis	Cane use in extension
	Cane use with extreme pain
	Thoracic extension exercises
	Low-impact weight-bearing activity

Precautions and Contraindications

Patients with unstable medical and surgical conditions, including unhealed fractures, unstable angina, and uncompensated cardiac, pulmonary, hypertensive, and thrombotic disorders, should not participate in strengthening, endurance, or flexibility exercises.

Precautions for resistive exercises include cardiovascular factors, overwork, osteoporosis, and immediate muscle soreness associated with exercise. A specific complication of isometric exercise is the potential for a significant increase in blood pressure.[77]

Behavioral Modification Approach to Exercise

We suggest that physical medicine techniques done in conjunction or along with a behavioral modification approach should produce a better outcome,

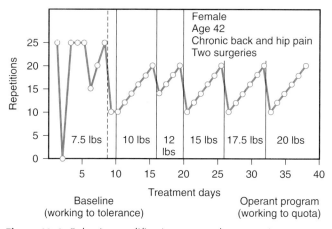

Figure 40–9. Behavior modification approach to exercise.

especially in patients with chronic pain. Figure 40–9 graphically depicts using exercise within a behavioral concept.[9]

Appropriate exercises specific for the pain area and general conditioning exercises such as bicycling, walking, or swimming are usually indicated. Fordyce[78] has noted that appropriate exercise in a behavior modification program must be relevant to the patient's pain and limitations, as well as being quantifiable, visible, and accessible. The patient's baseline exercise level is determined by asking the patient to exercise to tolerance (until pain, weakness, or fatigue necessitates stopping) over a few days.[9] Once the patient's baseline has been established, the initial goal of exercise is set within the patient's tolerance and then gradually increased, with new goals being set every few days.[9] Rewards and reinforcement are given when established goals are accomplished without demonstration of pain behavior.[79] In some patients, however, it is necessary to reduce excessive activity levels by teaching them to pace themselves more appropriately.[9]

This concept makes sense, because among the treatment goals of pain management are the decrease in illness behavior (reduced drug use and visits to physicians) and the increase in well behavior (increased physical activities, mobility, and return to gainful employment).[80] This may be accomplished by blocking noxious sensory input, decreasing tension and depression, rearranging reinforcement contingencies, or assisting in the learning of new behaviors.[81] Biofeedback, cognitive behavior modification, operant approaches, hypnosis, operant pain hypnosis, and relaxation techniques can assist in the treatment of chronic pain behavior.[82-85]

CONCLUSION

In this chapter, we discussed the physical medicine techniques used in treating pain. We presented the concept that although there are a number of approaches to the treatment of patients with pain, a multidisciplinary or interdisciplinary approach is recommended as the symptom becomes more chronic.

Additionally, treatment modalities used should be more successful if carried out within a behavioral modification approach.

Before treatment is undertaken, a comprehensive evaluation is necessary, including a functional evaluation and setting treatment goals that need to be delineated and agreed on by all involved in the treatment program. Physical modalities, manual techniques, and exercise can modify pain symptoms but probably will not cure them; this is especially true for patients with chronic pain. The appropriate use of medications, injections, and psychosocial intervention, in conjunction with physical medicine techniques, are often required to achieve the maximum outcome.

References

1. Linchitz RM, Sorell PJ: Physical Methods of Pain Management. In Raj PP (ed): Practical Management of Pain, 3rd ed. St. Louis, Mosby, 2000, pp 529-543.
2. Higby GJ: Heroin and medical reasoning: The power of analogy. N Y State J Med 1986;83:137-142.
3. Stanos SP, Tyburski MD, Harden RN: Management of chronic pain. In Braddom RL (ed): Physical Medicine and Rehabilitation, 3rd ed. Philadelphia, WB Saunders, 2006, pp 951-988.
4. Becker E, Horn S, Hussla B, et al: [Guidelines for the sociomedical assessment of performance in patients suffering from discopathy or associated diseases.] Gesundheitswesen 2003;65:19-39.
5. Turk DC: Clinical effectiveness and cost effectiveness of treatment for patients with chronic pain. Clin J Pain 2002;18:355-365.
6. Grabois M: Pain clinic cost-effectiveness and efficacy. In Editore M (ed): Proceedings of the Eighth World Congress—The Pain Clinic. Bologna, Italy, Moduzzi Editore, 1998, pp 75-85.
7. Bloodworth D, Calvillo O, Smith K, et al. Chronic pain syndromes: Evaluation and treatment. In Braddom RL (ed): Physical Medicine and Rehabilitation, 2nd ed. Philadelphia, WB Saunders, 2000, pp 913-933.
8. Schramm D: Applications of physical and occupational therapy in chronic pain syndrome. J Back Musculoskel Rehabil 1977;8:225.
9. Bloodworth D, Grabois M: Physical rehabilitation in chronic pain syndrome. In Miller RI, Abram SE (eds): Atlas of Anesthesia, vol VI. Philadelphia, Churchill Livingston, 1998, pp 13.1-13.15.
10. King JC: Chronic pain medicine rehabilitation for diagnostic groups. In Grabois M, Garrison SJ, Hart KA, et al (eds): Physical Medicine and Rehabilitation: The Complete Approach. New York, Blackwell Science, 2000, pp 1016-1034.
11. Fordyce WE, Fowler RS, Lehman JF, et al: Ten steps to help patients with chronic pain. Patient Care 1978;12:263.
12. Schonstein E, Kenny DT, Keating J, et al: Work conditioning, work hardening and functional restoration for workers with back and neck pain. Cochrane Database Syst Rev 2003;(3):CD001822.
13. Velozo CA: Work evaluations: Critique of the state of the art of functional assessment of work. Am J Occup Ther 1991;47:203-209.
14. Tramposh AK: The functional capacity evaluation: Measuring maximal work abilities. Occup Med Art Rev 1992;7:113-124.
15. Pransky GS, Dempsey PG: Practical aspects of functional capacity evaluations. J Occup Rehabil 2004;14:217-229.
16. King PM, Tuckwell N, Barrett TE: A critical review of functional capacity evaluations. Phys Ther 1998;78:852-866.
17. Rutkove SB, Lichtenstein SH: Role of electrodiagnostics in pain assessment. In Warfield CA, Bajwa ZH (eds): Principles and Practice of Pain Medicine. Philadelphia, McGraw-Hill, 2004, pp 112-120.

18. Haig AJ, Tong HC, Yamakawa KS, et al: Predictors of pain and function in persons with spinal stenosis, low back pain, and no back pain. Spine 2006;31:2950-2957.

19. Chan L, Turner JA, Comstock BA, et al: The relationship between electrodiagnostic findings and patient symptoms and function in carpal tunnel syndrome. Arch Phys Med Rehabil 2007;88:19-24.

20. Drory VE, Korczyn AD: The sympathetic skin response in reflex sympathetic dystrophy. J Neurol Sci 1995;128:92-95.

21. Sanders SH, Rucker KS, Anderson KO, et al: Clinical practice guidelines for chronic non-malignant pain syndrome patients. J Back Musculoskel Rehabil 1995;5:15-20.

22. Loeser JD: Pain because of nerve injury. Spine 1985;10: 232-235.

23. Grabois M: Comprehensive evaluation and management of patients with chronic pain. Cardiovasc Res Center Bull 1981;19:113-117.

24. Joshi GP: Multimodal analgesia techniques and postoperative rehabilitation. Anesthesiol Clin North Am 2005;23:185-202.

25. Upton RN, Semple TJ, Macintyre PE: Pharmacokinetic optimization of opioid treatment in acute pain therapy. Clin Pharmacokinet 1997;33:225-244.

26. Macintyre P: Intravenous patient-controlled analgesia: One size does not fit all. Anesthesiol Clin North Am 2005;23: 109-123.

27. Zorowitz RD, Smout RJ, Gassaway JA, et al: Usage of pain medications during stroke rehabilitation: The Post-Stroke Rehabilitation Outcomes Project (PSROP). Top Stroke Rehabil 2005;12:37-49.

28. Abramson DI: Physiologic basis for the use of physical agents in peripheral vascular disorders: Arch Phys Med Rehabil 1965; 46:216.

29. Fields HL, Basbaum AI: Brainstem control of spinal pain-transmission neurons. Annu Rev Physiol 1978;40:217-248.

30. Michlovitz SL, von Nieda K: Therapeutic heat and cold. In Behrens BJ, Michlovitz SL (eds): Physical Agents: Theory and Practice, 2nd ed. Philadelphia, FA Davis, 2006, pp 37-54.

31. Weinberger A, Fadilah R, Lev A et al: Intra-articular temperature measurements after superficial heating. Scand J Rehabil Med 1989;21:55-57.

32. Nussbaum EL. Behrens BJ: Therapeutic ultrasound. In Behrens BJ, Michlovitz SL (eds): Physical Agents: Theory and Practice, 2nd ed. Philadelphia, FA Davis, 2006, pp 57-79.

33. Maxwell L: Therapeutic ultrasound: Its effect on the cellular and molecular mechanisms of inflammation and repair. Physiotherapy 1992;79:421-426.

34. Soto-Quijano DA, Grabois M: Hydrotherapy. In Waldman SD (ed): Pain Management, vol 1. Philadelphia, WB Saunders, 2006, pp 1043-1051.

35. Behrens BJ, Kenna KM: Pain management with electrical stimulation. In Behrens BJ, Michlovitz SL (eds): Physical Agents: Theory and Practice, 2nd ed. Philadelphia, FA Davis, 2006, pp 209-219.

36. Sluka KA, Walsh D: Transcutaneous electrical nerve stimulation: Basic science mechanisms and clinical effectiveness. J Pain 2003;4:109-121.

37. Milne S, Welch V, Brosseau L, et al: Transcutaneous electrical stimulation (TENS) for chronic low back pain. Cochrane Database Syst Rev 2004;(4):CD00.

38. Melzack R, Coderre TJ, Katz, J, et al: Central neuroplasticity and pathological pain. Ann N Y Acad Sci 2001;933:157-174.

39. Gurney B: Soft tissue treatment techniques: Traction. In Behrens BJ, Michlovitz SL (eds): Physical Agents: Theory and Practice, 2nd ed. Philadelphia, FA Davis, 2006, pp 99-115.

40. Van der Heijden GJ, Beurskens AJ, Koes BW, et al: The efficacy of traction for back and neck pain: A systematic, blinded review of randomized clinical trial methods. Phys Ther 1995;75:93-104.

41. Harte AA, Baxter GD, Gracey JH: The efficacy of traction for back pain: A systematic review of randomized controlled trials. Arch Phys Med Rehabil 2003;84:1542-1553.

42. Graham N, Gross AR, Goldsmith C, et al: Mechanical traction for mechanical neck disorders: A systematic review. J Rehabil Med 2006;38:145-152.

43. Clarke J, van Tulder M, Blomberg S, et al: Traction for low back pain with or without sciatica: An updated systematic review within the framework of the Cochrane collaboration. Spine 2006;31:1591-1599.

44. Zylbergold RS, Piper MC: Cervical spine disorders: A comparison of three types of traction. Spine 1985;10:867-871.

45. Craig EJ, Kaelin D: Physical modalities. In Grabois M, Garrison SJ, Hart KA, et al (eds): Physical Medicine and Rehabilitation. The Complete Approach. Oxford, England, Blackwell Science, 2000, pp 440-457.

46. Ballantyne BA, Bryon T, Reser MD, et al: The effects of inversion traction on spinal column configuration, heart rate, blood pressure, and perceived discomfort. J Orthop Sports Phy Ther 1986;7:254-260.

47. Greenman PE: Principles of Manual Medicine, 2nd ed. Baltimore, Williams & Wilkins, 1996.

48. Haldeman S: Manipulation and massage for the relief of pain. In Melzack R, Wall PD (eds): Textbook of Pain, 2nd ed. New York, Churchill Livingstone, 1989, pp 942-951.

49. Bigos S, Bowyer O, Braen G, et al: Acute Low Back Problems in Adults. Clinical Practice Guideline (Publ. No. 95-0643, Quick Reference Guide No. 14). Rockville, Md, U.S. Department of Health and Human Services, Agency for Health Care Policy and Research, 1994.

50. Bronfort G: Spinal manipulation: Current state of research and its indications. Neurol Clin 1999;17:91-111.

51. Van Tulder MW, Koes BW, Bouter LM: Conservative treatment of acute and chronic nonspecific low back pain: A systemic review of randomized controlled trials of the most common interventions. Spine 1997;22:2128-2156.

52. Aure OF, Nilsen JH, Vasseljen O: Manual therapy and exercise therapy in patients with chronic low back pain: A randomised, controlled trial with 1-year follow-up. Spine 2003;28: 525-532.

53. Geisser M, Wiggert E, Haig A, et al: A randomized, controlled trial of manual therapy and specific adjuvant exercise for chronic low back pain. Clin J Pain 2005;21:463-470.

54. Skyba DA, Radhakrishnan R, Rohling JJ, et al: Joint manipulation reduces hyperalgesia by activation of monoamine receptors but not opioid or GABA receptors in the spinal cord. Pain 2003;106:159-168.

55. DiGiovanna EL: Somatic dysfunction. In DiGiovanna EL, Schiowitz S (eds): An Osteopathic Approach to Diagnosis and Treatment. Philadelphia, JB Lippincott, 1991, pp 6-12.

56. Vernon HJ, Dhami MSI, Howley TP, et al: Spinal manipulation and beta endorphin: A controlled study of the effect of a spinal manipulation on plasma beta-endorphin levels in normal males. J Manipulative Physiol Ther 1986;92:115-123.

57. Haldeman S, Hooper PD: Mobilization, manipulation, massage and exercise for the relief of musculoskeletal pain. In Wall PD, Melzak R (eds): Textbook of Pain. St. Louis, Churchill Livingston, 1999, pp 1399-1418.

58. Assendelft WJJ, Morton SC, Yu EI, et al: Spinal manipulative therapy for low back pain: A meta-analysis of effectiveness relative to other therapies. Ann Intern Med 2003;138:71-81.

59. Colachis SC Jr, Strohm BR: A study of tractive forces and angle of pull on vertebral interspaces in the cervical spine. Arch Phys Med Rehabilitation 1965;46:820-830.

60. Colachis SC Jr, Strohm BR: Cervical traction: Relationship of traction time to varied tractive force with constant angle of pull. Arch Phys Med Rehabil 1965;46:815-819.

61. Wong AMK, Leong CP, Chen C: The traction angle and cervical intervertebral separation. Spine 1992;17:136-138.

62. Farrell JP, Jensen GM: Manual therapy: A critical assessment of role in the profession of physical therapy. Phys Ther 1992; 72:843-852.

63. Callaghan MJ: The role of massage in the management of the athlete: A review. Br J Sports Med 1993;27:28-33.

64. Tappan FM: Healing massage techniques: Holistic, classic, and emerging methods. Norwalk, Conn, Appleton and Lange, 1988, pp 3-33.

65. Goats GC, Keir KA: Connective tissue massage. Br J Sports Med 1991;25:131-133.

66. Melzak R, Wall PD: Pain mechanisms: A new theory. Science 1965;150:971-977.

67. Melzak R: The gate control theory 25 years later: New perspectives in phantom limb pain. In Bond MR, Charlton JE, Woolf CJ (eds): Proceedings of the Sixth World Congress on Pain. Amsterdam, Elsevier, 1991, pp 9-21.
68. Bloodworth D: Exercise and physical reconditioning. In Waldman SD (ed): Pain Management, vol 1. Philadelphia, WB Saunders, 2006, pp 1055-1068.
69. Hayden JA, van Tulder MW, Malmivaara A, et al: Exercise therapy for treatment of non-specific low back pain. Cochrane Database Syst Rev 2005;(3):CD000335.
70. Deyo RA, Diehl AM, Rosenthal M: How many days of bed rest for acute low back pain? A randomized clinical trial. N Engl J Med 1986;315:1064-1070.
71. Kellett J: Acute soft tissue injuries—a review of the literature. Med Sci Sports Exerc 1986;18:489-500.
72. Hagen KB, Hilde G, Jamtvedt G, et al: Bed rest for acute low back pain and sciatica. Cochrane Database Syst Rev 2000;(2): CD001254.
73. Khalil TM, Asfour SS, Martinez LM, et al: Stretching in the rehabilitation of low back pain patients. Spine 1992;17: 311-317.
74. Takemasa R, Yamamoto H, Tani T: Trunk muscle strength in and effect of trunk muscle exercises for patients with chronic low back pain. Spine 1995;20:2522-2530.
75. Davies JE, Gibson T, Tester L: The value of exercises in the treatment of low back pain. Rheumatol Rehabil 1979;18: 243-247.
76. Detorri JR, Bullock SH, Sutlive TG, et al: The effects of spinal flexion and extension and their associated postures in patients with acute low back pain. Spine 1995;21:2303-2312.
77. Donald KW, Lind AR, McNichol GW, et al: Cardiovascular response to sustained (static) contractions. Circ Res 1967; 1(Suppl 1):15-30.
78. Fordyce WE: Behavioral Methods for Chronic Pain and Illness. St. Louis, Mosby-Year Book, 1967.
79. Walsh NE, Dumitru D, Schoenfeld LS, et al: Treatment of patients with chronic pain. In Delisa JA (ed): Physical Medicine and Rehabilitation: Principles and Practice, 4th ed. Philadelphia, Lippincott Williams & Wilkins, 2005, pp 493-529.
80. Fulton WM: Psychological strategies and techniques in pain management. Semin Anesth 1985;4:247-254.
81. Malone MD, Strube MJ: Meta-analysis of non-medical treatments for chronic pain. Pain 1988;34:231-244.
82. France R, Krishnau KRR: Chronic Pain. Washington DC, American Psychiatric Press, 1988.
83. Elmer BN, Freeman A: Pain Management Psychotherapy: A Practical Guide. New York, John Wiley & Sons, 1998.
84. Gatchel RJ, Turk DC: Psychological Approaches to Pain Management: A Practitioner's Guide. New York, Guilford Press, 1998.
85. Miller L: Psychotherapeutic approaches to chronic pain. Psychotherapy 1993;30:115-124.

41 Physical Rehabilitation for Patients with Chronic Pain

Harriët Wittink and Jeanine A. Verbunt

Ideally, patients with chronic pain are treated by a team of health professionals, commonly consisting of physicians, psychologists, physical and occupational therapists, social workers, and nurses, to address the biopsychosocial nature of pain. Within the interdisciplinary team, the physical therapist is responsible for comprehensive assessment, with emphasis on the musculoskeletal system, including assessment of strength, flexibility, and physical endurance, functional activities, and behavioral factors that may influence physical functioning, and management of the physical rehabilitation process. Physical therapists are thus intimately involved in pain management, not pain treatment.

Patients come to our clinics with certain expectations of evaluation and treatment. One study has investigated the expectations of patients with chronic pain on their first outpatient visit to a pain management program.[1] Most patients expected an explanation or an improved understanding of their pain problem. The most common satisfying outcome was relief or control of pain and the most common disappointing outcome was being told that nothing could be done. Most patients expected further medical investigation and changes to their prescribed medication. There was no mention of patients expecting a referral for pain management and only a small percentage of patients wanted advice on coping with pain, or self-management of pain. Although this study needs to be duplicated in other centers, it has a great deal of apparent validity. Many patients with chronic pain resist referral to physical therapy. Part of the difficulty lies in the history of treatment failures of the conditions with which patients often present. A number of factors may be responsible for past treatment failures, including persistent failure of physical therapists to recognize and treat the differences between acute and chronic pain states, past treatment that did not address the emotional and cognitive aspects of chronic pain, and an inability of the patient to recognize anything less than total

pain relief as success.[2] It is therefore important to identify patient expectations at the initial visit to prevent disappointment with referrals for pain management.

PHYSICAL THERAPY EVALUATION

In evidence-based practice, clinical decisions must first include consideration of the patient's clinical and physical circumstances to establish what is wrong and determine which treatment options are available. Second, the latter need to be tempered by research evidence concerning the efficacy, effectiveness, and efficiency of the options. Third, given the likely consequences associated with each option, the clinician must consider the patient's preferences and likely actions in terms of what interventions she or he is ready and able to accept. Clinical expertise is needed to bring these considerations together and recommend treatment that the patient is agreeable to accepting.[3] Accordingly, the purposes of a physical therapy evaluation are to establish a baseline from which to plan and begin interventions, assist in the selection of appropriate interventions, and evaluate the efficacy of interventions.

As described in the biopsychosocial model of pain introduced by Fordyce,[4] contributing factors to disability can be biologic and psychological, as well as social. Essential to this model is the idea that factors maintaining the pain problem are not necessarily the same as those initiating pain. To establish a baseline, therefore, a thorough inventory of all factors contributing to a patient's perceived level of disability is important. The World Health Organization has published the International Classification of Functioning, Disability and Health (ICF),[5] which provides a biopsychosocial model that identifies three concepts described from the perspective of body systems, the individual, and society. Within the context of health, the ICF has defined "bodily functions and structures" as physiologic functions of body systems or anatomic

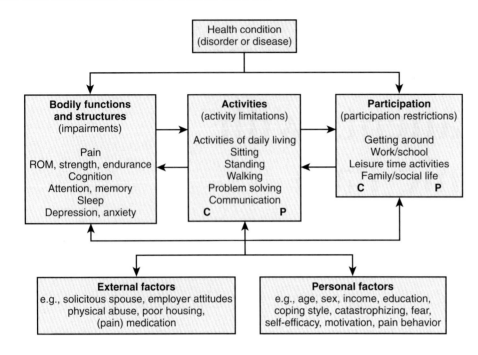

Figure 41–1. Example of International Classification of Functioning, Disability, and Health (ICF) framework. C, capacity; P, performance; ROM, range of motion. (Adapted from Ustun TB, Chatterji S, Bickenbach J, et al: The International Classification of Functioning, Disability and Health: A new tool for understanding disability and health. Disabil Rehabil 2003;25: 565-571.)

elements, such as organs, limbs, and their components. "Activity" is defined as the execution of specific tasks or actions by an individual, whereas "participation" is envisioned as encompassing involvement in a life situation. In the ICF, "functioning" refers to all body functions, activities, and participation. Disability is the ICF umbrella term for impairment, activity limitation, and participation restrictions. Contextual factors are provided within the ICF framework (Fig. 41–1), consisting of external environmental factors (e.g., significant others, employers, medications, and health care providers) and personal factors (e.g., age, education, income, worry that activity will exacerbate pain or injury, resulting in avoidance of activity to prevent anticipated negative consequences).

Qualifiers for the activities and participation classification make it possible to separate clearly the patient's inherent capacity to perform actions within a domain and performance in his or her actual environmental context.[5] Capacity refers to the environmentally adjusted inherent ability of the individual or, in other words, the highest probable functioning of a person in a given domain at a given point in time in a standardized environment. Capacity can be measured by physical tests or by questionnaires that ask, "Can you?" Performance describes what a person actually does in her or his current environment and thus describes the person's functioning as observed or reported in the person's real life environment, with the existing facilitators and barriers.[6] Performance can be measured by direct observation. As this is often highly impractical, self-report measures can be substituted that ask, "Do you?"

The Rehabilitation Problem-Solving (RPS) form is based on the ICF[7] and is a practical tool to help visualize the patient's state of functioning and disability.

The form is used to specify specific and relevant target problems, discern factors that cause or contribute to these problems, and plan the most appropriate intervention. In addition, the form was designed as a tool to facilitate intra- and interprofessional communication and improve the communication between health care professionals and their patients.[7] The form is divided into three parts: (1) header for basic information; (2) upper part, which describe the patient's perspective; and (3) lower part for analysis by the health care professionals. The form can help visualize the current understanding of the patient's state of activities and participation, his or her target problems, and how the health care team relates them to hypothetical mediators and contextual factors (Fig. 41–2).

Using the information obtained through carefully selected questionnaires, an interview, physical examination, and physical tests, most of the information needed to develop an appropriate treatment plan should be obtained.

Patient Interview

The Joint Commission (formerly the Joint Commission on Accreditation of Health Care Organizations) requires that all patients have the right to an adequate pain assessment, including documentation of pain location, intensity, quality, onset, duration, variations, rhythms, manner of expressing pain, pain relief, what makes it worse, effects of pain, and a pain plan. In addition to questions about the location, intensity, frequency, and duration of pain, questions such as "What do you think causes your pain?" and "What is the worst thing you think might happen to you because of your pain?" will give insight into the patient's belief system (especially important if the

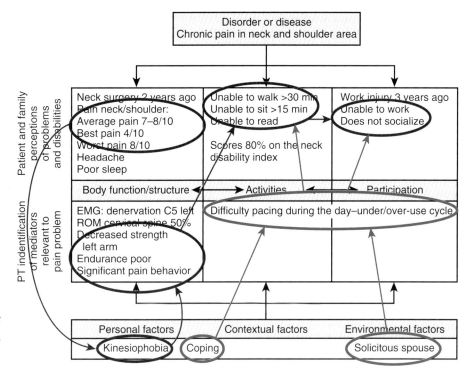

Figure 41–2. Rehabilitation Problem-Solving (RPS) form used for a patient with chronic neck and shoulder pain. EMG, electromyelogram; PT, physical therapist; ROM, range of motion. (Adapted from Steiner WA, Ryser L, Huber E, et al: Use of the ICF model as a clinical problem-solving tool in physical therapy and rehabilitation medicine. Phys Ther 2002;82:1098-1107.)

patient comes from a different culture) and the presence of catastrophizing. In addition, the physical therapist focuses on determining how (much) the pain interferes with activities and participation, activities of daily living such as housework, grocery shopping, getting around in the community, recreational and social activities, and ability to work and sleep. The number of hours lying down because of pain during a day is noted. Patients are further asked about significant others, partners, parents, and children—do they help out, ignore the patient, or prevent the patient from doing things because they fear the patient might "harm" him or herself?

Unfortunately, there are no perfect measures of physical activity or activity limitations. Comparison measures include subjective measures (based on self-report) and objective measures (based on direct measurement). Self-report measures can be self-administered or interviewer-administered in person, on the telephone, or both. However, self-report on physical functioning can reflect a difference between how patients function and how they believe they function, resulting in a different reported physical activity level compared with actual observed active behavior.[8] In an experimental setting, it appeared that patients in pain in particular had difficulties judging their own performance.[9]

Relatively few comparison studies have been performed between self-report and objective measures; the studies that are available seem to indicate a gap between them.[10] In rehabilitation practice, there is a tendency to use objective as well as self-report measures to assess physical activity. Objective measures include functional capacity tasks, markers of move-

ment (accelerometers), and observed or videotaped activity (direct observation). Self-reported status often involves outcomes of most relevance and importance to patients and their loved ones because they capture patient experience and perspective.[11] Psychosocial factors have been found to have a significant impact on functional activity, particularly in persons with chronic pain. The physical therapist's observations on a patient's mood and behavior should be communicated clearly to the rest of the team, which can then direct appropriate psychological and psychiatric treatment.

Psychological screening by means of history taking has been shown to have low sensitivity and predictive value for identifying distressed patients; thus, some type of formal screening, such as with a questionnaire, is recommended.[12] Psychosocial factors contributing to a patient's pain disability level that can be assessed by a questionnaire include fear of movement (Tampa Scale of Kinesiophobia,[13] catastrophizing,[14] depression (Beck Depression Inventory),[15] and other factors that otherwise might not be determined. Consideration of the patient's views is associated with greater satisfaction with care,[16] improved compliance with treatment programs,[17] and maintenance of continuous relationships in health care.[18]

Particularly important are questions about what the patient expects from treatment. Increasingly, there is evidence that patient beliefs play a large role in treatment outcome. For example, a patient who is looking for pain relief only and insists on medication management as the sole treatment for the pain is not likely going to be compliant with a rehabilitation program. Studies have shown that high patient expectations may influence clinical outcome independently of the treatment itself.[19] In one study, patients who preferred one type of treatment and received another actually got worse during treatment.[20]

Physical Examination

The traditional rehabilitation-oriented physical examination assesses impairments in joint range of motion (ROM), strength, neurologic integrity, and gait. Diagnostic procedures should focus on the identification of potentially serious "red flag" conditions that require prompt medical evaluation. The main objective is to determine whether there is a relationship between pain reports and objective physical findings, or whether the patient presents with intractable pain (chronic pain syndrome). In the former, rehabilitation might focus more specifically on impairments related to pain that interfere with the ability to function, whereas in the latter, rehabilitation might focus on improving physical functioning in general and have a more significant behavioral approach.

Patient anxiety may complicate the physical examination. Catastrophic cognition, behavioral displays of pain, and somatic sensations measured during examination have been shown to predict anxiety experienced during examination.[21] Muscle guarding and pain behaviors are often displayed during physical examination; these include moaning, sighing, rubbing, reluctance to perform any active movement (ROM), and the presence of telltale weakness and nonorganic signs. Nonorganic or behavioral signs[22] in patients with back pain can be assessed through palpation and simulation tests, including axial loading (pressure applied to the top of the patient's head), simulated rotation (moving shoulders and hips together so that no rotation occurs in the trunk), inconsistency between the straight-leg raise in a sitting versus supine position, telltale weakness with resisted muscle testing, and regional sensory changes. These tests have been validated in white patients only and may not be applicable in patients from ethnic minorities or those who are older than 60 years.

Studies in patients with chronic pain have identified discrepancies between self-report of physical activity and actual level of physical activity, so capacity testing is performed in addition to traditional impairment examination. This involves direct observation of patient performance of specific tasks and assessment of whether the patient is willing to move or fears performing specific tasks. Baseline functional ability assessment can provide objectively verifiable information about a patient's quality of life and ability to participate in normal life activities.

Some functional tests that have been used in a chronic pain population include the Back Performance Scale[23,24] and the physical performance test battery. The Back Performance Scale is a condition-specific performance measure of activity limitation in patients with back pain. It includes five tests of daily activities requiring mobility of the trunk: sock test, pick-up test, roll-up test, fingertip-to-floor test, and lift test. This test is reliable and valid, and discriminative ability and responsiveness to important change have been demonstrated.[23,24] The physical performance test battery is a generic test battery that includes nine physical performance tests: the time taken to complete various tasks (e.g., picking up coins, tying a belt, reaching up, putting on a sock, standing from sitting, 50-foot fast walk, 50-foot walk at preferred speed), the distance walked in 6 minutes, and the distance reached forward while standing. The test battery is reliable and has discriminant ability.[25] Aerobic fitness can be estimated from submaximal bicycle ergometer tests or measured using a treadmill test.[26]

In the assessment of work-related performance, a functional capacity evaluation (FCE) is often used.[27] The purpose of an FCE is to test a person's physical abilities to the maximum to produce objective documentation regarding work and activities of daily life. FCE has become part of the accepted practice in work injury prevention and rehabilitation.[28] During an FCE, the patient has to complete a standard protocol of physical tasks while a trained observer records the performance and limitations. Assessment includes ability to lift weights from floor to waist and from the waist to overhead, carry, crawl, squat, sit, stand, walk, climb stairs, and push and pull weights. Aerobic fitness may be determined from a (submaximal) bicycle or treadmill test. Additional specific tests may be performed, such as fine motor skills for the hands and handgrip strength. Practical data on the use of FCEs to determine an individual's physical capacities have been available since the 1990s, but research to justify the use of FCEs is still lacking. Although the term *capacity* is included in its name, FCE is a performance test rather than a capacity test. An FCE is not fully objective, because an observer has to decide whether a patient performed maximally or submaximally during the test. The influence of psychological factors is also assumed to be present in an FCE, but this can only be assessed by observation.

A number of studies have shown that self-report and performance and capacity tests, although related, appear to tap into different aspects of the physical functioning domain.[29] For example, patients with chronic low back pain (CLBP) have shown considerable differences in limitations when comparing self-report, clinical examination, and functional testing for assessing work-related limitations. Professional health care workers should be aware of these differences when using them in daily practice.[30,31]

THERAPY FOR CHRONIC PAIN

An important difference between patients with acute and chronic pain is the presence of any relationship between pain, activity limitations, and participation restrictions. For patients with acute pain, nociception, perceived pain, activity limitations, and participation restrictions are often closely related. Therefore, treatment in the acute phase will be focused on eliminating the causal factor of the pain, resulting in a reduction of activity limitations and prevention of disability. For patients with chronic pain, however, this treatment strategy will not be sufficient. Patients with chronic pain may never return to work, even when the only impairment identified is pain. Treatments that address chronic pain as a warning of tissue damage do not alter the illness and disability behavior of patients with chronic pain, nor will they improve their health-related quality of life. The focus of therapy should be to help these patients regain control over their lives by active participation in their pain management program and independent management of their pain. To achieve this, an active partnership is needed between the patient and therapist. As for other patients, patients with chronic pain want a confidence-based association that includes understanding, listening, respect, and being included in decision making.[32]

Patients with chronic pain are not a homogeneous group and there is no one type of treatment applicable to all patients with pain. Because each patient has a unique set of circumstances, psychosocial issues, and physical findings, treatment must be individualized and based on the comprehensive assessment of the patient and his or her individual goals.

In general, chronic pain management should include the following, as noted by Von Korff and collleagues[33]:

- Collaboration between physical therapist and patient
- Personalized rehabilitation plan
- Tailored education of the patient on the nature of the problem
- Resolution of treatable barriers related to functional goal attainment
- Tailored instruction in independent management of pain
- Instruction in methods to prevent future problems
- Monitoring of outcome (achievement of patient goals)
- Monitoring of adherence to treatment
- Planned follow-up

Collaboration between Physical Therapist and Patient

To decrease the negative impact of chronic pain on functioning and health-related quality of life, patients must adopt self-management skills. To do so, patients should have accepted the diagnosis of chronic pain and have an active orientation regarding self-management. Not all patients are ready for this, however, and attempts are being made to predict which patients will benefit from pain management programs.[34] The stages of change model is thought to map the process of behavior change, but needs further validation in the chronic pain population. Patients in the precontemplation stage are not moti-

vated to adopt self-management skills, whereas patients in the contemplation stage think about it. Patients in the preparation stage are planning to change and are already trying some (parts) of the skills required. Patients in the action stage are actively learning to engage in self-management, whereas patients in the maintenance stage keep on working to stabilize the new behavior pattern.[34] For an effective collaboration between the physical therapist and patient, the patient must at least be planning to take an active orientation approach toward self-management and the therapist should support and encourage this.

The physical therapist should include the following in practice: (1) a dynamic, multidimensional knowledge base that is patient-centered; (2) a clinical reasoning process that is embedded in a collaborative, problem-solving venture with the patient; (3) a central focus on movement assessment linked to patient function; and (4) a consistently caring attitude and commitment to patients, which have been shown to be central to expert physical therapy care.[35]

Not only do patients bring expectations about treatment, but the provider does as well. Treatment decisions are often based on the beliefs of the provider. Houben and colleagues[36] have used the Pain Attitudes and Beliefs Scale for Physiotherapists (PABS-PT) to measure provider-perceived harmfulness of physical activities and treatment recommendations for common low back pain. The PABS-PT differentiates between biomedical versus biopsychosocial treatment orientation with regard to common low back pain. Providers who scored high on the biomedical orientation were more likely to use a pain-contingent treatment approach and focus on "curing" impairments. Providers who scored high on the biopsychosocial orientation were more likely to use a time-contingent treatment approach and focus on increasing activities. Linton and associates[37] have investigated the level of fear avoidance beliefs in practicing general practitioners and physical therapists. Compared with providers with low fear avoidance, providers with high levels of fear avoidance had an increased risk for believing sick leave to be a good treatment (relative risk [RR] = 2.0), not providing good information about activities (RR = 1.7), and being uncertain about identifying patients at risk for developing persistent pain problems (RR = 1.5). They concluded that some providers hold beliefs reflecting fear avoidance and that these beliefs may influence treatment practice. The combination of a high fear-avoidant provider with a high fear-avoidant patient seems to be a recipe for disaster in chronic pain management and should be avoided.

Personalized Rehabilitation Plan

To win the collaboration of patients and their families, physical therapists need to negotiate and agree on a definition of the problem that they are working on with each patient. They must then agree on the targets and goals for management and develop an individualized collaborative self-management plan.[33] The patient and physical therapist need to agree on the goals of treatment to prevent confusion and disappointment and to establish a collaborative relationship. Appropriate goal setting is an important skill that patients must learn. Establishing specific but attainable goals can facilitate task performance. In contrast, unrealistic goals can lead to decreased motivation and a sense of failure. Self-efficacy facilitates goal setting; those with high self-efficacy choose to perform more challenging tasks.[38] They set themselves higher goals and stick to them. Self-efficacy can be understood as the confidence in one's ability to deal with certain life stressors. High self-efficacy is related to better treatment outcomes, such as higher levels of physical functioning and the use of pain coping strategies related to better adjustment to chronic pain.

Goals must be measurable so that treatment can be time-limited and have an observable end point. Return to a pain-free state is an example of an unrealistic goal. Common (realistic) goals are associated with a reduction of the impact of pain on the patient's life (i.e., increased level of activities and participation), independent pain management, and the attainment of functional goals. Functional goals include being able to walk for 1 hour, sitting through a meal or a movie, being able to carry and lift a certain amount of weight, playing with the children, going out with the family, and being able to perform essential job components. Return to work or vocational rehabilitation should be part of the treatment plan, when appropriate. A directive return to work approach has been shown to be successful in patients with chronic pain.[39] Goals must be realistic and attainable within a reasonable time. It is helpful to determine the number of treatments per week and the number of weeks of treatment before initiating treatment (e.g., treatment will occur three times a week for 6 weeks). Having a definite end point increases patient adherence and provides a framework on which the patient and treatment team can achieve goals. A treatment contract that includes goals, intensity and frequency of treatment, and expected compliance with treatment can be helpful.

During treatment, the use of goal-setting charts is recommended. Patients set a target for activities each week, record their achievements on the chart, note the nature of any difficulties and how these will be tackled next time, and make other comments. Patients may comment on their performance or on the appropriateness of the goals that they have set. Thus, they can monitor their progress and improve their accuracy when setting goals.

Education on the Nature of the Problem

A number of studies have shown that most patients expect an explanation or an improved understanding of their pain problem, a clear diagnosis of the cause of their pain, information, and instructions. They expect confirmation from the health care provider that their pain is real.[1,32] For patients attending pain clinics, the explanation of their pain problem is rated as important as the cure or relief of their pain.[1] Education on the neurophysiology of pain is important and may be considered a precondition for pain management success. Unfortunately, the underestimation of patients' ability to understand current scientific information about the neurophysiology of pain represents barriers to reconceptualization of the problem in chronic pain within the clinical and lay arenas.[40] Patients are capable of understanding the complexities of pain if explained well. The main goals of education are reassurance and empowerment. Studies that have used an approach to education that emphasizes the cognitive, behavioral, and neurophysiologic aspects of chronic pain have reported reduced disability, lowered use of health care services, normalization of pain understanding, and increased self-efficacy.

When treating patients in a group, education can be given by other patients as well. They may share solutions to functional problems, explain ways to pace their activities better, and describe independent pain management techniques that they have found helpful.

Resolution of Treatable Barriers Related to Functional Goal Attainment

Barriers related to the attainment of functional goals in patients with chronic pain are usually the result of a combination of physical factors and patient beliefs and understanding. Physical conditioning programs, given and supervised by a physical therapist or a multidisciplinary team, seem to be effective in reducing the number of sick days for some workers with chronic back pain when compared with usual care.[41] The program should include a cognitive-behavioral approach plus intensive physical training (specific to the job or not) targeted to aerobic capacity, muscle strength, endurance, and coordination. Ideally, exercise therapy is combined with a cognitive-behavioral approach in a chronic pain rehabilitation program.

Exercise Therapy

The "deconditioning syndrome"[42,43] was postulated in the mid-1980s as a factor contributing to the intolerance to physical activities and subsequent further loss of function and disability in patients with chronic pain. More recently, physical disuse has been presented as a factor that perpetuates chronic pain in theoretical pain research models. Although there is no conclusive evidence this is correct, it is still one of the theoretical frameworks used in pain rehabilitation.[44]

Exercise training can reverse the sequelae of physical disuse and help patients achieve functional goals.

Clinical trials have provided strong evidence for the efficacy of muscle conditioning and aerobic exercise to lessen symptoms in persons with osteoarthritis of the knee.[45-47] Others have reported that exercise is an important tool for reducing pain, stiffness, and joint tenderness in rheumatoid arthritis[48,49] and fibromyalgia syndrome patients.[50] Exercise has been shown to be effective for short-term pain relief in patients with rotator cuff disease, and provides a longer term benefit with respect to functional measures.[51] Exercise may be helpful for patients with CLBP, enhancing return to normal daily activities and work.[52,53] Supervised exercise therapy that consists of individually designed programs, including stretching or strengthening, may relieve pain and improve function for those with chronic nonspecific low back pain.[54] There is strong evidence that exercise therapy and multidisciplinary treatment programs and moderate evidence that nonsteroidal anti-inflammatory drugs, back schools, and behavioral therapy are effective for those with CLBP.[55]

Guzman[56] has reviewed the efficacy of multidisciplinary treatment of chronic back pain and concluded there is strong evidence that *intensive* multidisciplinary biopsychosocial rehabilitation with a functional restoration approach improves function when compared with inpatient or outpatient nonmultidisciplinary treatments. There was moderate evidence that intensive multidisciplinary biopsychosocial rehabilitation with a functional restoration approach improved pain when compared with outpatient nonmultidisciplinary rehabilitation or usual care.

Therefore, exercise therapy encompasses a heterogeneous group of interventions and, although the studies cited found beneficial effects of exercise on pain and function, there continues to be uncertainty about the most effective exercise approach. In most studies, there were insufficient data to provide useful guidelines for optimal exercise type or dosage, although some evidence exists that "sicker" patients may benefit from more intensive treatment. Haldorsen and associates[57] have shown that patients with poor prognosis for return to work returned to work at significantly higher rates when treated with a more intense multidisciplinary treatment program, whereas patients with a good return to work prognosis benefited equally from ordinary treatment as multidisciplinary treatment. Patients consequently do not all benefit from the same exercise program. Exercise programs need to be individually designed and tailored to the individual needs of the patient.

There is little evidence that supports the use of passive modalities in the treatment of patients with chronic pain. Spinal manipulative therapy has no statistically or clinically significant advantage over general practitioner care, analgesics, physical therapy, exercises, or back school in patients with CLBP.[58] Massage, on the other hand, might be beneficial for patients with subacute and chronic nonspecific LBP, especially when combined with exercises and education.[59]

Cognitive-Behavioral Approach

Cognitive-behavioral therapy is a combination of cognitive and behavioral therapy. Behavioral therapy addresses the relationships between certain situations and patients' habitual reactions to them (e.g., walking with a limp because it gets positive attention from the spouse). Cognitive therapy addresses patients' thoughts or beliefs that cause them to feel and act the way they do: "If I use my back, my legs will be paralyzed, so the safest thing for me is to lie on the couch and do nothing." Therefore, if patients exhibit unwanted behaviors, it is important to identify the beliefs that cause the behaviors and to teach patients how to replace or modify the beliefs so that more desirable behavior might ensue. Cognitive-behavioral modification can be accomplished in a number of ways, including the following: talking about beliefs (usually done in a group setting with other patients), being exposed to avoided activities, increasing the number and duration of usual activities, providing a reward system in which healthy behavior is rewarded and encouraged and nonhealthy behavior is ignored, and obtaining feedback from other patients about the behavior.

Many chronic pain patients have a tendency to do more on days when they feel well and to do less on days when they feel more pain and fatigue. This pain-contingent behavior results in a cycle of overdoing and underdoing, with the patient doing too much one day and nothing at all the next. Self-pacing during activity attempts to even out the activity peaks and troughs controlled by pain to achieve a moderate activity-rest cycle. Appropriate pacing requires that daily activities be regulated and structured. Gradual controlled increases in the general activity level will avert triggering sudden increases of pain that lead to reduction of activity. Activities are paced by timing or the introduction of exercise quotas interspersed with periods of rest or a different activity. In graded activity, the patient is started at a level of exercise that is easy enough to ensure success and thus provide positive reinforcement and increased patient self-confidence. The number and intensity of exercises and physical activities are then gradually and steadily increased. The home exercise program is progressive and quota-based, beginning at a submaximal level to ensure early success, with an appropriate rate of increase built in. This structure allows for achievement of functional goals and the disconnection of activities from pain. Chronic pain levels have been shown to stay the same or decrease despite significant increases in activity levels.

Pain-related fear has been consistently associated with initiation and maintenance of chronic pain disability.[60] Repeated exposure to avoided activities decreases anxiety and fear about them. For patients with high levels of pain and activity-related fear, behavioral methods such as quota-based progressive exercise programs, education on hurt versus harm, and performance-contingent rewards can be used.[61]

Exposure to in vivo treatment for chronic pain patients with high levels of fear and avoidance shows promise.[62] This entails patients being challenged to perform physical activities that they believe will harm them. Usually, exposure treatment is carried out as combined therapy with a physical therapist and behavioral therapist.

These methods may have adverse effects on patients with low levels of fear avoidance, however. One study has shown that patients with elevated fear-avoidance beliefs appear to have less disability from fear-avoidance–based physical therapy and patients with lower fear-avoidance beliefs appear to have more disability from this type of therapy when compared with those receiving standard physical therapy.[63]

It is still unknown which patients benefit most from certain types of behavioral treatment, although a number of systematic reviews have demonstrated efficacy of behavioral treatment for patients with chronic pain. Although multidisciplinary programs have shown effectiveness for patients with chronic pain, which component is most effective and whether combining treatment approaches has a cumulative effect remains obscure. For example, in a recent study, Smeets and coworkers[64] studied the effectiveness of three rehabilitation interventions—active physical, cognitive-behavioral, and combined treatment for nonspecific CLBP. The three interventions were compared with each other and a waiting list control group. All three active treatments were effective in comparison with no treatment, but no clinically relevant differences between the combined and single-component treatments were found.

Self-Management Techniques

Self-management ensures active patient participation in managing pain and achieving reasonable goals of functional restoration. Self-management ensures active patient participation and includes the following:

- Use of pain control modalities (e.g., ice, heat, self-massage, relaxation, cognitive-behavioral)
- Use of a graded gradually progressive exercise program to encourage overall fitness, activity, and healthy lifestyle

Passive modalities (e.g., transcutaneous electrical nerve stimulation [TENS], ultrasound, massage, corsets, traction, acupuncture) should be limited and used only in combination with an active exercise program.

There is increasing evidence that self-management programs are helpful in reducing pain and disability. Positive results on health-related quality of life outcomes (e.g., self-reported outcomes, health distress, disability, activity limitation, global health, pain, fatigue), health behaviors (e.g., practice of mental stress management, stretching and strength exercise, aerobic exercise), self-efficacy, and use of health care services (e.g., physician visits, hospitalizations) have been reported with self-management programs.[65]

Instruction in Methods to Prevent Future Problems

It is almost inevitable that a patient with chronic pain will experience an exacerbation of the pain problem at some time. The incidence of relapse following initially successful treatment of persistent pain also appears to be high, ranging from 30% to 60%.[66] Relapse may be the result of an individual physical event or it may result from cumulative physical and psychological stresses that challenge a patient's coping resources. The physical therapist can help identify challenging situations and develop strategies to cope with them. These may include setting criteria to visit health professionals, using pain medication, or encouraging the patient to rest and relax briefly. Plans for resumption of activity following such an exacerbation are critical.[67] If returning a patient to work is an important goal, including a detailed job description provides important ergonomic information. Implementing components of the job description can be practiced with the physical therapist and at home.

The goal of ergonomics is to ensure that the workplace is designed to prevent work-induced injuries. Non-neutral postures, forceful exertions, constrained or static postures, repetitive work, use of pinch grip, work over shoulder height, prolonged periods with the trunk inclined forward, heavy lifting, twisting while lifting, and whole body vibration are risk factors for work-related musculoskeletal disorders. A common type of ergonomic instruction during physical therapy involves educating the patient about manual handling and lifting, optimal seated postures and activities, and relationship of the chair to the workbench or desk. The patient is taught to take stretch breaks during work and to alternate job components.

At the end of treatment, an FCE should be performed to determine the safe physical performance limits for the patient.[68] The FCE results are then matched with the job description. Recommendations for return to work are based on this evaluation. Changes in the job that would enable the patient to return to work may be suggested. If possible, a workplace analysis also should be performed to help identify risks to the patient and to suggest changes in the work environment to accommodate the patient. Three major classes of risk factors can be identified—the force exerted on the job, positioning of the arms and trunk, and time elements of the job (frequency and duration of activities).

For return to work, a less demanding type of job, gradual increase in the hours worked per day, or both is usually recommended. One review[69] has shown that there is moderate evidence suggesting that back schools, in an occupational setting, reduce pain and improve function and return to work status in the short and intermediate term. Back schools were compared with exercise, manipulation, myofascial therapy, advice, placebo, or waiting list controls for patients with chronic and recurrent LBP. Future trials should improve methodologic quality and clinical relevance and evaluate the cost-effectiveness of back schools.

Some therapists offer a work-hardening program, in which a pain patient gradually works up to a simulated 8-hour work day. After discharge from these programs, full time return to work is appropriate.

Monitoring of Outcome (Achievement of Patient Goals)

Generic and disease specific measurement tools have been developed; many of these are discussed in Chapter 68. The treatment goals established with patients before therapy is initiated can serve as outcome measures to determine treatment efficacy and a simple Visual Analogue Scale (VAS) can visualize progress. For example, the patient can be asked the following question:

In the past week, were you able to walk a mile?

COMPLETELY UNABLE *COMPLETELY ABLE*

Because outcome is measured on individualized treatment goals, this type of measurement is most likely to be more sensitive to change than a tool that measures items that are not of interest to the patient. Goal attainment scaling, a technique to objectify and evaluate the achievement of patient-specific goals for treatment, can be used to evaluate treatment outcome in clinical practice and research.[70] A generic tool used in conjunction with the VAS to facilitate comparison with other patients is recommended.

Monitoring of Adherence to Treatment

Adherence is significantly related to treatment outcome levels, such as pain levels and functional abilities. As early as 1991, Turk and Rudy[66] reported that nonadherence to therapeutic recommendations during treatment and subsequent to treatment termination are neglected topics in regard to the treatment of patients with chronic pain. Almost 2 decades later, the topic remains underinvestigated.

The IMMPACT statement might change this. The Initiative on Methods, Measurement and Pain Assessment in Clinical Trials (IMMPACT)[71] statement recommends core outcome domains of the efficacy and effectiveness of treatments for chronic pain that should be considered by investigators conducting clinical trials. One of the core domains includes participant disposition (e.g., adherence to the treatment regimen and reasons for premature withdrawal from the trial). Adherence to pain management treatment recommendations and the number of "no shows" should be monitored in clinical practice as well.

Physical therapists need to offer an appropriate behavioral framework by maintaining a clear structure, consistent rules, and rewards for positive patient response during treatment. When a patient is persistently nonadherent, this should be addressed and the reasons for nonadherence explored. These can

include poor satisfaction with treatment results or a patient-provider relationship that does not work well.

Planned Follow-up

There is a paucity of literature on planned follow-up after multidisciplinary treatment. Planned follow-up can be done on an individual basis or in group settings and serves to prevent the implementation of crisis management strategies. It can also serve as an external motivator ("they are going to know I did not do my exercise"; self-management techniques). To date, there is no evidence about the optimal frequency or duration of follow-up visits.

CONCLUSION

Generally, the evaluation and treatment of chronic pain patients is a difficult task that is best performed in an interdisciplinary team setting, because both biomedical and psychosocial aspects related to the pain problem must be addressed. The role of the physical therapist is to form a close partnership with patients, help patients set and attain individual goals at activity and participation levels, and teach patients self-management skills. Ultimately, patients should become experts on managing their own chronic pain so that they can enjoy the best health-related quality of life possible.

SUMMARY

- Multidisciplinary care of patients with chronic pain has proven to be of significant value.
- A collaborative relationship between patient and therapist is essential.
- The pain management treatment plan must be tailored to the individual patient.
- Treatment goals, education, exercise, and behavioral techniques are at the core of physical therapy pain management.
- Active involvement of patients and treatment compliance are necessary.

References

1. Petrie KJ, Frampton T, Large RG, et al: What do patients expect from their first visit to a pain clinic? Clin J Pain 2005;21:297-301.
2. Wittink HM, Dodds A: Physical rehabilitation for patients with chronic pain. In Lipman A (ed): Pain Management for Primary Care Clinicians. Bethesda, Md, American Society of Health System Pharmacists, 2004, pp 107-122.
3. Haynes RB, Devereaux PJ, Guyatt GH: Physicians' and patients' choices in evidence-based practice. BMJ 2002;324:1350.
4. Fordyce WE: Operant conditioning: An approach to chronic pain. In Jacox A (ed): Pain Source Book for Nurses and Other Health Professionals. Boston, Little Brown, 1977, pp 275-284.
5. Ustun TB, Chatterji S, Bickenbach J, et al: The International Classification of Functioning, Disability and Health: A new tool for understanding disability and health. Disabil Rehabil 2003;25:565-571.

6. Stucki G, Cieza A, Ewert T, et al: Application of the International Classification of Functioning, Disability and Health (ICF) in clinical practice. Disabil Rehabil 2002;24:281-282.

7. Steiner WA, Ryser L, Huber E, et al: Use of the ICF model as a clinical problem-solving tool in physical therapy and rehabilitation medicine. Phys Ther 2002;82:1098-1107.

8. Fordyce WE, Lansky D, Calsyn DA, et al: Pain measurement and pain behavior. Pain 1984;18:53-69.

9. Schmidt AJ: Performance level of chronic low back pain patients in different treadmill test conditions. J Psychosom Res 1985;29:639-645.

10. Verbunt JA, Westerterp KR, van der Heijden GJ, et al: Physical activity in daily life in patients with chronic low back pain. Arch Phys Med Rehabil 2001;82:726-730.

11. Patrick DL, Chiang YP: Measurement of health outcomes in treatment effectiveness evaluations: Conceptual and methodological challenges. Med Care 2000;38:II14-II25.

12. Grevitt M, Pande K, O'Dowd J, et al: Do first impressions count? A comparison of subjective and psychologic assessment of spinal patients. Eur Spine J 1998;7:218-223.

13. Vlaeyen JW, Kole-Snijders AM, Boeren RG, et al: Fear of movement/(re)injury in chronic low back pain and its relation to behavioral performance. Pain 1995;62:363-372.

14. Sullivan MJL, Bishop SR, Pivik J: The Pain Catastrophizing scale: Development and validation. Psychol Assess 1995; 524-532.

15. Beck AT, Ward CH, Mendelson M, et al: An inventory for measuring depression. Arch Gen Psychiatry 1961;4:561-571.

16. Hall JA, Roter DL, Katz NR: Meta-analysis of correlates of provider behavior in medical encounters. Med Care 1988;26: 657-675.

17. Becker MH: Patient adherence to prescribed therapies. Med Care 1985;23:539-555.

18. Kaplan SH, Greenfield S, Ware JE: Assessing the effects of physician-patient interactions on the outcomes of chronic disease. Med Care 1989;7(Suppl):S110-S127.

19. Kalauokalani D, Cherkin DC, Sherman KJ, et al: Lessons from a trial of acupuncture and massage for low back pain: Patient expectations and treatment effects. Spine 2001;26:1418-1424.

20. Klaber Moffett JA, Jackson DA, Richmond S, et al: Randomised trial of a brief physiotherapy intervention compared with usual physiotherapy for neck pain patients: Outcomes and patients' preference. BMJ 2005;330:75.

21. Hadjistavropoulos HD, LaChapelle DL: Extent and nature of anxiety experienced during physical examination of chronic low back pain. Behav Res Ther 2000;38:13-29.

22. Waddell G: The Back Pain Revolution. Edinburgh, Churchill Livingstone, 1998.

23. Magnussen L, Strand LI, Lygren H: Reliability and validity of the Back Performance Scale: Observing activity limitation in patients with back pain. Spine 2004;29:903-907.

24. Strand LI, Moe-Nilssen R, Ljunggren AE: Back Performance Scale for the assessment of mobility-related activities in people with back pain. Phys Ther 2002;82:1213-1223.

25. Simmonds MJ, Olson SL, Jones S, et al: Psychometric characteristics and clinical usefulness of physical performance tests in patients with low back pain. Spine 1998;23:2412-2421.

26. Wittink HM: Physical fitness, function and physical therapy in patients with pain: Clinical measures of aerobic fitness and performance in patients with chronic low back pain. In Max M (ed): Pain 1999—An Updated Review. Refresher Course Syllabus. Seattle, IASP Press, 1999, pp 137-145.

27. Reneman MF, Brouwer S, Meinema A, et al: Test-retest reliability of the Isernhagen Work Systems Functional Capacity Evaluation in healthy adults. J Occup Rehabil 2004;14: 295-305.

28. King PM, Tuckwell N, Barrett TE: A critical review of functinal capacity evaluations. Phys Ther 1998;78:852-866.

29. Wittink H, Rogers W, Sukiennik A, et al: Physical functioning: Self-report and performance measures are related but distinct. Spine 2003;28:2407-2413.

30. Brouwer S, Dijkstra PU, Stewart RE, et al: Comparing self-report, clinical examination and functional testing in the assessment of work-related limitations in patients with chronic low back pain. Disabil Rehabil 2005;27:999-1005.

31. Van Heuvelen MJ, Kempen GI, Brouwer WH, et al: Physical fitness related to disability in older persons. Gerontology 2000;46:333-341.

32. Verbeek J, Sengers MJ, Riemens L, et al: Patient expectations of treatment for back pain: A systematic review of qualitative and quantitative studies. Spine 2004;29:2309-2318.

33. Von Korff M, Glasgow RE, Sharpe M: Organising care for chronic illness. BMJ 2002;325:92-94.

34. Dijkstra A: The validity of the stages of change model in the adoption of the self-management approach in chronic pain. Clin J Pain 2005;21:27-37.

35. Jensen GM, Gwyer J, Shepard KF: Expert practice in physical therapy. Phys Ther 2000;80:28-43.

36. Houben RM, Ostelo RW, Vlaeyen JW, et al: Health care providers' orientations towards common low back pain predict perceived harmfulness of physical activities and recommendations regarding return to normal activity. Eur J Pain 2005;9: 173-183.

37. Linton SJ, Vlaeyen J, Ostelo R: The back pain beliefs of health care providers: Are we fear-avoidant? J Occup Rehabil 2002; 12:223-232.

38. Bandura A: Self-efficacy in Changing Societies. New York, Cambridge University Press, 1995.

39. Catchlove R, Cohen K: Effects of a directive return to work approach in the treatment of workman's compensation patients with chronic pain. Pain 1982;14:181-191.

40. Moseley L: Unraveling the barriers to reconceptualization of the problem in chronic pain: The actual and perceived ability of patients and health professionals to understand the neurophysiology. J Pain 2003;4:184-189.

41. Schonstein E, Kenny DT, Keating J, et al: Work conditioning, work hardening and functional restoration for workers with back and neck pain. Cochrane Database Syst Rev 2003;(1): CD001822.

42. Mayer TG, Gatchel RJ, Kishino N, et al: Objective assessment of spine function following industrial injury. A prospective study with comparison group and one-year follow-up. Spine 1985;10:482-493.

43. Mayer TG, Gatchel RJ, Kishino N, et al: A prospective short-term study of chronic low back pain patients utilizing novel objective functional measurement. Pain 1986;25:53-68.

44. Verbunt JA, Seelen HA, Vlaeyen JW, et al: Fear of injury and physical deconditioning in patients with chronic low back pain. Arch Phys Med Rehabil 2003;84:1227-1232.

45. Brosseau L, MacLeay L, Robinson V, et al: Intensity of exercise for the treatment of osteoarthritis. Cochrane Database Syst Rev 2003;(2):CD004259.

46. Fransen M, McConnell S, Bell M: Exercise for osteoarthritis of the hip or knee. Cochrane Database Syst Rev 2003;(3): CD004286.

47. Roddy E, Zhang W, Doherty M: Aerobic walking or strengthening exercise for osteoarthritis of the knee? A systematic review. Ann Rheum Dis 2005;64:544-548.

48. Hakkinen A, Sokka T, Kotaniemi A, et al: A randomized two-year study of the effects of dynamic strength training on muscle strength, disease activity, functional capacity, and bone mineral density in early rheumatoid arthritis. Arthritis Rheum 2001;44:515-522.

49. Hakkinen A, Sokka T, Kautiainen H, et al: Sustained maintenance of exercise-induced muscle strength gains and normal bone mineral density in patients with early rheumatoid arthritis: A 5-year follow up. Ann Rheum Dis 2004;63:910-916.

50. Busch A, Schachter CL, Peloso PM, et al: Exercise for treating fibromyalgia syndrome. Cochrane Database Syst Rev 2002;(3): CD003786.

51. Green S, Buchbinder R, Hetrick S: Physiotherapy interventions for shoulder pain. Cochrane Database Syst Rev 2003;(2): CD004258.

52. Van Tulder MW, Malmivaara A, Esmail R, et al: Exercise therapy for low back pain. Cochrane Database System Rev 2000;(2):CD000335.

53. Hayden JA, van Tulder MW, Malmivaara AV, et al: Meta-analysis: Exercise therapy for nonspecific low back pain. Ann Intern Med 2005;142:765-775.

54. Hayden JA, van Tulder MW, Tomlinson G: Systematic review: Strategies for using exercise therapy to improve outcomes in chronic low back pain. Ann Intern Med 2005;142:776-785.

55. van Tulder MW, Koes BW, Assendelft WJ, et al: [Chronic low back pain: Exercise therapy, multidisciplinary programs, NSAIDs, back schools and behavioral therapy effective; traction not effective; results of systematic reviews]. Ned Tijdschr Geneeskd 2000;144:1489-1494.

56. Guzman JE: Multidisciplinary bio-psycho-social rehabilitation for chronic low back pain. Cochrane Database Syst Rev 2002;(1):CD000963.

57. Haldorsen EM, Grasdal AL, Skouen JS, et al: Is there a right treatment for a particular patient group? Comparison of ordinary treatment, light multidisciplinary treatment, and extensive multidisciplinary treatment for long-term sick-listed employees with musculoskeletal pain. Pain 2002;95:49-63.

58. Assendelft WJ, Morton SC, Yu EI, et al: Spinal manipulative therapy for low back pain. A meta-analysis of effectiveness relative to other therapies. Ann Intern Med 2003;138: 871-881.

59. Furlan AD, Brosseau L, Imamura M, et al: Massage for low-back pain: A systematic review within the framework of the Cochrane Collaboration Back Review Group. Spine 2002;27: 1896-1910.

60. Vlaeyen JW, Linton SJ: Fear-avoidance and its consequences in chronic musculoskeletal pain: A state of the art. Pain 2000;85:317-332.

61. Fordyce WE, Fowler RS, Lehmann JF, et al: Operant conditioning in the treatment of chronic pain. Arch Phys Med Rehabil 1973;54:399-408.

62. Boersma K, Linton S, Overmeer T, et al: Lowering fear-avoidance and enhancing function through exposure in vivo.

A multiple baseline study across six patients with back pain. Pain 2004;108:8-16.

63. George SZ, Fritz JM, Bialosky JE, et al: The effect of a fear-avoidance-based physical therapy intervention for patients with acute low back pain: Results of a randomized clinical trial. Spine 2003;28:2551-2560.

64. Smeets RJ, Vlaeyen JW, Hidding A, et al: Active rehabilitation for chronic low back pain: Cognitive-behavioral, physical, or both? First direct post-treatment results from a randomized controlled trial [ISRCTN22714229]. BMC Musculoskelet Disord 2006;7:5.

65. Lorig K, Ritter PL, Plant K: A disease-specific self-help program compared with a generalized chronic disease self-help program for arthritis patients. Arthritis Rheum 2005;53:950-7.

66. Turk DC, Rudy TE: Neglected topics in the treatment of chronic pain patients—relapse, noncompliance, and adherence enhancement. Pain 1991;44:5-28.

67. Harding V, Simmonds MJ, Watson P: Physical therapy for chronic pain. Pain: Clinical Updates 1998;6:1-2.

68. Reneman M, Wittink H: Functional performance testing. In Nordin M, Andersson G, Pope M (eds): Musculoskeletal Disorders in the Workplace: Principles and Practice, 2nd ed. St. Louise, Mosby, 2006, pp 397-408.

69. Heymans MW, van Tulder MW, Esmail R, et al: Back schools for nonspecific low back pain: A systematic review within the framework of the Cochrane Collaboration Back Review Group. Spine 2005;30:2153-2163.

70. Fisher K, Hardie RJ: Goal attainment scaling in evaluating a multidisciplinary pain management programme. Clin Rehabil 2002;16:871-877.

71. Turk DC, Dworkin RH, Burke LB, et al: Initiative on Methods, Measurement, and Pain Assessment in Clinical Trials: Developing patient-reported outcome measures for pain clinical trials: IMMPACT recommendations. Pain 2006;125:208-215.

CHAPTER
42 Acupuncture

Yuan-Chi Lin

Acupuncture, a modality of traditional Chinese medicine, is a therapy that involves the inserting of special needles into the skin at specific points, known as acupuncture points, to achieve the desired response. The *Huang Di Nei Jing (Yellow Emperor's Internal Classic)*, 100 BC, described the practice of acupuncture. Called *jin jiao*, acupuncture generally consists of the practices of needling and moxibustion. Moxibustion is a warming sensation produced by moxa (*Artemisia vulgaris*) over the acupuncture points. The practice of acupuncture also includes electroacupuncture, laser acupuncture, cupping, Chinese tui na massage, acupressure, and so on.

One of the essential theories of traditional Chinese medicine is the concept of yin and yang. The principle of yin and yang is simple, but its implication is philosophical. It was first mentioned in *The Book of Changes and Simplicity (Yi Jing)*, from about 700 BC. Yin and yang are interdependent, can be transformed into each other, and are natural phenomena that exist within the body. They are present in a constant state of dynamic balance. Yang is related to bright, hot, activity, light, outward, increase, dry, and male. Yin is present in the qualities of dark, cold, rest, passivity, inward, decrease, wet, and female. Optimal physical condition requires a balance of yin and yang within the body; disease is associated with a disharmony or imbalance between yin and yang. Acupuncture can be used to balance and promote yin and yang energy within the body.

There are more than 365 identifiable acupuncture points in the human body. There are also pathways, called meridians, connecting acupuncture points to each other. Qi (pronounced "chee") is the energy flow through these meridians. Difficult to define, qi represents power and movement, and is similar to energy. Qi is a functional, dynamic force that resides in living creatures, is the result of the interaction between heaven and earth, and is an energy that manifests concurrently on the physical and spiritual levels of humans.

Qi flows throughout the meridians of the body, maintaining our life and health. These meridians are not defined by physical structures such as blood or lymphatic vessels, but by their function. The body is viewed as a dynamic system of organs connected by the flow of qi within the meridians.

When there is stagnation or inadequate flow of qi through the meridians, pain or illness may result.

The flow of qi may be restored by the insertion of the very fine needles into a combination of appropriate acupuncture points along the meridians. The manual twirling of these needles produces a sore, heavy, or numb sensation known as "de qi" (obtaining qi). Acupuncture practitioners have observed that stimulating specific acupuncture points results in predictable responses in patients, with a given pattern of signs and symptoms. Practitioners of acupuncture routinely request the patient's detailed history and present illness in pursuing the diagnosis. Physical attention is also focused on the disposition of the pulse and appearance of the tongue. In traditional Chinese medicine, there are six pathologic factors that cause disease—wind, cold, heat, dampness, dryness, and fire. The goal of the history and physical examination is to assess the patient's balance of yin and yang, and to gain insight into other symptoms.

There are eight principal classifications of symptoms, which include yin or yang, external or internal, cold or hot, and deficient or excess. The aim of acupuncture therapy is to restore deficiencies or correct excesses in qi, thus restoring health. It is frequently used for preventive care, as well as for therapeutic purposes.

A Treatise on Acupuncturation, written by James Morss Churchill in 1823, was the first text about acupuncture published in English. Dr. Churchill described his success using acupuncture for rheumatic conditions, sciatica, and back pain. Sir William Osler's *Principles and Practice of Medicine*, first published in 1892, recommended the use of acupuncture for the treatment of sciatica and lumbago. Public awareness and use of acupuncture increased in the United States following *New York Times* writer James Reston's account of his emergency appendectomy in a Chinese hospital; his article described how physicians eased his postsurgical abdominal pain with acupuncture.[1]

BASIC RESEARCH

There are numerous reports confirming that acupuncture has reproducible neurobiologic effects. Acupuncture inhibits the transmission of pain according to the gate control theory put forth by Wall and Melzack in 1965.[2] Acupuncture may act by stimulating sensory A-beta fibers, directly inhibiting the spinal transmission of pain by smaller A-delta and C fibers.[3]

Researchers have also been paying attention to the relationship between acupuncture and the production of endogenous opioid peptides, such as the endorphins and enkephalins, and the stimulation of the endogenous descending inhibitory pathways. In an analysis of human cerebrospinal fluid, Sjolund and colleagues[4] have determined that endorphin levels in subjects become elevated following electroacupuncture. Acupuncture analgesia is mainly caused by the activation of the endogenous antinociceptive system to modulate pain transmission and pain response.[5]

Electroacupuncture at 2 Hz accelerates the release of enkephalin, β-endorphin, and endomorphin, whereas that of 100 Hz selectively increases the release of dynorphin. A combination of the two frequencies produces a simultaneous release of all four opioid peptides, resulting in a maximal therapeutic effect.[6] Peripheral stimulation of the skin or deeper structures activates various brain structures, spinal cord, or a combination via specific neural pathways.[7] A human study by Mayer and associates[8] indicated that acupuncture analgesia can be reversed by naloxone.

Several serotonin antagonists inhibit the effects of electroacupuncture. Electroacupuncture attenuates behavioral hyperalgesia and stress-induced colonic motor dysfunction in rats.[9] Electroacupuncture also attenuates behavioral hyperalgesia and stress-induced colonic motor dysfunction in rats via serotonergic pathways.

Neuronal correlation to acupuncture stimulation in the human brain has been investigated by functional magnetic resonance imaging (fMRI). Acupuncture needle manipulation on the LI 4 (he gu) point modulates the fMRI activity of the limbic system and subcortical structure.[10] Acupuncture stimulation at analgesic points involving the pain-related neuromatrix have been studied. Acupuncture stimulation at the GB 34 (yang ling quan) acupuncture point has elicited significantly higher activation than sham acupuncture over the hypothalamus and primary somatosensory motor cortex and deactivation over the rostral segment of the anterior cingulated cortex.[11]

SIDE EFFECTS

The use of disposable sterile acupuncture needles avoids the risk of cross-contamination. After the acupuncture, occasionally, a patient may have some bruising at an acupuncture site. Mild transient drowsiness may occur. Pneumothorax is the most frequently reported serious complication related to acupuncture.[12,13] In a study of cases of 78 acupuncturists, involving 31,822 acupuncture treatments in the United Kingdom, the most common adverse events reported were bleeding (310/10,000 consultations) and needling pain (110/10,000 consultations).[14] The York acupuncture safety study surveyed 34,000 treatments by traditional acupuncturists. Aggravation of symptoms occurred in 96 cases/10,000 consultations. There was a subsequent improvement in the presenting complaint in 70% of these cases.[15] None of these events were serious; major adverse consequences of acupuncture seem to be extremely rare.[16] Acupuncture as a method of treatment can be considered to be safe in the hands of a competent and experienced acupuncturist.[17]

CLINICAL USE OF ACUPUNCTURE

Acupuncture as a therapeutic intervention is currently a widely practiced discipline in the United States. In 1997, the National Institutes of Health[18] concluded that there are promising results supporting the efficacy of acupuncture for adult postoperative and chemotherapy-related nausea and vomiting and for postoperative dental pain. There are reasonable studies that conclude that the use of acupuncture results in satisfactory treatment for addiction, stroke rehabilitation, headache, menstrual cramps, tennis elbow, fibromyalgia, myofascial pain, osteoarthritis, low back pain, carpal tunnel syndrome, and asthma. Depending on the situation, acupuncture may be used as an adjunct treatment, acceptable alternative therapy, or integrated into a comprehensive management program.

Clinical research into the use of acupuncture for the treatment of pain has consisted primarily of uncontrolled trials. Although beneficial results have frequently been demonstrated, the flawed design of many of the studies places limited value on the outcomes. Systematic reviews of randomized controlled trials (RCTs) have provided the best evidence and the least bias in assessing the efficacy of any medical intervention. Several difficulties are inherent in the design of valid blinded RCTs of acupuncture.[19,20] An appropriate placebo for the acupuncture control group is difficult to determine. Various studies have used the placement of needles placed at nonmeridian sites, called "sham" acupuncture, to model acupuncture in control group patients.

Thirty percent of study subjects may respond positively to placebos. There are very few criteria in the current literature for the use of placebo in acupuncture research. Sham acupuncture is frequently used as the control treatment in research trials involving acupuncture; however, it presents a unique problem as a placebo. The well-outlined energy channels of the acupuncture meridian systems cover the entire body, linking wei-qi (defense qi), rong-qi (growth and development qi), and yuan-qi (the original qi inherited at birth). As the meridian systems affect the entire body, the sham acupuncture does still provide some acupuncture effect, and therefore cannot be considered to produce a true placebo effect. To attempt to address this problem, a placebo acupuncture needle has been developed, which retracts back into the handle of the acupuncture needle and does not penetrate the skin.[21]

Richardson and Vincent[22] have reviewed 27 controlled studies of acupuncture for the treatment of acute and chronic pain, as well as several large uncontrolled studies. In 50% to 80% of the patients studied, they noted that it was difficult to assess the long-term effectiveness of acupuncture, based on the collected data. In a meta-analysis of 14 RCTs of acupuncture for chronic pain in adults, Patel and coworkers[23] found that although few of the individual trials demonstrated statistically significant benefit from acupuncture, the pooled results for several subgroups did, in fact, attain statistical significance in favor of acupuncture.

Postoperative Pain

Acupuncture may be more useful in predictable situations involving acute pain, such as dental procedures and postoperative pain, or in the setting of medical conditions with recurrent episodes of acute pain, such as sickle cell crisis and recurrent abdominal pain. Although effective treatment is available in many cases (e.g., local anesthetics for dental procedures, opioids for severe postoperative pain), side effects such as respiratory depression may be seen. Taub and colleagues[24] used acupuncture for the treatment of dental pain in a single blinded, RCT in 39 adult patients undergoing dental restoration for cavities. Patients were randomized between real and sham acupuncture groups. Seventy percent of the experimental group reported good or excellent pain reduction, whereas 53% of the control group reported good or excellent pain reduction. The results for the two groups showed no statistical significance.

Systematic review has shown that acupuncture is effective in relieving dental pain.[25] Also, a study of the effect of acupuncture for pain after lower abdominal surgery revealed that preoperative treatment with low- or high-frequency electroacupuncture reduced the postoperative analgesic requirement and decreased the side effects of systemic opioids.[26]

Acupuncture has been shown to reduce postoperative opioid dose requirements in patients and to decrease their discomfort. In a randomized, controlled, double-blind study of patients scheduled for elective upper and lower abdominal surgery, acupuncture was found to reduce postoperative pain. Consumption of supplemental intravenous morphine was reduced 50%, and the incidence of postoperative nausea was reduced 20% to 30%. Plasma cortisol and epinephrine concentrations were reduced 30% to 50% in the acupuncture group.[27] In an RCT of electroacupuncture in 100 women undergoing lower abdominal surgery, the incidence of nausea and dizziness during the first 24 hours after surgery was significantly reduced in the electroacupuncture group compared with the control and sham groups. Preoperative treatment with low and high levels of electroacupuncture reduced postoperative analgesic requirements and associated side effects.[28] A study of electroacupuncture in the management of early postthoracotomy pain revealed that electroacupuncture may reduce narcotic analgesic usage in the early postoperative period.[29]

Nausea and Vomiting

Acupuncture using acupuncture needles, electrical apparatus, pressure, or magnets is commonly used for the management of nausea and vomiting caused by surgery or chemotherapy. Stimulation of the PC 6 (Nei guan) acupuncture point is also used to treat nausea and vomiting caused by sea sickness or pregnancy or to treat side effects of surgery or chemotherapy. A systematic review revealed beneficial results in 27 out of 33 RCTs of acupuncture, acupressure, or both, on the treatment of nausea and vomiting.[30] An RCT of pediatric patients that underwent tonsillectomy using electroacupuncture showed a significant reduction in the occurrence of nausea when compared with the sham and control groups. This study demonstrated that the efficacy of acupuncture for postoperative nausea and vomiting prevention is similar to commonly used pharmacotherapies.[31] Acupuncture is as effective as droperidol in controlling early postoperative nausea and vomiting in children.[32] A double-blind, randomized, placebo-controlled study revealed that hand acupressure is an effective method for reducing postoperative vomiting in children after strabismus repair.[33] However, in RCTs conducted by Yentis and colleagues[34] and Lewis and associates,[35] acupuncture and acupressure were found to be ineffective in preventing nausea and vomiting associated with strabismus repair.

PC 6 acupuncture point stimulation can be superior to antiemetic medication for nausea and vomiting. These results have been the most consistent in its use for postoperative nausea and vomiting. In 26 trials studying the care of more than 3000 patients, stimulation of the PC 6 acupuncture point was superior to sham acupuncture for the treatment of nausea and vomiting in both adults and children.[36]

Low Back Pain

In a meta-analysis of 12 RCTs, acupuncture was found to be superior to various control interventions for the management of low back pain.[37] An RCT of acupuncture versus transcutaneous electrical nerve stimulation for chronic low back pain in the elderly revealed that both are equally effective, with acupuncture improving spinal flexion.[38] An RCT of 50 patients with low back pain showed a significant decrease in pain intensity at 1 and 3 months in the acupuncture groups as compared with the placebo group. The acupuncture treatment significantly shortened the time the patients were out of work, improved their quality of sleep, and decreased analgesic intake.[39]

An RCT has revealed significant improvement from traditional acupuncture in chronic low back pain over physiotherapy, but not over sham acupuncture. The benefits included decreased pain intensity, pain disability, and psychological distress at the end of 12 weeks of treatment. At the 9-month follow-up, the superiority of acupuncture over the control group had lessened.[40] An RCT of 298 patients with low back pain revealed that acupuncture was more effective in improving pain than no acupuncture treatment, but there were no significant differences between acupuncture and minimal acupuncture.[41] An RCT of 241 patients with low back pain revealed that a short course of treatment by a qualified traditional acupuncturist is a safe and acceptable method of pain management.[42] Additionally, acupuncture care for low back pain is a cost-effective therapy in the long term.[43]

Headache

Several studies have shown the efficacy of acupuncture therapy for migraine headache.[44,45] In an RCT of 168 women with migraine, acupuncture was shown to be adequate for migraine prophylaxis. Relative to flunarizine, acupuncture treatment exhibited greater effectiveness in the first months of therapy and superior tolerability.[46] A prospective, randomized double-blind study has shown the efficacy of acupuncture for migraine prophylaxis. The reduction of migraine days in patients receiving acupuncture treatment were statistically significant compared with baseline. The treatment outcomes for migraine do not differ between patients treated with acupuncture or standard therapy.[47] A systematic review of 22 trials, involving a total of 1042 patients, concluded that acupuncture has a role in the treatment of recurrent headaches.[48] Acupuncture and sumatriptan were more effective than placebo injection for the early treatment of an acute migraine attack. When an attack could not be prevented, sumatriptan was more effective than acupuncture at relieving headache.[49] Supplementing medical management with acupuncture can result in improvements in health-related quality of life and the perception by patients that they suffer less from their headaches.[50]

Temporomandibular Joint Dysfunction

Three RCTs of acupuncture treatment of 205 patients with temporomandibular joint dysfunction had positive results. Acupuncture appears to be an effective treatment for painful dysfunction of the temporomandibular joint, but the results still require confirmation from more rigorous methods of trials.[51,52]

Neck Pain

Several clinical reports have suggested that acupuncture can be useful for the treatment of patients with neck pain. However, 14 RCTs involving 724 subjects with various causes of neck pain did not provide significant evidence in support of acupuncture for the treatment of neck pain.[53] There have been too few studies for chronic neck pain of sufficient quality and homogeneity to be able to draw conclusions about the effectiveness of the treatment. A scoring system to gauge the effects of acupuncture on neck pain has been proposed, but there are problems with its usage.[54] An RCT of 177 patients with chronic neck pain were randomly assigned treatment over a period of 3 weeks of acupuncture (56 patients), massage (60 patients), or "sham" laser acupuncture (61 patients). The patients received five treatments of acupuncture during this three-week period, and the acupuncture was found to be an effective short-term treatment.[55] Acupuncture was an effective short-term treatment for patients. An RCT of acupuncture for 123 patients with chronic neck pain, with 6 months of follow up, revealed that acupuncture is more effective than placebo treatment. The acupuncture treatment improved the patient's quality of life from a physical aspect, improved active neck mobility, and reduced the need for rescue medication.[56] There is some evidence that acupuncture relieves neck pain better than sham treatment or no treatment.[57]

Myofascial Pain Syndrome

Acupuncture may be useful for the treatment of chronic myofascial pain. In an uncontrolled study, Lewit reported immediate relief in 87% of cases and long-term benefit in at least 92 of 288 cases.[58] Melzack and colleagues reported a 71% correlation between acupuncture points and trigger points used for the treatment of myofascial pain.[59]

Knee Pain and Osteoarthritis

Knee pain and osteoarthritis is a common joint disorder, especially among women, more than 50 years of age. In a randomized controlled trial of 570 patients with osteoarthritis of the knee, acupuncture seems to provide improvement in function and pain relief as an adjunctive therapy for osteoarthritis of the knee when compared with sham acupuncture and education control groups.[60] Another study of 1007 patients with osteoarthritis of the knee compared conservative physiotherapy and as-needed anti-inflammatory drugs with added acupuncture treatment. The addition of either acupuncture or sham acupuncture led to greater improvement of pain and function at 26 weeks.[61] A systematic review and meta-analysis of randomized controlled trials of acupuncture for knee pain revealed acupuncture was superior to sham acupuncture for both pain and function. The differences were still significant at long-term follow-up.[62]

Carpal Tunnel Syndrome

Carpal tunnel syndrome is a common entrapment neuropathy of the median nerve. Eleven mild to moderate carpal tunnel syndrome patients were randomized into groups receiving real or sham laser acupuncture treatment. Significant decreases in the McGill Pain Questionnaire score, median nerve sensory latency, and Phalen's and Tinel's signs after the actual laser acupuncture treatment series were observed, but not in the placebo group.[62] A study of fMRI in patients with carpal tunnel syndrome revealed that hyperactivity in contralateral sensorimotor cortex diminishes after acupuncture treatment.[63]

Neuropathic Pain

The efficacy of acupuncture in patients with peripheral neuropathy is unclear. Peripheral neuropathy is common in patients infected with human immunodeficiency virus (HIV). Neither acupuncture nor amitriptyline was found to be more effective than placebo in relieving pain caused by HIV-related peripheral neuropathy.[64] Reports are available on the benefits of traditional acupuncture therapy and auricular therapy in treating complex regional pain syndrome, formerly known as reflex sympathetic dystrophy (RSD).[65,66] However, each of these reports involved only one to five patients in uncontrolled studies.

REFERRING PATIENTS FOR ACUPUNCTURE TREATMENT

Differentiating between disease and illness is important. A disease is what the physician diagnoses, whereas an illness is what the patient feels or suffers. There are many diseases for which there is no cure, but acupuncture can be used as a complementary medicine for the associated illnesses or for the side effects related to conventional medical therapies.

Licensing guidelines for the practice of acupuncture are determined by each state. The National Commission for the Certification of Acupuncturists has developed standards for training and for certification of licensed acupuncturists, and the American Board of Medical Acupuncture has established the guidelines and qualification requirements for physicians to practice medical acupuncture.

Over the past several years, the use of traditional Chinese medicine has become more common and accepted in the United States. Some health maintenance organization (HMO) insurance plans have begun to cover acupuncture treatments for their patients. Some workmen's compensation boards and personal injury insurance policies will also cover acupuncture. If there is an increase in the number of insurers willing to reimburse acupuncture therapy, patients will be more likely to seek acupuncture treatment in the future.[67]

How can we best advise patients with pain-related disorders who are interested in acupuncture? The pain service practitioner should discuss with the patients what their treatment preferences and outcome expectations are. It is essential to review with patients the safety and efficacy of acupuncture therapy thoroughly. Patients should be referred to qualified acupuncture providers, and follow-up appointments should also be scheduled to monitor the treatment response.

Acupuncture is steadily becoming an integral part of the health care delivery system. Research on acupuncture has allowed for its integration into conventional Western medical practice. More prospective, randomized, and controlled studies on acupuncture are needed to better understand its mechanisms, efficacy, and side effects.

ACUPUNCTURE POINTS

Acupuncture points are generally found in the deep depressions of the muscles, joints, or bones and are often sensitive to pressure. When determining the locations of acupuncture points on the body, a unit of measurement called a *cun* is used to pinpoint the locations. The measurement of a cun is relative to the patient's own body. One cun (about 1 inch) is equal to the space between the distal interphalangeal joint and the proximal interphalangeal joint on the middle finger.

- CV 12 (zhong guan; "central venter")—located in the midline, 4 cun above the umbilicus.
- LR 13 (zhang men; "camphor wood gate")—located on the lateral side of the abdomen, below the free end of the 11th rib, 2 cun above the navel and 6 cun on either side of the midline.
- GB 34 (yang ling quan; "young mound spring")—located in the deep depression 1 cun anterior and 1 cun inferior to the head of the fibula.
- GB 39 (xuan zhong or jue gu; "suspended bell or severed bone")—located 3 cun directly above the tip of lateral malleolus, in the depression between the posterior border of the fibula and the tendons of the peroneus longus and brevis.
- BL 17 (ge shu; "diaphragm shu")—located 1.5 cun lateral to the lower border of the spinous process of the seventh vertebrae.
- BL 11 (da zhu; "great shuttle")—located 1.5 cun lateral to the lower border of the spinous process of the first thoracic vertebra.
- LU 9 (tai yuan; "great abyss")—located at the transverse crease of the wrist, in the depression of the lateral side of the radial artery.
- CV 17 (tan chung; "chest center")—located in the midline of the sternum, between the nipples, at the level of the fourth intercostal space.
- LI 4 (he gu; "union valley")—located between the first and second metacarpal bones in the deep depression of the web space.
- PC 6 (nei guan; "internal gate")—located 2 to 3 cun above the transverse crease of the wrist, a deep depression between the tendons of the long palmar muscle and the radial flexor muscle of the wrist.
- ST 36 (zu san li; "leg three miles")—located 3 cun below the patella and 1 cun lateral to the crest of the tibia.
- SP 6 (san yin jiao; "three yin intersection")—located 3 cun above the tip of the medial malleolus, on the posterior border of the tibia.

References

1. Reston J: Now, let me tell you about my appendectomy in Peking. New York Times July 26, 1971.
2. Melzack R, Wall P: Pain mechanism: A new theory. Science 1965;150:971-979.

3. Lewith G, Kenyon, JN: Physiological and psychological explanations for the mechanism of acupuncture as a treatment for chronic pain. Soc Sci Med. 1984;19:1367-1378.

4. Sjolund B, Terenius L, Eriksson M: Increased cerebrospinal fluid levels of endorphins after electro-acupuncture. Acta Physiol Scand 1977;100:382-384.

5. He L: Involvement of endogenous opioid peptides in acupuncture alalgesia. Pain 1987;31:99-121.

6. Han JS: Acupuncture and endorphins. Neurosci Lett 2004; 361:258-261.

7. Han JS: Acupuncture: Neuropeptide release produced by electrical stimulation of different frequencies. Trend Neurosci 2003;26:17-22.

8. Mayer DJ, Price DD, Rafii A: Antagonism of acupuncture analgesia in man by the narcotic antagonist naloxone. Brain Res 1977;121:368-372.

9. Yonehara N: Influence of serotonin receptor antagonists on substance P and serotonin release evoked by tooth pulp stimulation with electro-acupuncture in the trigeminal nucleus cudalis of the rabbit. Neurosci Res 2001;40:45-51.

10. Hui K, Liu J, Makris N, et al: Acupuncture modulates the limbic system and subcortical gray structures of the human brain: Evidence from fMRI studies in normal subjects. Hum Brain Mapp 2000;9:13-25.

11. Wu MT, Sheen JM, Chuang KH, et al: Neuronal specificity of acupuncture response: A fMRI study with electroacupuncture. Neuroimage 2002;16:1028-1037.

12. Peuker E: Case report of tension pneumothorax related to acupuncture. Acupunct Med 2004;22:40-43.

13. von Riedenauer WB, Baker MK, Brewer RJ: Video-assisted thorascopic removal of migratory acupuncture needle causing pneumothorax. Chest 2007;131:899-901.

14. White A, Hayhoe S, Hart A, et al: Adverse events following acupuncture: Prospective survey of 32,000 consultations with doctors and physiotherapists. BMJ 2001;323:485-486.

15. MacPherson H, Thomas K, Walters S, et al: The York acupuncture safety study: Prospective survey of 34,000 treatments by traditional acupuncturists. BMJ 2001;323:486-487.

16. Melchart D, Weidenhammer W, Streng A, et al: Prospective investigation of adverse effects of acupuncture in 97,733 patients. Arch Intern Med 2004;164:104-105.

17. Ernst E, White A: Prospective studies of the safety of acupuncture: A systemic review. Am J Med 2001;110:481-485.

18. NIH Consensus Conference: Acupuncture. JAMA 1998;280: 1518-1524.

19. Vincent C, Richardson, PH: The evaluation of therapeutic acupuncture: Concepts and methods. Pain 1986;24:1-13.

20. Lewith G, Machin, D: On the evaluation of the clinical effects of acupuncture. Pain 1983;16:111-127.

21. Streitberger K, Kleinhenz J: Introducing a placebo needle into acupuncture research. Lancet 1998;352:364-365.

22. Richardson P, Vincent C: Acupuncture for treatment of pain. Pain 1986;24:15-40.

23. Patel M GF, Paccaud F, Marazzi A: A meta-analysis of acupuncture for chronic pain. Int J Epidemiol 1989;18:900-906.

24. Taub H, Beard, MC, Eisenberg L, et al: Studies of acupuncture for operative dentistry. J Am Dent Assoc 1977;99: 555-561.

25. Ernst E, Pittler M: The effectiveness of acupuncture in treating acute dental pain. Br Dent J 1998;184:443-447.

26. Barrows K, Jacobs B: Mind-body medicine. Med Clin North Am 2002;86:11-31.

27. Kotani N, Hashimoto H, Sato Y, et al: Preoperative intradermal acupuncture reduces postoperative pain, nausea and vomiting, analgesic requirement, and sympathoadrenal responses. Anesthesiology 2001;95:349-356.

28. Lin JG, Lo MW, Wen YR, et al: The effect of high- and low-frequency electroacupuncture in pain after lower abdominal surgery. Pain 2002;99:509-514.

29. Wong RH, Lee TW, Sihoe AD, et al:. Analgesic effect of electroacupuncture in postthoracotomy pain: A prospective randomized trial. Ann Thorac Surg 2006;81:2031-2036.

30. Vickers A: Can acupuncture have specific effects on health? A systematic review of acupuncture antiemetic trials. J Roy Soc Med 1996;89:303-311.

31. Rusy LM, Hoffman GM, Weisman SJ: Electroacupuncture prophylaxis of postoperative nausea and vomiting following pediatric tonsillectomy with or without adenoidectomy. Anesthesiology 2002;96:300-305.

32. Wang SM, Kain ZN: P6 acupoint injections are as effective as droperidol in controlling early postoperative nausea and vomiting in children. Anesthesiology 2002;97:359-366.

33. Schlager A, Boehler M, Puhringer F: Korean hand acupressure reduces postoperative vomiting in children after strabismus surgery. Br J Anaesth 2000;85:267-270.

34. Yentis SM, Bissonnette B: Ineffectiveness of acupuncture and droperidol in preventing vomiting following strabismus repair in children. Can J Anaesth 1992;39:151-154.

35. Lewis IH, Pryn SJ, Reynolds PI, et al: Effect of P6 acupressure on postoperative vomiting in children undergoing outpatient strabismus correction. Br J Anaesth 1991;67:73-78.

36. Ezzo J, Streitberger K, Schneider A: Cochrane systematic reviews examine P6 acupuncture-point stimulation for nausea and vomiting. J Altern Complement Med 2006;12:489-495.

37. Ernst E, White A: Acupuncture for back pain. Arch Intern Med 1998;158:2235-2241.

38. Grant D, Bishop-Miller J, Winchester D, et al: A randomized comparative trial of acupuncture versus transcutaneous electrical nerve stimulation for chronic back pain in the elderly. Pain 1999;82:9-13.

39. Carlsson C, Sjolund B: Acupuncture for chronic low back pain: A randomized placebo-controlled study with long-term follow-up. Clin J Pain 2001;17:296-305.

40. Leibing E, Leonhardtb U, Kösterc G, et al: Acupuncture treatment of chronic low-back pain—a randomized, blinded, placebo-controlled trial with 9-month follow-up. Pain 2002;96:189-196.

41. Brinkhaus B, Wltt CM, Jena S, et al: Acupuncture in patients with chronic low back pain: A randomized controlled trial. Arch Intern Med 2006;166:450-457.

42. Thomas KJ, Macpherson H, Thorpe L, et al: Randomised controlled trial of a short course of traditional acupuncture compared with usual care for persistent non-specific low back pain. BMJ 2006;333:623.

43. Ratcliffe J, Thomas KJ, Macpherson H, et al: A randomised controlled trial of acupuncture care for persistent low back pain: Cost-effectiveness analysis. BMJ 2006;333:626.

44. Dowson D, Lewith, GT, Machin, D: The effects of acupuncture versus placebo in the treatment of headache. Pain 1985;21: 35-42.

45. Loh L, Nathan, PW, Schott, GD, et al: Acupuncture versus medical treatment for migraine and muscle tension headaches. J Neurol Neurosurg Psychiatry 1984;47:333-337.

46. Allais G, De Lorenzo C, Quirico PE, et al: Acupuncture in the prophylactic treatment of migraine without aura: A comparison with flunarizine. Headache 2002;42:855-861.

47. Diener HC, Kronfeld K, Boewing G, et al: Efficacy of acupuncture for the prophylaxis of migraine: A multicentre randomised controlled clinical trial. Lancet Neurol 2006;5:310-316.

48. Melchart D, Linde K, Fischer P, et al: Acupuncture for recurrent headaches: A systematic review of randomized controlled trials. Cephalalgia 1999;19:779-786.

49. Melchart D, Thormaehlen J, Hager S, et al: Acupuncture versus placebo versus sumatriptan for early treatment of migraine attacks: A randomized controlled trial. J Intern Med 2003; 253:181-188.

50. Coeytaux RR, Kaufman JS, Kaptchuk TJ, et al: A randomized, controlled trial of acupuncture for chronic daily headache. Headache 2005;45:1113-1123.

51. Ernst E, White A: Acupuncture as a treatment for temporomandibular joint dysfunction: A systematic review of randomized trials. Arch Otolaryngol Head Neck Surg 1999;125: 269-272.

52. Fink M, Rosted P, Bernateck M, et al: Acupuncture in the treatment of painful dysfunction of the temporomandibular joint—a review of the literature. Forsch Komplementarmed 2006;13:109-115.

53. White A, Ernst E: A systemic review of randomized controlled trials of acupuncture for neck pain. Rheumatology 1999;38: 143-147.

54. White P, Lewith G, Berman B, et al: Reviews of acupuncture for chronic neck pain: Pitfalls in conducting systemic reviews. Rheumatology 2002;41:1224-1231.
55. Irnich D, Behrens N, Molzen H, et al: Randomised trial of acupuncture compared with conventional massage and"sham" laser acupuncture for treatment of chronic neck pain. Br Med J 2001;322:1574-1577.
56. Vas J, Perea-Milla E, Mendez C, et al: Efficacy and safety of acupuncture for chronic uncomplicated neck pain: A randomised controlled study. Pain 2006;126:245-255.
57. Trinh KV, Graham N, Gross AR, et al: Acupuncture for neck disorders. Cochrane Database Syst Rev 2006;(3):CD004870.
58. Lewit K: The needle effect in the relief of myofascial pain. Pain 1979;3:83-90.
59. Melzack T, Stillwell, DM, Fox, EJ: Trigger points and acupuncture points for pain: Correlations and implications. Pain 1977;3:3-23.
60. Scharf HP, Mansmann U, Streitberger K, et al: Acupuncture and knee osteoarthritis: A three-armed randomized trial. Ann Intern Med 2006;145:12-20.
61. White A, Foster NE, Cummings M, Barlas P: Acupuncture treatment for chronic knee pain: A systematic review. Rheumatology (Oxford) 2007;46:384-390.
62. Naeser MA, Hahn KA, Lieberman BE, Brauco KF: Carpal tunnel syndrome pain treated with low-level laser and microamperes transcutaneous electric nerve stimulation: A controlled study. Arch Phys Med Rehabil 2002;83:978-988.
63. Napadow V, Liu J, Li M, et al: Somatosensory cortical plasticity in carpal tunnel syndrome treated by acupuncture. Hum Brain Mapp 2007;28:159-171.
64. Shlay J, Chaloner K, Max M, et al: Acupuncture and amitriptyline for pain caused by HIV-related peripheral neuropathy. JAMA 1998;280:1590-1595.
65. Leo K: Use of electrical stimulation at acupuncture points for the treatment of reflex sympathetic dystrophy in a child: A case report. Phys Ther 1983;63:957-959.
66. Spoerel W, Varkey, M, Leung CY: Acupuncture in chronic pain. Am J Chin Med 1976;4:267-279.
67. Eisenberg D, Cohen M, Hrbek A, et al: Credentialing complementary and alternative medical providers. Ann Intern Med 2002;137:965-973.

43 Pain and Addictive Disorders: Challenge and Opportunity

Edward C. Covington

Why must a textbook of pain contain a chapter on addiction, given that most current data suggest that addictive disorders are no more prevalent in patients with pain than in the general adult population? The answer is that pain and addiction are often intricately interwoven. Addictive disorder is common in pain clinics, where it obscures diagnosis and impedes treatment. In fact, the treatments for chronic pain and for addiction may seem incompatible. Additionally, there is considerable fear among pain physicians of causing addiction or of being accused of doing so. Addicts are likely to occupy a disproportionate portion of the pain clinician's time and, unless skillfully managed, will have worse outcomes than other patients.

DEFINITIONS

"Addiction is a primary, chronic, neurobiologic disease, with genetic, psychosocial, and environmental factors influencing its development and manifestations. It is characterized by behaviors that include one or more of the following: impaired control over drug use, compulsive use, continued use despite harm, and craving."[1] This definition, taken from a joint statement of the American Academy of Pain Medicine, the American Pain Society, and the American Society of Addiction Medicine, was designed to provide clarity and consistency in communications concerning this disease, and to address perceived deficiencies in extant definitions and terms that promote misunderstanding.

Dependence

The term *dependence*, which is preferred by the American Psychiatric Association and the World Health Organization,[2] risks confusing physical dependence with addiction. Additional confusion arises from the fact that some states (e.g., Ohio[3]) have used the term *medication dependence* to simply indicate that a person's health requires the chronic use of a medication. Standard psychiatric nomenclature, codified in the *Diagnostic and Statistical Manual of Mental Disorders* (DSM)[4] lists tolerance and withdrawal as the first two of seven criteria for "substance dependence." These phenomena are, of course, normal and to be expected in prolonged use of opioids and do not indicate the presence of any disorder. They are also to be expected in the prolonged use of many antidepressants, anticonvulsants, and antihypertensives, among other drugs that have little or no capacity to elicit addictive behavior. Furthermore, withdrawal can be elicited in normal subjects following a single dose of morphine,[5] which reduces the value of this phenomenon as a diagnostic criterion. Although the term *dependence* has been promoted as less pejorative than addiction, the Liaison Committee on Pain and Addiction[1] has concluded that the costs in terms of miscommunication and loss of diagnostic precision are unacceptable, and that stigmatization of the terms *addict* and *addiction* need to be addressed in other ways.

Other definitions are more idiosyncratic. The Controlled Substances Act defines an "addict" as a person who "habitually uses any narcotic drug so as to endanger the public morals, health, safety, or who is so far addicted to the use of narcotic drugs as to have lost power of self-control with reference to his addiction."[6] Other governmental and nongovernmental organizations have their own definitions.

Tolerance

"Tolerance is a state of adaptation in which exposure to a drug induces changes that result in a diminution of one or more of the drug's effects over time."[1] Like dependence, it can be detected after a single dose of an opioid and, like dependence, may be mistaken for addiction. It develops differently for differing drug effects; for example, tolerance to opioid-induced respiratory depression and sedation develops much more rapidly than tolerance to analgesia and constipation. It also develops differently among individuals, occurring rapidly in some and slowly in others. It does not indicate the presence of an addictive disorder per se.

Prevalence

There is reason to believe that substance abuse is far more prevalent in health care consumers than has been commonly recognized and that even when recognized, it is often ignored. In a 1989 study of adults admitted to Johns Hopkins Hospital, screens for alcoholism were positive in 25% of medicine admissions, 30% of psychiatric admissions, 19% of neurology patients, 12.5% of obstetric-gynecologic (OBG) admissions, and 23% of surgical admissions. Detection rates by house staff and faculty were lower than 25% in surgery and OBG, 25% to 50% in neurology and medicine, and more than 50% in psychiatry. Physicians were more likely to overlook alcoholism in those with higher incomes and education, private medical insurance, and women. When physicians did diagnose active alcoholism, they often failed to initiate treatment.[7]

Estimates of the prevalence of addictive disorder in those with pain have varied widely. Disparities result from varying definitions of addiction, sometimes cursory evaluations for addiction, evaluations performed by personnel lacking addiction training and experience, failure to obtain collateral information, and varying rates of addiction in different populations. Most studies of addiction in those with pain have addressed prescription or street drugs; however, alcohol and nicotine have also been studied. Atkinson and colleagues,[8] using a structured interview in a primary care clinic, found higher lifetime rates of alcohol use disorders in those with chronic low back pain (64.9%) than in controls (38.8%). That the drinking was not a response to pain was demonstrated by finding that the disparity in risk was present only during the time prior to pain onset. Katon and associates[9] studied inpatients with chronic pain and found that of those with a history of alcohol abuse, the onset of abuse was almost 15 years (mean) prior to the pain treatment. Kaila-Kangas and coworkers,[10] among others, have confirmed an association between nicotine dependence and spinal disk disease.

Long[11] has reported that up to 90% of chronic pain patients (in an inpatient pain treatment center) misuse drugs and that 50% obtain opiates from multiple physicians; however, he did not report criteria for drug misuse. Maruta and colleagues[12] have studied 144 consecutive referrals for management of chronic noncancer pain (CNCP), and found that 41% have comorbid substance abuse and 24% have dependence. This is an unusually high percentage and is probably explained by the diagnostic criteria used, which would likely lead to numerous false-positive results. In 1992, Fishbain and associates[13] reviewed 24 studies of addiction in pain patients, but found only three that included compulsive use in the

definition of addiction; they reported a prevalence of 3.2% to 18.9%. Kouyanou and coworkers,[14] using strict diagnostic criteria in a population of 125 South London pain clinic patients, found that 12% met DSM-III criteria for active abuse or dependence and an additional 10% met criteria for a substance use disorder in remission. Hoffmann and colleagues[15] administered a structured diagnostic interview to 414 chronic pain patients at the Åre Hospital in Sweden and found that 23.4% met DSM-III-R criteria for active misuse or dependency, and an additional 9.4% met criteria for remission. The most prevalent drugs of dependence were analgesics (12.6%), alcohol (9.7%), and sedatives (7.0%). Among 200 chronic low back pain patients entering functional restoration, Polatin and associates[16] found that 19% had substance abuse disorders.

Prevalence figures must be examined closely to ascertain the denominator. For example, Chabal and coworkers[17] have found that 27.6% of chronic opioid users met three of five criteria for abuse; however, abusers represented only 5.2% of all chronic pain patients. They also noted that studies that include only patients who remained in treatment may be misleading, because most drug abusers in their study had dropped out of treatment by 18 months.

The 2004 National Survey on Drug Use and Health found that 9.4% of Americans aged 12 or older in 2004 were classified with substance dependence or abuse in the past year, about the same number as in 2002 and 2003.[18] Among users of pain relievers, 12.3% were classified with dependence or abuse. These figures did not include those in remission during the prior year.

Smothers and Yahr[19] have found that 5% of U.S. general hospital admissions are chronic drug users (14% of 18- to 44-year-olds). In an earlier study,[20] they found that about 25% of admissions who identified themselves as drinkers met research criteria for alcohol use disorders; of these, 40% to 42% were detected, as reflected by medical records.

It is reasonable to conclude that chemical dependence (excluding nicotine) is approximately as common in pain patients as in those without. The prevalence is probably considerably higher in pain clinics and general medical facilities. The vulnerability of those with addictive disorders to various traumas and illnesses would be expected to lead to their disproportionate representation in medical facilities. It is also likely that among those with chronic pain, patients with addiction are less likely to respond to treatment at the primary or specialty level, and therefore more likely to be referred to pain clinics.

DIAGNOSTIC CONSIDERATIONS

Identification of substance use disorders presents two difficulties. One is that criteria vary and some are of questionable validity when applied in a pain population. Another is that unlike most medical conditions, the patient is as likely to seek to obscure the diagnosis as to elucidate it. Perhaps because of these difficulties, some pain specialists have disclaimed responsibility for making the diagnosis. This practice is unacceptable, because it not only ignores a potentially devastating disease, but also subjects the patient to unwarranted treatment risks in a setting of diminished likelihood of benefit.

A more understandable but equally unacceptable reason for avoiding the diagnosis is that it literally adds insult to injury, given that the diagnosis is so stigmatized. Nevertheless, addiction is an often fatal condition, and the physician is obligated to inform the patient when a substance use problem is suspected.

It is important to distinguish the question of how to detect a condition (i.e., the diagnostic criteria) from what the disease actually is—its essence. By analogy, schizophrenia is detected by the presence of such signs as hallucinations and delusions, but they are likely to be only epiphenomena of a structural or metabolic brain disorder. The essence of addiction is likely to be a change in brain chemistry that leads to inordinate valuation of substance use, relative devaluation of other things, and diminished ability to control impulses related to substance use and acquisition.[21-23] Physical dependence is often erroneously thought of as a major factor in addiction treatment,

when the true challenge is relapse prevention. In animals and humans, relapse is typically precipitated by exposure to the previous drug of use, stress, and environmental cues associated with drug use. Much of relapse prevention consists of helping patients identify and avoid triggers that precipitate use and helping them learn to cope with such triggers when they occur.

Without the ability to detect the brain changes of addiction, it must be diagnosed based on behavioral abnormalities and reported alterations of thoughts and feelings. The standard criteria are those of the DSM-IV.[24] Its term, *substance dependence disorder*, closely approximates what is generally considered to be addiction; however, accurate diagnosis is contingent on vigilant attention to the paragraph preceding the bulleted criteria, which specifies that there must be "a maladaptive pattern of substance use" that leads to "clinically important distress or impairment." Without this, many pain patients on chronic opioid therapy would meet the requisite criteria for a substance use diagnosis. The criteria for dependence and abuse are listed in Box 43–1. These and other criteria not only risk diagnosing addiction in its absence, but can also contribute to failure to diagnose the condition when present, because the usual detrimental effects of drug use on lifestyle and

---

BOX 43–1. CRITERIA FOR DEPENDENCE AND ABUSE

Dependence
The patient's maladaptive pattern of substance use leads to clinically important distress or impairment as shown in a single 12-month period by three or more of the following:
- Tolerance, shown by either
  - Markedly increased intake of the substance is needed to achieve the same effect
  or
  - With continued use, the same amount of the substance has markedly less effect.
- Withdrawal, shown by either
  - The substance's characteristic withdrawal syndrome
  or
  - The substance (or one closely related) is used to avoid or relieve withdrawal symptoms.
- The amount or duration of use is often more than intended.
- The patient repeatedly tries without success to control or reduce substance use.
- The patient spends much time using the substance, recovering from its effects, or trying to obtain it.
- The patient reduces or abandons important social, occupational, or recreational activities because of substance use.

- The patient continues to use the substance, despite knowing that it has probably caused physical or psychological problems.

Dependence may be further categorized as in remission (early or sustained, full or partial), on agonist therapy, or in a controlled environment.

Abuse
The patient's maladaptive substance use pattern causes clinically important distress or impairment as shown in a single 12-month period by one or more of the following:
- Because of repeated use, the patient fails to carry out major obligations at work or at home.
- The patient uses substances, even when it is physically dangerous.
- The patient repeatedly has legal problems from substance use.
- Despite knowing that it has caused or worsened social or interpersonal problems, the patient continues to use the substance.
- For this class of substance, the patient has never fulfilled criteria for substance dependence.

From American Psychiatric Association: Diagnostic and Statistical Manual of Mental Disorders, 4th ed, text revision (DSM-IV-TR). Washington, DC, American Psychiatric Association, 2000.

psychosocial functioning may be less evident in pain patients and, when they do occur, are likely not to be ascribed to drug use.

Thus, it is simply more difficult to diagnose addictive disorders when the substances involved are prescribed for patients with CNCP. Compulsive use, for example, may not be apparent when opioids are prescribed for pain and increased in response to reports of inadequate analgesia. Legal problems rarely occur, and it is not necessary for patients to engage in criminal activity to obtain drugs.[25] Personality changes and regression, common in those with addictive disorders, are likely to be ascribed to the pain disorder rather than to the addiction. Family members may not complain, either because they fail to recognize drugs as having become a liability or because they are more comfortable with the patient intoxicated than complaining. Medical complications may be subtle, and criteria that help identify "recreational" addicts, such as cirrhosis, nasal septal perforations, hepatitis, and convictions for driving while intoxicated, are unlikely to be found in those addicted to prescribed opioids or sedatives.

Nevertheless, the essence of the disease of addiction is the same whether it originates through licit or illicit use, even though some manifestations differ. For example, loss of control may be demonstrated through an inability to ration the drug, so that handfuls are taken or a week's supply is used in 1 day, despite knowing that refills may be unavailable. Adverse consequences may include dozing off in midsentence or midmeal, and functional deficits may be seen when opioids lead to intoxication, inability to drive, or behavioral regression when the goal was to enhance function.

Numerous authors have listed clues to the presence of addiction in patients with pain, and others have identified "predictors" of substance abuse in those prescribed opioids. Obviously, these overlap substantially. Most have not been subjected to scientific scrutiny and their sensitivity and specificity, alone or in the aggregate, are unknown. They are, however, characteristics that appropriately alert the clinician to investigate more thoroughly, and as such, are useful.

It has been noted that the therapeutic user of opioids often shows appropriate concern, wants to know the risks of addiction, and is grateful for a discussion of the topic. In contrast, the addict is more likely to defend his or her use and may seem closed to input regarding it. Although therapeutic use, when effective, leads to an improved quality of life, addictive use, by definition, is harmful.

It seems that opioid use is rarely neutral and that if it is not part of the solution, it is likely to be part of the problem. Experience has suggested that development of an addiction is associated with functional regression.[26] The findings of worse physical and vocational performance in high scorers on the Pain Medicine Questionnaire by Adams and colleagues supports this.[27] Thus, failure to show functional improvement despite aggressive opioid therapy may be a clue to the presence of an addictive disorder.

Manifestations of problematic opioid use include such obvious behaviors as losing medications and prescriptions, multisourcing, polysubstance abuse, injecting or snorting oral medications, reporting prescription theft, calling after hours when house staff (unknown to them) may be induced to prescribe, drug-focused office visits, and lack of interest in non-opioid treatments or diagnostic evaluations. More extreme behaviors, such as prescription fraud, buying street drugs, and experiencing legal consequences ("deception to obtain controlled substances") are usually late-stage signs.

Reid and associates[28] have found that a prior history of a substance use disorder, along with younger age, predicts abuse of prescribed opioids; however, their definition of such abuse was highly inclusive. Michna and coworkers[29] have noted the importance of a history of drug abuse in the patient or family, psychiatric history, motor vehicle accidents, smoking and needing a cigarette within the first hour of awakening, higher doses of opioids, and lack of reported adverse effects from opioids. Savage[30] has suggested that opioid addiction could be present in patients who are unwilling to taper opioids to try alternative treatments, who have diminished function despite apparent analgesia, and who often request early refills.

Chabal and colleagues[17] have identified five criteria suggesting substance abuse:

1. A focus on opiate issues during visits that impedes progress with other treatments and persists beyond the third appointment
2. A pattern of early refills or escalating drug use in the absence of clinical change
3. Multiple calls or visits about opiate prescriptions
4. A pattern of prescription problems (e.g., lost, spilled, stolen)
5. Supplemental sources of opioids

Portenoy[31] has categorized aberrant behaviors into those determined to be more and less predictive of drug misuse. The more predictive behaviors include the following:

1. Forging prescriptions
2. Stealing or borrowing drugs
3. Frequently losing prescriptions
4. Resisting changes to pain treatment, despite adverse side effects

The less predictive behaviors include the following:

1. Aggressive complaining about the need for more drugs
2. Drug hoarding
3. Unsanctioned dose escalation or other forms of noncompliance

Several authors have noted that functional deterioration associated with analgesic therapy is suggestive of addiction. This is not surprising when one recalls that addictive disorders are diseases, and patients are impaired when they have them.

An important false-positive finding in the diagnosis of addiction has been referred to as *pseudoaddiction*.[32] This term describes a situation in which aberrant behaviors are erroneously attributed to addiction when in fact they result from inadequate treatment. It is not surprising that a patient experiencing severe pain who is treated with doses of opioids that are too small or far apart will watch the clock, display drug-seeking behavior, or obtain opioids from inappropriate sources.

Lusher and associates[33] have purported to distinguish addiction from pseudoaddiction on the basis of eight criteria, most of which relate to whether the use of opioids is for pain reduction or psychoactive effects. It is unclear, however, how to determine that patients requesting opioids are seeking euphoria, relaxation, or changes in mood, for example, rather than analgesia.

The prescription drug use questionnaire (PDUQ) was developed by Compton and colleagues[34] to facilitate the diagnosis of addictive disorder in chronic pain patients. It requires 20 minutes to administer, and thus is not practical for screening purposes; however, it does show good discrimination, because patients scoring lower than 11 did not meet criteria for a substance use disorder, and those scoring above 15 met these criteria. Scores above 25 indicate substance dependence. Three items correctly classified 92% of participants. These reflect the tendency to increase opioid dose or frequency, have a preferred route of administration, and consider themselves addicted.

Screening Tools

There is a need for screening instruments that will alert the clinician to the likelihood that a patient has or will have drug-related difficulties. Unfortunately, simple questioning may fail to reveal substance use disorders, because patients often give inaccurate reports.[35] In a study of 109 CNCP patients, Berndt and associates[36] have found that 21% concealed drug use, 2% were not taking prescribed medications, and 9% were uninterpretable. Robinson and coworkers[37] have

reviewed early initiatives to develop screening instruments for opioid abuse and found the field in its infancy, with no suitable instruments.

The simple four-item CAGE inventory[38] (Box 43–2) has been modified for use in detecting drug abuse.[39] The drug abuse screening test (DAST), although not developed for patients taking prescribed drugs, does contain several items that screen for drug use problems[40] (Appendix 43–1).

Prediction

Although conceptually distinct from instruments designed to detect existing addictive disorder, those whose purpose is to predict aberrant drug-related behavior in pain patients are closely related. Many seem to predict the past, in the sense that they detect signs of existing addictive disorder, which predicts future behavior to some extent.[41] Nevertheless, these screening instruments do predict patient difficulty with appropriate opioid use, which is useful. Webster and Webster[42] have developed the Opioid Risk Tool (ORT) (Table 43–1), which has yet to be evaluated by

---

BOX 43–2. CAGE* QUESTIONS ADAPTED TO INCLUDE DRUGS (CAGE-AID)

1. Have you felt you ought to cut down on your drinking or drug use?
2. Have people annoyed you by criticizing your drinking or drug use?
3. Have you felt bad or guilty about your drinking or drug use?
4. Have you ever had a drink or used drugs first thing in the morning to steady your nerves or to get rid of a hangover (eye opener)?

*C, cut down; A, annoyed; G, guilty; E, eye opener.
From Mayfield D, McLeod G, Hall P: The CAGE questionnaire: Validation of a new alcoholism screening instrument. Am J Psychiatry 1974;131:1121-1123.

Table 43–1. Opioid Risk Tool

RISK FACTOR	MARK EACH BOX THAT APPLIES	ITEM SCORE IF FEMALE	ITEM SCORE IF MALE
1. Family history of substance abuse:			
Alcohol	☐	1	3
Illegal drugs	☐	2	3
Prescription drugs	☐	4	4
2. Personal history of substance abuse:			
Alcohol	☐	3	3
Illegal drugs	☐	4	4
Prescription drugs	☐	5	5
3. Age (mark box if 16-45 yr)	☐	1	1
4. History of preadolescent sexual abuse	☐	3	0
5. Psychological disease:			
Attention-deficit disorder, obsessive compulsive disorder, bipolar disorder, schizophrenia	☐	2	2
Depression	☐	1	1

Developed by Webster LR, Webster RM: Predicting aberrant behaviors in opioid-treated patients: Preliminary validation of the Opioid Risk Tool. Pain Med 2005;6:432-442.

Table 43–2. SOAPP Questions Found to Predict Substance Use Problems

QUESTION	SCORE*
1. How often do you have mood swings?	__
2. How often do you smoke a cigarette within an hour after you wake up?	__
3. How often have any of your family members, including parents and grandparents, had a problem with alcohol or drugs?	__
4. How often have any of your close friends had a problem with alcohol or drugs?	__
5. How often have others suggested that you have a drug or alcohol problem?	__
6. How often have you attended an AA or NA meeting?	__
7. How often have you taken medication other than the way that it was prescribed?	__
8. How often have you been treated for an alcohol or drug problem?	__
9. How often have your medications been lost or stolen?	__
10. How often have others expressed concern over your use of medication?	__
11. How often have you felt a craving for medication?	__
12. How often have you been asked to give a urine screen for substance abuse?	__
13. How often have you used illegal drugs—for example, marijuana, cocaine—in the past 5 years?	__
14. How often, in your lifetime, have you had legal problems or been arrested?	__

*Scoring: 0 = never; 1 = seldom; 2 = sometimes; 3 = often; 4 = very often. In the initial study, a score of 7 or higher identified 91% of those who were later found to have aberrant behaviors.
Developed by Butler SF, Budman SH, Fernandez K, Jamison RN: Validation of a screener and opioid assessment measure for patients with chronic pain. Pain 2004;112:65-75.

independent investigators; however, it has shown excellent success at categorizing patients into low (score, 3 or lower), moderate (score, 4 to 7), or high (score, 8 or higher) risk for aberrant drug-related behaviors. Although clinicians may not use the ORT in practice, it may still be useful for detecting the traits captured by the test and to increase vigilance and cautions to patients when they are present.

The Screener and Opioid Assessment for Patients with Pain (SOAPP) was developed by Butler and colleagues[43] and was demonstrated to have acceptable sensitivity and specificity (Table 43–2). Like many screening instruments, it does not contain questions designed to detect dissimulations and reflects the patient's willingness to answer questions in a forthright manner.

Scammers

There are individuals, mostly addicts or drug dealers, who feign a pain problem to obtain opioids. The U.S. Drug Enforcement Administration (DEA) has provided clues to the identification of the drug abuser, which seems to refer to these people.[44] The following characteristics were noted:

- Unusual behavior in the waiting room
- Often demanding immediate action
- Unusual appearance—slovenly or overdressed
- Unusual knowledge of controlled substances
- Reluctant to provide access to information
- Will not give name of primary care provider
- May request a specific drug, resist others (don't work, allergic)
- Little interest in diagnosis—fails to keep appointments for tests, consultation
- Cutaneous signs of drug abuse
- Calls after regular hours
- Just passing through town
- Lost or stolen prescriptions
- Pressures the physician by eliciting sympathy or guilt, or by direct threats

It should be noted that requesting a specific opioid arouses less suspicion than it did in the past as a result of advances in understanding of mu (μ) receptor polymorphism, which results in genetic variations in response to different opioids.[45] Thus, some people derive more effective analgesia from morphine than from hydromorphone, for example, as well as the converse.

Iatrogenic Addiction

A question that troubles most who treat pain is, "How likely am I to cause harm?" Generally, this is not so much an expression of worry about respiratory depression or organ toxicity as about addiction. Additionally, there has been a plethora of litigation in which plaintiffs have claimed that physicians caused them to suffer lifelong consequences of their addictive disorder. Thus, physicians not only have concerns about the safety of patients, but also about their own safety.

Although most pain specialists agree that iatrogenic addiction is uncommon, there are few data available for establishing its exact incidence. Extant studies are largely poorly done and brief. Data are often difficult to obtain and there is often ambiguity not only about the presence of addiction, but also the time of its onset.

Nevertheless, available data suggest that the risk of inducing addictive disorder is minimal in short-term opioid therapy. Based on case reviews, it is likely that the overwhelming majority of individuals claiming iatrogenic addiction (1) are not addicted at all, but merely physically dependent, or (2) were addicted long before receiving legitimately prescribed opioids. It is clear that most patients addicted to prescribed opioids had an addictive disorder that preceded opioid therapy.

Porter and Jick, as part of the Boston Collaborative Drug Surveillance Program, examined files of 39,946 hospitalized medical patients monitored consecutively.[46] Among 11,882 who received one narcotic dose, there were four cases of apparently new addiction, and only one was considered major.

Perry and Heidrich[47] sent questionnaires to burn facilities to investigate methods of analgesia commonly provided for débridement. The authors noted that none of the 181 respondents, who had knowledge of at least 10,000 hospitalized burn patients, reported a single case of iatrogenic addiction. They further stated that "The 22 patients reported to abuse drugs after discharge all had a prior history of drug abuse."

Both these studies[46,47] suffer from serious deficiencies in how addiction was defined and assessed, and neither followed patients after hospitalization to determine whether evidence of addiction surfaced following discharge. In addition, they have been widely cited as evidence for the safety of *chronic* opioid therapy, which they do not address. They do suggest that *acute* opioid therapy has only a remote chance of inducing obvious addiction.

In a retrospective study of 48 patients hospitalized for addiction to oxycodone (OxyContin), Potter and associates[48] found that 31% began using OxyContin via a legitimate prescription; however, 77.1% reported prior non-opioid substance use problems (including alcohol) and 48% had prior problems with other opioids.

Similarly, in a sample of 200 chronic low back pain patients, substance abuse was found to have preceded pain in 94% of patients with substance abuse.[49] In a highly selected group of patients undergoing pain rehabilitation, our group found that of those with addictive disorder, 33% attributed their addiction to medical exposure, 64% to recreational use, and 3% to undetermined causes.[50] The proportion of patients in a pain clinic who were iatrogenically addicted would be expected to be much higher than the proportion of addicts in society whose addiction originated in this way.

Studies of iatrogenic addiction often fail to address the question of iatrogenic relapse. Animal[51] and human[52] studies have demonstrated that one of the most powerful stimuli for eliciting resumption of dormant drug-seeking behavior is exposure to the drug of choice. A case came to our attention of a heroin addict treated in a chemical dependence program who maintained sobriety for longer than 1 year until he was exposed to intravenous midazolam for procedural sedation. He experienced immediate onset of drug craving, obtained and injected heroin, to which he was no longer tolerant, and died. Studies are lacking to clarify the risk of relapse if, for example, a patient who has been sober from alcoholism for a number of years is exposed to chronic opioid therapy.

Another question that remains unanswered is the extent to which development of an addictive disorder is a function of time. It is known that there are "instant alcoholics" and "instant addicts" who manifest extreme addictive behavior after an initial exposure (also typically seen after intercranial self-stimulation in animals); however, most chemically dependent persons used the substance for some time in a non-addictive fashion prior to losing control. How can the reassuring data regarding the low risk of inducing opioid addiction be extrapolated? These data usually come from studies of less than 18 months' duration, yet they are applied to the clinical situation in which patients may be placed on opioids for decades. If addiction is in part a function of time, prolonged studies may be required to clarify the risk.

It is important to note in the current climate of headlines regarding prescription drug abuse that not all abuse of *prescription* drugs is abuse of *prescribed* drugs. Although the news media feature physicians who have prescribed inappropriately or the patients who have duped them, information from the DEA demonstrates that much of the street presence of analgesics is a result of theft from pharmacies, physicians, manufacturers, and distributors (i.e., this has nothing to do with prescribing).[53] Also, drugs are stolen from the medicine cabinets of presumably actual patients by laborers in their home and teenage visitors, among others.

SIGNIFICANCE OF ADDICTIVE DISORDERS IN CHRONIC PAIN

It is often said that addiction is like war in that its first casualty is the truth. Dishonesty is a moderate challenge in acute pain—there are numerous objective confirmations of pathology or the lack of it. However, it can be almost insurmountable in the case of chronic pain, in which there is often no demonstrable peripheral pathology or in which demonstrable pathology (e.g., disk disease) bears an unclear relationship to symptoms.[54] Functional imaging studies have lent scientific credence to the compassionate definition of pain as "whatever the patient says it is" by demonstrating greater cortical activation in patients who report high levels of pain than in those who report less pain.[55] This principle, however, is valid only when the patient has no major incentive to prevaricate. If one considers an addicted person who has undergone implantation of a spinal cord stimulator, it is apparent that she or he can report almost complete pain relief and still obtain opioids of unknown quality and high price on the street, or can report marginal relief and obtain safe opioids from a prescriber for the cost of a copay.

It seems likely that addiction will affect both the true and reported outcomes of various interventions for pain. Maruta and associates[12] have found that chronic pain patients who are comorbid for substance dependence have worse outcomes. Kouyanou and coworkers[56] have also noted that those with chemical dependence have more disability and depression. Addiction is associated with various forms of functional impairment and will likely impede the functional restoration that is an important goal of pain management. In addition, risks of trauma and medical complications of addiction may worsen outcome. It could be argued that interventions for pain in those with an active chemical dependence should be contingent on their participation in a recovery or other addiction treatment program, whether based on abstinence or agonist therapy.

TREATMENT OF PAIN IN THE PATIENT WITH ADDICTION

A number of authors have emphasized the importance of differentiating pain patients from addicts. However, the two conditions are not mutually exclusive and occur concurrently more frequently than would be expected by chance, because chemically dependent persons are at increased risk for trauma and illness and are overrepresented in numerous medical conditions. Mertens and colleagues,[57] for example, have studied 747 Kaiser Permanente patients admitted for chemical dependence treatment and found that they are much more likely than other patients to have such chronic conditions as low back pain, headache, and arthritis, along with more injuries. Jamison and associates[58] interviewed 248 patients at methadone maintenance centers and found that 61.3% reported chronic pain as a primary medical condition. Rosenblum and coworkers[59] found that severe chronic pain was present in 37% of 390 methadone maintenance treatment patients and in 24% of 531 chemically dependent inpatients. Thus, documentation of the prevalence of pain in addicts and the prevalence of addiction in those with pain makes it clear that it is often necessary to treat persons with both conditions.

Numerous authorities and professional organizations agree that it is unethical to withhold opioid analgesia from addicts. For example, the American Society for Pain Management Nursing has upheld this principle, and described strategies for dealing with patients at different stages of the addictive disease process.[60] However, no one argues that patients are entitled to treatment that is harmful, and all agree that opioids are not helpful for all cases of chronic pain. Thus, there will be some patients with pain complaints who seek opioids and who should be denied. Although there are almost no data clarifying the risks and benefits of chronic opioid analgesia in addicts, it is clear that such therapy has hazards that exceed those of opioid therapy in non-addicts.

It is a truism in addiction medicine that a patient's former drug of choice will have the most power to elicit cravings and relapse, which probably explains the clinical impression that opioid therapy with recovering alcoholics is often more successful and less likely to lead to adverse outcomes than for recovering opioid addicts. Nevertheless, the concept of cross-addiction suggests that a patient with *any* prior addiction is at heightened risk for new addiction, even to unrelated substances. Thus, the chronic marijuana user may be at special risk for developing opioid addiction, even though the substances are unrelated. It is therefore essential that the clinician not only identify preexisting problems with opioid abuse, but with all rewarding or reinforcing substances. A distinction must be made between acute pain and chronic nonmalignant pain, and between the patient who is actively engaging in substance abuse and the patient in recovery.

Acute Pain

Substance abuse is associated with trauma.[61] Acute injuries in addicts, even those with sustained recovery, often require more aggressive analgesia than in patients with no addiction history because of the presence of tolerance. (It is commonly observed that a period of abstinence eliminates apparent drug tolerance; however, on resumption of use, tolerance is rapidly reestablished in the once-tolerant person or animal.) The postoperative situation is similar. At times, this need for what may seem to be excessive medication can collide with staff desires to limit opioid use in those with an addictive disorder. The result is likely to be a dissatisfied and uncomfortable patient, perhaps a vociferous one, and an unpleasant experience for staff. Management is facilitated by recognizing that a patient who is loudly demanding analgesia is unlikely to be overmedicated. It may be helpful to rotate opioids to identify a medication with incomplete cross-tolerance with the patient's drug of choice. Methadone and buprenorphine will often provide satisfactory analgesia in these conditions.

Mehta and Langford[62] have reviewed recommendations for treatment of acute and postoperative pain in patients maintained on opioid agonists. These include continuing the patient's maintenance opioids and supplementing them with additional analgesia, multimodal when possible, such as short-acting opioids, local anesthetics, and adjuvant nonsteroidal anti-inflammatory drugs (NSAIDs). They also recommended use of patient-controlled analgesia with higher than usual bolus doses and shorter than usual lockout intervals. Transdermal opioids and implantable pumps were noted as alternatives.

A special problem is created by the emergency department (ED) frequent flyer; this is the patient who is known to all the ED staff in the area, who habitually shows up, usually on nights and weekends, demanding opioids for some chronic (e.g., pancreatitis) or recurrent (e.g., migraine, sickle cell disease) condition. The lack of continuity of care, because the person engages different shifts at different hospitals, presents a severe challenge to the development of a rational treatment plan; however, such a plan is mandatory. It is useful to establish a liaison with a nonemergency provider in the relevant field and to arrange for consultation, so that a plan of management for pain, addiction, or both can be developed. Assessment for addictive disorder should also be arranged. It is useful to recall that unrewarded behaviors are not repeated for long, so that patients who resist daytime consultation should be limited, when possible, to noneuphorigenic medications in the ED (e.g., parenteral phenothiazines for migraine, ketorolac for other pains) until they accept appropriate consultation.

Patients in Recovery

Patients who are recovering from an addictive disorder often face elective surgery with great trepidation, because they fear having to choose between unrelieved pain and relapse of their addiction. Many will even refuse analgesia in an effort to preserve their hard-won sobriety. Experience suggests that this is unnecessary. Patients should be encouraged to advise the surgeon and anesthesiologist well in advance of an elective procedure that they are in recovery and will probably require higher than average doses of analgesics, but wish to preserve their sobriety by avoiding their previous drug of choice, transitioning to long-acting oral agents as soon as possible, and making arrangements for safe use of opioids after discharge. These patients should increase their recovery work (e.g., 12-step meetings, meetings with addiction counselor) and notify their treating professionals and sponsor of their pending surgery so that support is in place. It is sometimes helpful to have a spouse, friend, or sponsor hold opioids and bring a supply each day, so that the patient is protected from the temptation of a bottle full of opioids in easy reach.

Patients on Pharmacotherapy for Addiction

Patients whose addiction is under treatment with opioid agonists (e.g., methadone, buprenorphine) require special consideration when they experience trauma or acute painful illness. The dose of methadone provided will not provide analgesia, but must be continued to prevent withdrawal. In addition, usual or higher doses of μ-opioid agonist therapy are required for the acute pain. Partial antagonists should, of course, be avoided to prevent causing an abstinence syndrome. Buprenorphine, a partial μ agonist, may antagonize effects of other μ agonists, requiring higher than normal doses.

Alcohol and opioid addiction are frequently treated with naltrexone, a long-acting μ antagonist, as a relapse prevention strategy. When such patients require acute therapy, much higher than normal opioid doses are required. Close observation is necessary because these doses may be toxic as the naltrexone level decreases over time.

Chronic Pain

Appropriate treatment of comorbid pain and addiction remains controversial and there is little data on which to base therapy.[63] Discussions center on opioid-based and non-opioid–based therapies. There are recommendations from clinicians in the field based on understandings of the two disorders and on clinical experience, and these must guide us for now; however, it must be recalled how often clinical wisdom has been proved wrong when data became available. Among the most notable was the recommendation 30 years ago to avoid opioids for chronic nonmalignant pain because tolerance would render them ineffective.

Opioid-based Treatment

In a 1991 survey of state medical board members, Joranson and colleagues[64] found that 58% considered it a probable violation of federal or state laws and regulations to prescribe opioids for CNCP in a person with a history of opioid abuse. A subsequent survey demonstrated a marked liberalization of this attitude[65]; however, many remain reluctant to prescribe opioids for those with substance abuse disorders.

There is a paucity of data on the outcome of chronic opioid therapy in patients with addictive disorder, and most studies have been small. In 20 patients with CNCP and a comorbid history of substance abuse who were treated for more than 1 year, Dunbar and Katz[66] found that those who abused treatment did so early, and those who did not abuse were more likely to be active in Alcoholics Anonymous and have stable support systems, and were less likely to be recent polysubstance abusers. Those who did not abuse treatment were more likely to benefit from it.

Kennedy and Crowley[67] used methadone and weekly psychotherapy to treat four patients with chronic pain and comorbid substance abuse disorders. Three patients remained in treatment (19 to 21 months), stopped needle use or markedly decreased substance abuse, and demonstrated functional improvement; all three had significant psychopathology requiring psychotropics.

Currie and associates[68] treated 44 patients with comorbid chronic pain and addiction in cognitive-behavioral groups with emphasis on substance abuse education and relapse prevention. Some chose to discontinue opioids because they felt unable to control their use. Those who continued opioids were transitioned to longer acting medications (excluding methadone). PRN opioids were prohibited and, once titrated to the optimal dosage, patients could not obtain additional medication. There were significant improvements in pain, emotional functioning, and medication reliance. At 12-month follow-up, 50% of the patients were opioid-free, and the remainder had reduced their use from 17 to 12 days/month. There was no significant difference in outcomes for opioid and non-opioid users, although those who continued to take opioids appeared to function better overall. The authors suggested that long-acting opioids may provide both analgesia and reduction of cravings for this population.

From these studies, as well as clinical reports, it is reasonable to conclude that chronic opioid analgesic therapy will help some patients with CNCP if managed optimally. The issue of ensuring that addiction is being adequately treated is often key to the management of the patient with comorbidity. For the reader interested in understanding the treatments being proposed, the *Textbook Of Substance Abuse Treatment*[69] provides an excellent summary, including psychodynamic, network, cognitive-behavioral, motivational, individual, group, and family psychotherapy and 12-step–based approaches.

Miotto and coworkers have suggested useful recommendations for treating the patient with chronic pain and addiction[25]:

1. Wean opioids if pain can be managed with non-opioids, although detoxification alone is ineffective treatment for addiction.
2. Do not withhold opioids from addicts, but integrate them into a plan to relieve pain and treat addictive disease.
3. Address the false promise that opioids enable a person to avoid pain.
4. Provide treatment in a pain center if the primary physician is reluctant to prescribe opioids.
5. Require a treatment contract to establish treatment boundaries.
6. Educate patients about tolerance, dependence, withdrawal, and interactions among opioids, other medications, and alcohol.
7. Optimize adjunctive medications and non-pharmacologic strategies (e.g., physical conditioning, coping skills, daily time management skills, and lifestyle modifications).
8. Address psychiatric disorders and risk factors; survivors of childhood trauma may require psychotherapy.
9. Involve families in rehabilitation efforts.
10. Consider random urine testing.
11. Require drug abuse treatment. (Most recommend that it be provided during or after pain treatment.)
12. Slowly titrate opioids to the point of maximum function.
13. Monitor analgesic misuse.
14. Reevaluate addictive disease if drug seeking persists despite increased dosing in the absence of disease progression.
15. Provide multiple dated small prescriptions to those who cannot adhere to instructions.
16. Do not replace lost medication.
17. Do not expect addiction-controlling doses of methadone to manage pain effectively.
18. Expect relapse, especially early in treatment, during stress, or with unrelieved pain. Treat relapse; do not abandon the patient.
19. Terminate opioids in the case of selling prescriptions.

Passik and Kirsh[70] have echoed several of these suggestions and emphasized the importance of strict contracts and frequent follow-ups with urine toxicology screening to maximize the likelihood of a good outcome. Savage[71] has suggested that chronic opioid analgesia be tried in addicts whose pain is distressing and opioid-responsive, and when other therapies fail or are impracticable. Also, stable, relatively high blood levels of opioids could treat addiction and pain. Risks must be balanced against risks of no treatment, because unrelieved pain may promote addictive relapse or use of street drugs.

Weaver and Schnoll[72] have highlighted the difficulty of distinguishing an addict seeking euphoria from a nonaddict with pseudoaddiction, because both exhibit drug-seeking behaviors. They suggest prompt upward titration of medication, in response to which the nonaddict or addict in solid recovery will stop increasing the dose when the pain is controlled. Because tolerance to analgesia develops more slowly than tolerance to euphoria, the person with active addiction is likely to continue to escalate the opioid dose, despite being impaired. They further suggest that patients with recent active addiction should be in active chemical dependence treatment, including 12-step meetings and work with an addiction counselor. They advocate clear rules and boundaries, use of an opioid contract, and withholding opioids until medical records can be obtained to confirm patient history. Patients should be limited to one pharmacy for controlled substances and required to bring in their prescription bottles at each visit for pill counts and confirmation of the pharmacy being used. Random urine toxicology screening should be performed, and there must be permission for communication with family, significant others, pharmacists, and other health care providers.

Toxicology Screening

It is helpful to know whether patients are (1) consuming the drugs that are prescribed and (2) using illicit drugs. Urinary drug testing (UDT) can help provide the clinician with this information and can help the patient maintain sobriety by assuring him or her that there is accountability. Additionally, UDT results can be of value to the patient who needs to document treatment adherence for reasons that range from child custody to narcotic investigations. There are, however, several caveats.

The clinician must maintain a relationship with the testing laboratory, because substances assessed, cutoff levels, and other factors may vary. The physician must understand what is being tested for. Most dipstick immunoassays, for example, test for the "federal five," drugs that must be tested for in federal employees and those in federally regulated industries; they include marijuana, cocaine, opiates, phencyclidine (PCP), and amphetamines. The opiates screen detects morphine, which is present in users of codeine and heroin, but usually does not detect synthetics or semisynthetics. Thus, a negative screening result does not indicate that a patient is noncompliant with hydrocodone, oxycodone, hydromorphone, fentanyl, methadone, or buprenorphine therapy. Drugs detected by other routine screening tests may include methadone, propoxyphene, benzodiazepines, barbiturates, and EDDP (a methadone metabolite). Some tests are highly cross-reactive. For example, assays for amphetamines detect sympathomimetic amines such as ephedrine and pseudoephedrine, leading to false-positive results. In contrast, a finding of cocaine or tetrahydrocannabinol (THC) is reliable and, in the case of THC, cannot be caused by being in a room in which a great deal of marijuana is being smoked. Immunoassays should be confirmed by gas chromatography and mass spectroscopy, and the laboratory will need to be informed what the physician is looking for. A negative urine screening result may indicate that the patient is diverting medication. It can also mean that the patient exhausted the supply of medication several days before the test, or that the patient used someone else's urine sample to conceal the use of illicit drugs. Positive results can occur because of metabolic products. For example, hydrocodone and morphine can be converted in part to hydromorphone.

Testing should be performed randomly, not just on patients suspected of abuse, because this strategy is open to bias (e.g., disproportionate testing of minorities) and has been shown to miss 50% of those using nonprescribed or illicit drugs.[73] Reasonable care should be taken that the sample not be obtained in a room with access to water for dilution, and that the color and temperature are appropriate. Testing laboratories can screen for adulterants, which can conceal abused drugs, and for the presence of a creatinine concentration compatible with that of urine.

Without getting into a dispute about patients' rights to use substances or the benefits of the use of medical marijuana, it is reasonable for the physician to make access to opioid therapy contingent on the patient's willingness to relinquish the use of illicit substances. This can be presented simply as a way to ensure the patient's access to treatment and the physician's continued ability to prescribe. If the person is *unwilling* to relinquish recreational use, it suggests that the pain problem does not warrant chronic opioid therapy. If the patient is *unable* to relinquish the drugs, then addiction treatment is indicated. An excellent review of the subject of UDT has been presented by the Alaska Academy of Family Physicians.[74]

Opioid Selection

The major goal of opioid selection is to achieve optimal analgesia with minimal risk of addictive relapse. Busto and Sellers[75] have noted that pharmacokinetic factors that promote persistent self-administration include rapid absorption and high bioavailability, rapid delivery to the central nervous system, low protein and peripheral tissue binding, small volume of distribution, short half-life, and high free drug clearance. Thus, drugs that are "fast in," with a bolus into the neuron, and "fast out," other things being equal, will be most subject to abuse.[76] This is consistent with informal observations that alternate delivery systems developed by addicts are almost invariably in the direction predicted by these factors. For example, smoked cocaine is profoundly more rewarding than chewed coca leaves, and transdermal nicotine has little appeal to the cigarette smoker.

Mironer and coworkers[77] have reviewed records of pain patients dismissed from treatment because of opioid misuse and active patients continuing to receive opioids. They compared the frequency of prescription of various opioids with the frequency of their abuse to determine a relative risk of misuse. Their results, from highest to lowest risk of abuse, are as follows: butorphanol (4.4), propoxyphene (2.5),

hydrocodone (1.61), codeine with acetaminophen (1.45), oxycodone, immediate release (1.35), oxycodone, delayed release (0.73), morphine, 12-hour (0.66), transdermal fentanyl (0.23), and methadone (0.08). Brookoff asked patients with a history of prescription drug abuse to estimate the street prices of various opioids.[78] Of participants who had tried controlled-release preparations, 60% found them to be of little use, and estimated their street value to be lower than that of other opioids.

It seems reasonable to conclude that when abuse is a concern, there should be a preference for opioids with delayed and prolonged action and an avoidance of rapid-onset drugs and those that are inhaled or injected.

Several other strategies have been proposed to help therapeutic opioid users remain in control of their use. It is common to request that patients always bring their pill bottles to office visits so that pill counts can be performed. Some clinicians will telephone patients and have them bring in the bottle at random times, the idea being that the unpredictable oversight will help the patient to take the drugs as prescribed. Addicts have been prescribed transdermal fentanyl and required to turn in used patches to receive a prescription for new patches, thereby demonstrating that they were not sold, opened, or cut into pieces.

Intrathecal analgesia is somewhat appealing as a strategy for providing opioid therapy to patients who have difficulty controlling their use of opioids. This route of administration seems resistant to abuse, although there are a few reports of this. Two patients withdrew opioid from the pump and injected it intravenously,[79,80] and one injected illicit drugs into the pump port.[81]

Additional Medications

The presence of comorbid psychiatric symptoms is more the rule than the exception in those with significant chronic pain problems and in those with addictive disorders. It is reasonable to assume that a preponderance of patients with both chronic pain and addictive disorder will additionally have psychiatric symptoms, most commonly anxiety or depression. There is often reasonable justification for taking the risk of chronic opioid therapy for such persons, because there may not be effective alternative options for pain control; however, there seems to be little justification for prescribing controlled substances for anxiety, muscle spasm, and insomnia. Most antidepressants have anxiolytic properties and are not subject to abuse.[82-85] This is equally true of the antiepileptic drugs (AEDs) commonly used for pain treatment.[86] Most so-called muscle relaxants are not habituating, with the exception of carisoprodol, which therefore has no role in the addicted patient. When needed, drugs from both categories (antidepressants and AEDs) that have sedative properties can be selected to minimize polypharmacy and unnecessary exposure of vulnerable patients to addicting substances.[87]

Non-Opioid–based Treatment

A number of pharmacologic and nonpharmacologic interventions have proved useful for chronic pain, and are effective in addition to or in lieu of opioids. It has been compellingly demonstrated over the course of several decades that there is a group of patients with chronic pain who are more comfortable and more functional without opioids. To date, we lack accurate predictors of patients who will do well with opioids and are essentially limited to a therapeutic trial to ascertain patients who will show improved function, mood, and relief of pain and to assess side effects and aberrant behavior. It is likely that patients with addiction will be overrepresented in the group who are better without opioids, because their risks are clearly increased.

In 1986, Finlayson and colleagues[88] admitted 50 patients with CNCP and comorbid substance dependence to an inpatient chemical dependency treatment facility and provided standard addiction treatment, without specific attention to pain. Of those completing treatment ($n = 34$), pain scores were essentially unchanged; however, patients reported that relief of their pain was better and, at follow-up, had increased ability to work and improved marital relationships.

Rome and associates[89] treated CNCP patients in a cognitive-behavioral program that included opioid withdrawal and physical reconditioning. Patients reported significant reductions of pain severity, interference caused by pain, affective distress, depression, and catastrophizing, as well as increased perceived life control and general activity level. Outcome did not differ among those taking lower doses, higher doses, or no opioids at admission.

Our group studied 527 patients treated in a 3- to 4-week chronic pain rehabilitation program, approximately one third of whom (182) suffered from active comorbid addictive disorder.[90] Most had failed to rehabilitate with opioid therapy, which was weaned. Benzodiazepines were weaned as well. We found that those with addiction were twice as likely to drop out of treatment as were those without such comorbidity (31% vs. 16%); however, of those who completed treatment, outcome was equally good. In this group, whose treatment included active physical reconditioning, various cognitive-behavioral therapies, and aggressive treatment with such adjuvants as antidepressants and anticonvulsants, mean pain decreased by 40% (6.7 to 4.05 on a 0 to 10 scale), mean Beck Depression Inventory decreased from 21 (severely depressed) to 7 (normal), and mean Pain Disability Index decreased from 44.7/70 (markedly impaired) to 20/70 (mild impairment). In all these variables, patients with addictive disorder did not differ from those without. This suggests that there is a viable option to treating patients with addictive disorder who respond poorly to opioids.

Previously, we had demonstrated that patients who fail to respond to moderate- to high-dose opioids may have pain reduction with opioid elimination as part of a comprehensive treatment approach, as described earlier.[50] In this report, 228 consecutive admissions to a chronic pain rehabilitation program were studied. Patients in this program typically have dysfunction that is discordant with pathology (i.e., they have become debilitated because of pain rather than anatomic deficits), inordinate suffering and dysphoria, or substance use problems. Of these patients, 56 were taking 100 mg PO morphine equivalents/day or more on admission (mean, 456 mg/day), and were selected for study. Opioids and benzodiazepines were completely eliminated. Data were available on 46, of whom 43 (93%) experienced a reduction in pain with opioid elimination (from 7.2 to 4.0/10). Three experienced an increase in pain. Depression and functional impairment also improved. Several patients believed that they were benefiting from chronic opioid therapy, but improved after opioid elimination. They commonly described "getting myself back" after elimination of opioids. Significantly, two thirds of the high-dose opioid patients had a diagnosis of addictive disorder, demonstrating again that some patients with comorbid chronic noncancer pain and addiction may have optimal comfort and function with non-opioid–based therapies.

Not all studies are positive, and Tennant and Rawson found poor results with detoxification.[91] They studied patients who had become dependent on opioids prescribed for chronic pain and found that detoxification plus psychotherapy is less effective than detoxification followed by opioid maintenance; 76.2% of those in the former group dropped out of treatment by 3 weeks, as compared to less than 5% of those given opioid maintenance. The authors noted that pain that emerges during detoxification "proved to be an insurmountable barrier to total withdrawal in the majority of patients." It is likely that our more favorable results[50] were in part the result of aggressive use of antidepressants and anticonvulsants, which reduce both pain and symptoms, or protracted withdrawal, such as anxiety and insomnia.

Although most studies of opioid therapy are short term,[92] those that extend beyond 18 months typically show dropout rates of 50% or higher,[93-96] and pain reductions of less than 30% of baseline,[93] even when used intrathecally.[97] Thus, it is apparent that even when opioids are necessary, they are rarely sufficient for the treatment of chronic pain patients in general, and this is even more true for those with comorbid addiction. Fitness, psychological counseling, and use of adjuvant analgesics are essential for most patients.

PROTECTING THE CLINICIAN

A medical text should properly concern itself primarily with the well-being of patients, which is the goal of health care. However, it must be noted that one impediment to such care is physicians' appropriate concern with their own protection and the protection of their livelihood. This obviously affects patient access to care.

Physicians may face sanctions for treating addicts with opioids, and addicts may seek compensation from physicians whom they claim caused their addiction. The fact that addiction is much more likely to have arisen from recreational drug use does not alter the fact that iatrogenic addiction does occur and may constitute a compensable injury. A greater risk, however, is that a patient who had a preexisting addiction may falsely believe or claim that the physician caused it.

Personal knowledge of physicians who have been sanctioned or sued for issues related to opioid prescribing suggests that the problems are most likely to occur during treatment of those with an addictive disorder. Although it is critical to recognize that addiction is a disease that no one desires to have, once present, antisocial behaviors often emerge to which the physician must not allow himself or herself to be vulnerable. Thus, patients must be held accountable. Addicts making a sincere effort to recover will appreciate being held accountable, like being weighed at Weight Watchers, because this helps reduce the likelihood of a relapse.

Protection of the physician's interests is promoted by diligent documentation and diagnosis of a preexisting addictive disorder. Some states require that chronic opioid therapy for those with a prior addiction be treated only after consultation with an addiction specialist, presumably one who concurs with the treatment plan and is willing to comanage the patient. It is equally critical that the physician meticulously document treatment response (perhaps with spousal confirmation) or the lack thereof, and terminate opioids unless they are clearly beneficial.

Physicians may assume that patients will accept a small risk of developing addiction to have a substantial likelihood of pain relief. This should not be assumed, because that decision belongs to the patient. It should be clearly documented that the patient understood the risk of potential addiction and opted for chronic opioid therapy prior to its institution.

CONCLUSION

The pain-addiction interface is complex. It poses special challenges and requires special techniques. Accurate diagnosis in this population is critical and at times difficult. A guiding principle is that although patients with addictive disorders are entitled to whatever relief physicians can provide, they are not always entitled to opioids, because no patient is entitled to demand harmful or ineffective therapy. There is the potential for excellent outcome in these cases—most patients with addictive disorder and chronic pain can be restored to good function and comfort, sometimes with and sometimes without opioids. Such an outcome is unlikely unless the clinician exercises due diligence in identifying preexisting substance use disorders

A particular challenge is the apparent fact that excellent pain or addiction treatment will be of little value to these patients unless they have both. The pain specialist is in a unique position to ensure that this occurs.

References

1. Savage SR, Joranson DE, Covington EC, et al: Definitions related to the medical use of opioids: Evolution towards universal agreement. J Pain Symptom Manage 2003;26:656-666.
2. World Health Organization: The ICD-10 Classification of Mental and Behavioral Disorders: Clinical Descriptions and Diagnostic Guidelines. Geneva, World Health Organization, 1992.
3. Ohio Department of Job and Family Services: Ohio Medicaid Provider Handbook: General Information for Medicaid Providers, 2002. Available at http://jfs.ohio.gov/ohp/bhpp/handbook/Ch3334.pdf.
4. American Psychiatric Association: Diagnostic and Statistical Manual of Mental Disorders, 4th ed. Washington, DC, American Psychiatric Association, 1994.
5. Azolosa JL, Stitzer ML, Greenwald MK: Opioid physical dependence development: Effects of single versus repeated morphine pretreatments and of subjects' opioid exposure history. Psychopharmacology (Berl) 1994;114:71-80.
6. U.S. Department of Justice: Controlled Substances Act. Pub L No. 91-513, 84 Stat 1242 (1970); Title 21, Chapter 13, U.S. Code Service §802 (1996). Available at www.usdoj.gov/dea/pubs/csa/802.htm.
7. Moore RD, Bone LR, Geller G, et al: Prevalence, detection, and treatment of alcoholism in hospitalized patients. JAMA 1989;261:403-407.
8. Atkinson JH, Slater MA, Patterson TL, et al: Prevalence, onset, and risk of psychiatric disorders in men with chronic low back pain: A controlled study. Pain 1991;45:111-121.
9. Katon W, Egan K, Miller D: Chronic pain: Lifetime psychiatric diagnoses and family history. Am J Psychiatry 1985;142:1156-1160.
10. Kaila-Kangas L, Leino-Arjas P, Riihimaki H, et al: Smoking and overweight as predictors of hospitalization for back disorders. Spine 2003;28:1860-1868.
11. Long DM: A comprehensive model for the study and therapy of pain: Johns Hopkins Pain Research and Treatment Program. In Ng LKY (ed): New Approaches to Treatment of Chronic Pain: A Review of Multidisciplinary Pain Clinics and Centers (NIDA monograph, vol 36). Bethesda, Md, National Institute of Disability 1981, pp 66-75.
12. Maruta T, Swanson DW, Finlayson RE: Drug abuse and dependency in patients with chronic pain. Mayo Clin Proc 1979;54:241-244.
13. Fishbain DA, Rosomoff HL, Rosomoff RS: Drug abuse, dependence, and addiction in chronic pain patients. Clin J Pain 1992;8:77-85.
14. Kouyanou K, Pither CE, Wessely S: Medication misuse, abuse and dependence in chronic pain patients. J Psychosom Res 1997;43:497-504.
15. Hoffmann NG, Olofsson O, Salen B, et al: Prevalence of abuse and dependency in chronic pain patients. Int J Addictions 1995;30:919-927.
16. Polatin PB, Kinney RK, Gatchel RJ, et al: Psychiatric illness and chronic low-back pain. The mind and the spine—which goes first? Spine 1993;18:66-71.
17. Chabal C, Erjavec MK, Jacobson L, et al: Prescription opiate abuse in chronic pain patients: Clinical criteria, incidence, and predictors. Clin J Pain 1997;13:150-155.
18. U.S. Department of Health and Human Services, Substance Abuse and Mental Health Services Administration, Office of Applied Studies: Results from the 2004 National Survey on Drug Use and Health: National Findings, 2005 (rev). Available at http://oas.samhsa.gov/nsduh/2k4nsduh/2k4results/2k4results.pdf.
19. Smothers BA, Yahr HT: Alcohol use disorder and illicit drug use in admissions to general hospitals in the United States. Am J Addict 2005;14:256-267.

20. Smothers BA, Yahr HT, Ruhl CE: Detection of alcohol use disorders in general hospital admissions in the United States. Arch Intern Med 2004;164:749-756.

21. Goldstein RZ, Volkow ND: Drug addiction and its underlying neurobiological basis: Neuroimaging evidence for the involvement of the frontal cortex. Am J Psychiatry 2002; 159:1642-1652.

22. Kalivas PW, Volkow ND: The neural basis of addiction: A pathology of motivation and choice. Am J Psychiatry 2005; 162:1403-1413.

23. Nestler EJ, Malenka RC: The addicted brain. Sci Am 2004; 290:78-85.

24. American Psychiatric Association: Diagnostic and Statistical Manual of Mental Disorders, 4th ed, text revision. Washington, DC. American Psychiatric Association, 2000.

25. Miotto K, Compton P, Ling W, et al: Diagnosing addictive disease in chronic pain patients. Psychosomatics 1996;37: 223-235.

26. Savage SR: Preface: Pain medicine and addiction medicine—controversies and collaboration. J Pain Symptom Manage 1993;8:254-256.

27. Adams, LL, Gatchel RJ, Robinson RC, et al: Development of a self-report screening instrument for assessing potential opioid medication misuse in chronic pain patients. J Pain Symptom Manage 2004;27:440-459.

28. Reid MC, Engles-Horton LL, Weber MB, et al: Use of opioid medications for chronic noncancer pain syndromes in primary care. J Gen Intern Med 2002;17:173-179.

29. Michna E, Ross EL, Hynes WL, et al: Predicting aberrant drug behavior in patients treated for chronic pain: Importance of abuse history. J Pain Symptom Manage 2004;28:250-258.

30. Savage SR: Long-term opioid therapy: Assessment of consequences and risks. J Pain Symptom Manage 1996;1:274-286.

31. Portenoy RK: Opioid therapy for chronic nonmalignant pain: A review of the critical issues. J Pain Symptom Manage 1996;11:203-217.

32. Weissman DE, Haddox JD: Opioid pseudoaddiction—an iatrogenic syndrome. Pain 1989;36:363-366.

33. Lusher J, Elander J, Bevan D, et al: Analgesic addiction and pseudoaddiction in painful chronic illness. Clin J Pain 2006;22:316-324.

34. Compton PJ, Darakjian J, Miotto K: Screening for addiction in patients with chronic pain and "problematic" substance use: Evaluation of a pilot assessment tool, J Pain Symptom Manage 1998;16:355-363.

35. Fishbain DA, Cutler RB, Rosomoff HL, et al: Validity of self-reported drug use in chronic pain patients. Clin J Pain 1999;15:184-191.

36. Berndt S, Maier C, Schütz HW: Polymedication and medication compliance in patients with chronic non-malignant pain. Pain 1993;52:331-339.

37. Robinson RC, Gatchel RJ, Polatin P, et al: Screening for problematic prescription opioid use. Clin J Pain 2001;17: 220-228.

38. Mayfield D, McLeod G, Hall P: The CAGE questionnaire: Validation of a new alcoholism screening instrument. Am J Psychiatry 1974;131:1121-1123.

39. Brown RL, Rounds LA: Conjoint screening questionnaires for alcohol and drug abuse. Wisconsin Med J 1995;94:135-140.

40. Skinner HA: The drug abuse screening test. Addict Behav 1982;7:363-371.

41. Schnoll SH, Finch J: Medical education for pain and addiction: Making progress toward answering a need. J Law Med Ethics 1994;22:252-256.

42. Webster LR, Webster RM: Predicting aberrant behaviors in opioid-treated patients: Preliminary validation of the Opioid Risk Tool. Pain Med 2005;6:432-442.

43. Butler SF, Budman SH, Fernandez K, Jamison RN: Validation of a screener and opioid assessment measure for patients with chronic pain. Pain 2004; 112:65-75.

44. U.S. Department of Justice: Don't Be Scammed By A Drug Abuser, 1999. Available at www.deadiversion.usdoj.gov/pubs/brochures/drugabuser.htm.

45. Uhl GR, Sora I, Wang Z: The mu opiate receptor as a candidate gene for pain: Polymorphisms, variations in expression, noci-ception, and opiate responses. Proc Natl Acad Sci USA 1999;96:7752-7755.

46. Porter J, Jick H: Addiction rare in patients treated with narcotics. N Engl J Med 1980;302:123.

47. Perry S, Heidrich G: Management of pain during debridement: A survey of U.S. burn units. Pain 1982;13:267-280.

48. Potter JS, Hennessy G, Borrow JA, et al: Substance use histories in patients seeking treatment for controlled-release oxycodone dependence. Drug Alcohol Depend 2004;76:213-215.

49. Polatin PB, Kinney RK, Gatchel RJ, et al: Psychiatric illness and chronic low-back pain. The mind and the spine–which goes first? Spine 1993;18:66-71.

50. Covington EC, Kotz MM: Pain reduction with opioid elimination. Presented at the Annual Meeting of the American Academy of Pain Medicine, Feb 13, 2002, San Francisco.

51. Gardner EL: What we have learned about addiction from animal models of drug self-administration. Am J Addict 2000;9:285-313.

52. Daley DC, Marlatt GA, Spotts CE: Relapse prevention: Clinical models and intervention strategies. In Graham AW, Schultz TK, Mayo-Smith M, et al (eds): Principles of Addiction Medicine, 3rd ed. Washington, DC, American Society of Addiction Medicine, 2003, pp 467-485.

53. Joranson DE, Gilson AM: Drug crime is a source of abused pain medications in the United States. J Pain Symptom Manage 2005;30:299-301.

54. Boden SD, Davis DO, Dina TS, et al: Abnormal magnetic resonance scans of the lumbar spine in asymptomatic subjects. J Bone Joint Surg 1990;72A:403-408.

55. Coghill RC, McHaffie JG, Yen YF: Neural correlates of inter-individual differences in the subjective experience of pain. Proc Natl Acad Sci U S A 2003;100:8538-8542.

56. Kouyanou K. Pither CE. Wessely S: Medication misuse, abuse and dependence in chronic pain patients. J Psychosom Res 1997;43:497-504.

57. Mertens JR, Lu YW, Parthasarathy S, et al: Medical and psychiatric conditions of alcohol and drug treatment patients in an HMO: Comparison with matched controls. Arch Intern Med 2003;163:2511-2517.

58. Jamison RN, Kauffman J, Katz NP: Characteristics of methadone maintenance patients with chronic pain. J Pain Symptom Manage 2000;19:53-62.

59. Rosenblum A, Joseph H, Fong C, et al: Prevalence and characteristics of chronic pain among chemically dependent patients in methadone maintenance and residential treatment facilities. JAMA 2003;289:2370-2378.

60. American Society for Pain Management Nursing: ASPMN position statement: Pain management in patients with addictive disease. J Vasc Nurs 2004;22:99-101.

61. Levy RS, Hebert CK, Munn BG, et al: Drug and alcohol use in orthopedic trauma patients: A prospective study. J Orthop Trauma 1996;10:21-27.

62. Mehta V, Langford RM: Acute pain management for opioid dependent patients. Anaesthesia 2006;61:269-276.

63. Nedeljkovic SS, Wasan A, Jamison RN: Assessment of efficacy of long-term opioid therapy in pain patients with substance abuse potential. Clin J Pain 2002;18:S39-S51.

64. Joranson DE, Cleeland CS, Weissman DE, Gilson AM: Opioids for chronic cancer and non-cancer pain: A survey of state medical board members. Fed Bull: J Med Licensure Discipline 1992;79:15-49.

65. Gilson AM, Joranson DE: Controlled substances and pain management: Changes in knowledge and attitudes of state medical regulators. J Pain Symptom Manage 2001;21:227-237.

66. Dunbar, MB, Katz NP: Chronic opioid therapy for non-malignant pain in patients with a history of substance abuse: Report of 20 cases. J Pain Symptom Manage 1996;11:163-171.

67. Kennedy JA, Crowley TJ: Chronic pain and substance abuse: A pilot study of opioid maintenance. J Subst Abuse Treat 1990;7:233-238.

68. Currie SR, Hodgins DC, Crabtree A, et al: Outcome from integrated pain management treatment for recovering substance abusers. J Pain 2003;4:91-100.

69. Galanter M, Kleber HD (eds): Textbook of Substance Abuse Treatment, 3rd ed. Washington, DC, American Psychiatric Publishing, 2004, pp 337-443.

70. Passik SD, Kirsh KL: Opioid therapy in patients with a history of substance abuse. CNS Drugs 2004;18:13-25.

71. Savage SR: Opioid therapy of chronic pain: Assessment of consequences. Acta Anaesth Scand 1999;43:909-917.

72. Weaver M, Schnoll S: Abuse liability in opioid therapy for pain treatment in patients with an addiction history. Clin J Pain 2002; 18:S61-S69.

73. Katz NP: Behavioral monitoring and urine toxicology testing in patients on long-term opioid therapy. Presented at the 17th Annual Meeting of the American Academy of Pain Medicine, Feb 14-18, 2001, Miami, Fla.

74. Alaska Academy of Family Physicians: Urine Drug Testing in Primary Care, 2002. Available at www.alaskaafp.org/urine_test.htm.

75. Busto U, Sellers EM: Pharmacokinetic determinants of drug abuse and dependence: A conceptual perspective. Clin Pharmacokinet 1986:11:144-153.

76. Quinn DI, Wodak A, Day RD: Pharmacokinetic and pharmacodynamic principles of illicit drug use and treatment of illicit drug users. Clin Pharmocokinet 1997;33:344-403.

77. Mironer YE, Brown C, Satterthwaite J, et al: Relative misuse potential of different opioids: A large pain clinic experience. Presented at the 19th Annual Scientific Meeting of the American Pain Society, November 2-5, 2000, Atlanta.

78. Brookoff D: Abuse potential of various opioid medications. J Gen Intern Med 1993;8:688-690.

79. Kittelberger KP, Buchheit T, Rice SF: Self-extraction of intrathecal pump opioid. Anesthesiology 2004;101:807.

80. Gock S, Wong S, Stormo K, et al: Self-intoxication with morphine obtained from an infusion pump. J Anal Toxicol 1999;23:130-133.

81. Burton AW, Conroy B, Garcia E, et al: Illicit substance abuse via an implanted intrathecal pump. Anesthesiology 1998;89:1264-1267.

82. d'Elia G, von Knorring L, Marcusson J, et al: A double-blind comparison between doxepin and diazepam in the treatment of states of anxiety. Acta Psychiatr Scand Suppl 1974;255:35-46.

83. Bianchi GN, Phillips J: A comparative trial of doxepin and diazepam in anxiety states. Psychopharmacologia 1972;25:86-95.

84. Rickels K, Downing R, Schweizer E, et al: Antidepressants for the treatment of generalized anxiety disorder: A placebo-controlled comparison of imipramine, trazodone, and diazepam. Arch Gen Psychiatry 1993;50:884-895.

85. Kapczinski F, Lima MS, Souza JS, et al: Antidepressants for generalized anxiety disorder. Cochrane Database Syst Rev 2003;(2):CD003592.

86. Van Ameringen M, Mancini C, Pipe B, et al: Antiepileptic drugs in the treatment of anxiety disorders: Role in therapy. Drugs 2004;64:2199-2220.

87. Saletu-Zyhlarz GM, Abu-Bakr MH, Anderer P, et al: Insomnia related to dysthymia: Polysomnographic and psychometric comparison with normal controls and acute therapeutic trials with trazodone. Neuropsychobiology 2001;44:139-149.

88. Finlayson RE, Maruta T, Morse RM, et al: Substance dependence and chronic pain: Experience with treatment and follow-up results. Pain 1986;26:175-180.

89. Rome JD, Townsend CO, Bruce BK, et al: Chronic noncancer pain rehabilitation with opioid withdrawal: Comparison of treatment outcomes based on opioid use status at admission. Mayo Clinic Proc 2004;79:759-768.

90. Scheman J, Van Keuren C, Smith S, et al: Treatment response to chronic pain rehabilitation program among those with an active addictive disorder. Presented at the 6th International Conference on Pain and Chemical Dependency, Feb 7, 2004, Brooklyn, NY.

91. Tennant FS Jr, Rawson RA: Outpatient treatment of prescription opioid dependence: Comparison of two methods. Arch Intern Med 1982;142:1845-1847.

92. Ballantyne JC, Mao J: Medical progress: Opioid therapy for chronic pain. N Engl J Med 2003;349:1943-1953.

93. Roth SH, Fleischmann RM, Burch FX, et al: Around the clock, controlled-release oxycodone therapy for osteoarthritis-related pain: Placebo-controlled trial and long-term evaluation. Arch Intern Med 2000;160:853-860.

94. Robbins L: Long-acting opioids for severe chronic daily headache. Headache Q 1999;10:135-139.

95. Saper JR, Lake AE 3rd, Hamel RL, et al: Daily scheduled opioids for intractable head pain: Long-term observations of a treatment program. Neurology 2004;62:1687-1694.

96. Kalso E , Edwards JE, Moore RA, et al: Opioids in chronic noncancer pain: Systematic review of efficacy and safety. Pain 2004;112:372-380.

97. Brown J, Klapow J, Doleys D, et al: Disease-specific and generic health outcomes: A model for the evaluation of long-term intrathecal opioid therapy in noncancer low back pain patients. Clin J Pain 1999;15:122-131.

43–1 Drug Abuse Screening Test (DAST)

1. Have you used drugs other than those required for medical reasons? (Yes/No)
2. Have you abused prescription drugs? (Yes/No)
3. Do you abuse more than one drug at a time? (Yes/No)
4. Can you get through the week without using drugs (other than those required for medical reasons)? (Yes/No)
5. Are you always able to stop using drugs when you want to? (Yes/No)
6. Do you abuse drugs on a continuous basis? (Yes/No)
7. Do you try to limit your drug use to certain situations? (Yes/No)
8. Have you had "blackouts" or "flashbacks" as a result of drug use? (Yes/No)
9. Do you ever feel bad about your drug abuse? (Yes/No)
10. Does your spouse (or parents) ever complain about your involvement with drugs? (Yes/No)
11. Do your friends or relatives know or suspect you abuse drugs? (Yes/No)
12. Has drug abuse ever created problems between you and your spouse? (Yes/No)
13. Has any family member ever sought help for problems related to your drug use? (Yes/No)
14. Have you ever lost friends because of your use of drugs? (Yes/No)
15. Have you ever neglected your family or missed work because of your use of drugs? (Yes/No)
16. Have you ever been in trouble at work because of drug abuse? (Yes/No)
17. Have you ever lost a job because of drug abuse? (Yes/No)
18. Have you gotten into fights when under the influence of drugs? (Yes/No)
19. Have you ever been arrested because of unusual behavior while under the influence of drugs? (Yes/No)
20. Have you ever been arrested for driving while under the influence of drugs? (Yes/No)
21. Have you engaged in illegal activities to obtain drugs? (Yes/No)
22. Have you ever been arrested for possession of illegal drugs? (Yes/No)
23. Have you ever experienced withdrawal symptoms as a result of heavy drug intake? (Yes/No)
24. Have you had medical problems as a result of your drug use (e.g., memory loss, hepatitis, convulsions, or bleeding)? (Yes/No)
25. Have you ever gone to anyone for help for a drug problem? (Yes/No)
26. Have you ever been in hospital for medical problems related to your drug use? (Yes/No)
27. Have you ever been involved in a treatment program specifically related to drug use? (Yes/No)
28. Have you been treated as an outpatient for problems related to drug abuse? (Yes/No)

PART
VI

Nerve Block Techniques
H. T. Benzon and J. Rathmell

44 Local Anesthetics for Regional Anesthesia and Pain Management

Francis V. Salinas, Khalid Malik, and Honorio T. Benzon

Regional anesthesia and postoperative analgesia involve the administration of an appropriate mass of local anesthetic agent at targeted sites within the central neuraxial space or along major plexus or peripheral nerves to produce surgical anesthesia, manage acute pain, or both. Local anesthetic agents may also be administered systemically or topically to provide analgesia for acute or chronic pain syndromes.

Achievement of surgical anesthesia with a single-injection technique requires safely producing an adequate level of reversible neural conduction block within an appropriate period while minimizing the potential risk of local anesthetic systemic toxicity. Surgical anesthesia may not only require an adequate depth of sensory anesthesia, but also motor blockade to provide optimal surgical conditions. In contrast, the goals of acute postoperative analgesia (or labor analgesia) via continuous administration of local anesthetics are achievement of an adequate depth of sensory analgesia while minimizing the degree of motor blockade, thereby facilitating postoperative functional recovery.

This chapter will provide an overview of the pharmacology of local anesthetics commonly used for acute and chronic pain management. A detailed review of the mechanism of action of local anesthetics is followed by a review of the physiochemical properties that determine the pharmacodynamic and pharmacokinetic profiles of individual local anesthetic agents. The potential for systemic toxicity of local anesthetics is followed by an overview of the clinical applications of the most commonly used local anesthetics for regional anesthesia and pain management. The last section, focusing on regional anesthesia and acute pain management, will cover the most commonly used analgesic adjuvants. Lastly, local anesthetics for chronic pain management will focus on the clinical applications of intravenous local

anesthetic infusions, oral mexiletine, and topical lidocaine (patch).

MECHANISM OF ACTION OF LOCAL ANESTHETICS

Electrophysiologic Basis of the Resting Membrane Potential

An understanding of normal neuronal conduction is essential to the understanding of the mechanism of action of local anesthetics. The neuronal cell membrane is composed of a hydrophobic lipid bilayer embedded with transmembrane proteins. This lipid bilayer allows the passage of small nonpolar molecules, but is relatively impermeable to polar ions. Charged ions must traverse the cell membrane via ion-specific protein channels that permit the passage of certain ions across the cell membrane while excluding others. The semipermeable nature of the lipid bilayer serves as a barrier to ion movement, allowing it to separate ionic charges electrically between the intracellular and extracellular aqueous milieu. Movement through these ion-specific channels is primarily based on two forces: (1) the relative concentration of the ions (concentration gradient); and (2) the relative charge (electrical potential gradient) on each side of the cell membrane. Therefore, ions will tend to diffuse from areas of higher concentration to areas of lower concentration, as well as to areas of opposite polarity (electrical charge).

The resting membrane potential of neuronal cells is usually about −60 to −70 mV, with the inside of the cell interior more negatively charged relative to the cell exterior. The resting membrane potential is a result of ionic disequilibrium created by a special transmembrane protein (the Na^+,K^+-ATPase ion pump) and the diffusion potential of ions. The Na^+,K^+ pump actively cotransports three Na^+ ions out of the cell and two K$^+$ ions into the cell powered by adenosine triphosphate (ATP) hydrolysis. The result is an intracellular-to-extracellular K$^+$ ratio of 120 to 4 mM (30:1) and an extracellular-to-intracellular Na$^+$ ratio of 140 to 15 mM (10:1). The separation of the positive and negative charges carried by the net movement of these ions creates an electrical field across the cell membrane described as individual diffusion potentials (or transmembrane voltages) for Na$^+$ and K$^+$. The transmembrane voltage exerts a force on an ion toward the opposite polarity in a magnitude proportional to the voltage difference. The Nernst equation for a specific ion mathematically describes the magnitude of the transmembrane voltage (Nernst potential) that exerts a force matching the diffusional force, thereby resulting in cessation of ion flow (equilibrium) through the channel.

At rest, the neuronal cell membrane predominantly demonstrates a selective permeability for K$^+$ ions. These K$^+$ channels are called nongated or leak channels, indicating that they are always open, regardless of the membrane potential.[1] Thus, the resting cell membrane behaves primarily as a K$^+$ electrode, with the Nernst equation predicting a resting membrane potential of –88 mV. The simplified Nernst equation can be described as follows:

$$E_K = (-58.1\ mV)\ \log[K^+]_i/[K^+]_o$$

where E_K = potassium equilibrium potential, $[K^+]_i$ = potassium ion concentration inside the cell, and $[K^+]_o$ = potassium ion concentration outside the cell.

K$^+$ equilibrium, however, is not the only factor in determining the resting membrane potential. In addition to K$^+$ channels, neuronal cell membranes have additional voltage-independent channels that allow leak currents of Na$^+$, Cl$^-$, and other ions (each with their respective Nernst potentials), which also contribute to the final resting membrane potential of –60 to –70 mV.[2]

Electrophysiologic Basis of the Action Potential

Generation of the Action Potential

The excitability of neurons, the ability to generate a large, rapid change of membrane voltage in response to a very small stimulus, is based on the action potential. It is the action potential that leads to the process of rapid depolarization—loss of the negative transmembrane potential because of inward current of positive charges—usually progressing to a positive transmembrane potential, and then rapidly repolarizing back to a negative transmembrane potential (Fig. 44–1). In contrast to the dependence of the resting membrane potential on K$^+$ disequilibrium

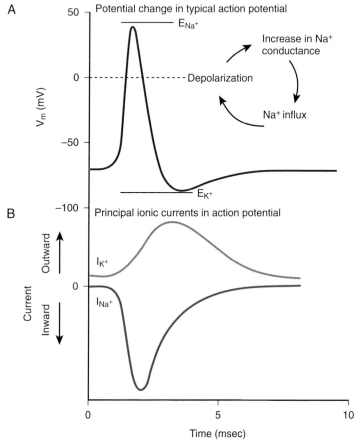

Figure 44–1. The action potential. **A,** The membrane potential change for a typical action potential rapidly rises from a resting membrane potential of –70 mV, reaching a maximum near the Nernst potential for Na$^+$ (E_{Na^+}) and then declining, with the negative undershoot near the Nernst potential for K$^+$ (E_{K^+}). The action potential is triggered by a positive feedback loop, in which the initial depolarizing stimulus leads to further depolarization. V$_m$, membrane potential. **B,** Two principal ionic currents give rise to the action potential. Note that the outward K$^+$ current has a slower rate of increase in amplitude and is slightly delayed in onset compared with the rapidly rising inward Na$^+$ current. (Used with permission from Study RE: The structure and function of neurons. In Hemmings H, Hopkins P [eds]: Foundations of Anesthesia Basic Sciences for Clinical Practice, 2nd Ed. Philadelphia, Elsevier, 2006, p 229.)

(and diffusion across nonvoltage-gated K^+ channels), the action potential depends on both Na^+ and K^+ disequilibrium that is maintained by the Na^+,K^+ pump, and ionic currents across voltage-gated Na^+ and K^+ channels.[2]

Voltage-gated Na^+ channels progress though several conformations based on temporal changes in the membrane potential. These channels are in a resting (closed) conformation at the resting membrane potential, but are suddenly activated (opened) if membrane depolarization reaches a threshold potential. Because the equilibrium potential for Na^+ is approximately +50 mV, activation of voltage-gated Na^+ channels, which now confers a relative selectivity of the cell membrane for Na^+ ions, transforms the cell membrane into Na^+ electrode, and allows a large inward current of Na^+ ions because of the large electrochemical gradient generated by the $Na+,K+$ pump (see Fig. 44–1B). The initial inward current of Na^+ through the voltage-gated channels leads to more depolarization and thus more channel opening, initiating a positive feedback loop until all the Na^+ channels that can be potentially activated are activated and the membrane potential reaches the equilibrium potential for Na^+ (see Fig. 44–1A).

Following activation of Na^+ channels and initiation of the action potential, the process must be terminated in order for the membrane to return to its resting potential. After a few milliseconds of suddenly opening, the Na^+ channels spontaneously undergo another conformational change to an inactivated state. Almost simultaneously, the K^+ gated channels also become activated and open in response to depolarization produced by the action potential, but do so with a small delay and at a slower rate compared with the Na^+ channels. Because the equilibrium potential for K^+ is approximately –90 mV, when the K^+ channels (during an action potential) open, the positive membrane potential creates a very strong electrochemical gradient for K^+ ions that leads to a positive outward ionic current, which will tend to return the membrane potential back to its negative resting state (see Fig. 44–1A). Because of the slight delay in the opening of the K^+ channels, the outward current of K^+ does not oppose the earlier inward current of Na^+ until after the action potential has been generated (see Fig. 44–1B). The positive feedback loop that generated the action potential continues until some of the Na^+ channels have become inactivated and enough of the K^+ channels have opened to change the balance of current to a net outward positive current, which results in membrane repolarization. During the process of repolarization, inactivated Na^+ channels and open K^+ channels revert to resting (closed) conformations.

Thus, a three-state kinetic scheme conceptually describes the changes in Na^+ channel conformation that accounts for the changes in Na^+ conductance during depolarization and repolarization.[2] The resting (closed), activated (open), and inactivated conformations correspond to the state of the Na^+ channel during the resting membrane potential, during the

action potential when the channel rapidly conducts an inward Na^+ current, and when the Na^+ channel stops conducting the inward Na^+ current immediately following the activated state, respectively. As a result of the voltage- and time-dependent conformational changes of the Na^+ and K^+ channels, the net movement of positive current is inward during the depolarizing phase of the action potential and outward during the phase of repolarization.

The initial change in membrane potential required to reach the activation threshold necessary to initiate the regenerative and self-sustaining process of the action potential is not an absolute value, but rather depends on the dynamic interactions between the voltage-gated Na^+ and K^+ channels. If the depolarizing stimulus is inadequate in duration, there will be insufficient time for Na^+ channels to become activated. If the rate of Na^+ channel activation is inadequate, there will not be enough activated Na^+ channels at one time to reach the threshold potential. Furthermore, voltage-gated K^+ channels would begin to increase their outward current, thereby preventing the membrane from reaching the activation threshold. Thus, successful generation of an action potential requires a depolarizing stimulus of adequate speed, amplitude, and duration such that the depolarizing effect of the activated Na^+ channels becomes sufficiently self-sustaining to overcome the opposing influences of Na^+ channel inactivation and the hyperpolarizing effects of K^+ channel activation.

Structural and Functional Anatomy of Peripheral Nerves

The structure of neurons is fairly uniform, consisting of a cell body, dendrites, which receive input from other neurons via synapses, and an axon, which transmits output from the neuron in the form of a propagated action potential to other neurons. As axons course through the body, they are intimately associated with non-neural glial cells. Oligodendrocytes are glial cells located predominantly in the white matter of the spinal cord, where they provide electrical insulation around central nervous system (CNS) axons in the form of myelin. In the peripheral nervous system, glial cells associated with axons are termed Schwann cells, and together they form a nerve fiber (Fig. 44–2A). The nerve fiber is the basic structural and functional unit of peripheral nerves. Individual nerve fibers are embedded within a loose, delicate connective tissue called the endoneurium, and are arranged in parallel bundles (nerve fascicles) of varying size, number, and arrangement, depending on type and location of a particular nerve. In turn, each fascicle is surrounded by a second connective tissue sheath, the perineurium, which consists of multiple concentric layers of flattened cells, whose number depends on the size of the fascicle (see Fig. 44–2B). Finally, the epineurium is the outermost connective sheath that serves to bind and encase the fascicles into a peripheral nerve (see Fig. 44–2C).

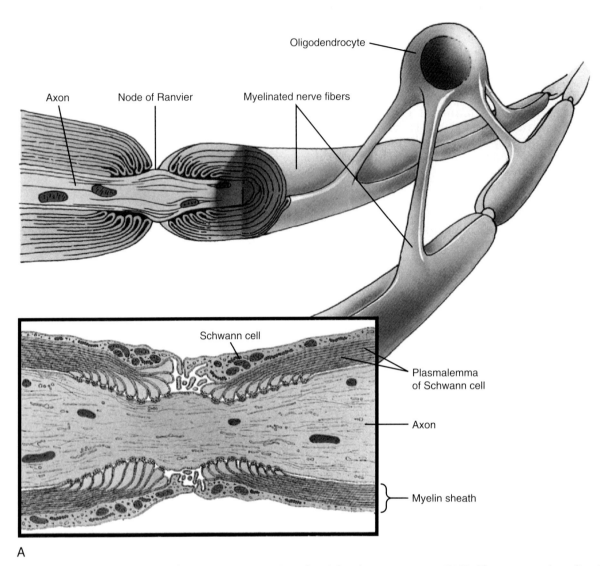

A

Figure 44–2. A, Myelination in the central nervous system (CNS) and peripheral nervous system (PNS). The purpose of myelination is to provide axons with electrical insulation, which significantly increases nerve conduction velocity. The lipid-rich membranes of the myelinating glial cells are wrapped around the axons to produce this insulation. Schwann cells *(figure insert)* myelinate axons in the PNS, whereas oligodendrocytes form myelin in the CNS.

Axons with a diameter greater than 1 μm are encased by the lipid bilayer plasma membrane of its associated Schwann cell. The cell membrane spirals around the axon, arranging the membranes in concentric layers and resulting in the formation of a myelin sheath (see Figs. 44–2A, B, and D). In a myelinated nerve fiber, a single axon is enclosed by a series of Schwann cells arranged along its length. The region where two adjacent Schwann cells are adjoined and the myelin is interrupted is referred to as a node of Ranvier (see Fig. 44–2D). Axons smaller than 1 μm in diameter indent the plasma membrane of a Schwann cell and become entrenched in separate troughs, but are not encased by myelin (see Fig. 44–2B). All axons in the peripheral nervous system are insulated by Schwann cell surfaces, but myelin only forms around larger axons. Thus, it is apparent that individual axons are surrounded by multiple

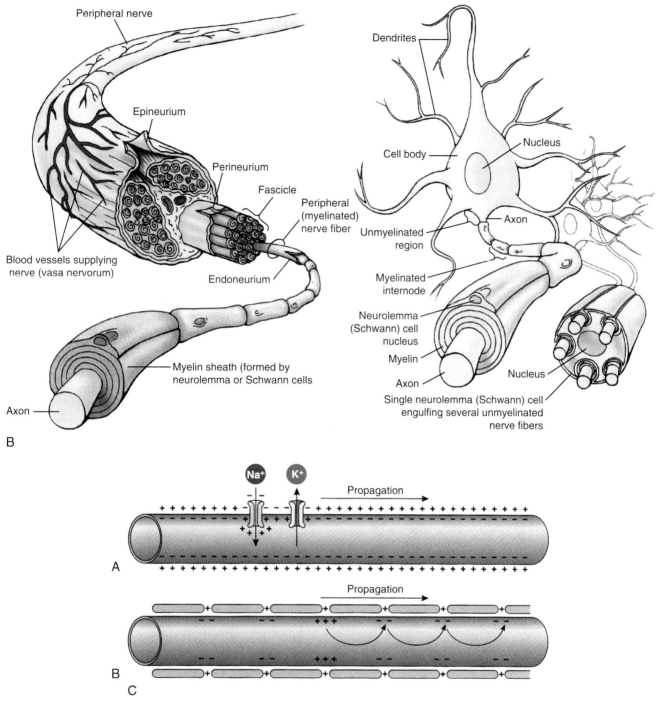

Figure 44–2, cont'd. B, The structure and function of a peripheral nerve. The nerve fiber is the basic structural and functional unit of peripheral nerves. Individual nerve fibers are embedded within a loose, delicate connective tissue called the endoneurium, arranged in parallel bundles (nerve fascicles) of varying size, number, and configuration, depending on the type and location of a particular nerve. In turn, each fascicle is surrounded by a second connective tissue sheath, the perineurium, which consists of multiple concentric layers of flattened epithelial cells connected by tight junctions. The number of layers depends on the size of the fascicle. The perineurium isolates the milieu of the axon from the surrounding endoneurial space, thereby preventing potentially harmful substances from entering the axon. The perineurium is one of the tissue barriers that must be penetrated so local anesthetics can reach their target sites within the axonal membrane. Finally, the epineurium is the outermost connective tissue sheath that serves to bind and encase the fascicles into a peripheral nerve. In the PNS, a single Schwann cell may encase multiple axons if the peripheral nerves are nonmyelinated. If the peripheral nerve is myelinated, one Schwann cell always wraps around one axon. **C,** In the PNS, the node of Ranvier (see *A*) is the site where two adjoining Schwann cells come together. This site is marked by small gaps in the myelin sheath, which forms the structural basis for saltatory conduction, allowing nerve impulses to be conducted at a higher velocity. (**A and C,** adapted from Gartner LP and Hiatt JL (eds): Color Textbook of Histology, 3rd edition. Philadelphia, Saunders, 2007, pp 185-218; and **B,** adapted from Moore KL, Dalley AF (eds): Clinically Oriented Anatomy, 5th edition. Philadelphia, Lippincott, Williams & Wilkins, 2006, pp 47-58.)

protective layers of connective tissue and lipid membranes, which may serve as substantial barriers for local anesthetic to reach the axon.

Propagation of the Action Potential

Once an action potential is generated, propagation of the electrical impulse along the axon is required for the information to be transmitted. Both the action potential and impulse propagation exhibit an all-or-none behavior. This is particularly important in the case of impulse propagation, because either the locally generated action potential generates a threshold potential at adjacent membrane segments and causes propagation along the axon, or local depolarization ceases. The action potential is propagated along the axon by continuous coupling between excited and nonexcited regions of the cell membrane.

The conduction velocity of the propagated impulse varies tremendously among neurons and, depending on their physiologic function, ranges from several meters per second (m/sec) to as much as 75 to 120 m/sec. The primary determinants of conduction velocity are axon diameter and myelination. The conduction velocity of an axon increases in proportion to the square root of the radius. Myelination can increase conduction velocity up to 10-fold over that achieved in nonmyelinated axons and all mammalian nerves with a diameter larger than 1 to 2 μm are myelinated. Myelin is a tight, multilayered wrapping of the Schwann cell lipid bilayer membrane that encloses individual myelinated axons. Although the myelin layer can account for over half the thickness of a neuron's diameter, it is not continuous along the length of the axon. Separating the myelinated regions, usually every 1 to 2 mm along the axon, are very short distances where the neuronal cell membrane is exposed to the extracellular aqueous milieu. Na^+ channels are highly concentrated at the nodes of Ranvier but, in contrast, are distributed along the entire length of an unmyelinated axon.[3]

An action potential generated from an adjacent node causes a depolarization sufficient to trigger the opening of enough Na^+ channels in the next node, resulting in an action potential that is then conducted to the next node. The process of an action potential propagated from node to node is called saltatory conduction, which allows very high conduction velocities along relatively small axons. The presence of myelin also accelerates conduction velocity because of increased electrical insulation of the axon. Thus, in contrast to nonmyelinated axons, which increase conduction velocity only with the square root of the diameter, conduction velocity increases directly with the axon diameter of myelinated axons. In summary, the action potential propagation along nonmyelinated axons requires achievement of the threshold potential at immediately adjacent membranes, whereas myelinated axons require generation of the threshold potential at a subsequent node of Ranvier.

Classification of Nerve Fibers

The diameter and myelination of a neuron not only correlate with conduction velocity, but also with message-carrying function. Because different functions require different conduction velocities along axons, conduction velocity can be used to classify neurons. Most nerves (including the dorsal root ganglia) in the peripheral nervous system that transmit information between their axons and the CNS contain a mixture of myelinated and nonmyelinated neurons that carry out both afferent and efferent functions. Neurons are categorized into three major classes, designated A, B, and C, corresponding to peaks in the temporal distribution of their conduction velocities (Table 44–1).[4] Group A includes large, myelinated, somatic afferent and efferent axons, group B includes smaller myelinated, preganglionic, autonomic efferent axons, and group C includes the smallest and nonmyelinated afferent axons.

Group A axons are further subdivided based on decreasing conduction velocity and diameter (see Table 44–1):
- A-delta fibers include both sensory afferent axons from proprioceptors of skeletal muscle and motor efferent axons to skeletal muscle responsible for motor function and reflex activity.
- A-beta afferent fibers include cutaneous mechanoreceptors responsible for touch and pressure.
- A-gamma efferent fibers to muscle spindles control muscle tone.

Table 44–1. Classification of Afferent and Efferent Nerve Fibers Based on Axon Diameter and Conduction Velocity

FIBER CLASS	DIAMETER (μm)	MYELIN	CONDUCTION VELOCITY (m/sec)	INNERVATION	FUNCTION
A alpha	12-20	+++	75-120	Afferent from muscle spindle proprioceptors Efferent to skeletal muscle	Motor and reflex activity
A beta	5-12	+++	30-75	Afferent from cutaneous mechanoreceptors	Touch and pressure
A gamma	3-6	++	12-35	Efferent to muscle spindles	Muscle tone
A delta	1-5	++	5-30	Afferent pain and thermoreceptors	"Fast" pain, touch, and temperature
B	<3	+	3-15	Preganglionic sympathetic efferent	Autonomic function

Data from Stranding S: Nervous system. In Stranding S, Ellis H, Healy JC, et al (eds): Gray's Anatomy, 39th ed. Edinburgh, Elsevier Churchill Livingstone, 2005, p 55.

- A-delta afferent fibers are responsible for temperature sensation and pain, typically described as sharp, intense, or lancinating.

Group C fibers carry information about temperature as well as pain, particularly pain that is perceived as dull, burning, or aching. Thus, afferent sensory axons have two separate conduction pathways that carry pain-related information. The myelinated A-delta fibers conduct signals (fast pain) rapidly and the nonmyelinated C fibers conduct signals (slow pain) relatively slower.

Refractory Period

An important characteristic of the action potential is the refractory period, which is the time after initiation of an action potential when it is impossible or more difficult to generate a second action potential. The absolute refractory period is the time from initial depolarization to when repolarization is almost complete. The basis for the absolute refractory period is Na^+ channel inactivation, when it is impossible to recruit a sufficient number of Na^+ channels to generate a second depolarizing stimulus until the previously activated Na^+ channels have recovered from inactivation, which takes several milliseconds.

The relative refractory period, when a stronger than predicted stimulus is required to generate a second action potential, follows the absolute refractory period. The basis for the relative refractory period is K^+ channel activation, when the repolarizing outward current of K^+ ions results in a brief period of hyperpolarization, such that a stronger depolarizing stimulus is required to activate the population of Na^+ channels that in the meantime have "reprimed" for activation. The refractory period limits the rate at which action potentials can be generated, which is an important aspect of neuronal signaling. Additionally, the refractory period facilitates unidirectional propagation of the action potential along the axon. Because the membrane on each side of the action potential is refractory, a second action potential approaching behind the first action potential will be terminated.

Molecular Mechanism of Action

Local anesthetics render neurons less excitable by directly binding to and inhibiting the ability of voltage-gated Na^+ channels to conduct Na^+ currents.[5,6] They do so by inhibiting the conformational changes that form the basis of Na^+ channel activity. Therefore, local anesthetics fundamentally inhibit the generation and propagation of the action potential. Understanding the concepts of local anesthetic ionization, the three-state kinetic scheme of the Na^+ channel, and tonic versus phasic block provide the basis for understanding the mechanism of reversible local anesthetic–induced conduction blockade.

The most commonly used local anesthetics are tertiary amines that exist in a dynamic equilibrium between an electrically neutral base form and a posi-

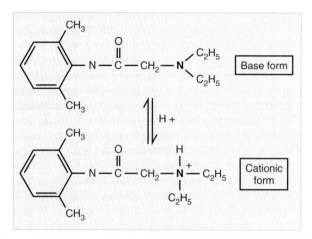

Figure 44-3. The equilibrium between the basic (neutral) lipid-soluble form and cationic (charged) form of lidocaine. The amount of the neutral basic form available for diffusion across the neural membrane is governed by the pK_a of the lidocaine and of the other local anesthetics and the pH of the surrounding milieu. (Adapted from Cosmo A, Difazio AM, Woods JC: Drugs commonly used for nerve blocking. In Abrams BC, Benzon HT, Hahn MB, et al (eds): Raj's Practical Management of Pain, 3rd Edition. St. Louis, Mosby, 2000, pp 557-573. With permission.)

tively charged protonated (cationic) form, depending on the pK_a and the pH of the aqueous milieu where local anesthetics are deposited (Fig. 44–3). The ratio of the charged (ionized) form (LAH^+) to the neutral form (LA) is described by the Henderson-Hasselbalch equation:

$$LAH^+/LA = 10^{pK_a - pH}$$

Thus, the pK_a is the hydrogen ion concentration at which concentration of the neutral form is equal to the concentration of the charged cation. Both ionized and nonionized drugs with local anesthetic activity can inhibit Na^+ channels. Permanently neutral local anesthetics (e.g., the secondary amine, benzocaine) freely permeate the hydrophobic neuronal membrane and inhibit Na^+ conductance and impulse conduction, whether applied directly intracellularly or deposited extracellularly, demonstrating that ionization is not absolutely essential for local anesthetic activity.

In contrast, quaternary derivatives of local anesthetics, which are permanently charged, have very little membrane permeability and exhibit potent inhibition of Na^+ conductance and conduction blockade only when they are directly infused into the neuronal cytoplasm.[7] Tertiary amines, which have pK_a values from about 7.7 to 8.9, exhibit more potent Na^+ channel inhibition when applied in an external alkaline pH, or when applied directly within neuronal cytoplasm at a neutral or slightly acidic pH. Thus, tertiary amine local anesthetics must first traverse the hydrophobic milieu of the neuronal membrane in the neutral form and, having reached the cytoplasm, become ionized to bind more avidly to the Na^+ channel.

The neutral local anesthetic benzocaine exhibits little change in Na^+ channel inhibition with an increased frequency of stimulation, whereas tertiary amine local anesthetics exhibit different degrees of Na^+ channel inhibition based on the frequency of neuronal stimulation. In the presence of local anesthetics, measures of Na^+ channel activity—either Na^+ currents or action potential amplitude—are decreased by 30% to 50% with low-frequency stimulation, which is known as tonic block. If the stimulation is repeatedly applied at a higher frequency, Na^+ channel activation is decreased incrementally for each stimulus until a new steady-state level of Na^+ channel inhibition is reached. This is called frequency-dependent, or phasic, block. The degree of Na^+ channel inhibition produced by the phasic block is quickly reversed to tonic levels when frequency of stimulation is decreased or stopped.

The differences in the degree of Na^+ channel inhibition exhibited by tertiary amine local anesthetics during tonic block compared with phasic block are best explained by the presence of a single local anesthetic receptor site within the Na^+ channel that demonstrates differing affinities for local anesthetics based on the specific Na^+ channel conformation.[5,6] Specifically, open and inactivated Na^+ channel conformations possess much higher affinities for local anesthetics as compared with the resting conformation. With each successive depolarization, the percentages of local anesthetic bound to Na^+ channels incrementally increase and conversely, the percentages of resting Na^+ channels incrementally decrease. Local anesthetic binding to the Na^+ channels exhibits a dynamic equilibrium; dissociation occurs in the time interval between successive depolarizations, which is exemplified by an increase in Na^+ channel activity when the frequency of stimulation is decreased. However, the process of local anesthetic dissociation, which would allow the Na^+ channel to return to a resting conformation, occurs at a slower rate compared with the rapid voltage-regulated return to a resting Na^+ channel conformation that occurs during the physiologic process of repolarization.

PHYSIOCHEMICAL PROPERTIES AND RELATIONSHIP TO ACTIVITY AND POTENCY

The clinically useful local anesthetics share the same basic structure, consisting of a lipophilic, substituted aromatic (benzene) ring linked to a hydrophilic tertiary amino group (except for benzocaine, which has a secondary amino group) via an intermediate alkyl chain consisting of either an amide or ester linkage. The type of linkage separates the local anesthetics into two chemically distinct classes based on their primary site of metabolism: (1) the aminoamides (Fig. 44–4A and B) are metabolized in the liver by microsomal enzymes; and (2) the aminoesters (see Fig. 44–4C) undergo rapid hydrolysis in the blood by pseudocholinesterase enzymes. The clinical activity of local anesthetics is determined by several intrinsic physiochemical properties (Table 44–2)[8]: lipid solubility, ionization, protein binding, and chirality.

Lipid Solubility

The aromatic ring is the major determinant of the lipophilic (lipid solubility) nature of local anesthetics. Lipid solubility correlates with the tendency of the local anesthetic molecule to associate with and pass through the membrane lipid bilayer into the axoplasm. Lipid solubility is increased by the type of alkyl substitution, either on the aromatic ring or the remaining structure. For example, in the aminoester class, a butyl substitution on the aromatic ring of procaine converts the compound to tetracaine (see Fig. 44–4C), increasing the lipid solubility nearly 60-fold. In the mepivacaine family (N-alkylpiperidine xylidide) of aminoamides, a change from a methyl to a butyl substitution on the tertiary amino group converts mepivacaine to bupivacaine (see Fig. 44–4B), which increases the lipid solubility 26-fold. A minor shortening of the four-carbon butyl group of bupivacaine to the three-carbon substitution (propyl) converts the compound to ropivacaine (see Fig. 44–4B), which is approximately 4.5 times less lipid soluble compared with bupivacaine.

Lipid solubility is an important determinant of local anesthetic potency and duration of action. The larger and more lipophilic local anesthetics are able to permeate the neural membrane more readily and thus can bind Na^+ channels with greater affinity. Although increasing lipid solubility may hasten penetration of neural membranes, it may also result in increased uptake and sequestration of local anesthetics in myelin and other lipid-soluble perineural compartments. Thus, the net effect of increasing lipid solubility is usually a decreased speed of onset of action.[9] Additionally, the duration of action is also increased as sequestration of local anesthetic molecules within the myelin and surrounding perineural compartments creates a depot for slow release of local anesthetics. Lastly, increased lipid solubility parallels intrinsic local anesthetic potency.[5,10] This observation may be explained by the correlation between lipid solubility and both Na^+ channel affinity and the ability to alter Na^+ channel conformation by directly affecting the fluidity of the neuronal lipid bilayer membrane.[11]

Ionization

Local anesthetics in solution are weak bases that exist in equilibrium between the lipid-soluble neutral form, or as the charged hydrophilic form. The pK_a, or dissociation constant, of a local anesthetic is the pH at which the different forms are present in equivalent amounts. The combination of the perineural and intraneural pH and pK_a of a particular local anesthetic determines the percentage of each compound that exists in each form (see Table 44–2).[8] The primary site of action of local anesthetics appears to be within the intracellular side of the transmembrane voltage-gated sodium channel, and the charged form appears to be the predominantly active form.[5,6] Thus, pK_a generally correlates with the speed of onset, because penetration by the neutral lipid-soluble form across the

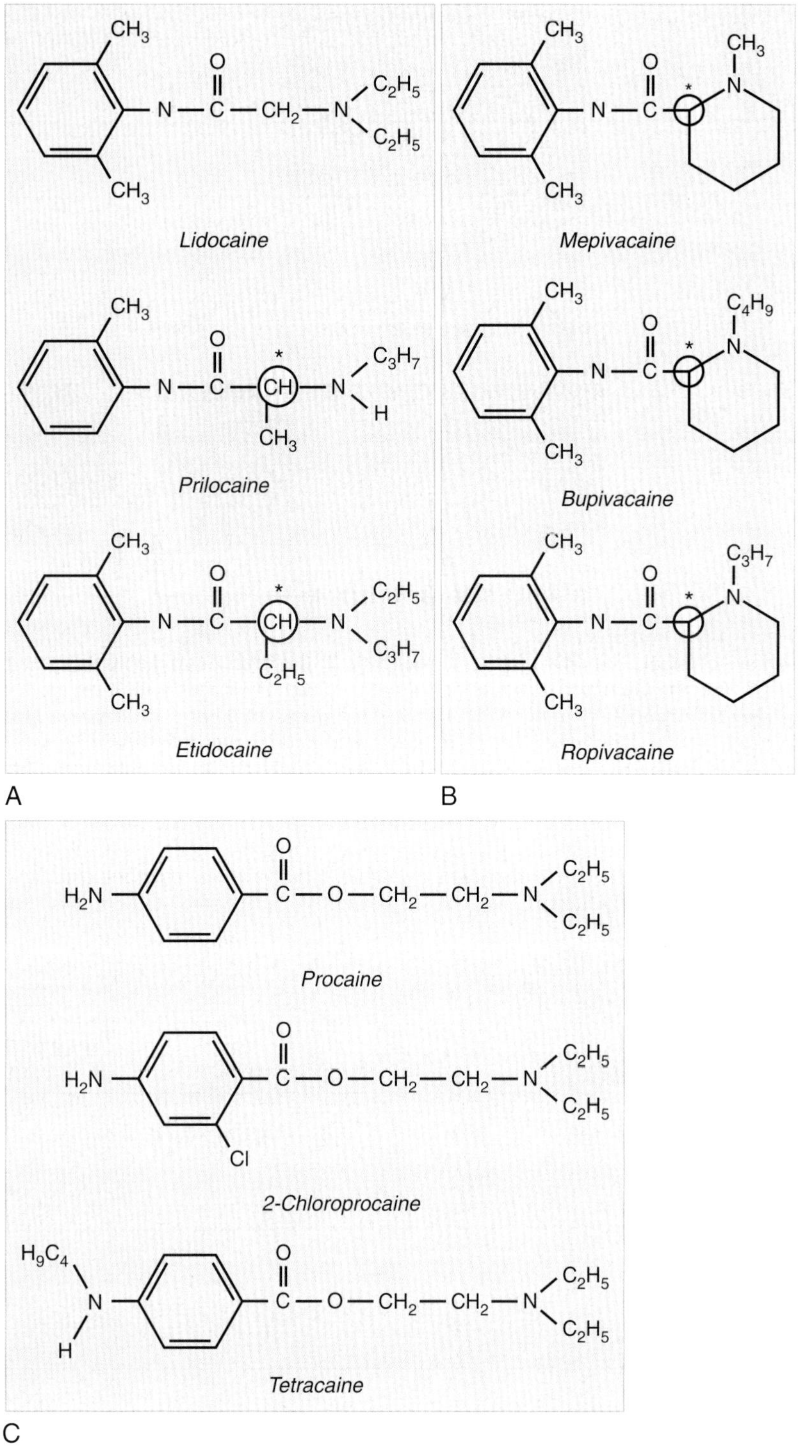

Figure 44–4. Chemical structures of local anesthetics. **A,** Group 1 aminoamides. **B,** Group 2 aminoamides. This group is characterized by the addition of a piperidine ring (basic xylidine component of lidocaine), resulting in the basic pipecolyl xylidine structure of mepivacaine, bupivacaine, and ropivacaine. **C,** Aminoesters. Note the location of the asymmetric carbons, when present *(asterisk)*. (Adapted from Cosmo A, Difazio AM, Woods JC: Drugs commonly used for nerve blocking. In Abrams BC, Benzon HT, Hahn MB, et al (eds): Raj's Practical Management of Pain, 3rd Edition. St. Louis, Mosby, 2000, pp 557-573. With permission.)

neural membrane is the primary mechanism for local anesthetics to gain access to the local anesthetic binding site. Once in the axoplasm, the neutral base form of the local anesthetic can accept a hydrogen cation and equilibrate into the active cationic form (Fig. 44–5).[12] The percentage of local anesthetics existing in the neutral lipid-soluble form at the physiologic pH of 7.4 is inversely proportional to the pK$_a$ of a specific local anesthetic. Thus, the lower the pK$_a$ is for a local anesthetic within a specific local tissue pH, the higher the percentage of local anesthetic exists in the lipid-soluble neutral form, which will hasten the penetration of the neural membrane and onset of action (see Fig. 44–5). For example, the local environmental milieu within inflamed tissue may often be acidic and hyperemic. The lower pH will drive the equilibrium toward a higher percentage of the lipid-insoluble cationic form and decrease the penetration across the neural membrane. Also, the increased vascularity may increase the systemic absorption of local anesthetics and further impair the clinical activity of the administered local anesthetic. Given that the pK$_a$

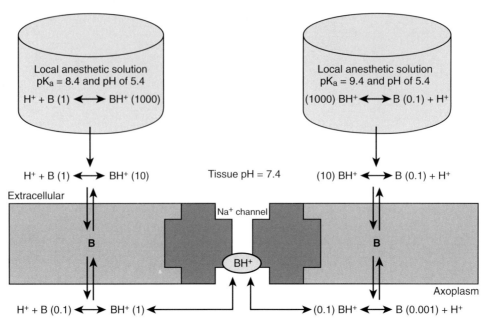

Figure 44–5. The primary site of action of local anesthetics appears to be within the intracellular side of the transmembrane voltage-gated sodium channel. The ratio of a local anesthetic in the neutral (lipid-soluble) base form and the ionized (lipophobic) form is dependent on its pK_a and the pH of the surrounding solution. A local anesthetic with a pK_a of 8.4 is 3 pH units (10^3) away from its 50% equilibrium state when contained in a commercially prepared solution at a pH of 5.4, with an approximate ionized-to-nonionized molecule ratio of 1000:1. When the local anesthetic is injected into normal body tissues (physiologic pH of 7.4) and subsequently gains access to the axoplasm, the ratio decreases by a factor of 10^2 to 10:1. For a local anesthetic with a pK_a of 9.4, the ratio of nonionized to ionized molecule in a commercially prepared solution at a pH of 5.4 is even higher (1000:0.1 or 10,000:1), with a subsequent ratio in normal body tissue of 100:1. The difference in the pK_a between the two local anesthetic solutions results in a 10-fold difference in the amount of nonionized lipid-soluble local anesthetic available to diffuse across the lipid membrane, and subsequently a 10-fold difference in the amount of the ionized active form of local anesthetic available to bind the Na^+ channel. (Adapted from Salinas FV: Pharmacology of drugs used for spinal and epidural anesthesia and analgesia. In Wong CW [ed]: Spinal and Epidural Anesthesia. New York, McGraw Hill, 2007, pp 75-109.)

Table 44–2. Physiochemical Properties of Clinically Useful Local Anesthetics and Opioids for Spinal and Epidural Anesthesia

LOCAL ANESTHETIC	pK_a	IONIZED (%)*	PARTITION COEFFICIENT (LIPID SOLUBILITY)	PROTEIN BINDING (%)
Amides				
Lidocaine	7.9	76	366	64
Mepivacaine	7.6	61	130	77
Bupivacaine	8.1	83	3420	95
Levobupivacaine	8.1	83	3420	>97
Ropivacaine	8.1	83	775	94
Etidocaine	7.7	66	7317	94
Esters				
Chloroprocaine	8.7	95	810	—
Procaine	8.9	97	100	6
Tetracaine	8.5	93	5822	94

*At pH 7.4.
From Salinas FV: Analgesic: Ion channel ligands, sodium channel blockers, local anes thetics. In Evers AS, Maze M (eds): Anesthetic Pharmacology: Physiologic Principles and Clinical Practice. Philadelphia, Elsevier, 2003, p 507.

of most local anesthetics is between 7.7 and 8.9, one may anticipate that bicarbonate would have the most pronounced effect when added to a local anesthetic solution into which epinephrine was added by the manufacturer. Such prepackaged solutions are in a more acidic form than plain (epinephrine) local anesthetic solutions so as to prolong shelf life.

Protein Binding

Protein binding also influences the clinical activity of local anesthetics, because only the unbound form is able to diffuse across neural membranes and exert pharmacologic activity. In general, increased lipid solubility is associated with increased protein binding to tissue and plasma proteins.[10,13] It has been erroneously assumed that increased protein binding correlates with increased duration of activity because of increased binding at the Na^+ channel receptor. However, the degree of protein binding does not correlate with binding to the protein structure of the Na^+ channel. Studies have suggested that the binding and dissociation of local anesthetic molecules from the Na^+ channel occurs in matters of seconds, regardless of the degree of protein binding.[14] Plasma protein binding is believed to correlate closely with the degree of protein binding on the neuronal membrane. It is likely that highly protein-bound local anesthetics are removed from the nerve at a slower rate, resulting in slower uptake and systemic absorption and prolonged duration of action. Thus, the duration of action associated with increased protein binding is primarily determined by the relatively slow diffusion of local anesthetics into and out of the nerve.

The most important binding proteins of local anesthetics in plasma are albumin and α_1-acid glycoprotein (AAG). Local anesthetics exhibit a low-affinity and high-capacity association with albumin and a high-affinity but low-capacity association with AAG. Although local anesthetics bind to AAG preferentially, binding to AAG is easily saturated with a clinically relevant dose of local anesthetic.[15] Once AAG saturation occurs, additional local anesthetic binding is to albumin. Because the binding capacity of albumin is very high, albumin can bind local anesthetics without saturation at concentrations in plasma exceeding clinically desired levels. Despite the high-capacity capability of albumin, high plasma concentrations of local anesthetics increase the risk for systemic toxicity by increasing the amount of the active unbound form. This is because the degree of protein binding is concentration-dependent and, as the transition from AAG binding to albumin binding occurs, the degree of protein binding consistently decreases. Plasma protein binding is also affected by plasma pH, such that the percentage of local anesthetic that is bound decreases as pH decreases. This is clinically relevant because with the development of acidosis (e.g., as occurs with significant seizure activity secondary to CNS toxicity), the amount of unbound active drug increases, even though the total plasma concentration of local anesthetic remains the same. Other clinical factors also influence the degree of plasma protein binding. AAG plasma concentrations are decreased in pregnancy and in the newborn.[16] In contrast, AAG plasma concentrations are increased as a result of various pathophysiologic conditions such as surgery, trauma, and certain disease states (e.g., uremia), with a subsequent increase in plasma protein binding.[17,18]

Chirality

Clinically useful local anesthetics, with the exception of lidocaine (which is achiral), ropivacaine (the *S*-enantiomer of a bupivacaine homologue, with a propyl rather than a butyl chain at the tertiary amino group), and levobupivacaine (the *S*-enantiomer of bupivacaine) are formulated as racemic mixtures.[19,20] Racemic drugs are 1:1 mixtures of two types of molecules (stereoisomers) bearing identical chemical composition and binding, but with a different three-dimensional spatial orientation around an asymmetric carbon chiral carbon (Fig. 44–6A).[21] Local anesthetics exhibit a specific type of stereoisomerism termed *enantiomerism*, in which the pair of stereoisomers in three-dimensional projection cannot be superimposed on each other.[21] Although enantiomers of local anesthetics have identical physiochemical properties, they exhibit potentially different clinically pharmacodynamic (e.g., potency and potential for systemic toxicity) and pharmacokinetic activity because of differences in their interaction with biologic receptors (Na^+ channel). For example, *R*-enantiomers appear to have increased in vitro potency for conduction blockade of both neuronal and cardiac Na^+ channels, and thus would have greater therapeutic efficacy as well as the potential for systemic toxicity. In contrast, *S*-enantiomers have been demonstrated to have lower potential for systemic toxicity compared with racemic mixtures and the *R*-enantiomer.[22]

PHARMACOKINETICS

Local anesthetics are not metabolized when administered in perineural compartments such as the central neuraxial space or along a major plexus or

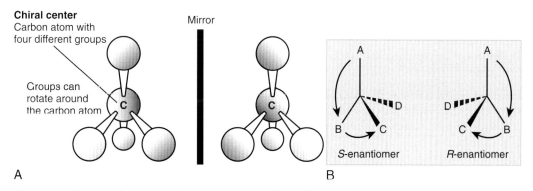

Figure 44–6. A, Molecule with a chiral center and it enantiomers. **B,** Three-dimensional projection of a pair of enantiomers that cannot be superimposed on each other. Bonds represented as solid lines are in the plane of the paper, those drawn with a dotted lines project away, and those represented by a wedge project toward the reader. (Adapted from Burke D, Henderson DJ: Chirality: A blueprint for the future. Br J Anaesth 2002;83:563-576.)

peripheral nerve. Instead, they are eliminated from these perineural spaces almost completely via vascular absorption into the systemic circulation. Once absorbed into the systemic circulation, the dose and duration of local anesthetic administration, the rate of tissue distribution, and the rate of biotransformation and elimination determine the concentration of local anesthetics in the blood and the potential for systemic toxicity.

Systemic Absorption

In general, the local anesthetics with decreased systemic absorption will have an increased margin of safety for clinical use. The rate and extent of systemic absorption are determined by a number of factors, including the tissue perfusion at the site of injection, the dose and duration of local anesthetic administration, the physiochemical characteristics of the local anesthetic agent, and the addition of epinephrine.

The relative amounts of fat and tissue perfusion surrounding the site of local anesthetic administration will interact with the local anesthetic agent because of its physiochemical properties to affect the rate of systemic uptake. In general, areas with more tissue perfusion will have a more rapid and complete uptake compared with those with more fat, irrespective of the specific local anesthetic agent. Thus, the rates of absorption from various sites of local anesthetic administration generally decrease in the following order: interpleural > intercostal > caudal > epidural > brachial plexus > lumbar plexus > femoral or sciatic. The higher the total dose of local anesthetic administered, the greater the systemic absorption and resulting maximum blood levels (C_{max}). Within the clinical range of doses used for local anesthetics, this relationship is almost linear and is relatively unaffected by local anesthetic concentration or volume and speed of administration.[12]

Physiochemical properties of local anesthetic agents will influence systemic absorption. Thus, the more potent agents, with higher lipid solubility and protein binding, will result in a slower rate of systemic absorption and C_{max}. Increased binding to neural and non-neural tissue probably account for this clinical observation.

The effects of epinephrine have been discussed earlier. Epinephrine decreases the rate of systemic absorption by counteracting the inherent vasodilating property of most local anesthetics. The reduction in C_{max} with the addition of epinephrine is most effective for the less lipid-soluble, less potent, shorter acting agents, because increased tissue binding rather than local tissue perfusion may be the greater determinant of systemic absorption for long-acting agents (Table 44–3).[12]

Distribution

After systemic absorption, local anesthetics are rapidly distributed throughout all body tissues, but the relative concentrations in different tissues depend on organ perfusion, partition coefficient of local anesthetic between different tissue compartments, and plasma protein binding. There is an initial rapid uptake from plasma by highly perfused tissues and a relatively slower uptake, primarily into skeletal muscle and fat. Thus, the end-organs of main concern for toxicity are the cardiovascular (heart) and central nervous (brain) systems, because both are considered members of the vessel-rich group and will have local anesthetic rapidly distributed to them. Despite the high tissue perfusion, regional blood flow and tissue levels of local anesthetics within these organ systems will not initially correlate with systemic blood levels because of hysteresis.[22] Regional and not systemic pharmacokinetics determines the subsequent pharmacodynamic effects, so systemic blood levels may not correlate with clinical effects of local anesthetics on end-organs.[23,24] Regional pharmacokinetics of local anesthetics for the heart and brain has not been fully elucidated; thus, the volume of distribution at steady state (VD_{ss}) is often used to describe local anesthetic distribution. However, VD_{ss} describes the extent of total body distribution and may be inaccurate for specific tissue groups.

Table 44–3. Effects of Addition of Epinephrine to Local Anesthetics

EFFECT	INCREASE DURATION OF ACTION	DECREASE BLOOD LEVELS (%)	CONCENTRATION OF EPINEPHRINE
Peripheral Nerve Blocks			
Bupivacaine	++	10-20	1:200,000
Lidocaine	++	20-30	1:200,000
Mepivacaine	++	20-30	1:200,000
Ropivacaine	––	0	1:200,000
Epidural Anesthesia			
Bupivacaine	++	10-20	1:200,000-1:300,000
Levobupivacaine	––	0	1:200,000-1:300,000
Lidocaine	++	20-30	1:200,000-1:600,000
Mepivacaine	++	20-30	1:200,000
Ropivacaine	––	0	1:200,000

++, overall supported; ––, overall not supported.
Adapted from Salinas FV: Analgesic: Ion channel ligands, sodium channel blockers, local anesthetics. In Evers AS, Maze M (eds): Anesthetic Pharmacology: Physiologic Principles and Clinical Practice. Philadelphia, Elsevier, 2003, p 507.

The main plasma proteins involved in local anesthetic binding are AAG and albumin. As noted, local anesthetics exhibit a high-affinity, low-capacity binding with AAG and a low-affinity, high-capacity binding with albumin. The clinical observation that AAG increases as a result of surgical trauma, with a subsequent rise in plasma protein binding, influences the potential toxicity of continuous perineural infusions of local anesthetics. This is because the possibility of accumulation, and the associated potential risk of toxicity, depend primarily on drug concentration, route of administration, and duration of infusion.

Continuous epidural infusions of dilute long-acting amide local anesthetics are commonly used to provide postoperative analgesia. Over the time course of continuous epidural infusion, total local anesthetic plasma concentration may progressively increase, raising the concern for systemic toxicity. Pharmacokinetic data have confirmed that total local anesthetic plasma concentrations increase steadily during 48 to 72 hours of continuous epidural[25-27] and peripheral perineural[28] local anesthetic administration. However, despite the progressive increase in total plasma concentration, the unbound concentration reaches peak steady-state levels well below the thresholds for systemic toxicity. During continuous infusion, postoperative increases in plasma protein levels (predominantly AAG) enhance the capacity of plasma protein binding, resulting in the divergence of total and unbound pharmacodynamically active concentrations. Thus, the pharmacokinetic data support the clinical experience of the safety of continuous epidural and peripheral perineural infusions of dilute local anesthetic solutions.

Elimination

Aminoesters are metabolized via the rapid hydrolysis of the ester bond by plasma pseudocholinesterase. The rate of enzymatic degradation varies, with chloroprocaine being degraded most rapidly, tetracaine the least rapidly, and procaine being intermediate. The aminoesters are metabolized to p-aminobenzoic acid (PABA), which is responsible for allergic reactions associated with this class of local anesthetics. Aminoamide metabolism occurs via enzymatic degradation, primarily in the liver. Thus, clearance of amide local anesthetics is highly dependent on hepatic perfusion, hepatic extraction, hepatic enzymatic function, and plasma protein binding. Excretion of metabolites of aminoamides occurs via renal excretion, with less than 5% of the unchanged drug excreted into urine. In general, local anesthetics with higher rates of clearance will have a greater margin of safety.

Clinical Pharmacokinetics

The primary benefit of understanding the systemic pharmacokinetics of local anesthetics involves two considerations—administration of the minimum effective dose to provide the appropriate degree of conduction blockade balanced against the desire to minimize the risk of systemic toxicity. Both physical and pathophysiologic characteristics will influence an individual patient's pharmacokinetics, making it difficult to estimate C_{max}. There is evidence for increased systemic levels of local anesthetics in newborn infants and older adults secondary to decreased clearance and increased systemic absorption.[29] The correlation of resultant systemic levels between dose of local anesthetics administered and patient weight is often inconsistent. The effects of gender on clinical pharmacokinetics have not been well defined, although pregnancy may decrease clearance.

Pathophysiologic states such as low cardiac output, right-to-left cardiac shunting, and decreased hepatic clearance because of decreased hepatic perfusion or impaired hepatic enzyme function can substantially decrease elimination; lower doses of local anesthetics should be administered in these clinical conditions. Excretion of the metabolites of the aminoamide local anesthetics occurs via the kidney, with less than 5% of the unchanged drug excreted into the urine. In contrast to previous theories, renal disease may have a potentially significant effect on the pharmacokinetics of aminoamide local anesthetics. Pharmacokinetic studies have demonstrated decreased clearance of lidocaine and ropivacaine, as well as their metabolites, in patients with severe renal insufficiency not receiving hemodialysis.[18] However, in patients with end-stage renal disease undergoing regular hemodialysis, there was no demonstrable evidence of decreased local anesthetic clearance.[30]

TOXICITY OF LOCAL ANESTHETICS

Systemic Toxicity

Local anesthetic systemic toxicity occurs because of unintentional intravascular (intra-arterial or intravenous) injection or because of unexpected excessive systemic absorption after perineural administration, both of which result in excessive blood levels of local anesthetics. In general, the central nervous system (CNS) is more susceptible to local anesthetic toxicity than the cardiovascular system (CVS). Thus, the dose and blood level of local anesthetic required to produce characteristic manifestations of early CNS toxicity (e.g., lightheadedness, aural symptoms, muscular tremors, myoclonic jerking) are typically lower than those required to produce signs of CVS toxicity (e.g., dysrhythmias, contractile dysfunction, and ultimately cardiovascular collapse).

Since Albright first reported patients manifesting cardiac arrest after administration of potent long-acting amide local anesthetics (primarily bupivacaine and etidocaine),[31] the overall incidence of CNS toxicity has decreased from 0.2% to 0.01%, although the data to support these incidences are probably incomplete. Based on two large prospective case series from France, the estimated incidence of CNS toxicity (seizures) with epidural anesthesia has stayed constant over the past decade, at 0.01%.[32,33] In contrast, the estimated incidence of CNS toxicity with peripheral nerve blocks has decreased from 0.07% to 0.01% over the same interval.[32,33]

Central Nervous System Toxicity

Local anesthetics readily cross the blood-brain barrier and produce a dose-dependent pattern of CNS manifestations. Signs of generalized CNS local anesthetic toxicity are dependent on the absolute and rate of rise of the plasma concentration of the specific local anesthetic agent. CNS toxicity is typically manifested as a two-stage pathophysiologic process. At lower toxic concentrations, an excitatory phase occurs (early auditory phenomenon, muscle tremors and twitching, and generalized tonic-clonic seizures) because of blockade of central inhibitory neuronal pathways. As the plasma concentration of local anesthetic progressively increases, blockade of central inhibitory and excitatory neurons leads to generalized CNS depression (hypoventilation and respiratory arrest). The incidence and temporal course of CNS toxicity vary after different regional anesthetic techniques, as would be expected because of differences in the likelihood of unintentional intravascular injection or unexpected systemic absorption, as well as the effect of CNS depressant drugs commonly administered while these techniques are being carried out.[34] A more rapid rate of intravascular administration of local anesthetic will also affect the manifestations of CNS toxicity, because the accelerated rate of increases in plasma concentration will decrease the plasma concentration required to induce seizures.[35,36]

The potential for systemic CNS toxicity approximately parallels the intrinsic anesthetic potency of the specific local anesthetic agents.[37] In general, decreased local anesthetic protein binding and clearance will increase the potential for CNS toxicity. Other clinical factors that can influence the potential for CNS toxicity include the acid-base status of the patient and the addition of epinephrine to local anesthetic solutions. Acidosis and hypercapnia increase the risk for CNS toxicity. An elevation in $PaCO_2$ enhances cerebral blood perfusion, which augments local anesthetic delivery to the CNS.[38] In addition, intracellular acidosis facilitates conversion of the neutral form of the local anesthetic agent to the cationic form. Because the cationic form does not diffuse across the lipid bilayer membrane, intracellular accumulation of the active cationic form will enhance Na^+ channel binding and the apparent CNS toxicity of local anesthetics. In addition, hypercapnia and acidosis decrease plasma protein binding of local anesthetics and increase the free fraction available for diffusion across neuronal membranes.

Epinephrine is frequently added to local anesthetic solutions to decrease the rate and extent of systemic absorption, as well as to provide an early clinical indicator of unintentional direct intravascular admin-

istration. The reduction in C_{max}, as well as the ability to detect unintentional intravascular administration, should contribute to an increased margin of safety. However, the convulsive threshold for systemically administered local anesthetics with epinephrine is significantly decreased compared with that of plain local solutions. The mechanisms by which epinephrine increases systemic toxicity have not been fully elucidated and may likely be multifactorial.[39] Epinephrine results in hypertension via peripheral vasoconstriction, and the resulting hyperdynamic circulation may augment systemic toxicity via increased perfusion and local anesthetic delivery to the CNS.[38] A study in rats has demonstrated that epinephrine added to local anesthetic solution significantly increases the unbound plasma concentration of local anesthetic compared with plain solutions. Moreover, the increase in unbound plasma concentration of local anesthetic with epinephrine solutions was reflected by comparable increases in the extracellular local anesthetic concentration in the brain compared with animals given only plain solutions.[40] Thus, epinephrine may augment CNS toxicity by increasing the percentage of the unbound, pharmacologically active fraction available for transport across intracerebral neuronal cells.

Cardiovascular System Toxicity

In general, substantially larger doses of local anesthetics are required to produce CVS toxicity compared with CNS toxicity. The pattern of CVS toxicity has indirect and direct effects. With the initial excitatory phase that accompanies early CNS toxicity, the activated sympathetic nervous system response results in tachycardia and hypertension. However, with increasingly toxic plasma concentrations, direct local anesthetic–mediated arrhythmogenicity and negative ionotropic effects supersede the CNS-mediated sympathetic effects.

Similar to CNS toxicity, the potential for CVS toxicity parallels the anesthetic potency of the agent. The more potent and lipid-soluble local anesthetics that are clinically useful (levobupivacaine, ropivacaine, and especially bupivacaine) demonstrate an inherently higher cardiotoxicity profile than less potent (and less lipid-soluble) agents.[37] Also, the more potent local anesthetics appear to have different patterns and concentration thresholds for local anesthetic CVS toxicity compared with the less potent agents. For example, increasingly toxic doses of lidocaine lead to cardiovascular collapse secondary to progressive myocardial depression, from which resuscitation is uniformly successful with ongoing pharmacologic support with epinephrine (Fig. 44–7).[41] In contrast, increasingly toxic doses of the long-acting amides often lead to fatal cardiovascular collapse as a result of ventricular fibrillation resistant to resuscitation.

The more potent local anesthetics consistently possess greater potential for arrhythmogenicity. Although all local anesthetics block the cardiac con-

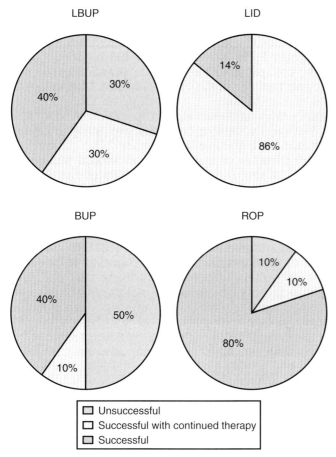

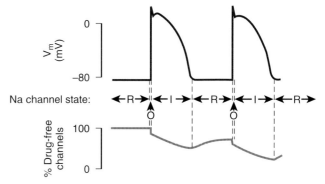

Figure 44–8. Relationship between cardiac action potential *(top),* sodium channel state *(middle),* and sodium channel block *(bottom)* by bupivacaine. Sodium channels are predominantly in the resting (R) form during diastole, open (O) transiently during the upstroke of the action potential, and are in the inactivated (I) form during the plateau of the action potential. Block of sodium channels by bupivacaine accumulates during the action potential (systole), with recovery during diastole. Vm, membrane potential.

Figure 44–7. Pie diagram representing resuscitative outcomes for each group of anesthetized dogs after incremental overdosage with levobupivacaine (LBUP), lidocaine (LID), bupivacaine (BUP), and ropivacaine (ROP). (Adapted from Groban L, Deal DD, Vernon JC, et al: Cardiac resuscitation after incremental overdose with lidocaine, bupivacaine, levobupivacaine, and ropivacaine in anesthetized dogs. Anesth Analg 2001;92:37-43.)

duction system through a dose-dependent blockade of Na⁺ channels, two features of bupivacaine's Na⁺ channel blocking characteristics may enhance its arrhythmogenicity. First, bupivacaine exhibits a much stronger binding affinity to resting and inactivated sodium compared with lidocaine. Second, local anesthetics bind to Na⁺ channels during systole and dissociate during diastole. Bupivacaine dissociates from Na⁺ channels much more slowly than lidocaine. Furthermore, bupivacaine dissociates so slowly that duration of diastole at a physiologic heart rate (60 to 180 beats/min) does not allow enough time for complete recovery of Na⁺ channels and, as a result, conduction block accumulates (Fig. 44–8).[42] In contrast, lidocaine fully dissociates from Na⁺ channels during diastole, with little accumulation of conduction block. Thus, enhanced arrhythmogenicity of the potent long-acting local anesthetics, especially bupivacaine, on the cardiac conduction system may explain their increased potential to produce sudden cardiovascular collapse through malignant arrhythmias.

Increased potency for direct depression of myocardial contractility from the more potent local anesthetics may also contribute to cardiovascular collapse. Dose-dependent reductions in myocardial contractility occur with local anesthetic systemic toxicity and their potential for negative ionotropy roughly parallels their potency for neuronal conduction block.[43] A number of mechanisms may account for the negative ionotropic effect of the potent long-acting local anesthetics. Bupivacaine has been shown to interfere with myocardial calcium uptake.[44] Additionally, the larger butyl substitutions responsible for the increased nerve conduction blocking potency have also been shown to increase affinity for binding to β₂-adrenergic receptors, which inhibits intracellular cyclic adenosine monophosphate (cAMP) production.[45] CNS-mediated mechanisms may also be involved in the increased CVS toxicity of bupivacaine. The nucleus tractus solitarius in the medulla is an important region for autonomic control of the CVS. Neuronal activity in the nucleus tractus solitarius of rats is profoundly diminished by intravenous administration of bupivacaine immediately preceding the development of hypotension.[46] Peripheral effects of bupivacaine on the autonomic and vasomotor systems may also augment its CVS toxicity. Bupivacaine possesses potent peripheral inhibitory effects on sympathetic reflexes[47] and direct vasodilating properties,[48] which may also exacerbate CVS collapse. Thus, multiple direct effects of the potent local anesthetic agents directly on the myocardium, autonomic nervous system, and peripheral vasculature may explain the increased CVS toxicity, as well as the refractoriness to standard resuscitation measures.

Management of Local Anesthetic Systemic Toxicity

Management of local anesthetic systemic toxicity depends on the severity of the clinical presentation. Because plasma levels of local anesthetics associated with minor adverse reactions decrease rapidly, as long as normal physiologic processes are maintained, such reactions may be allowed to resolve spontaneously, provided that attention is paid to maintaining airway patency, adequate oxygenation, and hemodynamic support. Seizures may be terminated with small intravenous doses of midazolam (0.05 to 0.1 mg/kg), sodium thiopental (1 to 2 mg/kg), or propofol (0.5 to 1.5 mg/kg). If generalized tonic-clonic seizures are not terminated with these intravenous anesthetics, intravenous administration of succinylcholine (0.5 to 1.0 mg/kg) followed by endotracheal intubation is indicated. Prompt termination of seizure activity is important to prevent the rapid development of severe metabolic acidosis associated with tonic-clonic muscular activity.[49]

Because the vast majority of systemic toxic reactions are secondary to unintentional intravascular administration or, less commonly, to systemic absorption of excessive doses of local anesthetics, efforts should be made to minimize the potential risks. The clinician must be cognizant of the risk factors associated with the regional analgesic technique selected and the physiologic status of the patient that may predispose to clinically significant systemic toxic reactions. Proper patient preparation includes appropriate monitoring of vital signs (e.g., heart rate, blood pressure, oxygenation) as well as continuous electrocardiography. Evidence has demonstrated the added value of monitoring changes in T-wave amplitude (decrease)[50] associated with the traditional epinephrine intravascular test dose, as well as S-wave amplitude (increase),[51] which may provide earlier detection of bupivacaine-induced cardiac depression.

Techniques that reduce the likelihood of unintentional intravascular administration should be used, as well as the lowest effective dose of local anesthetic. Although no single measure is completely reliable in preventing severe systemic toxicity, the following guidelines should be used[52]:

- The administered dose should be fractionated, with frequent aspiration to assess for possible intravascular placement of the needle or catheter.
- When large doses of long-acting local anesthetics are planned for a peripheral nerve block, epinephrine (in the absence of contraindications) should be added to local anesthetic solutions to help identify unintentional intravascular administration (the test dose) and to decrease systemic absorption.[53]
- Be aware of the different clinical criteria and their limitations for a positive test dose during different clinical situations.[52]
- For techniques with a higher potential risk of unintentional intravascular administration or excessive systemic absorption, consider using a long-acting agent (e.g., ropivacaine) with the least potential for cardiotoxicity.

When local anesthetic systemic toxicity progresses to cardiovascular collapse, the guidelines for advanced cardiac life support (ACLS) should be followed.[54] Because hypotension is usually the result of a combination of direct myocardial depression and peripheral vasodilation, vasoactive agents with both β_1 and α_1 (ephedrine, phenylephrine, or both) activity should be considered in incremental doses until the desired response is obtained. In case of cardiovascular collapse associated with malignant ventricular dysrhythmias, studies have indicated that vasopressin and amiodarone may be superior alternatives to epinephrine and lidocaine, respectively.[55,56]

With unresponsive cardiovascular collapse, cardiopulmonary bypass or, more practically, intravenous administration of lipid emulsion should be considered. A canine model has demonstrated the remarkable ability of intravenous lipid administration to effect resuscitation from bupivacaine-induced cardiac toxicity, even after 10 minutes of unsuccessful open cardiac massage.[57] The mechanisms by which intravenous lipid emulsion results in successful resuscitation of local anesthetic-induced cardiac toxicity are not yet fully elucidated. It is likely that the lipid emulsion provides an additional compartment into which excessive plasma local anesthetic can partition and facilitate removal of local anesthetic from the myocardium,[58] although improved direct myocardial mitochondrial metabolism may also play a role.[59] Subsequent to the promising animal data, case reports have confirmed the remarkable ability of intravenous lipid administration to help patients with severe local anesthetic-induced toxicity reverse rapidly.[60,61] Based on animal data, human case reports, and lack of toxicity of lipid emulsion infusions, intravenous lipid treatment for severe CVS local anesthetic toxicity should be considered if conventional measures fail, and certainly before cessation of resuscitative efforts.

CLINICAL APPLICATIONS

Local anesthetics may be administered as a single injection, usually as a large volume of a concentrated long-acting local anesthetic solution, with the goal of providing an extended duration of postoperative analgesia. Although this technique is less complex, it has the disadvantage of a fixed duration of analgesia determined by the physiochemical profile and anatomic administration of the specific agent, as well an increased potential risk of local anesthetic toxicity when a relatively large amount of drug is administered over a relatively short period of time.[35] More commonly, dilute solutions of local anesthetics (with or without analgesic adjuvants such as opioids, epinephrine, or clonidine) are now administered via a central neuraxial (epidural or, less commonly, spinal) or a peripheral nerve or plexus catheter.[62,63] Selection of a local anesthetic for pain management will depend on several factors:

- The decision to use the specific regional anesthetic technique for operative or postoperative analgesia, or both
- Time estimate of the need for postoperative analgesia, which determines the decision to use a single-injection or continuous catheter technique

- The need for motor blockade or, more commonly in the postoperative setting, the need for adequate motor function to facilitate ambulation and acceleration of functional recovery

This section will provide an overview of the clinical characteristics of the different classes of drugs (esters and amides) and individual local anesthetic agents that may be used for acute postoperative pain management.

Aminoester Agents

As a group, the aminoester local anesthetics are not commonly used for acute postoperative pain management.

Procaine

Procaine is the oldest aminoester local anesthetic in clinical use. It is a derivative of PABA, with a relatively high pK_a and low lipid solubility, which gives it a slow onset and a short duration of action. This reduces its usefulness when compared with other short-acting local anesthetics, such as lidocaine. It may be used for spinal anesthesia, but is no longer used as frequently because of its poorer quality of spinal anesthesia compared with lidocaine and its higher incidence of nausea and pruritus when combined with low-dose intrathecal fentanyl.

2-Chloroprocaine

2-Chloroprocaine (2-CP) is a derivative of procaine, with a rapid onset of action and an even more rapid degree of elimination (plasma half-life, less than 30 seconds) via plasma cholinesterase metabolism. It is most commonly used at 2% to 3% concentrations for rapid onset of epidural anesthesia or peripheral nerve block. The most common clinical application for 2-CP is epidural anesthesia for cesarean delivery because of its rapid onset of action and low potential for systemic toxicity in both the parturient and fetus. Older preparations of 2-CP contained sodium metabisulfite as a preservative, which has been linked to severe neurologic injury following unintentional intrathecal administration of doses intended for epidural anesthesia.[64] Subsequently, 2-CP was reformulated with ethylenediaminetetraacetic acid (EDTA) as the preservative but, in doses larger than 40 mL, the chelating action of EDTA has been implicated as the cause of severe paravertebral muscle spasm that occurs after resolution of the epidural anesthesia.[65] More recently, preservative-free 2-CP has been shown to provide a rapid onset of reliable spinal anesthesia, with a predictably dose-dependent short duration of action. This may potentially allow it to replace lidocaine as the drug of choice for short-duration ambulatory spinal anesthesia.[66,67]

Tetracaine

Tetracaine is the butylaminobenzoic acid derivative of procaine. Its marked lipid solubility makes it a potent long-acting agent that produces a dense sensory and motor block. It remains a popular choice for spinal anesthesia, with a relatively rapid onset (3 to 5 minutes) and duration of action of 2 to 3 hours, which may be extended to 4 to 6 hours with the addition of epinephrine. It has excellent topical analgesic properties and remains the agent of choice for topical ophthalmic anesthesia. The use of tetracaine for epidural anesthesia or peripheral nerve blocks is limited, because the larger doses required increase the risk for systemic toxicity.

Aminoamide Agents

Lidocaine

Lidocaine was the first aminoamide local anesthetic introduced into clinical practice. Its physiochemical profile allows rapid neural membrane penetration and produces a rapid onset of anesthesia, usually with an intermediate duration of action (1 to 2 hours, depending on the site of administration). Lidocaine remains a popular choice for epidural anesthesia, providing dense sensory and motor block of the trunk and lower extremities. Lidocaine use for peripheral nerve and plexus anesthesia is also common, but has the disadvantage of providing only a limited duration of analgesia into the postoperative recovery period. Because lidocaine has poorer sensorimotor dissociation (as compared with the long-acting amides), it is not commonly used for postoperative analgesic infusions, in which preserved motor function is desired to facilitate ambulation and active range of motion of extremities. Although lidocaine had been an ideal choice in the past for outpatient spinal anesthesia, concerns regarding its association with a limited duration of buttock and bilateral lower extremity discomfort, occasionally painful enough to interfere with normal activity, has significantly decreased its use over the past decade.[68]

Although continuous perineural infusions of lidocaine have limited usefulness because of the poor separation of sensorimotor block, continuous intravenous administration of lidocaine has been shown to be a useful adjunct for acute postoperative pain management. Prospective, randomized, double-blind studies have demonstrated that perioperative intravenous administration of lidocaine (bolus followed by a continuous infusion until the end of the surgery) results in clinically significant improvement in analgesia, faster return of bowel function, and sparing of postoperative systemic opioid requirements after major abdominal surgical procedures.[69,70] In a more recent study, perioperative intravenous lidocaine infusion not only significantly decreased intraoperative analgesic requirements and improved postoperative analgesia, but also accelerated functional recovery after laparoscopic colectomy, leading to a clinically significant reduction in hospital length of stay.[71] It is noteworthy that during all these studies, the low-dose analgesic infusions (usually 1 to 2 mg/kg/hr) did not result in plasma levels or clinical signs of systemic toxicity. Intravenous lidocaine not only has analgesic properties, but also has antihyperalgesic and anti-inflammatory properties, which are mediated at multiple sites including sodium channel blockade, inhibition of guanine (G) protein–coupled receptors, and N-methyl-D-aspartate receptors, which all probably contribute to its favorable acute postoperative analgesic properties.

Mepivacaine

Mepivacaine is the prototypical pipecolyl xylidine local anesthetic in the group II aminoamides (see Fig. 44–4B). It is similar to lidocaine with regard to clinical applicability for regional anesthesia. It has a rapid onset of action and intermediate duration of action slightly longer than lidocaine. The use of a 1.5% to 2.0% solution will provide 70 to 90 minutes of epidural anesthesia before the onset of two-dermatome regression and approximately 2 to 4 hours of anesthesia for peripheral nerve blocks, depending on the site of administration. The addition of epinephrine prolongs the duration of action by approximately 75% to 85% when used for brachial plexus or epidural anesthesia. Its low pK_a allows for excellent diffusion properties through tissues, allowing a rapid onset of block, and its lower lipid solubility (compared with lidocaine and bupivacaine) confers a lower risk of severe systemic toxic reactions. It also provides a dense motor block, which may be indicated for various surgical procedures. These properties make mepivacaine an excellent choice for establishing a surgical block via an epidural or peripheral perineural catheter, prior to initiating an infusion of a dilute long-acting amide to extend postoperative analgesia. Randomized clinical trials and a large case series have indicated that mepivacaine may prove to be a suitable alternative to lidocaine for short-duration spinal anesthesia, because its incidence of transient neurologic symptoms is significantly lower compared with that of lidocaine.[72,73] In contrast, mepivacaine is usually avoided for obstetric epidural anesthesia. The fetus poorly metabolizes mepivacaine, and the doses required for surgical anesthesia may lead to accumulation of high levels of mepivacaine in the fetal circulation, resulting in decreased fetal muscle tone.[74]

Bupivacaine

Bupivacaine belongs to the N-alkyl substituted family of aminoamides and is structurally similar to mepivacaine and ropivacaine (see Fig. 44–4B). Despite their structural similarities, the four-carbon butyl substitution on the hydrophilic nitrogen confers a significant increase in lipid solubility, nerve-blocking potency, and duration of action compared with the single-carbon methyl group for mepivacaine.

After its introduction into clinical practice, bupivacaine rapidly gained widespread use because of its clinical profile. It possesses a significantly longer duration of action compared with 2-chloroprocaine or lidocaine. The extended duration of action after a single injection of a relatively large dose provides surgical anesthesia and, depending on the site of administration, also provides a fixed duration of extended postoperative analgesia.

Bupivacaine has become widely used for obstetric anesthesia and analgesia because its longer duration of action allows for less frequent supplemental dosing, although this advantage is now less important with the widespread use of continuous epidural infusion techniques. Also, placental transfer of bupivacaine is limited by its high pK_a and lipid solubility. One of the most advantageous characteristics of bupivacaine compared with 2-CP or lidocaine is the sensorimotor dissociation provided by bupivacaine, especially at the lower concentrations commonly used for epidural analgesia during labor and acute postoperative analgesia. The ability of bupivacaine to provide adequate sensory analgesia with relatively little motor blockade allows for the ability to ambulate during labor and maintain expulsive efforts during the second stage of labor. Typical infusion regimens for labor analgesia are bupivacaine, 0.0625% to 0.25%, given at a rate of 8 to 15 mL/hr. Furthermore, bupivacaine has excellent compatibility with neuraxial opioids and may allow for bupivacaine concentrations as low as 0.05%. In the acute postoperative setting, postoperative analgesia provided by dilute solutions of bupivacaine, usually in conjunction with fentanyl or hydromorphone, via continuous epidural or peripheral perineural catheter infusions enhances early mobilization and contributes to an accelerated functional recovery.

The disadvantage of bupivacaine is its lower margin of safety compared with the shorter acting local anesthetic agents (e.g., 2-CP, lidocaine, mepivacaine), especially when administered in larger doses for surgical anesthesia. It is generally accepted that the CNS is more sensitive to local anesthetic toxicity than the CVS. Thus, signs and symptoms of CNS toxicity usually manifest before signs of CVS toxicity. Additionally, clinical experience prior to the introduction of bupivacaine had been that significant CVS toxicity after unintentional intravascular administration of less potent, shorter acting local anesthetics could be prevented with adequate oxygenation, ventilation and, if needed, hemodynamic support.

In 1979, Albright's report alerted anesthesiologists to the increased, severe, CVS toxicity (sudden cardiac arrest) with the newer (at that time) potent long-acting aminoamide local anesthetics, bupivacaine and etidocaine.[31] Albright highlighted the fact that unintentional intravascular administration with bupivacaine or etidocaine could manifest as almost simultaneous onset of seizures and cardiovascular collapse. Subsequently, the CVS toxicity of bupivacaine has been shown to be different compared with the short-acting local anesthetics in two important aspects: (1) the ratio of the doses or plasma concentrations required to produce cardiovascular collapse compared with those required to produce seizures is lower for bupivacaine; and (2) bupivacaine toxicity is associated with malignant ventricular dysrhythmias and cardiovascular collapse that are often resistant to standard resuscitation measures. Heightened awareness of the potential severe toxicity of bupivacaine led to withdrawal of U.S. Food and Drug Administration (FDA) approval of high concentrations of bupivacaine (0.75%) for obstetric use and for surgical patients as well. Subsequently, changes in clinical practice, such as administration of an epinephrine test dose, incremental dosing with frequent intermittent aspiration, limitations of dosing, and increased vigilance and monitoring during regional block, have decreased the incidence of significant CNS and CVS toxicity.[52] Unfortunately, serious CNS and CVS toxicity may still occur, even with improvements in injection technique equipment, preventive safety steps, and lower dosing, because unintentional intravascular administration of local anesthetics can rapidly lead to acute toxicity.[35]

Ropivacaine

In response to the need for a long-acting amino-amide local anesthetic with the same favorable neuronal blocking properties of bupivacaine but with a greater margin of safety, ropivacaine was released for widespread clinical use in 1996.[19] Ropivacaine is a homologue of bupivacaine (see Fig. 44–4B), but has a lower toxicity profile compared with bupivacaine because of two important characteristics.[37] Ropivacaine has a three-carbon (propyl) substitution rather than the four-carbon (butyl) group of bupivacaine on the tertiary amine, which makes ropivacaine significantly less lipid-soluble compared with bupivacaine (see Table 44–2). Furthermore, ropivacaine is formulated as the pure S-enantiomer, and it is well established that the pure S-enantiomer possesses a decreased toxicity profile compared with the racemic mixture or the pure R-enantiomer.[21,22] The lower lipid solubility of ropivacaine may also explain the in vitro and clinical observations that at more dilute concentrations generally used for continuous analgesic infusions, it produces less motor block than bupivacaine.[74,75]

Animal studies and human volunteer studies have consistently demonstrated that ropivacaine is approximately 30% to 40% less cardiotoxic than bupivacaine. In both animal[41,76,77] and human studies,[78,79] ropivacaine has been shown to induce less prolongation of the QRS duration, less depression of myocardial contractility, and less depression of myocardial mitochondrial activity compared with equivalent doses of bupivacaine. Clinical experience has shown that serious CVS toxicity with ropivacaine is extremely rare with several case reports to date, with one

responding to moderate vasopressor support[80] and the other responding to intravenous lipid emulsion.[61] In a remarkable case report, a patient inadvertently received an intravenous administration of 300 mg ropivacaine over 5 minutes, with seizures, hypotension, and respiratory arrest with no dysrhythmias observed, as well as an uneventful recovery.[81]

Overall, ropivacaine appears clinically equivalent to bupivacaine for surgical anesthesia, labor epidural analgesia, and postoperative analgesia. Epidural anesthesia with 0.5% ropivacaine is as clinically effective as 0.5% bupivacaine for cesarean delivery,[82] lower limb orthopedic surgery,[83] and urologic surgery,[84] with minimal differences in onset, duration of action, and intensity of motor block. Clinical data have shown that continuous epidural infusions of equivalent concentrations of ropivacaine and bupivacaine (0.08% to 0.1%) provide comparable labor analgesia, with ropivacaine providing less motor block, but with no clinically relevant differences in operative delivery or neonatal outcome.[85,86] Similarly, postoperative epidural infusions of equivalent concentrations of dilute ropivacaine and bupivacaine after hip arthroplasty have demonstrated comparable analgesia, but with less motor block for ropivacaine.[87] Studies of brachial plexus and peripheral nerve block anesthesia have demonstrated equivalent clinical outcomes with comparable doses of ropivacaine and bupivacaine.[88-90] As with continuous epidural analgesia, equivalent and equipotent dilute concentrations of ropivacaine and bupivacaine have provided comparable analgesia delivered via continuous interscalene catheters.[74,91]

Levobupivacaine

Levobupivacaine is the S-enantiomer of racemic bupivacaine. Its physiochemical characteristics are virtually identical to those of bupivacaine.[20] Clinical evidence has confirmed that levobupivacaine has similar nerve blocking potency and anesthetic-analgesic profile compared with bupivacaine. Clinical studies have established that levobupivacaine has a similar pharmacodynamic and pharmacokinetic profile compared with equivalent doses of bupivacaine when used for spinal anesthesia[92,93] and epidural anesthesia for cesarean delivery,[94] and for lumbar spine[95] and lower abdominal surgery.[96] Compared with bupivacaine or ropivacaine, levobupivacaine in equivalent concentrations from 0.1% to 0.25% has been shown to provide equianalgesic potency for lumbar epidural labor analgesia.[97,98]

Levobupivacaine appears to have a decreased affinity for cardiac Na^+ channels and lower arrhythmogenicity potential in isolated heart preparations when compared with racemic bupivacaine or the single R-enantiomer.[99,100] Based on animal studies, levobupivacaine results in a clinically significant lower incidence of seizures, malignant ventricular dysrhythmias, and fatal cardiovascular collapse compared with equivalent doses of bupivacaine.[99,100]

Furthermore, in volunteers subjected to intravenous infusions of the long-acting aminoamides until the onset of early CNS toxicity, levobupivacaine caused less myocardial depression than bupivacaine,[101] but with no difference compared with ropivacaine.[79]

Analgesic Adjuvants in Regional Anesthesia and Pain Management

Afferent nociception in the peripheral and central nervous system involves multiple receptors and pathways that are not easily targeted by the use of a single drug or mode of delivery. The use of multiple analgesic agents targeting transduction, transmission, and modulation of afferent pain signals at the site of injury, peripheral nerve, spinal cord, and supraspinal receptors allows for a multimodal approach to regional anesthesia and acute pain management.[102] Often, analgesic adjuvants are combined with local anesthetic solutions with the goal of decreasing local anesthetic requirements and, more important clinically, enhancing analgesia and reducing the risk for local anesthetic toxicity. The most common analgesic adjuvants used for central neuraxial and peripheral anesthesia and analgesia include epinephrine, α_2 agonists (e.g., clonidine), and opioids.

Epinephrine

The reported benefits of epinephrine include prolongation and increased intensity of local anesthetic block and decreased systemic absorption of local anesthetics.[103] The mechanism by which epinephrine prolongs and augments local anesthetic action is thought be secondary to its α_1-mediated vasoconstrictive effects, which antagonize the inherent vasodilating properties of most local anesthetics. The resulting decrease in local perineural tissue perfusion slows clearance from the site of local anesthetic administration, thus allowing for an increased amount of local anesthetic available for neuronal blocking activity.[104] Epinephrine may also slow clearance from within the superficial neural compartments and allow more local anesthetic to reach the deeper perineural, axon-containing compartments,[105] which may contribute to increased intensity of the block. Additional analgesic effects from epinephrine may also occur via interactions with α_2 receptors in the brain and spinal cord,[106] especially because local anesthetics increase the vascular uptake of epinephrine.[107]

Most commonly, epinephrine is added at a dose of 5 µg/mL (1:200,000 concentration) to a relatively large amount of local anesthetic solution intended to provide regional anesthesia and a fixed duration of postoperative analgesia. Epinephrine may also be added to continuous epidural infusions of dilute concentration local anesthetic–lipophilic opioid mixtures, resulting in a clinically relevant increase in epidural analgesia and a decrease in systemically mediated opioid side effects.[108] The lowest effective dose should be used, because epinephrine in combination with local anesthetics may have toxic affects on tissue,[109] the cardiovascular system,[110] and the spinal cord.[111]

α_2-Adrenergic Agonists and Clonidine

Clonidine is an α_2 agonist that produces analgesia via multiple mechanisms. Stimulation of α_2 receptors in the dorsal horn of the spinal cord produces analgesic effects by inhibition of the presynaptic release of excitatory neurotransmitters, such as substance P and glutamate.[112] Clonidine possesses local anesthetic properties and has been shown to inhibit peripheral nerve conduction of A-alpha and C fibers tonically.[113] More recently, animal studies have demonstrated that clonidine prolongs peripheral nerve block primarily via hyperpolarization-activated cationic currents and not via α-adrenergic mechanisms.[114] Thus, addition of clonidine may have multiple routes of action, depending on the specific analgesic application.

Overall, clinical trials have indicated that clonidine is a beneficial analgesic adjuvant when administered for central neuraxial anesthesia,[115,116] peripheral nerve blocks,[117] and intra-articular[118] and intravenous regional anesthesia,[119] without evidence of neurotoxicity. However, stimulation of α_2 receptors produces hypotension, bradycardia, and sedation in a dose-dependent fashion, and these effects overshadow the beneficial analgesic effects provided by clonidine. The addition of clonidine to continuous peripheral perineural infusions may potentially enhance analgesia, but clinical studies have failed to demonstrate any improvement in postoperative analgesia after upper or lower extremity surgery.[120,121]

Opioids (Peripheral)

This discussion will focus on peripherally administered opioids for postoperative analgesia. For a more comprehensive discussion on central neuraxial opioids, the reader is referred to the chapter on neuraxial agents (Chapter 37) and neuraxial anesthesia (Chapter 51). Opioids have traditionally been thought to mediate analgesia exclusively by activation of spinal and surpraspinal receptors. Over the last decade, an increasing body of knowledge has described the ability of inflammatory processes to stimulate the intra-axonal movement of opioid receptors, synthesized in the dorsal root ganglion, to peripheral sensory nerve terminals at the site of injury.[122] Once at the sensory nerve terminals, opioid receptors are incorporated within the neuronal membrane and thereby possibly mediate peripheral opioid analgesia. These changes do not occur immediately after tissue injury and may take days to become manifest. Inflammatory tissue injury is an important aspect of peripherally mediated opioid analgesia, because inflammation increases the number of sensory nerve terminals and also disrupts the perineural barrier, thereby allowing passage of opioids to their respective receptors.[123]

The most promising clinical studies for peripherally mediated opioid analgesia have been with the intra-articular administration of local anesthetics and opioids for postoperative analgesia. Although one meta-analysis has concluded that intra-articular administration of morphine after knee arthroscopy provides clinically relevant improvements in postoperative analgesia,[124] a more recent systematic review has concluded that the negative trials of higher quality counter the evidence from numerous positive trials of low quality.[125] In contrast, two systematic reviews have concurred that there is little evidence for adding opioids to local anesthetics for peripheral nerve blocks.[126,127] There may be several reasons for the expected lack of peripherally mediated effect of coadministration of opioids and local anesthetics for peripheral nerve blocks. Anatomically, peripheral opioid receptors are incorporated into the terminal processes of sensory afferent neurons, whereas nerve (plexus) trunks and peripheral nerves are traditionally blocked by the administration of local anesthetics proximal to these terminal processes. Additionally, lack of inflammation at the site of the peripheral nerve or plexus block, as well as the multiple layers of perineural and intraneural connective tissue, limit access of the opioid to the intra-axonal opioid receptors in transit, which may not be functional until they reach the terminal portion of the afferent sensory neuron. In summary, there may be analgesic benefit for intra-articular administration of morphine after arthroscopic knee surgery, whereas there is little theoretical reason or clinical evidence to support the use of local anesthetic–opioid mixtures for peripheral nerve block.

LOCAL ANESTHETICS FOR CHRONIC PAIN

Neuropathic Pain

Pain that originates from injury or dysfunction of the peripheral or central nervous system is termed *neuropathic pain*. This type of pain is often chronic and poorly responsive to traditional analgesics.[128] Neuropathic pain symptoms are typically treated with antidepressants,[129] anticonvulsants,[130] and opioid analgesics[131]; the side effects of these drugs, however, may be significant. Patients with neuropathic pain syndromes are often older adults who may have decreased liver and renal function and concomitant medical conditions that require them to take several medications. The use of these drugs may not be well tolerated in these patients, and drug-drug interactions and variable pharmacokinetics may further limit their usefulness.[132] Patients with neuropathic pain who cannot tolerate the side effects of these first-line drugs, those who do not respond to these medications, or those who do not want to take opioids are candidates for intravenous, oral, or topical local anesthetic treatment.

The mechanisms responsible for neuropathic pain generation and perpetuation are protean.[128] Neuropathic pain is attributed to primary afferent nociceptive or non-nociceptive input or to spontaneous ectopic discharges without activation of peripheral nociceptors.[133,134] The spontaneous ectopic nerve impulse generation and resultant neuropathic pain symptoms may be the result of abnormally developed sodium channels at the site of neuronal injury.[135] Persistent spontaneous ectopic discharges not only occur along an injured peripheral nerve but also in neuromas and in the dorsal root ganglion, maintaining a central hyperexcitable state.[136-138] The repeated activation of peripheral nociceptors eventually leads to central sensitization, resulting in hyperalgesia and allodynia, typical of neuropathic pain.[139] Lidocaine, by binding to the abnormally developed sodium channels, reduces the frequency of these ectopic discharges.[137] Local anesthetics inhibit these aberrant discharges at concentrations below those necessary to produce blockade of conduction.[133,137,140-142] Blockade of sodium channels also occurs at the dorsal horn of the spinal cord.[143] Certain types of neuropathic pain syndromes are caused by pathologic lesions of nerve fibers in or near the skin; topically administered lidocaine produces analgesia by local sodium channel blockade and not via systemic effects.[144]

Intravenous, Oral, or Topical Local Anesthetics

Intravenous Lidocaine

The early reports of intravenous local anesthetics for pain management involved their use for the treatment of cancer and postoperative pain. More recently, local anesthetic infusions have been used in the treatment of neuropathic pain and numerous studies have shown its efficacy in this syndrome.[134,145-148] A meta-analysis has reviewed randomized clinical trials and examined the efficacy and safety of systemic local anesthetics compared with placebo or active drugs in patients with neuropathic pain.[149] Of 41 studies, 10 intravenous lidocaine trials were included in the meta-analysis. The patients studied included those with peripheral neuropathic pain secondary to cancer, metabolic (diabetic polyneuropathy), infectious (human immunodeficiency virus [HIV] neuropathy, postherpetic neuralgia), posttraumatic, and mixed causes, and central neuropathic pain (spinal cord injury, stroke, postamputation). The median dose used in the studies was 5 mg/kg of intravenous lidocaine given over 30 minutes. The meta-analysis showed intravenous lidocaine to be superior to placebo and equal to morphine, gabapentin, amitriptyline, and amantadine.[149] The beneficial effect was noted to be more consistent for patients with peripheral pain secondary to trauma and diabetes and central pain. Intravenous lidocaine appeared to be ineffective against HIV-related polyneuropathy and plexopathy from tumor infiltration.[149] Although intravenous lidocaine and systemic morphine appeared to be equally effective for postherpetic neuralgia and postamputation stump pain, morphine was more effective than intravenous lidocaine for phantom pain.[150,151]

The adverse effects of intravenous lidocaine include nausea, vomiting, abdominal pain, diarrhea, dizziness, and perioral numbness. Less common side effects are tremor, dry mouth, metallic taste, insomnia, and tachycardia. The side effects are more common than placebo but equivalent to those of morphine, gabapentin, and amitriptyline.[149]

Different dose regimens have been used for intravenous lidocaine. Wu and colleagues[151] used a 1-mg/kg bolus followed by a 4-mg/kg infusion, to a maximum dose of 400 mg, and Ferrante and associates[152] administered 500 mg of intravenous lidocaine at a rate of 8.36 mg/min over 60 minutes. Most clinicians infuse 5 mg/kg of lidocaine over 30 to 60 minutes (5 to 10 mg/min), adjusting the rate to minimize the occurrence of symptoms of local anesthetic toxicity (e.g., drowsiness, circumoral numbness, slurring of speech). The number of treatments in the studies ranged from two[153] to three,[151] with intervals between treatments ranging from 1 day[151] to 3 weeks.[154] There appears to be no correlation between the lidocaine concentration and the onset or attainment of analgesia, and large increases in pain relief tend to occur from minimal increases in dosage.[152] The duration of pain relief may last for longer than 1 week,[153] and patients who respond favorably to intravenous lidocaine are placed on mexiletine for maintenance therapy. Although one study has shown the ability of intravenous lidocaine to predict the patient's response to mexiletine,[155] this predictability has not been the common experience of clinicians.

Oral Mexiletine

Mexiletine is an oral bioavailable analogue of lidocaine and a class IB antiarrythmic agent. It has been used in neuropathic pain syndromes secondary to cancer, diabetes, and other causes. In animal models of neuropathic pain, mexiletine has been shown to have significant antinociceptive effect compared with control treatment (e.g., saline, vehicle injection, or no treatment.[156-158] Mexiletine blocks transmission of nerve impulses by blocking the voltage-gated sodium channels (preferentially the open and inactivated channels) and impedes impulse generation or transmission in damaged nerve fibers in the peripheral nervous system.[137] In diabetic mice, mexiletine has been shown to reduce the potassium-mediated release of substance P from the spinal cord.[159]

The efficacy of mexiletine in neuropathic pain syndromes has been evaluated in several studies. Similar to the studies on intravenous local anesthetic infusions, most of these enrolled few patients, used varied dose regimens, had different experimental designs, and assessed different end points at different time periods.[149,160] In addition to reviewing the available clinical data on intravenous local anesthetics, the

meta-analysis study of Tremont-Lukats and coworkers[149] also reviewed the data on mexiletine. Of the retrieved clinical studies on mexiletine, 9 of 41 were suitable for meta-analysis. The median dosage used in the studies was 600 mg of mexiletine daily. Similar to intravenous lidocaine, mexiletine was noted to be equally effective as morphine, gabapentin, and amitriptyline and more effective than placebo.[149]

Similar to intravenous lidocaine, mexiletine appears to be more effective in patients with neuropathic pain secondary to diabetes, trauma, and central causes. Although Tremont-Lukats and colleagues[149] performed an excellent job of analyzing and interpreting the available data with regard to the analgesic efficacy of systemic local anesthetics, they were less useful in comparing the side effects.[160] The side effects of mexiletine are generally similar to those of intravenous lidocaine infusions. Compared with intravenous lidocaine, mexiletine causes more nausea and vomiting and fewer CNS symptoms, such as dizziness and tremors. One bothersome but rare reaction to mexiletine is a severe cutaneous reaction that consists of generalized skin reaction, fever, eosinophilia, lymphocytosis, and liver dysfunction.[161]

The oral bioavailability of mexiletine is approximately 90% and the time to reach peak serum concentration is 1.5 to 4 hours.[162,163] Its volume of distribution is large and variable. At physiologic pH, approximately 40% of mexiletine is bound to plasma proteins, mainly albumin and AAG. It is eliminated primarily by hepatic metabolism; approximately 5% of the dose is recovered unchanged in the urine. The elimination of mexiletine is therefore impaired in patients with hepatic dysfunction but, in patients with renal problems, is only slightly affected and rarely requires dosage adjustments. The enzyme mainly responsible for the hydroxylation of mexiletine, cytochrome P-450 2D6 (CYP2D6), is absent in some people. Those who lack this enzyme are called poor metabolizers and their clearance of hydroxylated metabolites is significantly lower.[164] The terminal elimination half-life ranges from 6.7 to 17.2 hours.[165]

The plasma concentration–effect relationship of mexiletine in ventricular arrhythmias is well established, with a therapeutic range of 0.5 to 2 mg/mL.[162] This dose-response relationship is not seen in patients with neuropathic pain. Nishiyama and Sakuta[166] have noted that the minimum effective plasma concentration of mexiletine in patients with alcohol neuropathy is 0.66 μg/mL. Wallace and associates[167] used dosages higher than those used by Nishiyama and Sakuta, 900 versus 300 mg/day, yet noted peak concentrations of 0.54 μg/mL. Galer and coworkers[155] have noted that the mean highest tolerated dose is 878 mg (range, 400 to 1200 mg), with a mean serum level of 0.76 μg/mL. These studies[155,166,167] show the lack of correlation among the mexiletine dose, serum level, and pain relief scores. In a study of volunteers,[168] it was noted that the mean maximum daily tolerated dose is 859 mg (range, 300 to 1350 mg), side effects occur at an average daily dose of 993 mg (range, 600 to 1350 mg), and peak plasma levels of 0.36 ± 0.21 µg/mL are reached at day 10. The lack of a predictable dose-response relationship for mexiletine makes it reasonable to start it at low dosages and to titrate it slowly, over a period of days to weeks, until pain relief is obtained or adverse effects are bothersome.[162,169]

Another clinical application of mexiletine is for perioperative pain management. Perioperative mexiletine, 600 mg given the night before breast cancer surgery and for 10 days after the surgery, has been shown to reduce the analgesic requirements by 50% from postoperative days 2 to 10.[170] This effect was similar to gabapentin, 1200 mg/day, given over the same time periods as mexiletine. Both drugs reduced the pain at rest and on movement on postoperative day 3. Gabapentin, but not mexiletine, also reduced the pain on movement from postoperative days 2 to 5. Neither drug, however, decreased the incidence or severity of pain at 3 months after surgery.

Lidocaine Patch

The lidocaine patch (LP) 5% (Lidoderm, Endo Pharmaceuticals, Chadds Ford, Pa) delivers lidocaine locally at the site of neuropathic pain generation, limiting its systemic effects and reducing its interactions with other concomitantly administered medications. After its efficacy was demonstrated in postherpetic neuralgia,[171] LP was the first agent approved for the treatment of this condition by the FDA. The patch measures 10×14 cm and contains 700 mg of lidocaine mixed with an adhesive, which is applied to a nonwoven polyethylene backing. The manufacturer's recommendations are for a maximum of three patches applied to the intact skin—the available formulation is not sterile—to cover the painful area fully for 12 hours/day; dose titration and escalation are not necessary. Most patients who are responsive to LP experience pain relief within a few days of patch application[172]; in some patients, however, the response may be delayed[173] and a trial period of 2 weeks is therefore recommended. One third of responsive patients will continue to experience pain relief throughout the day, including during the time when the patch is not applied, whereas the remaining patients report return of their pain after the patch is removed. Some clinicians therefore recommend using the patch for longer durations, up to 20 hours/day.

Pharmacokinetics
The pharmacokinetic profile of lidocaine absorption, peak levels, and elimination from the LP are similar in healthy volunteers, patients with postherpetic neuralgia, and patients with acute herpes zoster.[174] The absorption of lidocaine from the application site is limited, and only $3\% \pm 2\%$ of the total dose applied is absorbed systemically.[174] Maximum plasma lido-

caine concentration (130 ng/mL) is typically achieved by day 2 of patch application, 12 hours/day,[175] and is significantly lower than concentrations that have cardiac effects (1500 ng/mL) or are cardiotoxic (5000 ng/mL).[176] Even when the patch is applied for extended periods, up to 24 hours/day, the plasma lidocaine concentration (186 to 225 ng/mL) is similar to 12 hours/day of patch application, well below toxic levels.[177,178] Systemically absorbed lidocaine is primarily metabolized in the liver and the primary active metabolite, monoethylglycinexylidide, is approximately 25% of maximum plasma lidocaine concentration.

Tolerability and Adverse Reactions
The LP is generally well tolerated and few patients report any systemic side effects; interaction with other concomitantly administered drugs is also minimal.[172,174] Patients can continue to receive other treatments for neuropathic pain while they are being treated with the patch. Even when four patches are applied simultaneously and application times are extended to 24 hours/day, the LP is well tolerated and few patients report any adverse systemic effects.[178,179] The LP may be used indefinitely and there have been no reports of tolerance, physical dependence, or addiction. Local skin irritation or rash is the most common adverse reaction reported by about 28% of patients[176,178,179]; this dermal reaction, however, typically resolves spontaneously once the therapy is discontinued.

Efficacy
The efficacy of the LP has been most extensively scrutinized in patients with postherpetic neuralgia,[173,174] and these studies have shown that it is more effective than a placebo patch or no treatment. Pain relief with the placebo patch, however, was also superior to no treatment, and may be attributed to the protection offered to the area of hyperalgesia and allodynia by the placebo patch, but no studies have compared the LP with other treatment modalities for postherpetic neuralgia. The LP has also been used in patients with other painful conditions such as myofascial pain,[179] low back pain,[180] osteoarthritis,[181] and diabetic[182] and nondiabetic polyneuropathy.[183] These studies were either small case series or uncontrolled open-label studies, so the efficacy of LP in these conditions remains to be validated.

CONCLUSION

The pain medicine physician ought to be aware of the clinical pharmacology of the different local anesthetics, especially their maximum dosages and relative cardiovascular and CNS toxicities. The physician should know signs and symptoms and the management of local anesthetic toxicity. Local anesthetics are being used in the management of chronic pain; this include intravenous infusions, oral mexiletine, and the lidocaine patch.

SUMMARY

- Bupivacaine and ropivacaine are usually used in post-operative epidural infusions and continuous peri-neural catheter infusions because of their duration and their ideal sensory-motor dissociation. Ropivacaine appears to cause less motor block than bupivacaine and has a better cardiovascular safety profile.

- Guidelines to decrease systemic toxicity of local anesthetics include fractionation of the administered dose with frequent aspiration, addition of epinephrine when large doses are injected, knowledge of the signs of intravascular injection, and, the preferential use of ropivacaine when a long-acting agent is considered.

- Clonidine is a useful adjuvant to local anesthetic in neuraxial anesthesia/analgesia, peripheral nerve blocks, intra-articular, and intravenous regional anesthesia. However, it may cause hypotension, bradycardia, and sedation.

- The peripheral application of opioid, in conjunction with a local anesthetic, appears to be most useful in intra-articular injections. This may be related to the presence of inflammation in the area. In contrast, the efficacy of opioid-local anesthetic combination in peripheral nerve blocks is not convincing.

- Intravenous lidocaine infusions, usually 5 mg/kg over 30 minutes, are used in the treatment of peripheral pain secondary to trauma and diabetes and in central pain. It appears to be less effective in HIV polyneuropathy and tumor-related plexopathy.

- Mexiletine, at a median dose of 6500 mg daily, also appears to be effective in neuropathic pain secondary to trauma, diabetes, and central etiologies. The side effects are similar to IV lidocaine infusions although it may cause more nausea and vomiting and less CNS symptoms such as tremors and dizziness.

- Lidocaine patch can be applied over the painful area for 12-20 hours a day; the maximum plasma concentrations are below the toxic levels of lidocaine. Because some patients have a delayed response, a two-week trial period is recommended. It is FDA-approved for postherpetic neuralgia; studies describing its efficacy in other conditions were either case series and open-labeled.

References

1. Wann KT: Neuronal sodium and potassium channels: Structure and function. Br J Anaesth 1993;71:2-14.
2. Catterall WA: Structure and function of voltage-gated ion channels. Annu Rev Biochem 1995;64:493-351.
3. Waxman SG, Ritchie JM: Molecular dissection of the myelinated axon. Ann Neurol 1993;33:121-136.
4. Stranding S: Nervous system. In Stranding S, Ellis H, Healy JC, et al (eds): Gray's Anatomy, 39th ed. Edinburgh, Elsevier Churchill Livingstone, 2005, pp 43-68.
5. Butterworth JF, Strichartz GR: Molecular mechanisms of local anesthetics: A review. Anesthesiology 1990;72:711-734.
6. Catterall WA: From ionic currents to molecular mechanisms: The structure and function of voltage-gated sodium channels. Neuron 2000;26:13-25.
7. Strichartz GR: The inhibition of sodium currents in myelinated nerve by quaternary derivatives of lidocaine. J Gen Physiol 1973;62:37-57.
8. Salinas FV: Analgesics: Ion channel ligands, sodium channel blockers, local anesthetics. In Evers AS, Maze M (eds): Anesthetic Pharmacology: Physiologic Principles and Clinical Practice. Philadelphia, Elsevier, 2003, pp 507-537.
9. Gissen AJ, Covino BG, Gregus J: Differential sensitivity of fast and slow fibers in mammalian nerve. II. Margin of safety for nerve transmission. Anesth Analg 1982;61:561-569.
10. Strichartz GR, Sanchez V, Arthur GR, et al: Fundamental properties of local anesthetics. II. Measured octanol:buffer partition coefficients and pKa values of clinically used drugs. Anesth Analg 1990;71:158-170.
11. Yun I, Cho ES, Jang HO, et al: Amphophilic effects of local anesthetics on rotational mobility in neuronal and model membranes. Biochem Biophys Acta 2002;1564:123-132.
12. Salinas FV: Pharmacology of drugs used for spinal and epidural anesthesia and analgesia. In Wong CW (ed): Spinal and Epidural Anesthesia. New York, McGraw Hill, 2007, pp 75-109.
13. Taheri S, Cogswell LP 3rd, Gent A, et al: Hydrophobic and ionic factors in the binding of local anesthetics to the major variant of human alpha1-acid glycoprotein. J Pharmacol Exp Ther 2003;71:71-80.
14. Ulbricht WL: Kinetics of drug action and equilibrium results at the node of Ranvier. Physiol Rev 1981;61:785-828.
15. Denson D, Coyle D, Thompson G, et al: Alpha 1-acid glycoprotein and albumin in human serum bupivacaine binding. Clin Pharmacol Ther 1984;35:409-415.
16. Wulf H, Munstedt P, Maier C: Plasma protein binding of bupivacaine in pregnant women at term. Acta Anaesthesiol Scand 1991;35:129-133.
17. Wulf H, Winckler K, Denzer D: Plasma concentrations of alpha 1-acid glycoprotein following operations and its effect on the plasma protein binding of bupivacaine. Prog Clin Biol Res 1989;300:457-460.
18. Pere P, Salonen M, Jokinen M, et al: Pharmacokinetics of ropivacaine in uremic and nonuremic patients after axillary brachial plexus block. Anesth Analg 2002;96:563-569.
19. Simpson D, Curran MP, Oldfield V, et al: Ropivacaine: A review of its use in regional anesthesia and acute pain management. Drugs 2005;65:2675-2717.
20. Foster RH, Markham A: Levobupivacaine: A review of its pharmacology and use as a local anesthetic. Drugs 2000;59:551-579.
21. Burke D, Henderson DJ: Chirality: A blueprint for the future. Br J Anaesth 2002;83:563-576.
22. Casati A, Putzu M: Bupivacaine, levobupivacaine, and ropivacaine: Are they clinically different? Best Pract Res Clin Anaesthesiol 2005;19:247-268.
23. Huang YF, Upton RN, Runciman WB: IV bolus administration of subconvulsive doses of lignocaine to conscious sheep: Myocardial pharmacokinetics. Br J Anaesth 1993;70:326-332.
24. Huang YF, Upton RN, Runciman WB: IV bolus administration of subconvulsive doses of lignocaine to conscious sheep: Relationship between myocardial pharmacokinetics and pharmacodynamics. Br J Anaesth 1993;70:556-561.
25. Emanuelsson BMK, Zaric D, Nydahl PA, et al: Pharmacokinetics of ropivacaine and bupivacaine during 21 hours of continuous epidural infusion in healthy volunteers. Anesth Analg 1995;81:1163-1168.
26. Burm AGL, Stienstra R, Brouwer RP, et al: Epidural infusion of ropivacaine for postoperative analgesia after major orthopedic surgery. Anesthesiology 2000;93:395-403.
27. Veering BT, Burm AGL, Feyen HM, et al: Pharmacokinetics of bupivacaine during postoperative epidural infusion. Anesthesiology 2002;96:1062-1069.
28. Ekatodramis G, Borgeat A, Huledal G, et al: Continuous interscalene analgesia with ropivacaine 2 mg/ml after major shoulder surgery. Anesthesiology 2003;98:143-150.
29. Tucker GT, Mather LE: Properties, absorption, and disposition of local anesthetic agents. In Cousins MJ, Bridenbaugh PO (ed): Neural Blockade in Clinical Anesthesia and Management of Pain, 3rd ed. Philadelphia, Lippincott-Raven, 1998, pp 55-96.
30. De Martin S, Orlando R, Bertoli M, et al: Differential effect of chronic renal failure on the pharmacokinetics of lidocaine

in patients receiving and not receiving hemodialysis. Clin Pharmacol Ther 2000;80:597-606.

31. Albright GA: Cardiac arrest following regional anesthesia with etidocaine and bupivacaine. Anesthesiology 1979; 51:285-287

32. Auroy Y, Narchi P, Messiah A, et al: Serious complications related to regional anesthesia: Results of a prospective survey in France. Anesthesiology 1997;87:479-486.

33. Auroy Y, Benhamou D, Bargues L, et al: Major complications of regional anesthesia in France: The SOS regional anesthesia hotline service. Anesthesiology 2002;97:1274-1280.

34. Moore JM, Liu SS, Neal JM: Premedication with fentanyl and midazolam decreases the reliability of intravenous lidocaine test dose. Anesth Analg 1998;86:1015-1017.

35. Mather LE, Copeland SE, Ladd LA: Acute toxicity of local anesthetics: Underlying pharmacokinetic and pharmacodynamic concepts. Reg Anesth Pain Med 2005;30:553-566.

36. Shibata M, Shingu K, Murakawa M, et al: Tetraphasic actions of local anesthetics on central nervous system electrical activities in cats. Reg Anesth 1994;19:255-263.

37. Groban L: Central nervous system and cardiac effects from long-acting amide local anesthetic toxicity in the intact animal model. Reg Anesth Pain Med 2003;28:3-11.

38. Yamauchi Y, Kotania J, Ueda Y: The effects of exogenous epinephrine on a convulsive dose of lidocaine: Relationship with cerebral circulation. J Neurosurg Anesthesiol 1998; 10:178-187.

39. Yokoyama M, Hirakawa M, Goto H: Effect of vasoconstrictive agents added to lidocaine on intravenous lidocaine-induced convulsions in rats. Anesthesiology 1995;82:574-580.

40. Takahashi R, Oda Y, Tanaka K, et al: Epinephrine increases the extracellular lidocaine concentration in the brain: A possible mechanism for increased central nervous systemic toxicity. Anesthesiology 2006;105:984-989.

41. Groban L, Deal DD, Vernon JC, et al: Cardiac resuscitation after incremental overdose with lidocaine, bupivacaine, levobupivacaine, and ropivacaine in anesthetized dogs. Anesth Analg 2001;92:37-43.

42. Clarkson CW, Hondeghem LM: Mechanism for bupivacaine depression of cardiac conduction: Fast block of sodium channels during the action potential with slow recovery from block during diastole. Anesthesiology 1985;62:396-405.

43. Groban L, Deal DD, Vernon JC, et al: Does local anesthetic stereoselectivity or structure predict myocardial depression in anesthetized canines? Reg Anesth Pain Med 2002;27: 460-468.

44. Mio Y, Fukuda N, Kusakari Y, et al: Bupivacaine attenuates contractility by decreasing sensitivity of myofilaments to Ca^{2+} in rat ventricular muscle. Anesthesiology 2002;97: 1168-1177.

45. Butterworth J, James RL, Grimes J: Structure-affinity relationships and stereospecificity of several homologous series of local anesthetics for the β_2-adrenergic receptor. Anesth Analg 1997;85:336-342.

46. Denson DD, Behbehani MM, Gregg RV: Effects of intravenously administered arrhythmogenic dose of bupivacaine at the nucleus tractus solitarius in the conscious rat. Reg Anesth 1990;15:76-80.

47. Szocik JF, Gardener CA, Webb RC: Inhibitory effects of bupivacaine and lidocaine on adrenergic neuroeffector junctions in the rat-tail artery. Anesthesiology 1993;78:911-917.

48. Hogan QH, Stadnicka A, Bosnjak ZJ, et al: Effects of lidocaine and bupivacaine on isolated rabbit mesenteric veins. Reg Anesth Pain Med 1998;23:109-117.

49. Lipka K, Bulow HH: Lactic acidosis following convulsions. Acta Anaesthesiol Scand 2003;47:616-618.

50. Tanaka M, Goyagi T, Kimura T, et al: The efficacy of hemodynamic changes and T wave criteria for detecting intravascular injection of epinephrine test doses in anesthetized adults: A dose-response study. Anesth Analg 2000;91: 1196-1202.

51. Kim JT, Jung JY, Jung CW, et al: S-wave in lead III is helpful for the early detection of bupivacaine-induced cardiac depression in dogs. Can J Anesth 2005;52:864-869.

52. Mulroy MF: Systemic toxicity and cardiotoxicity from local anesthetics: Incidences and preventative measures. Reg Anesth Pain Med 2002;27:556-561.

53. Moore DC, Batra MS: The components of an effective test dose prior to epidural block. Anesthesiology 1981;55: 693-696.

54. Weinberg GL: Current concepts in resuscitation of patients with local anesthetic toxicity. Reg Anesth Pain Med 2002; 27:568-575.

55. Simon L, Kariya N, Pelle-Lancien E, et al: Bupivacaine-induced QRS prolongation is enhanced by lidocaine and phenytoin in rabbit hearts. Anesth Analg 2002;94:203-207.

56. Mayr VD, Raedler C, Wenzel V, et al: A comparison of epinephrine and vasopressin in a porcine model of cardiac arrest after rapid injection of bupivacaine. Anesth Analg 2000;98: 1426-1431.

57. Weinberg GL, Ripper R, Feinstein DL, et al: Lipid emulsion infusion rescues dogs from bupivacaine-induced cardiac toxicity. Reg Anesth Pain Med 2003;28:198-202.

58. Weinberg GL, Ripper R, Murphy P, et al: Lipid infusion accelerates removal of bupivacaine and recovery from bupivacaine toxicity in the isolated rat heart. Reg Anesth Pain Med 2006;31:296-303.

59. Stehr SN, Ziegeler JC, Pexa A, et al: The effects of lipid infusion on myocardial function and bioenergetics in L-bupivacaine toxicity in the isolated rat heart. Anesth Analg 2007;104:186-192.

60. Rosenblatt MA, Abel M, Fischer GW, et al: Successful use of a 20% lipid emulsion to resuscitate a patient after a presumed bupivacaine-related cardiac arrest. Anesthesiology 2006;105: 217-218.

61. Litz RJ, Popp M, Stehr SN, et al: Successful resuscitation of a patient with ropivacaine-induced asystole after axillary brachial plexus block using lipid infusion. Anaesthesia 2006;61: 800-801.

62. Boezaart AP: Perineural infusion of local anesthetics. Anesthesiology 2006:104:872-880.

63. Liu SS, Salinas FV: Continuous plexus and peripheral nerve blocks for postoperative analgesia. Anesth Analg 2003;96: 263-72.

64. Wang BC, Hillman DE, Speidholz NI, et al: Chronic neurologic deficits and Nesacaine-CE: An effect of the anesthetic, 2-chloroprocaine, or the antioxidant sodium bisulfite? Anesth Analg 1984:63:445-447.

65. Stevens RD, Urmey WF, Urquhart BL, et al: Back pain after epidurally anesthesia with chloroprocaine. Anesthesiology 1993;78:492-497.

66. Kouri ME, Kopacz DJ: Spinal 2-chloroprocaine: A comparison with lidocaine in volunteers. Anesth Analg 2004;98:75-80.

67. Casati A, Danelli G, Berti M, et al: Intrathecal 2-chloroprocaine for lower limb outpatient surgery: A prospective, randomized, double-blind clinical evaluation. Anesth Analg 2006;103:234-238.

68. Zaric D, Christiansen C, Pace NL, et al: Transient neurologic symptoms after spinal anesthesia with lidocaine versus other local anesthetics: A systematic review of randomized, controlled trials. Anesth Analg 2005;100:1811-1816.

69. Groudine SB, Fisher HAG, Kaufman RP, et al: Intravenous lidocaine speeds the return of bowel function, decreases postoperative pain, and shortens hospital stay in patients undergoing radical retropubic prostatectomy. Anesth Analg 1998;86:235-239.

70. Koppert W, Weigand M, Neumann F, et al: Perioperative intravenous lidocaine has preventive effects on postoperative pain and morphine consumption after major abdominal surgery. Anesth Analg 2004;98:1050-1055.

71. Kaba A, Laurent SR, Detroz BJ, et al: Intravenous lidocaine infusion facilitates acute rehabilitation after laparoscopic colectomy. Anesthesiology 2007;106:11-18.

72. Ligouri GA, Zayas VM, Chisolm MF: Transient neurological symptoms after spinal anesthesia with mepivacaine and lidocaine. Anesthesiology 1998;619-623.

73. YaDeau JT, Liguori GA, Zayas VM: The incidence of transient neurological symptoms after spinal anesthesia with mepivacaine. Anesth Analg 2005:101:661-665.

74. Borgeat A, Kalberer F, Jacob H, et al: Patient-controlled inter-scalene analgesia with ropivacaine 0.2% versus bupivacaine 0.15% after major open shoulder surgery: The effects on hand motor function. Anesth Analg 2001;92:218-223.

75. Casati A, Vinciguerra F, Cappelleri G, et al: Levobupivacaine 0.2% or 0.125% for continuous sciatic nerve block: A pro-spective randomized, double-blind comparison with 0.2% ropivacaine. Anesth Analg 2004;99:919-923.

76. Dony P, Dewinde V, Vanderick B, et al: The comparative toxicity of ropivacaine and bupivacaine at equipotent doses in rats. Anesth Analg 2000;91:1489-1492.

77. Morrison SG, Dominquez JJ, Frascarolo P, et al: A comparison of the electrophysiologic cardiotoxic effects of racemic bupi-vacaine, levobupivacaine, and ropivacaine in anesthetized swine. Anesth Analg 2000;90:1308-1314.

78. Knudsen K, Suurkula MB, Blomberg S, et al: Central nervous system and cardiovascular effects of i.v. infusions of ropiva-caine, bupivacaine, and placebo in volunteers. Br J Anaesth 1997;78:570-574.

79. Stewart J, Kellett N, Castro D: The central nervous system and cardiovascular system effects of levobupivacaine and ropivacaine in healthy volunteers. Anesth Analg 2003;97:412-416.

80. Reutsch YA, Fattinger KE, Borgeat A: Ropivacaine induced convulsions and severe cardiac dysrhthmia after sciatic block. Anesthesiology 1999;90:1784-1788.

81. Dernedde M, Furlan D, Verbesselt R, et al: Grand mal convul-sions after an accidental intravenous injection of ropiva-caine. Anesth Analg 2004;98:521-523.

82. Griffin RP, Reynolds F: Extradural anaesthesia for cesarean section: A double-blind comparison of 0.5% ropivacaine with 0.5% bupivacaine. Br J Anesth 1995;74:512-516.

83. McGlade DP, Kalpokas MV, Mooney PH, et al: Comparison of 0.5% ropivacaine and 0.5% bupivacaine in lumbar epi-dural anaesthesia for lower limb orthopedic surgery. Anaesth Intens Care 1997;25:262-266.

84. Kerkamp HE, Gielen MJ, Edstrom HH: Comparison of 0.75% ropivacaine with epinephrine and 0.75% bupivacaine with epinephrine in lumbar epidural anesthesia. Reg Anesth 1990;15:204-207.

85. Halpern SH, Breen TW, Campbell DC, et al: A multicenter, randomized, controlled trial comparing bupivacaine with ropivacaine for labor analgesia. Anesthesiology 2003;98:1431-1435.

86. Lee BB, Ngan Kee WD, Ng FF, et al: Epidural infusions of ropivacaine and bupivacaine for labor analgesia: A random-ized, double-blinded study of obstetric outcome. Anesth Analg 2004;98:1145-1152.

87. Bertini L, Mancini S, DiBenedetto P, et al: Postoperative anal-gesia by combined continuous infusions and patient-controlled epidural analgesia following hip replacement: Ropivacaine vs. bupivacaine. Acta Anaesthesiol Scand 2001;45:782-785.

88. Casati A, Fanelli G, Albertin A, et al: Interscalene brachial plexus anesthesia with either 0.5% ropivacaine or 0.5% bupi-vacaine. Minerva Anestesiol 2000;66:39-44.

89. McGlade DP, Kalpokas MV, Mooney PH, et al: A comparison of 0.5% ropivacaine and 0,5% bupivacaine for axillary brachial plexus anesthesia. Anesth Intens Care 1998;26:515-520.

90. Casati A, Fanelli G, Magistris L, et al: Minimum local anes-thetic volume blocking the femoral nerve in 50% of cases: A double blinded-comparison between 0.5% ropivacaine and 0.5% bupivacaine. Anesth Analg 2001;92:205-208.

91. Eroglu A, Uzunlar H, Sener M, et al: A clinical comparison of equal concentration and volume of ropivacaine and bupiva-caine for interscalene brachial plexus anesthesia and analge-sia in shoulder surgery. Reg Anesth Pain Med 2004;29:539-543.

92. Alley EA, Kopacz DJ, McDonald SB, Liu SS: Hyperbaric spinal levobupivacaine: A comparison to racemic bupivacaine in volunteers. Anesth Analg 2002;94:188-93.

93. Glaser C, Marhofer P, Zimpfer G, et al: Levobupivacaine versus racemic bupivacaine for spinal anesthesia. Anesth Analg 2002;94:194-198.

94. Faccenda KA, Simpson AM, Henderson DJ, et al: A compari-son of levobupivacaine and racemic bupivacaine for extradu-ral anesthesia for cesarean section. Reg Anesth Pain Med 2003;28:394-400.

95. Kopacz DJ, Helman JD, Nussbaum CE, et al: A comparison of epidural levobupivacaine 0.5% with or without epineph-rine for lumbar spine surgery. Anesth Analg 2001;93:755-760.

96. Kopacz DJ, Allen HW, Thompson GE: A comparison of epi-dural levobupivacaine 0.75% with racemic bupivacaine for lower abdominal surgery. Anesth Analg 2000;90:642-648.

97. Purdie NL, McGrady EM: Comparison of patient-controlled epidural bolus administration of 0.1% ropivacaine and 0.1% levobupivacaine, both with 0.0002% fentanyl, for analgesia during labor. Anaesthesia 2004;59:133-137.

98. Burke D, Henderson DJ, Simpson AM, et al: Comparison of 0.25% S(−)-bupivacaine with 0.25% RS-bupivacaine for epi-dural analgesia in labour. Br J Anaesth 1999;83:750-755.

99. Valenzuela C, Snyders DJ, Bennet PB, et al: Stereoselective block of cardiac sodium channels by bupivacaine in guinea-pig ventricular myocytes. Circulation 1995;92:3014-3024.

100. Mazoit JX, Boico O, Samii K: Myocardial uptake of bupiva-caine II. Pharmacokinetics and pharmacodynamics of bupivacaine in the isolated perfused heart. Anesth Analg 1993;77:477-482.

101. Bardsley H, Gristwood R, Baker H, et al: A comparison of the cardiovascular effects of levobupivacaine and rac-bupivacaine following intravenous administration to healthy volunteers. Br J Clin Pharmacol 1998;46:245-249.

102. Kelly DJ, Ahmad M, Brull SJ: Preemptive analgesia I: Physio-logic pathways and pharmacological modalities. Can J Anaesth 2001;48:1000-1010.

103. Neal JM: Effects of epinephrine in local anesthetics on the central and peripheral nervous systems: Neurotoxicity and neural blood flow. Reg Anesth Pain Med 2003;28:124-134.

104. Bernards CM, Kopacz DJ: Effect of epinephrine on lidocaine clearance in vivo: A microdialysis study in humans. Anesthe-siology 1999;91:962-968.

105. Sinnot CJ, Cogswell LP, Johnson A, et al: On the mechanism by which epinephrine potentiates lidocaine's peripheral nerve block. Anesthesiology 2003;98:181-188.

106. Curatolo M, Petersen-Felix S, Arendt-Nielsen L, et al: Epidural epinephrine and clonidine: Segmental analgesia and effects on different pain modalities. Anesthesiology 1997;87:785-794.

107. Ueda W, Hirakawa, Mori K: Acceleration of epinephrine absorption by lidocaine. Anesthesiology 1985;63:717-720.

108. Niemi G, Breivik H: Adrenaline markedly improves thoracic epidural analgesia produced by a low-dose infusion of bupi-vacaine, fentanyl, and adrenaline after major surgery. Acta Anaesthesiol Scand 1998;42:897-909.

109. Magee C, Rodeheaver GT, Edgerton MT, et al: Studies of the mechanisms by which epinephrine damages tissue defenses. J Surg Res 1977;23:126-131.

110. Hall JA, Ferro A: Myocardial ischaemia and ventricular arrhythmias precipitated by physiologic concentrations of adrenaline in patients with coronary artery disease. Br Heart J 1992;67:419-420.

111. Hodgson PH, Neal JM, Pollock JE, et al: The neurotoxicity of drugs given intrathecally (spinal). Anesth Analg 1999;88:797-809.

112. Eisenach JC, De Kock M, Klimscha W: Alpha (2)-adrenergic agonists for regional anesthesia: A clinical review of cloni-dine (1984-1995). Anesthesiology 1996;85:655-674.

113. Butterworth JF, Strichartz GR: The α_2-adrenergic agonists clonidine and guanfacine produce tonic and phasic block of conduction in rat sciatic nerve fibers. Anesth Analg 1993;76:295-301.

114. Kroin JS, Buvanendran A, Beck DR, et al: Clonidine prolonga-tion of lidocaine analgesia after sciatic nerve block in rats is mediated via the hyperpolarization-activated cation current, not by alpha-adrenoreceptors. Anesthesiology 2004;101:488-494.

115. Dobrydnjov I, Axelsson K, Gupta A, et al: Improved analgesia with clonidine when added to local anesthetic during

combined spinal-epidural anesthesia for hip arthroplasty: A double-blind randomized and placebo-controlled study. Acta Anaesthesiol Scand 2005;49:538-545.

116. van Tuijl I, van Klei WA, van der Werff DB, et al: The effect of addition of intrathecal clonidine to hyperbaric bupivacaine on postoperative pain and morphine requirements after caesarean section: A randomized controlled trial. Br J Anesth 2006;97:365-370.

117. Singelyn FJ, Dangoissse M, Bartholomee S, et al: Adding clonidine to mepivacaine prolongs the duration of anesthesia and analgesia after axillary brachial plexus block. Reg Anesth 1992;17:148-150.

118. Tan PH, Buerkle H, Cheng JT, et al: Double-blind parallel comparison of multiple doses of apraclonidine, clonidine, and placebo administered intra-articularly to patients undergoing arthroscopic knee surgery. Clin J Pain 2004;20:256-260.

119. Reuben SS, Steinberg RB, Klatt JL, et al: Intravenous regional anesthesia using lidocaine and clonidine. Anesthesiology 1999;91:654-658.

120. Casati A, Vinciquera F, Cappelleri G, et al: Adding clonidine to the induction bolus and postoperative infusion during continuous femoral nerve block delays recovery of motor function after total knee arthroplasty. Anesth Analg 2005;100:866-872.

121. Ilfeld BM, Morey TE, Thannikary LJ, et al: Clonidine added to a continuous interscalene ropivacaine perineural infusion to improve postoperative analgesia: A randomized, double-blind, controlled study. Anesth Analg 2005;100:1172-1178.

122. Janson W, Stein C: Peripheral opioid analgesia. Curr Pharm Biotechnol 2003;4:270-274.

123. Stein C, Schafer M, Machelska H: Attacking pain at its source: New perspective on opioids. Nat Med 2003;9:1003-1008.

124. Kalso E, Smith L, McQuay HJ, et al: No pain, no gain: Clinical excellence and scientific rigor-lessons learned from IA morphine. Pain 2002;98:269-275.

125. Rosseland LA: No evidence for analgesic effect of intra-articular morphine after knee arthroscopy: A qualitative systematic review. Reg Anesth Pain Med 2005;30:83-98.

126. Picard PR, Tramer MR, McQuay HJ, et al: Analgesic efficacy of peripheral opioids (all except intra-articular): A qualitative systemic review of randomized controlled trials. Pain 1997;72:309-318.

127. Murphy DB, McCartney CJ, Chan VW: Novel analgesic adjuncts for brachial plexus block: A systematic review. Anesth Analg 2000;90:1122-1128.

128. Bouhassira D. Neuropathic pain: The clinical syndrome revisited. Acta Neurol Belg 2001;101:47-52.

129. Watson CP, Evans RJ, Reed K, et al: Amitriptyline versus placebo in postherpetic neuralgia. Neurology 1982;32:671-673.

130. Rowbotham M, Harden N, Stacey B, et al: Gabapentin for the treatment of postherpetic neuralgia: A randomized controlled trial. JAMA 1998;280:1837-1842.

131. Rowbotham MC, Twilling L, Davies PS, et al: Oral opioid therapy for chronic peripheral and central neuropathic pain. N Engl J Med 2003;348:1223-32.

132. Leipzig RM, Cumming RG, Tinetti ME: Drugs and falls in older people: A systematic review and meta-analysis. I: psychotropic drugs. J Am Geriatr Soc 1999;47:30-9.

133. Devor M: Neuropathic pain and injured nerve: Peripheral mechanisms. Br Med Bull 1991;47:631-647.

134. Mao J, Chen LL: Systemic lidocaine for neuropathic pain relief. Pain 2000;87:7-17.

135. Devor M, Govrin Lippmann R, Angelides K: Na+ channel immunolocalization in peripheral mammalian axons and changes following nerve injury and neuroma formation. J Neurosci 1993; 13:1976-1992.

136. Wall PD, Gutnick M: Properties of afferent nerve impulses originating from a neuroma. Nature 1974;248:740-743.

137. Chabal C, Russell RC, Burchiel KJ. The effect of intravenous lidocaine, tocainide, and mexiletine on spontaneously active fibers originating in rat sciatic neuromas. Pain 1989;38:333-338.

138. Kajander KC, Wakisaka S, Bennett GJ: Spontaneous discharge originates in the dorsal root ganglion at the onset of a painful peripheral neuropathy in the rat. Neurosci Lett 1992;138:225-228.

139. Baron R: Peripheral neuropathic pain: From mechanisms to symptoms. Clin J Pain 2000; 16:S12-S20.

140. Omaha-Zapata I, Khabbaz MA, Hunter JC: QX-314 inhibits ectopic nerve activity associated with neuropathic pain. Brain Res 1997;771:228-237.

141. Abdi S, Lee DH, Chung JM: The anti-allodynic effects of amitriptyline, gabapentin, and lidocaine in a rat model of neuropathic pain. Anesth Analg 1998;87:1360-1366.

142. Devor M, Wall PD, Catalan N: Systemic lidocaine silences ectopic neuroma and DRG discharge without blocking nerve conduction. Pain 1992;48:261-268.

143. Woolf CJ, Wiesenfled-Hallin Z: The systemic administration of local anaesthetics produces a selective depression of C-afferent fibre evoked activity in the spinal cord. Pain 1985;23361-23374.

144. Rowbotham MC, Davies PS, Fields HL: Topical lidocaine gel relieves postherpetic neuralgia. Ann Neurol 1995;37:246-253.

145. Tanelian DL, MacIver MB: Analgesic concentrations of lidocaine suppress tonic A-delta and C fiber discharges produced by acute injury. Anesthesiology 1991;74:934-936.

146. Abram SE, Yaksh TL: Systemic lidocaine blocks nerve-injury induced hyperalgesia and nociceptor-driven spinal sensitization in the rat. Anesthesiology 1994;80:383-391.

147. Yaksh TL: Regulation of spinal nociceptive processing: Where we went when we wandered unto the path marked by the gate. Pain 1999;6:S49-S52.

148. Kalso E, Tramer MR, McQuay HJ, et al: Systemic local anesthetic-type drugs in chronic pain: A systematic review. Eur J Pain 1998;2:3-14.

149. Tremont-Lukats IW, Challapalli V, McNicol ED, et al: Systemic administration of local anesthetics to relieve neuropathic pain: A systematic review and meta-analysis. Anesth Analg 2005;101:1738-1749.

150. Rowbotham MC, Resiner-Keller LA, et al: Both intravenous lidocaine and morphine reduce the pain of postherpetic neuralgia. Neurology 1991;41:1024-1028.

151. Wu CL, Tella P, Staats PS, et al: Analgesic effects of intravenous lidocaine and morphine on postamputation pain. Anesthesiology 2002;96:841-848.

152. Ferrante FM, Paggioloi J, Cherukuri S, et al: The analgesic response to intravenous lidocaine in the treatment of neuropathic pain. Anesth Analg 1996;82:91-97.

153. Edwards WT, Habib F, Burney RG, et al: Intravenous lidocaine in the management of various chronic pain states: A review of 211 cases. Reg Anesth 1985;10:1-6.

154. Attall N, Gaude V, Brasseur L, et al: Intravenous lidocaine in central pain. A double-blind, placebo-controlled, psycho-physical study. Neurology 2000;54:564-574.

155. Galer BS, Harle J, Rowbotham MC: Response to intravenous lidocaine infusion predicts subsequent response to oral mexiletine: A prospective study. J Pain Symptom Manage 1996;12:161-167.

156. Kamei J, Hitosugi H, Kasuya Y: Effects of mexiletine on formalin-induced nociceptive responses in mice. Res Commun Chem Pathol Pharmacol 1993;80:153-162.

157. Khandwala H, Hodge E, Loomis CW: Comparable dose-dependent inhibition of AP-7 sensitive strychnine-induced allodynia and paw pinch-induced nociception by mexiletine in the rat. Pain 1997;72:299-308.

158. Jett MF, McGuirk J, Waligora D, et al: The effects of mexiletine, desipramine, and fluoxetine in rat models involving central sensitization. Pain 1997;69:161-169.

159. Kamei J, Hitosugi H, Kawashima N, et al: Antinociceptive effect of mexiletine in diabetic mice. Res Commun Chem Pathol Pharmacol 1992;77:24524-8.

160. Rathmell JP, Ballantyne JC: Local anesthetics for the treatment of neuropathic pain: On the limits of meta-analysis. Anesth Analg 2005;101:1736-1737.

161. Higa K, Hirata K, Dan K: Mexiletine-induced severe skin eruption, fever, eosinophilia, atypical lymphocytosis, and liver dysfunction. Pain 1997;73:97-99.

162. Jarvis B, Coukell AJ: Mexiletine. A review of its therapeutic use in painful diabetic neuropathy. Drugs 1998;56:691-707.

163. Campbell RWF: Mexiletine. New Engl J Med 1987;316: 29-34.

164. Turgeon J, Fiset C, Giguere R, et al: Influence of debrisoquine phenotype and of quinidine on mexiletine disposition in man. J Pharmacol Exp Ther 1991;259:789-798.

165. Monk JP, Brogden RN: Mexiletine: A review of its pharmacodynamic and pharmacokinetic properties, and therapeutic use in the treatment of arrythmias. Drugs 1990;40:374-411.

166. Nishiyama K, Sakuta M: Mexiletine for painful alcoholic neuropathy. Intern Med 1995;34:577-579.

167. Wallace M, Maguson S, Ridgeway B: Efficacy of oral mexiletine for neuropathic pain with allodynia: A double-blind placebo-controlled, crossover study. Reg Anesth Pain Med 2000;25:459-467.

168. Ando K, Wallace MS, Braun J, et al: Effect of oral mexiletine on capsaicin-induced allodynia and hyperalgesia: A double-blind, placebo-controlled, crossover study. Reg Anesth Pain Med 2000;25:468-474.

169. Galer BS: Painful polyneuropathy: Diagnosis, pathophysiology, and management. Semin Neurol 1994;14:237-246.

170. Fassoulaki A, Patris K, Sarantopoulos C, et al: The analgesic effect of gabapentin and mexiletine after breast surgery for cancer. Anesth Analg 2002;95:985-991.

171. Rowbotham MC, Davies PS, Verkempinck C, et al: Lidocaine patch: Double-blind controlled study of new treatment method for postherpetic neuralgia. Pain 1996;65:39-44.

172. Galer BS: Effectiveness and safety of lidocaine patch 5%. J Fam Pract 2002; 51: 867-868.

173. Katz NP, Gammaitoni AR, Davis MW, et al: Lidocaine patch 5% reduces pain intensity and interference with quality of life in patients with postherpetic neuralgia: An effectiveness trial. Pain Med 2002;3:324-332.

174. Campbell BJ, Rowbotham M, Davies PS, et al: Systemic absorption of topical lidocaine in normal volunteers, patients with post-herpetic neuralgia, and patients with acute herpes zoster. J Pharm Sci 2002;91:1343-1350.

175. Lidoderm prescribing information. Chadds Ford, Pa, Endo Pharmaceuticals, 2000.

176. Benowitz NL, Meister W: Clinical pharmacokinetics of lignocaine. Clin Pharmacokinet 1978;3:177-1201.

177. Gammaitoni AR, Davis MW: Pharmacokinetics and tolerability of lidocaine patch 5% with extended dosing. Ann Pharmacother 2002;36:236-240.

178. Gammaitoni AR, Alvarez NA, Galer BS: Pharmacokinetics and safety of continuously applied lidocaine patches 5%. Am J Health Syst Pharm 2002; 59: 2215-2220.

179. Dalpiaz AS, Lordon SP, Lipman AG: Topical lidocaine patch therapy for myofascial pain. J Pain Palliat Care Pharmacother 2004;18:15-34.

180. Hines R, Keaney D, Moskowitz MH, et al: Use of lidocaine patch 5% for chronic low back pain: A report of four cases. Pain Med 2002;3:361-365.

181. Galer BS, Sheldon E, Patel N, et al: Topical lidocaine patch 5% may target a novel underlying pain mechanism in osteoarthritis. Cur Med Res Opin 2004;20:1455-1458.

182. Barbano RL, Herrmann DN, Hart-Gouleau S, et al: Effectiveness, tolerability, and impact on quality of life of the 5% lidocaine patch in diabetic polyneuropathy. Arch Neurol 2004;6:914-918.

183. Herrmann DN, Barbano RL, Hart-Gouleau S, et al: An open-label study of the lidocaine patch 5% in painful idiopathic sensory polyneuropathy. Pain Med 2005;6:379-384.

45 Neurolytic Blocking Agents: Uses and Complications

Robert E. Molloy and Honorio T. Benzon

SCOPE OF NEUROLYTIC BLOCK

Neurolytic blockade is a valuable tool designed to produce prolonged interruption of neural transmission. In contrast to the action of local anesthetic block, which is measured in hours, neurolytic block aims to alter neural function for weeks to months. The common rationale for neurolytic block is prolonged relief of intractable pain, most often in patients with a malignancy. Neurolytic blocks can be used to treat visceral and somatic pain. Their use for chronic, nonmalignant pain, such as for chronic pancreatitis, is controversial. Additional analgesic applications may include relief of ischemic pain in occlusive vascular disease. Neurolytic block may also provide prolonged relief of muscle spasticity in patients with neurological disease. Raj[1] has recommended the following criteria before performing an analgesic neurolytic block: (1) pain is severe; (2) pain persists with less invasive techniques; (3) pain is well localized; (4) pain is relieved with diagnostic local anesthetic blocks; and (5) there are no undesirable effects after the local anesthetic block (Box 45–1).

Neurolytic blocks are particularly indicated for patients suffering from intractable pain, after failure to control the pain with the application of all available less invasive methods, and with short anticipated life expectancy. The risk of serious life-altering complications must be weighed against the anticipated benefit of pain reduction. For example, neurolytic intrathecal block may provide profound analgesia for a patient with an invasive tumor originating in the pelvis, but this method also often produces loss of bladder and bowel control as well as lower extremity weakness that interferes with ambulation. Because the typical patient with cancer pain has multiple sources of discomfort, this block may fail to relieve pain caused by metastatic disease or other pain mechanisms completely.

Clinical experience has suggested that the current role for neurolytic block is extremely restricted (Box 45–2). Neurolytic block is never the first treatment of choice and most often not an option in managing most pain syndromes. There are many reasons for this. The quality of sustained analgesia after neurolytic block often does not reproduce that obtained with initial, prognostic local anesthetic blockade. The duration of symptom relief is limited and often less than desired. Therapeutic tools used before the block must often be used again, although at lower doses, rather than discontinued after the procedure, to maintain desired symptom control.

Newer pharmacologic and other therapeutic tools are now available and are often effective when used in combination. Neurolytic blockade requires the effort and skills of highly trained practitioners, which may not be easily available. Neurolytic blockade places demands on the patient, including time, discomfort, and expense. It may produce complications that are significant and long-lasting. Randomized controlled trials documenting the efficacy and safety of these procedures are usually not available. A common exception to this statement are reports describing the use of neurolytic celiac plexus block in the management of visceral pain in patients with pancreatic cancer.

Specific neurolytic blocks may include any form of neural blockade in which local anesthetic injection produces a transient but desirable result. These procedures may include peripheral nerve blocks located in the head and neck, trunk, or extremity areas; visceral sympathetic ganglion block; paravertebral sympathetic chain block; neuraxial blockade; and motor nerve or muscle injections. Peripheral neurolytic blocks are rarely performed, for several reasons. The procedure can cause unwanted motor block when mixed nerves are blocked. The patient may find that numbness after the block is bothersome. Neuritis and deafferentation pain are undesirable side effects, occasionally more severe than the preexisting pain. Also, analgesic block is not predictably long-lasting or permanent.[1]

BOX 45–1. CRITERIA FOR NEUROLYSIS: INDICATIONS FOR NEUROLYTIC BLOCK

Pain is severe, intractable, or persists after less invasive treatments

Intolerable side effects of analgesic therapy

Intrathecal catheter not a preferred option

Advanced or terminal malignancy

Pain well localized:

    Unilateral pain, localized to the trunk

    Involves only a few dermatomes or one peripheral nerve

Primary somatic pain mechanism

Absence of intraspinal tumor spread

Pain relieved with prognostic local anesthetic block

No undesirable effects after local anesthetic block

Realistic expectations by patient and family

Informed consent clearly explains potential complications

BOX 45–2. LIMITATIONS OF NEUROLYTIC BLOCK

Quality of analgesia less than after local anesthetic block

Duration of analgesia limited, not permanent

Opioid titration required to a lower maintenance dose

Requires time, talent of skilled physicians

Demands on patient—time, discomfort, expense

Potential for long-term complications

    Weakness interfering with function, ambulation

    Numbness and secondary traumatic injury

    Neuropathic pain and dysesthesias

    Skin ulceration, soft tissue, muscle injury

    Phlebitis, thrombosis, tissue ischemia

Analgesic failure

    Incomplete block, wrong neural target

    New pain at distant site

Neurolytic spinal and epidural blocks with alcohol or phenol are rarely used today. Neuraxial opioids have proven to be an effective modality for the management of cancer pain. Cancer patients may develop new pain syndromes related to new sites of metastatic disease following a successful neurolytic block. It is not practical to perform additional intrathecal neurolytic injections at new levels, with their attendant risks. However, an indwelling intrathecal drug delivery system may be equally effective for the new source of pain or continue to be useful after minor modifications. Visceral neurolytic blocks are particularly effective and still in common use for cancer patients. The abdominal viscera are usually supplied by a plexus of sympathetic nerves, such as the celiac plexus, which are amenable to neurolytic block. With ideal application, visceral neurolytic blocks produce gratifying analgesia without attendant motor weakness or bothersome somatic sensory loss.

Patient selection is critical. A thorough assessment of the patient's overall condition must include an accurate diagnosis, the mechanism of pain symptoms, psychological background, social environment, level of comprehension, and current drug therapy. Application of a multimodal approach to therapy is required. Appropriate drug therapy, use of adjuvant drugs, and consideration of other invasive therapies, including the benefits and risks of each intervention, are essential. Once a neurolytic block is considered, there must be a thorough discussion of reasonable expectations for the procedure, limitations to any expected pain relief, probable need for use of analgesics and other drugs in reduced doses, and an honest description of potential complications. Prognostic local anesthetic block is desirable to demonstrate potential benefits to the patient and physician. However, concern for the patient's overall condition, comfort, and economic considerations may suggest elimination or combination of the prognostic block with the neurolytic procedure at the discretion of the physician. Obtaining informed consent from the patient is essential, and this must be carefully documented. The patient and family must understand and accept all potential complications. The patient's response should be monitored by assessment of pain levels, symptom relief, activity levels, appetite, sleep, mood, and drug intake before and after neurolytic block. The physician must anticipate an altered response to previously taken medications. For example, the potential for respiratory depression after sudden cessation of pain or for narcotic withdrawal syndrome requires carefully titrated opioid withdrawal.[2] The agents used for neurolytic block, and the complications that may result from their application, are considered in this chapter.[3-5]

PHARMACOLOGY OF NEUROLYTIC AGENTS

The neurolytic agents most commonly used are ethyl alcohol and phenol (Table 45–1). Glycerol and modified local anesthetic agents have been used occasionally.

Alcohol

Ethyl alcohol is commercially available in undiluted (absolute or 100%) vials. When exposed to the atmosphere, it absorbs water. The effective concentration is 50% to 100%. Alcohol is the classic neurolytic agent, first reported for subarachnoid injection by Dogliotti in 1931. Alcohol produces destruction of nerve fibers and subsequent wallerian degeneration of axonal fibers and Schwann cells. The basal lamina of the Schwann cell sheath may remain intact. This allows for new Schwann cell proliferation and provides a framework for subsequent nerve fiber growth. As a result, regeneration of axons can occur unless

Table 45–1. Agents for Neurolytic Block

PARAMETER	ALCOHOL	PHENOL
Physical properties	Low water solubility	Absorbs water from air
Stability at room temperature	Unstable	Stable
Intrathecal concentration (%)	100	4-7
Intrathecal diluent	None	Glycerin
Density relative to cerebrospinal fluid	Hypobaric	Hyperbaric
Sensation on injection	Immediate burning pain	Painless, warmth
Nerve block concentration (%)	50-100	4-10
Nerve block diluent	Local anesthetic	Water, saline, contrast dye
Safe dose for nerve block (g)	30	1
Mechanism of action	Extracts lipids; precipitates proteins	Coagulates proteins
Systemic toxicity	Disulfiram-like reaction	Convulsions; cardiovascular collapse

the cell bodies of these nerves have been completely destroyed.[2] Schlosser has demonstrated degeneration and absorption of the entire trigeminal nerve, except for the neurolemma, after alcohol block.[6] More dilute solutions produce less complete neural destruction of somatic neurons. The concentration of alcohol needed to provide adequate relief of pain with somatic block appears to be 50% to 70%. Attempts to find a relatively low concentration of alcohol capable of producing complete sensory loss without any motor deficits have not been ultimately successful.

Merrick has described the effects of alcohol injection on sympathetic nerves.[7] Injection of the sympathetic ganglion cells produces permanent nerve destruction, whereas injection of preganglionic and postganglionic fibers produces axonal degeneration, with limited destruction of ganglionic cell bodies and recovery of many neurons. Sympathetic neurons regenerate over the course of 3 to 5 months or longer.

Alcohol produces neurolysis by extracting neural cholesterol, phospholipids, and cerebrosides and by precipitating lipoproteins and neuropeptides.[8] Injection into a peripheral nerve results in wallerian degeneration, with damage to the nerve cell and the Schwann cell. In wallerian degeneration, the axon breaks down and the myelin sheath retracts, forming ellipsoids of myelin.[9] The axoplasm becomes enclosed within the ellipsoids of myelin, followed by hydrolysis within the ellipsoids by lysosomal enzymes. Regeneration begins during the first week of injury when Schwann cells start to multiply and macrophages ingest the debris. By the end of the first week, Schwann cells may develop a chain within the endoneurium. Macrophages disappear after 2 weeks while endoneurial tubes are filled with Schwann cells. This eventually results in sclerosis of the nerve fibers and myelin sheath.

Alcohol is readily soluble in body fluids, and spreads from the injection site rapidly. This may limit the ability to restrict the injectate to the target area and alters the volume required to produce adequate neurolysis. An alcohol block requires a larger volume than phenol.[5] Large volumes may favor spread of the agent to adjacent sites. Alcohol is readily absorbed into the bloodstream after celiac plexus

block. Alcohol blood levels have been measured after celiac plexus block using 50 mL of 50% ethyl alcohol. Thompson and colleagues[10] have found that blood alcohol levels rise acutely over the first 20 minutes to a peak level of 0.021 g/dL. This is only 25% of the common legal limit for alcohol intoxication.

Intrathecal alcohol injection also results in rapid uptake of alcohol, resultant destruction of the dorsal roots, and variable injury to the surface of the spinal cord and the posterior columns.[11] Alcohol is rapidly absorbed from cerebrospinal fluid (CSF). Matsuki and associates[12] have found that only 10% of the injected dose remains in the CSF after 10 minutes, and 4% after 30 minutes. Alcohol is hypobaric with respect to CSF and quickly floats to the top when injected into CSF. The patient must be positioned semiprone with the painful side uppermost to direct alcohol to the target dorsal roots. Denervation and pain relief occur a few days after injection and are complete after 1 week. The effective concentration is almost 100% for intrathecal use and 50% for celiac plexus block. Alcohol is injected undiluted for peripheral nerve block. Accidental intravascular injection of 30 mL of 100% ethanol will result in a blood alcohol level that is transiently above the legal limit for intoxication, without any danger for severe systemic toxicity. Intravenous injection may cause vessel thrombosis.[13]

Alcohol has been used most commonly for visceral sympathetic block, lumbar sympathetic block, intrathecal neurolysis, and trigeminal ganglion block. It has also been used for hypophysectomy in patients with metastatic breast or prostate cancer. Clinically, alcohol produces significant pain on injection, requiring the prior injection of a local anesthetic into tissues. Severe burning pain on injection persists for about 1 minute; it is then gradually followed by numbness and warmth. Alcohol is also commonly diluted with a local anesthetic prior to injection. Alcohol injection may be followed by burning or shooting neuropathic pain, which can last for weeks or months. This may occur after peripheral nerve block or with spread to somatic nerve roots after lumbar sympathetic block. Unintended spread of alcohol to adjacent tissues can produce cellular injury or necrosis. Alcohol may also produce arterial vasospasm. This may be related to a potential ischemic cause of paraplegia after celiac plexus block.[5] The effects of injection may be initially assessed after 12 to 24 hours.

Alcohol neurolytic injection may induce a disulfiram-like toxic reaction in patients being treated with drugs that inhibit the enzyme alcohol dehydrogenase. In a case report, the patient experienced a reaction with temporary flushing, sweating, dizziness, vomiting, and hypotension following an alcohol celiac plexus block with 15 mL of 67% alcohol.[14] The patient had received the antibiotic moxalactam, an inhibitor of this enzyme. Other agents that have this property include disulfiram, metronidazole, chloramphenicol, tolbutamide, chlorpropamide, and β-lactam–type antibiotics.[5]

Phenol

Mandl[15] reported the use of phenol for sympathetic ganglion block in animals in 1947; complete necrosis was observed within 24 hours, progressive degeneration over 45 days, and regeneration in less than 3 months. Maher[16] described the results of intrathecal phenol in humans in 1955. In essence, phenol appears to be just as neurotoxic as alcohol, producing nonselective damage to neural tissues. Phenol coagulates proteins as its primary mechanism of injury. At lower concentrations, it acts as a local anesthetic.

Stewart and Lourie[17] have observed nonselective degeneration of spinal nerve roots after phenol, suggesting that nerve damage is proportional to the concentration used. In studies of intrathecal injection in cats and humans, Smith[18] has demonstrated that hyperbaric phenol primarily destroys axons in posterior sensory rootlets, in the posterior columns of the cord, and to a lesser extent in the anterior root axons; this is essentially the same pattern as intrathecal alcohol. Phenol produces nonselective destruction by denaturing proteins of axons and adjacent blood vessels. Degeneration occurred over 2 weeks, and regeneration progressed over 14 weeks.[18] Maher and Mehta[19] have observed mostly sensory block after intrathecal injection of 5% phenol, but motor block also at higher concentrations. Phenol has a strong affinity for vascular tissue, and injury to blood vessels near nerve tissue may contribute to neurotoxicity.[20]

Injected phenol in glycerin appears to fix rapidly within the subarachnoid space. Ichiyanagi and colleagues[21] have found that phenol concentrations decrease to 30% of the initial concentration within 1 minute and to 0.1% by 15 minutes. Phenol injection near peripheral nerves produces protein coagulation, axonal degeneration, and subsequent wallerian degeneration. The degree of damage after peripheral nerve block is concentration-dependent, and the changes range from segmental demyelination to wallerian degeneration.[22] Axonal regeneration occurs more rapidly than after alcohol. Gregg and coworkers[23] have performed in vivo electrophysiological studies of the effects of alcohol and phenol peripheral nerve injections in cats. Alcohol produced significant depression of compound action potentials at 2 months; the effects of phenol seen at 2 weeks had returned to normal by 8 weeks.[24]

Phenol is usually prepared by the hospital pharmacy for clinical use. Various concentrations are prepared with saline, distilled sterile water, glycerin, and contrast dyes. Phenol is relatively insoluble in water. At room temperature, the maximum aqueous concentration achieved is 6.7%. Phenol is highly soluble in organic solvents such as alcohol and glycerol. Supersaturated solutions of 10% phenol prepared in distilled water or in bupivacaine are also used. A concentration of 12% phenol is easily prepared in renografin.[25] When mixed with water, phenol spreads widely, extending the area of destruction. The aqueous solution is more potent than a glycerol solution. The aqueous solution of phenol has a greater ability to penetrate the rat sciatic nerve perineurium and produce endoneurial damage than the glycerin preparation, but results are identical with intraneural injections.[26] Phenol in glycerin is hyperbaric relative to CSF. The patient must be positioned in the semisupine position with the painful side down to guide the injectate toward the target dorsal roots. A biphasic action is observed clinically. An initial local anesthetic effect produces warmth and numbness that diminishes over 24 hours, leaving a less intense neurolytic effect. This is an advantage during intrathecal neurolysis, because the painless warmth and numbness provide early feedback on the area being affected by the block. The eventual neurolytic effect is evident after 3 to 7 days.

Concentrations between 4% and 10% phenol are typically used for neurolytic block. Phenol is used clinically for lumbar sympathetic, celiac plexus, hypogastric plexus, somatic nerve, epidural, and intrathecal neurolytic blocks. Phenol is used not only for the management of pain but also in the treatment of spasticity.[27-29] The relative potencies of these two neurolytic agents are such that 3% phenol is roughly equivalent to 40% alcohol.[30] The intravascular injection of phenol may result in convulsions secondary to an increase in the excitatory neurotransmitter acetylcholine in the central nervous system.[31] Large systemic doses of phenol (more than 8.5 g) cause potentially lethal effects similar to those seen with local anesthetic overdose—generalized seizures and cardiovascular collapse. Clinical doses up to 1000 mg are unlikely to cause serious toxicity, if accidental intravenous injection is avoided.

Vascular Effects of Phenol and Alcohol

Vascular effects of neurolytic agents are of concern. An added risk is incurred when a neurolytic agent is injected near a prosthetic vascular graft. Dacron woven grafts exhibited diminished tensile strength after 72-hour exposure to 50% alcohol or 6% phenol, whereas Gore-Tex grafts were unchanged. Electron microscopy has demonstrated significant fiber degeneration of Dacron and much less degradation of Gore-Tex by higher concentrations of these agents.[32] Reported cases of paraplegia after neurolytic celiac plexus block have been postulated to occur because of spinal cord ischemia. Vasospasm of segmental lumbar arteries has been induced in dogs after exposure to ethanol and phenol.[33] This appears to be unrelated to synaptic neurotransmitters or to sodium channels. Johnson and colleagues[34] have demonstrated that low concentrations of ethanol induce significant contractile effects in human aortic smooth muscle cells, along with increased intracellular concentration of cytoplasmic ionized calcium. The fact remains that phenol and alcohol will destroy all types of tissue and may cause a contractile response in blood vessels which may lead to loss of neural function. Therefore, extreme care is required when they are used.

Glycerol

Glycerol, a trihydric alcohol that absorbs water from the atmosphere, is a mild neurolytic agent. It has been used primarily for trigeminal ganglion block. Glycerol injection was frequently effective in patients with trigeminal neuralgia in multiple reports, often with preservation of facial sensation.[35-38] Gasserian ganglion block is performed using 100% glycerol. Glycerol injection near nerve tissue produces localized perineural damage, whereas intraneural injection results in edema, axonal destruction, and wallerian degeneration.

UNDESIRABLE EFFECTS OF NEUROLYTIC AGENTS

Neurolytic agents may produce widespread, indiscriminate tissue injury.[13] Skin ulceration and soft tissue and muscle injury may occur, with severe pain at the injection site. Superficial injection and failure to flush the needle before removal predispose to these complications. Diffusion from the site of injection may lead to additional tissue damage and fibrosis. Undesirable nerve injury may occur with resultant numbness, burning neuropathic pain, and motor weakness. Neuropathic pain related to partial nerve destruction and regeneration may be more likely after peripheral rather than intrathecal neurolytic block. Additional tissue trauma may occur in areas of denervated tissue. Vascular complications may include phlebitis, vessel thrombosis, vasospasm, tissue ischemia, and damage to the microcirculation around small nerves. Pain on injection is characteristic of ethyl alcohol. Phenol injection may also be uncomfortable, but its initial local anesthetic effects tend to limit local pain. Accidental intravenous injection of neurolytic agents may cause undesirable systemic effects. Phenol toxicity may include convulsions, central nervous system depression, and cardiovascular collapse. Systemic toxicity from alcohol should produce the typical symptoms of intoxication. Systemic toxicity caused by overdose, in the absence of intravenous injection, is unlikely if total dose limits

are observed. A total systemic dose of 30 mL of 100% ethyl alcohol (30 g) should be easily tolerated. Clinical doses of phenol up to 1000 mg (20 mL 5% phenol) are unlikely to cause serious toxicity.[29]

Complications from Specific Neurolytic Blocks

Neurolytic agents can be injected into peripheral nerves, along the neuraxis within the intrathecal or epidural spaces, or adjacent to visceral sympathetic nerves. Each of these sites of injection is associated with specific complications (Table 45–2). Peripheral neurolysis includes injection into cranial, truncal, upper and lower extremity nerves, and trigger points, and for spasticity.[1]

Complications from Neuraxial Neurolysis

Subarachnoid neurolytic blocks are used in patients with short life expectancy resulting from malignancy, with somatic pain limited to two or three dermatomes, poorly controlled by analgesic and adjuvant drugs, and completely relieved by prognostic local anesthetic blocks.[39] The recommended dose of intrathecal alcohol and phenol is very small; 0.1-mL increments are injected, up to a total of 0.8 mL. The

Table 45–2. Complications of Neurolytic Blocks

COMPLICATION	TYPE OF NEUROLYTIC BLOCK
Weakness of limb	PNB, SAB, EPID
Numbness of limb	PNB, SAB, EPID, LSB, CPB
Dysesthesia, neuropathic pain	All blocks
Intravascular injection, systemic toxicity	All blocks except SAB
Skin slough, soft tissue injury	All blocks
Vascular injury, hematoma	LSB, CPB, SHPB
Accidental epidural or spinal	ICB, CPB, GGB
Somatic nerve root block	LSB, CPB
Foot ischemia	SHPB
Back pain	LSB, CPB, SHPB
Pneumothorax, chylothorax, chest pain, ejaculatory dysfunction	CPB
Renal injury, ureteral injury	CPB, LSB
Hypotension	CPB, SAB, EPID
Paraplegia, spinal infarct	CPB
Horner's syndrome, hoarseness, spinal infarct, brachial plexus block	SGB
Cranial nerve deficits; anesthesia of cornea, cheek, nose; nasal or corneal ulceration; keratitis, diplopia	GGB
Endocrine defects, CSF rhinorrhea, meningitis, visual loss	PA

CPB, celiac plexus block; CSF, cerebrospinal fluid; EPID, epidural block; GGB, gasserian ganglion block; ICB, intercostal nerve block; LSB, lumbar sympathetic block; PA, pituitary ablation; PNB, peripheral nerve block; SAB, subarachnoid block; SGB, stellate ganglion block; SHPB, superior hypogastric plexus block.

patient is immobilized for at least 30 minutes after the injection, and air is injected to clear the needle before it is withdrawn. Complications of intrathecal neurolytic block include heningeal puncture headache, aseptic meningitis, numbness, muscle weakness, bowel and bladder dysfunction, and dysesthesia.[39,40] The incidence of these complications ranges from 1% to 26% for rectal and urinary dysfunction, 1% to 14% for lower extremity weakness, 1% to 21% for sensory loss, and 0.3% to 4% for paresthesia/neuritis.[41] The nature of potential complications is related to the level of injection. Motor weakness involving limb function is noted when injection is performed at a cervicothoracic or lumbar site. Bladder and bowel complications usually follow when the injection occurs below the thoracic nerve roots. Because these complications are severe, it is important that the patients be carefully selected and fully informed of the complications that may interfere with quality of life. During the procedure, patients must be properly positioned, and the spinal needle must be inserted at the interspace corresponding to the target nerve roots.

An epidural approach to neurolytic block has been advocated for improved efficacy at the thoracic level and cervicothoracic junction, increased safety, ease of repeated injections, and relief of bilateral pain.[42,43] Placement of a thoracic epidural catheter is less demanding than positioning multiple needles just barely into the subarachnoid space without entering the spinal cord.[44] In contrast to intrathecal neurolysis, positioning with respect to the baricity of the alcohol or phenol is not a consideration in epidural neurolysis. An epidural catheter is inserted at the vertebral level corresponding to the painful area. Confirmation of catheter placement with injection of radiopaque dye is recommended to confirm the spread of the injectate. Three to 4 mL of local anesthetic is injected and the patient's response to prognostic block is evaluated. The same volume (2 to 5 mL) of 5.5% phenol in saline, or ethyl alcohol, is injected over 20 to 30 minutes in 0.2-mL increments. The injections are given daily for up to 3 days[42] or until the patient has significant pain relief.[43] Analgesic action persists for 1 to 3 months.

There are no studies that have compared the efficacy of subarachnoid and epidural neurolytic blocks. Although no serious complications were noted in previous reports, the safety of epidural neurolysis has been questioned. In primates, lower extremity weakness has been noted clinically and posterior nerve root damage was demonstrated histologically.[45] Autopsy studies in one patient showed destruction at the outer third of the dura, with no abnormality of the spinal cord or the nerve roots.[46] More detailed descriptions of the neural block procedures mentioned in this chapter have been presented by Raj[1] and Bonica and associates.[2]

Subarachnoid neurolytic block is rarely used now for patients with cancer pain. Implanted intrathecal morphine pumps have supplanted these blocks. Intrathecal pumps can be used to manage recurrent pain when the disease progresses, including painful metastases at distant sites.

SPECIFIC NEUROLYTIC BLOCKS

Visceral Sympathetic Neurolysis

Celiac plexus block effectively relieves pain from intra-abdominal malignancy by denervating the abdominal viscera, except for the left colon and pelvic viscera. The efficacy of neurolytic celiac plexus block has been demonstrated in a randomized controlled trial of 100 patients with advanced pancreatic cancer; neurolytic celiac plexus block was compared to systemic analgesic therapy.[47] The systemic analgesic group received a sham celiac plexus block that included subcutaneous bupivacaine injection. Patients were assessed on a weekly basis for 1 year unless death intervened. The pain severity and quality-of-life scores improved following treatment in both groups after 1 week. However, there was a larger decrease in pain scores in the celiac plexus group after 1 week and over time. There were no significant differences in opioid consumption, quality-of-life scores, or survival between the two treatment groups.[47]

Neurolysis of the celiac plexus can be performed through several approaches, including the transaortic,[48,49] transcrural,[50] and anterior approaches,[51] as well as bilateral splanchnicectomy.[52] Three percutaneous neurolytic celiac plexus block techniques—transcrural approach, transaortic approach, and bilateral splanchnicectomy—have been compared. There do not appear to be differences in analgesic efficacy or attendant complications among the various approaches.[52]

The complications of neurolytic celiac plexus block can be classified as neurologic and vascular injury, pulmonary or metabolic complications, and visceral injury.[53] Neurologic complications include accidental epidural or dural puncture, somatic nerve block resulting in weakness, paralysis, or numbness of the thigh,[10,54] and accidental injection into a radicular artery supplying the spinal cord, producing paraplegia.[55] Exposure to phenol or alcohol results in vasospasm of the segmental lumbar arteries in dogs,[33] and alcohol has been shown to have contractile effects in human aortic muscle cells by increasing the intracellular concentration of ionized calcium.[34] Vascular injury is possible because of the proximity of several blood vessels, including the aorta and inferior vena cava. The transaortic approach to celiac plexus block requires double penetration of the aortic wall.[52,56] Hematoma formation, aortic dissection, and injury to a preexisting aortic aneurysm or vascular graft may occur.[57,58] Intravascular injection may result in convulsions when phenol is used.[31] Intravascular alcohol injection does not result in toxicity because of the relatively low blood levels attained. Acetaldehyde toxicity may occur in Asians who lack the enzyme aldehyde dehydrogenase; this results in palpitations, facial flushing, and hypotension.[59]

Visceral injury may include hematuria caused by renal trauma and renal infarction after accidental neurolytic injection.[60] Injury to the kidney is more likely when needle insertion is more than 7.5 cm from the midline, a higher vertebral level is targeted (T11-12), or needle position is lateral to the vertebral body.[61] Pancreatic injury and pancreatitis might occur, but minimal elevations of the amylase level are noted after celiac plexus block.[62] Pulmonary trauma may also occur, particularly when higher vertebral body levels are targeted. Pneumothorax and pleural effusion have been reported after celiac plexus block. The latter complication may result from diaphragmatic irritation by a neurolytic agent injected into or superficial to the diaphragm.[63] Chylothorax and ejaculatory dysfunction have also been reported after celiac plexus block.[64,65] The frequency of complications after 104 celiac plexus blocks was as follows[65]: weakness or numbness in the T10-L2 distribution (8%), lower chest pain (3%), postural hypotension (2%), failure of ejaculation (2%), difficult urination (1%), and warmth and fullness of the leg (1%). The overall incidence of major complications from neurolytic celiac plexus block, such as paraplegia and bladder and bowel dysfunction, was 1 in 683 procedures. This was based on a review of 2730 patients having blocks performed from 1986 to 1990.[66] Meticulous technique and advanced imaging are used to minimize most complications. Fluoroscopy, contrast dye, and computed tomography have been used for this purpose.[67]

Superior hypogastric plexus block is used to manage the visceral component of pelvic pain caused by malignancy.[67-70] These retroperitoneal neural structures are present bilaterally, just anterior to the vertebral column between the lower third of the L5 and upper third of the S1 vertebral bodies. Vascular complications may include traumatic retroperitoneal hematoma or distal ischemia caused by iliac artery trauma that dislodges atherosclerotic plaque.[67] No neurologic complications were detected following this neurolytic block in 200 patients.

Ganglion impar block is performed in the midline, just anterior to the sacrococcygeal junction, to relieve persistent burning perineal pain associated with a pelvic malignancy.[71,72] Published reports on the outcome after neurolytic ganglion impar block are sparse, but no complications have been reported.

Lumbar Paravertebral Sympathetic Neurolysis

Thoracic paravertebral neurolytic blocks are not performed because of the potential for pneumothorax. *Lumbar sympathetic block* has been used to treat symptomatic peripheral vascular disease, complex regional pain syndrome, phantom limb pain, and hyperhidrosis. Needles are placed at the anterolateral surface of the L2 and L3 vertebral bodies using fluoroscopy to identify the intended vertebral levels, the desired depth of needle insertion, and adequate spread of contrast material into the appropriate space.[73] The use of two needles, 1- to 2-mL local

anesthetic test doses, and confirmation of sympathetic block should precede injection of 3 to 4 mL neurolytic agent at each level (L2 and L3).

Complications of lumbar sympathetic block include paresthesia, backache, sensory and motor loss after nerve root injury, and subarachnoid spread caused by injection of a dural cuff at the intervertebral foramen.[13] Ureteral injury may occur from direct needle trauma or neurolytic-induced thrombosis of its blood supply by a branch of the ovarian artery.[74] Genitofemoral neuralgia may occur in 7% to 20% of patients and persist for 4 to 5 weeks.[75] Postsympathectomy numbness and pain in the thigh may last several months. The use of fluoroscopy is mandatory to improve accuracy and safety when neurolytic block of the sympathetic chain is performed. Phenol neurolysis has provided more complete sympathetic block than radiofrequency rhizotomy of the lumbar sympathetic chain.[76] However, the incidence of postsympathectomy neuralgia was also higher in the phenol group (33% versus 11%).

Cervical Paravertebral Sympathetic Neurolysis

The lowest cervical sympathetic ganglion is usually fused with the first thoracic ganglion, forming the cervicothoracic (stellate) ganglion. The cervical sympathetic chain lies anterior to the prevertebral fascia and anterolateral to the longus colli muscle. Its alar fascial plane may communicate with the brachial plexus and the vertebral artery and it is in close proximity to the carotid sheath, phrenic nerve, and recurrent laryngeal nerve. These anatomic relationships may explain potential side effects of stellate ganglion block.[77] Cervical sympathetic chain block is often performed at the C6 level. Relatively large volumes (5 to 20 mL) are injected 2 mm superficial to the C6 tubercle; the intent is to spread solution downward to reach the stellate and upper thoracic ganglia.[78] Injection at the C7 level requires a smaller volume, but this approach increases the risk of vertebral artery injection and pneumothorax. The posterior paravertebral approach involves walking a needle off the upper thoracic lamina; fluoroscopy and contrast dye are required to confirm appropriate needle placement.

Stellate ganglion block using local anesthetic has been used to manage patients with complex regional pain syndrome, vascular insufficiency of the upper extremities,[79] and hyperhidrosis of the face and upper extremities. Neurolytic stellate ganglion blockade has been used for patients with complex regional pain syndrome when repeated local anesthetic blocks provide consistent short-term pain relief without prolonged benefit. Reported complications include Horner's syndrome, brachial plexus block, hoarseness, epidural or subarachnoid spread, and spinal cord infarct.[80,81] Ptosis associated with Horner's syndrome can be corrected by surgical suspension of the upper eyelid. The incidence of all complications has been reported to be 0.17%.[82] However, the severity of these potential complications renders neurolytic stellate ganglion block a relatively unattractive option. Radiofrequency rhizotomy and thoracoscopic sympathectomy have been used to avoid these complications of neurolytic stellate ganglion block.

Intercostal and Thoracic Paravertebral Somatic Neurolysis

Intercostal nerve blocks are used to treat thoracic and abdominal wall pain as a result of surgical procedures or local malignancy.[83-86] Complications include pneumothorax, neuraxial spread, intravascular injection, and intrapulmonary injection, with consequent bronchospasm. The incidence of pneumothorax detected by radiography is 0.082% to 2%.[87,88] Significant pneumothorax occurs less often, and chest tube insertion is rarely necessary. Total spinal anesthesia has been reported after intraoperative intercostal block during a thoracotomy, probably secondary to injection into a dural cuff or directly into the nerve with retrograde spread.[89] Intrapulmonary injection of phenol may produce bronchospasm.[90]

When multiple spinal nerve levels are involved, *paravertebral somatic nerve block* is used to limit the number of injections, because one injection may block several ipsilateral segments. Paravertebral somatic block serves as an alternative approach to epidural or intercostal block for unilateral, multisegmental acute or chronic chest wall pain.[91-93] Reported complications include pneumothorax, vascular injection, epidural spread, hypotension, and urinary retention. Fluoroscopy should be used when these truncal nerve blocks are performed. It is valuable to minimize and subsequently rule out the presence of a pneumothorax, particularly in an outpatient clinic setting.

Ilioinguinal and *iliohypogastric nerve blocks* are used in the perioperative management of pain after inguinal hernia repair[94] and cesarean section.[95] These blocks are also performed for diagnosis and treatment of inguinal and suprapubic pain after inguinal hernia repair or lower abdominal surgery. Reported complications include accidental block of the lateral femoral cutaneous and femoral nerves, but their frequency is not known. Pulsed radiofrequency rhizotomy has been used rather than neurolytic blockade when prognostic local anesthetic blocks have provided temporary pain relief.[96]

Neurolytic Blocks of the Head and Neck

Neurolytic block of nerves in the head and neck is performed for various reasons. These include the following: trigeminal ganglion block for trigeminal neuralgia unresponsive to medical management and for relief of cancer pain secondary to invasive tumors in the distribution of the trigeminal nerve; pituitary neurolysis for metastatic cancer (specifically breast and prostate cancers); and neurolytic block of peripheral cranial nerves.

The gasserian ganglion is formed from two trigeminal roots that leave the brainstem at the midpontine level.[97] The roots pass through the posterior cranial fossa and eventually enter Meckel's cave in the middle cranial fossa. The gasserian ganglion contains ophthalmic, maxillary, and mandibular sensory divisions, and the mandibular division acquires a motor root as it exits the foramen ovale. The trigeminal cistern, which contains CSF, lies behind the trigeminal ganglion. In *gasserian ganglion block,* the needle is inserted from a point lateral to the side of the mouth and directly caudad to the pupil; it is advanced in a cephalad direction toward the auditory meatus.[98] After contacting the base of the skull, the needle is withdrawn and walked posteriorly toward the foramen ovale. Fluoroscopy is required to confirm correct needle placement. After noting free flow of CSF, the injection is performed in a fashion similar to that for neurolytic subarachnoid block. Very small amounts of local anesthetic or neurolytic agent are injected in 0.1-mL increments to a total of 0.4 to 0.5 mL. Absolute alcohol or 6.5% phenol in glycerin may be used as the neurolytic agent. The patient remains supine when alcohol is used but placed in a sitting position with the chin on the chest before injection of phenol. This patient position aims to localize phenol around the maxillary and mandibular divisions of the trigeminal nerve and to minimize spread to the ophthalmic division, avoiding resultant corneal anesthesia.

The most common complications of gasserian ganglion block[13] include anesthesia of the cheek and nose (66%) and corneal anesthesia (20% to 69%). Additional complications include bleeding caused by vascular injury. Subscleral bleeding, significant facial hematoma, and hemorrhage in the temporal fossa may occur. Local anesthetic injection can produce spinal anesthesia, because the ganglion lies within the cerebrospinal fluid. Abnormal mastication may occur after block of trigeminal motor fibers.[99] Diplopia and strabismus occur as a result of oculomotor or abducens nerve injury. This is usually temporary, but permanent lateral rectus palsy has been reported.[13] Spread to the facial nerve results in paralysis of facial muscles and inability to close the eyelid. Eye trauma, keratitis, and corneal ulceration may follow.[100,101] Absence of tear formation and conjunctivitis result from damage to the greater superficial petrosal nerve. Acoustic nerve injury may result in deafness or dizziness. Delayed effects of gasserian ganglion neurolytic block include keratitis, nasal ulcerations, and oral erosions, usually after trauma to denervated areas. Anesthesia dolorosa may also occur. These complications may disrupt vision and oral nutrition, produce severe neurologic distress, and prove devastating to patients.[13,101] Radiofrequency rhizotomy of the gasserian ganglion has been used, with a similar technique of needle placement, to avoid the complications of chemical neurolysis, including spread of neurolytic agent into the CSF. The complications of thermal radiofrequency rhizotomy of the trigeminal ganglion and their incidences include masseter weakness (18%), paresthesia or dysesthesia (20%), diplopia (1.5%), and keratitis (3%).[102]

Chemical ablation of the pituitary with alcohol injection was used in the late 1970s and early 1980s to treat pain caused by metastatic breast and prostate cancer.[103,104] Results seemed to be better in patients with hormone-dependent tumors. The technique was modified and designed to minimize cerebrospinal fluid leak.[103,105,106] In *pituitary ablation,* the needle is inserted through the nose and advanced to the anterior wall of the sella turcica. General anesthesia and biplanar fluoroscopic guidance are necessary. Phenol or alcohol, in aliquots of 0.2 mL, is injected to a total of 4 to 6 mL. The pupils are monitored during the injection for signs of dilation, indicating spread of injectate outside the sella and oculomotor block; this requires replacement of the needle in a more anterior position before further drug injection. Cyanomethacrylate resin, 0.5 mL, is injected before the needle is withdrawn to prevent CSF leak. Cryoneurolysis and radiofrequency lesions of the pituitary gland have also been described.[107,108]

Endocrine effects of pituitary gland destruction include hypothyroidism, diabetes insipidus, adrenal insufficiency, abnormal temperature regulation, and loss of libido.[103,104,109,110] Additional complications include temporary headache, CSF rhinorrhea, visual field defects, ocular nerve palsy, air embolism, meningitis, and altered consciousness.[13] The incidence of these complications has been reported by Waldman.[111] Hormone replacement therapy is required to treat the expected endocrine deficiencies. Meticulous needle placement with fluoroscopic guidance is essential to limit complications. Sterile technique and preoperative antibiotics prevent infectious complications.

Individual neurolytic *cranial nerve blocks* have been performed, and each may produce unwanted sensory or motor deficits. Block of the maxillary nerve at the foramen rotundum or neurolytic infraorbital nerve block may cause ulceration and slough of the nasal ala and cheek, ischemic palatal necrosis, or slough of the posterior portion of the superior maxillary ridge.[13] Neurolytic mandibular nerve block at the foramen ovale may cause unilateral weakness of the muscles of mastication. Facial nerve block produces paralysis of the facial muscles. Glossopharyngeal nerve block produces pharyngeal muscle paralysis and there is also sensory loss in the nasopharynx, eustachian tube, uvula, tonsil, soft palate, base of tongue, and external auditory canal.[1] Neurolytic glossopharyngeal nerve block is also not performed because of its close proximity to the vagus, accessory, and hypoglossal nerves, which may be affected by this nerve block. Neurolytic block of cranial nerves may not be feasible because of the extent of patient disease and severity of potential complications. Neuraxial opioid therapy via an implanted cervical epidural catheter may be considered instead.

Neurolysis of Peripheral Nerves

Neurolytic block of peripheral nerves in the extremities may produce localized analgesia but also extremity paralysis, which is rarely acceptable. Neurolytic brachial plexus block with phenol has provided short-term pain relief without significant paralysis in a patient with arm pain caused by a Pancoast tumor.[112] The complications from neurolytic block of peripheral nerves include painful dysesthesias and sensory and motor blockade. The exact incidences of these complications are not known. Motor deficits may be beneficial to patients with muscle pain and spasticity caused by neurologic disease.

Neurolytic Blocks for Treatment of Spasticity

Patients with spasticity caused by neurologic disease experience discomfort, interference with nursing care, and resistance to therapeutic muscle lengthening. Management includes physical therapy, drug therapy, and neurolytic injections. Four approaches to neurolytic block include subarachnoid block, peripheral nerve block, motor nerve block, and intramuscular injection.[29] Intrathecal alcohol has successfully treated spasticity in patients with progressive multifocal leukoencephalopathy or spinal cord injury.[113,114] Intrathecal phenol has also been used for relief of spasticity in patients with multiple sclerosis or paraplegia.[115,116]

Neurolytic blocks of peripheral nerves are useful for patients with acquired spasticity. The blocks facilitate rehabilitation, improve gait and balance, and can restore normal position of the limb. Examples of these blocks include obturator nerve block to relieve hip adduction,[117] musculocutaneous nerve block for elbow flexion,[118,119] sciatic nerve block for hamstring spasticity,[120] and posterior tibial nerve block for plantar flexion.[121]

Diagnostic blocks with local anesthetic are usually performed before neurolytic injection to assess the effect of peripheral nerve block on muscle tone. In this technique, motor nerves or mixed nerves are targeted preferentially. A nerve stimulator is recommended for precise needle localization. Distal motor nerve injection aims to decrease focal motor tone and minimize unpleasant sensory loss. Injections of small volumes of 3% to 5% phenol are effective in relieving motor points in affected muscles.[122] Relaxation of the muscle usually lasts 2 months and functional training of the limb is performed during this time. The reported complications include focal motor weakness in 15% and dysesthesias in 10% of patients. The motor weakness usually lasts 1 week and the dysesthesias last several days to weeks.[123] The duration of reported effect after phenol injections has been widely variable (1 to 36 months). In general, the average duration of clinical benefit is approximately 6 months.[124] Direct intramuscular infiltration of alcohol in patients with cerebral palsy has suggested that reduction in spasticity may result without marked decrease in strength.[125] A series of intramuscular phenol injections (0.5 to 4 mL per muscle) has relieved cervical dystonia in 55 torticollis patients; 45% had at least moderate relief, and 27% had mild improvement.[126]

Complications reported after peripheral nerve and intramuscular injections include pain, edema, dysesthesia, motor weakness, intravascular injection, and toxicity.[29] A reported complication after phenol block of the brachioradialis muscle and the musculocutaneous nerve was arterial occlusion of the patient's upper limb.[127]

Neurolytic trigger point injections have been reported to be useful in patients with palpable painful neuromas (0.2 to 0.5 mL of 5% phenol),[128] in patients with poststernotomy pain secondary to scar neuroma (2 to 3 mL of 6% phenol),[129] and in patients with painful surgical scars (1 mL of absolute alcohol).[130] Neuritis has not been reported after these trigger point injections.

CONCLUSION

Neurolytic blocks have a restricted role in the management of pain. Prognostic local anesthetic blocks are required before these blocks can be performed, technical expertise is required in their performance, complications can result in a marked decrease in the patient's quality of life, and beneficial effects last a few months. Neuraxial neurolytic blocks can be used in cases of localized and segmental pain from cancer, at the thoracic vertebral levels; it is not recommended at the lumbar and sacral levels because of the potential development of lower extremity paralysis and bowel and bladder incontinence. Intrathecal opioid pump is better suited in these cases to control the pain from the tumor and from future metastases. Peripheral neurolytic blocks are rarely used because of the occurrence of painful dysesthesia secondary to neuritis. Visceral sympathetic neurolytic blocks are most efficacious in the treatment of abdominal and pelvic pain secondary to cancer; the performance of these blocks can be very gratifying in patients with a short life expectancy.

References

1. Raj PP: Peripheral neurolysis in the management of pain. In Waldman SD, Winnie AP (eds): Interventional Pain Management. Philadelphia, WB Saunders, 1996, pp 392-400.
2. Bonica JJ, Buckley FP, Moricca G, et al: Neurolytic blockade and hypophysectomy. In Bonica JJ, Chapman CR, et al (eds): The Management of Pain, 2nd ed. Philadelphia, Lea & Febiger, 1990, pp 1980-2039.
3. Jain S, Gupta R: Neurolytic agents in clinical practice. In Waldman SD (ed): Interventional Pain Management. Philadelphia, WB Saunders, 2001, pp 220-225.
4. Myers RR: Neuropathology of neurolytic agents. In Cousins MJ, Bridenbaugh PO (eds): Neural Blockade in Clinical Anesthesia and Management of Pain, 3rd ed. Philadelphia, Lippincott-Raven, 1998, pp 985-1006.
5. De Leon-Casasola OA, Ditonio E: Drugs commonly used for nerve blocking: Neurolytic agents. In Raj PP (ed): Practical Management of Pain, 3rd ed. St. Louis, Mosby, 2000, pp 575-578.
6. Schlosser H: Erfahrungen in der neuralgiebehandlung mit alkoholeinspritzungen. Verh Cong Innere Med 1907;24: 49.
7. Merrick RL: Degeneration and recovery of autonomic neurons following alcoholic block. Ann Surg 1941;113:298.
8. Rumsby MG, Finean JB: The action of organic solvents on the myelin sheath of peripheral nerve tissue-II (short chain and aliphatic alcohols). J Neurochem 1966;13:1509-1511.
9. Jain S, Gupta R: Neurolytic agents in clinical practice. In Waldman SD, Winnie AP (eds): Interventional Pain Management. Philadelphia, WB Saunders, 1996, pp 167-171.
10. Thompson GE, Moore DC, Bridenbaugh DL, et al: Abdominal pain and alcohol celiac plexus nerve block. Anesth Analg 1977;56:1-5.
11. Gallagher HS, Yonezawa T, Hay RC, et al: Subarachnoid alcohol block. II: Histological changes in the central nervous system. Am J Pathol 1961;35:679-693.
12. Matsuki M, Kato Y, Ichiyanagi K: Progressive changes in the concentration of ethyl alcohol in the human and canine subarachnoid spaces. Anesthesiology 1972;36:617-621.
13. Swerdlow M: Complications of neurolytic neural blockade. In Cousins MJ, Bridenbaugh PO (eds): Neural Blockade in Clinical Anesthesia and Management of Pain, 2nd ed. Philadelphia: JB Lippincott, 1988, pp 719-735.
14. Umeda S, Arai T: Disulfiram-like reaction to moxalactam after celiac plexus alcohol block.
15. Mandl F: Aqueous solution of phenol as a substitute for alcohol in sympathetic block. J Int Coll Surg, 1950;13: 566-568.
16. Maher RM: Relief of pain in incurable cancer. Lancet 1955;268:18-20.
17. Stewart WA, Lourie H: An experimental evaluation of the effects of subarachnoid injections of phenol-Pantopaque in cats. J Neurosurg 1963;20:64-72.
18. Smith MC: Histological findings following intrathecal injections of phenol solutions for the relief of pain. Br J Anaesth 1964;36:387-406.
19. Maher RM, Mehta M: Spinal (intrathecal) and extradural analgesia. In Lipton S (ed): Persistent Pain: Modern Methods of Treatment. New York, Grune & Stratton, 1977, p 61.
20. Wood KM: The use of phenol as a neurolytic agent. Pain 1978;5:205-229.
21. Ichiyanagi K, Matsuki M, Kinefuchi J, et al: Progressive changes in the concentration of phenol and glycerin in the human subarachnoid space. Anesthesiology 1975;42: 622-624.
22. Schaumburg HH, Byck R, Weller RO: The effect of phenol in peripheral nerve: A histological and physiologic study. J Neuropathol Exp Neurol 1970;29:615-630.
23. Gregg RV, Constantini CH, Ford DJ, et al: Electrophysiologic and histopathologic investigation of alcohol as a neurolytic agent. Anesthesiology 1985;63:A250.
24. Gregg RV, Constantini CH, Ford DJ, et al: Electrophysiologic and histopathologic investigation of phenol in renografin as a neurolytic agent. Anesthesiology 1985;63:A239.
25. Rauck R: Sympathetic nerve blocks. In Raj PP: Practical Management of Pain, 3rd ed. St. Louis, Mosby, 2000, pp 651-682.
26. Westerlund T, Vuorinen V, Kirvela O, et al: The endoneurial response to neurolytic agents is highly dependent on the mode of application. Reg Anesth Pain Med 1999;24: 294-302.
27. Khalili AA, Betts HB: Peripheral nerve block with phenol in the management of spasticity: Indications and complications. JAMA 1967;200:1155-1157.
28. Katz J, Knott LW, Feldman DJ: Peripheral nerve injections with phenol in the management of spastic patients. Arch Phys Med Rehabil 1967;48:97-99.
29. Zafonte RD, Munin MC: Phenol and alcohol blocks for the treatment of spasticity. Phys Med Rehabil Clin N Am 2001;12:817-832.
30. Moller JE, Helweg-Larson J, Jacobsen G: Histopathological lesions in the sciatic nerve of the rat following perineural application of phenol and alcohol solutions. Dan Med Bull 1969;16:116-119.
31. Benzon HT: Convulsions secondary to intravascular phenol: A hazard of celiac plexus block. Anesth Analg 1979;58: 150-151.
32. Gale DW, Valley MA, Rogers JN, et al: Effects of neurolytic concentrations of alcohol and phenol on Dacron and

Gore-Tex vascular prosthetic grafts. Reg Anesth 1994;19: 395-401.

33. Brown DL, Rorie DK: Altered reactivity of isolated segmental lumbar arteries of dogs following exposure to ethanol and phenol. Pain 1994;56:139-143.

34. Johnson ME, Sill JC, Brown DL, et al: The effect of the neurolytic agent ethanol on cytoplasmic calcium in arterial smooth muscle and endothelium. Reg Anesth 1996;21: 6-13.

35. Sweet WH, Poletti CE, Macon JB: Treatment of trigeminal neuralgia and other facial pains by retrogasserian injection of glycerol. Neurosurgery 1981;9:647-653.

36. Bennett MH, Lunsford LD: Percutaneous retrogasserian glycerol rhizotomy for tic doloreaux: Part 2. Results and implications of trigeminal evoked potentials. Neurosurgery 1984;14: 431-435.

37. Lumsford LD, Bennett MH: percutaneous retrogasserian glycerol rhizotomy in the treatment of trigeminal neuralgia. Part 1. Technique and results in 112 patients. Neurosurgery 1984;14:424-430.

38. Feldstein GS: Percutaneous retrogasserian glycerol rhizotomy in the treatment of trigeminal neuralgia. In Racz GB (ed): Techniques of Neurolysis. Boston. Kluwer Academic Publishers, 1988, pp 125-128.

39. Winnie AP: Subarachnoid neurolytic blocks. In Waldman SD, Winnie AP (eds): Interventional Pain Management. Philadelphia, WB Saunders, 1996, pp 401-405.

40. Gerbershagen HU: Neurolysis: Subarachnoid neurolytic blockade. Acta Anaesthesiol Belg 1981;32:45-47.

41. Cousins MJ: Chronic pain and neurolytic neural blockade. In Cousins MJ, Bridenbaugh PO (eds): Neural Blockade in Clinical Anesthesia and Management Of Pain, 2nd ed. Philadelphia, JB Lippincott, 1988, pp 1053-1084.

42. Korevaar WC: Transcatheter thoracic epidural neurolysis using ethyl alcohol. Anesthesiology 1988;69:989-993.

43. Racz GB, Sabongy M, Gintautas J, et al: Intractable pain therapy using a new epidural catheter. JAMA 1982;248: 579-581.

44. Molloy RE: Intrathecal and epidural neurolysis. In Benzon HT, Raja S, Molloy RE, et al (eds): Essentials of Pain Medicine and Regional Anesthesia, 2nd ed. New York, Elsevier-Churchill Livingstone, 2005, pp 550-557.

45. Katz JA, Selhorst S, Blisard KS: Histopathological changes in primate spinal cord after single and repeated epidural phenol administration. Reg Anesth 1995;20:283-290.

46. Hayashi I, Odashiro M, Sasaki Y: Two cases of epidural neurolysis using ethyl alcohol and histopathologic changes in the spinal cord. Masui 2000;49:877-880.

47. Wong GY, Schroeder DR, Carns PE, et al: Effect of neurolytic celiac plexus block on pain relief, quality of life, and survival in patients with unresectable pancreatic cancer: A randomized controlled trial. JAMA 2004;291:1092-1099.

48. Ischia S, Luzzani A, Ischia A, et al: A new approach to the neurolytic block of the coeliac plexus: The transaortic technique. Pain 1983;16:333-341.

49. Lieberman RP, Waldman SD: Celiac plexus block neurolysis with the modified transaortic approach. Radiology 1990;175: 274-276.

50. Singler RC: An improved technique for alcohol neurolysis of the celiac plexus. Anesthesiology 1981;56:137-141.

51. Romanelli DF, Beckman CF, Heiss FW: Celiac plexus block: Efficacy and safety of the anterior approach. Am J Roentgenol 1993;160:497-500.

52. Ischia S, Ischia A, Polati E, et al: Three posterior percutaneous celiac plexus block techniques. Anesthesiology 1992;76: 534-540.

53. Waldman SD, Patt RB: Celiac plexus block and splanchnic nerve block. In Waldman SD, Winnie AP (eds): Interventional Pain Management. Philadelphia, WB Saunders, 1996, pp 360-373.

54. Bell SN, Cole R, Roberts-Thomson IC: Coeliac plexus block for control of pain in chronic pancreatitis. Br Med J 1980; 281:1604.

55. Galizia EJ, Lahiri SK: Paraplegia following coeliac plexus block with phenol. Br J Anaesth 1974;46:539-540.

56. Lieberman RP, Waldman SD: Celiac plexus block neurolysis with the modified transaortic approach. Radiology 1990;175: 274-276.

57. Sett SS, Taylor DC: Aortic pseudoaneurysm secondary to celiac plexus block. Ann Vasc Surg 1991;5:88-91.

58. Kaplan R, Schiff-Keren B, Alt E: Aortic dissection as a complication of celiac plexus block. Anesthesiology 1995;83: 632-635.

59. Noda J, Umeda S, Mori K, et al: Acetaldehyde syndrome after celiac plexus block. Anesth Analg 1986;65:1300-1302.

60. Leung JWC, Bowen-Wright M, et al: Coeliac plexus block for pancreatitis. Br J Surg 1983;70:730-732.

61. Moore DC: Celiac (splanchnic) plexus block with alcohol for cancer pain of the upper intra-abdominal viscera. In Bonica JJ, Ventafridda V (eds): Advances in Pain Research and Therapy, vol 2. New York, Raven Press, 1979, pp 357-371.

62. Lubenow TR, Ivankovich AD: Serum alcohol, CPK, and amylase levels following celiac plexus block with alcohol. Reg Anesth 1988;13S:64.

63. Fujita Y, Takori M: Pleural effusion after CT-guided alcohol celiac plexus block. Anesth Analg 1987;66:911-912.

64. Fine PG, Bubela C: Chylothorax following celiac plexus block. Anesthesiology 1985;63:454-456.

65. Black A, Dwyer B: Coeliac plexus block. Anaesth Intens Care 1973;1:315-318.

66. Davis DD: Incidence of major complications of neurolytic coeliac plexus block. J R Soc Med 1993;86:264-266.

67. de Leon-Casasola O, Molloy RE, Lema M: Neurolytic visceral sympathetic blocks. In Benzon HT, Raja S, Molloy RE, et al (eds): Essentials of Pain Medicine and Regional Anesthesia, 2nd ed. New York, Elsevier-Churchill Livingstone, 2005, pp 542-549.

68. Plancarte R, Amezcua C, Patt RB, et al: Superior hypogastric plexus block for cancer pain. Anesthesiology 1990;73: 236-239.

69. de Leon-Casasola OA, Kent E, Lema MJ: Neurolytic superior hypogastric plexus block for chronic pelvic pain associated with cancer. Pain 1993;54:145-151.

70. Rosenberg SK, Tewari R, Boswell MV, et al: Superior hypogastric plexus block successfully treats penile pain after transurethral resection of the prostate. Reg Anesth Pain Med 1998;23:618-620.

71. Plancarte R, Amezcua C, Patt RB: Presacral blockade of the ganglion impar (ganglion of Walther). Anesthesiology 1990; 73:A751.

72. Wemm K, Saberski L: Modified approach to block the ganglion impar (ganglion of Walther). Reg Anesth 1995;20: 544-545.

73. Umeda S, Arai T, Hatano Y, et al: Cadaver anatomic analysis of the best site for chemical lumbar sympathectomy. Anesth Analg 1987;66:643-646.

74. Fraser I, Windle R, Smart JG, et al: Ureteric injury following chemical sympathectomy. Br J Surg 71:349, 1984.

75. Cherry DA: Chemical lumbar sympathectomy. Curr Concepts Pain 1984;2:12-15.

76. Haynsworth RF, Noe CE: Percutaneous lumbar sympathectomy: A comparison of radiofrequency denervation versus phenol neurolysis. Anesthesiology 1991;74;459-463.

77. Nader A, Benzon HT: Peripheral sympathetic blocks. In Benzon HT, Raja SN, Molloy RE, et al (eds): Essentials of Pain Medicine and Regional Anesthesia, 2nd ed. Philadelphia, Elsevier, 2005, pp 689-693.

78. Christie JM, Martinez CR: Computerized axial tomography to define the distribution of solution after stellate ganglion nerve block. J Clin Anesth 1995;7:306-311.

79. Lagade M, Poppers PJ: Stellate ganglion block: A therapeutic modality for arterial insufficiency of the arm in premature infants. Anesthesiology 1984;61:203-204.

80. Superville-Sovak B, Rasminsky M, Finlayson MH: Complications of phenol neurolysis. Arch Neurol 1975;32:226-228.

81. Keim HA: Cord paralysis following injection into traumatic cervical meningocele: Complication of stellate ganglion block. NY State J Med 1970;70:2115-2116.

82. Marples IL, Atkin RE: Stellate ganglion block. Pain Rev 2001;8:3-11.

83. Moore DC, Bridenbaugh LD: Intercostal nerve block in 4,333 patients: Indications, techniques, and complications. Anesth Analg 1962;41:1-11.

84. Bunting P, McGeachie JF: Intercostal nerve blockade producing analgesia after appendectomy. Br J Anaesth 1988;61:169-172.

85. Engberg G, Wiklund L: Pulmonary complications after upper abdominal surgery: Their prevention with intercostal blocks. Acta Anaesthesiol Scand 1988;32:1-9.

86. Molloy RE: Truncal blocks: Intercostal, paravertebral, interpleural, suprascapular, ilioinguinal, and iliohypogastric nerve blocks. In Benzon HT, Raja S, Molloy RE, Liu SS, et al (eds): Essentials of Pain Medicine and Regional Anesthesia, 2nd ed. New York, Elsevier-Churchill Livingstone, 2005, pp 636-644.

87. Moore DC, Bridenbaugh LD: Pneumothorax: Its incidence following intercostal nerve block. JAMA 1960;174:842-847.

88. Bridenbaugh PO, Dupen SL, Moore DC, et al: Postoperative intercostal nerve block analgesia versus narcotic analgesia. Anesth Analg 1973;52:81-85.

89. Benumof JF, Semenza J: Total spinal anesthesia following intrathoracic intercostal nerve blocks. Anesthesiology 1975;43:124-125.

90. Atkinson GL, Shupack RC: Acute bronchospasm complicating intercostal nerve block with phenol. Anesth Analg 1989;68:400-401.

91. Purcell-Jones G, Pither CE, Justins DM: Paravertebral somatic nerve block: A clinical radiographic, and computed tomographic study in chronic pain patients. Anesth Analg 1989;68:32-39.

92. Weltz CR, Greengrass RA, Lyerly HK: Ambulatory surgical management of breast carcinoma using paravertebral block. Ann Surg 1995;222:19-26.

93. Perttunen K, Nilsson E, Heinonen J, et al: Extradural, paravertebral and intercostal nerve blocks for post-thoracotomy pain. Br J Anaesth 1995;75:541-547.

94. Tverskoy M, Cozacov C, Ayache M, et al: Postoperative pain after inguinal herniorraphy with different types of anesthesia. Anesth Analg 1990;70:29-35.

95. Bunting P, McConachie I: Ilioinguinal nerve blockade for analgesia after cesarean section. Br J Anaesth 1988;61:773-775.

96. Cohen SP, Foster A: Pulsed radiofrequency as a treatment for groin pain and orchialgia. Urology 2003;61:645-647.

97. Waldman SD: Blockade of the gasserian ganglion and the distal trigeminal nerve. In Waldman SD, Winnie AP (eds): Interventional Pain Management. Philadelphia, WB Saunders, 1996, pp 230-241.

98. Brown DL: Trigeminal (gasserian) ganglion block. In Brown DL (ed): Atlas of Regional Anesthesia. Philadelphia, WB Saunders, 1992, pp 135-140.

99. Crimeni R: Clinical experience with mepivacaine and alcohol in neuralgia of the trigeminal nerve. Acta Anaesthesiol Scand Suppl 1966;24:173-176.

100. Mousel LH: Treatment of intractable pain of the head and neck. Anesth Analg 1967;46:705-710.

101. Henderson WR: Trigeminal neuralgia: The pain and its treatment. Br Med J 1967;1:7-15.

102. Loeser JD, Sweet WH, Tew JM, et al: Neurosurgical operations involving peripheral nerves. In Bonica JJ (ed): The Management of Pain, 2nd ed. Philadelphia, Lea & Febiger, 1990, pp 2044-2066.

103. Katz J, Levin AB: Treatment of diffuse metastatic cancer pain by instillation of alcohol into the sella turcica. Anesthesiology 46:115-121, 1977.

104. Corssen G, Holcomb MC, Moustapha I, et al: Alcohol-induced adenolysis of the pituitary gland: A new approach to control of intractable cancer pain. Anesth Analg 1977;56:414-421.

105. Levin AB, Katz J, Benson RC, et al: Treatment of pain of diffuse metastatic cancer by stereotactic chemical hypophysectomy: Long-term results and observations on mechanisms of action. Neurosurgery 1980;6:258-562.

106. Waldman SD, Feldstein GS: Neuroadenolysis of the pituitary: Description of a modified technique. J Pain Symptom Manage 1987;2:45-49.

107. Yanagida H, Corssen G, Trouwborst A, et al: Relief of cancer pain in man: Alcohol-induced neuroadenolysis vs. electrical stimulation of the pituitary gland. Pain 1984;19:133-141.

108. Duthie AM: Pituitary cryoablation. Anaesthesia 1983;38:495-497.

109. Katz J, Levin AB: Long-term follow-up study of chemical hypophysectomy and additional cases. Anesthesiology 1979;51:167-169.

110. Lloyd JW, Rawlinson WAL, Evans PJD: Selective hypophysectomy for metastatic pain. Br J Anaesth 1981;53:1129-1133.

111. Waldman SD: Neuroadenolysis of the pituitary: Indications and technique. In Waldman SD, Winnie AP (eds): Interventional Pain Management. Philadelphia, WB Saunders, 1996, pp 519-525.

112. Mullin V: Brachial plexus block with phenol for painful arm associated with Pancoast syndrome. Anesthesiology 1980;53:341-342.

113. Asensi V, Asensi J, Carton J, et al: Successful intrathecal ethanol block for intractable spasticity of AIDS related progressive multifocal leukoencephalopathy. Spinal Cord 1999;37:450-452.

114. Sangwan S, Chand S, Siwach R, et al: Treatment of intractable spasticity in spinal cord injured patients. Indian J Med Sci 1992;46:169-173.

115. Browne RA, Catton DZ: The use of intrathecal phenol for muscle spasms in multiple sclerosis: A description of two cases. Can Anaesth Soc J 1975;22:208-218.

116. Scott B, Weinstein Z, Chiteman R, et al: Intrathecal phenol and glycerin in metrizamide for treatment of intractable spasms in paraplegia. J Neurosurg 1985;63:125-127.

117. Kong K, Chua K: Outcome of obturator nerve block with alcohol for treatment of hip adductor spasticity. Int J Rehabil Res 1999;22:327-329.

118. Keenan MA, Tomas ES, Stone L, et al: Percutaneous phenol block of the musculocutaneous nerve to control elbow flexor spasticity. J Hand Surgery 1990;15A:340-346.

119. Kong K, Chua K: Neurolysis of the musculocutaneous nerve with alcohol to treat poststroke elbow flexor spasticity. Arch Phys Med Rehabil 1999;80:1234-1236.

120. Chua K, Kong K: Alcohol neurolysis of the sciatic nerve in the treatment of hemiplegic knee flexor spasticity: Clinical outcomes. Arch Phys Med Rehabil 2000;81:1432-1435.

121. Petrillo CR, Knoplock S: Phenol block of the tibial nerve for spasticity: A long-term follow-up study. Int Disabil Stud 1988;10:97-100.

122. Garland D, Lilling M, Keenan M: Percutaneous phenol block to motor points of spastic forearm muscles in head-injured adults. Arch Phys Med Rehabil 1984;65:243-245.

123. Moritz U: Phenol block of peripheral nerves. Scand J Rehabil Med 1973;5:160-163.

124. Gracies JM, Nance P, Elovic E, et al: Traditional pharmacologic treatments for spasticity Part I: Local treatments. Muscle Nerve 1997;20(Suppl 6):S61-S91.

125. Carpenter EB, Seitz DG: Intramuscular alcohol as an aid in management of spastic cerebral palsy. Dev Med Child Neurol 1980;22:497-501.

126. Massey JM: Treatment of spasmodic torticollis with intramuscular phenol injection. J Neurol Neurosurg Psychiatry 1995;58:258-259.

127. Gibson II: Phenol block in the treatment of spasticity. Gerontology 1987;33:327-330.

128. Ramamurthy S, Walsh NE, Schenfeld LS, et al: Evaluation of neurolytic blocks using phenol and cryogenic block in the management of chronic pain. J Pain Symptom Manage 1989;4:72-75.

129. Todd DP: Poststernotomy neuralgia: A new pain syndrome. Anesth Analg 1989;69:81-82.

130. Defalque RJ: Painful trigger points in surgical scars. Anesth Analg 1982;61:518-520.

46 Nerve Blocks of the Head and Neck

Kenneth D. Candido and Mani Batra

The primary indication for nerve blocks of the head and neck is for diagnostic and therapeutic purposes in cases of head and neck pain. Some of the more common indications are discussed in detail here, including the rationale for selecting regional nerve blocking techniques in the care and management of these patients.

HEADACHES

Differentiating the cause for headaches is a vexing task, often requiring the skill and experience of multiple clinicians from diverse specialties. The pain physician and skilled regional block specialist are well suited to the task by virtue of their respective experiences in performing conduction blockade of the greater and lesser occipital nerves (occipital neuralgic headache), cervical medial branches of the facet joints (cervicogenic headache), cervical epidural nerve block (nonspecific headache), and atlantoaxial joint (suboccipital headache). Therefore it is by use of the various modalities of regional block that a diagnostic or therapeutic block of the respective structures implicated in a given patient's pain may be discernible. The anatomic method is a more scientific method of pursuing the source of a headache than that of solely relying on historical information presented by the patient.

Atlantoaxial Joint Block

The primary indication for performing atlantoaxial (AA) nerve block is for the diagnostic and therapeutic evaluation of suboccipital pain that occasionally radiates into the temporomandibular joint (TMJ) area that is exacerbated by head rotation. Whiplash injuries and cervicogenic headaches are two of the more common indications for this block. The AA joint (Figs. 46–1 and 46–2) lacks posterior articulations and therefore is neither a bona fide facet joint nor a true zygapophyseal joint. Also there is neither an intervertebral disk between the atlas (C1) and the axis (C2) nor an intervertebral foramen at that level to accommodate an exiting nerve root. At the AA joint, the head flexes, extends, and rotates in a hori-

zontal plane, up to 60 degrees, giving the joint significant responsibility for the stability as well as the mobility of the head and neck. The joint can be injured by seemingly trivial insults and trauma. The resulting pain syndrome can be significant, manifesting as dull, continual, and achy pain in the posterior neck and suboccipital region. More severe injuries, such as those caused by motor vehicle accidents, might subject the joint to acceleration-deceleration–type injuries, with sequelae exceeding pain and dysfunction. Indeed, paralysis and even death could result from ligamentous disruption, analogous to an odontoid fracture. The fibers of the respective spinal nerves C1 and particularly C2 contribute to the formation of the occipital nerves (greater and lesser), which are a frequent target for the practicing pain physician in contemporary practice. An extremely important anatomic concept involves the relationship of the vertebral artery to the AA joint; whereas the artery is medial to the atlanto-occipital (AO) joint,[1] it is found lateral to the AA joint. Therefore, needles directed at the joint during nerve block need to be oriented slightly more medially, cognizant of the danger of aiming toward the interlaminar space or even toward the foramen magnum.

Technique of Atlantoaxial Nerve Block

Blockade of the AA joint requires fluoroscopic assistance to ascertain that the advancing needle does not encroach on the critical anatomic structures such as the vertebral artery and spinal cord. Patients are placed prone after obtaining the appropriate medical history, performing a targeted physical examination, and establishing that there are no bleeding problems or infectious issues related to the target for intended needle placement. Baseline vital signs are obtained and recorded. It is recommended that an intravenous peripheral line be established for prophylactic purposes. Bolsters are typically placed beneath the chest to elevate the shoulders off the procedure table, permitting the patient to flex the neck and rest the forehead on a neurosurgical doughnut or pillow. After performing a careful sterile skin preparation and draping, the fluoroscopic unit is oriented in an

Atlantoaxial joints

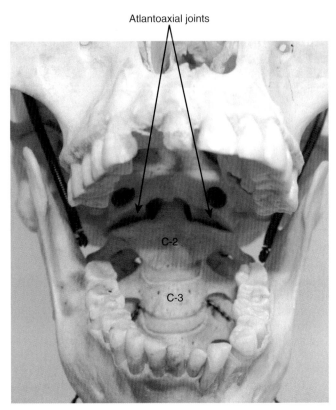

Figure 46–1. Demonstration of the mouth open view to reveal the anterior atlantoaxial (C1-2) joint.

Atlantoaxial joints

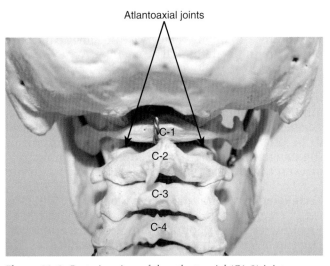

Figure 46–2. Posterior view of the atlantoaxial (C1-2) joint.

anteroposterior (AP) direction to identify the atlas and the foramen magnum, implementing a moderate craniad tilt of the unit until all structures are clearly visualized. The AA joint is located lateral and inferior to both the foramen magnum and the atlas (see Fig. 46–2). A local anesthetic skin wheal is made over the intended injection site using a small-gauge, 1.5-inch needle and injecting about 2 to 3 mL of 1% lidocaine solution without epinephrine (or equivalent). Next, an 18-gauge skin core is made using a sharp cutting needle to permit the passage of a blunt 22-gauge, styletted Whitacre-type subarachnoid

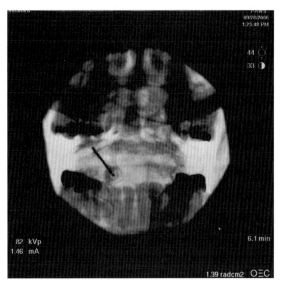

Figure 46–3. Posteroanterior radiograph demonstrating correct needle placement using a posterior approach to the left atlantoaxial joint.

needle. A curve is placed at its distal tip to allow steering of the needle once it has been advanced through the skin and subcutaneous tissues. The needle is advanced under continual fluoroscopic guidance, rotating the beam of the unit until the needle appears in tunnel or "gun barrel" view, which is represented as a dot advancing toward the posterolateral aspect of the AA joint. The needle should be directed slightly medially, to avoid the vertebral artery situated laterally, but not too medially because this could engage the spinal cord. Occasionally, but not always, a "popping" sensation will be appreciated as the needle traverses the joint and enters it from posterior to anterior (Fig. 46–3). The fluoroscopic unit must then be rotated laterally (Fig. 46–4) to confirm the needle placement at the appropriate depth between the atlas and axis. Once placement has been verified, gentle aspiration of the needle will assess for the presence of cerebrospinal fluid (CSF) or blood. If none is present, a small (i.e., 1 mL) volume of radiocontrast medium may be incrementally injected under real-time fluoroscopy. If the needle is indeed situated within the confines of the joint, a bilateral concavity will be demonstrated, which is indicative of an intact joint capsule. However, if the joint capsule has been ruptured, the dye may be seen to spread into the peridural space, and care should be taken not to inject long-acting, highly protein–bound, lipophilic local anesthetics (bupivacaine, ropivacaine) through the needle. Rapid runoff of the dye may signify vascular injection, and is to be guarded against, particularly if it is suspected that the needle may have entered the laterally situated vertebral artery. If this occurs, the needle should be redirected medially, reaspiration of the needle in four quadrants undertaken, and reinjection of contrast material before considering injecting local anesthetics or adjuvants. Even without directly injecting into the vertebral artery (even minuscule volumes of

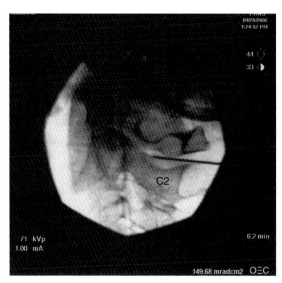

Figure 46–4. Lateral radiograph demonstrating appropriate needle placement for an atlantoaxial joint injection. Note the prominent spinous process of the second cervical vertebra (C_2).

Midpoint of the waists of the articular pillars

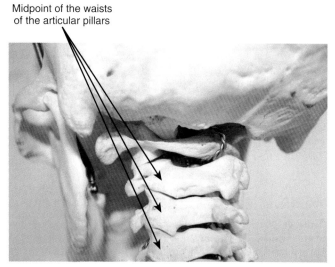

Figure 46–5. Lateral oblique view demonstrating close-up of the atlanto-occipital (AO) and atlantoaxial (AA) joints on the left. Also demonstrated is a close-up of the needle insertion points for medial branch blocks and radiofrequency ablation techniques of cervical facet joint denervation.

dilute local anesthetics injected here can lead to grand mal seizures), ataxia following AA block is not uncommon[2] and is likely caused by vascular uptake of local anesthetics in this extremely vascular region.

Cervical Facet Block and Medial Branch Block

The cervical facet joints and medial branches are commonly implicated in the cause of cervicogenic headache. C2 and C3 blocks are often undertaken to effectively disrupt neural pathways, giving rise to greater and lesser occipital nerve dysfunction. Blockade of the joints via the medial branches is typically undertaken for such headaches as well as for the treatment of nonspecific neck pain, degenerative arthropathies of the cervical spine, degenerative disk disease, cervical sprain, and trauma-related pain. Pain may be localized to the neck or radiate in a capelike fashion from the neck over the shoulders, with extension to the suboccipital area and supraclavicular area. The cervical facet joints are present from C2 and C3 caudally because the AO and AA joints are not true zygapophyseal joints, as described earlier. From C2 and C3 caudally, the joints are lined by synovium and possess a true joint capsule that is generously innervated and may be a source of neck pain and headache pain in certain individuals. The joints themselves may be injured in acceleration-deceleration types of insults, or may be affected by chronic degenerative arthritic changes. Pain results from synovial joint inflammation because of irritation from repetitive motion at an injured segment. The cervical facet joints, like the thoracic and lumbar facet joints, receive innervation from two adjacent spinal levels. The dorsal ramus from the level above and that at the joint provide fibers that invest the joint. This forms the foundation for the principle of blocking both the affected level, as well as the supe-

Midpoint of the waists of the articular pillars

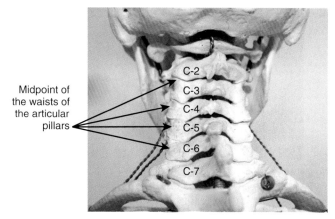

Figure 46–6. Posterior view of the scalloped areas representing the waists of the cervical articular pillars, site of needle placement for both local anesthetic medial branch facet joint block, as well as for radiofrequency ablation procedures and pulsed-radiofrequency techniques of denervating or neuromodulating the cervical facet joint nerves. The C7-T1 interlaminar opening is more capacious than more proximal levels, and is the site frequently chosen for cervical epidural needle placement.

rior level, to completely denervate the facet joint. Each dorsal ramus then innervates two facet joints, and each facet joint receives its innervation from two separate nerves. The medial branch, which wraps around the waist of the articular pillars of the vertebral bodies (Figs. 46–5 to 46–7), is the site for peripheral nerve block as well as for neuromodulation techniques of radiofrequency at the joint (Figs. 46–8 and 46–9). These nerves are held against the bone by a fascial envelope and are anchored there by tendons of the semispinalis capitis. The medial branch is consistently found at this anatomic location between C4 and C7, making needle placement for these levels a

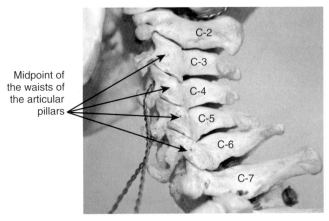

Figure 46–7. Lateral oblique view demonstrating the waists of the articular pillars in consideration of medial branch blocks of the cervical facet joints. Also demonstrated is the interlaminar space at C7-T1 for cervical epidural block needle placement.

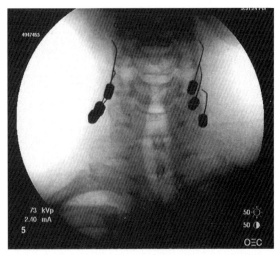

Figure 46–9. Posteroanterior radiograph using cephalad tilt of the fluoroscopy unit, with patient in prone position demonstrating needles appropriately placed for blockade of C3, C4, and C5 medial branch nerves, bilaterally (see Figs. 46–6 and 46–8). The needles are aligned much like the posts of a picket fence.

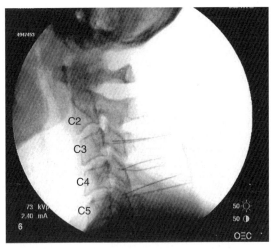

Figure 46–8. Lateral radiograph demonstrates bilateral placement of 22-gauge, 3.5-inch Whitacre subarachnoid needles at the middle of the waist of the articular pillars for C3, C4, and C5 blocks of the medial branches (see Figs. 46–5, 46–7, and 46–9). Notice the parallel nature of the respective needles at each site for bilateral medial branch block.

relatively simple task to accomplish. For example, at the C4-5 facet joint, the medial branches of C4 and C5 are blocked at their respective articular pillars to anesthetize the joint. At C2-3, the joint receives innervation from the third occipital nerve (one of two median branches of the C3 dorsal ramus), and somewhat by the C2 dorsal ramus. The medial branch of the C2 dorsal ramus is the greater occipital nerve (see later). The C2-3 facet joint innervation is a complex anatomic scheme, and for practical purposes our technique of blocking the third occipital nerve at the C3 articular process waist is sufficient for denervating or anesthetizing this joint (see Figs. 46–8 and 46–9).

Technique of Blocking the Medial Branches for Cervical Facet Joint Pain

Our technique of blocking the medial branches requires the use of fluoroscopic guidance (see Figs.

46–8 and 46–9). We believe this is essential to minimize the likelihood of advancing our needles too far ventrally with the patient in the prone position. Advancing too far ventrally could cause injury or irritation to the exiting cervical spinal nerve roots or to the more ventrally situated vertebral artery. Also if strict adherence to maintaining needle-to-bone contact is not maintained, it's possible for advancing needles to stray too far medially toward the interlaminar or transforaminal spaces, or too far laterally with a resultant failure of accessing the medial branches, which are secured to the waists of the articular pillars by a fascial sheath and the semispinalis capitis tendons. Appropriately screened candidates (i.e., no coagulation problems, no infection at the intended insertion site, etc.) are placed in the prone position, with a bolster placed under the chest to permit flexion of the head on the neck. The forehead is supported using a ring neurosurgical doughnut or pillow, with unrestricted breathing and with minimal to no sedation. Vital signs are monitored using standard American Society of Anesthesiologists–suggested monitors, and an intravenous cannula is placed in a distal extremity for purposes of administering resuscitative medications or adjuvants, as indicated. A careful sterile skin prep and drape is performed using a generic antiseptic solution. The fluoroscope is oriented anterior to posterior with a moderate to steep cephalad orientation. This is an essential step, which if not performed, inhibits or impairs the ability to visualize the periarticular osseous structures because of the obstruction imposed by the thick mandible. Scout films are obtained using sterile needles placed over the skin of the intended needle entry sites, and local anesthetic skin wheals are raised using a 27-gauge short (1.5 inches) needle with a short-acting local anesthetic agent (e.g., lidocaine 1% without epinephrine), in doses of 2 to 3 mL per site. Next a

22-gauge, 3.5-inch blunt (Whitacre type or equivalent) subarachnoid or block needle is advanced completely perpendicular to the skin toward the lateral-most edge of the vertebral body on the side selected. In this position it may not be practical to gauge the exact site (e.g., C3 vs. C4) where the needle is being directed. It is essential that when no more than 2 cm of needle have been introduced to switch to a straight lateral view to observe the depth of needle advancement, as well as to ascertain which anatomic segment is being addressed. This is usually of little concern because two levels (the level at the joint and the level cephalad to the joint) are being blocked to anesthetize a single level. So even if C4 is chosen, and the needle is seen as advancing toward the trapezoid body articular pillar at C3, the second needle may merely need to be placed caudad to the first to block both medial branches. Once the needle is seated at the appropriate depth, as seen on lateral fluoroscopy (see Fig. 46–8), and is not encroaching on either the visible neural foramen or too far ventral still toward the anatomic site of the vertebral artery, the needle is checked to be certain that the tip is touching bone. Again, using a curve-tipped needle helps realign the needle in cases in which the depth appears appropriate, but the needle tip is laterally directed away from bone. In this case a mere twisting of the needle hub will usually suffice to turn and steer the tip toward and subsequently against the bone, where the medial branches are situated in their respective fascial planes and are anchored by the semispinalis capitis tendons. When all needles are in the appropriate position for a given individual, they should be aligned like a picket fence. Then the lateral fluoroscopic image should demonstrate almost perfect parallel lines derived from the needles. An alternative technique, used by some interventionalists, is to place patients prone and to advance the needle from lateral to medial toward the bone under fluoroscopic guidance. This technique is clearly fraught with greater danger of striking the vertebral artery or an exiting cervical spinal nerve root than the technique described previously because of the direction of the needle toward the central neuraxis. Additionally, and potentially more than a mere nuisance, if the clinician subsequently determines that the patient might benefit from a radiofrequency (RF) or neurodestructive procedure of the cervical medial branches, he or she is then faced with the prospect of performing the procedure with the active tip of any RF needle, making minimal and insignificant contact with the target area or nerve of interest. Contrast this with the approach described herein, in which the RF needle active tip will be hugging the bone through its entire length, making the likelihood of success inherently much greater. Additionally there is less muscle in the pathway of the advancing needle using the lateral approach. This increases the likelihood that needles will not be firmly seated against the target and will be easily displaced once the second and possibly third or fourth needle is inserted at a given level.

Whichever technique is chosen, once the needles are situated and once there has been no paresthesia or blood from the needle during aspiration, a small (typically 0.5 to 1 mL) volume of radiocontrast medium may be injected to verify that no arterial cannulation has occurred. If this injection proves negative for such a cannulation, the same volume of a short-acting (i.e., lidocaine, mepivacaine) local anesthetic with or without corticosteroid may be added. We prefer to use the nonparticulate steroid dexamethasone acetate for this purpose, in doses of 2 mg per medial branch (up to 12 mg total) because the particulate agents such as methylprednisolone acetate tend to flocculate or clump when added to lidocaine, with the potential for neurologic compromise if such a phenomenon occurs in an end artery.

If RF procedures are anticipated to ameliorate recalcitrant symptoms, we typically perform double-diagnostic blocks as a prelude to RF, accepting a 60% or better response (somewhat arbitrarily) before doing the actual RF. Pulsed RF techniques have largely replaced radiofrequency ablation (RFA) lesioning in the neck for the most part. These are performed by applying 42° to 45° C temperatures for 120 seconds to each nerve in question.

Occipital Nerve Block

The greater occipital nerve (GON) arises from the dorsal primary rami of C2, with occasional contributions from C3 (Figs. 46–10 and 46–11). The nerve penetrates the fascia inferior to the superior nuchal crest, where it runs alongside the occipital artery for

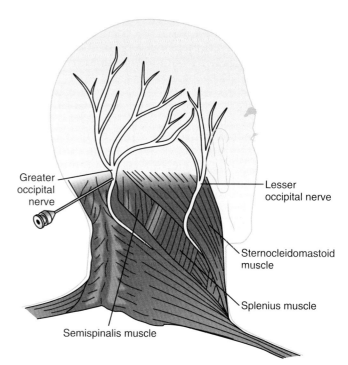

Figure 46–10. The anatomy and site of nerve blocking for the greater occipital nerve (GON).

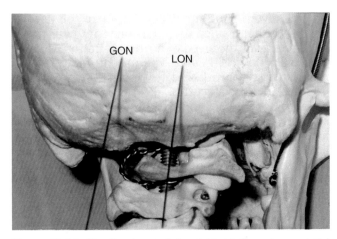

Figure 46–11. Needles inserted for right-sided greater occipital nerve (GON) block and for lesser occipital nerve (LON) block.

a variable distance. The sensory area innervated by the nerve includes the medial portion of the posterior scalp, with radiation ventrally up to the vertex. The lesser occipital nerve (LON) arises from the ventral primary rami of C2 and C3, and passes superiorly and laterally from the occiput to the lateral edge of the sternocleidomastoid muscle (Fig. 46–11). Here the nerve divides into cutaneous branches that innervate the lateral portion of the posterior scalp and cephalad surface of the ear pinna. Along with the great auricular nerve, the GON and LON provide the majority of sensory afferent information for the occipital area, and are responsible for transmitting information derived from C2-3 facet joint derangements to the referral area described.

Occipital nerve blocks have become increasingly popular methods of managing headaches of diverse causes, even though the scientific support for doing so is limited. GON blocks have been shown to be ineffective for chronic tension-type headache when prilocaine and dexamethasone were used in a group of 15 patients.[3] They have been used with various degrees of success for postconcussive headaches[4] (80% successful in these patients), atypical orofacial pain,[5] and especially for migraine headaches, when they are often combined with trigger point injections[6] or supraorbital nerve blocks,[7] in both cases affording a very high degree of success for ameliorating pain and brush allodynia. A novel use of GON block has been in the successful treatment of patients with abnormal head movements who also suffered from tinnitus and dizziness, associated with a previous history of trauma.[8] Whereas often the diagnosis of headache caused by occipital neuralgia is not too difficult to make,[9] there are cases of refractory headache that require advanced evaluation techniques. Some suggest performing CT-guided C2-3 nerve blocks as a prelude to considering patients candidates for percutaneous rhizotomy[10]; in our experience, fluoroscopically guided techniques of C2-3 nerve block have been extremely useful and have precluded the requirement to seek more advanced imaging for guidance (see Figs. 46–8 and 46–9).

Technique of Blocking the Greater and Lesser Occipital Nerves

Occipital nerve blocks have been erroneously described by some to be merely a field block of local anesthetic and steroid layered somewhere in the posterior part of the occiput, without regard to anatomic landmarks or consequences of errantly placed medications. Indeed there are cases of sudden unconsciousness reported following LON block, some a result of occipital artery injection, and at least one caused by unintentionally injecting local anesthetic into a previous bone defect from a craniotomy.[11] Also it is possible that unconsciousness might occur after a GON block that has been made too far inferiorly toward the foramen magnum. Additionally, if physicians are not careful and discriminating in their choices of frequency of GON block and use judicious doses of agents including corticosteroids, complications such as Cushing syndrome may result.[12] Our technique of blockade of the occipital nerves is to perform the procedure with the patient in the sitting position, with the forehead forward, resting on either a Mayo stand, the edge of a padded table, or a gurney. If possible, the occipital artery is palpated at the superior nuchal ridge. Occasionally using a Doppler probe may help identify the artery, which is often not robust or bounding, and subsequently not always readily discernible as a distinct structure. Because it is virtually impossible to completely disinfect the scalp without first performing a depilation at the intended injection site, we use alcohol wipes or a povidone-iodine (Betadine)–soaked pledget to soak the area with disinfectant before inserting the needle, without expectations of complete asepsis. Next we insert a fine-gauge (25 gauge, 1.5 inches) cutting needle, immediately medial to the artery and advance it perpendicular to the skin until the needle tip touches periosteum. Once the occipital bone has been contacted, the needle is retracted about 1 mm and is redirected slightly cephalad (Fig. 46–12). After gently aspirating, 5 mL of local anesthetic (0.5% bupivacaine or ropivacaine) with 4 mg of dexamethasone or 6 mg of betamethasone is injected in a fanlike manner, taking care not to direct the needle too far medially toward the foramen magnum. The LON may be blocked, as can the greater auricular nerve, by removing the needle, and placing it into the skin about 3 to 4 cm lateral to the entry point for GON block while also directing it inferiorly instead of superiorly as for GON block. After gentle aspiration, 5 mL of the same combination of local anesthetic with or without corticosteroid as noted previously may be injected, again in a fanlike distribution to block the nerve. After completing GON and LON blocks, it is important to gently massage the tissues of the scalp to spread the agents while maintaining pressure over the injection site(s). This will minimize ecchymosis or hematoma formation from this highly vascular area. Often an ice pack is applied for 20 to 30 minutes postprocedure to further minimize swelling and inhibit vascular absorption of

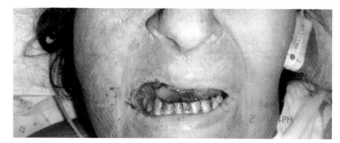

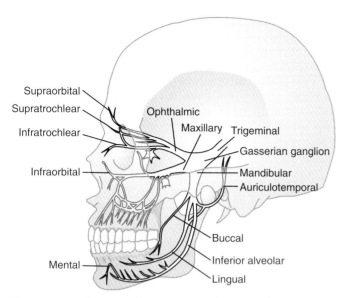

Figure 46–12. Anatomy of gasserian ganglion with demonstration of three rami of the trigeminal nerve.

Figure 46–13. Patient suffering from severe intraoral malignancy with invasion of the gasserian ganglion, requiring computed tomography–guided gasserian ganglion nerve block using ethanol.

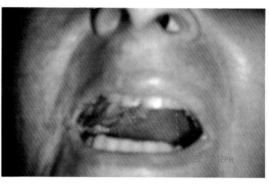

Figure 46–14. Another severely immunocompromised individual with leukoplakia in the mouth, who was suffering from metastatic malignancy with invasion of the gasserian ganglion; the patient also underwent uneventful gasserian ganglion block using absolute alcohol.

the local anesthetic agents, particularly if bilateral blocks have been performed.

FACIAL PAIN

Trigeminal Nerve Block and Gasserian Ganglion Block

Gasserian ganglion block is an underused technique for managing chronic face pain caused by trigeminal neuralgia (TGN) and for persistent pain caused by conditions such as recalcitrant herpes zoster ophthalmicus and postherpetic neuralgia. It also has been used for diagnostic purposes to differentiate pain originating from somatic structures from those mediated by sympathetic mechanisms. By far the most common indication, however, remains pain as a result of malignancy with invasion of neural structures of the head and face (Figs. 46–13 and 46–14). In these cases, local anesthetic nerve blocks may be accomplished as prognostic blocks before subjecting patients to alcohol or phenol blocks or to radiofrequency or cryoneurolysis of the gasserian ganglion. Some of the more common malignancies involving the respective structures innervated by the trigeminal nerve include tumors of the orbit, maxillary sinus, and mandible. Gasserian ganglion block may be undertaken when neurosurgical management (i.e., Janetta's procedure) is not feasible or practical. Occasional uses of the block and of neurodestruction of the gland include intractable cluster headache and ocular pain as a result of glaucoma. Idiopathic TGN is caused by vascular contact at the proximal portion of the preganglionic segment of the trigeminal nerve with preganglionic deformity and observed in up to 97% of individuals so affected,[13] with the remedy often being gasserian ganglion block. For individuals suffering from isolated dysfunction of either the maxillary (V2) or mandibular (V3) division of the

trigeminal nerve, it is often more feasible to perform single nerve injections on these structures because the success rate of performing blocks at the foramen rotundum (maxillary) and foramen ovale (mandibular) have been shown to be 84% and 92%, respectively, for chronic facial pain.[14] When compared with peripheral nerve procedures, however, ganglion level procedures (RF thermocoagulation, balloon compression, glycerolysis) are more effective overall, and should probably be attempted by skilled interventionalists if long-term success is sought.[15] The median pain-free interval that may be expected after percutaneous retrogasserian glycerol injection is 32 months, although the complication rate (hypesthesias, dysesthesias, anesthesia dolorosa) may approach 50% or more using this technique.[16] In another study using the same technique, the success rate, as defined by complete pain relief, at 3.5 years, was 71.4%, with 32% rate of mild hypesthesias, 19% paresthesias, and 3% dysesthesias.[17] The choice of whether to perform percutaneous neurodestructive ganglion procedures using fluoroscopic guidance, or computed tomography (CT) scan guidance is operator dependent. The largest case series to date have included more than 2000 percutaneous ethanol or RFA blocks over a 13-year period using fluoroscopy with excellent success.[18]

However, visualization of the foramen ovale is often difficult to accomplish using fluoroscopy alone. In recent times, CT-guided or CT fluoroscopy–guided gasserian ganglion thermolysis procedures have become increasingly popular because of the ability to more readily identify osseous structures (see Fig. 46–15).[19] In the evolving practice of using CT scanning for head and neck nerve blocks, determinations are being made for the most appropriate skull-rotation angles in which the foramen ovale is best visualized, for the relationship between the virtual puncture point and anatomic landmarks, and for the distance between the virtual puncture point and foramen.[20]

Technique of Blocking the Trigeminal Nerve via the Gasserian Ganglion

The gasserian or trigeminal ganglion lies in the cranium in an outpouching known as Meckel's cave, near the petrous part of the temporal bone (Fig. 46–16). Medially lies the cavernous sinus; superiorly is the inferior surface of the temporal lobe; posteriorly is the brainstem. Anteriorly the three major nerves of the ganglion are derived (ophthalmic, maxillary, mandibular). The ophthalmic (V1) and maxillary (V2) nerves are medially situated, and are sensory nerves, whereas the laterally situated nerve, the mandibular (V3), has motor as well as sensory function.

All patients considered candidates for either diagnostic or therapeutic block, or for neurolysis procedures, need to be evaluated to rule out the presence of coagulation disorders or historical use of medications that might impair platelet aggregation and adhesiveness. All procedures are performed using radiologic assistance, either CT scan or fluoroscopy. After securing intravenous access and placing patients supine, a full complement of noninvasive hemodynamic monitors is applied, and baseline vital signs are obtained and recorded. Oxygen is typically

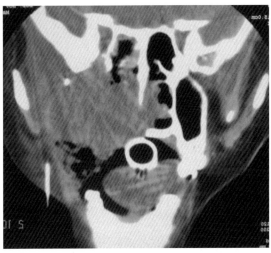

Figure 46–15. Computed tomography scan–guided gasserian ganglion block; the needle can be seen entering the tissues from the right side of the patient (*left side of the image*).

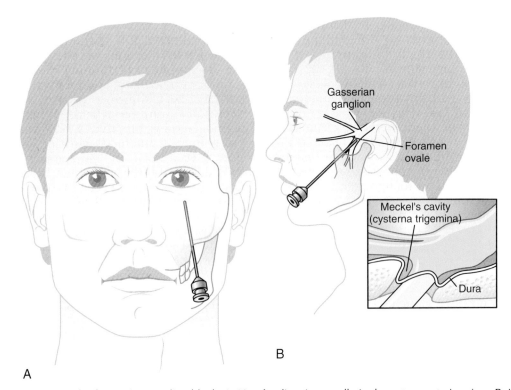

Figure 46–16. Anterior approach of gasserian ganglion block. **A,** Line for directing needle in the anteroposterior view. **B,** Line for directing needle in the lateral view. Inset shows the details of Meckel's cave.

administered via a nasal cannula. Modest amounts of sedative-hypnotic medication may be used to allay fears and limit apprehension in appropriate individuals. The head of the patient is kept in a neutral position, and a site 2 to 3 cm lateral to the corner of the mouth on the ipsilateral side is chosen as the needle entry point. The needle direction is toward the ipsilateral pupil, with a slight mesiad direction taken beneath the zygoma (Fig. 46–17). The fluoroscope should be used to obtain anteroposterior (AP) images. Then the beam should be oriented in a steep cephalad direction to attempt to visualize the foramen ovale. Even using this or the submental view does not guarantee that the foramen will be visualized. In the submental view, the orbital line and petrous ridge are visualized through the orbits using an AP image. Then the C-arm is moved slightly laterally and obliquely. The foramen ovale should appear medial to the medial edge of the mandible. Once the anatomic boundaries have been identified, the skin of the lateral area of the cheek is prepped and draped. A skin wheal is raised at the point chosen, using 1% lidocaine plain, 3 mL. Then, a 22-gauge, blunt nerve block or Whitacre subarachnoid needle is advanced toward the foramen ovale as described earlier. Usually a paresthesia in the distribution of the mandibular nerve is obtained after the foramen is entered. Once the needle appears to be in proximity to the foramen, the C-arm is switched to lateral to show the needle approximating the angle made by the clivus and petrous ridge of the temporal bone. This is an area close to the pituitary fossa and sphenoid sinus as well as the external auditory canal, so obviously every

effort must be made to ascertain that the needle is situated where intended. If the needle tip has entered Meckel's cave, it is not unusual for the dura to be punctured and cerebrospinal fluid (CSF) to be aspirated through the needle. In fact, some authorities suggest that not obtaining CSF implies that the block was incorrectly performed. Nevertheless, the next step in the block sequence is to inject 0.1 to 0.5 mL of water-based contrast medium into the space, to verify that no vascular structure has been entered and that the needle is still not in the subarachnoid space. If a diagnostic block is being performed, then 0.1 mL of lidocaine without epinephrine can be incrementally injected using a tuberculin syringe, to a total volume of about 0.5 mL, with continual intermittent aspiration. If neurolysis is desired, the same volume of 6.5% phenol in glycerin or absolute alcohol may be incrementally injected using a tuberculin syringe in the manner as described previously for local anesthetic injection. When using hyperbaric phenol solutions, the patient should be placed in the sitting position with the chin aiming toward the chest before injecting the agent; this will help maximize the likelihood that the phenol will spread preferentially to V2 and V3, and avoid the ophthalmic division of the TGN. For absolute alcohol, the patient should be left in the supine position. The same approach to gasserian ganglion block can be undertaken for RF, cryolesioning, balloon compression, or even for placing stimulating electrode leads for subsequent attachment to an implanted pulse generator.

Maxillary and Mandibular Nerve Blocks

The trigeminal nerve branches may also be blocked using a coronoid approach, although this technique does not ensure blockade of the ophthalmic (V1) nerve, and so is considered less of a gasserian ganglion block than of a V2-3 nerve block. The benefit of accessing the V2 and V3 nerves using this approach is the facility in doing so, the ease of reproducibility, and the possibility, albeit not recommended, of doing the procedure absent the requirement for radiologic guidance. The V2 nerve exits the middle cranial fossa through the foramen rotundum and crosses the pterygopalatine fossa. It then passes through the inferior orbital fissure, enters the orbit, and exits the face by way of the infraorbital foramen (Figs. 46–18 to 46–20). V2 can therefore be blocked just above the ventral margin of the lateral pterygoid plate. The maxillary nerve is a pure sensory nerve, providing innervation to the dura and middle cranial fossa, temporal and lateral zygomatic areas, and the mucosa of the maxillary sinus. V2 also supplies sensory fibers to the dentition of the upper jaw, and to the cheek, upper lip, side of the nose, and lower eyelid. The coronoid approach is a useful technique of accessing V2 as it leaves the foramen rotundum. From a technical ease standpoint, coronoid trigeminal block far surpasses the classic technique of gasserian ganglion block, and so is probably our technique of

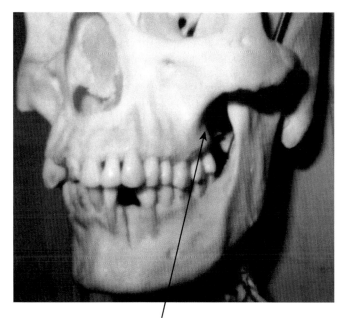

Needle entry point and
direction for GG block

Figure 46–17. Target for needle insertion and direction of needle advancement using the percutaneous anterior approach to left-sided gasserian ganglion block (GG).

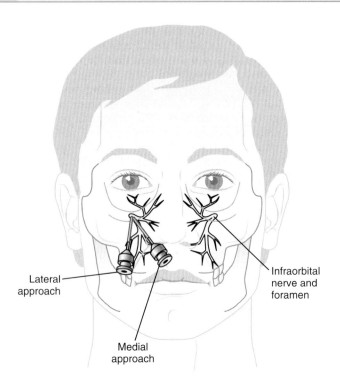

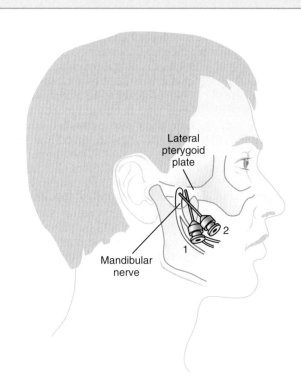

Figure 46–18. Anatomy of the infraorbital nerve block; lateral and medial approach.

Figure 46–20. Anatomy of the mandibular nerve block. The needle contacts the lateral pterygoid plate (*1*) and is withdrawn 2 mm to block the nerve (*2*).

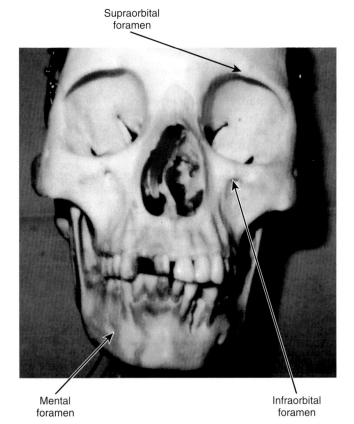

Figure 46–19. Anterior view of the facial skeleton revealing three foramina—supraorbital, infraorbital, and mental—for needle placement.

choice in all situations in which a V1 block is not essential for diagnosis or management of facial pain. With the patient in the supine position, the head is turned to the side opposite the intended block. The coronoid notch is easily identified by asking the patient to open and close the mouth, and with palpation anterior and inferior to the external auditory meatus. Once the landmarks are identified, the patient is asked to maintain the mouth in a neutral position while a 22-gauge, 3.5-inch Whitacre or other blunt-tipped block needle is advanced perpendicular to the skin of the side of the face, just below the zygomatic arch directly in the center of the coronoid arch. Once the lateral pterygoid plate is contacted (at about 4 to 5 cm from the skin), the needle is withdrawn about 2 mm. Withdrawing the needle slightly as such improves the likelihood of successfully blocking the mandibular nerve (V3) in addition to V2. A total of 5 to 10 mL of local anesthetic, with or without corticosteroid, is used for diagnostic or therapeutic block, whereas the same volume of alcohol may be carefully injected using the same approach if neurolysis is desired. The mandibular (V3) branch may be separately blocked here, or may be blocked in tandem with V2 as described previously. V3 has a large sensory and a smaller motor root, both of which leave the middle cranial fossa together via the foramen ovale. Sensory innervation is to the dura and mucosal lining of the mastoid sinus, as well as to the tragus and helix of the ear, skin over the muscles of mastication, posterior TMJ, chin, and anterior two thirds of the tongue (via the lingual nerve branch of the mandibular nerve, which sends diverging branches to the chorda tympani branch of the facial nerve). The motor elements, which are smaller overall, provide innervation to the masseter, external pterygoid, and temporalis muscle. If the nerve is to be blocked as noted above for the V2 block, the simplest and likeliest chance for success is via the coronoid approach. If it is desired to block the nerve separately, then once the needle contacts the lateral pterygoid plate, it should be redirected posteriorly and inferiorly until it passes the inferior aspect of the plate. At a point corresponding to approximately 1 cm deeper than the contact point of the lateral pterygoid plate, typically a V3 paresthesia is elicited. A usual dose of local anesthetic, or of neurolytic agent, is 3 to 5 mL using continual intermittent aspiration tests because of the high degree of vascularity in the area. Because the mandibular nerve (V3) has motor branches, it is not inconceivable that a well-performed local anesthetic or neurolytic procedure might result in paresis or weakness of the muscles of mastication, as well as some facial asymmetry caused by muscle weakness. This may be more than a nuisance, and should be clearly described during the informed consent process with the patient.

Mandibular and maxillary nerve blocks are typically used for ameliorating pain related to TGN, but indications for surgical analgesia, including using mandibular block as an adjunct for cervical plexus block (CPB) for carotid endarterectomy surgery, have been described.[21] Although most physicians continue to use fluoroscopic guidance in most cases of mandibular nerve block, the technique of CT-guided block has been described, and may be a suitable alternative if this modality is considered necessary to delineate the relevant anatomy.[22] Continuous catheter techniques of mandibular block also have been described for cancer pain management[23] as well as for analgesia after mandibular fracture repair.[24] Neural complications after mandibular nerve injury are not uncommon, and involve the lingual nerve (Fig. 46–21) more commonly than the inferior alveolar nerve, often lasting much longer than other common peripheral nerve injuries such as neuropraxias.[25] These injuries may represent neurotoxicity as a central cause, according to one recent review undertaken in 52 patients who had received these blocks.[25] Otherwise, intravascular injection, hematoma, dizziness, and ataxia occur with some frequency after these procedures, and should be discussed with patients during the informed consent process.[26]

For maxillary nerve block using the coronoid approach, it is important to not advance the block needle more than 0.25 cm once the pterygoid plate has been contacted, to minimize the chance of causing neural injury.[27] As for mandibular nerve block (described earlier), a CT-guided technique and a continuous catheter technique of maxillary nerve block have been described—the former to increase the likelihood of success[28] and the latter to extend the duration of analgesia in a group of patients undergoing radical maxillary sinusotomy.[29]

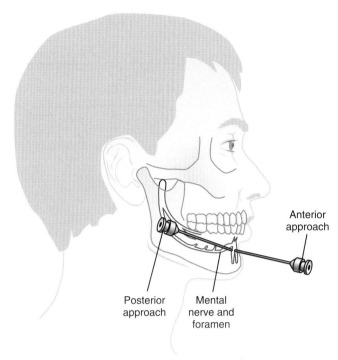

Figure 46–21. Anatomy and block of the inferior alveolar branch of the mandibular nerve (mental nerve).

Supraorbital, Infraorbital, and Mental Nerve Blocks

Peripheral branches of the trigeminal system may be readily accessible through percutaneous needle techniques.

Supraorbital Nerve Block

This is useful in treating painful conditions of the frontal nerve, a branch of V1. The nerve leaves the superior orbital fissure to enter the orbit, passing ventrally under the periosteum of the roof of the orbit. The frontal nerve gives off two corollary branches; the supraorbital and supratrochlear nerves. The supraorbital nerve is larger and more laterally situated than the supratrochlear nerve, and supplies sensory fibers to the forehead, upper eyelid, and anterior scalp. The nerve is typically blocked using a small volume of dilute local anesthetic with or without corticosteroid added, by injecting into the supraorbital foramen (see Fig. 46–19; Fig. 46–22). A 22- to 25-gauge, 1.5-inch sharp needle is typically used for the block, which is readily accomplished once the foramen is palpated, and after a sterile skin prep is performed. The goal of needle insertion is to avoid placing the needle tip through the foramen, which would assuredly elicit a paresthesia of the supraorbital nerve as it pins the nerve against the periosteum. Instead, guide the needle toward the foramen; once periosteum is contacted, the needle should be slid slightly medially so that its tip is abutting the rim of the foramen. Following a negative aspiration, 3 to 4 mL of local anesthetic with 2 mg of dexa-

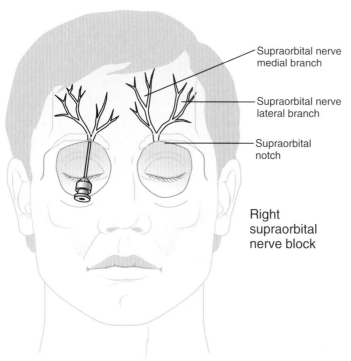

Supraorbital nerve
medial branch

Supraorbital nerve
lateral branch

Supraorbital
notch

Right
supraorbital
nerve block

Figure 46–22. Anatomy of the supraorbital nerve and the technique of nerve blocking.

methasone or 6 mg of betamethasone may be incrementally injected. The needle should be flushed and withdrawn, and a dressing applied over the injection site. Supraorbital nerve block has been successfully used in the treatment of hemicrania continua.[30] Supratrochlear nerve block may be performed at a point slightly medial to the insertion site described for supraorbital nerve block, using the same needle types and volumes and concentrations of local anesthetics and adjuvants. The indications, contraindications, complications, and side effects of this block are virtually identical to those aforementioned.

Infraorbital Nerve Block

Infraorbital nerve block (see Figs. 46–18 and 46–19) is used to block the peripheral contribution of the maxillary nerve, typically affected by conditions of chronic facial pain such as those caused by a complex regional pain syndrome (discussed later), and occasionally herpes zoster. The infraorbital nerve enters the orbit via the infraorbital fissure and passes along the floor of that structure in the infraorbital groove. It exits the skull through the infraorbital foramen, innervating the lower eyelid, lateral nose, and part of the superior lip. A branch of the nerve, the superior alveolar nerve, innervates the upper incisors, canines, and contiguous soft tissue.

Infraorbital block is performed with the patient in the supine position, and with the head maintained in a neutral position. The infraorbital foramen is palpated, and a mark is placed over it using a marking

pen. A sterile skin prep is performed, after which a fine-gauge (25 or 27 gauge), 1.5-inch needle is advanced into the foramen while maintaining a slight medial direction of the advancing needle tip. This maneuver helps minimize the pinning of the infraorbital nerve against bone, and potentially traumatizing the nerve. Even taking such precautions, the nerve may be stimulated, resulting in a paresthesia to the teeth or lateral naris. After aspirating for the presence of blood (difficult, at best through a 27-gauge needle), a small volume (3 mL) of local anesthetic, with or without a nonparticulate corticosteroid, is incrementally injected. After clearing the needle, it is withdrawn, and a small adhesive bandage is applied over the injection site. The patient should be observed for 20 minutes and examined for an expanding hematoma of the face, which is usually readily treated with pressure and occasionally with an ice pack.

Inferior Alveolar (Mental) Nerve Block

The inferior alveolar nerve is a distal branch of the mandibular nerve. The nerve exits the mental foramen at the level of the second molar tooth, having divided into an incisor branch and a mental branch. After exiting the foramen, the nerve sends a ramus superiorly, innervating the lower lip, inferior oral mucosa, and the chin (mental branch). This nerve block has been used in the treatment of mental neuralgia, facial herpes zoster, and in cases of TGN of the V3, in which the nerve is readily accessible for cryolesioning (see Figs. 46–19 and 46–21).[31] As in the infraorbital nerve block technique, there is both an extraoral and intraoral technique of mental nerve block. It appears that the intraoral technique is less painful for patients while providing a similar degree of successful block compared with the latter.[32] When evaluated in 123 patients using a standardized alveolar nerve block method, the block provided analgesia and anesthesia to the first molar (92%), first premolar (55.3%), and canine (38.2%) teeth of the lower jaw.[33] Additionally, levobupivacaine 0.5% with epinephrine 1:200,000 (5 μg/mL) was shown to be equipotent and equieffective to the same concentration and dose of bupivacaine when used for inferior alveolar nerve block. Because of its inherent reduced systemic and cardiac toxicity, perhaps levobupivacaine will replace the latter agent for peripheral nerve blocks of the trigeminal system.[34]

Inferior alveolar nerve block is performed with the patient in the supine position, and the head maintained in a neutral position. After palpating the mental foramen and performing a sterile skin prep, a small (25 or 27 gauge) 1.5-inch needle is advanced toward the foramen using a slight medial approach as for infraorbital nerve block, to minimize the likelihood of pinning the exiting nerve against periosteum. A paresthesia may nevertheless be obtained while performing the needle insertion, and patients need to be apprised of this possibility. After a negative aspiration test, 3 mL of local anesthetic with or without a nonparticulate corticosteroid is incrementally injected. The needle is cleared and withdrawn, and a small adhesive bandage is applied over the injection site. The patient should be observed for approximately 20 minutes to guard against the development of a hematoma, which is typically amenable to compression or the application of an ice pack.

Glossopharyngeal, Vagus, and Facial Nerve Blocks

Less commonly performed nerve blocks for facial and head pain include the glossopharyngeal, vagus, and facial nerve blocks.

Glossopharyngeal Nerve Block

The glossopharyngeal nerve (GPN) (cranial nerve IX) is infrequently implicated in painful conditions of the face and neck. Nevertheless, because of the lack of familiarity of many pain physicians with the anatomy and implications of glossopharyngeal nerve dysfunction, it is an important entity to consider in cases of recalcitrant pain particularly of the tongue, mouth, and pharynx. GPN block may be suitable for conditions such as glossopharyngeal neuralgia, and pain caused by malignancy. The nerve may be affected by tumors of the tongue, hypopharynx, and palatine tonsils. The block is also used during the anatomic evaluation method of differential nerve block. The GPN is a mixed cranial nerve carrying both motor and sensory fibers. The nerve is attached by three or four filaments to the medulla oblongata in a groove between the olive and inferior peduncle. Motor fibers, from cells of the nucleus ambiguus, innervate the stylopharyngeus muscle, whereas the sensory branches, from cells of the superior and petrous ganglia, innervate the tongue (posterior one third), palatine tonsil, fauces, and mucous membranes of the mouth and pharynx. A branch of the GPN, the carotid sinus nerve, is important in the regulation of blood pressure, pulse, and respiration because this branch innervates the carotid body and carotid sinus. Sympathetic efferent fibers from the nucleus ambiguus are preganglionic motor fibers as well as preganglionic secretory fibers of the sympathetic system. Parasympathetic fibers pass to the otic ganglion, and postganglionic fibers innervate the parotid gland. In conjunction with the vagus and spinal accessory nerves (cranial nerves X and XI), the GPN exits the jugular foramen near the internal jugular vein. All three cranial nerves lie between the internal jugular vein and the internal carotid artery. The styloid process of the temporal bone is a major landmark for successfully blocking the GPN (Fig. 46–23). GPN block is performed with the patient in the supine position, with the head turned slightly opposite to the affected side. Our practice includes the use of fluoroscopic imaging to delineate and define the ipsilateral mastoid and the ipsilateral angle of the mandible, as the styloid process is typically found

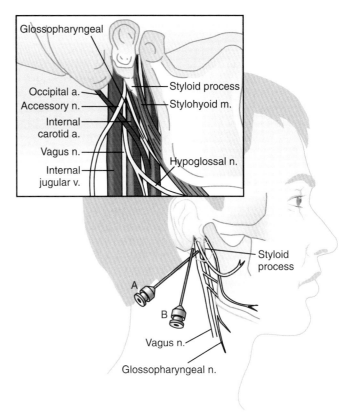

Figure 46–23. Anatomy and technique of blocking the glossopharyngeal and vagus nerves at the styloid process. The inset shows the details of the anatomy of the structures coursing through from the base of the skull in the posterior cranial fossa. a., artery; m., muscle; n., nerve; v., vein.

equidistant between these two respective structures. Fluoroscopy also permits real-time imaging of the pattern of injection of contrast media, so that in cases in which the needle tip has penetrated either the carotid or jugular systems, this activity should be observable and intravascular injection subsequently preventable. Once baseline scout films have been obtained, intravenous access ensured, and baseline vital signs documented, the skin overlying the styloid process should be prepped and draped in sterile fashion. A small skin wheal may be made over the styloid process using a 25-gauge, 1.5-inch needle and 1% plain lidocaine, 3 to 4 mL. Next, a 22-gauge, 1.5- to 2-inch blunt-tipped block needle may be advanced perpendicular to the skin toward the process, aiming for its posterior aspect. The usual depth of contact of the styloid varies from about 1.5 to 4 cm. Once the needle tip has slipped posteriorly off of the process, 1 mL of iodinated contrast media should be incrementally injected under live continuous fluoroscopy. Then, barring any intravascular spread, a short-acting (lidocaine; mepivacaine) and dilute (1% concentration) local anesthetic with epinephrine 1:200,000 (5 µg/mL) in a volume of 5 to 8 mL should be incrementally injected in divided doses. If indicated, a modest dose of nonparticulate corticosteroid (dexamethasone; betamethasone) may be added to the injectate. Patients need to be monitored for a minimum of 30 minutes following the block to verify that there has been no systemic response to the injected local anesthetic solution. Even taking these precautions and using fluoroscopic guidance does not completely eliminate the possibility of local anesthetic spillover onto the vagus nerve (with resultant ipsilateral vocal cord paralysis) or onto the spinal accessory nerve (weakness of the trapezius muscle).

Vagus Nerve Block

The tenth cranial nerve, the vagus, is also infrequently a source of chronic facial and neck pain. When it is involved, the syndromes underlying the pain are usually oncologic, but vagal neuralgia is also a recognized pain entity. Invasive tumors of the hypopharynx, larynx, and pyriform sinus are implicated in vagal nerve invasion and subsequent pain. The vagus, like the glossopharyngeal nerve, is a mixed motor and sensory nerve and has a more extensive course and distribution than any of the other cranial nerves because it passes through the neck and thorax to the abdomen. The vagus is attached by 8 to 10 filaments to the medulla oblongata in the groove between the olive and inferior peduncle, below the GPN. The superior and recurrent laryngeal nerves originate from the vagus. Sensory fibers from the vagus arise from cells of the jugular ganglion and ganglion nodosum (sympathetic afferent fibers) and innervate the posterior fossa dura mater, posterior external auditory meatus, inferior tympanic membrane, and mucosa of the larynx below the vocal cords. There are also sympathetic efferent fibers innervating the heart, lungs, bronchial tree, and associated vasculature. The vagus nerve sits behind the GPN, superficial to the internal jugular vein, in a sheath of dura mater that also houses the spinal accessory nerve (cranial nerve XI). This dural sheath is the septum that separates the vagus from the GPN at the jugular foramen. Vagal nerve blockade is accomplished in a manner analogous to GPN block, and in fact, spillover of local anesthetic when performing the latter block often results in partial or complete vagal nerve block as well. The styloid process of the temporal bone is the primary landmark, and because it is not always palpable, our technique uses fluoroscopic guidance (as for GPN block) to accomplish vagal nerve block. Appropriate candidates are queried as to the presence of bleeding problems, the use of medications that interfere with platelet aggregation, or other anticoagulants. Intravenous access is accomplished, and the block is performed with the patient supine. The head is rotated slightly toward the contralateral side, and the fluoroscope is aimed in a slightly oblique tilt to define the angle of the mandible and the mastoid process. The styloid should be approximately equidistant between these two structures. Because the nerve sits caudad to the GPN, the block technique is almost identical to that described with the major exception being that

once the needle slips posteriorly off the styloid process, it should be directed slightly caudad to the process, by approximately 0.5 cm. After careful aspiration for blood, 3 to 5 mL of local anesthetic with or without corticosteroid is incrementally injected. Successful block is often accompanied by dysphonia because of blockade of the recurrent or the superior laryngeal branches of the vagus. Spillover of local anesthetic to block the hypoglossal, GPN, or spinal accessory nerves may result in weakness of the tongue, ipsilateral trapezius muscle, or sensory changes in the posterior third of the tongue, palatine tonsil, or mucous membranes of the mouth and pharynx.

Facial Nerve Block

Facial nerve block is an uncommonly performed technique of cranial nerve blockade reserved for conditions involving documented dysfunction of the seventh cranial nerve. Cranial nerve VII consists of two roots: a motor root from the facial nucleus, and the nervus intermedius, which in turn consists of sensory afferents to the skin and for taste (to the nucleus tractus solitarius), as well as the preganglionic parasympathetics from the superior salivatory nucleus. Branches from cranial nerve VII include the large petrosal nerve that influences lacrimation and salivation, the nerve to the stapedius muscle, the chorda tympani nerve (taste to the anterior two thirds of the tongue), sensory articular branches (sensation from the external auditory canal and inferior pinna of the ear), and motor fibers to the muscles of facial expression. Herpes simplex type 1 may cause Bell's palsy, a condition amenable to facial nerve block. Diabetics and pregnant women also are at risk for developing Bell's palsy, which results in painful paralysis of the facial muscles over a 3- to 72-hour period in up to 50% of those afflicted.[35] Hemifacial spasm, petrous bone fracture, middle ear, mastoid or parotid surgery, or tumors (especially neuromas, meningiomas, hemangiomas or cholesteatomas) all can result in facial pain in the distribution of the facial nerve. Ramsay Hunt syndrome (herpes zoster of the geniculate ganglion), leprosy, Lyme disease, and otitis media can lead to painful syndromes of the nerve, amenable in certain cases to nerve block. Once the nerve emerges from the brainstem with the nerve of Wrisberg (nervus intermedius) it courses across the cerebellopontine angle next to cranial nerve VIII (vestibulocochlear nerve). These three nerves (cranial nerves VII and VIII, and the nervus intermedius) then enter the internal auditory canal (IAC). The facial nerve runs superiorly along the roof of the IAC. It then travels though the petrous temporal bone in a bony canal, the fallopian canal. At the geniculate ganglion, the facial nerve and the nervus intermedius coalesce into a common trunk. The distal segment of the facial nerve then exits the middle ear between the external auditory canal (EAC) and the horizontal semicircular canal. A constant landmark for the nerve is the inferior relationship of the nerve to the lateral

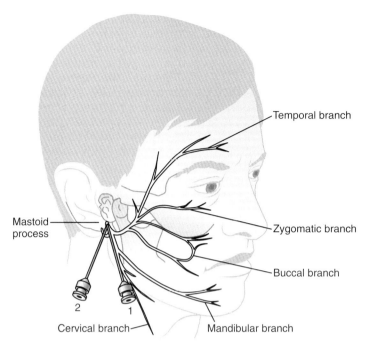

Figure 46–24. Anatomy of the facial nerve as it courses to the face. Needle placement for blocking the facial nerve between the mastoid process and the angle of the mandible is demonstrated.

semicircular canal. The nerve exits the fallopian canal via the stylomastoid foramen, between the digastric muscle and the stylohyoid muscle, before entering the parotid gland.

For facial nerve block, the patient is placed in the supine position with the head turned somewhat to the contralateral side. Intravenous access is obtained, and baseline vital signs documented. After palpating the mastoid process, or after identifying that structure using fluoroscopic guidance (preferred), a sterile skin prep is performed over the intended injection site. A 25- or 22-gauge, 1.5-inch blunt-tipped block needle is advanced through a local anesthetic skin wheal toward the anterior border of the mastoid process, directly beneath the external auditory meatus at the level of the ramus of the mandible (Fig. 46–24). Once the needle makes contact with the periosteum of the mastoid, it is advanced slightly more medially past the margin of that structure, until it is situated at the approximate point of where the facial nerve exits the stylomastoid foramen, at a depth of about 1 cm past the original bony contact. After aspirating for the presence of blood, 0.5 to 1 mL of radiocontrast is incrementally injected under continuous fluoroscopic guidance to verify that indeed no vascular structure has been encroached upon. Then, 3 to 5 mL of short-acting local anesthetic with or without nonparticulate corticosteroid is incrementally injected. The needle is cleared and withdrawn, and an adhesive bandage is applied over the injection site while observing the patient for the presence of any facial swelling that could result from vascular laceration.

ADDITIONAL TECHNIQUES FOR HEADACHE AND FACIAL PAIN MANAGEMENT

Cervical Epidural Block, Stellate Ganglion Block, and Sphenopalatine Ganglion Block

Cervical Epidural Block

Epidural nerve block is covered in the neuraxial section of this textbook, and is briefly included here for completeness. In the context of chronic head or neck pain, or headache, cervical epidural steroid injection block (CESI) is a technique that occasionally is used for diagnostic and therapeutic purposes. CESI is a valuable modality when performing a differential neural blockade for chronic undiagnosed pain. It is also valuable as a treatment option for the pain of acute herpes zoster or postherpetic neuralgia. Cancer-related pain, complex regional pain syndromes of the head (see later), and vascular insufficiency states are treated with local anesthetic or corticosteroid CESI. Tension-type headaches and those not responding to conventional medication management or conventional nerve block may also be successfully treated using this technique.

The technique is performed with the patient in the sitting, prone, or lateral decubitus position. Fluoroscopic guidance is not essential, but is clearly becoming the technique of choice because of reports of serious and often permanent neurologic injuries sustained by errantly placed injections or idiosyncratic reactions to procedurally given medications. Knowledge of the distance from the skin to the cervical epidural space at various levels may be helpful when performing these procedures, and has been determined in a study of 816 subjects.[36] (The depth to the epidural space in males at C5-6 was 4.7 ± 0.6 cm; at C6-7 it was 5.1 ± 0.6 cm; and at C7-T1 it was 5.6 ± 0.8 cm. In females the depth at C5-6 was 4 ± 0.6 cm; at C6-7 it was 4.6 ± 0.6 cm; and at C7-T1 it was 5 ± 0.6 cm [means $\pm$ standard deviations.])[36]

Our technique of choice is to perform the CESI with patients in the seated position, and to use fluoroscopic guidance whenever possible. Intravenous access is attained in all individuals to mitigate against the vasovagal syncope that occurs in up to 10% of patients in our experience. After obtaining and documenting baseline vital signs, the patient is placed with the head flexed forward and forehead resting against an immovable fluoroscopy table or Mayo stand that has been stabilized. The arms are placed comfortably at the sides, and the fluoroscopy C-arm is rotated into position over the head to enable the beam to be directed across the neck, obtaining a lateral image (Fig. 46–25). After palpating the anatomic midline and performing a sterile prep and drape, a skin wheal is raised at the chosen interspace, typically C5-6, C6-7, or C7-T1, using lidocaine 1% plain, 2 to 3 mL via a 25-gauge, 1.5-inch needle. Next, a 20-gauge Tuohy-type winged epidural needle is advanced from posterior to anterior between the spinous processes of the selected interspace, using

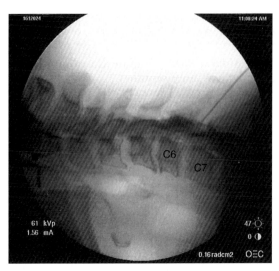

Figure 46–25. Lateral radiograph demonstrating needle placement at C6-7 for interlaminar cervical epidural steroid injection.

the hanging drop technique of Gutierrez.[37] In this technique, a drop of normal saline or local anesthetic solution is placed into the hub of the needle after the stylet has been removed once the needle is engaged in the interspinous ligament. As the needle approaches and then traverses the ligamentum flavum, the drop should be sucked into the epidural space as a result of the negative pressure found therein. If there is an equivocal response to the hanging drop approach, and on lateral fluoroscopy the needle appears to be at the level of the ligamentum flavum, then further advancement should not occur without verification of a midline position of the needle. This could represent a midline-placed needle that is seated between the interspinous ligament and the dura, in a patient for whom the ligamentum flavum is not fused in the midline. If by fluoroscopy the needle appears to be in the center of the interlaminar space, and the hanging drop has still not been sucked into the epidural space, a loss of resistance to air or saline test should be used before further needle advancement is attempted. After ascertaining that the needle tip is indeed within the epidural space (which varies from about 3 to 4 mm at the C7-T1 level, with the neck flexed), a 3-mL syringe with radiocontrast media should be attached to an extension tubing and subsequently to the hub of the needle ("immobile needle"), and 1 to 2 mL of contrast should be injected to delineate the confines of the space. In most cases, the dye will be predominantly localized to the posterior epidural space. Indeed, one study demonstrated that in only 28% of cases of CESI was injected contrast noted in the anterior or ventral epidural space.[38] After aspirating and noting the absence of cerebrospinal fluid (CSF) or blood, and demonstrating that no paresthesias have been elicited, a nonparticulate corticosteroid (i.e., dexamethasone 8 mg, or equivalent) in 1 mL of 1% lidocaine plain and 1 mL of normal saline solution may now be injected incrementally with intermittent aspiration every 1 mL. Next, the needle should be cleared using 0.5 mL of

normal saline, and then it should be removed and a sterile dressing applied over the injection site. The patient should be observed a minimum of 30 minutes to rule out a delayed syncopal response or a delayed allergic reaction to injected agents. Alternative techniques of CESI include performing the procedure with the patient prone, and using a continuous catheter technique placed through an epidural needle inserted at C7-T1 in an attempt to fluoroscopically guide the catheter into the ventral epidural space toward an exiting nerve root. This technique, however, has limited use in the management of chronic facial pain syndromes or in the palliation of headache pain.

Stellate Ganglion Block

Stellate ganglion block (SGB) is covered extensively in chapters on sympathetic nerve blocks. Because the block is occasionally used for syndromes other than those related to upper extremity pain, or pain caused by myocardial ischemia, including facial and head pain conditions, it is briefly included here. The technique is extremely useful for treating acute herpes zoster ophthalmicus, frostbite of the nose and face, sympathetically mediated pain of the head and neck (see later), and some types of vascular headaches. Appropriately performed, SGB has diverse effects on the sweating and cutaneous vascular responses of the face and head, although the response is not consistent in all cases.[39] Intraocular pressure, however, is consistently reduced by injecting 5 mL of 1% mepivacaine on the ipsilateral C7 transverse process for SGB in patients suffering from Bell's palsy.[40] After SGB, the blood flow of the optic nerve head and the peripapillary retina increases, although the implication of this finding in chronic pain syndromes is unclear.[41] When 6 to 8 mL of 1% mepivacaine was used for SGB, blood flow velocity assessment using MRI and the direct bolus tracking method in the common carotid artery increased, whereas blood flow velocity in the vertebral arteries was unchanged. This implies that blood flow changes occur in extracerebral but not intracerebral vessels, following SGB.[42] Using 10 mL of 2% plain lidocaine for SGB, however, was shown to decrease middle cerebral artery flow velocity, increase estimated cerebral perfusion pressure, and decrease zero flow pressure. This implies that SGB induces a decrease in cerebral vascular tone without affecting the capacity of the vessels to autoregulate, and may be one explanation for why cerebral vasospasm is amenable to reversal by SGB.[43] Using CT scan evaluation following C6 SGB and a 20-mL volume of local anesthetic showed that the bulk of solution remains sequestered near the head (i.e., medially) and not the neck of the rib at T1, implying that contact with the ganglion is not the mechanism of upper extremity sympathectomy.[44] Unlike the technique of interscalene brachial plexus block performed at C6, SGB does not inhibit ipsilateral hemidiaphragmatic function unless the local spills over onto the phrenic nerve via the brachial plexus[45] (see Fig. 46–28). Using the head-up tilt test, it was determined that right-sided SGB had minimal effects on systemic blood pressure or heart rate,[46] whereas it did increase QT interval, QTc interval (rate corrected QT), and QTcD (rate corrected QT dispersion) after head-up tilt.[47] These changes did not occur after left-sided SGB. The implications of these findings are that right-sided SGB is associated with a potentially increased risk of ventricular dysrhythmias and cardiac events, in distinction to the absence of these findings after left-sided SGB.[47]

The stellate ganglion is composed of the fused cervicothoracic (C7 and T1) sympathetic ganglia. Although some advocate performing an SGB at the most prominent palpable transverse process in the cervical spine (C6; Chassaignac's tubercle), anatomically it is more appropriate to inject local anesthetic at C7 (Figs. 46–26 to 46–28). Our technique is to use fluoroscopic guidance and perform a lateral paratracheal approach at C7. After determining the absence of coagulation problems or use of antiplatelet medication, the patient is placed supine and an intravenous cannula is placed in a distal extremity. Noninvasive hemodynamic monitors are applied, and after obtaining baseline vital signs a sterile skin prep is performed over the ipsilateral neck. The fluoroscopic unit is oriented anteroposteriorly, with a steep craniad tilt to remove the obstruction imposed by the mandible. A skin wheal is raised over the transverse process of C7 using 1% lidocaine, 2 mL via a 25-gauge 1.5-inch needle. Then a 22-gauge blunt needle with a curved tip is advanced directly perpendicular to the skin while advising the patient not to cough, swallow, or speak throughout the procedure. The patient is permitted to raise one finger to indicate "stop," the implication being that the procedure should be immediately halted to assess a change in comfort or the presence of a paresthesia. Once the

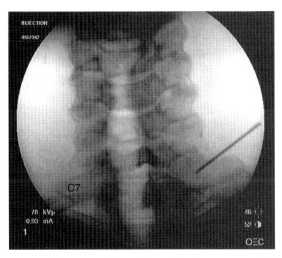

Figure 46–26. Anteroposterior radiograph using steep cephalad tilt (to remove the obstruction of the mandible in the figure) demonstrating a "finder" needle placed on the skin over the transverse process of C7.

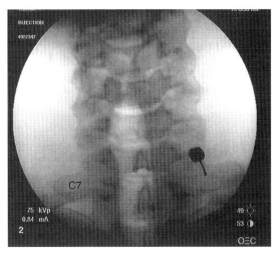

Figure 46–27. Needle tip (blunt 22-gauge, 3.5-inch Whitacre-type subarachnoid needle) advanced from anterior to posterior until it abuts the transverse process of C7.

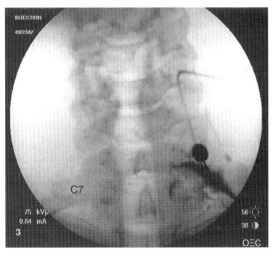

Figure 46–28. Injection of radiocontrast medium through the needle placed against the transverse process of C7 for stellate ganglion block, demonstrating some spread medially as well as along the brachial plexus (no sequelae demonstrated from the spillover onto the plexus).

C7 transverse process has been contacted, the needle is withdrawn 1 mm to clear the longus colli muscle, and a lateral image is obtained. If subsequent aspiration tests are negative for blood or CSF, 1 mL of radiocontrast media is incrementally injected under direct imaging. If there is no vascular spread or neuraxial dye pattern, a short-acting (i.e., 1% mepivacaine or lidocaine with epinephrine, 1:200,000) with or without a nonparticulate corticosteroid, may be incrementally injected after first giving a 0.5-mL test dose. This volume should be sufficient, if injected into the vertebral artery, to cause symptoms and signs of toxicity, even in the face of a negative dye study. A volume of 7 to 10 mL of solution is acceptable and typically provides effective blockade of relevant structures. It is important to observe the patient for up to 30 minutes after completion of the block to evaluate for any signs of brachial plexus or epidural spillover, and to monitor distal extremity temperature between ipsilateral and contralateral sides.

MISCELLANEOUS BLOCKS: SPHENOPALATINE AND CERVICAL PLEXUS

The sphenopalatine ganglion (SPG) block is useful for treating acute migraine headaches, acute cluster headaches, and facial neuralgias including Sluder, Vail, and Gardner syndromes.[48] Some have suggested that SPG block using 4% viscous lidocaine is not superior to placebo in the analgesic management of patients suffering from myofascial pain of the head.[49] Others have found that RF of the SPG relieved the symptoms of episodic cluster headache in 60.7% of 56 patients and in 30% of 10 patients with chronic cluster headache. An infrazygomatic approach was used, and complications were transient in all cases.[50] The SPG is located in the pterygopalatine fossa, posterior to the middle nasal turbinate. It is covered by a 1- to 1.5-mm-thick layer of connective tissue and mucous membrane. The SPG is approximately 5 mm in size and triangular in shape, and sends nerve fibers to the gasserian ganglion, trigeminal nerves, carotid plexus, facial nerve, and superior cervical ganglion. Our technique is to block the ganglion using the topical application instead of an intraoral approach. With the patient in the supine position and the head maximally extended, as in the sniffing position, 3 mL of 4% viscous lidocaine absorbed onto cotton-tipped pledgets are placed through the nostrils, one side at a time so as not to induce bulking. These are advanced slowly and deliberately to minimize epistaxis, in a direction that is directly perpendicular to the floor. The path taken with the pledgets is along the superior border of the middle turbinate of each nostril until the tip contacts the mucosa overlying the SPG. The pledgets are left in place for 30 minutes while the patient's vital signs are monitored, and they are then removed and discarded. Side effects are typically related to iatrogenic epistaxis, because local anesthetic toxicity is exceedingly rare using this approach.

Cervical plexus block is a technique of blocking the cervical nerve roots C2-4 for surgical analgesia and for chronic pain syndromes like spasmodic torticollis and cervical dystonias. One of the more common indications is to use cervical plexus block (CPB) for the intraoperative management of patients undergoing carotid endarterectomy surgery (CEA), because it permits an awake patient to give immediate feedback in the event of a neurologic compromise associated with shunting or with embolic phenomena.[51,52] CPB is also useful for the care and treatment of painful conditions of the neck when a differential diagnosis has failed to elicit a cause for the pain.[53] Finally, in cases of intractable hiccups, we have used CPB successfully to abort several cases of phrenic nerve irritation resulting from invasive malignancies. CPB has not been demonstrated to reduce pain or analgesic requirements following thyroid surgery, even when performed as a bilateral technique.[54,55] Essentially,

deep CPB is performed in a manner analogous to interscalene brachial plexus block (BPB), the difference being that the needle is inserted at the level of the thyroid cartilage (C4) instead of at the level of the cricoid cartilage (C6). By virtue of this technical alteration in approaches, however, instead of deriving sensory and motor blockade of the nerve roots destined to arborize into the three trunks of the brachial plexus (superior, middle, inferior), CPB blocks the structures innervated by more cephalad spinal nerve roots C2, C3, and C4. If the brachial plexus is prefixed, then theoretically at least the local anesthetic may result in blockade of the superior trunk with some motor weakness noted in the proximal upper extremity. The block is performed with the patient in the supine position and with the head turned to the opposite side. Monitors are applied and intravenous access is secured in the contralateral distal upper extremity. A sterile skin prep is performed, after which a 22-gauge, short-beveled, 1.5- to 2-inch block needle is advanced between the anterior and middle scalene muscles, remaining closer to the middle scalene than to the anterior one. The needle is advanced perpendicular to the skin with a slight medial, dorsal, and caudal approach to minimize the likelihood of entering one of the intervertebral foramina. After carefully aspirating and noting the absence of blood or cerebrospinal fluid, 15 to 20 mL of local anesthetic is incrementally injected with continual intermittent aspiration of the needle (via an extension tubing connected to the syringe—the "immobile needle") every 2 mL. Alternatively, a superficial CPB may be performed while increasing the volume to 30 mL because there is a communication between the superficial and deep plexuses that permits the spread of injected solution to reach the cervical nerve roots by some unknown mechanism.[56] Side effects and complications are as described in the section of this text dedicated to BPBs and include the potential for hemidiaphragmatic paralysis, subarachnoid and epidural block, peripheral nerve injury, vertebral arterial injection, embolization, hoarseness and dysphonia, and dysphagia. At least one case of bilateral vocal cord palsy has been described following use of this block in a patient who previously had undergone previous thyroid surgery and who had residual ipsilateral vocal cord paresis.[57]

UNUSUAL SOURCES OF HEAD AND NECK PAIN AMENABLE TO REGIONAL BLOCK

Complex regional pain syndromes (CRPS) of the head and neck are gratefully rare entities that require a high index of suspicion to identify.[58] As of this writing, there are fewer than two dozen cases in the published literature that meet the International Association for the Study of Pain (IASP) criteria. Most of the information concerning this entity arises in the form of isolated case reports.[59,60] The diagnosis is particularly difficult to make because the clinical features typically lack the vasomotor and sudomotor phenomena often seen in extremity CRPS. On the positive side, in most cases, facial pain syndromes with features of CRPS that meet the diagnostic criteria are often amenable to treatment with sympathetic ganglion blocks, regardless of the duration of symptoms. This implies that this unusual entity may be an independent syndrome masquerading as CRPS by virtue of its satisfying the diagnostic criteria.[61] Every effort should be made to identify these patients and treat them aggressively with standard techniques of peripheral nerve block that have been described in this chapter.

CONCLUSION

Facial, head, and neck pain remains a diagnostic and therapeutic challenge for many pain physicians. The anatomic considerations are almost overwhelming, and the critical relationship between neural and vascular structures makes precise treatment remedies essential. Our heavy reliance on radiographic guidance is congruent with these discordant processes, placing a targeted treatment into an area fraught with danger. Appropriate patient selection, monitoring, proper injection technique, and knowledge of the pharmacokinetics and pharmacodynamics of agents used are mandatory. The possible drug-drug interactions, increasing use of antiplatelet agents by individuals at high risk, and anatomic variation found in clinical practice serve to confound the picture even further.[62] Fortunately many patients do ultimately improve when dogged efforts are made to delineate the pain pathways subserving a given problem, and to then address those pathways with the tools of the contemporary interventionalist.[63]

References

1. Dreyfuss P, Rogers J, Dreyer S, Fletcher D: Atlanto-occipital joint pain: A report of three cases and description of an intraarticular joint block technique. Reg Anesth 1994;19:344-351.
2. Dieterich M, Pollmann W, Pfaffenrath V: Cervicogenic headache: Electronystagmography, perception of vertically and posturography in patients before and after C2-blockade. Cephalalgia 1993;13:285-288.
3. Leinisch-Dahlke E, Jurgens T, Bogdahn U, et al: Greater occipital nerve block is ineffective in chronic tension type headache. Cephalalgia 2005;25:704-708.
4. Hecht JS: Occipital nerve blocks in postconcussive headaches: A retrospective review and report of ten patients. J Head Trauma Rehabil 2004;19:58-71.
5. Sulfaro MA, Gobetti JP: Occipital neuralgia manifesting as orofacial pain. Oral Surg Oral Med Oral Pathol Oral Radiol Endod 1995;80:751-755.
6. Ashkenazi A, Young WB: The effects of greater occipital nerve block and trigger point injection on brush allodynia and pain in migraine. Headache 2005;45:350-354.
7. Caputi CA, Firetto V: Therapeutic blockade of greater occipital and supraorbital nerves in migraine patients. Headache 1997;37:174-179.
8. Matsushima JI, Sakai N, Uemi N, Ifukube T: Effects of greater occipital nerve block on tinnitus and dizziness. Int Tinnitus J 1999;5:40-46.
9. Gawel MJ, Rothbart PJ: Occipital nerve block in the management of headache and cervical pain. Cephalalgia 1992;12:9-13.
10. Kapoor V, Rothfus WE, Grahovac SV, et al: Refractory occipital neuralgia: Preoperative assessment with CT-guided nerve block

11. Okuda Y, Matsumoto T, Shinohara M, et al: Sudden unconsciousness during a lesser occipital nerve block in a patient with the occipital bone defect. Eur J Anaesthesiol 2001;18:829-832.
12. Lavin PJ, Workman R: Cushing syndrome induced by serial occipital nerve blocks containing corticosteroids. Headache 2001;41:902-904.
13. Kuroiwa T, Matsumoto S, Kato A, et al: MR imaging of idiopathic trigeminal neuralgia: Correlation with non-surgical therapy. Radiat Med 1996;14:235-239.
14. Stajcic Z, Todorovic L: Blocks of the foramen rotundum and the oval foramen: A reappraisal of extraoral maxillary and mandibular nerve injections. Br J Oral Maxillofac Surg 1997;35:328-333.
15. Peters G, Nurmikko TJ: Peripheral and gasserian ganglion-level procedures for the treatment of trigeminal neuralgia. Clin J Pain 2002;18:28-34.
16. Fujimaki T, Fukushima T, Miyazaki S: Percutaneous retrogasserian glycerol injection in the management of trigeminal neuralgia: Long-term follow-up results. J Neurosurg 1990;73:212-216.
17. Ischia S, Luzzani A, Polati E: Retrogasserian glycerol injection: A retrospective study of 112 patients. Clin J Pain 1990;6:291-296.
18. Delfino U, Beltrutti DP, Clemente M: Trigeminal neuralgia: Evaluation of percutaneous neurodestructive procedures. Clin J Pain 1990;6:18-25.
19. Sekimoto K, Koizuka S, Saito S, Goto F: Thermogangliolysis of the gasserian ganglion under computed tomography fluoroscopy. J Anesth 2005;19:177-179.
20. Horiguchi J, Ishifuro M, Fukuda H, et al: Multiplanar reformat and volume rendering of a multidetector CT scan for path planning a fluoroscopic procedure on gasserian block—A preliminary report. Eur J Radiol 2005;53:189-191.
21. Bourke DL, Thomas P: Mandibular nerve block in addition to cervical plexus block for carotid endarterectomy. Anesth Analg 1998;87:1034-1036.
22. Okuda Y, Takanishi T, Shinohara M, et al: Use of computed tomography for mandibular nerve block in the treatment of trigeminal neuralgia. Reg Anesth Pain Med 2001;26:382.
23. Kohase H, Umimo M, Shibaji T, Suzuki N: Application of a mandibular nerve block using an indwelling catheter for intractable cancer pain. Acta Anaesthesiol Scand 2004;48:382-383.
24. Singh B, Bhardwaj V: Continuous mandibular nerve block for pain relief: A report of two cases. Can J Anaesth 2002;49:951-953.
25. Hillerup S, Jensen R: Nerve injury caused by mandibular block analgesia. Int J Oral Maxillofac Surg 2006;35:437-443.
26. Konishi R, Mitsuhata H, Akazawa S, Shimizu R: Temporary severe vertigo associated with mandibular nerve block with absolute alcohol for treatment of trigeminal neuralgia. Anesthesiology 1997;87:699-700.
27. Singh B, Srivastava SK, Dang R: Anatomic considerations in relation to the maxillary nerve block. Reg Anesth Pain Med 2001;26:507-511.
28. Okuda Y, Okuda K, Shinohara M, Kitajima T: Use of computed tomography for maxillary nerve block in the treatment of trigeminal neuralgia. Reg Anesth Pain Med 2000;25:417-419.
29. Kohase H, Miyamoto T, Umino M: A new method of continuous maxillary nerve block with an indwelling catheter. Oral Surg Med Oral Pathol Oral Radiol Endod 2002;94:162-166.
30. Antonaci F, Pareja JA, Caminero AB, Sjaastad O: Chronic paroxysmal hemicrania and hemicrania continua: Anaesthetic blockades of pericranial nerves. Funct Neurol 1997;12:11-15.
31. Juniper RP: Trigeminal neuralgia—Treatment of the third division by radiologically controlled cryoblockade of the inferior dental nerve at the mandibular lingual: A study of 31 cases. Br J Oral Maxillofac Surg 1991;29:154-158.
32. Syverd SA, Jenkins JM, Schwab RA, et al: A comparative study of the percutaneous versus intraoral technique for mental nerve block. Acad Emerg Med 1994;1:509-513.

33. Lai TN, Lin CP, Kok SH, et al: Evaluation of mandibular block using a standardized method. Oral Surg Oral Med Oral Pathol Oral Radiol Endod 2006;102:462-468.

34. Branco FP, Ranali J, Ambrosano GM, Volpato MC: A double-blind comparison of 0.5% bupivacaine with 1:200,000 epinephrine and 0.5% levobupivacaine with 1:200,000 epinephrine for the inferior alveolar nerve block. Oral Surg Oral Med Oral Pathol Oral Radiol Endod 2006;101:442-447.

35. Ahmed A: When is facial paralysis Bell's palsy? Current diagnosis and treatment. Cleve Clin J Med 2005;72:398-401.

36. Han KR, Kim C, Park SK, Kim JS: Distance to the adult cervical epidural space. Reg Anesth Pain Med 2003;28:95-97.

37. Gutierrez A: Valor de la aspiracion liquida en el espacio peridural en la anesthesia peridural. Rev Cir Buenos Aires 1933; 12:225-227.

38. Stojanovic MP, Vu TN, Caneris O, et al: The role of fluoroscopy in cervical epidural steroid injections: An analysis of contrast dispersal patterns. Spine 2002;27:509-514.

39. Drummond PD: The effect of sympathetic blockade on facial sweating and cutaneous vascular responses to painful stimulation of the eye. Brain 1993;116:233-241.

40. Nagahara M, Tamaki Y, Araie M, Umeyama T: The acute effects of stellate ganglion block on circulation in human ocular fundus. Acta Opthalmol Scand 2001;79:45-48.

41. Yu HG, Chung H, Yoon TG, et al: Stellate ganglion block increases blood flow into the optic nerve head and the peripapillary retina in humans. Auton Neurosci 2003;109:53-57.

42. Nitahara K, Dan K: Blood flow velocity changes in carotid and vertebral arteries with stellate ganglion block: Measurement by magnetic resonance imaging using a direct bolus tracking method. Reg Anesth Pain Med 1998;23:600-604.

43. Gupta MM, Bithal PK, Dash HH, et al: Effects of stellate ganglion block on cerebral haemodynamics as assessed by transcranial Doppler ultrasonography. Br J Anaesth 2005;95:669-673.

44. Christie JM, Martinez CR: Computerized axial tomography to define the distribution of solution after stellate ganglion nerve block. J Clin Anesth 1995;7:306-311.

45. Sawyer RJ, Turnbull D, Richmond MN, et al: Assessment of diaphragm function after stellate ganglion block using magnetic stimulation. Anaesthesia 2002;57:70-76.

46. Koyama S, Sato N, Nagashima K, et al: Effects of right stellate ganglion block on the autonomic nervous function of the heart: A study using the head-up tilt test. Circ J 2002;66:645-648.

47. Fujii K, Yamaguchi S, Egawa H, et al: Effects of head-up tilt after stellate ganglion block on QT interval and QT dispersion. Reg Anesth Pain Med 2004;29:317-322.

48. Waldman SD: Sphenopalatine ganglion block: Transnasal approach. In Waldman SD (ed): Atlas of Interventional Pain Management (2nd ed). Philadelphia, Saunders Elsevier, 2004, pp 11-13.

49. Ferrante FM, Kaufman AG, Dunbar SA, et al: Sphenopalatine ganglion block for the treatment of myofascial pain of the head, neck and shoulders. Reg Anesth Pain Med 1998;23:30-36.

50. Sanders M, Zuurmond WW: Efficacy of sphenopalatine ganglion blockade in 66 patients suffering from cluster headache: A 12- to 70-month follow-up evaluation. J Neurosurg 1997;87:876-880.

51. Sindjelic R, Davidovic L, Vlajkovic G, et al: Pain associated with carotid artery surgery performed under carotid plexus block: Preemptive analgesic effect of ketorolac. Vascular 2006;14:75-80.

52. Messner M, Albrecht S, Lang W, et al: The superficial cervical plexus block for postoperative pain therapy in carotid artery surgery: A prospective randomized controlled study. Eur J Vasc Endovasc Surg 2007;33:50-54.

53. Shinozaki T, Sakamoto E, Shiiba S, et al: Cervical plexus block helps in diagnosis of orofacial pain originating from cervical structures. Tohoku J Exp Med 2006;210:41-47.

54. Eti Z, Irmak P, Gulluoglu BM, et al: Does bilateral superficial cervical plexus block decrease analgesic requirement after thyroid surgery? Anesth Analg 2006;102:1174-1176.

55. Herbland A, Cantini O, Reynier P, et al: The bilateral superficial cervical plexus block with 0.75% ropivacaine administered before or after surgery does not prevent postoperative pain after total thyroidectomy. Reg Anesth Pain Med 2006;31:34-39.

56. Pandit JJ, Dutta D, Morris JF: Spread of injectate with superficial cervical plexus block in humans: An anatomical study. Br J Anaesth 2003;91:733-735.

57. Kwok AO, Silbert BS, Allen KJ, et al: Bilateral vocal cord palsy during carotid endarterectomy under cervical plexus block. Anesth Analg 2006;1022:376-377.

58. Candido KD: Reflex sympathetic dystrophy of the face. In Waldman SD (ed): Pain Management. Philadelphia, Saunders Elsevier, 2007, pp 552-560.

59. Jaeger B, Singer E, Kroening R: Reflex sympathetic dystrophy of the face: Report of two cases and a review of the literature. Arch Neurol 1986;43:693-695.

60. Saxen MA, Campbell RL: An unusual case of sympathetically maintained facial pain complicated by telangiectasia. Oral Surg Oral Med Oral Pathol Oral Radiol Endod 1995;79:455-458.

61. Arden RL, Bahu SJ, Zuazu MA, Berguer R: Reflex sympathetic dystrophy of the face: Current treatment recommendations. Laryngoscope 1998;108:437-442.

62. Rosenberg M, Phero JC: Regional anesthesia and invasive techniques to manage head and neck pain. Otolaryngol Clin North Am 2003;36:1201-1219.

63. Gale G, Nussbaum D, Rothbart P, et al: A randomized treatment study to compare the efficacy of repeated nerve blocks with cognitive therapy for control of chronic head and neck pain. Pain Res Manage 2002;7:185-189.

CHAPTER
47 Upper Extremity Blocks

Joseph M. Neal

Regional anesthetic approaches to the brachial plexus are a mainstay of surgical anesthesia practice and play an increasingly important role in postoperative analgesia. Only in recent years have well-designed outcome studies confirmed the benefits of regional anesthesia for upper extremity surgery patients. When compared with traditional opioid-based postoperative analgesia for patients undergoing outpatient shoulder, arm, or hand surgery, single-shot regional techniques provide superior analgesia, reduce opioid-related side effects, improve patient satisfaction, and reduce the number of unplanned admissions. Although these benefits are generally limited to the day of surgery, they nevertheless represent a valuable alternative over general anesthetic and postoperative opioid techniques.[1-4] Furthermore, limited comparative studies have shown that interscalene or suprascapular block provides better analgesia than injection or infusion of intra-articular local anesthetic.[5,6] Continuous perineural catheter techniques provide superior analgesia for total shoulder arthroplasty and various ambulatory shoulder surgeries. Similar to single-shot techniques, the prolonged analgesia afforded by continuous perineural catheters is associated with fewer opioid-related side effects and higher patient satisfaction. What remains unclear is whether these techniques substantially improve economic outcomes such as faster rehabilitation or return to work.[7-11] This chapter offers a brief review of brachial plexus anatomy and pharmacology, with a primarily focus on the techniques and complications of upper extremity blocks.

BRACHIAL PLEXUS ANATOMY

The ventral primary rami of cervical nerves C5 to C8 and thoracic nerve T1 comprise the brachial plexus, with occasional contributions from C4 and T2 (Fig. 47–1). Understanding the complex interdigitations that define the brachial plexus is important for two reasons. First, brachial plexus approaches are directed towards its various anatomic divisions. For example, the interscalene approach is placed at the level of the distal roots and proximal trunks, whereas the infraclavicular approach is placed at the level of the cords. This anatomic subarchitecture in turn determines the expected motor response to peripheral nerve stimulation and which nerves are expected to become anesthetized consequent to that particular approach. Second, supplemental anesthetizing procedures are often necessary for nerves that are distinct from the brachial plexus or are intermediary branches. For example, the intercostobrachial nerve is primarily derived from T2, which is not part of the brachial plexus and must therefore be blocked separately if anesthesia of the upper medial arm is desired. Therefore, basic knowledge of brachial plexus anatomy is crucial for understanding the advantages and limitations of the various approaches to upper extremity regional anesthesia.

The functional neuroanatomy of the upper extremity is critically important for determining block selection and assessment. Motor function is generally well correlated with an observed motor response after electrical stimulation of a specific terminal nerve; for example, distal stimulation of the radial nerve consistently elicits wrist and finger extension. In contrast, as one moves proximally along the brachial plexus, stimulation yields muscle movements of a mixed nature. As an example of this concept, electrical stimulation of the superior trunk during the interscalene approach results in mixed muscle stimulation that produces shoulder elevation (Table 47–1).

Sensory innervation of the upper extremity is inconsistent and widely overlapping (Fig. 47–2). Certain areas of the arm, such as the distal palmar forearm, have overlapping sensory innervation from the medial and lateral antebrachial cutaneous nerves, plus occasional contributions from the median nerve. A practical implication of this neuroanatomic overlap is that most areas of the upper extremity require anesthesia of two or more terminal nerves, which speaks for the efficacy of plexus-based regional anesthesia rather than selectively approaching multiple nerves at the elbow or wrist. Furthermore, overlapping cutaneous sensory fields and motor function can be problematic for assessing anesthesia, which is best accomplished by testing end functions that can only be attributed to a single nerve. The "four Ps"[12] is an example of such a tool (Table 47–2).

BRACHIAL PLEXUS PHARMACOLOGY

Selection of a local anesthetic for brachial plexus anesthesia is based on expected surgical duration and the optimal duration of postoperative analgesia.

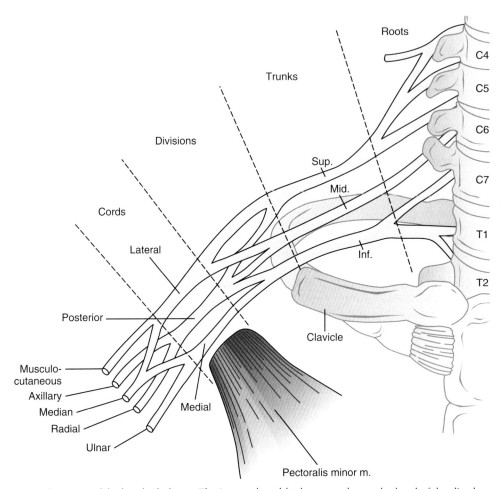

Figure 47–1. Anatomic architecture of the brachial plexus. The interscalene block approaches at the level of the distal roots–proximal trunks, the supraclavicular block approaches at the level of the distal trunks' proximal divisions, the infraclavicular block approaches at the level of the cords, and the axillary block approaches at the level of the terminal nerves. Inf., inferior; Mid., middle; Sup., superior. (Adapted from Rathmell JP, Neal JM, Viscomi CM: Requisites in Anesthesiology: Regional Anesthesia. Philadelphia, Elsevier-Mosby, 2004, p 60.)

Table 47–1. Brachial Plexus Stimulation: Expected Motor Response

APPROACH	STIMULATED PORTION OF THE BRACHIAL PLEXUS	EXPECTED MOTOR RESPONSE
Interscalene	Superior trunk	Shoulder abduction, elbow flexion
Supraclavicular	Middle and inferior trunk	Hand movement
Infraclavicular	Lateral cord	Forearm flexion, hand pronation (little finger moves laterally)
	Posterior cord	Wrist extension (little finger moves posteriorly)
	Medial cord	Finger flexion, thumb opposition (little finger moves medially)
Axillary	Musculocutaneous nerve	Forearm flexion, hand supination
	Median nerve	Forearm pronation, wrist flexion
	Ulnar nerve	Finger flexion, thumb opposition
	Radial nerve	Wrist extension

Adapted from Rathmell JP, Neal JM, Viscomi CM: Regional Anesthesia: The Requisites in Anesthesiology. Philadelphia, Elsevier-Mosby, 2004, Table 6-1.

When considering block duration, anesthesiologists should be cognizant of the expected degree of postoperative pain. For mildly painful procedures, some patients may interpret prolonged arm numbness as bothersome, whereas dense analgesia may mask early signs of impaired circulation in crush injuries or surgeries with the potential for developing compartment syndrome. Thus, local anesthetic selection for upper extremity block is best individualized to achieve specific therapeutic goals.

Potency studies of long-acting local anesthetics administered to the brachial plexus have suggested that bupivacaine, 0.5%, is equipotent to ropivacaine, 0.75%.[13,14] This equivalence is important, because a tendency to use more ropivacaine to attain the same effect as bupivacaine will likely negate the lower

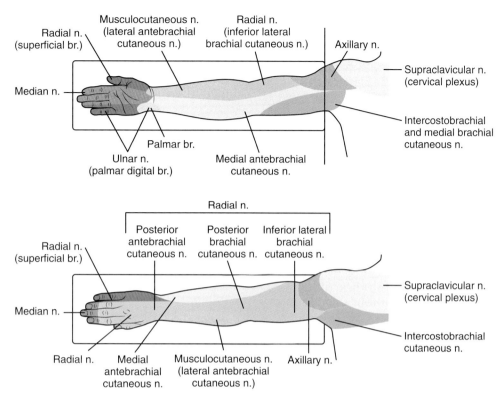

Figure 47–2. Cutaneous innervation of the upper extremity. In practice, cutaneous sensory zones are not distinct, but instead are widely overlapping. br., branch; n., nerve. (Adapted from Rathmell JP, Neal JM, Viscomi CM: Requisites in Anesthesiology: Regional Anesthesia. Philadelphia, Elsevier-Mosby, 2004, p 61.)

Table 47–2. Assessing Upper Extremity Nerve Block: The Four Ps

P	ACTION	NERVE ASSESSED
Push	Extend forearm against resistance.	Radial
Pull	Flex forearm against resistance.	Musculocutaneous
Pinch	Pinch palmar base of index finger.	Median
Pinch	Pinch palmar base of little finger.	Ulnar

cardiotoxicity properties of ropivacaine. When considering the total mass (dose) of a local anesthetic, decisions are best skewed toward using lower volume, concentration, and dose. Although it may appear counterintuitive, the work of Vester-Andersen and colleagues[15-17] and others have clearly demonstrated that block onset, quality, and duration are not improved by using larger volumes or concentrations of local anesthetic. Indeed, doing so risks local anesthetic concentration-dependent neurotoxicity and dose-dependent systemic toxicity. Therefore, local anesthetic volumes for upper extremity plexus block generally should be between 20 and 40 mL, depending on the approach chosen, and concentrations should be lower than 1.5% for lidocaine or mepivacaine, 0.75% or less for ropivacaine, and 0.5% or less for bupivacaine.[18]

Four local anesthetic additives have proven value when applied to the brachial plexus. Epinephrine, 2.5 μg/mL (1:400,000), prolongs duration, acts as a marker of intravascular injection, and decreases systemic uptake of local anesthetic.[18] The ability of epinephrine to prolong local anesthetic block is a consequence of reduced clearance from the injection site[19] and is unlikely to involve a significant α_2-adrenergic agonist effect.[20] Clonidine, 0.5 μg/kg, prolongs anesthesia and analgesia by 50% without systemic side effects such as hypotension or sedation.[21,22] Clonidine does not improve block quality during continuous perineural catheter techniques.[23] Buprenorphine, 0.3 mg, also prolongs anesthesia and analgesia,[24] as does dexamethasone, 2 mg.[25] The effect of these four additives is significant for intermediate-acting local anesthetics, but rarely prolongs the duration of long-acting local anesthetics. Other opioids, neostigmine, calcium channel blockers, and hyaluronidase do not improve local anesthetic block or have unresolved toxicity issues.[18]

Alkalinization of intermediate-acting local anesthetics facilitates faster block onset during epidural anesthesia, but does not have the same effect at the brachial plexus. Onset is not hastened by adding sodium bicarbonate to plain local anesthetic or to local anesthetic freshly mixed with epinephrine.[18] Animal models have shown that alkalinization of local anesthetic reduces block intensity and duration.[26]

TECHNIQUES TO INCREASE BLOCK SUCCESS

Optimal localization of neural structures along the brachial plexus should lead to more successful blockade. No studies have proven the superiority of a paresthesia-seeking technique versus peripheral nerve stimulation versus (for axillary block) a transarterial or perivascular technique. The best reported success rates for any of these techniques are approximately 90% to 95%[27,28]; all are superior to older techniques, such as identifying a fascial click or maximizing needle movement in unison with pulsation of the axillary artery.[18] Rather than by how a nerve is localized, block success is most affected by the number of injections made near the targeted neural structures. Single injection works well for blocks above the clavicle, but multiple injections provide faster onset and more complete anesthesia when using the infraclavicular or axillary approaches. Studies of axillary block have suggested that three or four injections are superior to one or two, although four injections may increase operator time but not always overall success.[18,29-36] The nerve that is stimulated and subsequently injected is also important. Axillary block is maximized when local anesthetic injection is made near the radial nerve (after obtaining extension of the hand and wrist, rather than the triceps[37]), the musculocutaneous nerve, and the median nerve. Placing local anesthetic near the ulnar nerve is not essential during multiple injection techniques.[38]

The use of ultrasonography to localize nerves holds great promise for improved brachial plexus block dynamics. Reports have described ultrasound-guided techniques for several approaches to the brachial plexus[39-41] (Fig. 47–3). Less certain is whether the use of ultrasound improves the technical qualities of upper extremity block, such as faster performance or onset.[42-44] The use of ultrasound appears to hold special promise for patients with abnormal anatomy or extremes of body habitus.[45] No adequately powered studies have proven any safety advantage linked to the use of ultrasound nerve localization. Initial studies have demonstrated that ultrasound has the ability to enhance our understanding of important research topics, such as needle-to-nerve proximity.[46] Such information may ultimately alter current concepts related to nerve localization and local anesthetic dosing.

Other techniques have been proposed to improve brachial plexus block. Exercising the arm after local anesthetic injection,[47] mixing short-acting with long-acting local anesthetics,[48] or adducting the arm after axillary block[49] have been proposed to hasten block onset or improve anesthetic spread, but all have minor, if any, practical effects.[18] Similarly, the application of digital pressure to improve block spread characteristics[50,51] or reduce the incidence of hemidiaphragmatic paresis[50,52] is ineffective (Fig. 47–4).

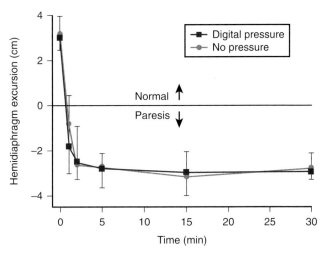

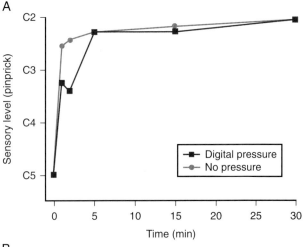

B

Figure 47–4. The use of digital pressure during interscalene block neither reduces the incidence of hemidiaphragmatic paresis **(A)** nor limits cephalad sensory anesthesia spread **(B).** (Redrawn from Rathmell JP, Neal JM, Viscomi CM. Requisites in Anesthesiology: Regional Anesthesia, Elsevier-Mosby, Philadelphia, 2004, p. 72.)

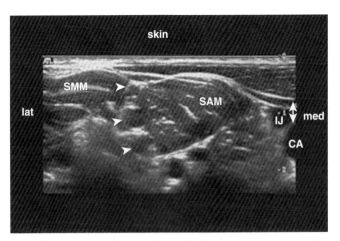

Figure 47–3. Transverse ultrasound of interscalene region. The nerves are hypoechoic *(arrows)*. CA, carotid artery; IJ, internal jugular; SAM, scalenus anticus muscle; SMM, scalenus medius muscle. (Adapted with permission from Chan VWS: Applying ultrasound imaging to interscalene brachial plexus block. Reg Anesth Pain Med 2003;28:341.)

BLOCK TECHNIQUES FOR MAJOR APPROACHES TO THE BRACHIAL PLEXUS

A number of techniques may be used for successful brachial plexus blocks.

Interscalene Block

Indications

The interscalene block approaches the brachial plexus at the level of its distal roots–proximal trunks. Because a block needle typically first encounters the superior trunk, the most consistent effect from this approach involves anesthesia of the shoulder and upper arm (Fig. 47–5). The inferior trunk (C8, T1) is unaffected by local anesthetic in approximately 50% of cases,[53] so the interscalene block is not recommended for surgeries involving ulnar nerve distribution.

Technique

The brachial plexus traverses the interscalene groove, which is bordered by the anterior and middle scalene muscles. The classic technique of Winnie[54] described the patient's head being turned 30 degrees to the contralateral side, and a 50-mm or smaller needle placed into the interscalene groove at the level of the sixth cervical vertebra. The needle is oriented perpendicular to all planes of the skin and then advanced with a slightly caudad angulation, which lessens the risk of entering the intervertebral foramen and encountering spinal nerves or the vertebral artery (Fig. 47–6). The end point for needle advancement is paresthesia or a motor response in the arm or anterior shoulder.[55,56] Movement of the posterior shoulder indicates that the needle is too posterior, whereas a diaphragmatic motor response indicates needle placement that is too anterior. Once paresthesia or motor response at approximately 0.5 mA is obtained, a 1-mL test dose of local anesthetic is injected to rule out intravascular injection, followed by incremental injection of 20 to 30 mL of local anesthetic.

An alternative lateral interscalene approach[57] has reportedly facilitated perineural catheter placement by reducing the angle that a catheter must make as it exits the block needle and enters the perineural area. Because the lateral approach directs the needle away from the vertebral column, this approach theoretically reduces the risk of vertebral artery injection or needle contact with the spinal cord or perispinal neural elements.

Supraclavicular Block

Indications

The supraclavicular approach aims to encounter the brachial plexus at the juncture of the distal trunks or proximal divisions as the plexus dips under the clavicle and across the first rib (Fig. 47–7). This area represents the most compact architecture of the brachial plexus, which has been postulated (but never proven) to explain the propensity of supraclavicular blocks for rapid onset and almost complete anesthesia of the upper extremity. This block is indicated for any surgery of the arm (see Fig. 47–5), although shoulder surgery may require supplementation of the supraclavicular nerve (C3-C4) to ensure anesthesia of the cape area around the shoulder. Supraclavicular block is successful in approximately 95% of patients, even obese patients.[58]

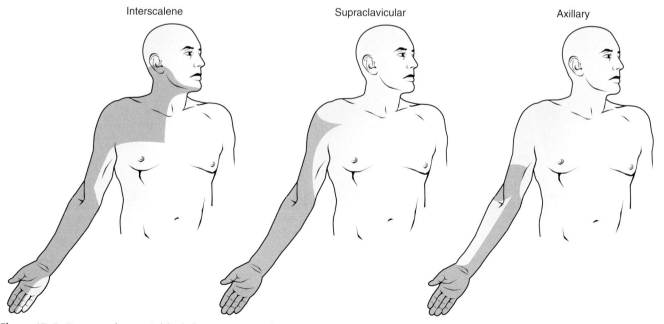

Figure 47–5. Patterns of sensory block from an interscalene, supraclavicular, or axillary approach to the brachial plexus. (Adapted from Rathmell JP, Neal JM, Viscomi CM: Requisites in Anesthesiology: Regional Anesthesia. Philadelphia, Elsevier-Mosby, 2004, p 62.)

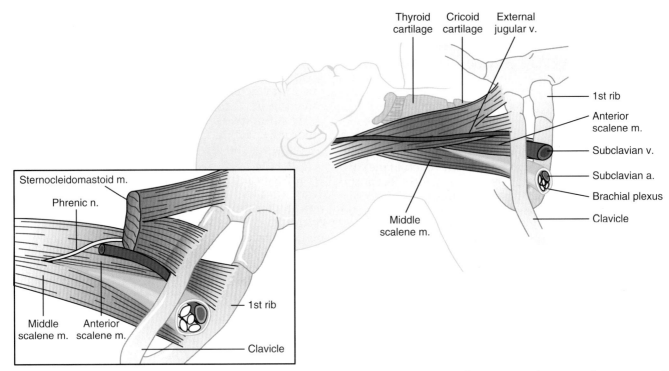

Figure 47–6. Interscalene approach of Winnie. The brachial plexus traverses through the interscalene groove, where a needle can approach it at the C6 level. Note that the phrenic nerve lies on the anterior scalene muscle, which exposes it to unintended stimulation. a., artery; m., muscle; n., nerve; v., vein. (Adapted from Rathmell JP, Neal JM, Viscomi CM: Requisites in Anesthesiology: Regional Anesthesia. Philadelphia, Elsevier-Mosby, 2004, p 63.)

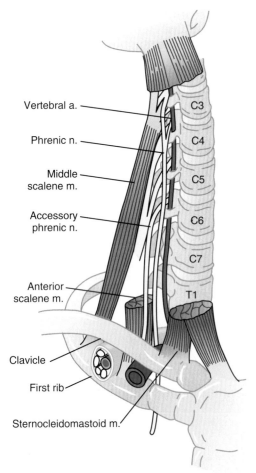

Figure 47–7. The supraclavicular approach takes advantage of the compactness of the brachial plexus as it goes under the clavicle and over the first rib. Note that the plexus resides posteriorly and laterally to the subclavian artery. a., artery; m., muscle; n., nerve. (Adapted from Rathmell JP, Neal JM, Viscomi CM: Requisites in Anesthesiology: Regional Anesthesia. Philadelphia, Elsevier-Mosby, 2004, p 65.)

Technique

A variety of techniques have been described for supraclavicular block.[59-61] The plumb bob technique places the needle just above the clavicle at the lateral border of the sternocleidomastoid muscle. The original description by Brown and associates[59] involved directing the needle straight downward, similar to a brick mason's plumb bob (Fig. 47–8). If a motor response or paresthesia is not elicited, the needle is incrementally fanned 20 degrees cephalad and then 20 degrees caudad in the parasagittal plane until the desired response is attained. A modification of this technique describes making the initial needle pass 45 degrees cephalad, followed by incremental caudad angulation until a suitable paresthesia or motor response is obtained. The logic of this modification is that it reduces the risk of contact with the lung copula in tall individuals.[62] If during the course of supraclavicular block the needle encounters the subclavian artery, it should be redirected posteriorly and laterally to identify the brachial plexus. Injecting 20 to 30 mL of local anesthetic after a single paresthesia or motor response to the arm or shoulder at less than 0.9 mA[63] completes the block procedure.

Infraclavicular Block

Indications

The infraclavicular block, which is indicated for surgery of the arm distal to the shoulder, approaches the brachial plexus at the level of the cords. This block anesthetizes the axillary and musculocutaneous nerves more reliably than the axillary approach.[64,65] Infraclavicular block techniques have the advantage of not requiring a specific arm position during placement, which is useful for patients with limited arm motion because of pain, casts, or dressings.[66] The infraclavicular approach is frequently used for continuous perineural catheter placement because the catheters reliably remain in place during use.

Technique

Similar to the supraclavicular approach, there have been several techniques described for infraclavicular block; none are inherently superior. The coracoid approach[67] begins with identifying the lateral aspect of the coracoid process in a supine patient. From this point, an entry point 2 cm caudad and 2 cm medial is marked (Fig. 47–9). A stimulating needle is directed posteriorly, perpendicular to all planes. Stimulation of the various cords can be ascertained by their resulting motor response—"at the cords, the pinkie towards." Stimulation of the posterior cord causes the little finger to move posteriorly, stimulation of the medial cord results in medial movement, and stimulation of the lateral cord results in lateral movement.[68] The posterior cord occupies the middle position and is the deepest of the three cords. Block success is maximized when two cords are identified and subsequently bathed with local anesthetic[69,70];

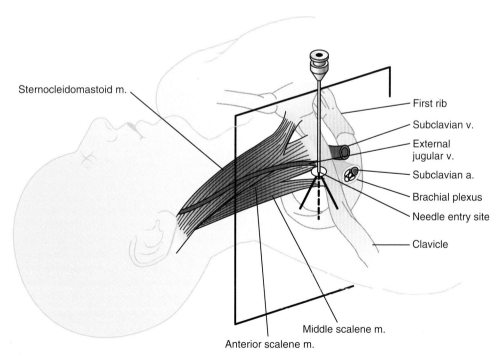

Figure 47–8. The plumb bob supraclavicular approach. The needle is placed above the clavicle, next to the lateral border of the sternocleidomastoid muscle, and directed toward the floor (as a brick mason's plumb bob would be directed). The needle is incrementally fanned 20 degrees cephalad, then 20 degrees caudad while seeking a paresthesia or motor response. In tall slender individuals, initially directing the needle 45 degrees cephalad helps avoid the pleural dome. a., artery; m., muscle; v., vein. (Adapted from Rathmell JP, Neal JM, Viscomi CM: Requisites in Anesthesiology: Regional Anesthesia. Philadelphia, Elsevier-Mosby, 2004, p 66.)

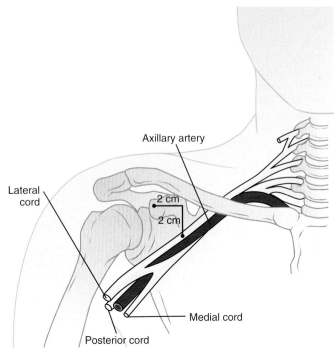

Axillary artery

Lateral cord

2 cm

2 cm

Medial cord

Posterior cord

Figure 47–9. The infraclavicular approach. The entry point is marked after identifying the lateral edge of the coracoid process and then moving 2 cm medial and 2 cm caudad. A needle is then directed posteriorly toward the three cords of the brachial plexus and the axillary artery, which is approximately 4 ± 1.5 cm from the skin. (Adapted from Rathmell JP, Neal JM, Viscomi CM: Requisites in Anesthesiology: Regional Anesthesia. Philadelphia, Elsevier-Mosby, 2004, p 67.)

injection around the posterior cord is the most important.[71] A total of 30 to 40 mL of local anesthetic is sufficient for infraclavicular block.

Axillary Block

Indications

The axillary block anesthetizes the brachial plexus at the level of the four terminal nerves, the radial, ulnar, median, and musculocutaneous. It is indicated for surgeries distal to and including the elbow[72] (see Fig. 47–5). With the exception of very proximal approaches high in the axilla, the axillary block is not as ideally suited for continuous catheter techniques as the infraclavicular approach and approaches above the clavicle.

Techniques

In the axilla, the terminal nerves closely surround the axillary artery, which is the main surface landmark for accomplishing this block. Classic descriptions of axillary architecture place the radial nerve nearly posterior to and slightly inferior to the artery; the ulnar nerve more superficial, but also inferior to

the artery; the median nerve superficial and superior to the artery; and the musculocutaneous nerve superior to the artery and residing deeper within the belly of the coracobrachialis muscle (Fig. 47–10). However, anatomic variation is frequent, especially with regard to nerve position relative to the axillary artery. These inherent variations may partially explain why the various techniques for axillary block have similar success rates.

The transarterial technique generally achieves higher success rates with two 10- to 20-mL local anesthetic injections anterior and posterior to the axillary artery.[73] Success rates are similar with paresthesia versus peripheral nerve stimulation techniques.[18,28] Either technique's success is enhanced by identifying and subsequently injecting local anesthetic nearby three or four terminal nerves rather than using a single injection. Four injections may increase performance time without appreciably affecting success rates.[18,34,35] Expected motor responses for each nerve are listed in Table 47–1. Further technical refinement suggests that success is most dependent on identifying and subsequently injecting local anesthetic near the radial and median nerves, and least dependent on injection around the ulnar nerve.[35,36] Clinical trials have suggested that axillary block should require less than 40 mL of local anesthetic.[17] Because the musculocutaneous nerve diverges from the plexus at the level of the axilla, it can remain unanesthetized during transarterial or single-injection techniques. If not localized by ultrasound or nerve stimulation, the musculocutaneous nerve is easily blocked by infiltrating 5 mL of local anesthetic into the belly of the coracobrachialis muscle. The perivascular infiltration technique[74] uses a continuously moving needle to fan 10 to 15 mL of local anesthetic next to the superior border of the axillary artery in three progressively outward needle passes, with the process being repeated along the inferior aspect of the artery. Because of this outward fanning technique, the musculocutaneous nerve is usually anesthetized.

Accessory Blocks

Indications

Nerves that arise separately from the brachial plexus or are inconsistently anesthetized by a brachial plexus block innervate select upper extremity sensory fields. The supraclavicular nerve block (C3-4) is a useful adjunct to supraclavicular brachial plexus block when surgery is performed around the cape of the shoulder. The suprascapular nerve (C5-6) branches from the superior trunk of the brachial plexus to supply the posterior two thirds of the shoulder joint and the acromioclavicular joint. Blocking it prolongs analgesia after shoulder arthroscopy performed under general anesthesia,[4] but adds no value to interscalene block for open anterior shoulder surgery.[75] Suprascapular block with local anesthetic and steroid also

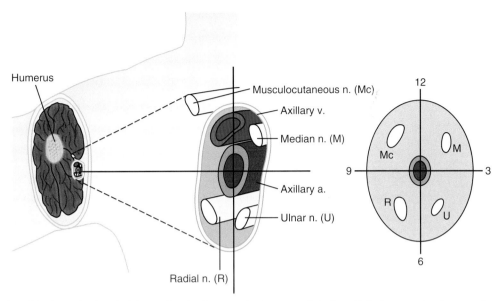

Figure 47–10. Axillary block. At the level of the axilla, the four terminal nerves of the brachial plexus maintain a quadrant-like relationship to the axillary artery. Although there is substantial variation among patients, the radial and ulnar nerve are typically inferior (6-o'clock position) to the artery, with the radial artery being deeper. The median nerve is typically superficial and superior (12-o'clock position) to the artery. The musculocutaneous nerve most often lies within the belly of the coracobrachialis muscle, and thus requires a separate anesthetizing procedure. a., artery; n., nerve; v., vein. (Adapted from Rathmell JP, Neal JM, Viscomi CM: Requisites in Anesthesiology: Regional Anesthesia. Philadelphia, Elsevier-Mosby, 2004, p 67.)

provides prolonged pain relief for chronic degenerative shoulder conditions.[76] The intercostobrachial nerve (T2) is separate from the brachial plexus and provides sensory innervation to the upper medial arm and anterior axilla. Supplemental anesthesia of this nerve is indicated for blocking upper extremity tourniquet sensation or for anterior arthroscopic port placement in patients anesthetized only with an interscalene block. The medial antebrachial cutaneous nerve is an intermediary branch from the medial cord; the lateral antebrachial cutaneous nerve is the cutaneous terminus of the musculocutaneous nerve. Both can be blocked for primary or incomplete anesthesia of the forearm.[77]

Techniques

Suprascapular nerve block is accomplished by depositing local anesthetic near the suprascapular notch. Drawing a line along the scapular spine and bisecting it with a second line drawn parallel to the vertebral spine outlines the surface landmarks. The resultant upper outer quadrant is then bisected with a third line, with a point noted about 2 to 3 cm from the intersection of the first two lines (Fig. 47–11). A needle oriented parallel to the patient's back is placed at this point and directed toward the scapular spine. Once contact is made, the needle is gently directed anterior to barely enter the suprascapular notch; 10 mL of local anesthetic is subsequently injected.

The supraclavicular nerve is anesthetized by injecting a subcutaneous wheal of local anesthetic along the posterior border of the sternocleidomastoid muscle from the clavicle to the mastoid (Fig. 47–12). The intercostobrachial nerve is anesthetized by injecting a subcutaneous wheal of local anesthetic along the axillary crease. The medial antebrachial cutaneous nerve is anesthetized by injecting subcutaneous local anesthetic in a semicircular manner around the medial arm, about one fourth the distance from the elbow to the axilla. The lateral antebrachial cutaneous nerve is anesthetized by injecting local anesthetic just deep to the lateral border of the biceps tendon, followed by injecting a subcutaneous wheal toward the lateral epicondyle[77] (Fig. 47–13). None of these blocks requires more than 5 mL of local anesthetic.

Selective Nerve Blocks at the Elbow and Wrist

Indications

There are few indications for selective nerve blocks of the upper extremity, because innervation of the forearm and hand manifests extensive crossover of cutaneous sensory distribution; therefore, single nerve blockade is rarely adequate. Selective blocks at the elbow or wrist are also problematic if prolonged pneumatic tourniquet use is required. The best indication for selective block is using a median nerve block at the wrist for carpal tunnel release.[78]

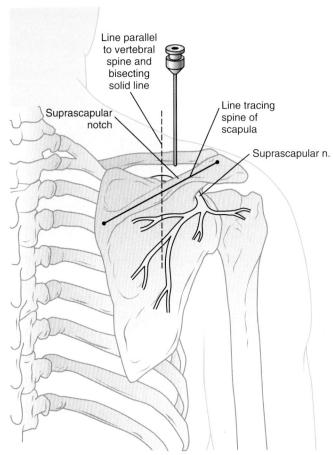

Figure 47–11. Suprascapular nerve block. A line is drawn along the scapular spine and then bisected by a second line parallel to the vertebral spine. The entry point is 2 to 3 cm into the upper outer quadrant. The needle is directed from the top to avoid deep entry into the suprascapular notch, which could risk pneumothorax. n., nerve. (Adapted from Rathmell JP, Neal JM, Viscomi CM: Requisites in Anesthesiology: Regional Anesthesia. Philadelphia, Elsevier-Mosby, 2004, p 69.)

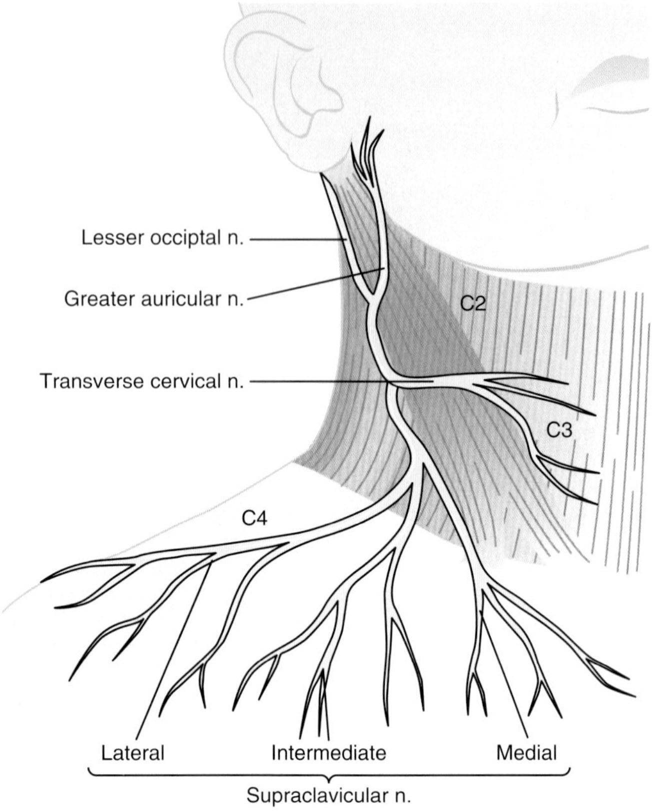

Figure 47–12. Supraclavicular nerve block. This block anesthetizes the cutaneous cape around the shoulder. Simple subcutaneous infiltration of local anesthetic along the posterior border of the sternocleidomastoid muscle accomplishes this block. A 1-mL injection of local anesthetic into the midbelly of the sternocleidomastoid muscle will anesthetize the supraclavicular nerve fibers as they make their way to the surface. n., nerve. (Modified from Brown DL: Atlas of Regional Anesthesia, 3rd ed. Philadelphia, WB Saunders, 2006, p 191.)

Techniques

At the elbow, the radial and median nerves are blocked at the level of the humeral epicondyles. The radial nerve is deep; the median and ulnar nerves are relatively superficial (Fig. 47–14). A needle inserted just lateral to the biceps tendon is used to access the radial nerve. A motor response (see Table 47–1) can be elicited or the block can be accomplished by fanning local anesthetic in proximity of the nerve without seeking a paresthesia (Fig. 47–15). A needle placed just medial to the brachial artery is used to access the median nerve, which is identified by seeking an appropriate motor response (see Table 47–1) or anesthetized by simply infiltrating local anesthetic (see Fig. 47–15). Five mL of local anesthetic is adequate for either block. Blocking the ulnar nerve at the olecranon fossa is not recommended because, at this level, its sensory fibers only innervate the hand. Therefore, blocking the ulnar nerve at the

wrist avoids concern of pressure injury secondary to injecting local anesthetic under the tight olecranon retinaculum. Cutaneous anesthesia of the ulnar forearm is best accomplished with a medial antebrachial cutaneous nerve block.

At the wrist, the radial nerve requires two injections for complete anesthesia. The first injection is placed radially and next to the radial artery 2 cm proximal to the radius styloid process; a second superficial injection is then directed across the top of the wrist to anesthetize the superficial radial nerve (Fig. 47–16). The median nerve is approached at the wrist flexor crease with a needle directed between the palmaris longus and flexor carpi radialis tendons, deep to the carpal retinaculum. A paresthesia, motor response, or simple infiltration technique provides adequate localization. The ulnar nerve is anesthetized at the level of the ulnar styloid process by a deep injection between the flexor carpi ulnaris tendon and the ulnar artery, after which a superficial injection is directed around the ulnar wrist (Fig. 47–17).

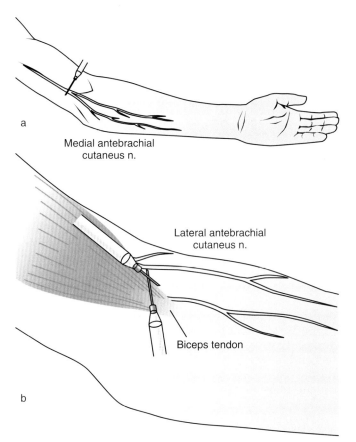

a

Medial antebrachial
cutaneus n.

Lateral antebrachial
cutaneus n.

Biceps tendon

b

Figure 47–13. The medial antebrachial cutaneous nerve is blocked by a simple subcutaneous injection of local anesthetic **(a)** in a semicircle approximately one fourth the distance from the elbow to the axilla, in the medial upper arm. Injecting 1 to 2 mL of local anesthetic just lateral to the biceps tendon **(b)**, and then extending a subcutaneous wheal toward the lateral epicondyle, anesthetizes the lateral antebrachial cutaneous nerve. n., nerve. (Adapted with permission from Viscomi CM, Reese J, Rathmell JP: Medial and lateral antebrachial cutaneous nerve blocks: An easily learned regional anesthetic for forearm arteriovenous fistula surgery. Reg Anesth 1996;21:2-5.)

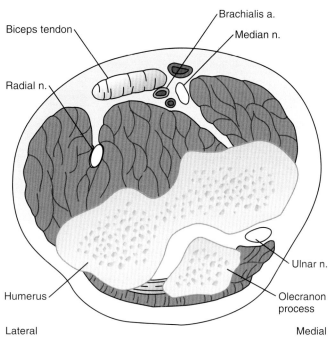

Biceps tendon

Brachialis a.

Median n.

Radial n.

Ulnar n.

Humerus

Olecranon process

Lateral

Medial

Figure 47–14. Cross section of the arm at the elbow. Note that the radial nerve is relatively deep, the median nerve is relatively superficial and just medial to the brachial artery, and the ulnar nerve is in the olecranon fossa. a., artery; n., nerve. (Adapted from Rathmell JP, Neal JM, Viscomi CM: Requisites in Anesthesiology: Regional Anesthesia. Philadelphia, Elsevier-Mosby, 2004, p 69.)

Continuous Perineural Catheters

Indications

Prolonged analgesia of the upper extremity can be accomplished using continuous perineural catheter techniques. Surgeries expected to cause prolonged moderate to severe pain are appropriate for catheter placement. These include total shoulder arthroplasty, rotator cuff repair, and major reconstructive operations of the elbow, wrist, or hand. Accumulated evidence has suggested that perineural catheters can be efficiently managed in the ambulatory setting with a high degree of patient acceptance.[7,8,10,79-81] Key to successful management is establishing clear lines of contact between the physician and patient.[10,80] Preliminary reports have suggested that even major surgeries such as total shoulder arthroplasty can be managed on an outpatient basis when perineural

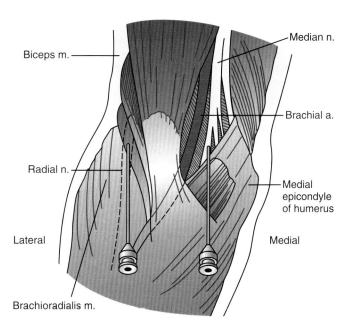

Biceps m.

Median n.

Brachial a.

Radial n.

Medial epicondyle of humerus

Lateral

Medial

Brachioradialis m.

Figure 47–15. Approaches to the radial and median nerves at the elbow. A needle placed laterally to the biceps tendon accesses the radial nerve. A needle placed medially to the brachial artery accesses the median nerve. a., artery; m., muscle; n., nerve. (Adapted from Rathmell JP, Neal JM, Viscomi CM: Requisites in Anesthesiology: Regional Anesthesia. Philadelphia, Elsevier-Mosby, 2004, p 70.)

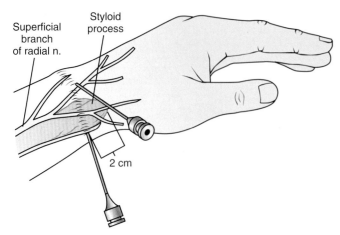

Figure 47–16. Radial nerve block at the wrist. Approximately 2 cm proximal to the radius styloid process, a first injection is placed just lateral to the radial artery, followed by a superficial injection laterally across the top of the wrist. n., nerve. (Adapted from Rathmell JP, Neal JM, Viscomi CM: Requisites in Anesthesiology: Regional Anesthesia. Philadelphia, Elsevier-Mosby, 2004, p 70.)

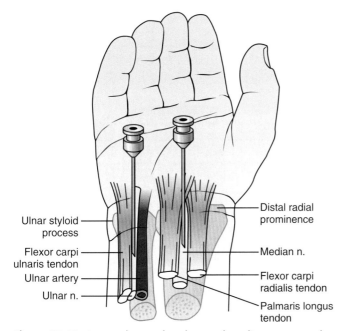

Figure 47–17. Approaches to the ulnar and median nerves at the wrist. The ulnar nerve is accessed by a needle placed between the flexor carpi ulnaris tendon and the ulnar artery, at the level of the ulnar styloid process. A second superficial injection is directed around the medial wrist. A needle placed at the wrist flexor crease and directed between the flexor carpi radialis and palmaris longus tendons accesses the median nerve. n., nerve. (Adapted from Rathmell JP, Neal JM, Viscomi CM: Requisites in Anesthesiology: Regional Anesthesia. Philadelphia, Elsevier-Mosby, 2004, p 70.)

catheters are used to control pain and facilitate rehabilitation.[11]

Techniques

The ideal technique for placement of upper extremity perineural catheters has not been identified.[9] Some authors prefer the use of stimulating catheters, particularly for the posterior paravertebral approach,[82] whereas others prefer nonstimulating catheters.[79] More direct approaches that do not require the catheter to make an acute angle after exiting the needle are touted (without benefit of comparative studies) to facilitate catheter threading. Various experts have therefore recommended the posterior paravertebral,[82] lateral interscalene,[57] supraclavicular,[43] and intersternocleidomastoid approaches.[83] Despite requiring the catheter to bend at nearly a right angle on exiting the needle, the infraclavicular approach is also popular for arm surgeries, in part because it is easier to fix the catheter in position. Limited data have suggested that patient-controlled perineural analgesia techniques are superior to continuous infusion techniques, but these recommendations vary depending on the relative painfulness of the surgery.[7,81]

COMPLICATIONS OF UPPER EXTREMITY BLOCK

Nerve Injury

Permanent nerve injury after upper extremity block is extremely rare, probably occurring in 0 to 16/10,000 patients (95% confidence interval [CI]).[84] Nerve dysfunction, particularly persistent paresthesia or numbness, is relatively common (up to 19%) immediately after surgery, but the vast majority of these symptoms resolve within 4 weeks.[18,85] Warning signs that an injury may be particularly worrisome include complete absence of nerve function immediately after surgery, probably indicating nerve transection or ischemia, motor deficit, worsening symptoms over time, or failure to show early signs of resolution. Particularly in these cases, early neurologic consultation is recommended to rule out reversible causes, establish bilateral baseline function, and coordinate further diagnostic workup and rehabilitation.[86]

Whether brachial plexus blocks should be attempted in anesthetized or heavily sedated patients is controversial. Especially in the case of interscalene block, a series of case reports[87,88] have clearly pointed to the risk of intramedullary injection with devastating consequences. As the approach moves away from the neck, the risk of spinal cord injury probably lessens, but the risk of unrecognized intraneural (specifically, intrafascicular) injection remains poorly quantified. Some peripheral nerve injuries have occurred in non-anesthetized patients without a preceding warning such as pain on injection or severe paresthesia, whereas other patients have noted these warnings and still sustained injury. Yet another subset of patients has experienced pain on injection but no subsequent injury.[84,89-91] Until our understanding of peripheral nerve injury and premonitory symptoms becomes clearer, it is my recommendation to give the patient every chance of recognizing potential injury by not placing brachial plexus blocks in anesthetized patients. Furthermore, it is important for clinicians to recognize that using a peripheral nerve stimulator does not protect against injury.[87,92,93] There is also circumstantial evidence[73,94] that performing selective nerve block at the elbow or wrist in patients with an incomplete proximal brachial plexus block places the patient at higher risk for perioperative nerve injury.[18]

Whether brachial plexus block is contraindicated in patients with preexisting nerve injury is unclear. Patients who have undergone ulnar nerve transposition are no more likely to sustain a postoperative exacerbation or new symptoms, regardless of whether they received general anesthesia or a brachial plexus block.[95] In contrast to this reassuring data, patients with preexisting nerve dysfunction, even of a subclinical nature, have developed postoperative dysfunction.[96]

Intravascular Injection

Brachial plexus blocks are relatively low risk for delayed systemic local anesthetic toxicity compared with epidural or intercostal block, but there are no reliable data on which to base maximum recommended doses of local anesthetic.[97] The risk of seizure secondary to intravascular injection is five times higher with peripheral nerve blocks than with epidural block.[84] This risk is particularly relevant to brachial plexus regional anesthesia because of the proximity of the vertebral, carotid, and subclavian (via retrograde flow) arteries to direct injection during the placement of interscalene or supraclavicular block.[98]

Unintended Destinations of Local Anesthetics

Because the neck contains so many vital structures, it is common for local anesthetics intended for the brachial plexus to affect other structures. Most serious is when local anesthetic is unintentionally placed near the neuraxis, causing epidural or spinal anesthesia during attempted interscalene anesthesia. The C6 foramen is only 23 mm from the skin in the average patient,[99] so it is easy to conceive how excessively deep needle placement could result in this complication. Neuraxial injection of local anesthetic is manifested by rapid (total spinal anesthesia) or delayed (massive epidural anesthesia) appearance of bilateral upper and lower extremity block that is often associated with hypotension, bradycardia, and apnea. This complication must be diagnosed and treated rapidly with airway control, volume expansion, and early provision of exogenous epinephrine to counteract blockade of the cardioaccelerator fibers and absent vascular tone.[18]

Local anesthetics intended for the brachial plexus during blocks above the clavicle and infraclavicular blocks can also spread to the cervical sympathetic chain, where they cause Horner's syndrome. Another unintended effect is anesthesia of the recurrent laryngeal nerve, which results in hoarseness or difficulty swallowing. Both these nuisance side effects resolve in unison with anesthetic block resolution.[18]

Hemidiaphragmatic Paresis

Impairment of diaphragmatic function is common during above the clavicle approaches. Hemidiaphragmatic paresis occurs in all patients who undergo interscalene block, and some of these patients will develop a 25% to 32% reduction in spirometric measures of pulmonary function.[100-102] The incidence of hemidiaphragmatic paresis is lower (14% to 86%, 95% CI) in patients undergoing supraclavicular block. Although healthy volunteers experienced no diminution of pulmonary function during the supraclavicular approach, this may not hold true for patients with underlying pulmonary disease.[75] It is therefore recommended that any patient unable to withstand a 25% or more reduction in pulmonary function not be given brachial plexus block above the clavicle. The incidence of hemidiaphragmatic paresis is lower with infraclavicular approaches, and may be approach-specific. For example, 26% of patients given a vertical infraclavicular block developed reduced or paradoxical hemidiaphragmatic function that was accompanied by an approximately 30% diminution of spirometric values.[103] Conversely, no ventilatory dysfunction was observed with the more distal coracoid approach.[104] Hemidiaphragmatic paresis during continuous perineural infusion appears to lessen over time. In a study of patient-controlled perineural interscalene catheter analgesia with ropivacaine 0.2%, diaphragmatic function and spirometric values were no different than those observed in patients randomized to receive opioid patient-controlled analgesia.[105]

Pneumothorax

The incidence of pneumothorax associated with supraclavicular block has likely decreased with the advent of procedures such as the plumb bob technique, which were in part designed to avoid needle contact with the pleural dome. Nevertheless, there remains a small (less than 1%) but poorly defined risk of pneumothorax with the supraclavicular and intersternocleidomastoid approaches. Even though extremely rare, pneumothorax has been reported with the interscalene and coracoid infraclavicular approaches. Clinicians should recognize that symptoms of pneumothorax are typically delayed 6 to 12 hours after initial needle puncture, and are more likely to consist of pleuritic chest pain rather than dyspnea.[18]

SUMMARY

Upper extremity regional anesthesia is a valuable part of the anesthesiologist's armamentarium, particularly for providing superior analgesia and improved early outcome measures after ambulatory surgery. This chapter has described common techniques for accomplishing neural blockade at various approaches along the brachial plexus. It has also reviewed basic anatomy and pharmacology of the brachial plexus, plus the more common and/or serious complications of these useful blocks.

- Upper extremity regional anesthetic techniques can improve analgesia in the immediate postoperative period, reduce opioid-related side effects, improve patient satisfaction, and reduce unplanned hospital admissions. Brachial plexus blockade does not affect outcome measures beyond the first 24 hours.
- The functional anatomy of the upper extremity is variable. Relying on a single cutaneous distribution to plan which nerve requires blockade or to assess adequacy of anesthesia is unreliable.
- The primary determinant in local anesthetic selection for upper extremity block is anesthetic or analgesic duration. Epinephrine, clonidine, dexamethasone, or buprenorphine extend the duration of intermediate-acting local anesthetics, but not long-acting ones.
- As one proceeds distally along the brachial plexus, multiple-injection techniques improve block success. There is no evidence that any regional anesthetic technique—paresthesia, peripheral nerve stimulation, perivascular, ultrasound, or transarterial—is inherently more effective or safer than another.
- Shoulder surgery is best accomplished with interscalene block, arm or hand surgery is amenable to infraclavicular block, and arm surgery, including and distal to the elbow, is a classic indication for axillary block. The supraclavicular block is most likely to anesthetize the entire upper extremity, although it will occasionally not anesthetize the ulnar nerve.
- Accessory blocks are valuable for surgeries that involve a cutaneous sensory distribution outside the brachial plexus. A suprascapular block adds value to general anesthesia for shoulder arthroscopy, a supraclavicular nerve block anesthetizes the cape distribution around the shoulder, the intercostobrachial block anesthetizes the upper medial arm, and medial and lateral antebrachial cutaneous blocks are excellent supplements for primary or incomplete anesthesia of the forearm.
- The practice of supplementing incomplete brachial plexus blocks by anesthetizing terminal nerves at the elbow or wrist has been associated with perioperative nerve injury.
- Continuous perineural catheter techniques provide superior analgesia compared with placebo or opioid techniques. Data are as yet insufficient to show meaningful improvement in other outcomes, such as rehabilitation or earlier return to work.
- Permanent anesthesia-related nerve injury after brachial plexus block is distinctly rare. Particularly when using the interscalene approach, it is recommended to avoid placing these blocks in sleeping or heavily sedated patients.
- Local anesthetic systemic toxicity in conjunction with brachial plexus regional anesthesia is relatively common, at least in part because of unintentional injection into arteries that directly supply the brain.
- Anesthesiologists must be vigilant for the rare complication of neuraxial anesthesia during the course of interscalene brachial plexus block. Signs and symptoms of high spinal or massive epidural anesthesia require prompt airway control and aggressive treatment of hypotension and bradycardia with potent α-adrenergic agonists, such as epinephrine.
- Blocks above the clavicle are not recommended for patients who are unable to withstand a 25% to 30% reduction in pulmonary function.

References

1. Hadzic A, Karaca PE, Hobeika P, et al: Peripheral nerve blocks result in superior recovery profile compared with general anesthesia in outpatient knee arthroscopy. Anesth Analg 2005;100:976-981.
2. Hadzic A, Williams BA, Karaca PE, et al: For outpatient rotator cuff surgery, nerve block anesthesia provides superior same-day recovery after general anesthesia. Anesthesiology 2005;102:1001-1007.
3. McCartney CJ, Brull R, Chan VW, et al: Early but no long-term benefit of regional compared with general anesthesia for ambulatory hand surgery. Anesthesiology 2004;101:461-467.
4. Ritchie E, Tong D, Chung F, et al: Suprascapular nerve block for postoperative pain relief in arthroscopic shoulder surgery: A new modality? Anesth Analg 1997;84:1306-1312.
5. Singelyn FJ, Lhotel L, Fabre B: Pain relief after arthroscopic shoulder surgery: A comparison of intraarticular analgesia, suprascapular nerve block, and interscalene brachial plexus block. Anesth Analg 2004;99:589-592.
6. Delaunay L, Souron V, Lafosse L, et al: Analgesia after arthroscopic rotator cuff repair: Subacromial versus interscalene continuous infusion of ropivacaine. Reg Anesth Pain Med 2005;30:117-122.
7. Ilfeld BM, Enneking FK: Continuous peripheral nerve blocks at home: A review. Anesth Analg 2005;100:1822-1833.
8. Klein SM, Greengrass RA, Gleason DH, et al: Major ambulatory surgery with continuous regional anesthesia and a disposable infusion pump. Anesthesiology 1999;91:563-565.
9. Boezaart AP: Perineural infusion of local anesthetics. Anesthesiology 2006;104:872-880.
10. Ilfeld BM, Esener DE, Morey TE, et al: Ambulatory perineural infusion: The patients' perspective. Reg Anesth Pain Med 2003;28:418-423.
11. Ilfeld BM, Wright TW, Enneking FK, et al: Joint range of motion after total shoulder arthroplasty with and without a continuous interscalene nerve block: A retrospective, case-control study. Reg Anesth Pain Med 2005;30:429-433.
12. Thompson GE, Brown DL: The common nerve blocks. In Nunn JF, Utting JE, Brown BR (eds): General Anaesthesia, 5th ed. London, Butterworths, 1989, pp 1068-1069.
13. Raeder JC, Drosdahl S, Klaastad O, et al: Axillary brachial plexus block with ropivacaine 7.5 mg/mL. A comparative study with bupivacaine 5 mg/mL. Acta Anaesthesiol Scand 1999;43:794-798.
14. Vaghadia H, Chan V, Ganapathy S, et al: A multicentre trial of ropivacaine 7.5 mg × ml^{-1} vs bupivacaine 5 mg × ml^{-1} for supraclavicular brachial plexus anaesthesia. Can J Anaesth 1999;46:946-951.
15. Vester-Andersen T, Christiansen C, Sorensen M, et al: Perivascular axillary block II: Influence of injected volume of local anesthetic on neural blockade. Acta Anaesthesiol Scand 1983;27:95-98.
16. Vester-Andersen T, Eriksen C, Christiansen C: Perivascular axillary block III: Blockade following 40 ml of 0.5%, 1% or 1.5% mepivacaine with adrenaline. Acta Anaesthesiol Scand 1984;28:95-98.

17. Vester-Andersen T, Husum B, Lindeburg T, et al: Perivascular axillary block IV: Blockade following 40, 50 or 60 ml of mepivacaine 1% with adrenaline. Acta Anaesthesiol Scand 1984;28:99-105.

18. Neal JM, Hebl JR, Gerancher JC, et al: Brachial plexus anesthesia: Essentials of our current understanding. Reg Anesth Pain Med 2002;27:402-428.

19. Bernards CM, Kopacz DJ: Effect of epinephrine on lidocaine clearance *in vivo*: A microdialysis study in humans. Anesthesiology 1999;91:962-968.

20. Sinnott CJ, Cogswell III LP, Johnson A, et al: On the mechanism by which epinephrine potentiates lidocaine's peripheral nerve block. Anesthesiology 2003;98:181-188.

21. Singelyn FJ, Dangoisse M, Bartholomee S, et al: Adding clonidine to mepivacaine prolongs the duration of anesthesia and analgesia after axillary brachial plexus block. Reg Anesth 1992;17:148-150.

22. Singelyn FJ, Gouverneur J-M, Robert A: A minimum dose of clonidine added to mepivacaine prolongs the duration of anesthesia and analgesia after axillary brachial plexus block. Anesth Analg 1996;83:1046-1050.

23. Ilfeld BM, Morey TE, Wang RD, et al: Continuous popliteal sciatic nerve block for postoperative pain control at home. Anesthesiology 2002;97:959-965.

24. Candido KD, Winnie AP, Ghaleb AH, et al: Buprenorphine added to the local anesthetic for axillary brachial plexus block prolongs postoperative analgesia. Reg Anesth Pain Med 2002;27:162-167.

25. Movafegh A, Razazian M, Hajimaohamadi F, et al: Dexamethasone added to lidocaine prolongs axillary brachial plexus blockade. Anesth Analg 2006;102:263-267.

26. Sinnott CJ, Garfield JM, Thalhammer JG, et al: Addition of sodium bicarbonate to lidocaine decreases the duration of peripheral nerve block in the rat. Anesthesiology 2000;93:1045-1052.

27. Foss NB, Kristensen BB, Jensen PS, et al: Effect of postoperative epidural analgesia and pain after hip fracture surgery: A randomized, double-blind, placebo-controlled trial. Anesthesiology 2005;102:1197-1204.

28. Goldberg ME, Gregg C, Larijani GE, et al: A comparision of three methods of axillary approach to brachial plexus blockade for upper extremity surgery. Anesthesiology 1987;66:814-816.

29. Baranowski AP, Pither CE: A comparison of three methods of axillary brachial plexus anaesthesia. Anaesthesia 1990;45:362-365.

30. Lavoie J, Martin R, Tetrault JP, et al: Axillary plexus block using a peripheral nerve stimulator: Single or multiple injections. Can J Anaesth 1992;39:583-586.

31. Koscielniak-Nielsen ZJ, Stens-Pedersen HL, Lippert FK: Readiness for surgery after axillary block: Single or multiple injection techniques. Eur J Anaesthesiol 1997;14:164-171.

32. Sia S, Bartoli M, Lepri A, et al: Multiple-injection axillary brachial plexus block: A comparison of two methods of nerve localization–nerve stimulation versus paresthesia. Anesth Analg 2000;91:647-651.

33. Sia S, Lepri A, Ponzecchi P: Axillary brachial plexus block using peripheral nerve stimulator: A comparison between double- and triple-injection techniques. Reg Anesth Pain Med 2001;26:499-503.

34. Handoll HHG, Koscielniak-Nielsen ZJ: Single, double or multiple injection techniques for axillary brachial plexus block for hand, wrist or forearm surgery. Cochrane Database Syst Rev 2006;(1):CD003842.

35. Koscielniak-Nielsen ZJ: Multiple injections in axillary block. Where and how many? [editorial]. Reg Anesth Pain Med 2006;31:192-195.

36. Rodriguez J, Taboada M, Valino C, et al: A comparison of stimulation patterns in axillary block: Part 2. Reg Anesth Pain Med 2006;31:202-205.

37. Sia S, Lepri A, Magherini M, et al: A comparison of proximal and distal radial nerve motor responses in axillary block using triple stimulation. Reg Anesth Pain Med 2005;30:458-463.

38. Sia S, Bartoli M: Selective ulnar nerve localization is not essential for axillary brachial plexus block using a multiple nerve stimulation technique. Reg Anesth Pain Med 2001;26:12-16.

39. Kapral S, Krafft P, Eibenberger K, et al: Ultrasound-guided supraclavicular approach for regional anesthesia of the brachial plexus. Anesth Analg 1994;78:507-513.

40. Perlas A, Chan VWS, Simons M: Brachial plexus examination and localization using ultrasound and electrical stimulation. Anesthesiology 2005;99:429-435.

41. Arcand G, Williams SR, Chouinard P, et al: Ultrasound-guided infraclavicular versus supraclavicular block. Anesth Analg 2005;101:886-890.

42. Gray AT: Ultrasound-guided regional anesthesia: Current state of the art. Anesthesiology 2006;104:368-373.

43. Williams SR, Chouinard P, Arcand G, et al: Ultrasound guidance speeds execution and improves the quality of supraclavicular block. Anesth Analg 2003;97:1518-1523.

44. Sandu NS, Capan LM: Ultrasound-guided infraclavicular brachial plexus block. Br J Anaesth 2002;89:254-259.

45. De Andres J, Sala-Blanch X: Ultrasound in the practice of brachial plexus anesthesia. Reg Anesth Pain Med 2002;27:77-89.

46. Perlas A, Niazi A, Mccartney C, et al: The sensitivity of motor response to nerve stimulation and paresthesia for nerve localization as evaluated by ultrasound. Reg Anesth Pain Med 2007; 32:41-45.

47. Okasha AS, El Attar AM, Soliman HL: Enhanced brachial plexus blockade: Effect of pain and muscular exercise on the efficiency of brachial plexus blockade. Anaesthesia 1988;43:327-329.

48. Covino BG, Wildsmith JAW: Clinical pharmacology of local anesthetic agents. In Cousins MJ, Bridenbaugh PO (eds): Neural Blockade in Clinical Anesthesia and Management of Pain, 3rd ed. Philadelphia, Lippincott-Raven, 1998, pp 97-128.

49. Yamamoto K, Tsubokawa T, Ohmura S, et al: The effects of arm position on central spread of local anesthetics and on quality of the block with axillary brachial plexus block. Reg Anesth Pain Med 1999;24:36-42.

50. Urmey WF, Grossi P, Sharrock NE, et al: Digital pressure during interscalene block is clinically ineffective in preventing anesthetic spread to the cervical plexus. Anesth Analg 1996;83:366-370.

51. Vester-Andersen T, Christiansen C, Sorensen M, et al: Perivascular axillary block I: Blockade following 40 mL 1% mepivacaine with adrenaline. Acta Anaesthesiol Scand 1982;26:519-523.

52. Sala-Blanch X, Lazaro JR, Correa J, et al: Phrenic nerve block caused by interscalene brachial plexus block: Effects of digital pressure and a low volume of local anesthetic. Reg Anesth Pain Med 1999;24:231-235.

53. Lanz E, Theiss D, Jankovic D: The extent of blockade following various techniques of brachial plexus block. Anesth Analg 1983;62:55-58.

54. Winnie AP: Interscalene brachial plexus block. Anesth Analg 1970;49:455-466.

55. Roch JJ, Sharrock NE, Neudachin L: Interscalene brachial plexus block for shoulder surgery: A proximal paresthesia is effective. Anesth Analg 1992;75:386-388.

56. Silverstein WB, Saiyed MU, Brown AR: Interscalene block with a nerve stimulator: A deltoid motor response is a satisfactory endpoint for successful block. Reg Anesth Pain Med 2000;25:356-359.

57. Borgeat A, Dullenkopf A, Ekatodramis G, et al: Evaluation of the lateral modified approach for continuous interscalene block after shoulder surgery. Anesthesiology 2003;99:436-442.

58. Franco CD, Gloss FJ, Voronov G, et al: Supraclavicular block in the obese population: An analysis of 2020 blocks. Anesth Analg 2006;102:1252-1254.

59. Brown DL, Cahill DR, Bridenbaugh LD: Supraclavicular nerve block: Anatomic analysis of a method to prevent pneumothorax. Anesth Analg 1993;76:530-534.

60. Hickey R, Garland TA, Ramamurthy S: Subclavian perivascular block: Influence of location of paresthesia. Anesth Analg 1989;68:767-771.

61. Winnie AP, Collins VJ: The subclavian perivascular approach of brachial plexus anesthesia. Anesthesiology 1964;25:353-363.

62. Klaastad O, VadeBoncouer TR, Tillung T, et al: An evaluation of the supraclavicular plumb bob technique for brachial plexus block by magnetic resonance imaging. Anesth Analg 2003;96:862-867.

63. Franco CD, Domashevich V, Voronov G, et al: The supraclavicular block with a nerve stimulator: To decrease or not to decrease, that is the question. Anesth Analg 2004;98:1167-1171.

64. Kapral S, Jandrasits O, Schabernig C, et al: Lateral infraclavicular plexus block vs. axillary block for hand and forearm surgery. Acta Anaesthesiol Scand 1999;43:1047-1052.

65. Koscielniak-Nielsen ZJ, Rotboll Nielsen P, Risby Mortensen C: A comparison of coracoid and axillary approaches to the brachial plexus. Acta Anaesthesiol Scand 2000;44:274-279.

66. Minville V, Fourcade O, LIdabouk L, et al: Infraclavicular brachial plexus block versus humeral block in trauma patients: A comparison of patient comfort. Anesth Analg 2006;102:912-916.

67. Wilson JL, Brown DL, Wong GY: Infraclavicular brachial plexus block: Parasagittal anatomy important to the coracoid technique. Anesth Analg 1998;87:870-873.

68. Borene SC, Edwards JN, Boezaart AP: At the cords, the pinkie towards: Interpreting infraclavicular motor responses to neurostimulation. Reg Anesth Pain Med 2004;29:125-129.

69. Rodriguez J, Barcena M, Taboada-Muniz M, et al: A comparison of single versus multiple injections on the extent of anesthesia with coracoid infraclavicular brachial plexus block. Anesth Analg 2004;99:1225-1230.

70. Weller RS, Gerancher JC: Brachial plexus block: "Best" approach and "best" evoked response—where are we [editorial]? Reg Anesth Pain Med 2004;29:520-523.

71. Lecamwasam H, Mayfield J, Rosow L, et al: Stimulation of the posterior cord predicts successful infraclavicular block. Anesth Analg 2006;102:1564-1568.

72. Schroeder LE, Horlocker TT, Schroeder DR: The efficacy of axillary block for surgical procedures about the elbow. Anesth Analg 1996;83:747-751.

73. Stan TC, Krantz MA, Solomon DL, et al: The incidence of neurovascular complications following axillary brachial plexus block using a transarterial approach. Reg Anesth 1995;20:486-492.

74. Thompson G: The multiple compartment approach to brachial plexus anesthesia. Tech Reg Anesth Pain Manage 1997;1:163-168.

75. Neal JM, McDonald SB, Larkin KL, et al: Suprascapular nerve block prolongs analgesia after nonarthroscopic shoulder surgery, but does not improve outcome. Anesth Analg 2003;96:982-986.

76. Shanahan EM, Ahern M, Smith M, et al: Suprascapular nerve block (using bupivacaine and methylprednisolone acetate) in chronic shoulder pain. Ann Rheum Dis 2003;62:400-406.

77. Viscomi CM, Reese J, Rathmell JP: Medial and lateral antebrachial cutaneous nerve blocks: An easily learned regional anesthetic for forearm arteriovenous fistula surgery. Reg Anesth 1996;21:2-5.

78. Gebhard RE, Al-Samsam T, Greger J, et al: Distal nerve blocks at the wrist for outpatient carpal tunnel surgery offer intraoperative cardiovascular stability and reduce discharge time. Anesth Analg 2002;95:351-355.

79. Klein SM, Grant SA, Greengrass RA, et al: Interscalene brachial plexus block with a continuous catheter insertion system and a disposable infusion pump. Anesth Analg 2000;91:1473-1478.

80. Klein SM, Nielsen KC, Greengrass RA, et al: Ambulatory discharge after long-acting peripheral nerve blockade: 2382 blocks with ropicacaine. Anesth Analg 2002;94:65-70.

81. Singelyn FJ, Suguy S, Gouverneur JM: Interscalene brachial plexus analgesia after open shoulder surgery: Continuous versus patient-controlled infusion. Anesth Analg 1999;89:1216-1220.

82. Boezaart AP, De Beer JF, Nell ML: Early experience with continuous cervical paravertebral block using a stimulating catheter. Reg Anesth Pain Med 2003;28:406-413.

83. Pham-Dang C, Gunst JP, Gouin F, et al: A novel supraclavicular approach to brachial plexus block. Anesth Analg 1997;85:111-116.

84. Auroy Y, Benhamou D, Bargues L, et al: Major complications of regional anesthesia in France. The SOS regional anesthesia hotline service. Anesthesiology 2002;97:1274-1280.

85. Candido KD, Sukhani R, Doty R, et al: Neurologic sequelae after interscalene brachial plexus block for shoulder/upper arm surgery: The association of patient, anesthetic, and surgical factors to the incidence and clinical course. Anesth Analg 2005;100:1489-1495.

86. Sorenson EJ: Neurologic injuries associated with regional anesthesia. Reg Anesth Pain Med (in press).

87. Benumof JL: Permanent loss of cervical spinal cord function associated with interscalene block performed under general anesthesia. Anesthesiology 2000;93:1541-1544.

88. Passannante AN: Spinal anesthesia and permanent neurologic deficit after interscalene block. Anesth Analg 1996;82:873-874.

89. Auroy Y, Narchi P, Messiah A, et al: Serious complications related to regional anesthesia: Results of a prospective survey in France. Anesthesiology 1997;87:479-486.

90. Cheney FW, Domino KB, Caplan RA, et al: Nerve injury associated with anesthesia: A closed claims analysis. Anesthesiology 1999;90:1062-1069.

91. Lee LA, L PK, Domino KB, et al: Injuries associated with regional anesthesia in the 1980s and 1990s. Anesthesiology 2004;101:143-152.

92. Choyce A, Chan VWS, Middleton WJ, et al: What is the relationship between paresthesia and nerve stimulation for axillary brachial plexus block? Reg Anesth Pain Med 2001;26:100-104.

93. Neal JM: How close is close enough? Defining the "paresthesia chad" [editorial]. Reg Anesth Pain Med 2001;26:97-99.

94. Selander D, Edshage S, Wolff T: Paresthesiae or no paresthesiae? Nerve lesions after axillary blocks. Acta Anaesth Scand 1979;23:27-33.

95. Hebl JR, Horlocker TT, Sorenson EJ, et al: Regional anesthesia does not increase the risk of postoperative neuropathy in patients undergoing ulnar nerve transposition. Anesth Analg 2001;93:1606-1611.

96. Hebl JR, Horlocker TT, Pritchard DJ: Diffuse brachial plexopathy after interscalene blockade in a patient receiving cisplatin chemotherapy: The pharmacologic double-crush syndrome. Anesth Analg 2001;92:249-251.

97. Rosenberg PH, Veering BT, Urmey WF: Maximum recommended doses of local anesthetics: A multifactorial concept. Reg Anesth Pain Med 2004;29:564-575.

98. Brown DL, Ransom DM, Hall JA, et al: Regional anesthesia and local anesthetic-induced systemic toxicity: Seizure frequency and accompanying cardiovascular changes. Anesth Analg 1995;81:321-328.

99. Lombard TP, Couper JL: Bilateral spread of analgesia following interscalene brachial plexus block. Anesthesiology 1983;58:472-473.

100. Urmey WF, Gloeggler PJ: Pulmonary function changes during interscalene brachial plexus block: Effects of decreasing local anesthetic injection volume. Reg Anesth 1993;18:244-249.

101. Urmey WF, McDonald M: Hemidiaphragmatic paresis during interscalene brachial plexus block: Effects on pulmonary function and chest wall mechanics. Anesth Analg 1992;74:352-357.

102. Urmey WF, Talts KH, Sharrock NE: One hundred percent incidence of hemidiaphragmatic paresis associated with interscalene brachial plexus anesthesia as diagnosed by ultrasonography. Anesth Analg 1991;72:498-503.

103. Rettig HC, Gielen MJM, Boersma E, et al: Vertical infracla-vicular block of the brachial plexus: Effects on hemidiaphrag-matic movement and ventilatory function. Reg Anesth Pain Med 2005;30:529-535.

104. Rodriguez J, Barcena M, Rodriguez V, et al: Infraclavicular brachial plexus block effects on respiratory function and extent of block. Reg Anesth Pain Med 1998;23:564-568.

105. Borgeat A, Perschak H, Bird P, et al: Patient-controlled inter-scalene analgesia with ropivacaine 0.2% versus patient-controlled intravenous analgesia after major shoulder surgery: Effects on diaphragmatic and respiratory function. Anesthe-siology 2000;92:102-108.

CHAPTER

48 Lower Extremity Peripheral Nerve Blocks

Bonnie Deschner, Christopher Robards, Daquan Xu, and Admir Hadzic

Unlike upper extremity nerve blocks, more than one injection site is required to anesthetize the entire lower extremity. Because of their deeper location, lower extremity blocks can be more technically challenging than upper extremity nerve blocks. Despite these challenges, lower extremity peripheral nerve blocks are becoming an increasingly more common method for providing anesthesia and analgesia of the lower extremities. They are particularly useful in procedures resulting in greater tissue trauma when analgesia significantly facilitates postoperative management.[1,2] Because of the increasing prevalence of age-related joint diseases, the number of lower extremity orthopedic and vascular procedures requiring peripheral nerve blockade will also continue to increase.

When continuous peripheral nerve blockade of the lower extremity is used, prolonged anesthesia and analgesia can be obtained, lasting well into the postoperative period. Patients can be discharged from the hospital with peripheral nerve catheters and local anesthetic infusion pumps that deliver local anesthetic to the patient at home. An important advantage of peripheral nerve blockade is the improved postoperative analgesia and decreased opioid-related side effects.[2,3] Evidence has suggested that outpatient continuous peripheral nerve blocks have analgesic potential beyond that obtained with postoperative single-injection blocks.[2] A recent meta-analysis found that patient satisfaction is significantly improved, and that patients benefit with better sleep patterns, shorter hospital stays, and improved rehabilitation.[4]

ANATOMY

Lumbar Plexus

The lumbar plexus (L1-L5) consists of six nerves—iliohypogastric, ilioinguinal, genitofemoral, lateral femoral cutaneous, femoral, and obturator. The first nerve emerges between the first and second lumbar vertebrae, and the last exits between the last lumbar vertebra and the base of the sacrum (Fig. 48–1).

The iliohypogastric and ilioinguinal nerves are primarily sensory nerves that arise from L1 and supply innervation to the skin of the suprapubic and inguinal regions. The genitofemoral nerve arises from L1 and L2 to supply motor innervation to the cremaster muscle and additional sensory innervation to the inguinal area. The lateral femoral cutaneous, femoral and, to a lesser degree, obturator nerves are important nerves to block when surgical anesthesia or analgesia of the lower extremity is sought.

The lateral femoral cutaneous nerve is formed from the L2 and L3 nerve roots and, as its name suggests, is a sensory nerve. It provides sensation to the lateral aspect of the thigh. The femoral nerve (L2-L4) is the major motor nerve of the thigh, providing extension at the knee through innervation of the rectus femoris, vastus medialis, vastus intermedius, and vastus lateralis muscles of the thigh. It also provides cutaneous sensory innervation to much of the anterior and medial thigh, as well as the medial portion of the leg distal to the knee. The obturator nerve (L2-L4) provides sensory innervation to a portion of the leg proximal to the knee as well as motor innervation to the adductor muscles of the thigh (Fig. 48–2).

Sacral Plexus

The sacral plexus is formed from the nerve roots L4-S3. Because of this overlap with the lumbar plexus, the two are sometimes referred to as the lumbosacral plexus. The sacral plexus gives rise to one major nerve and many small nerve branches. The sciatic nerve is the major nerve of the sacral plexus, and it is the most important nerve of concern for lower extremity peripheral nerve blocks below the knee (Fig. 48–3). It forms on the anterior surface of the piriformis muscle and exits the pelvis through the greater sciatic notch. It consists of the tibial and common peroneal branches, which provide the entire motor and sensory innervation to the leg below the knee with the exception of the cutaneous portion medially, supplied by the saphenous nerve.

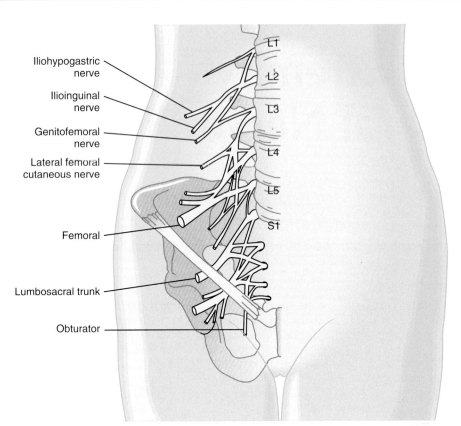

Figure 48–1. Schematic representation of the lumbar plexus and its individual nerve branches. For lower extremity nerve blocks, the lateral femoral cutaneous, femoral, and obturator nerves are of greatest concern. (Adapted with permission from Hadzic A, Vloka JD: Peripheral Nerve Blocks: Principles and Practice. New York, McGraw-Hill, 2004, p 20.)

Labels on figure:
- Iliohypogastric nerve
- Ilioinguinal nerve
- Genitofemoral nerve
- Lateral femoral cutaneous nerve
- Femoral
- Lumbosacral trunk
- Obturator
- L1, L2, L3, L4, L5, S1

PHARMACOLOGY FOR LOWER EXTREMITY NERVE BLOCKADE

This review of pharmacology focuses only on practical issues relating to lower extremity nerve blockade. A more extensive review of pharmacologic considerations and the potential value of adjuvants can be found elsewhere in this text (see Chapters 44 and 47). Specific local anesthetics for a nerve block are chosen by considering the patient and surgical procedure. It is important to predict with reasonable certainty the duration of desired surgical anesthesia, expected severity of postoperative pain associated with the particular procedure, and whether the patient is required to ambulate. For longer acting agents, bupivacaine and ropivacaine are used. Ropivacaine, 0.2% and bupivacaine, 0.25%, were shown to be clinically comparable when used for femoral nerve block for postoperative analgesia following total knee arthroplasty.[5] For prolonged surgical anesthesia, ropivacaine, 0.5% to 0.75%, and bupivacaine, 0.5%, are typically used.

Although they are not free from systemic toxicity, the lower cardiotoxic profile of levobupivacaine and ropivacaine may warrant their preferential use over bupivacaine as the longer-acting agents of choice.[6] For short procedures not associated with severe postoperative pain and procedures performed on an ambulatory basis, short- and intermediate-acting local anesthetics are the agents of choice. For example, femoral nerve block has been shown to be preferred by patients over spinal anesthesia using alkalinized 3% 2-chloroprocaine for long saphenous vein stripping.[7] Also, a superior recovery profile has been demonstrated when compared with general anesthesia in patients receiving lumbar plexus block with 3% 2-chloroprocaine for knee arthroscopy.[8] Other options for intermediate-acting agents are 1% prilocaine and 2% mepivacaine, which have both been shown to produce adequate sensory and motor block for knee arthroscopy.[9] Mepivacaine 2% has even been shown to decrease recovery room stay when used during combined sciatic-femoral nerve block for knee arthroscopy.[10] Although there are generalized recommendations, the maximum allowable dose of local anesthetic to be injected during peripheral nerve block is an issue that has not yet been resolved.[11] A recent randomized controlled trial, however, has shown that nontoxic plasma concentrations can be maintained with injections of up to 60 mL of ropivacaine, 0.5%, with epinephrine, 1:400,000, during combined lumbar plexus–sciatic nerve blockade.[12]

Adding epinephrine, 2.5 µg/mL, can help identify intravascular injection and aid block prolongation by decreasing drug clearance,[13] but at the risk of potentially worsening neurologic injury in case of intraneural injection.[14,15] Clonidine as an additive to continuous femoral nerve catheter infusions has been shown to prolong the return of motor function without improving the quality of the block.[16] Clonidine administered in femoral-sciatic nerve blocks did not improve analgesia, patient satisfaction, or decrease the postoperative consumption of opiates.[17] Studies using neostigmine, hyaluronidase, and tramadol as adjuvants have reported disappointing results in upper extremity blocks. Similar studies on lower extremity nerve blocks have not been performed. Age and physiologic characteristics (e.g.,

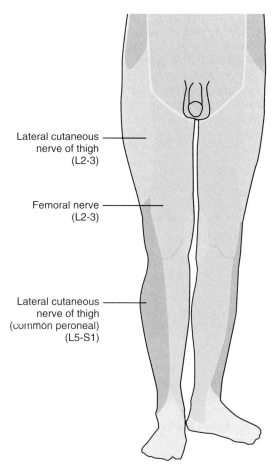

Figure 48–2. Schematic representation of the dermatomal distribution of the lumbar plexus. Note that the saphenous nerve is a branch of the lumbar plexus (femoral nerve) and extends to the level of the foot.

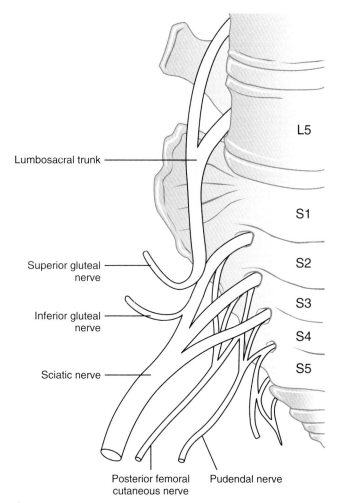

Figure 48–3. Schematic representation of the sacral plexus and its individual nerve branches. The main branch of the sacral plexus is the sciatic nerve, which gives rise to all innervation below the knee, except for the saphenous nerve. (Adapted with permission from Hadzic A, Vloka JD: Peripheral Nerve Blocks: Principles and Practice. New York, McGraw-Hill, 2004, p 22.)

drug clearance) of the patient may influence block duration, but no studies have addressed these commonly held assumptions. Furthermore, recent studies of combined lumbar plexus–sciatic blocks have found that maximum safe ropivacaine plasma concentrations are independent of patient age, weight, or body mass index.[12,18]

BLOCK TECHNIQUES FOR MAJOR LUMBOSACRAL PLEXUS APPROACHES

In all block descriptions, a short bevel needle is assumed to be used unless otherwise specified. The 1.5- to 2-inch needles are typically 22-gauge needles and the 4-inch needle is typically a 21-gauge needle. The choice of needle length varies, depending on patient body habitus. However, in general, the relationship is as follows: lumbar plexus block, 4-inch needle; obturator block, 2-inch needle; femoral block, 1.5- to 2-inch needle; sciatic block, 4-inch needle; and popliteal block, 2-inch (intertendinous) or 4-inch (lateral) needle (Table 48–1). Also, with all nerve stimulation techniques, a constant current nerve stimulator delivering a 0.1-msec current is assumed unless otherwise specified.

Table 48–1. Lower Extremity Nerve Blocks and Appropriate Needle Length

TYPE OF BLOCK	NEEDLE LENGTH
Lumbar plexus	4 inches (100 mm)
Obturator	2 inches (50 mm)
Femoral	1.5-2 inches (37.5-50 mm)
Sciatic	4 inches (100 mm)
Popliteal	2 inches (50 mm, intertendinous approach)
	4 inches (100 mm, lateral approach)

Posterior Lumbar Plexus Block (Psoas Compartment Block)

Indications

The lumbar plexus block (LPB) was first described in 1976 by Chayen and colleagues.[19] However, the original landmarks led to a risk of epidural anesthesia. The subsequent modification by Winnie and associates have resulted in a needle insertion site that is overly lateral.[20] The newer techniques use landmarks with the needle insertion site more medial at the junction of the lateral third and medial two thirds of a line between the spinous process of L4 and a line parallel to the spinal column passing through the posterior superior iliac spine (PSIS).[21] LPB can provide anesthesia or analgesia to the anterolateral and medial thigh, knee, and medial leg below the knee. When combined with a sciatic nerve block, anesthesia of almost the entire leg can be achieved.[22,23] The LPB is commonly used for analgesia following total hip arthroplasty[24,25] and total knee arthroplasty,[23,26] and in the treatment of chronic hip pain.[27]

Technique

The LPB is a deep block, and the needle traverses several layers of structures from posterior to anterior—posterior lumbar fascia, paraspinous muscles, anterior lumbar fascia, quadratus lumborum, and psoas muscle.[15] The patient is placed in the lateral decubitus position, operative side up, with a slight forward tilt. The foot on the side to be blocked is positioned over the dependent leg so that twitches of the quadriceps muscle can be easily seen. Although several needle insertion sites have been suggested, locating the transverse process of the lumbar vertebral body with the needle tip after insertion is common to all techniques. The two surface anatomic landmarks of importance for determining the insertion point for the needle are the iliac crest and the midline spinous processes. The top of the iliac crest correlates with the body of the L4 vertebral body or the L4-L5 interspace in most patients. The point 3 to 4 cm lateral to the intersection of the iliac crest and the midline spinous processes marks the needle insertion site (Fig. 48–4).

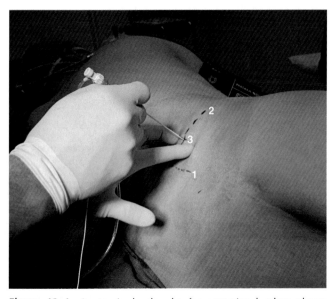

Figure 48–4. Anatomic landmarks for posterior lumbar plexus block: midline *(1)*; iliac crest line *(2)*; needle insertion site, 4 cm lateral to midline *(3)*. The figure demonstrates how a continuous lumbar plexus block is performed.

A nerve stimulator is set at an initial current of 1.5 mA. The needle is advanced at an angle perpendicular to all skin planes. As the needle is advanced, local twitches of the paravertebral muscles are first obtained. As the needle is further advanced, the transverse process may be encountered. Contact with the transverse process is not routinely sought but, when present, it provides a consistent landmark to avoid excessive needle penetration during LPB.[20] The distance from the skin to the lumbar plexus ranges from 6.1 to 10.1 cm in men and 5.7 to 9.3 cm in women.[20] This distance correlates gender and body mass index (BMI). The distance from the transverse process to the lumbar plexus is usually less than 2 cm, independent of BMI or gender. Contraction of the quadriceps muscle is usually obtained at a depth of 6 to 8 cm. The nerve stimulator current is reduced to produce stimulation of the quadriceps muscle between 0.5 to 1.0 mA, and 25 to 35 mL of local anesthetic is injected incrementally with negative aspiration every 5 mL.[21] It is important to avoid too deep a needle penetration and the resultant complications that may arise, such as renal hematoma and total spinal anesthesia.[15] The anesthesiologist performing the block should be aware that epidural spread of local anesthetic has been reported to occur in up to 16% of cases.[15]

Continuous Lumbar Plexus Block

A continuous LPB can be performed to provide prolonged postoperative analgesia. The landmarks and technique are similar to the single-shot technique with the exception that an 18-gauge 4-inch long Tuohy needle is used instead of a 21-gauge short-bevel needle, and that a catheter is inserted through the needle 5 to 10 cm beyond the tip when the needle is determined to be in correct position.[21] A stimulating or nonstimulating nerve block catheter kit can be used to perform the block. The benefit of the stimulating catheter kit is that one can confirm correct positioning of the catheter in situ with a nerve stimulator prior to dosing local anesthetic through it. With the nonstimulating catheter, local anesthetic is typically dosed through the needle, as with a single-shot technique, and the catheter is inserted without confirmation of its final positioning. The assumption with a nonstimulating catheter kit is that if the needle is held steady during slow and smooth injection of local anesthetic, the needle-nerve relationship is maintained and the catheter should be positioned in proximity to the nerve. No published data have firmly supported stimulating catheter placement over nonstimulating catheters when performing a continuous LPB.

After an initial bolus dose of local anesthetic, levobupivacaine, 0.125%, or ropivacaine, 0.2%, provides excellent postoperative analgesia when given as a continuous infusion through a peripheral nerve catheter. Although there is disagreement concerning maximum safe doses, infusions of 12 mL/hr of ropivacaine, 0.2%, for longer than 48 hours theoretically can lead to accumulation of local anesthetic and a risk for potential toxicity.[28,29] Typically, an infusion rate of 8 to 10 mL/hr is used with a patient-controlled bolus dose of 5 to 8 mL/hr.[21]

Obturator Block

The obturator nerve block was first described by Labat in 1922. The obturator nerve has both anterior and posterior branches. Only the anterior branch carries the highly variable cutaneous innervation, whereas the posterior branch carries sensory innervation to the knee joint. Both branches carry motor innervation to the adductors of the thigh. Much of the distribution previously attributed to obturator block when performing a three-in-one block has actually been found to be cutaneous innervation from the femoral nerve.[30] Therefore, proper assessment of the obturator nerve block involves testing adductor muscle strength rather than sensory coverage.[30]

Indications

Indications for obturator nerve block are to treat hip pain, relieve adductor muscle spasm, and occasionally, during urologic surgery, suppress the obturator reflex.[31-33] The classic approach consists of carrying out consecutive movements of the needle until the tip of the needle is placed over the top of the obturator foramen, where the nerve runs before splitting into its two terminal branches. The technique involves contacting the pubic tubercle and redirecting the needle along the anterior pubic wall (2 to 4 cm), after which it is redirected anteriorly and posteriorly. The needle is then withdrawn again and slightly redirected (cephalically and laterally) at an angle of 45 degrees for another 2 to 3 cm until contractions of the thigh adductor muscles are observed. The more recently developed interadductor approach is well tolerated by the patient and may be a simpler approach to accomplish obturator nerve block.[32]

Technique

With the patient placed in extreme leg abduction, the femoral artery and the tendon of the adductor longus muscle at the pubic tubercle are identified and a line is drawn over the inguinal crease from the pulse of the femoral artery to the tendon of the adductor longus muscle. The needle is inserted at the midpoint of this line at a 30-degree angle cephalad. Twitch responses from the long adductor and gracilis muscles are easily detectable on the posterior and medial aspect of the thigh. If the needle is inserted deeper (0.5 to 1.5 cm) and slightly laterally over the short adductor muscle, a motor response from the major adductor muscle is obtained and can be seen as a twitch on the posteromedial aspect of the thigh. Following successful nerve localization, 5 to 7 mL of local anesthetic is injected.

Femoral Block

The femoral nerve is the largest branch of the lumbar plexus arising from the second, third, and fourth lumbar nerves eventually dividing into anterior and posterior divisions. Femoral nerve block is classified as an intermediate nerve block technique; it is relatively easy to master and has a low risk of complications and many clinical applications for surgical anesthesia and postoperative analgesia.[15,21] Stimulation of the femoral nerve is indicated by patellar ascension as the quadriceps muscle contracts. Needle insertion just lateral to the femoral pulse at the level of the femoral crease results in the highest frequency of needle–femoral nerve contacts.[34] The *anterior* part of the femoral nerve containing the sartorius muscle branches is usually identified first.[34] Stimulation of these branches leads to contraction of the sartorius muscle on the medial aspect of the thigh, but this should not be considered the correct needle position. The articular and muscular branches arise from the *posterior* aspect of the femoral nerve.

Indications

Indications for single-injection femoral nerve block (FNB) include anesthesia for knee arthroscopy, anesthesia and analgesia for femoral shaft fractures, anterior cruciate ligament (ACL) reconstruction, and total knee reconstruction.[35-37]

Technique

The only anatomic landmarks needed for femoral nerve block are the femoral crease and femoral artery pulse. The needle insertion site is immediately lateral to the femoral artery, introduced in the sagittal, slightly cephalad plane (Fig. 48–5). When the sartorius muscle twitch is first obtained, the needle is simply redirected laterally and advanced several millimeters deeper. Quadriceps muscle twitch at 0.2 to

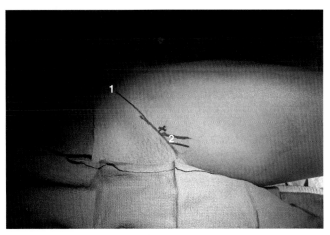

Figure 48–5. Anatomic landmarks for femoral nerve block: femoral crease *(1)*; femoral artery *(2)*; point of needle insertion *(x)*.

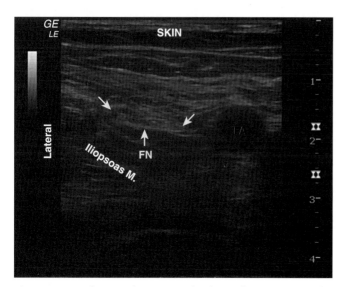

Figure 48–6. Ultrasound image at the femoral crease. Note the proximity of the femoral nerve to the femoral artery. FA, femoral artery; FN, femoral nerve.

0.5 mA is ideal, and injection of 15 to 30 mL of local anesthetic provides adequate blockade injected incrementally, with negative aspiration every 5 mL. Ultrasound imaging can delineate the femoral nerve and vessels at the level of the femoral crease (Fig. 48–6). Ultrasound can be useful in certain subsets of patients when landmarks are difficult to identify, such as obese patients, and in patients with a history of femoral artery revascularization.

Continuous Femoral Nerve Block

A continuous femoral bock can be performed to provide prolonged postoperative analgesia. The landmarks and technique are similar to the single-shot technique except that an 18-gauge Tuohy needle is used instead of a 21-gauge short-bevel needle, the needle is angulated slightly more cephalad at insertion to facilitate catheter advancement, and the catheter is inserted through the needle 5 to 10 cm beyond the needle tip when the needle is determined to be in the correct position.[21] The bevel of the Tuohy needle should be directed cephalad to facilitate proximal threading of the catheter. Although both stimulating and nonstimulating catheters have been used with success for femoral blocks, a convincing benefit of using stimulating catheters has not been shown.[38-40] Similar to continuous LPB, after an initial bolus dose of local anesthetic, ropivacaine, 0.2%, bupivacaine, 0.125%, and levobupivacaine, 0.125%, can be used for continuous infusion at a rate of 8 to 10 mL/hr. However, in this case, a patient-controlled bolus dose of 5 mL every 30 minutes is added.[21]

The "3-in-1 block" refers to a modification of the standard femoral block, in which a larger volume of local anesthetic is injected, with pressure being held distal to the needle injection site.[41] It is believed that this firm pressure will force local anesthetic to spread proximally and subsequently block the lateral femoral cutaneous and obturator branches of the lumbar plexus, along with the femoral nerve. Unfortunately, it has been shown that blockades of the obturator and lateral femoral cutaneous nerves are inconsistent.[42-45]

Fascia Iliaca Block

The fascia iliaca block was first described by Dalens and coworkers[46] in pediatric patients undergoing lower extremity surgery. This block has been shown to produce faster onset of lateral femoral cutaneous nerve blockade compared with femoral nerve block.[44] It is an excellent alternative to femoral nerve block in the anticoagulated patient because the needle insertion site is lateral and away from the femoral artery.

Indications

Because the result of a successful fascia iliaca block is femoral nerve blockade, the indications are similar and include analgesia for knee arthroscopy, analgesia for femoral shaft fractures, ACL reconstruction, and total knee reconstruction. The traditional fascia iliaca block is a "blind" technique and there are no reports of its use for surgical anesthesia.

Technique

The fascia iliaca block is traditionally performed using a double-pop technique. A nerve stimulator is not used because the needle insertion site is lateral to the femoral nerve. The needle insertion site is determined by drawing a line from the anterior superior iliac spine to the pubic tubercle and dividing it into thirds. The needle insertion site is 1 cm inferior to this line at the intersection of the lateral one third and medial two thirds. A short-bevel needle should be used to facilitate feeling the pop as the fascia lata and fascia iliaca are penetrated. After the second pop, 30 mL of local anesthetic is injected incrementally, with negative aspiration every 5 mL. The advent of high-resolution ultrasound machines is likely to make this technique more objective and reproducible (see Fig. 48–6).

Sciatic Block

The sciatic nerve is the largest nerve of the sacral plexus, innervating almost the entire leg below the knee. The primary indications are for foot and ankle surgery; however, a sciatic nerve block can be combined with a lumbar plexus block to obtain anesthesia of the entire lower extremity.

There are several approaches to block the sciatic nerve. When the decision is made to perform the block, the level at which it should be blocked depends on the surgical site. As a general rule, an ankle block can be used for surgical procedures involving the lower half to third of the foot. A popliteal sciatic block is indicated for surgical procedures involving the foot, ankle, and lower half of the leg below the knee. If the surgical site involves the knee or thigh, a more proximal block of the sciatic nerve is required.

Parasacral Approach

When blocked at this proximal location, sciatic nerve block not only provides anesthesia for foot and ankle surgery, but can also provide anesthesia to other branches of the sacral plexus, including the superior and inferior gluteal nerves, pudendal nerve, and posterior cutaneous nerve of the thigh.[15,47] Successful continuous block at this level has also been shown by Gaertner and colleagues,[47] who demonstrated correct catheter placement with radiopaque dye. Block at this level may not be desirable for certain distal procedures because of the possibility of adductor weakness and subsequent immobility[15,48] The block of the obturator nerve is not consistent when a parasacral sciatic nerve block is performed.[1]

The technique was first described by Mansour[49] in 1993. With the patient in a semiprone position, the parasacral approach to the sciatic nerve is initiated by drawing a line from the posterior superior iliac spine to the lowest point of the ischial tuberosity. The point of needle insertion is 6 cm caudal to the posterior superior iliac spine along this line.[49] The needle should be inserted perpendicular to all planes. Twitches of the muscles below the knee, particularly the foot, indicate good needle placement. When twitches are obtained at 0.2 to 0.5 mA, 20 mL of local anesthetic is injected incrementally, with negative aspiration every 5 mL.

Transgluteal Approach

Labat first described the sciatic nerve block, now referred to as the classic approach of Labat, at the beginning of the 20th century. This approach is based on the geometric relationship of the PSIS and greater trochanter to the sciatic nerve, with the patient positioned in a modified Sims position.[15] Winnie modified the original description by adding another landmark, the sacral hiatus, to account more precisely for the variability in body habitus.[50]

A line is drawn from the PSIS to the greater trochanter. A second line is drawn perpendicular from the midpoint of the first line drawn and extended 4 cm. This point is the site of needle insertion (Fig. 48–7). When a muscle twitch of the feet or toes is obtained from 0.2 to 0.5 mA, 20 mL of local anesthetic is injected incrementally, with negative aspiration every 5 mL.

Subgluteal Approaches

Anterior, lateral, supine flexed hip, and posterior positions have all been described as approaches to

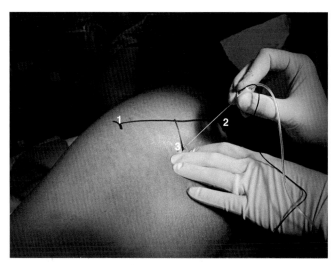

Figure 48–7. Anatomic landmarks for transgluteal sciatic nerve block: greater trochanter *(1)*; posterior superior iliac spine *(2)*; needle insertion site *(3)*, 4 cm caudad to midpoint of *1* and *2*.

the sciatic nerve at the subgluteal region,[51-53] with each having its own advantages. The advantage of the anterior approach is the fact that the patient is able to remain supine, and both the femoral and sciatic nerve scan be blocked with one sterile preparation. The advantage of the lateral approach is a reported 83% success rate of block of the posterior cutaneous nerve of the thigh.[15] The advantages of the supine flexed hip position, referred to as the Raj approach,[52] are that the sciatic nerve is made more superficial by stretching the gluteal muscles and the ease of its landmark identification. However, the posterior approach has been reported to produce less discomfort in patients while still being highly successful.[54]

Anterior Approach Technique

A line is drawn over the femoral crease. The femoral artery is palpated, and a second line is drawn perpendicular from the first line originating at the femoral pulse. The line is extended 4 to 5 cm from the femoral crease. The end of this line marks the needle entry site.[21] Muscle twitch of the foot or toes should be obtained from 0.2 to 0.5 mA and 20 mL of local anesthetic is injected incrementally, with negative aspiration every 5 mL. Internal rotation of the leg can greatly facilitate finding the sciatic nerve because it moves the lesser trochanter from the path of the needle.[55,56] Using magnetic resonance imaging, Ericksen and associates[57] have found that the sciatic nerve is inaccessible in 65% of patients at the level of the lesser trochanter and suggested approaching the sciatic nerve 4 cm caudad, where the lesser trochanter is rarely an obstruction.

Lateral Approach Technique

The lateral approach to the sciatic nerve was first described in 1959 by Ichniyanagi; it uses the greater trochanter of the femur as a landmark for the needle insertion.[15] Muscle twitch of the foot or toes should be obtained from 0.2 to 0.5 mA and 20 mL of local anesthetic is injected incrementally, with negative aspiration every 5 mL.

Supine Flexed Hip (Raj) Approach Technique

Raj and coworkers[52] described this technique in 1975; it overcomes some of the disadvantages of other methods. With the patient in the supine position, the hip is flexed to bring the knee toward the abdomen. The greater trochanter of the femur and the ischial tuberosity are palpated and a line is drawn to connect the two. The midpoint of that line is the needle insertion site, perpendicular to the skin. Muscle twitch of the foot or toes should be obtained with a current intensity of 0.2 to 0.5mA and 20 mL of local anesthetic is injected incrementally, with negative aspiration every 5 mL.

Subgluteal Approach Technique

The subgluteal approach is highly successful, and is an excellent alternative to the transgluteal approach to the sciatic nerve.[54,58] A line is drawn from the greater trochanter to the ischial tuberosity of the femur. Then, from the midpoint of this line, a second line is drawn perpendicularly and extended caudally for 4 cm. The end of this line represents the entry point of the needle. Muscle twitch of the foot or toes should be obtained at 0.2 to 0.5 mA and 20 mL of local anesthetic is injected incrementally, with negative aspiration every 5 mL.

Popliteal Approach

Popliteal approaches to the sciatic nerve block are performed from the lateral or posterior aspect of the leg. The lateral approach offers the benefit of maintaining the patient in the supine position and the posterior approach offers the benefit of easily identifiable landmarks and simplicity to perform. The level in the thigh at which the sciatic nerve branches into the tibial and common peroneal nerves varies greatly; to block both components, a more proximal needle insertion site should be chosen than was originally suggested.[59]

Lateral Approach Technique

The landmarks for the lateral approach to the popliteal block are the popliteal fossa crease, vastus lateralis muscle, and biceps femoris muscle (Fig. 48–8). The needle insertion site is 7 cm cephalad to the popliteal fossa crease, between the two muscles. The needle is inserted perpendicular to the skin and advanced to touch the femur. The depth is marked and the needle is withdrawn to the skin and advanced at a 30-degree angle posterior to the angle that produced contact with the femur initially[59,60] (Fig. 48–9). The needle is advanced up to 2 cm past the skin-femoral distance, because puncture of the popliteal artery or vein is possible with deeper needle insertion. Muscle twitches of the foot and toes at 0.2 to 0.5 mA indicate good needle position, and 35 to 45 mL of local anesthetic

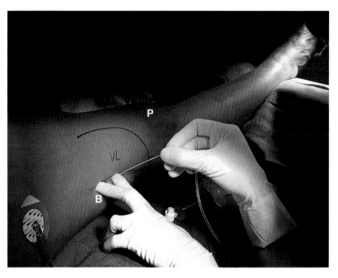

Figure 48–8. Anatomic landmarks for lateral popliteal nerve block. B, biceps femoris muscle; P, patella; VL, vastus lateralis muscle.

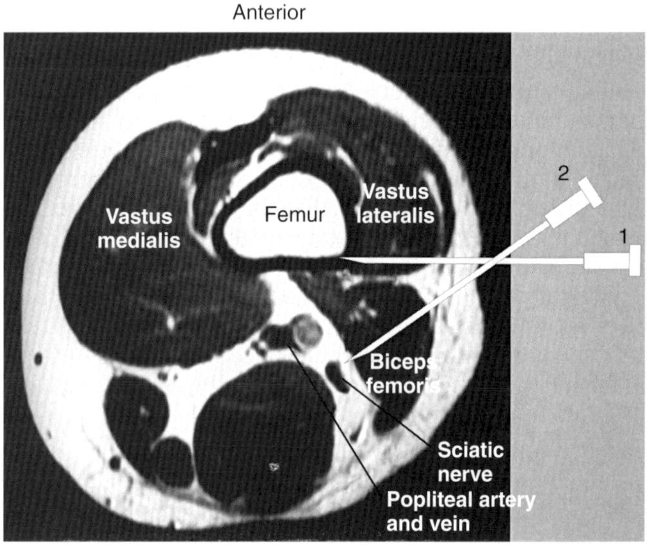

Figure 48–9. Axial magnetic resonance image of the thigh at the level of a lateral popliteal nerve block. Note that the artery and vein lie deep to the nerve as it is approached by the needle. The angle of needle redirection after the femur is contacted is approximately 30 degrees. (Adapted with permission from Hadzic A, Vloka JD: Peripheral Nerve Blocks: Principles and Practice. New York, McGraw-Hill, 2004, p 307.)

is injected incrementally, with negative aspiration every 5 mL. A double-injection technique with slightly caudal needle orientation that requires stimulation of both the tibial and common peroneal components of the sciatic nerve has been described.[61] When compared with ankle block and subcutaneous infiltration, lateral popliteal block has shown significant prolongation of analgesia in the postoperative period.[62,63]

Posterior Approach Technique

Originally, the sciatic nerve was approached at a level 5 cm above the popliteal fossa (classic approach).[64] More recent studies have determined that the sciatic

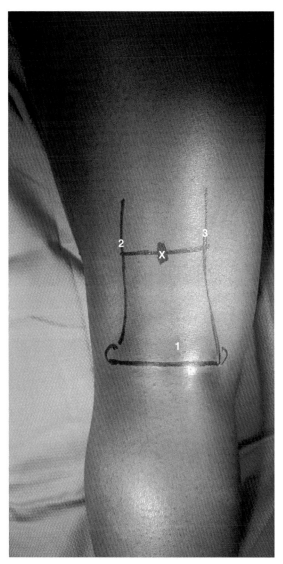

Figure 48–10. Anatomic landmarks for posterior popliteal nerve block: popliteal fossa crease *(1)*; biceps femoris tendon *(2)*; semitendinosus tendon *(3)*; point of needle insertion *(x)*.

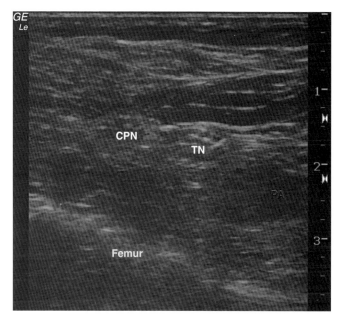

Figure 48–11. Ultrasound-guided sciatic nerve block, single injection. Shown is the sciatic nerve with its components, tibial nerve (TN) and common peroneal nerve (CPN), lateral to the popliteal artery (PA). (Reproduced with permission from J N Y School Reg Anesth. Available at nysora.com/techniques_ultrasound/femoral, Fig. 7.)

nerve diverges into the common peroneal and tibial nerves more proximally in the thigh (7 to 12 cm). Using the tendons of the biceps femoris, the semitendinosus and semimembranosus muscles provide consistent landmarks for identifying the needle insertion site.[59,65] Once the popliteal crease and the tendons of the hamstring muscles have been identified, the needle insertion site is labeled 7 cm proximal to the popliteal crease at the midpoint between the two tendons (Fig. 48–10). Note that the sciatic nerve lies lateral to the popliteal artery in this image (Fig. 48–11). Muscle twitches of the foot or toes should be visible between 0.2 and 0.5 mA, and 35 to 45 mL of local anesthetic is injected incrementally, with negative aspiration every 5 mL.

Continuous Sciatic Block

A continuous sciatic nerve block can be performed to provide prolonged postoperative analgesia at all

levels at which a single-injection sciatic nerve block can be performed. The landmarks and technique are similar to those of single-injection techniques, except that an 18-gauge Tuohy needle is used instead of a 21- or 22-gauge short-bevel needle, and a catheter is threaded through the needle 5 to 10 cm beyond the needle tip when the needle is determined to be in correct position.[21] The bevel of the Tuohy needle should be directed cephalad to facilitate proximal threading of the catheter. Similar to continuous LPB and femoral blocks, after an initial bolus dose of local anesthetic, ropivacaine, 0.2%, bupivacaine, 0.125%, and levobupivacaine, 0.125%, can be used for continuous infusion at a rate of 8 to 12 mL/hr.[21,28] A lower basal infusion rate should be used if the patient-controlled analgesia function on the infusion pump is initiated.[21] Stimulating catheters have been shown to provide faster onset of sensory and motor blockade, as well as provide superior analgesia, when compared with nonstimulating techniques.[66,67]

Ankle Block

An ankle block is a basic peripheral nerve block that is easy to perform, carries a low risk of systemic complications, and is effective for a wide variety of procedures on the foot and toes.[68,69]

Indications

Indications for blockade include various surgical procedures of the foot.[68] All terminal nerves to the foot are branches of the sciatic nerve (deep peroneal,

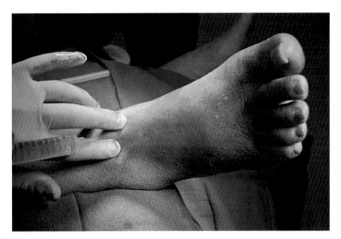

Figure 48–12. Block of the deep peroneal nerve.

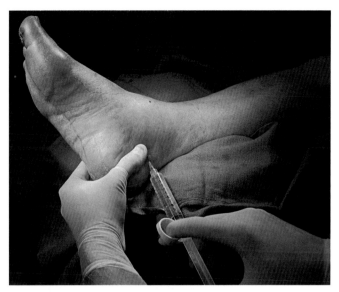

Figure 48–13. Block of the posterior tibial nerve.

superficial peroneal, posterior tibial, sural) except the saphenous nerve, a branch of the femoral nerve. Because of variations in the distribution of sensory innervation provided by each nerve, some have recommended blocking all five nerves for any procedure of the foot.[70] A 1.5-inch, 25- to 27-gauge needle, with a control syringe, is ideal for performing this block.

Technique

Deep Peroneal Nerve
The needle insertion site is immediately lateral to the dorsalis pedis artery, lateral to the tendon of the extensor hallucis longus muscle. The needle is advanced through the skin until bone is contacted. The needle is then withdrawn back 1 to 2 mm, and 2 to 3 mL of local anesthetic is injected. A fan technique is then used, redirecting the needle 30 degrees medially and laterally, with additional injections of 2 to 3 mL of local anesthetic in both directions (Fig. 48–12).

Posterior Tibial Nerve
This nerve is anesthetized by injecting local anesthetic just behind the medial malleolus, followed by a fan technique similar to that described for the deep peroneal nerve (Fig. 48–13).

Superficial Peroneal, Sural, and Saphenous Nerves
These three nerves are superficial cutaneous extensions of the sciatic and femoral nerves. A block of all three nerves is accomplished using a simple circumferential injection of local anesthetic subcutaneously at the level of the medial and lateral malleolus (Fig. 48–14).

Lower Extremity Perineural Catheters

Perineural catheters for continuous infusion of local anesthetic can be placed at almost any site at which a single-injection peripheral nerve block can be performed. The benefit of having a continuous catheter

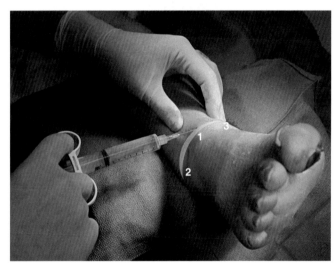

Figure 48–14. Block of superficial peroneal nerve *(1)*, sural nerve *(2)*, and saphenous nerve *(3)*.

is that anesthesia and analgesia are not limited by the duration of effect of the local anesthetics administered with a single injection.[71,72] Several studies have documented improvement in the postoperative course (e.g., decreased opioid-related side effects, decreased pain scores) after placing a peripheral nerve catheter,[4] and a multicenter prospective analysis of 1416 patients has shown that perineural catheters provide effective analgesia 96.3% of the time, with almost no adverse clinical consequences.[73] Studies have shown statistically and clinically significant improvement in postoperative course at all times after surgery in terms of pain scores and opioid-related side effects when using continuous perineural catheters.[20,74] Continuous lumbar plexus block has been used for postoperative analgesia following total hip arthroplasty,[75] total knee arthroplasty,[76] and ACL reconstruction.[77,78]

Unlike some other perineural catheters, lumbar plexus catheters are less likely to become dislodged because of the large mass of muscle traversed while placing them. Continuous femoral nerve block has been shown to improve outcomes after major knee surgery.[40,73,79,80] Continuous fascia iliaca catheters have also been shown to increase range of motion and decrease opioid usage postoperatively in patients undergoing total knee arthroplasty.[47,81] Continuous sciatic catheters can be placed at any point along the nerve, and successful continuous sciatic blockade has been reported at the parasacral, subgluteal, and popliteal levels.[82] The future of perineural catheters may lie in the results of ongoing studies concerning liposomal local anesthetic formulations. One study has shown that analgesia lasts 48 hours after a single injection of 2% liposomal bupivacaine.[82] If liposomal methods of drug delivery prove to be efficacious, the indications and use of continuous perineural catheters may decrease.

TECHNIQUES TO IMPROVE BLOCK SUCCESS

Most physicians now localize nerves using a nerve stimulator. Although there are no studies conclusively demonstrating an increased success rate over paresthesia techniques, nerve stimulator techniques do improve patient comfort.[15] In addition, whereas paresthesia techniques can still be used for upper extremity nerve blocks, these are rarely used and are impractical for lower extremity nerve blocks because of the large motor fiber component of these nerves. For example, there are no reports of the use of a paresthesia technique for lumbar plexus, femoral nerve, or popliteal block in the literature but there was a report comparing localization techniques for sciatic nerve block. Out of 100 sciatic nerve blocks, paresthesia was found in only 44 cases, whereas a positive response to the nerve stimulator was achieved in 95 cases.[83] Both techniques had similar success rates once the nerve was localized, but this suggests that nerve stimulators are better than paresthesia techniques at localizing nerves. Studies comparing single versus multiple stimulation techniques, specifically with the sciatic nerve block at the popliteal level, have shown that multiple stimulation techniques may be more successful.[84] Although the greater number of needle passes and injections could potentially increase the likelihood for nerve injury, this has not been borne out in studies.[85]

The most recent advances in nerve localization for peripheral nerve blockade have been with ultrasound imaging. Accurate ultrasound-guided needle placement in the lumbar plexus has been demonstrated,[86] and visualization of the lumbar paravertebral region has also been shown to be possible in most patients using a curved array transducer operating at 4 to 5 MHz.[87] However, in the patients studied, delineation of the lumbar plexus itself was not possible. Furthermore, the lumbar paravertebral region is difficult to visualize in obese patients and male patients because of their anthropometrically tall iliac crests.

Because of its deep location and resultant poor visualization with ultrasound probes, ultrasound-guided LPB is difficult to perform. Ultrasound-guided femoral nerve block, however, has been shown to improve onset time, quality of block, and decreased incidence of vascular puncture when compared with a nerve stimulator technique.[88] Furthermore, it has also been shown that successful femoral nerve block using ultrasound can be performed using less local anesthetic compared with a nerve stimulator technique.[89] Ultrasound-guided posterior popliteal blocks allow direct visualization of sciatic nerve anatomy, the point at which it divides, and the spatial relationship between the peroneal and tibial nerves distally. Visualization of local anesthetic spread within the fascial sheath after injection has been shown to correlate with a rapid onset and completeness of sciatic nerve block and may facilitate accurate localization of the sciatic nerve in patients with peripheral neuropathy.[90,91] Improvement in ultrasound technology with compound imaging has made visualization of structures more straightforward, but the future role of ultrasound for peripheral nerve blockade will be established when more studies confirm its validity and specify indications for its use.

COMPLICATIONS OF LOWER EXTREMITY BLOCKS

Nerve Injury

There are relatively little data on the incidence of peripheral nerve injury directly attributed to anesthesia, but the current estimate is that severe nerve injury occurs in 0.02% to 0.4% of cases.[85,92,93] Neurologic injury following peripheral nerve block and surgery can be attributed to various causes, including needle trauma, intraneuronal injection, neuronal ischemia, patient positioning, retractor injury, and hematoma formation.[15] It is likely that many postoperative nerve injuries result from a combination of these factors.

Mechanisms of neuronal injury related to peripheral nerve block fall into one of four categories (Table 48–2). Direct needle trauma to the nerves is a subject that has been studied with mixed results. In one study, the risk of perforating a nerve fascicle was significantly lower when using a short-bevel compared with a long-bevel needle.[94] However, in another study, in which needles were deliberately advanced through rat sciatic nerves in vitro, short-bevel needles

Table 48–2. Mechanisms of Neuronal Injury Related to Peripheral Nerve Blocks

TYPE OF INJURY	MECHANISM
Mechanical, acute	Laceration; stretch; intraneural injection
Vascular	Acute ischemia; hemorrhage
Pressure	Extraneural; intraneural; compartment syndrome
Chemical	Injection of neurotoxic solutions

were associated with more neural trauma on histologic examination compared with the cleaner cutting long-bevel needles.[95] Despite these conflicting results, most commercially manufactured peripheral nerve block needles are of the short-bevel type.

Intraneural injection of local anesthetic is believed to play a role in neuronal injury by disrupting the nerve fascicle and neural anatomy. Several studies have documented an association of intraneural injection with abnormal resistance (pressure) on injection.[14,96,97] Theoretically, objective inline pressure monitoring can help avoid excessive injection pressure and standardize injection technique, given the individual variations of injection pressure among anesthesiologists.[98] However, there are currently no clinical data documenting any benefit of routine injection pressure monitoring. The addition of vasoconstrictors is believed to worsen nerve ischemia potentially by decreasing blood flow,[14] but this been shown not to be a risk factor for postoperative nerve dysfunction in patients undergoing lower extremity surgery.[85]

Pain on injection has long been regarded as a principal sign of intraneural injection. Although this would suggest not performing peripheral nerve blocks on heavily sedated patients or those under general anesthesia,[99] numerous reports have demonstrated that pain may not occur during injection, despite a subsequent nerve injury.[100-103]

Finally, there is the possibility of preexisting subclinical neurologic disease that can be made worse by peripheral nerve blockade. Originally described by Upton and McComas in 1973,[104] a double-crush phenomenon suggests that two separately occurring minor injuries to a nerve can ultimately lead to a severe nerve injury. A case report of a patient receiving cisplatin therapy who developed a brachial plexus injury addressed the concept of a pharmacologic double-crush syndrome, in which the first minor injury was caused by cisplatin and the second was caused by local anesthetic administered during interscalene block.[105] This should be kept in mind when considering peripheral nerve blockade for patients with any type of preexisting peripheral neuropathy.

Intravascular Injection

Intravascular injection of local anesthetic during performance of a peripheral nerve block can lead to serious complications, including seizure and cardiac arrest.[106-108] Most cases have been reported following upper extremity peripheral nerve block, but the likelihood of toxicity would seem to be more closely associated with intrinsic vascularity at the injection site more than any other factor. Therefore, lumbar plexus block should carry a higher risk of systemic toxicity than other lower extremity blocks. Although there are few case reports of lower extremity peripheral nerve block–associated systemic toxicity, many of them occurred after lumbar plexus blockade.[109-111] Aspiration prior to injection to ensure that there is no blood return and incremental dosing are most efficacious for avoiding these potentially devastating complications.

Unintended Needle Placement

When compared with upper extremity nerve blocks, unintended needle placement is of relatively minor concern for most lower extremity blocks. However, the posterior lumbar plexus block, in particular, has the potential for serious consequences if precautions are not taken.[93] Cases of subcapsular renal hematoma and total spinal anesthesia have been reported with lumbar plexus block.[112,113] With a grossly misplaced needle, there is the chance of bowel perforation. Use of the correct needle length and intentionally seeking the transverse process when performing this block can help avoid these complications.

The Anticoagulated Patient

Although it might be expected that there would be a significant number of hemorrhagic complications associated with lower extremity peripheral nerve blocks because of their deep location, this is not the case. Unlike centroneuraxial blockade, there is no consensus as to what is considered a safe coagulation profile for peripheral nerve blockade. Most hemorrhagic complications have been reported following lumbar plexus block, and in many of these cases the patients were anticoagulated postoperatively.[114-117] It is wise to consider alternative anesthetic plans for patients with known coagulopathy, particularly when considering a block in which the nerves have a deep anatomic location.

Pressure Ulcers

There have been cases of pressure ulcers developing in some patients receiving peripheral nerve blocks because of a lack of sensation in the foot.[118,119] Most of these have been reported in conjunction with sciatic nerve block, and this complication can be avoided by padding pressure points and improved teaching of the nursing staff caring for these patients. Similarly, indications for and relative analgesic value of long-acting or continuous sciatic nerve blocks should be carefully considered.

SUMMARY

- Unlike the upper extremity, more than one injection is required to anesthetize the entire lower extremity.
- When considering anatomy, it is important to realize that with the exception of a medial strip of cutaneous sensation (saphenous nerve), all sensation below the knee is derived from the sciatic nerve.
- Lower extremity peripheral nerve block techniques have been well documented to improve analgesia and decrease opioid-related side effects. They also result in increased patient satisfaction and rehabilitation, and faster hospital discharge.

- Ropivacaine is less cardiotoxic than bupivacaine and is a good choice for a long-acting local anesthetic. Chloroprocaine and mepivacaine are good choices for shorter ambulatory procedures and when severe postoperative pain is not anticipated.
- Adding epinephrine to local anesthetics can prolong duration of action by decreasing clearance. Clonidine has been shown to prolong blockade when used with intermediate-acting local anesthetics. Other adjuvants are either ineffective or not well studied.
- Continuous perineural catheters have been shown to result in improved pain scores and decreased opioid-related side effects in the postoperative period.
- Nerve stimulator techniques are preferred over paresthesia techniques for lower extremity nerve blocks.
- Because lower extremity blocks require deeper levels of sedation and lower extremity nerves have a large motor component, paresthesia techniques are now essentially obsolete for lower extremity peripheral nerve blocks.
- Ultrasound-guided nerve blocks have the advantage of visualizing the local anesthetic spread in proximity of the nerves and potentially speeding nerve localization.
- Abnormal resistance on injection (more than 20 psi) and severe pain on injection may herald an intraneural injection and should be avoided.
- Underlying subclinical neurologic disease can contribute to the development of neurologic injury through the double-crush phenomenon.
- The best maneuvers to decrease the risk of intravascular injections are frequent aspiration for blood, incremental dosing, and avoidance of forceful injections.
- There is no consensus on what is considered a safe coagulation profile prior to performing a peripheral nerve block. Avoidance of deep blocks—for example, a lumbar plexus block—is wise in patients with coagulopathy.

References

1. Jochum D, Iohom G, Choquet O, et al: Adding a selective obturator nerve block to the parasacral sciatic nerve block: An evaluation. Anesth Analg 2004;99:1544-1559.
2. Klein SM, Evans H, Nielsen KC, et al: Peripheral nerve block techniques for ambulatory surgery. Anesth Analg 2005;101:1663-1676.
3. Ilfeld BM, Enneking FK: Continuous peripheral nerve blocks at home: A review. Anesth Analg 2005;100:1822-1833.
4. Richman JM, Liu SS, Courpas G, et al: Does continuous peripheral nerve block provide superior pain control to opioids? A meta-analysis. Anesth Analg 2006;102:248-257.
5. Ng HP, Cheong KF, Lim A, et al: Intraoperative single-shot "3-in-1" femoral nerve block with ropivacaine 0.25%, ropivacaine 0.5% or bupivacaine 0.25% provides comparable 48-hr analgesia after unilateral total knee replacement. Can J Anaesth 2001;48:1102-1108.
6. Ohmura S, Kawada M, Ohta T, et al: Systemic toxicity and resuscitation in bupivacaine-, levobupivacaine-, or ropivacaine-infused rats. Anesth Analg 2001;93:743-748.
7. Vloka JD, Hadzic A, Mulcare R, et al: Femoral and genito-femoral nerve blocks versus spinal anesthesia for outpatients undergoing long saphenous vein stripping surgery. Anesth Analg 1997;84:749-752.
8. Hadzic A, Karaca PE, Hobeika P, et al: Peripheral nerve blocks result in superior recovery profile compared with general anesthesia in outpatient knee arthroscopy. Anesth Analg 2005;100:976-981.
9. Marsan A, Kirdemir P, Mamo D, et al: Prilocaine or mepivacaine for combined sciatic-femoral nerve block in patients receiving elective knee arthroscopy. Minerva Anestesiol 2004;70:763-769.
10. Casati A, Cappelleri G, Berti M, et al: Randomized comparison of remifentanil-propofol with a sciatic-femoral nerve block for out-patient knee arthroscopy. Eur J Anaesthesiol 2002;19:109-114.
11. Rosenberg PH, Veering BT, Urmey WF: Maximum recommended doses of local anesthetics: A multifactorial concept. Reg Anesth Pain Med 2004;29:564-575.
12. Vanterpool S, Steele SM, Nielsen KC, et al: Combined lumbar-plexus and sciatic-nerve blocks: An analysis of plasma ropivacaine concentrations. Reg Anesth Pain Med 2006;31:417-421.
13. Bernards CM, Kopacz DJ: Effect of epinephrine on lidocaine clearance in vivo: A microdialysis study in humans. Anesthesiology 1999;91:962-968.
14. Selander D, Mansson LG, Karlsson L, et al: Adrenergic vasoconstriction in peripheral nerves of the rabbit. Anesthesiology 1985;62:6-10.
15. Enneking FK, Chan V, Greger J, et al: Lower-extremity peripheral nerve blockade: Essentials of our current understanding. Reg Anesth Pain Med 2005;30:4-35.
16. Casati A, Vinciguerra F, Cappelleri G, et al: Adding clonidine to the induction bolus and postoperative infusion during continuous femoral nerve block delays recovery of motor function after total knee arthroplasty. Anesth Analg 2005;100:866-872.
17. Couture DJ, Cuniff HM, Maye JP, et al: The addition of clonidine to bupivacaine in combined femoral-sciatic nerve block for anterior cruciate ligament reconstruction. AANA J 2004;72:273-278.
18. Hanks RK, Pietrobon R, Nielsen KC, et al: The effect of age on sciatic nerve block duration. Anesth Analg 2006;102:588-592.
19. Chayen D, Nathan H, Chayen M: The psoas compartment block. Anesthesiology 1976;45:95-99.
20. Capdevila X, Macaire P, Dadure C: Continuous psoas compartment block for postoperative analgesia after total hip arthroplasty: New landmarks, technical guidelines and clinical evaluation. Anesth Analg 2002;94:1606-1613.
21. Hadzic A, Vloka, JD: Peripheral Nerve Blocks: Principles and Practice. New York, McGraw-Hill, 2004.
22. Ho A, Karmakar M: Combined paravertebral lumbar plexus and parasacral sciatic nerve block for reduction of hip fracture in a patient with severe aortic stenosis. Can J Anesth 2002;49:946-950.
23. Luber M, Greengrass R, Vail TP: Patient satisfaction and effectiveness of lumbar plexus and sciatic nerve block for total knee arthroplasty. J Arthroplasty 2001;16:17-21.
24. Turker G, Uckunkaya N, Yavascaoglu B: Comparison of catheter-technique psoas compartment block and the epidural block for analgesia in partial hip replacement surgery. Acta Anaesthesiol Scand 2003;47:30-36.
25. Stevens RD, Van Gessel E, Flory N, et al: Lumbar plexus block reduces pain and blood loss associated with total hip arthroplasty. Anesthesiology 2000;93:115-121.
26. Watson MW, Mitra D, McLintock TC, et al: Continuous versus single-injection lumbar plexus blocks: Comparison of the effects on morphine use and early recovery after total knee arthroplasty. Reg Anesth Pain Med 2005;30:541-547.
27. Goroszeniuk T, di Vadi P: Repeated psoas compartment blocks for the management of long-standing hip pain. Reg Anesth Pain Med 2001;26:376-378.
28. Casati A, Vinciguerra F, Cappelleri G, et al: Levobupivacaine 0.2% or 0.125% for continuous sciatic nerve block: A prospective, randomized, double-blind comparison with 0.2% ropivacaine. Anesth Analg 2004;99:919-923.
29. Kaloul I, Guay J, Cote C, et al: Ropivacaine plasma concentrations are similar during continuous lumbar plexus blockade using the anterior three-in-one and the posterior psoas compartment techniques. Can J Anaesth 2004;51:52-56.

30. Bouaziz H, Vial F, Jochum D, et al: An evaluation of the cutaneous distribution after obturator nerve block. Anesth Analg 2002;94:445-449.

31. Trainer N, Bowser BL, Dahm L: Obturator nerve block for painful hip in adult cerebral palsy. Arch Phys Med Rehabil 1986;67:829-830.

32. Wassef MR: Interadductor approach to obturator nerve blockade for spastic conditions of adductor thigh muscles. Reg Anesth 1993;18:13-17.

33. Akata T, Murakami J, Yoshinaga A: Life-threatening haemorrhage following obturator artery injury during transurethral bladder surgery: A sequel of an unsuccessful obturator nerve block. Acta Anaesthesiol Scand 1999;43:784-788.

34. Vloka J, Hadzic A, Drobnik L: Anatomic landmarks for femoral nerve block: A comparison of four needle insertion sites. Anesth Analg 1999;89:1467-1470.

35. Goranson B, Lang S, Cassidy J: A comparison of three regional anaesthesia techniques for outpatient knee arthroscopy. Can J Anesth 1997;44:371-376.

36. Fletcher A, Rigby A, Heyes F: Three-in-one femoral nerve block as analgesia for fractures neck of femur in the emergency department: A randomized, controlled trial. Ann Emerg Med 2003;41:227-233.

37. Mulroy M, Larkin K, Batra M: Femoral nerve block with 0.25% or 0.5% bupivacaine improves postoperative analgesia following outpatient arthroscopic anterior cruciate ligament repair. Reg Anesth Pain Med 2001;26:24-29.

38. Morin AM, Eberhart LH, Behnke HK, et al: Does femoral nerve catheter placement with stimulating catheters improve effective placement? A randomized, controlled, and observer-blinded trial. Anesth Analg 2005;100:1503-1510.

39. Pham-Dang C, Kick O, Collet T, et al: Continuous peripheral nerve blocks with stimulating catheters. Reg Anesth Pain Med 2003;28:83-88.

40. Salinas FV, Neal JM, Sueda LA, et al: Prospective comparison of continuous femoral nerve block with nonstimulating catheter placement versus stimulating catheter-guided perineural placement in volunteers. Reg Anesth Pain Med 2004;29:212-220.

41. Winnie AP, Ramamurthy S, Durrani Z: The inguinal paravascular technic of lumbar plexus anesthesia: The "3-in-1 block." Anesth Analg 1973;52:989-996.

42. Lang SA, Yip RW, Chang PC, et al: The femoral 3-in-1 block revisited. J Clin Anesth 1993;5:292-296.

43. Cauhepe C, Oliver M, Colombani R, et al: [The "3-in-1" block: Myth or reality?] Ann Fr Anesth Reanim 1989;8:376-378.

44. Capdevila X, Biboulet P, Bouregba M, et al: Comparison of the three-in-one and fascia iliaca compartment blocks in adults: Clinical and radiographic analysis. Anesth Analg 1998;86:1039-1044.

45. Marhofer P, Oismuller C, Faryniak B, et al: Three-in-one blocks with ropivacaine: Evaluation of sensory onset time and quality of sensory block. Anesth Analg 2000;90:125-128.

46. Dalens B, Vanneuville G, Tanguy A: Comparison of the fascia iliaca compartment block with the 3-in-1 block in children. Anesth Analg 1989;69:705-713.

47. Gaertner E, Lascurain P, Venet C, et al: Continuous parasacral sciatic block: A radiographic study. Anesth Analg 2004;98:831-834.

48. Morris GF, Lang SA, Dust WN, et al: The parasacral sciatic nerve block. Reg Anesth 1997;22:223-228.

49. Mansour NY: Reevaluating the sciatic nerve block: Another landmark for consideration. Reg Anesth 1993;18:322-323.

50. Winnie A: Regional anesthesia. Surg Clin North Am 1975;55:861-862.

51. Beck GP: Anterior approach to sciatic nerve block. Anesthesiology 1963;24:222-224.

52. Raj PP, Parks RI, Watson TD, et al: A new single-position supine approach to sciatic-femoral nerve block. Anesth Analg 1975;54:489-493.

53. Guardini R, Waldron BA, Wallace WA: Sciatic nerve block: A new lateral approach. Acta Anaesthesiol Scand 1985;29:515-519.

54. Di Benedetto P, Casati A, Bertini L, et al: Posterior subgluteal approach to block the sciatic nerve: Description of the technique and initial clinical experiences. Eur J Anaesthesiol 2002;19:682-686.

55. Vloka JD, Hadzic A, April E, et al: Anterior approach to the sciatic nerve block: The effects of leg rotation. Anesth Analg 2001;92:460-462.

56. Moore CS, Sheppard D, Wildsmith JA: Thigh rotation and the anterior approach to the sciatic nerve: A magnetic resonance imaging study. Reg Anesth Pain Med 2004;29:32-35.

57. Ericksen ML, Swenson JD, Pace NL: The anatomic relationship of the sciatic nerve to the lesser trochanter: Implications for anterior sciatic nerve block. Anesth Analg 2002;95:1071-1074.

58. di Benedetto P, Bertini L, Casati A, et al: A new posterior approach to the sciatic nerve block: A prospective, randomized comparison with the classic posterior approach. Anesth Analg 2001;93:1040-1044.

59. Vloka JD, Hadzic A, April E, et al: The division of the sciatic nerve in the popliteal fossa: Anatomical implications for popliteal nerve blockade. Anesth Analg 2001;92:215-217.

60. Vloka JD, Hadzic A, Kitain E, et al: Anatomic considerations for sciatic nerve block in the popliteal fossa through the lateral approach. Reg Anesth 1996;21:414-418.

61. Zetlaoui PJ, Bouaziz H: Lateral approach to the sciatic nerve in the popliteal fossa. Anesth Analg 1998;87:79-82.

62. McLeod DH, Wong DH, Claridge RJ, et al: Lateral popliteal sciatic nerve block compared with subcutaneous infiltration for analgesia following foot surgery. Can J Anaesth 1994;41:673-676.

63. McLeod DH, Wong DH, Vaghadia H, et al: Lateral popliteal sciatic nerve block compared with ankle block for analgesia following foot surgery. Can J Anaesth 1995;42:765-769.

64. Rorie DK, Byer DE, Nelson DO, et al: Assessment of block of the sciatic nerve in the popliteal fossa. Anesth Analg 1980;59:371-376.

65. Hadzic A, Vloka JD, Singson R, et al: A comparison of intertendinous and classical approaches to popliteal nerve block using magnetic resonance imaging simulation. Anesth Analg 2002;94:1321-1324.

66. Rodriguez J, Taboada M, Carceller J, et al: Stimulating popliteal catheters for postoperative analgesia after hallux valgus repair. Anesth Analg 2006;102:258-262.

67. Casati A, Fanelli G, Koscielniak-Nielsen Z, et al: Using stimulating catheters for continuous sciatic nerve block shortens onset time of surgical block and minimizes postoperative consumption of pain medication after halux valgus repair as compared with conventional nonstimulating catheters. Anesth Analg 2005;101:1192-1197.

68. Schurman DJ: Ankle-block anesthesia for foot surgery. Anesthesiology 1976;44:348-352.

69. Pinzur M, Morrison C, Sage R: Syme's two-stage amputation in insulin-requiring diabetics with gangrene of the forefoot. Foot Ankle Int 1991;11:394-396.

70. Delgado-Martinez AD, Marchal-Escalona JM: Supramalleolar ankle block anesthesia and ankle tourniquet for foot surgery. Foot Ankle Int 2001;22:836-838.

71. Singelyn FJ, Deyaert M, Joris D, et al: Effects of intravenous patient-controlled analgesia with morphine, continuous epidural analgesia, and continuous three-in-one block on postoperative pain and knee rehabilitation after unilateral total knee arthroplasty. Anesth Analg 1998;87:88-92.

72. Capdevila X, Barthelet Y, Biboulet P, et al: Effects of perioperative analgesic technique on the surgical outcome and duration of rehabilitation after major knee surgery. Anesthesiology 1999;91:8-15.

73. Capdevila X, Pirat P, Bringuier S, et al: Continuous peripheral nerve blocks in hospital wards after orthopedic surgery: A multicenter prospective analysis of the quality of postoperative analgesia and complications in 1,416 patients. Anesthesiology 2005;103:1035-1045.

74. Turker G, Uckunkaya N, Yavascaoglu B, et al: Comparison of the catheter-technique psoas compartment block and the epidural block for analgesia in partial hip replacement surgery. Acta Anaesthesiol Scand 2003;47:30-36.

75. Luber MJ, Greengrass R, Vail TP: Patient satisfaction and effectiveness of lumbar plexus and sciatic nerve block for total knee arthroplasty. J Arthroplasty 2001;16:17-21.

76. Matheny JM, Hanks GA, Rung GW, et al: A comparison of patient-controlled analgesia and continuous lumbar plexus block after anterior cruciate ligament reconstruction. Arthroscopy 1993;9:87-90.

77. Chelly JE, Greger J, Gebhard R, et al: Continuous femoral blocks improve recovery and outcome of patients undergoing total knee arthroplasty. J Arthroplasty 2001;16:436-445.

78. Yazigi A, Madi-Gebara S, Haddad F, et al: Intraoperative myocardial ischemia in peripheral vascular surgery: General anesthesia vs combined sciatic and femoral nerve blocks. J Clin Anesth 2005;17:499-503.

79. Ganapathy S, Wasserman RA, Watson JT, et al: Modified continuous femoral three-in-one block for postoperative pain after total knee arthroplasty. Anesth Analg 1999;89: 1197-1202.

80. Eledjam J, Cuvillon P, Capdevila X, et al: Postoperative analgesia by femoral nerve block with ropivacaine 0.2% after major knee surgery: Continuous versus patient-controlled techniques. Reg Anesth Pain Med 2002;27:604-611.

81. di Benedetto P, Casati A, Bertini L, et al: Postoperative analgesia with continuous sciatic nerve block after foot surgery: A prospective, randomized comparison between the popliteal and subgluteal approaches. Anesth Analg 2002;94: 996-1000.

82. Grant GJ, Barenholz Y, Bolotin EM, et al: A novel liposomal bupivacaine formulation to produce ultralong-acting analgesia. Anesthesiology 2004;101:133-137.

83. Davies MJ, McGlade DP: One hundred sciatic nerve blocks: A comparison of localisation techniques. Anaesth Intens Care 1993;21:76-78.

84. Paqueron X, Bouaziz H, Macalou D, et al: The lateral approach to the sciatic nerve at the popliteal fossa: One or two injections? Anesth Analg 1999;89:1221-1225.

85. Fanelli G, Casati A, Garancini P, et al: Nerve stimulator and multiple injection technique for upper and lower limb blockade: Failure rate, patient acceptance, and neurologic complications. Study Group on Regional Anesthesia. Anesth Analg 1999;88:847-852.

86. Kirchmair L, Entner T, Kapral S, et al: Ultrasound guidance for the psoas compartment block: An imaging study. Anesth Analg 2002;94:706-710.

87. Kirchmair L, Entner T, Wissel J, et al: A study of the paravertebral anatomy for ultrasound-guided posterior lumbar plexus block. Anesth Analg 2001;93:477-481.

88. Marhofer P, Schrogendorfer K, Koinig H, et al: Ultrasonographic guidance improves sensory block and onset time of three-in-one blocks. Anesth Analg 1997;85:854-857.

89. Marhofer P, Schrogendorfer K, Wallner T, et al: Ultrasonographic guidance reduces the amount of local anesthetic for 3-in-1 blocks. Reg Anesth Pain Med 1998;23:584-588.

90. Sinha A, Chan V: Ultrasound imaging for popliteal sciatic nerve block. Reg Anesth Pain Med 2004;29:130-134.

91. Sites B, Gallagher J, Sparks M: Ultrasound-guided popliteal block demonstrates an atypical motor response to nerve stimulation in 2 patients with diabetes mellitus. Reg Anesth Pain Med 2003;28:479-482.

92. Auroy Y, Narchi P, Messiah A, et al: Serious complications related to regional anesthesia: Results of a prospective survey in France. Anesthesiology 1997;87:479-486.

93. Auroy Y, Benhamou D, Bargues L, et al: Major complications of regional anesthesia in France: The SOS Regional Anesthesia Hotline Service. Anesthesiology 2002;97:1274-1280.

94. Selander D, Dhuner KG, Lundborg G: Peripheral nerve injury caused by injection needles used for regional anesthesia: An experimental study of the acute effects of needle point trauma. Acta Anaesthesiol Scand 1977;21:182-188.

95. Rice AS, McMahon SB: Peripheral nerve injury caused by injection needles used in regional anaesthesia: Influence of bevel configuration, studied in a rat model. Br J Anaesth 1992;69:433-438.

96. Hadzic A, Dilberovic F, Shah S, et al: Combination of intraneural injection and high injection pressure leads to fascicular injury and neurologic deficits in dogs. Reg Anesth Pain Med 2004;29:417-423.

97. Kapur E, Dilberovic F, Zaciragic A, et al: Neurologic and histologic outcome after intraneural injections of lidocaine in canine sciatic nerves. Acta Anaesthesiol Scand 2006;50: 1-7.

98. Claudio R, Hadzic A, Shih H, et al: Injection pressures by anesthesiologists during simulated peripheral nerve block. Reg Anesth Pain Med 2004;29:201-205.

99. Benumof JL: Permanent loss of cervical spinal cord function associated with interscalene block performed under general anesthesia. Anesthesiology 2000;93:1541-1544.

100. Fremling MA, Mackinnon SE: Injection injury to the median nerve. Ann Plast Surg 1996;37:561-567.

101. Bashein G, Robertson HT, Kennedy WF, Jr: Persistent phrenic nerve paresis following interscalene brachial plexus block. Anesthesiology 1985;63:102-104.

102. Lim EK, Pereira R: Brachial plexus injury following brachial plexus block. Anaesthesia 1984;39:691-694.

103. Gillespie JH, Menk EJ, Middaugh RE: Reflex sympathetic dystrophy: A complication of interscalene block. Anesth Analg 1987;66:1316-1317.

104. Upton AR, McComas AJ: The double crush in nerve entrapment syndromes. Lancet 1973;2:359-362.

105. Hebl JR, Horlocker TT, Pritchard DJ: Diffuse brachial plexopathy after interscalene blockade in a patient receiving cisplatin chemotherapy: The pharmacologic double-crush syndrome. Anesth Analg 2001;92: 249-251.

106. Crews JC, Rothman TE: Seizure after levobupivacaine for interscalene brachial plexus block. Anesth Analg 2003;96: 1188-1190.

107. Errando CL, Peiro CM: Cardiac arrest after interscalene brachial plexus block. Acta Anaesthesiol Scand 2004;48: 388-389.

108. Huet O, Eyrolle LJ, Mazoit JX, et al: Cardiac arrest after injection of ropivacaine for posterior lumbar plexus blockade. Anesthesiology 2003;99:1451-1453.

109. Pham-Dang C, Beaumont S, Floch H, et al: [Acute toxic accident following lumbar plexus block with bupivacaine.] Ann Fr Anesth Reanim 2000;19:356-359.

110. Breslin DS, Martin G, Macleod DB, et al: Central nervous system toxicity following the administration of levobupivacaine for lumbar plexus block: A report of two cases. Reg Anesth Pain Med 2003;28:144-147.

111. Mullanu C, Gaillat F, Scemama F, et al: Acute toxicity of local anesthetic ropivacaine and mepivacaine during a combined lumbar plexus and sciatic block for hip surgery. Acta Anaesthesiol Belg 2002;53:221-223.

112. Aida S, Takahashi H, Shimoji K: Renal subcapsular hematoma after lumbar plexus block. Anesthesiology 1996;84:452-455.

113. Pousman RM, Mansoor Z, et al: Total spinal anesthetic after continuous posterior lumbar plexus block. Anesthesiology 2003;98:1281-1282.

114. Weller RS, Gerancher JC, Crews JC, et al: Extensive retroperitoneal hematoma without neurologic deficit in two patients who underwent lumbar plexus block and were later anticoagulated. Anesthesiology 2003;98:581 585.

115. Aveline C, Bonnet F: Delayed retroperitoneal haematoma after failed lumbar plexus block. Br J Anaesth 2004;93: 589-591.

116. Hsu DT: Delayed retroperitoneal haematoma after failed lumbar plexus block. Br J Anaesth 2005;94:395.

117. Klein SM, D'Ercole F, Greengrass RA, et al: Enoxaparin associated with psoas hematoma and lumbar plexopathy after lumbar plexus block. Anesthesiology 1997;87:1576-1579.

118. Todkar M: Sciatic nerve block causing heel ulcer after total knee replacement in 36 patients. Acta Orthop Belg 2005; 71:724-725.

119. Apsingi S, Dussa CU: Can peripheral nerve blocks contribute to heel ulcers following total knee replacement? Acta Orthop Belg 2004;70:502-504.

49 Truncal Blocks

Patrick Narchi, François Singelyn, and Xavier Paqueron

As peripheral nerve blocks of the upper or lower limb, truncal blocks provide excellent postoperative pain relief, avoid the risk of the catastrophic complications associated with central nerve blockade (thoracic epidural analgesia) such as epidural hematoma or abscess, and can be used as an anesthetic technique for different types of surgery. However, their use in daily practice remains limited. Considering the many advantages they offer, the truncal blocks described in this chapter should have a place in the armamentarium of any anesthesiologist involved in the management of postoperative analgesia, particularly in the outpatient setting. In this chapter, we will discuss the following truncal blocks—paravertebral, intercostal, ilioinguinal, iliohypogastric, and genitofemoral, and rectus sheath blocks.

PARAVERTEBRAL NERVE BLOCKADE

The renewed interest for paravertebral blocks in the late 1970s[1] was related to many factors: involvement of the anesthesiologist in postoperative pain control; the development of ambulatory surgery; and the need to use simpler and more reliable techniques that would decrease the need for postoperative intensive care unit (ICU) stay. Paravertebral block is the injection of a local anesthetic close to the vertebra where the spinal nerves exit the intervertebral foramina. This injection leads to a unilateral somatic and sympathetic blockade extending longitudinally above and below the injected interspace. It is indicated for acute pain treatment and chronic unilateral pain syndromes. The paravertebral block provides a unilateral analgesia of the trunk without any major cardiovascular or respiratory effects.

ANATOMY

The paravertebral space is a triangular-shaped space bounded posteriorly by the superior costotransverse ligament, anterolaterally by the parietal pleura, and superiorly and inferiorly by the head and neck of adjacent ribs. This space is in continuity with the epidural space through the intervertebral foramen, with the intercostal space, and with the contralateral paravertebral space anteriorly. It contains the dorsal and ventral rami and the sympathetic chain. Hence,

infiltration of this space with local anesthetic results in unilateral sensory, motor, and sympathetic blockade (Fig. 49–1).

In the paravertebral space, the endothoracic fascia is firmly applied to the ribs and fuses medially on the vertebral body.[2] This fascia thus divides the paravertebral space into two compartments, the anterior extrapleural and the posterior subendothoracic. Naja and colleagues[3] have claimed that there is better longitudinal spread of the local anesthetic when an injection is performed ventral to the endothoracic fascia, whereas an injection dorsal to this fascia leads to a localized spread. However, others, such as Lang, Fitzgerald, and Harmon[4,5] have questioned the importance of such a fascia. Whether the injection of local anesthetics in the low paravertebral thoracic segments may spread to the lumbar levels has been debated by many authors.[2,6-8] Although some authors have questioned the anatomic barrier created by the psoas muscle, others have stressed that the local anesthetic can spread through the posterior insertion of the diaphragm when the solution is injected deeper to the endothoracic fascia[9] or along the lateral border of the psoas muscle.

Technique

As for any regional technique, standard assessment includes electrocardiography, pulse oximetry, and noninvasive blood pressure (NIBP) monitoring.

Position

To facilitate palpating the landmarks, the sitting position is usually preferred. However, the lateral decubitus position is also acceptable during the performance of this block.

Approaches

Different approaches have been suggested in the performance of the block.

Blind Approach
Once the transverse process is contacted (usually at a maximum distance of 4 to 5 cm from the skin), the

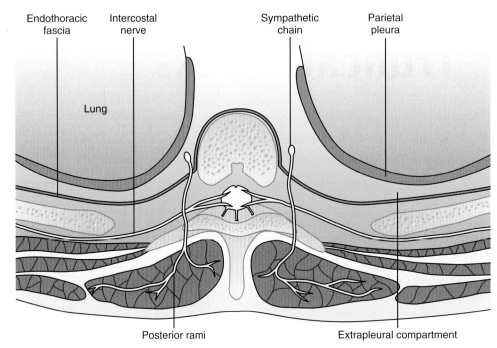

Endothoracic fascia   Intercostal nerve   Sympathetic chain   Parietal pleura

Lung

Posterior rami   Extrapleural compartment

Figure 49–1. Cross section of the paravertebral space at the thoracic level.

needle is withdrawn to the subcutaneous tissue, reoriented caudally (but sometimes cephalad when caudal insertion is impossible because of bone contact), and advanced 1 to 1.5 cm deeper to the transverse process.

Loss of Resistance Approach

Loss of resistance (a syringe filled with saline and/or air is connected to the needle) is felt once the paravertebral space is entered. This may be associated with the blind approach just described.

Nerve Stimulator Approach

This remains a matter of debate.[8] The use of a peripheral nerve stimulator appears to improve the needle-nerve position as assessed by many clinical studies.[3,4,10]

Ultrasound Approach

Ultrasonography has been used to measure the depth of needle insertion during paravertebral block.[11] However, it is not commonly used at present.

Equipment

An 8- to 10-cm needle is needed to perform this block. It can be a 22-gauge spinal , a 19-gauge Touhy epidural, or a stimulating needle connected to a peripheral nerve stimulator.

Puncture Sites

The block has to cover the site of surgical analgesia. At the thoracic level, breast surgery requires blockade of the T1 to T6 dermatomes, whereas thoracotomy requires lower dermatomal blockade (T4 to T10). At the lumbar level, an extensive block (T10 to L2) is needed. Adequate sedation and a local anesthetic infiltration of all puncture sites are mandatory because needle insertion through the different muscular structures and bone contact are painful.

Single-Injection Technique

The needle entry site is marked 2.5 to 3 cm lateral to the cephalad border of each spinous process ipsilateral to the operative side (Fig. 49–2). The needle, attached via an extension tubing to a syringe, is advanced anteriorly in the parasagittal plane until it contacts the transverse process. It is then withdrawn to the subcutaneous tissue and reoriented to walk off the caudad edge of the transverse process. The needle is advanced anteriorly approximately 1 to 1.5 cm deeper to the transverse process. Naja and associates[12] have shown that the distance from skin to the paravertebral space, when confirmed by a nerve stimulator, is longer in the upper and lower thoracic levels compared with the midthoracic level (T4 to T8). In addition, whereas their median needle insertion depth was 55 mm, it was determined that the body mass index (BMI) influences the depth at the upper and lower thoracic levels but not at the midthoracic level.[12] After negative aspiration, 4 to 5 mL of a long-acting local anesthetic (e.g., 0.5% ropivacaine or levobupivacaine) is injected at each level, without exceeding a total volume of 0.3 mL/kg. The onset of sensory loss and surgical anesthesia typically occurs at 10 and 20 to 30 minutes, respectively, after injection. Intraoperative sedation is provided by titrated doses of propofol (20 to 40 µg/kg/min).

Reports have suggested[13-16] that a single-injection technique is as effective as a multiple-injection

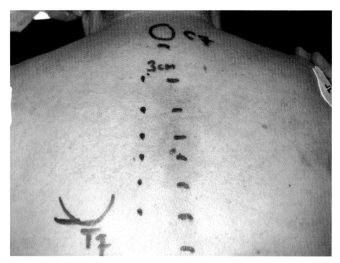

Figure 49–2. Landmarks for high thoracic paravertebral block.

technique (average of five dermatomes blocked) as long as the total volume of 0.3 mL/kg is used. These results were confirmed in a thermographic study by Cheema and coworkers,[17] who showed that a single-injection paravertebral block leads to a unilateral somatic and sympathetic block,[17] and in a volunteer study performed by Saito and colleagues[7] that showed unilateral block after a single-injection technique.[7] It is preferable, however, to use a multiple-injection technique instead of injecting a greater volume through a single-injection site when an extensive spread of local anesthetic is needed[18] because of the risk of bilateral or epidural spread, or both, with large-volume injections.

Catheter Technique

The catheter is inserted 2 to 3 cm once the paravertebral space has been identified. Typically, 20 mL of long-acting local anesthetic is injected as a bolus dose for surgery—an average of six to eight segments are blocked—and followed by a continuous infusion of a dilute long-acting local anesthetic (e.g., 0.125% levobupivacaine or 0.2% ropivacaine) at a rate of 5 mL/hr. Catheters have the advantage of providing surgical anesthesia and postoperative analgesia.[19] Bilateral paravertebral block catheters have been shown to be effective after bilateral thoracotomy in children,[20] major abdominal vascular surgery,[17] and outpatient bilateral reduction mammoplasty.[21]

Drugs and Additives

A bolus dose of 2 mg/kg of ropivacaine can be safely used, as demonstrated in the pharmacokinetic study of Karmakar and associates.[22] They recommended the addition of epinephrine, 1/200,000, to ropivacaine to decrease C_{max}, delay T_{max}, and the bioavailability of the rapid absorption phase. The measured venous plasma concentrations of ropivacaine (2.83 ± 1.31 µg/mL) did not exceed the toxic threshold when a con-

tinuous infusion rate of 0.1 mL/kg/hr of 0.5% solution was used.[23]

Indications

Paravertebral block is associated with a complete loss of somatosensory evoked potentials (SSEPs), which explains the excellent analgesia during and after surgery[24] and its efficacy in reducing the incidence and severity of chronic pain syndrome after surgery.[25] The block has been used effectively for several surgical indications and chronic pain syndromes (Box 49–1).

Major Breast Surgery

In addition to postoperative pain, a high incidence of nausea and vomiting has been reported after general anesthesia during the 24 hours following breast cancer surgery. Paravertebral block results in effective anesthesia for operative procedures of the breast and axilla,[15] reduces postoperative nausea and vomiting, and provides prolonged postoperative sensory block minimizing narcotic requirements. As opposed to a standard analgesic regimen, which requires a single overnight hospital stay, paravertebral block allows discharge on the same day; this can result in a total cost savings of up to 22%.[26]

Paravertebral blocks performed as a multiple-injection technique have been shown to be effective for breast surgery.[13,26] In conjunction with sedation, adequate anesthesia for the vast majority of patients having breast cancer operations is provided.[13] Pusch and coworkers[27] have shown that a single-injection paravertebral block (T4 level) is a good alternative to general anesthesia for breast surgery. It provides adequate intra- and postoperative analgesia as well as early mobilization in 93% of patients. Moreover, Buggy and Michael[28] have shown that the unilateral sympathetic blockade induced by a paravertebral block improves flap tissue oxygenation after breast reconstruction with latissimus dorsi; theoretically, this should improve healing of the flap.

Breast surgery may result in a postmastectomy syndrome. Its incidence varies, from 20% to 50% of patients.[29,30] Many factors, including the severity of postoperative pain, anxiety, and younger age, favor its occurrence. Interestingly, preincisional paravertebral block has been shown to reduce the prevalence of motion-related and chronic pain 1 year after this type of surgery.[31,32] However, it should be noted that, because of specific complications, such as pneumothorax or epidural spread, its risk-benefit ratio does not favor its use for minor breast surgery. Even if paravertebral block provides better pain relief than general anesthesia after such surgery, the relatively low pain scores and the very low incidence of postoperative nausea and vomiting observed with general anesthesia do not warrant the use of paravertebral block in these situations.[33]

Thoracic Surgery

Marret and associates[23] have shown that continuous paravertebral block using 0.5% ropivacaine (0.1 mL/kg/hr) as part of a multimodal approach is more effective in relieving pain at rest and on coughing and results in decreased side effects when compared with IV patient-controlled analgesia (PCA) with morphine. Although thoracic epidural analgesia is still considered the gold standard for postoperative analgesia after thoracic surgery, continuous paravertebral analgesia has been shown to be as effective as epidural analgesia[17,34-39] whether the catheter is inserted blindly by the anesthesiologist or under direct vision by the surgeon before wound closure. Moreover, a paravertebral catheter avoids the potential major risks observed with epidural analgesia, such as epidural hematoma, infection, or spinal cord injury. A recent meta-analysis of thoracic epidural analgesia and paravertebral block after thoracic surgery has shown that although the quality of pain relief is comparable during the first 48 hours postoperatively, the incidence of side effects (e.g., hypotension, urinary retention), failed blocks, and pulmonary complications are significantly lower after paravertebral block.[36] When compared with interpleural analgesia, use of paravertebral block catheters result in better ventilatory parameters, lower respiratory morbidity, and shorter duration of stay.[17] Chronic pain after thoracotomy may occur in 20% to 50% of cases.[40] The occurrence of this syndrome is significantly reduced when effective and intense postoperative pain treatment (e.g., epidural analgesia, paravertebral block) is provided.[41,42]

Cardiac Surgery

Unilateral continuous paravertebral block has been shown to be effective in managing pain after major unilateral thoracic surgeries, such as minimally invasive coronary artery bypass surgery.[43]

Inguinal Hernia Repair

The effectiveness of paravertebral block in providing adequate and long-lasting postoperative pain relief after hernia surgery is well documented in the literature.[10,12,14,18,44-46] In this setting, the paravertebral block should be performed between the T10 and L2 levels. In pediatric surgery, paravertebral block with a mixture of 2% lidocaine, epinephrine, and clonidine provided better postoperative analgesia during the first 48 hours compared with standard general anesthesia.[12] In adults, Hadzic and colleagues[44] have shown that paravertebral block (T9 to L1) using 20 mL of 0.75% ropivacaine is more effective than the combination of general anesthesia and wound infiltration:, resulting in more postanesthesia care unit bypass, less supplemental analgesia, and earlier home discharge.

Multiple Rib Fractures

Paravertebral block provides effective pain relief after multiple rib fractures.[1,2,8,47,48] It can be performed either as a single-shot (bolus of 15 to 20 mL of long-acting local anesthetic) or continuous technique. It has been shown to improve ventilatory parameters and arterial blood gas levels.

Neuralgias and Pleuritic Pain

Paravertebral block has been used to treat chronic pain after thoracotomy or mastectomy. It is effective in relieving pain after thoracic surgery.[1,17,24,50-52] A low thoracic paravertebral block (T9) catheter is effective in relieving severe pleuritic pain after acute pancreatitis.[54]

Contraindications

The contraindications to paravertebral block include local infection, empyema, allergy to local anesthetics, major chest deformity, previous ipsilateral thoracic surgery, and coagulation abnormalities.

Failure Rate

Paravertebral block is an easy technique to learn. Even in inexperienced hands, it rapidly provides a high success rate.[13,51] It has been shown that the success rate is significantly improved after a cutoff of 15 paravertebral blocks. The failure rate with this technique varies, between 6% and 15%, depending on the experience of the operator.[9,13,27,55]

Complications

Many studies[13,17,51,55,56] have described the incidence of complications after paravertebral blocks as varying between 2% and 5%. The complications are shown in Box 49–2. The incidence of hypotension requiring

BOX 49–2. COMPLICATIONS FROM PARAVERTEBRAL BLOCKS

Pneumothorax (0.5%-1.5%)
Hypotension vascular puncture (6%)
Intrathecal spread (1%)
Toxic seizures
Horner's syndrome
Epidural spread

a low dose of a vasopressor, such as ephedrine, is 4%. The hypotension may be the result of sympathetic blockade (unilateral or bilateral) or a vasovagal event during the procedure. Horner's syndrome can result because of the cephalad spread of the local anesthetic after a high thoracic paravertebral block. With regard to epidural spread, dye injection studies have shown the incidence of unilateral epidural spread to be as high as 70%. However, its clinical effects are negligible because of the small amount of local anesthetic injected.[55,57]

INTERCOSTAL NERVE BLOCKADE

Anatomy

The intercostal nerves are the anterior divisions of the thoracic spinal nerves from T1 to T11. They are distributed mainly to the thoracic pleura and abdominal peritoneum. The first two nerves supply fibers to the upper limb in addition to their thoracic branches, the next four are limited in their distribution to the parietal pleura of the thorax, and the lower five supply the parietal pleura of the thorax and abdomen. The seventh intercostal nerve terminates at the xyphoid process. The tenth intercostal nerve terminates at the umbilicus. The 12th thoracic nerve (subcostal) is distributed to the abdominal wall and groin.

First Intercostal Nerve

The anterior division of the first thoracic nerve divides into two branches; one leaves the thorax in front of the neck of the first rib, and enters the brachial plexus; the other, the first intercostal nerve, runs along the first intercostal space and ends on the front of the chest as the first anterior cutaneous branch of the thorax.

Second to Sixth Intercostal (Upper) Nerves

The anterior divisions of the second, third, fourth, fifth, and sixth thoracic nerves are confined to the parietal pleura of the thorax. They pass forward in the intercostal spaces below the intercostal vessels. At the back of the chest, they lie between the pleura and the posterior intercostal membranes, but soon pierce the latter and run between the two planes of intercostal muscles as far as the middle of the rib. They then enter the substance of the intercostales interni, gain the inner surfaces of the muscles, and lie between them and the pleura. Near the sternum, they cross in front of the internal mammary artery and transversus thoracis muscle, pierce the intercostales interni, anterior intercostal membranes, and pectoralis major, and supply the integument of the front of the thorax and over the breast.

About midway between the vertebrae and sternum, they give off lateral cutaneous branches. The anterior division runs forward to the side and the anterior chest, supplying the skin and the breast. The posterior division runs backward and supplies the skin over the scapula and latissimus dorsi. The lateral cutaneous branch of the second intercostal nerve, the intercostobrachial nerve, does not divide into an anterior and posterior branch. It pierces the intercostalis externus and serratus anterior, crosses the axilla to the medial side of the arm, and joins with the medial brachial cutaneous nerve. It supplies the skin of the upper half of the medial and posterior part of the arm.

Intercostal (Lower) Nerves 7 to 11

The anterior divisions of thoracic intercostal nerves 7 to 11 are continued anteriorly from the intercostal spaces into the abdominal wall. They have the same arrangement as the upper intercostal nerves as far as the anterior ends of the intercostal spaces, where they pass behind the costal cartilages and between the obliquus internus and transversus abdominis to the sheath of the rectus abdominis, which they perforate. They supply the skin of the front of the abdomen.

Thoracic Nerve 12

Its anterior division (subcostal nerve) runs along the lower border of the 12th rib, runs in front of the quadratus lumborum, perforates the transversus, and passes forward between it and the obliquus internus to be distributed in the same manner as the lower intercostal nerves. It communicates with the iliohypogastric nerve of the lumbar plexus. Its lateral cutaneous branch perforates the obliquus internus and externus, descends over the iliac crest in front of the lateral cutaneous branch of the iliohypogastric, and is distributed to the skin of the front part of the gluteal region, extending as low as the greater trochanter.

Technique and Drugs

The intercostal nerve block (ICB) is generally performed transcutaneously at the level of the posterior axillary line (Fig. 49–3). The needle is inserted until a bone contact with the rib is obtained. It is then

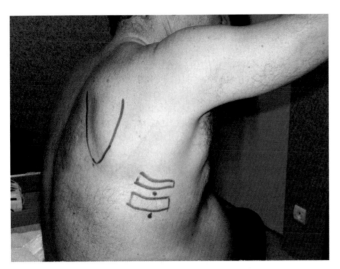

Figure 49–3. Landmarks for intercostal nerve block.

partially withdrawn, reoriented caudally, and advanced less than 0.5 cm deeper than the bone contact. The use of a stimulating needle connected to a peripheral nerve stimulator may be helpful. Eliciting intercostal muscle contractions indicates adequate needle location. Usually, it is preferable to block two proximal and two distal adjacent nerves to the selected level simultaneously to cover all the areas affected by the surgical incision. During thoracotomy, the block may be performed by the surgeon under direct vision at the beginning or more frequently at the end of the operation, before skin closure.

The vast majority of authors use 0.5% bupivacaine as the local anesthetic of choice. In continuous techniques, the rate of infusion is 5 to 7 mL/hr for an average-size adult. Many studies have shown that C_{max} occurs rapidly, within 3 to 20 minutes after the block.[58-60] The administration of 16 mL of 0.5% plain bupivacaine or 1.5% lidocaine with epinephrine results in an acceptable range of local anesthetic plasma concentration (1.44 ± 0.2 µg/mL for bupivacaine and 2.78 ± 0.2 µg/mL for lidocaine).

Indications

The indications for intercostal nerve blocks include the relief of postoperative pain after breast surgery, thoracotomy, video-assisted thoracic surgery, and coronary artery bypass surgery. The blocks have been used for the relief of pain after rib fractures and chronic pain syndromes involving the chest. For minor breast surgery, multiple ICBs (T3 to T6), performed with 0.5% bupivacaine, result in significantly greater quality and duration of postoperative analgesia compared with general anesthesia alone.[58]

Many studies have confirmed the effectiveness of ICB in relieving pain after thoracic surgery.[60-62] It has been noted that ICB performed at five levels with 20 mL of 0.5% bupivacaine results in effective analgesia, similar to thoracic epidural analgesia, during the first 6 hours after thoracotomy. In contrast, inter-

pleural analgesia was found to be ineffective in providing adequate pain relief.[60,62] In a recent prospective study, D'Andrilli and coworkers[63] have observed better pain relief during the first 48 hours postoperatively and better surgical outcome after minithoracotomy when intercostal nerve blocks (a total dose of 20 mL of 0.75% ropivacaine injected at five levels) are added to opioid analgesia. Debreceni and colleagues[64] have shown that continuous intercostal block, with a catheter inserted by the surgeon at the end of surgery, is significantly less effective than thoracic epidural analgesia during the first 12 postoperative hours. Despite the analgesic superiority of thoracic epidural analgesia, the alteration of respiratory parameters was comparable between the groups, suggesting that respiratory disturbances are more likely because of tissue trauma (ribs, muscles, and nerves) than inadequate pain control. A study by Luketich and associates[65] has shown that the combination of IV PCA with a continuous intercostal catheter (inserted by the surgeon) is as effective as thoracic epidural analgesia, with a lower failure rate and avoidance of side effects and serious complications related to epidural analgesia. Thus, continuous intercostal nerve blockade after thoracotomy using an extrapleural catheter results in better pain relief and preservation of pulmonary function compared with systemic narcotics, and appears to be at least as good as an epidural approach.

Video-assisted thoracic surgery is less invasive than open thoracotomy but is still followed by postoperative pain and impairment of lung function.[66] The administration of bilateral ICB of the second, third, and fourth intercostal nerves, under direct vision during surgery, was shown to be safe and effective for reducing postoperative pain and analgesic requirements.[67,68] However, another study[66] was unable to show any difference between intercostal blocks, intrapleural analgesia, and opioid analgesia.

A number of studies have confirmed the efficacy of intercostal nerve blocks in relieving pain and improving ventilatory parameters after multiple rib fractures.[69-71] For minimally invasive coronary bypass surgery, it has been demonstrated that ICB (four levels, 5 mL 0.1% ropivacaine/level), compared with opioid analgesia, provides better pain relief in the early period after surgery and allows an earlier patient discharge to the intermediate care ward.[72] In chronic pain syndromes, case reports have shown significant and long-lasting pain relief, up to 9 months, when intercostal blocks are performed with a high concentration of local anesthetic.[73]

Contraindications and Complications

Contraindications to intercostal nerve blocks include the presence of local infection and contralateral pneumothorax. The major complication of intercostal blocks is pneumothorax. Its incidence is estimated to be 1.4% for each intercostal nerve blocked,[74] with the overall incidence per patient depending on the number of blocks performed.

ILIOINGUINAL, ILIOHYPOGASTRIC, AND GENITOFEMORAL NERVE BLOCKADES

Anatomy

The iliohypogastric (IH) and ilioinguinal (II) nerves originate from the T12 (subcostal nerve) and L1 (ilioinguinal, iliohypogastric) nerve roots of the lumbar plexus. Both nerves pass through the fascia lumborum at the lateral border of the quadratus lumborum muscle and then extend to the area between the obliquus internus abdominis and transversus abdominis muscles. The iliohypogastric nerve is located superiorly and medially to the ilioinguinal nerve. In the area of the anterior superior iliac spine, it bifurcates into the lateral and medial cutaneous rami as its two terminal branches. The lateral cutaneous ramus passes through the obliquus internus abdominis and externus abdominis muscles and provides sensory innervation to the skin in the region of the anterior buttock. The medial cutaneous ramus passes through the obliquus internus abdominis muscle and the aponeurosis of the obliquus externus abdominis muscles and supplies the skin of the abdominal wall region above the symphysis. The ilioinguinal nerve supplies the skin region of the superomedial aspect of the thigh, as well as the anterior region of the scrotum in the male or mons pubis and labium majus in the female.

The genitofemoral (GF) nerve is mainly a sensory nerve. It is formed from L1 to L2 in the substance of the psoas major muscle. At the level of L3 to L4, it emerges on the ventral surface of the muscle along its medial border. It runs downward on the muscular surface and divides into the genital and femoral branches above the inguinal ligament. The genital branch enters the inguinal canal through the deep inguinal ring. It supplies motor fibers to the cremasteric muscle and sensory fibers to the skin over the male scrotum and to the female mons pubis and labia majora. The femoral branch accompanies the external iliac artery and, below the inguinal ligament, remains enveloped by the femoral vascular sheath lateral to the femoral artery. It supplies the skin over the femoral triangle.

Indications

Iliohypogastric and Ilioinguinal Nerve Blocks

In conjunction with genitofemoral nerve blockade, these blocks are indicated as anesthetic and analgesic techniques for inguinal herniorrhaphy, orchiopexy, or hydrocelectomy. Combined IH and II nerve blocks significantly reduce pain scores after inguinal herniorrhaphy and supplemental analgesia after discharge.[75] Compared with spinal anesthesia, general anesthesia and II-IH blocks allow a shorter time to home discharge, lower pain scores at discharge, higher satisfaction scores at 24-hour follow-up, and lower costs.[76,77] The combined blocks have been suggested as an alternative anesthetic technique for strangulated hernia repair in high-risk patients who are unsuitable candidates for general or neuraxial anesthesia.[78] In children, the effectiveness of the blocks appear to be similar to that of caudal blocks.[79,80]

The amount of postoperative IV morphine usage during the first 24 hours after cesarean section has been noted to be significantly reduced after bilateral ilioinguinal nerve blocks.[81] However, there appears to be no difference in the incidence of opioid-related adverse effects.[82] Ilioinguinal nerve blocks have been recommended for patients with persistent pain and paresthesia after inguinal herniorrhaphy, appendectomy, cesarean section, or hysterectomy. Successful relief of symptoms after a diagnostic II nerve block may indicate an ilioinguinal nerve entrapment and surgery may be a suitable treatment.[83,84]

Genitofemoral Nerve Block

In conjunction with ilioinguinal and iliohypogastric nerve blocks, this block is indicated for inguinal herniorrhaphy, orchidopexy, or hydrocelectomy. The benefit of the additional genitofemoral nerve block to II-IH nerve block is limited during the traction of the sac, however; it has no additional postoperative analgesic effect.[85] In addition to femoral nerve block, blockade of the genitofemoral nerve is an efficient anesthetic and analgesic technique for stripping of the long saphenous vein.[86] Finally, isolated genitofemoral nerve block is recommended as a diagnostic procedure in cases of chronic inguinal pain syndrome. Relief of symptoms indicates a genitofemoral neuralgia or nerve entrapment.[84]

Contraindications and Drugs

Local infection and previous II, IH, and/or GF nerve injury are the only contraindications. Bupivacaine has been the most commonly used local anesthetic. However, it is more rapidly absorbed from the injection site and leads to higher plasma concentrations compared with the less cardiotoxic ropivacaine.[87] Thus, ropivacaine or levobupivacaine 0.5% appears to be the more appropriate local anesthetic solution. Both drugs combine a rapid onset of anesthesia and prolonged postoperative analgesia, up to 12 hours.[66,88] The addition of triamcinolone[89] or clonidine[90,91] appears to offer no advantages over plain local anesthetic solution in prolonging the duration of analgesia.

Technique

Ilioinguinal and Iliohypogastric Nerve Blockades

Classic Approach
The patient lies supine. The landmarks are the umbilicus, ipsilateral anterosuperior iliac spine, and pubic tubercle (Fig. 49–4). A line is drawn between the anterior superior iliac spine and the umbilicus, and

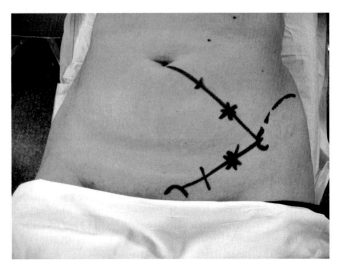

Figure 49–4. Landmarks for ilioinguinal and iliohypogastric nerve blocks.

another line is drawn between the anterior superior iliac spine and the pubic tubercle; both lines are divided into three equal segments. On each line, the site of puncture is located at the junction of the lateral and medial thirds. At both puncture sites, the short bevel needle is inserted at a 50- to 70-degree angle to the skin in an anteroposterior and caudal direction. It is advanced until a loss of resistance is felt, which occurs as the aponeurosis of the external oblique muscle is pierced. After negative aspiration, 5 mL of local anesthetic is injected. The needle is then advanced deeper to pierce the internal oblique muscle aponeurosis, and a similar amount of local anesthetic is administered.

Ultrasound-Guided Technique

The classic approach can be inaccurate and it is not surprising that ilioinguinal-iliohypogastric nerve blocks yield failure rates of 20% to 30%.[92] Furthermore, severe complications, such as intestinal perforation,[93] have been reported. The safety and effectiveness of the blocks can be greatly improved by direct visualization with ultrasonography.[94-96] The ultrasound examination should be performed with a high-frequency linear probe. The ilioinguinal nerve is best visualized immediately medial to the anterior superior iliac spine. It is located at a mean distance of 6 mm from this bony landmark. The iliohypogastric nerve is close (less than 1 cm) to the ilioinguinal nerve and both nerves are located close to the peritoneum.[96] The needle is inserted transverse to the ultrasound probe and placed between the obliquus internus abdominis and transversus abdominis muscles. The volume of local anesthetic required to anesthetize both nerves is 0.075 mL/kg in a child[95] or 0.2 mL/kg in an adult,[96] a dose much smaller than that recommended with the blind technique. The ultrasound-guided technique yields a 96% success rate[94,96] and avoids potential complications such as accidental intestinal puncture.

Genitofemoral Nerve Blockade

With the patient in the supine position, the following landmarks are identified—the pubic tubercle, inguinal ligament, inguinal crease, and femoral artery. The femoral branch of the nerve is blocked by inserting the needle at the lateral border of the femoral artery at the inguinal crease. A fanlike infiltration of the subcutaneous tissue is performed in a medial, caudal, and cephalad direction with 10 to 15 mL of local anesthetic solution. The genital branch of the nerve is blocked by infiltration of 10 mL of local anesthetic just lateral to the pubic tubercle, below the inguinal ligament.

Complications

Transient femoral nerve palsy,[97-100] pelvic[101] or bowel[102] hematoma, and small bowel[103] or colonic[93] puncture have been described. The complications can be avoided when an ultrasound-guided technique is performed. However, additional large-scale studies are required to confirm the safety of the technique.[94,96]

RECTUS SHEATH BLOCKADE

Anatomy

The umbilical area is innervated by the tenth thoracoabdominal intercostal nerves from the right and left sides. Each nerve passes between the transverse abdominis muscle and the internal oblique muscle. It runs between the sheath and the posterior wall of the rectus abdominis muscle and ends as the anterior cutaneous branch supplying the skin of the umbilical area. The rectus abdominis muscles extend between the xyphoid and the pubic tubercle. They are enclosed in the rectus sheath, which is formed by the aponeurosis of the external and internal oblique and transverse muscles.

Indications, Contraindications, and Drugs

The rectus sheath block is indicated as an analgesic technique after umbilical or epigastric hernia repair.[104-106] It also decreases pain after laparoscopy and midline laparotomy.[107,108] Local infection is the only specific contraindication. Bupivacaine has been the most commonly used local anesthetic. Less cardiotoxic drugs, such as ropivacaine or levobupivacaine 0.5%, are currently used, especially when high doses are required.

Technique

Classic Approach
The aim of the block is to inject the local anesthetic solution between the muscle and posterior aspect of the rectus sheath. The needle is inserted 0.5 cm medial to the linea semilunaris in a perpendicular plane, just above or below the umbilicus (Fig. 49–5).

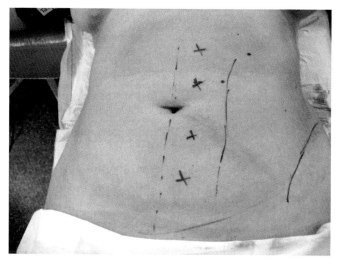

Figure 49–5. Landmarks for rectus sheath block.

The anterior rectus sheath is identified by moving the needle with a back and forth motion until a scratching sensation is felt. The rectus sheath and belly of the muscle are entered. The needle is then further advanced until the posterior aspect of the rectus sheath is appreciated with a scratching sensation as the needle is moved, again with a back and forth motion. Once the sheath is felt, it is entered and, after a negative aspiration test for blood, 10 to 15 mL of local anesthetic is injected on each side.

Ultrasound-Guided Technique

An ultrasound-guided technique has been described. It appears to be beneficial, especially in children, in whom the depth of the posterior rectus sheath is unpredictable. The use of ultrasound has a high success rate, with minimal complications.[107]

Complications

Intravascular injection is a potential complication. A case of retroperitoneal hematoma has been reported.[109]

SUMMARY

- Paravertebral block provides excellent pain relief after thoracotomy and major breast surgery. A continuous catheter technique could be used in this setting. The incidence of side effects and complications remains low compared with parenteral or thoracic epidural analgesia.
- Intercostal blocks are effective for relieving pain after unilateral thoracic or abdominal surgery. However, the need to block multiple intercostal nerves limits their wider use in clinical practice.
- Minor blocks, such as ilioinguinal, iliohypogastric, and rectus sheath blocks, are helpful in managing postoperative pain after ambulatory procedures such as inguinal or umbilical hernia repair. These blocks have a low incidence of complications and side effects.

References

1. Eason MJ, Wyatt R: Paravertebral thoracic block—a reappraisal. Anaesthesia 1979;34:638-642.
2. Karmakar MK, Chung DC: Variability of a thoracic paravertebral block: Are we ignoring the endothoracic fascia? Reg Anesth Pain Med 2000;25:325-327.
3. Naja MZ, Ziade MF, El Rajab M, et al: Varying anatomical injection points within the thoracic paravertebral space: Effect on spread of solution and nerve blockade. Anaesthesia 2004;59:459-463.
4. Lang SA: The use of a nerve stimulator for thoracic paravertebral block. Anesthesiology 2002;7:521.
5. Fitzgerald K, Harmon D: Thoracic paravertebral blockade. Anaesthesia 2004;59:1028-1029.
6. Lonnqvist PA: Continuous paravertebral block in children: Initial experience. Anaesthesia 1992;47:607-609.
7. Saito T, Den S, Cheema SP, et al: A single-injection, multi-segmental paravertebral block-extension of somatosensory and sympathetic block in volunteers. Acta Anaesthesiol Scand 2001;45:30-33.
8. Karmakar MK: Thoracic paravertebral block. Anesthesiology 2001;95:771-780.
9. Najarian MM, Johnson JM, Landercasper J, et al: Paravertebral block: An alternative to general anesthesia in breast cancer surgery. Am Surg 2003;69:213-8.
10. Naja MZ, el Hassan MJ, Oweidat M, et al: Paravertebral blockade vs general anesthesia or spinal anesthesia for inguinal hernia repair. Middle East J Anesthesiol 2001;16:201-210.
11. Pusch F, Wildling E, Klimscha W: Sonographic measurement of needle insertion depth in paravertebral blocks in women. Br J Anaesth 2000;85:841-843.
12. Naja MZ, Gustafsson AC, Ziade MF, et al: Distance between the skin and the thoracic paravertebral space. Anaesthesia 2005;60:680-684.
13. Coveney E, Weltz CR, Greengrass R, et al: Use of paravertebral block anesthesia in the surgical management of breast cancer: Experience in 156 cases. Ann Surg 1998;227:496-501.
14. Weltz CR, Klein SM, Arbo JE, et al: Paravertebral block anesthesia for inguinal hernia repair. World J Surg 2003;27:425-429.
15. Klein SM, Bergh A, Steele SM, et al: Thoracic paravertebral block for breast surgery. Anesth Analg 2000;90:1402-1405.
16. Greengrass R, O'Brien F, Lyerly K, et al: Paravertebral block for breast cancer surgery. Can J Anaesth 1996;43:858-861.
17. Cheema SP, Ilsley D, Richardson J, et al: A thermographic study of paravertebral analgesia. Anaesthesia 1995;50:118-121.
18. Buckenmaier CC, Steele SM, Nielsen KC, et al: Paravertebral somatic nerve blocks for breast surgery in a patient with hypertrophic obstructive cardiomyopathy. Can J Anaesth 2002;49:571-574.
19. Boezaart AP, Raw RM: Continuous thoracic paravertebral block for major breast surgery. Reg Anesth Pain Med 2006;31:470-476.
20. Karmakar MK, Booker PD, Franks R: Bilateral continuous paravertebral block used for postoperative analgesia in an infant having bilateral thoracotomy. Paediatr Anaesth 1997;7:469-471.
21. Buckenmaier CC, Steele S, Nielsen KC: Bilateral continuous paravertebral catheters for reduction mammoplasty. Acta Anaesthesiol Scand 2002;46:1042-1045.
22. Karmakar MK, Ho AM, Law BK, et al: Arterial and venous pharmacokinetics of ropivacaine with and without epinephrine after thoracic paravertebral block. Anesthesiology 2005;103:704-711.
23. Marret E, Bazelly B, Taylor G, et al: Paravertebral block with ropivacaine 0.5% versus systemic analgesia for pain relief after thoracotomy. Ann Thorac Surg 2005;79:2109-2113.
24. Richardson J, Jones J, Atkinson R: The effect of thoracic paravertebral blockade on intercostal somatosensory evoked potentials. Anesth Analg 1998;87:373-376.
25. Richardson J, Sabanathan S, Mearns A: Post-thoracotomy neuralgia. The Pain Clinic 1994;7:87-97.

26. Weltz CR, Greengrass RA, Lyerly HK: Ambulatory surgical management of breast carcinoma using paravertebral block. Ann Surg 1995;222:19-26.

27. Pusch F, Freitag H, Weinstabl C, et al: Single-injection paravertebral block compared to general anaesthesia in breast surgery. Acta Anaesthesiol Scand 1999;43:770-774.

28. Buggy DJ, Michael K: Paravertebral analgesia with levobupivacaine increases postoperative flap tissue oxygen tension after immediate latissimus dorsi breast reconstruction compared with intravenous opioid analgesia. Anesthesiology 2004;100:375-380.

29. Perkins FM, Kehlet H: Chronic pain as an outcome of surgery. Anesthesiology 2000;93:1123-1133.

30. Tasmuh T, Kataja M, Blomqvist C: Treatment-related factors predisposing to chronic pain in patients with breast cancer. Acta Oncologica 1997;36:625-630.

31. Kairaluoma PM, Bachmann MS, Rosenberg PH, et al: Preincisional paravertebral block reduces the prevalence of chronic pain after breast surgery. Anesth Analg 2006;103:703-708.

32. Iohom G, Abdalla H, O'Brien J, et al: The associations between severity of early postoperative pain, chronic postsurgical pain and plasma concentration of stable nitric oxide products after breast surgery. Anesth Analg 2006;103:995-1000.

33. Terheggen MA, Wille F, Borel Rinkes IH, et al: Paravertebral blockade for minor breast surgery. Anesth Analg 2002;94:355-359.

34. Richardson J, Sabanathan S, Jones J, et al: A prospective, randomized comparison of preoperative and continuous balanced epidural or paravertebral bupivacaine on post-thoracotomy pain, pulmonary function and stress responses. Br J Anaesth 1999;83:387-392.

35. Kelly FE, Murdoch JA, Sanders DJ, et al: Continuous paravertebral block for thoraco-abdominal oesophageal surgery. Anaesthesia 2005;60:98-99.

36. Davies RG, Myles PS, Graham JM: A comparison of the analgesic efficacy and side-effects of paravertebral vs epidural blockade for thoracotomy—a systematic review and meta-analysis of randomized trials. Br J Anaesth 2006;96:418-426.

37. Downs CS, Cooper MG: Continuous extrapleural intercostal nerve block for post-thoracotomy analgesia in children. Anaesth Intensive Care 1997;25:390-397.

38. Eng J, Sabanathan S: Continuous paravertebral block for postthoracotomy analgesia in children. J Pediatr Surg 1992;27:556-557.

39. Karmakar MK, Booker PD, Franks R, et al: Continuous extrapleural paravertebral infusion of bupivacaine for postthoracotomy analgesia in young infants. Br J Anaesth 1996;76:811-5.

40. Dajczman E, Gordon A, Kreisman H: Long-term postthoracotomy pain. Chest 1991;99:270–274.

41. Tiipana E, Nilsson E, Kalso E: Post-thoracotomy pain after thoracic epidural analgesia: A prospective follow-up study. Acta Anaesthesiol Scand 2003;47:433-438.

42. Senturk M, Ozca P, Talu G: The effects of three different analgesia techniques on long-term postthoracotomy pain. Anesth Analg 2002;94:11-15.

43. Dhole S, Mehta Y, Saxena H, et al: Comparison of continuous thoracic epidural and paravertebral blocks for postoperative analgesia after minimally invasive direct coronary artery bypass surgery. J Cardiothorac Vasc Anesth 2001;15:288-292.

44. Hadzic A, Kerimoglu B, Loreio D, et al: Paravertebral blocks provide superior same-day recovery over general anesthesia for patients undergoing inguinal hernia repair. Anesth Analg 2006;102:1076-1081.

45. Naja ZM, El-Rajab M, Al-Tannir MA, et al: Thoracic paravertebral block: Influence of the number of injections. Reg Anesth Pain Med 2006;31:196-201.

46. Wassef MR, Randazzo T, Ward W: The paravertebral nerve root block for inguinal herniorrhaphy—a comparison with the field block approach. Reg Anesth Pain Med 1998;23:451-456.

47. Gilbert J, Hultman J: Thoracic paravertebral block: A method of pain control. Acta Anaesthesiol Scand 1989;33:142-145.

48. Karmakar MK, Critchley LA, Ho AM, et al: Continuous thoracic paravertebral infusion of bupivacaine for pain management in patients with multiple fractured ribs. Chest 2003;123:424-431.

49. Nair V, Henry R: Bilateral paravertebral block: A satisfactory alternative for labour analgesia. Can J Anaesth 2001;48:179-184.

50. Ferrandiz M, Aliaga L, Catala E, et al: Thoracic paravertebral block in chronic postoperative pain. Reg Anesth 1994;19:221-222.

51. Kirvela O, Antila H: Thoracic paravertebral block in chronic postoperative pain. Reg Anesth 1992;17:348-350.

52. Antila H, Kirvela O: Neurolytic thoracic paravertebral block in cancer pain: A clinical report. Acta Anaesthesiol Scand 1998;42:581-585.

53. Culp WC, McCowan TC, DeValdenebro M, et al: Paravertebral block: An improved method of pain control in percutaneous transhepatic biliary drainage. Cardiovasc Intervent Radiol 2006;29:1015-1021.

54. Paniagua P, Catala E, Villar-Landeira JM: Successful management of pleuritic pain with thoracic paravertebral block. Reg Anesth Pain Med 2000;25:651-653.

55. Lonnqvist PA, MacKenzie J, Soni AK, et al: Paravertebral blockade: Failure rate and complications. Anaesthesia 1995;50:813-815.

56. Tenicela R, Pollan SB: Paravertebral-peridural block technique: A unilateral thoracic block. Clin J Pain 1990;6:227-234.

57. Purcell-Jones G, Pither CE, Justins DM: Paravertebral somatic nerve block: A clinical, radiographic, and computed tomographic study in chronic pain patients. Anesth Analg 1989;68:32-39.

58. Atanassoff PG, Alon E, Weiss BM: Intercostal nerve block for lumpectomy: Superior postoperative pain relief with bupivacaine. J Clin Anesth 1994;6:47-51.

59. Moore DC, Mather LE, Bridenbaugh LD: Arterial and venous plasma levels of bupivacaine following peripheral nerve blocks. Anesth Analg 1976;55:763–8.

60. Bachmann-Mennenga B, Biscoping J, Kuhn DF, et al: Intercostal nerve block, interpleural analgesia, thoracic epidural block or systemic opioid application for pain relief after thoracotomy? Eur J Cardiothorac Surg 1993;7:12-18.

61. Galway JE, Caves PK, Dundee JW: Effect of intercostal nerve blockade during operation on lung function and the relief of pain following thoracotomy. Br J Anaesth 1975;47:730-735.

62. Perttunen K, Nilsson E, Heinonen J, et al: Extradural, paravertebral and intercostal nerve blocks for post-thoracotomy pain. Br J Anaesth 1995;75:541-547.

63. D'Andrilli A, Ibrahim M, Ciccone AM, et al: Intrapleural intercostal nerve block associated with mini-thoracotomy improves pain control after major lung resection. Eur J Cardiothorac Surg 2006;29:790-794.

64. Debreceni G, Molnar Z, Szelig L, et al: Continuous epidural or intercostal analgesia following thoracotomy: A prospective randomized double-blind clinical trial. Acta Anaesthesiol Scand 2003;47:1091-1095.

65. Luketich JD, Land SR, Sullivan EA, et al: Thoracic epidural versus intercostal nerve catheter plus patient-controlled analgesia: A randomized study. Ann Thorac Surg 2005;79:1845-1849.

66. Leger R, Ohlmer A, Scheiderer U, et al: Pain therapy after thoracoscopic interventions: Do regional analgesia techniques (intercostal block or interpleural analgesia) have advantages over intravenous patient-controlled opioid analgesia (PCA)? Chirurg 1999;70:682-689.

67. Bolotin G, Lazarovici H, Uretzky G, et al: The efficacy of intraoperative internal intercostal nerve block during video-assisted thoracic surgery on postoperative pain. Ann Thorac Surg 2000;70:1872-1875.

68. Temes RT, Won RS, Kessler RM, et al: Thoracoscopic intercostal nerve blocks. Ann Thorac Surg 1995;59:787-788.

69. Seddon SJ, Doran BR: Alternative method of intercostal blockade: A preliminary study of the use of an injector gun for intercostal nerve blockade. Anaesthesia 1981;36:304-306.

70. Watson DS, Panian S, Kendall V, et al: Pain control after thoracotomy: Bupivacaine versus lidocaine in continuous extrapleural intercostal nerve blockade. Ann Thorac Surg 1999;67:825-828.

71. Osinowo OA, Zahrani M, Softah A: Effect of intercostal nerve block with 0.5% bupivacaine on peak expiratory flow rate and arterial oxygen saturation in rib fractures. J Trauma 2004;56:345-347.

72. Behnke H, Geldner G, Cornelissen J, et al: Postoperative pain therapy in minimally invasive direct coronary arterial bypass surgery: IV opioid patient-controlled analgesia versus intercostal block. Anaesthesist 2002;51:175-179.

73. Doi K, Nikai T, Sakura S, et al: Intercostal nerve block with 5% tetracaine for chronic pain syndromes. J Clin Anesth 2002;14:39-41.

74. Shanti CM, Carlin AM, Tyburski JG: Incidence of pneumothorax from intercostal nerve block for analgesia in rib fractures. J Trauma 2001;51:536-539.

75. Ding Y, White P: Post-herniorrhaphy pain in outpatients after pre-incision ilioinguinal-hypogastric nerve block during monitored anaesthesia care. Can J Anaesth 1995;42:12-15.

76. Yilmazlar A, Bilgel H, Donmez C, et al: Comparison of ilioinguinal-hypogastric nerve block versus spinal anesthesia for inguinal herniorrhaphy. South Med J 2006;99:48-51.

77. Song D, Greilich NB, White P, et al: Recovery profiles and costs of anesthesia for outpatient unilateral inguinal herniorrhaphy. Anesth Analg 2000;91:876-881.

78. Carré P, Mollet J, Le Poultel J, et al: Ilio-inguinal iliohypogastric nerve block with a single puncture: An alternative for anesthesia in emergency inguinal surgery. Ann Fr Anesth Reanim 2001;20:643-646.

79. Markham S, Tomlinson J, Hain W: Ilioinguinal nerve block in children: A comparison with caudal block for intra- and postoperative analgesia. Anaesthesia 1986;41:1098-1103.

80. Findlow D, Aldridge LM, Doyle E: Comparison of caudal block using bupivacaine and ketamine with ilioinguinal nerve block for orchidopexy in children. Anaesthesia 1997;52:1110-1113.

81. Ganta R, Samra SK, Maddineni VR, et al: Comparison of the effectiveness of bilateral ilioinguinal nerve block and wound infiltration for postoperative analgesia after caesarean section. Br J Anaesth 1994;72:229-230.

82. Bell A JB, Olufolabi A, Dexter F, et al: Iliohypogastric-ilioinguinal nerve block for post-Cesarean delivery analgesia decreases morphine but not opioid-related side effects. Can J Anesth 2002;49:694-700.

83. Starling J, Harms BA, Schroeder M, et al: Diagnosis and treatment of genitofemoral and ilioinguinal entrapment neuralgia. Surgery 1987;102:581-586.

84. Harms BA, DeHaas DR, Starling JR: Diagnosis and management of genitofemoral neuralgia. Arch Surg 1984;119:339-341.

85. Sasaoka N, Kawaguchi M, Yoshitani K, et al: Evaluation of genitofemoral nerve block, in addition to ilioinguinal and iliohypogastric nerve block, during inguinal hernia repair in children. Br J Anaesth 2005;94:243-246.

86. Vloka JD, Hadzi A, Mulcare R, et al: Femoral nerve block versus spinal anesthesia for outpatients undergoing long saphenous vein stripping surgery. Anesth Analg 1997;84:749-752.

87. Ala-Kokko TI, Karinen J, Raiha E, et al: Pharmacokinetics of 0.75% ropivacaine and 0.5% bupivacaine after ilioinguinal-iliohypogastric nerve block in children. Br J Anaesth 2002;89:438-441.

88. Gunter JB, Gregg T, Varughese AM, et al: Levobupivacaine for ilioinguinal/iliohypogastric nerve block in children. Anesth Analg 1999;89:647-679.

89. McCleane G, Mackle E, Stirling I: The addition of triamcinolone acetonide to bupivacaine has no effect on the quality of analgesia produced by ilioinguinal nerve block. Anaesthesia 1994;49:819-820.

90. Kaabachi O, Zerelli Z, Methamem M, et al: Clonidine administered as adjuvant for bupivacaine in ilioinguinal-iliohypogastric nerve block does not prolong postoperative analgesia. Paediatr Anaesth 2005;15:586-590.

91. Beaussier M, Weickmans H, Abdelhalim Z, Lienhart A: Inguinal herniorrhaphy under monitored anesthesia care with ilioinguinal-iliohypogastric block: The impact of adding clonidine to ropivacaine. Anesth Analg 2005;101:1659-1662.

92. Ho AM, Lim HS, Yim AP, et al: The resolution of ST segment depressions after high right thoracic paravertebral block during general anesthesia. Anesth Analg 2002;95:227-228.

93. Johr M, Sossai R: Colonic puncture during ilioinguinal nerve block in a child. Anesth Analg 1999;88:1051-1052.

94. Willschke H, Marhofer P, Bösenberg A, et al: Ultrasonography for ilioinguinal/iliohypogastric nerve blocks in children. Br J Anaesth 2005;95:226-230.

95. Willschke H, Bosenberg A, Marhofer P, et al: Ultrasonographic-guided ilioinguinal/iliohypogastric nerve block in pediatric anesthesia: What is the optimal volume? Anesth Analg 2006;102:1680-1684.

96. Eichenberger U, Greher M, Kirchmair L, et al: Ultrasound-guided blocks of the ilioinguinal and iliohypogastric nerve: Accuracy of a selective new technique confirmed by anatomical dissection. Br J Anaesth 2006;97:238-243.

97. Shivashanmugam T, Kundra P, Sudhakar S: Iliac compartment block following ilioinguinal iliohypogastric nerve block. Paediatr Anaesth 2006;16:1084-1086.

98. Rosario DJ, Jacob S, Luntley J, et al: Mechanism of femoral nerve palsy complicating percutaneous ilioinguinal field block. Br J Anaesth 1997;78:314-316.

99. Hadzic A, Vloka JD, Saff GN, et al: The "three-in-one block" for treatment of pain in a patient with acute herpes zoster infection. Reg Anesth 1997;22:575-578.

100. Derrick JL, Aun CS: Transient femoral nerve palsy after ilioinguinal block. Anaesth Intensive Care 1996;24:115.

101. Vaisman J: Pelvic hematoma after an ilioinguinal nerve block for orchialgia. Anesth Analg 2001;92:1048-1049.

102. Frigon C, Mai R, Valois-Gomez T, et al: Bowel hematoma following an iliohypogastric-ilioinguinal nerve block. Paediatr Anaesth 2006;16:993-996.

103. Amory C, Mariscal A, Guyot E, et al: Is ilioinguinal/iliohypogastric nerve block always totally safe in children? Paediatr Anaesth 2003;13:164-166.

104. Courreges P, Poddevin F, Lecoutre D: Para-umbilical block: A new concept for regional anaesthesia in children. Paediatr Anaesth 1997;7:211-214.

105. Ferguson S, Thomas V, Lewis I: The rectus sheath block in paediatric anaesthesia: New indications for an old technique? Paediatr Anaesth 1996;6:463-466.

106. Isaac LA, McEwen J, Hayes JA, et al: A pilot study of the rectus sheath block for pain control after umbilical hernia repair. Paediatr Anaesth 2006;16:406-409.

107. Azemati S, Khosravi MB: An assessment of the value of rectus sheath block for postlaparoscopic pain in gynecologic surgery. J Minim Invasive Gynecol 2005;12:12-15.

108. Yentis SM, Hills-Wright P, Potparic O: Development and evaluation of combined rectus sheath and ilioinguinal blocks for abdominal gynaecological surgery. Anaesthesia 1999;54:475-479.

109. Yuen PM, Ng PS: Retroperitoneal hematoma after a rectus sheath block. J Am Assoc Gynecol Laparosc 2004;11:448.

50 Neurolysis of the Sympathetic Axis for Cancer Pain Management

Oscar de Leon-Casasola

Neurolytic blocks of sympathetic axis were procedures that were once widely used for the control of upper abdominal or pelvic pain in patients with cancer. However, recent studies have suggested that these blocks are not effective in treating pain that is not visceral in origin. Consequently, when there is evidence of disease outside the viscera, which in the simplest form translates to lymphadenopathy, the success rate decreases significantly. Moreover, a controlled randomized study has shown that even in the best case scenario, the duration of full pain control is no longer than 2 months. Thus, we should reconsider our indications for these procedures and, when indicated, they should be performed early in the course of the disease.

Stretching, compressing, invading, or distending visceral structures can result in a poorly localized noxious visceral pain. Patients experiencing visceral pain often describe the pain as vague, deep, squeezing, crampy, or colicky. Other signs and symptoms include referred pain (e.g., shoulder pain that appears when the diaphragm is invaded with tumor) and nausea and vomiting caused by vagal irritation.

Visceral pain associated with cancer may be relieved by oral pharmacologic therapy that includes combinations of nonsteroidal anti-inflammatory drugs (NSAIDs), opioids, and coadjuvant therapy. In addition to pharmacologic therapy, neurolytic blocks of the sympathetic axis are also effective in controlling visceral cancer pain and should be considered as important adjuncts to pharmacologic therapy for the relief of severe visceral pain. These blocks rarely eliminate cancer pain because patients frequently experience somatic and neuropathic pain as well. Therefore, oral pharmacologic therapy must be continued for the majority of patients with advanced stages of their disease. The goals of performing a neurolytic block of the sympathetic axis are to maximize the analgesic effects of opioid or nonopioid analgesics and reduce the dosage of these agents to alleviate side effects.

Because neurolytic techniques have a narrow risk-benefit ratio, undesirable side effects and complications from neurolytic blocks can be minimized by sound clinical judgment and by assessment of the potential therapeutic effect of the technique on each patient. This chapter will discuss pertinent information regarding neurolysis of the celiac plexus block, superior hypogastric block, and ganglion impar.

CELIAC PLEXUS BLOCK

The celiac plexus is situated retroperitoneally in the upper abdomen. It is at the level of the T12 and L1 vertebrae, anterior to the crura of the diaphragm. The celiac plexus surrounds the abdominal aorta and the celiac and superior mesenteric arteries. The plexus is composed of a network of nerve fibers from the sympathetic and parasympathetic systems. It contains two large ganglia that receive sympathetic fibers from the three splanchnic nerves (greater, lesser, and least). The plexus also receives parasympathetic fibers from the vagus nerve. Autonomic nerves supplying the liver, pancreas, gallbladder, stomach, spleen, kidneys, intestines, and adrenal glands, as well as blood vessels, arise from the celiac plexus.

Neurolytic blocks of the celiac plexus have been used for malignant and chronic nonmalignant pain. In patients with acute or chronic pancreatitis, the celiac plexus block has been used with variable success.[1] Similarly, patients with cancer in the upper abdomen who have a significant visceral pain component have responded well to this block.[2]

Three approaches to block nociceptive impulses from the viscera of the upper abdomen include the retrocrural (or classic) approach, anterocrural approach, and neurolysis of the splanchnic nerves.[3] Regardless of the approach, the needle(s) are inserted at the level of the first lumbar vertebra, 5 to 7 cm from the midline. Then, the tip of the needle is directed toward the upper third of the body of L1 for the retro-

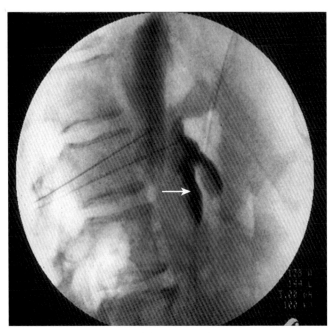

Figure 50–1. Neurolysis of the celiac plexus. Retrocrural versus anterocrural tip needle positions in the lateral view are shown. Note that the tip of the needle is in the upper third of L1 and about 1 cm beyond its anterior border for a retrocrural technique. Moreover, the contrast medium spread is cephalad. In contrast, the tip of the needle is in the lower third of L1 and about 3 cm beyond its anterior border for an anterocrural technique. In this case, the contrast medium spread occurs caudad. Note the inferior spread and distribution of contrast in front of the aorta (*arrow*).

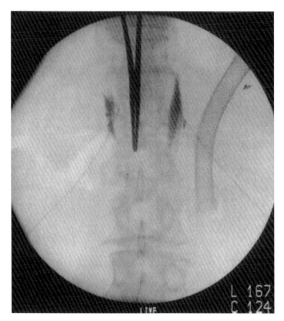

Figure 50–2. Neurolysis of the splanchnic nerves. Needle positioning is shown in the anteroposterior view. Note that the contrast medium spread is limited to the lateral portion of T12.

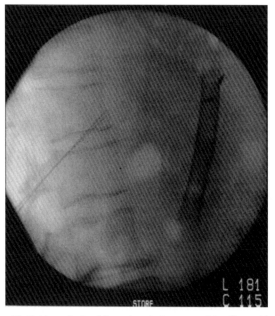

Figure 50–3. Neurolysis of the splanchnic nerves. Needle positioning is shown in the lateral view. Note that the tip of the needle is advanced until it is at the same level of the anterior border of T12 to avoid potential pleural puncture.

crural approach and the lower third of the body of L1 for an anterocrural technique (Fig. 50–1). In the case of the retrocrural approach, the tip of the needle is advanced no more than 0.5 cm anterior to the anterior border of L1. In the case of the anterocrural approach, the tip of the needle is advanced through the aorta on the left side until no more blood flow is noted through the needle, which is why the anterocrural approach is also known as the transaortic approach. In the case of splanchnic nerve block, the needle is directed toward the body of T-12 (Fig. 50–2). Perfect needle positioning in this case is achieved when the tip of the needle is at the anterior portion of the T12 vertebral body in the lateral view (Fig. 50–3).

More recently, computed tomography (CT) and ultrasound techniques have allowed pain specialists to perform neurolysis of the celiac plexus via a transabdominal approach. This approach is frequently used when patients are unable to tolerate the prone or lateral decubitus position or when their liver is so enlarged that a posterior approach is not feasible. Moreover, CT guidance will allow an anterocrural technique to be performed without piercing the aorta, adding an element of safety in this case (see later, "Complications").

Drugs and Dosing

For neurolytic blocks using the retrocrural or anterocrural approaches, 50% to 100% alcohol is used.

Injected by itself, alcohol can produce severe pain. Thus, it is recommended first to inject 5 to 10 mL of 0.25% bupivacaine, 3 to 5 minutes prior to the injection of alcohol or at the time of the injection, by diluting 100% alcohol to a 50% concentration with the same amount of local anesthetic (0.25% bupivacaine). Phenol in a 10% final concentration may also be used; this has the advantage of being painless on injection, and both agents seem to have the same clinical efficacy. The dose of alcohol or phenol administered varies with the approach to be used. For the retrocrural approach, 20 to 25 mL of alcohol is used on each side. Consequently, the need to inject this high volume precludes the use of phenol in the retrocrural approach. For the anterocrural approach, 8 to 10 mL of either neurolytic agent is used per side. For splanchnic nerve blocks, 6 to 8 mL of phenol per side is recommended.

Complications

Complications associated with celiac plexus blocks appear to be related to the technique used—retrocrural,[4] transcrural,[5] or transaortic.[6] In a prospective randomized study of 61 patients with cancer of the pancreas, Ischia and colleagues[3] compared the efficacy and incidence of complications associated with these three approaches with celiac plexus neurolysis. Orthostatic hypotension occurred more often when the retrocrural (50%) or splanchnic (52%) technique was used, suggesting an associated sympathetic chain neurolysis. In contrast, the anterocrural approach produced a 10% incidence of hypotension. Conversely, transient diarrhea was more frequent with the anterocrural approach (65%) than with the splanchnic nerve block technique (5%) but not the retrocrural approach (25%). The incidence of dysesthesia, interscapular back pain, reactive pleurisy, hiccups, or hematuria was not statistically different among the three groups.

The incidence of complications from neurolytic celiac plexus blocks was evaluated by Davis[7] in 2730 patients having blocks performed from 1986 to 1990. The overall incidence of major complications (e.g., paraplegia, bladder and bowel dysfunction) was 1 in 683 procedures. However, the report did not describe which approach or approaches were used to perform the blocks.

Following are several considerations in the diagnosis and management of specific complications.

Malposition of the needle is avoided with radiologic imaging prior to the injection of a neurolytic agent, because the tip of the needle may be intravascular, in the peritoneal cavity, or in a viscus. Imaging techniques currently used include biplanar fluoroscopy, CT, or ultrasound guidance. However, no study has evaluated the superiority of one technique over the others. Wong and Brown[8] have suggested that the use of radiologic imaging does not alter the quality of the block or the incidence of complications; this was based on a retrospective study of 136 patients with pancreatic cancer pain treated with a celiac plexus block with or without radiologic control of the position of the needle's tip. However, it is unclear how many of those patients had radiologic imaging. Assuming that 50% of patients did not, the upper 95% confidence interval (CI) for complications is 5%.[9]

Orthostatic hypotension may occur up to 5 days after the block. Treatment includes bed rest, avoidance of sudden changes in position, and replacement of fluids. Once compensatory vascular reflexes are fully activated, this side effect disappears. Wrapping the lower extremities from the toes to the upper thighs with elastic bandages has been successful in patients who developed orthostatic hypotension; they were then able to walk during the first week after the block.

Backache may result from local trauma during needle placement, resulting in a retroperitoneal hematoma, or from alcohol irritation of the retroperitoneal structures. Patients with a backache should have at least two hematocrit measurements at a 1-hour interval. If there is a decrease in the hematocrit value, radiologic imaging is indicated to rule out a retroperitoneal hematoma. A urinalysis positive for red blood cells suggests renal injury.

Retroperitoneal hemorrhage is rare; however, in patients who present with orthostatic hypotension, the possibility of hemorrhage must be ruled out before assuming that it is a physiologic response to the block. Patients who present with backache and orthostatic hypotension after a celiac plexus block should be admitted to the hospital for serial hematocrit monitoring. If the hematocrit level is low or decreasing, patients should undergo radiologic evaluation to rule out injury to the kidneys, aorta, or other vascular structures. A surgical consult should be obtained as soon as feasible.

Diarrhea may occur as a result of sympathetic block of the bowel. Treatment includes hydration and antidiarrheal agents. Oral loperamide is a good choice, although any anticholinergic agent may be used. Matson and colleagues[10] have reported near-fatal dehydration from diarrhea following this block. In debilitated patients, diarrhea must be treated aggressively.

Abdominal aortic dissection has also been reported.[11,12] The mechanism of aortic injury is direct damage by the needle during performance of the block. As expected, the anterocrural approach is more frequently associated with this complication. Thus, this approach should be avoided if atherosclerotic disease of the abdominal aorta is present.

Paraplegia and *transient motor paralysis* have occurred after celiac plexus block.[13-19] These neurologic complications may occur because of a spasm of the lumbar segmental arteries that perfuse the spinal cord.[20] In fact, canine lumbar arteries undergo contraction when exposed to both low and high concentrations of alcohol.[20] Thus, these data suggest that alcohol should not be used if there is evidence of significant atherosclerotic disease of the aorta, because the circulation to the spinal cord may also be impaired and is only dependent on lumbar artery flow. However, there was also a report of paraplegia after phenol use,[13] thus suggesting that other factors (e.g., direct vascular or neurologic injury or retrograde spread to the spinal cord) may be involved. These complications further support the need for the use of radiologic imaging during performance of these blocks.

Efficacy

To date, only three randomized controlled trials[3,21,22] and one prospective study[23] have evaluated the efficacy of celiac plexus neurolysis in pain caused by cancer of the upper abdomen. In a prospective randomized study, Ischia and associates[3] have evaluated the efficacy of three different approaches to celiac plexus neurolysis in pancreatic cancer. Of 61 patients with pancreatic cancer pain, 29 (48%) experienced *complete* pain relief after the neurolytic block. The remaining 32 patients (52%) required further therapy for residual visceral pain caused by technical failure in 15 patients and neuropathic or somatic pain in 17 patients. The second trial,[21] which compared the procedure with oral pharmacologic therapy in 20 patients, concluded that neurolytic celiac plexus block (NCPB) results in an equal reduction in the Visual Analogue Pain Scale (VAPS) as therapy with a combination of NSAIDs and opioids. However, opioid consumption was significantly lower in the group of patients who underwent neurolysis when compared with the group receiving oral pharmacologic therapy during the 7 weeks of the study. Moreover, the incidence of side effects was higher in patients who received oral pharmacologic therapy when compared with those who underwent neurolysis block. Regarding the third randomized, controlled study by Wong and coworkers,[22] the authors are to be congratulated for designing and completing this study. Their results are welcome in light of a lack of properly designed comparative studies between neurolytic techniques and comprehensive medical management (CMM). However, there are several issues in the design and the results of this study that need to be highlighted:

1. Patients enrolled in the study did not have severe pain at study entry. Mean pain scores at baseline were 4.4 ± 1.7 in the NCPB group and 4.1 ± 1.8 in the CMM group. This is a surprising finding in patients with this type of malignancy, and may reflect ethnic and racial differences in pain perception and reporting by the population enrolled in the study.

2. Although the authors reported a significant statistical reduction in pain scores 1 week after therapy when comparing the NCPB group with the CMM group, the difference between the two groups may not be clinically important. Patients assigned to the NCPB group reported mean pain scores of 2.1 ± 1.4, whereas those randomized to the CMM group reported pain scores of 2.7 ± 2.1 during that interval. Moreover, a statistical difference was noted when the percentage reduction from baseline for the NCPB and the CMM group was analyzed separately (53% reduction from baseline for the NCPG group, $P = 0.05$, versus the 27% reduction observed in the CMM group, $P = 0.01$).

3. In analyzing these results, it is critically important to note that most patients (93%) used opioids during the first week of therapy, with similar amounts of opioids being administered to the two treatment groups. In fact, opioid consumption increased over time, with no differences between groups at the different intervals during the study. Moreover, the incidence of side effects was no different between the two treatment groups at any point in time.

4. Similarly, quality-of-life measurements and the physical and functional well-being subscales of the Functional Assessment of Cancer Therapy-Pancreatic Cancer (FACT-PA) did not differ between the two groups at any evaluation point.

Two important questions stem from these results:

1. Can the authors actually conclude that the major finding of the study is that NCPB significantly improves pain relief in patients with advanced pancreatic cancer compared with those who received optimized CMM?

2. Based on these results, is it justifiable to submit a patient with advanced pancreatic cancer to an NCPB, considering the potential side effects and complications associated with this procedure?

In response to the first question, I do not believe that the authors can conclude that NCPB significantly improves pain relief in patients with advanced pancreatic cancer. This is partly because the levels of analgesia achieved by the patients assigned to either group after 1 week of therapy can be considered clinically acceptable. Additionally, the only statistical difference was found when the authors analyzed the percentage reduction of pain from baseline by each of the treatment groups. Thus, I do not believe that, based on these results, I would recommend NCPB to a patient with advanced pancreatic cancer, because complications do occur, as has been noted.

Considering these reservations, should NCPB not be performed in patients with pancreatic malignancies? As with every clinical study, the results of Wong and colleagues[22] only applied to the population studied and under the conditions of the study protocol design. The critical issue is that all patients had nonresectable disease, which suggests that patients were likely to have other pain components, such as somatic or neuropathic pain, or both, which are not responsive to NCPB.[3] This is because neurolytic blocks of the sympathetic axis are effective in treating visceral pain only. Moreover, previous studies have suggested that when there is evidence of disease outside the pancreas, such as celiac or portal adenopathy, or both, the success rate of this block decreases significantly.[24] In the study by De Cicco and associates,[23] long-lasting pain relief was described in 9/9 patients (95% CI, 60 to 100) when contrast medium spread in the four quadrants and in 10/21 patients (95% CI, 26 to 70) when contrast spread was in three quadrants. None of the 75 patients with contrast spread in one or two quadrants experienced long-lasting pain relief.[24] Thus, the presence of adenopathy because of metastasis is a poor prognostic factor to success of the block.

The results of the study by Wong and coworkers[22] further support the notion that NCPB should not be performed in patients with advanced unresectable carcinomas of the pancreas. This block should be reserved for those patients without evidence of disease outside the viscera, in which it is guaranteed that the patient has a visceral pain component only.

A prospective nonrandomized study[24] compared 41 patients treated according to the World Health Organization (WHO) guidelines for cancer pain relief with 21 patients treated with a neurolytic celiac plexus block. It was concluded that this technique can play an important role in managing pancreatic cancer pain.

Because one of the three randomized controlled studies compared different approaches to the celiac plexus and had no control group,[3] and the other study compared the procedure with an analgesic drug,[21] it is not possible to estimate the success rate of this technique. In contrast, the results of a meta-analysis that evaluated the results of 21 retrospective studies in 1145 patients concluded that adequate to excellent pain relief can be achieved in 89% of patients during the first 2 weeks following the block.[25] Partial to complete pain relief continued in approximately 90% of the patients who were alive at the 3-month interval and in 70% to 90% of the patients during the 3-month interval before death. Moreover, the efficacy was similar in patients with pancreatic cancer compared with those with other intra-abdominal malignancies of the upper abdomen. However, these results are based on retrospective evaluations that may not yield reliable information or may be subject to publication bias. In addition, the statistical techniques used for the analysis must take into account factors such as the heterogeneity produced by the patients' selection criteria, technical differences in the performance of the blocks, choice of neurolytic agents and doses used, diversity in the tools for the evaluation of pain, and goals of therapy. Thus, the meta-analysis must be interpreted with caution, because the report may be overly enthusiastic.

New Perspectives

As previously discussed, oral pharmacologic therapy with opioids, NSAIDs, and coadjuvants is frequently used for the treatment of cancer pain. However, the evidence suggests that chronic use of high doses of opioids may have a negative effect on immunity.[26] Thus, analgesic techniques that lower opioid consumption may have a positive effect on patient outcomes. In a prospective, randomized trial, Lillemoe and colleagues[27] have shown that patients with non-resectable cancer of the pancreas who receive a splanchnic neurolysis live longer than patients who do not. These findings may be the result of lower opioid use in the neurolysis patients who not only had better preserved immune functions, but also experienced fewer side effects (e.g., nausea and vomiting), thus allowing them to eat better. Although the study by Wong and associates[22] did not show that patients randomized to the neurolytic arm of the

study lived longer, this may be explained by their high intake of opioids during the study period, thus negating the effect of the blocks. Consequently, the effects of this procedure on long-term survival are unclear.

SUPERIOR HYPOGASTRIC PLEXUS BLOCK

Cancer patients with tumor extension into the pelvis may experience severe pain unresponsive to oral or parenteral opioids. Also, excessive sedation or other side effects may limit the acceptability and usefulness of oral opioid therapy. Therefore, a more invasive approach is needed to control pain and improve the quality of life for these patients.

Pelvic pain associated with cancer and chronic nonmalignant conditions may be alleviated by blocking the superior hypogastric plexus.[28,29] Analgesia to the organs in the pelvis is possible because the afferent fibers innervating these structures travel in the sympathetic nerves, trunks, ganglia, and rami. Thus, a sympathectomy for visceral pain is analogous to a peripheral neurectomy or dorsal rhizotomy for somatic pain. One study[29] has suggested that visceral pain is an important component of the cancer pain syndrome experienced by patients with cancer of the pelvis, even in advanced stages. Thus, percutaneous neurolytic blocks of the superior hypogastric plexus should be considered more often for patients with advanced stages of pelvic cancer.

The superior hypogastric plexus is situated in the retroperitoneum, bilaterally extending from the lower third of the fifth lumbar vertebral body to the upper third of the first sacral vertebral body. The technique for the blockade has been described elsewhere.[28-30] The patient is placed in the prone position, with a pillow under the pelvis to flatten the lumbar lordosis. Two 7-cm needles are inserted, with the bevel directed medially 45 and 30 degrees caudad so that the tips lay anterolateral to the L5-S1 intervertebral disk space. Aspiration is important to avoid injection into the iliac vessels. If blood is aspirated, a transvascular approach can be used (see later, "Complications"). Accurate placement of needle is verified by biplanar fluoroscopy. Anteroposterior (AP) views should reveal the tip of the needle at the level of the junction of the L5 and S1 vertebral bodies. This is an important safety step to avoid potential spread of the neurolytic agent toward the L5 roots (see later, "Complications"). Lateral views will confirm placement of the needle's tip just beyond the vertebral body's anterolateral margin. The injection of 3 to 5 mL of water-soluble contrast medium is used to verify accurate needle placement and to rule out intravascular injection. In the AP view, the spread of contrast should be confined to the midline region. In the lateral view, a smooth posterior contour corresponding to the anterior psoas fascia indicates that the needle is at the appropriate depth. For a prognostic hypogastric plexus blockade or for patients with noncancer-related pain, local anesthetic alone is used. For therapeutic purposes in patients with

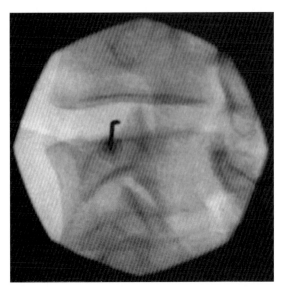

Figure 50–4. Transdiskal positioning of the needle at L5-S1 for superior hypogastric plexus block (oblique view).

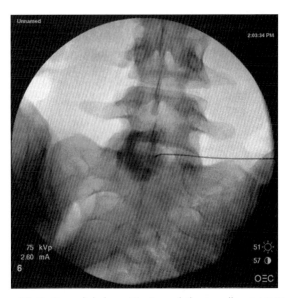

Figure 50–6. Transdiskal positioning of the needle at L5-S1 for superior hypogastric plexus block (anteroposterior view).

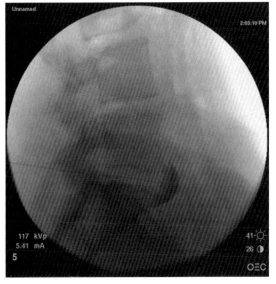

Figure 50–5. Transdiskal positioning of the needle at L5-S1 for superior hypogastric plexus block (lateral view).

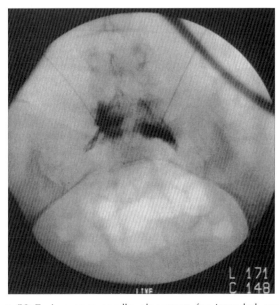

Figure 50–7. Improper needle placement for intended superior hypogastric neurolysis. Note that the contrast medium spread is to the L5 nerve root.

cancer-related pain, phenol is typically used as the neurolytic solution.

Mastering this technique is not easy, because the transverse process of L5 makes it difficult to access the anterior portion of the L5-S1 region. Consequently, a transdiskal approach has been suggested (Figs. 50–4 to 50–6). However, this approach may be associated with the inherent risks of puncturing the intervertebral disk.

Complications

The combined experience of more than 200 cases from the Mexican Institute of Cancer, Roswell Park Cancer Institute, and M.D. Anderson Cancer Center has indicated that neurologic complications have not

occurred as a result of this block.[30] However, extreme care should be exercised, because placing the tip of the needle in the upper middle of L5 may be associated with retrograde spread to the nerve roots. If the spread is not recognized, the injection of neurolytic agents could result in predicted neurologic deficit (Figs. 50–7 and 50–8).

Efficacy

The effectiveness of the block was originally demonstrated by a significant decrease in pain via VAPS scores. In their study, Plancarte and coworkers[28] showed that the block is effective in reducing VAPS

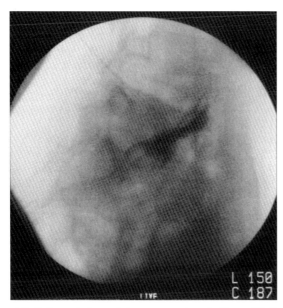

Figure 50–8. Lateral view of the same patient in Figure 50–7.

scores in 70% of patients with pelvic pain associated with cancer. Most of the enrolled patients had cervical cancer. In a subsequent study,[29] 69% of patients experienced a decrease in VAPS scores. Moreover, a mean daily opioid morphine reduction of 67% was seen in the success group (736 ± 633 reduced to 251 ± 191 mg/day), and 45% in the failure group (1443 ± 703 reduced to 800 ± 345 mg/day).[29] In a more recent multicenter study,[30] 159 patients with pelvic pain associated with cancer were evaluated. Overall, 115 patients (72%) had satisfactory pain relief after one or two neurolytic procedures. Mean opioid use decreased by 40%, from 58 ± 43 to 35 ± 18 mg/day of morphine equivalents 3 weeks after treatment in all patients studied. This decrease in opioid consumption was significant for both the success group (56 ± 32 reduced to 32 ± 16 mg/day) and the failure group (65 ± 28 reduced to 48 ± 21 mg/day).[30] Success was defined in the two studies as the ability to reduce opioid consumption by at least 50% in the 3 weeks following the block and a decrease in the VAPS scores.[29,30]

In a case report, Rosenberg and colleagues[31] have reported on the efficacy of superior hypogastric plexus block in a patient with severe chronic non-malignant penile pain after transurethral resection of the prostate. Although the patient did not receive a neurolytic agent, a diagnostic block performed with 0.25% bupivacaine and 20 mg of methylprednisolone acetate was effective in relieving the pain for more than 6 months. The usefulness of this block in chronic benign pain conditions has not been adequately documented.

GANGLION IMPAR BLOCK

The ganglion impar is a solitary retroperitoneal structure located at the level of the sacrococcygeal junction. This unpaired ganglion marks the end of the two sympathetic chains. Visceral pain in the perineal area associated with malignancies may be effectively treated with neurolysis of the ganglion impar (Walther's).[32] Patients who will benefit from this block frequently present with a vague, poorly localized pain that is frequently accompanied by sensations of burning and urgency. However, the clinical value of this block is unclear, because the published experienced is limited.

Anatomy

The ganglion impar is a solitary retroperitoneal structure located anteriorly to the sacrococcygeal junction. This ganglion marks the end of the two sympathetic chains and is the only unpaired autonomic ganglion in the body. Ganglion impar has gray nerve fiber communication from the ganglion to the spinal nerve, but appears to lack white nerve fibers, which communicate the spinal nerves to the ganglion in the thoracic and upper lumbar regions.[32] Visceral afferents innervating the perineum, distal rectum, anus, distal urethra, vulva, and distal third of the vagina converge at the ganglion impar. The original technique was described by Plancarte and associates.[32] The technique requires the patient to be positioned in the lateral decubitus position, with the hips fully flexed. A standard 22-gauge, 3.5-inch spinal needle is bent 1 inch from its hub to form a 30-degree angle. The needle is then introduced under local anesthesia through the anococcygeal ligament, with its concavity oriented posteriorly; under fluoroscopic guidance, it is directed along the midline at or near the sacrococcygeal junction while placing a finger in the rectum to avoid puncturing this structure. Retroperitoneal location is verified by observation of the spread of 2 mL of water-soluble contrast medium. An alternative needle geometry, bending the needle to the shape of an arc, has been proposed by Nebab and Florence.[33]

An easier technique is the trans-sacrococcygeal approach,[34] in which the tip of the needle is directly placed into the retroperitoneal space by inserting a 20-gauge, 1.5 inch needle through the sacrococcygeal ligament under fluoroscopic guidance, so that the tip of the needle is just anterior to the anterior portion of the sacrum. This technique avoids the invasion of more caudal structures (rectum) with the needle and avoids the need to insert a finger in the rectal lumen.

For diagnostic blocks, local anesthetic alone is used. For neurolytic blocks, phenol 6% is recommended. Cryoablation of the ganglion impar has been also described for repeated procedures via a trans-sacrococcygeal approach in a patient with chronic benign pain after abdominoperineal resection.[35]

Efficacy

Three studies have evaluated the efficacy of ganglion impar block in a prospective, nonrandomized, noncontrolled fashion. Plancarte and colleagues[32] have evaluated 16 patients with advanced cancer (cervical, 9; colon, 2; bladder, 2; rectum, 1; endometrial cancer, 2) and persistent pain despite treatment (pharmacologic management resulted in a 30% global reduction in pain). Localized perineal pain was present in all cases, characterized as burning and urgent in 8 patients and of mixed character in 8 patients. Pain was referred to the rectum (7 patients), perineum (6 patients), or vagina (3 patients). After a neurolytic block with a transanococcygeal approach, 8 patients reported complete pain relief, whereas the remainder experienced significant pain reduction (60% to 90%). Blocks were repeated in 2 patients and follow-up was carried out for 14 to 120 days, depending on survival.

Swofford and Ratzman[36] have reported on the efficacy of the trans-sacrococcygeal approach. Twenty patients with perineal pain unresponsive to previous intervention were studied, 18 with a bupivacaine-steroid block and 2 with a neurolytic block. In the bupivacaine-steroid group, 5 patients reported complete (100%) pain relief, 10 patients reported more than 75% pain reduction, and 3 patients reported more than 50% pain reduction. Both neurolytic blocks resulted in complete pain relief. Duration of the pain relief varied from 4 weeks to long-term relief.

Vranken and colleagues[37] have studied the effect of the ganglion impar block in long-lasting, treatment-resistant coccydynia. Twenty patients, 17 women and 3 men, with a diagnosis of coccydynia (spontaneous, 7; fracture, 3; injury, 10) received a 5-mL injection of 0.25% bupivacaine. There was no pain reduction or increase in quality of life associated with the procedure. Thus, based on this study, it would appear that this block is ineffective for the treatment of coccydynia.

Complications

Although there is always the risk of damaging adjacent structures to the ganglion impar, there have been no complications reported from this technique. Plancarte and associates[38] have reported one case in which epidural spread of contrast within the caudal canal was observed. In this case, needle repositioning resolved the problem. Although published experience is limited and criteria to predict success or failure is unavailable, patients with poorly localized perineal pain, with a burning character, are considered candidates for the block. The procedure is considered safe.

CONCLUSION

Neurolysis of the celiac plexus or splanchnic nerves, superior hypogastric plexus, or ganglion impar may be used for patients with visceral pain of the upper abdomen, pelvis, and perineal region, respectively. The presence of disease in the corresponding lymph nodes is a marker of poor prognosis for these blocks. The incidence of reported complications is low.

However, they may occur and have significant implications for the quality of life of the patient. Thus, strict adherence to the technique is important to prevent potential problems. Again, the use of this technique in patients who do not have a significant visceral pain component is unwarranted.

References

1. Rykowski JJ, Hilgier M: Continuous celiac plexus block in acute pancreatitis. Reg Anesth 1995;20:528-532.
2. Wong GY, Brown DL: Regional anesthetic techniques for the management of cancer pain. In Urmey W (ed): Techniques in Regional Anesthesia and Pain Management, vol 1. Philadelphia, WB Saunders, 1997, pp 18-26.
3. Ischia S, Ischia A, Polati E, et al: Three posterior percutaneous celiac plexus block techniques: A prospective randomized study in 61 patients with pancreatic cancer pain. Anesthesiology 1992;76:534-540.
4. Singler RC: An improved technique for alcohol neurolysis of the celiac plexus block. Anesthesiology 1982;56:137-141.
5. Hilgier M, Rykowski JJ: One-needle transcrural celiac plexus block: Single shot, or continuous technique, or both. Reg Anesth 1994;19:277-283.
6. Ischia S, Luzzani A, Ischia A, et al: A new approach to the neurolytic block of the coeliac plexus: The transaortic technique. Pain 1983;16:333-341.
7. Davis DD: Incidence of major complications of neurolytic coeliac plexus block. J R Soc Med 1993;86:264-266.
8. Wong GY, Brown DL: Celiac plexus block for cancer pain. In Urmey W (ed): Techniques in Regional Anesthesia and Pain Management, vol 1. Philadelphia, WB Saunders, 1997, pp 18-26.
9. Hanley JA, Lippman-Hand A: If nothing goes wrong, is everything all right? Interpreting zero numerators. JAMA 1983;249:1743-1745.
10. Matson JA, Ghia JN, Levy JH: A case report of a potentially fatal complications associated with Ischia's transaortic method of celiac plexus block. Reg Anesth 1985;10:193-196.
11. Sett SS, Taylor DC: Aortic pseudoaneurysm secondary to celiac plexus block. Ann Vasc Surg 1991;5:88-91.
12. Kaplan R, Schiff-Keren B, Alt E: Aortic dissection as a complication of celiac plexus block. Anesthesiology 1995;83:632-635.
13. Galizia EJ, Lahiri SK: Paraplegia following coeliac plexus block with phenol: Case report. Br J Anaesth 1974;46:539-540.
14. Lo JN, Buckley JJ: Spinal cord ischemia a complication of celiac plexus block. Reg Anesth 1982;7:66-68.
15. Cherry DA, Lamberty J: Paraplegia following coeliac plexus block. Anaesth Intens Care 1984;12:59-61.
16. Woodham MJ, Hanna MH: Paraplegia after coeliac plexus block. Anaesthesia 1989;44:487-489.
17. van Dongen RT, Crul BJ: Paraplegia following coeliac plexus block. Anaesthesia 1991;46:862-863.
18. Jabbal SS, Hunton J: Reversible paraplegia following coeliac plexus block. Anaesthesia 1992;47:857-858.
19. Wong GY, Brown DL: Transient paraplegia following alcohol celiac plexus block. Reg Anesth 1995;20:352-355.
20. Brown DL, Rorie DK: Altered reactivity of isolated segmental lumbar arteries of dogs following exposure to ethanol and phenol. Pain 1994;56:139-143.
21. Mercadante S: Celiac plexus block versus analgesics in pancreatic cancer pain. Pain 1993;52:187-192.
22. Wong G, Schoeder DR, Carns PE, et al: Effect of neurolytic celiac plexus block on pain relief, quality of life, and survival in patients with unresectable pancreatic cancer. JAMA 2004;291:1092-1099.
23. De Cicco M, Matovic M, Bortolussi R et al: Celiac plexus block: Injectate spread and pain relief in patients with regional anatomic distortions. Anesthesiology 2001;94:561-565.
24. Ventafridda GV, Caraceni AT, Sbanotto AM, et al: Pain treatment in cancer of the pancreas. Eur J Surg Oncol 1990; 16:1-6.

25. Eisenberg E, Carr DB, Chalmers TC: Neurolytic celiac plexus block for treatment of cancer pain: A meta-analysis. Anesth Analg 1995;80:290-295.
26. Yeager MP: Morphine inhibits spontaneous and cytokine-enhanced natural killer cell cytotoxicity in volunteers. Anesthesiology 1995;83:500-508.
27. Lillemoe KD, Cameron JL, Kaufman HS, et al: Chemical splanchnicectomy in patients with unresectable pancreatic cancer: A prospective randomized trial. Ann Surg 1993;217:447-457.
28. Plancarte R, Amescua C, Patt RB, et al: Superior hypogastric plexus block for pelvic cancer pain. Anesthesiology 1990;73:236-239.
29. de Leon-Casasola OA, Kent E, Lema MJ: Neurolytic superior hypogastric plexus block for chronic pelvic pain associated with cancer. Pain 1993;54:145-151.
30. Plancarte R, de Leon-Casasola OA, El-Helaly M, et al: Neurolytic superior hypogastric plexus block for chronic pelvic pain associated with cancer. Reg Anesth 1997;22:562-568.
31. Rosenberg SK, Tewari R, Boswell MV, et al: Superior hypogastric plexus block successfully treats severe penile pain after transurethral resection of the prostate. Reg Anesth Pain Med 1998;23:618-620.
32. Plancarte R, Amescua C, Patt RB: Presacral blockade of the ganglion of Walther (ganglion impar). Anesthesiology 1990;73:A751.
33. Nebab EG, Florence IM: An alternative needle geometry for interruption of the ganglion impar. Anesthesiology 1997;86:1213-1214.
34. Wemm KJ, Sabersky L: Modified approach to block the ganglion impar (ganglion of Walther). Reg Anesth 1995;20:544-545.
35. Loev MA, Varklet VL, Wilsey BL: Cryoablation: A novel approach to neurolysis of the ganglion impar. Anesthesiology 1998;88:1391-1393.
36. Swofford JB, Ratzman DM: A transarticular approach to blockade of the ganglion impar (ganglion of Walther). Reg Anesth Pain Med 1998;23(Suppl 3):103.
37. Vranken JH, Bannink IMJ, Zuurmond WWA: Invasive procedures in patients with coccygodynia: Caudal epidural infiltration, pudendal nerve block and blockade of the ganglion impar. Reg Anesth Pain Med 2000;25(Suppl 2):25.
38. Plancarte R, Velazquez R, Patt RB: Neurolytic blocks of the sympathetic axis. In Patt RB (ed): Cancer Pain. Philadelphia, Lippincott-Raven, 1993, pp 419-442.

CHAPTER
51 Neuraxial Anesthesia

Daniel T. Warren and Spencer S. Liu

More than a century has passed since Corning injected cocaine between the spinous processes of a dog, delivering perhaps the first neuraxial anesthetic. Spinal anesthesia has been used clinically since 1898, when Augustus Bier used the technique for lower extremity orthopedic surgery. The use of epidural anesthesia for labor pain maintained the interest of the medical community amidst the rapid advancement of general anesthesia in the middle of the last century. Further progress in continuous catheter techniques, use of neuraxial anesthetic adjuvants, and enhanced safety of neuraxial anesthesia has provided opportunities for advancing care for our patients.

ANATOMY

Vertebrae, Intervertebral Disks, and Ligaments

The neural structures of the spinal cord are housed by the bony vertebral column comprised of 7 cervical, 12 thoracic, 5 lumbar, 5 fused sacral, and 4 fused coccygeal vertebrae. The cervical and lumbar lordosis and thoracic kyphosis of the normal spine allow functional spinal movements and appropriate distribution of mechanical forces. A typical vertebra is comprised of a cylindric vertebral body joined via the pedicles to the posterior elements—the laminae, spinous process, transverse processes, and superior and inferior articular processes. The regional characteristics of the vertebrae are pertinent to the techniques used to access the neuraxis in clinical situations. Relevant features of represen-tative thoracic and lumbar vertebrae are shown in Figure 51–1.

Between the end plates of successive vertebral bodies are the intervertebral disks, consisting of the outer annulus fibrosus and inner nucleus pulposus. Further structural support comes from the anterior and posterior longitudinal ligaments running along the ventral and dorsal aspects of the vertebral bodies, respectively. Along with the more superficial supraspinous ligament, the deeper interspinous ligament joins the spinous processes to one another. The ligamentum flavum connects adjacent lamina, thus forming the posterior wall of the spinal canal. The embryologic origin of this ligament is from two (right and left) individual neural crest structures. These ligaments are expected to join in the midline, but have an inconsistent extent of fusion. Sagittal gaps result from incomplete fusion, which are variable not only among individuals, but also among spinal levels within a given patient. Cervical and upper thoracic levels show a higher rate of sagittal gaps in the ligamentum flavum (Table 51–1) compared with levels below T3-4 (as high as 50% to 70%), and are thus perhaps more troublesome for relying on loss of resistance techniques for epidural access.[1]

Neural Structures

The spinal cord begins at the base of the brainstem and continues caudad, terminating as the conus medullaris, typically at the level of L1-2 in the adult. At each spinal level, the ventral and dorsal roots of the spinal nerves are formed from the converging rootlets from the respective aspects of the cord. The spinal cord and portions of the spinal nerves are bathed in the cerebrospinal fluid (CSF), which is secreted mainly by the choroid plexuses located on the roofs of the lateral, third, and fourth ventricles. Normal daily production of CSF is approximately 550 mL. CSF is reabsorbed mainly through the arachnoid villi and, to a much lesser extent, through the epidural veins of the vertebral column. It typically has a density range of 1.00028 to 1.00100 g/mL.[2]

The spinal cord, nerve roots, and CSF are enveloped by three membranes, the pia mater, arachnoid mater, and the dura mater, which are contiguous with the coverings of the brain by the same names. The innermost of these is the highly permeable and vascular pia mater, which intimately lines the surface of the cord and nerve roots. The arachnoid mater approximates the outermost membrane, the dura mater. Within the boundaries of the arachnoid is the subarachnoid space, containing the CSF, trabecular network, and dentate ligaments. The subarachnoid space, with the accompanying CSF, extends laterally as far as the dorsal root ganglion with the dural nerve root sleeves. The spinal dura mater begins at the level of the foramen magnum, where it is contiguous with cranial dura. It extends caudally to the level of S2 in most adults, where the dura fuses with the filum terminale (extension of the pia), and coccygeal periosteum. Between the dura mater and arachnoid mater

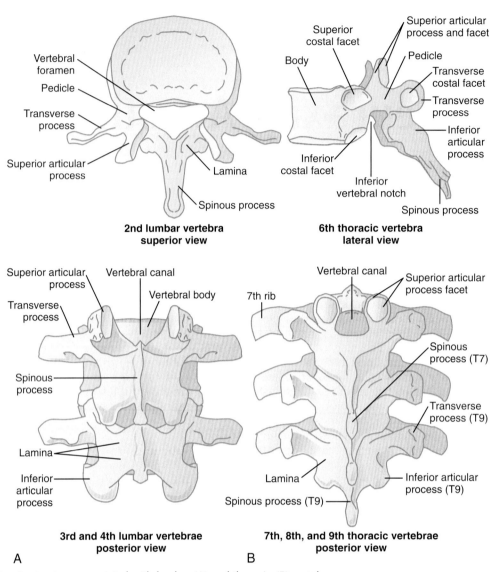

Figure 51–1. Anatomic structures associated with lumbar **(A)** and thoracic **(B)** vertebrae.

Table 51–1. Rates of Incomplete Fusion of Ligamentum Flavum

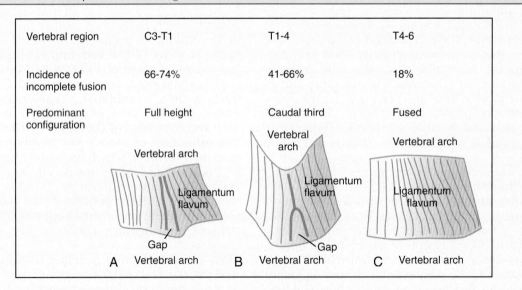

Vertebral region	C3-T1	T1-4	T4-6
Incidence of incomplete fusion	66-74%	41-66%	18%
Predominant configuration	Full height	Caudal third	Fused

A, Gaps spanning the full height of the midline are more common in the cervical region.
B, Caudal gaps are predominant in the upper thoracic interspaces.
C, Complete fusion is more reliable below T4.
Data summarized from Lirk P, Kolbitsch C, Putz C: Cervical and high thoracic ligamentum flavum frequently fails to fuse in the midline. Anesthesiology 2003;99:1387-1390.

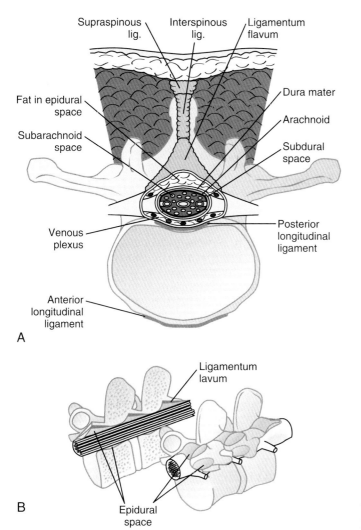

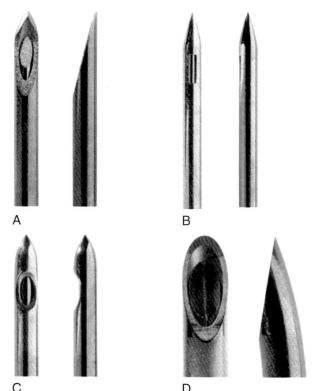

Figure 51–3. Close-up views of the tips of a cutting tip spinal needle, Quincke **(A),** and two pencil point needles, Whitacre **(B)** and Gertie-Marx **(C).** Also shown is the tip of a common epidural needle, a 17-gauge Tuohy **(D).**

Figure 51–2. A, Cross-sectional view of the lumbar region depicting the location of the epidural space and other anatomic structures associated with neuraxial procedures. **B,** The epidural space is somewhat compartmentalized but is continuous via potential space pathways that expand with injection of liquid.

resides the subdural space, which contains little more than a small amount of serous fluid. This space is often implicated in some occurrences of failed spinal anesthetics and total spinal following intended epidural administration of local anesthetic solutions.

Epidural Space

The epidural space (Fig. 51–2) is bordered by the posterior longitudinal ligament and vertebral lamina, with adjoining ligamentum flavum. The spinal epidural space runs from the level of the foramen magnum to the sacral hiatus, where it is bound by the sacrococcygeal ligament. The lateral borders of the epidural space are partially delineated by the vertebral pedicles, but this space extends laterally through the intervertebral foramina to communicate with the paravertebral spaces on each side. Although the epidural space is somewhat compartmentalized by the sections of the dura abutting the ligamentum

flavum, vertebral lamina, and other borders of the vertebral canal, these compartments are joined by a potential space. The contents of the epidural space include epidural fat, venous plexus, and segmental arteries. The plexus of epidural veins (Batson's plexus) is predominantly within the anterior and lateral portions of the epidural space, with rare presence in the posterior aspect. The epidural fat, principally located in the posterior and lateral aspects of the epidural space, provides a site for depot sequestration of epidurally administered local anesthetics and opioids related to the lipid solubility of the drug.[3]

EQUIPMENT

Spinal Needles

Several needle designs have been used throughout the history of spinal anesthesia, but the needles in common practice today are classified as cutting needles or pencil point needles (Fig. 51–3). The Quincke style needle, one of the most frequently used cutting needles, has a medium-length bevel, coming to a sharp point, which cuts through dural and arachnoid structures as it passes to the subarachnoid space. In contrast, the Green, Whitacre, Sprotte, and Gertie-Marx pencil point needles (often called atraumatic) have a rounded, noncutting tip. The latter three have openings on the side rather than at the tip. Needle gauge usually ranges from 27 to 18, with the smaller gauge needles requiring an introducer needle. Efforts to minimize the incidence of postdural puncture headache have driven the advancement of needle design. More recent designs include tapered needles and the reintroduction of stylet-point needles, such as the Ballpen needle (Rusch, Betschdorf, France).

Epidural Needles and Catheters

Needles used for accessing the epidural space are designed to facilitate catheter insertion and techniques for identification of the epidural space. Presently, the most commonly used needle is the Tuohy style needle (see Fig. 51–3D), characterized by a curved Huber tip. This curved tip decreases coring of tissue during insertion, but has been used mainly to attain directional control of catheter insertion. Epidural needles are typically 16 to 20 gauge and are accompanied by a tight-fitting stylet. Larger gauge needles are less likely to be deflected by firm ligaments and osseous structures and may provide a more reliable loss of resistance for identification of the epidural space.[4]

Several variations of catheters are available with options for multiorifice tips, metal stylets, and varying stiffness. Commercially available catheters for cannulation of the epidural space are composed of polyurethane, nylon, or silicone-based material. Catheters with wire-wound reinforcement are designed to prevent kinking of the lumen and increase durability, thus making them useful for postoperative analgesic infusions.

PATIENT SELECTION AND CONTRAINDICATIONS

It is imperative that the patient be able to cooperate and tolerate the experience, from placement of the block to block resolution. The surgical procedure should be able to be performed with a sensory block level that is tolerable and safe for the patient under the required positioning, monitoring, and supplemental medication and sedation for the patient's condition. Lower extremity, pelvic, and lower abdominal procedures can be suited for spinal or epidural anesthesia. Upper abdominal procedures usually require sensory levels that are not comfortably attainable with regional techniques alone, and would require supplementation with light general anesthesia. Procedures involving the perineum usually are more suited to spinal anesthesia, recognizing the potential for sacral nerve sparing with epidural anesthesia because of the large size of the sacral roots.

Although the issue of contraindications to neuraxial anesthesia remains controversial, the single absolute contraindication may be patient refusal. Strong relative contraindications that would preclude neuraxial anesthesia in most clinical circumstances include significant hypovolemia, infection at the site of needle entrance, increased intracranial pressure, sepsis or bacteremia, and significant coagulopathy. Each clinical scenario requires analysis of the risk-benefit ratio for a given patient and situation, often with consideration of the current medicolegal environment. Generally, declarations that preexisting neurologic conditions such as peripheral neuropathy and multiple sclerosis and other demyelinating processes are contraindications to neuraxial anesthesia are not data-driven. Rather, these statements reflect concern that the anesthetic agent or technique may be inappropriately implicated in any deterioration in the patient's condition following neuraxial blockade.

TECHNIQUE

Accessing the Subarachnoid Space

A standard approach should begin with identifying the midline and palpating the iliac crests. The intercrest line is usually described as crossing the level of the fourth lumbar vertebra or the L3-4 or L4-5 interspace. The midline approach offers advantages of simplicity and the stability provided by an interspinous ligament. The spinal needle is passed through skin, subcutaneous tissue, supraspinous ligament, interspinous ligament, ligamentum flavum, epidural space, dura, and arachnoid into the CSF of the subarachnoid space. When the midline approach is difficult, the paramedian approach may still allow access to the subarachnoid space when presented with a heavily calcified interspinous ligament, midline osteophytes, or positional lordosis (Fig. 51–4).

Accessing the Epidural Space

Both midline and paramedian approaches can be used for needle placement, and the epidural space theoretically can be accessed at any vertebral level. The most common method for identification of the epidural space is the loss of resistance (LOR) technique using saline or air, although saline may be preferred given the risk of headache if air is unintentionally injected into the subarachnoid space. A dramatic loss of resistance is reassuring of the passage of the needle tip just beyond the ligamentum flavum and into the epidural space.

Other techniques for identifying the epidural space have been described. The use of electrical nerve stimulation via a stimulating catheter can provide evidence of placement within the epidural space by confirming the appropriate stimulation threshold.[5] Furthermore, information regarding the spinal level of the catheter tip can be inferred by observing the myotomal distribution of the stimulation. Lechner and colleagues[6] have described an apparatus for use in epidural access that produces audible and visual indications of the pressure encountered at the tip of an attached epidural needle. Beyond providing information via two senses to indicate the drop in pressure characteristic of entering the epidural space, this device allows a two-handed advancement of the epidural needle. Additional clinical investigation is needed to establish the appropriate usefulness of these methods.

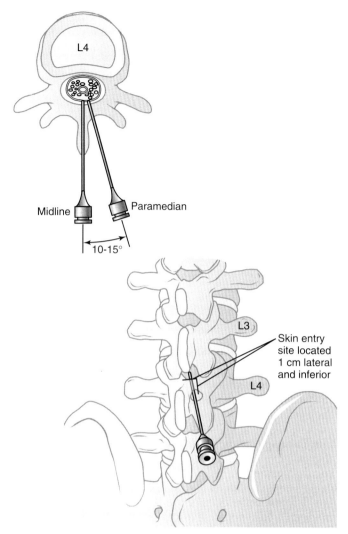

Figure 51–4. In the paramedian approach for neuraxial access, an entrance site is identified 1 cm lateral and caudad to the inferior aspect of the superior spinous process. After appropriate local anesthetic is infiltrated, the needle is typically inserted to touch down on the lamina; it is walked first medially and then cranially to step off the lamina.

PHARMACOLOGY

Factors Affecting Block Height

Spinal Anesthesia

Numerous variables have been investigated as potential determinants of block height (Box 51–1). The most significant physiologic parameter related to block height is CSF volume. Unfortunately, easily measurable physical features, such as height, weight, gender, and age do not correlate well with CSF volume, although it has been observed that obese individuals have lower CSF volumes than those who are nonobese.[7] Some studies have shown a minor influence of age and height on peak block levels,[8,9] but these correlations are weak and have inadequate predictive power to influence clinical practice.

BOX 51–1. FACTORS PROPOSED AS DETERMINANTS OF SPINAL BLOCK HEIGHT

Patient Characteristics
Age
Height
Weight
Gender
Intra-abdominal pressure

Characteristics of Local Anesthetic Solution
Baricity
Drug dose (mass)
Concentration of solution
Volume of injection
Temperature

Technical Variations
Patient positioning
Site of injection
Speed of injection
Direction of bevel
Barbotage

CSF Characteristics
Volume
Density
Velocity, circulation

Table 51–2. Baricity Reported for Spinal Anesthesia Preparations[10-13]

AGENT	BARICITY
Hyperbaric	
Bupivacaine, 0.75%, in 8.25% dextrose	1.0227
Tetracaine, 0.5%, in 5% dextrose	1.0133
Lidocaine, 5%, in 7.5% dextrose	1.0265
Procaine, 10%, in water	1.0104
2-Chloroprocaine, 2%, in saline	1.0012
Isobaric	
Bupivacaine, 0.5%, in saline	0.9983
Bupivacaine, 0.75%, in saline	0.9988
Tetracaine, 0.5%, in saline	0.9997
Lidocaine, 2%, in saline	0.9986
Hypobaric	
Bupivacaine, 0.3%, in water	0.9946
Tetracaine, 0.2%, in water	0.9922
Lidocaine, 0.5%, in water	0.9985

Data from references 10-13.

Baricity, drug dose (mass), and patient position relative to baricity of the agent are the most significant factors influencing block height. Solutions with a density higher than 1.0015 g/mL (3 standard deviations [SDs] above mean patient CSF density) can be expected to work well in a hyperbaric solution (Table 51–2). Although hyperbaric agents are usually formulated with dextrose, it should be noted that plain 2-chloroprocaine behaves in a hyperbaric fashion. In the supine patient, hyperbaric agents injected at or above the apex of the lumbar lordotic curvature will migrate to the thoracic kyphosis—hence, the tendency for a peak block of T4-6 in most supine patients. Manipulation of patient position after subarachnoid injection of hyperbaric solutions can enhance migration of the agent to the thoracic region (head-down position), or to the sacral region (head-up or sitting position).

Isobaric solutions, which have a density clinically equivalent to that of CSF, neither sink nor float after injection into the intrathecal space, and thus patient position does not affect block height. In this case, peak block height is most determined by dose of anesthetic agent (mass effect); still, individual CSF density and volume contribute.[14]

Hypobaric solutions offer an advantage in perianal surgery or other procedures that require a head-down or jackknife position, or for lateralized procedures when the patient cannot lie on the operative side. These preparations are formed by diluting anesthetic agents in distilled water, achieving a density lower than 0.9990 g/mL. After intrathecal injection, a hypo-baric agent floats to the nondependent region of the spinal column; thus, the patient must remain in the head-down position long enough to avoid inadvertent rise of the block.

Epidural Anesthesia

In contrast to spinal anesthesia, epidural anesthesia produces a segmental block that is a function of the site of injection of local anesthetic. Most procedures amenable to spinal anesthesia could also be served by epidural anesthesia that obtains a similar block height (Table 51–3). However, unless a caudal technique is used, the potential for sacral nerve sparing with epidural blockade, because of increased epidural fat and nerve root size in the low lumbar and sacral regions, may preclude its use for perineal procedures.

Injection of local anesthetic into the lumbar epidural space is typically suited for lower extremity and lower abdominal procedures, but increasing the dose and volume is necessary to get extension to midthoracic levels. In general, one can think of administering 2 mL of local anesthetic solution for each additional dermatome to be blocked. Thoracic epidural injections tend not to extend caudally to the degree seen with lumbar injections; thus, these are reserved for procedures in the thorax and upper abdomen. When administering anesthetic to the thoracic region, the dose is typically reduced by 30% to 50% compared with the lumbar region to accommodate the decreased volume and compliance of the thoracic epidural space and avoid unwanted cephalad spread.

For the ranges that are typically used for surgical anesthesia, concentration of the anesthetic solution has little effect on extent of the epidural block, but increased block density is observed with higher concentrations. Increasing the volume of solution injected for a given total dose will have a minor effect on cephalad spread (about four dermatomes when increasing from 10 to 30 mL), but will compromise density and quality of the block. Although it is often used clinically, patient position also has no demonstrable effect on lateralization of the block or cephalad spread.

The effect of patient age on epidural block height and dose requirement seems to be clinically relevant only in extremes of age,[15] attributed to the increased likelihood of spinal canal stenosis and decreased epidural compliance in the aged population. In similar scale, the influence of height and weight on the spread of epidural block is small and usually clinically insignificant unless considering the extremes of the spectrum.[16]

Clinical Aspects of Neuraxial Agents

Local Anesthetics

Local anesthetic agents are discussed in Chapter 44 in detail, but some clinical points relating to neuraxial anesthesia will be addressed here. The choice of neuraxial agents is determined by the nature and estimated time of the surgical procedure, as well as postoperative issues such as disposition. Representative durations for doses of spinal and epidural agents are presented in Tables 51–4 and 51–5. For spinal anesthesia, increasing the dose of agent administered will prolong the block and, unless counteracted by positioning and baricity, may also increase peak block height.

Long-acting Agents

Bupivacaine and levobupivacaine have the benefit of having a very low incidence of transient neurologic symptoms (TNS; see later, "Neurologic Complications")[17] when used for low-dose spinal anesthesia. However, the variability in time to complete resolution of the block and achievement of discharge criteria provides a challenge in the ambulatory setting. The addition of epinephrine to bupivacaine or levobupivacaine may provide increased motor block, as well as increased duration. Levobupivacaine is approximately equipotent to bupivacaine, with the exception of less systemic toxicity.

Ropivacaine was developed to reduce the risk of cardiotoxicity with bupivacaine and was released for clinical use in 1996. When used as a spinal agent, ropivacaine has a clinical profile similar to bupiva-

Table 51–3. Block Height Requirements for Common Surgical Procedures

SURGICAL PROCEDURE	BLOCK HEIGHT
Upper abdominal surgery, cesarean section	T4-5
Lower abdominal procedures (inguinal herniorrhaphy, appendectomy), pelvic surgery	T6-8
Transurethral resection of prostate, hip, and lower extremity (with thigh tourniquet), obstetric vaginal delivery	T10
Lower extremity	L2-3
Perineal procedures (limited to exterior)	S1-2

Table 51–4. Typical Dose Response for Local Anesthetics Used for Spinal Anesthesia

LOCAL ANESTHETIC	DOSE (mg)	PEAK BLOCK (mg)	DURATION OF SENSORY BLOCK (min)	DURATION OF MOTOR BLOCK (min)	TIME UNTIL DISCHARGE (min)	ANESTHETIC SUCCESS RATE (%)
Bupivacaine*	5	T5 (T4-7)	123 (27)	50 (20)	181 (30)	75
	7.5	T8 (T4-11)	144 (25)	75 (24)	202 (28)	100
	10	T8 (T6-10)	194 (26)	100 (24)	260 (30)	100
	15	T5 (T4-7)	343 (28)	150 (24)	471 (35)	100
Ropivacaine	8	T9 (T4-L1)	130 (27)	107 (25)	165 (45)	63
	10	T8 (T4-L2)	152 (44)	135 (31)	174 (38)	83
	12	T8 (T4-L1)	176 (42)	162 (37)	199 (52)	93
	14	T9 (T3-L1)	192 (48)	189 (44)	233 (52)	100
Lidocaine	30					0
	40	T4 (T2-10)	130 (26)	93 (24)	178 (34)	90
	60	T3 (T2-10)	162 (32)	128 (31)	216 (33)	90
	80	T3 (T1-7)	170 (24)	142 (32)	236 (46)	97
Mepivacaine	30	T9 (T2-L5)	158 (32)	116 (38)	180 (34)	72
	45	T6 (T2-12)	182 (38)	142 (37)	191 (29)	100
	60	T5 (T2-L1)	203 (36)	168 (36)	203 (35)	100
Prilocaine	50	T6 (T1-10)	128 (38)	165 (37)	253 (55)	100
Procaine	100	T5 (T1-10)	120 (23)	100 (30)	244 (43)	83
2-Chloroprocaine[†]	30	T8 (T6-L1)	103 (12)	54 (23)	103 (12)	NA
	40	T7 (T3-T10)	114 (14)	69 (16)	113 (14)	NA
	60	T4 (C6-T6)	132 (23)	100 (13)	141 (21)	NA

*Levobupivacaine is equipotent.
†2-chloroprocaine spinal anesthesia is currently an off-label use.
NA, clinical data not available.
Dose response data allow selection of appropriate dose for planned anesthetic duration. Increasing doses of spinal local anesthetics increases the duration of both anesthesia and recovery. Hyperbaric solutions contain glucose or dextrose; isobaric solutions are glucose-free.
Data from Halpern SH, Walsh V: Epidural ropivacaine versus bupivacaine for labor: A meta-analysis. Anesth Analg 2003;96:1473-1479. † data from Kopacz DJ: Spinal 2-chloroprocaine: Minimum effective dose. Reg Anesth Pain Med 2005;30:36-42.

Table 51–5. Expected Duration of Sensory Block for Local Anesthetics Commonly Used for Epidural Anesthesia

LOCAL ANESTHETIC	CONCENTRATION (%)	TIME UNTIL TWO-DERMATOME REGRESSION (min)	TIME FOR COMPLETE RESOLUTION (min)
Bupivacaine	0.5-0.75	120-240	300-460
Levobupivacaine	0.5-0.75	105-290	390-780
Ropivacaine	0.5-1	90-180	240-420
Lidocaine	1.5-2	60-100	160-200
Mepivacaine	1.5-2	60-100	160-200
2-Chloroprocaine	2-3	45-60	100-160

caine at equipotent doses (ropivacaine is 60% as potent as bupivacaine), with little risk of TNS.[18] There is some evidence that ropivacaine may have less motor block when compared with bupivacaine when used for labor analgesia.[19]

Although tetracaine is used less commonly at present, it is still the agent that provides the most reliable hypobaric spinal block (tetracaine 0.2% in water). It should be noted that the use of vasoconstrictors might increase the risk of TNS with tetracaine.[20]

Intermediate-acting Agents

Lidocaine has enjoyed widespread popularity and safety as a neuraxial agent, but has undergone increasing scrutiny regarding neurotoxicity given the high incidence of TNS seen when used for ambulatory spinal anesthesia (see later, "Neurologic Complications"). In an effort to avoid this problem, because this seems to be a dose-dependent phenomenon, lower doses of lidocaine have been investigated, usually requiring adjuvant agents to provide suitable

reliability of spinal blockade. Lidocaine is used in concentrations of 1.5% and 2% for epidural anesthesia to provide reliable single-shot blockade for procedures lasting less than 120 minutes. However, continuous catheter techniques commonly use lidocaine, with reinjection usually required every 60 to 90 minutes.

Mepivacaine has a similar clinical profile to lidocaine when used as a neuraxial agent, although it has higher potency (1.3 to 1 compared with spinal lidocaine). Although 4% mepivacaine appears to have a similar incidence of TNS as lidocaine, a recent survey of 1273 patients using 1.5% mepivacaine reported only a 6% incidence of TNS.[21] It is used in concentrations of 1% to 2% for epidural anesthesia, again with similar effects as lidocaine.

Prilocaine is an amide local anesthetic with pharmacologic properties similar to lidocaine when used as a spinal anesthetic. However, it shows a much lower incidence of TNS compared with spinal lidocaine[22] and thus may be a favorable agent for ambulatory spinal anesthesia. Currently, prilocaine is not widely available in the United States, but it is used commonly in Europe.

Short-acting Agents

Procaine has been used since the early 1900s to provide brief spinal anesthesia, but currently has limited clinical usefulness given the rate of block failure (see Table 51–4) and incidence of side effects. For reasons that are poorly understood, spinal procaine carries a higher risk of nausea than other local anesthetics (odds ratio, 3:1). Although it has a lower incidence of TNS than spinal lidocaine (see later, "Neurologic Complications"), spinal procaine is not an ideal agent for outpatient spinal anesthesia.

2-Chloroprocaine has been receiving increased attention in the focus of current issues in ambulatory anesthesia and concerns of relative neurotoxicities of neuraxial agents. After introduction into clinical use, 2-chloroprocaine enjoyed increasing popularity as an agent for epidural anesthesia, particularly in obstetric anesthesia. This lasted until the 1980s, with the appearance of several reports of apparent neurotoxicity, with lower extremity paralysis and sacral nerve dysfunction resulting from accidental intrathecal injection of large volumes of 2-chloroprocaine in the form of Nesacaine-CE (intended for the epidural space). The combination of the antioxidant sodium bisulfite in the presence of a low pH was assumed to be responsible for the neurotoxicity,[23] and the formulation of 2-chloroprocaine was changed. Currently, two of the three commercially available formulations of 2-chloroprocaine (Nesacaine-MPF and generic chloroprocaine) are preservative-free and antioxidant-free. Given the availability of these new preparations and growing concerns about the TNS associated with lidocaine, 2-chloroprocaine has been reinvestigated for off-label use as a short-acting spinal anesthetic. Work by Kopacz and associates[24-29] has shown 2-chloroprocaine to provide a reliable spinal anesthesia with consistent time to resolution and achievement of discharge criteria without identifiable occurrence of TNS. It should be noted that 2% 2-chloroprocaine behaves in a hyperbaric fashion,[27] and that the addition of epinephrine to spinal 2-chloroprocaine is not recommended because of consistent and disturbing reports of flulike symptoms in volunteers receiving this combination.[24] Also, a laboratory study in a rat model has observed direct neurotoxicity from high doses of preservative-free 2-chloroprocaine that was equivalent to 2% lidocaine.[30] Thus, the complete risk-benefit ratio of the off-label use of spinal 2-chloroprocaine is not known completely.

The use of 2% and 3% 2-chloroprocaine is an appropriate choice for epidural anesthesia of short duration. Following the release of Nesacaine-MPF, which contains EDTA, reports of back pain on block resolution were associated with high volumes of injected agent (more than 40 mL).[31] This is thought to occur because of tetanic spasm of the paraspinous muscles resulting from chelation of calcium by the EDTA. Given these concerns, it may be prudent to use 2-chloroprocaine preparations that are preservative- and antioxidant-free for neuraxial blockade.

Analgesic Adjuncts

Early use of adjuvant medications for neuraxial anesthesia centered around increasing the duration and intensity of blockade. With the increasing percentage of surgeries being performed in the ambulatory setting, interest has turned to finding adjuncts that will allow faster recovery without compromising anesthetic reliability (Table 51–6).

Table 51–6. Common Adjuvants for Neuraxial Anesthesia

AGENT	DOSE	TYPICAL ANESTHETIC EFFECT	COMMENTS
Fentanyl	Spinal, 10-25 µg	33% increase in anesthetic success with small doses of local anesthetic; 25% increase in duration of surgical anesthesia; 60% incidence of easily treated pruritus	No delay of anesthetic recovery
	Epidural, 1-2 µg/kg	Twofold reduction in volatile anesthetic requirements; decreased visceral pain with cesarean section	Bolus administration may act at spinal level, infusions act systemically
Clonidine	Spinal, 15-45 µg	37% increase in anesthetic success with small doses of local anesthetic; 29% increase in duration of motor block; decrease in heart rate and blood pressure; mild perioperative sedation	No delay of anesthetic recovery
	Epidural, 150 µg	Two- to threefold increase in duration of sensory anesthesia; increased time to first analgesic request	Less oxygen desaturation, pruritus, urinary retention compared with opioids
Epinephrine	Spinal, 0.1-0.6 mg	Dose-related increase in surgical anesthesia and motor block	Dose-related increase in time until recovery of the same or greater magnitude
	Epidural, 5 µg/mL	Increased duration, intensity of block with lidocaine and 2-chloroprocaine; will intensify block, but less effect on duration with bupivacaine; minimal effect with ropivacaine	Decreased plasma levels with lidocaine and bupivacaine, but not ropivacaine

Data from references 32, 34-36, 38, 41-49.

Opioids

The potent analgesic effects of neuraxial opioids have been exploited to improve perioperative analgesia and reduce the supraspinal side effects of sedation and respiratory depression seen with systemic opioids. Neuraxial opioids that diffuse into the spinal cord exert spinal analgesia by modulating A-delta and C fibers to decrease afferent nociceptive input,[32] inhibiting Ca^{2+} influx presynaptically and increasing K^+ conductance and hyperpolarize ascending neurons postsynaptically.[33]

Because of its hydrophilic nature, neuraxial morphine provides highly selective, prolonged spinal analgesia but is not generally used to augment intraoperative anesthesia because of its slow onset. The lipophilic opioids, such as fentanyl, are more suited for intraoperative use in the intrathecal space because of rapid onset, modest duration, and lower risk of delayed respiratory depression. The addition of 10 to 25 µg fentanyl to low-dose lidocaine and bupivacaine spinal anesthetics has been shown to improve anesthetic success dramatically without delaying achievement of discharge criteria for ambulatory patients.[34] However, when used with the ultrashort-acting spinal anesthetic 2-chloroprocaine, fentanyl can delay discharge slightly (95 vs. 104 minutes) and increase pruritus.[26]

The administration of epidural fentanyl can reduce volatile anesthetic requirements more than intravenous fentanyl (more than twofold at 2 µg/kg).[35] The method of delivery of epidural fentanyl may be important for optimal effect. Ginosar and coworkers[36] have demonstrated that epidural fentanyl given as a bolus imparts segmental analgesia consistent with its spinal level of action but, if given as an infusion, the analgesia is mediated through systemic uptake and a supraspinal effect, as is seen with sufentanil and alfentanil.[37]

α_2 Agonists

Clonidine and related α_2 agonists are receiving increased interest in the field of regional anesthesia because of their ability to enhance neuraxial analgesia without the respiratory depression and pruritus common to opioids. As with analgesia, the sedation, hypotension, and bradycardia seen with neuraxial clonidine are dose-dependent.[38] Clonidine exerts its analgesic effects by binding to α_2 adrenoreceptors (on primary afferent, substantia gelatinosa, and several brainstem nuclei, attributed to analgesic mechanisms), attenuating A-delta and C-fiber nociception, producing conduction blockade via increased potassium conductance, and increasing acetylcholine and norepinephrine levels in the CSF, inhibiting the release of substance P.[39] Although clonidine rapidly redistributes systemically to the periphery after epidural or spinal administration because of lipophilicity, the analgesic effect is spinally mediated, as evidenced by the lack of correlation between time of analgesia and peripheral blood levels.

Although previously investigated as a sole anesthetic, intrathecal clonidine is clinically used in com-

bination with various local anesthetics to produce dose-dependent prolongation of sensory and motor block.[40,41] Showing a promising role in ambulatory anesthesia, De Kock and coworkers[42] have demonstrated that the addition of as little as 15 µg of clonidine to ropivacaine, 8 mg, for spinal anesthesia in outpatients undergoing knee arthroscopy produces a considerable increase in anesthetic success, from 70% to 90%, without significant effect on recovery time. However, increasing the dose to 45 µg increases resolution of motor and sensory block and time to void from 170 to 215 minutes. Adding clonidine to local anesthetics intensifies and prolongs epidural blockade and can reduce the local anesthetic dose requirement.[43] The benefits of clinical doses of neuraxial clonidine usually persist for about 3 hours; these can be achieved without increasing hemodynamic instability more than local anesthetic alone or significantly altering responsiveness to resuscitation drugs.[38,44] The typical dose of clonidine for addition to local anesthetics for epidural bolus administration is 150 µg, or 2 µg/kg. Klimscha and colleagues have demonstrated that the addition of 150 µg of clonidine to 10 mL of 0.5% bupivacaine for epidural anesthesia increases the mean duration of anesthesia from 1.8 to 5.3 hours, reduces pain scores, and increases time to first postoperative analgesic request.[45]

Vasoconstrictors

Epinephrine and phenylephrine are added to local anesthetic solutions in an attempt to prolong the anesthetic effect, provide more reliable block, and intensify anesthesia and analgesia.[46,47] Vasoconstriction results in decreased blood flow, reducing uptake of local anesthetics into the circulation. This maintains concentrations at the site of injection and reduces peak plasma concentrations. Additionally, intrinsic analgesic effects of epinephrine are exerted via stimulation of presynaptic α_2 adrenoreceptors.

The typical dose of epinephrine used in spinal anesthesia is 0.2 mg (although doses of 0.1 to 0.6 mg have been described), which, when added to a bupivacaine spinal anesthetic, will increase the time of regression to L2 by 25%.[48] The addition of epinephrine to spinal anesthetics prolongs motor block and delays the return of bladder function, which is problematic for ambulatory surgery patients trying to achieve discharge criteria.[49]

For epidural anesthesia, the typical use of epinephrine is in concentrations of 1:200,000, or 5 µg/mL. The clinical effect of epinephrine on duration of anesthesia depends on the local anesthetic used. Epinephrine is more effective at prolonging the anesthetic duration of shorter acting agents, such as lidocaine and 2-chloroprocaine. Adding 1:200,000 epinephrine to 2% lidocaine will nearly double the time to resolution of blockade.[50] Agents with longer duration of action show much less prolongation of anesthesia with the addition of epinephrine. Adding epinephrine to ropivacaine will intensify the block, but will not prolong the duration of epidural anesthesia or affect plasma levels,[51] likely because of the innate vasoconstricting effects of ropivacaine. Other agents do show reduction of plasma levels when epinephrine is added.[46] Epinephrine 1:200,000 will decrease plasma lidocaine and chloroprocaine levels by 20% to 30%, but will decrease plasma bupivacaine levels by only 10% to 20%. The effect of epinephrine on plasma levels of local anesthetics has long been thought to be caused by constriction of the epidural venous plexus, and therefore reduced blood flow and slower uptake of local anesthetics. Other studies, however, have suggested that reduced dural blood flow and increased hepatic clearance may be more important in this phenomenon.[52] The potential to prolong discharge times and delay bladder function limits the usefulness of adding epinephrine to epidural agents for ambulatory surgery.

PHYSIOLOGY

Neurophysiology

Neural blockade by local anesthetics is discussed in Chapter 44; therefore, this section will highlight some clinical aspects specific to neuraxial blockade. After intrathecal injection, the local anesthetic is found in the spinal cord as well as in the spinal nerve rootlets in the CSF. Following epidural injection, local anesthetic is found in spinal nerves in the epidural space, spinal nerve rootlets in the CSF, and in the spinal cord. Thus, conduction blockade may take place at multiple sites along the neural pathway for both spinal and epidural anesthesia, although exact mechanisms have not been delineated.[53] Previous studies have provided some insight into primary sites of action. With spinal anesthesia, somatosensory evoked potentials from the tibial nerve (peripheral nervous system) are abolished, whereas direct spinal cord stimulation remains unchanged,[54,55] consistent with the theory that the spinal nerve rootlets are the primary site of action of spinal anesthesia, not the spinal cord. Similarly, measurement of evoked potentials in monkeys again has indicated that the primary site of action of epidural anesthesia is the spinal nerve rootlets.[56] However, measurement of somatosensory evoked potentials from the tibial nerve are only modestly changed following induction of epidural anesthesia, and the magnitude of change in somatosensory evoked potentials does not correlate with intensity of epidural block.[57] These observations provide objective support for the clinical impression that spinal anesthesia is more intense and complete than epidural anesthesia.

The term *differential* (or *graduated*) *spinal block* has been used to describe the practice of administering increasing amounts of local anesthetic to the subarachnoid space to produce first sympathetic blockade, then sensory blockade, and finally motor blockade. This is usually done in an effort to help identify the type of pain pathways involved in a complicated pain syndrome, theoretically differentiating among sympathetically mediated pain, noci-ceptive somatic pain, and central pain. This concept is founded on the presumption that nerve fibers of different types and sizes are susceptible to blockade at different concentrations of local anesthetic. Thus, in theory, low doses of local anesthetic would block the small preganglionic sympathetic fibers, but spare the larger A-delta somatic sensory fibers, which would then be blocked with proper additional dose of local anesthetic that would yet spare the A-alpha and A-beta motor fibers. This can be observed clinically in surgical patients with spinal blockade, in whom sympathetic blockade can extend two to six dermatomes higher than sensory block, which may extend two or three dermatomes higher than the level of motor blockade. This phenomenon is postulated to result from a gradual reduction in the CSF concentration of local anesthetic at increasing distance from the level of subarachnoid injection. Although it has long been thought that nerve fiber sensitivity to blockade is a function of fiber size, some studies have suggested that fiber diameter may not be the principal determinant of blockade.[58]

Beyond direct conduction blockade within the CNS, spinal and epidural anesthesia produce sedation that correlates with block height, but is unrelated to systemic pharmacologic levels.[59] Animal studies using electroencephalographic monitoring and direct brain stimulation during spinal anesthesia have suggested that this occurs because of a decrease in reticular activating system activity caused by decreased tonic afferent input from the anesthetized region.[60] Clinical studies have indicated that spinal anesthesia decreases sedative requirements for propofol and midazolam by approximately 30% to 50% with clinically relevant spinal block heights.[61,62] Similarly, the use of epidural anesthesia or analgesia reduces volatile anesthetic requirements by 20% to 30% during surgery when general anesthesia is titrated to hemodynamics or bispectral index (BIS) monitoring.[63,64]

Respiratory Physiology

With spinal or epidural blockade to midthoracic levels in patients without preexisting respiratory disease, pulmonary function, gas exchange, and control of breathing are generally preserved.[65] Sedative medications used to facilitate neuraxial blockade are more likely to affect the patient's respiratory status than the blockade itself.[66] The rare respiratory arrest after spinal anesthesia is thought to result from brainstem hypoperfusion secondary to decreased cardiac output rather than to the direct effects of local anesthetics on the brainstem. Under normal conditions, the concentration of local anesthetic in the ventricular fluid is not high enough to cause medullary depression.

Cardiovascular Physiology

In the nonobstetric population, the incidence of hypotension and bradycardia after spinal anesthesia are approximately 33% and 13%, respectively.[16,67] Large epidemiologic studies from France, Scandinavia, and the United States have indicated that the risk of cardiac arrest after spinal anesthesia is approximately 0.1 to 1/1,000 and 1/10,000 after epidural anesthesia.[68] Although cardiac arrest after spinal anesthesia appears to be disturbingly frequent, one study has suggested that survival is better for cardiac arrest during neuraxial block as opposed to cardiac arrest during general anesthesia (65% vs. 31%).[69] This may be the result of enhanced vigilance, because several risk factors for bradycardia and hypotension have been identified for spinal anesthesia (Table 51–7). Although probably similar, the risk factors for epidural anesthesia have not been fully identified because of the decreased frequency of occurrence. Understanding the mechanisms involved in these physiologic derangements will allow early recognition and prompt treatment to avoid untoward outcomes in neuraxial anesthesia.

Cardiovascular changes seen with spinal anesthesia occur because of blockade of the sympathetic efferent fibers, and are thus generally related to block height.[70] Arterial and venous relaxation contributes to hypotension, resulting in decreased systemic vascular resistance (SVR) and cardiac output (CO). SVR has been shown to decrease more in older patients (26% from baseline) than in young healthy subjects (13% to 18% from baseline).[71] Venodilation causes increased pooling of blood in the capacitance vessels, thus reducing central blood volume. This decreases venous return to the heart, resulting in reduced preload and therefore reduced CO.

Although heart rate is typically maintained, bradycardia can occur with spinal anesthesia in 10% to 15% of cases, and unexpected circulatory collapse remains a dreaded complication with potentially grave outcome. In addition to the risk factors of age younger than 50 years, American Society of Anesthesiology status, and concomitant use of beta blockers, the incidence of bradycardia increases with increased block height, with 75% associated with sensory block above T5[72] (see Table 51–7). Sympathetic blockade

above T5 is thought to inhibit cardioaccelerator fibers (T1-4) and allow parasympathetic predominance over heart rate, mediated via the vagus nerve. However, some studies of heart rate variability have suggested that sympathetic and parasympathetic systems can remain in balance, even with high thoracic blockade.[73,74] Reports of bradycardia or asystole and circulatory collapse in patients with blocks too low to be attributed solely to sympathectomy further indicates that other factors likely play important roles. Bradycardia may be induced by an increase in baroreceptor reflex activity.[75] With redistribution of blood to capacitance vessels, decreased venous return to the heart, and the resulting decreased filling pressures, intracardiac stretch receptors in the right atrium and left ventricle have been suggested to participate in a bradycardic response (Bezold-Jarisch reflex).[76,77] Thus, maintaining preload and aggressively treating bradycardia may help improve the safety of spinal anesthesia.[78]

The practice of administering a crystalloid bolus prior to spinal anesthesia, in an effort to maintain central blood volume, has been a traditional method for preventing hypotension induced by neuraxial blockade. However, some studies have noted a more complex interaction between fluid loading, hemodynamic effects, and efficacy for prevention of hypotension in the nonobstetric population. For example, a prophylactic bolus of 500 to 1500 mL of crystalloid may be ineffective for prevention of hypotension in normovolemic patients if given prior to induction of spinal anesthesia[79] but may be effective if administered later, during the actual performance of spinal anesthesia.[80] This may occur because of the pharmacokinetics of crystalloids, resulting in a rapid redistribution out of the intravascular compartment, and thus providing only a fleeting contribution to venous return.[81] Furthermore, crystalloid bolus does not adequately address other factors contributing to hypotension—heart rate and SVR—and may actually decrease SVR.[82] In contrast, the administration of colloid solutions is more effective in maintaining intravascular volume because of favorable pharmacokinetics[82,83] and may actually increase SVR.[82] Prophylactic administration of 500 to 1000 mL of colloid solution prior to induction of spinal blockade has been shown to prevent hypotension more effectively but can grossly affect fluid balance in the patient. In regard to treatment of hypotension in the setting of established hypovolemia, crystalloid remains a suitable choice because of altered volume kinetics in this setting.[84]

Appropriate pharmacologic treatment of hypotension should be tailored to the clinical situation at hand, with consideration of alterations in SVR and CO. Vasopressors with α-adrenergic agonist activity, such as phenylephrine and metaraminol, are effective for increasing SVR, but possibly at the expense of a decrease in CO resulting from increased afterload.[85] Therefore, it is believed that the use of mixed α-adrenergic and β-adrenergic agonist drugs such as ephedrine may be more appropriate for the treat-

Table 51–7. Risk Factors for Hypotension and Moderate Bradycardia (Pulse <50 bpm) During Spinal Anesthesia[65,72]

RISK FACTOR	ODDS RATIO
Hypotension	
Sensory level above T5	3.8
Age >40 yr	2.5
Baseline SBP < 120 mm Hg	2.4
Spinal puncture above L2-3	1.8
Bradycardia	
Baseline heart rate <60 bpm	4.9
ASA physical status I (versus ASA physical status III or IV)	3.5
Prolonged PR interval	3.2
Use of beta-blocking drugs	2.9
Sensory level above T5	1.7

ASA, American Society of Anesthesiology; bpm, beats/min; SBP, systolic blood pressure.

ment of hypotension induced by neuraxial blockade because of their ability to augment heart rate and CO and SVR. Atropine in doses of 0.4 to 1 mg intravenously can be used to treat moderate bradycardia if ephedrine is not effective. In case of precipitous bradycardia or situations not responsive to these interventions, one should not hesitate to use epinephrine. Closed claims data analysis has suggested that the lack of early administration of epinephrine is a management pattern in spinal anesthesia leading to cardiac arrest, with poor outcome.[86]

Although similar hemodynamic changes are seen with epidural anesthesia, these tend to be better tolerated than those seen with spinal anesthesia, perhaps because of a more gradual and titratable onset. Even so, sudden bradycardic cardiac arrest has been described with epidural anesthesia. Risk of sudden cardiovascular collapse from epidural anesthesia may be influenced by the addition of epinephrine to the epidural solution. With the typical dose range used for epidural anesthesia, systemic levels of epinephrine remain low, producing a β-adrenergic effect of vasodilation and increased heart rate and myocardial contractility. Ward and colleagues[87] have evaluated the cardiovascular effects of epidural blockade to T5 using lidocaine with and without epinephrine. Mean arterial pressure decreased 20% in the epinephrine group compared with 10% in the lidocaine-only group. However, the group with epinephrine also showed a 20% to 30% increase in cardiac output. Bonica and associates[88] have suggested that this systemic β-adrenergic effect of epinephrine might prevent the potential cardiovascular collapse from epidural blockade.

Gastrointestinal, Hepatic, and Genitourinary Physiology

Neuraxial anesthesia produces a sympathectomy and parasympathetic dominance, resulting in relaxation of sphincters, constriction of the bowel, and an increase in secretions. This imbalance of the autonomic nervous system has also been implicated in the occurrence of nausea seen with neuraxial blockade. Hepatic blood flow is related to mean arterial pressure, and thus is maintained if the patient is hemodynamically stable. Similarly, renal blood flow and renal function are preserved during spinal anesthesia when perfusion pressure is adequate. Urinary retention after spinal anesthesia is the most noteworthy and clinically significant concern in regard to the genitourinary system. Postoperative urinary retention occurs in about 16% of patients in the recovery unit.[89] The ability to void normally does not return until sensory anesthesia has regressed to the S3 sacral segment. Prolonged inhibition of normal detrusor function with the use of long-acting local anesthetics such as bupivacaine may allow bladder overdistention and urinary retention. Factors such as age (older than 50 years), volume of intraoperative fluid administration, and type of surgical procedure influence the rate of urinary retention.[89]

COMPLICATIONS

Postdural Puncture Headache

Postdural puncture headache (PDPH) remains a common complication of spinal anesthesia. It is seen in as many as 50% of cases of inadvertent dural puncture during epidural anesthesia. Although the incidence of PDPH following spinal anesthesia varies greatly, depending on the types of needles used and patient population, rates as high as 40% are seen with 22-gauge bevel-tipped needles. The introduction of smaller gauge pencil point needles for spinal anesthesia has decreased the incidence of PDPH to approximately 1%.[90] The mechanism of PDPH is thought to involve sagging of the brain while standing or sitting upright, resulting from loss of CSF from the thecal sac. This is believed to result in traction on the meninges, meningeal vessels, and, at times, traction on the cranial nerves, leading to cranial nerve palsy. Magnetic resonance imaging (MRI) studies demonstrating reduced CSF volume[91] and postgadolinium meningeal enhancement during PDPH[92] have lent support to this theory of CSF loss and meningeal irritation. The headache is classically positional, being most pronounced while the patient is standing and almost eliminated when the patient is supine. Patients usually experience a bandlike aching pain in the frontal and occipital regions, posterior neck pain, and occasionally nausea, tinnitus, photophobia, and diplopia. Differentiation from infectious meningitis is important; this is usually based on the positional nature of symptoms, lack of fever and, if necessary, normal peripheral white cell count and CSF profile.

Whereas the incidence of PDPH declines with increasing patient age, factors that may be controlled by the clinician to reduce its occurrence include the use of smaller gauge needles, pencil point needles, and longitudinal orientation of the bevel if a cutting needle is used. The mechanisms involved in bevel orientation are unclear. It has been traditionally believed that more dural fibers are cut by a transversely oriented cutting bevel, and thus a more substantial hole in the dura is made. However, given that dural fibers are not longitudinally arranged, but are in a random orientation, the number of fibers cut should not depend on bevel direction. It has been suggested that the longitudinal tension placed on the meninges tends to pull open a transversely oriented defect, allowing more CSF leakage, and explaining this observation. As for pencil point needles, the supposition that they cause less trauma to the meninges is questionable. Reina and coworkers[91] have suggested that Whitacre needles produce more trauma, as evidenced by electron microscopy images, and that the reduced loss of CSF may be due to an "edematous plug" resulting from a more substantial inflammatory reaction.

Patients should be reassured that the symptoms of PDPH are likely to resolve within 1 week and be encouraged to use bed rest, oral analgesics, adequate hydration, and caffeine. If the patient does not respond adequately to conservative treatment or has prolonged symptoms, an epidural blood patch can be considered. This is typically performed by accessing the epidural space within one interspace of the suspected dural tear and injecting 10 to 20 mL of autologous blood in a sterile fashion. This is intended to form a clot, or patch, over the dural defect, preventing further leakage of CSF. Additionally, this volume will tamponade the dural sac and restore buoyant support to the brain, accounting for the near-immediate relief that many patients report. Success of the epidural blood patch has been reported to be from 70% to 95%, with those who fail to improve with an initial patch showing the same range of response to a repeat procedure. The effectiveness of prophylactic blood patch administration is controversial; some studies have shown no benefit and others have reported more than 50% success in preventing PDPH.[93] It appears that it may be reasonable and effective if larger volumes (15 to 20 mL) are used for high-risk patients.[94]

Infectious Complications

In large retrospective review, Moen and associates[95] have estimated the incidence of meningitis to be lower than 1/50,000 following spinal anesthesia and about 1/90,000 after epidural procedures; the incidence of epidural abscess is 1/37,000 following epidural block. Sources of microorganisms include contaminated equipment or injected solutions or from patients—namely, bacteremia. Lumbar puncture is thought to disrupt the blood-brain barrier and allow transfer of bloodborne bacteria into the spinal space. Animal studies have supported this theory, but also have shown that pretreatment with antibiotics drastically reduces this risk.[96]

Epidural anesthesia for surgical procedures may have a similar risk profile, but the use of indwelling epidural catheters for continuous analgesic infusions provides an additional risk; these serve as a wick for surface infections to migrate along the tract, and perhaps become a deep infection or epidural abscess. However, surveillance studies and investigation of rates of bacterial contamination of epidural catheter tips have indicated that this risk is low.[95,97] Patients with postoperative catheters should be observed for signs of infection, with the catheter site being inspected daily. If signs of surface infection are present, the catheter should be removed and the site monitored for improvement, with or without the initiation of antibiotics (as deemed suitable). If the patient presents with severe back pain or new neurologic deficits that are not explained by the analgesic infusion, the diagnosis of epidural abscess must be considered and MRI or computed tomography (CT) performed if appropriate.

Hemorrhagic Complications

With neuraxial procedures, hematoma can develop in the epidural, subdural, or intrathecal space, with potential for devastating neurologic outcome. The usual presenting symptoms are back pain and motor or sensory deficit not explained by the administration of anesthetic or analgesic agents. In patients with such symptoms, especially in the setting of anticoagulants, definitive diagnosis should be sought without delay. A review by Vandermeulen and associates[98] has indicated that early identification by MRI or CT and surgical decompression performed within 4 to 6 hours of presentation is associated with good neurologic recovery.

The estimated incidence of spinal hematoma in the absence of anticoagulant and antiplatelet medications is lower than 1 in 150,000 central neuraxial blocks.[99] Most cases of spinal hematoma are in patients receiving anticoagulants or with impaired hemostatic function from hepatic dysfunction or thrombocytopenia. The American Society of Regional Anesthesia and Pain Medicine has released a consensus statement about the issues related to neuraxial procedures in patients receiving anticoagulant and antiplatelet medications.[99]

Neurologic Complications

Although the overall incidence of persistent neurologic injury associated with neuraxial blocks is reported to be approximately 0.08% to 0.16%, the vast majority of these reported cases fail to show evidence that the block was directly causative.[100] Potential mechanisms of neurologic injury following neuraxial anesthesia include direct needle or catheter trauma, neurotoxicity of injected substances (intended agents or unintended chemicals), infectious complications, hemorrhagic complications, or spinal cord ischemia. Most perceived injuries are related to persistent paresthesia or motor weakness, but cauda equina syndrome is also rarely reported.

Paresthesia is reported in as many as 6% of patients during needle placement for spinal anesthesia, but this rarely results in persistent neurologic deficit.[100] Similarly, most paresthesias associated with indwelling epidural catheters are likely to dissipate following removal of the catheter. Despite its rare occurrence, paresthesia during block placement is considered a risk factor for persistent paresthesia. Patients experiencing this should be reassured and queried postoperatively regarding their neurologic status.

Despite a long history of relative safety, animal data suggest that all local anesthetics have some potential to cause neural injury; however, lidocaine and tetracaine appear to have a greater potential for neurotoxicity than bupivacaine at clinically relevant concentrations.[101] Attention has been focused on the issues surrounding neurotoxicity of local anesthetics and common additives because of identification of several cases of cauda equina syndrome associated with continuous spinal anesthesia via microcatheters. Although injuries in these cases have been attributed to pooling and maldistribution of the local anesthetic within the thecal sac because of how it was administered through a catheter, there have

Table 51–8. Reported Incidence of Transient Neurologic Symptoms (TNS) with Spinal Anesthesia for Ambulatory Surgery

LOCAL ANESTHETIC	PATIENT POSITION	INCIDENCE (%)
Bupivacaine, 0.25-0.75%	Supine	0-1
	Knee arthroscopy	0-1
	Lithotomy	0-1
Ropivacaine, 0.25%	Supine	1
Ropivacaine, 0.2-0.35%	Knee arthroscopy	0
Lidocaine, 2-5%	Supine	6
Lidocaine, 3%	Prone	0.4
Lidocaine, 0.5%	Knee arthroscopy	17
Lidocaine, 5%	Knee arthroscopy	16
Lidocaine, 5%	Lithotomy	24
Mepivacaine, 1.5%	Knee arthroscopy, mixed	6-8
Mepivacaine, 4%	Mixed	30
Procaine, 5%	Knee arthroscopy	6
Prilocaine, 2-5%	Mixed	3-4%

Bupivacaine and ropivacaine reliably have a low incidence of TNS, whereas lidocaine typically exhibits the highest incidences. Other local anesthetics are intermediate in incidence of TNS.

Data from Liu SS, McDonald SB: Current issues in spinal anesthesia. Anesthesiology 2001;94:888-906; YaDeau JT, Liguori GA, Zayas VM: The incidence of transient neurologic symptoms after spinal anesthesia with mepivacaine. Anesth Analg 2005;101:661-665.

Table 51–9. Test Dose with Epinephrine to Detect Intravascular Injection*

CLINICAL SCENARIO	HEMODYNAMIC CRITERIA FOR INTRAVASCULAR INJECTION OF EPINEPHRINE, 15 µg
Healthy surgical patient	HR increase >20 bpm SBP increase >15 mm Hg T-wave amplitude decrease by >25% on ECG
General anesthesia	HR increase >8 bpm SBP increase >13 mm Hg
Spinal anesthesia	HR increase >20 bpm SBP unreliable
Age >60 yr	HR increase >9 bpm SBP increase >15 mm Hg
β-adrenergic blockade	HR unreliable SBP increase >15 mm Hg

*Responses expected to occur within 2 minutes of injection.
bpm, beats/min; ECG, electrocardiogram; HR, heart rate; SBP, systolic blood pressure.
Data from Liu SS, McDonald SB: Current issues in spinal anesthesia. Anesthesiology 2001;94:888-906; YaDeau JT, Liguori GA, Zayas VM: The incidence of transient neurologic symptoms after spinal anesthesia with mepivacaine. Anesth Analg 2005;101:661-665.

been reports of similar injuries from single-shot lidocaine spinal anesthetics using relatively high doses (more than 75 mg) with epinephrine.[102]

A much more frequent complication following neuraxial anesthesia is transient neurologic symptoms (TNS). These symptoms, initially termed *transient radicular irritation*, are described as back pain radiating to the buttocks or the lower extremities. Although TNS have been reported following spinal anesthesia with all local anesthetics, they are more common with lidocaine; the incidence in prospective studies is between 4% and 36%.[17] Wide disparity in the observed rates of TNS (Table 51–8) indicates that multiple factors are involved in its development. Factors demonstrated to contribute to the incidence of TNS include the use of lidocaine (relative risk of 4.35 compared with other local anesthetics), lithotomy position, knee arthroscopy, and early ambulation (as in outpatient surgery) (see Table 51–8).[103]

The cause of TNS continues to be elusive. Although direct neurotoxicity of local anesthetics would seem to be the obvious suspect, evidence against neurotoxicity being the principal cause of TNS includes lack of motor deficit and electrophysiologic changes during acute symptoms,[104] as well as response to nonsteroidal anti-inflammatory drugs (NSAIDs) and other modalities treating muscular discomfort. Other proposed mechanisms include stretching of neural structures via positioning and muscle relaxation, needle trauma, and muscular spasm.

Systemic Toxicity and Epidural Test Dose

Verification of correct placement of needles and catheters in the epidural space prior to initiating epidural anesthesia is required to avoid unintentional subdural, subarachnoid, and intravascular complications. Subdural injection is rare and may be difficult to recognize, because CSF will not be aspirated from the needle or catheter. The clinical pattern is of an unusually high block after administration of local anesthetic.[105] Inadvertent subarachnoid injection is a more frequent event, with the incidence of total spinals ranging from 0.3% to 0.6%. Unintentional intravascular injection is probably more common; the incidence of systemic toxic reactions, ranging from mild CNS symptoms to seizures, is from 2% to 0.01%.[105] It is important to realize that an epidural catheter may migrate into the intravascular or subarachnoid space at any time during use.

Although it is standard practice to administer a test dose prior to initiating full epidural anesthesia in an effort to detect unintentional placement of the needle or catheter into the subarachnoid or intravascular space, the efficacy of the epidural test dose varies, depending on components and patient population (Table 51–9). A 3-mL volume of local anesthetic is the primary component of a test dose. Theoretically, subarachnoid injection of this local anesthetic will produce a much more rapid and profound sensory and motor block than epidural injection. However, changes can be subtle and require time to develop. One study has indicated that 2 to 4 minutes are required prior to the development of sensory or motor block after subarachnoid injection of 3 mL of 1.5% lidocaine.[105] Subarachnoid injection of a bupivacaine test dose (3 mL, 0.25% to 0.5%) produces spinal blocks with highly variable onset time and spread and is probably not a reliable indicator.[105] Use of a test dose to detect subarachnoid placement is not without risk, because high spinal anesthesia requiring tracheal intubation after 3 mL of 1.5% lidocaine or 0.5% bupivacaine has been noted.[105] The local anesthetic component can also be used to detect intravascular injection by assessing symptoms of CNS irritability such as tinnitus, perioral tingling, metallic taste, and dizziness. Detection ability is limited, because the standard 3-mL test dose (45 mg lidocaine or 15 mg bupivacaine) contains insufficient local anesthetic to produce such symptoms reliably. Previous studies have suggested that larger doses, such as 100 mg, or 1 mg/kg of lidocaine, or more than 25 mg of bupivacaine, levobupivacaine, and ropivacaine re required in the nonsedated patient.[105,106] Administration of even modest doses of sedation will further reduce the ability of patients to report these symptoms (40% reduction in sensitivity).[107]

Epinephrine is commonly added to the local anesthetic dose to increase sensitivity for detection of intravascular injection. Addition of 15 µg is the standard dose of epinephrine and will consistently produce increases in heart rate and systolic blood pressure and reduction in T-wave amplitude within 60 to 120 seconds in healthy patients[105] (see Table 51–9). Use of beta blockers, advanced age, and addition of general or spinal anesthesia will decrease the hemodynamic response to this dose of epinephrine and reduced criteria should be applied in these circumstances.[105] Intravascular injection of epinephrine may be of concern in patients with hypertension, those at risk for myocardial ischemia, and obstetric patients, and potential hazards should be considered in these situations.

CONCLUSION

Through the years, neuraxial anesthesia has continuously endured controversy, which is likely to be true in the foreseeable future as well. In the hands of a skilled anesthesiologist, a properly performed neuraxial block customized for the appropriate patient is an elegant option for many common surgical procedures. In some clinical situations, this may be an important tool to help affect patient outcome positively. Further understanding of the benefits, risks, and nature of neuraxial anesthesia through well-structured research will allow clinicians to serve the needs of diverse patients more effectively.

SUMMARY

- A detailed three-dimensional understanding of neuraxial anatomy will allow a methodic and rational approach for accessing the subarachnoid and epidural spaces.
- For a given clinical scenario, the choice of anesthetic dose, agents, and combinations of agents should be individualized to optimize neuraxial blockade.
- Early recognition and appropriate treatment of hypotension and bradycardia associated with neuraxial anesthesia are essential to prevent cardiovascular collapse and untoward outcomes.

- Understanding the nature of transient neurologic symptoms and potential neurotoxicity of local anesthetics is continuing to evolve. However, there is growing consensus that TNS may not represent direct neural toxicity.
- For patients receiving anticoagulant and antiplatelet medications, assessing the risk-benefit ratio is challenging. Clinicians should be familiar with the recommendations presented by the American Society of Regional Anesthesia and Pain Management in the consensus statement addressing these issues.[99]

References

1. Lirk P, Kolbitsch C, Putz C: Cervical and high thoracic ligamentum flavum frequently fails to fuse in the midline. Anesthesiology 2003;99:1387-1390.
2. Richardson MG, Wissler RN: Density of lumbar cerebrospinal fluid in pregnant and nonpregnant humans. Anesthesiology 1996;85:326-330.
3. Bernards CM, Shen DD, Sterling ES, et al: Epidural, cerebrospinal fluid, and plasma pharmacokinetics of epidural opioids. Part 1: Differences among opioids. Anesthesiology 2003;99:455-465.
4. Liu SS, Melmed AP, Klos JW, et al: Prospective experience with a 20-gauge Tuohy needle for lumbar epidural steroid injections: Is confirmation with fluoroscopy necessary? Reg Anesth Pain Med 2001;26:143-146.
5. Goobie SM, Montgomery CJ, Basu R, et al: Confirmation of direct epidural catheter placement using nerve stimulation in pediatric anesthesia. Anesth Analg 2003;97:984-988.
6. Lechner TJ, van Wijk MG, Maas AJ, et al: Clinical results with the acoustic puncture assist device, a new acoustic device to identify the epidural space. Anesth Analg 2003;96:1183-1187.
7. Hogan QH, Prost R, Kulier A, et al: Magnetic resonance imaging of cerebrospinal fluid volume and the influence of body habitus and abdominal pressure. Anesthesiology 1996; 84:1341-1349.
8. Pitkanen M, Haapaniemi L, Tuominen M, et al: Influence of age on spinal anaesthesia with isobaric 0.5% bupivacaine. Br J Anaesth 1984;56:279-284.
9. Taivainen T, Tuominen M, Rosenberg PH: Influence of obesity on the spread of spinal analgesia after injection of plain 0.5% bupivacaine at the L3-4 or L4-5 interspace. Br J Anaesth 1990;64:542-546.
10. Horlocker TT, Wedel DJ: Density, specific gravity, and baricity of spinal anesthetic solutions at body temperature. Anesth Analg 1993;76:1015-1018.
11. Bodily MN, Carpenter RL, Owens BD: Lidocaine 0.5% spinal anaesthesia: A hypobaric solution for short-stay perirectal surgery. Can J Anaesth 1992;39:770-773.
12. Greene NM: Distribution of local anesthetic solutions within the subarachnoid space. Anesth Analg 1985;64:715-730.
13. Na KB, Kopacz, DJ: Spinal chloroprocaine solutions: Density at 37 degrees C and pH titration. Anesth Analg 2004;98:70-74.
14. Higuchi H, Hirata J, Adachi Y, et al: Influence of lumbosacral cerebrospinal fluid density, velocity, and volume on extent and duration of plain bupivacaine spinal anesthesia. Anesthesiology 2004;100:106-114.
15. Hirabayashi Y, Shimizu R: Effect of age on extradural dose requirement in thoracic extradural anaesthesia. Br J Anaesth 1993;71:445-446.
16. Liu SS, McDonald SB: Current issues in spinal anesthesia. Anesthesiology 2001;94:888-906.
17. Freedman JM, Li DK, Drasner K, et al: Transient neurologic symptoms after spinal anesthesia: An epidemiologic study of 1,863 patients. Anesthesiology 1998;89:633-641.

18. McDonald SB, Liu SS, Kopacz DJ, et al: Hyperbaric spinal ropivacaine: A comparison to bupivacaine in volunteers. Anesthesiology 1999;90:971-977.

19. Halpern SH, Walsh V: Epidural ropivacaine versus bupivacaine for labor: A meta-analysis. Anesth Analg 2003;96:1473-1479.

20. Sakura S, Sumi, M, Sakaguchi Y, et al: The addition of phenylephrine contributes to the development of transient neurologic symptoms after spinal anesthesia with 0.5% tetracaine. Anesthesiology 1997;87:771-778.

21. YaDeau JT, Liguori GA, Zayas VM: The incidence of transient neurologic symptoms after spinal anesthesia with mepivacaine. Anesth Analg 2005;101:661-665.

22. Martinez-Bourio R, Arzuaga M, Quintana JM, et al: Incidence of transient neurologic symptoms after hyperbaric subarachnoid anesthesia with 5% lidocaine and 5% prilocaine. Anesthesiology 1998;88:624-628.

23. Gissen AJ, Datta S, Lambert D: The chloroprocaine controversy. II: Is chloroprocaine neurotoxic? Reg Anesth 1984;9:135-145.

24. Smith KN, Kopacz DJ, McDonald SB: Spinal 2-chloroprocaine: A dose-ranging study and the effect of added epinephrine. Anesth Analg 2004;98:81-88.

25. Yoos JR, Kopacz DJ: Spinal 2-chloroprocaine for surgery: An initial 10-month experience. Anesth Analg 2005;100:553-558.

26. Vath JS, Kopacz DJ: Spinal 2-chloroprocaine: The effect of added fentanyl. Anesth Analg 2004;98:89-94.

27. Warren DT, Kopacz DJ: Spinal 2-chloroprocaine: The effect of added dextrose. Anesth Analg 2004;98:95-101.

28. Kouri ME, Kopacz DJ: Spinal 2-chloroprocaine: A comparison with lidocaine in volunteers. Anesth Analg 2004;98:75-80.

29. Kopacz DJ: Spinal 2-chloroprocaine: Minimum effective dose. Reg Anesth Pain Med 2005;30:36-42.

30. Taniguchi M, Bollen AW, Drasner K: Sodium bisulfite: Scapegoat for chloroprocaine neurotoxicity? Anesthesiology 2004;100:85-91.

31. Stevens RA, Urmey WF, Urquhart BL, et al: Back pain after epidural anesthesia with chloroprocaine. Anesthesiology 1993;78:492-497.

32. Hamber EA, Viscomi CM: Intrathecal lipophilic opioids as adjuncts to surgical spinal anesthesia. Reg Anesth Pain Med 1999;24:255-563.

33. Schneider SP, Eckert WA, Light AR: Opioid-activated postsynaptic, inward rectifying potassium currents in whole cell recordings in substantia gelatinosa neurons. J Neurophysiol 1998;80:2954-2962.

34. Liu S, Chiu AA, Carpenter RL, et al: Fentanyl prolongs lidocaine spinal anesthesia without prolonging recovery. Anesth Analg 1995;80:730-734.

35. Harukuni I, Yamaguchi H, Sato S, et al: The comparison of epidural fentanyl, epidural lidocaine, and intravenous fentanyl in patients undergoing gastrectomy. Anesth Analg 1995;81:1169-1174.

36. Ginosar Y, Riley ET, Angst MS. The site of action of epidural fentanyl in humans: The difference between infusion and bolus administration. Anesth Analg 2003;97:1428-1438.

37. Coda BA, Brown MC, Schaffer R, et al: Pharmacology of epidural fentanyl, alfentanil, and sufentanil in volunteers. Anesthesiology 1994;81:1149-1161.

38. Eisenach JC, De Kock M, Klimscha W: Alpha(2)-adrenergic agonists for regional anesthesia: A clinical review of clonidine (1984-1995). Anesthesiology 1996;85:655-674.

39. De Kock M, Eisenach J, Tong C, et al: Analgesic doses of intrathecal but not intravenous clonidine increase acetylcholine in cerebrospinal fluid in humans. Anesth Analg 1997;84:800-803.

40. Strebel S, Gurzeler JA, Schneider MC, et al: Small-dose intrathecal clonidine and isobaric bupivacaine for orthopedic surgery: A dose-response study. Anesth Analg 2004;99:1231-1238.

41. Davis BR, Kopacz DJ: Spinal 2-chloroprocaine: The effect of added clonidine. Anesth Analg 2005;100:559-565.

42. De Kock M, Gautier P, Fanard L, et al: Intrathecal ropivacaine and clonidine for ambulatory knee arthroscopy: A dose-response study. Anesthesiology 2001;94:574-578.

43. Aveline C, El Metaoua S, Masmoudi A, et al: The effect of clonidine on the minimum local analgesic concentration of epidural ropivacaine during labor. Anesth Analg 2002;95:735-740.

44. Wu CT, Jao SW, Borel CO, et al: The effect of epidural clonidine on perioperative cytokine response, postoperative pain, and bowel function in patients undergoing colorectal surgery. Anesth Analg 2004;99:502-509.

45. Klimscha W, Chiari A, Krafft P, et al: Hemodynamic and analgesic effects of clonidine added repetitively to continuous epidural and spinal blocks. Anesth Analg 1995;80:322-327.

46. Niemi G, Breivik H: Epinephrine markedly improves thoracic epidural analgesia produced by a small-dose infusion of ropivacaine, fentanyl, and epinephrine after major thoracic or abdominal surgery: A randomized, double-blinded crossover study with and without epinephrine. Anesth Analg 2002;94:1598-1605.

47. Sakura S, Sumi M, Morimoto N, et al: The addition of epinephrine increases intensity of sensory block during epidural anesthesia with lidocaine. Reg Anesth Pain Med 1999;24:541-546.

48. Moore JM, Liu SS, Pollock JE, et al: The effect of epinephrine on small-dose hyperbaric bupivacaine spinal anesthesia: Clinical implications for ambulatory surgery. Anesth Analg 1998;86:973-977.

49. Chiu AA, Liu S, Carpenter RL, et al: The effects of epinephrine on lidocaine spinal anesthesia: A cross-over study. Anesth Analg 1995;80:735-739.

50. Liu SS, Hodgson PS: Local anesthetics. In Barash PG, Cullen BF, Stoelting RF (eds): Clinical Anesthesia. Philadelphia, Lippincott-Raven, 2001, pp 449-472.

51. Lee BB, Ngan Kee WD, Plummer JL, et al: The effect of the addition of epinephrine on early systemic absorption of epidural ropivacaine in humans. Anesth Analg 2002;95:1402-1147.

52. Sharrock N, Go G, Mineo R: Effect of I.V. low-dose adrenaline and phenylephrine infusions on plasma concentrations of bupivacaine after lumbar extradural anaesthesia in elderly patients. Br J Anaesth 1991;67:694-698.

53. Cohen E: Distribution of local anesthetic agents in the neuraxis of the dog. Anesthesiology 1968;29:1002-1005.

54. Boswell MV, Iacono RP, Guthkelch AN: Sites of action of subarachnoid lidocaine and tetracaine: Observations with evoked potential monitoring during spinal cord stimulator implantation. Reg Anesth 1992;17:37-42.

55. Lang E, Krainick JU, Gerbershagen HU: Spinal cord transmission of impulses during high spinal anesthesia as measured by cortical evoked potentials. Anesth Analg 1989;69:15-20.

56. Cusick JF, Myklebust JB, Abram SE: Differential neural effects of epidural anesthetics. Anesthesiology 1980;53:299-306.

57. Zaric D, Hallgren S, Leissner L, et al: Evaluation of epidural sensory block by thermal stimulation, laser stimulation, and recording of somatosensory evoked potentials. Reg Anesth 1996;21:124-138.

58. Fink BR: Mechanisms of differential axial blockade in epidural and subarachnoid anesthesia. Anesthesiology 1989;70:851-858.

59. Gentili M, Huu PC, Enel D, et al: Sedation depends on the level of sensory block induced by spinal anaesthesia. Br J Anaesth 1998;81:970-971.

60. Antognini JF, Jinks SL, Atherley R, et al: Spinal anaesthesia indirectly depresses cortical activity associated with electrical stimulation of the reticular formation. Br J Anaesth 2003;91:233-238.

61. Ben-David B, Vaida S, Gaitini L: The influence of high spinal anesthesia on sensitivity to midazolam sedation. Anesth Analg 1995;81:525-528.

62. Tverskoy M, Fleyshman G, Bachrak L, et al: Effect of bupivacaine-induced spinal block on the hypnotic requirement of propofol. Anaesthesia 1996;51:652-653.

63. Morley AP, Derrick J, Seed PT, et al: Isoflurane dosage for equivalent intraoperative electroencephalographic suppression in patients with and without epidural blockade. Anesth Analg 2002;95:1412-1418.
64. Casati L, Fernandez-Galinski S, Barrera E, et al: Isoflurane requirements during combined general/epidural anesthesia for major abdominal surgery. Anesth Analg 2002;94:1331-1337.
65. Salinas FV, Sueda LA, Liu SS: Physiology of spinal anaesthesia and practical suggestions for successful spinal anaesthesia. Best Pract Res Clin Anaesthesiol 2003;17:289-303.
66. Yamakage M, Kamada Y, Toriyabe M, et al: Changes in respiratory pattern and arterial blood gases during sedation with propofol or midazolam in spinal anesthesia. J Clin Anesth 1999;11:375-379.
67. Curatolo M, Scaramozzino P, Venuti FS, et al: Factors associated with hypotension and bradycardia after epidural blockade. Anesth Analg 1996;83:1033-1040.
68. Auroy Y, Benhamou D, Bargues L, et al: Major complications of regional anesthesia in France: The SOS Regional Anesthesia Hotline Service. Anesthesiology 2002;97:1274-1280.
69. Kopp SL, Horlocker TT, Warner ME, et al: Cardiac arrest during neuraxial anesthesia: Frequency and predisposing factors associated with survival. Anesth Analg 2005;100:855-865.
70. Defalque RJ: Compared effects of spinal and extradural anesthesia upon the blood pressure. Anesthesiology 1962;23:627-630.
71. Rooke GA, Freund PR, Jacobson AF: Hemodynamic response and change in organ blood volume during spinal anesthesia in elderly men with cardiac disease. Anesth Analg 1997;85:99-105.
72. Carpenter RL, Caplan RA, Brown DL, et al: Incidence and risk factors for side effects of spinal anesthesia. Anesthesiology 1992;76:906-916.
73. Kimura T, Komatsu T, Hirabayashi A, et al: Autonomic imbalance of the heart during total spinal anesthesia evaluated by spectral analysis of heart rate variability. Anesthesiology 1994;80:694-698.
74. Introna R, Yodlowski E, Pruett J, et al: Sympathovagal effects of spinal anesthesia assessed by heart rate variability analysis. Anesth Analg 1995;80:315 321.
75. Gratadour P, Viale JP, Parlow J, et al: Sympathovagal effects of spinal anesthesia assessed by the spontaneous cardiac baroreflex. Anesthesiology 1997;87:1359-1367.
76. Campagna JA, Carter C: Clinical relevance of the Bezold-Jarisch reflex. Anesthesiology 2003;98:1250-1260.
77. Kinsella SM, Tuckey JP: Perioperative bradycardia and asystole: Relationship to vasovagal syncope and the Bezold-Jarisch reflex. Br J Anaesth 2001;86:859-868.
78. Pollard JB: Cardiac arrest during spinal anesthesia: Common mechanisms and strategies for prevention. Anesth Analg 2001;92:252-256.
79. Arndt JO, Bomer W, Krauth J, et al: Incidence and time course of cardiovascular side effects during spinal anesthesia after prophylactic administration of intravenous fluids or vasoconstrictors. Anesth Analg 1998;87:347-354.
80. Mojica JL, Melendez HJ, Bautista LE: The timing of intravenous crystalloid administration and incidence of cardiovascular side effects during spinal anesthesia: The results from a randomized controlled trial. Anesth Analg 2002;94:432-437.
81. Svensen C, Hahn RG: Volume kinetics of ringer solution, dextran 70, and hypertonic saline in male volunteers. Anesthesiology 1997;87:204-212.
82. Marhofer P, Faryniac B, Oismuller C, et al: Cardiovascular effects of 6% hetastarch and lactated Ringer's solution during spinal anesthesia. Reg Anesth Pain Med 1999;24:399-404.
83. Sharma SK, Gajraj NM, Sidawi JE: Prevention of hypotension during spinal anesthesia: A comparison of intravascular administration of hetastarch versus lactated Ringer's solution. Anesth Analg 1997;84:111-114.
84. Drobin D, Hahn RG: Volume kinetics of Ringer's solution in hypovolemic volunteers. Anesthesiology 1999;90:81-91.
85. Critchley LA, Conway F: Hypotension during subarachnoid anaesthesia: Haemodynamic effects of colloid and metaraminol. Br J Anaesth 1996;76:734-736.
86. Lee LA, Posner KL, Domino KB, et al: Injuries associated with regional anesthesia in the 1980s and 1990s: A closed claims analysis. Anesthesiology 2004;101:143-152.
87. Ward RJ, Bonica JJ, Freund FG, et al: Epidural and subarachnoid anesthesia: Cardiovascular and respiratory effects. JAMA 1965;25:275-278.
88. Bonica JJ, Akamatsu TJ, Berges PU, et al: Circulatory effects of epidural block: II. Effects of epinephrine. Anesthesiology 1971;34:514-522.
89. Ketia H, Diouf E, Tubach F, et al: Predictive factors of early postoperative urinary retention in the postanesthesia care unit. Anesth Analg 2005;101:592-596.
90. Lambert DH, Hurley RJ, Hertwig L, et al: Role of needle gauge and tip configuration in the production of lumbar puncture headache. Reg Anesth 1997;22:66-72.
91. Reina MA, de Leon-Casasola OA, Lopez A, et al: An in vitro study of dural lesions produced by 25-gauge Quincke and Whitacre needles evaluated by scanning electron microscopy. Reg Anesth Pain Med 2000;25:393-403.
92. Hannerz J, Ericson K, Bro Skejo HP: MR imaging with gadolinium in patients with and without post-lumbar puncture headache. Acta Radiol 1999;40:135-141.
93. Cheek TG, Banner R, Sauter J, et al: Prophylactic extradural blood patch is effective: A preliminary communication. Br J Anaesth 1988;61:340-342.
94. Colonna-Romano P, Shapiro BE: Unintentional dural puncture and prophylactic epidural blood patch in obstetrics. Anesth Analg 1989;69:522-523.
95. Moen V, Dahlgren N, Irestedt L: Severe neurological complications after central neuraxial blockades in Sweden 1990-1999. Anesthesiology 2004;101:950-959.
96. Carp H, Bailey S: The association between meningitis and dural puncture in bacteremic rats. Anesthesiology 1992;76:739-742.
97. Steffen P, Seeling W, Essig A, et al: Bacterial contamination of epidural catheters: Microbiological examination of 502 epidural catheters used for postoperative analgesia. J Clin Anesth 2004;16:92-97.
98. Vandermeulen EP, Van Aken H, Vermylen J: Anticoagulants and spinal-epidural anesthesia. Anesth Analg 1994;79:1165-1177.
99. Horlocker TT, Wedel DJ, Benzon HT, et al: Regional anesthesia in the anticoagulated patient: Defining the risks (the Second ASRA Consensus Conference on Neuraxial Anesthesia and Anticoagulation). Reg Anesth Pain Med 2003;28:172-197.
100. Horlocker TT, McGregor DG, Matsushige DK, et al: A retrospective review of 4767 consecutive spinal anesthetics: Central nervous system complications. Anesth Analg 1997;84:578-584.
101. Hodgson PS, Neal JM, Pollock JE, et al: The neurotoxicity of drugs given intrathecally (spinal). Anesth Analg 1999;88:797-809.
102. Gerancher JC: Cauda equina syndrome following single spinal administration of 5% hyperbaric lidocaine through a 25-gauge Whitacre needle. Anesthesiology 1997;87:687-689.
103. Zaric D, Christiansen C, Pace NL: Transient neurologic symptoms after spinal anesthesia with lidocaine versus other local anesthetics: A systematic review of randomized, controlled trials. Anesth Analg 2005;100:1811-1816.
104. Pollock JE, Burkhead D, Neal JM, et al: Spinal nerve function in five volunteers experiencing neurologic symptoms after lidocaine subarachnoid anesthesia. Anesth Analg 2000;90:658 665.
105. Mulroy MF, Norris MC, Liu SS: Safety steps for epidural injection of local anesthetics: Review of the literature and recommendations. Anesth Analg 1997;85:1346-1356.
106. Owen MD, Gautier P, Hood DD: Can ropivacaine and levobupivacaine be used as test doses during regional anesthesia? Anesthesiology 2004;100:922-925.
107. Moore JM, Liu SS, Neal JM: Premedication with fentanyl and midazolam decreases the reliability of intravenous lidocaine test dose. Anesth Analg 1998;86:1015-1017.

52 Intrathecal Drug Delivery: Overview of the Proper Use of Infusion Agents

Timothy R. Deer

Chronic pain is pain that endures after the expected time of healing. Millions of Americans suffer from this problem and seek medical treatment.[1] These syndromes, caused by a wide range of disease states, can lead to suffering, poor quality of life, and disability. In addition to the expense of direct patient care, a significant toll is placed on society in the areas of disability, social services, and ancillary costs. A secondary price is the effect on the family, social relationships, and substance abuse disorders.

Low back pain is the most common cause of chronic pain in the United States in those presenting for medical care. Most adults have suffered from an acute low back symptom in their lifetime, but most resolve in 6 weeks with minimal treatment. Those who persist with pain use a tremendous amount of resources and have extremely high health care expenditures.[2] The most symptomatic 6% of pain patients have been estimated to use 85% of the dollars spent on this problem. To treat the complicated pain patient more effectively, many physicians have begun to use an algorithmic approach when choosing applicable therapies. The role of intrathecal drug delivery varies significantly based on the disease state and the patient's individual characteristics.[3]

In patients with pain related to cancer or the effects of cancer treatment, intrathecal drug delivery systems (IDDSs) are a valuable option. In these patients, the use of intrathecal agents is appropriate if oral or transdermal opioids cause unacceptable side effects or prove to be ineffective at reasonable doses. In most of these patients, a nociceptive or mixed pain picture is present and spinal cord stimulation is not an option. In patients with pain unrelated to cancer, the use of intrathecal medications is often considered when the factors discussed are noted, but also after surgical intervention or failed spinal cord stimulation.

DISEASE STATES FOR INFUSION

To understand the current state of infusion therapy and drug choice, we must also understand the type of patients chosen for implantation. Cancer pain patients have been the primary group for intrathecal pumps in the past.[4] Up to 75% of all cancer patients suffer from pain as a component of their disease or from the side effects of treatment. Many of these patients can achieve pain control with other routes of opioid delivery, but as many as 15% do not have acceptable relief, even with aggressive attempts by the treating physician with comprehensive medical management.[5] This group is the primary treatment population for many implanting physicians.[6] In recent years, the use of pumps in the noncancer population has outpaced that for cancer-related pain syndromes. The largest group of patients in this complex of disease states has pain of spinal origin.[3]

Many patients who suffer from pain of the lower back or cervical spine eventually undergo spinal surgery. These chronic spine-related pain syndromes have become a problem of epidemic proportions in the United States, with more than 600,000 spinal surgeries performed annually. The number of these patients who fail to have their pain symptoms alleviated is significantly higher than those who do not have successful mechanical results. Another large group of spine-related disease patients is those with osteoporotic fractures that cause debilitation.[7] As many as 700,000 patients annually suffer from spinal compression fractures. In many of these patients, who are primarily female, the use of kyphoplasty or vertebroplasty has eliminated the need for pumps. Despite this new procedure, many of these patients still have such severe pain that intrathecal pumps are needed.[8]

Other diseases of the spine lead to severe pain, including spinal stenosis, spondylosis, and spondylolisthesis. In addition to spinal disorders, other diseases can cause severe pain that requires intrathecal drugs.[9] These problems include neuropathies, complex regional pain syndrome, rheumatoid arthritis, connective tissue disorders, chronic pancreatitis, and other visceral pain diseases. Many of these conditions can be treated with interventional procedures such as epidural injections, facet or sacroiliac joint injections, radiofrequency ablation, pulsed radiofrequency, or spinal cord stimulation. Unfortunately, in many cases, these procedures fail to give acceptable results.[10] Because of the prevalence of patients suffering from pain and the increasing societal awareness of treatment possibilities, the use of oral opioids has increased in recent years. This has led to a new focus on appropriate prescribing and regulation. Since 2000, the U.S. Drug Enforcement Administration (DEA) has clarified its position on these important issues, and the American Academy of Pain Medicine and American Pain Society have issued a consensus statement on the appropriate use of these substances.[11]

With new interventional techniques and recommendations for proper opioid use, the number of patients who fail all other options and are referred for consideration of an intrathecal pump is still considerable. The use of these devices for cancer pain has become part of the standard of care for those who fail conservative treatment. The use of intrathecal agents in noncancer pain is growing in popularity and many patients who may have failed the treatment in the past are now being reconsidered because of advances in the understanding of intrathecal drug options.

PRINCIPLES OF INTRATHECAL USE

In the 1980s, when pioneers such as Penn, Coombs, Mueller, North, and others began administering morphine into the spinal fluid for pain and baclofen for spasticity from cerebral palsy, the process was novel.[12] The U.S. Food and Drug Administration (FDA) approved preservative-free morphine for moderate to severe pain and baclofen for intractable spasticity based on these early research endeavors. The basic premise was to infuse the drug through an indwelling spinal catheter that received the drug from an indwelling subcutaneous pump. The pump is filled with the desired drug(s) and then infused by a computer-programmed rotor or a hydraulically driven continuous flow pump. The device itself requires skill to implant, refill, reprogram, and manage. The device is not helpful and may be harmful if the correct medications are not chosen; they should be selected based on the pain pattern, disease state, and patient's medical history.

Many implanters in the late 1980s and early 1990s began to notice that morphine alone was not an acceptable option for many chronic pain patients. Krames[3] noted that morphine as a solo agent often caused side effects and allergies and failed to produce the desired result. The desire to achieve better outcomes has led to a large body of evidence supporting the use of other agents to treat pain. New research has focused on bupivacaine, ziconotide, clonidine, midazolam, ketamine, tetracaine, hydromorphone, fentanyl, sufentanil, gabapentin, and other drugs. Animal toxicity data and human safety information have been studied for many of these agents. Neurotoxicity and adverse outcome reports have led to an understanding of these agents and to an algorithmic approach of how these medications should be used. This chapter will review the key points in regard to thinking algorithmically when selecting intrathecal drugs.

The Science behind Intrathecal Drugs

Intrathecal drug infusion allows drugs to be directly deposited near the spinal cord receptors. This avoids of the first-pass effect and eliminates the need for the agent to travel across the blood-brain barrier.[13] By this direct access to the receptors, an equianalgesic dose becomes markedly diminished as compared with alternative routes, resulting in a marked reduction of side effects and adverse events.

Access to spinal receptors may not be the only reason for the efficacy of intrathecal agents, because the process may be more complicated. Studies have shown that spinal opioid delivery results in adenosine release in the cerebrospinal fluid.[14] This effect appears to be related to an opioid-adenosine interaction. The possibility of other chemical mediators being released has been considered and ongoing research is studying nitric oxide, serotonin, and catecholamines.

In addition to the action at the spinal cord level, the use of intrathecal drug infusion also affects the receptors in the supraspinal region. This can lead to nausea, fatigue, and other adverse side effects, despite the low dose of medication.[15]

Outcomes Based on Disease

Much of the early work involving intrathecal therapy involved patients suffering from spasticity. This led to an interest for use in patients suffering from cancer pain. In the only prospective randomized multicenter study, Smith and colleagues[5] compared intrathecal drug infusion with comprehensive medical management (CMM). In the study, the patients were randomized to intrathecal drug trial with CMM or the comprehensive use of medications, nerve blocks, radiation, or other routine measures. The data were evaluated in an intent to treat manner, with the patient's results remaining in the original randomized group regardless of the results of the pump trial. The intrathecal treatment group had a significantly better result in regard to fatigue, level of consciousness, and quality of life for the patient and caregiver. There was also a strong trend toward improved survival in the intrathecal pump group. The difference did not reach statistical significance ($P = 0.6$) as randomized, but would have been significant had the groups been analyzed based on those actually receiving a permanent pump. This study, combined with many retrospective reports and case series, suggests that intrathecal infusions should be the standard of care for patients suffering from cancer. However, in many areas of the country, the referral to a specialist capable of placing these devices is often delayed until the last few weeks of life, which makes patients poor candidates for the therapy. This difficulty with the proper request for consultation has led cancer pain to become a secondary reason for pump implantation.

Most pumps placed in the United States for pain indications are implanted for diseases related to the spine. The most common diagnosis in this group is failed back surgery syndrome. Other reasons for implantation include compression fracture, spinal stenosis, radiculitis, spondylosis, and spondylolisthesis. The combination of opioid and baclofen has been administered in patients in whom a significant spinal cord injury has occurred, or in whom significant spasm is part of the clinical picture. There are no significant studies on the results of these combined infusions.

Although spinal diseases are the most common reason for placing an intrathecal pump, other disease states have had reports of positive outcomes with the IDDS. Diseases that have been successfully treated include peripheral neuropathy, interstitial cystitis, chronic abdominal pain, postherpetic neuralgia, postmastectomy syndrome, post-thoracotomy syndrome, and systemic diseases such as rheumatoid arthritis.[16] It should be noted that the disease state is only one component to consider when choosing an appropriate patient for intrathecal therapy. Patient factors that affect outcomes must also be considered.

Patient Selection for IDDS

The proper selection of a pump candidate is extremely important for achieving an acceptable outcome. Poor patient selection cannot be overcome with good technique or by using drug algorithms to salvage a proper response. In selecting a suitable patient, the implanter must consider several factors (Box 52–1).

If the patient has an acceptable profile meeting each of these factors, he or she is an ideal candidate for implantation. If not all criteria are met, but other reasonable options have been exhausted, the physician may move forward as a measure of last resort.[17]

Psychological Assessment

The patient suffering a from cancer-related pain syndrome does not require a psychological clearance, but may benefit from counseling to deal with chronic disease and death and dying issues. All patients receiving intrathecal drug infusions for noncancer pain should be evaluated for psychological stability.

BOX 52–1. QUESTIONS TO CONSIDER BEFORE INTRATHECAL PUMP PLACEMENT

Are the pain complaints related to an objective physiologic diagnosis?

Have less invasive therapies been tried or considered?

Is the patient's life expectancy 3 months or longer?

Is the patient's function limited by the pain symptoms?

Is the patient psychologically stable? Is there uncontrolled psychosis, severe depression, intractable anxiety, or significant personality disorders?

Is the patient compliant with other treatment recommendations?

Does the patient have any contraindications to pump placement, such as bacteremia, bleeding disorders, or localized infection?

Has an acceptable trial been performed to document adequate pain response and controllable side effects?

Is the patient aware of the expectations of the procedure?

Is the patient agreeable to permanent pump placement despite the risks of the procedure and the long-term risks of the drugs to be infused?

This can be done in several fashions, but the literature does not show any particular method as being superior to other tools. Options include interviewing analysis, multiphasic testing, intelligence testing, pain inventories, and overall impression of the patient by the mental health professional. There are no prospective studies that show a difference in outcome at 1 year or longer based on psychological assessment. It is widely believed that the chance of a good outcome may be diminished by untreated severe depression, anxiety disorder, or drug addiction, suicidal or homicidal ideation, or significant personality disorders. If any of these problems are present, they should be addressed and stabilized prior to placement of the permanent implant. Those with personality disorders have not been shown to be responsive to treatment and the presence of a diagnosis of borderline, antisocial, or multiple personality disorder should be approached with extreme caution.[18]

Pump Trialing

The choice of intrathecal infusion agents begins with the trial. The type of trial the patient undergoes is at the discretion of the physician who must decide several factors (Box 52–2).

A consensus group of 19 experienced physicians has recommended guidelines on intrathecal pump trial.[19] The overall recommendation was to use the results of the trial to help guide drug selection for the permanent pump placement.

In a large, prospective, multicenter analysis, Deer and colleagues[20] have compared trialing methods in patients selected for an intrathecal drug delivery system. An analysis of the results was performed at time of implant, at 3-month intervals, and at the end of 1 year. Factors that were used for analysis included functional ability, pain scores, quality of life, and patient satisfaction. Trialing was performed at 34 centers based on the usual practice of the implanting physician. Pain was also classified by each physician as nociceptive, neuropathic, or mixed pain syndrome based on preselected pain-descriptive terms such as aching, burning, shooting, or stabbing. Trialing was performed by single-shot, continuous infusion, or intermittent bolus.

In the analysis of the data, there was no statistical difference in outcomes at 1 year, regardless of the method of trialing used.[20] There was a difference in the outcome of the trial in patients who received monodrug therapy, which was usually an opioid, versus those who received two or more agents during the trial. There was an 11% reduction in the success rate when polyanalgesia was not used. This was statistically evident in patients who had neuropathic or mixed pain syndromes. The study showed that opioids, when used as sole agents, may not be adequate to treat complex neuropathic or mixed pain syndromes properly. This observation may even be more significant in treatments extending longer than 1 year, because a significant number of patients develop tolerance to opioids.

INTRATHECAL INFUSION AGENTS

FDA Approval and Off-Label Use

The FDA has approved two drugs for continuous intrathecal infusion for the treatment of pain, preservative-free morphine and ziconotide. Because of this regulatory approval, morphine is often the initial choice for the trialing process and permanent implantation. In many patients with burning, stabbing, or lancinating pain, morphine alone does not provide acceptable relief. Because of this problem, many physicians have routinely used second-line agents as adjuvants. These drugs include local anesthetics, drugs that work at the alpha receptors, and alternative opioids. The use of these drugs is termed *off-label use*. This is an acceptable practice as long as certain criteria are met (Box 52–3).

Scientific Evidence for the Use of Intrathecal Infusion Agents

The agents approved by the FDA for intrathecal use are helpful to a number of patients suffering from chronic pain. A survey of physician practice has shown that these drugs are not being used as sole agents in many clinical settings. The initial report was published prior to the approval of ziconotide. Hassenbusch and Portenoy[21] have surveyed physician implanters in North America, Europe, and Australia in regard to their choice of drugs for infusion and found that only 65% of patients have acceptable results when using morphine as a sole agent. Most physicians used other drugs as additives to morphine or changed to an alternate opioid, such as hydromorphone.

After this survey was published, a consensus conference of invited experts was held. The physicians represented a wide range of geographic locations, primary specialties, and academic or private settings. The goal of the conference was to give a consensus opinion on the evidence for use of the different intrathecal agents and to create an algorithm for their proper intrathecal use. An extensive search of the literature from 1965 to 1999 was performed to gather information; the data included animal and human studies on drugs injected into the intrathecal space. A Cochrane analysis was then done on the literature and the strength of evidence for each paper was evaluated. The results, published in 2000,[22] were supported at the time by the literature and clinical experience of the group. The algorithm created from that consensus panel suggested only morphine as a first-line agent, based on clinical data and safety information.

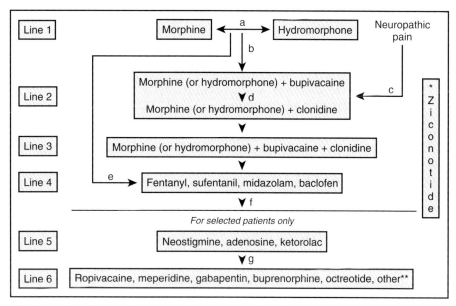

Figure 52–1. Recommended algorithm for intrathecal drug therapy. *a,* If side effects occur, switch to other opioid. *b,* If maximum dosage is reached without adequate analgesia, add adjuvant medication (Line 2). *c,* If patient has neuropathic pain, consider starting with opioid monotherapy (morphine or hydromorphone) or, in selected patients, with pure or predominant neuropathic pain, consider opioid plus adjuvant medication (Line 2). *d,* Some of the panel advocated the use of bupivacaine first because of concern about clonidine-induced hypotension. *e,* If side effects or lack of anesthesia on second first-line opioid, may switch to fentanyl (Line 4). *f,* There are limited preclinical data and limited clinical experience; therefore, caution in the use of these agents should be considered. *g,* There are insufficient preclinical data and limited clinical experience; therefore, extreme caution in the use of these agents should be considered. *,* This specific line to be determined after FDA review. **Potential spinal analgesics: methadone, oxymorphone, *N*-methyl-D-aspartate (NMDA) antagonists. (With permission from Hassenbusch SJ, Portenoy RK, Cousins M, et al: PolyAnalgesic Consensus Conference 2003: An update on the management of pain by intraspinal drug delivery—report of an expert panel. J Pain Symptom Manage 2004;27:540-563.)

The consensus conference reconvened in 2003 to reassess the literature that had been published since the first meeting. The recommended algorithm (Fig. 52–1) that came from the second meeting is often used as a guideline for ongoing medical care in patients with intrathecal pumps.[23] The algorithm changed slightly from the initial publication; morphine and hydromorphone were considered acceptable as first-line agents. The use of hydromorphone was supported by acceptable safety data, evidence of efficacy, and some information suggesting that it may be slightly less likely to cause an inflammatory mass. In case either one of the two first-line agents does not produce relief or cause side effects, then the second line of the algorithm is followed. This recommendation is to switch to the other first-line drug in patients with primary nociceptive pain or add clonidine or bupivacaine for patients with primary neuropathic or mixed pain syndromes. If these changes do not create an acceptable response, a third line of therapy is initiated, which involves using one of the primary opioids along with clonidine and bupivacaine. Another alternative is to substitute the opioid with a third choice, such as fentanyl or sufentanil, which are more lipophilic and potent.[22]

The use of local anesthetics in the spinal fluid is not a new concept and has been reported since the 1880s. The decision to add a local anesthetic to an infusion on a chronic basis is usually based on pain characteristics that are burning or lancinating. Of the available local anesthetics, only bupivacaine has been supported in the literature for continuous intrathecal infusion. Clinical studies have shown improved pain relief and a reduction in opioid dose when compared with opioid alone. The dosage most commonly studied has ranged from 1 to 20 mg/day.[24] Laboratory investigations have also supported the use of this drug. Data have shown bupivacaine to be stable in infusion systems, compatible with other drugs, and safe in animal models.[25] No other local anesthetic is currently supported by the literature for continuous infusion. Tetracaine is neurotoxic at high doses. Ropivacaine has been used in an anecdotal fashion, but recent studies do not support its use.[26]

In an elegant study, Staats and colleagues[27] studied the effects of intrathecal ziconotide. In this prospective, randomized, double-blind multicenter study, the efficacy of this drug was compared with that of saline in patients suffering from pain related to cancer and AIDS. The study showed statistically significant improvements in the treatment group in regard to analgesia, quality of life, and global satisfaction. Ziconotide, a modified snail toxin, works at the calcium channels in the neuraxis. At this level, the drug acts to block the N-type voltage channels selectively. By working at a target site that differs from that of opioids, this drug may provide relief in those who have failed morphine or hydromorphone. The possibility of using ziconotide as an adjuvant in combination with opioids is based on receptor differences. It is extremely sensitive to oxygen and, because of this, may have some limitations as an admixture. Current research is being undertaken to evaluate the efficacy of these combination therapies.[28]

Ziconotide was not included in the 2003 consensus algorithm but was discussed at that meeting. The decision was to await the results of the pivotal studies that were being evaluated by the FDA. After the paper by Staats and associates,[27] the FDA approved the drug for intrathecal use.

In addition to the pivotal study by Staats and coworkers,[27] there are additional data that support the use of ziconotide. Presley[29] has conducted a prospective double-blind, placebo-controlled study on 257 patients with pain of noncancer origin. In this study, efficacy was assessed after 10 to 12 days. The results showed statistically significant improvement in the treatment group in regard to pain relief ($P = 0.0002$) and improved mood, sleep, and quality of life. The ziconotide group also was able to reduce their oral opioid use as compared with placebo ($P = 0.001$).[29]

In most research settings, opioids have been grouped together for analysis, making it difficult for the results of any specific drug to be evaluated. The cancer studies and multicenter analysis have been discussed earlier in this chapter. Other studies have been performed with opioids as the sole agent. A small retrospective analysis evaluated 29 patients with intrathecal opioid infusion. Fentanyl was the drug infused in 8 of 29 patients, with an average time of infusion of 31 months. Results showed a 68.4% improvement in pain, with a statistically significant improvement in global satisfaction.[30] In another retrospective analysis, patients who received fentanyl alone were compared with patients on combination therapy with fentanyl and bupivacaine.[31] No adverse events were seen in either group, but the combination had a statistically significant reduction in pain compared to opioid alone.[31]

Methadone has been considered by some physicians as an ideal option for intrathecal infusion because of its properties as an oral agent. Oral methadone has been shown to have some efficacy for nociceptive and neuropathic pain secondary to action at opioid and N-methyl-D-aspartate (NMDA) receptors. Three studies considered the efficacy of methadone for intrathecal therapy; two of the three studies were done in a prospective fashion. The patients involved, who suffered from cancer and noncancer disease states, received a total dosage of 5 to 60 mg/day. The duration of treatment ranged from 3 days to 37 months. The authors noted a significant reduction in pain and improvement in the quality of life in each study. Adverse events included blurred vision and somnolence. There have been animal reports of NMDA receptor drugs creating spinal cord injury; it is recommended that the use of methadone be withheld until additional specific animal safety testing is performed.[32-34]

Deer and colleagues and others[35,36] have reviewed the use of bupivacaine as a sole agent and as an adjuvant to opioids. All previous studies using bupivacaine as a chronic infusion agent were analyzed. It was concluded that the literature supports stability of the drug in solution, absence of neurotoxicity, and safe clinical use of bupivacaine. The intrathecal administration of bupivacaine as a sole agent is not well supported in the literature with regard to efficacy, but it does appear to be safe. The drug is efficacious when used in combination with opioids and has synergistic effects resulting in opioid sparing.

Hassenbusch and colleagues[37] performed a 20-month prospective open-label analysis of clonidine for cancer and noncancer pain syndromes. In this phase II analysis of 31 patients, clonidine was used at doses ranging from 144 to 1200 µg. The results were favorable in the 22 patients who completed at least 1 year of follow-up. In this group, 59% were considered as achieving long-term success. The investigators noted that once an effective dose is achieved, tolerance rarely occurs and dose escalation is not reported. Equally important was that functional improvement is stable in the group that had pain relief, with minimal problems (e.g., somnolence, hypotension). In the patients who did not achieve good results, the limiting factor was hypotension, drowsiness, impotence, and urinary retention.[37] Other studies on clonidine have been retrospective in design.

The addition of clonidine, in the same dose range, to morphine or hydromorphone also provided limited improvement in efficacy compared with opioid alone.[38] Adverse events were numerous and included hypotension, sedation, pruritus, and catheter complications. The catheter complication involved a patient who received a long-term opioid infusion prior to the addition of clonidine. The patient developed an inflammatory mass attributed to the infusion but clonidine was not considered as a causative agent for the lesion. The other adverse events in this study are impossible to differentiate in regard to cause between the two drugs.[38]

Uhle and colleagues[39] have performed a prospective evaluation of 10 patients who received clonidine for neuropathic pain. In this study, the average dose of clonidine was 44 µg. The combination of clonidine with morphine or buprenorphine resulted in a significant reduction of patients' pain. Side effects were minor and easily controlled. It was also noted that buprenorphine has limited animal or human data on long-term safety as a chronic spinal agent. Clonidine stability studies have shown the drug to be stable in combination with morphine and with a combination of morphine and bupivacaine for longer than 90 days.[40]

In Australia and parts of Asia, the use of intrathecal midazolam has become a common practice; it should be noted that the drug in those areas is preservative-free.[41] The neurotoxicity data on preservative-free midazolam is acceptable in pig and sheep models. The sheep model also showed improved thresholds in regard to toleration of painful stimuli.[42]

Deer and Hassenbusch reconvened a third meeting of the consensus group to evaluate new studies and clinical data. This meeting, held in 2007,[43] will result in an update of the algorithm. The rest of this chapter will give recommendations for clinical practice based on the current literature. All treatment should be individualized based on patient history and relevant factors.

RECOMMENDATIONS FOR THE USE OF INTRATHECAL AGENTS FOR PAIN TREATMENT

Based on a review of the evidence and previous algorithms, several clinical decisions can be made in a logical progression based on patient responses and physician experience (Fig. 52–2).

Complications of intrathecal drug delivery can be related to the device or the infused drug. If a physician chooses to use an algorithmic approach to drug infusion, she or he must be able to recognize and treat adverse events. In a large retrospective analysis, Paice and colleagues[44] considered the issue of infusion system complications. In their analysis, 21.6% of patients showed some form of pump malfunction. The most common cause of problems in these patients

was catheter failure.[45] In a retrospective report, Coombs and associates[45] reported no complications in infusions of less than 3 months.

Long-term infusion of intrathecal opioids can influence hormonal function. This is also true for opioids delivered by other routes and is seen with naturally occurring opioids. The escalation of opioid dose should prompt the physician to consider changing the drug or using adjuvant medications to reduce the opioid dose.[46]

The effect of long-term intrathecal opioids in male patients was examined by Willis and Doleys[47] over a period of 12 months or longer. The overall effect seen in a large number of patients was decreased testosterone levels and small gonads. The treatment of this problem includes transdermal or injectable testosterone. Prior to supplementation with testosterone, the patient should undergo a prostate examination and have serum testosterone and prostate-specific antigen levels determined.

In addition to the hormonal effect of intrathecal opioids, another concern that has surfaced is the creation of an inflammatory mass. This noninfectious reaction usually occurs at the catheter tip and can lead to significant problems within the spinal

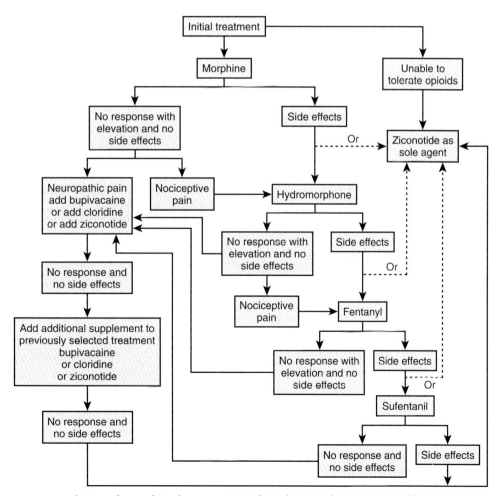

Figure 52–2. Treatment protocol. Note that a clinical reassessment of condition and symptom should be completed at each step in the decision tree. Other treatments may be assessed in extreme cases, such as end-of-life care.

cord. A consensus panel was created to make recommendations about the cause and prevention of these lesions.[48] Some of the panels' conclusions were to avoid concentrations of morphine or hydromorphone of more than 30 mg/mL, whenever possible. Coffey and Burchiel, who were both members of this panel, published an article recommending monitoring of the patient by intermittent physical examination.[49]

The data on inflammatory masses indicate that they may occur in clusters in individual practices. McMillan and colleagues[50] reported a significant cluster in their practice, with more than 40% of patients developing inflammatory masses and one having left lower extremity paralysis. Deer[51] performed magnetic resonance imaging in 208 consecutive patients presenting for follow-up; in this screening study, the incidence of granuloma was only 3%, with no significant sequelae being observed.

Yaksh and associates[52,53] performed studies using dog and sheep models and showed that the creation of the inflammatory mass is secondary to a localized inflammatory reaction to some opioids. A mitogen-activated protein kinase appears to play a role in the development of lymphocyte recruitment, resulting in a severe buildup of fibrous tissue. The body's response appears to resolve once the offending drug is discontinued. The most common offending agent was morphine. Hydromorphone appears to be able to cause the same problem, although not to the same extent as morphine. Other drugs, including fentanyl and baclofen, have been associated with infrequent reports of inflammatory mass formation.[49,51-53]

Some studies have theorized that clonidine may have an intrinsic effect on preventing inflammatory mass formation. Although this information is exciting, no prospective comparative study has shown this to be true. If the dose and concentration of the opioid can be reduced by a synergistic effect of clonidine, then the dose-sparing attribute of this drug may result in fewer inflammatory masses in patients receiving combination therapy.[53,54] Most of these have developed in patients receiving morphine at concentrations of 40 mg/mL or higher.

A similar concentration effect has been seen with hydromorphone, although it was reported at low concentrations, below 4 mg/mL. The presence of inflammatory masses in patients receiving low concentrations of opioid suggests the need for vigilance in all patients with intermittent neurologic examinations, which should be performed at the time of follow-up or pump refill.[55]

Peripheral edema can occur after intrathecal opioid infusion. This problem has been theorized to occur as a result of opioid action on the pituitary leading to changes in antidiuretic hormone levels. Previous retrospective analyses of patients who experience this problem noted that many of the patients had a history of pedal edema. Such patients should therefore be monitored for the development of this problem. Treatments include diuretics, compression stockings, and extremity elevation. If these treatments fail, the infused drug should be rotated.[56]

COMPOUNDING

Preservative-free morphine sulfate sterile solution (Infumorph) is the only drug currently approved and labeled by the FDA for the intrathecal treatment of pain. As noted, many patients fail to respond to morphine alone and require an admixture of two or more agents. Other patients require a concentration of medication that is not commercially available. To satisfy both these requirements, many implanters use a compounding pharmacist to mix the desired drug because most off-label medications for intrathecal use are not available in commercial form. Many commercial drugs are prepared with preservatives or excipients or have improper solubility properties for intrathecal use. Several factors should be considered by the compounding pharmacist when mixing these agents (Box 52–4).

The U.S. Pharmacopoeia and the American Society of Health System Pharmacists have issued guidelines on compounded sterile drugs that may be infused into the spinal fluid. These guidelines are helpful and apply to patients undergoing intrathecal drug infusions.[52,57,58] Once the implanter has chosen a compounding pharmacist, the physician should ask for documentation that the guidelines are being followed and should also visit the compounding center, if possible.

INTRATHECAL DRUG INFUSIONS: FUTURE CONSIDERATIONS

Advances in the area of spinal cord stimulation have been largely based on equipment development. The same potential for advances in devices exist for pumps. These possibilities include more durable catheters, smaller pumps, improved programming capabilities, and better sensing mechanisms. Even though these possibilities are exciting, most advances in drug delivery will be in the arena of new infusion agents. Criteria for developing new drugs are strict and include chemical stability, compatibility with catheters and pumps, acceptable animal toxicology data, and viable pharmacokinetic drug formulations.[59] The next agent to make a critical difference

---

BOX 52–4. IDEAL PROPERTIES OF COMPOUNDED DRUGS FOR INTRATHECAL USE

The drug should:
- Be labeled "preservative-free" and contain no contaminants and toxins
- Have an acceptable pH
- Be soluble at body temperature
- Be compatible with intrathecal devices
- Be tested for accuracy of concentration and be documented

clinically is as yet unknown, but several agents have shown some promise.

Deer and colleagues[60,61] have examined the use of the growth hormone analogue octreotide in a randomized, prospective, double-blind study. The results showed the drug to be safe, with minimal adverse effects. The efficacy of the drug was not statistically significant when compared with placebo; however the lack of side effects led the authors to question appropriate dosing. Additional analysis with a more aggressive dosing schedule should be considered to evaluate the potential of this drug fully.

Another promising agent is gabapentin, which has been used extensively via oral administration to treat neuropathic pain. The analgesic efficacy of intrathecal gabapentin has been evaluated in humans. Initial pilot studies showed no adverse events.[23] Gabapentin has also been evaluated in rat models. In a bolus dosing protocol, the drug reduced mechanical allodynia, diminished hyperalgesia, and reduced neuropathic pain.

Gabapentin has shown no ability to affect nociceptive pain based on formalin and hot-plated paw testing. Intrathecal gabapentin was much more effective and potent than when given by any other route.[62-64] In addition to being a potentially efficacious drug for monotherapy, animal models have also shown potential for combination therapy. Gabapentin may work synergistically when combined with clonidine or with agents working on NMDA receptors.

Rat models using these drug combinations[65] have shown a much more effective response when given with two or more of these agents than any of the drugs alone. Tizanidine also has potential as a long-term drug. In a comparative dog study, clonidine had similar efficacy as tizanidine for acute pain when both drugs were given intrathecally. The clonidine group had a significantly higher number of adverse events.[66]

Possible intrathecal drugs include conopeptides, hormonal analogues, anticonvulsants, free radical scavengers, and drugs that affect nitric oxide. Future studies will reveal whether any of these agents will result in a new armamentarium to use in treating this difficult group of patients.

CONCLUSION

Intrathecal drug delivery is a valuable tool for patients suffering from moderate to severe pain that has not responded to more conservative measures. The use of these therapies requires a commitment on the part the physician, nursing staff, compounding pharmacist, and the other members of the pain management team. Good outcomes can be achieved when patients are chosen correctly, the proper drug is used, and a logical algorithmic approach to infusion therapy is followed. The physician should remain vigilant, and be aware of possible adverse events that can occur as a result of intrathecal drug infusions. Future studies

are needed; investment in new drug research will be critical to ensuring the advancement of intrathecal therapy.

References

1. Argoff CE: Pharmacologic management of chronic pain. J Am Osteopath Assoc 2002:102:S21-S27.
2. Long DM, Ben Debba M, Torgerson WS, et al: Persistent back pain and sciatica in the United States: Patient characteristics. J Spinal Disord 1996;9:40-58.
3. Krames ES: Intrathecal infusional therapies for intractable pain: Patient management guidelines. J Pain Symptom Manage 1993;8:36-46.
4. Hassenbusch SJ, Pillay PK, Magdinec M, et al: Constant infusion of morphine for intractable cancer pain using an implanted pump. J Neurosurgery 1990;73:405-409.
5. Smith TJ, Staats PS, Deer T, et al:. Randomized clinical trial of an implantable drug delivery system compared with comprehensive medical management for refractory cancer pain: Impact on pain, drug-related toxicity, and survival. J Clin Oncol 2002;18:4040-4049.
6. Foley KM: The treatment of cancer pain. N Engl J Med 1985; 313:84-95.
7. Deer T: Injections for the diagnosis and treatment of spinal pain. Anesthesiology 2004;32:53-69.
8. Wu SS, Lachmann E, Nagler W: Current medical, rehabilitation, and surgical management of vertebral compression fractures. J Womens Health 2003;12:17-26.
9. Pahl MA, Brislin B, Boden S, et al: The impact of four common lumbar spine diagnoses upon overall health status. Spine J 2006;6:125-130.
10. Burton AW, Hassenbusch SJ 3rd, Warneke C, et al: Complex regional pain syndrome (CRPS): Survey of current practices. Pain Pract 2004;4:74-83.
11. American Academy of Pain Medicine and the American Pain Society: Consensus Statement: The Use of Opioids for the Treatment of Chronic Pain. Glenview, Ill, American Pain Society and American Academy of Pain Medicine, 1997.
12. Coombs DW, Saunders RL, Gaylor MS, et al: Relief of continuous chronic pain by intraspinal narcotics infusion via an implanted reservoir. JAMA 1983;250:2336-2339.
13. Onofrio BM: Treatment of chronic pain of malignant origin with intrathecal opiates. Clin Neurosurg 1983;31:304-315.
14. Eisenach JC, Hood DD, Curry R, et al: Intrathecal but not intravenous opioids release adenosine from the spinal cord. Pain 2004;5:64-68.
15. Goodchild C, Nadeson R, Cohen E: Supraspinal and spinal cord opioid receptors are responsible for antinociception following intrathecal morphine injections. Eur J Anesthesiol 2004;21:179-185.
16. Manchikanti L, Staats PS, Singh V, et al: Evidence-based practice guidelines for the interventional techniques in the management of chronic spinal pain. Pain Physician 2003;6:3-81.
17. Shetter AG, Hadley MN, Wilkinson E: Administration of intraspinal morphine sulfate for the treatment of intractable cancer pain. J Neurosurg 1986;18:740-747.
18. Brown J, Klapow J, Doleys D, et al: Disease-specific and generic health outcomes: A model for the evaluation of long-term intrathecal opioid therapy in noncancer low back pain patients. Clin J Pain 1999;15:122-131.
19. Katz N: The impact of pain management on quality of life. J Pain Symptom Manage 2002;24:S38-S47.
20. Deer T, Chapple I, Classen A, et al: Intrathecal drug delivery for treatment of chronic low back pain: Report from the National Outcomes Registry for Low Back Pain. Pain Med 2004;5.6-13.
21. Hassenbusch SJ, Portenoy RK: Current practices in intraspinal therapy—a survey of clinical trends and decision making. J Pain Symptom Manage 2000;20:S4-S11.
22. Bennett G, Burchiel K, Buchser E, et al: Clinical guidelines for intraspinal infusion: A report of an expert panel. PolyAnalgesic Consensus Conference 2000. J Pain Symptom Manage 2000;20:S37-S43.

23. Hassenbusch SJ, Portenoy RK, Cousins M, et al: PolyAnalgesic Consensus Conference 2003: An update on the management of pain by intraspinal drug delivery—report of an expert panel. J Pain Symptom Manage 2004;27:540-563.

24. Deer T, Caraway DL, Kim CK, et al: Clinical experience with intrathecal bupivacaine in combination with opioid for the treatment of chronic pain related to failed back surgery syndrome and metastatic cancer pain of the spine. Spine J 2002;2:274-8.

25. Hildebrand K, Elsberry D, Deer T: Stability, compatibility, and safety of intrathecal bupivacaine administered chronically via an implantable delivery system. Clin J Pain 2001;17:239-244.

26. Dahm P, Lundborg C, Janson M, et al: Comparison of 0.5% intrathecal bupivacaine with 0.5% intrathecal ropivacaine in the treatment of refractory cancer and noncancer pain conditions: Results from a prospective, crossover, double-blind, randomized study. Reg Anesth Med 2000;25:480-487.

27. Staats P, Yearwood T, Charapata SG, et al: Intrathecal ziconotide in the treatment of refractory pain in patients with cancer or AIDS: A randomized controlled trial. JAMA 2004;291:63-70.

28. Deer T, Kim C, Bowman R, et al: A case analysis of safety for patients receiving opioids plus ziconotide for noncancer pain [abstract]. Presented at the American Academy of Pain Medicine Annual Meeting, Feb 6-10, 2007, New Orleans, La.

29. Presley RW: Intrathecal ziconotide in the treatment of opioid-refractory neuropathic and nonmalignant pain: A controlled clinical trial. (submitted for publication).

30. Roberts LJ, Finch PM, Goucke CR, et al: Outcome of intrathecal opioids in chronic noncancer pain. Eur J Pain 2001;5:353-361.

31. Mironer YE, Grumman S: Experience with alternative solutions in intrathecal treatment of chronic nonmalignant pain. Pain Digest 1999;9:299-302.

32. Mironer YE, Tollison CD: Methadone in the intrathecal treatment of chronic nonmalignant pain resistant to other neuroaxial agents: The first experience. Int Neuromod Soc 2001;4:25-31.

33. Mironer YE, Haasis JC III, Chappleet ET: Successful use of methadone in neuropathic pain: A multicenter study by the National Forum of Independent Pain Clinicians. Pain Digest 1999;9:191-193.

34. Shir Y, Shapira SS, Shenkman Z, et al: Continuous epidural methadone treatment for cancer pain. Clin J Pain 1991;7:339-341.

35. Bennett G, Serafini M, Burchiel K, et al: Evidence-based review of the literature on intrathecal delivery of pain medication. J Pain Symptom Manage 2000;20:S12-S36.

36. Deer TR, Serafini M, Buchser E, et al: Intrathecal bupivacaine for chronic pain: A review of current knowledge. Neuromodulation 2002;4:196-207.

37. Hassenbusch SJ, Gunes S, Wachsman S, et al: Intrathecal clonidine in the treatment of intractable pain: A phase I/II study. Pain Med 2002;3:85-91.

38. Ackerman LL, Follett KA, Rosenquist RW: Long-term outcomes during treatment of chronic pain with intrathecal clonidine or clonidine/opioid combinations. J Pain Symptom Manage 2003;26:668-677.

39. Uhle EI, Becker R, Gatscher S, et al: Continuous intrathecal clonidine administration for the treatment of neuropathic pain. Stereotact Funct Neurosurg 2000;75:167-175.

40. Bennett G, Deer T, Du Pen S, et al: Future directions in the management of pain by intraspinal drug delivery. J Pain Symptom Manage 2000;20:S44-S50.

41. Yaksh TL, Allen JW: The use of intrathecal midazolam in humans: A case study of process. Anesth Analg 2004;98:1536-1545.

42. Johansen MJ, Satterfield WC, Baze WB, et al: Toxicity and efficacy of intrathecal midazolam. Pain Med 2002;3:188-189.

43. 2007 Polyanalgesic Consensus Panel, Jan 18-21, 2007, Miami, Fla.

44. Paice J, Penn R, Shott S: Intraspinal morphine for chronic pain: A retrospective, multicenter study. J Pain Symptom Manage 1996;11:71-80.

45. Coombs, D, Maurer L, Saunders R: Outcomes and complications of continuous intraspinal narcotic analgesia for cancer pain control. J Clin Oncol 1984;2:1414-1420.

46. Daniell H: Hypogonadism in men consuming sustained-action oral opioids. J Pain 2002;3:377-384.

47. Willis KD, Doleys DM: The effects of long-term intraspinal infusion therapy with noncancer pain patients: Evaluation of patient, significant-other, and clinic staff appraisals. Neuromodulation 1999;2:241-253.

48. Hassenbusch S, Burchiel K, Coffey RJ, et al: Management of intrathecal catheter-tip inflammatory masses: A consensus statement. Pain Med 2002;3:313-323.

49. Coffey R, Burchiel K: Inflammatory mass lesions associated with intrathecal drug infusion catheters: Report and observations on 41 patients. Neurosurgery 2002;50:78-86.

50. McMillan M, Doud T, Nugent W: Catheter-associated masses in patients receiving intrathecal analgesic therapy. Anesth Analg 2003;96:186-190.

51. Deer T: A prospective analysis of intrathecal granuloma in chronic pain patients: A review of the literature and report of a surveillance study. Pain Physician 2004;7:225-228.

52. Yaksh TL, Hassenbusch S, Burchiel K, et al: Inflammatory masses associated with intrathecal drug infusion: A review of preclinical evidence and human data. Pain Med 2002;3:300-312.

53. Yaksh TL, Horais KA, Tozier NA, et al: Chronically infused intrathecal morphine in dogs. Anesthesiology 2003;99:174-87.

54. Walker SM, Goudas LC, Cousins MJ, et al: Combination spinal analgesic chemotherapy: A systematic review. Anesth Analg 2002;95:674-715.

55. Gradert TL, Baze WB, Satterfield WC, et al: Safety of chronic intrathecal morphine infusion in a sheep model. Anesthesiology 2003;99:188-198.

56. Aldrete JA, Couto da Silva JM: Leg edema from intrathecal opiate infusions. Eur J Pain 1997;4:361-365.

57. Grouls RJE, Korsten EHM, Yaksh TL: General considerations for the formulation of drugs for spinal delivery. In Yaksh TL (ed): Spinal Drug Delivery. Amsterdam, Elsevier Science, 1999, pp 371-393.

58. Yaksh TL, Rathbun ML, Provencher JC: Preclinical safety evaluation for spinal drugs. In Yaksh TL (ed): Spinal Drug Delivery. Amsterdam, Elsevier Science, 1999, pp 417-437.

59. Bennett G, Deer T, Du Pen S, et al: Future directions in the management of pain by intraspinal drug delivery. J Pain Symptom Manage 2000;20:S44-S50.

60. Deer TR, Kim CK, Bowman RG II, et al: The use of continuous intrathecal infusion of octreotide in patients with chronic pain of noncancer origin: An evaluation of side effects and toxicity in a prospective double blind fashion. Neuromodulation 2005;8:171-175.

61. Deer TR, Penn R, Kim CK, et al: The use of continuous intrathecal infusion of octreotide in patients with chronic pain of noncancer origin: An evaluation of efficacy in a prospective double blind fashion. Neuromodulation 2006;8:284-289.

62. Yoon MH, Yaksh TL: The effect of intrathecal gabapentin on pain behavior and hemodynamics on the formalin test in rats. Anesth Analg 1999;89:434-439.

63. Wallin J, Cui JG, Yakhnitsa V, et al: Gabapentin and pregabalin suppress tactile allodynia and potentiate spinal cord stimulation in a model of neuropathy. Eur J Pain 2002;6:261-272.

64. Lu C, Westlund K: Gabapentin attenuates nociceptive behaviors in an acute arthritis model in rats. J Pharmacol Exp Ther 1999;290:214-219.

65. Cheng JK, Pan HL, Eisenach JC: Antiallodynic effect of intrathecal gabapentin and its interaction with clonidine in a rat model of postoperative pain. Anesthesiology 2000;92:1126-1131.

66. Kroin JS, McCarthy RJ, Penn RD, et al: Intrathecal clonidine and tizanidine in conscious dogs: Comparison of analgesic and hemodynamic effects. Anesth Analg 1996;82:627-635.

CHAPTER
53 Intra-articular Analgesia

Anil Gupta and Kjell Axelsson

An ideal analgesic should provide analgesia locally at the site of trauma without any systemic or local side effects, preferably as long as the pain persists. Scientists have searched for this ideal analgesic over several centuries, but as yet no such drug exists. Local anesthetics (LAs) are a good example of drugs that provide excellent analgesia with minimal toxicity when they are used in the correct doses. However, LAs have a short duration of effect,[1] which limits their usefulness to the immediate postoperative period, unless injected intermittently or continuously in traumatized tissues. Therefore the search for LAs enclosed in microspheres or infusions through catheters in order to prolong their duration of effect, continues.[2] Opiates have been used a long time and are efficacious, specifically following major surgery. Following the discovery and isolation of opioid receptors on peripheral nerves and joints in the late 1980s,[3] an intensive search began for the use of opiates peripherally to obtain pain relief without their well-known side effects. Thus analgesia for postoperative pain relief following arthroscopy and arthroscopic knee surgery has been the focus of more than 50 publications during the past 15 years, when the first reports described clinically beneficial effects of morphine injected intra-articularly. Although most authors have studied the knee joint as a model for research, other joints including the ankle, shoulder, and elbow, also have been studied. A variety of drugs and combinations of drug have been injected intra-articularly in order to provide analgesia, including LAs and opioids, nonsteroidal anti-inflammatory drugs (NSAIDs), α_2-adrenergic agonists, anticholinergics, and steroids, as well as ketamine (Table 53–1).

Despite the notoriously large number of publications on these issues, a well-designed study recruiting a sufficient number of patients and asking the relevant questions has yet to be performed. This review of the literature summarizes the findings of some of the studies published and focuses on the drawbacks, limitations, and problems that surround this complex but interesting question of the efficacy of IA (intra-articular) analgesics in the clinical setting.

VARIATIONS IN PAIN INTENSITY AND METHODS OF MEASUREMENT

Intensity of Postoperative Pain

In order to study the efficacy of drugs following surgery, it is important to know the intensity of anticipated pain. Studying efficacy of analgesics following procedures associated with only mild pain are likely to be either unsuccessful (i.e., not show analgesic efficacy) or require a forbiddingly large number of patients in order to show statistical significance. In addition, even when statistical difference is seen, it may not be clinically meaningful, and sometimes ethically questionable. Therefore, when assessing the efficacy of drugs injected intra-articularly, it is important to study procedures associated with moderate to severe postoperative pain. In this way, it is estimated that 20% to 30% fewer patients may need to be studied, to provide meaningful assessment of drug efficacy.[4] Because of the variation in the pain intensity between procedures, a group of international experts have started working on procedure-specific pain management and analyzing the best evidence available to date for the management of postoperative pain. More information on this is available on their home page (www.postoppain.org).

Biologic Variations in Pain Intensity

Recent evidence seems to suggest that women have more pain following arthroscopic surgery compared with men and may account for some of the differences between men and women. In one study, Taenzer and colleagues studied 736 patients undergoing arthroscopic anterior cruciate ligament reconstruction and found that women seem to experience greater intensity of pain that is associated with a decrease in an intermediate measure of functional outcome.[5] They concluded that these differences might result from differences in either response to analgesics or neuron processing. In another study, Rosseland and associates showed that gender differ-

Table 53–1. Intra-articular Analgesics

DRUG	DOSES USED	NUMBER OF STUDIES PUBLISHED	NUMBER OF SYSTEMATIC REVIEWS PUBLISHED
Local anesthetics		>20	1
Opioids			4
Morphine*	0.5, 1, 2, 3, 4, 5, 10 mg	>50	
Pethidine	10, 50, 100, 200 mg	5	
Fentanyl	10, 50 µg	<5	
Sufentanil	5, 10 µg	<5	
NSAIDs			0
Ketorolac	5, 30, 60 mg	5-10	
Tenoxicam	20 mg	5-10	
α₂ Agonists			0
Clonidine	150, 1 µg/kg	5-10	
Others			0
Neostigmine	500 µg	<5	
Ketamine	0.5 mg/kg		
Oxycodone	5 mg	1	
Diamorphine	5 mg	1	

*For studies on IA morphine, the reader is referred to the already published systematic reviews with extensive reference lists.[4,44-46]
NSAIDs, nonsteroidal anti-inflammatory drugs.

ences might account for the differences in analgesia experienced by women after arthroscopic knee surgery, with women experiencing more pain than men.[6] Finally, Cepeda and Carr found that women had more intense pain and required 30% more morphine to achieve a similar degree of analgesia compared with men.[7] In addition to sex variation in pain intensity, variation of pain intensity during the different phases of the menstrual cycle also should be considered in studies on analgesic efficacy, because some evidence seems to suggest that the analgesic consumption is greater in women during the luteal phase of the menstrual cycle.[8] There also is a clinically significant reduction in the intensity of pain perception or symptoms with age so that older people appear to perceive less pain than do younger patients.[9] This could be related to the decrease in Aδ and C-fiber nociceptive function, delay in central sensitization, or an increase in pain thresholds.[10-12]

Assessment of Pain

Pain is a subjective sensation and varies tremendously among individuals. Consequently the methods used to measure pain, as well as the scales described in the literature, are numerous. Although the Visual Analogue Scale (VAS) and the numeric rating scale (NRS) are well described and validated in the literature,[13] other scales may not be properly evaluated; therefore, it is extremely important to use standard and validated methods for pain assessment. In addition, it also is important to specify whether pain has been assessed during rest or during movement, particularly when movement may aggravate pain intensity. Varying terminology is used to describe pain on movement such as "dynamic pain," "pain on coughing," "pain on movement," or pain during "knee flexion" or "leg elevation." As long as the parameter being measured is correctly described and constant in all patients, the exact terminology can remain

descriptive in relation to the type of surgery. Measuring pain intensity at fixed intervals after the operation may sometimes give inaccurate results because of its relationship to the last intake of analgesics. Thus not only the pain intensity but also the total consumption of analgesics may be relevant to the conclusions drawn. Sometimes, the "area under the curve" for pain intensity assessment may be more relevant than the pain intensity at fixed times. Finally, in studies on postoperative pain and analgesics, it may be more relevant to measure pain relief rather than intensity. Although the latter is an indirect measure of pain, relief of pain is more relevant for the patient. However, pain relief is somewhat more difficult to measure because VAS or NRS may incorrectly describe pain relief as pain intensity.

Saline, a Placebo Analgesic

In a randomized controlled trial, Rosseland and associates showed that pain after knee arthroscopy is modest and short-lived and can successfully be treated with intra-articular saline 10 mL or 1 mL (placebo).[14] The same group also found that the addition of 2 mg morphine to 10 mL saline did not improve the analgesia following arthroscopic knee surgery in patients with moderate to severe pain.[15] This could be explained because saline may produce a local analgesic effect by cooling or by diluting IA algogenic substances. Indeed, this may represent a true therapeutic effect attributable to the removal or dilution of pain-mediating substances in the wound as suggested by Thomas and colleagues.[16] Similarly, Axelsson and associates showed analgesia following the injection of saline subacromially.[17] Alford and Fadale found that saline infusions intra-articularly provided similar pain relief as bupivacaine infusion following anterior cruciate ligament repair.[18] These were both better than no infusion, suggesting that pain mediators locally may be washed away by the infusion of saline. The dilution of histamine, potassium, or vasoactive polypeptides, which mediate pain, has been suggested to be one explanation for this effect.[16] Placebo effect is well defined in the literature in studies on analgesics, and therefore it is important to include a placebo group in randomized, double-blind trials, specifically when studying new analgesics or techniques.

DRUGS USED INTRA-ARTICULARLY

Local Anesthetics

Single doses of LA administered intra-articularly are used frequently. LAs have been used successfully as the sole anesthetic for minor arthroscopic procedures (Fig. 53–1) and, used in this way, provide adequate analgesia of short duration. In the only systematic review published in the literature on the efficacy of LAs injected intra-articularly, Møiniche and coworkers evaluated double-blind, randomized controlled trials comparing LAs with placebo or no treatment in the relief of postoperative pain following

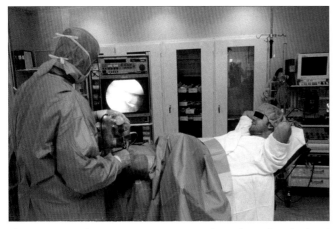

Figure 53–1. Arthroscopy is now commonly performed under local anesthetic.

arthroscopic knee surgery.[1] They found a significant prolongation of pain relief lasting between 30 and 50 minutes in only 2 of 6 studies. In addition, these authors also found that in 9 (of 20) studies, the consumption of supplementary analgesics was reduced by 10% to 50% during the observation periods of up to 4 hours (Fig. 53–2). However, in most cases, the analgesic requirements were small to moderate, reflecting on the mild intensity of postoperative pain in these studies. They concluded that the pain relief obtained using LAs injected intra-articularly is mild to moderate, and of short duration. However, this may be of clinical significance in outpatient surgery. LAs have been used via catheters as intermittent injections or continuous infusion intra-articularly into the knee joint,[19] subacromially,[17] intra-abdominally following hysterectomy,[20] subcutaneously following cesarean section,[21] and during peripheral nerve blocks,[22] with variable success.

Major Knee Surgery

A summary of the articles published and the conclusions drawn by the authors during knee surgery are summarized in Table 53–2. The anterior synovium, infrapatellar fat pad, and joint capsule are sensitive to pain stimuli.[23] Chew and colleagues tested the analgesic efficacy of 0.25% or 0.5% bupivacaine administered into the infrapatellar fat pad via a catheter after anterior cruciate ligament reconstruction (ACLR).[24] A self-administered infusion pump (50 mL) allowed the patients to administer 4-mL doses of bupivacaine. The authors found no significant difference between 0.5% and 0.25% bupivacaine in the amount of bupivacaine infused and VAS scores. However, patients given 0.5% bupivacaine infusion required significantly lower opioid (requirements) than historical controls. Continuous catheter techniques have been used for pain relief after knee replacement (TKR) in three studies. In one study, DeWeese and associates compared continuous infu-

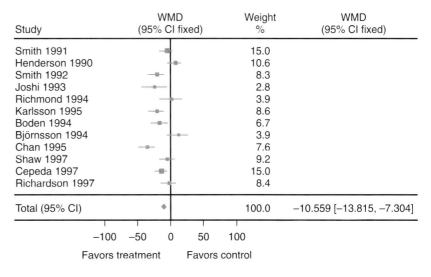

Figure 53–2. Meta-analysis of all studies using a single dose of local anesthetic injected intra-articularly. Weighted mean difference (WMD) with 95% confidence intervals (95% CI, horizontal lines) in Visual Analogue Scale (VAS) pain scores early postoperatively (1-4 hours) between the intra-articular local anesthetic and control groups. (Data from Møiniche S, Mikkelsen S, Wetterslev J: A systematic review of intraarticular local anesthesia for postoperative pain relief after arthroscopic knee surgery. Reg Anesth Pain Med 1999;24:430-437.)

Study	WMD (95% CI fixed)	Weight %	WMD (95% CI fixed)
Smith 1991		15.0	
Henderson 1990		10.6	
Smith 1992		8.3	
Joshi 1993		2.8	
Richmond 1994		3.9	
Karlsson 1995		8.6	
Boden 1994		6.7	
Björnsson 1994		3.9	
Chan 1995		7.6	
Shaw 1997		9.2	
Cepeda 1997		15.0	
Richardson 1997		8.4	
Total (95% CI)		100.0	−10.559 [−13.815, −7.304]

−100 −50 0 50 100

Favors treatment   Favors control

Table 53–2. Local Anesthetics in Knee Surgery

DRUG/CONCENTRATION	METHOD OF DRUG DELIVERY	TYPE OF SURGERY	TYPE OF STUDY	EFFECT (VAS OR ANALGESIC INTAKE)	REFERENCE
Bupivacaine 0.25% and 0.5%	Intermittent injection via catheter	ACLR	Open	No difference between 0.25% and 0.5%	24
Bupivacaine 0.5%	Continuous infusion	TKR	Open	Epidural better than IA LA	25
Bupivacaine 0.25%	Continuous infusion	TKR	Double-blind	Lower morphine requirement in IA LA group	26
Bupivacaine 0.25%	Continuous infusion	ACLR	Double-blind	Lower VAS and analgesic needs	27
Bupivacaine 0.25%	Continuous infusion	TKR	Double-blind	No difference between saline and LA	28

ACLR, anterior cruciate ligament repair; IA, intra-articular; LA, local anesthetic; TKR, total knee replacement; VAS, Visual Analogue Scale.

Table 53–3. Local Anesthetics in Shoulder Surgery*

DRUG/CONCENTRATION	METHOD OF DRUG DELIVERY	TYPE OF SURGERY	TYPE OF STUDY	EFFECT (VAS OR ANALGESIC INTAKE)	REFERENCE
0.25% bupivacaine 2 mL/hr	Continuous infusion	Subacromial decompression	Double-blind	Lower VAS scores; lesser analgesic consumption	29
0.5% ropivacaine 2 mL/hr	Continuous infusion	Unilateral shoulder arthroscopy	Double-blind	Lower VAS at rest and movement	30
0.2% and 0.375% ropivacaine	Continuous infusion	Cuff repair	Double-blind	Lower VAS scores; lesser analgesic consumption	31
0.5% bupivacaine 2 mL/hr	Continuous infusion	Rotator cuff repair	Double-blind	Lower VAS scores	32
0.25% bupivacaine 2 mL/hr	Continuous infusion	Subacromial surgery	Double-blind	Mild analgesic effect	33
ropivacaine 6 mL/hr	Continuous infusion	Acromioplasty	Double-blind	No benefit	34
0.2% ropivacaine	Continuous infusion and bolus	Rotator cuff repair	Open	Interscalene block better than IA infusion of LA	35
0.5% ropivacaine	Intermittent injection	Subacromial decompression	Double-blind	Lower VAS score and analgesic consumption	17
0.125% bupivacaine 2.5-10 mL/hr	Intermittent injection	Subacromial decompression	Open	Good analgesia	36
2% lidocaine 2 mL/hr plus bolus	Continuous infusion plus intermittent injection	Subacromial decompression	Open	Better pain relief than placebo	37
0.2% ropivacaine plus bolus	Continuous infusion plus intermittent injection	Subacromial decompression	Double-blind	Lower VAS score by 44%	38

*Effect of LA injected IA on postoperative pain following shoulder surgery. The list of studies shown is not exhaustive.
VAS, Visual Analogue Scale.

sion of 0.5% bupivacaine 2 mL/hr, administered intra-articularly with a historical group in which patients were given controlled epidural analgesia of 0.125% bupivacaine plus fentanyl 2 μg/mL.[25] The IA infusion was less efficient and higher analgesic consumption was registered during the 24-hour test period. In a double-blind study, bupivacaine 0.25%, 5 mL/hr was compared with saline during a 48-hour IA infusion. The authors found that there was a significant reduction in opioid consumption, which resulted in less nausea, fatigue, and malaise, and even enhanced rehabilitation and increased satisfaction.[26] In another study, Hoenecke and colleagues found that surgical knee patients receiving local anesthetic infusion postoperatively experienced less pain and required fewer narcotics.[27] They also found that the disposable

pump allowed administration of the medication on an outpatient basis. In one recent study, the authors found that injection of warmed lidocaine improves intraoperative anesthetic and postoperative analgesic conditions.[28] In summary, IA infusion of local anesthetic after total knee replacement and anterior cruciate ligament reconstruction seems to have some analgesic effect.

Shoulder Surgery

A summary of the articles published and the conclusions drawn by the authors using continuous LA infusions during shoulder surgery are summarized in Table 53–3. To treat the postoperative pain after

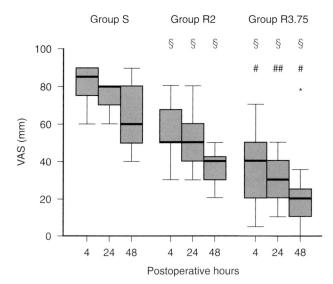

Figure 53–3. Comparison of 0.2% or 0.375% ropivacaine with saline infusion during 48 hours postoperatively. VAS, Visual Analogue Scale. * >3 times quartile range; #P < 0.05 versus GpR$_2$; §P < 0.005 versus GpS. (Data from Gottschalk A, Burmeister M-A, Radtke P, et al: Continuous wound infiltration with ropivacaine reduces pain and analgesic requirement after shoulder surgery. Anesth Analg 2003;97:1086-1091.)

acromioplastic surgery, LAs administered subacromially have recently been found to be effective. In six studies[29-35] continuous infusion was used, and in four studies the patient-controlled regional analgesia (PCRA) technique was used.[17,36-38] Savoie and coworkers[29] found that 0.25% bupivacaine with an infusion rate of 2 mL/hr decreased not only the VAS scores during 48 hours of administration of LAs but also the administered analgesic consumption during the first 5 postoperative days. Others reported significantly decreased VAS scores compared with saline when 0.5% bupivacaine was administered with an infusion rate of 2 mL/hr.[32] The analgesic effect was dose dependent when ropivacaine 0.2% and 0.375% was compared.[31] Both ropivacaine concentrations resulted in significantly lower pain scores and analgesic consumption than saline during 48 hours (Fig. 53–3). In two other studies, however, continuous IA bupivacaine infusion resulted in only minor analgesic effects. In the first study, 0.25% bupivacaine with infusion rate 2 mL/hr for 50 hours resulted in only a 30-minute shorter stay in the postanesthesia care unit (PACU) compared with placebo.[33] In the second study, an infusion of ropivacaine 6 mL/hr for 48 hours did not improve pain relief in comparison with saline.[34] The use of chilled compressive dressings and NSAID medication[33] as well as a subcutaneous drain[34] could contribute to diminishing the difference between the test drug and placebo.

Klein and associates[30] evaluated the postoperative pain relief when long-acting preoperative interscalene block (0.5% ropivacaine) was compared with IA continuous infusion of 0.5% ropivacaine, 2 mL/hr for

24 hours. Intra-articular ropivacaine resulted in lower VAS scores both at rest and on movement. Delaunay and colleagues compared interscalene block with subacromial LA infusion following arthroscopic rotator cuff repair.[35] Continuous interscalene block provides better analgesia compared with continuous subacromial infusion but with an increased incidence of minor side effects. In an open study, Mallon and coworkers[37] described a patient-controlled catheter technique based on both continuous subacromial infusion of 2% lidocaine, 2 mL/hr, and 1-mL lidocaine boluses self-administered at 15-minute intervals as needed. During the 72-hour infusion, the pain relief was significantly increased (improved) in the lidocaine group compared with the placebo group. In another PCRA study, 0.2% ropivacaine at 5 mL/hr was combined with 2-mL boluses of 0.2% ropivacaine and a 15-minute lockout time.[38] The authors reported significant decrease of VAS scores by 44% during 48 hours. We have tested the combined analgesic effect of LA administration both into subacromial bursa and intra-articularly via PCRA[17] (Fig. 53–4); 20 mL of 1% prilocaine adrenaline was injected into the subacromial bursa and 10-mL boluses of 0.5% ropivacaine per hour were self-administered via an elastomeric pump. Patients given local anesthetics in the bursa as well as subacromially had significantly lower VAS scores early postoperatively and lower morphine consumption than those administered saline. A great variation of pain was found in the groups and the range of ropivacaine administration varied from one to eight in the groups (median five or six administrations); 10 mL of 0.5% ropivacaine via an elastomeric pump produced pain relief within 20 minutes. However, the infusion of saline reduced the pain at rest by 25%, which could be considered a placebo effect.[14] A combination of preoperative intrabursal and subacromial local anesthetic infusion was recommended.

Pitfalls in Studies on Intra-articular Local Anesthetics

Intermittent versus Continuous Techniques

The intermittent injection of drugs offers advantage in that it prevents overdosing because pain is not continuous but exacerbated during certain maneuvers, such as movement, and can be either prevented or treated by the self-injection of fixed amounts of drugs intra-articularly through a catheter and an infusion pump. This technique, called patient-controlled regional analgesia and originally described by Rawal and colleagues,[36] has been used effectively in several studies for postoperative analgesia following shoulder surgery,[17] hand surgery,[39] laparoscopic cholecystectomy,[40] and cesarean sections.[21] In contrast, the continuous infusion of LAs or other analgesic combinations has advantage in that pain does not arise suddenly during an unplanned movement, but this is at the cost of overdosing the drugs because the infusion continues despite the absence of any pain. Also, there is a potential for drug toxicity. Lastly, this method may have the disadvantage that

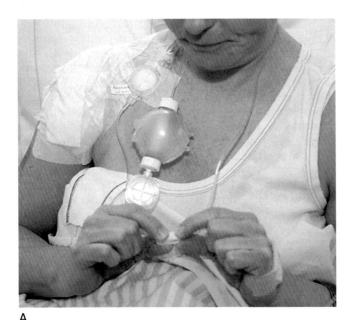

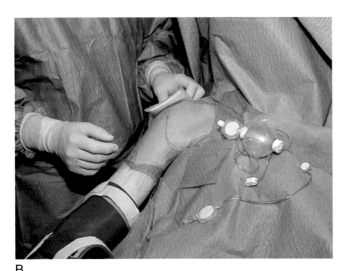

Figure 53–4. Postoperative pain management using elastometric pump **(A)**, and patient-controlled regional analgesia (PCRA) following subacromial decompression **(B)**.

during maximal pain intensity, the total analgesic drug concentration may be inadequate. Perhaps a combination of low-dose infusion combined with intermittent larger dose injections such as before exertion, may best solve this problem.[38] Depending on the procedure and the anticipated pain intensity, one method may have advantages over another.

Site of Injection of Local Anesthetics

Injections of LAs at portal sites may reduce postoperative pain for short periods in a similar way as has been shown for IA injections. However, the anterior synovium, infrapatellar fat pad, and joint capsule are very sensitive to pain stimuli,[23] and injections into these areas may provide better pain relief. Subacromial injections of LAs have been found to provide good pain relief compared with placebo following shoulder surgery.[17,38,41] No studies on IA analgesia have been published in which the authors have compared the site of LA injection during IA procedures, in relation to postoperative pain and analgesic requirements.

Use of Adrenaline

Although adrenaline has been known to have analgesic efficacy for more than 100 years and recent evidence suggests that its pharmacodynamic effect is via α_2 adrenoceptors in the substantia gelatinosa in the dorsal horn of the spinal cord,[42] controlled studies on the use of adrenaline as an analgesic when administered intra-articularly are lacking in the literature. Axelsson and coworkers found lower postoperative pain scores and analgesic requirements in patients undergoing subacromial decompression who were given prilocaine-adrenaline preoperatively as opposed to saline-adrenaline.[17] Whether adrenaline has a preemptive pharmacologic effect or physiologic effect (decrease in blood flow) to produce analgesia remains uncertain. Certainly, epidurally administered adrenaline with LAs and fentanyl provides better pain relief than LAs and fentanyl alone.[43] More studies are warranted on this important subject.

Volume and Dose of Local Anesthetics
Injected Intra-articularly

The volume as well as the dose (mg) of LAs injected intra-articularly may play a role in the analgesic efficacy of LAs postoperatively. Small volumes of LAs injected intra-articularly may theoretically leak out of the IA space, limiting its usefulness. It is difficult to fill the entire joint with LA because of the sensitive joint capsule. Similarly, small doses of LA may not have the desired effects. In one study, Gottschalk and colleagues found a reduction in pain intensity postoperatively at some points in patients receiving 3.75 mg/mL compared with 2 mg/mL ropivacaine[31] (see Fig. 53–3). In the systemic analysis of IA LAs on postoperative pain by Møiniche and colleagues, a mean dose of 90 mg bupivacaine was recommended with an injection volume between 20 and 40 mL.[1] However, it remains unclear whether the dose or the volume plays an important role in determining efficacy of IA local anesthetics.

Morphine

Stein and associates first described peripheral morphine receptors in 1988. Their first clinical study in 1991 on the efficacy of morphine injected intra-articularly found a reduction in pain intensity during the first 6 postoperative hours following minor arthroscopic surgery.[3] This analgesic effect could be confirmed to be that of morphine via peripheral receptors because the injection of naloxone intra-articularly reversed the analgesic effect.[3] Since then, the interest in the IA effects of morphine has grown by leaps and bounds, with more than 50 studies having been published assessing the efficacy of morphine injected intra-articularly into the knee joint. The results and conclusions have, however, been contradictory in these studies. In a systematic review of the literature in 1997, Kalso and colleagues concluded that "intra-articular morphine may have some effect in reducing postoperative pain intensity and consumption of analgesics" (p. 127).[44] Gupta and coworkers evaluated 45 studies in a meta-analysis of the literature, and found a definite but mild analgesic effect, which could be dose-dependent (Fig. 53–5). However, these authors could not completely exclude a systemic effect of IA morphine.[45] Another systemic review by Kalso and colleagues found that 5 mg of IA morphine injected into the knee joint provides postoperative pain relief for up to 24 hours.[46] They also concluded that when there is "no pain, there is no gain," suggesting that pain intensity must be at least moderate in order to detect any significant analgesic effects of morphine intra-articularly. Rosseland and associates confirmed that postoperative analgesic effect of IA morphine was found only in a subgroup of patients with greater pain intensity in the immediate postoperative period.[47] They also found that women perceived greater pain than men and therefore it was important to consider sex differences in studies on pain, thus adding another dimension to this complex problem. In a systematic review, the author showed that when only high-quality studies in which the pain intensity was moderate to severe were considered, 5 mg IA morphine provided no significant analgesia postoperatively.[4] This was in contrast with the findings of Kalso and colleagues presented earlier.[46]

Pitfalls in Studies on Intra-articular Morphine

Use of Systemic Opioids Intraoperatively

A substantial number of studies used intraoperative analgesics like fentanyl intraoperatively, which complicates the issue because analgesic efficacy (when seen) could be a result of the preemptive or pharmacologic effect of these opiates in the early postoperative period. Studies in which only LAs are used intraoperatively without general anesthesia (GA) or is given without opioids, may be more important in order to exclude this possibility. In two studies, the authors assessed postoperative pain following arthroscopy performed under LA, without intraoperative opioids. In one study, Gupta and colleagues found no benefit of morphine 3 mg injected intra-articularly compared with saline.[48] In another study published recently, Ng and coworkers found improved analgesia when morphine and ketorolac were combined with ropivacaine compared with ropivacaine or bupivacaine alone.[49] Whether this effect was caused by ketorolac alone or its combination with morphine remains unclear.

Method of Injection of Drugs Intra-articularly

Variations in techniques of injection of drugs intra-articularly may account for some of the differences seen among studies. For instance, drugs have been injected via the arthroscope under direct vision or at the end of surgery intra-articularly via a needle. Injection of drugs through the arthroscope before its removal may result in some of the drug either "running out" from the site of injection into tissue planes or, in the worst scenario, coming out through

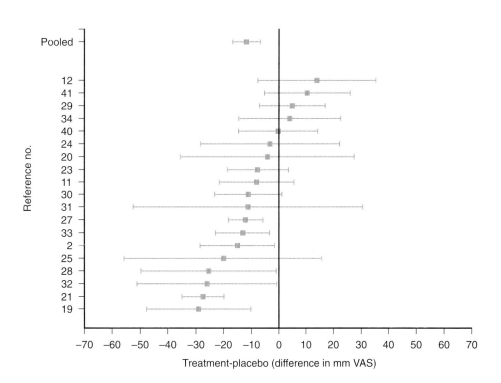

Figure 53–5. Early (0 to 2 hr) postoperative pain following intra-articular morphine. VAS, Visual Analogue Scale. (Data extracted from Gupta A, Bodin L, Holmstrom B, et al: A systematic review of the peripheral analgesics effects of intraarticular morphine. Anesth Analg 2001;93:761-770.)

the incision sites. This depends naturally on the volume of the injectate and the meticulousness of the operator. A small volume of injectate that leaks out of the incision site would not have any meaningful effect, whereas large volumes may not remain in the limited IA space. Similarly, a quick injection through the arthroscope and immediate removal may not ensure that the drugs remain where they are intended. Thus the volume of drug remaining in the IA space may vary and may account for some of these differences. Injections of drugs postoperatively through a catheter placed intra-articularly via an arthroscope may enable the entire volume of the drug to remain IA, but very few studies have used this simple but effective method. Intermittent or continuous infusion of drugs via a catheter may prolong analgesic effects and has been used recently in many studies. This technique, as opposed to a single injection of the drug via the arthroscope or needle, needs to be further evaluated.

Systemic Effect of Intra-articular Morphine

Many studies have been done to assess whether the analgesic effect is the result of the systemic absorption of intra-articularly injected morphine. In one set of studies, the authors injected a similar dose of morphine intramuscularly or intravenously, as a comparator.[3,50-54] Results were equivocal with some studies documenting equianalgesic effect,[51,52,54] whereas others showed better analgesia with IA morphine.[3,50,53] No clear relationship appears to exist between the dose of morphine and analgesia when comparing IA with IM/IV morphine. Plasma concentrations of morphine were measured after intra-articular injections of 1 and 5 mg morphine in one study[50] and after IV and intra-articular injection (5 mg) in another study[53] The plasma concentration of morphine 2 hours after 5 mg morphine injected intra-articularly was approximately 50% of the concentration achieved after IV injection.[53] In the other study,[50] of the 10 patients studied, 2 had spuriously large concentrations and 2 others had undetectable levels (<1 ng/mL). In the remaining 6 patients, the authors found smaller concentrations of morphine than are usually described after systemic morphine. In a third study, although the maximum plasma concentration following IA injection has been lower compared with IV injection, the area under the curve during 0 to 6 hours for 5 mg morphine intra-articularly or intravenously was similar, suggesting that substantial amounts of morphine are absorbed into the systemic circulation over time.[55] The authors, however, concluded that the analgesic effects of morphine appear to be via peripheral receptors. In conclusion, whether there is a systemic effect of morphine following its IA injection remains unclear.

Dose-Response Effect

A few studies are published in the literature in which the authors have studied the effects of increasing doses of morphine intra-articularly on postoperative analgesia.[56,57] The majority of these studies suggest that increasing the dose to 5 mg has resulted in improved postoperative analgesia. Denti and associates found that 2 mg morphine was adequate for minor arthroscopic procedures but 5 mg was necessary for anterior cruciate ligament surgery.[57] Although low doses of morphine (<1 mg) injected intra-articularly should theoretically produce a high concentration of IA morphine,[44] a dose-response effect was demonstrated by Likar and colleagues[56] in doses of 1 to 4 mg intra-articularly, whereas Kalso and associates[46] demonstrated in their systematic review of the literature that all studies in which 5 mg morphine was injected intra-articularly showed a positive result at all time periods. Thus the data seem to suggest that a larger dose of morphine would probably result in better pain relief.

Use of Tourniquet

Following drug injection, the use of a tourniquet on the thigh has been proposed to reduce pain intensity and may account for the differences in results. The role of the tourniquet, however, remains controversial. Whitford and colleagues suggested that retaining the tourniquet for 10 minutes after the injection of morphine postoperatively provides better pain relief than if it is released immediately,[58] a finding that has not been confirmed by others.[59] Many surgeons do not use a tourniquet while performing arthroscopic procedures on the knee. Some joints are not accessible to a tourniquet and therefore this method, even if it is effective, may not be universally applicable.

Role of Inflammation

Marchal and coworkers classified procedures a priori into low inflammatory (diagnostic arthroscopy, partial meniscectomy) or high inflammatory (synovial plicae removal, patellar shaving, anterior cruciate ligament repair) and found that operative procedures associated with low inflammatory states responded best to bupivacaine, whereas those with high inflammatory states respond better to IA morphine, thus supporting the theory that inflammation is a prerequisite for the peripheral analgesic effect of opioids[60] (Fig. 53–6). Others have suggested that the upgrading of morphine receptors during states of inflammation may account for its improved efficacy during inflammatory states, a phenomenon well documented in a rat model.[61]

Pethidine

In addition to being an opioid, pethidine is unique in having some LA effects and has been used as the sole anesthetic during spinal analgesia.[62] Therefore analgesia following IA injection of pethidine may have an effect as a local anesthetic as well as via peripheral morphine receptors. IA pethidine 5% with adrenaline was found to be comparable to lidocaine 5% with adrenaline during arthroscopy of the ankle. However, postoperatively, pethidine resulted in a lower pain score at rest than prilocaine.[63] In another

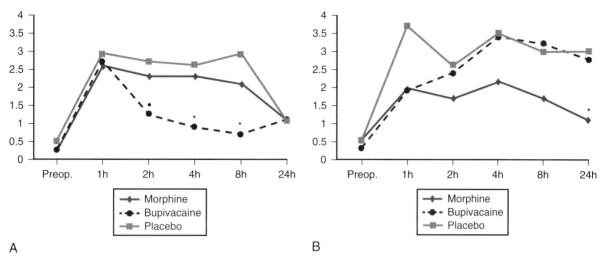

Figure 53–6. The effect of intra-articular morphine in patients with low and high inflammation. **A,** Postoperative pain. Lower inflammatory group. Mean Visual Analogue Scale (VAS) values obtained at different intervals. $*P < 0.05$; $\bullet P = 0.06$ (n.s.). **B,** Postoperative pain. High inflammatory group. Mean VAS values obtained at different intervals. $*P < 0.05$. (Data from Marchal JM, Delgado-Martinez AD, Poncela M, et al: Does the type of arthroscopic surgery modify the analgesic effect of intraarticular morphine and bupivacaine? A preliminary study. Clin J Pain 2003;19:240-246.)

Table 53–4.   Intra-articular Pethidine

DRUG/CONCENTRATION	COMPARATOR DRUG	TYPE OF SURGERY	TYPE OF STUDY	EFFECT (VAS OR ANALGESIC INTAKE)	REFERENCE
Pethidine 5%	Local anesthesia	Ankle surgery	Double-blind	Lower pain scores in pethidine compared with LA group	63
Pethidine 10 mg	Fentanyl, morphine, saline injected IA or systemically	Arthroscopic knee joint surgery	Double-blind	Similar analgesia as morphine or fentanyl, and similar to systemic drug	64
Pethidine 50 mg	Morphine or saline	Arthroscopic knee joint surgery	Double-blind	Early, short lasting analgesia (0.5-2 hr) from pethidine	65
Pethidine 200 mg	LA (prilocaine plus adrenaline)	Arthroscopic knee joint surgery	Double-blind	Good analgesia from pethidine IA during 1-4 hr	66
Pethidine 50, 100, 200 mg	LA (prilocaine plus adrenaline)	Arthroscopic knee joint surgery	Double-blind	Pethidine 100-200 mg provided good postoperative analgesia	120

IA, intra-articular; LA, local anesthetic; VAS, Visual Analogue Scale.

study, 1 mg morphine, 10 mg pethidine, or 10 µg fentanyl provided similar pain relief and similar analgesic consumption if the drugs were administered intra-articularly or systemically.[64] The authors concluded that the analgesia seen following IA pethidine may be identical to that provided by its systemic administration. Lyons and colleagues compared the effects of morphine, pethidine, and placebo and concluded that the local anesthetic effect of pethidine may be responsible for the improved early analgesia, but its duration of action was shorter than that of morphine.[65] Finally, Ekblom and associates found that pethidine 200 mg intra-articularly provided the best analgesia and the effect was not potentiated by the addition of adrenaline and prilocaine.[66] However,

used in this large dose, a systemic effect of pethidine cannot be ruled out. A summary of the studies on pethidine intra-articularly is shown in Table 53–4.

Fentanyl

Fentanyl, like pethidine, has been shown to have some LA effect.[66] In contrast to morphine, however, it is highly fat soluble and therefore may cross the synovial membrane quickly, thus providing systemic analgesia, similar to its effect when injected epidurally.[67] In a randomized double-blind study, IA fentanyl 50 µg was compared with IA bupivacaine after knee arthroscopy.[68] During the first 2 postoperative hours, IA bupivacaine 0.25% produced superior anal-

Table 53–5.   Intra-articular Fentanyl and Sufentanil

DRUG/CONCENTRATION	METHOD OF DRUG DELIVERY	TYPE OF SURGERY	TYPE OF STUDY	EFFECT (VAS OR ANALGESIC INTAKE)	REFERENCE
Fentanyl	Bupivacaine	Knee arthroscopy	Double-blind	IA bupivacaine better during 0-2 hr	68
Fentanyl 50 µg	Morphine or saline	Arthroscopic surgery	Double-blind	Fentanyl better than morphine 3 mg	69
Sufentanil 5 or 10 µg	Sufentanil 5 or 10 µg IV	Arthroscopic procedures	Double-blind	Lower VAS scores in sufentanil groups compared with IV sufentanil	70
Sufentanil 10 µg	Methylprednisolone plus sufentanil or saline	Arthroscopic knee surgery	Double-blind	Lower pain scores and analgesic consumption in combined group	71
Sufentanil 2.5 µg/hr	Epidural, femoral nerve block	ACLR	Not blinded	Epidural or femoral nerve block better than IA sufentanil for ACLR	72

ACLR, anterior cruciate ligament repair; IA, intra-articular; IV, intravenous; LA, local anesthetic; VAS, Visual Analogue Scale.

gesia compared to IA fentanyl. However, VAS pain scores during the next 18 hours were similar between IA bupivacaine and fentanyl. In another study 50 µg fentanyl was compared with placebo. Pain scores were lower during 8 hours in the IA fentanyl group compared with placebo.[69] Thus fentanyl in a dose of 50 µg does appear to provide analgesia, which is better than placebo but similar to bupivacaine. However, more studies are warranted on this important drug, which is commonly administered intravenously. Also plasma concentrations of fentanyl have not been measured following its IA injection in order to exclude a systemic effect. Studies published on IA fentanyl are summarized in Table 53–5.

Sufentanil

Sufentanil is fat soluble and can therefore cross membranes easily. When IA sufentanil 10 µg was compared with placebo or IV 5 µg sufentanil after arthroscopic knee surgery, it was found that VAS at rest and on movement was significantly lower in the sufentanil groups compared with control group postoperatively and at day 1.[70] In addition, the analgesic consumption was significantly lower and the time until home discharge from the PACU was significantly shorter in the sufentanil groups. However, there was no significant difference between IA or IV sufentanil. Therefore, a systemic effect of sufentanil could not be ruled out. In another study, Kizilkaya and coworkers injected sufentanil 10 µg intra-articularly and found it to produce better analgesia and less analgesic consumption compared with saline following knee arthroscopy.[71] In one final study,[7] a continuous infusion of 5 mL/hr of ropivacaine 2 mg/mL plus sufentanil 0.2 mg/mL combined with patient-controlled analgesia boluses of 5 mL each with a lock-out period of 2 hours was administered intra-articularly.[72] This analgesic technique was compared with epidural analgesia and continuous femoral blockade with the same infusion regimen postopera-

tively. The analgesic effect of the IA infusion was insufficient, with higher pain scores and higher additional analgesic requirements. Studies published on IA sufentanil are summarized in Table 53–5.

STEROIDAL AND NONSTEROIDAL ANTI-INFLAMMATORY DRUGS (NSAIDS)

Several studies published in the literature have assessed the effects of NSAIDs, specifically ketorolac and tenoxicam, injected intra-articularly on postoperative pain following arthroscopic surgery (Table 53–6). Studies on IA methylprednisolone are few and mostly in chronic pain states, which does not allow any definite conclusions to be drawn. In one study on acute pain, the authors injected methylprednisolone combined with LA and morphine into the ankle joint and compared it to placebo. This combination reduced pain, joint swelling, time of immobilization, duration of sick leave, and return to sports after the arthroscopic procedure. However, 1 of 18 patients had transitory purulent arthritis requiring antibiotics, and arthroscopic synovectomy occurred.[73] In another study, sufentanil or sufentanil-methylprednisolone were compared during arthroscopic meniscectomy surgery. The combined use of IA sufentanil (10 µg) and methylprednisolone (40 mg) in surgery reduced both postoperative pain scores and the use of additional analgesics.[71] The use of steroids intra-articularly following arthroscopy can lead to postoperative infections with an incidence of 2% as was shown by Armstrong and Bolding.[74] In this study the initial phase of the outbreak of infection correlated with the use of intraoperative IA corticosteroids.

Ketorolac

Reuben and Connelly found that the use of IA ketorolac improves the comfort in patients undergoing arthroscopic meniscus repair.[75] In another study in which Reuben and Connelly studied the effects of

Table 53–6. Intra-articular Nonsteroidal Anti-inflammatory Drugs

DRUG/CONCENTRATION	COMPARATOR DRUG	TYPE OF SURGERY	TYPE OF STUDY	EFFECT (VAS OR ANALGESIC INTAKE)	REFERENCE
Ketorolac 60 mg	Morphine, and combination	Arthroscopic meniscus repair	Double-blind	Ketorolac or morphine equally good; combination not better	75
Ketorolac 60 mg	Bupivacaine, and combination	Arthroscopic surgery	Double-blind	Combination of bupivacaine and ketorolac was best	76
Ketorolac 30 and 60 mg	Morphine, placebo	Arthroscopic surgery	Double-blind	Ketorolac 60 mg better than 30 mg and placebo	48
Ketorolac 60 mg	Bupivacaine, morphine, saline	Arthroscopic meniscectomy	Double-blind	Ketorolac better than bupivacaine or morphine	77
Ketorolac 5 mg	Ketorolac 10 mg IV	Arthroscopy of knee	Double-blind	Ketorolac IA better than IV	78
Tenoxicam 20 mg	Tenoxicam 20 mg IV	Arthroscopy of knee	Double-blind	Tenoxicam IA provided better analgesia	79
Tenoxicam 20 mg IA	Tenoxicam 20 mg IV	Arthroscopy of knee	Double-blind	Tenoxicam IA provided better analgesia	80
Tenoxicam 20 mg	Morphine or saline	ACLR	Double-blind	Tenoxicam IA provided better analgesia	81
Tenoxicam 20 mg	Bupivacaine or combination	Arthroscopic knee surgery	Double-blind	Combination of tenoxicam and bupivacaine provided best analgesia	82
Tenoxicam 20 mg	Bupivacaine or saline	Arthroscopy of knee	Double-blind	Lower analgesic requirements but no difference in pain intensity	83

ACLR, anterior cruciate ligament repair; IA, intra-articular; IV, intravenous; LA, local anesthetic; VAS, Visual Analogue Scale.

ketorolac and bupivacaine, they found that the group which received a combination of IA bupivacaine and IA ketorolac had decreased postoperative pain, a decreased need for postoperative analgesics, and an increased analgesic duration.[76] Gupta and associates found a dose-dependent reduction in pain intensity following ketorolac injected intra-articularly with maximal effect at 60 mg.[48] Calmet and coworkers found that 60 mg ketorolac provided better analgesic effect than 10 mL bupivacaine 0.25% or 1 mg morphine when injected intra-articularly.[77] In another study, Convery and associates showed that ketorolac 5 mg intra-articularly provides similar analgesia compared with 10 mg intravenously following knee arthroscopy, which may discount the theory on systemic absorption of ketorolac.[78] It is possible that the large doses of ketorolac administered intra-articularly by Gupta and colleagues[48] and Calmet and associates[77] may exert their effects via systemic absorption of the drug injected intra-articularly. However, as in the case of morphine, it is not known whether therapeutic plasma concentrations of ketorolac can be achieved, which may suggest a systemic, as well as a peripheral effect.

Tenoxicam

Colbert and coworkers showed that IA tenoxicam provides superior postoperative analgesia and reduces postoperative analgesic requirements compared with IV tenoxicam in patients undergoing day case knee arthroscopy.[79] Elhakim and associates showed that IA tenoxicam 20 mg provided better analgesia and decreased the requirements for postoperative analgesic compared with IV tenoxicam 20 mg.[80] Guler and colleagues found that IA tenoxicam provided better analgesia than that in the control group.[81] Talu and colleagues found that injection of IA tenoxicam 20 mg and bupivacaine was a simple, safe, and effective method of analgesia after arthroscopic meniscectomy with high patient satisfaction.[82] Cook and coworkers showed that the use of IA tenoxicam 20 mg at the end of arthroscopy reduced oral analgesic requirements during the first day after the operation but did not alter patients' perception of pain.[83]

Finally, in a systematic review of the literature, Rømsing and associates found four studies comparing IA NSAIDs with systemic administration (Fig. 53–7). Results showed a statistically significant effect in favor of IA NSAIDs. The authors concluded that there was evidence for a clinically relevant peripheral analgesic action of IA NSAIDs.[84]

In summary, when comparing ketorolac or tenoxicam with placebo injected intra-articularly, all studies found a better analgesic effect of these drugs. The duration of postoperative analgesia varied in these studies. Several studies reported better pain relief following IA compared with IV tenoxicam, which would suggest that this is mediated via peripheral IA receptors.

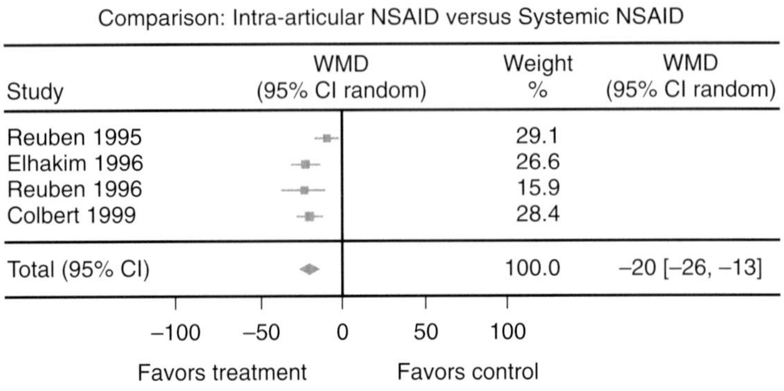

Comparison: Intra-articular NSAID versus Systemic NSAID

Study	WMD (95% CI random)	Weight %	WMD (95% CI random)
Reuben 1995		29.1	
Elhakim 1996		26.6	
Reuben 1996		15.9	
Colbert 1999		28.4	
Total (95% CI)		100.0	−20 [−26, −13]

−100 −50 0 50 100

Favors treatment   Favors control

Figure 53–7. Pooled data on the efficacy of intra-articular nonsteroidal anti-inflammatory drug (NSAID) on postoperative pain following arthroscopic surgery. CI, confidence interval; WMD, weighted mean difference. (Data extracted from Rømsing J, Møiniche S, Ostergaard D, et al: Local infiltration with NSAIDs for postoperative analgesia: Evidence for a peripheral analgesic action. Acta Anaesth Scand 2000;44: 672-683.)

Table 53–7. Intra-articular Clonidine*

DRUG/CONCENTRATION	METHOD OF DRUG DELIVERY	TYPE OF SURGERY	TYPE OF STUDY	EFFECT (VAS OR ANALGESIC INTAKE)	REFERENCE
Clonidine 150 μg	Clonidine 150 μg subcutaneous, saline or morphine	Arthroscopic knee surgery	Not blinded	Clonidine IA provided better analgesia	85
Clonidine 150 μg	Morphine 2 mg, combination	Arthroscopy of knee	Double-blind	Similar analgesia	86
Clonidine 150 μg	Morphine, combination or saline	Arthroscopic knee surgery	Double-blind	Combination of clonidine and opiate best	87
Clonidine 150 μg	Morphine 5 mg or saline	Arthroscopic knee surgery	Double-blind	Clonidine IA provided better analgesia	88
Clonidine 1 μg/kg	Bupivacaine, morphine 3 mg, combination	Arthroscopic meniscus repair	Double-blind	Combination of clonidine and morphine was best	89
Clonidine 1 μg/kg	Bupivacaine, combination, clonidine subcutaneous	Arthroscopic knee surgery	Not blinded	Combination of clonidine and bupivacaine was best	90
Clonidine 1 μg/kg	Morphine, neostigmine, tenoxicam, bupivacaine	Arthroscopic knee surgery	Double-blind	Clonidine or neostigmine provided best analgesia	91

*The list of studies is not exhaustive.
IA, intra-articular; VAS, Visual Analogue Scale.

CLONIDINE

α_2-Adrenergic agonists have been shown to have a central effect via the dorsal horn of spinal cord and a supratentorial, as well as a peripheral effect.[85] The IA injection of clonidine has been assessed in several studies published to date. All studies have universally found clonidine to produce improved analgesia alone or in combination with other drugs (Table 53–7). Gentili and coworkers found that 150 μg IA clonidine produces analgesia unrelated to vascular uptake of the drug because subcutaneous administration of a similar dose was not equally effective.[85] In a second study comparing the effects of 150 μg clonidine with 2 mg morphine, Gentili and coworkers found similar analgesic effects in the doses used.[86] Buerkle and associates found that that the peripheral codelivery of an opioid and an α_2 agonist resulted in improved postoperative pain relief when compared with each single agent given alone.[87] Iqbal and colleagues found that

IA administration of 150 μg of clonidine resulted in longer-lasting pain relief postoperatively as compared with 5 mg of preservative-free morphine.[88] Joshi and colleagues found that the combination of morphine (3 mg) and clonidine (1 μg/kg) resulted in decreased postoperative pain and analgesic use, as well as an increased analgesic duration compared with either drug alone in patients undergoing knee arthroscopy[89] (Fig. 53–8). There also was a significant benefit from the individual IA administration of both clonidine and morphine compared with placebo. Reuben and associates found that the IA administration of clonidine along with bupivacaine resulted in a significant improvement in analgesia compared with either drug alone.[90] There was an increased time to first analgesic request and a decreased need for postoperative analgesics. Finally, in a comparative study of five different analgesics injected intra-articularly, Alagol and associates found that clonidine and neostigmine offered the best analgesia.[91]

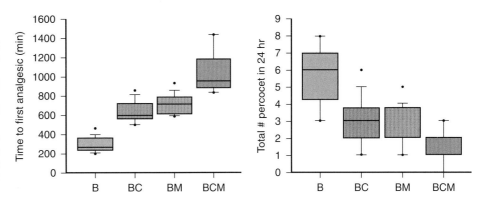

Figure 53–8. The effect of combining bupivacaine, clonidine, and morphine combined to individual drugs is shown. B, bupivacaine; BC, bupivacaine and clonidine; BCM, bupivacaine, clonidine, and morphine; BM, bupivacaine and morphine. (Data extracted from Joshi W, Reuben SS, Kilaru PR, et al: Postoperative analgesia for outpatient arthroscopic knee surgery with intraarticular clonidine and/or morphine. Anesth Analg 2000; 90:1102-1106.)

In summary, clonidine produces analgesia when injected intra-articularly, and the effects are probably comparable to that of morphine or neostigmine alone. Combination with morphine appears to increase analgesia but not with neostigmine. However, hypotension can be a problem when using 150 μg clonidine intra-articularly.

KETAMINE

In an animal study, Zhou and associates found that peripheral injections of ketamine and other N-methyl D-aspartate (NMDA) receptor antagonists reduced glutamate-induced pain.[92] In humans, Dal and colleagues[93] found long-lasting analgesia following IA ketamine, which was comparable with IA neostigmine, but less effective than IA bupivacaine. Rosseland and coworkers[94] studied patients with moderate to severe pain after IA arthroscopy. In these patients IA saline with and without ketamine produced pain relief, but there was no significant difference between the two groups. Intramuscular ketamine showed significantly better early pain relief in comparison with IA administration. This was also the finding of Huang and associates, who injected ketamine 0.5 mg/kg intra-articularly and found a similar effect as saline intra-articularly.[95] In another study, Batra and coworkers found that an IA bupivacaine-ketamine combination provides better pain relief than IA ketamine alone after out-patient arthroscopic knee surgery.[96] Thus the evidence of any significant analgesia from ketamine intra-articularly is minimal and cannot be recommended for postoperative pain management following arthroscopic surgery.

TRAMADOL

Tramadol is a weak μ agonist and serotonin antagonist. In three studies, IA tramadol has been studied and found to be equianalgesic to fentanyl or morphine intra-articularly. In a dose-response study, 20, 50, and 100 mg IA tramadol was studied and compared with IV tramadol of the same doses. IA administration prolonged the duration of analgesia and 100 mg IA tramadol produced the longest duration

(700 minutes).[97] Side effects such as nausea and vomiting were most frequent after 100 mg IV tramadol. In one study, IA tramadol 1.5 mg/kg resulted in pain relief comparable with IA fentanyl 1.5 μg/kg.[98] In another study it was reported that 50 mg IA tramadol provided analgesia equivalent to 5 mg IA morphine.[99] In summary, mild analgesic effects of tramadol comparable to morphine intra-articularly have been demonstrated but side effects including postoperative nausea and vomiting (PONV) dominate when the dose is greater than 100 mg.

NEOSTIGMINE

Cholinergic agonists and cholinesterase inhibitors administered systemically display a dose-dependent analgesic effect mediated through the activation of ascending and descending cerebral cholinergic pathways.[100,101] These effects are even more profound when the drugs are administered spinally.[102] Neostigmine has been injected intra-articularly in several studies. Altough Gentili and associates found that neostigmine 500 μg was equianalgesic to clonidine 150 μg but better than placebo,[103] Lauretti and coworkers found no analgesic effect of peripheral neostigmine compared with placebo, but had an excellent effect when injected epidurally.[104] In another study, neostigmine intra-articularly was found to be equianalgesic to ketamine.[93] Alagol and colleagues compared the analgesic efficacy of neostigmine to clonidine, tenoxicam, bupivacaine, morphine, or placebo and reported that the best analgesia was produced by neostigmine or clonidine.[91] In a dose-response study, Yang and associates found that 500 μg neostigmine produced moderate but significant analgesia.[105] Although analgesia has been shown with IA neostigmine, Schafer argues that acetylcholine release does not occur at the nerve endings within the IA space and therefore neostigmine cannot have an effect via anticholinesterase activity.[106] However, Yang and associates suggest that several mechanisms such as the hyperpolarization of neurons, reduction in the release of pronociceptive neurotransmitters, or activation of the nitric oxide–cyclic guanosine monophosphate pathway might mediate this peripheral cholinergic antinociception by elevating endogenous acetylcholine.[105]

It is difficult to draw any definite conclusions on the effects of neostigmine injected intra-articularly because of opposing results in the studies published in the literature. Although several studies have shown it to be reasonably effective, the theoretic explanation for its analgesic effect is, at the moment, lacking.

DRUG COMBINATIONS

Many drugs have been used in combination in numerous studies to potentiate the effects of single agents, which was discussed earlier. Combining different analgesics with differing mechanisms of action has the advantage of reducing side effects of individual drugs, and therefore several combinations have been used, with in most cases, advantages. However, few studies have compared these combinations with similar drugs and doses administered intravenously to exclude a systemic effect.

Intra-articular Injections without Catheters

Ketorolac has been combined with morphine and ropivacaine to provide improved analgesia after arthroscopic knee surgery by some[107] but not others.[75] In a recent study, Ng and coworkers compared analgesic efficacy of a combination of ropivacaine, morphine, and ketolorac to ropivacaine alone intra-articularly and found that morphine and ketolorac enhanced analgesia produced by LAs alone, reduced postdischarge analgesic consumption, and improved activities of daily living (ADL) without increasing side effects after ambulatory arthroscopic knee surgery.[49] Ketorolac has also been combined with local anesthetics to provide better pain relief than ketorolac alone.[76] Similarly, clonidine has been combined with morphine,[87,89] as well as local anesthetics,[90] resulting in improved analgesia. In another study comparing the effects of clonidine with neostigmine, the authors found that IA administration of 150 µg of clonidine, 500 µg neostigmine, or both produce postoperative analgesia, and the combination was not more effective.[103] However, 45% of the patients who had received clonidine in this study had at least one episode of hypotension versus 4% of those who did not ($P < 0.01$). The incidence of bradycardia was 20% and 0%, respectively ($P = 0.01$). The combination of lidocaine, pethidine, and tenoxicam given intra-articularly provided superior analgesia and reduced oral analgesic requirement during the first day after arthroscopy, compared with lidocaine and pethidine alone.[108] Finally, Lombardi and colleagues showed that soft tissue and IA injection of long-acting local anesthetic with epinephrine and morphine provides better pain control in the immediate postoperative period, decreases blood loss, and decreases the need for rescue narcotics and reversal agents.[109]

Intra-articular Injections via Catheters

In contrast with single injections that may provide short-term pain relief, intermittent injections or infusions have been used in order to prolong the analgesia. Thus, in one study, ropivacaine 0.2% was combined with sufentanil 0.2 µg/mL as an infusion (5 mL/hr) during arthroscopic anterior cruciate ligament reconstruction (ACLR).[72] The authors concluded that either epidural or continuous femoral nerve block provides adequate pain relief in patients who undergo ACLR. However, IA analgesia seemed insufficient for the analgesic requirements of this surgical procedure. In contrast to this study, Rasmussen and associates used a continuous infusion of a combination of ropivacaine and morphine following total knee replacement in a nonrandomized, non-blinded study and found that it reduced pain and enhanced rehabilitation after total knee replacement.[73] Thus the literature is somewhat controversial in this area. Morphine administered intra-articularly combined with other drugs may increase the postoperative analgesic effects. In one study, morphine combined with ketorolac for IA pain relief following minor arthroscopic procedures provided a synergistic effect.[48] Recently we have reported that addition of morphine and ketorolac to ropivacaine intra-articularly enhances analgesic efficacy of LA, reduces postdischarge analgesic consumption, and improves ADLs without increasing side effects in patients undergoing arthroscopy.[17] When using the patient-controlled regional analgesia system, the combination of IA ropivacaine, morphine, and ketorolac has also been demonstrated to be superior in comparison to control (saline) or to a combination of ropivacaine and morphine intra-articularly in reducing morphine consumption after anterior cruciate ligament repair.[107] A continuous infusion of morphine and bupivacaine also has been used for pain relief after subacromial arthroscopy.[41] These authors studied the analgesic effect of a continuous subacromial infusion of bupivacaine 2.5 mg/hr combined with morphine 0.2 mg/hr for 3 postoperative days. Analgesic infusion decreased the pain scores at rest and reduced supplemental requirements for 4 days postoperatively compared with saline infusion.

In summary, combination of drugs may be used to provide pain relief postoperatively after knee surgery with the following results: ketorolac combined with morphine and/or local anesthesia appears to provide better pain relief than either drug alone. Clonidine combined with morphine or LA provides better pain relief in some studies but not all. Morphine and LA combined together have mild benefits but are not as efficacious as when these are combined with NSAIDs.

SAFETY OF INTRA-ARTICULAR ANALGESICS

Safety of Delivery Systems

For ambulatory practice, the IA catheters are connected to either disposable elastomeric pumps

(Homepump, I-Flow Corp., Lake Forest, Cal; Infusor, Baxter, Deerfield, Ill.) (Fig. 53–9) or electronic pumps (Graseby PCA, Microject Sorensen Medical). The IA analgesic techniques are based on continuous, patient-controlled, or continuous and patient-controlled infusion. When the continuous infusion technique with elastomeric pumps is used, the rate of flow is controlled by the lumen of the catheter. By using simple techniques, that is, opening a clamp (Homepump) or pressing a button (Infusor or Homepump), the patient can self-administer pain treatment. Ilfeld and colleagues[110] tested different pumps for continuous regional analgesia and found that the accuracy differed significantly among the pumps exhibiting flow rates within plus or minus 15% of their expected rate. An increase in temperature also affected pumps to differing degrees with infusion rates increasing from 0% to 25% for each model tested. Capdevila and colleagues[111] compared an elastomeric pump (Infusor) and electronic pumps (Graseby and Microject) and found that the elastomeric pump was as effective as the electronic pumps, was less expensive, had fewer technical problems, and gave better patient satisfaction.

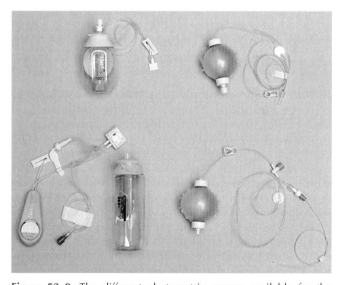

Figure 53–9. The different elastometric pumps available for the delivery of local anesthetic into the wound or intra-articularly.

Technical Problems with Catheters

In some studies it has been reported that the catheter can be dislodged,[17] disconnected,[112] or partially blocked at the outlet.[24] Better methods need to be explored in order to retain the catheter firmly in position while allowing easy removal. With the older elastomeric balloon pump technique there was a risk that the patient would fail to close the clamp, resulting in the contents of the pump emptying within 1 hour. However, no case of systemic toxicity of LA has been reported in the literature. The risk of systemic toxicity is low as the absorption of LA from the joint structure is slow, resulting in low plasma concentrations of LAs[17,31,49,113] (see later for details). Also newer and safer elastometric pumps allow delivery of LAs only if the patient presses a button. Long-acting and low-toxic LAs such as ropivacaine or levobupivacaine are therefore recommended.

Local and Systemic Infections

Infections at the site of drug injection or systemic infections are a major concern but the reported incidence is low. A summary of the studies published in the literature in which cultures were taken from the catheter tip following IA placement is shown in Table 53–8. In two studies, positive isolated bacterial cultures from the catheter tip have been reported in a few patients without any sign of clinical infections.[17,107] In one of these studies,[107] although there was an increase in body temperature and a higher C-reactive protein, the patient responded well to antibiotics, and wound healing was considered normal. However, in two other studies,[25,73] two patients were reported to have deep infection, which required long antibiotic therapy. Thus proper aseptic catheter technique using bacterial filters and sterile preparation and injection of drugs is important, particularly during orthopedic surgery.

Local Anesthetic Toxicity

Several studies have been published in which the plasma concentration of an LA was measured following its IA injection (Table 53–9). Both free and total plasma concentrations were much lower than known toxic plasma concentrations despite sufficiently high

Table 53–8. Risk of Infection

CONTROL/LOCAL ANESTHETIC	SURGERY	POSITIVE CULTURE	GROWTH	CLINICAL WOUND INFECTION	REFERENCE
Saline	Subacromial decompression	30%	Coagulase-negative staphylococcus	Negative	17
Bupivacaine plus fentanyl	Knee replacement	0.6%	*Streptococcus pneumoniae*	Positive	25
Ropivacaine plus morphine	Knee replacement	1%	?	Deep infection	19
Ropivacaine plus morphine	Anterior cruciate ligament repair	7.8%	*Staphylococcus epidermidis*	Negative	107

Table 53–9. Systemic Toxicity of Local Anesthetic

LOCAL ANESTHETIC*	DOSE	SURGERY	TOTAL CONCENTRATION µG/ML	FREE CONCENTRATION µG/ML	REFERENCE
Ropivacaine	225 mg	Shoulder	1.42	0.08	113
Ropivacaine	500 mg (1 hr)	Subacromial compression	2.23	0.12	17
Ropivacaine	225 mg plus 900 mg/48 hr	Shoulder/rotator cuff	—	<0.6	31
Lidocaine-adrenaline	400 mg	Knee arthroscopy	0.8	0.2	49
Ropivacaine	150 mg	Knee arthroscopy	1.2	0.06	49
Ropivacaine	200 mg	Knee arthroscopy	1.29	0.047	114

*Systemic toxicity of LA is shown using different drugs and at different sites of injection. Mild toxic symptoms: Free concentration 0.6 mg/mL.[115]

doses of LAs.[17,49,113,114] Single injections of up to 500 mg ropivacaine subacromially have not produced toxic symptoms in humans.[17] In the only study published during continuous infusion of ropivacaine following shoulder surgery, greater than 1000 mg resulted in free plasma concentrations less than 0.6 µg/mL, which is far below known toxic concentrations in humans.[115] Therefore the likelihood of any significant LA toxicity when the drugs are used in these doses appears to be small.

Side Effects and Complications

For a new technique to be acceptable in clinical practice, it is important to show not only efficacy but also a low incidence of side effects and complications in relation to existing techniques. Although the IA technique has been used extensively, reports of side effects and complications have been few. This could be from one of two reasons: authors have either not adequately documented side effects in their studies, or there is a true low incidence of side effects with this technique. Among the reported side effects of IA morphine, itching is probably the most frequent but the least worrisome. Other side effects have included nausea and vomiting and redness at the injection site when catheters have been used. There also has been a serious concern in the use of NSAIDs intra-articularly and the effect on bone healing. Although this has been shown to be true in animal studies, there is lack of evidence in human studies, particularly during single-dose administration. A single dose of ketorolac injected intra-articularly in rats was found to result in significantly more inflammation than saline on histologic examination after 5 days, which was not attributable to the alcohol in the injectate.[116] Morphine and ketorolac have been found to produce mild histopathologic changes in rabbit knee joints, morphine causing more than ketorolac.[117] However, the authors concluded that both these drugs can be used intra-articularly with safety. In another study by the same group, IA bupivacaine and neostigmine also were found to cause histopathologic changes in rabbit knee joints, with neostigmine having a greater effect than bupivacaine.[118] More studies are, however, needed on this important question. Until more studies are available to show the opposite, we do not use NSAIDs intra-articularly following traumatic bone injury because any delay in healing in this group of patients could have disastrous consequences. Operative site bleeding following the administration of NSAIDs is a real risk when these drugs are administered systemically. However, apart from spontaneous IA bleeding following the use of clopidogrel or aspirin,[119] no significant bleeding complications have been reported following IA injection of NSAIDs. Other minor side effects do not appear to be significantly different among patients given IA neostigmine, morphine, tenoxicam, clonidine, or bupivacaine.[91]

FUTURE STUDIES

Despite the large volume of information available as well the enormous number of studies published on the subject, the effect of individual drugs on postoperative pain management remains unclear. The combination of drugs has been shown to produce maximum benefit with the lowest risk and more studies on the different combinations and doses need to be established through well-designed studies including a sufficiently large number of patients. The question of analgesic efficacy of morphine following IA surgery is still unclear because of deficiencies in study designs and choice of patient population. The ideal opioid for pain relief intra-articularly needs to be identified and perhaps more specific drugs effective on the peripheral receptors developed. Prolonging the effects of LA opioids as well as other IA analgesics through the use of IA catheters needs further documentation. Considering the enormous costs involved in the development and marketing of pumps for use with the catheter techniques, the safety as well as the cost effectiveness of these techniques need to be analyzed. The risk of infections in joints has been one of the concerns of orthopedic surgeons when LAs are injected via catheters intra-articularly. Therefore, and considering that insertion of a catheter at the end of the operation is a simple procedure, it would be important to exclude this major concern of surgeons. Specifically, IA analgesia should be assessed during procedures associated with moderate to severe pain such as anterior cruciate ligament repair or total knee replacement, assessing not only the efficacy of this technique but even the side effects and complications, such as postoperative infections. The answer to many of these questions cannot be given by retrospective analysis of data and by systematic reviews but by a well-designed large prospective study that has taken into consideration some of the problems presented here. Safety is only in numbers, and authors should therefore be asked to report not only efficacy variables but also any and all adverse effects. An analysis of the side effect of drugs injected intra-articularly should be obligatory in future studies on IA analgesia to confirm that they have indeed advantages that conclusively overweigh their disadvantages. Issues relating to costs of drugs and equipment in relation to the benefits offered also should be documented.

CONCLUSION

IA analgesics have been used for more than a decade with variable results. In studies in which IA morphine has provided analgesia, the effects have been mild and it has been difficult to exclude systemic effects. On the other hand, NSAIDs (ketorolac and tenoxicam) have consistently shown efficacy. However, the important question on the effect of NSAIDs on bone healing has not been answered. Combination of several drugs including LAs, ketorolac, adrenaline, and even morphine have shown efficacy in several studies. However, the exact drug combination and doses need to be studied. It is difficult to draw any conclusions on other drugs including clonidine, neostigmine, ketamine, fentanyl, and pethidine because of the limited number of studies published in a varying patient population. The use of catheters intra-articularly has the major advantage of prolonging analgesia when LAs or a combination of drugs are used, and this method needs to be further developed.

References

1. Møiniche S, Mikkelsen S, Wetterslev J: A systemic review of intraarticular local anesthesia for postoperative pain relief after arthroscopic knee surgery. Reg Anesth Pain Med 1999; 24:430-437.
2. Colombo G, Padera R, Langer R, Kohane DS: Prolonged duration of local anesthesia with lipid protein-sugar particles containing bupivacaine and dexamethasone. J Biomed Mater Res A 2005;75:458-464.
3. Stein C: Peripheral analgesic actions of opioids. J Pain Symptom Manage 1991;6:119-124.
4. Rosseland LA: No evidence for analgesic effect of intraarticular morphine after knee arthroscopy: A qualitative systematic review. Reg Anesth Pain Med 2005;30:83-98.
5. Taenzer AH, Clark C, Curry CS: Gender affects report of pain and function after arthroscopic anterior cruciate ligament reconstruction. Anesthesiology 2000;93:670-675.
6. Rosseland LA, Stubhaug A: Gender is a confounding factor in pain trials: Women report more pain than men after arthroscopic surgery. Pain 2004;112:248-253.
7. Cepeda MS, Carr DB: Women experience more pain and require more morphine than men to achieve a similar degree of analgesia. Anesth Analg 2003;97:1464-1468.
8. Sener EB, Kocamanoglu S, Cetinkaya MB, et al: Effects of menstrual cycle on postoperative analgesic requirements, agitation, incidence of nausea and vomiting after gynecological laparoscopy. Gynecol Obstet Invest 2005;59:49-53.
9. Gibson SJ, Helme RD: Age-related differences in pain perception and report. Clin Geriatr Med 2001;17:433-456.
10. Chakour MC, Gibson SJ, Bradbeer M, Helme RD: The effect of age on A delta- and C-fibre thermal pain perception. Pain 1996;64:143-152.
11. Harkins SW, Davis MD, Bush FM, Kasberger J: Suppression of first pain and slow temporal summation of second pain in relation to age. J Gerontol A Biol Sci Med Sci 1996;51: M260-M265.
12. Zheng Z, Gibson SJ, Khalil Z, et al: Age-related differences in the time course of capsaicin-induced hyperalgesia. Pain 2000;85:51-58.
13. Gagliese L, Weizblit N, Ellis W, Chan VW: The measurement of postoperative pain: A comparison of intensity scales in younger and older surgical patients. Pain 2005;117:412-420.
14. Rosseland LA, Helgesen KG, Breivik H, Stubhaug A: Moderate-to-severe pain after knee arthroscopy is relieved by intraarticular saline: A randomised controlled trial. Anesth Analg 2004;98:1546-1551.
15. Rosseland LA, Stubhaug A, Grevbo F, et al: Effective pain relief from intraarticular saline with or without morphine 2 mg in patients with moderate-to-severe pain after knee arthroscopy: A randomized, double-blind controlled clinical study. Acta Anaesthesiol Scand 2003;47:732-738.
16. Thomas DF, Lambert WG, Williams KL: The direct perfusion of surgical wounds with local anaesthetic solution: An approach to postoperative pain? Ann R Coll Surg Engl 1983;65:226-229.
17. Axelsson K, Nordensson U, Johanzon E, et al: Patient controlled regional analgesia (PCRA) with ropivacaine after arthroscopic subacromial decompression. Acta Anaesthesiol Scand 2003;47:993-1000.
18. Alford JW, Fadale PD: Evaluation of postoperative bupivacaine infusion for pain management after anterior cruciate ligament reconstruction. Arthroscopy 2003;19:855-861.
19. Rasmussen S, Kramhøft MU, Sperling KP, Pedersen JHL: Increased flexion and reduced hospital stay with a continuous intraarticular morphine and ropivacaine after primary total knee replacement: Open intervention study of efficacy and safety of 154 patients. Acta Orthop Scand 2004;75: 606-609.
20. Gupta A, Perniola A, Axelsson K, et al: Postoperative pain after abdominal hysterectomy: A double-blind comparison between placebo and local anesthetic infused intraperitoneally. Anesth Analg 2004;99:1173-1179.
21. Givens VA, Lipscomb GH, Meyer NL: A randomized trial of postoperative wound irrigation with local anesthetic for pain after cesarean delivery. Am J Obstet Gynecol 2002;186: 1188-1191.
22. Eledjam JJ, Cuvillon P, Capdevila X, et al: Postoperative analgesia by femoral nerve block with ropivacaine 0.2% after major knee surgery: Continuous versus patient-controlled techniques. Reg Anesth Pain Med 2002;27:604-611.
23. Dye SF, Vaupel GL, Dye CC: Conscious neurosensory mapping of the internal structures of the human knee without intraarticular anesthesia. Am J Sports Med 1998; 773-777.
24. Chew HF, Evans NA, Stanish WD: Patient-controlled bupivacaine infusion into the infrapatellar fat pad after anterior cruciate ligament reconstruction. Arthroscop Rel Surg 2003: 19:500-505.
25. DeWeese FT, Akbari Z, Carline E: Pain control after knee arthroplasty: Intraarticular versus epidural anesthesia. Clin Orthop Rel Res 2001;392:226-231.
26. Colwell CW Jr: The use of a pain pump and patient-controlled analgesia in joint reconstruction. Am J Orthop 2004;33:10-12.
27. Hoenecke HR Jr, Pulido PA, Morris BA, Fronek J: The efficacy of continuous bupivacaine infiltration following anterior cruciate ligament reconstruction. Arthroscopy 2002;18:854-858.

28. Nechleba J, Rogers V, Cortina G, Cooney T: Continuous intra-articular infusion of bupivacaine for postoperative pain following total knee arthroplasty. J Knee Surg 2005;18: 197-202.

29. Savoie FH, Field LD, Nan Jenkins R, et al: The pain control infusion pump for postoperative pain control in shoulder surgery. Arthroscopy 2000;16:339-342.

30. Klein SM, Nielsen KC, Martin A, et al: Interscalene brachial plexus block with continuous intraarticular infusion of ropivacaine. Anesth Analg 2001;93:601-605.

31. Gottschalk A, Burmeister M-A, Radtke P, et al: Continuous wound infiltration with ropivacaine reduces pain and analgesic requirement after shoulder surgery. Anesth Analg 2003; 97:1086-1091.

32. Barber FA, Herbert MA: The effectiveness of an anesthetic continuous-infusion device of postoperative pain control. J Arthrosc Rel Surg 2002;18:76-81.

33. Quick BC, Guanche CA, Prairie E: Evaluation of anesthetic pump for postoperative care after shoulder surgery. J Shoulder Elbow Surg 2003;12:618-621.

34. Boss AP, Maurer T, Seiler S, et al: Continuous subacromial bupivacaine infusion for postoperative analgesia after open acromioplasty and rotator cuff repair: Preliminary results. J Shoulder Elbow Surg 2004;13:630-634.

35. Delaunay L, Souron V, Lafosse L, et al: Analgesia after arthroscopic rotator cuff repair: Subacromial versus interscalene continuous infusion of ropivacaine. Reg Anesth Pain Med 2005;30:117-122.

36. Rawal N, Axelsson K, Hylander J, et al: Postoperative patient-controlled local anaesthetic administration at home. Anesth Analg 1998;86:86-89.

37. Mallon WJ, Thomas CW: Patient-controlled lidocaine analgesia for acromioplasty surgery. J Shoulder Elbow Surg 2000; 9:85-88.

38. Harvey GP, Chelly JE, Samsam TA, Coupe K: Patient-controlled ropivacaine analgesia after arthroscopic subacromial decompression. Arthroscop Rel Surg 2004;20: 451-455.

39. Rawal N, Allvin R, Axelsson K, et al: Patient-controlled regional analgesia (PCRA) at home: Controlled comparison between bupivacaine and ropivacaine brachial plexus analgesia. Anesthesiology 2002;96:1290-1296.

40. Gupta A, Thorn SE, Axelsson K, et al: Postoperative pain relief using intermittent injections of 0.5% ropivacaine through a catheter after laparoscopic cholecystectomy. Anesth Analg 2002;95:450-456.

41. Park JY, Lee G-W, Kim Y, Yoo M-O: The efficacy of continuous intrabursal infusion with morphine and bupivacaine for postoperative analgesia after subacromial arthroscopy. Reg Anesth Pain Med 2002;27:145-149.

42. Yaksh TL, Reddy SV: Studies in the primate on the analgetic effects associated with intrathecal actions of opiates, alpha-adrenergic agonists and baclofen. Anesthesiology. 1981;54: 451-467.

43. Niemi G, Breivik H: Adrenaline markedly improves thoracic epidural analgesia produced by a low-dose infusion of bupivacaine, fentanyl and adrenaline after major surgery: A randomised, double-blind, cross-over study with and without adrenaline. Acta Anaesthesiol Scand 1998;42:897-909.

44. Kalso E, Tramer M, Carroll D, et al: Pain relief from intra-articular morphine after knee surgery: A qualitative systematic review. Pain 1997;71:127-134.

45. Gupta A, Bodin L, Holmstrom B, et al: A systematic review of the peripheral analgesics effects of intraarticular morphine. Anesth Analg 2001;93:761-770.

46. Kalso E, Smith L, McQuay HJ, et al: No pain, no gain: Clinical excellence and scientific rigour—lessons learned from IA morphine. Pain 2002;98:269-275.

47. Rosseland LA., Stubhaug A, Skoglund A, et al: Intra-articular morphine for pain relief after knee arthroscopy. Acta Anaesth Scand 1999;43:252-257.

48. Gupta A, Axelsson K, Allvin R, et al: Postoperative pain following knee arthroscopy: The effects of intra-articularly ketorolac and/or morphine. Reg Anesth Pain Med 1999; 24:225-230.

49. Ng H-P, Nordström U, Axelsson K, et al: Efficacy of intra-articular bupivacaine, ropivacaine or a combination of ropivacaine, morphine and ketorolac on postoperative pain relief following ambulatory arthroscopic knee surgery: A randomized double-blind study. Reg Anesth Pain Med 2006;31: 26-33.

50. Joshi GP, McCarroll SM, Cooney CM, et al: Intra-articular morphine for pain relief after knee arthroscopy. J Bone Joint Surg Br 1992;74:749-751.

51. Björnsson A, Gupta A, Vegfors M, et al: Intraarticular morphine for postoperative analgesia following knee arthroscopy. Reg Anesth 1994;19:104-108.

52. Dierking GW, Östergaard HT, Dissing CK, et al: Analgesic effects of intra-articular morphine after arthroscopic meniscectomy. Anaesthesia 1994;49:627-629.

53. Richardson MD, Bjorksten AR, Hart JAL, McCullough K: The efficacy of intra-articular morphine for postoperative knee arthroscopy analgesia. Arthroscopy 1997;13:584-589.

54. Hege-Scheuing G, Michaelsen K, Buhler A, et al: Analgesie durch intraartikulares Morphin nach Kniegelenks-arthroskopien? Eine doppelblinde, randomisierte Studie mit patientenkontrollierter Analgesie. Anaesthesist 1995;44:351-358.

55. Brandsson S, Karlsson J, Morberg P, et al: Intraarticular morphine after arthroscopic ACL reconstruction: A double-blind placebo-controlled study of 40 patients. Acta Orthop Scand 2000;71:280-285.

56. Likar R, Mousa SA, Philippitsch G, et al: Increased numbers of opioid expressing inflammatory cells do not affect intra-articular morphine analgesia. Br J Anaesth 2004;93:375-380.

57. Denti M, Randelli P, Bigoni M, et al: Pre- and postoperative intra-articular analgesia for arthroscopic surgery of the knee and arthroscopy-assisted anterior cruciate ligament reconstruction. A double-blind randomized, prospective study. Knee Surg Sports Traumatol Arthrosc 1997;5:206-212.

58. Whitford A, Healy M, Joshi GP, et al: The effect of tourniquet release time on the analgesic efficacy of intraarticular morphine after arthroscopic knee surgery. Anesth Analg 1997; 84:791-793.

59. Klinken C: Effects of tourniquet time in knee arthroscopy patients receiving intraarticular morphine combined with bupivacaine. CRNA 1995;6:37-42.

60. Marchal JM, Delgado-Martinez AD, Poncela M, et al: Does the type of arthroscopic surgery modify the analgesic effect of intraarticular morphine and bupivacaine? A preliminary study. Clin J Pain 2003;19:240-246.

61. Keates HL, Cramond T, Smith MT: Intraarticular and peri-articular opioid binding in inflamed tissue in experimental canine arthritis. Anesth Analg 1999;89:409-415.

62. Ngan Kee WD: Intrathecal pethidine: Pharmacology and clinical applications. Anaesth Intensive Care 1998;26:137-146.

63. Westman L, Valentin A, Engström B, et al: Local anesthesia for arthroscopic surgery of the ankle using pethidine or prilocaine Arthroscopy 1997;13:307-312.

64. Söderlund A, Westman L, Ersmark H, et al: Analgesia following arthroscopy—A comparison of intra-articular morphine, pethidine and fentanyl. Acta Anaesth Scand 1997;41:6-11.

65. Lyons B, Lohan D, Flynn CG, et al: Intra-articular analgesia for arthroscopic meniscectomy. Br J Anaesth 1995;75:552-555.

66. Ekblom A, Westman L, Soderlund A, et al: Is intra-articular pethidine an alternative to local anaesthetics in arthroscopy? A double-blind study comparing prilocaine with pethidine. Knee Surg Sports Traumatol Arthrosc 1993;1:189-194.

67. Ginosar Y, Columb MO, Cohen SE, et al: The site of action of epidural fentanyl infusions in the presence of local anesthetics: A minimum local analgesic concentration infusion study in nulliparous labor. Anesth Analg 2003;97: 1439-1445.

68. Pooni JS, Hickmott K, Mercer D, et al: Comparison of intra-articular fentanyl and intra-articular bupivacaine for postoperative pain relief after knee arthroscopy. Eur J Anaesth 1999;16:708-711.

69. Varkel V, Volpin G, Ben-David B, et al: Intraarticular fentanyl compared with morphine for pain relief following arthroscopic knee surgery. Can J Anaesth 1999;46:867-871.

70. Vranken JH, Vissers KC, de Jongh R, et al: Intraarticular sufentanil administration facilitates recovery after day-case knee arthroscopy. Anesth Analg 2001;92:625-628.

71. Kizilkaya M, Yildirim OS, Dogan N, et al: Analgesic effects of intraarticular sufentanil and sufentanil plus methylprednisolone after arthroscopic knee surgery. Anesth Analg 2004; 98:1062-1065.

72. Dauri M, Polzoni M, Fabbi E, et al: Comparison of epidural continuous femoral block and intraarticular analgesia after anterior cruciate ligament reconstruction. Acta Anaesth Scand 2003;74:20-25.

73. Rasmussen S, Kehlet H: Intraarticular glucocorticoid, morphine and bupivacaine reduces pain and convalescence after arthroscopic ankle surgery: A randomized study of 36 patients. Acta Orthop Scand 2000;71:301-304.

74. Armstrong RW, Bolding F: Septic arthritis after arthroscopy: the contributing roles of intraarticular steroids and environmental factors. Am J Infect Control 1994;22:16-18.

75. Reuben SS, Connelly NR: Postarthroscopic meniscus repair analgesia with intraarticular ketorolac or morphine. Anesth Analg 1996;82:1036-1039.

76. Reuben SS, Connelly NR: Postoperative analgesia for out-patient arthroscopic knee surgery with intraarticular bupivacaine and ketorolac. Anesth Analg 1995;80:1154-1157.

77. Calmet J, Esteve C, Boada S, Gine J: Analgesic effect of intra-articular ketorolac in knee arthroscopy: Comparison of morphine and bupivacaine. Knee Surg Sports Traumatol Arthrosc 2004;12:552-555.

78. Convery PN, Milligan KR, Quinn P, et al: Low-dose intra-articular ketorolac for pain relief following arthroscopy of the knee joint. Anaesthesia 1988;53:1117-1129.

79. Colbert ST, Curran E, O'Hanlon DM, et al: Intra-articular tenoxicam improves postoperative analgesia in knee arthroscopy. Can J Anaesth 1999;46:653-657.

80. Elhakim M, Fathy A, Elkott M, et al: Intra-articular tenoxicam relieves post-arthroscopy pain. Acta Anaesth Scand 1996;40: 1223-1226.

81. Guler G, Karaoglu S, Velibasoglu H, et al: Comparison of analgesic effects of intra-articular tenoxicam and morphine in anterior cruciate ligament reconstruction. Knee Surg Sports Traumatol Arthrosc 2002;10:229-232.

82. Talu GK, Ozyalcin S, Koltka K, et al: Comparison of efficacy of intra-articular application of tenoxicam, bupivacaine and tenoxicam: Bupivacaine combination in arthroscopic knee surgery. Knee Surg Sports Traumatol Arthrosc 2002;10: 355-360.

83. Cook TM, Tuckey JP, Nolan JP: Analgesia after day-case knee arthroscopy: Double-blind study of intra-articular tenoxicam, intra-articular bupivacaine and placebo. Br J Anaesth 1997;78:163-168.

84. Rømsing J, Møiniche S, Ostergaard D, et al: Local infiltration with NSAIDs for postoperative analgesia: Evidence for a peripheral analgesic action. Acta Anaesth Scand 2000;44: 672-683.

85. Gentili M, Juhel A, Bonnet F: Peripheral analgesic effect of intra-articular clonidine. Pain 1996;64:593-596.

86. Gentili M, Houssel P, Osman M, et al: Intra-articular morphine and clonidine produce comparable analgesia but the combination is not more effective. Br J Anaesth 1997;79: 660-661.

87. Buerkle H, Huge V, Wolfgart M, et al: Intra-articular clonidine analgesia after knee arthroscopy. Eur J Anaesthesiol 2000;17:295-299.

88. Iqbal J, Wig J, Bhardwaj N, Dhillon MS: Intra-articular clonidine vs. morphine for post-operative analgesia following arthroscopic knee surgery (a comparative evaluation). Knee 2000;7:109-113.

89. Joshi W, Reuben SS, Kilaru PR, et al: Postoperative analgesia for outpatient arthroscopic knee surgery with intraarticular clonidine and/or morphine. Anesth Analg 2000;90:1102-1106.

90. Reuben SS, Connelly NR: Postoperative analgesia for out-patients arthroscopic knee surgery with intraarticular clonidine. Anesth Analg 1999;89:802-803.

91. Alagol A, Calpur OU, Usar PS, et al: Intraarticular analgesia after arthroscopic knee surgery: Comparison of neostigmine, clonidine, tenoxicam, morphine and bupivacaine. Knee Surg Sports Traumatol Arthrosc 2005;13:658-663.

92. Zhou S, Bonasera L, Carlton SM, et al: Peripheral administration of NMDA, AMPA, or KA results in pain behaviors in rates. Neurol Report 1996;7:895-900.

93. Dal D, Tetik O, Altunkaya H, et al: The efficacy of intra-articular ketamine for postoperative analgesia in outpatient arthroscopic surgery. Arthroscopy 2004;20:300-305.

94. Rosseland LA, Stughaug A, Sandberg L, et al: Intra-articular (IA) catheter administration of postoperative analgesics. A new trial design allows evaluation of baseline pain, demonstrates large variations in need of analgesics, and finds no analgesic effect of IA ketamine compared with IA saline. Pain 2003;104:25-34.

95. Huang GS, Yeh CC, Kong SS, et al: Intra-articular ketamine for pain control following arthroscopic knee surgery. Acta Anaesthesiol Sin 2000;38:131-136.

96. Batra YK, Mahajan R, Bangalia SK, et al: Bupivacaine/ketamine is superior to intra-articular ketamine analgesia following arthroscopic knee surgery. Can J Anaesth 2005; 52:832-836.

97. Alagol A, Calpur OU, Kaya G, et al: The use of intraarticular tramadol for postoperative analgesia after arthroscopic knee surgery: A comparison of different intraarticular and intravenous doses. Knee Surg Sports Traumatol Arthrosc 2004; 12:184-188.

98. Cagney B, Williams O, Jennings L, et al: Tramadol or fentanyl analgesia for ambulatory knee arthroscopy. Eur J Anaesthesiol 1999;16:182-185.

99. Akinci SB, Saricaoglu F, Atay OM, et al: Analgesic effect of intra-articular tramadol compared with morphine after arthroscopic knee surgery. Arthroscopy 2005;9:1060-1065.

100. Beilin B, Nemirovsky AY, Zeidel A, et al: Systemic physostigmine increases the antinociceptive effect of spinal morphine. Pain 1997;70:217-221.

101. Hartvig P, Gillberg PG, Gordh T Jr, Post C: Cholinergic mechanisms in pain and analgesia. Trends Pharmacol Sci 1989;Suppl:75-79.

102. Krukowski JA, Hood DD, Eisenach JC, et al: Intrathecal neostigmine for post-cesarean section analgesia: Dose response. Anesth Analg 1997;84:1269-1275.

103. Gentili M, Dominique E, Szymskiewicz O, et al: Postoperative analgesia by intraarticular clondine and neostigmine in patients undergoing knee arthroscopy. Reg Anesth Pain Med 2001;26:342-347.

104. Lauretti GR, de Oliveira R, Perez MV, Paccola CA: Postoperative analgesia by intraarticular and epidural neostigmine following knee surgery. J Clin Anesth 2000;12:444-448.

105. Yang LC, Chen LM, Wang CJ, Buerkle H: Postoperative analgesia by intra-articular neostigmine in patients undergoing knee arthroscopy. Anesthesiology 1998;88:334-339.

106. Schafer M: Analgesic effects of neostigmine in the periphery. Anesthesiology 2000;92:1207-1208.

107. Vintar N, Rawal N, Veselko M: Intraarticular patient-controlled regional anesthesia after arthroscopically assisted anterior cruciate ligament reconstruction: Ropivacaine/morphine/ketorolac versus ropivacaine/morphine. Anesth Analg 2005;101:573-578.

108. Elhakim M, Nafie M, Eid A, et al: Combination of intra-articular tenoxicam, lidocaine and pethidine for outpatient knee arthroscopy. Acta Anaesthesiol Scand 1999;43:803-808.

109. Lombardi AV Jr, Berend KR, Mallory TH, et al: Soft tissue and intra-articular injection of bupivacaine, epinephrine, and morphine has a beneficial effect after total knee arthroplasty. Clin Orthop Relat Res 2004;428:125-130.

110. Ilfeld BM, Morey TE, Enneking FK: The delivery rate accuracy of portable infusion pumps used for regional analgesia. Anesth Analg 2002;95:1331-1336.

111. Capdevila X, Macaire P, Aknin P, et al: Patient-controlled perineural analgesia after ambulatory orthopedic surgery: Evaluation and comparison of three pumps. Anesth Analg 2003;96:414-417.

112. Ganapathy S, Amendola A, Lichfield R, et al: Elastomeric pumps for ambulatory patient controlled regional analgesia. Can J Anaesth 2000;47:897-902.
113. Horn EP, Schroeder F, Wilhelm S, et al: Wound infiltration and drain lavage with ropivacaine after major shoulder surgery. Anesth Analg 1999;89:1461-1466.
114. Convery PN, Milligan KR, Quinn P, et al: Efficacy and uptake of ropivacaine and bupivacaine after single intra-articular injection in the knee joint. Br J Anaesth 2001;87:570-576.
115. Knudsen K, Beckman Suurkula M, et al: Central nervous and cardiovascular effects of i.v. infusions of ropivacaine, bupivacaine and placebo in volunteers. Br J Anaesth 1997;78:507-514.
116. Irwin MG, Cheung KM, Nicholls JM, Thompson N: Intra-articular injection of ketorolac in the rat knee joint: Effect on articular cartilage and synovium. Br J Anaesth 1998;80:837-839.
117. Dogan N, Erdem AF, Gundogdu C, et al: The effects of ketorolac and morphine on articular cartilage and synovium in the rabbit knee joint. Can J Physiol Pharmacol 2004;82:502-505.
118. Dogan N, Erdem AF, Erman Z, Kizilkaya M: The effects of bupivacaine and neostigmine on articular cartilage and synovium in the rabbit knee joint. J Int Med Res 2004;32:513-519.
119. Gille J, Bernotat J, Bohm S, et al: Spontaneous hemarthrosis of the knee associated with clopidogrel and aspirin treatment. Z Rheumatol 2003;62:80-81.
120. Soderlund A, Boreus LO, Westman L, et al: A comparison of 50, 100 and 200 mg of intra-articular pethidine during knee joint surgery; a controlled study with evidence for local demethylation to norpethidine. Pain 1999;80:229-238.

54 Spinal Cord and Peripheral Nerve Stimulation

Allen W. Burton

SPINAL CORD STIMULATION

Spinal cord stimulation (SCS), sometimes called dorsal column stimulation, describes the use of pulsed electrical energy near the spinal cord to control pain.[1] This technique was first applied in the intrathecal space and finally in the epidural space as described by Shealy and associates in 1967.[2] In the present day, neurostimulation most commonly involves the implantation of leads in the epidural space to transmit this pulsed energy across the spinal cord or near the desired nerve roots. This technique has notable analgesic properties for neuropathic pain states, anginal pain, and peripheral ischemic pain. The same technology can be applied in deep brain stimulation, cortical brain stimulation, and peripheral nerve stimulation.[3-5] These techniques are mainly in the realm of the neurosurgeon, although more pain specialists are revisiting peripheral stimulation techniques. This chapter concentrates on the modality of spinal cord stimulation.

Mechanism of Action

Neurostimulation began shortly after Melzack and Wall proposed the gate control theory in 1965.[6] This theory proposed that painful peripheral stimuli carried by C-fibers and lightly myelinated A-delta fibers terminated at the substantia gelatinosa of the dorsal horn (the gate). Large myelinated A-beta fibers responsible for touch and vibratory sensation also terminated at "the gate" in the dorsal horn. It was hypothesized that their input could be manipulated to "close the gate" to the transmission of painful stimuli. As an application of the gate control theory, Shealy implanted the first spinal cord stimulator device for the treatment of chronic pain.[2] This technique was noted to control pain, and has undergone numerous technical and clinical refinements in the ensuing years.

Although the gate theory was initially proposed as the mechanism of action, the underlying neurophysiologic mechanisms are not clearly understood. Recent research has given us insight into effects occurring at the local and supraspinal levels and through dorsal horn interneuron and neurochemical mechanisms.[7,8] Linderoth and colleagues[8] have noted that the mechanism of analgesia when SCS is applied in neuropathic pain states may be very different from those involved in analgesia as a result of limb ischemia or angina. Experimental evidence points to SCS having a beneficial effect at the dorsal horn level by favorably altering the local neurochemistry, thereby suppressing the hyperexcitability of the wide dynamic range interneurons. Specifically, there is some evidence for increased levels of gamma-aminobutyric acid (GABA) release, serotonin, and perhaps suppression of levels of some excitatory amino acids including glutamate and aspartate. In the case of ischemic pain, analgesia seems to be obtained through restoration of a favorable oxygen supply and demand balance, perhaps through alteration of sympathetic tone.

Patient Selection

Appropriate patients for neurostimulation must meet the following criteria: the diagnosis must be amenable to this therapy (that is, neuropathic pain syndromes), the patient has failed conservative therapy, significant psychological issues have been ruled out, and a trial has demonstrated pain relief.[9] Pure neuropathic pain syndromes are relatively less common than the mixed nociceptive and neuropathic disorders including failed back surgery syndrome (FBSS), and clear selection criteria based on the type and pattern of pain are not readily apparent. Many patients with chronic pain will have some symptoms of depression, but psychological screening can be extremely helpful for avoiding failed implants in patients with major psychological disorders. An interesting study by Olson and colleagues revealed a high correlation between many items on a complex psychological testing battery and favorable response to trial stimulation.[10] It appears that overall mood state is an important predictor of outcomes.

Despite the recent increase in the number of agents available to treat neuropathic pain, a substantial number of patients still suffer from poorly controlled neuropathic pain. Puig estimates as many as 50% of neuropathic pain patients have ineffective pain relief even with appropriate pharmacologic management.[11] Recommended selection criteria from this author include (1) confirmed diagnosis of neuropathic pain; (2) chronicity of greater than 6 months; (3) failed trials of polypharmacy including anticonvulsants, antidepressants, and other drugs (such as opioids) because of lack of efficacy or side effects; (4) the lemniscate pathway (spinal connection to painful site) must be preserved so that stimulation induced paresthesias can be felt; and (5) the absence of contraindications including nociceptive pain syndromes.

A careful trial period is essential to avoid the failed implant. Trials of different lengths have been advocated; the risk of a longer trial is mainly infection, whereas the primary risk of too short a trial is misreading success. I use a 5- to 7-day trial and encourage patients to be as active as possible in their usual environment, with the exception of limiting bending and twisting movements. Despite advances in understanding of diagnoses that respond to neurostimulation, an increased understanding of and improved psychological screening and availability of improved multilead systems, clinical failures of implanted neurostimulator devices remain all too common. Pain physicians must critically evaluate their own outcomes and adhere to the strict selection criterion outlined here. Simpson has recently published a neurosurgeon's perspective on the use of SCS in treating chronic pain.[12] To paraphrase Simpson, "The mindset of the public and many physicians favors drugs over physical treatments such as surgery and neurostimulation . . . and many physicians exhibit a 'protective' reluctance to refer for these procedures, but are prepared to persist with polypharmacy despite the real risks of mental impairment, nausea, constipation, weight gain, and addiction. The worst thing a neurostimulator can do is fail to work" (p. 54). Many pain specialists are beginning to side with Simpson on this issue, preferring a trial of SCS before committing a patient to chronic opioid therapy.

Technical Considerations

SCS is a technically challenging interventional/surgical pain management technique. It involves the placement of an electrode array (leads) in the epidural space, a trial period, anchoring the lead(s), positioning and implantation of the pulse generator or radiofrequency (RF) receiver, and the tunneling and connection of the connecting wires. I advocate a col-

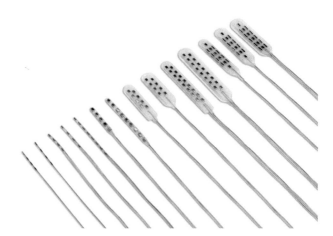

Figure 54–1. *Left to right:* Neurostimulator leads: percutaneous type to paddle type. (Courtesy of ANS, Inc., Plano, Tex.)

laborative effort between a surgeon and anesthesiologist for optimal success with neurostimulation.

Electrodes are of two types: catheter or percutaneous versus paddle or surgical (Fig. 54–1). These electrodes are connected to an implanted pulse generator (IPG) or an RF unit (Fig. 54–2A-C). Currently, three companies—Medtronic, Inc., American Neuromodulation Systems, Inc., and Advanced Bionics, Inc.—make neurostimulation equipment (Appendix 54–1). Interested readers are directed to these companies for further specific information on the equipment.

A stimulation trial may be accomplished in two ways: straight percutaneous or implanted lead. In both trial methods, under fluoroscopy and sterile conditions, a lead is introduced into the epidural space with a standard epidural needle. In order to facilitate threading of the lead cephalad in the dorsal midline region it is imperative to have the needle at a fairly shallow angle. It is important to *avoid* perpendicular needle placement into the epidural space because of the consequent 90-degree bend then required to introduce the stimulator lead. The lead is directed under fluoroscopic imaging into the posterior or dorsal paramedian epidural space up to the desired anatomic location—generally the low thoracic cord region to "cover" the lower extremities (i.e., the lead is moved cephalad and caudad in the epidural space until the pattern of resulting electrical stimulation overlies the painful region; Fig. 54–3). Trial stimulation is undertaken to attempt to cover the painful area with an electrically induced paresthesia. After the painful area is captured either with one or two leads, the two techniques differ.

In the straight percutaneous trial, the needle is withdrawn, an anchoring suture is placed into the skin, and a sterile dressing is applied. The lead passes from the epidural space, through the skin to the external pulse generator throughout the trial period. When the patient returns after a several day trial, the dressing is removed, the suture is clipped, and the

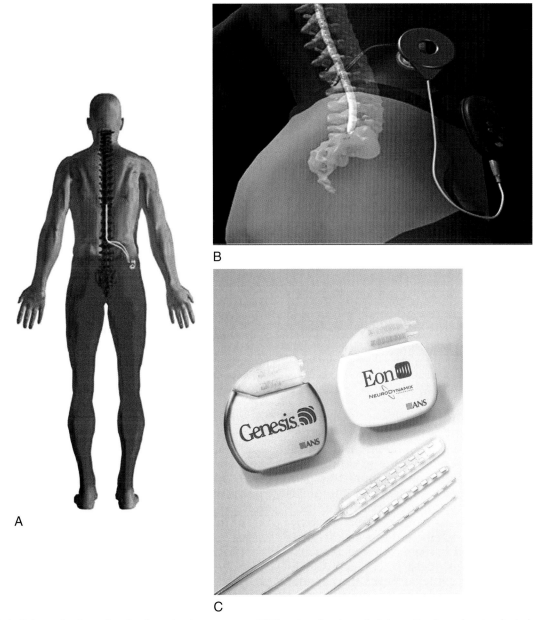

Figure 54–2. A, Schematic view of an implanted pulse generator (IPG) system in place. **B,** Schematic view of an implanted radiofrequency (RF) system. RF systems transmit the energy needed for neurostimulation from an external battery through a surface antenna to an internal receiver. RF systems have the advantage of using an external power source, which is easily replaced; the disadvantage of RF systems is their size and the need to wear an adhesive antenna on the skin. **C,** Representative IPG neurostimulation units with leads. (**A,** Courtesy of Medtronic, Inc. Minneapolis, Minn.; **B** and **C,** courtesy of ANS, Inc., Plano, Tex.)

lead is removed and discarded *regardless* of the success of the trial. When the patient returns for an implant, a new lead is placed in the location of the trial lead and connected to an IPG.

In the "implanted lead" trial, after successful positioning of the trial lead(s), local anesthetic is infiltrated around the needle(s) and an incision is made, cutting down to the supraspinous fascia to anchor the leads securely using nonabsorbable suture. The anchoring device should be placed as closely as possible to the fascia entry site, ideally with the "nose" of the anchor protruding into the fascia. The anchor is secured using nonabsorbable suture, such as 2.0

silk. Then a temporary extension wire is tunneled away from the back incision and out through the skin. This exiting connector is secured to the skin using a suture, antibiotic ointment, and a sterile dressing. If the trial is successful, at the time of implant the back incision is opened and the percutaneous lead extension is cut, pulled out through the skin site, and discarded. The permanent lead(s) that was used for the trial is hooked to new sterile extension(s) and tunneled to the IPG.

The "implanted lead" method has the advantages of saving the cost of new electrodes at implant and ensuring that the implanted lead position matches

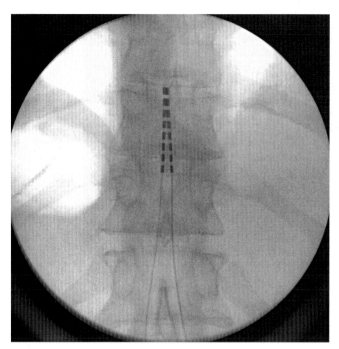

Figure 54–3. Anteroposterior radiograph of dual-eight contact stimulator leads centered over the T-10 level. (Courtesy A. Burton, MD.)

the trial lead position. Advantages of the "percutaneous lead" approach include avoiding the costs of two trips to the operating room (even for an unsuccessful trial, this is necessary to remove the anchored trial lead); avoiding an incision and postoperative pain during the trial, which may confuse trial interpretation by the patient; and avoiding the risk of infection associated with the percutaneous temporary extension. The percutaneous extension must be anchored and meticulously dressed or the risk of infection may be higher than with the straight percutaneous technique.[13] The majority of clinicians favor the percutaneous trial method. Most consider 50% or more pain relief to be indicative of a successful trial, although the ultimate decision also should include other factors such as activity level and medication intake. Some combination of pain relief, increased activity level, and decreased medication intake is indicative of a favorable trial.

A trial with paddle-type electrodes requires the implanted lead approach with the significant addition of a laminotomy to slip the flat plate electrode into the epidural space. Some physicians trial the patient with the straight percutaneous approach and if successful send the patient to a neurosurgeon for a paddle-type implant. My preference is to do a straight percutaneous trial, with an implant using non–paddle-type electrodes.

The IPG/RF unit is generally implanted in the lower abdominal area or in the posterior superior gluteal area. It should be in a location the patient can access with the dominant hand for adjustment of the settings with the patient-held remote control unit. The decision to use a fully implantable IPG or an RF unit

is based on several considerations. If the patient's pain pattern requires the use of many anode or cathode settings with high power requirements during the trial, consider an RF unit. The IPG battery life largely depends on the power settings used, but the newer IPG units generally last several years at average power settings. All three manufacturers offer rechargeable IPG systems with two significant advantages over the previous IPG devices: (1) the patient may use higher voltage settings without worry of prompt battery depletion, allowing more flexibility in programming and (2) the promise of a much longer interval until replacement is required, perhaps 10 years or more. Recharging is done via external recharger every 7 to 14 days as needed.

Complications

Complications associated with spinal cord stimulation range from simple, easily correctable problems, such as lack of appropriate paresthesia coverage, to devastating paralysis, nerve injury, and death. Prior to implantation of the trial lead, an educational session should occur with the patient and family members. This meeting should include a discussion of possible risks and complications. In the postoperative period, the caregiver should be involved in identifying problems and alerting the health care team.

North and colleagues at Johns Hopkins reported their experience in 320 consecutive patients treated with SCS between 1972 and 1990.[14] A 5% rate of subcutaneous infection was seen, which is consistent with other published trials. The most frequent complication was lead migration or breakage, and that remains the predominant weakness of neurostimulation. In an earlier series, bipolar leads required electrode revision in 23% of patients. The revision rate for patients with multichannel devices was 16%. Failure of the electrode lead was observed in 13% of patients and steadily declined over the course of the study. When analyzed by implant type (single-channel percutaneous, single-channel laminectomy, and multichannel), the lead migration rate for multichannel devices was approximately 7%. Analysis of hardware reliability for 298 permanent implants showed that technical failures (particularly electrode migration and malposition) and clinical failures had become significantly less common as implants had evolved into programmable, multichannel devices.

In a 5-year experience at the Cleveland Clinic, Rosenow and colleagues reported a 43% revision or removal rate among 289 patients implanted with SCS systems.[15] Thirty-three percent of all leads required revision, with the most common reasons being lead breakage, poor pain coverage, migration, and infection in descending order of frequency. Ten percent of patients had a lead migration requiring revision. Paddle-type leads broke twice as often as percutaneous leads. Twenty-two percent of all patients required more than one revision procedure; 49% requiring at least one lead revision underwent multiple revisions. Anatomically, cervical leads were the most likely to

Table 54–1. Spinal Cord Stimulation Complications in Order of Decreasing Frequency

COMPLICATION	REPORTED FREQUENCY (BY REFERENCE)
Lead migration with need for revision	7%,[18] 10%,[19] 5%,[20] 14%,[21] 11%[22]
Lead breakage with need for revision	13%,[18] 23%,[19] 0%,[20] 13%,[21] 6%[22]
Infection	4%,[19] 7%,[20] 3%,[21] 5%[22]
Neurologic injury	Case reports, rare [24,25]

require revision. Their overall infection rate was 3.6%.

Barolat and associates and May and coworkers reported lead revision rates caused by lead migration of 4.5% and 13.6% and breakage of 0% and 13.6%, respectively.[16,17] Infections occurred in 7% and 2.5% of cases, respectively. No serious complications were seen in either study. These studies are representative of the complication rate of neurostimulation therapy (Table 54–1). Kumar and colleagues in Saskatchewan have quantified the costs of SCS complications and published suggestions to improve outcomes.[18] Their series included 160 patients treated over 10 years with SCS implantation. They noted 42 patients with 51 complications classified as hardware related (39) or biologic (12) with the range of costs of treatment from $130 (hematoma aspiration) to $22,406 (system reimplantation) (in 2005 Canadian dollars). Their most common hardware failures were lead displacement (11% of patients), followed by fractured electrode (5.6% of patients). Their most common biologic complication was wound infection at 4.4% overall, with subcutaneous hematoma next at 3% overall. These authors present an analysis of engineering work done at Medtronic, Inc. with regard to lead migration and fracture. This manufacturer recommends use of a silicon anchor (not hard plastic) with the tip of the anchor pushed through the deep fascia to reduce the pressure point or fatigue point on the anchor with repeated bending. Further, they recommend a strain relief loop between the anchor and the IPG, with the abdomen being the preferred site of IPG implant because of less stress on the leads during bending. Another poorly understood phenomenon described by Kumar is late tolerance to stimulation in 16 of 160 patients (10%).

Infections range from simple infections at the surface of the wound to epidural abscess. The patient should be instructed on wound care and recognition of signs and symptoms indicative of infection. Many superficial infections can be treated with oral antibiotics or simple surgical incision and drainage followed by wound irrigation. For an excellent review on infectious complications of SCS the reader is referred to Follet and colleagues' recent review of 114 cases with recommendations for avoidance.[19] They found that the most common site of infection was the IPG (54%), the connector tract (17%), the back incision (8%), and others. *Staphylococcus* species were the most common pathogen, cultured in 18% of cases, with system explant required in 82% of cases. There has been one death related to infection and one case of epidural abscess leading to paralysis caused by SCS reported.[20,21] My standard practice includes prophylactic preoperative antibiotics (30 minutes preincision) and oral coverage postoperatively for 3 days.

If infection reaches the tissues involving the devices, in most cases the implant should be removed. In such cases, one should have a high index of suspicion for an epidural abscess. Abscess of the epidural space can lead to paralysis and death if not identified quickly and treated aggressively. In the case of temporary epidural catheters (*somewhat analogous* to a percutaneous stimulator trial), Sarubbi and Vasquez discovered only 20 well-described cases.[22] The mean age of these 22 patients was 49.9 years, the median duration of epidural catheter use was 3 days, and the median time to onset of clinical symptoms after catheter placement was 5 days. The majority of patients (63.6%) had major neurologic deficits, and 22.7% had concomitant meningitis. *Staphylococcus aureus* was the predominant pathogen. Despite antibiotic therapy and drainage procedures, 38% of patients continued to have neurologic deficits. These unusual but serious complications of temporary epidural catheter use require timely and accurate diagnostic evaluation and treatment because the consequences of delayed therapy can be substantial. Schuchard and Clauson reported an infection with *Pasteurella* during an implanted lead trial, which required explanting the system.[23] I have experienced one similar case with *S. aureus* requiring removal of the entire system.

Programming

There are four basic parameters in neurostimulation that may be adjusted to create stimulation paresthesias in the painful areas thereby mitigating the patient's pain. They are amplitude, pulse width, rate, and electrode selection.[24]

Amplitude is the intensity or strength of the stimulation measured in volts. Typically, voltage may be set from 0 to 10 volts, with lower settings used over peripheral nerves and with paddle-type electrodes. Pulse width is a measure in microseconds (μs) of the duration of a pulse. Pulse width is usually set between 100 and 400 μs. A larger pulse width typically gives the patient a broader coverage. Rate is measured in hertz (Hz) or cycles per second, between 20 and 120 Hz. At lower rates the patient feels more of a thumping, whereas at higher Hz, the feeling is more of a buzzing. Electrode selection is a complex topic that has been the subject of some research by Barolet and colleagues, who provided mapping data of coverage patterns based on lead location in 106 patients.[25] The primary target is the cathode (–), with electrons flowing from the cathode(s) (–) to the anode(s) (+). The newest stimulator systems allow for partial anode and cathode arrangements at the different contacts, which has been termed *current steering* by some. This expands the ability to cover most painful areas with a well-placed lead or leads, and makes the number of possible configurations available for programming almost infinite. Thus a programming strategy is important, and each company has developed computer-assisted programming to narrow down the possible choices. Most patients' stimulators are programmed with electrode selection changed until the patient obtains anatomic coverage, then the pulse width and rate are adjusted for maximal comfort. The patient is left with full control to (1) turn the stimulator on and off, (2) choose between numerous "programs" in their device (which have different effects), and (3) adjust the intensity of stimulation up and down to comfort.

The lowest acceptable settings on all parameters are generally used to conserve battery life unless using the newer rechargeable systems. Other programming modes that save battery life include a cycling mode during which the stimulator cycles full on and off at patient-determined intervals (minutes, seconds, or hours). The patient's programming may change over time, and reprogramming needs are common. The neurostimulator manufacturing companies are helpful to clinicians with patient reprogramming assistance. Many busy pain practices designate a nurse practitioner or physician's assistant to handle patient reprogramming needs.

Outcomes

The most common use for SCS in the United States is failed back surgery syndrome (FBSS), whereas in Europe, peripheral ischemia is the predominant indication. With respect to clinical outcomes it makes sense to subdivide the outcomes based on diagnosis (Table 54–2). In a review of the available SCS literature, most evidence falls within the level III (limited) category, as a result of the invasiveness of the modality and difficulties inherent in blinding treatment with SCS, because much of the available literature used older technologies. Recognition must also be given to the time frame within which a study was performed because of rapidly evolving SCS technology. Basic science knowledge, implantation techniques, lead placement locations, contact array designs, and programming capabilities have changed dramatically from the time of the first implants. These improvements have led to decreased morbidity and much greater probability of obtaining adequate paresthesia coverage with subsequent improved outcomes.[26] However, the SCS literature remains scant in terms of high-quality evidence. Coffey and Lozano call for future study designs to include unambiguous entry criteria, randomization, parallel control groups receiving sham treatment, and blinding of patients, investigators, and programmers. They also suggest minimum follow-up time of 1 year for chronic pain conditions, with a Kaplan-Meier–type analysis of ongoing pain relief.[27,28]

Table 54–2.   A Summary of Outcomes of Spinal Cord Stimulation By Disease

Failed back surgery syndrome	Grade B supportive evidence (favorable pain relief, functional capacity, health-related quality of life, and return to work all favorably affected)[39]
Complex regional pain syndrome	Grade A supportive evidence (favorable global perceived effect, pain reduction, and a variety of other quality of life/disability measures)[37]
Peripheral ischemia	Grade A supportive evidence (favorable limb salvage rates and quality of life measures)[50]
Angina pectoris	Substantial supportive evidence from prospective controlled studies (fewer anginal attacks, lower nitrate requirements, improved exercise capacity and equivalent cardiovascular outcomes to revision coronary bypass surgery, and lower complication rate—no meta-analysis done)[53,54]

SPINAL CORD STIMULATION OUTCOMES: FAILED BACK SURGERY SYNDROME

Van Buyten has reviewed this topic extensively and found significant supportive literature for SCS in the patient with FBSS.[29] Specifically, he points out sufficient evidence for sustained long-term pain relief with medication reduction, improvement in quality of life, increased ability to return to work, increased patient satisfaction, minimal side effects, and cost effectiveness compared with alternative therapies. Further advantages noted include the trial period for SCS, which limits treatment failures and the reversibility of the technique.

There has been one recent prospective randomized study looking specifically at reoperation versus SCS in patients with FBSS. North and associates[30] selected 51 patients as candidates for repeat laminectomy. All the patients had undergone previous surgery and were excluded from randomization if they presented with severe spinal canal stenosis, extremely large disk fragments, a major neurologic deficit such as footdrop, or radiographic evidence of gross instability. In addition, patients were excluded for untreated dependency on narcotic analgesics or benzodiazepines, major psychiatric comorbidity, the presence of any significant or disabling chronic pain problem, or a chief complaint of low back pain exceeding lower extremity pain. Crossover between groups was permitted. The 6-month follow-up report included 27 patients. At this point they became eligible for crossover. Of the 15 patients who had undergone reoperation, 67% (10 patients) crossed over to SCS. Of the 12 who had undergone SCS, 17% (2 patients) opted for crossover to reoperation. For 90% of the patients, long-term (3-year follow-up) evaluation has shown that spinal cord stimulation continues to be more effective than reoperation, with significantly better outcomes for SCS. Overall 47% of patients in the SCS group achieved 50% or greater pain relief compared with 12% in the reoperation group ($p < 0.01$). Additionally, patients randomized to reoperation used significantly more opioids than those randomized to spinal cord stimulation. Other measures assessing activities of daily living and work status did not differ significantly.[30]

Two recent, prospective case series have been done. The first, by Barolat and colleagues examined the outcomes of patients with intractable low back pain treated with epidural spinal cord stimulation (SCS) using paddle electrodes and an RF stimulator.[31] In four centers, 44 patients were implanted and followed with the Visual Analogue Scale (VAS), the Oswestry Disability Questionnaire, the Sickness Impact Profile (SIP), and a patient satisfaction rating scale. All patients had back and leg pain, and all had at least one previous back surgery, with most (83%) having two or more back surgeries, and 51% having had a spinal fusion. Data were collected at baseline, at 6 months, 12 months, and 2 years. All patients showed a reported mean decrease in their 10-point VAS scores compared with baseline. The majority of patients reported fair to excellent pain relief in both the low back and legs. At 6 months 91.6% of the patients reported fair to excellent relief in the legs and 82.7% of the patients reported fair to excellent relief in the low back. At 1 year 88.2% of the patients reported fair to excellent relief in the legs and 68.8% reported fair to excellent relief in the low back. Significant improvement in function and quality of life was found at both the 6-month and 1-year follow-ups using the Oswestry and SIP, respectively. The majority of patients reported that the procedure was worthwhile (92% at 6 months, 88% at 1 year). The authors concluded that SCS proved beneficial at 1 year for the treatment of patients with chronic low back and leg pain.

The second multicenter prospective case series was published by Burchiel and coworkers in 1996.[32] The study included 182 patients with a permanent system after a percutaneous trial. Patient evaluation of pain and functional levels was performed before and 3, 6, and 12 months after implantation. Complications, medication use, and work status also were monitored. A 1-year follow-up evaluation was available for 70 patients. All pain and quality-of-life measures showed statistically significant improvement, whereas medication use and work status did not significantly improve during the treatment year. Complications requiring surgical intervention were experienced by 17% (12 of 70) of the patients.

There have been two older systematic review articles on neurostimulation and one recent meta-analysis by Taylor.[35] Turner and colleagues completed a meta-analysis from the articles related to the treatment of FBSS by spinal cord stimulation, from 1966 to 1994.[33] They reviewed 39 studies that met the inclusion criteria. The mean follow-up period was 16 months, with range of 1 to 45 months. Pain relief exceeding 50% was experienced by 59% of patients, with a range of 15% to 100%. Complications occurred

in 42% of patients, with 30% of patients experiencing one or more stimulator-related complications. However, all the studies were case control investigations. Based on this review, the authors concluded that there was insufficient evidence from the literature for drawing conclusions about the effectiveness of spinal cord stimulation relative to no treatment or other treatments, or about the effects of spinal cord stimulation on patient work status, functional disability, and medication use.

The second systematic review, done by North and Wetzel, consisted of a review of case control studies and two prospective control studies.[34] They concluded that if a patient reports a reduction in pain of at least 50% during a trial, as determined by standard rating methods, and demonstrates improved or stable analgesic requirements and activity levels, significant benefit may be realized from a permanent implant. The authors conclude the bulk of the literature appears to support a role for spinal cord stimulation in neuropathic pain syndromes, but caution that the quality of the existing literature is marginal.

Taylor reviewed the literature on SCS in the treatment of FBSS and found Grade B evidence for this therapy based on the review of 382 articles, out of which 1 randomized control trial (RCT), 1 cohort study, 72 case series, and 4 cost series met criteria for the meta-analysis.[35] Taylor's careful review of 72 case series of SCS in FBSS showed 62% of patients obtaining at least 50% or better pain relief, with 53% no longer requiring analgesics. Furthermore, functional capacity and health-related quality of life (HRQL), as well as return to work were all favorably affected. Seventy percent of patients expressed satisfaction with their SCS system.

SPINAL CORD STIMULATION OUTCOMES: COMPLEX REGIONAL PAIN SYNDROME

Research of high quality regarding SCS and complex regional pain syndrome (CRPS) is limited, but existing data are positive in terms of pain reduction, quality of life, analgesic use, and function.

Kemler and colleagues published a prospective, randomized, comparative trial to compare SCS versus conservative therapy for CRPS.[36] Patients with a 6-month history of CRPS of the upper extremities were randomized to undergo trial SCS (and implant if successful) plus physiotherapy versus physiotherapy alone. In this study, 36 patients were assigned to receive a standardized physical therapy program together with spinal cord stimulation, whereas 18 patients were assigned to receive therapy alone. In 24 of the 36 patients, randomized to spinal cord stimulation along with physical therapy, the trial was successful, and permanent implantation was performed. At a 6-month follow-up assessment, the patients in the spinal cord stimulation group had a significantly greater reduction in pain, and a significantly higher percentage rated themselves as much improved for the global perceived effect. However, there were no clinically significant improvements in functional status. The authors concluded that in the short term, spinal cord stimulation reduces pain and improves the quality of life for patients with CRPS involving the upper extremities.

Several important case series have been published on the use of neurostimulation in the treatment of CRPS. Calvillo and coworkers reported a series of 36 patients with advanced stages of complex regional pain syndrome (at least 2 years' duration) who had undergone successful SCS trial (>50% reduction of pain).[37] They were treated with either spinal cord stimulation or peripheral nerve stimulation, and in some cases with both modalities: 36 months after implantation the reported pain measured on VAS was an average of 53% better; this change was statistically significant. Analgesic consumption decreased in the majority of patients. Forty-one percent of patients had returned to work on a modified duty. The authors concluded that in the late stages of complex regional pain syndrome, neurostimulation (with SCS or PNS) is a reasonable option when alternative therapies have failed.

Another case series reported by Oakley and Weiner is remarkable in that it used a sophisticated battery of outcomes tools to evaluate treatment response in CRPS using spinal cord stimulation.[38] The study followed 19 patients and analyzed the results from the McGill Pain Rating Index, the Sickness Impact Profile, Oswestry Disability Index, Beck Depression Inventory, and VAS. Nineteen patients were reported as a subgroup enrolled at two centers participating in a multicenter study of efficacy and outcomes of spinal cord stimulation. Specific preimplant and postimplant tests to measure outcome were administered. Statistically significant improvement in the Sickness Impact Profile physical and psychosocial subscales was documented. The McGill Pain Rating Index words chosen and sensory subscale also improved significantly as did VAS scores. The Beck Depression Inventory trended toward significant improvement. All patients received at least partial relief and benefit from their device, with 30% receiving full relief. Eighty percent (80%) of the patients obtained at least 50% pain relief through the use of their stimulators. The average percent of pain relief was 61%. The authors concluded that patients with CRPS benefit significantly from the use of spinal cord stimulation, based on average follow-up of 7.9 months.

A literature review by Stanton-Hicks of SCS for CRPS consisted of seven case series. These studies ranged in size from 6 to 24 patients. Results were noted as good to excellent in greater than 72% of patients over 8 to 40 months. The review concluded that SCS has proven to be a powerful tool in the management of patients with CRPS (Fig. 54–4).[39]

A retrospective, 3 year, multicenter study of 101 patients by Bennett and colleagues evaluated the effectiveness of SCS applied to complex regional pain syndrome I (CRPS I) and compared the effectiveness of octapolar versus quadrapolar systems, as well as high-frequency and multiprogram parameters.[40] VAS was significantly decreased in the group using the dual-octapolar system, with reductions in overall VAS approaching 70%. Of the dual-octapolar group, 74.8% used multiple arrays to maximize paresthesia coverage. VAS reduction in the group using quadrapolar systems approached 50%; 86.3% of quadrapolar systems and 97.2% of dual-octapolar systems continued to be used. Overall satisfaction with stimulation was 91% in the dual-octapolar group and 70% in the quadrapolar group ($p < 0.05$). The authors concluded that SCS is effective in the management of chronic pain associated with CRPS I and that use of dual-octapolar systems with multiple-array programming capabilities appeared to increase the paresthesia coverage and thus, further reduce pain. High-frequency stimulation (>250 Hz) was found to be essential in obtaining adequate analgesia in 15% of the patients using dual-octapolar systems (this frequency level was not available to those with quadrapolar systems).

Taylor recently performed a meta-analysis on the use of SCS to treat CRPS and concluded that Grade A (highest level) evidence is available supporting the use of SCS to treat CRPS.[35] Stanton-Hicks recently expanded upon the usefulness on SCS in the treatment of CRPS in the context of an overall treatment strategy, which included analgesics, physiotherapy, psychological therapies, and other interventions in a time-contingent manner because of the progressive debility of untreated or undertreated CRPS, stressing a step up in aggressiveness of therapy every 12 to 16 weeks in the face of lack of response.[41] This treatment algorithm is from a 2002 consensus panel and review of the literature (see Fig. 54–3).[42]

SPINAL CORD STIMULATION OUTCOMES: PERIPHERAL ISCHEMIA AND ANGINA

Cook and associates reported in 1976 that SCS effectively relieved pain associated with peripheral ischemia.[43] This result has been repeated and noted to have particular efficacy in conditions associated with vasospasm such as Raynaud's disease.[44] Many studies have shown impressive efficacy of SCS to treat intractable angina.[45] Reported success rates are consistently high and these indications, already widely used in other countries, are certain to expand within the United States.

Ubbink and Vermeulen recently performed a meta-analysis on the world's literature on SCS for peripheral ischemia or critical leg ischemia (CLI).[46] The authors used Cochrane Review criteria for inclusion of an article into their analysis. They found 9 reports describing 6 clinical trials, 5 of which were randomized. The overall sample size was 444 patients and a variety of end points were evaluated, but consistently the primary end point was limb salvage at 12 months. The limb amputation rate was 11% lower in the SCS group versus the conservative treatment group. Overall, SCS-treated patients showed higher quality of life indices and less analgesic consumption. Only 2 of these 6 trials used capillary microscopy laser Doppler measurements of tissue oxygenation ($Tcpo_2$)

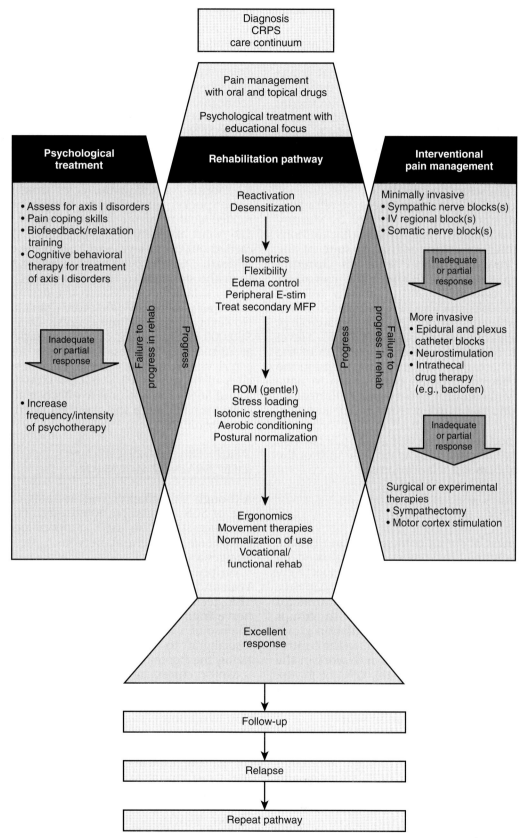

Figure 54–4. Treatment algorithm for complex regional pain syndrome (CRPS). IV, intravenous; MFP, myofascial pain; ROM, range of motion. (From Stanton-Hicks M, Burton AW, Bruehl SP, et al: An updated interdisciplinary clinical pathway for CRPS: Report of an expert panel. Pain Pract 2002;2[1]:1-16.)

measurements, which should lead to optimal outcomes. One of the latter trials suggested a $TcpO_2$ of less than 10 is likely to require amputation regardless of treatment, and $TcpO_2$ of greater the 30 is likely to improve regardless of treatment. Further, that group advocates an increase in $TcpO_2$ of at least 10 mm Hg during the SCS trial.[47] By using this selection criteria, limb salvage rates approach 83% versus conservative care rates, which run between 20% and 64%. Thus existent high-level Grade A evidence exists for the use of SCS in CLI. Further RCTs should show higher success rates (versus conservative therapy) based on the refined $TcpO_2$ selection criteria.

SCS has been used in the treatment of refractory angina pectoris states since first reported by Murphy and Giles in Australia.[48] It is estimated that millions of patients suffer refractory angina in spite of the endoluminal revascularization strategies currently used in clinical cardiology. Buchser and coworkers have recently reviewed the topic and in spite of numerous favorable studies, little support for this technique has been forthcoming in the cardiology realm.[49] The lead or leads are placed at the T1-2 level just to the left of midline with manipulation of the lead until the chest is covered with paresthesia in the usual anginal region. SCS has been shown to have similar efficacy to coronary bypass surgery in treating refractory angina, but with lower morbidity and mortality rates acutely.[50] The mechanism of action of SCS in the angina pectoris patient, as with the CLI patient, is a relief of the ischemia with a favorable shift of the oxygen supply demand relationships.

Cost Effectiveness

Cost effectiveness of spinal cord stimulation (in the treatment of chronic back pain) was evaluated by Kumar and colleagues in 2002.[51] They prospectively followed 104 patients with FBSS. Of the 104 patients, 60 were implanted with a spinal cord stimulator using a standard selection criterion. Both groups were monitored over 5 years. The stimulation group annual cost was $29,000 versus $38,000 in the control group. The authors found 15% return to work in the stimulation group versus 0% in the control group. The higher costs in the nonstimulator group were in the categories of medications, emergency center visits, x-rays, and ongoing physician visits.

Bell and North performed an analysis of the medical costs of SCS therapy in the treatment of patients with FBSS.[52] The medical costs of SCS therapy were compared with an alternative regimen of surgeries and other interventions. Externally powered (external) and fully internalized (internal) SCS systems were considered separately. No value was placed on pain relief or improvements in the quality of life that successful SCS therapy can generate. The authors concluded that by reducing the demand for medical care by FBSS patients, SCS therapy can lower medical costs and found that on average SCS therapy pays for itself within 5.5 years. In those patients for whom SCS therapy is clinically efficacious, the therapy pays for itself within 2.1 years.

Kemler and Furnee performed a similar study but looked at "chronic reflex sympathetic dystrophy (RSD)" using outcomes and costs of care before and after the start of treatment.[53] This essentially is an economic analysis of the outcomes paper. Fifty-four patients with chronic RSD were randomized to receive either SCS together with physical therapy (SCS + PT; $n = 36$) or physical therapy alone (PT; $n = 18$). Twenty-four SCS and PT patients responded positively to trial stimulation and underwent SCS implantation. During 12 months of follow-up, costs (routine RSD, SCS, out-of-pocket) and effects (pain relief by VAS, health-related quality of life [HRQL] improvement by EQ-5D) were assessed in both groups. Analyses were carried out up to 1 year and up to the expected time of death. SCS was both more effective and less costly than the standard treatment protocol. As a result of high initial costs of SCS, in the first year, the treatment per patient is $4000 more than control therapy. However, in the lifetime analysis, SCS per patient is $60,000 cheaper than control therapy. In addition, at 12 months, SCS resulted in pain relief (SCS + PT [−2.7] vs. PT [0.4] [$p < 0.001$]) and improved HRQL (SCS + PT [0.22] vs. PT [0.03] [$p = 0.004$]). The authors found SCS to be both more effective and less expensive compared with the standard treatment protocol for chronic RSD.

PERIPHERAL, CORTICAL, AND DEEP BRAIN STIMULATION

Although this chapter concentrates on the technique of SCS, it must be noted that neurostimulation can successfully be used at other locations in the peripheral and central nervous systems to provide analgesia.

Peripheral nerve stimulation was introduced by Wall and Sweet as well as others in the mid-1960s.[54] This technique has shown efficacy for peripheral nerve injury pain syndromes as well as CRPS, with the use of a carefully implanted paddle lead using a fascial graft to help anchor the lead without traumatizing the nerve.[55]

Motor cortex and deep brain stimulation have been explored to treat highly refractory neuropathic pain syndromes including central pain, deafferentation syndromes, trigeminal neuralgia, and others.[56] Deep brain stimulation has become a widely used technique for movement disorders and much less so for painful indications, although there have been many case reports in treating highly refractory central pain syndromes.[57]

CONCLUSION

Spinal cord stimulation is an invasive, interventional surgical procedure that is useful in refractory chronic pain syndromes. Meyerson and Linderoth have written some principles of neurostimulation that are cornerstones of SCS theory and practice (Box 54–

BOX 54–1. PRINCIPLES OF NEUROSTIMULATION

- Spinal cord stimulation (SCS) mechanism of action is not completely understood but influences multiple components and levels within the central nervous system (CNS) with both interneuron and neurochemical mechanisms.
- SCS therapy is effective for many neuropathic pain conditions. Stimulation-evoked paresthesia must be experienced in the entire painful area.
- Stimulation should be applied with low intensity, just suprathreshold for the activation of the low-threshold, large-diameter fibers, and should be of nonpainful intensity. To be effective SCS must be applied continuously (or in cycles) for at least 20 minutes before the onset of analgesia. This analgesia develops slowly and typically lasts several hours after cessation of the stimulation.
- SCS has demonstrated clinical and cost effectiveness in limb ischemia, failed back surgery syndrome (FBSS), and complex regional pain syndrome (CRPS). Clinical effectiveness also has been shown in angina pectoris, with favorable preliminary reports in visceral pain states as well as occipital neuralgia.
- Multicontact, multiprogram systems improve outcomes and reduce the incidence of surgical revisions. The role of the paddle versus percutaneous leads is uncertain with islands of support for each.
- Serious complications are exceedingly rare but can be devastating. Meticulous care must be taken during implantation to minimize procedural complications. The most frequent complications are lead breakage or migration (approximately 13% for permanent percutaneous leads and higher for paddle leads) and wound infections (approximately 5% or less).

1).[58,59] The evidence for spinal cord stimulation in properly selected populations with neuropathic pain states is good to moderate. According to recent analyses outlined earlier, Grade A evidence exists for the treatment of critical limb ischemia and CRPS, with Grade B evidence for FBSS. Clearly this technique should be reserved for patients who have failed more conservative therapies. With appropriate selection and careful attention to technical issues, the clinical results are overwhelmingly positive.

The frequent need for revision procedures as outlined in this chapter is important in many ways. Although the revision procedures entail relatively minimal risk, there are numerous costs for the patient and health system. The patient's analgesia is interrupted, entailing the expense and time of lost work or productivity, increased medication use, SCS hardware expenses, operative expenses, and other direct costs. Correction of this high hardware failure rate must be addressed in future technology systems in the face of increased scrutiny over shrinking health care resources if this expensive therapy is to remain a viable choice.

References

1. Kumar K, Nath R, Wyant GM: Treatment of chronic pain by epidural spinal cord stimulation: A 10-year experience. J Neurosurg 1991;5:402-407.
2. Shealy CN, Mortimer JT, Resnick J: Electrical inhibition of pain by stimulation of the dorsal columns: Preliminary reports. J Int Anesth Res Soc 1967;46:489-491.
3. Kumar K, Toth C, Nath RK: Deep brain stimulation for intractable pain: A 15 year experience. Neurosurgery 1997;40:736-746.
4. Nguyen JP, Lefaucher JP, Le Guerinel C, et al: Motor cortex stimulation in the treatment of central and neuropathic pain. Arch Med Res 2000;31:263-265.
5. Campbell JN, Long DM: Stimulation of the peripheral nervous system for pain control. J Neurosurg 1976;45:692-699.
6. Melzack R, Wall PD: Pain mechanisms: A new theory. Science 1965;150:971-979.
7. Oakley J, Prager J: Spinal cord stimulation: Mechanism of action. Spine 2002;22:2574-2583.
8. Linderoth B, Foreman R: Physiology of spinal cord stimulation: Review and update. Neuromodulation 1999;3:150-164.
9. Burchiel KJ, Anderson VC, Wilson BJ, et al: Prognostic factors of spinal cord stimulation for chronic back and leg pain. Neurosurgery 1995;36:1101-1111.
10. Olson KA, Bedder MD, Anderson VC, et al: Psychological variables associated with outcome of spinal cord stimulation trials. Neuromodulation 1998;1:6-13.
11. Puig MM: When does chronic pain become intractable and when is pharmacological management no longer appropriate? The pain specialist's perspective. J Pain Symptom Manage 2006;31:S1-S2.
12. Simpson BA: The role of neurostimulation: The neurosurgical perspective. J Pain Symptom Manage 2006;S4:S3-S5.
13. May MS, Banks C, Thomson SJ: A retrospective, long-term, third-party follow-up of patients considered for spinal cord stimulation. Neuromodulation 2002;3:137-144.
14. North RB, Kidd DH, Zahurak M, et al: Spinal cord stimulation for chronic, intractable pain: Two decades' experience. Neurosurgery 1993;32:384-395.
15. Rosenow JM, Stanton-Hicks M, Rezai AR, Henderson JM: Failure modes of spinal cord stimulation hardware. J Neurosurg Spine 2006;5:183-190.
16. Barolat G, Oakley J, Law J, North R: Epidural spinal cord stimulation with a multiple electrode paddle lead is effective in treating low back pain. Neuromodulation 2001;2:59-66.
17. May MS, Banks C, Thomson SJ: A retrospective, long-term, third-party follow-up of patients considered for spinal cord stimulation. Neuromodulation 2002;3:137-144.
18. Kumar K, Wilson JR, Taylor RS, Gupta S: Complications of spinal cord stimulation, suggestions to improve outcome, and financial impact. J Neurosurg Spine 2006;5:191-203.
19. Follet KA, Boortz-Marx RL, Drake JM, et al: Prevention and management of intrathecal drug delivery and spinal cord stimulator system infections. Anesthesiology 2004;100:1582-1594.
20. Torrens K, Stanley PJ, Ragunathan PL, Bush DJ: Risk of infection with electrical spinal cord stimulation. Lancet 1997;349:729.
21. Meglio M, Cioni B, Rossi GF: Spinal cord stimulation in management of chronic pain. A 9-year experience. J Neurosurg 1989;70:519-524.
22. Sarubbi F, Vasquez J: Spinal epidural abscess associated with the use of temporary epidural catheters: Report of two cases and review. Clin Infect Dis 1997;25:1155-1158.
23. Schuchard M, Clauson W: An interesting and heretofore unreported infection of a spinal cord stimulator: Smitten by a kitten revisited. Neuromodulation 2001;2:67-71.
24. Alfano S, Darwin J, Picullel B: Programming Principles in Spinal Cord Stimulation: Patient Management Guidelines for Clinicians. Minneapolis, Medtronic, 2001, pp 27-33.

25. Barolat G, Massaro F, He J, et al: Mapping of sensory responses to epidural stimulation of the intraspinal neural structures in man. J Neurosurg 1993;78:233-239.

26. North RB, Kidd DH, Zahurak M, et al: Spinal cord stimulation for chronic, intractable pain: Experience over two decades. Neurosurgery 1993;32:384-394.

27. Coffey RJ, Lozano AM: Neurostimulation for chronic noncancer pain: An evaluation of the clinical evidence and recommendations for future trial design. J Neurosurg 2006;105:175-189.

28. Burchiel K: Neurostimulation for chronic noncancer pain (Editorial). J Neurosurg 2006;105:174.

29. Van Buyten JP: Neurostimulation for chronic neuropathic back pain in failed back surgery syndrome. J Pain Symptom Manage 2006;31:S25-S29.

30. North RB, Kidd DH, Farrokhi F, Piantadosi SA: Spinal cord stimulation versus repeated lumbosacral spine surgery for chronic pain: A randomized controlled trial. Neurosurgery 2005;51:106-116.

31. Barolat G, Oakley J, Law J, North R: Epidural spinal cord stimulation with a multiple electrode paddle lead is effective in treating low back pain. Neuromodulation 2001;2:59-66.

32. Burchiel KJ, Anderson VC, Brown FD, et al: Prospective, multicenter study of spinal cord stimulation for the relief of chronic back and extremity pain. Spine 1996;21:2786-2794.

33. Turner JA, Loeser JD, Bell KG: Spinal cord stimulation for chronic low back pain: A systematic literature synthesis. Neurosurgery 1995;37:1088-1095.

34. North R, Wetzel T: Spinal cord stimulation for chronic pain of spinal origin. Spine 2002;22:2584-2591.

35. Taylor RS: Spinal cord stimulation in complex regional pain syndrome and refractory neuropathic back and leg pain/failed back surgery syndrome: Results of a systematic review and meta-analysis. J Pain Symptom Manage 2006;31:S13-S19.

36. Kemler MA, Barendse GA, van Kleef M, et al: Spinal cord stimulation in patients with chronic reflex sympathetic dystrophy. N Engl J Med 2000;343:618-624.

37. Calvillo O, Racz G, Didie J, Smith K: Neuroaugmentation in the treatment of complex regional pain syndrome of the upper extremity. Acta Orthop Bel 1998;1:57-63.

38. Oakley J, Weiner R: Spinal cord stimulation for complex regional pain syndrome: A prospective study of 19 patients at two centers. Neuromodulation 1999;1:47-50.

39. Stanton-Hicks M: Spinal cord stimulation for the management of complex regional pain syndromes. Neuromodulation 1999;3:193-201.

40. Bennett D, Alo K, Oakley J, Feler C: Spinal cord stimulation for complex regional pain syndrome I (RSD): A retrospective multicenter experience from 1995-1998 of 101 patients. Neuromodulation 1999;3:202-210.

41. Stanton-Hicks M: Complex regional pain syndrome: Manifestations and the role of neurostimulation in its management. J Pain Symptom Manage 2006;31:20-24.

42. Stanton-Hicks M, Burton AW, Bruehl SP, et al: An updated interdisciplinary clinical pathway for CRPS: Report of an expert panel. Pain Pract 2002;2:1-16.

43. Cook AW, Oygar A, Baggenstos P, et al: Vascular disease of extremities: Electrical stimulation of spinal cord and posterior roots. N Y State J Med 1976;76:366-368.

44. Broseta J, Barbera J, De Vera JA: Spinal cord stimulation in peripheral arterial disease. J Neurosurg 1986;64:71-80.

45. Eliasson T, Augustinsson LE, Mannheimer C: Spinal cord stimulation in severe angina pectoris-presentation of current studies, indications, and clinical experience. Pain 1996;65:169-179.

46. Ubbink DTh, Vermeulen H: Spinal cord stimulation for critical leg ischemia: A review of effectiveness and optimal patient selection. J Pain Symptom Manage 2006;31:S30-S35.

47. Gersbach P, Hasdemir MG, Stevens RD, et al: Discriminative microcirculatory screening of patients with refractory limb ischemia for dorsal column stimulation. Eur J Vasc Enovasc Surg 1997;13:464-471.

48. Murphy DF, Giles KE: Dorsal column stimulation for pain relief from intractable angina pectoris. Pain 1987;28:365-368.

49. Buchser E, Durrer A, Albrecht E: Spinal cord stimulation for the management of refractory angina pectoris. J Pain Symptom Manage 2006;31:S36-S42.

50. Ekre O, Eliasson T, Norrsell H, et al: Long-term effects of spinal cord stimulation and coronary bypass grafting on quality of life and survival in the ESBY study. Eur Heart J 2002;23:1938-1945.

51. Kumar K, Malik S, Demeria D: Treatment of chronic pain with spinal cord stimulation versus alternative therapies: Cost-effectiveness analysis. Neurosurgery 2002;51:106-115.

52. Bell G, North R: Cost-effectiveness analysis of spinal cord stimulation in treatment of failed back surgery syndrome. J Pain Symptom Manage 1997;5:285-296.

53. Kemler M, Furnee C: Economic evaluation of spinal cord stimulation for chronic reflex sympathetic dystrophy. Neurology 2002;59:1203-1209.

54. Wall PD, Sweet WH: Temporary abolition of pain in man. Science 1967;155:108-109.

55. Hassenbusch SJ, Stanton-Hicks M, Shoppa D: Long-term results of peripheral nerve stimulation for reflex sympathetic dystrophy. J Neurosurg 1996;84:415-23.

56. Tsubokawa T, Katayama Y, Yamamoto T, et al: Chronic motor cortex stimulation in patients with thalamic pain. J Neurosurg 1993;78:393-401.

57. Limousin P, Krack P, Pollack P, et al: Electrical stimulation of the subthalamic nucleus in advanced Parkinson's disease. N Engl J Med 1998;339:1105-1111.

58. Linderoth B, Meyerson B: Spinal cord stimulation: Mechanisms of action in surgical management of pain. In Burchiel K (ed): Surgical Management of Pain. New York, Thieme Medical Pub, 2002, pp 505-526.

59. Meyerson BA, Linderoth B: Mode of action of spinal cord stimulation in neuropathic pain. J Pain Symptom Manage 2006;31:S6-S12.

54–1 Neurostimulator Companies

- Medtronic Inc., 710 Medtronic Parkway, Minneapolis, MN 55432-5604; (763) 514-5604; www.medtronic.com.
- American Neuromodulation Systems, Inc., 6501 Windcrest Drive, Ste. 100, Plano, TX 75024; 800-727-7846. www.ans-medical.com.
- Advanced Bionics, Inc., 25129 Rye Canyon Loop, Valencia, CA 91355; 800-678-2575; www.advancedbionics.com.

CHAPTER

55 Interlaminar and Transforaminal Epidural Steroid Injections

Jon B. Obray and Marc A. Huntoon

Low back pain and associated radicular pain are prevalent in the United States, and are responsible for significant health care expenditures and lost workdays that adversely affect patients socially, emotionally, and financially.[1] *Radiculopathy* is a syndrome of neurologic conduction loss (sensory or motor) arising secondary to compressive phenomena (e.g., disk impingement on the foraminal spinal nerve, spondylosis, vertebral subluxation, ligamentum flavum cyst, infections, or other causes).[2] Neural compression, as evidenced by an experiment using a silk thread to reproduce the effects of lumbar disk protrusion, produces sensory and motor conduction deficits.[3] *Radicular pain,* or pain in the distribution of a spinal nerve, likely requires a combination of both pathologic compression and irritation of the nerve plus the release of some neurochemical factor(s). Radiculopathy and radicular pain can thus occur simultaneously—a patient may manifest both conduction deficits and pain, or as mutually exclusive events.[2]

Surgical treatment has been the mainstay of treatment of intractable radicular pain for several decades, but few large-scale comparison studies with comprehensive nonsurgical care have been reported.[4-6] The efficacy of surgical procedures for many spinal conditions has come under greater scrutiny though because of significant geographic differences in practice and inconsistent outcomes.[7] Previous studies suggested that radicular pain is effectively treated by diskectomy.[4,5] These studies also demonstrated a favorable natural history with lumbar radicular pain syndromes,[4,5] which compare well with the previous epidemiologic study of cervical radicular pain.[8] Recent data from the Spine Pain Outcomes Research Trial (SPORT) trial looking at nonsurgical versus surgical care for lumbar disk herniation[6] demonstrated no statistically significant superiority of surgical diskectomy over conservative care for primary study outcomes though, and thus conservative treatments such as injections for radicular pain will likely continue to increase (Fig. 55–1A-C). In addition, the SPORT trial agreed with previous trials[4,5] that the

natural history of discogenic radicular pain is one of slow improvement over time. Recent 5-year follow-up data from an earlier controlled trial of transforaminal epidural steroid injections suggest that conservative care may be effective in decreasing the need for disk surgery over time, with potentially lower morbidity.[9]

During the past decade from 1993 to 1999, the number of injections billed to the U.S. Medicare system steadily increased to 680,000 epidural steroid procedures per year, with a large number of other spinal injections increasing as well. Cervical and thoracic epidural procedures increased the most, from 10,105 procedures to 48, 210 (377%).[10] Because large studies suggest that the natural history of radiculopathy secondary to disk herniation is favorable,[4-7] the challenge of successful treatment of radicular pain is to effect pain reduction while minimizing risk or harm to the patient. Uncertainty regarding nonsurgical best practice with a seemingly increasing number of serious complications[11] poses a significant challenge to interventional pain physicians.

HISTORY

Mixter and Barr were the first to suggest that intervertebral disk herniations might be responsible for mechanical compression on the exiting spinal nerve root causing radicular pain.[12] Four years prior to the idea that the disk was somehow involved, Evans had proposed treatment for the syndrome of *primary or idiopathic sciatica* with injections via the trans-sacral canal of 120 mL of 2% procaine (Novocaine).[13] Kelly[14] later suggested that the production of inflammatory changes on the nerve might be the cause of pathophysiologic injury. Building on those ideas, Lindahl and Rexed[15] demonstrated that inflammation, evidenced by lymphocyte infiltration and edema, could be seen on histologic section of dorsal root nerve biopsies in 7 of their 10 patients at the time of surgical diskectomy.

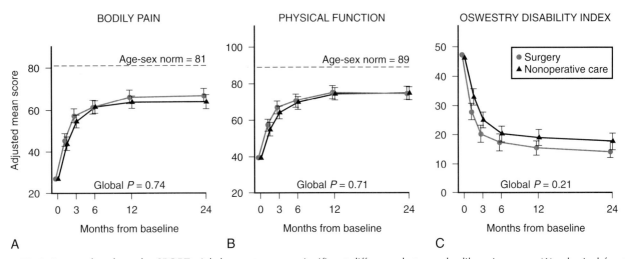

Figure 55–1. Recent data from the SPORT trial demonstrates no significant difference between bodily pain scores (**A**), physical function (**B**), and Oswestry Disability Index (**C**) over a 2-month study period comparing surgery and conservative care of patients with radicular pain. (From Weinstein JN, Tosteson TD, Lurie JD, et al. Surgical vs nonoperative treatment for lumbar disk herniation: The Spine Patient Outcomes Research Trial [SPORT]: A randomized trial. JAMA 2006;296:2441-2450.)

Early work on injectable corticosteroids by Hench and colleagues led to the eventual development of hydrocortisone.[16] Later, Thorn (unpublished data) injected compound F into a rheumatoid arthritic patient's knee, followed by a larger series of knee joint injections by Hollander and associates.[17] Theorizing that inflammation might be amenable to injection in the epidural space, the first injection of epidural corticosteroids was in Europe in 1952 by Robecchi and Capra.[18] Then in 1953, Li'evre and associates described their results in 20 patients receiving hydrocortisone in the epidural space.[19]

In 1961, Goebert and colleagues discussed their results of 121 injections in 113 patients over the preceding 5-year period. Of the total, all but 27 of these injections were caudal, and only 3 were cervical. Injections consisted of a mixture of 1% procaine in 30-mL volumes with 125 mg of hydrocortisone acetate, usually on 3 consecutive days.[20] Between 1960 and the late 1980s, interlaminar and caudal approaches to the epidural space predominated, largely via nonimage-guided techniques using surface landmarks and "loss of resistance" techniques. In 1988, el Khoury and coworkers[21] published a study suggesting that a large percentage of these "blind" epidural injections were not appropriately placed, either not being in the epidural space or not properly communicating with the target area of the injection. In a subsequent large review, Johnson and colleagues described their experience in 5489 consecutive injections that resulted in only four complications. They proposed that the use of a contrast medium epidurogram allowed one to provide accurate localization within the epidural space while also demonstrating that the injectate reached the target area. Further, only 10 patients in the entire series required sedation, suggesting the procedure was thus exceedingly safe on an outpatient basis.[22]

Epidural steroid injections are most widely used for radicular pain caused by herniated or extruded disk material. Guidelines from organizations, such as the International Spinal Intervention Society (ISIS), which are evidence based, have become accepted by some practices.[23]

PATHOPHYSIOLOGY

Inflammation of the spinal nerve root caused by proinflammatory mediators such as prostaglandins and cytokines, and mechanical compression are now thought to be key inciting events of radicular symptoms.[24] Corticosteroids, through their anti-inflammatory effects, may reduce these inflammatory changes in or around the nerve,[25] decreasing pain and improving function.

Until recently the pathophysiology of nociceptive pain emanating from the disk has been poorly understood. Nociceptive neural structures have been demonstrated with modern immunohistochemistry techniques in the outer third of the annulus fibrosis. The nociceptive neural fibers are small unmyelinated C-fibers that are activated by peptidergic neurotransmitters such as calcitonin gene-related peptide (CGRP) or substance P. In discography-proven pathologic disks, nerve ingrowth in the disk may extend farther into the disk matrix, usually accompanied by neovascularization, and with further degradation of the disk matrix.[26] These nerves appear to be originating from the vertebral end plate region, which may be the progenitor of pathologic pain attributed to the disk itself.[27] The disk is relatively avascular, and homeostatic attempts to improve disk nutrition may explain why new blood vessels (and associated nerve fibers) invade the disk from the vertebral end plate region. Blood flow is predominantly via passive diffusion. Circulation in the end plate is likely controlled by local neurotransmitters, which suggests that neural fibers are present as well.

The processes that lead to disk degeneration and disease may ultimately lead to herniation of the disk. Herniated nucleus pulposus results in local release of cytokines and other inflammatory mediators that cause a chemical radiculitis. Burke and associates[28] found increased levels of the inflammatory cytokines interleukin (IL)-6 and IL-8 in disk material taken from patients with known disk disease. Olmarker and coworkers[29] found that the application of disk material onto spinal nerve roots induced functional and morphologic changes in those nerves. Others have shown that disk cells express tumor necrosis factor-alpha (TNF-α), which, when applied to spinal nerve roots, causes similar changes to those seen after application of disk material[30] and that selective inhibition of TNF-α may reduce the intraneural edema seen in this context.[31]

Systemic delivery of specific anti-inflammatory agents for the treatment of radicular syndromes in humans has shown early promise. Korhonen and colleagues[32] treated patients with disk herniation and radicular pain with intravenous infliximab, a TNF-α inhibitor, and found that pain scores were reduced at 1-year follow-up when compared with controls. Etanercept, another TNF-α inhibitor, also has shown promising but preliminary efficacy as systemic treatment for lumbosacral radicular syndromes.[33] Precise delivery of anticytokines to the site of inflammation has not been studied.

EVIDENCE-BASED THERAPY

Many reviews of trials of epidural steroid injections suggested the early studies either were not well controlled or had methodologic deficiencies.[34-36] The efficacy of epidural corticosteroid injections in treating radicular pain syndromes overall appears to be a transient improvement in steroid treatment patients.[37] There are multiple examples in which controlled trials of procedural therapies demonstrated little significant clinical benefit when previous noncontrolled observational studies and case series had suggested benefit.[38-40] Furthermore, "epidural" describes an anatomic space, which can be accessed via injection from different routes: interlaminar, transforaminal, and caudal. The different technical approaches to the epidural space further complicate study because different approaches may have different efficacy and risks.[35] Further complicating the clinical scenario is whether the pathology is cervical or lumbar, given significant pathologic differences between the cervical and lumbar spine.[11]

Several well-designed studies have corroborated a short-term benefit with epidural steroid injections. These short-term benefits must be recognized when selecting a technique for the injection, as further discussed in the complications section. Given the favorable natural history of the majority of patients with radicular pain syndromes, especially those related to a disk protrusion, a thorough understanding of benefit and risks of epidural steroid injections for radicular pain syndromes is needed. A selection of these studies with respect to interlaminar, transforaminal, and caudal epidural steroid injections is reviewed in this section.

Carette and colleagues[37] performed a randomized, placebo-controlled trial looking at the efficacy of lumbar interlaminar epidural steroid injections (up to three) for sciatica (Table 55–1). The study group included 158 patients with unilateral or bilateral lower extremity pain, signs of nerve root irritation or compression, and computed tomography (CT) evidence of nerve root compression at the appropriate levels. A total of 78 patients were allocated to the methylprednisolone group (80 mg) and 80 to the placebo group (saline). The primary outcome was patient function measured by the Oswestry Disability Index. The epidural injections were not fluoroscopically guided, which may lead to misplaced injections at a significant frequency.[21] The treatment group received 80 mg of methylprednisolone acetate mixed with 8 mL of isotonic saline or 1 mL of isotonic saline in the epidural space. The study did not show a statistically significant change in functional improvement as assessed by the Oswestry scores, but did find a reduction in leg pain as assessed by the Visual Analogue Scale (VAS) at 6 weeks in the corticosteroid treatment group (difference in mean change of –0.11, 95% confidence interval, –21.1 to –0.9, $P = 0.03$), but this improvement was no longer significant at 3 months.

Arden and colleagues[41] performed a randomized, placebo-controlled trial looking at the efficacy of lumbar interlaminar epidural steroid injections (up to three) for sciatica as well. The study group included 228 patients with unilateral lower extremity pain and signs of nerve root irritation. A total of 120 patients

Table 55–1.   Selected Studies—Interlaminar Epidural Steroid Injections

AUTHORS	PATIENTS	DESIGN/TECHNIQUE	OUTCOME MEASURE	CONCLUSION
Arden, et al[41]	C = 108 T = 120	RA, DB, PC No fluoroscopic guidance	1—Oswestry 2—VAS, others	Improvement at 3 wk with ESI, but not thereafter
Wilson-MacDonald, et al[53]	C = 48 T = 44	RA, DB, PC No fluoroscopic guidance	1—Oswestry 2—Oxford pain chart	Improvement at 35 days with ESI, but not thereafter
Carette, et al[37]	C = 80 T = 78	RA, DB, PC No fluoroscopic guidance	1—Oswestry 2—VAS, others	Improvement in leg pain at 6 wk, but not thereafter
Cuckler, et al[54]	C = 31 T = 42	RA, DB, PC No fluoroscopic guidance	1—subjective improvement >75%	No significant improvement

C, cervical; DB, double-blind; ESI, epidural steroid injection; PC, prospective controlled; RA, randomized; T, thoracic; VAS, Visual Analogue Scale.

were allocated to the triamcinolone group (80 mg), with 108 allocated to the placebo (saline) group. The primary outcome was patient function measured by the Oswestry Disability Questionnaire (ODQ). A number of secondary outcomes were collected, including a 100-mm VAS for leg and back pain. The epidural injections were not fluoroscopically guided. The treatment group received 80 mg of triamcinolone and 10 mL 0.25% bupivacaine at weeks 0, 3, and 6. The placebo group received injections of 2 mL of normal saline into the interspinous ligament. The treatment group reported a statistically significant improvement in self-reported function compared with placebo at 3 weeks (improvement in ODQ adjusted for baseline (10.3 [14.8] vs. 6.6 [15.6]; $P = 0.017$). The number of patients achieving a 75% improvement in the ODQ was greater in the active group compared with the placebo group (15 [12.5%] vs. 4 [3.7%]; $P = 0.016$). At 3 weeks the number needed to treat to achieve a 75% improvement in the ODQ over and beyond placebo injection was 11.4. There were no statistically significant differences between the groups at 6 weeks or beyond on any outcome measure.

In response to the review of Koes and coworkers,[34] Karppinen and colleagues[42] hypothesized that the poor efficacy reported may be a result of insufficient penetration of corticosteroids to the locus of nerve root irritation administered via an interlaminar approach (Table 55–2). They completed a randomized double-blind trial to test the efficacy of periradicular corticosteroid injection for sciatica. The study group included 163 patients with unilateral lower extremity pain. Magnetic resonance imaging (MRI) was performed, but nerve root compression was not part of the inclusion criteria. Eighty patients were randomized to a single injection of methylprednisolone-bupivacaine, along with 80 allocated to a saline injection, for a total of 160 patients. Three patients were not randomized because of inability to produce a neurogram with fluoroscopic guidance. The primary outcome measure was back and leg pain on a 100-mm VAS. Transforaminal epidural injections were performed using fluoroscopic guidance, with injection of contrast dye to produce a neurogram. The injectate was 2 to 3 mL depending on the

level, using either methylprednisolone (40 mg/mL)-bupivacaine (5 mg/mL) or isotonic (0.9%) saline. The results showed that the treatment effect on leg pain was significantly better in the steroid-bupivacaine group at 2 weeks with pain reduction of 45% versus 24% for placebo ($P < 0.01$), but not thereafter. Back pain was better in the steroid group at 3 months. Back and leg pain was better in the saline group versus the steroid group at 6 months (difference −16.2 [−26.8 to −5.6], $P = 0.003$ for leg pain). No difference in groups was noted at 1 year. However, only one injection was used for the study. Interestingly, they noted that a single transforaminal corticosteroid injection seemed to be associated with a rebound phenomenon at 3 and 6 months.

Ng and colleagues[43] performed a randomized double-blind controlled trial of transforaminal epidural steroid injections for sciatica as well. The study group included 88 patients with unilateral leg pain. Symptoms had to be consistent with the MRI diagnosis of nerve root compression secondary to either lumbar disk herniation or foraminal stenosis. Two patients were withdrawn because of blinding failure. A total of 43 patients were allocated to treatment with a transforaminal injection of 40 mg methylprednisolone and bupivacaine, along with 43 patients allocated to the placebo group (local anesthetic injection only). The primary outcome was a 10% change in the Oswestry Disability Index. Secondary outcomes assessed included the VAS (100 mm, with 20% change regarded as significant), change in walking distance, and the patient's level of satisfaction. The study demonstrated no statistically significant difference in the outcome measures among groups assessed at 3 months.

Riew and colleagues[44] published a prospective randomized trial of lumbar transforaminal epidural steroid injections versus local anesthetic injection using lumbar spine surgery as a primary outcome. The study group included 55 patients with lower extremity pain and MRI- or CT-confirmed disk herniation or spinal stenosis. A total of 28 patients were allocated to a bupivacaine-betamethasone injection, with 27 patients allocated to the transforaminal bupivacaine injection only. Injections were performed with fluoroscopic guidance. They found a

Table 55–2.   Selected Studies—Transforaminal Epidural Steroid Injections

AUTHORS	PATIENTS	DESIGN/TECHNIQUE	OUTCOME MEASURES	CONCLUSION
Karppinen, et al[42]	C = 80 T = 80	RA, DB, PC Fluoroscopic guidance—1 injection	1—VAS 2—Oswestry, others	Improved leg pain at 2 wk, no difference at 4 wk Increased back and leg pain at 6 mo in steroid group
Riew, et al (ref both RCT and 5-yr follow-up data)[9,44]	C = 27 T = 28	RA, DB, PC Fluoroscopic guidance, up to 4 injections	1—rate of operative intervention	Reduced surgical rates in corticosteroid plus LA group
Ng, et al[43]	C = 43 T = 43	RA, DB, PC Fluoroscopic guidance, 1 injection	1—Oswestry 2—VAS	No significant difference between the groups

C, cervical; DB, double-blind; ESI, epidural steroid injection; L, local anesthetic; PC, prospective controlled; RA, randomized; RCT, randomized controlled trial; T, thoracic; VAS, Visual Analogue Scale.

Table 55–3. Selected Studies—Caudal Epidural Steroid Injections

AUTHORS	PATIENTS	DESIGN/TECHNIQUE	OUTCOME MEASURE	CONCLUSION
Bush and Hillier[45]	C = 11 T = 12	RA, DB, PC No fluoroscopic guidance	1—VAS 2—Grogono and Woodgate Symptomatology Questionnaire	Improved leg pain and lifestyle at 4 wk, no significant difference at 1 yr
Dashfield, et al[46]	Caudal = 33 Endoscopy = 27	RA, DB Caudal ESI versus targeted endoscopic delivery of steroid Fluoroscopy utilized	1—McGill Pain Questionnaire 2—Hospital Anxiety and Depression Scale 3—VAS	Reduction in pain intensity and anxiety in caudal group at 6 wk, 3 mo, and 6 mo

C, cervical; DB, double-blind; ESI, epidural steroid injection; PC, prospective controlled; RA, randomized; T, thoracic; VAS, Visual Analogue Scale.

significant reduction in lumbar spine surgery in patients treated with up to four trans-foraminal epidural steroid injections. Recently, Riew and colleagues[9] reported 5-year follow-up data on the patients who avoided operative treatment in their 2000 randomized trial. The majority of these patients still had not undergone operative treatment. There was no statistically significant difference in the number of patients in the bupivacaine versus bupivacaine-betamethasone groups with regard to lumbar spine surgery in the interval period since the original trial.

Bush and Hillier[45] studied caudal epidural corticosteroid injections for patients with intractable sciatica in a double-blind, placebo-controlled fashion (Table 55–3). Patients with lower extremity pain and a positive straight-leg raise were included in the study. Patients with suspected cauda equina syndrome or symptoms less than 4 weeks' duration were excluded. The study group included 23 patients with lower extremity pain with signs of lumbar nerve root irritation. A total of 12 patients were allocated to the steroid group, with 11 allocated to the placebo group. The caudal epidural injection was performed without fluoroscopic guidance, with 25 mL of injectate administered, including 80 mg triamcinolone and 0.5% procaine hydrochloride. The placebo group received 25 mL saline. Outcome measures studied included a symptomatology questionnaire and a VAS. The treatment group showed statistically-significant improvement in lifestyle and reduction of pain at 4 weeks (VAS 16 vs. 45, $P = 0.02$). At 1 year, both groups showed a statistically significant resolution of symptoms. No major side effects were reported.

Dashfield and colleagues[46] performed a prospective, randomized, double-blind trial comparing caudal steroid injection with targeted steroid placement during spinal endoscopy for chronic sciatica. The study group included 60 patients with lower extremity pain in the distribution of a lumbar nerve root. A total of 30 patients were allocated to the caudal injection group and 30 assigned to the endoscopy-guided targeted injection group. Spinal endoscopy could not be performed in 3 patients, who then were assigned to the caudal injection group. Injections were not fluoroscopically confirmed. The caudal injection group received 10 mL of 1% lidocaine with 40 mg triamcinolone. The endoscopy group had 10 mL 1% lidocaine with 40 mg triamcinolone injected at the painful nerve root. The primary outcome measure was the visual analogue score. Additional outcome measures included the short-form McGill Pain Questionnaire (SF-MPQ) and anxiety and depression using the Hospital Anxiety and Depression Scale (HADS). The results showed no significant difference between the groups. A significant reduction in pain as recorded by VAS was reported at 6 weeks ($P = 0.034$), 3 months ($P = 0.026$), and 6 months ($P = 0.01$) in the caudal injection group. Postprocedure adverse events included nonpersistent low back discomfort in both groups, which was insufficient to require hospitalization. Otherwise, no serious complications were reported.[46]

No randomized placebo-controlled studies of cervical epidural steroid injections, interlaminar or transforaminal, have been conducted to date.[47] Retrospective studies have suggested clinical improvement in radicular symptoms with interlaminar epidural steroid injections.[48,49] A number of prospective cohort studies and retrospective analyses have demonstrated benefit with transforaminal cervical epidural steroid injection.[50-52] No studies have been identified comparing interlaminar to transforaminal administration of corticosteroid.[47]

In summary, the evidence seems to support the use of interlaminar, caudal, and transforaminal corticosteroid injections for radicular pain as a result of spinal stenosis or disk pathology for short-term analgesia. Most studies suggest modest benefits for variable periods of 2 weeks to perhaps 3 months. The short-term benefit from epidural injections and the natural history of radicular pain may complement each other in regard to patient clinical improvement. The impact of other aggressive conservative therapies such as medications, exercise, physical therapies, and cognitive behavioral strategies combined with epidural corticosteroids has not been studied. Significant complications of epidural steroid administration can occur (see "Complications"). Certain safety measures may reduce these complications, but their effect is unclear and difficult to study, given the relative rarity of these serious complications. No head-to-head studies have been performed comparing interlaminar to transforaminal to caudal approaches to the epidural space, which may be relevant given the unique risks to the patient with each approach.

SELECTED EPIDURAL INJECTION TECHNIQUES

Cervical Transforaminal

For cervical transforaminal injections, the patient is supine and the head is elevated and turned slightly opposite to the side being targeted. Great care is taken to mark the great vessels of the neck, to avoid placement of needles through these areas. The skin is prepped with chlorhexidine solution and sterilely draped. A subcutaneous skin wheal is raised, and a 25- or 22-gauge bent-tipped needle is selected for a coaxial fluoroscopic technique. An oblique lateral radiograph is adjusted to maximize the optimal transverse view of the intervertebral foramen. The superior articular process is seen at the posterior aspect of the foramen, and is optimally seen as a straight line. The needle is introduced laterally in the neck aiming toward the superior articular process (SAP) in the posterior foramen, when the foramen is viewed in maximal breadth. From the SAP, the needle is "walked" into the posterior aspect of the foramen at its midpoint, making sure that an anteroposterior (AP) projection does not show the needle tip extending beyond the midsagittal plane of the cervical articular pillar.[47] Once the needle is in position, various safety measures are used, as are discussed in the complications section, including local anesthetic test dosing, real-time fluoroscopic contrast injections, and digital subtraction techniques.

Transforaminal Lumbar Epidural

The patient is placed prone on the fluoroscopy table, and an oblique view is obtained with the SAP at the desired injection level noted. The target point, the lateral surface of the SAP, along a line that bisects the sagittal plane of the pedicle is marked. The target is thus at approximately the 6 o'clock position of the pedicle at the same level[53] (Fig. 55–2). A chlorhexidine-based prep solution is applied in a circular fashion and sterile drapes applied. A skin wheal and deeper subcutaneous infiltration are provided, usually with 1% lidocaine, and the needle is usually gently bent at the tip to allow greater steerability. Either a Quincke-type needle or a blunt needle with side port opening may be used depending on preference, with some authors contending that a blunt needle may be less apt to enter blood vessels.[55] The needle is advanced with incremental fluoroscopic images until the tip approaches the appropriate depth. AP and lateral images are obtained to verify the needle is either within the "safe triangle area" as proposed by Bogduk and Cherry,[56] or is dorsal to the dorsal root ganglion (Fig. 55–3). Nonionic contrast injection of 0.2 to 1 mL should demonstrate a neurogram as well as epidural spread medially and outlining the pedicle (Fig. 55–4). Digital subtraction fluoroscopy at eight frames per second is useful to substantiate absent vascular uptake (Fig. 55–5). Local anesthetic test-dosing with 1 mL of 1% lidocaine is

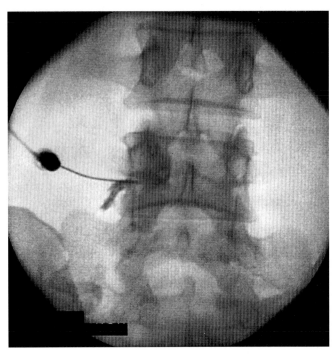

Figure 55–2. A needle for left L4 transforaminal epidural placement. The needle has been "walked off" the lateral edge of the superior articular process and is at approximately the midsagittal plane relative to the pedicle above.

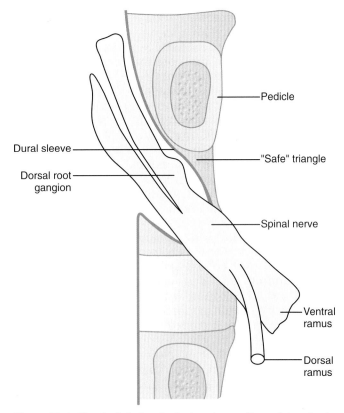

Figure 55–3. The *"safe"* triangle depicts the confines of the classic transforaminal epidural technique. The needle is safely placed inferior to the pedicle's inferior border, superior to the tangentially exiting spinal nerve, and lateral to the dural sleeve.

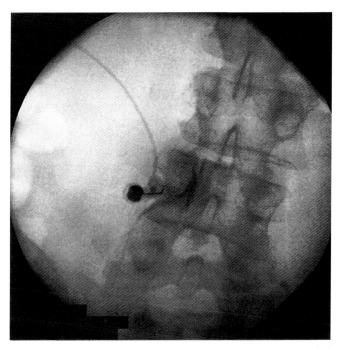

Figure 55–4. The contrast spread is seen following the medial border of the pedicle and outlining the exiting spinal nerve.

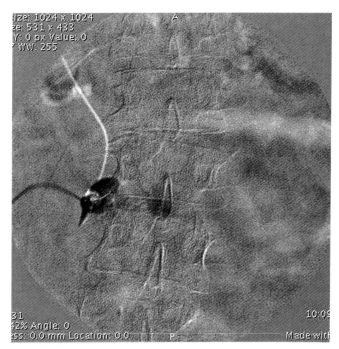

Figure 55–5. A digital subtraction sequence of a left L2 transforaminal epidural injection. The contrast outlines the exiting spinal nerve and displays no vascular uptake in spite of the high likelihood of proximity to the great segmental medullary artery of Adamkiewicz (see Fig. 55–9).

also useful to prevent accidental administration of corticosteroid particulate into a spinal segmental medullary artery. Once confirmation of a safe needle location is achieved, the injection of corticosteroid or other agent can commence.

Cervical Interlaminar Epidural

Generally the cervical interlaminar approach is most safely performed at the C7-T1 or T1-2 levels. The epidural space is widest at these levels and may be 1.5 to 2 mm. There are occasionally discontinuous areas of the cervical epidural space[57,58] and often the width is drastically narrowed by underlying disease, such as spinal stenosis or intervertebral disk herniation that can produce significant compression of the posterior epidural space.[59] It is almost always advisable to have MRI imaging available before performing any cervical epidural injections. Once the safety of potential interlaminar approach is verified, a chlorhexidine-alcohol prep is performed and sterile drapes placed. The interlaminar opening is viewed in maximal diameter, usually with a caudocephalad angulation of the image intensifier. The lamina immediately inferior to the interlaminar opening target is marked. An epidural needle is chosen, generally with a Tuohy or otherwise blunted tip. A skin wheal and subcutaneous infiltration is performed with 1% lidocaine. The epidural needle is advanced slowly down to the inferior laminar bone using intermittent fluoroscopy. Once the inferior laminar bone is contacted, the needle is gradually walked superiorly and medially into the center of the interlaminar opening until it just slips superiorly past the lamina.

At this point, a glass syringe containing 3 mL or less of saline is attached, and a lateral fluoroscopic view is obtained. The needle is then slowly advanced while the operator is correlating the tactile loss of resistance technique with the lateral fluoroscopic view until reaching the anterior extent of the spinous processes. A subtle loss of resistance will be detected as the needle enters the epidural space. A paresthesia or cerebrospinal fluid aspirate should prompt abandonment of the procedure. Once the needle is in position, 0.5 mL of nonionic contrast will demonstrate cervical epidural spread of the contrast. The corticosteroid or other agent can then be injected. An alternative to the direct injection technique above uses a curved needle and 20-gauge catheter that can be threaded cephalad through the needle. A very flat 45-degree or less epidural needle angle with a paramedian direction aiming toward the targeted site can aid in threading the catheter without paresthesia.[60]

Interlaminar Lumbar Epidural

After informed consent is obtained, the patient should be positioned prone on the fluoroscopic table. With the use of fluoroscopic guidance, the interlaminar space of interest is identified and marked. Our practice is to favor the side of pathology, given the relative frequency of unilateral contrast dye spread with epidurography (Fig. 55–6). A skin wheal is raised with local anesthetic after sterile preparation and draping of the injection site. An epidural needle, typically Hustead or Tuohy, is advanced using a

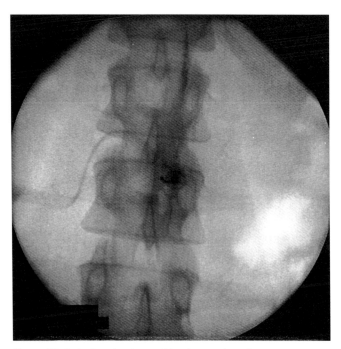

Figure 55–6. An interlaminar epidural procedure demonstrates one-sided spread at the same level and cephalad to the injection.

coaxial fluoroscopic technique. The epidural space is typically identified with loss of resistance to fluid or air. Contrast dye approved for intrathecal use is injected to confirm epidural placement with characteristic dye spread. Both AP and lateral fluoroscopic views provide additional support for correct needle placement. Once proper location is verified, the injectate can consist of 2 to 4 mL total volume, including corticosteroid, preservative-free normal saline, or local anesthetic.

COMPLICATIONS

Complications from epidural steroid injections can generally be categorized as follows: (1) specifically relative to the technique used (interlaminar, caudal, or transforaminal); (2) related to needle trauma, that is, whether a direct neural injury has occurred, any accidental puncture of the dura (postdural puncture cerebrospinal hypotension); (3) vasospastic or ischemic (accidental injection into a vascular structure causing ischemia (anterior spinal artery syndrome); (4) infectious (epidural abscess, meningitis, diskitis); (5) complication related to the drug injected; or (6) related to the drug diluent or additives, for example, benzyl alcohol or polyethylene glycol. Injected corticosteroids have been associated with multiple complications including osteoporosis and osteopenia, avascular necrosis, steroid-induced myopathy, arachnoiditis, cushingoid signs and symptoms (stria, truncal obesity, weight gain, hirsutism, edema, increased blood sugar), cataracts, infection risk, and many others.[61] In order to minimize these adverse

effects, recommendations to either arbitrarily limit corticosteroid exposure or use steroid-sparing treatments have become common clinical practice. Early studies of epidural or intrathecal corticosteroids used one to four doses of 80 mg methylprednisolone over the course of days to weeks until symptom improvement.[62] Recommendations still persist to give no more than three doses in 6 months.[63]

Many studies have evaluated the effects of certain commercial preparations of corticosteroids. Polyethylene glycol (PEG) can cause nerve damage, but only concentrations of 20% or higher did so in an isolated nerve preparation, which responded within an hour to washout of the PEG.[64] Several studies have examined the effects of various preparations containing benzyl alcohol 0.9%, but none of these animal models demonstrated irreparable harm to tissues.[65-67] It is becoming more common for various compounding pharmacies to make steroid solutions to the specifications of client physicians, which may lessen issues of unwanted substances added as preservatives, but raise the specter of infectious agents or errors in compounding to the surface. Therefore, alternative interventions with reproducible beneficial effects in the treatment of radicular pain and lacking significant systemic toxicity with repeated administration would potentially represent a significant therapeutic advance over the corticosteroids.

A large review of the literature from 1960 to 1994 of complications of cervical and lumbar epidural steroid injections documented 6947 cases of patients receiving one or more epidural steroid injections. Overall, the incidence of complications was very low.[68] Another large study of 1214 patients receiving predominantly lumbar interlaminar epidurals at two university pain clinics, demonstrated no major complications resulting in neurologic damage, and an incidence of postdural puncture headache of only 0.8%.[69] Other authors have proposed that the transforaminal technique may be safer, arguing that dural puncture is less likely. For example, Botwin and colleagues[70] studied 322 patients and noted no dural punctures, but a 3.1% incidence of transient nonpositional headache. Cervical interlaminar epidural injections with or without fluoroscopic guidance were similarly successful in treating radicular symptoms in approximately two thirds of patients with no major neurologic complications in past studies.[48] Case reports of spinal cord injury[71,72] illustrated the potential for catastrophic neural injury from spinal cord puncture in sedated or anesthetized patients, as well as the fact that fluoroscopic imaging is not necessarily protective. The American Society of Anesthesiology closed claims reports from 5475 total claims during the years 1970 to 1999 revealed the increasing occurrence reporting of injuries from chronic pain procedures. Epidural steroids made up most of the total number (83%) of all injections, but accounted for 40% of the claims. Thirty percent of the chronic pain claims leading to payment were associated with a disabling injury, and increased from the previous two decades by 17%.[73]

Infectious Complications

Until recently many of the cases of epidural abscess and meningitis in the literature were reported in the context of perioperative epidural catheter infusions, which is not necessarily similar to the incidence after a single corticosteroid injection. Gaul and associates[74] reviewed every case admitted to their neurologic unit with meningitis during the years 1992 to 2000. This review yielded 128 patients, of whom 8 had received prior corticosteroid spinal injections. Review of the cases reported in the literature[75] yielded a total number of 11 abscesses, and 3 abscesses plus meningitis reported after spinal injections of corticosteroid. The cases of abscess and meningitis associated with injections appear to be overwhelmingly staphylococcus species, with 9 of 15 cases occurring in immunocompromised patients (mostly patients with diabetes and metastatic cancer).The patients usually presented within the first 2 weeks after injection with back pain as the most prominent symptom. A high clinical index of suspicion and laboratory findings (erythrocyte sedimentation rate, and C-reactive protein) may be more helpful than the white blood cell count in screening. Ultimately, magnetic resonance imaging (MRI) is necessary to make the diagnosis (Fig. 55–7).

Ischemic Injury (Anterior Spinal Artery Syndrome)

Carette and Fehlings have called for further studies on cervical epidural steroid injections because of the increasing performance of these techniques that have less evidence of efficacy than lumbar procedures but a substantial number of complications.[11] Several recent reports of anterior spinal artery syndrome during cervical transforaminal epidural steroid injections have raised safety concerns.[47,76-81] Anatomic studies have demonstrated that there may be vulnerability of segmental medullary arteries that supply the anterior spinal artery. These arteries could be branches from the vertebral artery, ascending cervical artery, or deep cervical arteries.[81] Branches entering the posterior aspect of the cervical intervertebral foramen (Figs. 54–8 and 54–9) or anastomosing with the vertebral artery may explain some complications.[81] Likewise, a lumbar safe zone may not protect one from a catastrophic injection into a tributary of the artery of Adamciewicz.[82]

SUMMARY

- The natural history of discogenic radicular pain is favorable for conservative management.
- Randomized, placebo-controlled trials show short-term benefit with epidural steroid injection via multiple techniques.
- Best practice of nonsurgical radicular pain syndromes is yet to be defined. Few comparative, nonsurgical trials have been conducted.
- Devastating complications of epidural steroid injection, especially in the cervical spine, have occurred.
- Because of the rare, but catastrophic, nature of some of these complications with the favorable natural history of discogenic radicular pain, optimization of safety should be of primary concern.
- Future directions in research could look at alternative pharmacologic agents or techniques to address the pathophysiology of radicular pain syndromes.

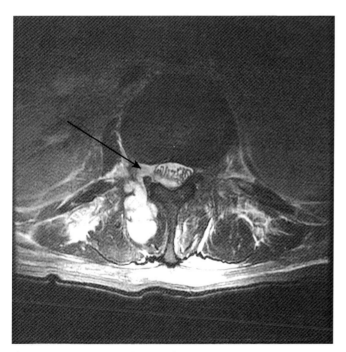

Figure 55–7. An accumulation of abscess material *(arrow)* is seen tracking epidurally and into the perispinal soft tissues. (From Hooten WM, Kinney MO, Huntoon MA: Epidural abscess and meningitis after epidural corticosteroid injection. Mayo Clin Proc 2004;79: 682-686.)

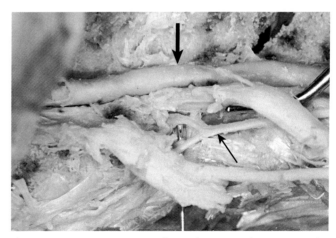

Figure 55–8. An anatomic cadaver dissection demonstrates the vertebral artery *(pink, large arrow)* and the exiting left C5 spinal nerve lifted by the probe. A needle tip is pushing on a spinal branch of the ascending cervical artery *(small arrow)* at the outer aspect of the C4-5 intervertebral foramen.

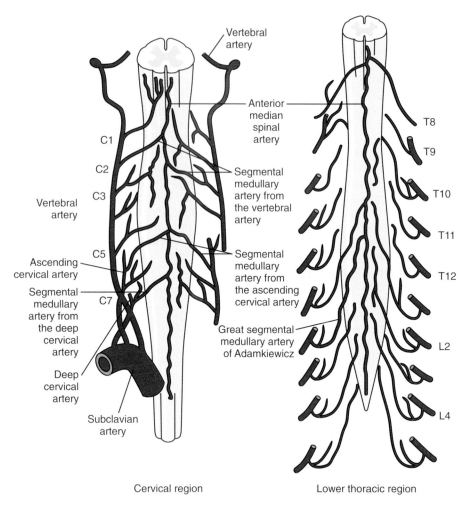

Vertebral artery

Anterior median spinal artery

C1

C2

C3

Vertebral artery

Segmental medullary artery from the vertebral artery

C5

Ascending cervical artery

Segmental medullary artery from the ascending cervical artery

C7

Segmental medullary artery from the deep cervical artery

Deep cervical artery

Great segmental medullary artery of Adamkiewicz

Subclavian artery

Cervical region

T8

T9

T10

T11

T12

L2

L4

Lower thoracic region

Figure 55–9. An artist's adaptation of an earlier drawing from Gillilan. *Left panel* shows the contributions of several segmental medullary vessels to the anterior median spinal artery. *Right panel* demonstrates the great segmental medullary artery of Adamkiewicz entering at the L2 intervertebral foramen on the left side. (From Gillilan LA: The arterial blood supply of the human spinal cord. J Comp Neurol 1958: 110:75-103.)

References

1. Deyo RA, Tsui-Wu YJ: Descriptive epidemiology of low-back pain and its related medical care in the United States. Spine 1987;12:264-268.
2. Bogduk N: Clinical Anatomy of the Lumbar Spine and Sacrum (3rd ed). Edinburgh, Churchill Livingstone, 1997.
3. Smyth MB, Wright V: Sciatica and the intervertebral disc: An experimental study. J Bone Joint Surg (Am)1959;40:1401-1418.
4. Weber H: Lumbar disc herniation: A controlled, prospective study with ten years of observation. Spine 1983;8:131-140.
5. Atlas S, Keller R, Wu Y, et al: Long-term outcomes of surgical and nonsurgical management of sciatica secondary to lumbar disc herniation: 10 year results from the Maine Lumbar Spine Study. Spine 2005;30:927-935.
6. Weinstein JN, Tosteson TD, Lurie JD, et al: Surgical vs non-operative treatment for lumbar disk herniation. The Spine Patient Outcomes research Trial (SPORT): A randomized trial. JAMA 2006;296:2441-2450.
7. Deyo RA, Nachemson A, Mirza SK: Spinal-fusion surgery—The case for restraint. New Engl J Med 2004;350:722-726.
8. Radhakrishnan K, Litchy WJ, O'Fallon WM, Kurland LT: Epidemiology of cervical radiculopathy. Brain 1994;117:325-335.
9. Riew KD, Park JB, Cho YS, et al: Nerve root blocks in the treatment of lumbar radicular pain: A minimum 5 year followup. J Bone Joint Surg (Am) 2006;88:1722-1725.
10. Carrino JA, Morrison WB, Parker L, et al: Spinal injection procedures: Volume, providers' distribution and reimbursement in the US Medicare population from 1993-1999. Radiology 2002;225:723-729.
11. Carette S, Fehlings MG: Cervical radiculopathy. N Engl J Med 2005;353:392-399.
12. Mixter WJ, Barr JS: Rupture of the intervertebral disc with involvement of the spinal canal. N Engl J Med 1934;211:210-215.
13. Evans W: Intrasacral epidural injection in the treatment of sciatica. Lancet 1930; Dec 6:1225-1229.
14. Kelly M: Is pain due to pressure on nerves? Spinal tumors and the intervertebral disc. Neurology 1956;6:32-36.
15. Lindahl O, Rexed D: Histologic changes in the spinal nerve roots of operated cases of sciatica. Acta Orthop Scand 1951;20:215.
16. Hench PS, Kendall EC, Slocumb CH, et al: The effect of a hormone of the adrenal cortex (17-hydroxy-11-dehydrocorticosterone: Compound E) and of pituitary adrenocorticotropic hormone on rheumatoid arthritis. Proc Staff Meet Mayo Clin 1949;24:181-197.
17. Hollander JL, Brown EM, Jessar RA, et al: Hydrocortisone and cortisone injected into arthritic joints. JAMA 1951;147:1629-1635.
18. Robecchi A, Capra R. L idrocortisone (composto F): Prime esperienze cliniche in campo reumatologico. Minerva Med 1952;98:1259-1263.
19. Li'evre JA, Bloch-Michel H, Pean G, et al: L hydrocortisone en injection locale. Rev Rhum 1953;20:310-311.
20. Goebert HW, Jallo SJ, Gardner WJ, et al: Painful radiculopathy treated with epidural injections of procaine and hydrocortisone acetate: Result in 113 patients. Anesth Analg 1961;140:130-134.

21. el-Khoury GY, Ehara S, Weinstein JN, et al: Epidural steroid injection: A procedure ideally performed with fluoroscopic control. Radiology 1988;168:554-557.
22. Johnson BA, Schellhas KP, Pollei SR: Epidurography and therapeutic epidural injections: Technical considerations and experience with 5334 cases. Am J Neuroradiol 1999;20:697-705.
23. ISIS practice guidelines, 2004. International Spine Intervention Society.
24. Kjell D, Myers RR: Pathogenesis of sciatic pain: Role of herniated nucleus pulposus and deformation of spinal nerve root and dorsal root ganglion. Pain 1998;78:99-105.
25. Lee HM, Weinstein JN, Meller ST, et al: The role of steroids and their effects on phospholipase A$_2$: An animal model of radiculopathy. Spine 1998;23:1191-1196.
26. Freemont AJ, Jeziorska M, Hoyland JA, et al: Mast cells in the pathogenesis of chronic back pain: A hypothesis. J Pathol 2002;197:281-285.
27. Brown MF, Hukkanen MVJ, McCarthy ID, et al: Sensory and sympathetic innervation of the vertebral endplate in patients with degenerative disc disease. J Bone Joint Surg (Br) 79:147-153.
28. Burke JG, Watson RWG, McCormack D, et al: Intervertebral discs which cause low back pain secrete high levels of proinflammatory mediators. J Bone Joint Surg (Br) 2002;84:196-201.
29. Olmarker K, Rydevik B, Nordborg C: Autologous nucleus pulposus induces neurophysiologic and histologic changes in porcine cauda equine nerve roots. Spine 1993;18:1425-1432.
30. Igarashi T, Kiduchi S, Shubayev V, et al: Exogenous tumor necrosis factor-alpha mimics nucleus pulposus-induced neuropathology: Molecular, histologic, and behavioural comparisons in rats. Spine 2000;25:2975-2980.
31. Olmarker K, Rydevik B: Selective inhibition of tumor necrosis factor-alpha prevents nucleus induced thrombus formation, intraneural edema, and reduction of nerve conduction velocity: Possible implications for future pharmacologic treatment strategy of sciatica. Spine 2001;26:863-869.
32. Korhonen T, Karppinen J, Malmivaara A, et al: Efficacy of infliximab for disc herniation–induced sciatica. One-year follow-up. Spine 2004;29:2115-2119.
33. Genevay S, Stingelin S, Gabay C: Efficacy of etanercept in the treatment of acute severe sciatica: A pilot study. Ann Rheum Dis 2004;63:1120-1123.
34. Koes BW, Scholten RJPM, Mens JMA, et al: Efficacy of epidural steroid injections for low back pain and sciatica: A systematic review of randomized clinical trials. Pain 1995;63:279-288.
35. Watts RW, Silagy CA: A meta-analysis on the efficacy of epidural corticosteroids in the treatment of sciatica. Anaesth Intensive Care 1995;23:564-569.
36. Boswell MV, Shah RV, Everett CR, et al: Interventional techniques in the management of chronic spinal pain: Evidence-based practice guidelines. Pain Physician 2005;8:1-47.
37. Carette S, Leclaire R, Marcoux S, et al: Epidural corticosteroid injections for sciatica due to herniated nucleus pulposus. N Engl J Med 1997;336:1634-1640.
38. Cobb LA, Thomas GI, Dillard DH, et al: An evaluation of internal-mammary-artery ligation by a double-blind technique. N Engl J Med 1959;260:1115-1118.
39. Moseley JB, O'Malley K, Petersen NJ, et al: A controlled trial of arthroscopic surgery for osteoarthritis of the knee. N Engl J Med. 2002;347:81-88.
40. Bradley JD, Heilman DK, Katz BP: Tidal irrigation as treatment for knee osteoarthritis: A sham-controlled, randomized, double-blinded evaluation. Arthritis Rheum 2002;46:100-108.
41. Arden NK, Price C, Reading I, et al: A multicentre randomized controlled trial of epidural corticosteroid injections for sciatica: The WEST study. Rheumatology 2005;44:1399-1406.
42. Karppinen J, Malmivaara A, Kurunlahti M, et al: Periradicular infiltration for sciatica: A randomized controlled trial. Spine 2001;26:1059-1067.
43. Ng L, Chaudhary N, Sell P: The efficacy of corticosteroids in periradicular infiltration for chronic radicular pain: A randomized, double-blind, controlled trial. Spine 2005;30:857-862.
44. Riew KD, Yin Y, Gilula L, et al: The effect of nerve-root injections on the need for operative treatment of lumbar radicular pain: A prospective, randomized, controlled, double-blind study. J Bone Joint Surg (Am) 2000;82:1589-1593.
45. Bush K, Hillier S: A controlled study of caudal epidural injections of triamcinolone plus procaine for the management of intractable sciatica. Spine 1991;15:572-575.
46. Dashfield AK, Taylor MB, Cleaver JS, Farrow D: Comparison of caudal epidural steroid with targeted steroid placement during spinal endoscopy for chronic sciatica: A prospective, randomized, double-blind trial. Br J Anaesth 2005;94:514-519.
47. Rathmell JP, Aprill C, Bogduk N: Cervical transforaminal injection of steroids. Anesthesiology. 2004;100:1595-1600.
48. Rowlingson JC, Kirschenbaum LP: Epidural analgesic techniques in the management of cervical pain. Anesth Analg 1986;65:938-942.
49. Cicala RS, Westbrook L, Angel JJ: Side effects and complications of cervical epidural steroid injections. J Pain Symptom Manage 1989;4:64-66.
50. Bush K, Hillier S: Outcome of cervical radiculopathy treated with periradicular/epidural corticosteroid injections: A prospective study with independent clinical review. Eur Spine J 1996;5:319-325.
51. Vallée JN, Feydy A, Carlier RY, et al: Chronic cervical radiculopathy: Lateral approach periradicular corticosteroid injection. Radiology 2001;218:886-892.
52. Slipman CW, Lipetz JS, Jackson HB, et al: Therapeutic selective nerve root block in the nonsurgical treatment of atraumatic cervical spondylitic radicular pain: A retrospective analysis with independent clinical review. Arch Phys Med Rehabil 2000;81:741-746.
53. Wilson-MacDonald J, Burt G, Griffen D, Glynn C: Epidural steroid injection for nerve root compression: A randomized, controlled trial. J Bone Joint Surg (Br) 2005;87:352-355.
54. Cuckler JM, Bernini PA, Wiesel SW, et al: The use of epidural steroids in the treatment of lumbar radicular pain. J Bone Joint Surg (Am) 1985;67:63-66.
55. Heavner JE, Racz GB, Jenigiri B, et al: Sharp versus blunt needle: A comparative study of penetration of internal structures and bleeding in dogs. Pain Pract 2003;3:226-231.
56. Bogduk N, Cherry D: Epidural corticosteroid agents for sciatica. Med J Aust 143:402-406, 1985.
57. Hogan QH: Epidural anatomy examined by cryomicrotome section. Influence of age, vertebral level, and disease. Reg Anesth 1996;21:395-406.
58. Lirk P, Kolbitsch C, Putz G, et al: Cervical and high thoracic ligamentum flavum frequently fails to fuse in the midline. Anesthesiology 2003;99:1387-1390.
59. Field J, Rathmell JP, Stephenson JH, Katz NP: Neuropathic pain following cervical epidural steroid injection. Anesthesiology 2000;93:885-888.
60. Larkin TM, Carragee E, Cohen S: A novel technique for delivery of epidural steroids and diagnosing the level of nerve root pathology. J Spinal Disorders Tech 2003;16:186-192.
61. Huntoon MA: Steroid complications. In Neal J, Rathmell JP (eds): Complications in Regional Anesthesia and Pain Medicine. New York, Elsevier, 2006, pp 331-339.
62. Winnie AP, Hartman JT, Meyers HL Jr, et al: Pain clinic II: Intradural and extradural corticosteroids for sciatica. Anesth Analg 1972;51:990-999.
63. DeSio JM: Epidural steroid injections. In Warfield CA, Bajwa ZH (eds): Principles and Practice of Pain Medicine (2nd ed). New York, McGraw-Hill, 2004, pp 655-656.
64. Benzon HT, Gissen AJ, Strichartz GR, et al: The effect of polyethylene glycol on mammalian nerve impulses. Anesth Analg 1987;66:353-359.
65. Cicala RS, Westbrook L, Angel JJ: Side effects and complications of cervical epidural steroid injections. J Pain Symptom Manage 1989;4:64-66.
66. Delaney TJ, Rowlingson JC, Carron H, et al: Epidural steroid effects on nerves and meninges. Anesth Analg 1980;59:610-614.
67. Latham J, Fraser RD, Moore RJ, et al: The pathologic effects of intrathecal betamethasone. Spine 1997;22:1558-1562.

68. Abram SE, O'Connor TC: Complications associated with epidural steroid injections. Reg Anesth 1996;21:149-162.

69. Horlocker TT, Bajwa ZH, Zubaira A, et al: Risk assessment of neurologic complications associated with antiplatelet therapy in ambulatory pain clinic patients undergoing epidural steroid injection. Anesth Analg 2002;95:1691-1697.

70. Botwin KP, Gruber RD, Bouchlas CG, et al: Complications of fluoroscopically guided transforaminal lumbar epidural injections. Arch Phys Med Rehabil 2000;81:1045-1050.

71. Bromage PR, Benumof JL: Paraplegia following intracord injection during attempted epidural anesthesia under general anesthesia. Reg Anesth Pain Med 1998;23:104-107.

72. Hodges SD, Castleberg RL, Miller T, et al: Cervical epidural steroid injection with intrinsic spinal cord damage. Spine 1998;23:2137-2142.

73. Fitzgibbon DR, Posner KL, Domino KB, Caplan RA: American Society of Anesthesiologists Closed Claims Project: Chronic pain management. Anesthesiology 2004;100:98-105.

74. Gaul C, Neundorfer B, Winterholler M: Iatrogenic (para-)spinal abscesses and meningitis following injection therapy for low back pain. Pain 2005;116:407-410.

75. Hooten WM, Kinney MO, Huntoon MA: Epidural abscess and meningitis after epidural corticosteroid injection. Mayo Clin Proc 2004;79:682-686.

76. Brouwers PJAM, Kottink EJBL, Simon MAM, Prevo RL: A cervical anterior spinal artery syndrome after diagnostic blockade of the right C6 nerve rood. Pain 2001;91:397-399.

77. Baker R, Dreyfuss P, Mercer S, Bogduk N: Cervical transforaminal injection of corticosteroids into a radicular artery: A possible mechanism for spinal cord injury. Pain 2003;103: 211-215.

78. Ludwig MA, Burns SP: Spinal cord infarction following cervical transforaminal epidural injection: A case report. Spine 2005;30: E266-E268.

79. Rozin L, Rozin R, Koehler SA, et al: Death during transforaminal epidural steroid nerve root block (C7) due to perforation of the left vertebral artery. Am J Forensic Med Pathol 2003;24:351-355.

80. Karasek M, Bogduk N: Temporary neurologic deficit after cervical transforaminal injection of local anesthetic. Pain Med 2004;5:202-205.

81. Huntoon MA: Anatomy of the cervical intervertebral foramina: Vulnerable arteries and ischemic neurologic injuries after transforaminal epidural injections. Pain 2005;117: 104-111.

82. Huntoon MA, Martin DP: Paralysis following transforaminal epidural injection and previous spinal surgery. Reg Anesth Pain Med 2004;29:494-495.

CHAPTER
56 Facet Joint Pain

Chad M. Brummett and Steven P. Cohen

Low back and neck pain represents an epidemic throughout the industrialized world. Although the prevalence of low back pain (LBP) varies greatly throughout the literature, some lifetime estimates are as high as 84% to 90%.[1,2] The lifetime prevalence of neck pain has been estimated to be about 67%.[3] Work absences and disability as a result of LBP have a serious economic impact on both individual patients and society as a whole, with annual costs ranging from $20 to $50 billion in the United States.[4] In the Netherlands, a country with 5% of the U.S. population, the cost of chronic neck pain exceeds $500 million per year.[5] As the population ages, the effects of low back and neck pain will continue to grow.

The zygapophysial (facet) joint is a potential source of neck, shoulder, mid-back, low back pain, and leg pain. In addition, cervical facet disease can cause headaches. Interventions to the zygapophysial joints (z-joint) are second only to epidural steroid injections as the most common type of procedure in pain management centers in the United States.[6] Although there has been a great deal of research into the diagnosis and treatment of facet pain, the issue still remains controversial. This chapter discusses the relevant anatomy, mechanisms of injury, prevalence, pain referral patterns, diagnosis, and treatment of facet arthropathy.

ANATOMY AND FUNCTION

The spine is normally composed of 7 cervical, 12 thoracic, and 5 lumbar vertebrae (Fig. 56–1). The z-joints are paired structures situated posterolaterally to the vertebral body. In conjunction with the intervertebral disk, they comprise the three-joint complex. Together these joints function to support and stabilize the spine and prevent injury by limiting motion in all planes of movement. The lumbar z-joints are true synovial joints formed from the superior articular process of one vertebra and the inferior articular process of the vertebra above. The volume capacity of these joints is approximately 1 to 1.5 mL in the lumbar region and 0.5 to 1 mL in the cervical region.[7] The articular surfaces are covered by hyaline cartilage and contain a fibrous capsule. The fibrous capsule is about 1 mm thick and formed mostly of collagenous tissue arranged in a transverse fashion to provide resistance to forward flexion.[8,9] The superior and infe-

rior joint borders are formed by the fibrous capsule. In the lumbar spine, the multifidus muscle serves as the posterior joint border, and the ligamentum flavum replaces the fibrous capsule at the anterior border.[10] The position of the joint relative to the sagittal and coronal planes helps determine the role that the joint plays in protecting the spine against excessive motion. Joints parallel to the sagittal plane provide little resistance to backward and forward shearing forces, but allow for a greater degree of rotation, flexion, and extension. Joints oriented closer to the coronal plane allow for less rotation, flexion, and extension, but serve as excellent protection against shearing forces. The cervical z-joints are inclined at roughly 45 degrees from the horizontal plane and angled 85 degrees from the sagittal plane. This alignment functions to prevent excessive anterior translation and assist the disks in weight-bearing.[11]

The medial branch of the posterior rami supplies sensory innervation to the facet joint. Each exiting spinal nerve splits into an anterior and posterior primary ramus (Fig. 56–2). The anterior ramus is the larger of the two branches and the main source of motor and sensory fibers. The posterior ramus divides into lateral, intermediate, and medial branches. In the lumbar region the lateral branch provides innervation to the paraspinous muscles, thoracolumbar fascia, sacroiliac joint, and variable sensory fibers to the skin overlying the spinous processes. The small intermediate branch supplies the longissimus muscle. The medial branch is the largest branch of the posterior primary ramus and innervates not only the lumbar z-joint but also the multifidus muscle, interspinal muscle and ligament, and the periosteum of the neural arch. Thus, to block sensory input from one facet joint, two adjacent medial branches must be anesthetized. In some people, facet joint innervation may come from other sources.

Facet joints are imbued with a rich innervation containing encapsulated (Ruffini-type endings, pacinian corpuscles), unencapsulated, and free nerve endings.[12] In addition to being a potential pain generator, the z-joint capsule is thought to serve in a proprioceptive capacity, as evidenced by the presence of low threshold, rapidly adapting mechanosensitive neurons. Kallakuri and associates used immunocytochemistry to characterize the presence of substance P and calcitonin gene-related peptide

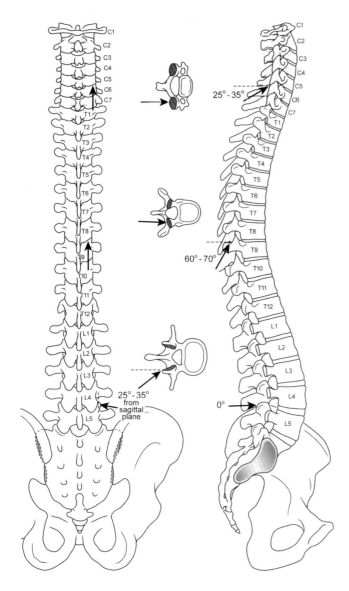

Figure 56–1. Anatomy of the facet joints. The plane of orientation of the facet joints varies significantly among cervical, thoracic, and lumbar levels. The axis of the joints and the plane of entry for intra-articular injection are shown for typical cervical, thoracic, and lumbar facet joints. (Reproduced with permission from Rathmell JP: Atlas of image-guided intervention in regional anesthesia and pain medicine. Lippincott, Philadelphia, 2006. Figure 7–1, page 67.)

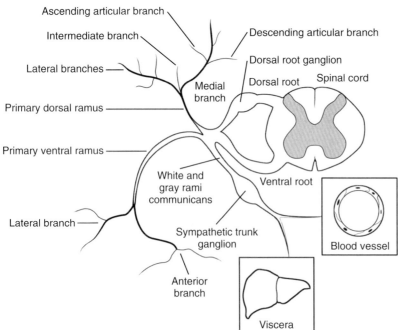

Figure 56–2. Schematic drawing of the spinal cord and segmental spinal innervation. (From Cohen SP, Raja SN: Pathogenesis, diagnosis, and treatment of lumbar zygapophysial [facet] joint pain. Anesthesiology 2007;106:591-614.)

reactive nerve fibers in the cervical facets of 12 human cadavers.[13] In addition to substance P and calcitonin gene-related peptide, a substantial percentage of nerve endings in facet capsules contains neuropeptide Y, indicating the presence of sympathetic efferent fibers.[14,15] Nerve fibers have been found in subchondral bone and intra-articular inclusions of facet joints, signifying that facet-mediated pain may originate in structures besides the joint capsule.[16,17] Inflammatory mediators such as prostaglandins,[18] and the inflammatory cytokines interleukin-6 and tumor necrosis factor-alpha[19] have been found in facet joint cartilage and synovial tissue in degenerative lumbar spinal disorders.

Lumbar Facet Joints

The lumbar facet joints are aligned lateral to the sagittal plane and vary in angle (Fig. 56–3). The inferior articular process faces anterolaterally, and the superior articular process faces posteromedially.[10,20] In an anatomic study published in 1940 by Horwitz and Smith,[21] the authors found that the L4-5 z-joints tended to be more coronally positioned (almost 70 degrees with respect to the sagittal plane), whereas the L2-3 and L3-4 joints were likely to be oriented more parallel (<40 degrees) to the sagittal plane. In more recent studies by Masharawi and colleagues[11] and Punjabi and coworkers,[22] the investigators found that the upper lumbar facet joints (T12-L2) were oriented closer to the midsagittal plane of the vertebral body (mean range 26 to 34 degrees), whereas the lower facet joints tended to be oriented away from that plane (40 to 56 degrees). In the upper lumbar spine, approximately 80% of the facet joints are curved and 20% are flat. In the lower lumbar spine these numbers are reversed.[21] Studies by Grobler and associates[23] and Boden and colleagues[24] found a positive association between degenerative spondylolisthesis and more sagitally oriented lower lumbar facet joints. The inferior articular processes of L5 combine with the superior articular processes of the sacrum to form the L5-S1 facet joints. The dip in the sacrum immediately lateral to the superior articular process is termed the sacral ala.

The sensory innervation of the facet joints comes from the medial branches arising from the posterior primary rami at the same level and the level above the facet joint.[25,26] For example, the L4-5 medial branch receives its innervation from the L3 and L4 medial branch nerves. The medial branches of L1 to L4 run across their respective transverse processes one level below the named spinal nerve (e.g., L4 crosses the transverse process of L5), traversing the dorsal leaf of the intertransverse ligament at the base of the transverse process. The nerve then proceeds along the junction of the superior articular process and the transverse process, coursing underneath the mamilloaccessory ligament and splitting into multiple branches as it crosses the vertebral lamina (Fig. 56–4). Calcification of the mamilloaccessory ligament can be a source of nerve entrapment.[27] This is

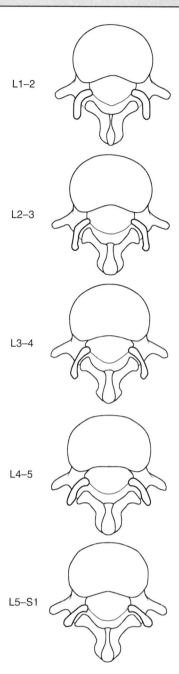

Figure 56–3. Segmental variation in lumbar zygapophysial joint orientation in the transverse plane. (From Cohen SP, Raja SN: Pathogenesis, diagnosis, and treatment of lumbar zygapophysial [facet] joint pain. Anesthesiology 2007;106:591-614.)

most common at the L5 (20%), but also occurs at L4 (10%) and L3 (4%). The L5 innervation amenable to blockade is actually the dorsal ramus itself, which runs along the junction of the superior articular process of the sacrum and the sacral ala.[28,29] Some authors have claimed that a branch from the S1 nerve root can run cephalad to supply a portion of the L5-S1 facet joint, although this point remains controversial.[30,31]

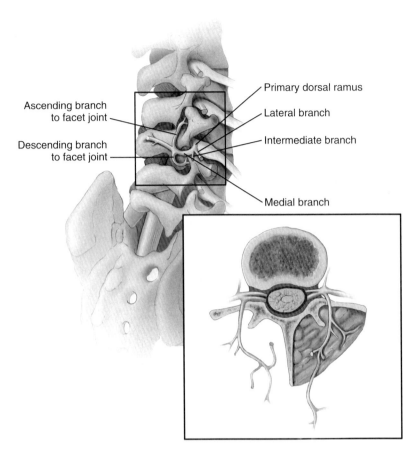

Ascending branch
to facet joint

Descending branch
to facet joint

Primary dorsal ramus

Lateral branch

Intermediate branch

Medial branch

Figure 56–4. Right lateral oblique view of the lumbar vertebral bodies and the dorsal rami medial branches. (From Cohen SP, Raja SN: Pathogenesis, diagnosis, and treatment of lumbar zygapophysial [facet] joint pain. Anesthesiology 2007;106:591-614.)

Thoracic Facet Joints

Thoracic facets are the most vertically oriented joints as noted in Figure 56–1, with the anterior portion of the joint located more cephalad.[11,32,33] The frontal orientation permits more lateral flexion at the expense of axial rotation. In the low thoracic spine, the angle transitions from a predominantly frontal orientation to the characteristic sagittal orientation of the lumbar facets. This transition varies, but generally occurs between T11-12 [11] and T12-L1.[22] Unlike the lumbar facet joints in which tropism is unusual,[10,34] asymmetry is the rule rather than the exception in the thoracic spine, with the right side generally oriented more vertically and frontally than the left.[11]

The sensory innervation of the thoracic facets is comparable to that found in the lumbar spine. At most levels, innervation comes from the medial branch from the same level and the level above. Exceptions to this rule sometimes occur at the uppermost thoracic z-joints, where the medial branches from C7 and C8 may travel caudad to levels as low as T3.[35] In a cadaveric study by Chua and Bogduk,[36] the authors showed that the thoracic medial branches assume different courses depending on the level. In the midthoracic levels they do not run on bone but are instead suspended in the intertransverse space. The thoracic medial branches also swing laterally to circumvent the multifidus muscle; therefore, motor stimulation of the multifidus muscle cannot be used to confirm needle placement during radiofrequency (RF) as it is in the lumbar spine. In none of the 84 medial branch dissections did authors find the nerve crossing the junction between the superior articular process and the transverse process, as occurs in the lumbar spine. Instead, the superolateral corner of the transverse process was noted to be a more accurate target point for diagnostic blockade and denervation (Figs. 56–5 and 56–6).

Cervical Facet Joints

In order to facilitate the complex motions of the neck, the position and shape of the cervical z-joints change greatly from the base of the occiput to the cervicothoracic junction.[22,37,38] The occiput sits on the C1 articular processes in an orientation nearly parallel to the axial plane. The superior articular process at C3 faces posteromedially, with a 70-degree angle in the sagittal plane and a 45-degree angle in the transverse plane. The relative position of the C2-3 facet inhibits rotation and serves to anchor the C2 vertebra as a rotational pivot for the atlantoaxial joint (C1-2). Between the C3-4 and C7-T1 facet joints, the orientation transitions to the consistent posterolateral position of the C7 superior articular process. The most frequent site of this transition is at the C5-6 joint. The position of the z-joints at this level allows

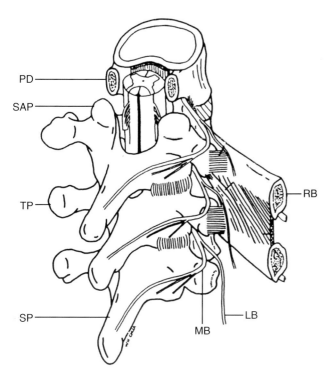

Figure 56–5. A sketch of the typical course of the thoracic medial branch from a right superior oblique view showing the target point of the superolateral corner of the transverse process. LB, lateral branch; MB, medial branch; PD, pedicle; RB, rib; SAP, superior articular process; SP, spinous process; TP, transverse process. (From Chua WH, Bogduk N: The surgical anatomy of thoracic facet denervation. Acta Neurochirugia 1995;136:140-144.)

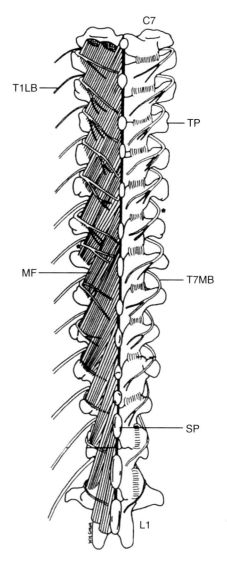

Figure 56–6. A posterior view of the course of the thoracic medial branches again showing the target points of the superolateral corners of the transverse processes. The multifidus and lateral branches are not shown on the right side. C, cervical vertebra; L, lumbar vertebra; LB, lateral branch; MB, medial branch; MF, multifidus; SP, spinous process; TP, transverse process. (From Chua WH, Bogduk N: The surgical anatomy of thoracic facet denervation. Acta Neurochirugia 1995;136:140-144.)

for flexion, extension, rotation, and lateral bending. Due to the enhanced mobility of this segment, the C5-6 level is also the most prone to facet dislocations and spondylosis. The C7 superior articular processes are oriented approximately 93 degrees to the sagittal plane and 65 degrees to the transverse plane. In addition, the shapes of the facet joints between C3 and C6 tend to be round and almost flat, whereas the C6-T1 z-joints are elliptical with a more concave surface. The combination of shape and orientation at the cervicothoracic junction is designed to maximize stability.

The innervation patterns of the cervical z-joints are slightly more complicated and varied than the lumbar and thoracic levels. There are eight cervical nerve roots, the first seven of which exit the intervertebral foramen above the vertebral body of the same number. Similar to the lumbar and thoracic z-joints, the C3-4 to C7-T1 facet joints receive dual innervation from the medial branches of the posterior rami from the same level and one level above.[39] The nerves curve around the waist of the articular pillars at their respective levels, then branch out to supply two joints. Tight fascia and the tendons of the semispinalis capitis muscle ensure that the medial branches cling closely to the periosteum, thereby making their position more predictable. On lateral projection the medial branches tend to lie in the center of the articular pillars.[40–42] Unlike in the lumbar spine, the pos-

terior rami in the cervical region provide little innervation to the paraspinous muscles (Fig. 56–7).

The cervical facet joints above the C3-4 level are slightly more complicated. The C2-3 facet joint receives the majority of its innervation from the C3 dorsal ramus. The C3 dorsal ramus normally divides into two separate medial branches. The larger superior branch is better known as the third occipital nerve, and the inferior branch is conventionally termed the deep median branch. Some innervation for the C2-3 level also derives from the C2 dorsal rami, which may form five distinct branches, the largest of which is the greater occipital nerve.[42,43] Along with the upper cervical z-joints themselves, the dorsal rami and their branches can also be a source of cervicogenic headaches.[44,45]

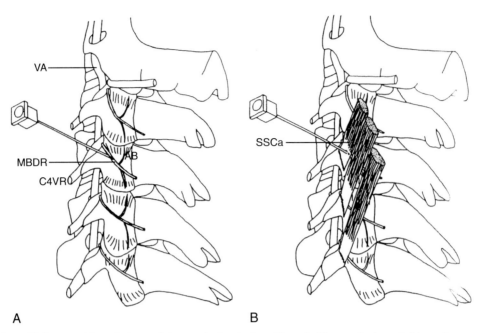

Figure 56–7. Sketches of left, posterolateral views of the cervical articular pillars. **A,** The cervical medial branches course across the waist of the articular pillars. A needle inserted from a lateral approach anesthetizes the medial branch proximal to the origin of its articular branches. **B,** The articular branches lie deep to the tendinous origin of the semispinalis capitis, which acts to hold the anesthetic in place against the medial branch. AB, articular branches; C, cervical vertebra; MBDR, medial branch; SSCa, semispinalis capitis; VA, vertebral artery. (From Barnsley L, Bogduk N: Medial branch blocks are specific for the diagnosis of cervical zygapophysial joint pain. Reg Anesth 1993;18:343-350.)

MECHANISMS OF INJURY

In the vast majority of cases, facet joint arthropathy is the product of years of repetitive strain, low-grade trauma, and stress from intervertebral disk degeneration. In some cases an inciting event or pathology can be identified. This is especially true in trauma patients with whiplash injuries.[41,45,46] In most patients, whiplash leads to chronic neck and shoulder pain. However, in some cases, rear impact injuries can result in cervical facet dislocations and fractures, causing radiculopathy or spinal cord injury.[47-55] In addition, high-impact trauma such as motor vehicle accidents (MVAs) or sports injuries may result in z-joint pain secondary to hyperflexion,[56] rotation, and distraction injuries.[57]

Cadaveric and Laboratory Studies

Cadaveric studies have shed some light into mechanisms of z-joint movement and displacement. Ianuzzi and coworkers found that joint movements occurring with any given motion are directly correlated with the magnitude of joint displacement, and tend to be greatest at the L4-5 and L5-S1 joints.[58] At the three most caudad joints (L3-S1), contralateral bending is associated with greater capsular strain than ipsilateral bending (i.e., the left facet joints are most strained during right lateral flexion). In contrast, the L1-2 and L2-3 joints undergo greater strain during ipsilateral

flexion. For the upper three facet joints, the maximum joint displacement and greatest strain are associated with lateral bending, usually to the right. For the two lowest joints, the greatest degree of strain occurs during forward flexion (Table 56–1).

Later work provides evidence that fusion of two vertebrae can lead to accelerated degeneration at adjacent levels.[59-63] Little and colleagues fixated human lumbar spine specimens with a single anterior thoracolumbar plate at L4-5 and measured capsular displacement and strains for a wide range of physiologic motions.[63] Motion was increased at the level of fixation and both adjacent levels. The fusion also increased intervertebral angulation at L3-4 and L5-S1, with decreased motion at L4-5. Although the fusion relieved anterior (ipsilateral) strain at L4-5, there was greater posterior strain at L4-5 and anterior and posterior strain at both adjacent levels.

The z-joints can respond to repetitive strain and inflammation by filling with fluid and distending, thereby stretching the capsule and causing pain.[64] The pain from capsular inflammation can spread beyond the joint area by compressing the exiting nerve root in the neural foramen or spinal canal. This is especially true of foramina that are already narrowed by facet joint hypertrophy, osteophytes, or herniated intervertebral disks.[65-68] Facet joint pain can therefore manifest in a radicular pattern. Irritation of the capsule also may cause reflex spasm of the erector spinae, multifidus, and other paraspinous muscles.[65,69,70]

Table 56–1. Motions Associated with the Largest
Intervertebral Angulation and Strain for the Lumbar
Facet Joints

FACET JOINT LEVEL	MOVEMENT ASSOCIATED WITH MAXIMAL IVA	LARGEST STRAIN
L1-2	Right bending	Right bending
L2-3	Left bending	Right bending
L3-4	Right bending	Right bending
L4-5	Forward flexion	Forward flexion
L5-S1	Extension	Forward flexion

IVA, intervertebral angle.
Modified from Ianuzzi A, Little JS, Chiu JB, et al: Human lumbar facet joint capsule strains: I. During physiological motions. Spine J 2004;4:141-152.

The pathophysiologic basis for persistent lumbar facet pain was established in a series of elegant experiments conducted by Cavanaugh and associates, Ozaktay and coworkers, and Yamashita and colleagues in New Zealand white rabbits. These studies showed that the application of proinflammatory and algesic mediators into facet joints resulted in inflammatory changes, including vasodilation, venous congestion, and the accumulation of polymorphonuclear leukocytes. The associated inflammatory response led to sensitization and reduced firing thresholds of both nociceptors and proprioceptive nerve fibers. The result was an increase in discharge rate and recruitment of previously silent units.[71-74] Persistent nociception is known to cause peripheral sensitization with the potential for central sensitization and neuroplasticity.[75] Later work by Chen and associates showed the presence of C- and A-delta fibers in the cervical facet joint capsules of goats.[76] C-fibers were more prevalent in the dorsolateral aspect of the z-joint capsule, where tendons and muscles attach. Whereas animal research plays a critical role in improving our understanding of the pathophysiology of facet pain, there are a wide array of anatomic and functional differences between animals and humans.[77] Therefore caution should be exercised when extrapolating the results of animal studies to humans.

These preclinical data do indicate that chronic facet pain is likely to occur with repetitive, chronic strain, or less commonly following any acute event that stretches the joint beyond its physiologic limits. Clinical studies indicating a higher prevalence of facet arthropathy in the elderly,[78-80] and case reports of facet pain following high-energy trauma,[45,57] support these preclinical findings.

Human Studies

In clinical studies chronic facet pain has been associated with several conditions. In LBP patients and asymptomatic individuals, sagittally oriented facet joints were associated with degenerative spondylolisthesis.[23,24] In these patients, recurrent rotational strains result in myriad changes to the disks and paired facet joints, including loss of disk height,

osteophyte formation, and degenerative joint hypertrophy.[81,82]

The intervertebral disk and paired facet joints work in concert. Therefore changes in any part of the three-joint unit will alter the motion and function of the others. Degenerative disk disease (DDD) has been shown to result in concomitant changes in the facet joints.[83-85] In the reverse scenario, degeneration and motion abnormalities of the facet joints can induce and accelerate intervertebral disk degeneration.[86-88] A magnetic resonance imaging (MRI) study evaluating the relationship between DDD and facet joint osteoarthritis concluded that DDD often precedes facet arthritis and is a more reliable indicator of aging than facet hypertrophy.[89] In addition, facet arthropathy tends to be most pronounced at spinal levels with advanced DDD. However, a clinical study investigating the relationship between injection-confirmed discogenic low back pain and facet joint arthropathy yielded conflicting findings.[90] Among 92 patients with axial LBP, 39% had at least one positive discogram with a negative control disk, and 9% received concordant pain relief following a series of diagnostic facet blocks. Yet only 3% of patients had both positive discography and diagnostic facet blocks.

A number of conditions besides osteoarthritis may affect the facet joint. These include inflammatory arthritides such as rheumatoid arthritis, ankylosing spondylitis, and reactive arthritis.[91-94] In addition, synovial impingement, meniscoid entrapment, chondromalacia facetae, pseudogout, synovial inflammation, villonodular synovitis, and acute and chronic infection may cause facetogenic pain.[94-99] Synovial pseudocysts within the facets can cause distention and pressure on adjacent structures, leading to calcification and asymmetric facet hypertrophy.[100-105] Pseudocysts typically present with axial pain and radiculopathy, but can also cause motor weakness, myelopathy, and cauda equina syndrome.[104,105] A retrospective review of MRI scans in 303 consecutive patients with LBP found 9.5% of the patients had z-joint synovial cysts, the majority located posteriorly.[106]

There are a number of reported cases of lumbar facetogenic pain secondary to traumatic dislocation from rapid deceleration injuries, mostly at L5-S1.[56,57,107-111] The purported mechanism of injury in these cases was hyperflexion, rotation, and distraction. By itself, hyperextension rarely leads to facet fractures.[56] Twomey and colleagues dissected the lumbar spines of 31 subjects that had died from trauma (mostly motor vehicle accidents).[112] They found occult bony fractures in the superior articular process or subchondral bone plate in 35% of subjects and facet capsular or articular cartilage damage in 77% of cases. These findings indicate that occult bony and soft tissue injuries to the facet joints may be a source of LBP after trauma.

For chronic post-traumatic neck pain, cervical z-joints have been estimated to account for upward of 60% of cases.[39,113] However, trauma causes only a small percentage of chronic neck pain. An epidemiologic study conducted in patients with chronic cervical pain found trauma to be the precipitating event in only 13% of cases.[114] Among patients with positive cervical facet blocks, the percentage of cases attributed to trauma varies significantly. In a small, controlled study evaluating RF denervation for cervicogenic headaches, 5 of 12 patients reported a previous inciting event.[115] However, in the largest cervical facet denervation outcome study, Cohen and coworkers[116] found that only 23% of the 92 subjects with a positive response to diagnostic z-joint blocks cited trauma as the principal cause. In rare cases, tumors may also cause facet joint pain.[117,118]

PREVALENCE

The prevalence of facet joint pain varies greatly throughout the literature. The lumbar facets are most commonly affected, followed in descending order by cervical and thoracic facet arthropathy.

Prevalence of Lumbar Facet Arthropathy

The prevalence rate of lumbar z-joint pain ranges from 5% to 90% in the literature.[119-126] Many of the studies investigating prevalence, however, have been flawed. Numerous reviews have found that diagnosing facet joint pain using history, physical examination, and radiologic findings is unreliable; the only reliable and valid method to diagnose a painful z-joint is by image-guided medial branch blocks (MBBs) or intra-articular injections with local anesthesia.[127-129] Diagnostic facet blocks without controls have been associated with false-positive rates ranging from 25% to 41%.[130-133]

This high false-positive rate has led some experts to advocate controlled or comparative blocks as the only reliable method to diagnose lumbar facetogenic pain.[134] The reported prevalence of facet pain using single local anesthetic (LA) blocks has ranged from 8% to 94%.[78,125] The addition of placebo-controlled LA blocks decreases prevalence rates significantly to between 9% and 42% (Table 56–2).[79,90,130-133,135-137] Not surprisingly, the estimated prevalence rates tend to increase with age.

Larger epidemiologic studies by primary care physicians and spine surgeons have found much lower rates of lumbar facet pain. Newton and colleagues[138] studied all cases of acute and chronic low back pain in a large health maintenance organization (HMO) population over a 9-month period and found a 6% prevalence of facet-mediated pain. In a comprehensive epidemiologic study by Long and coworkers, spine surgeons from eight academic medical centers in the United States collected demographic and clinical information on more than 4000 patients with LBP over a 5-year period.[123] Final diagnoses were rendered based on historical and physical examinations, radiologic and other diagnostic studies, and response to treatment or diagnostic injections. The diagnosis of facet joint arthritis was given to 4.8% of the 2374 patients that completed the study.

The more cephalad lumbar facet joints are infrequently found to be the main source of axial LBP. In descending order, the most frequently implicated painful facet joints are L5-S1, L4-5, and L3-4.[90,132,133]

There are a number of factors that make prevalence studies difficult to interpret. Most studies excluded patients with focal neurologic signs or symptoms, yet foraminal narrowing secondary to facet hypertrophy is a well-described cause of radiculopathy.[65,66,68] A second confounding factor is that the best studies investigating the prevalence of facet hypertrophy used comparative MBBs.[130] Although the medial branch is the largest branch of the primary dorsal ramus, the other two branches are the intermediate branch, which innervates the longissimus muscle, and the lateral branch, which supplies the iliocostalis muscle, thoracolumbar fascia, skin over the lower back and buttock, and sacroiliac joint.[28,139-141] The medial branches above L5 are most easily blocked at the superomedial border of the transverse process at its junction with the superior articular process. In these areas, local anesthetic will almost invariably block all three primary dorsal rami branches because of their proximity. Although it is difficult to infer the precise prevalence of lumbar facet joint pain, based on the available literature the best estimate is that it affects approximately 10% to 15% of patients with LBP.

Prevalence of Cervical and Thoracic Facet Arthropathy

Less is known about the prevalence of cervical and thoracic facet arthropathy, although there have been a few prospective trials. In one of the earliest cervical z-joint prevalence studies, Aprill and Bogduk performed provocative discography, intra-articular facet injections, or both in 318 patients with chronic nonradicular neck pain following injury. Based on concordant pain provocation to both sets of blocks, the authors estimated the prevalence of cervical z-joint pain to be 26%.[113] In addition to not using analgesic response to facet blocks as their primary diagnostic criteria, another flaw in this study is that only 52 of the 318 patients underwent diagnostic cervical facet blocks. In an observational study by Barnsley and associates conducted in 50 patients with chronic neck pain following whiplash injury, the authors found a prevalence rate of 54% based on double-blind comparative LA MBBs.[142]

In a prospective study conducted in 500 patients with nonradicular neck ($n = 255$) and mid- ($n = 72$) or low back pain, Manchikanti and colleagues[136] used a concordant response to LA MBBs done with 1% lidocaine and 0.25% bupivacaine to diagnose a painful thoracic or cervical facet joint. The authors found the prevalence of cervical facetogenic pain in neck pain patients to be 55%, whereas patients with mid- and upper back pain had a 42% prevalence of thoracic facet pain. The latter finding is consistent with a previous study done by the same group that found a 48% prevalence of thoracic facet pain in

Table 56–2. Results of Lumbar Facet Joint Pain Prevalence Studies Conducted Using Either Placebo-Controlled or Comparative Local Anesthetic Blocks

AUTHOR, YEAR	PATIENTS	INTERVENTIONS	RESULTS	FALSE-POSITIVE* RATE AND COMMENTS
Schwarzer et al, 1994[90]	92 patients with chronic LBP without neurologic deficit or prior surgery. All patients underwent comparative facet blocks and provocative discography.	Patients received either intra-articular (0.5 mL) or MBB (0.5 mL) with 2% lidocaine at 3 lowest facet levels. In patients who obtained ≥50% relief, blocks were repeated with 0.5% bupivacaine. A positive response was pain relief sustained for ≥3 hr.	39% (n = 36) of patients achieved definite pain relief after lidocaine blocks; 25% of patients who underwent confirmatory blocks with bupivacaine obtained had a positive response, for a 9% prevalence rate.	26% rate of FP blocks; 39% of patients had positive discography. Only 3 had both positive discography and positive response to facet blocks. Median age 37 yr. Male/female ratio was 2:1.
Schwarzer et al, 1994[132]	176 patients with chronic LBP without neurologic deficit or prior surgery.	Patients received either intra-articular or MBB (0.5 mL) with 2% lidocaine at 3 lowest levels. In patients who obtained ≥50% pain relief, blocks were repeated with 0.5% bupivacaine. A positive response was pain relief sustained for ≥3 hr.	47% (n = 83) of patients reported a definite or greater response after lidocaine, with 26 of 71 patients who underwent confirmatory blocks obtaining concordant relief for a prevalence rate of 15%.	FP rate of 38%. Median age 38 yr.
Schwarzer et al, 1995[133]	63 patients with chronic LBP without neurologic deficit or prior surgery.	Patients received placebo injections followed by single-level intra-articular facet injections (up to 1.5 mL of 0.5% bupivacaine) at 3 lowest levels, on separate occasions. A positive response was pain relief sustained for ≥3 hr only with bupivacaine.	40% obtained >50% pain relief with bupivacaine but not placebo. 37% had >90% pain relief.	32% of patients obtained >50% pain relief for ≥3 hr after placebo; 18 of 23 obtained relief at only 1 level. Median age 59 yr. Female/male ratio was 3:1.
Revel et al, 1998[79]	80 patients with chronic LBP not due to sciatica, without prior surgery.	Patients received either placebo or 1 mL of lidocaine injected into the 2 most caudad facet joints. A positive response was >75% pain relief.	31% of lidocaine group obtained significant pain relief after the injection.	18% of patients receiving intra-articular saline obtained significant pain relief. Mean age 58 years. Female/male ratio was 2:1.
Manchikanti, et al, 1999[30]	120 patients with chronic LBP without neurologic deficit.	Patients received MBB with 0.4-0.6 mL of 1% lidocaine and/or 0.25% bupivacaine. All patients: a positive response was ≥75% relief lasting longer with bupivacaine than lidocaine.	81 (67.5%) patients reported a definite response to lidocaine MBB. 54 of these reported definite pain relief after the bupivacaine block, for a prevalence rate of 45%.	FP rate was 41%. Patients who had previous surgery were less likely to have lumbar z-joint pain. Trauma was implicated as cause of pain in 53% of patients. Mean age 47 yr. 25% FP rate. Mean age was 48 yr.
Manchikanti et al, 2000[131]	180 patients with chronic LBP without neurologic deficits.	Patients received double MBB from L1-5 with 0.5 mL of lidocaine and bupivacaine, LA with pitcher plant extract (Sarapin), or LA with pitcher plant extract and steroid. A positive response was ≥75% relief lasting longer with bupivacaine than lidocaine.	74% (n = 133) of patients obtained a positive response to the lidocaine blocks, but only 65 reported definite pain relief after bupivacaine blocks for a 36% prevalence rate.	
Dreyfuss et al, 2000[135]	41 carefully chosen patients out of 138 screened by telephone interview with chronic LBP, no neurologic deficits and an absence of psychiatric or severe concomitant spinal pathology.	Patients received MBB with 2% lidocaine at maximally tender areas. Patients who obtained ≥80% pain relief underwent confirmatory blocks with bupivacaine. A positive response was definite pain relief lasting >2 hr.	22 patients obtained significant pain relief after lidocaine MBB, with 15 obtaining ≥80% after bupivacaine blocks for a 37% prevalence rate.	FP rate of 17%. Mean age 55 yr in 15 responders. Patients carefully chosen to evaluate outcomes for radiofrequency denervation.
Manchikanti et al, 2000[137]	200 patients with chronic LBP without neurologic deficits.	Patients received MBB with 1% lidocaine. All patients who obtained ≥75% relief underwent confirmatory blocks with 0.25% bupivacaine. A positive response was ≥75% relief lasting longer with bupivacaine.	64% (n = 127) reported a positive response to lidocaine blocks, with 84 obtaining definite pain relief after bupivacaine blocks for a 42% prevalence rate.	37% FP rate. Mean age 47 yr.
Manchikanti et al, 2004[136]	397 patients with chronic LBP without neurologic deficits.	Patients received MBB with 1% lidocaine. All patients who obtained ≥75% pain relief underwent confirmatory blocks with 0.25% bupivacaine. A positive response was ≥80% relief lasting longer with bupivacaine.	198 (50%) of patients obtained a positive response to lidocaine blocks, with 124 reporting definite pain relief with bupivacaine for a 31% prevalence rate.	FP rate was 27%. Mean age 47 yr.

*False-positive (FP) rate: if not mentioned, this was determined by dividing the number of patients who obtained pain relief with the lidocaine screening block but not by the confirmatory block by the total number of blocks.
LA, local anesthetic; LBP, low back pain; MBB, medial branch block.

patients with mid- and upper back pain.[143] Bilateral involvement was found in 69% of the patients in the cervical spine, 64% in the thoracic spine, and 72% in the lumbar spine.[136]

The estimated prevalence of cervical facetogenic pain in patients with chronic neck pain based on studies using comparative blocks has been estimated between 49% and 60% (Table 56–3).[41,45,136,142,144] The C2-3 and C5-6 levels were found to be the most prevalent levels in two studies of chronic neck pain patients.[45,142] The C2-3 facet joint also was found to have the highest rate of degenerative disease in a study of 196 excavated human skeletons from the sixth to eighth centuries from Germanic row graves in southwestern Germany.[145]

The majority of the well-designed cervical facet prevalence studies have been done in patients with whiplash injuries after an MVA, which makes it difficult to estimate the prevalence in neck pain patients without a history of trauma. It is well known that cervical facetogenic pain comprises a large percentage of cases of persistent whiplash injury. Based on the available literature, the prevalence of cervical facet pain is likely around 50% in patients with chronic neck pain. The prevalence of thoracic facet pain in patients with chronic axial mid-back pain is between 42% to 48%[136,143] (see Table 56–2).

DIAGNOSIS

History and Physical Examination

Researchers have tried for many years to delineate historical and physical examination findings pathognomonic for facet arthropathy (Table 56–4). Some information can be gleaned from the pain referral patterns discussed in the subsequent section. Historical and physical associations, however, have proven less reliable. The majority of the investigations have focused on lumbar z-joints, although there are some data available for cervical and thoracic z-joint pain.

Earlier studies were able to identify findings consistent with facet pain. Low-volume, intra-articular bupivacaine facet blocks done on 41 patients with LBP with or without leg pain found at least temporary pain relief in 14 of the 25 patients who completed the study.[146] When compared with nonresponders, subjects who responded positively to the blocks tended to have pain localized to the back and thigh and worsening pain with forward flexion. The "lumbar facet syndrome" was described by Helbig and Lee in 1988 based on a retrospective study of 22 patients.[147] Those patients who responded to intra-articular injections were more likely to have back pain associated with groin or thigh pain, paraspinal tenderness, and reproduction of pain with extension-rotation maneuvers. Pain radiating below the knee was found to be a negative predictor.

Larger and more methodologically sound studies have failed to validate the "lumbar facet syndrome." Prospective studies of 390 and 176 patients with chronic LBP were unable to correlate any historical or physical finding associated with a positive response to facet injections.[78,148] In both studies, only a small percentage (10% and 15%, respectively) of the patients responded to diagnostic blocks. A randomized, placebo-controlled study of 80 patients with chronic LBP by Revel and coworkers found seven factors associated with response to facet joint anesthesia: age greater than 65 and pain not exacerbated by coughing, not worsened by hyperextension, not worsened by forward flexion, not worsened when rising from forward flexion, not worsened by extension-rotation, and well-relieved by recumbency.[79] Yet subsequent investigations also failed to corroborate these findings. In summary, no historical or physical examination findings can reliably predict response to diagnostic facet blocks.

Few studies investigate the history and physical findings most consistent with cervical and thoracic facet pain. As noted, the prevalence of facet involvement in patients with chronic neck and thoracic pain is higher than for LBP. Therefore, prognostic factors may be somewhat less important. One study found that a blinded manipulative therapist was able to diagnose symptomatic cervical facet joint pain correctly in patients with positive diagnostic cervical MBBs by means of perceived passive displacement of the joint and its resistance to displacement.[149] However, a subsequent study conducted using controlled blocks as the gold standard for cervical z-joint pain found, whereas manual examination had a sensitivity of 88%, the low specificity (39%) precluded its use as a valid diagnostic tool.[150] Lord and associates found that patients with chronic neck pain who had a positive response to diagnostic cervical facet blocks were more likely to be female, victims of a rear-end collision, and have restricted neck movement, though the findings were not statistically significant.[45] Another study showed a 94% correlation between lumbar and cervical facet pain in patients with confirmed lumbar facet pain and concomitant neck pain.[151] The majority of cervical facet prevalence studies have been conducted on whiplash victims, thereby making it difficult to draw conclusions as to the association between neck pain in nontrauma patients and cervical facet disease.

Pain Referral Patterns

Many investigators have used a variety of techniques to map out pain referral patterns in facetogenic pain. Methods have included pain provocation via stimulation of the facet joint capsules and medial branches in both asymptomatic volunteers and pain patients, and pain patterns in patients who respond positively to facet or medial branch injections of LA, with or without steroid. The majority of these studies have failed to demonstrate any reliable pain referral patterns.[152,153] These discrepancies between pain provocation patterns and pain mapping or historical findings are consistent with previous studies done with sacroiliac joint and selective nerve root blocks.[154,155] As noted, pain from the facet joint is

Table 56–3. Results of Cervical and Thoracic Zygapophysial Joint Pain Prevalence Studies Conducted Using Either Placebo-Controlled or Comparative Local Anesthetic Blocks

AUTHOR, YEAR	PATIENTS	INTERVENTIONS	RESULTS	FALSE-POSITIVE RATE AND COMMENTS
Barnsley et al, 1993[41]	47 patients with chronic neck pain >3 mo after MVA.	Patients received cervical MBB with 0.5 mL of either 2% lidocaine or 0.5% bupivacaine. Patients with positive block received other agent; positive response required longer pain relief with bupivacaine.	27 patients had longer relief with bupivacaine compared with lidocaine, indicating a 60% prevalence rate.	13 patients (27%) had positive response to both LAs but in excess of expected duration. Average age 41 yr. Female/male ratio 1:1. All but 3 patients involved in litigation.
Barnsley et al, 1995[142]	50 patients with chronic neck pain >3 mo duration after whiplash injury from MVA.	Patients received cervical MBB with 0.5 mL of either 2% lidocaine or 0.5% bupivacaine at random. Patients with positive block received complementary anesthetic; positive response required longer pain relief with bupivacaine.	27 patients who completed study met criteria for a positive painful joint, indicating a 54% prevalence rate.	10 patients (20%) had longer pain relief from lidocaine than bupivacaine or no pain relief with repeat block. Average age 41 yr. Female/male ratio 1.5:1. C2-3 and C5-6 most frequently affected levels.
Lord et al, 1996[45]	68 patients with chronic neck pain >3 mo duration after whiplash injury from MVA.	Patients received diagnostic C2-3 block to rule out patients with third occipital headache. Placebo-controlled cervical facet blocks below C2-3 done with 0.5 mL of either 2% lidocaine or 0.5% bupivacaine. If negative, other levels were then attempted. If positive, patients received either NS or other LA at random, then had third block with remaining agent.	31 of 52 patients (60%) that completed study had cervical facet pain at C2-3 or below, indicating a 60% prevalence rate. Among patients with HA as dominant symptoms, 50% prevalence of C2-3 facet joint pain. In patients without C2-3 facet pain, prevalence of lower cervical facet pain was 49%.	Average age 41 yr. Female/male ratio 2:1. C2-3 and C5-6 were most commonly affected levels.
Manchikanti et al, 2002[44]	106 patients with chronic neck pain with or without HA or upper extremity pain.	Patients received diagnostic blocks using 0.5 mL of 1% lidocaine followed by 0.5 mL of 0.25% bupivacaine 2 wk apart.	64 of 81 patients with positive lidocaine blocks had longer relief with confirmatory bupivacaine blocks for a 60% prevalence rate.	40% FP rate. Mean age 43 yr. Female/male ratio 2:1; 15% of patients had previous neck surgery.
Manchikanti et al, 2004[136]	500 patients with chronic neck, thoracic and/or low back pain without neurologic symptoms; 255 patients had cervical symptoms and 72 patients had thoracic symptoms.	Patients received MBB with 1% lidocaine followed by confirmatory blocks with 0.25% bupivacaine. A positive response was ≥80% relief lasting longer with bupivacaine. Minimum of 2 levels blocked based on pain patterns.	55% prevalence rate of cervical facet joints in patients with cervical spine pain; 42% prevalence rate of thoracic facet joints in patients with thoracic pain.	FP rate 63% for cervical and 55% for thoracic MBB. Average age 47 yr. Female/male ratio 2:1 for both cervical and thoracic.
Manchikanti et al, 2002[143]	46 patients with chronic thoracic pain (>6 mo) without neurologic symptoms.	Patients received MBB with 1% lidocaine followed by confirmatory blocks with 0.5% bupivacaine. A positive response was >80% concordant pain relief.	22 of 36 patients with positive lidocaine blocks had longer relief with confirmatory bupivacaine blocks for a 48% prevalence rate.	FP rate 58%. Average age 46 yr.

FP, false-positive; HA, headache; LA, local anesthetic; MBB, medial branch block; MVA, motor vehicle accident; NS, normal saline.

Table 56–4. Studies Evaluating the Ability of Historical and Physical Examination Findings to Predict Response to Diagnostic Lumbar Facet Injections

AUTHOR, YEAR	PATIENTS AND INTERVENTIONS	RESULTS	COMMENTS
Fairbank et al, 1981[146]	25 patients with acute LBP received intra-articular facet injections at 2 levels with 0.5 mL of LA.	Responders had pain localized to back and thigh, whereas nonresponders had pain in lower leg. Responders tended to complain of more pain during forward flexion.	8 patients obtained relief lasting 1-48 hr and 6 obtained long-term relief. No difference between groups in duration of symptoms, disability scores, or psychological profile.
Helbig and Lee, 1988[147]	Retrospective study conducted in 22 patients with LBP and leg pain. Injection parameters not noted.	Back pain radiating to groin or thigh, paraspinal tenderness and reproduction of pain with extension-rotation associated with positive response. Pain extending below knee associated with negative response.	23% of patients had negative response, 27% had a temporary response, and 50% a prolonged response.
Lewinnek and Warfield, 1986[122]	Retrospective study conducted in 21 patients. Intra-articular injections done with LA and steroid.	Negative screening exam for other causes of LBP or sciatica and paraspinal tenderness over 1 or more facet joints associated with positive response.	75% of patients had an initial positive response, but only 33% had a response lasting >3 mo.
Jackson et al, 1988[28]	390 patients with LBP underwent intra-articular LA and steroid injections at L4-5 and L5-S1 with 1.5 mL.	Unable to identify a "facet syndrome." Factors associated with a positive response were older age, absence of leg pain, and absence of pain with Valsalva.	7.7% reported complete pain relief after injection.
Lilius et al, 1990[298]	109 patients with unilateral chronic LBP were randomized to receive either 8 mL of LA and steroid into 2 facet joints, around 2 facet joints, or NS into 2 facet joints.	No clinical finding was associated with outcome. The number of "inappropriate signs or symptoms" and previous back surgery were positively associated with failure.	Approximately 30% of patients showed significant improvement. Pain relief at 1 hr postinjection correlated with pain relief at 3 mo postinjection. No basis for large volumes injected.
Revel et al, 1992[80]	40 patients with chronic LBP underwent intra-articular facet injections with 1.5 mL of LA.	Factors associated with a positive response were older age, absence of exacerbation by coughing, relief when recumbent, absence of exacerbation by forward flexion and rising from flexion, and by hyperextension and extension-rotation.	55% had positive response to injection, of which 43% had >90% relief.
Schwarzer et al, 1994[132]	176 patients with chronic LBP underwent confirmatory medial branch or facet blocks with 0.5 mL of LA.	No statistically significant association between response to blocks found for any feature on history or physical exam.	15% responded with concordant relief to lidocaine and confirmatory bupivacaine blocks.
Schwarzer et al, 1995[133]	63 patients with chronic LBP underwent intra-articular facet injections with LA and NS.	No historical or physical exam finding could distinguish patients with positive response to blocks.	40% of patients obtained significant relief with LA but not NS.
Revel et al, 1998[79]	80 patients with chronic LBP underwent intra-articular facet injections with 1 mL of LA or NS.	Factors associated with a positive response were older age, absence of exacerbation by coughing, relief when recumbent, absence of exacerbation by forward flexion and rising from flexion, and by hyperextension and extension-rotation.	Results identical to previous uncontrolled study. Presence of 5 of 7 variables distinguished 92% of responders and 80% of nonresponders.
Manchikanti et al, 1999[130]	120 patients with chronic LBP underwent confirmatory MBB with 0.4-0.6 mL of LA.	Only historical or PE finding associated with a positive response was absence of back pain with straight leg raising.	45% of patients had a concordant positive response to lidocaine and bupivacaine blocks.
Manchikanti et al, 2000[131]	180 patients with chronic LBP underwent confirmatory MBB with 0.4-0.6 mL of LA mixed with or without pitcher plant extract (Sarapin) and steroid.	Only historical or PE finding associated with a positive response was absence of back or leg pain with straight leg raising.	36% had a concordant positive response to both blocks.
Manchikanti et al, 2000[137]	200 patients with chronic LBP underwent confirmatory MBB with 0.4-0.6 mL of LA.	Only clinical feature associated with positive response was relief of pain in supine position. Negative correlation between exacerbation of back pain with straight leg raising and positive block.	42% prevalence rate. Negative correlation between previous surgery, and positive response to blocks.
Young et al, 2003[299]	23 patients with chronic LBP underwent intra-articular facet injections with <1.5 mL of LA.	Only lack of pain provocation when rising from sitting was associated with positive response.	61% of patients experienced concordant pain during injection and relief after LA instillation.
Laslett et al, 2004[300]	111 patients underwent intra-articular or MBB with 0.5 mL of LA. Study designed to confirm Revel's findings.[23]	Only absence of pain with coughing and absence of pain exacerbation when rising from flexion showed a trend toward being associated with a positive response ($P = 0.07$).	23% of patients obtained ≥75% pain relief after block. Patients older than 65 years of age were more likely to obtain complete pain relief.
Laslett et al, 2006[301]	151 patients underwent confirmatory MBB or intra-articular injections with 0.5 mL of LA.	Factors associated with positive response were age >50, pain relieved by walking, pain relieved by sitting, onset of paraspinal pain, high somatization score, pain worsened by extension-rotation, and absence of "centralization" of pain.	31 patients excluded. Data missing in many patients. Utility of predictive factors diminished with decreasing pain reduction standards.

LA, local anesthetic; LBP, low back pain; MBB, medial branch block; NS, normal saline; PE, physical examination.

usually secondary to years of chronic strain and repetitive damage. Therefore pain provocation studies of the facet joint or its nerve supply may not simulate physiologic conditions.

When the existing data are synthesized, however, certain pain patterns do emerge (Fig. 56–8). The joint capsule appears more likely to generate pain than the synovium or articular cartilage. A great deal of overlap between neighboring facet joints exists. All lumbar levels are capable of producing groin pain, though it is most common in the lower levels (Table 56–5). Pain from the upper lumbar facets tends to extend into the flank, hip, and upper lateral thigh, whereas pain from the lower lumbar levels is likely to penetrate deeper into the thigh, usually in the lateral and posterior aspects. Infrequently, the L4-5 and L5-S1 facet joints can provoke pain in the lateral calf, and rarely into the foot. Patients with osteophytes, synovial cysts, or facet hypertrophy also may manifest radicular symptoms.

Clinical studies have been conducted in both healthy volunteers and patients with suspected cervical facet pain to determine pain referral patterns from the joints.[156-158] The results of these experiments are strikingly consistent. From C2-3, the pain pattern generally extends rostrally to the upper cervical region and suboccipital area. Infrequently, symptoms will extend toward the ear or further up the scalp. From C3-4, pain is referred to the upper and middle posterior neck, with occasional radiation into the lower occiput. From C4-5, the most common referral pattern is into the lower posterior cervical region, although in a significant percentage of people it extends into the middle posterior neck and supra-

scapular region. Pain from C5-6 is typically distributed to either the suprascapular region or lower neck, but can sometimes extend to the shoulder joint or midposterior neck. From C6-7, pain is usually referred into the upper scapula or lower neck. Pain from the C7-T1 z-joint most frequently extends farther down into the midscapula area. Later work by Windsor and colleagues[159] indicated that the pain referral patterns elicited by cervical medial branch stimulation tend to be smaller and slightly different from articular z-joint distention (Fig. 56–9).

Similar work has been done for thoracic z-joints. Dreyfuss and associates[160] mapped thoracic facet pain patterns based on intra-articular contrast injections of the T3-4 to T10-11 z-joints in nine asymptomatic volunteers (Fig. 56–10). Fukui and colleagues[35] later investigated pain referral patterns during intra-articular injection of the upper and lower-most thoracic z-joints. The resultant pain referral patterns were as follows: pain from the C7-T1 and T1-T2 z-joints typically radiates into the suprascapular region and superior angle of the scapula. Pain extending into the midscapular region may come from either C7-T1, T1-2, or T2-3, and pain from the T11-12 z-joint generally extends into the paravertebral region around the site of injection out to around the iliac crest area.

Radiologic Findings

The prevalence of facet joint disease as observed with radiologic imaging depends on the age, presence of symptoms, imaging modality used, and threshold for a diagnosis of "abnormal." In LBP patients, the

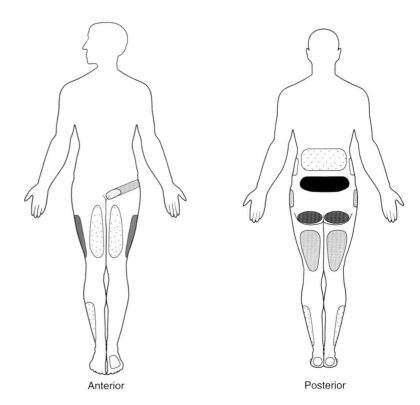

Figure 56–8. Pain referral patterns from the lumbar facet joints. In descending order, the most common referral patterns extend from the *darkest* (low back) to the *lightest* regions (flank and foot). The key at the bottom of the figure legend is listed in order of affected frequency (i.e., low back to foot). The *facet levels* next to each location represent the zygapophysial joints associated with pain in each region. Low back: L5-S1, L4-5, L3-4; buttock: L5-S1, L4-5, L3-4; lateral thigh: L5-S1, L4-5, L3-4, L2-3; posterior thigh: L5-S1, L4-5, L3-4; greater trochanter: L5-S1, L4-5, L3-4, L2-3; groin: L5-S1, L4-5, L3-4, L2-3, L1-2; anterior thigh: L5-S1, L4-5, L3-4; lateral lower leg: L5-S1, L4-5, L3-4; upper back: L3-4, L2-3, L1-2; flank: L1-2, L2-3; foot: L5-S1, L4-5. (From Cohen SP, Raja SN. Pathogenesis, diagnosis, and treatment of lumbar zygapophysial [facet] joint pain. Anesthesiology 2007;106:591-614.)

Anterior   Posterior

Table 56–5. Results of Studies Examining Pain Referral Patterns for Lumbar Zygapophysial Joint Pain

AUTHOR, YEAR	PATIENTS AND INTERVENTIONS	RESULTS
Hirsch et al, 1963[302]	Number of patients and characteristics not mentioned. Injected <0.3 mL of 11% hypertonic NS into one of the lower facet joints.	Pain distributed to SI joint and gluteal areas, then out to greater trochanter. Pain identical to typical LBP.
Mooney and Robertson, 1976[303]	5 controls and 15 patients with chronic LBP. Injected 1-3 mL of 5% hypertonic NS into L3-4 thru L5-S1 facet joints, and S1-2 in patients with lumbarization of the sacrum.	L3-4 produced pain radiating down lateral aspect of leg. L4-5 and L5-S1 produced pain radiating posteriorly down the leg, often below the knee in patients with LBP. If present, S1-2 produced pain radiating under buttock. Increasing volume increased amount of radiation. Patients with LBP had greater radiation than patients without back pain.
McCall et al, 1979[304]	Injected 0.4 mL of 6% hypertonic saline intracapsular and pericapsular into the L1-2 and L4-5 facet joints of 6 asymptomatic male volunteers.	There was little difference in pain distribution between intra- and pericapsular injections. Pain from L4-5 radiated to the flank, buttock, iliac crest, upper and lower groin, and thigh above the knee. Pain from L1-2 radiated to the flank, iliac crest, upper groin, and occasionally the abdomen. Pain never radiated contralaterally.
Fairbank et al, 1981[146]	25 patients with acute back or leg pain underwent lumbar z-joint injections at the area of maximal tenderness and 1 additional randomly chosen joint with 0.5 mL bupivacaine.	Responders had pain in the back and thigh, whereas nonresponders had pain in back and lower leg. Symptomatic pain reproduction occurred only in 6 patients.
Lippitt et all, 1984[227]	Retrospective review of 99 patients with LBP of varying duration who underwent lumbar z-joint injections with 1 mL of lidocaine and steroid.	No pattern of pain was noted to be more common in responders. Included patients with unilateral or bilateral hip pain, buttock pain, or pain localized to low back.
Lynch and Taylor, 1986[305]	50 patients with chronic LBP diagnosed by physical exam and x-rays as having facet pain underwent intra-articular steroid injections in 1 or 2 lower facet joints.	39 patients reported total (n = 11) or partial (n = 28) relief of pain after 2 weeks. More than 90% of patients reported low back pain during injection, with half reporting pain radiating into ipsilateral thigh and buttock. No patient reported pain below knee.
Helbig and Lee, 1988[147]	Retrospective review of 22 patients with chronic low back and leg pain. Injected lumbar z-joint(s) with LA and steroid. Divided patients into negative response (no relief), temporary response (relief lasted more than a few hr but less than 6 mo), and prolonged response (>6 mo relief).	80% of patients with groin or thigh pain had a prolonged response. No patient with groin pain and only 1 with thigh pain had negative response. Patients with pain below knee had 37% negative responses and only 25% prolonged responses.
Jackson et al, 1988[78]	390 patients with low back and no neurologic signs underwent L4-5 and L5-S1 z-joint injections with steroid and 1 mL of bupivacaine.	Postinjection pain relief was more likely to occur in patients without leg pain.

Study	Methods	Findings
Marks, 1989[306]	138 patients with chronic LBP underwent lumbar facet and MBB at the same levels. Blocks done with 1 mL of lidocaine, except at L5-S1, where 1.5 mL was used.	The pain produced at all levels was mostly local. The L4-5 and L5-S1 joints were also likely to radiate to buttock, greater trochanter, and all aspects of thigh. About 5% of time pain extended below knee. Pain from L2-5 sometimes extended to groin. Stimulation of nerves was more likely to produce distally referred pain than intra-articular provocation.
Kuslich et al, 1991[307]	193 patients undergoing decompression surgery under local anesthesia. Stimulated a variety of tissue, included lumbar z-joints by mechanical force or unipolar cautery.	Facet capsule stimulation produced pain in 30% of patients, but "significant pain" only 2.5% of time. Pain radiated into back and buttock, but never the leg.
Marks et al, 1992[171]	86 patients with chronic LBP receive either lumbar z-joint or MBB with steroid and 1 or 1.5 mL LA (at L5-S1 or the L5 dorsal ramus).	No pattern of pain predicted response to injection. Patients were included who had axial pain and pain radiating to the leg.
Schwarzer et al, 1994[153]	90 patients with chronic LBP underwent lumbar z-joint blocks with 0.8 mL of contrast and lidocaine at 3 levels.	Based on analgesic response to a single block, there was a significant association between concordant pain provocation and pain relief. However, based on concordant analgesic response to serial lidocaine and bupivacaine blocks, there was no association between pain provocation and pain relief.
Fukui et al, 1997[35]	48 patients with chronic LBP underwent lumbar z-joint blocks with contrast until pain was provoked, then received 0.5-1 mL of LA. Patients who obtained excellent but temporary relief proceeded to RF denervation, with electrical stimulation used to locate the target nerve.	Intra-articular contrast injection always reproduced a patient's pain. Pain from L1-2 joint always produced lumbar pain. In descending order, L2-3 joint produced pain in the lumbar region, hip, and buttock or lateral thigh. L3-4 produced pain mostly in the lumbar region, buttock, or lateral and posterior thigh. L4-5 elicited pain in the lumbar region, buttock, or lateral thigh. L5-S1 elicited pain in the lumbar region, buttock, lateral thigh, or posterior thigh. Pain relief from stimulation of medial branches was similar to that of lumbar z-joints.
Kaplan et al, 1998[199]	15 asymptomatic patients underwent painful facet capsular distension with up to 2.5 mL of contrast.	All subjects experienced a well-circumscribed area of pain without radiation into the inferior buttock or extremity.
Manchikanti et al, 1999[130]	120 patients with chronic LBP and no neurologic deficits underwent confirmatory MBB with 0.4-0.6 mL of lidocaine and bupivacaine.	No pattern of pain predicted response to injection. Patients were included who had axial pain only, thigh pain, groin pain, and leg pain.
Manchikanti et al, 2000[137]	200 patients with chronic LBP without neurologic deficits underwent confirmatory MBB with 0.4-0.6 mL of lidocaine and bupivacaine.	No pattern of pain predicted response to injection. Patients were included who had axial pain only, thigh pain, groin pain, and leg pain.
Young et al, 2003[299]	23 patients with chronic LBP and no neurologic deficits underwent lumbar z-joint injections with <1.5 mL of LA. A positive response was designated as both concordant pain provocation and relief with LA.	The location of pain (radiating toward or away from the spinal column) was not associated with a positive response.

LA, local anesthetic; LBP, low back pain; z-joint, zygapophysial (facet) joint; MBB, medial branch block; NS, normal saline; RF, radiofrequency; SI, sacroiliac.

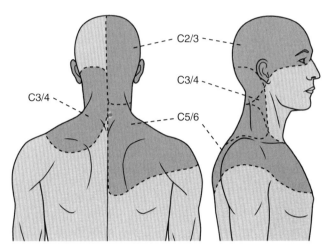

Figure 56–9. Pain referral patterns from the cervical facet joints. (From Bogduk N, Marsland A: The cervical zygapophysial joints as a source of neck pain. Spine 1988;13:615.)

Table 56–6. Levels of Degeneration of Facet Joints Based on Magnetic Resonance Imaging

GRADE	RADIOLOGIC FINDINGS
0	Normal zygapophysial joints (2-4 mm width)
1	Joint space narrowing or mild osteophyte formation or mild hypertrophy of the articular process
2	Narrowing of the joint space with sclerosis or moderate osteophyte formation or moderate hypertrophy of the articular process or mild subarticular bone erosions
3	Narrowing of the joint space with marked osteophyte formation or severe hypertrophy of the articular process or severe subarticular bone erosions or subchondral cysts

Adapted from Weishaupt D, Zanetti M, Boos N, et al: MR imaging and CT in osteoarthritis of the lumbar facet joints. Skeletal Radiol 1999;28: 215-219.

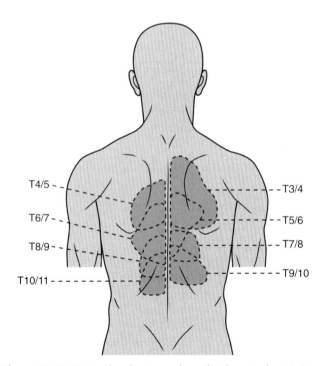

Figure 56–10. Pain referral patterns from the thoracic facet joints. (From Dreyfuss P, Tibiletti C, Dreyer SJ: Thoracic zygapophysial joint pain patterns. A study in normal volunteers. Spine 1994; 19:809.)

incidence of degenerative facet disease noted on computed tomography (CT) ranges from about 40% in some studies[119,161] to 85% in others.[125] Some studies found MRI to be less sensitive than CT in detecting degenerative facet changes,[125,162,163] whereas other studies done in LBP patients revealed MRI to be more than 90% sensitive and specific compared with CT (Table 56–6).[89,164] In a study of 14 patients with DDD, patients less than 40 years of age showed minimal osteoarthritic changes of the lumbar facets.[89] The prevalence increases significantly in patients older

than the age of 60 years; however, facet degeneration is not a universal change. In asymptomatic volunteers, the incidence of lumbar facet degeneration ranges from 8% to 14%.[163,165,166] In a study involving 60 asymptomatic individuals ages 20 to 50 years, MRIs were evaluated for degenerative disk changes, end plate abnormalities, and facet osteoarthritis by two independent radiologists. Although disk bulge (62%) and protrusion (67%) were frequently present, neither radiologist noted severe facet osteoarthritis.[163]

The use of radiologic imaging as a predictor for response to diagnostic facet blocks has been conflicting at best. Although some studies have found a positive association between CT, MRI, and other imaging and response to facet blocks,[119,122,147,161,167] an equal number have not.[78,80,125,146,154,168] In a study by Carrera and Williams, the response to high-volume (2 to 4 mL) diagnostic blocks was found to correlate with CT evidence of lumbar facet disease in 93 patients with LBP.[161] However, a larger study by Jackson and coworkers involving 390 patients found no relationship between x-ray findings and response to lumbar z-joint blocks.[78] Schwarzer and colleagues found no relationship between concordant analgesic response to placebo-controlled intra-articular facet blocks and CT findings of z-joint osteoarthritis in 63 patients with chronic axial LBP.[154] In a recent multi-center study by Cohen and associates involving 192 patients who underwent lumbar radiofrequency (RF) denervation based on a positive response to a single MBB, the authors found no association between MRI evidence of facet hypertrophy or degeneration and 6-month outcomes.[169] Kawaguchi and colleagues found no significant relationship between the degree of radiographic lumbar facet and LBP symptoms in a study of 106 patients with rheumatoid arthritis.[170] In the cervical and thoracic regions, there is a paucity of data evaluating the ability of radiologic imaging studies to predict response to diagnostic facet blocks. In the largest cervical facet denervation study ever conducted in 92 patients who underwent RF lesioning based on a positive response to a single, diagnostic MBB, Cohen and coworkers found no association between 6-month outcomes and MRI evidence of facet arthritis at three different hospitals.[116] In summary, the literature does not support the routine use of radiologic imaging in the diagnosis of facet arthropathy.

DIAGNOSTIC BLOCKS

The poor correlation between historical and physical examination findings and zygapophysial pain has led to widespread acceptance of the use of diagnostic blocks to confirm the facet joint as a primary pain generator. Whereas MBBs and intra-articular injections are widely touted to be equally effective diagnostic tools,[96,127,129,134] the evidence for this claim is based on two studies, neither of which used a crossover design, controlled blocks, or prescreened patients for z-joint pain.[171,172] There are several factors that undermine the diagnostic validity of MBBs. In a cadaveric study done in the 1930s, Kellegren showed that the injection of 0.5 mL of fluid spread into an area encompassing 6 cm^2 of tissue.[173] Therefore the injection of low-volume LA is likely to block the lateral and intermediate branches in addition to the medial branch. Because these nerves supply afferent innervation to multiple potential pain-generating structures including the paraspinal muscles, ligaments, sacroiliac (SI) joints, and skin, MBBs can relieve pain even in the presence of normal facet joints. In addition, false-positive rates have been found to be as high as 63% in the cervical region, 53% for thoracic facet blocks, and 27% for lumbar facet blocks.[136]

Although intra-articular facet injections inherently may be more accurate in diagnosing facet pain, these blocks can be technically challenging and fraught with their own limitations (Fig. 56–11). The injection of 1 to 2 mL of fluid will likely rupture the joint capsule, leading to the extravasation of local anesthetic onto other pain-generating structures. Depending on the point of rupture, these structures may include the epidural space, intervertebral foramen, ligamentum flavum, and paraspinal musculature.[64,124,126,171]

Medial Branch Blocks versus Intra-articular Injections

Only two studies have compared MBBs to intra-articular facet injections. In a prospective randomized study by Nash, 67 patients with LBP were randomized in pairs to receive either MBBs with 2 mL of LA or intra-articular injections with 1.5 mL of LA and steroid.[172] In the 26 pairs who completed the study, 12 reported MBBs to be more beneficial at their 1-month follow-up, 11 reported intra-articular injection to be better, and 3 reported no difference between the two. In the second study, Marks and coworkers randomized 86 LBP patients to receive either intra-articular injections or MBBs using 2 mL of LA and steroid.[171] Although no immediate post-

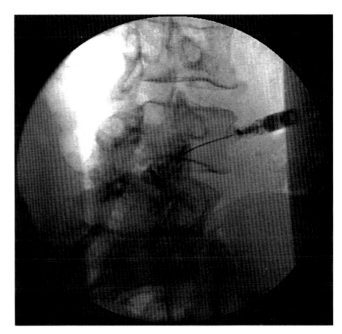

Figure 56–11. Oblique fluoroscopic image demonstrating right-sided L4-5 intra-articular facet joint block.

procedural difference was noted, patients in the intra-articular group experienced better pain relief at 1 month. At 3 months, however, no difference was noted.

It is difficult to draw conclusions based on these comparative studies because of the multitude of design flaws, the most prominent being the lack of a definitive diagnosis in the study populations. Studies investigating the prevalence and false-positive rates in chronic LBP patients (see Table 56–2) found comparable diagnostic value for MBB and intra-articular injections. Only one of three placebo-controlled studies evaluating the outcomes of lumbar RF denervation using intra-articular injections to "confirm" facetogenic pain demonstrated positive outcomes,[174-176] whereas the only study that screened patients with MBBs showed a positive outcome.[177] In a prospective randomized study comparing lumbar facet cryodenervation success rates between patients who underwent medial branch and pericapsular lumbar facet screening blocks, Birkenmaier and associates[178] found superior outcomes up to 6-months postprocedure in the MBB group. However, the excessive volumes used during both diagnostic procedures, the absence of controlled blocks, and the lack of proven validity for pericapsular injections all detract from the authors' conclusions.

Intra-articular injections can be technically more challenging, especially in the steep, frontally oriented thoracic facet joints. In addition, MBBs involve anesthetization of the nerves to be lesioned, and hence may serve as a "dry run" before the definitive treatment. Given the lack of evidence for intra-articular injections as a superior diagnostic tool and the technical ease of performing MBBs, it seems logical to use MBBs as a prognostic tool for subsequent denervation (Figs. 56–12 and 56–13).

False-Positive Blocks

Numerous studies have found a high false-positive rate of diagnostic facet blocks that appears to be unaffected by the type of block used (i.e., intra-articular or MBB). Rates have ranged from 25% to 40% in the lumbar spine,[128,131,132,136] 58% in the thoracic spine,[143] and 27% to 63% in the cervical spine.[41,136,144,151,179,180] Lord and colleagues conducted a randomized, double-blind study evaluating 50

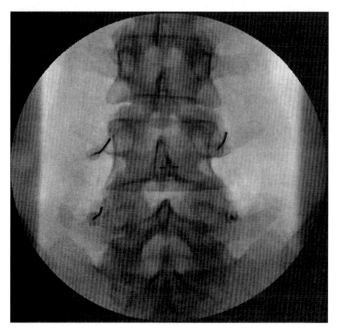

Figure 56–12. Anteroposterior fluoroscopic image demonstrating bilateral L3 and L4 medial branch blocks.

patients with chronic neck pain following an MVA with serial cervical MBB using normal saline, lidocaine, and bupivacaine in random order.[180] The authors found that the use of serial blocks using lidocaine and bupivacaine had a high degree of specificity (88%) but only marginal sensitivity (54%). Although a high specificity will result in a low false-positive rate, the low sensitivity predisposes patients to a false-negative diagnosis.

The reasons for false-positive facet blocks are multifactorial and include placebo-response (18% to 32%) to diagnostic interventions, use of sedation, the liberal use of superficial LA, and the spread of injectate to other pain-generating structures.[181] Although some investigators have disputed this assertion,[182-184] it is our belief that not only opioids but also sedatives such as midazolam can lead to false-positive blocks by interfering with the interpretation of analgesic response (i.e., preventing patients from engaging in normal activities) and by virtue of their muscle-relaxant properties.[185] If sedation is used, however, stricter standards for a positive block must be applied. Manchikanti and coworkers[184] showed that the administration of midazolam or fentanyl in the diagnosis of cervical facet joint pain using a double-block paradigm could be a confounding factor when 50% or greater pain relief was used as the cutoff for a positive response. However, when 80% or greater pain relief was used as the threshold for a positive response, the effect of sedation on validity was low. A recent large, multicenter study by Cohen and colleagues found no difference in lumbar facet denervation outcomes between patients who obtained more than 50% and those who obtained more than 80% pain relief after single diagnostic MBB.[186] In a recent survey of 500 patients scheduled for facet blocks or epidurals

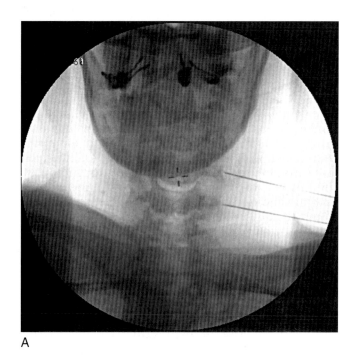

A

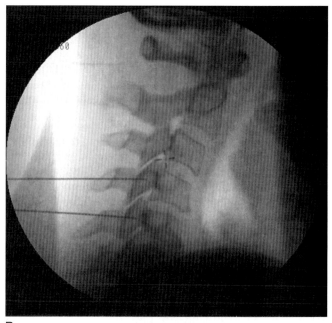

B

Figure 56–13. A, Anteroposterior and **B,** lateral fluoroscopic images demonstrating right-sided C4 and C5 medial branch blocks.

at an outpatient spine center, Cucuzzella and associates found that only 17% requested sedation.[187]

Even in patients with symptomatology consistent with unambiguous pathology, diagnostic blocks may lack specificity. North and coworkers conducted a prospective study on 33 patients with L5 or S1 radiculopathy and radiologic evidence of ongoing nerve root compression.[188] All patients underwent a battery of LA blocks that included selective nerve root block, sciatic nerve block, MBB, and subcutaneous control injections. The authors found that approximately 90% of patients obtained almost complete pain relief following the selective nerve root block, 70% obtained almost complete relief after the sciatic block, and a majority received at least 50% pain relief after the MBB. In contrast, the median degree of pain relief after the subcutaneous injection was around 30%. The authors concluded that uncontrolled LA blocks lack specificity in the diagnostic evaluation of referred pain syndromes.

Dreyfuss and associates used postprocedural CT scans following 120 fluoroscopically guided lumbar MBBs to assess specificity and contrast spread.[29] Two target points were chosen: one at the superomedial border of the transverse process, and a second lower site midway between the upper border of the transverse process and the mamilloaccessory ligament. In 16% of injections, contrast was noted to spread into the intervertebral foramen or epidural space, occurring more commonly at cephalad lumbar levels. When the lower target point was used, spread into the adjacent neural structures occurred only when the needle was inadvertently placed too high. In all cases, distal spread was noted into the cleavage plane between the multifidus and longissimus muscles. The injectate volume of 0.5 mL bathed the target in every case. The authors concluded that lower volumes may be adequate for MBB, and that using a more caudad target point may increase the specificity of lumbar MBB.

Following up on the Dreyfuss study, Cohen and colleagues[189] sought to determine whether spread into the epidural space or intervertebral foramina could account for a false-positive MBB by examining the relationship between clinical signs of radiculopathy, discographic findings, and RF outcomes in 78 patients with positive MBB who went on to fail RF denervation.[189] The authors found a negative correlation between discogenic pain and failed RF denervation, and no association between radicular pain and RF treatment outcomes. In contrast, a trend was noted whereby patients with failed back surgery syndrome experienced worse outcomes after facet denervation. The authors concluded that myofascial pain might be a significant cause of false-positive MBBs.

The evidence that the inadvertent treatment of myofascial pain may be a significant cause of false-positive MBB is circumstantial but multifaceted. In their large multicenter epidemiologic study involving more than 2000 patients, Long and colleagues found myofascial pain to be the second most common

cause of chronic LBP after herniated disk.[123] Controlled studies conducted in chronic LBP patients have shown efficacy for both muscle relaxants and low-volume botulinum toxin injections, and electromyographic evidence of increased paraspinal muscle activity compared with matched controls.[190-193] Ackerman and associates tested the hypothesis as to whether myofascial pain could account for the high rate of false-positive facet blocks in a double-blind study conducted in 75 men with chronic LBP.[194] Subjects received either intra-articular facet injections or MBB using two techniques, one in which LA was used to provide superficial anesthesia down to the target point, and a second in which saline was injected as the needle was advanced. The authors found that the incidence of postprocedure pain relief was significantly higher in patients who had LA injected into their musculature than in those who received saline injected superficially. The injection of LA into the skin and soft tissues may also reduce LBP by means other than the inadvertent treatment of myofascial pain. In studies by Woolf and colleagues, the authors found that the superficial injection of even small amounts of lidocaine reduced nociceptive behavior in animal models of neuropathic pain, a finding attributed to the systemic absorption of the sodium channel blocker (Box 56–1).[195,196]

In an effort to reduce the amount of superficial anesthesia used for MBB, Stojanovic and colleagues introduced a single-needle technique whereby multiple medial branches are blocked using a single skin entry point.[197] In a prospective crossover study comparing the single-needle and conventional multiple-needle techniques, the authors found the single-needle technique required significantly less superficial LA, resulted in less procedure-related pain, and was quicker to perform than the multiple-needle approach.[198] With regard to final needle position, contrast spread, and postprocedure pain relief, no differences were noted between the two techniques (Fig. 56–14).

BOX 56–1. INTERVENTIONS THAT MAY REDUCE THE INCIDENCE OF FALSE-POSITIVE LUMBAR FACET BLOCKS

---

1. Perform placebo-controlled blocks, or if not possible, comparative local anesthetic blocks.
2. Aim for a lower target point on the transverse process.
3. Reduce injectate volume to ≤0.5 mL.
4. Be judicious with the use of superficial anesthesia.
5. Consider a single-needle approach.
6. Consider using computed tomography guidance when doing intra-articular injections in patients with severe spondylosis.
7. Avoid the use of sedation or intravenous opioids.

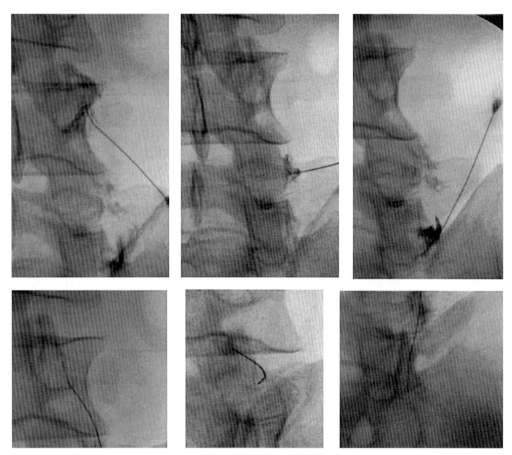

Figure 56–14. Anteroposterior fluoroscopic image showing contrast spread for L3 *(left)*, L4 *(middle)*, and L5 *(right)* medial branch blocks using the single-needle technique. Bottom figures show needle placement in an oblique fluoroscopic view for the same blocks.

False-Negative Blocks

The potential for a false-negative result from diagnostic lumbar facet injections has been estimated to be 11%.[199] This may be a result of a multitude of factors, although the predominant mechanism(s) remains unclear. Venous uptake of LA has been reported to occur in 8% of lumbar facet blocks in one study[29] and 33% in another.[199] It is believed that even following needle repositioning after positive venous aspiration, the false-negative rate may be as high as 50%. Therefore some experts suggest that if aspiration is positive during diagnostic facet blocks, it might be more advantageous to abort the procedure and repeat it later than risk a false-negative result.[199] Another factor that may play a significant role in a false-negative response is aberrant innervation from nerves other than branches of the dorsal rami.

Should Single or Double Diagnostic Blocks Be Used?

As noted, false-positive rates have been found to be as high as 63% for cervical, 53% for thoracic, and 27% for lumbar facet blocks.[136] Therefore numerous experts have advocated performing double blocks, using either saline controls or two different LAs, before proceeding to RF denervation.[128,132,133,136,148,200]

Yet this is seldom done in clinical practice, and there are no studies comparing outcomes or cost-benefit ratios between using single or double blocks. In an uncontrolled study assessing outcomes from medial branch denervation following comparative LA blocks, Dreyfuss and coworkers found that 60% of the 15 patients who proceeded with radiofrequency lesioning obtained at least 90% pain relief at 12 months, and 87% achieved at least 60% relief.[135] The criterion for participation in this study was at least 80% concordant pain relief following lidocaine and bupivacaine MBB. However, 460 patients were interviewed for this study, and after history, physical examination, and record review, only 41 were chosen to participate. If single blocks or less stringent criteria had been used, the success rate of RF denervation would probably have been lower, but the total number of successful treatments would have undoubtedly been higher.

A number of factors must be considered when determining the need for comparative LA blocks, including the patient's relative risk for a false-positive or false-negative diagnostic block, the complication rate of each diagnostic and RF procedure, the anticipated dropout rate, and cost effectiveness. Neuritis is the most common complication of medial branch RF denervation. Yet the incidence is low (<5%),[201] and can be reduced even further with the preemptive of steroid or pentoxifylline.[202] Therefore the serious complication rate associated with both diagnostic MBB and RF denervation is essentially the same. In a theoretical, systematic study examining the cost-effectiveness of using controlled facet blocks, Bogduk and Holmes[203] determined that the use of placebo-controlled injections in the cervical region cannot be justified in the United States based on financial considerations, and in only some circumstances can be justified for lumbar z-joint blocks. Given that a substantial percentage of patients will respond with long-term pain relief even to sham denervations,[175,176] it is unlikely that the routine use of confirmatory facet blocks will become standard of care anytime soon.

TREATMENT

Conservative Treatment and Pharmacotherapy

A multimodal approach for the treatment of facetogenic pain is essential. Although many patients presenting to interventional pain medicine clinics will receive a procedural approach to therapy, there is value in conservative therapy, medical management, and when indicated, psychotherapy. Pharmacotherapy and noninterventional treatments for spinal pain have been investigated, but no study has evaluated these alternatives specifically in patients with facet pain. Tailored exercise programs and yoga have been shown to reduce pain and prevent relapses in patients with chronic LBP.[204-207] Osteopathic manipulation has shown mixed results, with two studies indicating moderate relief for LBP patients[208,209] and another showing no difference between true and sham manipulations.[210] For subacute neck and back pain, a randomized study comparing conservative care (i.e., physical and pharmacotherapy) alone to conservative care with osteopathic manipulation three or four times per week found improved outcomes in the combined therapy group at 2 months but not 6 months postintervention.[211] In addition, some randomized trials have found significant benefit with acupuncture and acupressure in chronic low back and neck pain.[212-216] Similar to manipulation, however, one of the largest and most methodologically sound studies found no difference between true and sham acupuncture.[217]

Nonsteroidal anti-inflammatory drugs and acetaminophen are widely considered first-line drugs for the treatment of LBP, with little evidence to support one particular drug over another.[218-220] A comprehensive review of published clinical trials evaluating pharmacotherapy in LBP by Schnitzer and associates[221] found strong evidence for the use of antidepressants for chronic LBP and muscle relaxants in acute LBP. In addition to LBP, skeletal muscle relaxants have also shown efficacy in controlled trials for neck pain.[222] There is little doubt that untreated psychopathology can adversely affect back and neck pain treatment outcomes.[223,224] In a study by Polatin and colleagues[225] conducted in 200 chronic LBP patients, the authors found that 77% met lifetime criteria and 59% demonstrated current symptoms for at least one psychiatric diagnosis, with the most common being depression, substance abuse, and anxiety disorders.[223] In the only study assessing the influence of psychopathology on facet interventions, Lilius and coworkers[226] found a strong correlation between a negative response to intra- and periarticular LA and steroid injections and inappropriate signs and symptoms. The authors concluded that high levels of inappropriate signs and symptoms may be more indicative of psychosocial pathology than organic pathology.

The optimal management of facet joint pain should encompass both noninterventional and interventional treatment, although clinicians are encouraged to exercise caution when extrapolating the results of studies conducted in patients with nonspecific back and neck pain to those with clear-cut z-joint pathology.

Intra-articular Steroid Injections

There is some controversy regarding the use of intra-articular LA and steroid injections for the diagnosis and treatment of facet pain. In uncontrolled studies, the long-term relief of LBP after intra-articular steroid injection ranges from 18% to 63%, with most of these studies being conducted in patients who did not undergo previous diagnostic z-joint blocks.[120,122,123,125,126,161,227] Other studies have reported intermediate-term pain relief after intra-articular LA alone[146] and hyaluronic acid.[228]

Results in controlled trials have been mixed at best (Table 56–7). In a large study, Lilius and coworkers[229] found no significant difference in outcomes between 109 patients who received large-volume (8 mm) LA and steroid injected into two joints, the same mixture administered around the joints, or physiologic saline. In another study comparing intra-articular steroid and saline in 97 patients with chronic LBP, Carette and associates found a statistically significant benefit only at the 6-month mark in the steroid group.[230] Although this was a large and methodologically sound study whereby patients were prescreened with diagnostic intra-articular LA blocks, the control group received intra-articular normal saline. Normal saline has been shown on multiple occasions to provide better pain relief than a true placebo for a variety of invasive procedures.[231-233] Barnsley and colleagues randomized 41 patients with chronic neck pain following a motor vehicle accident to receive 1 mL of either intra-articular bupivacaine or betamethasone under double-blind conditions.[234] The median time to return of 50% of the patient's preinjection pain was 3 days in the steroid group and 3.5 days in the local anesthetic group, with less than one half of patients reporting pain relief greater than 1 week. All patients in this study were prescreened for cervical z-joint pain using comparative MBB.

Table 56–7. Prospective, Clinical Trials Evaluating Intra-articular Steroid Injections for Lumbar and Cervical Facet Joint Pain

AUTHOR, YEAR, METHODOLOGY SCORE	PATIENTS AND INTERVENTIONS	RESULTS	COMMENTS
Lynch and Taylor,[305] 1986; MQ score = 0*	50 patients with chronic low back pain underwent attempted intra-articular steroid injections at 2 most caudal lumbar z-joints. Failed "extra-articular" injections designated as "control" group.	Relief of pain at 2 wk and 6 mo was better in patients who had 2 intra-articular injections than the other groups. Patients who had 1 intra-articular injection had better relief than those who had no successful injections.	Flaws include lack of randomization, poor outcome assessment, failure to identify patients based on diagnostic injections, and failure to blind the examining physician.
Lilius et al, 1989[229]; MQ score = 1	109 patients with unilateral chronic LBP received 8 mL of LA and steroid injected into 2 lumbar z-joints (n = 28), around 2 joints (n = 39), or 8 mL of NS into 2 joints (n = 42).	All 3 groups demonstrated significant improvement in pain scores (at 3 mo), disability scores, clinical exam findings, and return to work at 6 wk postinjection. No differences were noted on any variable among groups.	Patients were not diagnosed with lumbar z-joint pain before injection. Large volumes used rendered injections nonspecific. Large standards of deviation were found for variables measured. Other flaws include suboptimal outcomes measures and lack of a blinded observer. Pain scores measured at 3 mo by questionnaire.
Nash, 1990[172]; MQ score = 2	67 patients with chronic LBP were randomized by pairs to receive either 1.5 mL of intra-articular LA and steroid or MBB with 2 mL of LA.	At 1-mo follow-up, 12 pairs reported MBB to be more beneficial, 11 reported intra-articular injection to be better, and 3 reported no difference.	11 patients lost to follow-up. Flaws include not using lumbar z-joint blocks for diagnosis, lack of a blinded observer, poor outcome measures, and no true control group.
Carette et al,[230] 1991[172]; MQ score = 5	97 patients with chronic LBP who reported immediate relief after LA facet injections received either 2 mL of steroid and saline (n = 49) or saline (n = 48) into L4-5 and L5-S1 lumbar z-joints.	42% of patients who received steroid and 33% who received placebo reported marked improvement for up to 3 mo (P = ns). At 6 mo the steroid group reported less pain and disability. Only 22% of patients in steroid group and 10% in placebo group had sustained improvement thru 6 mo.	Differences between groups at 6 mo reduced when cointerventions were taken into account. Although this is the only study that identified study patients based on diagnostic injections, these injections were not "controlled." NS is known to provide pain relief greater than that expected from placebo.
Marks et al, 1992[171]; MQ score = 3	86 patients with chronic LBP were randomized to receive either 1.5 mL of steroid and LA MBB or intra-articular injections (2 mL at lowest level).	Patients who had facet joint injections had better pain relief than those who had MBB at all follow-up visits up to 3 mo, but this was only significant at 1-month review.	Flaws include no true control group, failure to identify patients based on diagnostic injections, no monitoring of cointerventions, lack of a blinded observer, and poor outcome assessment.
Barnsley et al, 1994[234]; MQ score = 5	41 patients with chronic neck pain following MVA were randomized to receive either 1 mL of 0.5% bupivacaine or 5.7 mg betamethasone into painful cervical z-joints diagnosed by comparative LA MBB.	Less than half the patients reported relief for more than 1 wk, and fewer than 1 in 5 patients reported relief for more than 1 mo, irrespective of treatment group. Median time to return of 50% of preprocedure pain was 3 days in steroid group and 3.5 in LA group (P = ns).	All patients with neck pain following whiplash injury. May be different than chronic neck pain of other etiologies. Some patients with long-lasting benefit in both groups.
Fuchs et al, 2005[228]; MQ score = 1	60 patients with chronic LBP were randomized to receive either 1 mL of hyaluronic acid (HA) or steroid into the 3 lowest facet joints at weekly intervals times 6.	Patients who received HA injections experienced a 40% decrease in pain scores vs. a 56% reduction in those who received steroid (P = ns). Greatest pain reduction observed 3 mo post-treatment in HA group and 1 wk post-treatment in steroid group.	Inclusion criteria included at least moderate facet degeneration on radiologic imaging. Flaws include lack of a control group, failure to identify patients based on diagnostic injections, no monitoring of cointerventions, and multiple injections.
Pneumaticos et al, 2006[240]; MQ score = 3	47 patients with chronic LBP worse and radiologic evidence of lumbar z-joint abnormalities were randomized in a 2:1 ratio to undergo intra-articular LA and steroid injections (3 mL) based on SPECT scans or physical exam.	1 mo postinjection, 87% of patients with positive SPECT had significant pain improvement vs. 12.5% of patients with negative SPECT and 31% of patients who underwent injections based on physical exam.	Differences remained significant at 3 mo but not 6 mo postinjection. Pain scores obtained by mailed questionnaire. No functional assessment done. Use of SPECT was cost-effective.

*Methodologic quality (MQ) score based on the 5-point Jadad scale.[308] A score of ≥3 indicates high methodologic quality.
LA, local anesthetic; LBP, low back pain; MVA, motor vehicle accident; MBB, medial branch block; ns, not significant; SPECT, single photon emission computed tomography; z-joint, zygapophysial (facet) joint.

In six recent review articles, the authors have been evenly split as to the efficacy of intra-articular steroids.[128,200,235-238] Given the basic science studies demonstrating inflammatory mediators around degenerated facet joints,[18,19] we believe that intra-articular steroid injections may provide intermediate-term relief to a small subset of patients with an actively inflamed z-joint. Evidence to support this assertion is bolstered by several recent prospective and observational studies evaluating low to intermediate volume (1 to 3 mL) LA and steroid intra-articular lumbar facet joint injections performed in more than 160 patients with axial LBP.[167,239,240] In these studies patients with positive single photon emission computed tomography (SPECT) experienced dramatically better pain relief (>75% success rate) compared with those with negative or no single photon emission computed tomography (<40% success rate) up to 3 months postinjection. In the two studies that followed patients for 6 months postinjection, the beneficial effect wore off after the 3-month evaluation.[167,240] Radionuclide bone scintigraphy is capable of depicting synovial changes caused by inflammation, degenerative changes associated with bone remodeling, and increased metabolic function. In addition to radiological evidence of joint inflammation and degeneration, intra-articular steroid injections may be more effective in those patients who obtain definitive pain relief following a diagnostic screening block, and when LA is added to the injectate.

Therapeutic Medial Branch Blocks

In a series of prospective randomized evaluations of repeat therapeutic MBB with LA, LA plus Sarapin (pitcher plant extract), LA plus steroid, and LA plus steroid and Sarapin, Manchikanti and colleagues reported significant relief in all groups for up to 1 year in lumbar,[241] thoracic,[242] and cervical facet pain.[243] Patients in the studies were screened with comparative LA blocks. There were no differences found with either the addition of steroid or Sarapin to the LA. Whereas a small group of patients may derive extended relief from repeated MBBs, other studies have failed to corroborate these findings.[171,172] Nevertheless, there is likely a small subset of patients that will receive sustained benefit following LA MBB.

Radiofrequency Denervation

The first description of percutaneous RF for treatment of the "intervertebral disk syndrome" was by Rees in 1971.[244] Notwithstanding his greater than 99% reported success rate, it remains a subject of controversy as to whether his technique actually achieved "facet rhizolysis" because the instrument he used may not have been long enough to accomplish anything more than a myofasciotomy.[245] The technique of percutaneous RF lesioning is generally credited to Shealy, who was motivated by what he perceived to be an unacceptably high incidence of

local hemorrhagic complications.[246,247] Subsequently, it has been used to treat different forms of spinal pain, including whiplash,[248] sacroiliac joint pain,[140,249] discogenic pain[250] and intractable sciatica.[251] There are many uncontrolled trials touting the benefits of RF denervation for facet pain.[252] For lumbar facet RF denervation, most studies report sustained relief in 50% to 80% of patients without previous back surgery,[169,252-258] whereas 35% to 50% of subjects with failed back surgery syndrome obtain prolonged relief.[169,259-261] In the only study reporting outcomes based on prior surgery for cervical z-joint denervation, Cohen and coworkers found no difference in success rates between patients with failed neck surgery syndrome and those who had never undergone surgery.[116]

Only five placebo-controlled studies have been conducted evaluating RF denervation for lumbar z-joint pain (Table 56–8). In the first study, King and Lagger randomized 60 patients with low back and leg pain to receive empirical (without stimulation) RF denervation of the dorsal rami, an RF lesion made in the muscle, or a sham lesion after electrical stimulation.[245] At their 6-month follow-up, 27% of patients in the facet denervation group experienced satisfactory pain relief versus 53% in the myotomy group and 0% in the sham group. The main criticism in this study is that no diagnostic blocks were performed to screen people for lumbar z-joint pain. More than 15 years later, Gallagher and associates randomized 41 patients based on their response to diagnostic intra-articular blocks (equivocal or good response) to either sham or true denervation.[174] A statistically significant difference in outcomes was observed at 1 month only between sham and true RF denervation in those patients who obtained a definitive response to diagnostic blocks. This difference persisted for the duration of the 6-month follow-up period. In the smallest but most methodologically sound study among the five controlled trials, van Kleef and colleagues found a 46% pain reduction in the RF lesion group versus an 8% reduction in the placebo group.[177] At the 12-month follow-up, 7 of 15 patients continued to have a successful outcome versus only 2 of 16 in the sham group. Leclaire and coworkers conducted a placebo-controlled study in 70 patients with a putative diagnosis of facet arthropathy.[175] At their 4-week follow-up, the only outcome variable that favored the treatment group was an improvement in the mean Roland-Morris disability score. At 12 weeks no difference was noted between groups for pain levels or any measure of functional capacity. The key flaw in this study is that the authors used "significant pain relief lasting more than 24 h" after an intra-articular injection of LA and steroid as their main inclusion criterion. In addition to being ambiguous, the 24-hour threshold is inconsistent with the pharmacodynamics of lidocaine. In the largest controlled study evaluating RF denervation, van Wijk and colleagues[176] found the only difference between the treatment and control groups at three months was that more RF patients reported a greater than 50% diminution in back pain

Table 56–8. Outcomes for Randomized Controlled Studies Assessing Medial Branch Radiofrequency Denervation for Lumbar and Cervical Facet Joint Pain

STUDY, YEAR	NUMBER AND TYPE OF PATIENTS	FOLLOW-UP PERIOD AND METHODOLOGIC* SCORES	RESULTS	COMMENTS
King and Lagger, 1976[245]	60 patients with chronic low back and leg pain, and paraspinal tenderness were randomized to 3 groups. Group 1 had RF denervation of the primary posterior ramus, group 2 had RF performed using a 1.25-inch needle inserted within the area of maximum tenderness (assumed to be a myotomy), and group 3 received stimulation but no coagulation (control).	6 mo MQ = 2 CR = 5	In group 1, 27% had ≥50% relief at 6 mo vs. 53% in group 2 and 0% in group 3.	Did not use diagnostic blocks before randomization. Likely included many patients with sciatica. In some patients, 1.25 inches may be sufficient to reach medial branch. Used 120-sec lesion; 3 lesions were empirically made without electrical stimulation.
Gallagher et al, 1994[174]	Subjects were 41 patients with chronic LBP who obtained "clear-cut or equivocal" relief from single intra-articular facet joint injections with LA and steroid; 18 patients with a good response and 6 patients with an equivocal response underwent RF denervation; 12 patients with a good response and 5 with an equivocal response underwent sham denervation.	6 mo MQ = 2 CR = 6	Significant differences in pain scores noted only between patients with a good response to LA blocks who underwent true RF denervation (n = 18) and those with a good response who underwent sham treatment (n = 12). Differences were noted 1 and 6 mo after procedures.	Did not define "good" or "equivocal" response to diagnostic injections. Anatomic landmarks not well described. Observer not blinded. Electrode not placed parallel to nerve. In "Methods" stated only LA used, but in abstract stated LA and steroid were used. Used 90-sec lesions.
van Kleef et al, 1999[177]	Subjects were 31 patients with chronic LBP who obtained ≥50% pain relief after a single MBB (1 dropout). Compared true denervation with sham.	12 mo MQ = 5 CR = 8	After 3 mo, 9 of 15 patients in lesion group vs. 4 of 16 in sham group had ≥50% pain relief. At 1-yr follow-up, 7/15 in lesion group and 2/16 in sham group had ≥50% relief.	Used 0.75 mL of injectate for diagnostic blocks. Electrode not placed perpendicular to target nerve. Used multifidus rather than sensory stimulation to identify medial branch. Used 60-sec lesions.
Sanders and Zuurmond, 1999[309]	Subjects were 34 patients with chronic LBP who obtained ≥50% relief after single intra-articular injection with lidocaine. Half the patients received medial branch RF denervation and half intra-articular denervation.	3 mo MQ = 1 CR = 6	Both groups improved at 3-mo, but intra-articular denervation group improved more than medial branch RF group.	Used 1 mL for diagnostic blocks. Medial branch lesions done at inferolateral aspect of facet capsule and upper border of transverse process; 3 intra-articular facet lesions done. Used 60-sec lesions.

Study	Methods	Duration / MQ / CR	Results	Comments
Leclaire et al, 2001[175]	Subjects were 70 patients with chronic LBP who obtained "significant" pain relief lasting more than 24 hr after single intra-articular facet injection with lidocaine and steroid (4 dropouts). Compared true denervation with sham.	12 wk MQ = 4 CR = 8	At 4 wk there were modest improvements in Roland-Morris ($P = 0.05$) and VAS pain scores (P = ns), but not Oswestry score. No difference in any outcome measure at 12 wk.	Did not define "significant pain relief" with diagnostic injection. Inclusion criteria of greater than 24-hr pain relief is inconsistent with pharmacology of lidocaine. Performed 2 lesions, each for 90 sec. Anatomic landmarks not noted. Electrode not placed parallel to nerve.
Van Wijk et al, 2005[176]	81 patients with chronic LBP who obtained ≥50% pain relief after 2-level intra-articular facet injection with LA (no dropouts). Compared true denervation with sham.	12 mo MQ = 5 CR = 7	Combined outcome measure (pain score, physical activity and analgesic intake) showed no differences between groups at 3 mo. VAS pain score improved in both groups at 3 mo. Global perceived effect was greater in treatment than sham group at 3 mo.	Blinding ended at 3 mo in more than 70% of patients. Improvement in pain scores persisted throughout 12-mo follow-up. Used 60-sec lesions.
Lord et al, 1996[248]	24 patients (12 per group) with neck pain lasting more than 3 mo after MVA and failed conservative treatment. Included patients with positive response to placebo-controlled, diagnostic blocks. Randomized to have true RF at 80° C for 90 sec or 37° C (placebo treatment) between C3-C7° according to their response to diagnostic blocks.	3 mo (12 mo in patients with persistent relief) MQ = 5 CR = 8	Mean time to return of 50% of preoperative pain was 263 days in RF group and 8 days in placebo group ($p = 0.04$). At 27 wk, 7 patients in RF group and 1 in control group remained pain-free.	Excluded patients with solely C2-3 facet pain. Five patients in RF group with numbness in territory of treated nerves.
Stovner et al, 2004[115]	12 patients with unilateral cervicogenic HA received comparative LA blocks and a greater occipital nerve block. Randomized to cervical facet RF or sham procedure.	24 mo MQ = 4 CR = 7	At 3 mo, 4 of 6 RF patients had meaningful clinical response (≥30% improvement) as did 2 of the 6 in the sham group. 6 mo postprocedure, no differences noted between groups. Concluded cervical facet denervation is not effective for cervicogenic HA.	RF group had better response to diagnostic blocks. Only able to recruit 12 patients in 2.9 yr. Excluded patients with ongoing litigation.

*Methodologic quality (MQ) score based on the 5-point Jadad scale.[308] A score of ≥3 indicates high methodologic quality. Clinical relevance (CR) score based on patient selection parameters and RF technique description (0-9 scale) as described by Geurts et al.[295]

HA, headache; LA, local anesthetic; LBP, low back pain; MBB, medial branch block; MVA, motor vehicle accident; ns = not significant; R, radiofrequency; VAS, Visual Analogue Scale.

than sham patients (62% vs. 39%). For mean reduction in Visual Analogue Scale (VAS) pain scores, change in analgesic intake, and functional assessments, no differences were noted between groups.

A key flaw to many of these studies is the failure to select patients based on placebo-controlled or comparative LA blocks. In addition, needle positioning was likely suboptimal. Dreyfuss and associates[135] conducted the only placebo-controlled study evaluating outcomes from lumbar facet radiofrequency denervation in which patients were diagnosed with facet pain based on concordant response to serial LA blocks. They reported that 87% of 15 patients obtained at least 60% relief 12-months status post-radiofrequency denervation, with 60% of patients achieving at least 90% relief.

Whereas some may construe these findings as evidence that RF denervation is a fundamentally flawed treatment, a more plausible interpretation is that they indicate a strong need to optimize RF denervation techniques and better identify those candidates likely to obtain positive outcomes. Several investigators have determined that placing the electrode parallel, rather than perpendicular to the target nerve substantially increases the size of the lesion, thereby reducing the likelihood the treatment will miss or only partially coagulate the target nerve.[262,263] After a literature review and cadaveric study, Lau and colleagues[263] concluded the ideal electrode position to be along the lateral neck of the superior articular process rather than at the groove between the angle of the superior articular and transverse processes, as was used in most studies.[175,176] Other investigators found the maximal lesion size to be reached within 60 seconds of lesion time,[36,262,264] independent of whether the system is temperature or voltage controlled.[265] Studies conducted in human myocardium determined that irrigation fluid has either no effect or a slightly beneficial effect on lesion size.[266] Hence the use of LA to prevent procedure-related pain or steroid to reduce the incidence of neuritis[202] should theoretically have no adverse effects on the efficacy of RF denervation.

There have only been two randomized, double-blind trials evaluating percutaneous RF denervation for cervical facet pain. Lord and coworkers randomized 24 patients with whiplash injury following an MVA and a positive response to diagnostic, placebo-controlled cervical MBBs to receive either cervical medial branch denervation or a sham procedure.[248] Patients with pain stemming solely from the C2-3 z-joint were excluded. In order to establish a diagnosis of cervical facet pain, a series of three blocks were performed. The first block was done with either lidocaine or bupivacaine, the second block with either normal saline or the other local anesthetic, and the third block with the remaining agent. A block was deemed positive only if the patient had complete relief each time a local anesthetic was used but no relief when normal saline was administered. Except for needle temperature, all therapeutic aspects of the procedures were the same in both groups. The mean time to return to 50% of baseline pain was 263 days in the RF group and 8 days in the placebo group ($p = 0.04$). At 27 weeks, 7 patients in the RF group and 1 patient in the control group remained pain-free. Five of the patients in the RF group had numbness in the territory of the treated nerves, but none considered it troublesome.

In a more recent study, Stovner and associates randomized 12 patients diagnosed with cervicogenic headaches based on clinical symptoms and a positive response to comparative LA blocks to receive either cervical facet RF denervation or a sham procedure.[115] At their 3-month follow-up, 4 of 6 patients in the RF denervation group obtained a meaningful clinical response versus 2 of 6 patients in the sham group. At 6 months no differences were noted between groups. Two years postprocedure, patients in the sham group felt that they had more significant improvement than those in the RF group. The results of sham denervation in this study are comparable with that found in a previous uncontrolled study evaluating RF for cervicogenic headache, in which patients reported a 34% reduction in symptoms.[267] In an open-label prospective study comparing cervical z-joint RF results between litigant and nonlitigant patients with whiplash injuries, Sapir and Gorup found no significant differences between 1-year outcomes.[268] Potential reasons for limited RF success rates for chronic neck pain and cervicogenic headaches include technical difficulty denervating the most frequently affected C2-3 facet joint, concomitant sources of head pain, and the lack of specificity for diagnostic injections. In an observational study conducted in 56 patients with post-traumatic neck pain, provocative discography and MBB were positive at the same level in 41% of patients.[269]

Although there have only been two placebo-controlled trials assessing cervical facet denervation, several uncontrolled studies deserve mention. McDonald and colleagues prospectively studied patients diagnosed with cervical facet pain based on controlled diagnostic blocks, and found that 18 of 28 patients obtained significant pain relief lasting at least 90 days.[270] In those patients with a positive response, the median duration of relief was 421.5 days. A later study by Barnsley measured the duration of pain relief following cervical facet denervation in patients with a positive response to a controlled cervical MBB.[46] In the 45 patients studied, 36 (80%) experienced significant relief, with a mean duration of 36 weeks. In both studies, patients who experienced a good initial response to denervation obtained comparable relief following repeat procedures. In an uncontrolled prospective study involving 40 patients with refractory thoracic pain, Stolker and coworkers obtained good results following thoracic medial branch denervation.[271] Patients were diagnosed with thoracic facet pain based on clinical criteria and a transient response to diagnostic MBB. After 2 months 47.5% of patients were pain-free, 35% reported more than 50% pain relief, and 17.5% experienced minimal or no relief. At an average follow-up of 31 months (18 to 54 months), 44% of patients remained pain-free, 39% continued to have more than 50% pain relief, and 17% had poor outcomes. Although these results are encouraging, the diagnosis of thoracic facet joint pain was made with clinical predictors, which are inherently nonspecific, and single medial branch local anesthetic blocks, which are known to carry a high false-positive rate.[136] In addition, the long-term relief seen in many of the patients is beyond that typically observed in the cervical and lumbar spine.

The use of sensory stimulation to corroborate proximity to the targeted medial branch is another flaw of many RF studies. Generally, a threshold of ≤0.5 volts is deemed sufficient. Although sensory stimulation may indicate proximity to the target nerve at this voltage, it is our experience that many patients perceive concordant stimulation at ≤0.5 volts, even when the electrode is purposefully placed in muscle, as during a sham procedure. An attractive alternative or addition to sensory stimulation in the lumbar spine is to attempt to elicit multifidus muscle contraction because the same medial branch that innervates the lumbar facet joint also supplies this large paraspinal muscle. Both studies in which the medial branch was identified using motor stimulation demonstrated positive outcomes.[135,177]

In a large multicenter outcome study, Cohen and colleagues attempted to identify factors associated with successful RF treatment in 192 patients who underwent denervation at three teaching hospitals after a single, positive MBB.[169] Among the 15 variables analyzed for their association with treatment outcome, only paraspinal tenderness was found to predict a successful treatment. Factors associated with failed treatment included increased pain with hyperextension and axial rotation (i.e., facet loading), duration of pain, and previous back surgery. The latter two variables have been associated with treatment failure not only for radiofrequency denervation but also a host of other LBP interventions including epidural steroid injections and open surgery.[272-274] When pain returns following RF denervation, which typically occurs between 6 months and 1 year, repeated neurotomy can be performed with no diminution in efficacy.[275] In addition to continuous, high-temperature RF medial branch ablation, pulsed RF (2 to 6 months of effective pain relief),[276] cryodenervation (3 to 6 months of pain relief),[178,277-279] and phenol neurolysis[280,281] also have been reported to provide intermediate to long-term pain relief in uncontrolled studies.

Surgery

Surgery is occasionally performed to treat facet arthropathy despite a lack of evidence supporting fusion for degenerative spinal disorders.[282,283] Not surprisingly, the results of studies evaluating the use of lumbar z-joint blocks to predict lumbar arthrodesis outcomes are discouraging (Table 56–9). In the three studies that compared surgical outcomes between facet block responders and nonresponders, all failed to show a difference between groups.[284-286] Bough and associates conducted a retrospective review of 127 facet joints surgically removed from 84 patients in an attempt to correlate histologic evidence of facet degeneration with provocative response to preoperative facet arthrography.[152] Although the authors found the positive predictive value of concordant pain reproduction to be 85%, the negative predictive value was only 43%, leading them to conclude provocative facet arthrography was of little value as a presurgical screening tool. In a prospective case series, Lovely and Rastogi found that 83% of 23 patients who responded to bracing and three successive facet blocks achieved more than 90% pain relief after fusion surgery at the latest follow-up.[287] However, the large volumes used per block, the failure to exclude placebo responders, and the lack of any comparison group undermine the conclusions that can be drawn. One reason patients with lumbar z-joint pain might respond to arthrodesis is because some surgeons, either purposefully or inadvertently, perform medial branch rhizotomies during pedicle screw placement. In summary, there is no convincing evidence to support any surgical intervention for lumbar z-joint pain aside from that resulting from a traumatic dislocation.

COMPLICATIONS

Serious complications and side effects are extremely uncommon after facet interventions. The metabolic and endocrine sequelae of intrafacetal depot steroids have not been studied, but extrapolating from epidural steroid injections one would expect suppression of the hypothalamic-pituitary-adrenal axis lasting up to 4 weeks depending on the depot steroid used, and impaired insulin sensitivity manifesting as elevated glucose levels for less than a week.[288,289] Although rare, a host of infections have been reported after intra-articular injections including septic arthritis, epidural abscess, and meningitis.[290-292] Case reports of spinal anesthesia and postdural puncture headache also have been published.[293,294]

Numbness or dysesthesias have been reported after RF denervation, but tend to be transient and self-limiting.[36,249-257,259-266,272-281,288-297] Burns are rare with RF procedures and may result from electrical faults, insulation breaks in the electrodes, and generator malfunction.[246,256,257] The most common complication following facet joint RF is neuritis, with a reported incidence of less than 5%.[201] In one study the administration of corticosteroid or pentoxifylline was found to reduce the incidence of postprocedure pain following RF denervation.[202] There is also a theoretical risk of thermal injury to the ventral rami if an electrode slips ventrally over the lumbar transverse process.

Table 56–9. Studies Evaluating the Ability of Lumbar Facet Blocks to Predict Operative Results

AUTHOR, YEAR	PATIENTS AND METHODS	RESULTS	COMMENTS
Esses et al, 1989[310]	Prospective study evaluating the value of external fixation to predictive fusion outcome in 35 patients; 14 patients underwent preoperative facet blocks.	Among the 9 patients who reported temporary relief from facet blocks, 5 experienced relief from external fixation. In the 5 patients who had no relief with facet blocks, 4 experienced relief after fixation.	Study not designed to assess value of facet blocks in predicting outcome of spinal fixation.
Bough et al, 1990[152]	Retrospective study comparing results of surgical pathology and preoperative provocative facet arthrography in 84 patients who underwent spinal fusion.	The specificity of pain provocation for facet disease was 75%, sensitivity 59%, positive predictive value 85%, and negative predictive value 43%. The authors concluded symptom provocation during facet arthrography was of little value as a surgical screening tool.	Histopathology results reviewed for 127 lumbar z-joints. Clinical outcomes not discussed.
Jackson, 1992[311]	Retrospective review involving 36 patients who underwent posterolateral lumbar fusion after facet injections.	Both groups improved after fusion. The 26 patients who responded favorably to facet injections did no better clinically than the 10 patients who did not.	Mean follow-up 6.1 yr. Response to injection not a consideration for fusion.
Esses and Moro, 1993[285]	Retrospective review involving the results of spinal fusion (*n* = 82) and nonoperative treatment (*n* = 44) in 126 patients who underwent facet blocks.	15% of patients had complete relief, 41% partial relief, and 44% no relief after lumbar z-joint blocks. Response to facet blocks not predictive of surgical or nonsurgical success.	296 patients underwent facet blocks during index period, but only 126 had follow-up (mean 4.6 yr).
Lovely and Rastogi, 1997[265, 287]	Prospective case series involving 91 patients who responded to bracing and underwent 197 facet blocks. 28 patients who obtained greater than 70% pain relief on 3 separate occasions underwent spinal fusion.	Fusion was technically successful 77% of time; 83% of patients reported ≥90% relief, and 13% reported partial relief.	Mean follow-up 32 mo. No comparison group who either failed or did not receive preoperative lumbar z-joint blocks. Used 3-5 mL injectate per facet level.

z-joint, zygapophysial (facet) joint.

CONCLUSION

Pain originating from the facet joints has long been recognized as a potential source of back and neck pain. Anatomic studies suggest that with aging, the lumbar facet joints become weaker and their orientation changes from coronal to sagittal positioning, predisposing them to injury from rotational stress. The three most caudal lumbar facet joints—L3-4, L4-5 and L5-S1—are exposed to the greatest strain during lateral bending and forward flexion, and are thus more prone to repetitive strain, inflammation, joint hypertrophy, and osteophyte formation. In patients with chronic neck pain, the C2-3 and C5-6 facet joints are most commonly affected. Osteoarthritis of the facet joints is commonly found in association with degenerative disk disease. The exact prevalence of facet disease is unclear but may be as high as 10% to 15% in patients with axial LBP, 49% to 60% in patients with chronic neck pain, and 42% to 48% in patients with axial mid-back pain.

There are no discrete historical and physical findings pathognomonic for lumbar, thoracic, or cervical facet arthropathy. The referral patterns for pain arising from the facet joints at different levels overlap considerably. In addition to axial LBP, pathology arising from the lower facet joints is associated with referred pain to the buttock, thigh, groin, and sometimes lower leg, whereas that referred from the upper lumbar facet joints extends into the flank, hip, groin, and lateral thigh. Cervical facet disease tends to refer pain to the neck, head, shoulders, and mid-back. Reports on the correlation between CT and MRI evidence of facet arthropathy and the response to diagnostic lumbar facet blocks are conflicting. Because the facet joint is innervated by the medial branches arising from the posterior rami of the spinal nerve at the same level and a level above the joint, LA blocks of these nerves have been advocated for diagnostic and prognostic purposes. Intra-articular facet injections with LA also have been proposed as a method for diagnosing facet joint pain, with both procedures appearing to provide comparable diagnostic value. As with other blocks, the potential for false-positive and false-negative results needs to be considered, and steps taken to reduce their incidence.

In addition to providing short and occasionally intermediate-term pain relief, diagnostic blocks are considered predictive of the potential usefulness of subsequent neurolytic procedures such as RF denervation. In carefully selected patients who fail conservative treatments such as physical and pharmacologic therapies, intra-articular steroid injections and RF denervation are treatment options. Studies evaluating the long-term outcomes from these procedures have thus far provided conflicting evidence. The results of surgical therapies including arthrodesis for facet arthropathy are discouraging.

References

1. Levin KH, Covington EC, Devereaux MW: Neck and low back pain. Continuum (NY) 2001;7:1-205.
2. Walker BF: The prevalence of low back pain: A systematic review of the literature from 1966 to 1998. J Spinal Disord 2000;13:205-217.
3. Cote P, Cassidy JD, Carroll LJ, Kristman V: The annual incidence and course of neck pain in the general population: A population-based cohort study. Pain 2004;112:267-273.
4. Pai S, Sundaram LJ: Low back pain: An economic assessment in the United States. Orthop Clin North Am 2004;35:1-5.
5. Borghouts JA, Koes BW, Vondeling H, Bouter LM: Cost-of-illness of neck pain in the Netherlands in 1996. Pain 1999;80:629-636.
6. Manchikanti L: The growth of interventional pain management in the new millennium: A critical analysis of utilization in the Medicare population. Pain Physician 2004;7:465-482.
7. Glover JR: Arthrography of the joints of the lumbar vertebral arches. Orthop Clin North Am 1977;8:37-42.
8. Cyron BM, Hutton WC: The tensile strength of the capsular ligaments of the apophyseal joints. J Anat 1981;132:145-150.
9. Yahia LH, Garzon S: Structure on the capsular ligaments of the facet joints. Ann Anat 1993;175:185-188.
10. Bogduk N: Clinical Anatomy of the Lumbar Spine and Sacrum (3rd ed). Edinburgh, Churchill Livingstone, 1997.
11. Masharawi Y, Rothschild B, Dar G, et al: Facet orientation in the thoracolumbar spine: Three-dimensional anatomic and biomechanical analysis. Spine 2004;29:1755-1763.
12. Cavanaugh JM, Ozaktay AC, Yamashita HT, King AI: Lumbar facet pain: Biomechanics, neuroanatomy and neurophysiology. J Biomech 1996;29:1117-1129.
13. Kallakuri S, Singh A, Chen C, Cavanaugh JM: Demonstration of substance P, calcitonin gene-related peptide, and protein gene product 9.5 containing nerve fibers in human cervical facet joint capsules. Spine 2004;29:1182-1186.
14. Ashton IK, Ashton BA, Gibson SJ, et al: Morphological basis for back pain: The demonstration of nerve fibers and neuropeptides in the lumbar facet joint capsule but not in ligamentum flavum. J Orthop Res 1992;10:72-78.
15. el-Bohy A, Cavanaugh JM, Getchell ML, et al: Localization of substance P and neurofilament immunoreactive fibers in the lumbar facet joint capsule and supraspinous ligament of the rabbit. Brain Res 1988;460:379-382.
16. Beaman DN, Graziano GP, Glover RA, et al: Substance P innervation of lumbar spine facet joints. Spine 1993;18:1044-1049.
17. Giles LG, Taylor JR: Innervation of lumbar zygapophyseal joint synovial folds. Acta Orthop Scand 1987;58:43-46.
18. Willburger RE, Wittenberg RH: Prostaglandin release from lumbar disc and facet joint tissue. Spine 1994;19:2068-2070.
19. Igarashi A, Kikuchi S, Konno S, Olmarker K: Inflammatory cytokines released from the facet joint tissue in degenerative lumbar spinal disorders. Spine 2004;29:2091-2095.
20. Lewin T, Moffett B, Vidik A: The morphology of the lumbar synovial intervertebral joints. Acta Morphol Nederl Scand 1962;4:299-319.
21. Horwitz T, Smith RM: An anatomical pathological and roentgenological study of the intervertebral joints of the lumbar spine and of the sacroiliac joints. Am J Roentgenol 1940;43:173-186.
22. Punjabi MM, Oxland T, Takata K, et al: Articular facets of the human spine. Quantitative three-dimensional anatomy. Spine 1993;18:1298-1310.
23. Grobler LJ, Robertson PA, Novotny JE, Pope MH: Etiology of spondylolisthesis: Assessment of the role played by lumbar facet joint morphology. Spine 1993;18:80-91.
24. Boden SD, Riew KD, Yamaguchi K, et al: Orientation of the lumbar facet joints: Association with degenerative disc disease. J Bone Joint Surg Am 1996;78:403-411.
25. Bogduk N: Clinical Anatomy of the Lumbar Spine and Sacrum (3rd ed). Edinburgh, Churchill Livingstone, 1997, pp 127-144.
26. Pedersen HE, Blunck CF, Gardner E: The anatomy of lumbosacral posterior rami and meningeal branches of spinal nerve (sinu-vertebral nerves); with an experimental study of their functions. J Bone Joint Surg Am 1956;38-A:377-391.
27. Maigne JY, Maigne R, Guerin-Surville H: The lumbar mamillo-accessory foramen: A study of 203 lumbosacral spines. Surg Radiol Anat 1991;13:29-32.
28. Bogduk N, Wilson AS, Tynan W: The human lumbar dorsal rami. J Anat 1982;134:383-397.
29. Dreyfuss P, Schwarzer AC, Lau P, Bogduk N: Specificity of lumbar medial branch and L5 dorsal ramus blocks: A computed tomography study. Spine 1997;22:895-902.
30. Jerosch J, Castro WH, Liljenqvist U: Percutaneous facet coagulation: Indication, technique, results, and complications. Neurosurg Clin North Am 1996;7:119-134.
31. Paris SV: Anatomy as related to function and pain. Orthop Clin North Am 1983;14:475-489.
32. Ebraheim NA, Xu R, Ahmad M, Yeasting RA: The quantitative anatomy of the thoracic facet and the posterior projection of its inferior facet. Spine 1997;22:1811-1817; discussion 1818.
33. Malmivaara A, Videman T, Kuosma E, Troup JD: Facet joint orientation, facet and costovertebral joint osteoarthrosis, disc degeneration, vertebral body osteophytosis, and Schmorl's nodes in the thoracolumbar junctional region of cadaveric spines. Spine 1987;12:458-463.
34. Murtagh FR, Paulsen RD, Rechtine GR: The role and incidence of facet tropism in lumbar spine degenerative disc disease. J Spinal Disord 1991;4:86-89.
35. Fukui S, Ohseto K, Shiotani M: Patterns of pain induced by distending the thoracic zygapophyseal joints. Reg Anesth 1997;22:332-336.
36. Chua WH, Bogduk N: The surgical anatomy of thoracic facet denervation. Acta Neurochir (Wien) 1995;136:140-144.
37. Milne N: The role of zygapophysial joint orientation and uncinate processes in controlling motion in the cervical spine. J Anat 1991;178:189-201.
38. Pal GP, Routal RV, Saggu SK: The orientation of the articular facets of the zygapophyseal joints at the cervical and upper thoracic region. J Anat 2001;198:431-441.
39. Bogduk N, Marsland A: The cervical zygapophysial joints as a source of neck pain. Spine 1988;13:610-617.
40. Barnsley L, Bogduk N: Medial branch blocks are specific for the diagnosis of cervical zygapophyseal joint pain. Reg Anesth 1993;18:343-350.
41. Barnsley L, Lord S, Bogduk N: Comparative local anaesthetic blocks in the diagnosis of cervical zygapophysial joint pain. Pain 1993;55:99-106.
42. Santavirta S, Hopfner-Hallikainen D, Paukku P, et al: Atlanto-axial facet joint arthritis in the rheumatoid cervical spine. A panoramic zonography study. J Rheumatol 1988;15:217-223.
43. Bovim G, Berg R, Dale LG: Cervicogenic headache: Anesthetic blockades of cervical nerves (C2-C5) and facet joint (C2/C3). Pain 1992;49:315-320.
44. Lord SM, Barnsley L, Wallis BJ, Bogduk N: Third occipital nerve headache: A prevalence study. J Neurol Neurosurg Psychiatry 1994;57:1187-1190.
45. Lord SM, Barnsley L, Wallis BJ, Bogduk N: Chronic cervical zygapophysial joint pain after whiplash. A placebo-controlled prevalence study. Spine 1996;21:1737-1744; discussion 1744-1745.
46. Barnsley L: Percutaneous radiofrequency neurotomy for chronic neck pain: Outcomes in a series of consecutive patients. Pain Med 2005;6:282-286.

47. Beyer CA, Cabanela ME, Berquist TH: Unilateral facet dislocations and fracture-dislocations of the cervical spine. J Bone Joint Surg Br 1991;73:977-981.
48. Cotler HB, Cotler JM, Alden ME, et al: The medical and economic impact of closed cervical spine dislocations. Spine 1990;15:448-452.
49. Hadley MN, Fitzpatrick BC, Sonntag VK, Browner CM: Facet fracture-dislocation injuries of the cervical spine. Neurosurgery 1992;30:661-666.
50. Key A: Cervical spine dislocations with unilateral facet interlocking. Paraplegia 1975;13:208-215.
51. Lintner DM, Knight RQ, Cullen JP: The neurologic sequelae of cervical spine facet injuries: The role of canal diameter. Spine 1993;18:725-729.
52. Mahale YJ, Silver JR: Progressive paralysis after bilateral facet dislocation of the cervical spine. J Bone Joint Surg Br 1992;74:219-223.
53. Pick RY, Segal D: C7-T1 bilateral facet dislocation: A rare lesion presenting with the syndrome of acute anterior spinal cord injury. Clin Orthop Relat Res 1980;150:131-136.
54. Shanmuganathan K, Mirvis SE, Levine AM: Rotational injury of cervical facets: CT analysis of fracture patterns with implications for management and neurologic outcome. AJR Am J Roentgenol 1994;163:1165-1169.
55. Wolf A, Levi L, Mirvis S, et al: Operative management of bilateral facet dislocation. J Neurosurg 1991;75:883-890.
56. Nabeshima Y, Iguchi T, Matsubara N, et al: Extension injury of the thoracolumbar spine. Spine 1997;22:1522-1525; discussion 1525-1526.
57. Song KJ, Lee KB: Bilateral facet dislocation on L4-L5 without neurologic deficit. J Spinal Disord Tech 2005;18:462-464.
58. Ianuzzi A, Little JS, Chiu JB, et al: Human lumbar facet joint capsule strains: I. During physiological motions. Spine J 2004;4:141-152.
59. Chow DH, Luk KD, Evans JH, Leong JC: Effects of short anterior lumbar interbody fusion on biomechanics of neighboring unfused segments. Spine 1996;21:549-555.
60. Esses SI, Doherty BJ, Crawford MJ, Dreyzin V: Kinematic evaluation of lumbar fusion techniques. Spine 1996;21:676-684.
61. Lee CK: Accelerated degeneration of the segment adjacent to a lumbar fusion. Spine 1988;13:375-377.
62. Lee CK, Langrana NA: Lumbosacral spinal fusion. A biomechanical study. Spine 1984;9:574-581.
63. Little JS, Ianuzzi A, Chiu JB, et al: Human lumbar facet joint capsule strains: II. Alteration of strains subsequent to anterior interbody fixation. Spine J 2004;4:153-162.
64. Dory MA: Arthrography of the lumbar facet joints. Radiology 1981;140:23-27.
65. Gray DP, Bajwa ZH, Warfield CA: Facet block and neurolysis. In Waldman SD (ed): Interventional Pain Management, 2nd ed. Philadelphia, Saunders, 2001, pp 446-483.
66. Oudenhoven RC: Lumbar monoradiculopathy due to unilateral facet hypertrophy. Neurosurgery 1982;11:726-727.
67. Pape E, Eldevik P, Vandvik B: Diagnostic validity of somatosensory evoked potentials in subgroups of patients with sciatica. Eur Spine J 2002;11:38-46.
68. Wilde GP, Szypryt EP, Mulholland RC: Unilateral lumbar facet joint hypertrophy causing nerve root irritation. Ann R Coll Surg Engl 1988;70:307-310.
69. Indahl A, Kaigle A, Reikeras O, Holm S: Electromyographic response of the porcine multifidus musculature after nerve stimulation. Spine 1995;20:2652-2658.
70. Kang YM, Choi WS, Pickar JG: Electrophysiologic evidence for an intersegmental reflex pathway between lumbar paraspinal tissues. Spine 2002;27:E56-E63.
71. Cavanaugh JM, Ozaktay AC, Yamashita T, et al: Mechanisms of low back pain: A neurophysiologic and neuroanatomic study. Clin Orthop Relat Res 1997;335:166-180.
72. Ozaktay AC, Cavanaugh JM, Blagoev DC, et al: Effects of a carrageenan-induced inflammation in rabbit lumbar facet joint capsule and adjacent tissues. Neurosci Res 1994;20:355-364.
73. Ozaktay AC, Cavanaugh JM, Blagoev DC, King AI: Phospholipase A2-induced electrophysiologic and histologic changes in rabbit dorsal lumbar spine tissues. Spine 1995;20:2659-2668.
74. Yamashita T, Cavanaugh JM, Ozaktay AC, et al: Effect of substance P on mechanosensitive units of tissues around and in the lumbar facet joint. J Orthop Res 1993;11:205-214.
75. Woolf CJ, Salter MW: Neuronal plasticity: Increasing the gain in pain. Science 2000;288:1765-1769.
76. Chen C, Lu Y, Kallakuri S, et al: Distribution of A-delta and C-fiber receptors in the cervical facet joint capsule and their response to stretch. J Bone Joint Surg Am 2006;88:1807-1816.
77. Boszczyk BM, Boszczyk AA, Putz R: Comparative and functional anatomy of the mammalian lumbar spine. Anat Rec 2001;264:157-168.
78. Jackson RP, Jacobs RR, Montesano PX: 1988 Volvo award in clinical sciences. Facet joint injection in low-back pain: A prospective statistical study. Spine 1988;13:966-971.
79. Revel M, Poiraudeau S, Auleley GR, et al: Capacity of the clinical picture to characterize low back pain relieved by facet joint anesthesia. Proposed criteria to identify patients with painful facet joints. Spine 1998;23:1972-1976; discussion 1977.
80. Revel ME, Listrat VM, Chevalier XJ, et al: Facet joint block for low back pain: Identifying predictors of a good response. Arch Phys Med Rehabil 1992;73:824-828.
81. Farfan HF: Effects of torsion on the intervertebral joints. Can J Surg 1969;12:336-341.
82. Kirkaldy-Willis WH, Farfan HF: Instability of the lumbar spine. Clin Orthop Relat Res 1982:110-123.
83. Gotfried Y, Bradford DS, Oegema TR Jr: Facet joint changes after chemonucleolysis-induced disc space narrowing. Spine 1986;11:944-950.
84. Kirkaldy-Willis WH, Wedge JH, Yong-Hing K, Reilly J: Pathology and pathogenesis of lumbar spondylosis and stenosis. Spine 1978;3:319-328.
85. Punjabi MM, Krag MH, Chung TQ: Effects of disc injury on mechanical behavior of the human spine. Spine 1984;9:707-713.
86. Adams MA, Freeman BJ, Morrison HP, et al: Mechanical initiation of intervertebral disc degeneration. Spine 2000;25:1625-1636.
87. Adams MA, Hutton WC: The effect of posture on the role of the apophysial joints in resisting intervertebral compressive forces. J Bone Joint Surg Br 1980;62:358-362.
88. Haher TR, O'Brien M, Dryer JW, et al: The role of the lumbar facet joints in spinal stability. Identification of alternative paths of loading. Spine 1994;19:2667-2670; discussion 2671.
89. Fujiwara A, Tamai K, Yamato M, et al: The relationship between facet joint osteoarthritis and disc degeneration of the lumbar spine: An MRI study. Eur Spine J 1999;8:396-401.
90. Schwarzer AC, Aprill CN, Derby R, et al: The relative contributions of the disc and zygapophyseal joint in chronic low back pain. Spine 1994;19:801-806.
91. Ball J: Enthesopathy of rheumatoid and ankylosing spondylitis. Ann Rheum Dis 1971;30:213-223.
92. de Vlam K, Mielants H, Verstraete KL, Veys EM: The zygapophyseal joint determines morphology of the enthesophyte. J Rheumatol 2000;27:1732-1739.
93. Guillaume MP, Hermanus N, Peretz A: Unusual localisation of chronic arthropathy in lumbar facet joints after parvovirus B19 infection. Clin Rheumatol 2002;21:306-308.
94. Glaser JA, El-Khoury GY: Unknown case. Diagnosis: Facet joint septic arthritis T12-L1 on the left with extension of the infection into the spinal canal producing a large epidural abscess. Spine 2001;26:991-993.
95. Campbell AJ, Wells IP: Pigmented villonodular synovitis of a lumbar vertebral facet joint. J Bone Joint Surg Am 1982;64:145-146.
96. Dreyfuss PH, Dreyer SJ, Herring SA: Lumbar zygapophysial (facet) joint injections. Spine 1995;20:2040-2047.
97. Eisenstein SM, Parry CR: The lumbar facet arthrosis syndrome. Clinical presentation and articular surface changes. J Bone Joint Surg Br 1987;69:3-7.

98. Fujishiro T, Nabeshima Y, Yasui S, et al: Pseudogout attack of the lumbar facet joint: A case report. Spine 2002;27: E396-E398.

99. Smida M, Lejri M, Kandara H, et al: Septic arthritis of a lumbar facet joint case report and review of the literature. Acta Orthop Belg 2004;70: 290-294.

100. Hemminghytt S, Daniels DL, Williams AL, Haughton VM: Intraspinal synovial cysts: Natural history and diagnosis by CT. Radiology 1982;145:375-376.

101. Howington JU, Connolly ES, Voorhies RM: Intraspinal synovial cysts: 10-year experience at the Ochsner Clinic. J Neurosurg 1999;91:193-199.

102. Rapin PA, Gerster JC: Calcified synovial cyst of a zygapophyseal joint. J Rheumatol 1993;20:767-768.

103. Sabo RA, Tracy PT, Weigner JM: A series of 60 juxtafacet cysts: Clinical presentation, the role of spinal instability, and treatment. J Neurosurg 1996;85:860-865.

104. Christophis P, Asamoto S, Kuchelmeister K, Schachenmayr W: "Juxtafacet cysts," a misleading name for cystic formations of mobile spine (CYFMOS). Eur Spine J 2007, Jan 4.

105. Stoodley MA, Jones NR, Scott G: Cervical and thoracic juxtafacet cysts causing neurologic deficits. Spine 2000; 25:970-973.

106. Doyle AJ, Merrilees M: Synovial cysts of the lumbar facet joints in a symptomatic population: Prevalence on magnetic resonance imaging. Spine 2004;29:874-878.

107. Das De S, McCreath SW: Lumbosacral fracture-dislocations. A report of four cases. J Bone Joint Surg Br 1981;63-B: 58-60.

108. Fabris D, Costantini S, Nena U, Lo Scalzo V: Traumatic L5-S1 spondylolisthesis: Report of three cases and a review of the literature. Eur Spine J 1999;8:290-295.

109. Kaplan SS, Wright NM, Yundt KD, Lauryssen C: Adjacent fracture-dislocations of the lumbosacral spine: Case report. Neurosurgery 1999;44:1134-1137.

110. Verlaan JJ, Oner FC, Dhert WJ, Verbout AJ: Traumatic lumbosacral dislocation: Case report. Spine 2001;26:1942-1944.

111. Levine AM, Bosse M, Edwards CC: Bilateral facet dislocations in the thoracolumbar spine. Spine 1988;13:630-640.

112. Twomey LT, Taylor JR, Taylor MM: Unsuspected damage to lumbar zygapophyseal (facet) joints after motor-vehicle accidents. Med J Aust 1989;151:210-212, 215-217.

113. Aprill C, Bogduk N: The prevalence of cervical zygapophyseal joint pain. A first approximation. Spine 1992;17:744-747.

114. Frank AO, De Souza LH, Frank CA: Neck pain and disability: A cross-sectional survey of the demographic and clinical characteristics of neck pain seen in a rheumatology clinic. Int J Clin Pract 2005;59:173-182.

115. Stovner LJ, Kolstad F, Helde G: Radiofrequency denervation of facet joints C2-C6 in cervicogenic headache: A randomized, double-blind, sham-controlled study. Cephalalgia 2004; 24:821-830.

116. Cohen SP, Bajwa ZH, Kraemer JJ, et al: Factors predicting success and failure for cervical facet radiofrequency denervation: A multi-center analysis. American Society of Regional Anesthesia & Pain Medicine Annual Fall Meeting, San Francisco, CA, 2007.

117. Furlong MA, Motamedi K, Laskin WB, et al: Synovial-type giant cell tumors of the vertebral column: A clinicopathologic study of 15 cases, with a review of the literature and discussion of the differential diagnosis. Hum Pathol 2003;34:670-679.

118. Kulkarni AG, Goel A, Muzumdar D: Solitary osteochondroma arising from the thoracic facet joint—Case report. Neurol Med Chir (Tokyo) 2004;44:255-257.

119. Carrera GF: Lumbar facet joint injection in low back pain and sciatica: Preliminary results. Radiology 1980;137: 665-667.

120. Destouet JM, Gilula LA, Murphy WA, Monsees B: Lumbar facet joint injection: Indication, technique, clinical correlation, and preliminary results. Radiology 1982;145:321-325.

121. Lau LS, Littlejohn GO, Miller MH: Clinical evaluation of intra-articular injections for lumbar facet joint pain. Med J Aust 1985;143:563-565.

122. Lewinnek GE, Warfield CA: Facet joint degeneration as a cause of low back pain. Clin Orthop Relat Res 1986: 216-222.

123. Long DM, BenDebba M, Torgerson WS, et al: Persistent back pain and sciatica in the United States: Patient characteristics. J Spinal Disord 1996;9:40-58.

124. Moran R, O'Connell D, Walsh MG: The diagnostic value of facet joint injections. Spine 1988;13:1407-1410.

125. Murtagh FR: Computed tomography and fluoroscopy guided anesthesia and steroid injection in facet syndrome. Spine 1988;13:686-689.

126. Raymond J, Dumas JM: Intraarticular facet block: Diagnostic test or therapeutic procedure? Radiology 1984;151:333-336.

127. Dreyer SJ, Dreyfuss PH: Low back pain and the zygapophysial (facet) joints. Arch Phys Med Rehabil 1996;77:290-300.

128. Dreyfuss PH, Dreyer SJ: Lumbar zygapophysial (facet) joint injections. Spine J 2003;3:50S-59S.

129. Sowa G: Facet-mediated pain. Dis Mon 2005;51:18-33.

130. Manchikanti L, Pampati V, Fellows B, Bakhit CE: Prevalence of lumbar facet joint pain in chronic low back pain. Pain Physician 1999;2:59-64.

131. Manchikanti L, Pampati V, Fellows B, Bakhit CE: The diagnostic validity and therapeutic value of lumbar facet joint nerve blocks with or without adjuvant agents. Curr Rev Pain 2000;4:337-344.

132. Schwarzer AC, Aprill CN, Derby R, et al: The false-positive rate of uncontrolled diagnostic blocks of the lumbar zygapophysial joints. Pain 1994;58:195-200.

133. Schwarzer AC, Wang SC, Bogduk N, et al: Prevalence and clinical features of lumbar zygapophysial joint pain: a study in an Australian population with chronic low back pain. Ann Rheum Dis 1995;54:100-106.

134. Bogduk N: International Spinal Injection Society guidelines for the performance of spinal injection procedures. Part 1: Zygapophysial joint blocks. Clin J Pain 1997;13:285-302.

135. Dreyfuss P, Halbrook B, Pauza K, et al: Efficacy and validity of radiofrequency neurotomy for chronic lumbar zygapophysial joint pain. Spine 2000;25:1270-1277.

136. Manchikanti L, Boswell MV, Singh V, et al: Prevalence of facet joint pain in chronic spinal pain of cervical, thoracic, and lumbar regions. BMC Musculoskel Disord 2004;5:15.

137. Manchikanti L, Pampati V, Fellows B, Baha AG: The inability of the clinical picture to characterize pain from facet joints. Pain Physician 2000;3:158-166.

138. Newton W, Curtis P, Witt P, Hobler K: Prevalence of subtypes of low back pain in a defined population. J Fam Pract 1997;45:331-335.

139. Cohen SP: Sacroiliac joint pain: A comprehensive review of anatomy, diagnosis, and treatment. Anesth Analg 2005;101: 1440-1453.

140. Cohen SP, Abdi S: Lateral branch blocks as a treatment for sacroiliac joint pain: A pilot study. Reg Anesth Pain Med 2003;28:113-119.

141. Johnston HM: The cutaneous branches of the posterior primary divisions of the spinal nerves, and their distribution in the skin. J Anat Physiol 1908;43:80-92.

142. Barnsley L, Lord SM, Wallis BJ, Bogduk N: The prevalence of chronic cervical zygapophysial joint pain after whiplash. Spine 1995;20:20-25;discussion 26.

143. Manchikanti L, Singh V, Pampati V, et al: Evaluation of the prevalence of facet joint pain in chronic thoracic pain. Pain Physician 2002;5:354-359.

144. Manchikanti L, Singh V, Rivera J, Pampati V: Prevalence of cervical facet joint pain in chronic neck pain. Pain Physician 2002;5:243-249.

145. Weber J, Czarnetzki A, Spring A: Paleopathological features of the cervical spine in the early middle ages: natural history of degenerative diseases. Neurosurgery 2003;53:1418-1423; discussion 1423-1424.

146. Fairbank JC, Park WM, McCall IW, O'Brien JP: Apophyseal injection of local anesthetic as a diagnostic aid in primary low-back pain syndromes. Spine 1981;6:598-605.

147. Helbig T, Lee CK: The lumbar facet syndrome. Spine 1988; 13:61-64.

148. Schwarzer AC, Aprill CN, Derby R, et al: Clinical features of patients with pain stemming from the lumbar zygapophysial joints. Is the lumbar facet syndrome a clinical entity? Spine 1994;19:1132-1137.

149. Jull G, Bogduk N, Marsland A: The accuracy of manual diagnosis for cervical zygapophysial joint pain syndromes. Med J Aust 1988;148:233-236.

150. King W, Lau P, Lees R, Bogduk N: The validity of manual examination in assessing patients with neck pain. Spine J 2007;7:22-26.

151. Manchikanti L, Singh V, Pampati V, et al: Is there correlation of facet joint pain in lumbar and cervical spine? An evaluation of prevalence in combined chronic low back and neck pain. Pain Physician 2002;5:365-371.

152. Bough B, Thakore J, Davies M, Dowling F: Degeneration of the lumbar facet joints: Arthrography and pathology. J Bone Joint Surg Br 1990;72:275-276.

153. Schwarzer AC, Derby R, Aprill CN, et al: The value of the provocation response in lumbar zygapophyseal joint injections. Clin J Pain 1994;10:309-13

154. Schwarzer AC, Wang SC, O'Driscoll D, et al: The ability of computed tomography to identify a painful zygapophysial joint in patients with chronic low back pain. Spine 1995;20:907-912.

155. Slipman CW, Plastaras CT, Palmitier RA, et al: Symptom provocation of fluoroscopically guided cervical nerve root stimulation. Are dynatomal maps identical to dermatomal maps? Spine 1998;23:2235-2242.

156. Aprill C, Dwyer A, Bogduk N: Cervical zygapophyseal joint pain patterns. II: A clinical evaluation. Spine 1990;15:458-461.

157. Dwyer A, Aprill C, Bogduk N: Cervical zygapophyseal joint pain patterns. I: A study in normal volunteers. Spine 1990;15:453-457.

158. Fukui S, Ohseto K, Shiotani M, et al: Referred pain distribution of the cervical zygapophyseal joints and cervical dorsal rami. Pain 1996;68:79-83.

159. Windsor RE, Nagula D, Storm S, et al: Electrical stimulation induced cervical medial branch referral patterns. Pain Physician 2003;6:411-418.

160. Dreyfuss P, Tibiletti C, Dreyer SJ: Thoracic zygapophyseal joint pain patterns. A study in normal volunteers. Spine 1994;19:807-811.

161. Carrera GF, Williams AL: Current concepts in evaluation of the lumbar facet joints. Crit Rev Diagn Imaging 1984;21:85-104.

162. Leone A, Aulisa L, Tamburrelli F, et al: [The role of computed tomography and magnetic resonance in assessing degenerative arthropathy of the lumbar articular facets]. Radiol Med (Torino) 1994;88:547-52.

163. Weishaupt D, Zanetti M, Hodler J, Boos N: MR imaging of the lumbar spine: Prevalence of intervertebral disk extrusion and sequestration, nerve root compression, end plate abnormalities, and osteoarthritis of the facet joints in asymptomatic volunteers. Radiology 1998;209:661-666.

164. Weishaupt D, Zanetti M, Boos N, Hodler J: MR imaging and CT in osteoarthritis of the lumbar facet joints. Skeletal Radiol 1999;28:215-219.

165. Jensen MC, Brant-Zawadzki MN, Obuchowski N, et al: Magnetic resonance imaging of the lumbar spine in people without back pain. N Engl J Med 1994;331:69-73.

166. Wiesel SW, Tsourmas N, Feffer HL, et al: A study of computer-assisted tomography. I. The incidence of positive CAT scans in an asymptomatic group of patients. Spine 1984;9:549-551.

167. Dolan AL, Ryan PJ, Arden NK, et al: The value of SPECT scans in identifying back pain likely to benefit from facet joint injection. Br J Rheumatol 1996;35:1269-1273.

168. Raymond J, Dumas JM, Lisbona R: Nuclear imaging as a screening test for patients referred for intraarticular facet block. J Can Assoc Radiol 1984;35:291-292.

169. Cohen SP, Hurley RW, Christo PJ, et al: Clinical predictors of success and failure for lumbar facet radiofrequency denervation. Clin J Pain 2007;23:45-52.

170. Kawaguchi Y, Matsuno H, Kanamori M, et al: Radiologic findings of the lumbar spine in patients with rheumatoid arthritis, and a review of pathologic mechanisms. J Spinal Disord Tech 2003;16:38-43.

171. Marks RC, Houston T, Thulbourne T: Facet joint injection and facet nerve block: A randomised comparison in 86 patients with chronic low back pain. Pain 1992;49:325-328.

172. Nash TP: Facet joints—Intra-articular steroids or nerve block? Pain Clin 1990;3:77-82.

173. Kellegren JH: On the distribution of pain arising from deep somatic structures with charts of segmental pain areas. Clin Sci 1939;4:35-46.

174. Gallagher J, Petriccione di Vadi PL, Wedley JR, et al: Radiofrequency facet joint denervation in the treatment of low back pain: A prospective controlled double-blind study to assess its efficiancy. Pain Clin 1994;7:193-198.

175. Leclaire R, Fortin L, Lambert R, et al: Radiofrequency facet joint denervation in the treatment of low back pain: A placebo-controlled clinical trial to assess efficacy. Spine 2001;26:1411-1416; discussion 1417.

176. van Wijk RM, Geurts JW, Wynne HJ, et al: Radiofrequency denervation of lumbar facet joints in the treatment of chronic low back pain: A randomized, double-blind, sham lesion-controlled trial. Clin J Pain 2005;21:335-344.

177. van Kleef M, Barendse GA, Kessels A, et al: Randomized trial of radiofrequency lumbar facet denervation for chronic low back pain. Spine 1999;24:1937-1942.

178. Birkenmaier C, Veihelmann A, Trouillier HH, et al: Medial branch blocks versus pericapsular blocks in selecting patients for percutaneous cryodenervation of lumbar facet joints. Reg Anesth Pain Med 2007;32:27-33.

179. Barnsley L, Lord S, Wallis B, Bogduk N: False-positive rates of cervical zygapophysial joint blocks. Clin J Pain 1993;9:124-130.

180. Lord SM, Barnsley L, Bogduk N: The utility of comparative local anesthetic blocks versus placebo-controlled blocks for the diagnosis of cervical zygapophysial joint pain. Clin J Pain 1995;11:208-2013.

181. Hogan QH, Abram SE: Neural blockade for diagnosis and prognosis. A review. Anesthesiology 1997;86:216-241.

182. Manchikanti L, Pampati V, Damron K: The role of placebo and nocebo effects of perioperative administration of sedatives and opioids in interventional pain management. Pain Physician 2005;8:349-355.

183. Manchikanti L, Pampati V, Damron KS, et al: A randomized, prospective, double-blind, placebo-controlled evaluation of the effect of sedation on diagnostic validity of cervical facet joint pain. Pain Physician 2004;7:301-309.

184. Manchikanti L, Pampati V, Damron KS, et al: The effect of sedation on diagnostic validity of facet joint nerve blocks: An evaluation to assess similarities in population with involvement in cervical and lumbar regions (ISRCTNo: 76376497). Pain Physician 2006;9:47-51.

185. Cohen SP, Mullings R, Abdi S: The pharmacologic treatment of muscle pain. Anesthesiology 2004;101:495-526.

186. Cohen SP, Stojanovic MP, Crooks M, et al: Lumbar facet radiofrequency denervation success as a function of pain relief during diagnostic medial branch blocks: A multi-center analysis. Spine J 2007; Accepted for publication.

187. Cucuzzella TR, Delport EG, Kim N, et al: A survey: Conscious sedation with epidural and zygapophyseal injections: Is it necessary? Spine J 2006;6:364-369.

188. North RB, Kidd DH, Zahurak M, Piantadosi S: Specificity of diagnostic nerve blocks: A prospective, randomized study of sciatica due to lumbosacral spine disease. Pain 1996;65:77-85.

189. Cohen SP, Larkin TM, Chang AS, Stojanovic MP: The causes of false-positive medial branch (facet joint) blocks in soldiers and retirees. Mil Med 2004;169:781-786.

190. Ambroz C, Scott A, Ambroz A, Talbott EO: Chronic low back pain assessment using surface electromyography. J Occup Environ Med 2000;42:660-669.

191. Browning R, Jackson JL, O'Malley PG: Cyclobenzaprine and back pain: A meta-analysis. Arch Intern Med 2001;161:1613-1620.

192. Foster L, Clapp L, Erickson M, Jabbari B: Botulinum toxin A and chronic low back pain: A randomized, double-blind study. Neurology 2001;56:1290-1293.

193. Geisser ME, Ranavaya M, Haig AJ, et al: A meta-analytic review of surface electromyography among persons with low back pain and normal, healthy controls. J Pain 2005; 6:711-726.

194. Ackerman WE, Munir MA, Zhang JM, Ghaleb A: Are diagnostic lumbar facet injections influenced by pain of muscular origin? Pain Pract 2004;4:286-291.

195. Woolf CJ, McMahon SB: Injury-induced plasticity of the flexor reflex in chronic decerebrate rats. Neuroscience 1985;16:395-404.

196. Woolf CJ, Wiesenfeld-Hallin Z: The systemic administration of local anaesthetics produces a selective depression of C-afferent fibre evoked activity in the spinal cord. Pain 1985;23:361-374.

197. Stojanovic MP, Zhou Y, Hord ED, et al: Single needle approach for multiple medial branch blocks: a new technique. Clin J Pain 2003;19:134-137.

198. Stojanovic MP, Dey D, Hord ED, et al: A prospective crossover comparison study of the single-needle and multiple-needle techniques for facet-joint medial branch block. Reg Anesth Pain Med 2005;30:484-490.

199. Kaplan M, Dreyfuss P, Halbrook B, Bogduk N: The ability of lumbar medial branch blocks to anesthetize the zygapophysial joint. A physiologic challenge. Spine 1998;23:1847-1852.

200. Berven S, Tay BB, Colman W, Hu SS: The lumbar zygapophyseal (facet) joints: A role in the pathogenesis of spinal pain syndromes and degenerative spondylolisthesis. Semin Neurol 2002;22:187-196.

201. Kornick C, Kramarich SS, Lamer TJ, Todd Sitzman B: Complications of lumbar facet radiofrequency denervation. Spine 2004;29:1352-1354.

202. Dobrogowski J, Wrzosek A, Wordliczek J: Radiofrequency denervation with or without addition of pentoxifylline or methylprednisolone for chronic lumbar zygapophysial joint pain. Pharmacol Rep 2005;57:475-480.

203. Bogduk N, Holmes S: Controlled zygapophysial joint blocks: The travesty of cost-effectiveness. Pain Med 2000;1:24-34.

204. Geisser ME, Wiggert EA, Haig AJ, Colwell MO: A randomized, controlled trial of manual therapy and specific adjuvant exercise for chronic low back pain. Clin J Pain 2005;21: 463-470.

205. Maul I, Laubli T, Oliveri M, Krueger H: Long-term effects of supervised physical training in secondary prevention of low back pain. Eur Spine J 2005;14:599-611.

206. Staal JB, Hlobil H, Twisk JW, et al: Graded activity for low back pain in occupational health care: A randomized, controlled trial. Ann Intern Med 2004;140:77-84.

207. Williams KA, Petronis J, Smith D, et al: Effect of Iyengar yoga therapy for chronic low back pain. Pain 2005;115:107-117.

208. Andersson GB, Lucente T, Davis AM, et al: A comparison of osteopathic spinal manipulation with standard care for patients with low back pain. N Engl J Med 1999;341: 1426-1431.

209. Giles LG, Muller R: Chronic spinal pain: a randomized clinical trial comparing medication, acupuncture, and spinal manipulation. Spine 2003;28:1490-1502; discussion 1502-1503.

210. Licciardone JC, Stoll ST, Fulda KG, et al: Osteopathic manipulative treatment for chronic low back pain: A randomized controlled trial. Spine 2003;28:1355-1362.

211. Williams NH, Wilkinson C, Russell I, et al: Randomized osteopathic manipulation study (ROMANS): Pragmatic trial for spinal pain in primary care. Fam Pract 2003;20:662-669.

212. Kerr DP, Walsh DM, Baxter D: Acupuncture in the management of chronic low back pain: A blinded randomized controlled trial. Clin J Pain 2003;19:364-370.

213. Meng CF, Wang D, Ngeow J, et al: Acupuncture for chronic low back pain in older patients: A randomized, controlled trial. Rheumatology (Oxford) 2003;42:1508-1517.

214. Tsukayama H, Yamashita H, Amagai H, Tanno Y: Randomised controlled trial comparing the effectiveness of electroacupuncture and TENS for low back pain: A preliminary study for a pragmatic trial. Acupunct Med 2002;20:175-180.

215. Hsieh LL, Kuo CH, Lee LH, et al: Treatment of low back pain by acupressure and physical therapy: Randomised controlled trial. BMJ 2006;332:696-700.

216. Trinh K, Graham N, Gross A, et al: Acupuncture for neck disorders. Spine 2007;32:236-243.

217. Brinkhaus B, Witt CM, Jena S, et al: Acupuncture in patients with chronic low back pain: A randomized controlled trial. Arch Intern Med 2006;166:450-457.

218. Mens JM: The use of medication in low back pain. Best Pract Res Clin Rheumatol 2005;19:609-621.

219. Videman T, Osterman K: Double-blind parallel study of piroxicam versus indomethacin in the treatment of low back pain. Ann Clin Res 1984;16:156-160.

220. Zerbini C, Ozturk ZE, Grifka J, et al: Efficacy of etoricoxib 60 mg/day and diclofenac 150 mg/day in reduction of pain and disability in patients with chronic low back pain: Results of a 4-week, multinational, randomized, double-blind study. Curr Med Res Opin 2005;21:2037-2049.

221. Schnitzer TJ, Ferraro A, Hunsche E, Kong SX: A comprehensive review of clinical trials on the efficacy and safety of drugs for the treatment of low back pain. J Pain Symptom Manage 2004;28:72-95.

222. Borenstein DG, Korn S: Efficacy of a low-dose regimen of cyclobenzaprine hydrochloride in acute skeletal muscle spasm: Results of two placebo-controlled trials. Clin Ther 2003;25:1056-1073.

223. Fayad F, Lefevre-Colau MM, Poiraudeau S, et al: [Chronicity, recurrence, and return to work in low back pain: common prognostic factors]. Ann Readapt Med Phys 2004;47: 179-189.

224. Tatrow K, Blanchard EB, Silverman DJ: Posttraumatic headache: an exploratory treatment study. Appl Psychophysiol Biofeedback 2003;28:267-278.

225. Polatin PB, Kinney RK, Gatchel RJ, et al: Psychiatric illness and chronic low-back pain. The mind and the spine—Which goes first? Spine 1993;18:66-71.

226. Lilius G, Laasonen EM, Myllynen P, et al: [Lumbar facet joint syndrome. Significance of non-organic signs. A randomized placebo-controlled clinical study]. Rev Chir Orthop Reparatrice Appar Mot 1989;75:493-500.

227. Lippitt AB: The facet joint and its role in spine pain. Management with facet joint injections. Spine 1984;9:746-750.

228. Fuchs S, Erbe T, Fischer HL, Tibesku CO: Intraarticular hyaluronic acid versus glucocorticoid injections for nonradicular pain in the lumbar spine. J Vasc Interv Radiol 2005;16:1493-1498.

229. Lilius G, Laasonen EM, Myllynen P, et al: Lumbar facet joint syndrome. A randomised clinical trial. J Bone Joint Surg Br 1989;71:681-684.

230. Carette S, Marcoux S, Truchon R, et al: A controlled trial of corticosteroid injections into facet joints for chronic low back pain. N Engl J Med 1991;325:1002-1007.

231. Blanchard J, Ramamurthy S, Walsh N, et al: Intravenous regional sympatholysis: A double-blind comparison of guanethidine, reserpine, and normal saline. J Pain Symptom Manage 1990;5:357-361.

232. Frost FA, Jessen B, Siggaard-Andersen J: A control, double-blind comparison of mepivacaine injection versus saline injection for myofascial pain. Lancet 1980;1:499-500.

233. Price DD, Long S, Wilsey B, Rafii A: Analysis of peak magnitude and duration of analgesia produced by local anesthetics injected into sympathetic ganglia of complex regional pain syndrome patients. Clin J Pain 1998;14:216-226.

234. Barnsley L, Lord SM, Wallis BJ, Bogduk N: Lack of effect of intraarticular corticosteroids for chronic pain in the cervical zygapophyseal joints. N Engl J Med 1994;330:1047-1050.

235. Cohen SP, Raja SN: Pathogenesis, diagnosis, and treatment of lumbar zygapophysial (facet) joint pain. Anesthesiology 2007;106:591-614.

236. Bogduk N: A narrative review of intra-articular corticosteroid injections for low back pain. Pain Med 2005;6:287-296.

237. Resnick DK, Choudhri TF, Dailey AT, et al: Guidelines for the performance of fusion procedures for degenerative disease of

the lumbar spine. Part 13: Injection therapies, low-back pain, and lumbar fusion. J Neurosurg Spine 2005;2:707-215.

238. Slipman CW, Bhat AL, Gilchrist RV, et al: A critical review of the evidence for the use of zygapophysial injections and radiofrequency denervation in the treatment of low back pain. Spine J 2003;3:310-316.

239. Holder LE, Machin JL, Asdourian PL, et al: Planar and high-resolution SPECT bone imaging in the diagnosis of facet syndrome. J Nucl Med 1995;36:37-44.

240. Pneumaticos SG, Chatziioannou SN, Hipp JA, et al: Low back pain: Prediction of short-term outcome of facet joint injection with bone scintigraphy. Radiology 2006;238:693-698.

241. Manchikanti L, Pampati V, Bakhit CE, et al: Effectiveness of lumbar facet joint nerve blocks in chronic low back pain: A randomized clinical trial. Pain Physician 2001;4:101-117.

242. Manchikanti L, Manchikanti KN, Manchukonda R, et al: Evaluation of therapeutic thoracic medial branch block effectiveness in chronic thoracic pain: A prospective outcome study with minimum 1-year follow up. Pain Physician 2006;9:97-105.

243. Manchikanti L, Manchikanti KN, Damron KS, Pampati V: Effectiveness of cervical medial branch blocks in chronic neck pain: A prospective outcome study. Pain Physician 2004;7:195-201.

244. Rees WE: Multiple bilateral subcutaneous rhizolysis of segmental nerves in the treatment of the intervertebral disc syndrome. Ann Gen Pract 1971;26:126-127.

245. King JS, Lagger R: Sciatica viewed as a referred pain syndrome. Surg Neurol 1976;5:46-50.

246. Shealy CN: Percutaneous radiofrequency denervation of spinal facets: Treatment for chronic back pain and sciatica. J Neurosurg 1975;43:448-451.

247. Shealy CN: Facet denervation in the management of back and sciatic pain. Clin Orthop Relat Res 1976:157-164.

248. Lord SM, Barnsley L, Wallis BJ, et al: Percutaneous radiofrequency neurotomy for chronic cervical zygapophyseal-joint pain. N Engl J Med 1996;335:1721-1726.

249. Yin W, Willard F, Carreiro J, Dreyfuss P: Sensory stimulation-guided sacroiliac joint radiofrequency neurotomy: Technique based on neuroanatomy of the dorsal sacral plexus. Spine 2003;28:2419-2425.

250. Barendse GA, van Den Berg SG, Kessels AH, et al: Randomized controlled trial of percutaneous intradiscal radiofrequency thermocoagulation for chronic discogenic back pain: Lack of effect from a 90-second 70 C lesion. Spine 2001;26:287-292.

251. Pevzner E, David R, Leitner Y, et al: [Pulsed radiofrequency treatment of severe radicular pain]. Harefuah 2005;144:178-180, 231.

252. Niemisto L, Kalso E, Malmivaara A, et al: Radiofrequency denervation for neck and back pain: A systematic review within the framework of the Cochrane Collaboration Back Review Group. Spine 2003;28:1877-1888.

253. Burton CV: Percutaneous radiofrequency facet denervation. Appl Neurophysiol 1976;39:80-86.

254. Houston JR: A study of subcutaneous rhizolysis in the treatment of chronic backache. J R Coll Gen Pract 1975;25:692-697.

255. McCulloch JA: Percutaneous radiofrequency lumbar rhizolysis (rhizotomy). Appl Neurophysiol 1976;39:87-96.

256. Ogsbury JS 3rd, Simon RH, Lehman RA: Facet "denervation" in the treatment of low back syndrome. Pain 1977;3:257-263.

257. Oudenhoven RC: The role of laminectomy, facet rhizotomy, and epidural steroids. Spine 1979;4:145-147.

258. Rashbaum RF: Radiofrequency facet denervation: A treatment alternative in refractory low back pain with or without leg pain. Orthop Clin North Am 1983;14:569-575.

259. McCulloch JA, Organ LW: Percutaneous radiofrequency lumbar rhizolysis (rhizotomy). Can Med Assoc J 1977;116:28-30.

260. North RB, Han M, Zahurak M, Kidd DH: Radiofrequency lumbar facet denervation: Analysis of prognostic factors. Pain 1994;57:77-83.

261. Schaerer JP: Radiofrequency facet rhizotomy in the treatment of chronic neck and low back pain. Int Surg 1978;63:53-59.

262. Bogduk N, Macintosh J, Marsland A: Technical limitations to the efficacy of radiofrequency neurotomy for spinal pain. Neurosurgery 1987;20:529-535.

263. Lau P, Mercer S, Govind J, Bogduk N: The surgical anatomy of lumbar medial branch neurotomy (facet denervation). Pain Med 2004;5:289-298.

264. Vinas FC, Zamorano L, Dujovny M, et al: In vivo and in vitro study of the lesions produced with a computerized radiofrequency system. Stereotact Funct Neurosurg 1992;58:121-133.

265. Buijs EJ, van Wijk RM, Geurts JW, et al: Radiofrequency lumbar facet denervation: A comparative study of the reproducibility of lesion size after 2 current radiofrequency techniques. Reg Anesth Pain Med 2004;29:400-407.

266. Demazumder D, Mirotznik MS, Schwartzman D: Comparison of irrigated electrode designs for radiofrequency ablation of myocardium. J Interv Card Electrophysiol 2001;5:391-400.

267. van Suijlekom HA, van Kleef M, Barendse GA, et al: Radiofrequency cervical zygapophyseal joint neurotomy for cervicogenic headache: A prospective study of 15 patients. Funct Neurol 1998;13:297-303.

268. Sapir DA, Gorup JM: Radiofrequency medial branch neurotomy in litigant and nonlitigant patients with cervical whiplash: A prospective study. Spine 2001;26:E268-E273.

269. Bogduk N, April C: On the nature of neck pain, discography and cervical zygapophysial joint blocks. Pain 1993;54:213-217.

270. McDonald GJ, Lord SM, Bogduk N: Long-term follow-up of patients treated with cervical radiofrequency neurotomy for chronic neck pain. Neurosurgery 1999;45:61-67; discussion 67-68.

271. Stolker RJ, Vervest AC, Groen GJ: Percutaneous facet denervation in chronic thoracic spinal pain. Acta Neurochir (Wien) 1993;122:82-90.

272. Benzon HT: Epidural steroid injections for low back pain and lumbosacral radiculopathy. Pain 1986;24:277-295.

273. North RB, Campbell JN, James CS, et al: Failed back surgery syndrome: 5-year follow-up in 102 patients undergoing repeated operation. Neurosurgery 1991;28:685-90; discussion 690-691.

274. Quigley MR, Bost J, Maroon JC, et al: Outcome after microdiscectomy: Results of a prospective single institutional study. Surg Neurol 1998;49:263-267; discussion 267-268.

275. Schofferman J, Kine G: Effectiveness of repeated radiofrequency neurotomy for lumbar facet pain. Spine 2004;29:2471-2473.

276. Mikeladze G, Espinal R, Finnegan R, et al: Pulsed radiofrequency application in treatment of chronic zygapophyseal joint pain. Spine J 2003;3:360-362.

277. Barlocher CB, Krauss JK, Seiler RW: Kryorhizotomy: An alternative technique for lumbar medial branch rhizotomy in lumbar facet syndrome. J Neurosurg 2003;98:14-20.

278. Staender M, Maerz U, Tonn JC, Steude U: Computerized tomography-guided kryorhizotomy in 76 patients with lumbar facet joint syndrome. J Neurosurg Spine 2005;3:444-449.

279. Schuster GD: The use of cryoanalgesia in the painful facet syndrome. J Neurol Orthopaed Surg 1982;3:271-274.

280. Silvers HR: Lumbar percutaneous facet rhizotomy. Spine 1990;15:36-40.

281. Selby HR, Paris SV: Anatomy of facet joints and its correlation with low back pain. Contemp Orthop 1981;312:1097-1103.

282. Deyo RA, Nachemson A, Mirza SK: Spinal-fusion surgery—The case for restraint. N Engl J Med 2004;350:722-726.

283. Gibson JN, Waddell G, Grant IC: Surgery for degenerative lumbar spondylosis. Cochrane Database Syst Rev 2000:CD001352.

284. Esses SI, Botsford DJ, Kostuik JP: The role of external spinal skeletal fixation in the assessment of low-back disorders. Spine 1989;14:594-601.

285. Esses SI, Moro JK: The value of facet joint blocks in patient selection for lumbar fusion. Spine 1993;18:185-190.

286. Jackson RP: The facet syndrome. Myth or reality? Clin Orthop Relat Res 1992:110-121.

287. Lovely TJ, Rastogi P: The value of provocative facet blocking as a predictor of success in lumbar spine fusion. J Spinal Disord 1997;10:512-517.

288. Kay J, Findling JW, Raff H: Epidural triamcinolone suppresses the pituitary-adrenal axis in human subjects. Anesth Analg 1994;79:501-505.

289. Ward A, Watson J, Wood P, et al: Glucocorticoid epidural for sciatica: Metabolic and endocrine sequelae. Rheumatology (Oxford) 2002;41:68-71.

290. Alcock E, Regaard A, Browne J: Facet joint injection: A rare form cause of epidural abscess formation. Pain 2003;103:209-210.

291. Gaul C, Neundorfer B, Winterholler M: Iatrogenic (para-) spinal abscesses and meningitis following injection therapy for low back pain. Pain 2005;116:407-410.

292. Orpen NM, Birch NC: Delayed presentation of septic arthritis of a lumbar facet joint after diagnostic facet joint injection. J Spinal Disord Tech 2003;16:285-287.

293. Cohen SP: Postdural puncture headache and treatment following successful lumbar facet block. Pain Digest 1994;4:283-284.

294. Goldstone JC, Pennant JH: Spinal anaesthesia following facet joint injection. A report of two cases. Anaesthesia 1987;42:754-756.

295. Geurts JW, van Wijk RM, Stolker RJ, Groen GJ: Efficacy of radiofrequency procedures for the treatment of spinal pain: A systematic review of randomized clinical trials. Reg Anesth Pain Med 2001;26:394-400.

296. Lora J, Long D: So-called facet denervation in the managment of intractable back pain. Spine 1976;1:121-126.

297. Tzaan WC, Tasker RR: Percutaeous radiofrequency facet rhizotomy—Experience with 118 procedures and reappraisal of its value. Can J Neurol Sci 2000;27:125-130.

298. Lilius G, Harilainen A, Laasonen EM, Myllynen P: Chronic unilateral low-back pain: Predictors of outcome of facet joint injections. Spine 1990;15:780-782.

299. Young S, Aprill C, Laslett M: Correlation of clinical examination characteristics with three sources of chronic low back pain. Spine J 2003;3:460-465.

300. Laslett M, Oberg B, Aprill CN, McDonald B: Zygapophysial joint blocks in chronic low back pain: A test of Revel's model as a screening test. BMC Musculoskel Disord 2004;5:43.

301. Laslett M, McDonald B, Aprill CN, et al: Clinical predictors of screening lumbar zygapophyseal joint blocks: Development of clinical prediction rules. Spine J 2006;6:370-379.

302. Hirsch C, Ingelmark BE, Miller M: The anatomical basis for low back pain: Studies on the presence of sensory nerve endings in ligamentous, capsular and intervertebral disc structures in the human lumbar spine. Acta Orthop Scand 1963;33:1-17.

303. Mooney V, Robertson J: The facet syndrome. Clin Orthop Relat Res 1976;115:149-156.

304. McCall IW, Park WM, O'Brien JP: Induced pain referral from posterior lumbar elements in normal subjects. Spine 1979;4:441-446.

305. Lynch MC, Taylor JF: Facet joint injection for low back pain. A clinical study. J Bone Joint Surg Br 1986;68:138-141.

306. Marks R: Distribution of pain provoked from lumbar facet joints and related structures during diagnostic spinal infiltration. Pain 1989;39:37-40.

307. Kuslich SD, Ulstrom CL, Michael CJ: The tissue origin of low back pain and sciatica: A report of pain response to tissue stimulation during operations on the lumbar spine using local anesthesia. Orthop Clin North Am 1991;22:181-187.

308. Jadad AR, Moore RA, Carroll D, et al: Assessing the quality of randomised clinical trials: Is blinding necessary? Control Clin Trials 1996;17:1-12.

309. Sanders M, Zuurmond WW: Percutaneous intra-articular lumbar facet joint denervation in the treatment of low back pain: A comparison with percutaneous extra-articular lumbar facet denervation. Pain Clinic 1999;11:329-335.

310. Esses SI, Botsford DJ, Kostuik JP: The role of external spinal skeletal fixation in the assessment of low-back disorders. Spine 1989;14:594-601.

311. Jackson RP: The facet syndrome: Myth or reality? Clin Orthop Relat Res 1992;279:110-121.

CHAPTER
57 Radiofrequency Treatment

M. van Kleef, Menno Sluijter, and J. Van Zundert

The use of electric current for pain management has a long history but its popularity has waxed and waned over time because of concerns about safety and until technical improvements made treatment feasible. As early as the second half of the 19th century, brain lesions in animals were made with direct current application, and empirical rules for quantifying lesion size based on current and time were developed.[1,2] One of the first uses in humans dates back to 1931, when direct current of 350 mA was delivered through a needle with a 10-mm uninsulated tip placed in the gasserian ganglion under radiologic control for the management of trigeminal neuralgia.[3] This technique produced lesions with unpredictable size.[4] The use of high-frequency electric current was found to produce lesions of predictable size.[5,6] Because frequencies of 300 to 500 kHz were also used in radio transmitters, the current was called radiofrequency (RF) current. Later, temperature monitoring was suggested to be the most important parameter in obtaining a standardized lesion size when performing stereotactic brain surgery with RF current.[7] The use of RF in pain management dates back to 1965 for percutaneous lateral cordotomy for unilateral pain in cancer patients.[6] A few years later RF treatment of trigeminal neuralgia was described.[8]

The first use of RF current for spinal pain was reported by Shealy,[9] who performed RF lesioning of the medial branch for lumbar zygapophyseal joint pain using a 14-gauge thermistor electrode introduced through a 12-gauge guide needle. This is a fairly large needle diameter that may produce mechanical lesions besides the desired thermal lesions.[10] Another application in spinal pain was introduced by Uematsu,[11] who described RF lesioning of the dorsal root ganglion (DRG) using the same electrode as used by Shealy for medial branch block. The recommended tip temperature of 75° C, combined with the large electrode diameter produced sizable lesions, causing deafferentation pain, and the technique was soon abandoned.[10]

At the end of the 1970s percutaneous cordotomy and RF treatment of the gasserian ganglion were the only widely accepted RF procedures. The use of RF for spinal pain was limited to a few enthusiasts who were regarded as eccentrics. A turning point came in 1980, when small-diameter electrodes, known as the Sluijter Mehta Kit (SMK) system, were introduced for the treatment of spinal pain.[12] The system consists of a 22-gauge disposable cannula with a fine thermocouple probe inside for temperature measurement. The smaller electrode size resulted in diminished discomfort during the procedure. Because there was now less risk for mechanical injury to major nerve trunks, targets in the anterior spinal compartment were no longer off-limits, and procedures such as the RF lesion adjacent to the DRG, the lesion of the communicating ramus,[13,14] and the sympathetic chain became part of the treatment armamentarium.

The RF lesion in the nucleus of the disk for discogenic pain dates back to 1991, and it was described in 1996.[15] This procedure was based on the idea that the low impedance inside the nucleus would cause a high-power deposition. This was theorized to lead to indirect heating of the annulus fibrosus because the disk space is heat insulated cranially and caudally. The initial positive findings were not substantiated in a subsequent randomized controlled trial (RCT).[16]

Over the years the concept that the clinical effect of RF was caused by the formation of heat had not been challenged. Thermocoagulation of nerve fibers would interfere with the conduction of nociceptive stimuli, and pain would be relieved when the nociceptive stimuli stopped reaching the spinal cord. A selective effect of heat on thin nerve fibers might play a role,[17] but that was as far as the discussion went. There were several reasons that the role of heat was finally questioned. First, the classical concept presupposes a strict configuration: the RF lesion must be made in between the nociceptive focus and the central nervous system (CNS). Yet RF lesions can be successfully used in very different situations. For example, in the treatment of acute radicular pain due to a herniated disk the electrode is placed distally to the nociceptive focus.[18] Secondly, RF lesioning adjacent to the DRG induces only transient sensory loss in the relevant dermatome, which can be considered as heat related, whereas the pain relief may be of much longer duration.[19] And third, the role of heat was also questioned by the publication that no differences in outcome were noted when two different tip temperatures (40° and 67° C) were applied to the cervical DRG in chronic cervical radicular pain.[20]

It is against this background that pulsed radiofrequency (PRF) was developed.[21] It is the aim of PRF to deliver strong, fluctuating electric fields while the temperature effects are kept to a minimum. In PRF, radiofrequency current is applied in pulses instead of continuously. Two bursts of 20 ms each are delivered in 1 second. Following the active phase of 20 ms, the silent period of 480 ms allows for washout of the generated heat. The output is usually set at 45 volts, which is much higher than the output used in continuous RF, which is 15 to 20 volts. (Concerning PRF, an extensive literature search is published by Cahana and associates.[22] This group could detect 58 reports on the clinical use of pulsed radiofrequency in different applications: 32 full publications and 26 abstracts. Because this is a new technique, a substantial part of these results is reported in the abstract books of international scientific congresses. Their number is increasing yearly and they are progressively published in peer-reviewed indexed journals.)

Radiofrequency Lesion Generator System

A modern RF-lesion generator (Fig. 57–1) has the following functions:
- Continuous online impedance measurement
- A nerve stimulator
- Monitoring of voltage, current, and wattage during the RF procedure
- Temperature monitoring
- Pulsed current delivery mode

These features are important for the following reasons:

Electrical impedance is measured to confirm the continuity of the electrical circuit. The impedance signal can be converted to a varying audible pitch by the generator, which allows the various tissue interfaces to be "heard" while the operator concentrates on the procedure. The impedance will vary from about 300 to 600 Ω in the extradural tissue. Impedance monitoring is of special interest in cordotomies and in RF disk lesions. In cordotomies the impedance increases above the level of 1000 Ω on entering the spinal cord,[23] thus indicating that the electrode is properly positioned. In RF disk lesions the impedance falls sharply as the electrode enters the disk,[15] below the level of 200 Ω.

Nerve stimulation is of great importance in RF procedures. After placement of the needle under fluoroscopic control, nerve stimulation is carried out to confirm the proper position of the electrode and to permit minor adjustments. Stimulation is carried out at 50 Hz to ensure the proximity of the electrode to the sensory fibers; 2-Hz stimulation is performed to detect muscle contractions, indicating needle placement that is too close to motor fibers. Ford and col-

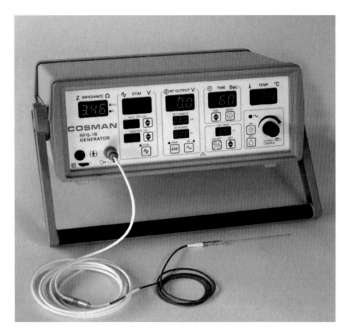

Figure 57–1. Radiofrequency generator.

leagues[24] have shown that if an electrode is actually resting on the nerve, the minimum stimulation level required to produce a discharge is 0.25 volt. As one moves away from the nerve, at a distance of 1 cm, 2 volts would be required. In this manner, the stimulation threshold is an indicator for the electrode nerve distance.

Temperature monitoring is performed using a thermocouple, which is capable of measuring temperature even in very small–diameter electrodes. The thermocouple consists of a junction of two dissimilar metal elements, producing a voltage, which is proportional to temperature. The thermocouple is placed at the tip of the electrode, which is in the hottest part of the lesion.

Theoretic Aspects of Radiofrequency Lesioning

Continuous Radiofrequency

The generator establishes a voltage gradient between the (active) electrode and the (dispersive) ground plate. The body tissues complete the circuit and RF current flows through the tissue, resulting in an alternating electric field. This electric field creates an electric force on the ions (electrolytes) in the tissue, causing them to move back and forth at a high rate. Frictional dissipation of the ionic movement within the fluid medium causes tissue heating. RF heat is therefore generated in the tissue and the electrode is heated by the tissue. The size of the lesion depends on the tip temperature, and the tip temperature depends on the power deposition. But there are other factors involved as well. Heat is also removed from the lesion area by conductive heat loss and by the blood circulation. This is referred to as heat "washout." The larger the heat washout, the smaller the lesion

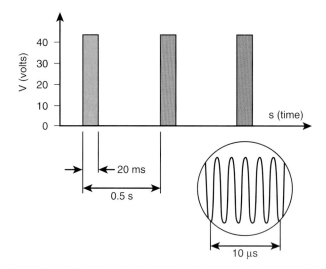

Figure 57–2. Schematic drawing of the duty cycle during pulsed radiofrequency. There are two active cycles/second of 20 msec each. During the active phase radiofrequency is delivered at the normal frequency of 500,000 Hz. (Based on Sluijter ME: Radiofrequency Part I. Meggen, Switzerland, Flivopress, 2001, with permission of the publisher.)

will be for a given tip temperature. Considerable variations of tissue factors influence the heat washout. For example, bone is an effective heat insulator with little water content. For this reason, radiofrequency lesions close to bone will not have the same degree of heat washout as they might have in more conductive tissue. Similarly, the segmental blood vessels, which lie in close relation to the dorsal root ganglion, may cause considerable heat washout, thereby reducing the size of the lesion.[25]

Pulsed Radiofrequency

Pulsed radiofrequency (PRF) (Fig. 57–2) is based on the dual effect of exposure of the tissue to RF fields. Besides the ionic friction that causes the production of heat, there is an independent, nonthermal effect that has the potential of producing modification of neural structures and neuronal behavior. Thermal and nonthermal effects must therefore be discussed separately.

Practical Considerations

When making a heat lesion with continuous RF adjacent to the DRG, it is customary to observe a minimum value of the sensory stimulation threshold of 0.4 volt at 50 Hz, in order to achieve effective denervation. This rule does not apply to PRF because despite the microscopic evidence for destruction, no alterations in nerve function have been reported in a clinical setting. Yet it may be wise to avoid the ultralow sensory thresholds (<0.05 volt) because such values may reflect intraneural electrode placement. A

very small area of necrosis around the needle tip does occur,[25] which is not desirable in an intraneural location.

In a small proportion of procedures the mean tip temperature exceeds 43° C at some point during the PRF procedure. In this case, as a precaution, the power output should be decreased. This can be done by lowering the voltage, or by decreasing either the duration of the active cycle (typically 20 to 30 msec) or the cycle frequency (typically 2 Hz).

It is undesirable to adjust the voltage during a PRF procedure to the mean tip temperature. The mean tip temperature does not affect the outcome of the procedure,[10] and because there is a large variation in heat washout such a practice will cause large and unpredictable variations in voltage. As long as the tip temperature does not exceed 43° C during the PRF procedure, then maintaining the voltage at 45 volts regardless of the resultant tip temperature appears to be the best course of action.

Mode of Action of Pulsed Radiofrequency

PRF was initiated as a method to explore the mode of action of RF, not as a discovery de novo. It is therefore not surprising that the mode of action is not yet clear. Much has been learned on the physical events around the electrode,[25] but it is not known yet how these events cause the clinical effect. There are presently two theories. First, there may be a mild but significant ablative effect, mainly affecting thin nerve fibers. This would not be in contradiction with the absence of sensory changes following PRF because in fact the situation is the same after application of continuous RF. Following a heat lesion sensory changes occur only during the period of postprocedural discomfort but they are absent once the period of pain relief has set in. Second, there might be an effect on the dorsal horn, where trans-synaptic induction of gene expression has been found, in both the short[26] and long term.[27] If this is the case, it is not yet clear how these changes are caused, because the RF is far above the physiologic range of stimulation that leads to nerve depolarization.

INDICATIONS AND CONTRAINDICATIONS FOR RADIOFREQUENCY TREATMENT

Radiofrequency Procedures of the Head

Radiofrequency of the Gasserian Ganglion

Trigeminal Neuralgia
Patients with trigeminal neuralgia have brief episodes of sharp, shooting pain in one or more of the trigeminal divisions, which are typically provoked by touch. This so-called trigger area need not be in the division where the patient experiences the pain. Many patients with first-division pain, for example, have the trigger zone in the second division. In the classic case, the patient is free of pain between painful episodes.

However, residual pain has been reported in 42% of cases.[28] These patients were described as having a combination of trigeminal neuralgia and atypical facial pain. Some of these patients even had a continuous type of pain before the onset of trigeminal neuralgia. Trigeminal neuralgia predominantly occurs in the older age-groups (>50 years old), but it may occasionally be seen in very young patients. It is thought to be caused by vascular compression of the trigeminal root. It occurs frequently in patients with multiple sclerosis, and may indeed be the first symptom of the disease, but more typically it occurs at a later stage, about 12 years after the diagnosis has been made. In a study evaluating the clinical characteristics of patients with trigeminal neuralgia, 22 patients had multiple sclerosis. Six of them had atypical trigeminal neuralgia and 16 patients had signs of brainstem involvement.[29] It is not clear if the pain is caused by plaques in the CNS in these patients, but clinically there was no distinction between patients with and without brainstem involvement. Trigeminal neuralgia also may be caused by a primary nerve tumor. This should always be excluded before symptomatic treatment is considered. A minority of the patients with trigeminal neuralgia report focal numbness in the affected region. But on examination with trigeminal-evoked potentials, abnormalities have been reported in as many as 35% of patients.[30] These figures are distinctly higher in symptomatic trigeminal neuralgia, 60% reporting sensory deficits or having an abnormal corneal reflex. Obviously the sensory deficit often goes unnoticed.

Treatment

In younger patients in otherwise good health, posterior fossa craniotomy with microvascular decompression is the treatment of choice. This treatment has a high success rate and it avoids the sensory loss that is one of the consequences of thermocoagulation of the ganglion. In experienced hands, the complication rate is low; however, when a complication occurs, this is usually a more serious neurologic injury.[31] In patients with multiple sclerosis, the procedure only works if it is combined with a partial section of the trigeminal nerve.[32] This could be an argument in favor of a more central mechanism of the condition in these patients. The duration of pain relief is substantially longer after microvascular decompression than after thermocoagulation of the ganglion. Once the pain recurs, however, there is a problem. Recurrent vascular compression is seldom found during reoperation.[33] Partial sectioning of the nerve is the procedure of choice. But generally other forms of treatment such as thermocoagulation are recommended because the incidence of complications is distinctly higher after reoperation.[33,34] The outcome of thermocoagulation is less favorable, however, in operated patients.[35] Thermocoagulation of the gasserian ganglion, first described by Sweet and Wepsic,[8] has its own advantages and disadvantages.

Procedure

The technique of placing a needle (preferably an SMK-C10) into the gasserian ganglion is as follows:

The oval foramen is visualized first by using a tunnel vision technique. In order to do this the direction of the x-rays should be reversed from the normal configuration because the image intensifier is too bulky to avoid contact with the patient's chest (Fig. 57–3). The C-arm position should be adjusted until the oval foramen is identified just medial to the mandibular processes and just lateral to the maxilla.

The shape of the foramen varies with the angle of the x-rays with the horizontal plane. A more vertical direction will transform the foramen into a round, almost circular shape. A more horizontal direction will make the foramen flat, like a split. The C-arm should be adjusted so that the foramen really has its oval shape. If the skin entry point is now marked over the target point, it will be seen that the variation from patient to patient, in relation to the corner of the mouth, is considerable. The entry point may be just superior to the mandible, but it also may be much more superior, close to the maxilla.

The division of the trigeminal nerve that is the target for treatment also determines the choice of the entry point. For the first division, the end position must be made medial, more superior and less deep (Fig. 57–4).

Adverse Events and Complications

The procedure has a very low morbidity and virtually no mortality. Reports vary considerably regarding recurrence of pain. This is caused by variation in technique. If a dense sensory loss is produced, there is a low incidence of recurrence.[8,36] There is a price to pay for this, however, because the loss of facial sensation and the accompanying paresthesia account for 80% of the side effects of the procedure. One must therefore choose between an earlier recurrence and a lower incidence of paresthesia and the reverse situation. Other complications involve masseter weakness and paralysis (4.1%), anesthesia dolorosa (1%), keratitis (0.6%), and transient paralysis of cranial nerves III and IV (0.8%).[37] A much less frequent complication is permanent palsy of the abducens nerve.[38] There is an extensive experience with RF treatment of trigeminal neuralgia. A review of 25 years' experience with 1600 patients receiving percutaneous RF trigeminal rhizotomy for idiopathic neuralgia indicates acute pain relief in 97.6% of the patients and continued complete pain relief at 5 years' follow-up in 57.7%.[37] Comparisons with other techniques are based mainly on retrospective evaluations.[39-45]

The effectiveness of PRF for trigeminal neuralgia is still a matter of debate.[46] However, a recent prospective randomized study demonstrated that PRF is not an effective method of pain treatment for idiopathic trigeminal neuralgia.[47]

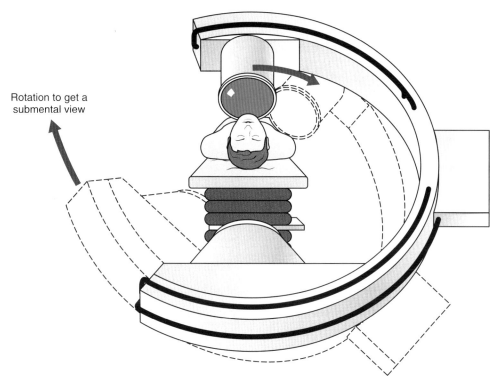

Figure 57–3. Schematic drawing of the fluoroscopy position for performing a radiofrequency procedure of the gasserian ganglion.

Rotation to get a submental view

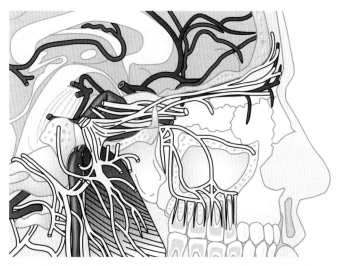

Figure 57–4. Anatomy of the gasserian ganglion and various trigeminal divisions. (From Sluijter ME: Radiofrequency Part II. Meggen, Switzerland, Flivopress, 2001, with permission of the publisher.)

Radiofrequency Treatment of the Sphenopalatine Ganglion

The sphenopalatine ganglion is a parasympathetic ganglion, located in the pterygopalatine fossa, just beneath the maxillary nerve. It is in, or close to, the foramen that connects the pterygopalatine fossa to the nasal cavity. Preganglionic fibers reach the ganglion from the facial nerve, through the greater superficial petrosal nerve and the nerve of the pterygoid canal. There are also connections through the deep petrosal nerve that joins with the greater superficial petrosal nerve to form the vidian nerve (Fig. 57–5). Many afferent fibers cross the ganglion, originating from the nasal mucosa, the soft palate, and the pharynx, on their way to the maxillary nerve and eventually to the gasserian ganglion.

Procedure

The patient is placed in supine position with the head immobilized. The pterygopalatine fossa is identified on the lateral fluoroscopic image, and a line overlying the fossa is drawn on the skin. The intersection of this line with the inferior edge of the zygomatic arch is the entry point. After anesthetizing the skin a 10-cm SMK cannula with a 5-mm active tip is inserted at this point and it is then carefully advanced under lateral fluoroscopic control in a superior and anterior direction, to enter the pterygopalatine fossa (Fig. 57–6). As soon as the fossa is entered, contact is usually made with the maxillary nerve, and the patient will report a paresthesia, then 1 to 2 mL of 2% lidocaine is injected and a pause is observed to allow for the local anesthetic to take effect. The cannula is then further advanced until the tip just passes through the sphenopalatine foramen, which is located in the anterior superior corner of the fossa. It is important that the tip actually passes the foramen, to prevent damage to the maxillary nerve during the lesion.

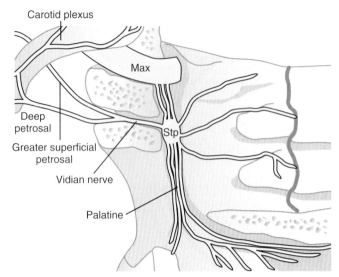

Figure 57–5. Connections of the sphenopalatine ganglion. (From Sluijter ME: Radiofrequency Part II. Meggen, Switzerland, Flivopress, 2001, with permission of the publisher.)

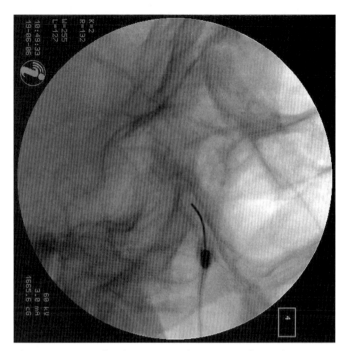

Figure 57–6. Needle placement in the pterygopalatine fossa.

The C-arm of the image intensifier is then placed in the anteroposterior (AP) position. The tip of the cannula should now be projected over the lateral wall of the nasopharynx (Fig. 57–7).

The stylet is removed and replaced by a thermocouple RF probe. The position of the electrode is verified by electrical stimulation at 50 Hz, and this usually results in paresthesia inside the nose at 0.2 to 1 volt. Paresthesia occurring at the outside of the cheek or upper lip indicates stimulation of the maxillary nerve, indicating a position that is too far lateral. If the patient reports paresthesia in the palate, the cannula is also advanced a few millimeters. The treatment consists of three consecutive lesions performed at 70° to 80° C during 60 seconds.[48] In between these lesions the cannula is slowly advanced (1 to 3 mm).

Adverse Events and Complications

Total destruction of the sphenopalatine ganglion causes dryness of the eye, an "open nose" because the mucosa has less inclination to swell, and numbness of the soft palate. Following a heat RF lesion, dryness of the eye is unusual. Numbness of the soft palate does occur, but the condition is usually temporary, with gradual recovery over a period of 4 to 6 weeks. It has been permanent in the occasional patient in whom taste is affected, causing a very unpleasant experience.

Results

There is a rationale for RF treatment of cluster headache because there are so many parasympathetic symptoms during an attack.[48] Also the treatment of atypical facial pain in the second division of the trigeminal nerve has been described.[49] A case report on the use of pulsed radiofrequency of the sphenopala-

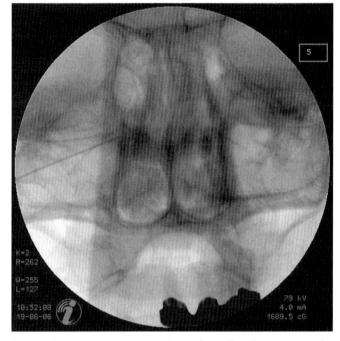

Figure 57–7. Anteroposterior view of needle placement in the pterygopalatine fossa.

tine ganglion for post-traumatic headache showed 17 months of pain relief.[50] An analysis of PRF treatment of the sphenopalatine ganglion in 30 patients suffering chronic head and face pain showed complete pain relief in 21% and mild to moderate pain relief in 65%. No side effects or complications were mentioned.[51] The evidence for the use of PRF is weak, but given the safer character of this treatment option the authors recommend to use PRF first.

Radiofrequency Procedures of the Cervical Spine

Cervical Zygapophyseal (Facet Joint) Pain

Patients with cervical zygapophyseal (facet) joint pain commonly present with a dull and aching bilateral neck pain. Pain emanating from the cervical facet joints can refer into the occiput, interscapular, or shoulder girdle regions depending on which cervical facet joint is involved.[52-55] Pain from the higher cervical facet joints may be at the origin of cervicogenic headache.[56] On physical examination one may find a reduced range of motion of the cervical spine if the higher facet joints are involved. Marked paravertebral tenderness to palpation suggests regional soft tissue changes in response to the underlying injured facet joint, but these findings are not pathognomonic. X-rays, computed tomography (CT), and magnetic resonance imaging (MRI) scans may reveal morphologic abnormalities of the facets; however, there is no direct relationship between anatomic findings and pain.[57,58]

The indications to perform RF denervation of the medial branches that innervate the cervical facet joints are both degenerative and post-traumatic neck pain, such as whiplash-associated pain. Periosteal tearing of the facet joints caused by muscle ligamentous sprain is thought to be the most common cause of whiplash-associated cervical pain.[59-61] Nontraumatic cervical pain can be caused either by progressive degenerative disease or postural changes.

Cervicogenic headache is another possible indication for performing RF treatment of the medial branches of the cervical facet joints. This is described as a unilateral headache localized in the neck and the occipital region and sometimes projecting to the forehead. The pain is presumed to originate from cervical structures, including the facet joints. The anatomy of the cervical spine is illustrated in Figure 57–8. This distinct headache syndrome was described as early as 1926 and Sjaastad and coworkers were the first to name it cervicogenic headache and to propose diagnostic criteria.[56,62] RF denervation of the cervical medial branches is aimed at reducing nociceptive signals from spinal facet joints and shows some promise for treatment of cervicogenic headache.[63] RF facet treatment is usually performed in at least three levels. The levels C2-5 are treated for cervicogenic headache and C4-6 for mid-localized cervical pain.

Procedure

Sedation is not used because of the need for continuous communication between physician and patient. Several approaches to reach the medial branch of the dorsal ramus at the upper and middle cervical area can be used.

The most commonly used approach by these authors is the posterolateral approach.[64] For this technique the patient is positioned supine on the operating table. The C-arm is positioned in a moderately oblique (±25 degrees) angle with the horizontal plane to secure a safe distance between the electrode

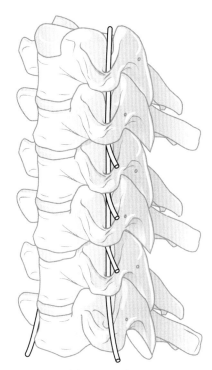

Figure 57–8. Anatomy of the cervical spine (artist's rendering).

tip and the exiting segmental nerve. In this position the direction of the x-rays is almost aligned with the axis of the intervertebral foramen, thus the segmental nerves exit approximately in a plane perpendicular to the image intensifier. The degree of obliquity should be such that the contralateral pedicles are projected a little anterior to 50% of the vertebral body (Fig. 57–9). Only slight caudal or cranial angulation of the C-arm will allow a clear view of the intervertebral disks and the neuroforamina. In this projection, the medial branch runs over the base of the superior articular process. Entry points are marked on the skin, somewhat posterior and caudal to the target points as seen on the monitor, that is, dorsal from the posterior border of the facet column and slightly caudal.

A cannula (50-mm SMK) is now introduced in the horizontal plane, and in a slightly cranial direction. The tip of the cannula should be projected over the bone of the facetal column, to prevent inadvertent passage of the cannula posterior to the facet joints. It should also stay posterior to a line connecting the posterior aspects of the intervertebral foramina, to prevent contact with the exiting segmental nerves. The cannula is carefully advanced, observing these rules, until contact is made with bone at the base of the superior articular process.

The most caudal cannula should be introduced first. This is because this is technically the most difficult level, and it is easier to do it while the other needles are not yet in the way. Once the first needle is in the proper position, the other needles are introduced in the same way as described earlier. We prefer

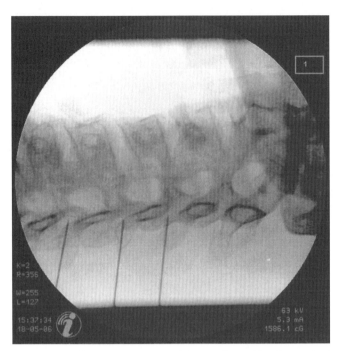

Figure 57–9. Fluoroscopic image of the needle position for cervical medial branch procedure.

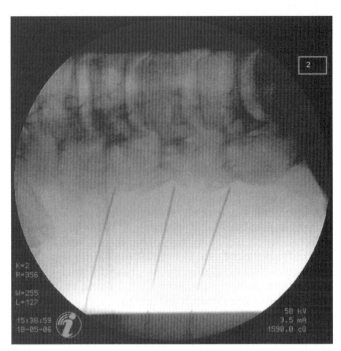

Figure 57–10. Anteroposterior view of the cervical spine—needle position for medial branch procedure.

to take advantage of the first needle serving as an indicator for the direction and depth for subsequent needles, which accounts for our recommendation of placing all needles before applying RF rather than lesioning a single medial branch and then placing the next needle.

The technique is identical for the medial branches from C3-6. The direction of the needle at the C2 level is different. It should be oriented toward the small branches of the greater occipital nerve that innervate the C2-3 facet joint and not toward the medial branch itself, which is in fact the greater occipital nerve. For the RF treatment of this facet joint, the needle should be placed at the arch of C2 at the level of the upper border of foramen of C3. The position of the C-arm is then changed to AP, and this should confirm the position of the needle tips adjacent to the concavity ("waist") of the articular pillars of the cervical spine at the corresponding level (Fig. 57–10). A heat lesion at the C2-3 level often causes severe postoperative discomfort. We therefore prefer to use PRF in this case.

When anatomic positioning is optimal, electrical stimulation is performed. First an electrical stimulation rate of 50 Hz should be performed, which should elicit a tingling sensation in the neck at less than 0.5 volt. Next, stimulation at 2 Hz is performed to confirm accurate needle position. Contractions of the paraspinal muscles will be noticed. Muscle contractions in the arm indicate a needle placement too close to the exiting nerve. In that case the needle should be repositioned more posteriorly. Once proper positioning of the needle is confirmed, the medial

branch of the dorsal ramus is anesthetized with 1 to 2 mL local anesthetic solution (lidocaine 1% or 2%). An 80° C RF thermo lesion is made for 60 seconds at each level.

A second approach, which is more popular in the United States, is the posterior approach of the facet joint. This was first introduced by Lord and associates in 1995.[65] In this technique the patient is positioned prone on the operating table, with the head flexed (about 5 to 10 degrees) and with the face resting on a padded ring. This is a "tunnel vision" technique, in which the target points are the posterior aspects of the waists of the articular pillars, and the levels to be blocked are the same as the entry points. The needle is introduced from the posterior aspect of the neck to make contact with each of the two nerves supplying each painful joint.

Adverse Events and Complications

To date, there are few reported complications from cervical facet joint denervation when performing the procedure using the posterolateral approach and systematically following the previously described steps.[66] Some postoperative burning pain is described in more than 30% of patients.[63] It disappears spontaneously after 1 to 3 weeks. A feeling of dizziness and vertigo is frequently described, especially after medial branch blocks at higher levels. Secondarily RF denervation of the third occipital nerve can partially block the upper cervical proprioceptive afferents and can result in transient ataxia and unsteadiness.[36,54,67] Thus patients undergoing RF treatment of the superior cervical facets should be advised not to drive a car or handle other dangerous machinery for 24 hours following the procedure. Some patients (13%) report a transient exacerbation of their pain, which they describe as burning in nature. This usually resolves in 2 to 6 weeks.[67] Vervest and Stolker also reported 4% of patients with occipital hypoesthesia that resolved in 3 months.[67] They supposed it was caused by a lesion of the third occipital nerve.

Results

A randomized, double-blind, controlled trial in patients with chronic pain of the lower cervical facet joints after whiplash injury, whose facet pain was confirmed with double-blind placebo controlled local anesthetic blocks, revealed that RF facet denervation could provide lasting pain relief that was not a placebo effect.[61] The long-term efficacy of percutaneous RF medial branch neurotomy in the treatment of chronic neck pain was assessed in a double-blind, controlled study.[68] Neurotomy (using the posterior parasagittal approach) was performed in patients with a positive response to either comparative or placebo-controlled blocks. Neck pain relief was clinically satisfying but of limited duration. The procedure can, however, be repeated when pain recurs, with similar success.

The efficacy of RF medial branch neurotomy for the treatment of facet joint pain in whiplash patients was evaluated in a prospective study. The patient population consisted of a group involved in litigation and a group with no litigation case pending. The response to RF treatment was not influenced by a potential secondary gain. The study showed that RF neurotomy is efficacious in the treatment of traumatic cervical facet arthropathy.[69] Van Suijlekom and coworkers evaluated the effect of radiofrequency lesioning of the medial branch of the dorsal ramus of the segmental nerve at the levels C3-6 in the treatment of cervicogenic headache.[63] In this study the lateral approach was used. They demonstrated that RF cervical facet denervation leads to a significant reduction in headache severity and number of days with headache and analgesic intake in patients with cervicogenic headache diagnosed according to the criteria of Sjaastad and colleagues.[56] In a randomized, double-blind, sham-controlled study on RF denervation of facet joints C2-3 for the treatment of cervicogenic headache, 12 patients were included and followed during 24 months. A slight improvement was noted in the RF group at 3 months, whereas no differences were noted during the remaining follow-up period. These findings led to the conclusion that the procedure is probably not beneficial in cervicogenic headache.[70]

Haspeslagh and associates[71] could not find evidence that RF treatment of cervical facet joints is better treatment than injection in the greater occipital nerve. However, a definite conclusion about the clinical efficacy of the procedure can only be drawn from a randomized controlled trial in a greater number of patients.

Cervical Radicular Pain

Cervicobrachialgia is a widespread pain syndrome. Bland estimates that 9% of all men and 12% of all women experience this pain at some time in their lives.[72] Later on, in 1994, Radhakrishnan and associates published a population-based survey.[73] In this epidemiologic survey, an annual incidence of cervical radiculopathy of 83.2 per 100,000 in a population between 13 and 91 years was found.

The pain in cervicobrachialgia is described as a continuous, dull aching pain in the neck (most commonly localized in the mid- and lower cervical area) radiating beyond the shoulder into the arm with referral to a particular spinal segment. Segmental pain in the upper extremity can be related to disk pathology, such as cervical disk protrusion with irritation of the spinal nerve. Spinal nerve irritation can also be caused by narrowing of the intervertebral foramen by spondylosis. The most common levels involved are C6, C7, and to a lesser extent C5. The levels C4 and C8 are uncommon. The involved spinal level can be estimated by the dermatome in which the pain is radiating[74] and can be determined by diagnostic nerve blocks.[66,75,76] Diagnosis of cervical radicular pain and radiculopathy requires a complete history taking; clinical diagnosis using standardized test methods of physical examination, medical imaging, electrophysiologic investigation, and determination of the causative level by means of selective nerve root blocks.

Procedure

To perform a diagnostic segmental nerve block a viewing technique is used with the C-arm positioned so that the x-rays are parallel to the axis of the intervertebral foramen. This axis points 25 to 35 degrees anterior and 10 degrees caudal. With the C-arm in this position the entry is found by projecting a metal ruler over the caudal part of the foramen. A 50-mm, 22-gauge neurography needle is carefully introduced parallel to the beam of the x-rays. Then the direction of the x-rays is changed to AP position and the cannula is further introduced until the tip is projected just lateral from the facetal column. After the segmental nerve has been identified with 0.4 mL iohexol contrast medium, 0.5 mL of 2% lidocaine is slowly infiltrated around the nerve. The resultant radiopaque mixture is closely observed during injection so that accidental overflow into the epidural space can be avoided.[75]

For the RF procedure, the same viewing technique is used. The entry point is found by projecting the metal ruler over the caudal and posterior parts of the foramen. The cannula (SMK-C5 with a 2-mm exposed tip) is introduced parallel to the beam of the x-rays and, if necessary, the approach is corrected while still in the superficial layers until the cannula is projected on the screen as a single dot (Fig. 57–11). In practice this dot should lie directly over the dorsal part of the intervertebral foramen at the transition between the

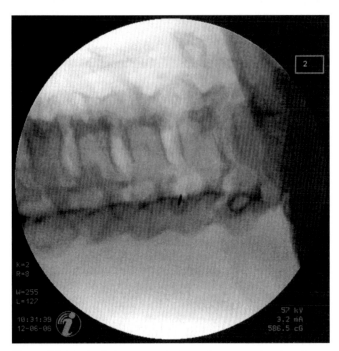

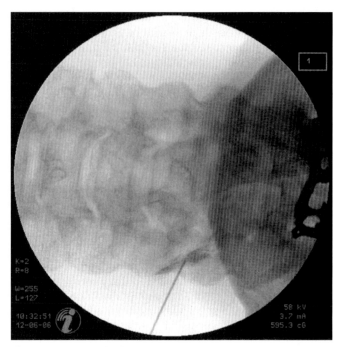

Figure 57–11. Radiofrequency lesion adjacent to the dorsal root ganglion 20 degrees oblique, 10 degrees craniocaudal projection. The needle is positioned in the posterior aspect of the foramen, at the junction of the middle and caudal third part. It is projected as a dot in tunnel vision.

Figure 57–12. Radiofrequency dorsal root ganglion (RF-DRG) anteroposterior view. The tip of the needle is projected over the facetal column.

middle and most caudal third. This dorsal position is chosen in order to avoid possible damage to the motor fibers of the segmental nerve and to the vertebral artery that runs anterior to the ventral part of the foramen. The direction of the x-rays is then changed to AP and the cannula is further introduced until the tip is projected over the middle of the facetal column (Fig. 57–12).

The stylet is now replaced by the RF probe. After checking the impedance, electrical stimulation is started at a rate of 50 Hz. The patient should feel a tingling sensation between 0.4 and 0.65 volt. The frequency is then changed to 2 Hz and the patient is observed for muscle contractions. These should not occur below a voltage of 1.5 times the sensory threshold. One half milliliter of iohexol is now injected to exclude an accidental intradural positioning of the electrode, and this is followed by 2 mL of 2% lidocaine. RF current is then passed through the electrode in order to increase the tip temperature to 67° C. This temperature is maintained for 60 seconds.

Adverse Events and Complications

A side effect that is often seen (40% to 60%) is a mild burning sensation (some deep neck soreness) in the treated dermatome that subsides spontaneously after 1 to 3 weeks.[75] Some sensory changes, such as a slight hypoesthesia may occur, but invariably disappears within 3 or 4 months.[19,20,75]

Known complications of a blockade of a cervical segmental nerve are the epidural intrathecal, intra-

vascular injection of local anesthetic. During this procedure, injectate can be placed in the adjacent venous plexus, in the vertebral artery or even in the carotid artery. Because of the proximity to the brain in the higher cervical levels, there is the risk of local anesthetic CNS toxicity (seizure), although only a low volume of local anesthetic is used.[77]

Results

In 1991, Vervest and Stolker published a retrospective study in 53 patients with prolonged cervical pain radiating to the occipital region, head, shoulder, or arm not responding to conservative treatment.[67] If there was local tenderness at the facet joints, a percutaneous cervical facet joint denervation was performed. If this was not successful and there was cervical pain with referral to the occipital region or arm, indicating segmental nerve irritation, diagnostic segmental nerve blocks were performed. A positive diagnostic block was followed by an RF-DRG. The results were good to excellent in 80.5% of treatments. After a follow-up of 1.5 years, 44 patients (84.5%) still had satisfactory pain relief.

In an open prospective study, 20 consecutive patients with chronic intractable pain in the cervical region with referral to the head, shoulder, or arm, RF-DRG provided pain relief in 75% of patients at 3 months and in 50% of patients at 6 months.[19] These results indicated an acceptable initial pain relief, but a tendency for pain recurrence at 3 to 9 months. A prospective double-blind, randomized, sham-controlled trial of RF lesions adjacent to the cervical DRG for the management of chronic cervical radicular pain, showed a positive outcome during the first

8 weeks after the procedure.[75] Slappendel and colleagues[20] found in a double-blind, randomized study with 3 months' follow-up that RF treatment adjacent to the cervical DRG at 40° C is equally effective as treatment at 67° C.

Despite these encouraging results, in a recent systematic review Geurts and associates[78] concluded that there is limited evidence that RF-DRG is more effective than placebo in chronic cervicobrachialgia. Niemisto and coworkers[79] in their systematic review came to the same conclusion.

In 2003, Van Zundert and colleagues published a clinical audit of 18 patients with cervicogenic headache or cervicobrachialgia who failed conservative treatment and underwent pulsed radiofrequency treatment adjacent to the cervical dorsal root ganglion.[80] In 72% of the patients there was a minimum pain reduction of at least 50% at 8 weeks. At 1 year 33% of the patients continued to rate the treatment outcome as good or very good. No neurologic side effects or complications were observed. The first RCT on PRF adjacent to the cervical DRG in patients with chronic cervical radicular pain was published. At 3 months the PRF group showed a significantly better outcome with regard to the global perceived effect (>50% improvement) and Visual Analogue Scale (VAS) (20-point pain reduction). The need for pain medication was significantly reduced in the PRF group after 6 months. No complications were observed during the study period.[81]

There is limited evidence that a PRF-DRG on a cervical level is as effective as an RF-DRG. But PRF-DRG is safer and has fewer side effects. Therefore the authors suggest against performing RF lesioning at this level.

Radiofrequency Procedures of the Thoracic Spine

Thoracic pain accounts for approximately 5% of all referrals to a pain clinic.[82,83] Thoracic pain may have many causes from cardiac to lung pathology in addition to pain referred to the chest from other affected organs (upper abdominal organs such as gallbladder and pancreas). In the lower thoracic regions pain must be differentiated from renal pathology.[84] Thoracic pain may have an underlying pathology such as disk herniations, aneurysms, tumors,[85] postoperative sternal wound infection,[86] trauma,[87] old fractures, or herpetic infections,[88] and stress fractures in athletes.[89,90] Chronic postsurgical pain has been described following many different operations, most notably thoracotomy, mastectomy, and coronary artery bypass grafting.[91-93] However in most cases, thoracic pain is judged to be of spinal origin, emanating from nociceptive nerve endings in the periosteum, ligaments, disks, or joints.[94]

Thoracic pain can be divided into thoracic mechanical joint pain and thoracic segmental pain. The thoracic spine is a relatively immobile section. The range of motion for both flexion and extension is of the order of 10 degrees, and lateral flexion is almost impossible. Rotation of the thoracic spine is the only meaningful movement of the thoracic spine.

Thoracic mechanical pain features pain in both thoracic facet joints as well as thoracic disks.[95,96]

Pain emanating from thoracic facet joints is usually related to degenerative processes, vertebral collapse, and continual mechanical strain.[94] The problem can be in the facet joint but may manifest elsewhere in the spine.[54] There are no specific pathognomonic criteria, whereby thoracic facet joint pain can be diagnosed based on a patient's history and physical examination. A diagnosis of thoracic facet joint pain can be made based on similarity of symptoms to lumbar and cervical facet syndromes. Extensive examination should be performed to rule out any pathology as a primary cause for symptoms and signs.

When thoracic spinal pain becomes chronic and resistant to conservative treatment modalities such as physical therapy, pharmacologic therapy, and transcutaneous electrical nerve stimulation (TENS), minimal invasive treatment modalities including radiofrequency lesioning of the facet joints can be considered.

The thoracic facet joints are more vertically oriented than the lumbar facet joints and lie almost parallel to the coronal plane (Fig. 57–13). They are oriented perpendicular to the sagittal plane and face directly anterior. The thoracic facet joints are innervated by medial branches of the posterior primary rami of the segmental nerves. Each thoracic facet joint is bisegmentally innervated by the medial branch of the same level and the medial branch of the level above. The thoracic medial branches pass through the intertransverse space and touch the superolateral corner of the transverse process. Then they run medially and inferiorly across posterior surfaces of the transverse processes before entering the posterior compartment of the back and innervating the multifidus muscles.[97] In that location they give

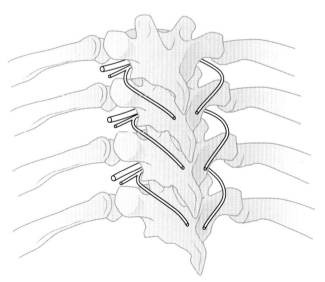

Figure 57–13. Anatomy of the thoracic spine.

ascending articular branches to the facet joint. An exception to this pattern occurs at the midthoracic levels (T5-8). Although the curved course remains essentially the same, inflection occurs at a point superior to the superolateral corner of the transverse process. This course is different than that seen with the lumbar medial branches, which are fixed at the junction of the superior articular process and the transverse process. The T11 and T12 medial branches have the same course as the lumbar medial branches.[98]

Procedure

The patient is placed in the prone position. Obtaining a fluoroscopic view is quite difficult for a variety of reasons. In this region one has to contend with overprojection of the ribs, the prominent transverse process that is directed slightly cranial and markedly posterior, and the size and orientation of the pedicles that can make them difficult to visualize. In addition, the orientation of the thoracic facet joints impedes the operator's ability to differentiate between superior and inferior articular processes.

In contrast to diagnostic thoracic intra-articular block, which has been well described,[99] expert opinion varies on RF lesioning of medial branches in the thoracic vertebrae. Nonetheless we describe how to perform an RF lesion of the medial branches at the thoracic level. Although we embrace this technique some authors have suggested that the needle tip is actually "too far anterior" to the medial branch to result in denervation. Using the junction between the superior articular process and the superior border of the transverse process as a target point for thoracic medial branch neurotomy, Stolker and colleagues reported that the medial branch of the dorsal ramus was never within reach of the electrodes.[100] The C-arm is positioned in the axial plane and an external radiopaque object such as a clamp is used to identify the proper level. A straight AP view of the vertebra at the anticipated target level is obtained. The end plates of the vertebra should be parallel without any visible end plate double contours. Then the C-arm is rotated slightly obliquely. This should facilitate the access to the target point that is the junction of the superior articular process and the transverse process. A proposed entry point is marked on the skin and local anesthetics (lidocaine 1%) are injected with a 23-gauge needle. The RF needle is then inserted parallel with the angle of the C-arm beam until bone contact at the junction of the superior articular process and the transverse process (Fig. 57–14A).

Subsequently, the needle is redirected slightly more cranially and laterally until it is just loses osseous contact. Then the needle position is checked in the lateral view. The needle tip should be just posterior to a line connecting the posterior aspects of the neuroforamina (see Fig. 57–14B).

Stimulation at 50 Hz is now performed. A paravertebral tingling sensation should be perceived with a current of less than 0.5 volt. Next, stimulation at 2 Hz should provoke paravertebral muscle contrac-

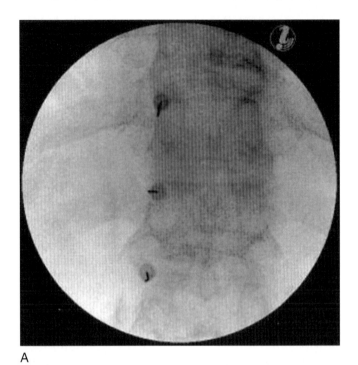

A

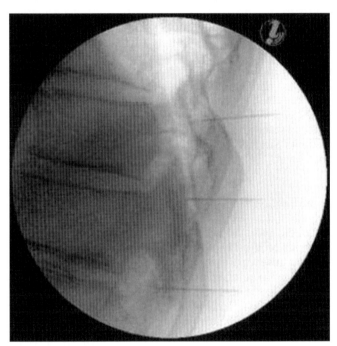

B

Figure 57–14. Thoracic facet joint and AP view **(A)** lateral view **(B).**

tions at less than or equal to 1 volt. Stimulation should be negative for anterior nerve root stimulation, which would be perceived as muscle contraction or pain in the anterior chest wall or abdominal region depending on the level undergoing RF. When proper needle positioning has been confirmed with fluoroscopic imaging and electrical stimulation, 0.5 mL of lidocaine 1% or 2% is administered at each level. After local anesthesia has taken effect RF lesioning is conducted for 60 seconds at 20 volts. We typically perform RF treatment of three levels because of the multisegmental innervation of the facet joints.

Adverse Events and Complications

As with any RF procedure there is always the possibility of postprocedure exacerbation of pain. A complication unique to the thoracic region is a pneumothorax. Proper technique and the use of fluoroscopic guidance for the placement of the needle will minimize the risk of this complication. The patient must be warned of the possibility of the development of a pneumothorax and should return to the hospital if shortness of breath or pain with inspiration develops.

Stolker and coworkers evaluated 40 patients with thoracic facet syndrome who underwent percutaneous facet joint denervation: 24 left sided, 21 right sided, and 6 bilateral. Seven study patients underwent two sessions and two patients had three facet joint denervation sessions; 82% of patients had 50% to 75% pain relief at 2 months. Four patients were lost to long-term follow-up (18 to 54 months, mean 31 months); 44% of study patients were pain-free and 39% had a 50% or greater reduction of their pain.[96] In line with these criteria being nonspecific in thoracic facet syndrome all patients in this study had positive diagnostic blocks performed prior to radiofrequency ablation. Stolker and coworkers attributed their results to the consistent course of the medial branch of the dorsal rami of the thoracic spinal nerves as they leave the intertransverse space; however, the anatomic target point (junction between the superior articular process and the transverse process) they used in their study is at variance with the anatomic course of thoracic medial branch described by Chua and Bogduk.[97] They reported that the medial branch crosses the superolateral corners of the transverse processes and then passes medially and inferiorly along the posterior surfaces of the transverse processes before ramifying into the multifidus muscle it supplies.[97] Bogduk has called for the need for a double-blind, controlled clinical trial of Stolker's approach to thoracic facet nerve denervation or modification of their procedure so as to be concordant with the surgical anatomy of the thoracic medial branches.[97]

In another study by Tzaan and Tasker in 2000, which evaluated 17 patients with thoracic facet syndrome, 15 patients had satisfactory pain relief at follow-up, with 2 patients having their procedure repeated.[101]

Thoracic Segmental Pain Syndromes

Thoracic segmental pain syndromes have many causes including disease or lesions of ribs, disorders of the thoracic skeletal spine (fractures, arthritis, metabolic disorders, and tumors), or neuropathies originating from spinal roots, spinal nerves, or intercostal nerves.[94]

Some thoracic segmental pain syndromes are iatrogenic, such as post-thoracotomy and postmastectomy syndromes as well as incisional pain after upper gastrointestinal surgery.[92,93,102]

Percutaneous thoracic sympathectomy is considered the most efficacious for sympathetic mediated pain, Raynaud's syndrome, hyperhidrosis, and vasculopathy.[103] Percutaneous radiofrequency adjacent to the thoracic dorsal root ganglion has been described for segmental nerve pain related to intercostal pain, rib tip syndrome, twelfth rib syndrome, vertebral collapse, and segmental peripheral neuralgia.

In the higher thoracic segments, it is difficult to reach the dorsal root ganglia because of overlying anatomic structures. Among the obstacles are the wide facet column, articulations of the transverse processes with the ribs, and most importantly the lungs. The pulmonary structures prevent adopting a very lateral approach, which would have been ideal to allow getting under the posterior osseous barriers. In successive lower thoracic segments, the anatomy gradually resembles the anatomy of the lumbar spine. This change creates an opportunity for lower thoracic DRG to be reached as if it were a lumbar DRG.

Procedure

Two or more diagnostic blocks at different levels must be performed to identify the segment involved because of the frequent overlapping of thoracic segmental pain from one segment to another. An intercostal block can be used as a test block of a thoracic segmental nerve.[104] The level that provides the best temporary pain reduction is then selected for RF lesioning of the dorsal root ganglion. As described, in the upper thoracic spine the classic approach (posterolateral approach) is not possible because the foramina face more anteriorly and accurate positioning of the needle is hindered by the angle of the ribs. Therefore an alternative technique is used to reach the DRG of T7 and above. The patient is placed in the prone position and a dorsal approach is used. The target point is the craniodorsal part of the intervertebral foramen and is thus the same as the target point in the classic dorsolateral approach. The entry point is the midpoint of the pedicle in the AP view (Figs. 57–15 and 57–16).

This entry point is checked in a lateral view, where it should aim for the superior dorsal quadrant of the foramina where the DRG is supposed to be lying. Under local anesthesia, a small hole is drilled through the lamina of the vertebra under fluoroscopic guidance in the AP view using a 16-gauge Kirschner wire. A potential danger is the piercing of the facet joint. The RF cannula is inserted through the hole into the proper position, which is checked in the lateral view and should be in the craniodorsal part of the intervertebral foramen (Fig. 57–17).

The stylet of the cannula is replaced with an RF probe and stimulation at 50 Hz is carried out. The patient should feel tingling sensations in the selected dermatome using a 0.4- to 1-volt stimulus. Stimulation at 2 Hz should not give contractions of the

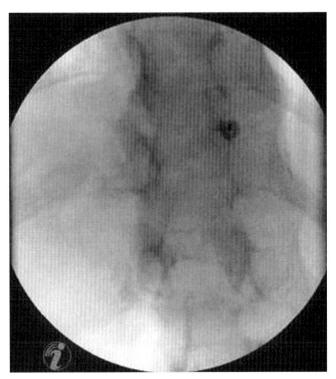

Figure 57–15. Thoracic pulsed radiofrequency dorsal root ganglion (PRF-DRG) entry point.

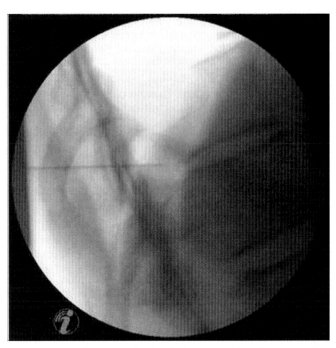

Figure 57–17. Thoracic pulsed radiofrequency-dorsal root ganglion (PRF-DRG) lateral view.

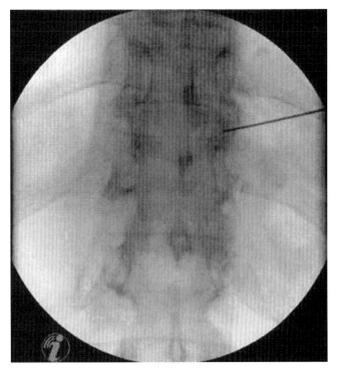

Figure 57–16. Thoracic pulsed radiofrequency dorsal root ganglion (PRF-DRG) anteroposterior view; note that the needle is in the middle of the facetal column.

intercostal muscles at a stimulation threshold below 1.5 times the sensory threshold. After satisfactory placement is achieved, 0.4 mL of iohexol contrast medium is injected to exclude intradural or intravascular spread. When correct position has been confirmed, 1 to 2 mL of lidocaine 1% or 2% is injected and a 60-second 67° C lesion is made.

At the lower levels the same approach can be used as at the lumbar level. The needle position, the stimulation, and the lesion parameters are identical. This technique is described under RF-DRG treatment in the lumbar region.

A 10-cm SMK 22-gauge cannula with a 5-mm active tip and an RF probe can be used. This needle can be manually curved to perform the parasagittal approach. For the dorsal approach, a 16-gauge Kirschner wire can be used the make a burr hole into the lamina.

Adverse Events and Complications

One of the most important complications is the possibility of damage to the nerve root or spinal cord during needle placement. Another common complication is neuritis. Again, there is a slight possibility of a pneumothorax and hemothorax. These particular complications should be described in detail to any prospective candidate for RF lesioning at the thoracic level. Other possible complications include infection, increased pain, bleeding, and bruising. It cannot be overemphasized that the absence of a pneumothorax should be clinically excluded. If any doubt remains then radiographs are mandatory.

Results

Radiofrequency treatment adjacent to the thoracic dorsal root ganglion was evaluated in 45 patients who underwent 53 PRFs adjacent to the dorsal root ganglion, 37 at one level, 1 patient bilaterally at one level, and 7 patients at two levels unilaterally. Clinical diagnoses included intercostal neuralgia, postthoracotomy pain syndrome, postmastectomy pain syndrome, twelfth rib syndrome, rib resection, osteoporosis, vertebral metastasis, and traumatic collapsed vertebra. At first follow-up 2 months postprocedure, 66.7% were pain-free, 24% obtained more than 50% pain relief, and 9% obtained no pain relief. Four patients were lost to long-term follow-up or died from their malignant disease. After a follow-up of 13 to 46 months (median 24 months) 49% were pain-free, 37% had good pain relief, and 14.6% had no pain relief.[105]

The authors in this study advocate prognostic blockade as essential to (1) confirm the diagnosis of segmental pain, (2) to determine appropriate level of treatment, and (3) to assess potential benefit of percutaneous RF adjacent to the dorsal root ganglion.

In a similar study Van Kleef and Spaans[19] evaluated effects of a single-level RF lesioning adjacent to the dorsal root ganglion in thoracic segmental pain. In this study 43 patients were evaluated with a minimum of a 6-month history of unilateral thoracic segmental pain unresponsive to conservative therapies. Twenty-seven of the patients had pain in the distribution of one or two segments (group 1) only, whereas 16 patients had pain in more than two segmental levels (group 2). Short-term analysis at 8 weeks postprocedure showed that 52% of patients in group 1 were pain-free or had good pain relief, whereas only 18% of patients in group 2 were pain-free or had good pain relief. Long-term follow-up (36 to 168 weeks, mean 99 weeks) illustrated that 37% of patients in group 1 were pain-free or had good pain relief, whereas only 18% of patients in group 2 had such a positive outcome at long-term follow-up (40 to 60 weeks, mean 128 weeks).

Conclusions

The data on RF facet and RF-DRG on thoracic levels published in the years 1994 to 1996 are all retrospectively collected. For that reason the level of evidence for the different procedures is low. In case of thoracic segmental radicular pain for which treatment of the DRG might be considered, we prefer a PRF-DRG as first step, in line with the policy on cervical level. In spite of the fact that there is no formal evidence for this procedure, PRF is safer on this level. When a PRF-DRG on the thoracic level has only a temporary effect an RF-DRG can be considered.

Radiofrequency Procedures of the Lumbar Spine

Introduction

The annual incidence of low back pain is 18.6% in an adult population, and most of it is mild.[106] The prognosis of this low back pain is not as good as we once believed. Spitzer[107] stated that 92% of these patients were recovered 6 months after the onset of this low back pain. Recent studies indicate that 62% of patients with low back pain still experienced pain after 12 months.[108,109] At this moment there are few interventions with long-term effect on chronic low back pain. However, there are some evidence-based interventions with minimal clinical short-term effect such as behavior therapy, back schools, manipulation and COX-inhibitors.[110] The minority of low back pain patients have specific causes of their pain such as herniated disk, spondylolisthesis, diskitis, or fractures. Most have undiagnosed low back pain. In those patients the back pain may emanate from potential painful structures including the lumbar facet joints, the intervertebral disks, or the sacroiliac joint(s). The anatomy of the lumbar spine is illustrated in Figure 57–18.

Lumbar Zygapophyseal (Facet Joint) Pain

The prevalence of facet joint pain is 15% to 32% of an adult population with low back pain.[111] Patients with lumbar facet joint pain may present with paramedian pain (one or both sides), absence of exacerbation by coughing ($P < 0.07$), absence of exacerbation by forward flexion and raising from this flexion ($P < 0.002$), absence of worsening by hyperextension, and pain immediately on standing and walking

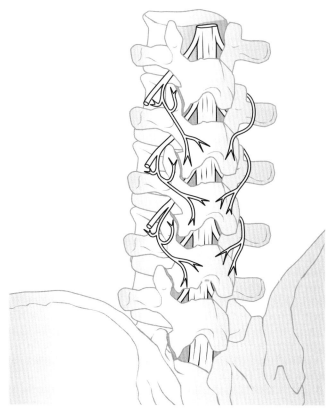

Figure 57–18. Anatomy of the lumbar spine.

$(P = 0.001).^{112,113}$ The diagnosis is confirmed by means of at least 50% pain reduction after a diagnostic local anesthetic nerve block of the dorsal ramus of L4-5.

Procedure

The patient assumes a prone position on the fluoroscopic table. A pillow is placed under the abdomen to diminish the physiologic lumbar lordosis. First, targeted levels are identified and a straight AP projection is obtained. Then the C-arm is rotated cranially or caudally until there are no double contours of the caudal end plate of the middle vertebra. The middle vertebra of the levels to be treated is used as the reference point prior to the searching for the optimal position of the C-arm. Subsequently, the C-arm is rotated to an approximately 15-degree oblique view until the spinous processes are projecting over the midline but well inside the contralateral facet joints. Then the entry point should be marked over the target point, which is the junction of the superior articular process and transverse process. To perform a diagnostic block, the target point should be approximately 1 mm under this junction to avoid unwanted spreading of local anesthetics to segmental nerves and creating false-positive results. After injection of local anesthetic (lidocaine 1%) into the skin, the needle is inserted at the entry point and slowly advanced using a tunnel vision technique until the tip makes contact with bone. For a diagnostic block, the position of the needle is then checked in the lateral view, and should be at the level of the inferior part of the intervertebral foramen in line with the facet joint column. When accurate positioning is confirmed and following a negative aspiration, 1 mL of local anesthetic (lidocaine 1%) is injected at each level. To perform RF lesioning of the medial branch, after making bone contact with the needle tip, the needle is redirected slightly more cephalad until bone contact is lost, and the cannula is advanced 1 to 2 mm farther anteriorly over the superior margin of the transverse process (Figs. 57–19 and 57–20).

The C-arm is then rotated into the lateral view to check the position of the needle tip, which should be in line with the facet joint column and at the level of the inferior part of the intervertebral foramen about 1 mm dorsal to the level of the line connecting the posterior aspects of the intervertebral foramina. It should be a little deeper and more cranial than the position of the needle for the diagnostic block. When this position is confirmed, stimulation at 50 Hz is conducted. The patient should feel new pressure or tingling in the back at less than 0.5 volt. If sensations are felt in the ipsilateral extremity, the needle tip is too close to the segmental nerve. It is imperative to withdraw the needle slightly and check stimulation again at 50 Hz. Subsequently stimulation at 2 Hz is performed. The patient should experience localized contractions of the multifidus muscle and not of muscles of the leg. These local contractions can be palpated by the operator. Similarly any contractions that occur in the leg may be detected by the operator or the assistant if a hand is placed over the muscles

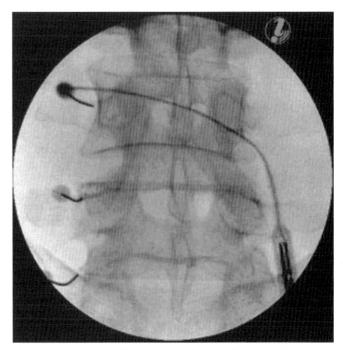

Figure 57–19. Needle position for medial branch lumbar procedure.

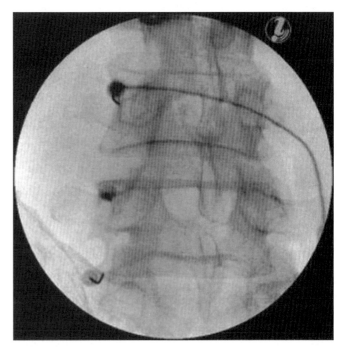

Figure 57–20. Rotated C-arm for lumbar facet procedure.

innervated by the exiting nerve root. If the patient perceives pain or contractions in the extremity or if muscular contractions are detected by an operator, then the needle must be repositioned. After accurate positioning of the needle tip and a negative aspiration is demonstrated, 1 mL of local anesthetic (lidocaine 1%) is injected at each level. RF lesioning at 67° C is performed for 60 seconds.

The fluoroscopic view for the L5-S1 facet joint and thus the medial branch of the L5 is different from the other lumbar levels because of the difference in anatomy. The L5 medial branch lies at the junction between the superior sacral articular process and the upper border of the sacrum. Because there is no pedicle at this level to use as a radiologic landmark, the C-arm is positioned so that the junction is seen as a round curved transition. The C-arm is rotated slightly oblique (about 15 degrees). The identified target point is the curve of the transition and is the same as the entry point. The needle is thus placed using tunnel vision.[25]

The depth of the needle is checked in a lateral radiograph: the tip must project over the posterior border of the facet column. Thereafter, the rest of the procedure is the same as described before. A 22-gauge, 10-cm SMK needle with a 5-mm active tip can be used to perform an RF lesioning.

The patient is allowed to go home immediately after the procedure. Driving a car or handling dangerous machinery is proscribed for the first 24 hours. In some cases there will be a transient numbness of the ipsilateral extremity because of overflow of local anesthetics into the intervertebral foramen.

Results

Technically, the two prerequisites for success of RF facet denervation include that the painful facet joints must be identified by using a diagnostic block, and that the nerve supply to the targeted facet joints is precisely localized and sectioned.[114] Techniques for RF facet denervation vary nevertheless.

Gallagher and associates[115] randomized 41 patients to receive RF facet denervation (27 patients) or sham treatment (14 patients) using the Shealy technique, and presented data showing 42% good relief from 1 to 4 weeks and 24% continued relief at 6 months. They concluded that radiofrequency facet denervation was efficacious for the management of low back pain originating from the facet joints.

Van Kleef and colleagues[116] included 31 patients, selected by a positive response to a diagnostic nerve block, to randomly receive RF facet denervation ($n = 15$) or sham treatment ($n = 16$). At 3, 6, and 12 months after treatment, there were significantly more successes in the RF group compared with the sham group. They conclude that RF facet denervation results in significant short- and long-term alleviation of pain and functional disability in a selected group of patients.

A 70-patient double-blinded, randomized, controlled trial by Leclaire and coworkers[114] found no efficacy for RF facet denervation. Suitable candidates were selected by diagnostic intra-articular facet joint block. However, in this study patient selection was done by means of a diagnostic facet block evaluated 1 week after this procedure by a general physician (family doctor). The prevalence of facet pain in this study is much too high (92 %) because of this methodologic flow. They reported that only the Oswestry

scale, but not Roland-Morris and VAS, was slightly improved at 4 weeks. At 12 weeks neither scale showed any treatment effect. They concluded that the efficacy of RF facet denervation has not been established.[114]

Van Wijk and associates[117] recently performed a trial involving 81 low back pain patients suffering from a lumbar facet syndrome, as confirmed by two-level diagnostic intra-articular facet joint block. Kaplan-Meier survival curves showed no significant differences between RF facet denervation and control group during 1 year follow-up. No differences in effect between RF and control could be found when measured by VAS-back, VAS-leg, physical activities, or analgesic intake. However, in both groups VAS-back was significantly reduced, and in the RF group VAS-leg. Global Perceived Effect measurement showed a significant difference in favor of RF treatment. The SF-36 questionnaire showed an improvement of "vitality" in the RF group.[117]

In conclusion, these four RCTs report conflicting results. Although the two smaller RCTs[115,116] found convincing proof for the efficacy of RF facet denervation, the two larger RCTs[114,117] reported no or mild efficacy. Of note, the target of diagnostic block (nerve versus joint) between the former and latter studies differed.

One other prospective study, although not an RCT, seems to be of additional importance when estimating the efficacy of RF facet denervation. Dreyfuss and associates[118] found that 60% of patients ($n = 9$) obtained at least 90% pain reduction at 12 months, and 87% obtained at least 60% pain relief from RF facet denervation. Relief was associated with denervation of the multifidus muscle.[118] This study differs in three important aspects from all previous studies of RF facet denervation. First, the authors used a different protocol for diagnostic block. Although initially, Lord and coworkers[59] advocated the use of double-blind, placebo-controlled blocks to reach a precise diagnosis of "cervical" facet pain, Dreyfuss and colleagues in their study used a modified comparative block protocol and omitted saline injections. For the first diagnostic nerve block 0.5 mL of 2% lidocaine was injected. Patients reporting at least 80% pain relief for longer than 1 hour returned for confirmatory blocks using 0.5% bupivacaine. Patients exhibiting at least 80% pain relief for longer than 2 hours were then offered RF treatment. Second, this study used a different operation technique for RF facet denervation. Differences in comparison with other studies include type of electrode (16-gauge Ray electrode), preoperative access to the target nerve, and coagulation of the targeted nerve 8 to 10 mm along its length needing multiple lesioning. The meaning of multifidus stimulation and denervation is unclear and is still a subject of discussion.[119,120]

Geurts and colleagues[78] in their systematic review concluded that there is moderate evidence that radiofrequency lumbar facet denervation is more effective for chronic low back pain than placebo, whereas the Cochrane Review Reports conflicting evidence on the effect of RF lesioning on pain and disability in chronic low back pain of zygapophyseal joint origin.[79]

Side Effects and Complications

A retrospective analysis of the incidence of complications associated with fluoroscopically guided percutaneous radiofrequency denervation of the lumbar facet joints yielded a 1% overall incidence of minor complications per lesion site. On a total of 616 RF facet denervations, three cases of localized pain lasting longer than 2 weeks (0.5%) and three cases of neuritic pain lasting less than 2 weeks (0.5%) were noted. No cases of infection, new motor deficits, or new sensory deficits were identified.[121]

Percutaneous Radiofrequency Lesion Adjacent to the Dorsal Root Ganglion

The placement of percutaneous radiofrequency lesions adjacent to the dorsal root ganglion (RF-DRG) was developed in the 1980s as an alternative to surgical rhizotomy for chronic refractory pain.[122] Although initially, surgical rhizotomy led to impressive short-term pain relief in various pain syndromes,[123] in the long term a dramatic loss of efficacy occurred, accompanied by severe adverse effects if substantial denervation had been carried out.[124]

The rationale for the use of RF-DRG in lumbosacral radicular pain is the concept that nociceptive input at the level of the primary sensory neuron might be reduced by coagulation of a small part of the DRG without causing a sensory deficit.[15] It has been stressed that RF-DRG should be restricted to "high-input" nociceptive spinal pain syndromes. In the presence of deafferentation symptoms, RF-DRG might lead to an aggravation of pain complaints.[12] Moreover, mechanical entrapment of the nerve in combined back pain and radiculopathy must be removed as a contributing factor before proceeding with RF-DRG. To minimize the risk of deafferentation pain, an RF-DRG heat lesion should not be used if there is a loss of reflexes or cutaneous sensation of the targeted spinal nerve. Thus, if diagnostic sleeve root injections were beneficial, surgical interventions eliminated, and more conservative interventional procedures had failed, RF-DRG can be considered.

Procedure

RF-DRG is aimed at creating a minimal lesion near the dorsal root ganglion for treating nerve root pain without neurologic deficits.[125] For this purpose, at lumbar levels, a 10-cm electrode (22-gauge, 5-mm active tip) is placed in the dorsal cranial quadrant of the intervertebral foramen (lateral view), and introduced with its tip between one third and about halfway across the midfacetal column in the AP projection (Fig. 57–21).

Sensory and motor stimulation is applied at 50 and 2 Hz. The electrode position is adjusted if necessary to reach a sensory stimulation threshold between 0.5

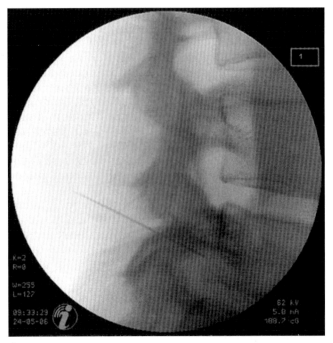

A

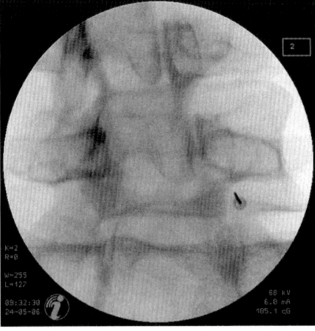

B

Figure 57–21. A, lateral view of the needle in the superior part of the intervertebral foramen L5. **B,** slightly oblique view of the needle position for lumbar radiofrequency of the dorsal root ganglion of L5. **C,** AP view of PRF-DRG. Note the spread of the contrast medium.

and 1 volt. Motor stimulation threshold is required to be at least 1.5 times the sensory stimulation threshold. A final check of the electrode position is made by injecting radiopaque contrast dye to visualize the nerve root and ganglion. Subsequently, a local anesthetic is injected through the cannula to obtain dense anesthesia. RF treatment is usually done at 65° to

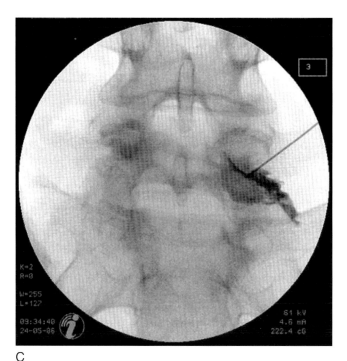

C

Figure 57–21, cont'd.

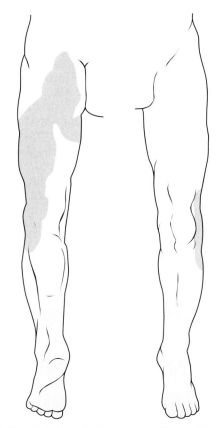

Figure 57–22. Typical radiation pattern of sacroiliac joint pain. (Adapted from van der Wurff P: Sacroiliac pain diagnosis and treatment [thesis]. University Hospital of Utrecht, Utrecht, Netherlands, 2004.)

67° C for 90 seconds. At the sacral level the position of the DRG is first visualized with radiopaque contrast dye, injected through a 22-gauge needle that is placed in the dorsal sacral foramen of the corresponding nerve root. Subsequently, a small hole is drilled through the overlying sacral bone, using a Kirschner wire and a pneumatic drill, to obtain access to the dorsal ganglion. The remainder of the procedure is identical to the one at the lumbar level.

Results

In radiating lower limb pain, one prospective,[126] and several retrospective studies[122,127-130] have reported beneficial effects of lumbosacral RF-DRG in between 32% and 76% of cases. One sham-lesion–controlled RCT to assess the efficacy of RF-DRG for lumbosacral radicular pain has been performed. In this study, lumbosacral RF-DRG failed to show advantage over sham treatment with local anesthetics with about 80% certainty.[131] In a previous retrospective study, 279 patients were treated with RF-DRG because of chronic spinal pain radiating to the leg and they reported an initial success rate of approximately 60%.[129] In successful patients, the mean duration of pain reduction was 3.7 years.

There is moderate evidence that an RF-DRG is not effective in the treatment of lumbar radicular pain. For that reason this procedure is performed.

Radiofrequency Sacroiliac Joint Denervation (RF-SIJ)

Sacroiliac (SI) joint pain may result from sacroiliitis (Bechterew's disease), infections, spondyloarthrop-athy, pyogenic or crystal arthropathy, fracture of the sacrum and pelvis, and diastasis.[132] Primary pain emanating from the SI joint in the absence of demonstrable pathology is thought to be of mechanical origin and is termed a sacroiliac syndrome. The extent and vagaries of SI joint innervation have led to controversies regarding the correct technique for RF denervation. The prevalence of this pain is estimated to be around 5% to 15% of patients with low back pain.

Patients with SI joint pain may present with a one-sided or two-sided low back pain below the level of L5. Clinical suspicion for this syndrome may increase when three out of five provocative tests for SI joint pain during physical examination are positive.[133-135] The typical radiation pattern of SI joint pain is illustrated in Figure 57–22. Currently the diagnosis is best confirmed by means of at least one diagnostic nerve block of L5 and the lateral branch blocks of S1-3.

Procedure

Presently, three techniques have been described, all of which differ substantially from one another.[132] We use the following technique: In patients with a positive diagnostic block, RF denervation is performed using fluoroscopic guidance and superficial anesthesia. With the C-arm intensifier positioned to confer either a slightly oblique (L4 dorsal ramus), AP (L5 dorsal ramus and lateral branches), or cephalocaudad (lateral branches) view, 22-gauge SMK-C10 cannulae with 5-mm active tips are inserted until bone is contacted at the locale of the targeted nerve. Correct placement is confirmed using electrostimulation at 50 Hz, with concordant pain being noted at or below 0.6 volt at all levels from L4 to S2. With right-sided lateral branch blocks at the S1-2 levels, the optimum stimulation pattern was found anywhere between 1:30 and 5:30 on the face of a clock directly outside the posterior foramen on the surface of the sacrum. For left-sided blocks, optimum stimulation was usually found between 7:00 and 10:00. In some patients a concordant stimulation pattern cannot be obtained at less than 0.8 volt for the S3 lateral branch. In such cases two empirically made lesions are recommended, at 2:30 and 4:30 for right-sided S3 lateral branch blocks, and 7:30 and 9:30 for left-sided lateral branch blocks. Prior to lesioning, the absence of contractions in leg muscles was verified at three times the stimulation threshold. When fluoroscopic images and stimulation parameters indicate correct electrode placement, 0.3 mL lidocaine 2% is injected through each cannula for local anesthesia. The RF probe is then reinserted, and a 90-second 80° C lesion is made.[136] Needle placement for RF-SI procedure is illustrated in Figure 57–23.

Results

Radiofrequency treatment of the SI joint was studied in a prospective trial. Thirty-three sequential patients with SI joint syndrome underwent 50 denervations by means of a "strip" lesion technique, combined with betamethasone injection.[132] Follow-up at 6 months revealed good results (≥50 % pain reduction) in 12 of 33 patients (36%). A retrospective study with 9 patients suffering SI joint pain confirmed by SI joint block reported a significant pain relief (≥50 %) in 8 of them. Although these results seem promising,

the efficacy of RF-SI joint for the treatment of the SI syndrome remains to be proven by future studies.

CONCLUSION

Radiofrequency treatment of chronic pain syndromes has seen a remarkable evolution over the past decade; RF current can now be applied in continuous and pulsed fashion. The former application method generates heat lesions, whereas the latter induces changes in the nerve cells. Besides studies on efficacy and safety, computer modeling, in vitro, and animal experiments have begun to shed a light on the potential mode of action of PRF. Evidence gathered in good quality studies demonstrates that continuous and PRF can be applied to effectively treat some chronic pain syndromes. When performed in well-selected patients, who often suffer pain refractory to conventional treatment, the degree of pain relief can be higher than with conventional treatment. Moreover, in contrast with drug studies, the follow-up period is much longer, providing proof of long-term efficacy. Radiofrequency treatment can produce minor, immediate side effects that typically resolve spontaneously within a short time. Major neurologic complications are rare, but have been reported with conventional heat lesioning, although not with PRF. Because of the low neurodestructive potential, pulsed radiofrequency is our choice for the treatment of the dorsal root ganglion. A randomized-controlled trial comparing PRF with sham intervention adjacent to the cervical DRG for cervical radicular pain showed a higher success rate in the PRF group at 3 months.[81] These encouraging results point to the urgent need for further studies on this promising nondestructive mode of treatment. In these studies attempts should be made to study a homogeneous patient population for the given pathology. Soon we hope to see evidence emerge for the following applications of RF and PRF for the treatment of lumbar radicular pain syndromes, sacroiliac pain, lumbar discogenic pain, and cervical facet pain.

References

1. Ahadian FM: Pulsed radiofrequency neurotomy: Advances in pain medicine. Curr Pain Headache Rep 2004;8(1):34-40.
2. Tepperman J: Horsley and Clarke: A biographical medallion. Perspect Biol Med 1970;13(3):295-308.
3. Kirschner M: Zür electrochirugie. Arch Klin Chir 1931;167:761.
4. Sweet WH, Mark VH: Unipolar anodal electrolyte lesions in the brain of man and rat: Report of five human cases with electrically produced bulbar or mesencephalic tractotomies. AMA Arch Neurol Psychiatry 1953;70:224-234.
5. Hunsperger RW, Wyss OAM: Quantitative ausschaltung van nervengewebe durch hochfrequenzkoagulation. Helv Physiol Acta 1953;11:283-304.
6. Rosomoff HL, Brown CJ, Sheptak P: Percutaneous radiofrequency cervical cordotomy: Technique. J Neurosurg 1965;23(6):639-644.
7. Mundinger F, Riechert T, Gabriel E: [Studies on the physical and technical bases of high-frequency coagulation with controlled dosage in stereotactic brain surgery]. Zentralbl Chir 1960;8510:51-63.

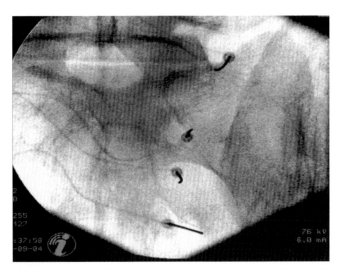

Figure 57–23. Needle position for radiofrequency-sacroiliac (RF-SI) procedure.

98. Bogduk N, Long DM: The anatomy of the so-called "articular nerves" and their relationship to facet denervation in the treatment of low-back pain. J Neurosurg 1979;51(2):172-177.

99. Date E, Gray L: Electrodiagnostic evidence for cervical radiculopathy and suprascapular neuropathy in shoulder pain. Electromyogr Clin Neurophysiol 1996;36(6):333-339.

100. Stolker RJ, Vervest AC, Groen GJ: The treatment of chronic thoracic segmental pain by radiofrequency percutaneous partial rhizotomy. J Neurosurg 1994;80(6):986-992.

101. Tzaan WC, Tasker RR: Percutaneous radiofrequency facet rhozotomy—Experience with 118 procedures and reappraisal of its value. Can J. Neurol Sci 2000;27(2):125-130.

102. Kalso E, Mennander S, Tasmuth T, Nilsson E: Chronic post-sternotomy pain. Acta Anaesthesiol Scand 2001;45(8):935-939.

103. Wenger C: Radiofrequency lesions for the treatment of spinal pain. Pain Digest 1998;81-16.

104. Dooley JF, McBroom RJ, Taguchi T, Macnab I: Nerve root infiltration in the diagnosis of radicular pain. Spine 1988;13(1):79-83.

105. Stolker RJ, Vervest ACM, Groen GJ: The treatment of chronic thoracic segmental pain by radiofrequency percutaneous partial rhizotomy. J Neurosurg 1994;80:986-992.

106. Cassidy JD, Cote P, Carroll LJ, Kristman V: Incidence and course of low back pain episodes in the general population. Spine 2005;30(24):2817-2823.

107. Spitzer W: Report on Quebec task force on low back pain. Spine 1987;S1-S59.

108. Hestbaek L, Leboeuf-Yde C, Manniche C: Low back pain: What is the long-term course? A review of studies of general patient populations. Eur Spine J 2003;12(2):149-165.

109. Wahlgren DR, Atkinson JH, Epping-Jordan JE, et al: One-year follow-up of first onset low back pain. Pain 1997;73(2):213-221.

110. Airaksinen O, Brox JI, Cedraschi C, et al: European guidelines for the management of chronic nonspecific low back pain. Eur Spine J 2006;15(Suppl 2):S192-S300.

111. Schwarzer AC, Wang SC, O'Driscoll D, et al: The ability of computed tomography to identify a painful zygapophysial joint in patients with chronic low back pain. Spine 1995;20(8):907-912.

112. Revel ME, Listrat VM, Chevalier XJ, et al: Facet joint block for low back pain: Identifying predictors of a good response. Arch Phys Med Rehabil 1992;73(9):824-828.

113. Revel M, Poiraudeau S, Auleley GR, et al: Capacity of the clinical picture to characterize low back pain relieved by facet joint anesthesia. Proposed criteria to identify patients with painful facet joints. Spine 1998;23(18):1972-1976.

114. Leclaire R, Fortin L, Lambert R, et al: Radiofrequency facet joint denervation in the treatment of low back pain: A placebo-controlled clinical trial to assess efficacy. Spine 2001;26(13):1411-1416.

115. Gallagher J, Vadi PLP, Wesley JR: Radiofrequency facet joint denervation in the treatment of low back pain—A prospective controlled double-blind study in assess to efficacy. Pain Clin 1994;7:193-198.

116. van Kleef M, Barendse GA, Kessels A, et al: Randomized trial of radiofrequency lumbar facet denervation for chronic low back pain. Spine 1999;24(18):1937-1942.

117. van Wijk RM, Geurts JW, Wynne HJ, et al: Radiofrequency denervation of lumbar facet joints in the treatment of chronic low back pain: A randomized, double-blind, sham lesion-controlled trial. Clin J Pain 2005;21(4):335-344.

118. Dreyfuss P, Halbrook B, Pauza K, et al: Efficacy and validity of radiofrequency neurotomy for chronic lumbar zygapophysial joint pain. Spine 2000;25(10):1270-1277.

119. Barendse G, Spaans F, Stomp-Van Den Berg S, et al: Local denervation of lumbar paraspinal muscles may not be used as criterion for the effectivity of radiofrequency lesions of the zygapophyseal joints. Pain Clin 2001;13(2):115-135.

120. Oudenhoven R: Paraspinal electromyography following facet rhizotomy. Spine 1977;2:299-304.

121. Kornick C, Kramarich SS, Lamer TJ, Todd Sitzman B: Complications of lumbar facet radiofrequency denervation. Spine 2004;29(12):1352-1354.

122. Pagura JR: Percutaneous radiofrequency spinal rhizotomy. Appl Neurophysiol 1983;46:138-146.

123. Loeser JD: Dorsal rhizotomy for the relief of chronic pain. J Neurosurg 1972;36(6):745-750.

124. North RB, Kidd DH, Campbell JN, Long DM: Dorsal root ganglionectomy for failed back surgery syndrome: A 5-year follow-up study. J Neurosurg 1991;74(2):236-242.

125. Kline M: Radiofrequency techniques in clinical practice. In Waldman S, Winnie A (eds): Interventional Pain Management. Philadelphia, Saunders, 1996, pp 185-217.

126. Nash TP: Percutaneous radiofrequency lesioning of dorsal root ganglia for intractable pain. Pain 1986;24:67-73.

127. Uematsu S, Udvarhelyi GB, Benson DW, Siebens AA: Percutaneous radiofrequency rhizotomy. Surg Neurol 1974;2(5):319-325.

128. Niv D, Chayen MS: Reduction of localized cancer pain by percutaneous dorsal root ganglia lesions. Pain Clin 1992;5:229-234.

129. van Wijk RM, Geurts JW, Wynne HJ: Long-lasting analgesic effect of radiofrequency treatment of the lumbosacral dorsal root ganglion. J Neurosurg 2001;94(2 Suppl):227-231.

130. Sluijter ME, Mehta M: Treatment of chronic back and neck pain by percutaneous thermal lesions. In Persistent Pain, Modern Methods of Treatment. London: Academic Press, 1981.

131. Geurts JWM, van Wijk RM, Wynne HJ, et al: Radiofrequency lesioning of dorsal root ganglia for chronic lumbosacral radicular pain. A randomised, double blind, controlled trial. Lancet 2003;361(9351):21-26.

132. Ferrante FM, King LF, Roche EA, et al: Radiofrequency sacroiliac joint denervation for sacroiliac syndrome. Reg Anesth Pain Med 2001;26(2):137-142.

133. Riddle DL, Freburger JK: Evaluation of the presence of sacroiliac joint region dysfunction using a combination of tests: A multicenter intertester reliability study. Phys Ther 2002;82(8):772-781.

134. Potter NA, Rothstein JM: Intertester reliability for selected clinical tests of the sacroiliac joint. Phys Ther 1985;65(11):1671-1675.

135. van der Wurff P: Clinical diagnostic tests for the sacroiliac joint: Motion and palpation tests. Aust J Physiother 2006;52(4):308.

136. Cohen SP, Abdi S: Lateral branch blocks as a treatment for sacroiliac joint pain: A pilot study. Reg Anesth Pain Med 2003;28(2):113-119.

58 Hip, Sacroiliac Joint, and Piriformis Injections

Honorio T. Benzon and Antoun Nader

HIP INJECTIONS

Intra-articular and intrabursal hip aspirations and injections are useful diagnostic and therapeutic tools in pain management. Although evidence-based reviews that support or refute their efficacy are few, substantial clinical experiences support their effectiveness. The most common diagnostic indications include the aspiration of fluid for evaluation and injection of a local anesthetic to confirm the pain generator source. Therapeutic indications are mostly to decrease pain and improve mobility, usually as an adjunct therapy. A corticosteroid mixed with a local anesthetic is most commonly injected. Therapeutic responses to corticosteroid injections are usually variable. Most patients who respond do so after the first injection. If no benefits are obtained after two injections, subsequent positive outcome after additional injections is rare. Therefore, further workup is warranted when symptoms are persistent after one or two injections. The benefit of subsequent injections should always be weighed against the concern that repeated steroid use may accelerate normal aging-related articular cartilage atrophy and weaken tendons and ligaments.[1]

Mechanisms of Action of Corticosteroids

An intra-articular injection of corticosteroids suppresses inflammation resulting in decreased edema, redness, and tenderness of the inflamed tissue. Several mechanisms of steroid effect have been reported (Box 58–1). Whether these are the same mechanisms of action that occur after parenteral or oral administration of corticosteroids is uncertain.

Selection of Corticosteroid

Few studies have investigated the efficacy and duration of action for various corticosteroids in joint and soft tissue injections. In general, the less soluble an agent (acetate suspensions as compared to sodium phosphate), the longer it remains in the joint and the more prolonged the effect. Consequently, steroids in suspension are longer acting; however, they are more likely to cause postinjection transient flare-ups. In addition, a low solubility agent is preferred for joint injections to avoid the risk of surrounding soft tissue atrophy. Methylprednisolone is often the agent selected for this type of injection. The dosage of corticosteroids is usually site dependent, with larger joints requiring more corticosteroids than smaller soft tissue sites. Usually corticosteroid preparations are mixed with a local anesthetic to avoid the injection of a highly concentrated suspension into a single area.

Complications

The complications after steroid injections are usually divided into local reactions at the injection site and systemic complications (Box 58–2). Local reactions are usually self-limited and may include swelling, tenderness, and warmth. They often present a few hours after the injection and can last up to 2 days. In addition, a poststeroid injection pain flare may occur within the first 24 to 36 hours after the injection. This is usually the result of crystal-induced synovitis and thought to be caused by preservatives in the injectable suspension. All of these reactions are usually self-limited and respond to application of ice packs. Other local complications include soft tissue atrophy, local depigmentation, periarticular calcifications, tendon rupture, and localized infection. Systemic effects after steroid injection are possible, the most common of which is elevation of blood sugar in patients who are diabetic. Other rare complications include water retention, taste alteration, adrenal suppression, and abnormal uterine bleeding.

Greater Trochanteric Bursa and Bursa Injections

Up to three trochanteric bursae have been described around the greater trochanter.[2] The largest one is the subgluteus maximus bursa, which lies lateral to the greater trochanter and located deep in the fibers of the tensor fascia lata and gluteus maximus muscle as they join to form the iliotibial tract. The second major bursa, the subgluteus medius bursa, is located

BOX 58–1. MECHANISMS OF ACTION OF CORTICOSTEROIDS

Cellular membrane stabilization
Alterations in synovial membrane permeability with resultant decrease in synovial fluid complement and changes in synovial fluid liquid cell counts and activity
Alterations in neutrophil function and chemotaxis
Alterations in hyaluronic acid synthesis

BOX 58–2. COMPLICATIONS AFTER HIP INJECTIONS

Local Complications
Swelling
Tenderness
Infection
Postinjection pain flare-up
Soft tissue atrophy
Depigmentation
Periarticular calcifications
Tendon rupture

Systemic Complications
Increase in blood glucose
Adrenal suppression
Abnormal uterine bleeding
Alteration of taste

BOX 58–3. CAUSES OF BURSITIS OF THE HIP

Chronic trauma
Arthritis
Leg length inequalities
Previous hip surgery
Lumbar spine disease

superior and posterior to the greater trochanter and lies beneath the gluteus medius muscle. The third bursa, the subgluteus minimus bursa, lies anterior and superior to the proximal surface of the greater trochanter.[2] Inflammation of any of these bursae may lead to trochanteric bursitis, which is the primary indication for the trochanteric bursae injection.

Bursitis is usually characterized by pain and tenderness over the greater trochanter. The pain may radiate down the lateral thigh to the knee or into the buttocks. It is usually worse when first standing from a seated position. It feels somewhat better after a few steps but may recur after walking for a half hour. Patients are unable to lie on the affected side. Trochanteric bursitis is usually associated with chronic pressure or trauma to the greater trochanter of the femur (Box 58–3). Other associated factors include lumbar spine disease, significant leg length inequalities, previous surgery around the hip, and arthritis. Point tenderness over the lateral greater trochanter is the essential finding. Occasionally, rounded or irregular specific deposits may be seen around the trochanter in lateral hip radiographs. There may be irregular bone spurs in the area. Corticosteroid injections, nonsteroidal anti-inflammatory drugs (NSAIDs), and lateral-bend stretching are usually successful in relieving pain in more than 90% of patients. Occasionally, repeat injections are required for symptomatic relief. Because of its efficacy, early steroid injections are usually preferred.

Technique of Trochanteric Bursa Injections

The patient is placed in the lateral decubitus position with the affected hip upward. The hip is usually flexed 30 to 50 degrees and the knee is flexed 60 to 90 degrees. A pillow is placed between the patient's knees to relax the iliotibial band and decrease the pressure required to inject the solution. The greater trochanter is identified and the point of maximum tenderness is localized. After standard monitors are placed and sterile preparation and draping is complete, a 22-gauge spinal needle is inserted at the most tender or swollen area, perpendicular to the skin until it contacts the greater trochanter. The needle is then withdrawn 1 to 2 mm so that the tip is in the bursa and not the bone. The needle should not be withdrawn too far, otherwise it will be above the fascia lata and outside the bursa. Fluoroscopy with injection of contrast media can be used to confirm correct needle placement (Figs. 58–1 and 58–2).[2] After aspiration, the solution is injected in 1- to 2-mL increments to confirm that the solution is not administered intravascularly. The needle is withdrawn and then reinserted in different directions to ensure that the area around the point of maximum tenderness is infiltrated. The puncture wound is then dressed with a sterile adhesive bandage. It has been noted that trochanteric bursa injections are less accurate in older adult and obese patients.[2]

Injectate and Patient Instructions

Usually 3 to 5 mL of a local anesthetic (lidocaine 1%, bupivacaine 0.25%) mixed with a corticosteroid (e.g., methylprednisolone 40 to 80 mg) is injected. The patient should be advised that after the local anesthetic wears off, pain may persist or become worse for a few days until the corticosteroid takes effect.

Hip Joint Injections

The hip joint is a ball-and-socket joint enveloped in the dense capsular tissue with a complex nerve supply[3]:
1. The femoral nerve supplies the joint, iliofemoral ligament, and superior capsule.
2. The obturator nerve supplies the joint and pubofemoral ligament.

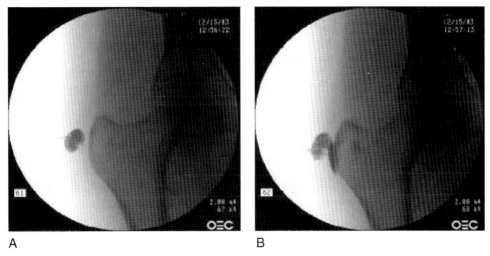

Figure 58–1. Injection into the subgluteus maximus bursa. Note that the image in **(A)** shows a soft tissue spread, whereas the image in **(B)** shows injection into the subgluteus maximus bursa after the needle was redirected inferiorly. (From Cohen SP, Narvaez, JC, Lebovits AH, Stojanovic MP: Corticosteroid injections for trochanteric bursitis: Is fluoroscopy necessary? A pilot study. Br J Anaesth 2005;94:100-106. Reprinted with permission.)

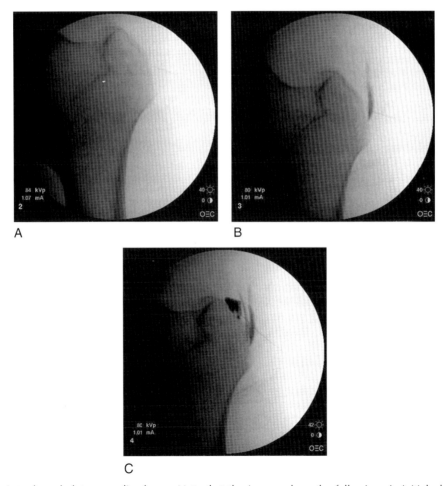

Figure 58–2. Injection into the subgluteus medius bursa. Note that the images show the following: **A,** initial placement of the needle; **B,** injection of contrast into the tendon of the gluteus medius muscle; and **C,** subgluteus medius bursagram. (From Cohen SP, Narvaez, JC, Lebovits AH, Stojanovic MP: Corticosteroid injections for trochanteric bursitis: Is fluoroscopy necessary? A pilot study. Br J Anaesth 2005;94:100-106. Reprinted with permission.)

3. The superior gluteal nerve supplies the joint, superior and lateral part of the joint capsule, and the gluteus medius and minimus muscles.
4. The nerve to the quadratus lumborum supplies the joint, posterior capsule, and ischiofemoral ligament.

A painful hip may present a diagnostic dilemma because 10% to 15% of patients may have coexistent hip arthritis and osteoarthritis of the spine. The patient may present with inguinal pain, referred pain below the knee, limitation of hip motion, back pain, and radiographic evidence of degenerative arthritis of both the hip and the spine. Intra-articular hip injections may help to pinpoint the intracapsular origin of the problem.

Techniques

Hip injections are commonly done with or without fluoroscopy, either through the anterior or lateral approach.[4] Injections under ultrasound guidance also have been described.

The Anterior Approach

The patient is placed in the supine position and the femoral artery is palpated and marked. A line is drawn from the anterosuperior iliac spine to the symphysis pubis. The spinal (3.5 cm) needle is inserted at a point 2.5 cm lateral and 2.5 cm distal to a point where the femoral pulse intersects the line from the anterosuperior spine to the symphysis. The needle is inserted in a 60-degree cephalad and medial direction until bone is contacted, then slightly withdrawn to allow a free flow of the injection.

Lateral Approach

With the patient in the supine position, the femur is rotated and turned in 10 degrees. A spinal needle is inserted just proximal to the tip of the greater trochanter in a horizontal direction until the bone is reached. The needle is withdrawn just enough to allow free flow of the injection.

Leopold and colleagues[5] compared the anterior and lateral approaches in human fresh-frozen cadaver specimens. They noted that both the anterior and lateral approaches were difficult to perform when based on anatomic landmarks, without fluoroscopic guidance. The anterior approach was successful in only 60% of the injections and the lateral technique in 80% of the injections. The anterior approach resulted in a greater risk of trauma to the femoral artery and nerve compared with the lateral approach.[5] They concluded that the lateral approach was safer and more effective than the anterior approach. To avoid neurovascular injury, they recommended fluoroscopic or ultrasound guidance for needle placements during hip injections and aspirations.

Fluoroscopic-Guided Anterior Approach

With the patient in the supine position, a marker is used to denote the course of the femoral artery. The insertion site of the needle is marked on the skin lateral to the vascular bundle, vertically on the midportion of the femoral neck. The needle is advanced in a straight direction until it reaches the anterior aspect of the base of the femoral neck (Fig. 58–3). A small amount of iodinated contrast is injected to verify the intra-articular position of the needle.

Fluoroscopic-Guided Lateral Approach

The lateral approach allows visualization of the needle at all times during the insertion of the needle. The entry site is immediately cephalad to the greater trochanter, at the midlevel of the anteroposterior dimension of the thigh.[6] A 5-inch, 22-gauge spinal needle is advanced under fluoroscopic guidance in a cephalad angle so that it enters the hip joint laterally at the junction of the femoral head and neck (Fig. 58–4). A small amount of iodinated contrast is injected to verify the intra-articular position of the needle.[6]

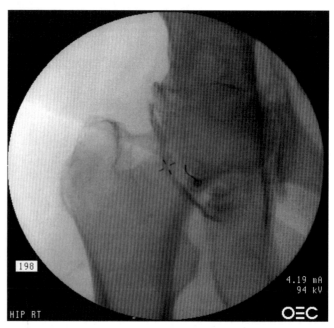

Figure 58–3. Anterior approach to injection of the hip joint. The needle is directed slightly downward until it makes contact with the anterior aspect of the femoral neck.

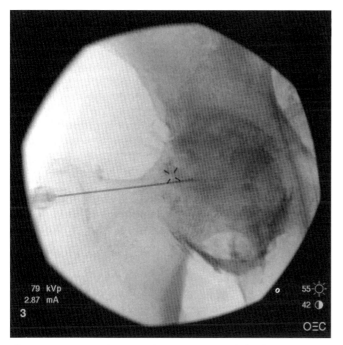

Figure 58–4. Lateral approach to injection of the hip joint. The needle is advanced so that it enters the hip joint laterally at the junction of the femoral head and neck.

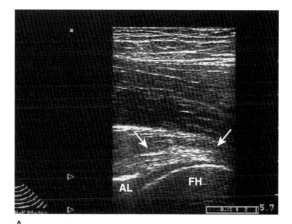

A

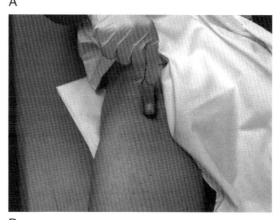

B

Figure 58–5. A, Sagittal ultrasound view showing the hyperechoic femoral head (FH), overlying iliofemoral ligament *(arrows)*, and triangular echo of the anterior labrum (AL). **B,** Orientation of the ultrasound to obtain the picture in **(A)**. (From Smith J, Hurdle MF: Office-based ultrasound-guided intra-articular hip injection: Technique for physiatric practice. Arch Phys Med Rehabil 2006; 87:296-298. Reprinted with permission.)

Ultrasound-Guided Hip Injections

The patient is placed in the supine position with the hip in neutral or slightly internal rotation.[7] The anterosuperior iliac spine is identified and the transducer is oriented in a sagittal plane with its superior end located just medial to the anterosuperior iliac spine. The transducer is moved medially until the rounded surface of the femoral head is visualized under ultrasound guidance, appearing as a rounded hyperechoic (bright) surface (Fig. 58–5). The transducer is moved medially to identify the femoral nerve and vessels. After confirming the position of the neurovascular structure, the transducer is moved back to the anterior hip joint. The inferior end of the transducer is rotated laterally while maintaining the superior end on the femoral head. The target is the femoral head–neck junction and overlying hyperechoic iliofemoral ligament and hip capsule. The transducer is placed as far laterally as possible on the junction of the head and neck of the femur. Under direct ultrasound visualization, a 22-gauge spinal needle is advanced to the junction of the femoral head and neck. An increase in resistance is felt as the needle traverses the iliofemoral ligament before it enters the hip joint.[7] Direct visualization of the needle tip and injection of 1 to 2 mL of solution confirms intra-articular placement. Additional injections are usually done while visualizing distention of the capsule; fluids appear anechoic (dark) on ultrasound. As the hip is injected the hyperechoic capsule and iliofemoral ligament are seen peeling away from the head and neck of the femur. The corticosteroid crystals are hyperechoic and can be clearly visualized spreading between the junction of the head and neck of the femur and the overlying capsule (Fig. 58–6).[7] A mixture of local anesthetic and steroid, or a steroid alone, or a local anesthetic alone can be injected.

Contraindications, Precautions, and Patient Instructions

The main contraindications to intra-articular hip corticosteroid injections are patients who have septic joint, unstable joint, intra-articular hip fracture, clotting disorder, and those patients on anticoagulants.

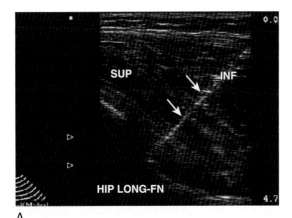

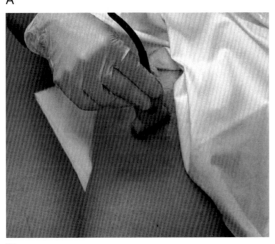

Figure 58–6. A, Ultrasound view with the transducer oriented along the long axis of the femoral neck (FN). The needle is seen piercing the hyperechoic iliofemoral ligament and entering the hip joint near the junction of the head and neck of the femur. A thin band of hyperechoic steroid crystals is seen outlying the curvilinear shape of the femoral head, deep to the iliofemoral ligament. SUP, superior; INF, inferior. **B,** Ultrasound transducer orientation used to obtain the picture in **(A).** (From Smith J, Hurdle MF: Office-based ultrasound-guided intra-articular hip injection: Technique for physiatric practice. Arch Phys Med Rehabil 2006;87:296-298. Reprinted with permission.)

Intra-articular steroids should not be injected before septic arthritis is ruled out.

Intra-articular hip injections should be done under strict aseptic conditions. Infection is rare with proper technique. Fitzgerald[8] reported 3000 joints and periarticular injections performed annually at the Mayo Clinic without a single case of a joint infection. A patient with diabetes can have an increase in blood glucose. There is always a potential for systemic effect from the absorbed corticosteroid resulting in suppression of the hypothalamic-adrenal axis for 2 to 7 days. It is recommended that only one joint be injected per visit, and injections should be spread out over as long a period as possible. It is advisable to rest the joint for a brief time after an injection of corticosteroid to reduce the possibility of postinjection

increase in pain and to decrease the absorption of steroid by the synovial membrane.[8]

Injectate: Steroid Alone versus Local Anesthetic Alone

In a prospective study by Kullenberg and associates,[9] 50 patients with osteoarthritis of the hip pain of more than 4 weeks' duration were randomized into two groups. One group received 80 mg of triamcinolone acetonide, and the other group received 2 mL of 1% mepivacaine injected into the hip. The authors noted that the patients who had the steroid injection improved significantly at 3 and 12 weeks in terms of pain, functional ability, and range of motion of the hip joint. Neither significant pain relief nor improvement in functional ability was noted in the patients who were injected with local anesthetic.[9]

Sacroiliac Joint Syndrome

The anatomy of the sacroiliac (SI) joint has been discussed.[10] It is considered a diarthrodial joint because it contains synovial fluid, the articulating bones have ligamentous connections, the outer fibrous joint capsule has an inner synovial lining, and the cartilaginous surfaces allow motion to occur.[11] The sacral side of the joint is thicker and made up of hyaline cartilage, whereas the iliac side is made up of thin fibrocartilage. The adult joint has irregular and coarse surfaces that increase with age reflecting the stresses and strains to which the joint is exposed.[12] The irregular contour of the joint contributes to its stability; the function of the joint is to transmit or dissipate the loading of the upper trunk to the lower extremities. Accessory SI joints have been reported.

The ligaments of the SI joint include the anterior sacroiliac ligament, interosseous ligament, and posterior sacroiliac ligament. The anterior sacroiliac ligament traverses the ilium to the sacrum, and the posterior sacroiliac ligament traverses the posterior iliac ridge to the sacrum; the interosseous ligament is responsible for the stability of the joint. The sacrotuberous ligament, which is superficial to the posterior SI ligament, has multiple muscle attachments including the gluteus maximus, piriformis, and long head of the biceps femoris. These multiple muscle attachments provide a potential for activities such as sitting, walking, and standing, which stress the sacroiliac joint.[11] The sacroiliac joint is innervated at its anterior and posterior aspects. Posteriorly, the joint is innervated by the lateral branches of the posterior primary ramus of the L4 to S4 dorsal rami.[13,14] The predominant innervation is from the dorsal ramus of S1[15] and there are isolated dorsal innervations from S1-4.[16] The anterior innervation is from the ventral rami of the L5 to S2 and via branches from the sacral plexus.[13] Its variable and extensive innervation accounts for the multiple presentations and variable referred pain patterns of sacroiliac joint pain.[17] The blood supply of the joint is from the anastomosis between the median sacral artery and lateral sacral branches from the internal iliac artery.

Sacroiliac Joint Dysfunction

The causes of SI joint dysfunction have been discussed in Chapter 17. The pathologic conditions that affect the sacroiliac joint include inflammatory, degenerative, traumatic, metabolic, infectious, tumor, iatrogenic conditions, and sacroiliac joint syndrome. *Sacroiliac joint dysfunction,* or *SI joint syndrome,* is pain from a sacroiliac joint that has no demonstrable lesion and is presumed to have some type of biochemical abnormality that causes the pain.[18] It can be initiated by trauma or pregnancy (caused by the hormone relaxin). There may be a history of lifting a heavy object with the patient in a twisted position, or the patient mis-stepping off a curb.[11] The incidence of SI joint dysfunction in patients with back pain ranges from 15% to 30%.

The location and referral patterns of SI joint dysfunction have been summarized by Benzon[10]; he based his composite pain diagram on the studies by Fortin, Schwarzer, Dreyfuss, and others.[18-21] The pain from SI joint dysfunction is usually located in the superior medial quadrant of the buttock, inferior to the posterosuperior iliac spine, and lateral buttock, with radiation to the greater trochanter and upper lateral thigh, and groin (Fig. 58–7). Two distinguishing features of the pain from SI joint dysfunction are the presence of groin pain[21] and absence of pain above the level of L5.[18] There may be radiation below the knee. In contrast to the pain pattern of SI joint dysfunction, the typical location of pain from a facet joint syndrome is pain that originates from the low back and radiates to the posterior thigh down to the knee while the pain from a herniated disk usually extends to the leg and foot.

As stated, the pain in sacroiliac joint dysfunction is associated with the following characteristics:

Location: Superior medial quadrant of the buttock, inferior to the posterior superior iliac spine. No pain above the level of L5 vertebra.[18]

Referral sites: Greater trochanter, groin, and upper lateral thigh; less often to the posterior thigh or below the knee (posterior leg)

Aggravating factors: Bending, sitting, and riding

Relief: Walking or standing

The physical examination of a patient with SI joint syndrome usually reveals tenderness over the posterior aspect of the joint and over the sacral sulcus. There are no neurologic symptoms such as numbness or weakness. The confirmation of sacroiliac joint dysfunction requires the presence of physical examination findings with commonly used tests including the FABER-Patrick test, Gaenslen test, Yeoman test[17] or extension test,[22] sacroiliac shear test or posterior shear test, and the Gillet test.[10,22,23] Although Yeoman's test stretches the femoral nerve and extends the lumbar spine, it appears to be the most specific and reliable test.[22] The FABER-Patrick test also stresses the hip joint, Gaenslen's stresses the hip joint and

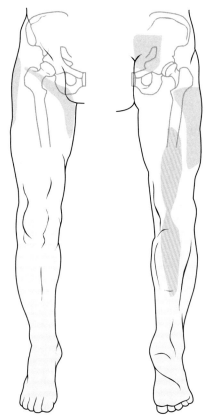

Figure 58–7. Pattern of pain from sacroiliac joint syndrome. (From Benzon HT: Pain originating from the buttock: Sacroiliac joint dysfunction and piriformis syndrome. In Benzon HT, Raja S, Molloy RE, et al [eds]: Essentials of pain medicine and regional anesthesia. New York, Elsevier Churchill Livingstone, 2005, pp 356-365, with permission.)

stretches the femoral nerve, and Gillet's can be difficult to perform.

The tests do not by themselves suggest the presence of SI joint dysfunction. Up to 2% of asymptomatic patients were found to have positive findings in one or more of these tests.[23] No historical feature, none of the screening tests that were evaluated, and no ensemble of the tests demonstrated worthwhile diagnostic value.[18] No aggravating or relieving factors were of value in diagnosing SI joint pain. The presence of tenderness over the sacral sulcus, pain over the SI joint, buttock pain, and the patient pointing to the posterior superior iliac spine as the main source of pain showed better sensitivity than the other tests evaluated.[18] It is obvious that the screening provocative tests do not rule in sacroiliac joint dysfunction or completely rule out other causes of pain. The tests are of added value in confirming the diagnosis of SI joint syndrome when the history and symptoms are suggestive of SI joint dysfunction and other causes of the patient's pain (e.g., piriformis syndrome, facet syndrome) have been eliminated.

The diagnosis of SI joint dysfunction can be based on the history, symptoms, and positive screening tests. Some experts require the presence of three positive screening tests to confirm SI joint dysfunction. The radiographic evaluation of the joint rarely adds value. Although provocation of pain on injection of the SI joint is not a suitable criterion of SI joint dysfunction, a diagnostic local anesthetic block of the joint is considered to be the standard criterion for SI joint pain.[21]

Technique of Sacroiliac Joint Injection

For diagnostic injections, patients are is asked to stop their pain medication on the day of the block. Sedation is usually not required but light sedation (1 to 2 mL midazolam) may be given in a very nervous patient. If sedation is to be given, the patient should be accompanied by a responsible adult. Contraindications to the injection include infection in the area, bleeding diathesis, and pregnancy. Allergy to the contrast media may require pretreatment with H_1 and H_2 antagonists, whereas allergy to local anesthetics may require identification of the appropriate local anesthetic to be used for the procedure.

The patient is prone and sterile precautions are observed during the procedure. Fluoroscopy guidance is recommended because blind SI injection rarely results in correct placement of the drug.[24] The *target point* lies along the inferoposterior aspect of the joint, in the area 1 to 2 cm cephalad from its most caudal end.[25] Under straight anteroposterior (AP) view, the SI joint presents several lines that course caudocranially in a semiparallel fashion. The lateral line represents the ventral or anterior margin of the joint, and the medial line represents the dorsal or posterior margin of the joint.[25,26] The C-arm is rotated across the patient (5 to 20 degrees of contralateral rotation) until the medial cortical line of the medial silhouette is maximally crisp[25] and the ventral and dorsal margins are superimposed. A 20- to 25-degree cephalad tilt, as recommended by Dussault and coworkers[27] helps in isolating the planes of the posterior and anterior joints. After skin infiltration, a 25- or 22-gauge, 3.5-cm spinal needle is inserted 0.5 to 1 cm below the inferior margin of the joint and directed into the *target* point. Entry into the joint is felt as a loss of bony resistance as the needle tip lies between the ilium and the sacrum; the needle is visualized as lying between the two bones on fluoroscopy. One mL of contrast medium is injected and the joint is outlined (Fig. 58–8). The volume of the joint ranges from 0.8 to 2.5 mL[28]; a maximum volume of 2.5 mL has been recommended for SI joint injections.[25]

Other approaches include placement of the needle at the inferior end where the posterior and anterior joints overlap, if a markedly lucent zone is noted in that area.[25] The midportion of the joint also can be cannulated. With 20 to 30 degrees of contralateral obliquity, the medial and lateral planes of the joint overlap. The needle entry is at the most lucent zone of the joint space; a 20- to 30-degree medial-to-lateral and 10- to 20-degree inferior direction of the needle approach has been recommended to gain entry into

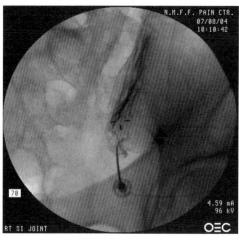

Figure 58–8. Sacroiliac joint injection; note the spread of the dye along the joint.

the midportion of the joint.[29] Finally, the superior aspect of the joint can be accessed with a cephalocaudad approach.

The response of the patient to the injection of contrast media is noted as either "no pain," "unfamiliar pain," or "similar pain" in comparison with the pain complaint.[21] After the joint is outlined, 1 to 2 mL of lidocaine or bupivacaine with steroid (6 mg betamethasone or 40 to 60 mg methylprednisolone) is injected. A greater than 75% reduction of pain over the SI joint is considered to be a "definite response."[21]

The complications of the procedure include bleeding, infection, transient lower extremity weakness, and transient difficulty in voiding.[26] The transient weakness of the lower extremity is secondary to partial block of the sciatic nerve that is located just anterior to the piriformis muscle that is at the same depth as the inferior aspect of the sacroiliac joint. Blockade of the sciatic nerve may be due to extravasation of the local anesthetic or to improper placement of the needle.

Immediate relief after an SI joint injection is usually seen in 50% to 80% of the patients; 90% have relief within 12 hours.[27,30] Follow-up of the patients who had the injection showed satisfactory relief for 9 months in 81% of patients.[14]

Computed Tomography–Guided Sacroiliac Joint Injection

Injection of the SI joint has been described under CT guidance.[30-32] The patient is prone and SI joint scanned. The section with the most suitable access to the joint is set and the gluteal injection site determined. The needle is inserted into the joint and steroid or local anesthetic injected. Success rates from CT-guided injections range from 75%[30] to 92.5%,[31] with the duration of relief lasting 14 days[30] to 10 months.[31] The lack of availability of CT in pain clinics restricts a wider application of this approach.

Radiofrequency Denervation of the Sacroiliac Joint

Ferrante and associates[33] reported the efficacy of thermal radiofrequency (RF) denervation of the SI joint. The rationale for their technique is neurolysis of the small, terminal sensory fibers that supply the posterior aspect of the joint. Their patients previously responded to a fluoroscopy-guided diagnostic injection of the SI joint with bupivacaine and betamethasone. Two probes were used to create a bipolar strip lesion. The first RF probe was inserted at the inferior margin of the joint and a second RF probe was placed more cephalad, at a distance of less than 1 cm from the first probe. The RF probe was heated to 80° C for 90 seconds, creating thermal strip lesions. Successive probes were placed less than 1 cm cephalad from the last probe, and multiple lesions were created in a repetitive "leapfrog" manner as high in the joint as possible, creating a "strip lesion" in the posterior joint.[33] A total of 50 SI joint denervations were performed in 33 patients, 12 of whom (36%) reported at least a 50% decrease in Visual Analogue Scores for pain for at least 6 months (the investigators' criterion for success). Despite the fact that it was a retrospective study, Ferrante and associates showed the efficacy of such technique.[33] The posterior superior iliac spine obscures access to the superior portion of the joint, making only the lower third portion of the joint accessible to the lesioning. It should be noted that some clinicians lesion the whole posterior border of the joint under heavy sedation: 100% relief is probably not achievable with the technique because no thermal lesions are created in the anterior aspect of the joint.

The ideal distance of the two probes to create a continuous strip lesion was studied by Pino and colleagues.[34] They compared the lesions created by two needles placed at 2, 4, 6, 8, and 10 mm from each other; egg white was used as the protein medium for easy visualization and measurement of the lesions. The temperatures of the probes were raised from 40° to 90° C and held at 90° C for 190 seconds. They noted that contiguous strip lesions were produced when the cannulas were spaced 6 mm or less apart—unipolar lesions resulted when the lesions were spaced more than 6 mm apart (Fig. 58–9).[34] Ninety

percent of the final lesion area was reached by 20 seconds and the final lesions reached by 150 seconds. They concluded that the probes should be placed between 4 and 6 mm apart to maximize the surface area of the thermal lesion and that the treatment duration should be between 120 and 150 seconds at 90° C.[34]

Radiofrequency Lesioning of the Lateral Branches

Two retrospective studies showed the efficacy of thermal RF lesioning of the lateral branches of the posterior primary ramus of the L4 to S3 dorsal rami in the treatment of SI joint syndrome.[35,36] In Cohen and Abdi's study,[35] 18 patients with SI joint pain had nerve blocks of the L4-5 primary dorsal rami and S1-3 lateral branches that innervate the posterior SI joint. Thirteen of the 18 patients obtained approximately 50% relief, 2 of the 13 had relief that lasted several months, 9 of the 13 patients underwent RF lesioning (80° C for 90 seconds) of the nerve, and 8 of the 9 patients who had the RF denervation experienced greater than 50% relief that persisted for at least 9 months.[35]

In Yin and associates' study,[36] 9 of 14 (64%) patients experienced a successful outcome (defined as >60% patient-perceived improvement with concurrent >50% decrease in visual integer pain score for 6 months), and 5 patients (36%) had complete relief at 6 months after thermal RF of the lateral branches of S1-3. Prior to the RF lesion, the patients had reproducible and consistent relief of their pain after two SI joint injections. Yin and associates also performed cadaver studies to follow the course of lateral branches. They noted that the lateral branches were located at the 2 to 6 o'clock positions at the right and at the 6 to 10 o'clock positions on the left side. The efficacy and rationale for lesioning of the lateral branches were questioned because the innervation of the ventral aspect of the SI joint was not lesioned. However, Yin and associates[36] as well as others[15,16] noted the predominant dorsal innervation of the SI joint.

Bipolar RF strip lesions adjacent to the lateral dorsal foramina of S1-3 combined with monopolar lesioning of the L5 dorsal ramus have been advocated by

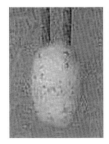
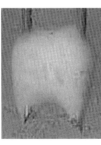
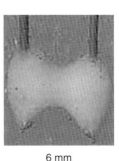
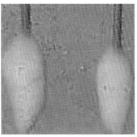
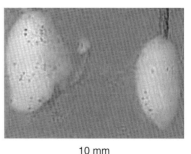

| 2 mm | 4 mm | 6 mm | 8 mm | 10 mm |

Figure 58–9. Bipolar lesions produced with the two cannulas at different distances. Note that a continuous lesion is produced when the cannulas are 6 mm or less. (From Pino CA Hoeft MA, Hofsess C, Rathmell JP: Morphologic analysis of bipolar radiofrequency lesions: Implications for treatment of the sacroiliac joint. Reg Anesth Pain Med 2005;30:335-338. Reprinted with permission.)

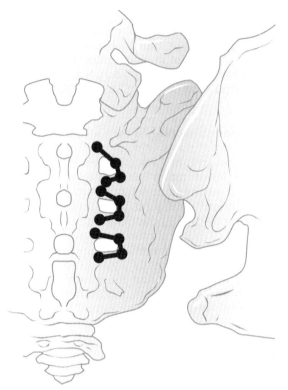

Figure 58–10. Bipolar lateral dorsal S1-3 periforaminal strip radiofrequency lesion. (From Burnham RS, Yasui Y: An alternative method of radiofrequency neurotomy of the sacroiliac joint: A pilot study of the effect on pain, function, and satisfaction. Reg Anesth Pain Med 2007;32:12-19. Reprinted with permission.)

Burnham and Yasui (Fig. 58–10).[37] In their technique, bipolar strip lesions were created approximately 5 mm lateral to the edge of the lateral half of the dorsal sacral foramina of S1, S2, and S3 by placing two 20-gauge, 10-mm exposed curved-tip RF cannulas 4 to 6 mm apart. The active probe was attached to the RF generator, and the other probe (passive) was attached to the ground through a bipolar adapter. For the right side, lesions were made at the 12 and 2 o'clock positions, then 2 and 4 o'clock positions (the needle at the 12 o'clock was removed and placed at the 4 o'clock position), and finally at the 4 and 6 o'clock positions (the needle at the 2 o'clock was removed and placed at the 6 o'clock position). On the left side, the same "leapfrog" technique was used to make bipolar strip lesions at the 12 and 10 o'clock, 10 and 8 o'clock, and 8 and 6 o'clock positions (Fig. 58–11). Their initial results showed 8 of 9 patients had significant reductions in the severity and frequency of their back and leg pain and in their analgesic intake.[37]

A combined RF lesioning of the SI joint and the dorsal branch of S5 under CT guidance has been described. Gevargez and colleagues lesioned the ventral and dorsal aspects of the joint.[32] However, only the area of the joint and only one nerve are lesioned. They reported that 34% of their patients had complete relief at 3 months and 32% had substantial pain reduction.

Note that it is customary to inject 0.5 to 1 mL local anesthetic (e.g., lidocaine) before the thermal RF lesion and to inject 0.5 mL of a mixture of local anesthetic (e.g., bupivacaine) and steroid (e.g., 8 mg/mL triamcinolone) after the lesioning for postoperative analgesia.

Piriformis Syndrome

Piriformis syndrome is another pain syndrome that originates in the buttock, and comprises 5% to 6% of patients referred for the treatment of back and leg pain.[38] It can occur after trauma, anatomic abnormalities, infection, or surgery (Box 58–4).[38-44] A history of trauma often is elicited in approximately 50% of cases; the trauma is usually not severe and the symptoms of piriformis syndrome may occur several months after trauma. Trauma to the buttock leads to inflammation and spasm of the piriformis muscle, and inflammatory substances are released from the inflamed muscle and irritate the sciatic nerve. The inflamed or hypertrophied piriformis muscle compresses the sciatic nerve between the muscle and the pelvis. A difference of $\frac{1}{2}$ inch or more in leg lengths may result in irritation of the sciatic nerve by the piriformis muscle in the shorter leg. The syndrome may occur after total hip replacement surgery or back surgery.[44,45] Laminectomy results in the formation of scar tissue that impinges on the nerve roots and "shortens" the sciatic nerve, rendering it prone to repeated tension and trauma by the piriformis muscle.

The piriformis muscle originates from the anterior surface of the S2-4 sacral vertebrae, capsule of the sacroiliac joint, and gluteal surface of the ilium near the posterior surface of the iliac spine. It runs laterally through the greater sciatic foramen, becomes tendinous, and inserts into the piriformis fossa at the medial aspect of the greater trochanter of the femur. The piriformis muscle is innervated by the branches of L5, S1, and S2 spinal nerves. The sciatic nerve, posterior femoral cutaneous nerve, gluteal nerves, and gluteal vessels pass below the piriformis muscle. There are several anatomic relationships between the piriformis and the sciatic nerve; the most common arrangement (90% to 98%) is the undivided sciatic nerve passing below the piriformis with the second most common arrangement a divided sciatic nerve passing below and through the muscle.[38,46] In rare cases in which the piriformis muscle is split and branches of the sciatic nerve have different courses, the tibial component usually passes below the piriformis and the common peroneal component passes through the piriformis muscle.

Anatomic abnormalities of the piriformis muscle and sciatic nerve can cause sciatica. Patients with split sciatic nerve, with one component passing through the muscle, may have symptoms similar to a radiculopathy (but with the pain originating in the buttock) secondary to irritation of the nerve. A case report described a patient with "sciatica" wherein the patient's symptoms were relieved after the lower

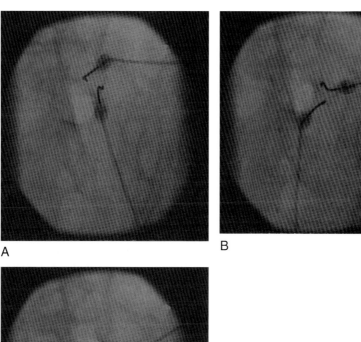

A

B

C

Figure 58–11. A, Right S1 lateral branch in the 12 to 2 o'clock position. **B,** Right S1 lateral branch in the 2 to 4 o'clock position. **C,** Right S1 lateral branch in the 4 to 6 o'clock position. (From Burnham RS, Yasui Y: An alternative method of radiofrequency neurotomy of the sacroiliac joint: A pilot study of the effect on pain, function, and satisfaction. Reg Anesth Pain Med 2007;32: 12-19. Reprinted with permission.)

BOX 58–4. CAUSES OF PIRIFORMIS SYNDROME

Trauma to the buttock or pelvis
Hypertrophy of the piriformis muscle
Anatomic abnormalities of the piriformis muscle or the sciatic nerve
Differences in leg lengths
Piriformis myositis
After total hip replacement surgery or laminectomy

BOX 58–5. CARDINAL FEATURES OF PIRIFORMIS SYNDROME

History of trauma to the sacroiliac and gluteal regions
Pain in the region of the sacroiliac joint, greater sciatic notch, and piriformis muscle, extending down the leg and causing difficulty in walking
Acute exacerbation of pain by stooping or lifting
Palpable sausage-shaped mass over the piriformis muscle, which is tender to palpation
Pain on flexion, adduction, and internal rotation of the ipsilateral hip
Possible gluteal atrophy

---

head of the bipartite piriformis muscle was resected.[41] Another report described a patient with a fascial constricting band around the sciatic nerve and a piriformis muscle lying anterior to the nerve.[42] The resection of the fibrous band and piriformis muscle restored the normal relationship between the sciatic nerve and piriformis, and relieved the patient's hip and buttock pain and sciatica. Several authors consider entrapment of the sciatic nerve by the piriformis as a cause of the syndrome and recommend surgical release of the muscle and its fascia as treatment of the syndrome.[41,42,47]

Patients with piriformis syndrome have cardinal features (Box 58–5).[38] They complain of buttock pain with or without radiation to the ipsilateral leg. The buttock pain usually extends from the sacrum to greater trochanter. Although some patients may have paralumbar pain, pain in the lower back is rare.[38] Irritation of the sciatic nerve results in the buttock pain radiating to the ipsilateral leg, whereas involvement of the posterior cutaneous nerve of the thigh only, which is very rare, causes the pain to radiate to the posterior thigh down to the knee. The pain is worse after sitting on a hard surface. Prolonged sitting, as in driving or biking, or when getting up from a sitting position, aggravates the pain.[39] Bowel movement may cause pain because of the proximity of the piriformis muscle to the lateral pelvic wall; female patients may complain of dyspareunia. Numbness in the foot occurs when the sciatic nerve is compressed by the piriformis muscle.

The patient may have a pelvic tilt or uneven scapulas. There may be tenderness in the buttock, from the medial edge of the greater sciatic foramen to the greater trochanter. A spindle-shaped mass might be felt in the buttock and tenderness may be felt in the area of the piriformis on rectal and pelvic examinations. The pain is aggravated by hip flexion, adduction, and internal rotation. Neurologic examination is usually negative. There might be leg numbness when the sciatic nerve is irritated; the straight-leg test may be normal or limited. Three physical examination signs help in confirming the presence of piriformis syndrome[46]:

Pace sign: pain and weakness on resisted abduction of the hip while the patient is seated (i.e., the hip is flexed)

Lasègue's sign: Pain on voluntary flexion, adduction, and internal rotation of the hip. Note that pain on straight-leg raise is also called a Lasèque's sign.

Freiberg's sign: Pain on forced internal rotation of the extended thigh. This is caused by stretching of the piriformis muscle and pressure on the sciatic nerve at the sacrospinous ligament.

Lasègue's and Freiberg's signs may appear contradictory. However, the piriformis has different functions when the hip is flexed and when it is extended. The piriformis muscle abducts the flexed thigh (this explains the pain with Lasègue's sign) and externally rotates the extended hip joint (causing pain with the Freiberg maneuver).

The diagnosis of piriformis syndrome is made on clinical grounds. Electromyography (EMG), computed tomography (CT), and magnetic resonance imaging (MRI) may aid in the diagnosis. EMG may detect myopathic and neuropathic changes including a delay in the H-reflex with the affected leg in a flexed, adducted, and internally rotated (FAIR) position as compared with the same H-reflex in the normal anatomic position. A three-standard deviation prolongation of the H-reflex has been recommended as the physiologic criterion for piriformis syndrome.[48] This EMG finding suggests entrapment of the nerve as it passes under the piriformis muscle. The CT of the soft tissues of the pelvis may show an enlarged piriformis muscle or abnormal uptake by the muscle, whereas MRI confirms the enlarged piriformis muscle.[49,50]

The differential diagnoses of piriformis syndrome include the causes of low back pain and radiculopathy. In contrast with foraminal stenosis or herniated disk, the patient with piriformis syndrome does not have neurologic deficits unless there is irritation of the sciatic nerve. Facet syndrome, sacroiliac joint dysfunction, myofascial pain syndrome, trochanteric bursitis, pelvic tumor, endometriosis, and conditions irritating the sciatic nerve should be considered in the differential diagnoses of syndrome. These conditions are usually ruled out by the medical history and physical examination of the patient. It should be noted that most patients with piriformis syndrome show the concomitant presence of other causes of back and leg pain. This is because piriformis syndrome usually occurs as a part of soft tissue injuries resulting from rotation or flexion movements of the hip and torso.

The treatments of piriformis syndrome include physical therapy combined with the use of medications such as muscle relaxants, anti-inflammatory drugs, and analgesics to reduce the spasm, inflammation, and pain.[46] Physical therapy includes stretching of the piriformis muscle with flexion, adduction, and internal rotation of the hip accompanied by pressure applied to the muscle.[38,39] Once the symptoms improve, strengthening of the hip abductors is added to the regimen. Abnormal biomechanics caused by bad posture, pelvic obliquities, and leg length discrepancies are corrected. Vapocoolant spray with soft-tissue stretch of the area also has been recommended and ultrasound treatments may help reduce the pain.[51,52]

Local anesthetic and steroid injections may break the pain/muscle spasm cycle and patients who do not respond to the conservative therapy are candidates for these injections. Previous injections were made at the focal point of pain and irritability deep in the belly of the muscle or at the medial or lateral aspects of the muscle. It should be noted that compression of the sciatic nerve usually occurs at the lateral aspect of the piriformis. Caudal local anesthetic and steroid injections may be effective as the injected solution diffuses along the nerve root sleeves and the proximal part of the sciatic nerve, blocking the nerves that innervate the piriformis muscle.[53]

Techniques of Piriformis Muscle and Perisciatic Nerve Injections

Piriformis injections can be performed blindly. More specific techniques involve identification of the piriformis muscle with a muscle EMG, with the guidance of CT, a nerve stimulator, or a combined fluoroscopy-nerve stimulator guidance. In the EMG-fluoroscopy–guided technique[54] the patient is in the prone position and the expected position of the piriformis muscle is identified using the greater trochanter of the femur and lateral border of the sacrum and the sacroiliac joint as landmarks. The muscle EMG is used to confirm the correct placement of the needle in the muscle. After the correct spread of the contrast media is shown on the fluoroscopy, the steroid is injected into the piriformis muscle. In the CT-guided technique, the piriformis muscle is identified and a needle is inserted under CT guidance. In Porta's technique,[55] local anesthetic (2 mL 0.5% bupivacaine) is injected into the muscle followed by 100 units of botulinum toxin type A. The unavailability of the EMG and CT equipments in most pain treatment centers limits a wider application of these techniques.

Hanania and Kitain[56,57] described the technique of periscatic injection. In their technique the patient is in the lateral or semiprone position with the non-dependent hip and knee flexed and the dependent extremity straight. A nerve stimulator is used to identify the location of the sciatic nerve. The needle is then withdrawn a few centimeters and 40 mg methylprednisolone in 5 to 10 mL dilute local anesthetic is injected. No fluoroscopy is used in this technique. In their paper, Hanania and Kitain described six patients who were previously unresponsive or partially responsive to blind piriformis muscle injections or epidural steroid injections. Their patients had relief of their pain for up to 18 months after their periscatic injection with the local anesthetic and steroid.

Benzon and coworkers[46] described a technique wherein fluoroscopy was combined with the nerve stimulator. The patient is prone and the lower border of the sacroiliac (SI) joint, greater sciatic foramen, and head of the femur are identified on fluoroscopy. The area is prepped and draped, and the entry site is anesthetized with local anesthetic. A 15-cm insulated needle, connected to a nerve stimulator is inserted at 1.5 plus or minus 0.8 cm (range: 0.5 to 3 cm) lateral and 1.2 plus or minus 0.6 cm (range: 0.5 to 2 cm) caudal to the lower border of the SI joint (Fig. 58–12A). The needle is advanced perpendicularly until a motor-evoked response of the sciatic nerve is obtained at less than 0.5 mA, usually at 9.2-cm (range: 7.5 to 13 cm) depth. The evoked motor response of the foot can be inversion, eversion, dorsiflexion, or plantar flexion.[58] The needle is pulled back 0.3 to 0.6 cm to avoid intraneural injection, and 40 mg methyl-prednisolone in 5 to 6 mL saline is injected. The needle is pulled back another 0.5 to 0.7 cm to place the tip of the needle at the belly of the piriformis muscle; 2 to 3 mL of contrast media is injected and the piriformis muscle is outlined (see Fig. 58–12B). Forty mg methylprednisolone in 6 to 8 mL local anesthetic is injected into the muscle. The injection of the local anesthetic into the belly of the muscle is important to avoid leakage of the local anesthetic into the sciatic nerve and cause sensory and motor blockade of the leg and foot. Note that saline is injected periscatically to avoid motor blockade of the patient's leg while local anesthetic is injected into the piriformis muscle to relax the muscle and break the spasm–pain cycle. The injection of steroid periscatically is recommended, whether there is "radicular" leg pain or not, because there is probably some irritation and inflammation of the sciatic nerve in cases of piriformis syndrome. The rationale for the steroid includes its anti-inflammatory and nociceptive-blocking properties.[59,60]

Botulinum toxin may be injected into the muscle if the patient has transient response to the steroid and local anesthetic injection. Botulinum toxin

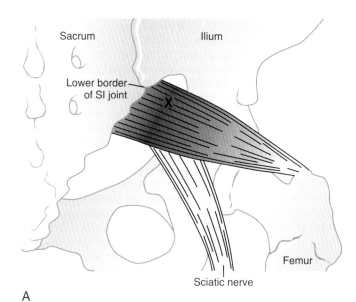

A

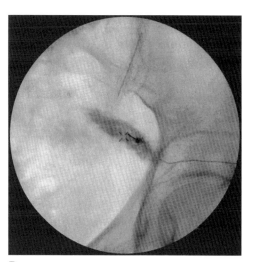

B

Figure 58–12. Piriformis injection. **A,** The needle is inserted 1 to 1.5 cm lateral and inferior to the lower border of the sacroiliac (SI) joint. *X* indicates the site of needle insertion. **B,** Note that the piriformis muscle is outlined by the dye. (From Benzon HT, Katz JA, Benzon HA, Iqbal MS: Piriformis syndrome: Anatomic considerations, a new injection technique, and a review of the literature. Anesthesiology 2003;98:1442-1448. Reprinted with permission.)

blocks the release of acetylcholine at the neuromuscular junction, resulting in the prolonged relaxation of the muscle.[61] Recovery of the muscle depends on neuromuscular sprouting and reinnervation of the muscle that may take several weeks to months. The doses of the botulinum toxin are100 mouse units for botulinum toxin type A (BTX-A; Botox) in 4 mL bupivacaine and 5000 to 10,00 units for botulinum toxin type B (Myobloc).[55] The reported complications of botulinum toxin injection include polyradiculoneuritis, brachial plexopathy, and local psoriasiform dermatitis.[62-65] Caution should be observed when botulinum toxin is injected into the piriformis muscle. It should be injected into the belly of the muscle to avoid leakage into the sciatic nerve.

A randomized study compared BTX-A and methylprednisolone injections in patients with piriformis syndrome.[55] Thirty days after the injection, the patients in both groups showed marked reduction in their pain scores with no significant difference between the two groups. At 60 days after the injection, the patients who had botulinum injection had significantly lower pain scores.[55] In our clinical experience, some of our patients who had the local anesthetic-steroid injections had sustained relief for up to 3 months. The prolonged relief in some of our patients may be due to the concomitant perisciatic injection of the steroid. The added perisciatic injection may break the cycle of pain and spasm better than the piriformis muscle injection alone.

Surgery may be entertained in patients who do not respond to the combined treatments of injection, physical therapy, and medications, or when there is documented anatomic abnormality of the piriformis muscle. The muscle may be excised, divided, or thinned.[38,39,41,42,47] The loss of piriformis muscle function is compensated by the obturator internus, gemelli, and quadratus femoris muscles because these muscles share common insertions with the piriformis.

CONCLUSION

Injections into the greater trochanteric bursa and into the hip joint are usually performed by orthopedic surgeons. Although a fair number of these injections are done blindly, an increasing number is being referred to the pain clinic for injections under fluoroscopy guidance. Sacroiliac joint and piriformis syndromes, in addition to myofascial syndrome, comprise the most common causes of pain in the buttock. The clinician should know not only the signs and symptoms of these syndromes but also the physical examination tests that help make the diagnosis. There have been many advances in the description of the techniques of injection into the SI joint, RF lesioning of the joint and the lateral branches of the posterior primary ramus of the L5-S3 nerves, and perisciatic and piriformis injections. These advances should help the clinician in managing these pain syndromes, conditions of which we had very little knowledge just a few years ago.

SUMMARY

- Hip injections are either diagnostic or therapeutic. They are used to decrease pain and improve mobility in the affected joint.
- Injection into the hip area is either into the trochanteric bursa or the joint. Bursa injections are best performed with fluoroscopy guidance. Injections into the hip joint can be performed through the lateral approach or anterior approach, and with fluoroscopy the lateral approach is more effective and poses less risk of trauma to the femoral artery and nerve. Injection with ultrasound guidance eliminates x-ray equipment and exposure to radiation.

- The pain of the SI joint syndrome is usually felt in the SI joint area and usually radiates to the groin, lateral thigh, posterior thigh, and leg. There is a characteristic picture of the pain from SI joint syndrome.
- The common tests that confirm the presence of SI joint syndrome include the FABER-Patrick, Gaenslen, Yeoman, shear, and Gillet tests.
- The diagnosis of SI joint syndrome is based on the patient's history, symptoms, positive confirmatory tests, elimination of the other causes of buttock pain, and a positive response to an SI joint injection.
- Relief from SI joint injection with local anesthetic and steroid can be temporary. More prolonged relief can be obtained by thermal RF lesioning of the SI joint or the lateral branches of the primary ramus of the L5-S3 nerves. Continuous RF lesions can be obtained by performing bipolar strip lesions.
- Piriformis syndrome can be caused by trauma, muscle hypertrophy, anatomic abnormalities, infection, previous hip or back surgery, or differences in leg lengths.
- The pain from piriformis syndrome originates from the buttock and radiates to the greater trochanter of the ipsilateral hip. The pain radiates to the posterior leg when there is irritation of the sciatic nerve. Pace, Lasègue, and Freiberg signs confirm the presence of the syndrome. The EMG may show a delay in the H reflex with the hip in the flexed, adducted, and internally rotated position.
- The treatment of piriformis syndrome includes physical therapy, medications, and injection into the piriformis muscle and around the irritated sciatic nerve.

References

1. Cardone DA, Tallia AF: Joint and soft tissue injection. Am Fam Physician 2002;66:283-288.
2. Cohen SP, Narvaez JC, Lebovits AH, Stojanovic MP: Corticosteroid injections for trochanteric bursitis: Is fluoroscopy necessary? A pilot study. Br J Anaesth 2005;94:100-106.
3. Morelli V, Weaver V: Groin injuries and groin pain in athletes: Part 1. Prim Care 2005;32:163-183.
4. Newberg AH: Anesthetic and corticosteroid joint injections: A primer. Semin Musculoskelet Radiol 1998;2:415-420.
5. Leopold SS, Battista V, Oliverio JA: Safety and efficacy of intraarticular hip injection using anatomic landmarks. Clin Orthop Relat Res 2001:192-197.
6. Kilcoyne RF, Kaplan P: The lateral approach for hip arthrography. Skeletal Radiol 1992;21:239-240.
7. Smith J, Hurdle MF: Office-based ultrasound-guided intraarticular hip injection: Technique for physiatric practice. Arch Phys Med Rehabil 2006;87:296-298.
8. Fitzgerald, RH: Intrasynovial injection of steroids uses and abuses. Mayo Clin Proc 1976;51:655-659.
9. Kullenberg B, Ruinesson R, Tuvhag R, et al: Intraarticular corticosteroid injection: Pain relief in osteoarthritis of the hip? J Rheumatol 2004;31:2265-2268.
10. Benzon HT: Pain originating from the buttock: Sacroiliac joint dysfunction and piriformis syndrome. In Benzon HT, Raja S, Molloy RE, et al (eds): Essentials of Pain Medicine and Regional Anesthesia. New York, Elsevier, 2005, pp 356-365.
11. Mooney V: Understanding, examining for, and treating sacroiliac pain. J Musculo Med 1993;10:37-49.
12. Walker JM: The sacroiliac joint: A critical review. Physical Ther 1992;72:903-916.
13. Ikeda R: Innervation of the sacroiliac joint: Macroscopic and histological studies. J Nippon Med School 1991;58:587-596.

14. Paris SV: Anatomy as related to function and pain: Symposium on evaluation and care of lumbar spine problems. Orthop Clin North Am 1983;14:475.
15. Grob K, Neuhuber W, Kissling R: Die innervation des sacriliacalgelenkes beim Menschen. Zeitsch Rheumatol 1995;27:117-122.
16. Fortin JD, Wahsington WJ, Falco JE: Three pathways between the sacroiliac joint and neural structures. Am J Neuroradiol 1999;20:14229-1434.
17. Bernard TN, Cassidy JD: The sacroiliac joint syndrome. In Frymoyer JW (ed): The Adult Spine. New York, Raven Press, 1991, pp 2107-2130.
18. Dreyfuss P, Michaelson M, Pauza K, et al: The value of medical history and physical examination in diagnosing sacroiliac joint pain. Spine 1996;21:2594-2602.
19. Fortin DO, Dwyer AP, West S, Pier J: Sacroiliac joint: Pain referral maps upon applying a new injection/arthrography technique. Part I: Asymptomatic volunteers. Spine 1994;19:1475-1482.
20. Fortin JD, Aprill CN, Ponthieux B, Pier J: Sacroiliac joint: Pain referral maps upon applying a new injection/arthrography technique. Part II: Clinical evaluation. Spine 1994;19:1483-1489.
21. Schwarzer AC, Aprill AN, Bogduk N: The sacroiliac joint in chronic low back pain. Spine 1995;20:31-37.
22. Kirkaldy-Willis WH, Burton CV: Managing Low Back Pain (3rd ed). New York, Churchill Livingstone, 1999, pp 121-148.
23. Dreyfus P, Dreyer S, Griffin J, et al: Positive screening tests in asymptomatic adults. Spine 1994;19:1138-1143.
24. Rosenberg J, Quint T, de Rosayro A: Computed tomographic localization of clinically-guided sacroiliac joint injections. Clin J Pain 2000;16:18-21.
25. Bogduk N (ed): Practice Guidelines. Spinal Diagnostic and Treatment Procedures. San Francisco, International Spine Intervention Society, 2004, pp 66-86.
26. Fenton DS, Czervionke LF: Image-guided spine intervention Philadelphia, Saunders, 2003, pp 127-139.
27. Dussault RG, Kaplan PE, Anderson MW: Fluoroscopy-guided sacroiliac joint injections. Radiology 2000;214:273-277.
28. Fortin JD, Tolchin RB: Sacroiliac joint provocation and arthrography. Arch Phys Med Rehabil 1993;74:125-129.
29. Ebraheim NA, Xu R, Naudad M, et al: Sacroiliac joint injection: A cadaver study. Am J Orthop 1997;26:338-341.
30. Pulisetti D, Ebraheim NA: CT-guided sacroiliac joint injections. J Spinal Disord 999;12:310-312.
31. Bollow M, Braun J, Taupitz M, et al: CT-guided intraarticular corticosteroid injection into the sacroiliac joints in patients with spondyloarthropathy: Indications and follow-up with contrast enhanced MRI. J Comput Assist Tomogr 1996;20:512-521.
32. Gevargez A, Groenemeyer D, Schirp S, Braun M: CT-guided percutaneous radiofrequency denervation of the sacroiliac joint. Eur Radiol 2002;12:1360-1365.
33. Ferrante FM, King LF, Roche EA, et al: Radiofrequency sacroiliac joint denervation for sacroiliac joint syndrome. Reg Anesth Pain Med 2001;26:137-142.
34. Pino CA, Hoeft MA, Hofsess C, Rathmell JP: Morphologic analysis of bipolar radiofrequency lesions: Implications for treatment of the sacroiliac joint. Reg Anesth Pain Med 2005;30:335-338.
35. Cohen SP, Abdi S: Lateral branch blocks as a treatment for sacroiliac joint pain: A pilot study. Reg Anesth Pain Med 2003;28:113-119.
36. Yin W, Willard F, Carreiro J, Dreyfuss P: Sensory stimulation guided sacroiliac joint radiofrequency neurotomy: Technique based on neuroanatomy of the dorsal sacral plexus. Spine 2003; 28:2419-2425.
37. Burnham RS, Yasui Y: An alternative method of radiofrequency neurotomy of the sacroiliac joint: A pilot study of the effect on pain, function, and satisfaction. Reg Anesth Pain Med 2007;32:12-19.
38. Parziale JR, Hudgins TH, Fishman LM: The piriformis syndrome. Am J Orthop 1996;25:819-823.
39. Barton PM: Piriformis syndrome: A rational approach to management. Pain 1991;47:345-352.
40. Durrani Z, Winnie AP: Piriformis syndrome: An undiagnosed cause of sciatica. J Pain Symptom Manage 1991;6:374-379.
41. Chen WS: Bipartite piriformis muscle: An unusual cause of sciatic nerve entrapment. Pain 1994;58:269-272.
42. Sayson SC, Ducey JP, Maybrey JB, et al: Sciatic entrapment neuropathy associated with an anomalous piriformis muscle. Pain 1994;59:149-152.
43. Chen WS: Sciatica due to piriformis pyomyositis. J Bone Joint Surg 1992;74-A:1546-1548.
44. Cameron HU, Noftal F: The piriformis syndrome. Can J Surg 1988;31:210.
45. Mizuguchi T: Division of the piriformis muscle for the treatment of sciatica: Postlaminectomy syndrome and osteoarthritis of the spine. Arch Surg 1976;111:719-722.
46. Benzon HT, Katz JA, Benzon HA, Iqbal MS: Piriformis syndrome: Anatomic considerations, a new injection technique, and a review of the literature. Anesthesiology 2003;98:1442-1448.
47. Solheim LF, Siewers P, Paus B: The priformis muscle syndrome: Sciatic nerve entrapment treated with section of the piriformis muscle. Acta Orthop Scand 1981;52:73-75.
48. Fishman LM, Zybert PA: Electrophysiologic evidence of piriformis syndrome. Arch Phys Med Rehabil 1992;73:359-364.
49. Jankiewicz JT, Hennrikus WL, Houkom J: The appearance of the piriformis muscle in computed tomography and magnetic resonance imaging: A case report and review of the literature. Clin Orthop 1991;262:205-209.
50. Karl RD, Yedinak MA, Hartshorne MF, et al: Scintigraphic appearance of the piriformis muscle syndrome. Clin Nucl Med 1985;10:361-363.
51. Steiner C, Staubs, Gannon M, Buhlinger C: Piriformis syndrome. Pathogenesis, diagnosis and treatment. J Am Osteopath Assoc 1987;87:318-323.
52. Simons D, Travell J: Myofascial origins of low back pain. Postgrad Med 1983;73:99-108.
53. Mullin V: Caudal steroid injection for treatment of piriformis syndrome. Anesth Analg 1990;71:705-707.
54. Fishman SM, Caneris OA, Bandman TB, et al: Injection of the piriformis muscle by fluoroscopic and electromyographic guidance. Reg Anesth Pain Med 1998;23:554-559.
55. Porta M: A comparative trial of botulinum toxin type A and methylprednisolone for the treatment of myofascial pain syndrome and pain from chronic muscle spasm. Pain 2000;85:101-105.
56. Hanania M: New technique for piriformis muscle injection using a nerve stimulator (letter). Reg Anesth Pain Med 1997;22:200-202.
57. Hanania M, Kitain E: Perisciatic injection of steroid for the treatment of sciatica due to piriformis syndrome. Reg Anesth Pain Med 1998;23:223-228.
58. Benzon HT, Kim C, Benzon HP, et al: Correlation between evoked motor response of the sciatic nerve and sensory blockade. Anesthesiology 1997;87:547-552.
59. Devor M, Govrin-Lippman R, Raber P: Corticosteroids suppress ectopic neural discharge originating in experimental neuromas. Pain 1985;22:127-137.
60. Johannsson A, Hao J, Sjolund B: Local corticosteroid application blocks transmission in normal nociceptive C-fibers. Acta Anaesthesiol Scand 1990;34:335-338.
61. Jankovic T, Brin MF: Therapeutic uses of botulinum toxin. N Engl J Med 1991;324:1186-1193.
62. Glanzman RL, Gelb DJ, Drury I, et al: Brachial plexopathy after botulinum toxin injections. Neurology 1990;40:1143.
63. Haug BA, Dressler D, Prange HW: Polyradiculoneuritis following botulinum toxin therapy. J Neurol 1990;237:62-63.
64. Bowden JB, Rapini RP: Psoriasiform eruption following intramuscular botulinum A toxin. Cutis 1992;50:415-416.
65. Sampaio C, Castro-Caldas A, Sales-Luis ML, et al: Brachial plexopathy after botulinum toxin administration for cervical dystonia (letter). J Neurol Neurosurg Psychiatry 1993;56:220.

59 Lumbar Discography

Steven P. Cohen and Thomas M. Larkin

LOW BACK PAIN OVERVIEW

Back pain has plagued mankind since time immemorial. In most cases the development of low back pain (LBP) is self-limiting and does not require operative intervention. Ninety percent of cases of LBP resolve without medical attention within 4 months; 50% resolve within a week.[1] However, the remaining cases exact an enormous toll on society in terms of personal suffering and economic impact. In recent years the prevalence of back pain disability has exploded in industrialized societies, accounting for an annual cost exceeding $50 billion in the United States. The statistics are even more unsettling when viewed from a personal and economic perspective. In patients with LBP who haven't worked in 6 months, the lifetime return-to-work rate is 50%. In those who have been off work for 1 year, only 25% will return to work. For those patients whose injury has left them unable to work for 2 years, the return to work rate is less than 5%.[2-4] This dramatic surge in the incidence and cost of chronic LBP has led to a concurrent rise in the use of diagnostic modalities and therapeutic interventions aimed at ameliorating this growing problem. Among the various types of LBP, internal disk disruption (IDD) is widely acknowledged to be the most common source of axial symptoms, and second only to herniated nucleus pulposus (HNP) overall.

Discography was first described in 1948 as a diagnostic tool for HNP.[5] Since then the development of simpler, safer, and more accurate imaging modalities has largely supplanted discography as an investigative technique for nerve root compression. Yet provocative lumbar discography continues to be a popular though controversial means for diagnosing axial LBP caused by IDD. This is because unlike magnetic resonance imaging (MRI) or computed tomography (CT) scanning, discography is not just an imaging modality but a provocative test purported to correlate symptoms with pathology. Although some studies have shown a high degree of correlation between discography results and histologic findings,[6,7] and discography and surgical outcomes,[8,9] others have failed to demonstrate such a relationship.[10,11]

Provocative Tests in Context

Much of the criticism surrounding discography stems from generalized disapproval about the diagnostic value of provocative procedures for other spinal disorders. In a study by Marks, no consistent segmental or sclerotomal referral patterns were found during 385 provocative lumbar facet blocks in 138 patients with chronic spinal pain.[12] Bough and associates assessed the histologic findings of 127 facet joints surgically removed based on preoperative provocative lumbar facet arthrography.[13] The authors found the specificity of degenerative facet joint changes to be 75%, but the sensitivity to be only 59%. They concluded that the reproduction of symptoms during facet arthrography was of little value as a presurgical screening procedure. Schwarzer and colleagues conducted a prospective study in 90 patients (203 joints) to determine the relationship between pain provocation and the analgesic response to lumbar zygapophysial joint blocks.[14] Using a single analgesic block as the diagnostic criterion, the production of similar or exact pain reproduction was found to predict subsequent response to analgesic facet blocks. However, when the more stringent criterion of concordant analgesic response to confirmatory blocks with lidocaine and bupivacaine was used, no significant association was found.

In 1994, Fortin and coworkers conducted two studies designed to evaluate sacroiliac (SI) joint pain referral maps generated by the distention of joints in asymptomatic volunteers. In the first study, the authors designed a pain referral map by distending the SI joint capsule in 10 asymptomatic subjects by injecting radiopaque contrast and lidocaine.[15] Similar to a set of previous studies done on cervical facet joints,[16,17] the authors found that the pain generated during the initial joint injection corresponded with the hypesthesia experienced after lidocaine was administered. In the second study, independent observers chose 16 patients with chronic LBP whose pain diagrams most closely resembled the pain referral maps generated in the first study, and injected their joints with bupivacaine.[18] Ten of the 16 patients obtained more than 50% pain relief after the installation of bupivacaine. Of note, the pain referral maps generated in the first Fortin study were significantly different from SI joint referral zones described by other authors based solely on analgesic blocks.[19]

Finally, Schwarzer and colleagues conducted an SI joint prevalence study in 43 patients with LBP principally below L5-S1.[20] Using analgesic response to local anesthetic blocks alone, 30% of patients were considered to have SI joint pain. Using pain relief combined with a ventral capsular tear on post-arthrography CT imaging, 21% of patients met the diagnostic criteria for SI joint pain. Using the three criteria of concordant pain provocation, abnormal imaging, and analgesic response to local anesthetic injection, only 16% were considered to have SI joint pain. Among the 27 patients with similar or exact pain reproduction during provocative testing, only 41% experienced "gratifying" pain relief following local anesthetic injection. The lack of strong validity for provocative facet and SI joint injections as diagnostic tools is consistent with the findings of Slipman and associates, who demonstrated distinct differences between dynatomal and dermatomal maps during provocative cervical nerve root blocks.[21] In summary, there seems to be little evidence to support the use of provocative injections to diagnose other sources of LBP.

Lumbar Intervertebral Disk Anatomy

The intervertebral disk complex is composed of the nucleus pulposus (NP), the annulus fibrosus (AF), and the vertebral end plates (VE). Lying above and below the disk are the vertebral bodies, or the sacrum below L5-S1. The disk is attached to the adjacent vertebral bodies via the vertebral end plates centrally, and the ligamentous attachments of the AF peripherally. Together, these components allow for the principal movements exhibited by the lumbar spine, which include axial compression, axial distraction, flexion, extension, axial rotation and lateral flexion. Horizontal translation does not generally occur as an isolated movement, but is involved in axial rotation. Posteriorly, the intervertebral disk is supported by the other two components of the three-part structure, the paired zygapophysial joints. Working in concert, these structures function to support and stabilize the spine, and prevent injury by limiting motion in all planes of movement.[22]

The nucleus pulposus consists primarily of water (70% to 90%) in a matrix composed of proteoglycan, a substance containing a very high water-binding capacity, and type II collagen. The dry weight of the intervertebral disk consists of approximately 65% proteoglycan; the remainder of the nucleus is composed largely of type II collagen. The high water content of the disk creates a broad, relatively noncompressible weight-bearing surface that serves to cushion the spine from the stress of the truncal load.[22]

The annulus fibrosus is composed of primarily type I collagen that is arranged in highly organized, concentric lamellae. These lamellae form 10 to 20 sheets surrounding the NP, being thicker toward the center of the disk. The AF is thick and strong anteriorly and laterally, but tends to be weaker posteriorly. This

anatomic incongruity accounts for the disproportionate percentage of disk herniations occurring posteriorly. Posteriorly, the AF is concave shaped in the lumbar spine. Like the NP, the AF contains a high water content, in the range of 60% to 70%; 50% to 60% of its dry weight is type I collagen.[22] The annulus functions to help stabilize the vertebral bodies, and acts as a ligament to limit excess motion.

The vertebral end plate is composed of hyaline cartilage close to the vertebral body and fibrocartilage near the NP. The fibrocartilage is formed as an extension of the annular fibers. This tough layer of fibrocartilage surrounds the NP. The end plates completely envelop the NP centrally, but taper off peripherally where the outermost AF lamellae directly attach to the vertebral bodies. The composition of the end plates resembles the annulus at its attachments to the vertebral bodies, and the NP centrally.

The healthy adult disk is basically avascular, with its nutrition being supplied through the VE and AF via passive diffusion. Whereas the periphery of the annulus is completely permeable, the bone-disk interface is only partially permeable to substrates.[23] The annulus contains blood vessels only in its most superficial lamellae. The nucleus itself contains no direct blood supply. The oxygen and nutrients that diffuse through the end plates come from branches of the lumbar arteries supplying the vertebral bodies.

The anabolic functions of the healthy disk are maintained by chondrocytes and fibroblasts, whereas catabolic functions depend on the matrix metalloproteinase enzymes collagenase (which degrades collagen) and stromelysin (which degrades proteoglycans). The metabolism of cells in the nucleus is exquisitely sensitive to changes in pH, being maximally active in the range of 6.9 and 7.2. Even in the presence of high oxygen concentrations, the metabolism of the disk is mainly anaerobic, with only 1.5% of glucose being converted to carbon dioxide.[24,25] Any number of factors can lead to a breakdown in the delicate metabolic function of the disk, including changes in pH, inflammatory mediators, and nutritional deficiencies.[22]

Functionally, the innervation to the lumbar intervertebral disks stems from two extensive nerve plexuses that accompany the posterior and anterior longitudinal ligaments.[22] These are known as the posterior and anterior plexuses. The anterior plexus consists of contributions from the anterior branches of gray rami communicantes, small medioventral branches of the sympathetic trunk, and perivascular nerve plexuses. The posterior plexus is a diffuse network of interconnecting fibers receiving somatic and autonomic input from multiple spinal levels.[26] Its visible components derive mainly from sinuvertebral nerves, formed from somatic roots arising from ventral rami, and autonomic contributions from gray ramus communicantes (which receive input from the sympathetic trunk), but the majority of its nerve fibers are actually microscopic. The posterior and anterior plexi are connected via a less prominent conglomeration of nerves known as the lateral plexus, formed by branches of the gray rami communicantes.[22,26] Together, these plexuses provide transmission of sensory information from the entire circumference of the intervertebral disk via a variety of different neural pathways.

In the newborn, the innervation of the lumbar intervertebral disk is dense, most likely because of the extensive blood supply.[27] This rich vascularization disappears around 4 years of age, and is accompanied by a concomitant diminution of nerve density.[28-30] However, in later years when degenerative processes set in, there is a recrudescence of blood vessels and nerve endings. Nerve fibers are typically sparse in lumbar intervertebral disks, innervating only the outer one third. But in patients with degenerative disk disease, herniated nucleus pulposus, and chronic low back pain, the innervation becomes both denser and deeper, frequently penetrating the inner AF and occasionally the NP.[31-35]

There is considerable evidence supporting the role lumbar sympathetic afferents play in the perception of LBP. This includes the provocation of LBP by stimulation of the sympathetic trunk and the relief of LBP following lumbar sympathetic block.[36,37] Moreover, the contribution of these sympathetic afferents appears mainly to be transmitted via the L2 nerve root, as evidenced by the work of Foerster,[38] who demonstrated that L2 is the dermatome corresponding to LBP, and Nakamura and coworkers,[39] who showed that LBP disappeared or significantly decreased after selective blockade of the L2 nerve root. The observation that the lumbar intervertebral disks and their adjacent ligaments are innervated by branches of the sympathetic nervous system does not necessarily mean that sensory input from these structures returns to the spinal cord via the sympathetic trunk. Rather, it has been suggested that somatic afferent fibers from the disks and surrounding pain-generating structures course with the rami communicantes to return to the central nervous system via ventral rami. Several different types of nonvascular nerve endings have been described including simple, cluster, partially, and fully encapsulated.[30] Although the exact role of each type of nerve ending is unknown, it is speculated that under nonpathologic conditions they primarily function as mechanoreceptors[33] (Fig. 59–1).

Pathogenesis of Discogenic Low Back Pain

Whether the lumbar intervertebral disks receive sensory innervation has been a controversial topic for many years. In the early and mid-20th century, anatomic studies failed to demonstrate nerve endings within lumbar intervertebral disks, and it was therefore believed that disks could not be a principal source of pain generation.[40-42] Subsequent studies have since disproved this contention. In normal human disks sensory nerves extend into the outer third of the annulus. In degenerated and herniated disks, the innervation is deeper and more extensive,

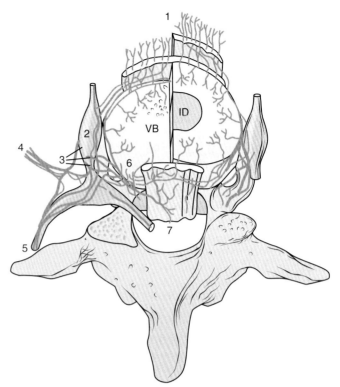

Figure 59–1. Schematic drawing of the nerve plexi surrounding the vertebral body (VB) and intervertebral disk (ID); 1 and 7 represent the anterior and posterior plexuses, respectively. The deep, extensive penetration of the nerves indicates degeneration has occurred; (2), sympathetic trunk; (3), rami communicantes; (4), ventral ramus of the spinal nerve; (5), dorsal ramus; (6), sinuvertebral nerves. (Drawing courtesy of Specialist Jennifer Sempsroft, U.S. Army.)

with some nerve fibers penetrating the nucleus pulposus.[31-35] It is now generally acknowledged that intervertebral disks do receive sensory innervation, and indeed can be a significant cause of LBP.[26,30,43-45]

Mechanical Changes

In the normal disk, mechanical interplay between the AF and NP distributes weight-bearing uniformly across the entire disk surface.[46,47] When a disk becomes physically stressed such as by activities involving flexion of the lumbar spine, the nucleus acts as a noncompressible mass, with its gelatinous contents bulging in the axial, sagittal, and coronal planes. A competent annulus tends to resist this outward bulging, resulting in an equitable force distribution throughout the disk plane.[22] In these circumstances, the annulus is not unduly stressed in the vertical direction because its broad surface area translates into the nucleus bearing the greatest share of the load.

Over time, age-related changes or an acute injury can lead to a breakdown in the normally smooth balance of load bearing. Histologic studies conducted in lumbar spine cadaver specimens reveal that as early as the second decade of life, a reduction in blood flow leads to diminished nutritional supply to the end plate. This in turn results in tissue breakdown within the disk, commencing in the NP and shortly thereafter, the vertebral end plates.[29] This progressive, macroscopic degeneration, in conjunction with either low-level repetitive stress or an acute traumatic event can lead to two possible sources of injury: a microfracture of the vertebral end plate or an annular tear from torsional overload.[48] When this occurs, the ability of the NP to evenly dissipate a compressive load becomes compromised. Unlike in normal disks, a compressive load in degenerated disks is not uniformly distributed. Instead, the preponderance of the weight-bearing burden is borne by the richly innervated AF.[46,47] Although this can be maintained for short periods, if the end plate fracture does not heal, the repetitive stress on the annulus can eventually lead to tearing of the fibers. These tears further decrease the load-bearing capacity of the disk because torn lamellae can no longer function as support apparatus. This initiates a vicious circle, causing even more stress on the remaining lamellae, leading to further tearing of the annular fibers, which can eventually result in the complete loss of annular integrity.[49] A denouement of this sequence of events is that the disk is now predisposed to nuclear herniation. The loss of disk height that inevitably ensues may then further deteriorate into continued narrowing of the disk, accompanied by the pathologic changes commonly seen in severe degenerative disk disease such as Modic changes, sclerosis of the end plates and bridging osteophytes[50,51] (Table 59–1). In severe cases, this manifests as autofusion and anklylosis of adjacent segments.[52]

Chemical Changes

Several changes may occur in degenerated disks whose end result is a decrease in the threshold of nociception. First, a break in an end plate can lead to the introduction of inflammatory cytokines into the nucleus, resulting in reduced oxygen diffusion, a rise in lactate levels, and a decrease in pH. This conglomeration of factors can result in a slowdown in metabolic and reparative processes, leading to increased degradative metalloproteinase activity and diminished chondrocyte activity, which in turn function to accelerate disk degradation.[25,53] In certain contexts, proinflammatory cytokines can be a direct source of pain. But in the context of a functional annulus, no pain should be experienced because the inflammatory mediators cannot reach the nociceptors present in the outer portion of the disk. However, when an annular tear develops, granulation tissue forms, through which nerve endings are able to extend through the annulus, sometimes penetrating as far centrally as the NP.[54] Thus in the presence of a compromised AF, chemical mediators are able to reach sensitized nerve endings, the by-product of which is LBP.[55]

The sensitization and irritation of nerve endings in the end plate may also result in pain.[49] This model of chemical nociception is supported by a multitude of studies showing disk immunoreactivity to a variety of substances including vasoactive intestinal polypeptide,[56] substance P and calcitonin gene-related peptide,[57,58] as well as elevated levels of nitric oxide,[53] prostaglandin E_2,[53,59] interleukin (IL)-2,[53] IL-6,[59] IL-8,[59] phospholipase A_2,[60-64] leukotriene B_4,[65] thromboxane B_2,[65] and tumor necrosis factor-alpha,[66,67] in diseased and herniated intervertebral disks.

Taken in concert, these factors provide a biochemical and mechanical rationale for performing discography. The generation of pain at low intradiskal pressures is best explained by a preponderance of inflammatory mediators around the sensitized disk; in medical terminology, this is referred to as "chemically sensitized" disks. When disk degeneration is less severe or the disruption less acute, the disk may react to stimulation only at higher pressures, at which point the nerve fibers of the degraded annulus are stretched to the point of pain induction. This scenario describes the "mechanically sensitized" disk. Perhaps an easier way to conceptualize these models is that a chemically sensitized disk is analogous to

Table 59–1. Modic Changes on Magnetic Resonance Imaging in Patients with Degenerative Disk Disease

CATEGORY OF SIGNAL INTENSITY CHANGE*	T1-WEIGHTED MRI	T2-WEIGHTED MRI	HISTOPATHOLOGIC CHANGES	SIGNIFICANCE AND COMMENTS
Type I	Decreased signal intensity	Unchanged or increased signal intensity	Disruption and fissuring of the end plate and vascularized fibrous tissue within the adjacent marrow	Changes signify edema. Type I changes tend to convert to type II changes over time.
Type II	Unchanged or increased signal intensity	Isointense or slightly hyperintense signal	End plate disruption with yellow marrow replacement in the adjacent vertebral body	Signifies fatty degeneration. This is the most common type, and tends to remain stable over time.
Type III	Decreased signal intensity	Decreased signal intensity	Extensive bony sclerosis, indicative of dense woven bone within the vertebral body rather than the marrow	No marrow to produce magnetic resonance imaging (MRI) signal

*Refers to signal intensity changes in the vertebral body marrow adjacent to the end plates of degenerative intervertebral disks.
Adapted from Modic MT, Masaryk TJ, Ross JS, et al: Imaging of degenerative disk disease. Radiology 1988;168:177-186.

the phenomenon of allodynia, whereas a mechanically sensitive disk is akin to hyperalgesia. In the latter stages of disk disease, the annulus may become functionally incompetent, in which case the injection of contrast may fail to generate intermediate to high pressures. This can result in an uninterpretable, or even false-negative pain response if manometry is not used. On CT imaging, severely degenerated disks are likely to show a diffuse pattern of contrast spread with extensive leakage into the epidural space, but small leaks are possible to miss using plain fluoroscopy. Normal disks resist pain provocation because they lack both the chemical hypersensitivity and mechanical overloading present in diseased disks. In clinical practice, these examples represent an ideal diagnostic paradigm that fails to account for the multitude of genetic, social, cultural, and psychological factors that affect pain perception. To optimize diagnosis and treatment outcomes, these factors must be considered when performing any pain-provoking procedure.

Lumbar Disk Pain Referral Patterns

The premise upon which discography is based is that controlled pressurization of a painful disk will reproduce a patient's symptoms. The limitations of this paradigm have been discussed previously. In addition to the flaws inherent with any provocative test, inaccuracies also may result from oversedation with anxiolytics or opioids, excessive administration of superficial anesthesia, anxiety, procedure-related pain, the ephemeral nature of disk pressurization, and the inability to distinguish concordant from noncordant pain in the fleeting moments when the disk pressure exceeds the nociceptive threshold. Nevertheless, several investigators have attempted to categorize the pain patterns for positive discograms. In a prospective study conducted in 187 LBP patients scheduled for diagnostic CT-discography, Ohnmeiss and colleagues found that L3-4 discograms were likely to be positive if patients described their pain as involving the lumbar region with radiation into the anterior but not posterior thigh, and often into the anterior leg.[68] For L4-5 disks, the most common pain referral pattern was lumbar pain involving more equivalent proportions of anterior and posterior thigh pain. In L5-S1 discogenic pain, the pain description generally encompassed the lumbar and posterior thigh regions, with fewer patients reporting anterior thigh or leg pain. Pain in the absence of disk pathology tended to be limited to the low back and buttocks (Fig. 59–2).

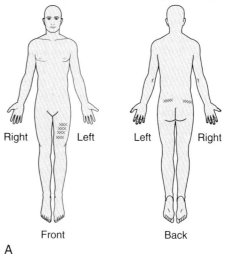

Pain referral pattern for L3-4 discogenic back pain

Right Left   Left Right

Front   Back

A

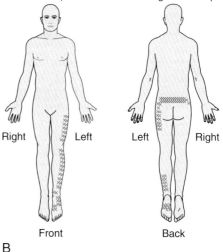

Pain referral pattern for L4-5 discogenic back pain

Right Left   Left Right

Front   Back

B

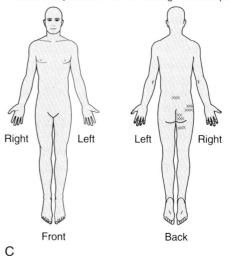

Pain referral pattern for L5-S1 discogenic back pain

Right Left   Left Right

Front   Back

C

Figure 59–2. A, Pain referral pattern for L3-4 discogenic back pain; **B,** pain referral pattern for L4-5 discogenic back pain; **C,** pain referral pattern for L5-S1 discogenic back pain. (Adapted from Ohnmeiss DD, Vanharanta H, Ekholm J. Relation between pain location and disk pathology: A study of pain drawings and CT/discography. Clin J Pain 1999;15:210-217.)

In the late 1980s, Vanharanta and colleagues performed a series of studies evaluating the effects various disk abnormalities have on pain referral patterns. In the first of these studies, the evaluation of CT-discograms in 91 patients showed a positive relationship between the occurrence of pain and the presence of annular ruptures.[69] The second study found that narrow disks were more likely to be associated with "exact pain reproduction" compared with disks of normal height.[70] In the same study, it was also suggested that the degree of pain concordance is influenced by spinal level. Specifically, severely degenerated L3-4 disks were less likely to result in concordant pain than comparable disks at the L4-5 and L5-S1 spinal levels. The third paper, a prospective multicenter study evaluating the results of 300 surgical candidates with a variety of clinical diagnoses, found no significant relationship between concordant pain provocation in the four diagnostic groups: disk herniation (82%), degenerative disk disease (81%), lumbar syndrome (56%), and radiculopathy (59%).[71] Disks that were deteriorated tended to be painful regardless of a patient's diagnostic classification. In the fourth study based partly on the same patient population, the authors found that the percentage of degenerated disks that elicited either "no pain" or "noncordant pain" was higher in older adult patients.[72] A later retrospective study by the same group of authors found that outer annular ruptures were the only predictors of concordant pain in a reanalysis of 833 discograms done in 306 LBP patients.[73]

Maezawa and Muro came to a different conclusion than Vanharanta and colleagues. In a retrospective analysis of 1477 discograms performed in 523 patients with axial or radicular LBP, the authors found the elicitation of pain was only weakly associated with IDD, whereas the presence of a herniated disk was strongly associated with pain provocation.[74] Saifuddin and coworkers performed a retrospective review of 260 lumbar discogram reports whose aim was to correlate morphologic disk abnormalities with pain referral patterns.[75] The authors demonstrated a highly significant association between annular tears and concordant back and radiating pain of any type. An association between isolated posterior tears and radiating pain also was found, but no relationship between anterior annular tears and any pain radiation was noted. No differences in pain referral patterns were identified when full-thickness and partial-thickness posterior tears were compared. There was an increased incidence of leg pain compared with groin, hip, or buttock pain during L4-5 and L5-S1 disk provocation, but this trend did not reach statistical significance. Finally, in a retrospective study by Slipman and colleagues, the authors found no correlation between the side of a patient's concordantly painful annular tear on CT discography and the side of their pain complaints.[76] To summarize these studies, the presence of degenerative changes of any type is more likely to be associated with pain than nondegenerated disks or disks with only minimal degradation. Pain provocation also may be more likely to occur in the presence of annular tears and nuclear herniations, with more evidence supporting the former assertion.

False-Positive Pain Provocation

In the past 30 years the use of discography for detecting disk pathology has been largely supplanted by more advanced radiologic studies such as MRI and CT scanning. The evidence that these newer modalities are not only safer, but also more accurate than plain discography in detecting herniated nuclear material is indisputable. In a prospective study by Jackson and colleagues comparing myelography, CT myelography, plain discography, and CT discography with surgical findings in 231 disks explored at surgery, the authors found CT discography to be the most accurate test (87%) and plain discography to be the least accurate (58%).[77] CT discography ranked highest in sensitivity for HNP (92%) compared with 78% for CT myelography, 72% for CT, 70% for myelography, and 81% for plain discography.[77] For specificity, CT discography was also the most accurate (81%), followed by CT (76%), CT myelography (76%), myelography (70%), and plain discography (31%).

Because discography is more invasive and unequivocally less sensitive in detecting most disk pathology than newer imaging techniques, the primary justification for its continued use lies in its ability to correlate pathology with symptoms. This rationale seems reasonable given the fact that close to two thirds of asymptomatic adults have abnormal findings on MRI scans of their lumbar spines, with the prevalence of these findings increasing with age.[78] LBP is an epidemic of unprecedented proportions in industrial societies, with the estimated lifetime prevalence ranging from 60% to more than 80%.[79,80] Without a corroborative test to validate these abnormal MRI findings, it is likely that many of these patients would be conferred with incorrect diagnoses, and subsequently undergo unnecessary surgical procedures. There is little doubt that unnecessary stabilization operations are performed far too frequently in the United States, but there is dissent as to whether discography prevents this from happening or facilitates it.[81] Proponents of discography believe that correlating pathology with symptoms prevents unnecessary surgical intervention, whereas opponents question both the significance of discographic pathology and the validity of provoked symptoms. These criticisms are bolstered by the relative lack of specificity of discography, the inherent difficulty in validating provoked symptomatology, the large number of studies showing false-positive pain provocation in patients without low back symptoms, and disparities compared with histologic findings on surgical specimens.

In phase I of a two-part experiment, Yasuma and associates studied 181 lower thoracic and lumbar disks discographically and histologically in 30 adult cadavers.[82] Their findings revealed 32 true-positive,

15 false-positive, 122 true-negative, and 12 false-negative discograms. Discograms were designated as false-positive when the injected contrast was noted to extend beyond the peripheral vertebral margin, but histologic sectioning of the disk was negative for protrusion. False-negatives were defined as a negative discogram despite a histologically confirmed disk protrusion. In the 32 true positive disks, both the discograms and histologic sections showed 10 anterior protrusions, 17 posterior protrusions, and 5 posterior herniations. Among the 15 false-positive discograms, 9 were misdiagnosed as a protrusion and 6 as a herniation. In part two of this study, the authors conducted a retrospective review of 77 discography patients subsequently found to have a herniated disk during surgical exploration.[82] The discograms were falsely interpreted as negative in 32% of the 59 patients with a protruding disk, and 56% of the 18 patients with a prolapse. In a previous study, the authors found that false-positive discograms were more likely to occur when fissures or cysts were present in a degenerated annulus, but did not establish continuity with the nuclear cavity.[83]

The first study to question the validity of discography was published in 1968 by Holt, who found false-positive results in 37% of 30 asymptomatic prisoners.[84] More than 20 years later, Walsh and colleagues performed CT discography in 10 asymptomatic male volunteers and 7 "control" patients with chronic LBP.[85] Sixty-five percent of the 20 disks injected in the back pain patients showed radiologic abnormalities, with all 7 patients having at least one degenerated disk. In the patients without back pain, CT discograms were interpreted as abnormal in 17% of the 35 disks injected and half of the 10 subjects. However, none of these 5 patients experienced concordant pain associated with pain-related behavior during the injections. Thus the false-positive rate in this study was zero.

In 1996, Block and associates conducted a landmark prospective study in 90 patients with low back and leg pain who underwent CT-discography at the three lowest lumbar levels.[86] Minnesota Multiphasic Personality Inventory (MMPI) was administered to each subject before discography, and scored independently. In the 72 patients with at least one nondisrupted disk, 34 reported discordant pain provocation at a normal level, with the remaining 38 patients reporting a "concordant negative response." In the 34 patients who reported pain during pressurization of normal disks, the mean hypochondriasis, hysteria, and depression scores were significantly higher than in patients for whom stimulation of normal disks did not elicit pain.

Between 1999 and 2000, Carragee and coworkers published a series of studies attempting to identify patients at high risk for false-positive discograms. In the first study, eight patients with no history of back problems or structural spinal abnormalities who had undergone recent iliac crest bone grafting for reasons unrelated to lumbar spine, hip, or pelvic pathology were studied with provocative discography of their 3 most caudal disks.[87] Four of the eight study subjects experienced severe LBP similar to the postoperative pain at their bone graft site during injection of at least one disk. All symptomatic disks had an abnormal morphologic appearance.

In the second study, the authors performed lumbar discography on 10 patients with neck and upper extremity pain but no lower back symptoms, 6 patients with somatization disorder, and 10 control patients devoid of pain symptoms.[88] The three most caudad lumbar disks were injected in all patients, with 5 patients having the L2-3 disk studied as well. Eighty-three percent of patients in the somatization group, 40% of the chronic cervical pain patients, and 10% of the control patients experienced moderate or severe pain during contrast injection in at least 1 disk. Pain was provoked in 11% of disks with intermediate grade disruptions and 37% of disks with annular tears. In contrast, none of the 31 radiographically normal disks were associated with pain during injection. In the last study, three-level discography was performed in 47 patients who had undergone a single-level diskectomy for sciatica.[89] Twenty subjects with no recurrent symptoms were designated as the "study" group, and 27 patients with persistent back or leg symptoms formed the "control" group. In the asymptomatic participants, positive injections occurred in 8 of 20 (40%) operated disks. In the control patients with symptoms, positive injections occurred in 17 of the 27 operative disks (63%), with the pain being concordant in 15. No significant differences were found in discography results between symptomatic and asymptomatic participants with normal psychometric scores. In contrast, patients with abnormal prediscography psychological test scores were more likely to rate their pain as unbearable during injection of both operative and nonoperative disks compared with patients in both groups with no psychopathology. All positive disks were radiographically abnormal.

There are several flaws in the studies assessing false-positive discograms in asymptomatic subjects, the main one being inherent in the study design: in subjects without preexisting LBP, one cannot provoke true concordant pain, which has become a hallmark of modern-day discography. The second major shortcoming is that although the Carragee studies used manometry to limit intradiskal pressures, pressure readings were not a determining factor in the designation of a positive disk. The guiding principle behind discography is the provocation of pain, but the application of excessive pressure to any bodily structure that contains nerves, including components of the spine besides disks,[15,16] will provoke pain in normal subjects.

In an effort to determine the effect objective pressure readings have on the incidence of positive disk injections in asymptomatic volunteers, Derby and colleagues performed 43 discograms in 13 subjects with either no history or infrequent episodes of LBP.[90] In the patients with occasional back pain, 35% of the 20 injected disks were painful, versus 52% in volunteers with no history of LBP. Most disks required high pressures before pain was elicited and even then, the pain was mild. There was no relationship between painful disk injections and MRI or discographic abnormalities. Controlling for the intensity of response and the pressures at which pain was elicited, the authors concluded the incidence of false-positive discograms was less than 10%. Some of the potential causes of false-positive discograms include inadvertent annular injection (Fig. 59–3),[118] contrast-induced irritation of nervous tissue, end plate deflection resulting from suboptimal needle placement, and stimulation of pressure receptors when excessively high pressures are generated.[91,92] Given the high propensity for false-positive findings in patients with previous back surgery, psychopathology, or somatization symptoms, positive discograms should be viewed with caution in these individuals. To optimize specificity, we suggest obtaining two adjacent control disks, a recommendation previously endorsed by Endres and Bogduk in an attempt to improve accuracy in patients at high risk for false-positive discography.[93] Although it may seem intuitive that this would enhance specificity or improve outcomes, these issues have yet to be addressed in the literature.

Prevalence of Discogenic Low Back Pain

Axial back pain is one of the most common yet challenging problems faced by pain physicians. Numerous structures besides degenerated disks can cause axial LBP; two of the more common ones are the lumbar facet joints and muscles. In a porcine study by Indahl and colleagues, the authors determined that there is significant overlap between the neuromuscular connections of the intervertebral disks, zygapophysial joints, and paraspinal muscles, such that the relative contributions to LBP of each of these structures may be difficult to estimate.[94] One may thus conclude that in many if not most patients with chronic LBP, the cause of pain is multifactorial.

The prevalence of discogenic LBP varies widely in medical literature. In one of the most cited studies, Schwarzer and associates found the incidence of discogenic pain to be 39% in 92 patients with chronic axial LBP and no focal neurologic findings or previous back surgery.[95] The authors based their diagnoses on exact pain reproduction during provocative disk stimulation, coupled with abnormal imaging on CT discography and the presence of an adjacent, negative control disk. Collins and coworkers conducted a prospective study comparing the use of MRI and discography in the evaluation of 29 patients with unremitting axial LBP without focal neurologic deficits.[96] The authors found exact reproduction of the patients' symptoms to be present in 13 disks in 12 patients, for a prevalence rate of 41%. In all 13 symptomatic disks, both MRI and discography showed degenerative changes. In another study comparing MRI and discography results, Horton and Daftari performed 63 discograms in 25 patients with nonradicular LBP.[97]

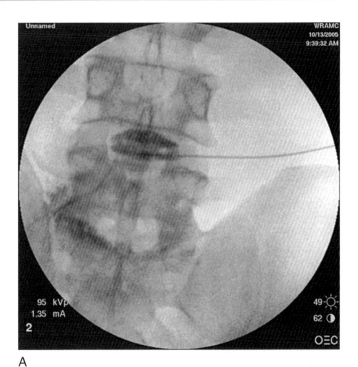

A

B

Figure 59–3. Anteroposterior (**A**) and lateral (**B**) fluoroscopic annulograms at L5-S1. **A,** Anteroposterior discogram showing annular injection at L5-S1. **B,** Lateral discogram showing annular injection at L5-S1.

Discography yielded moderate to severe pain at 26 levels, with 19 patients reporting similar or exact pain reproduction, for a prevalence rate of 76%. Only 1 of the 26 disks was morphologically normal. Finally, Long and associates conducted a very large epidemiologic study in 2374 patients with low back pain seen by spine surgeons at seven academic medical centers.[98] Final diagnoses were rendered after imaging studies were reviewed and treatment prescribed, and the ordered tests and therapies were performed at the discretion of the surgeon. Nonherniated degenerated disk was the concluding diagnosis in 6.1% of patients. Based on the conflicting evidence that does exist, discogenic LBP appears to be the major source of pain in approximately one third of patients with chronic LBP.

Correlation with Radiologic Studies

There is compelling evidence that discography, even without CT scanning, may overestimate the prevalence of clinically significant internal disk disruption, but it is equally clear that discography may fail to detect disk pathology seen with other radiologic studies. In a study by Gibson and associates comparing MRI and discography in the diagnosis of DDD, agreement between the two techniques was found in 44 of 50 disks studied.[99] In the six disks in which a discrepancy occurred, evidence of IDD was missed in five discograms and one MRI. In the five cases in which discography failed to detect disk pathology, two were a result of incorrect placement of the discography needle in the annulus, and failure to detect early signs of degeneration accounted for the other three. Although disk stimulation symptoms were recorded in the study, discography results were based only on radiographic findings.

Yoshida and coworkers sought to investigate the relationship between plain discography and T2-weighted and gadolinium-enhanced T1-weighted MRIs in 23 patients with chronic LBP.[100] A posterior annular tear was detected in 16 of the 17 positive disks using T2-weighted MRI and 10 of 14 positive disks using the gadolinium-enhanced T1 images. The T2 study also detected 11 annular tears in 39 negative disks versus 8 annular tears out of 32 negative disks for the T1- gadolinium study. The sensitivity, specificity, positive predictive value, and negative predictive value of the T2-weighted studies in detecting symptomatic disks were 94%, 71%, 59%, and 97%, respectively, which favorably compared with the T1-weighted images. The authors concluded that the high sensitivity and negative predictive value of T2 MRI make it a useful screening tool in avoiding unnecessary discography in chronic LBP patients.

Simmons and associates compared CT discography with MRI in 164 patients with chronic LBP, with or without radicular symptoms.[101] Correlation between the two techniques was seen in 55% of cases. In the 371 disks in which MRI and discography were concordant, 172 were normal and 199 abnormal. In the disks classified as abnormal based on MRI, 37% were asymptomatic during injection. In 13% ($n = 60$) of disks, MRIs were abnormal but discograms normal. In 7% of disks ($n = 34$), MRI showed normal and discography abnormal findings. In 21 of these 34 disks, injection of contrast into the disk elicited exact pain reproduction.

In a comparative study evaluating MRI and discography in patients with axial LBP, Collins and col-

leagues found that imaging characteristics for the two diagnostic procedures correlated in 65 of 73 disks.[96] In the other eight cases, four disk levels showed evidence of early degeneration on discography but appeared normal on MRI, whereas four disks showed decreased signal intensity on T2-weighted MRI but were discographically normal. In the 12 patients with concordant pain on discography, spinal fusion was performed. At their 9-month follow-up, 9 of 12 patients reported clinical improvement.

Aprill and Bogduk[102] performed CT discography on 41 patients with chronic LBP who demonstrated a high-intensity zone (HIZ) on T2-weighted MRI. In all patients, CT discography revealed either a grade 3 or 4 annular disruption in the affected disk. The sensitivity and specificity of an HIZ for detecting similar pain reproduction during disk provocation were 63% and 97%, respectively. For the detection of exact pain reproduction, the sensitivity was 82% and the specificity 89%. In the identification of a grade 4 annular disruption, the sensitivity of an HIZ was only 54%, but the specificity was 89% and the positive predictive value 90%.

Other studies have shown a much stronger correlation between MRI and discography. Linson and Crowe found the two investigative modalities to be in agreement in 91 of 97 disks studied in 50 patients.[103] In the six disks in which a discrepancy was present, five were read as normal by MRI but abnormal by discography. In an earlier study by Schneiderman and coworkers, MRI and discography positively correlated in 100 of 101 levels.[104] Overall, discography appears to be comparable or slightly more sensitive for the detection of IDD than MRI or CT scanning, especially with regard to radial annular fissures. Approximately 15% to 25% of degenerative disks on MRI will fail to provoke concordant pain on discography. The main problem with correlative studies is that when an incongruity exists, it is impossible to determine whether the discrepancy is from a lack of sensitivity (false-negatives) or specificity (false-positives) in one of the diagnostic procedures (Table 59–2).

Effect on Outcomes from Spinal Fusion

The value of spine surgery to treat DDD and axial LBP is a subject that has engendered passionate controversy in the medical and lay literature. Whereas operative results for spinal arthrodesis vary greatly depending on the success criteria and follow-up period, they are widely acknowledged to be less beneficial than surgery for radicular pain, with success rates ranging from less than 50% to more than 80%.[119-121] Moreover, these reported outcomes must be considered in light of the fact that no fusion studies have ever been conducted under controlled conditions. A recent Cochrane Database Review concluded there was no scientific evidence supporting any form of surgical decompression or fusion in the treatment of DDD,[122] and the few randomized, uncontrolled studies comparing spinal fusion to

Table 59–2. Studies Comparing Lumbar Discography with CT Scanning or Magnetic Resonance Imaging in Patients with Degenerative Disk Disease

AUTHOR, YEAR	NUMBER OF SUBJECTS	NATURE OF STUDY	RESULTS	COMMENTS
Gibson et al, 1986[99]	22 patients, 50 disks	Compared MRI and discography in patients with mechanical LBP	Agreement between studies in 44 of 50 disks	Discography results based on radiographic findings only as patients were sedated. In the 6 disks that didn't correlate, MRI was superior to discography.
Schneiderman et al, 1987[104]	36 patients with LBP, with or without leg pain, 101 discograms	Compared MRI and discography	MRI accurate in assessing disk morphology in 100 of 101 levels. Of 52 disks with normal MRI, only 1 had positive discogram. Of 49 disks with MRI signal, only 2 discograms normal.	Used only T2-weighted MRI. CT discography used on 39 levels.
Zucherman et al, 1988[105]	18 patients with LBP with or without radicular symptoms	Clinical case series. In most cases discography was followed by CT scanning.	All patients had normal MRI and abnormal discograms	Normal MRI and abnormal discograms were basis for inclusion
Yu et al, 1989[106]	8 cadavers, 36 disks	Compared MRI and discography against cryomicrotomy anatomic sectioning for detecting annular tears	Discography identified 15 radial fissures, 10 of which were seen on MRI. Two of the 15 annular fissures were missed on cryomicrotomy.	Included a newborn and 2-year-old. Considered only radial tears of annulus. Could not correlate findings with symptoms.
Bernard, 1990[107]	250 patients (725 disks) with chronic LBP who underwent CT discography	Retrospective study comparing accuracy of MRI, intrathecally enhanced or nonenhanced CT scan, or plain x-rays with CT discography. MRI was done before discography in 67 pts (190 disks).	A normal T2-weighted MRI correctly predicted 64 normal disks by CT discography, and incorrectly predicted 12 normal disks that were abnormal by CT discography. In 105 disks, abnormal T2 MRI correctly predicted abnormal disks by CT discography; 9 disks that were normal by CT discography had decreased signal intensity on T2-weighted MRI. Correlation between MRI and CT discography was 89%.	CT discography provided additional information affecting patient management in 93% of cases. In 94% of the 180 operations, CT discography correctly predicted the type of disk herniation.
Collins et al, 1990[96]	29 patients, 73 discograms	Compared MRI and discography in patients with axial LBP	57 disks were abnormal on discography, with 13 producing concordant pain in 12 patients. Discography findings correlated with MRI in 90% of cases; 4 disks showed degeneration on discography with normal MRI, and 4 had abnormal MRI with normal discography.	The 12 patients with positive discograms underwent spinal fusion, with 9 reporting clinical improvement at 9-month follow-up.
Linson and Crowe, 1990[103]	50 patients, 97 disks	Compared MRI and discography in patients with chronic LBP	91% correlation for disk degeneration between MRI and discography	5 of the 6 disks with negative correlation were read as normal by MRI and abnormal by discography. No mention of control disks during discography.
Simmons et al, 1991[101]	164 patients, 371 disks	Compared CT discography and MRI in patients with chronic LBP with or without radiculopathy	55% correlation based on patients; 80% based on disks	MRI normal and discogram abnormal in 34 disks. Discogram normal and MRI abnormal in 60 disks. 37% of disks abnormal on MRI were asymptomatic on discography. Do not include outcomes in 76 patients who underwent surgery.

Study	Patients/Disks	Description	Findings	Comments
Birney et al, 1992[108]	90 patients, 264 disks	Examined correlation between MRI and discography for DDD and HNP. Compared surgical findings with discography in 57 patients.	Agreement between MRI and discography in 86% of disks. MRI more accurate for DDD and slightly superior to MRI for HNP; discography slightly superior to MRI for DDD (MRI missed 1 disk, discography 100% sensitive)	Considered patients with LBP and radicular pain. Surgical findings correlated with diagnostic studies at 63 of 76 levels.
Osti and Fraser, 1992[109]	33 patients, 114 disks	Compared MRI and discography in patients with LBP	All 54 disks identified as abnormal on MRI showed abnormal discogram patterns; 6 of the 60 disks identified as normal on MRI were abnormal on discography. Of the 39 disks that provoked concordant pain on discography, 27 were abnormal on MRI; 33 of the 39 asymptomatic disks by discography had normal MRI signals, with 24 having normal discographic patterns.	Six of 46 disks classified as degenerate on MRI were asymptomatic at discography. Concluded discography is more accurate than MRI for detecting annular pathology. Patient population not well defined.
Aprill and Bogduk, 1992[102]	41 patients (105 disks) with chronic LBP with or w/o radicular symptoms.	Compared HIZ on T2-weighted MRI with CT discography.	In all patients who exhibited an HIZ on MRI, CT discography revealed either a grade 3 or 4 annular disruption. A grade 3 or 4 disruption was also present in 34 patients without an HIZ.	Concordant pain provocation with discography was present in 38 of 40 HIZ disks, and 22 of 78 disks without an HIZ. CT discography performed in only 41 out of 500 patients in whom MRI was examined.
Horton and Daftari, 1992[97]	25 patients with nonradicular LBP, involving 63 discograms	Comparative study between MRI and discography for discogenic LBP	19 patients had positive discograms. Of the different MRI patterns, only "dark/torn," "dark/bulged," or "speckled/flat" were more likely to be positive rather than negative discograms.	MRI findings classified by pattern, not presence or absence of pathology
Brightbill et al, 1994[6]	7 patients with LBP	Clinical case series involving patients with discrepancy between discography and MRI who underwent surgery and were found to have internal disk disruption	All 7 subjects had normal MR imaging and positive discography.	Did not consider surgical outcomes
Loneragan et al, 1994[110]	18 patients with chronic LBP thought to be discogenic (43 disks).	Compared MRI and CT discography in the diagnosis of DDD and HNP	MRI missed 3 of 10 disks with early degenerative changes, and 1 of 3 herniations	In no cases did MRI offer more information than CT discography.
Schellhas et al, 1996[111]	63 patients, 100 disks with HIZ on T2 MRI in pts with LBP and/or radicular pain	Retrospective analysis analyzing the significance of HIZ zones in predicting positive discography	All 100 disks with HIZ were discographically abnormal, with 87 showing concordant pain. In 17 asymptomatic control patients, MRI scans revealed only 1 HIZ disk.	37 patients had prior back surgery. Also included patients with radiculopathy.
Braithwaite et al, 1998[112]	58 patients with chronic, nonradicular LBP	Retrospective study comparing vertebral end plate changes on MRI with pain provocation during discography in 152 disks	Among 91 disks with degeneration on MRI, 78 elicited pain vs. only 12 of 61 disks without MRI degeneration. Among the 26 disks with vertebral end plate changes on MRI, 24 were painful during discography vs. 69 of 129 disks without end plate changes.	MRI revealed disk degeneration at 128 of 290 levels, and end plate changes were identified at 31 levels. All patients were being investigated for discogenic LBP as a precursor to spinal fusion; 138 disks evaluated by MRI were not injected.

Table 59–2. Studies Comparing Lumbar Discography with CT Scanning or Magnetic Resonance Imaging in Patients with Degenerative Disk Disease—cont'd

AUTHOR, YEAR	NUMBER OF SUBJECTS	NATURE OF STUDY	RESULTS	COMMENTS
Saifuddin et al, 1998[113]	58 patients (152 disks) with chronic, nonradicular LBP	Retrospective study determining the sensitivity of T2-weighted MRI in detecting painful posterior annular tears	There were 86 annular tears on discography, 54 of which were posterior and 26 that were anterior and posterior. The sensitivity, specificity, positive and negative predictive value of MRI in diagnosing concordantly painful posterior annular tears were 27%, 95%, 89%, and 47%, respectively.	Study evaluated the same patients as the Braithwaite study
Milette et al, 1999[114]	45 patients, 132 disks	Evaluated MRI and discography results in patients with chronic LBP	On MRI, 71% of disks showed normal contour, and 64% normal signal intensity. Only 40% of discograms were radiographically normal. Discography demonstrated stage 2 and 3 disk disruptions in 26% of disks w/normal contour on MRI, and 13% of disks with both normal contour and signal.	Used only T2-weighted MRI. Study was designed to assess differences between disk protrusions, bulges and loss of signal intensity on MRI, not to compare imaging studies.
Sandhu et al, 2000[115]	53 patients with LBP, 133 discograms	Retrospective analysis comparing discography with vertebral end plate signal changes on MRI	No significant correlation between discography and end plate signal changes.	41% of disks with positive end plate changes were positive discograms vs. 27% without. Among positive discograms, only 23% exhibited T2-weighted MRI end plate changes.
Yoshida et al, 2002[100]	23 patients, 56 disks	Examined correlation between MR images and pain response on discography	Sensitivity, specificity, positive predictive value, and negative predictive value of T2-MRI were 94%, 71%, 59%, and 97%, respectively	Did not specifically compare discography and MRI. T2-weighted MRI superior to gadolinium-enhanced images.
Kakitsubata et al, 2003[116]	24 disks from 5 cadavers	Compared MRI and MRI discography with anatomic correlation for detecting annular tears	Sensitivity of MR discography was 100%, 57%, and 21% for radial, transverse, and concentric tears in annulus, respectively vs. 67%, 71%, and 21% for conventional MRI	Could not correlate findings with symptoms
Lim et al, 2005[117]	66 patients with chronic LBP and no neural compression	Retrospective study comparing T1- and T2-weighted MRI findings with CT discography results (97 disks)	Concordant pain was more common with grade 4 or 5 degeneration on MRI, in disks with HIZ, and when the disk was fissured and ruptured on CT discography or contrast spread into or beyond the outer annulus	Concordant pain was not associated with decreased disk height, end plate abnormalities or facet joint arthritis

"Discography" refers to discograms performed without CT scanning.
CT, computed tomography; DDD, degenerative disk disease; HIZ, high intensity zone on MR; HN, herniated nucleus pulposus; IDD, internal disk disruption; LBP, low back pain; MRI, magnetic resonance imaging.
Adapted and updated from Cohen SP, Larkin TM, Barna SA, et al: Lumbar discography: A comprehensive review of outcome studies, diagnostic accuracy, and principles. Reg Anesth Pain Med 2005;30:163-183.

rehabilitation have been mixed.[121,123] The presence of concomitant pain sources in most patients with discogenic pain, along with the mixed clinical outcomes even when arthrodesis is technically successful,[121-123] are factors that must be considered when evaluating clinical studies examining the correlation between discography results and surgical outcomes.

Several investigators have attempted to correlate discography results with surgical findings and outcomes. Colhoun and colleagues evaluated surgical outcomes in 162 patients who underwent preoperative discography for axial LBP.[8] In the 137 patients with concordant pain on discography, 89% had a favorable outcome at the mean follow-up period of 3.6 years. In the 25 patients whose disks showed morphologic abnormalities but elicited no provocation of symptoms, only 52% reported significant benefit. Discography in this study was not accompanied by manometry, and the surgical treatments evaluated were mostly spinal fusions.

Esses and coworkers conducted a prospective study examining the role of external spinal fixation in predicting the success of spinal fusion in patients with chronic LBP.[124] Thirty-two of the 35 subjects underwent provocative discography prior to fixator placement. Of the 21 patients whose discography showed radiographically degenerated disks, 17 experienced complete or significant pain relief with the external fixator. In the 13 patients for whom results were available, 9 went on to obtain significant relief after spinal fusion.

In the 11 patients with normal-appearing disks, 8 experienced complete or significant relief with spinal fixation, with 6 of the 8 deriving clinical benefit from arthrodesis. Among the 15 patients with concordant pain on discography, 13 obtained either complete or significant relief after external spinal fixation. In the 10 patients who then proceeded to fusion, 6 obtained either complete or significant relief. Among the 17 patients with nonconcordant or no pain on discography, 12 experienced complete or significant relief following fixator placement. In the 12 patients in this group who went on to definitive surgery, 9 achieved either complete or significant pain relief. The follow-up period following posterior spinal fusion is not mentioned in the manuscript. Although determining the predictive value of discography on surgical success was not the main purpose of this study, the outcomes reported do not support a positive relationship between the results of discography and therapeutic response.

Madan and associates conducted a retrospective analysis aimed at determining the predictive value of provocative discography on surgical outcomes in 73 patients with chronic LBP.[10] The first 41 patients in this series underwent circumferential arthrodesis without preoperative discography, with the last 32 patients receiving surgery only if their pain was reproduced during disk provocation. In the discography group, 75.6% of patients had satisfactory outcomes at a minimum 2-year follow-up versus 81.2% in the group who did not undergo preoperative dis-

cography. Manometry readings were not considered as a criterion in the interpretation of discography results, and treatment outcomes were based on a modified Oswestry scoring system. In summary, the lack of strong evidence for the use of fusion to treat DDD,[121,122] and the methodologic flaws in the existing studies make the interpretation of data exceedingly difficult. For the existing data, the results are conflicting as to whether preoperative discography improves fusion outcomes in discogenic LBP patients. The results of studies evaluating discography as a predictive tool for surgery are presented in Table 59–3.

Correlation with Intradiskal Electrothermal Therapy and Disk Replacement Surgical Outcomes

The advent of new therapies for discogenic LBP such as intradiskal electrothermal therapy (IDET) and total disk replacement surgery has recently generated profound interest in the medical community. As a percutaneous, minimally invasive treatment for discogenic pain, the reported outcomes for IDET vary widely, ranging from minimal benefit[132] to almost 80% success rates.[133] Among the two published placebo-controlled studies, one reported significant improvement in both pain and disability scores[134] whereas the other failed to show a statistically significant difference compared to sham IDET.[135] Overall, the majority of studies report improvement rates in the 50% range in carefully chosen candidates.[136,137] Because all published studies have used preprocedure discography as a screening test for IDET candidates, it is not possible to determine the effect discography has on outcomes.

There have been numerous attempts dating back to the 1950s to design implants aimed at the functional reconstruction of a spinal segment. The concept of disk arthroplasty was first put into clinical use in 1966 by Fernstrom, who described using a stainless steel ball as a vertebral spacer to restore lost disk height and preserve motion.[138] Disk replacement surgery has been used in Europe as a treatment for DDD since the 1980s, but has only been approved in the United States since 2004 for single-level DDD. The reported success rates in these studies vary from around 50% to more than 80% improvement in medium-term follow-up (Table 59–4).

The studies evaluating disk replacement surgery are almost equally divided between those that have routinely used preoperative discography as a screening test and those that have not.[139-157] Unfortunately, methodologic flaws in these uncontrolled studies, wide variability in outcome criteria, and the absence of any direct comparisons between patients who underwent preoperative discography and those who did not, preclude any meaningful conclusions from being drawn. Taken in this limited context, the use of prediscography screening before disk replacement surgery does not seem to improve outcomes compared with choosing patients based solely on MRI and clinical presentation.

Table 59-3. Clinical Studies Evaluating the Effect of Preoperative Discography on Lumbar Spinal Arthrodesis Outcomes

STUDY, YEAR	NUMBER OF PATIENTS	TYPE OF STUDY	RESULTS	COMMENTS
Kostuik, 1979[125]	350 patients with painful scoliosis who underwent spinal instrumentation	Retrospective study	Preoperative discography improved success rate from 65%-70% to 85%	Used L5-S1 discography to determine whether anterior or posterior instrumentation should be used
Blumenthal et al, 1988[126]	34 patients with internal disk disruption at level 1 confirmed. All patients had normal CT scans, myelograms, and electromyograms.	Not indicated	Clinical success rate 74%. The successful fusion rate was 73% by plain x-ray, with an average time to union of 12 months. Fusion rate was higher in nonsmokers.	Success defined by the patient returning to work or resuming normal activities, and requiring no medications or only an anti-inflammatory drug Mean follow-up 3.6 years
Colhoun et al, 1988[8]	162 patients with axial LBP	Prospective observational study	Of 137 patients in whom discogram revealed DDD and provoked concordant pain, 89% had favorable outcome. Only 52% of those patients in whom discography showed DDD but provoked no pain had a favorable outcome.	
Esses et al, 1989[124]	35 patients with chronic LBP and FBSS who underwent ESF before arthrodesis	Prospective study evaluating effect of ESF prior to spinal fusion; 32 patients also underwent preop discography	Among the 15 patients with concordant pain on discography, 13 experienced significant or complete pain relief with ESF; 6 of these 10 patients had significant relief after arthrodesis	Study not designed to evaluate predictive value of discography on surgical success. Not all patients underwent preop discography.
Gill and Blumenthal, 1992[127]	53 patients with predominantly axial LBP and IDD at L5-S1.	Retrospective study involving L5-S1 fusion	50% of patients with type I discogram and normal MRI scans improved vs. 75% of patients with types II or III discogram and abnormal MRI.* Poor results in all 5 patients with level-2 fusions. In single-level fusions, 35% of pts had good results, 18% fair, and 47% poor outcomes.	Abnormal discogram was the basis for surgery. Average follow-up was 20 months.
Knox and Chapman, 1993[128]	22 patients who underwent anterior spinal fusion for discogram-concordant LBP	Retrospective study		Strong correlation between subjective (clinical improvement) and objective (fusion success) results CT discography used in all but 1 patient. Not all patients had a control disk (26 patients had single-level discography).
Wetzel et al, 1994[11]	48 patients with axial LBP who underwent lumbar arthrodesis following provocative discography	Retrospective study	At first follow-up (mean 5.3 wk), 66% had satisfactory outcome. At final follow-up (mean 35 months), 46% had satisfactory outcome.	
Parker et al, 1996[129]	23 patients with mechanical LBP and positive discography	Prospective case series involving spinal fusion and/or instrumentation	39% of patients reported good outcomes, 13% fair outcomes, and 48% had poor results	Abnormal discogram was basis for surgery. Mean follow-up was 47 months.
Vamvanij et al, 1998[130]	56 patients with discogenic LBP confirmed by CT discography who underwent 1 of 4 fusion techniques	Not indicated	Overall rate of patient satisfaction 46%	Success rate for patients who had anterior lumbar fusion with cage and facet fusion 63%. Success rates for the other 3 groups ranged from 36% to 46%.
Derby et al, 1999[131]	96 patients who underwent discography for LBP	Retrospective study	In patients with chemically sensitized disks (≥6/10 concordant pain at <15 psi more than opening pressure, $n = 36$), success rates were 89% for interbody/combined fusion, 20% for posterior intertransverse fusion and, 12% for no surgical therapy.	Mean follow-up for surgical patients was 28 months. No difference between outcomes for interbody/combined fusion and posterior intertransverse fusion for surgical sample as a whole.
Madan et al, 2002[10]	41 patients who underwent spinal arthrodesis without preop discography and 32 patients who underwent surgery based on positive discography	Not indicated	81% of patients who had surgery based on MRI and clinical findings had satisfactory outcome vs. 76% of patients who underwent arthrodesis based on positive discogram	Mean follow-up was 2.4 years in discography group and 2.8 years in MRI/clinical group

*Type I discogram designated as internal disk disruption without extravasation of contrast associated with concordant pain reproduction. Types II and III denote the presence of annular disruption with spread of contrast to the periphery and epidural space, respectively.
CT, computed tomography; DDD, degenerative disk disease; ESF, external spinal fixator; FBSS, failed back surgery syndrome; IDD, internal disk disruption; LB, low back pain; psi, pounds per square inch. Adapted and updated from Cohen SP, Larkin TM, Barna SA, et al: Lumbar discography: A comprehensive review of outcome studies, diagnostic accuracy, and principles. Reg Anesth Pain Med 2005;30:163-183.

Table 59-4. Summary of Outcome Data for Lumbar Disk Replacement Surgery Based on Preoperative Discography Screening*

STUDY, YEAR	PREOPERATIVE DISCOGRAPHY?	NUMBER OF DISK REPLACEMENT PATIENTS	TYPE OF SURGERY	OUTCOMES
Enker et al, 1993[139]	Yes	6	TDR	4 of 6 patients had satisfactory results (1 excellent, 2 good, 1 fair).
Zeegers et al, 1999[140]	In 36 of 50 patients	50	TDR	32 of 46 patients followed for 2 years had a positive clinical result. Do not provide separate data for patients having discography.
Bertagnoli and Kumar, 2002[141]	No	108	TDR	Results "excellent" in 91%, "good" in 7%, "fair" in 2%, and poor in no (0%) patients at 3-month to 2-year follow-up.
Hochshuler et al, 2002[142]	Yes	56	TDR	52.7% improvement in mean VAS scores at 6-week follow-up. In the 22 patients followed for ≥1 year, improvements in VAS and Oswestry Disability Index (ODI) scores were maintained.
Mayer et al, 2002[143]	No	34	TDR	Mean VAS score decreased from 6.3 preop to 3.4 at 1-year follow-up (not all patients followed for 1 year); 61% of patients "completely" satisfied, and 22% "satisfied."
Delmarter et al, 2003[144]	Not routinely	35	TDR	Mean VAS score decreased from 7.4 to 4.4, and ODI from 31 to 15 at 6-month follow-up. There were no significant differences between the patients who received TDR and the 18 randomized to fusion.
Blumenthal et al, 2003[145]	Yes	57	TDR	63% of patients improved at 2-year follow-up (based on >20 patients improvement on VAS score).
Shim et al, 2003[146]	In patients with DDD at more than 1 level	46	PDR	Mean VAS score 8.5 preop, 3.1 at 1-year follow-up; 11% had excellent and 67% good results.
Van Ooij et al, 2003[147]	Yes	27	TDR	Good outcome obtained in 12 to 26 patients, with variable follow-up period (range 1 month-10 years).
Tropiano et al, 2003[148]	No	53	TDR	87% of patients "entirely satisfied." Mean ODI 56 preop, 14 at last follow-up (mean 1.4 years).
McAfe et al, 2003[149]	Yes	41	TDR	Mean VAS score 73.5 preoperatively, and 30.4 at 1-3 years' follow-up.
Kim et al, 2003[150]	Not mentioned except for negative discogram being a contraindication	11 patients with juxtafusional DDD	TDR	Of the 5 patients followed for >6 months, mean ODI decreased from 64% to 24%.
Jin et al, 2003[151]	No	45	PDR	Mean ODI decreased from 52.2% to 16.5% in the 30 patients seen at their 6-month follow-up; 87% of patients were clinically improved.
Zigler et al, 2003[152]	Not routinely	28	TDR	Decrease in VAS score from approximately 7.8 to 5.6 after 6 months.
Guyer et al, 2004[153]	Yes	100	TDR	Mean ODI score decreased from 71 to 30 at 2-year follow-up vs. from 70 to 28 in 44 patients who received anterior interbody fusion.
Lemaire et al, 2005[154]	Yes	107	TDR	62% of patients had excellent results (≥70% resumption of activity), 28% had good results (>60% and ≤70%), and 10% poor outcomes at mean follow-up of 11.3 years.
Blumenthal et al, 2005[155]	Yes	205	Total	Mean reduction in VAS pain score 42.4% and mean reduction in ODI 48.5% at 24-month follow-up; 71.3% were satisfied. Study was designed to compared disk replacement with lumbar fusion.
Cakir et al, 2005[156]	Yes	29	TDR	VAS pain score decreased from a mean of 67 to 22 in 25 patients with physiologic segmental lordosis and from 71 to 23 in those with nonphysiologic lordosis. Minimum follow-up, 12 months. Study was not designed to measure outcomes. Main finding was that although total lumbar lordosis did not change significantly, segmental lordosis usually increased.
Tropiano et al, 2005[157]	No	55	TDR	60% of patients had excellent (>70% improvement) outcomes, 15% (60%-70%) good outcomes, and 25% a poor result. Mean follow-up, 8.7 years.

*Note: Table does not include studies lacking information about patient selection criteria.
DDD, degenerative disk disease; PDR, partial disk replacement; TDR, total disk replacement; VAS, Visual Analogue Scale.
Adapted and updated from Cohen SP, Larkin TM, Barna SA, et al: Lumbar discography: A comprehensive review of outcome studies, diagnostic accuracy, and principles. Reg Anesth Pain Med 2005;30:163-183.

Discography versus Bony Vibration Test

The main argument for discography is that it is the only available test that correlates symptoms with pathology.[158,159] In an attempt to find a less invasive replacement for discography, Yrjama and Vanharanta devised the bony vibration test (BVT), whereby a blunt, vibrating object such as the shaft of an electric toothbrush is compressed against the skin overlying successive spinous processes in order to provoke pain. In the pilot study conducted in 57 patients with LBP, the authors found the sensitivity and specificity of BVT to be 0.71 and 0.63, respectively, compared with provocative discography.[160] When patients with failed back surgery syndrome (FBSS) and painful disk herniations were excluded (n = 40), the sensitivity increased to 0.96 and the specificity to 0.72. The difference in accuracy resulted from the finding that prolapsed lumbar disks that provoked pain during discography were almost always painless during vibration testing. In two follow-up studies comparing BVT findings with MRI and CT discography, the authors found similarly high sensitivities and specificities when patients with previously operated backs and complete annular tears were excluded.[161,162]

In an attempt to combine vibration provocation with noninvasive imaging capability, Yrjama and colleagues added ultrasonic disk imaging to vibratory stimulation in the evaluation of 38 patients with chronic LBP.[163] In the 26 patients in whom pain was provoked during discography, BVT was painful in 17; in the 12 negative discographies, BVT was painless in 7. However, in the 14 patients in whom annular fissures were present, the combination of ultrasound and vibration testing yielded only 1 "false-positive" and 1 "false-negative" result in comparison with discography. To date, the findings of Yrjama and colleagues have yet to be replicated by other authors, and no studies exist correlating vibration provocation with surgical outcomes. Until these studies are conducted, it is unlikely BVT will supplant discography as a diagnostic tool for discogenic LBP.

Standardization of Discography

Several important variables should be assessed during discographic examination, including the volume of contrast injected, the degree and pattern of pain provocation, morphologic changes in the disk, and the pressure at which pain is elicited. One criticism of discography is that except for the volume injected and radiologic findings, all other parameters depend on the pain response of the patient. However, pain is always subjective, and what one person considers painful may be innocuous in another. In an attempt to standardize discography, several investigators have sought to objectify the criteria for a positive discography. In their prospective studies in asymptomatic patients, both Walsh and coworkers[85] and Carragee and associates[89] used a 0-to-5 pain-related behavior scale that was subsequently correlated with pain intensity and disk morphology. In the Walsh study,

disparities between reported pain and pain-related behavior occurred in 6 of 51 disks, with all cases involving patients reporting significant pain (>3/5) in the absence of corresponding pain behavior (<2/5 actions). In the three combined Carragee studies, the agreement between pain behavior and numerical pain score was greater than 90%. Both investigators videotaped the pain response for further review.

Stojanovic and colleagues performed a prospective analysis of discography-associated heart rate changes in 26 patients and 75 discograms.[164] The authors found that positive discograms were associated with greater heart rate changes than discograms that elicited no pain or nonconcordant pain, with all positive disks exhibiting pathologic radiographic changes. When more than 5 beats/minute increase from baseline was used as the cutoff value, the sensitivity of heart rate response was 85% and the specificity 100%. The rationale for the use of heart rate changes and pain behavior to validate reported pain response is based on numerous studies showing both variables to be valid indicators of pain perception.[165]

The problem with the use of secondary variables to corroborate discography interpretation is that although they may be useful in identifying the small subset of patients in whom secondary gain issues and extensive psychological overlay contribute to self-reported pain scores, their effects in treatment outcomes remain unknown.

Although numerous investigators have used manometry during disk stimulation, the use of discrete cutoff values for pressures that should and should not provoke pain have been surprisingly scarce. In 1999, Derby and coworkers introduced a three-tiered system whereby concordant pain greater than 6/10 in severity at less than 15 pounds per square inch (psi) above opening pressure was designated to be a chemically sensitized disk, concordant pain greater than 6/10 in intensity at between 15 and 50 psi above opening pressure was considered a mechanically sensitive disk, and concordant pain between 51 and 90 psi was termed indeterminate or normal[131] (Box 59-1). In a retrospective analysis, intermediate-term (mean 16 months) outcomes were assessed in 96 patients who were treated either conservatively or with spinal fusion. No differences in outcomes were found between patients who underwent interbody or combined fusions and those who received intertransverse fusions across the entire sample. However subgroup analysis found that patients with chemically sensitized disks who underwent interbody or combined fusions experienced better outcomes than those who underwent intertransverse fusions. One serious flaw in this diagnostic scheme is that it does not control for baseline pain differences between patients. Thus a discogram that provokes 5/10 in a patient with incapacitating 4/10 baseline pain would be considered negative, whereas a discogram that provokes 6/10 pain in a patient with 10/10 baseline pain would be positive. A second problem is that significant numerical differences may exist between manometric systems, so that a scale

BOX 59–1. DATA COLLECTION FOR DISCOGRAPHY

- Technical success of the procedure (are the needles properly positioned?)
- The pressure observed when contrast is first visible in the disk (opening pressure)
- The pressure at which pain is first noted
- The amount of contrast injected (maximum volume)
- The maximum pressure noted (peak pressure)
- Injection end point (reason injection was stopped)
  - High-pressure end point (firm)
  - Low-pressure end point
  - Volume end point
  - Pain end point
- The pattern of contrast distribution (e.g., diffuse, fissuring, extravasation into the epidural space)
- The pain response. Where does it hurt? Is it identical, similar, or different in location and character from your typical pain? On a 0 to 10 scale how do you rate the intensity?
- The presence of control disks. If none is obtained, the procedure is nondiagnostic.

developed for one system may not be valid when used in a different system.

Performing Discography

Patient Preparation

A detailed history and physical should be performed prior to the procedure even when the patient is being referred by another specialist for preoperative testing. It is the responsibility of the discographer to review all pertinent information including preprocedural laboratory tests, electromyography and nerve conduction study results, plain films, and MRIs. It may be helpful to record a description of the pain symptoms or create a pain diagram for reference during the procedure. Although discographers report their final diagnostic conclusions, it is the patient who ultimately communicates provoked symptoms and degree of concordance with typical pain. The patient who has a difficult time describing the typical pain syndrome may have an equally difficult time describing provoked symptoms. The indications for discography have previously been outlined in numerous guidelines and reviews[93,107,159,166-175] and include the following:

1. Evaluation of patients with unremitting spinal pain, with or without extremity pain, of greater than 4 months' duration that has been unresponsive to appropriate conservative therapy.
2. Patients with severe, persistent symptoms in whom other diagnostic tests have failed to reveal clear confirmation of a suspected disk as the source of pain.
3. Evaluation of persistent pain in the postsurgical patient whose symptoms may be arising from intervertebral disk degeneration, recurrent herniation, or pseudarthrosis of a spinal fusion.
4. To determine the number of levels to be fused in spinal surgery or determination of the primary symptomatic disk level.
5. To determine whether adjacent levels to a planned spinal arthrodesis are either normal or painful.
6. To diagnose lateral disk herniations.
7. If the patient prima facie satisfies the criteria for treatment by intradiskal electrothermal therapy, in which case pain is provoked to detect discogenic pain. In these cases, CT discography may be undertaken to assess disk morphology to determine whether an IDET electrode can be navigated in the disk and if so, where it should be placed.
8. For assessment of minimally invasive surgical candidates to confirm contained disk herniations, or to investigate dye distribution before chemonucleolysis or other percutaneous decompression procedures.

At our institutions, before the start of the procedure we review the MRI for levels demonstrating decreased signal intensity on T2-weighted images, increased signal consistent with a high-intensity zone, decreased disk height, or other evidence of degeneration with the idea that we will likely inject all abnormal levels. This notion is supported by studies that show that although MRI is sensitive for identifying disk pathology, it is less accurate in detecting the pattern of disk morphology.[99,104]

Current International Spinal Injection Society (ISIS) guidelines recommend that two control levels be obtained for optimal interpretation of disk stimulation.[93] However, many authors do not adhere to these stringent guidelines.[107,159,176] At our institutions, we consider one adjacent, unequivocal negative disk adequate for control purposes. For the most commonly symptomatic L5-S1 disk, only one adjacent control disk is possible.

Preparation of the patient for disk stimulation begins with the visit prior to discography. It is during this time that the patient is briefed on what to expect during the procedure. Patients must realize that discography is performed for diagnostic information rather than direct therapeutic benefit. Some patients may be surprised to learn that the short-term goal of discography is pain provocation rather than analgesia. They should be familiar with the use of the pain scale that will be utilized during the procedure, and prepared to note whether the pain induced by discography is concordant or dissimilar to their typical pain.

Absolute contraindications to the procedure include patient refusal, inability to adequately report response to the procedure, untreated localized infection over the operative field, untreated coagulopathy, and pregnancy. Relative contraindications include allergy to contrast medium, local anesthetic or antibiotics, systemic infection, and anatomic derangements that preclude safe and successful conduct of the procedure.

Procedural Preparation

The operative suite should be equipped with oxygen, emergency medications, resuscitative equipment, and all appropriate monitors. It is our practice that all individuals in the procedure room wear caps and masks, and operators wear sterile gowns and gloves, as is routinely practiced with open surgical procedures. Whereas ISIS recommends draping the entire patient as well as the image intensifier and remote console,[93] other discographers create only a small sterile field.

Discographers also vary in their use of sedation. Many different methods of sedation have been described, from none at all to benzodiazepines alone and in various combinations with opioids.[107,177,178] If used, sedation should be light enough to relieve anxiety and promote tolerance to the procedure without compromising the patient's ability to assess symptoms. The excessive use of sedation increases the risk for neurologic injury and other complications.

Because of the possibility of inadvertent intrathecal administration, only nonionic contrast material should be injected. Nonionic dye also minimizes the risk of allergic reaction, which can be delayed until contrast material is systemically absorbed from the disk. In patients with known prior contrast reactions, premedication is necessary. Some discographers use no contrast or contrast only to confirm placement of the needle in the NP, and inject saline to elevate intradiskal pressure. Another option is to use gadolinium as the contrast agent.[179]

Needle Placement

Discography is an invasive procedure that carries inherent risks and therefore should only be performed by experienced clinicians. ISIS recommends that anyone performing this procedure should have extensive experience with less technically challenging interventional procedures including facet blocks and epidural steroid injections. There are numerous different ways to perform this procedure,[93,107,159,176,177,180-182] and this section describes only one (Figs. 59–4 and 59–5).

Image guidance for needle placement is ideally achieved through C-arm or biplanar fluoroscopy. Interspinous and interlaminar approaches have been advocated following fusion with paraspinal bone graft, but are otherwise rarely used because of the necessity of dural penetration. Patients can be placed in the left lateral decubitus or prone position. In the prone position, the side of approach is usually determined by the preference of the discographer unless

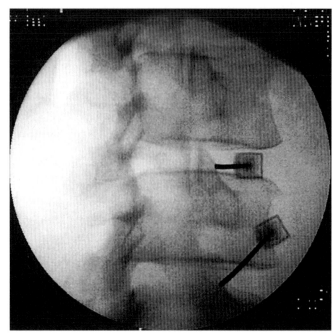

Figure 59–4. Oblique fluoroscopic view for discography needle placement using an extrapedicular approach.

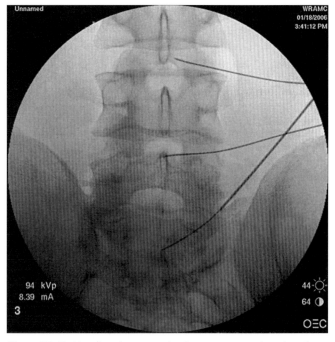

Figure 59–5. Needle placement in the anteroposterior view for a three-level discogram.

unilateral pathology or an anatomic obstacle is suspected. Although recommended by some authors,[93,182] we have shown that an approach from the side ipsilateral to a patient's symptomatology does not affect the rate of false-positive discograms.[183]

Assuming prone positioning, craniocaudal angulation is adjusted so that the imaging beam parallels the disk space at selected L1-2 to L4-5 levels. This can be done by lining up the image so that the x-ray beam passes parallel to the subchondral border of the inferior vertebral end plate of the disk. The C-arm is then rotated laterally until the superior articulating process of the lower vertebra is positioned just posterior to the geometric center of the disk. After superficial injection of local anesthesia, an 18-gauge introducer is advanced just lateral to the outside border of the superior articulating process, preferentially at the midpoint of the superior-inferior margin of the disk (see Fig. 59–4). At this point the fluoroscope is changed from an oblique to a standard lateral view. A 22- or 25-gauge (150 mm) discography needle is advanced through the introducer needle into the annulus. The annular fibers provide a firmer feel than the nucleus and surrounding soft tissue. The needle is then advanced through the annulus until it is situated halfway between the anterior and posterior borders of the disk. The end point should remain close to the midpoint of the superior-inferior margins of the disk because injection into the end plates can result in a false-positive response. When the needle is satisfactorily positioned on lateral imaging, the fluoroscope is rotated to an anteroposterior view in which the final needle position should be confirmed in the middle third of the disk. If the needle has not passed far enough on anteroposterior (AP) view, the entry point was too lateral; if the needle has passed clear to the opposite side of the disk, the entry point was too medial. In the normal disk, central needle placement is necessary to avoid injection into the richly innervated annulus fibrosus, which may result in a false-positive discogram. In degenerated disks, peripheral needle placement is sometimes feasible but never optimal.

At L5-S1, a modified double-needle technique is often necessary because of the iliac crests that prohibit a trajectory aimed directly at the center of the disk. Entry into this level is subject to higher failure rates, which may be substantially reduced by using a curved needle technique.[180] Target identification at this level begins with a sharp, caudal angulation of the beam that passes parallel to the subchondral plate of the inferior end plate of the disk. At this point the C-arm is rotated laterally, until either the superior articulating process of the S1 vertebra is positioned just posterior to the geometric center of the disk or the iliac crests begin to encroach on the target point. Usually, a small triangular window can be appreciated that is bordered laterally by the iliac crest, medially by the superior articulating process, and superiorly by the subchondral border of the superior end plate. Once the entry point is identified, an 18-gauge introducer is advanced toward the lateral margin of the superior articulating process of S1 and walked off just beyond its edge. The C-arm is then positioned in the lateral view. Especially at L5-S1, it is important to adjust the angulation of the camera so that the superior and inferior end plates appear sharp and discernible. A 22-gauge discography needle is then bent slightly about 1 cm from its tip and advanced through the introducer until it meets the outer edge of the annulus. A bend in the needle may facilitate steering the needle around bony obstacles and with proper rotation, may promote a more central placement of the needle tip. As the needle is advanced toward the edge of the disk, it is not uncommon to have the patient experience paresthesias. If this occurs, either the needle is withdrawn and approached at a different angle, or the position of the introducer is moved superiorly or inferiorly. As for the upper disks, the final needle position for L5-S1 should ideally be in the middle third of the disk, but it is not unusual at this level for it to end up in a more peripheral location.

Disk Stimulation and Interpretation

After all needles have been properly positioned, the patient is prepared for the injection. If the patient is still experiencing persistent effects of sedation, it is prudent to wait until he or she is more alert. Patients should be questioned again as to their pain level, taking care to ensure they can distinguish residual procedural pain from their typical low back and extremity pain. They should be able to respond appropriately to questions pertaining to the quality, intensity, location, and concordance of provoked pain, which will provide critical diagnostic information.

Responses may be more reliable if the patient is not informed that an injection is occurring. The patient should also be blinded to the level of injection. The sequence of disk injection depends on the discographer's expectation for pain provocation at each level. Once severe pain is produced, the patient may be less able to tolerate or judge subsequent injections. Therefore, the level considered likely to cause the most intense pain should be injected last. After injecting all levels, it is sometimes necessary to confirm initial reactions by injecting levels a second time.

Verbal and nonverbal reactions, including facial expressions, must be closely monitored and recorded using a discogram worksheet (Table 59–5). Besides pain response, other data that should be recorded include total volume of contrast, injection end point (reason that the injection was stopped), and nucleogram appearance. Normal disks take less than 1 mL of contrast before firm resistance is reached (high pressure end point).

Degenerated disks generally accept larger volumes of contrast and demonstrate moderate or soft resistance to injection (low-pressure end point). When the disk communicates with the epidural space as a result of complete annular disruption, unlimited contrast volume can be injected with little to no resistance (volume end point). When severe symptoms are provoked, the injection should be stopped even if minimal contrast has been injected (pain end point).[178]

Injection pressures can be measured using specialized, commercially available devices, and are recom-

Table 59–5. Interpretation of Disk Stimulation Data

DISK CLASSIFICATION	INTRADISKAL PRESSURE AT PAIN PROVOCATION	PAIN SEVERITY	PAIN TYPE	INTERPRETATION
Chemical	Immediate onset of pain occurring as <1 mL of contrast is visualized reaching the outer annulus, or pain provocation at <15 pounds per square inch (psi) more than opening pressure	≥6/10	Concordant	Positive
Mechanical	Pain noted between 15 and 50 psi at more than opening pressure	≥6/10	Concordant	Positive (but other pain generators may be present; further investigation is warranted)
Indeterminate	Pain noted between 51 and 90 psi	≥6/10	Concordant	Generally negative, but further investigation may be indicated
Normal	>90 psi	No pain or pressure	NA	Negative

Modified from Derby R, Howard MW, Grant JM, et al: The ability of pressure-controlled discography to predict surgical and nonsurgical outcomes. Spine 1999;24:364-372.

mended by ISIS.[93] Proponents of manometry state that a pressure-recording device allows for the objective designation of painful disks as either chemically or mechanically sensitive.[93,131] Others have not endorsed the use of these devices,[107,173,181] claiming that an experienced discographer can determine relative pressures using only a syringe. To date, there are no studies evaluating the effect of manometry on surgical outcomes or discographic results. However, it is our opinion that the proper use of manometry can enhance both the sensitivity and specificity of discography, and reduce the likelihood of inadvertent disk injury. Any bodily structure containing mechanoreceptors, whether diseased or normal, can be a source of pain when subjected to excessive pressure. This effect can be even more pronounced when the pressure is elevated too rapidly, resulting in false-positive discograms. Conversely, if pressure cannot be generated in a severely degenerated disk because of annular incompetence, a discogram may be mistakenly interpreted as negative. An additional benefit of pressure measurement is that it alerts the discographer to overpressurization of disks, which can result in permanent injury.

If manometry is used, one should first determine the opening pressure of the disk, which in practical terms is the pressure at which contrast is first visualized entering the disk (usually <15 psi). Once opening pressure is determined, the disk is slowly filled with contrast, in aliquots of 0.25 to 1 mL. The end point is usually a high-pressure end point at around 100 psi, or the point at which pain is experienced. In cases of severely degenerative disks, it may not be possible to achieve pressures greater than 50 psi. If either 100 psi or 50 psi above opening pressure is reached without pain being noted, the disk is considered negative and can serve as a control. Generating pressures greater than 100 psi greatly increases the risk of iatrogenic injury. If pain is noted at low pressures (<15 psi above opening pressure), the disk is considered chemically sensitive. If pain is noted between 15 and 50 psi above opening pressure, the disk is considered mechanically sensitive, and the discogram may or may not be positive. If pain is noted at greater than 50 psi above opening pressure the response is not clinically significant.[93] Pain at higher pressures may be a result of mechanical irritation, end-plate deflection, or the stimulation of mechanoreceptors (see Table 59–5).

Numerous discography classification systems have been advocated, including some devoid of pressure considerations.[93,131,177,178] No single set of criteria is universally accepted as standard (Box 59–2). In a large multicenter study, Derby and associates demonstrated that patients with chemically sensitized disks (i.e., concordant pain at <15 psi above opening pressure) were more likely to obtain good results with interbody fusion than intertransverse fusion surgery.[131]

Some authors have advocated videotaping to document patient reactions during disk injections.[107,177] Videotaped findings are later correlated with fluoroscopy, or compared with simultaneous changes in physiologic parameters such as heart rate and blood pressure. If relevant, the videotape can be made available to the referring surgeon.

Image Interpretation

For morphologic interpretation of fluoroscopic images, although plain discography is clearly inferior to CT discography, useful information may nevertheless be garnered from the overall appearance of the contrast spread. A small central "cotton ball" accumulation of contrast usually indicates a normal painless disk. Normal disks may also appear to have a central bilobular appearance, like a "hamburger in a bun." A thin line of contrast that extends to the posterior edge of the disk is consistent with an annular tear, and it is not unusual for patients to complain of pain when the contrast moves posteriorly. Small lines of anterior extravasation are sometimes seen but are less likely to elicit a painful

BOX 59–2. INTERPRETATION OF DISCOGRAMS

Unequivocal Discogenic Pain

1. Stimulation of the target disk reproduces concordant pain.
2. Pain intensity is rated as being at least 7 on a 10-point Visual Analogue Scale (VAS).
3. Pain is reproduced at a pressure of less than 15 pounds per square inch (psi) above opening pressure.
4. Presence of two adjacent control disks that are nonpainful.

Definite Discogenic Pain

1. Stimulation of target disk reproduces concordant pain.
2. Pain intensity is rated as being at least 7 on a 10-point VAS.
3. Pain is reproduced at a pressure of less than 15 psi above opening pressure.
4. Presence of one adjacent control disk that is nonpainful.

OR

1. Stimulation of the target disk reproduces concordant pain.
2. Pain intensity is rated as being at least 7 on a 10-point VAS.
3. Pain is reproduced at a pressure of less than 50 psi above opening pressure.
4. Presence of two adjacent control disks that are nonpainful.

Probable Discogenic Pain

1. Stimulation of the target disk reproduces concordant pain.
2. Pain intensity is rated as being at least 7 on a 10-point VAS.
3. Pain is reproduced at a pressure of less than 50 psi above opening pressure.
4. Presence of one adjacent control disk that is nonpainful, and a second adjacent control disk that produces nonconcordant pain at a pressure of greater than 50 psi.

Adapted from Endres S, Bogduk N: Practice guidelines and protocols: Lumbar disc stimulation. Presented at the International Spinal Injection Society 9th Annual Scientific Meeting, Boston, Sept 14-16, 2001, pp 56-75.

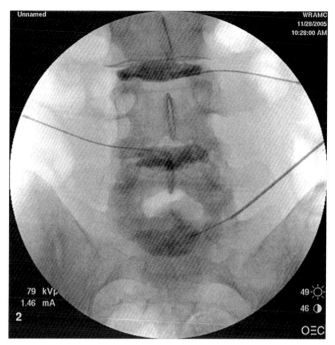

Figure 59–6. Anteroposterior view of a discogram showing early degenerative changes in the L3-4 and L4-5 intervertebral disks.

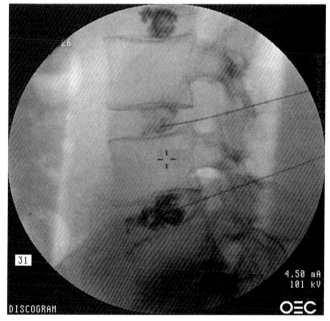

Figure 59–7. Lateral view of normal L3-4 and L4-5 discograms. The L5-S1 discogram reveals a partial tear in the anterior annulus that was clinically insignificant.

response. More diffuse posterior spread of contrast can indicate a large annular tear. Spread of contrast into the epidural space is consistent with a complete tear of the annulus and loss of integrity of the outer annular wall. Diffuse spread in all directions, with or without spread into the epidural space, is indicative of a severely degenerated disk (Figs. 59–6 to 59–8).

Fluoroscopy can show morphologic differences between normal and degenerated disks, but poorly characterizes the locations of annular tears and their relationship to nerve roots. Disk architecture is much better assessed by CT because of its cross-sectional acquisition of thin slices parallel to the disk spaces. Thus many annular tears seen on CT images are

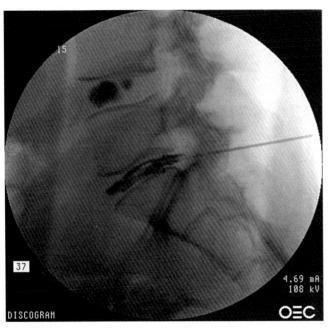

Figure 59–8. Lateral view of a two-level discogram revealing a normal L4-5 disk and a diffusely degenerated L5-S1 disk with a complete posterior annular tear. (Adapted from Bernard TN: Lumbar discography followed by computed tomography. Refining the diagnosis of low-back pain. Spine 1990;15:690-707; Sachs BL, Vanharanta H, Spivey MA, et al: Dallas discogram description: A new classification of CT/discography in low-back disorders. Spine 1987;12:287-294.)

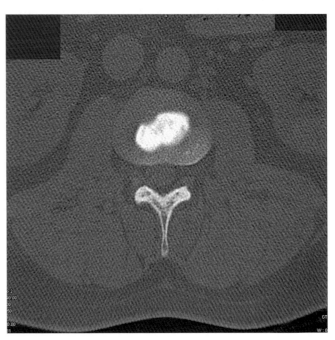

Figure 59–9. Axial view of a normal computed tomography (CT) discogram. Note the "cotton ball" appearance of the contrast within the confines of the nucleus pulposus.

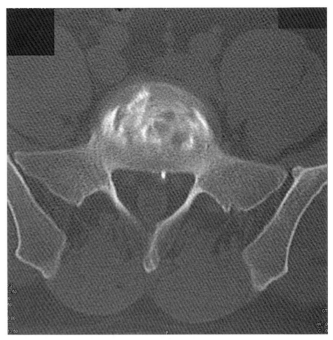

Figure 59–10. Axial computed tomography (CT) discogram of a diffusely degenerated L5-S1 disk.

invisible at fluoroscopy. For this reason, we perform procedures requiring a functional annulus, such as nucleoplasty, only after CT discography.[167] Contiguous helical CT images enable longitudinal reformations in the identical coronal and sagittal planes obtained in MRI. Coronal and sagittal CT reformations demonstrate the distribution of contrast in each disk relative to both the internal and external annulus, as well as focal contour abnormalities relative to the central spinal canal, lateral recesses, neural foramina, and nerve roots (Figs. 59–9 to 59–11).

The most commonly used terminology of disk disease was adapted for MRI. This terminology is difficult to apply to CT discography because it addresses only contour abnormalities, such as diffuse or focal disk bulge, protrusion, extrusion, and sequestration. Internal disk abnormalities that cannot be detected on MRI become obvious on CT because they are filled with contrast material. On CT discographic images, the morphologic analysis of disk architecture, including NP and annulus, can be applied to disks with normal MR imaging contours as well as herniated disks. The Dallas Discogram Scale was originally developed to describe and grade annular tears, and has sub-sequently undergone several modifications (Fig. 59–12).[107,178] The modified Dallas classification for disk morphology takes into account annular tears as well as extra-annular contrast leak and diffuse degenerative changes. Using this modified scheme, disk morphology is graded from 0 to 7[107] (Fig. 59–13; Box 59–3).

The final interpretation of lumbar discography should take into consideration not only disk stimulation data and morphology but also less tangible factors such as a patient's psychological profile, expectations, behavior, and physiologic parameters during pain provocation, and potential confounding factors such as secondary gain and return-to-work issues. In the well-chosen discography candidate, pain is infrequently reproduced in a disk that is mor-

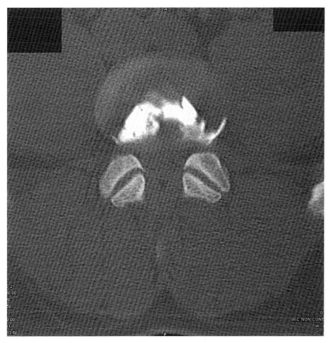

Figure 59–11. Axial view of a computed tomography (CT) discogram demonstrating bilateral posterolateral annular tears.

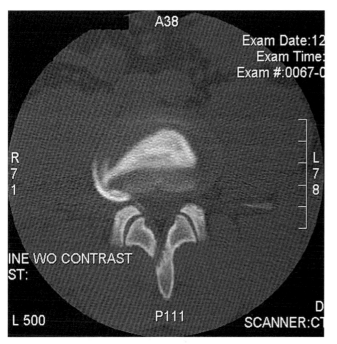

Figure 59–12. Computed tomography (CT) discogram demonstrating a large right posterolateral annular tear. On this axial image, the spread of contrast appears to be contained within the annulus.

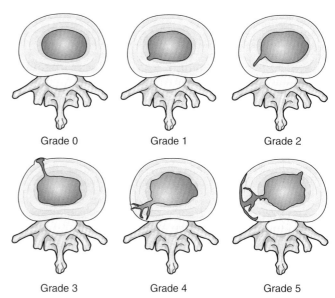

Grade 0   Grade 1   Grade 2

Grade 3   Grade 4   Grade 5

Figure 59–13. Modified Dallas discogram scheme for the classification of annular tears by computed tomography (CT) discography. (Drawings by Jee Hyun Kim. From Cohen SP, Larkin TM, Barna SA, et al: Lumbar discography: A comprehensive review of outcome studies, diagnostic accuracy, and principles. Reg Anesth Pain Med 2005;30:163-183.)

Postprocedural Care

At the conclusion of disk stimulation, the disks may be injected with a solution of local anesthetic. In a small case series by Kotilainen and colleagues, the authors found that 83% and 67% of patients who received intradiskal bupivacaine 0.5% obtained good pain relief 1 day and 2 weeks postprocedure, respectively.[184] In clinical practice, the amount injected into the disk is largely determined by the disk itself because trying to force fluid into a fully pressurized disk may do more harm than good. Typically, in a degenerative disk with an annular tear, 0.5 mL local anesthetic should safely help reduce postprocedural pain. It may also be helpful to reanesthetize the tract of the needle, but care must be taken to avoid unintentionally anesthetizing a nerve root. Although these measures are often sufficient to alleviate postprocedural pain, it is our practice to inject ketorolac 30 mg IV at the termination of the procedure. Occasionally a patient may require extra analgesic medications to treat postprocedural discography pain. Whereas a recent retrospective study concluded intradiskal steroids confer adequate pain relief,[185] two placebo-controlled trials failed to demonstrate any benefit.[186,187]

Complications and Disk Injury

Diskitis is the most feared complication of discography because infection can be extremely difficult to treat as a result of the poor blood supply intervertebral disks receive. Procedure-related pain is commonplace following discography, yet any patient who experiences a new neurologic finding or complains

phologically, manometrically, and volumetrically normal. In the rare instances when this does occur, the discographer must carefully consider the patient's entire clinical picture, including historical and physical examination findings, the presence of spinal and psychological pathology, additional radiologic and supplemental diagnostic tests, and the technical success of the discogram before deciding on a treatment course.

BOX 59–3. COMPUTED TOMOGRAPHY CLASSIFICATION OF DISCOGRAPHY

Type 1: The discogram is normal manometrically, volumetrically, radiologically, and produced no pain. The computed tomography (CT) discogram showed contrast to be centrally located in both axial and sagittal projections.

Type 2: Identical to type 1 except it is positive for pain reproduction.

Type 3: The annular tears lead to a radial fissure. This group can be further subdivided into:
—**Type 3a:** The radial fissure is posterior;
—**Type 3b:** The fissure radiates posterolaterally
—**Type 3c:** The fissure extends laterally to a line drawn from the center of the disk tangential to the lateral border of the superior articulating process.

Type 4: When the radial fissure reaches the periphery of the annulus fibrosus, nuclear material protrudes, causing the outer annulus to bulge.

Type 5: When the outer annular fibers rupture, nuclear material may extrude beneath the posterior longitudinal ligament directly contacting either the dura or a nerve root.

Type 6: When the extruded fragment is no longer in continuity with the interspace, it is said to be sequestrated. Manometrically, volumetrically, and radiologically, these discograms are always abnormal. Concordant pain may be reproduced only if enough pressure is generated against the free fragment to cause stimulation of pain sensitive structures.

Type 7: The end stage of the degenerative process is internal disk disruption, in which multiple annular tears occur. The discograms are abnormal manometrically and volumetrically, and familiar pain may or may not be reproduced. Radiologically, the contrast usually fills the entire interspace in a chaotic fashion. The CT discogram shows contrast extravasation throughout multiple annular tears.

Data from Bernard TN: Lumbar discography followed by computed tomography. Refining the diagnosis of low-back pain. Spine 1990;15:690-707; Sachs BL, Vanharanta H, Spivey MA, et al: Dallas discogram description. A new classification of CT/discography in low-back disorders. Spine 1987;12:287-294.

of increased pain 1 week after the procedure warrants reevaluation. At minimum the postdiscography workup should include a focused history, physical examination, and laboratory screening tests. Erythrocyte sedimentation rate (ESR) and C-reactive protein are the most sensitive indicators of diskitis, but elevation usually does not occur until 3 weeks after the procedure.[188,189] If the ESR is greater than 50, a bone scan or MRI is needed to rule out diskitis. The most common cause of postprocedure diskitis is *Staphylococcus aureus*.[189]

In a retrospective study conducted in 432 patients, Fraser and coworkers found that the incidence of diskitis was reduced from 2.7% to 0.7% when a through-and-through, double-needle technique was used.[190] A review by Guyer and Ohnmeiss found an overall incidence of diskitis of less than 0.15% by patient and less than 0.08% by disk, with most of the studies included not administering prophylactic antibiotics.[191] Osti and associates advocated mixing 1 mg/mL of cefazolin with the injected contrast as a safe and effective means of preventing diskitis following a two-part study.[192] In the first phase of the study, intradiskal cefazolin was found to be equivalent to parenteral antibiotics administered 30 minutes preprocedure in preventing diskitis in sheep inoculated with intradiskal *Staphylococcus epidermidis*. In the second phase of the study, none of 127 patients developed radiographic or clinical evidence of diskitis following discography conducted by mixing cefazolin 1 mg/mL with contrast. A recent in vitro study by Klessig supports the prophylactic use of intradiskal antibiotics in lieu of systemic therapy for patients undergoing provocative discography.[193]

The administration of prophylactic antibiotics is by no means universal. Willems and colleagues performed a literature review of postdiscography diskitis cases with and without the use of prophylactic antibiotics.[194] Inclusion criteria were use of the double-needle technique and stringent reporting of complications and dropouts. Including their own report on 200 patients who underwent 435 discograms, 11 studies were analyzed, of which only 1 administered prophylactic antibiotics. Among the 4981 patients included in the analysis who did not receive prophylactic antimicrobial therapy, the incidence of diskitis was 0.25% (0.09% of 12,770 discograms). The only study in which prophylactic antibiotics were administered was the Osti study,[192] which had no reported cases of diskitis. The authors concluded that the low risk of diskitis when the double-needle technique is used does not support the routine use of prophylactic antibiotics. Considering the inherent difficulties in treating diskitis and the fact that no serious complications have ever been reported from the use of low-dose intradiskal antibiotics, the authors feel the prophylactic use of intradiskal cefazolin or clindamycin is justified (Box 59–4). Collectively we have performed more than 3000 discograms using intradiskal antibiotics, with zero incidence of diskitis. If diskitis should occur, the mainstay of treatment is antibiotics and pain control; surgical intervention is not usually necessary. Potential complications of diskitis include epidural abscess, intervertebral fusion, and paralysis.[195]

A key question surrounding discography is whether artificial elevation of the intervertebral disk pressure can worsen existing LBP, or injure the intervertebral disk.

In an experimental biochemical model tested in 113 cadavers, Iencean determined that the amount of pressure required to rupture the annulus was inversely proportional to the degree of degeneration,

BOX 59–4. ANTIBIOTIC PROPHYLAXIS GUIDELINES

Intravenous

Cefazolin 1 g in 50 mL normal saline 30-60 minutes before procedure

or

Clindamycin (for cephalosporin or penicillin allergy) 900 mg in 50 mL normal saline 30-60 minutes before procedure

or

Ciprofloxacin (for cephalosporin or penicillin allergy) 400 mg in 50 mL normal saline 30-60 minutes before procedure

Intradiskal

Cefazolin 2-4 mg (10 mg/mL) either before start of the contrast injection or mixed with contrast

or

Clindamycin 1-2 mg (6 mg/10 mL) either before start of the contrast injection or mixed with contrast

---

and ranged from 108 to 188 psi.[196] However, vigilance should be exercised at all times during disk stimulation because there are many reports of discography-induced lumbar disk herniation occurring at lower pressures.[197]

Carragee and coworkers attempted to answer this question in a controlled prospective study examining whether provocative lumbar discography is associated with long-term low back symptoms in 26 subjects without low back complaints.[198] In the 10 patients who were pain-free after unrelated neck surgery, none reported persistent LBP 1 year following discography. In 10 patients with chronic neck or arm pain after cervical spine surgery, 2 of 10 reported persistent pain 1 year after discography. In the 6 patients with somatization disorder, two thirds (4 of 6) reported ongoing pain after discography. In two control groups composed of somatization patients who did not undergo discography and LBP patients with positive discograms but no other nondiscogenic spine abnormalities, no significant change in low back symptomatology was noted during the 1-year follow-up. In a 4-year follow-up study that included the same patients reported on earlier, the authors concluded that painful disk injections and annular disruptions were poor and weak predictors, respectively, of future low back problems in patients without preexisting low back complaints.[199] Conversely, the authors found psychological distress and preexisting pain complaints not involving the low back to be stronger predictors of the subsequent development of LBP. In three studies evaluating the clinical and anatomic sequelae of discography, Johnson,[200] Flanagan and Chung,[201] and Saifuddin and associates[202] found no evidence that discography causes

damage to intervertebral disks based on repeat discograms, clinical and radiographic findings, and MRI, respectively.

In a study analyzing 146 lumbar discograms in 52 patients, Tallroth and colleagues found that 2% of patients experienced nausea, 4% convulsions, and 6% severe back pain during the procedures.[203] Ten percent of patients reported severe headache and 81% worsening LBP 1 day postprocedure. The headaches were attributed to neuraxial leakage of contrast. In a retrospective study assessing complications in 4400 cervical discograms performed in 1357 patients, Zeidman and coworkers reported a complication rate of 0.6%, or 0.16% of disk injections.[204] Adverse events included seven cases of diskitis and one abscess. Prophylactic antibiotics were only administered to patients deemed to be at high risk for infection. Other possible complications of discography include meningitis, spinal headache, subdural or epidural abscess, intrathecal and retroperitoneal hemorrhage, arachnoiditis, nerve root injury, paravertebral muscle pain and contusions, postprocedural pain exacerbation, vasovagal reactions, allergic reactions, and damage to the disk including but not limited to herniation.[159,205-210]

CONCLUSION

Considering the long history of discography in diagnosing disk pathology and the advent of more advanced imaging techniques, what is the future of disk stimulation? Given that the lifetime prevalence of low back pain approaches 80% by some estimates and that various stages of disk degeneration can be detected in a majority of people—even without low back symptoms—it is clear that some sort of test is needed to determine whether a causative relationship exists between the two phenomena. Although it is true that discography, with or without computed tomography, remains the only imaging tool that ostensibly allows a clinician to relate pathology with symptoms, the significance of this remains unclear.

When assessing discographic pathology, proponents of discography argue that it is necessary to correlate provoked pain with anatomic abnormalities. In regards to symptomatic disk herniations, the enhanced accuracy and safety of MRI has rendered plain discography obsolete for this purpose. For internal disk disruption, CT discography is a more sensitive diagnostic tool than plain MRI, although T2-weighted MRIs may detect some pathology missed on plain discograms. Based on cadaveric studies, discography seems to be more accurate in identifying radial rather than transverse or concentric tears in the AF. Disk stimulation studies have consistently found that degenerated disks of all types are more likely to provoke pain than normal disks, and that annular disruption seems to be a prominent source of pain generation. However, the significance of these findings is limited by the high prevalence of these features, the fact that in clinical contexts discography is almost exclusively performed in disks already noted to be abnormal on CT or MRI, and the observation that a substantial percentage of LBP patients may be at increased risk for "false-positive" discograms.

As a diagnostic procedure that carries substantial risks, the critical question that will determine whether discography remains a viable preoperative screening tool or becomes merely another footnote in history is whether it improves patient outcomes, and presently the evidence for this is lacking. In the two studies directly comparing fusion outcomes between patients who underwent routine preoperative discography screening and those who didn't, the results are conflicting. For IDET, the controversy surrounding its efficacy and the fact that all published studies have consistently used preprocedure discography prevent any conclusions from being drawn. With disk replacement surgery, although the studies are almost evenly divided between those that routinely used preoperative discography and those that did not, the lack of direct comparison between groups, methodologic flaws, and differences in outcome measures, length of follow-up, and surgical technique used render any comparisons futile. Given the lack of evidence supporting any interventional treatment for discogenic LBP, even if prospective, randomized studies were to be conducted on the benefits of discography, they would be unlikely to definitively resolve this controversy.

What is clear is that there is a wide discrepancy in the use of lumbar discography to treat discogenic LBP. The routine use of discography as a screening tool before IDET, a minimally invasive surgical procedure, and the sporadic use of the procedure before spinal arthrodesis and disk replacement surgery, is inconsistent. After weighing the risks and benefits of discography, the authors believe that the procedure should be generally used before any invasive surgical procedure used to treat discogenic LBP except when the evidence implicating a particular disk(s) as the pain generator is compelling. Inherent in this recommendation is that the procedure be conducted according to evidence-based standards, which have yet to be agreed upon. These standards might include routine manometry, obtaining two adjacent control disks in patients at high risk for "false-positive" pain provocation, psychological screening similar to what is routinely used before spinal cord stimulation, a combination of concordant pain provocation, and pain relief after intradiskal local anesthetic injection (as is common when performing selective nerve blocks) to increase specificity, and requiring at least one objective measure to confirm a positive discogram, such as a significant heart rate increase or the elicitation of certain facial expressions. This recommendation is also contingent on the results of disk stimulation being considered in the context of other diagnostic screening tests, and with consideration to the propensity of patients with preexisting psychopathology and somatization symptoms to have false-positive pain provocation. One point in which there does seem to be a consensus is that clinical studies are needed to better elucidate the role discography

will assume in the diagnosis of disk pathology in the future, and to determine what effect, if any, it has on the surgical treatment of discogenic LBP.

References

1. Weinstein SM, Herring SA, Cole AJ: Rehabilitation of the patient with spinal pain. In DeLisa JA, Gans BM (eds): Rehabilitation Medicine: Principles and Practice (3rd ed). Philadelphia, Lippincott-Raven, 1998, pp 1423-1451.
2. Waddell G: Epidemiology. A new clinical model for the treatment of low back pain. In Weinstein JN, Wiesel SW (eds): The Lumbar Spine: The International Society for the Study of the Lumbar Spine. Philadelphia, Saunders, 1990, pp 38-56.
3. McGill CM: Industrial back problems. A control program. J Occup Med 1968;10:174-178.
4. Waddell G: The Back Pain Revolution. Edinburgh, Scotland, Churchill Livingstone, 1998, pp 103-107.
5. Lindblom K: Diagnostic puncture of intervertebral disks in sciatica. Acta Orthop Scand 1948;17:231-239.
6. Brightbill TC, Pile N, Eichelberger RP, Whitman M Jr: Normal magnetic resonance imaging and abnormal discography in lumbar disc disruption. Spine 1994;19:1075-1077.
7. Adams MA, Dolan P, Hutton WC: The stages of disc degeneration as revealed by discograms. J Bone Joint Surg (Br) 1986;68:36-41.
8. Colhoun E, McCall IW, Williams L, Cassar Pullicino VN: Provocation discography as a guide to planning operations on the spine. J Bone Joint Surg (Br) 1988;70:267-271.
9. Whitecloud TS 3rd, Seago RA: Cervical discogenic syndrome. Results of operative intervention patients with discography. Spine 1987;12:313-316.
10. Madan S, Gundanna M, Harley JM, et al: Does provocative discography screening of discogenic back pain improve surgical outcomes? J Spinal Disord Tech 2002;15:245-251.
11. Wetzel FT, LaRocca SH, Lowery GL, Aprill CN: The treatment of lumbar spinal pain syndromes diagnosed by discography. Lumbar arthrodesis. Spine 1994;19:792-800.
12. Marks R: Distribution of pain provoked from lumbar facet joints and related structures during diagnostic spinal infiltration. Pain 1989;39:37-40.
13. Bough B, Thakore J, Davies M, Dowling F: Degeneration of the lumbar facet joints. Arthrography and pathology. J Bone J Surg 1990;72:275-276.
14. Schwarzer AC, Derby R, Aprill CN, et al: The value of the provocation response in lumbar zygapophyseal joint injections. Clin J Pain 1994;10:309-313.
15. Fortin JD, Dwyer AP, West S, Pier J: Sacroiliac joint: Pain referral maps upon applying a new injection/arthrography technique. Part I: Asymptomatic volunteers. Spine 1994;19: 1475-1482.
16. Dwyer A, Aprill C, Bogduk N: Cervical zygaophyseal joint pain patterns. I: A study in normal volunteers. Spine 1990;15: 453-457.
17. Aprill C, Dwyer A, Bogduk N: Cervical zygapophyseal joint pain patterns. II: A clinical evaluation. Spine 1990;15: 458-461.
18. Fortin JD, Aprill CN, Ponthieux B, Pier J: Sacroiliac joint: Pain referral maps upon applying a new injection/arthrography technique. Part II: Clinical evaluation. Spine 1994;19: 1483-1489.
19. Slipman CW, Jackson HB, Lipetz JS, et al: Sacroiliac joint pain referral zones. Arch Phys Med Rehabil 2000;81:334-338.
20. Schwarzer AC, Aprill CN, Bogduk N: The sacroiliac joint in chronic low back pain. Spine 1995;20:31-37.
21. Slipman CW, Plastaras CT, Palmitier RA, et al: Symptom provocation of fluoroscopically guided cervical nerve root stimulation: Are dynatomal maps identical to dermatomal maps? Spine 1998;23:2235-2242.
22. Bogduk N: Clinical anatomy of the lumbar spine and sacrum (3rd ed). Edinburgh, Scotland, Churchill Livingstone, 1997, pp 205-212.

23. Urban JP, Holm S, Maroudas A, Nachemson A: Nutrition of the intervertebral disk. An in vivo study of solute transport. Clin Orthop Relat Res 1977;129:101-114.

24. Holm S, Maroudas A, Urban JP, et al: Nutrition of the intervertebral disc: Solute transport and metabolism. Connect Tissue Res 1981;8:101-119.

25. Ohshima H, Urban JP: The effect of lactate and pH on proteoglycan and protein synthesis rates in the intervertebral disc. Spine 1992;17:1079-1082.

26. Groen GJ, Baljet B, Drukker J: Nerves and nerve plexuses of the human vertebral column. Amer J Anat 1990;188:282-296.

27. Jackson HC, Winkelmann RK, Bickel WH: Nerve endings in the human lumbar spinal column and related structures. J Bone Joint Surg (Am) 1966;48:1272-1281.

28. Palmgren T, Gronblad M, Virri J, et al: An immunohistochemical study of nerve structures in the anulus fibrosis of human normal lumbar intervertebral discs. Spine 1999;24:2075-2079.

29. Boos N, Weissbach S, Rohrbach H, et al: Classification of age-related changes in lumbar intervertebral discs. Spine 2002;27:2631-2644.

30. Malinsky J: The ontogenic development of nerve terminations in the intervertebral discs of man. Acta Anat 1959;38:96-113.

31. Coppes MH, Marani E, Thomeer RT, et al: Innervation of annulus fibrosis in low back pain. Lancet 1990;36:189-190.

32. Coppes MH, Marani E, Thomeer RT, Groen GJ: Innervation of "painful" lumbar discs. Spine 1997;22:2342-2349.

33. Freemont AJ, Peacock TE, Goupille P, et al: Nerve ingrowth into diseased intervertebral disc in chronic back pain. Lancet 1997;350:178-181.

34. Palmgren T, Gronblad M, Virri J, et al: Immunohistochemical demonstration of sensory and autonomic nerve terminals in herniated lumbar disc tissue. Spine 1996;21:1301-1306.

35. Ashton IH, Roberts S, Jaffray DC, et al: Neuropeptides in the human intervertebral disc. J Orthop Res 1994;12:186-192.

36. Brena SF, Wolf SL, Chapman SL, Hammonds WD: Chronic back pain: Electromyographic, motion and behavioral assessments following sympathetic nerve blocks and placebos. Pain 1980;8:1-10.

37. White JC, Sweet WH: Pain. Its mechanisms and neurosurgical control. Springfield, Ill, Charles C Thomas, 1995, pp 67-98.

38. Foerster O: The dermatomes in man. Brain 1933;56:1-39.

39. Nakamura S, Takahashi K, Takahashi Y, et al: The afferent pathways of discogenic low-back pain. J Bone Joint Surg (Br) 1996;78:606-612.

40. Wiberg G: Back pain in relation to nerve supply of the intervertebral disc. Acta Orthop Scand 1947;19:211-221.

41. Ikari C: A study of the mechanism of low back pain. The neurohistological examination of the disease. J Bone Joint Surg 1954;36A:195.

42. Jung A, Brunschwig A: Recherches histologiques des articulations des corps vertebraux. Presse Med 1932;40:316-317.

43. Ehrenhaft JL: Development of the vertebral column as related to certain congenital and pathological changes. Surg Gynecol Obstet 1943;76:282-292.

44. Hirsch C, Ingelmark BE, Miller M: The anatomical basis for low back pain. Acta Orthop Scand 1963;33:1-17.

45. Jackson HC, Winkelmann RK, Bickel WM: Nerve endings in the human lumbar spinal column and related structures. J Bone Joint Surg (Am) 1966;48:1271-1281.

46. Adams MA, McNally DS, Dolan P: "Stress" distributions inside intervertebral discs. The effects of age and degeneration. J Bone Joint Surg (Br) 1996;78:965-972.

47. Adams MA, McNally DS, Wagstaff J, Goodship AE: Abnormal stress concentrations in the lumbar intervertebral discs following damage to the vertebral bodies: Cause of disc failure? Eur Spine J 1993;1:214-221.

48. Yoganandan N, Maiman DJ, Pintar F, et al: Microtrauma in the lumbar spine: A cause of low back pain. Neurosurgery 1988;23:162-168.

49. Heggeness MH, Doherty BJ: Discography causes end plate deflection. Spine 1993;18:1050-1053.

50. Modic MT, Masaryk TJ, Ross JS, et al: Imaging of degenerative disk disease. Radiology 1988;168:177-186.

51. Frobin W, Brinckmann P, Kramer M, Hartwig E: Height of lumbar discs measured from radiographs compared with degeneration and height classified from MR images. Eur Radiol 2001;11:263-269.

52. Vernon-Roberts B: Age-related and degenerative pathology of intervertebral discs and apophyseal joints. In Jayson MV (ed): The Lumbar Spine and Back Pain. Edinburgh, Scotland, Churchill Livingstone, 1992, pp 17-41.

53. Kang JD, Georgescu HI, McIntyre-Larkin L, et al: Herniated lumbar intervertebral discs spontaneously produce matrix metalloproteinases, nitric oxide, interleukin-6, and prostaglandin E2. Spine 1996;21:271-277.

54. Peng B, Wu W, Hou S, et al: The pathogenesis of discogenic low back pain. J Bone Joint Surg (Br) 2005;87:62-66.

55. Bogduk N, McGuirk B: Pain Research and Clinical Management. Medical Management of Acute and Chronic Low Back Pain. An Evidence Based Approach, Volume 13. Amsterdam, Elsevier Science, 2002, pp 119-122.

56. Ahmed M, Bjurholm A, Kreicbergs A, Schultzberg M: Neuropeptide Y, tyrosine hydroxylase and vasoactive intestinal polypeptide-immunoreactive nerve fibers in the vertebral bodies, discs, dura mater, and spinal ligaments of the rat lumbar spine. Spine 1993;18:268-273.

57. Konttinen YT, Gronblad M, Antti-Poika I, et al: Neuroimmunohistochemical analysis of peridiscal nociceptive neural elements. Spine 1990;15:383-386.

58. Ashton IK, Roberts S, Jaffray DC, et al: Neuropeptides in the human intervertebral disc. J Orthop Res 1994;12:186-192.

59. Burke JG, Watson RW, McCormack D, et al: Intervertebral discs which cause low back pain secrete high levels of proinflammatory mediators. J Bone Joint Surg (Br) 2002;84:196-201.

60. Lu GH, Li J, Zhou JN: Inflammatory-inducing effect of lumbar disc tissue: An experimental study. Hunan Yi Ke Da Xue Xue Bao 2001;26:531-533 (in Chinese).

61. Tanaka N, Ishida T, Hukuda S, Horiike K: Purification of a low-molecular-weight phospholipase A(2) associated with soluble high-molecular-weight acidic proteins from rabbit nucleus pulposus and its comparison with a rabbit splenic group IIa phospholipase A(2). J Biochem (Tokyo) 2000;127:985-991.

62. Miyahara K, Ishida T, Hukuda S, et al: Human group II phospholipase A2 in normal and diseased intervertebral discs. Biochim Biophys Acta 1996;1316:183-190.

63. Saal JS, Franson RC, Dobrow R, et al: High levels of inflammatory phospholipase A2 activity in lumbar disc herniations. Spine 1990;15:674-678.

64. Franson RC, Saal JS, Saal JA: Human disc phospholipase A2 is inflammatory. Spine 1992;17(6 Suppl):S129-S132.

65. Nygaard OP, Mellgren SI, Osterud B: The inflammatory properties of contained and noncontained lumbar disc herniation. Spine 1997;22:2484-2488.

66. Olmarker K, Rydevik B: Selective inhibition of tumor necrosis factor-alpha prevents nucleus pulposus–induced thrombus formation, intraneural edema, and reduction of nerve conduction velocity: possible implications for future pharmacologic treatment strategies of sciatica. Spine 2001;26:863-869.

67. Igarashi T, Kikuchi S, Shubayev V, Myers RR: Exogenous tumor necrosis factor-alpha mimics nucleus pulposus–induced neuropathology. Molecular, histologic, and behavioral comparisons in rats. Spine 2000;25:2975-2980.

68. Ohnmeiss DD, Vanharanta H, Ekholm J: Relation between pain location and disc pathology: A study of pain drawings and CT/discography. Clin J Pain 1999;15:210-217.

69. Vanharanta H, Sachs BL, Spivey MA, et al: The relationship of pain provocation to lumbar disc deterioration as seen by CT/discography. Spine 1987;12:295-298.

70. Vanharanta H, Sachs BL, Spivey MA, et al: A comparison of CT/discography, pain response and radiographic disc height. Spine 1988;13:321-324.

71. Vanharanta H, Guyer RD, Ohnmeiss DD, et al: Disc deterioration in low-back syndromes. A prospective, multi-center CT/discography study. Spine 1988;13:1349-1351.

72. Vanharanta H, Sachs BL, Ohnmeiss DD, et al: Pain provocation and disc deterioration by age. A CT/ discography study in a low-back pain population. Spine 1989;14:420-423.

73. Moneta GB, Videman T, Kaivanto K, et al: Reported pain during lumbar discography as a function of anular ruptures and disc degeneration. Spine 1994;19:1968-1974.

74. Maezawa S, Muro T: Pain provocation at lumbar discography as analyzed by computed tomography/discography. Spine 1992;17:1309-1315.

75. Saifuddin A, Emanuel R, White R, et al: An analysis of radiating pain at lumbar discography. Eur Spine J 1998;7:358-362.

76. Slipman CW, Patel RK, Zhang L: Site of symptomatic annular tear and site of low back pain: Is there a correlation? Spine 2001;26:E165-E169.

77. Jackson RP, Becker GJ, Jacobs RR, et al: The neuroradiographic diagnosis of lumbar herniated nucleus pulposus: I. A comparison of computed tomography (CT), CT-myelography, discography, and CT-discography. Spine 1989;14:1356-1361.

78. Jensen MC, Brant-Zawadzki MN, Obuchowski N, et al: Magnetic resonance imaging of the lumbar spine in people without back pain. N Engl J Med 1994;331:69-73.

79. Walker BF: The prevalence of low back pain: A systematic review of the literature from 1966 to 1998. J Spinal Disord 2000;3:205-217.

80. Manchikanti L: Epidemiology of low back pain. Pain Physician 2000;3:167-192.

81. Deyo RA, Nachemson A, Mirza SK: Spinal-fusion surgery—The case for restraint. N Engl J Med 2004;350:722-726.

82. Yasuma T, Ohno R, Yamauchi Y: False-negative discograms. J Bone Joint Surg (Am) 1988;70:1279-1290.

83. Yasuma T, Makino E, Saito S: A significance of the limited form of discography—A comparison with histological findings of the lumbar discs in the autopsy cases. Seikeigeka 1988;39:311-318 (in Japanese).

84. Holt EP Jr: The question of lumbar discography. J Bone Joint Surg (Am) 1968;50:720-726.

85. Walsh TR, Weinstein JN, Sprat KF, et al: Lumbar discography in normal subjects. A controlled, prospective study. J Bone Joint Surg (Am) 1990;72:1081-1088.

86. Block A, Vanharanta H, Ohnmeiss DD, Guyer RD: Discographic pain report: Influence of psychological factors. Spine 1996;21:334-338.

87. Carragee EJ, Tanner CM, Yang B, et al: False-positive findings on lumbar discography. Reliability of subjective concordance assessment during provocative disc injection. Spine 1999;24:2542-2547.

88. Carragee EJ, Tanner CM, Khurana S, et al: The rates of false-positive lumbar discography in select patients without low back symptoms. Spine 2000;25:1373-1380.

89. Carragee EJ, Chen Y, Tanner CM, et al: Provocative discography in patients after limited lumbar discectomy. Spine 2000;25:3065-3071.

90. Derby R, Lee SH, Kim BJ, et al: Pressure-controlled lumbar discography in volunteers without low back symptoms. Pain Med 2005;6:213-221.

91. Collis JS, Gardner WJ: Lumbar discography: An analysis of one thousand cases. J Neurosurg 1962;19:452-461.

92. Almen T: Experimental investigations with iohexol and their clinical relevance. Acta Radiol 1983;Suppl 366:9-19.

93. Endres S, Bogduk N: Practice guidelines and protocols: Lumbar disc stimulation. Presented at the International Spinal Injection Society 9th Annual Scientific Meeting, Boston, Sept 14-16, 2001, pp 56-75.

94. Indahl A, Kaigle AM, Reikeras O, Holm SH: Interaction between porcine lumbar intervertebral disc, zygapophyseal joints, and paraspinal muscles. Spine 1997;22:2834-2840.

95. Schwarzer AC, Aprill CN, Derby R, et al: The prevalence and clinical features of internal disc disruption in patients with chronic low back pain. Spine 1995;17:1878-1883.

96. Collins CD, Stack JP, O'Connell DJ, et al: The role of discography in lumbar disc disease: A comparative study of magnetic resonance imaging and discography. Clin Radiol 1990;42:252-257.

97. Horton WC, Daftari TK: Which disc as visualized by magnetic resonance imaging is actually a source of pain? Correlation between magnetic resonance imaging and discography. Spine 1992;17(6 Suppl):S164-S171.

98. Long DM, BenDebba M, Torgerson WS, et al: Persistent back pain and sciatica in the United States: Patient characteristics. J Spinal Disord 1996;9:40-58.

99. Gibson MJ, Buckley J, Mawhinney R, et al: Magnetic resonance imaging and discography in the diagnosis of disc degeneration. A comparative study of 50 discs. J Bone Joint Surg (Br) 1986;68:369-373.

100. Yoshida H, Fujiwara A, Tamai K, et al: Diagnosis of symptomatic disc by magnetic resonance imaging: T2-weighted and gadolinium-DPTA-enhanced T1-weighted magnetic resonance imaging. J Spinal Disord Tech 2002;15:193-198.

101. Simmons JW, Emery SF, McMillin JN, et al: Awake discography. A comparison study with magnetic resonance imaging. Spine 1991;16(6 Suppl):S216-S221.

102. Aprill C, Bogduk N: High-intensity zone: A diagnostic sign of painful lumbar disc on magnetic resonance imaging. Br J Radiol 1992;65:361-369.

103. Linson MA, Crowe CH: Comparison of magnetic resonance imaging and lumbar discography in the diagnosis of disc degeneration. Clin Orthop 1990;250:160-163.

104. Schneiderman G, Flannigan B, Kingston S, et al: Magnetic resonance imaging in the diagnosis of disc degeneration: Correlation with discography. Spine 1987;12:276-281.

105. Zucherman J, Derby R, Hsu K, et al: Normal magnetic resonance imaging with abnormal discography. Spine 1988;13:1355-1359.

106. Yu S, Haughton VM, Sether LA, Wagner M: Comparison of MR and discography in detecting radial tears of the annulus: A postmortem study. Am J Neuroradiol 1989;10:1077-1081.

107. Bernard TN: Lumbar discography followed by computed tomography: Refining the diagnosis of low-back pain. Spine 1990;15:690-707.

108. Birney TJ, White JJ Jr, Berens D, Kuhn G: Comparison of MRI and discography in the diagnosis of lumbar degenerative disc disease. J Spinal Disord 1992;5:417-423.

109. Osti OL, Fraser RD: MRI and discography of annular tears and intervertebral disc degeneration: A prospective clinical comparison. J Bone Joint Surg (Br) 1992;74:431-435.

110. Loneragan R, Khangure MS, McCormick C, Hardcastle P: Comparison of magnetic resonance imaging and computed tomographic discography in the assessment of lumbar disc degeneration. Australas Radiol 1994;38:6-9.

111. Schellhas KP, Pollei SR, Gundry CR, Heithoff KB: Lumbar disc high-intensity zone. Correlation of magnetic resonance imaging and discography. Spine 1996;21:79-86.

112. Braithwaite I, White J, Saifuddin A, et al: Vertebral end-plate (Modic) changes on lumbar spine MRI: Correlation with pain reproduction at lumbar discography. Eur Spin J 1998;7:363-368.

113. Saifuddin A, Braithwaite I, White J, et al: The value of lumbar spine magnetic resonance imaging in the demonstration of annular tears. Spine 1998;23:453-457.

114. Milette PC, Fontaine S, Lepanto L, et al: Differentiating lumbar disc protrusions, disc bulges, and discs with normal contour but abnormal signal intensity: Magnetic resonance imaging with discographic correlations. Spine 1999;24:44-53.

115. Sandhu HS, Sanchez-Caso LP, Parvataneni HK, et al: Association between findings of provocative discography and vertebral endplate signals as seen on MRI. J Spinal Disord 2000;13:438-443.

116. Kakitsubata Y, Theodorou DJ, Theodorou SJ, et al: Magnetic resonance discography in cadavers: Tears of the annulus fibrosus. Clin Orthop 2003;407:228-240.

117. Lim C-H, Jee W-H, Son BC, et al: Discogenic lumbar pain: Association with MR imaging and CT discography. Eur J Radiol 2005;54:431-437.

118. Cohen SP, Larkin TM, Barna SA, et al: Lumbar discography: A comprehensive review of outcome studies, diagnostic accuracy, and principles. Reg Anesth Pain Med 2005;30: 163-183.

119. Junge A, Frohlich M, Ahrens S, et al: Predictors of bad and good outcome of lumbar spine surgery: A prospective clinical study with 2 years' follow up. Spine 1996;21:1056-1064.

120. Zdeblick TA: The treatment of degenerative lumbar disorders. A critical review of the literature. Spine 1995;20(24 Suppl): 126S-137S.

121. Deyo RA, Nachemson A, Mirza SK: Spinal-fusion surgery— The case for restraint. N Engl J Med 2004;350:722-726.

122. Gibson JN, Waddell G, Grant IC: Surgery for degenerative lumbar spondylosis. Cochrane Database Syst Rev 2000;2: CD001352.

123. Carragee EJ: Persistent low back pain. N Engl J Med 2005; 352:891-898.

124. Esses SI, Botsford DJ, Kostuik JP: The role of external spinal skeletal fixation in the assessment of low-back disorders. Spine 1989;14:594-600.

125. Kostuik JP: Decision making in adult scoliosis. Spine 1979; 4:521-525.

126. Blumenthal SL, Baker J, Dossett A, Selby DK: The role of anterior lumbar fusion for internal disc disruption. Spine 1988;13:566-569.

127. Gill K, Blumenthal SL: Functional results after anterior lumbar fusion at L5-S1 in patients with normal and abnormal MRI scans. Spine 1992;17:940-942.

128. Knox BD, Chapman TM: Anterior lumbar interbody fusion for discogram concordant pain. J Spinal Disord 1993;6: 242-244.

129. Parker LM, Murrell SE, Boden SD, Horton WC: The outcome of posterolateral fusion in highly selected patients with discogenic low back pain. Spine 1996;21:1909-1917.

130. Vamvanij V, Fredrickson BE, Thorpe JM, et al: Surgical treatment of internal disc disruption: An outcome study of four fusion techniques. J Spinal Disord 1998;11:375-382.

131. Derby R, Howard MW, Grant JM, et al: The ability of pressure-controlled discography to predict surgical and nonsurgical outcomes. Spine 1999;24:364-372.

132. Spruit M, Jacobs WC: Pain and function after intradiscal electrothermal treatment (IDET) for symptomatic lumbar disc degeneration. Eur Spine J 2002;11:589-593.

133. Saal JA, Saal JS: Intradiscal electrothermal treatment (IDET) for chronic discogenic low back pain: A prospective outcome study with minimum 2-year follow-up. Spine 2002;27: 966-973.

134. Pauza KJ, Howell S, Dreyfuss P, et al: A randomized, placebo-controlled trial of intradiscal electrothermal therapy for the treatment of discogenic low back pain. Spine J 2004; 4:27-35.

135. Freeman BJ, Fraser RD, Cain CM, et al: A randomized, double-blind, controlled trial: Intradiscal electrothermal therapy versus placebo for the treatment of chronic discogenic low back pain. Spine 2005;30:2369-2378.

136. Cohen SP, Larkin T, Abdi S, et al: Risk factors for failure and complications of intradiscal electrothermal therapy: A pilot study. Spine 2003;28:1142-1147.

137. Karasek M, Bogduk N: Twelve-month follow-up of a controlled trial of intradiscal thermal anuloplasty for back pain due to internal disc disruption. Spine 2000;25:2601-2607.

138. Fernstrom U: Arthroplasty with intercorporeal endoprosthesis in herniated disc and in painful disc. Acta Chir Scand Suppl 1966;357:154S-159S.

139. Enker P, Steffee A, McMillin C, et al: Artificial disc replacement. Preliminary report with a 3-year minimum follow-up. Spine 1993;18:1061-1070.

140. Zeegers WS, Bohnen LM, Laaper M, Verhaegen MJ: Artificial disc replacement with the modular type SB Charite III: 2-year results in 50 prospectively studied patients. Eur Spine J 1999;8:210-217.

141. Bertagnoli R, Kumar S: Indications for full prosthetic disc arthroplasty: A correlation of clinical outcome against a variety of indications. Eur Spine J 2002;11(Suppl 2): S131-S136.

142. Hochschuler SH, Ohnmeiss DD, Guyer RD, Blumenthal SL: Artificial disc: Preliminary results of a prospective study in the United States. Eur Spine J 2002;11(Suppl 2):S106-S110.

143. Mayer HM, Wiechert K, Korge A, Qose I: Minimally invasive total disc replacement: surgical technique and preliminary clinical results. Eur Spine J 2002;(Suppl 2):S124-S130.

144. Delmarter RB, Fribourg DM, Kanim LE, Bae H: ProDisc artificial total lumbar disc replacement: Introduction and early results from the United States clinical trial. Spine 2003;28: S167-S175.

145. Blumenthal SL, Ohnmeiss DD, Guyer RD, Hochschuler SH: Prospective study evaluating total disc replacement: Preliminary results. J Spinal Disord Tech 2003;16:450-454.

146. Shim CS, Lee SH, Park CW, et al: Partial disc replacement with the PDN prosthetic disc nucleus device. J Spinal Disord Tech 2003;16:324-330.

147. van Ooij A, Oner FC, Verbout AJ: Complications of artificial disc replacement: A report of 27 patients with the SB Charite disc. J Spinal Disord Tech 2003;16:369-383.

148. Tropiano P, Huang RC, Girardi FP, Marnay T: Lumbar disc replacement: Preliminary results with ProDisc II after a minimum follow-up period of 1 year. J Spinal Disord Tech 2003;16:362-368.

149. McAfee PC, Fedder IL, Saiedy S, et al: SB Charite disc replacement: Report of 60 prospective randomized cases in a U.S. center. J Spinal Disord Tech 2003;16:424-433.

150. Kim WJ, Lee SH, Kim SS, Lee C: Treatment of juxtafusional degeneration with artificial disc replacement (ADR): Preliminary results of an ongoing study. J Spinal Disord Tech 2003;16:390-397.

151. Jin D, Qu D, Zhao L, et al: Prosthetic disc nucleus (PDN) replacement for lumbar disc herniation. J Spinal Disord Tech 2003;16:331-337.

152. Zigler JE, Burd TA, Vialle EN, et al: Lumbar spine arthroplasty: Early results using ProDisc II: A prospective randomized trial of arthroplasty versus fusion. J Spinal Disord Tech 2003;16:352-361.

153. Guyer RD, McAfee PC, Hochschuler SH, et al: Prospective randomized study of the Charite artificial disc: Data from two investigational centers. Spine J 2004;4(6 Suppl):252S-259S.

154. Lemaire JP, Carrier H, Ali EH, et al: Clinical and radiological outcomes with the Charite artificial disc. A 10-year minimum follow-up. J Spinal Disord Tech 2005;18:353-359.

155. Blumenthal S, McAfee PC, Guyer RD, et al: A prospective, randomized, multicenter Food and Drug Administration investigational device exemptions study of lumbar total disc replacement with the CHARITE artificial disc versus lumbar fusion. Part I. Evaluation of clinical outcomes. Spine 2005; 30:1565-1575.

156. Cakir B, Richter M, Kafer W, et al: The impact of total lumbar disc replacement on segmental and total lumbar lordosis. Clin Biomech 2005;20:357-364.

157. Tropiano C, Huang RC, Girardi FP, et al: Lumbar total disc replacement. Seven to eleven-year follow-up. Bone Joint Surg (Am) 2005;87:490-496.

158. Schellhas KP, Pollei SR: The role of discography in the evaluation of patients with spinal deformity. Orthop Clin North Am 1994;25:265-273.

159. Tehranzadeh J: Interventional procedures in musculoskeletal radiology: Discography 2000. Radiol Clin North Am 1998; 36:463-495.

160. Yrjama M, Vanharanta H: Bony vibration stimulation: A new, non-invasive method for examining intradiscal pain. Eur Spine J 1994;233-235.

161. Yrjama M, Tervonen O, Kurunlahti M, Vanharanta H: Bony vibration stimulation test combined with magnetic resonance imaging: Can discography be replaced? Spine 1997; 22:808-813.

162. Vanharanta H, Ohnmeiss DD, April CN: Vibration pain provocation can improve the specificity of MRI in the diagnosis of symptomatic lumbar disc rupture. Clin J Pain 1998; 14:239-247.

163. Yrjama M, Tervonen O, Vanharanta H: Ultrasonic imaging of lumbar discs combined with vibration pain provocation compared with discography in the diagnosis of internal

annular fissures of the lumbar spine. Spine 1996;21: 571-574.

164. Stojanovic MP, Cheng Z, Larkin TM, Cohen SP: Psychophysical measurements during lumbar discography: A heart rate response study. J Spinal Disord Tech 2007;20:387-391.

165. Cohen SP, Christo PJ, Moroz L: Pain management in trauma patients. Am J Phys Med Rehabil 2004;83:142-161.

166. Executive Committee of the North American Spine Society: Position statement on discography. Spine 1988;13: 1343.

167. Cohen SP, Williams S, Kurihara C, et al: Nucleoplasty with or without intradiscal electrothermal therapy (IDET) as a treatment for lumbar herniated disc. J Spinal Disord Tech 2005;18S:S119-S124.

168. Abdullah AF, Ditto EW, Byrd EB, Williams R: Extreme-lateral lumbar disc herniations: Clinical syndrome and special problems of diagnosis. J Neurosurg 1974;41:229-234.

169. Perey O: Contrast medium examination of the intervertebral disc of the lower lumbar spine. Acta Orthop Scand 1951; 20:237-334.

170. Edwards WC, Orme TJ, Orr-Edwards G: CT discography: Prognostic value in the selection of patients for chemonucleolysis. Spine 1987;12:792-795.

171. Trosier O, Cypel D: Discography: An element of decision: Surgery vs. chemonucleolysis. Clin Orthop 1986;206:70-78.

172. Singh V, Piryani S, Liao K: Evaluation of percutaneous disc decompression using coablation in chronic back pain with and without leg pain. Pain Physician 2002;6:273-280.

173. Guyer RD, Ohnmeiss DD: NASS: Lumbar discography. Spine J 2003;3(3 Suppl):11S-27S.

174. Guyer RD, Hochschuler SH: Laser disc decompression: The importance of proper patient selection. Spine 1994;19: 2054-2058.

175. Keck C: Discography: Technique and interpretation. Am Arch Surg 1960.

176. Tarver JM, Rathmell JP, Alsofrom GF: Lumbar discography. Reg Anesth Pain Med 2001;26:263-266.

177. Raj PP, Lou L, Serdar E, Staats PS: Lumbar discography. From Clinical Insights on MD Consult Online. Available at: www. mdconsult.com.

178. Sachs BL, Vanharanta H, Spivey MA, et al: Dallas discogram description: A new classification of CT/discography in low-back disorders. Spine 1987;12:287-294.

179. Falco FJ, Moran JG: Lumbar discography using gadolinium in patients with iodine contrast allergy followed by post-discography computed tomography scan. Spine 2003;28: E1-E4.

180. Kumar N, Agorastides ID: The curved needle technique for accessing the L5/S1 disc space. Br J Radiol 2000;73:655-657.

181. Fenton DS, Czervionke LF: Image-Guided Spine Intervention. Philadelphia, Saunders, 2003, pp 227-256.

182. Schellhas KP: Discography. Neuroimag Clin North Am 2000;10:579-596.

183. Cohen SP, Larkin T, Fant GV, et al: Does needle insertion site affect discography results? A retrospective analysis. Spine 2002;27:2279-2283.

184. Kotilainen E, Muittari P, Kirvela O: Intradiscal glycerol or bupivacaine in the treatment of low back pain. Acta Neurochir (Wien) 1997;139:541-545.

185. Benyahya R, Lefevre-Colau MM, Fayad F, et al: Intradiscal injection of acetate of prednisolone in severe low back pain: Complications and patients' assessment of effectiveness. Ann Readapt Med Phys 2004;47:621-626 (in French).

186. Simmons JW, McMillin JN, Emery SF, Kimmich SJ: Intradiscal steroids: A prospective double-blind clinical trial. Spine 1992;17(6Suppl):S172-S155.

187. Khot A, Bowditch M, Powell J, Sharp D: The use of intradiscal steroid therapy for lumbar spinal discogenic pain: A randomized controlled trial. Spine 2004;29:833-836.

188. Guyer RD, Collier R, Stith WJ, et al: Discitis after discography. Spine 1988;13:1352-1354.

189. Silber JS, Anderson DG, Vaccaro AR, et al: Management of postprocedural discitis. Spine J 2002;2:279-287.

190. Fraser RD, Osti OL, Vernon-Roberts B: Discitis after discography. J Bone Joint Surg (Br) 1987;69:26-35.

191. Guyer RD, Ohnmeiss DD: Lumbar discography: Position statement from the North American Spine Society Diagnostic and Therapeutic Committee. Spine 1995;20:2048-2059.

192. Osti OL, Fraser RD, Vernon-Roberts B: Discitis after discography: The role of prophylactic antibiotics. J Bone Joint Surg (Br) 1990;72:271-274.

193. Klessig HT, Showsh SA, Sekorski A: The use of intradiscal antibiotics for discography: An in vitro study of gentamycin, cefazolin and clindamycin. Spine 2003;28:1735-1738.

194. Willems PC, Jacobs W, Duinkerke ES, De Kleuver M: Lumbar discography: Should we use prophylactic antibiotics? A study of 435 consecutive discograms and a systematic review of the literature. J Spinal Disord Tech 2004;17:243-247.

195. Bajwa ZH, Ho C, Grush A, et al: Discitis associated with pregnancy and spinal anesthesia. Anesth Analg 2002;94: 415-416.

196. Iencean SM: Lumbar intervertebral disc herniation following experimental intradiscal pressure increase. Acta Neurochir (Wien) 2000;142:669-676.

197. Poynton AR, Hinman A, Lutz G, Farmer JC: Discography-induced acute lumbar disc herniation: A report of five cases. J Spinal Disord Tech 2005;18:188-192.

198. Carragee EJ, Chen Y, Tanner CM, et al: Can discography cause long-term back symptoms in previously asymptomatic subjects? Spine 2000;25:1803-1808.

199. Carragee EJ, Barcohana B, Alamin T, van den Haak E: Prospective controlled study of the development of lower back pain in previously asymptomatic subjects undergoing experimental discography. Spine 2004;29:1112-1117.

200. Johnson RG: Does discography injure normal discs? An analysis of repeat discograms. Spine 1989;14:424-426.

201. Flanagan MN, Chung BU: Roentgenographic changes in 188 patients 10-20 years after discography and chemonucleolysis. Spine 1986;11:444-448.

202. Saifuddin A, Renton P, Taylor BA: Effects on the vertebral end-plate of uncomplicated lumbar discography: An MRI study. Eur Spine J 1998;7:36-39.

203. Tallroth K, Soini K, Antti-Poika I, et al: Premedication and short term complications in iohexol discography. Ann Chir Gynaecol 1991;80:49-53.

204. Zeidman SM, Thompson K, Ducker TB: Complications of cervical discography: Analysis of 4400 diagnostic disc injections. Neurosurgery 1995;37:414-417.

205. Roosen K, Bettag W, Fiebach O: Complications of cervical discography. ROFO Fortschr Geb Rontgenstr Nuklearmed 1975;122:520-527 (in German).

206. Junila J, Niinimaki T, Tervonen O: Epidural abscess after lumbar discography: A case report. Spine 1997;22:2191-2193.

207. deSeze S, Levernieux J: Les accidents de la discographie. Rev Rhum Mal Osteoartic 1952;19:1027-1033.

208. Goldie I: Intervertebral disc changes after discography. Acta Chir Scand 1957;113:438-439.

209. Grubb SA, Lipscomb HJ, Guilford W: The relative value of lumbar roentgenograms, metrizamide myelography, and discography in the assessment of patients with chronic low-back syndrome. Spine 1987;12:282-286.

210. McCulloch JA, Waddell G: Lateral lumbar discography. Br J Radiol 1978;51:498-502.

CHAPTER

60 Intradiskal Procedures for the Management of Low Back Pain

Brock Gretter and Nagy Mekhail

Most people suffer significant enough back pain at some point in their lives that their normal daily activities will be disrupted.[1] Most of these cases resolve with conservative management but approximately 5% or more of these will suffer chronic pain and functional impairment.[2] As many as 60% of patients suffer recurrent or persistent low back pain (LBP).[3] An estimated 3% to 50% of all causes of LBP are "discogenic" from internal disk disruption (IDD). In this chapter, we discuss the anatomy, pathogenesis, diagnosis, and treatment of IDD.

DEFINITION

IDD is a pathologic condition in which the internal structure of the disk is disrupted while the external surface remains normal.[3]

ANATOMY

The intervertebral disk is composed of an inner nucleus pulposus and, surrounding that circumferentially, an outer annulus fibrosis. The disk is bounded superiorly and inferiorly by the vertebral end plates. The nucleus pulposus is not innervated—only the outer portion of the annulus fibrosis is normally innervated. Three types of nerves provide this innervation. The gray rami communicantes (from the sympathetic chain) innervate the lateral edges of the annulus fibrosis while the lumbar ventral rami innervate the anterior edges of the annulus fibrosis. The sinuvertebral nerves innervate the posterior wall of the annulus and posterior longitudinal ligament.[4,5] The sinuvertebral nerves contain a somatic component from the ventral ramus and an autonomic component from the gray ramus communicans.[5]

PATHOGENESIS

Mechanical loading to areas of degenerated and disrupted lamellae causes sensitization of the annular nociceptors.[6,7] In response, neovascularization, neuronal penetration with unmyelinated nerve fibers, and ingrowth of Schwann cells occurs.[8-10] The nucleus pulposus contains chemicals and peptides that may leak into the outer annular layers or beyond and irritate neuronal tissue. These inflammatory chemicals include tumor necrosis factor-alpha, matrix metalloproteinases, phospholipase A_2, cyclooxygenase, prostaglandins, nitric oxide, cytokines, and interleukins.[3,11] Granulation tissue, growing into the annular tear, also can irritate nerves.

DIAGNOSIS OF DISCOGENIC PAIN

Diagnosing IDD as the source of a patient's back pain is a challenge because there is no gold standard test that can confirm IDD as the primary cause. Imaging studies like magnetic resonance imaging (MRI) can detect disk abnormalities but MRI can not correlate anatomic changes with pain. Disks that appear abnormal on MRI may not be painful; disks that display degenerative morphology on the MRI occur in a similar frequency in symptomatic and asymptomatic patients.[12] Although MRI is quite sensitive, some disk abnormalities, such as annular tears, may not be detected on MRI. Discography appears to be useful in detecting such small tears in an attempt to correlate anatomic changes with pain.

The diagnosis of discogenic pain begins with history and physical examination. The symptoms of discogenic pain are nonspecific and classically include nonradicular back pain that is worsened in the sitting position (Box 60–1). Discogenic pain is often provoked by bending and may involve the buttock, hip, groin, and thighs. There is generally a notable lack of signs on physical examination. Conservative treatments such as stabilization exercise training, back education, activity modification, epidural steroid injections, and facet injections are often attempted at this stage.[4] If the pain is unresolved, subsequent diagnostic steps may be taken including imaging

BOX 60–1. CRITERIA FOR DIAGNOSIS OF DISCOGENIC PAIN

Lumbar spine pain greater than 6 months
Sitting intolerance
Normal neurologic examination
Negative straight-leg raise
Magnetic resonance imaging: no nerve root compression
Concordant pain on discography
Positive functional discography

Table 60–1. Classification of Levels of Evidence

Level I	Conclusive: research-based evidence with multiple relevant and high-quality scientific studies or consistent review of meta-analyses
Level II	Strong: research-based evidence from at least one properly designed randomized controlled trial; or research-based evidence from multiple properly designed studies of smaller size; or multiple low-quality trials
Level III	Moderate: (1) evidence obtained from well-designed pseudo-randomized controlled trials (alternate allocation or some other method); (2) evidence obtained from comparative studies with concurrent controls and allocation not randomized (cohort studies, case-controlled studies, or interrupted time series with a control group); (3) evidence obtained from comparative studies with historical control, two or more single-arm studies, or interrupted time series without a parallel control group
Level IV	Limited: evidence from well-designed nonexperimental studies from more than one center or research group; or conflicting evidence with inconsistent findings in multiple trials
Level V	Indeterminate: Opinions of respected authorities based on clinical evidence, descriptive studies, or report of expert committees

Data from reference 14.

studies such as computed tomography (CT) or MRI. For IDD, MRI is the morphologic imaging study of choice for low back pain.[13] Typically, a high-intensity zone is seen on T2 sagittal images, indicating an annular tear. The postcontrast T1 view also is used and considered to be the most sensitive for annular tears. On this image, granulation tissue may enhance. Often, the MRI is equivocal, so further diagnostic intervention, namely discography, is required.

Many authors agree that discography is indicated for chronic back pain that is unresponsive to conservative measures. Discography is a provocative and invasive diagnostic test that can help identify annular defects in a manner that can reproduce a patient's pain. It involves opacification of the nucleus pulposus by pressurized injection with contrast medium. This allows visualization of defects in the annulus fibrosis, which may simultaneously provoke a patient's back pain. When this correlation is found, the procedure is said to produce concordant pain. Concordancy is highly suggestive of an IDD cause. Discography is more sensitive than MRI, plain radiographs, or myelography in the diagnosis of anatomic disk abnormalities.[13] Discography has a significant false-positive rate. Healthy patients have been shown in several trials to exhibit false-positive results.[13] Often this is attributed to painless degenerative change, especially seen in the aging population. This emphasizes the need for demonstration of both morphologic abnormality and concordant pain to have a positive result. For a more detailed discussion, refer to Chapter 59.

A meta-analysis of 71 most relevant studies using Agency for Healthcare Research and Quality (AHRQ) and Quality of individual Articles of Diagnostic Studies (QUADAS) scoring systems reported "evidence is strong for the diagnostic accuracy of discography as an imaging tool. Evidence is also strong for the ability of discography to evoke pain. There is strong evidence supporting the role of discography in identifying that subset of patients with lumbar discogenic pain. There is moderate evidence supporting the role of discography in identifying a subset of patients with cervical discogenic pain. There is limited evidence supporting the role of discography in identifying a subset of patients with thoracic discogenic pain"(p. 203).[14] In this study, evidence was classified into five levels: conclusive (level I), strong, moderate, limited, and indeterminate (level V) (Table 60–1).

The American Society of Interventional Pain Physicians (ASIPP) has set forth the following guidelines to help physicians decide when to perform discography[11]:

- Further evaluation of demonstrably abnormal disks to help assess the extent of abnormality or correlation of the abnormality with clinical symptoms (in case of recurrent pain from a previously operated disk and a lateral disk herniation)
- Patients with persistent, severe symptoms in whom other diagnostic tests have failed to reveal clear confirmation of a suspected disk as the source of pain
- Assessment of patients who have failed to respond to surgical procedures to determine if there is painful pseudarthrosis or a symptomatic disk in a posteriorly fused segment, or to evaluate possible recurrent disk herniation
- Assessment of disks before fusion to determine if the disks within the proposed fusion segment are symptomatic and to determine if disks adjacent to this segment are normal
- Assessment of minimally invasive surgical candidates to confirm a contained disk herniation or to investigate contrast distribution pattern before intradiskal procedures

Technique

Discography should be performed in an outpatient surgical or radiologic suite under aseptic conditions. Antibiotic prophylaxis is recommended for all intradiskal procedures, and may be administered either intradiskally or intravenously.[15,16] Some of the suggested prophylactic doses are summarized in Table 60–2.

Subjects may be premedicated with midazolam. Patients are placed in a prone position. Monitoring should be performed, and this commonly includes blood pressure, pulse oximetry, and electrocardiogram (ECG) analysis. A fluoroscopic examination is performed to identify the segments to be tested. The segments to be included are the diseased segments and a control level. Local anesthetic is injected along the projected needle course and an introducer needle is inserted. Physicians vary in the type of introducer used. One protocol recommends using a 20-gauge, 3.5-inch introducer needle that is advanced toward the targeted disk.[17] Through the introducer, a 25-gauge, 6-inch needle is passed until its tip is located in the center of the disk. Annular resistance to the needle should be assessed subjectively and compared between levels. Position should be confirmed with perpendicular views (anteroposterior and lateral). Opening pressures (Table 60–3) are recorded if a pressure-measuring device is used. Nonionic contrast is then injected into the disk, ideally using a controlled injection system with pressure readout (Fig.

60–1). Manual injection is sometimes used with the operator subjectively recording resistance to injection. Patients should be awake and alert at the time of injection so they may report evoked pain. Patients are asked to rate the pain on a 0-to-10 scale before and during injection.

The suggested end points to injection include the following: pain severity of 5/10 or greater that lasts at least 30 seconds; intradiskal pressure of 80 to 100 pounds per square inch (psi); and a total of 3.5 mL of contrast medium injected.[17] On reaching an end point, anteroposterior (AP) and lateral images should be assessed to record the distribution of contrast medium. Specifically, the examiner determines if dye has leaked outside the disk through a fissure in the annulus fibrosis. After the control level and the test

Table 60–2. Proposed Antibiotic Coverage for Discography

DRUG	DOSE	SPECIAL USE
Cefazolin	1-2 g intravenous (IV) 30 minutes before procedure, or 1-10 mg/mL with intradiskal contrast	
Clindamycin	600 mg IV 30 minutes before procedure, or 7.5 mg/mL with intradiskal contrast	Beta lactam allergy
Vancomycin	1 g IV over 60 minutes before procedure	Documented methicillin-resistant *Staphylococcus aureus* (MRSA) carriers

Data from references 15 and 16.

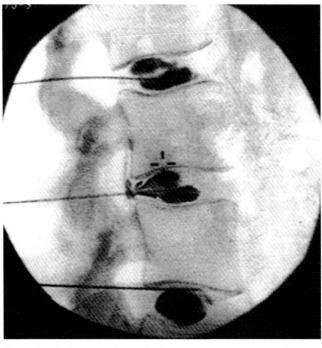

Figure 60–1. Discography under fluoroscopy. Lateral view showing control levels above and below with abnormal level between. The abnormal level demonstrates a posterior fissure.

Table 60–3. Discographic Diagnostic Categories

DISK CLASSIFICATION	INTRADISKAL PRESSURE AT PAIN PROVOCATION	PAIN SEVERITY	PAIN TYPE	RULING
Chemical	Immediate onset of familiar pain occurring as <1 mL of contrast is visualized reaching the outer annulus, or pain provocation at <15 pounds per square inch (psi) above opening pressure	≥6/10	Concordant	Positive
Mechanical	Between 15 and 50 psi (above opening pressure)	≥6/10	Concordant	Positive (but other pain generators may be present; further investigation may be warranted)
Indeterminate	Between 51 and 90 psi	≥6/10	Concordant	Further investigation warranted
Normal	>90 psi	No pain		Negative

Data from reference 50.

levels are completed, patients may be sent for post-discography CT scan, preferably within 4 hours of the discography.[17]

Additionally, functional discography may be performed to further aid diagnosis of concordant pain.[18] This procedure is a variant of discography as mentioned earlier. After the disk is pressurized and data recorded, a thin balloon-tipped catheter is advanced through the introducer into the nucleus pulposus. This catheter has one port to inject medications into the nucleus and another port attached to a balloon at the tip of the catheter. This catheter system is left in place while the introducer needle is withdrawn, and the patient is taken to the recovery room. While there, the balloon is inflated and the patient is instructed to perform pain-eliciting activities (such as sitting upright). At this point, a physician injects 0.5 to 0.7 mL of 4% lidocaine in an attempt to eliminate the patient's pain. This situation further confirms the diagnosis of IDD with concordant pain.

Complications

The incidence of complications during discography approximates 0.6%—the most feared is diskitis.[19] The intervertebral disks have poor blood supply, likely making them more susceptible to infectious complications. Willems and associates noted that the incidence of diskitis without prophylactic antibiotics was 0.25%.[20] Others reported a zero incidence of diskitis with prophylactic antibiotic use.[5] Recent published guidelines suggested the routine use of prophylactic antibiotics.[15] The diagnosis of postprocedural diskitis requires a high index of suspicion; it typically presents as worsening back pain in the week after discography. The most sensitive laboratory indicators of diskitis are erythrocyte sedimentation rate and C-reactive protein; these values peak 3 weeks after the procedure. The most common causative organism in diskitis is *Staphylococcus aureus*.[5,21,22]

Treatment

The initial conservative treatment for IDD generally includes the following modalities:
- Physical therapy
- Activity modification
- Rest
- Chiropractic care
- Manual therapy
- Medications

Treatments may also include epidural or intradiskal steroid injections and acupuncture. Invasively, surgical treatment is another option. Surgical arthrodesis commonly involves disk excision combined with instrumented interbody fusion to provide stabilization.[23]

INTRADISKAL ELECTROTHERMAL THERAPY

Intradiskal electrothermal therapy (IDET) is a minimally invasive technique in which a thermal resistance catheter is placed percutaneously in the posterolateral disk and converts radiofrequency energy to heat. Heat causes collagen of the annulus fibrosis to contract. On the molecular level, the triple helix of collagen fibers is cross-linked by hydrogen bonds that are heat sensitive. On exposure to heat these hydrogen bonds are disrupted, causing collapse of the molecular strands and resulting in a new contracted molecule; it appears to maximally contract at approximately 75 degrees. This technique has been used in other applications such glenohumeral joint capsule disease.[4] The heat also causes neural blockade, by the same mechanism that is therapeutic in radiofrequency lesioning of other neural structures, such as medial branch nerves in facet-mediated pain states. Intervertebral disks are excellent candidate structures for heating procedures because the disk is virtually avascular, so heat does not travel as easily in it as in other structures. This allows heat to be held in a specific area of the disk while peripheral structures, which are more vascularized, quickly dissipate any escaping heat.[4]

Technique

IDET should be performed in a similar setting to discography, with the same recommendations regarding antibiotic prophylaxis, positioning, monitoring, and premedication. A fluoroscopic examination is performed to identify the segments to be tested. Local anesthetic is injected along the projected needle course. The side entered is contralateral to the lesion. A 17-gauge introducer needle is inserted until it contacts the annulus fibrosis. Through the introducer, the flexible electrode is advanced until it assumes a circumferential position either within the annulus fibrosis or between the nucleus pulposus and the annulus fibrosis. Efforts should be made to avoid kinking the catheter because this can lead to breakage. The catheter contains proximal and distal radiopaque markers; the portion in between the markers should cover the posterior wall of the annulus and as much as possible of the lateral walls. When satisfactory placement is confirmed by AP and lateral images (Fig. 60–2), the electrode is gradually heated. The heating protocol suggested by one manufacturer, and used at our institution, is as follows: heat catheter to 90° C if tolerated, and maintain for 4 minutes at that temperature. The warm-up time to achieve 90° is 12.5 minutes, so the total heating duration is 16.5 minutes. If the patient does not tolerate 90° because of pain, heating is performed at 85° for 5 minutes. If that temperature is not tolerated, heating is performed at 80° for 5 minutes. Patients may be administered analgesics, but must be able to report radicular pain. If the patient has radicular pain then the heating should be stopped and the catheter repositioned. After the procedure, patients often experience an increase in their typical pain, which subsides in about a week.[24-26]

After the procedure, patients are advised to rest for 1 to 3 days. This includes limiting sitting or walking

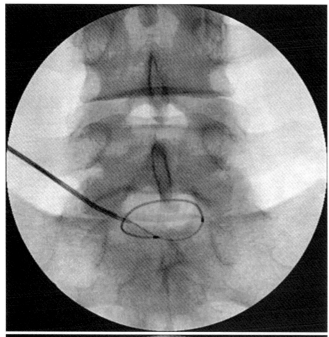

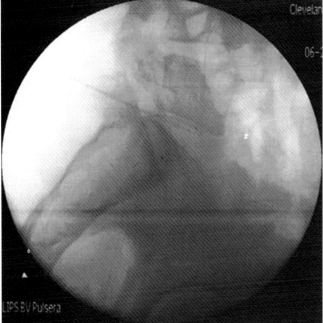

Figure 60–2. Intradiskal electrothermal therapy (IDET) images under fluoroscopy. Top image shows anteroposterior view of the IDET catheter placed in L5-S1 intervertebral disk. Lower image is a lateral view of the same catheter placement.

to 10 to 20 minutes at a time, and instead reclining or lying down. During the postprocedure period, until 6 to 8 weeks have elapsed, patients are instructed to wear a lumbar corset to restrict movement. One week postprocedure, patients may begin low-impact activities including sedentary work, driving with lumbar support for up to 20 to 30 minutes, and lifting up to 5 to 10 pounds. Until 6 weeks postprocedure, patients are advised to not bend or twist the low back; lift more than 5 to 10 pounds, or perform a formalized physical therapy program. Patients may return to sedentary work in 1 week. After this time they are to enter a formal physical therapy program.[4]

Complications

In a recent review, 23 complications were reported in 486 patients in 12 studies, with an overall incidence of complications as 0.8%.[25] As with discography, the most feared complication is diskitis. The following is a list of actual or theoretical complications[25,27,28]:

- Nerve root injury
- Radicular pain
- Headache
- Nondermatomal leg pain
- Dural puncture
- Worsening pain
- Catheter kinking or breakage
- Infection: osteonecrosis, epidural abscess, diskitis
- Cauda equina syndrome
- Bleeding
- Disk herniation
- Spinal cord damage

Efficacy

A meta-analysis of 17 studies using a random effects model showed IDET to be an efficacious procedure.[25] As shown in Table 60–4, IDET resulted in improvement across each of four outcome scales.[25-41] The Visual Analogue Scale (VAS) is a 0-to-10 ranking of pain. The mean decrease in VAS was 2.9. The physical function of Medical Outcomes Survey, SF-36 is a 1-to-100 assessment of a patient's ability to perform physical activities while the bodily pain of SF-36 is a 0-to-100 assessment of pain severity.[42] The mean improvement in SF-36 was 21.1. The Oswestry Dis-

Table 60–4. Summary of a Meta-analysis Study on the Efficacy of Intradiskal Electrothermal Therapy

OUTCOME	NUMBER OF SUBJECTS	MEAN IMPROVEMENT CHANGE	95% CI
Visual Analogue Scale	503	2.9	2.5, 3.4
Physical function of SF-36	196	21.1	13.4, 28.8
Bodily pain of SF-36	196	18	11.9, 24.1
Oswestry Disability Index	79	7	2.0, 11.9

Data from references 25 through 41.
SF-36, medical outcomes survey.

Table 60–5. Comparison of Intradiskal Electrothermal Therapy and Surgical Fusion in Patients with Internal Disk Disruption

	OUTCOMES	Spinal Fusion			Intradiskal Electrothermal Therapy		
		NO. (OF 33)	MEDIAN % CHANGE	RANGE	NO. (OF 18)	MEDIAN % CHANGE	RANGE
Pain severity (VAS)*	RCT	6	36	30-77	1	36	NA
	NCT	1	NA	37-52	2	63	NA
	BA	8	61	42-75	8	50	22-71
	CS	11	53	24-62	1	64	NA
Back-specific impairment (Oswestry)†	RCT	8	40	17-73	2	20	4-35
	NCT	1	NA	39-54	0	NA	7-24
	BA	2	NA	58-77	3	14	
	CS	6	42	17-49	0	NA	
Quality of life (e.g., SF-36)‡	RCT	5	43	21-123	2	17	7-27
	NCT	0	NA		0	NA	
	BA	1	110	NA	6	49	22-76
	CS	0	NA		0	NA	

*Pain severity is measured by VAS.
†Impairment is measured by Oswestry Disability Index.
‡Quality of life is measured by either SF-36 physical functioning domain or physical component summary score.
BA, prospective before-after trial; CS, retrospective case series; NA, not applicable; NCT, nonrandomized controlled trial; RCT, randomized controlled trial; VAS, Visual Analogue Scale.
Data from reference 39.

ability Index is a 0-to-100 assessment of limitation from pain.[43] The mean improvement in Oswestry index was 7.

Andersson and colleagues compared the efficacies of IDET and surgical fusion in patients with IDD.[44] This evaluation is particularly relevant because these two interventions are the more invasive treatments, used when more conservative measures have failed. In this review, symptoms were improved similarly after both IDET and surgical fusion. The complication rate appeared to be much less with IDET, and performing IDET does not prohibit surgical fusion in the future (Table 60–5).

Patient selection appears to play an important role in determining success of IDET. A study reported a mean decrease in VAS of five points in patients who were not involved in workers compensation cases.[40] This was a significant improvement compared to patients involved in workers compensation cases. Also, overweight patients or patients with multilevel degenerative disk disease with three or more degenerated levels shown on MRI are unlikely to benefit from IDET.[27,41] IDET is more likely to be beneficial in selected disks that have greater than 50% disk height compared with adjacent intervertebral disks.[40] The physician's experience may affect IDET success. It has been suggested that the current IDET catheter creates a lesion that may be too small to correct disk pathology.[45]

A new alternative to IDET is transdiskal biacuplasty. This procedure involves first inserting two electrodes posterolaterally in a diseased disk, positioned in the annulus fibrosis (Fig. 60–3). Then the electrodes are heated, creating lesions between the electrodes in the posterior annulus. While the heating proceeds, the electrodes are internally cooled. This procedure has the theoretical advantage of a more homogeneous and thorough heating of the annulus than what the IDET is able to accomplish.[46] There is no published data on its efficacy yet, but it is promising as a future alternative to IDET.

PERCUTANEOUS DISK DECOMPRESSION

Percutaneous disk decompression, or nucleotomy, is a procedure that removes central disk substance, with or without destruction of minute areas of that disk. Annular tears may permit leakage of nuclear material outside the disk. This leakage can initiate, promote, and continue the inflammatory process, causing a chronically painful condition. In addition, continued leakage can delay or stop resorption of the disk. Central nuclear decompression causes low pressure in the nucleus, permitting a herniated disk to more easily resorb so the painful inflammatory cycle is interrupted. The most common new decompressive technique is nucleoplasty. In nucleoplasty, a 17-gauge cannula is used to introduce a device with multiple small electrodes into the center of the disk. Radiofrequency (RF) energy is applied creating a small plasma field of ionized particles that are removed from the disk by suction. Variations of this procedure have been used since the 1960s but today's newer techniques use RF energy with the relatively small 17-gauge introducer cannula. The efficacy of nucleoplasty in reducing back pain is less well studied than for IDET.[3]

Discography is performed as part of the decision-making process to perform nucleotomy. Nucleoplasty has been performed to treat small- to moderate-sized disk herniations that cause compressive or inflammatory-type pathology. Nucleoplasty has also been performed to treat disks that have demonstrated annular tears on discography even when there is not a significant protrusion.[3] In such disks, it is thought

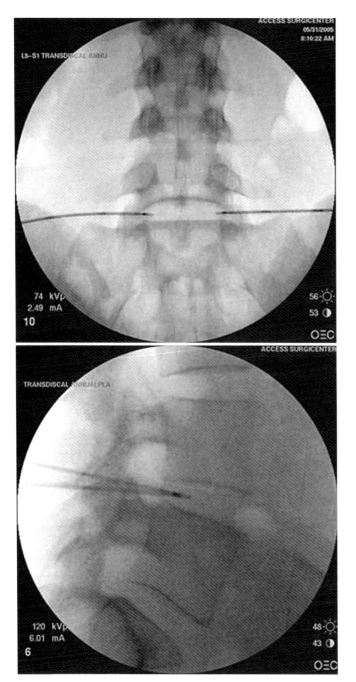

Figure 60–3. Transdiskal biacuplasty images under fluoroscopy. Top image shows anteroposterior view demonstrating correct placement of electrodes in the annulus fibrosus. Bottom image shows lateral view demonstrating correct electrode placements in the disk.

that there are subligamentous protrusions that are contributing to a patient's pain. In each of these conditions, physicians believe that a reduction in intradiskal pressure will likely improve symptoms.

Singh and Derby proposed the following as contra-indications to percutaneous disk decompression[3]:

- Large noncontained disk herniation, sequestration, or extrusion
- Equivocal results of provocative and analgesic discogram
- Infection
- Cauda equina syndrome or newly developed signs of neurologic deficit
- Patients unable to understand informed consent protocol
- Uncontrolled coagulopathy and bleeding disorders

Technique

For nucleoplasty, the patient preparation, antibiotic prophylaxis, monitoring, and positioning are similar for discography and IDET. Singh and colleagues used the following technique, which is similar that used at our institution: a 17-gauge cannula is used to access the disk space on the same side as the pain or lesion.[47] The cannula is advanced to approximately the junction of the annulus and the disk. The combined ablation and coagulation wand is advanced through the cannula into the nucleus. The wand is used in ablation mode and is advanced farther into the nucleus at approximately 0.5 cm/second. Then the wand is retracted in coagulation mode. This is done six times to create six channels. Postoperatively, activity is significantly restricted in a similar manner to after the IDET procedure.

Complications

The complications for nucleotomy are similar to that for the other percutaneous intradiskal procedures, mentioned in the discography and IDET sections. Complications that are specific to nucleoplasty include probe tip fracture as it is forced against an end plate, and occlusion of the probe by nuclear material during suctioning.[3]

Efficacy

Three prospective studies have evaluated the efficacy of nucleoplasty. Each has shown that nucleoplasty is beneficial in the majority of patients, with good short-term results.[11,47-49] The results at 1 year are favorable, but less so. This is shown in Table 60–6.

Table 60–6.   Efficacy of Percutaneous Disk Decompression

AUTHORS	NUMBER OF PATIENTS	INITIAL RELIEF	RELIEF AT 1 YEAR
Singh et al, 2002[48]	67	82%	56%
Sharps and Isaac 2002[49]	49	79%	79%
Singh et al, 2005[47]	47	80%	53%

CONCLUSION

Internal disk disruption is a condition in which the internal structure of the disk is disrupted. It is characterized by nonradicular low back pain aggravated by axial loading as in the sitting position. Discogenic pain is diagnosed by the presence of concordant pain on discography. IDET appears to be effective in patients with discogenic low back pain secondary to an annular tear. Percutaneous disk decompression, specifically nucleoplasty, has been used in the treatment of small to moderate-sized contained disk herniations. It appears to be effective in the short term but with decreased success rate at 1-year follow-up.

References

1. Deyo RA, Cherkin D, Conrad D, Violinn E: Cost, controversy, crisis: Low back pain and the health of the public. Annu Rev Public Health 1991;12:141-156.
2. Carey TS, Garrett JM, Jackman AM: Beyond the good prognosis: Examination of an inception cohort of patients with chronic low back pain. Spine 2000;25:115-120.
3. Singh V, Derby R: Percutaneous lumbar disc decompression. Pain Physician 2006;9(2):139-146.
4. Saal JA, Saal JS: Intradiscal electrothermal therapy for the treatment of chronic discogenic low back pain. Clin Sports Med 2002;21:167-187.
5. Cohen SP, Larkin TM, Barna SA, et al: Lumbar discography: A comprehensive review of outcome studies, diagnostic accuracy, and principles. Reg Anesth Pain Med 2005;30:163-184.
6. Osti OL, Vernon-Roberts B, Fraser RD: 1990 Volvo award in experimental studies. Annulus tears and intervertebral disc degeneration: An experimental study using an animal model. Spine 1990;15:762-767.
7. Osti OL, Vernon-Roberts B, Moore R, Fraser RD: Annular tears and disc degeneration in the lumbar spine: A post-mortem study of 135 discs. J Bone Joint Surg (Br)1992;74:678-682.
8. Coppes MH, Marani E, Thomeer RT, Groen GJ: Innervation of "painful" lumbar discs. Spine 1997;22:2342-2349.
9. Freemont AJ, Peacock TE, Goupille P, et al: Nerve ingrowth into diseased intervertebral disc in chronic back pain. Lancet 1997;350:178-181.
10. Johnson WE, Evans H, Menage J, et al: Immunohistochemical detection of Schwann cells in innervated and vascularized human intervertebral discs. Spine 2001;26:2550-2557.
11. Boswell MV, Shah RV, Everett CR, et al: Interventional techniques in the management of chronic spinal pain: Evidence-based practice guidelines. Pain Physician 2005;8:1-47.
12. Buirski G, Silberstein M: The symptomatic lumbar disc in patients with low-back pain: Magnetic resonance imaging appearances in both a symptomatic and control population. Spine 1993;18:1808-1811.
13. Resnick DK, Malone DG, Ryken TC: Guidelines for the use of discography for the diagnosis of painful degenerative lumbar disc disease. Neurosurg Focus 2002;13:E1-E6.
14. Shah RV, Everett CR, McKenzie-Brown AM, Sehgal N: Discography as a diagnostic test for spinal pain: A systematic and narrative review. Pain Physician 2005;8:187-209.
15. Rathmell JP, Lake T, Ramundo MB: Infectious risks of chronic pain treatments: Injection therapy, surgical implants, and intradiscal techniques. Reg Anesth Pain Med 2006;31:346-352.
16. Mangram AJ, Horan TC, Pearson ML, et al: Guideline for prevention of surgical site infection. Hospital Infection Control Practices Advisory Committee. Infect Control Hosp Epidemiol 1999;20:250-278.
17. Derby R, Lee SH, Kim BJ, et al: Pressure-controlled lumbar discography in volunteers without low back symptoms. Pain Med 2005;6:213-221.
18. Kyphon Inc: Product information brochure on Discyphor Catheter System for the functional anaesthetic discography procedure. Kyphon Inc, Sunnyvale, Calif.
19. Zeidman SM, Thompson K, Ducker TB: Complications of cervical discography: Analysis of 4400 diagnostic disc injections. Neurosurgery 1995;37:414-417.
20. Willems PC, Jacobs W, Duinkerke ES, DeKleuver M: Lumbar discography: Should we use prophylactic antibiotics? A study of 435 consecutive discograms and a systematic review of the literature. J Spinal Disord Technol 2004;17:243-247.
21. Guyer RD, Collier R, Stith WJ, et al: Discitis after discography. Spine 1998;13:1352-1354.
22. Silber JS, Anderson DG, Vaccaro AR, et al: Management of postprocedural discitis. Spine J 2002;2:279-287.
23. Hanley EN, Davis SM: Lumbar arthrodesis for the treatment of back pain. J Bone Joint Surg (Am) 1999;81:716-730.
24. Saal JA, Saal JS: Intradiscal electrothermal treatment for chronic discogenic low back pain: Prospective outcome study with a minimum 2-year follow-up. Spine 2002;27:966-974.
25. Appleby D, Andersson G, Totta M: Meta-analysis of the efficacy and safety of intradiscal electrothermal therapy (IDET). Pain Med 2006;7:308-316.
26. Pauza KJ, Howell S, Dreyfuss P, et al: A randomized, placebo-controlled trial of intradiscal electrothermal therapy for the treatment of discogenic low back pain. Spine J 2004;4:27-35.
27. Cohen SP, Larkin T, Abdi S, et al: Risk factors for failure and complications of intradiscal electrothermal theapy: A pilot study. Spine 2003;28:1142-1147.
28. Djurasovic M, Glassman S, Dimar J, Johnson J: Vertebral osteonecrosis associated with the use of intradiscal electrothermal therapy: A case report. Spine 2002;27:325-328.
29. Bogduk N, Karasek M: Two-year follow-up of a controlled trial of intradiscal electrothermal annuloplasty for chronic low back pain resulting from internal disc disruption. Spine J 2002;2:343-350.
30. Wetzel T, McNally T, Phillips F: Intradiscal electrothermal therapy used to manage chronic discogenic low back pain. Spine 2002;27:2621-2626.
31. Lutz C, Lutz GE, Cooke PM: Treatment of chronic lumbar discogenic pain with intradiskal electrothermal therapy: A prospective outcome study. Arch Phys Med Rehabil 2003;84:23-28.
32. Derby R, Bjorn E, Yung C, et al: Intradiscal electrothermal annuloplasty (IDET): A novel approach for treating chronic discogenic back pain. Neuromodulation 2000;3:82-88.
33. Spruit M, Jacobs WC: Pain and function after intradiscal electrothermal treatment (IDET) for symptomatic lumbar disc degeneration. Eur Spine J 2002;11:589-597.
34. Gerszten PC, Welch WC, McGrath PM, Willis SL: A prospective outcome study of patients undergoing intradiscal electrothermy (IDET) for chronic low back pain. Pain Physician 2002;5:360-364.
35. Singh V: Intradiscal electrothermal therapy: A preliminary report. Pain Physician 2000;3:367-373.
36. Endres SM, Fiedler GA, Larson K: Effectiveness of intradiscal electrothermal therapy in increasing function and reducing chronic low back pain in selected patients. Wisconsin Med J 2002;101:31-34.
37. Freedman BA, Cohen SP, Kuklo TR, et al: Intradiscal electrothermal therapy (IDET) for chronic low back pain in active-duty soldiers: 2-year follow-up. Spine J 2003;3:502-509.
38. Lee M, Cooper G, Lutz C, Hong H: Intradiscal electrothermal therapy (IDET) for treatment of chronic lumbar discogenic pain: A minimum 2-year clinical outcome study. Pain Physician 2003;6:443-448.
39. Davis TT, Delamarter RB, Sra P, Goldstein TB: The IDET procedure for chronic discogenic low back pain. Spine 2004;29:752-756.
40. Mekhail N, Kapural L: Intradiscal thermal annuloplasty for discogenic pain: An outcome study. Pain Pract 2004;4:84-90.
41. Kapural L, Mekhail N, Korunda Z, Basali A: Intradiscal thermal annuloplasty for the treatment of lumbar discogenic pain in patients with multilevel degenerative disc disease. Anesth Analg 2004;99:472-476.

42. Ware JE, Snow KK, Kosinski M, Gandek B: SF-36 Health Survey Manual and Interpretation Guide. Boston, New England Medical Center, The Health Institute, 1993.

43. Fairbank J, Couper J, Davies J, et al: The Oswestry low back pain questionnaire. Physiotherapy 1980;66:271-273.

44. Andersson GB, Mekhail NA, Block JE: Treatment of intractable discogenic low back pain: A systematic review of spinal fusion and intradiscal electrothermal therapy (IDET). Pain Physician 2006;9:237-248.

45. Bogduk N, Lau P, Govind J, Karasek M: Intraediscal electrothermal therapy. Tech Reg Anesth Pain Manage 2005;9:25-34.

46. Product information on transdiscal biacuplasty. Baylis Medical Corporation, Montreal, Canada. Available at: www.transdiscal.com.

47. Singh V, Piryani C, Liao K: Role of percutaneous disc decompression using coblation in managing chronic discogenic low back pain: A prospective, observational study. Pain Physician 2005;7:419-426.

48. Singh V, Piryani C, Liao K, Nieschultz S: Percutaneous disc decompression using coblation (nucleoplasty) in the treatment of discogenic pain. Pain Physician 2002;5:250-259.

49. Sharps LS, Isaac Z: Percutaneous disc decompression using nucleoplasty. Pain Physician 2002;5:121-126.

50. Derby R, Howard M, Grant JM, et al: The ability of pressure-controlled discography to predict surgical and nonsurgical outcomes. Spine 1999;24:364-371.

CHAPTER

61 Minimally Invasive Procedures for Vertebral Compression Fractures

Amol Soin and Nagy Mekhail

Osteoporosis is a common disease affecting older adults. A common complication of osteoporosis is vertebral compression fracture (VCF). Although the majority of fractures are asymptomatic, with two thirds of them found incidentally on a chest x-ray,[1] they are capable of creating debilitating pain. Symptomatic patients often report no history of trauma. Minor activities such as bending over suddenly, lifting objects, and coughing all have been associated with developing VCFs.[2] An estimated 700,000 vertebral fractures occur annually in the United States.[3] VCFs occur at various vertebral levels, but most commonly at the thoracolumbar junction.[4]

In addition to being a common cause of chronic pain, VCFs have significant socioeconomic impact. It has been estimated that the annual costs of osteoporotic fractures are as high as $13.8 billion.[5-7] Clinically, patients with untreated VCFs suffer from a decrease in vertebral body height, kyphosis, decreased mobility leading to atelectasis, pneumonia, deep venous thrombosis, and loss of independence sometimes necessitating nursing home stays or hospital admission. The prevalence reaches as high as 40% in 80-year-old women,[8] and 26% in women older than age 50.

Two of the newer modalities to treat VCFs include vertebroplasty and kyphoplasty. Vertebroplasty involves the injection of the vertebral body with polymethylmethacrylate (PMMA), whereas kyphoplasty involves the creation of a cavity prior to cement injections with the use of balloons in an inflation and deflation sequence. It is believed that these procedures lead to restoration of some of the lost vertebral height and decrease the stress placed on the vertebrae below, which in turn produces analgesia. Both of these procedures can be done percutaneously.[9] One of the newer modalities for percutaneous vertebral augmentation is a central cavity creation. This variation of vertebroplasty involves manually creating a cavity to inject a more viscous form of cement and may produce some height restoration.

One of the advantages of the percutaneous technique is the fact that it is minimally invasive and requires little or no hospital stay. The majority of patients suffering from vertebral compression fractures are older adults. As such, they often have comorbidities that place them at a higher risk for anesthetic complications from more invasive surgical interventions. These patients often are poor surgical candidates for surgical fixation and therefore are without options for treatment, which may lead to sequelae associated with immobility (Box 61–1). Additionally, there is significant socioeconomic impact to fixing the vertebral compression fractures, by increasing patient mobility, general mood, and saving future health care dollars devoted to pain relief. Percutaneous vertebral augmentation techniques provide a minimally invasive way to stabilize painful vertebral compression fractures.

PATIENT SELECTION

Clinical history is one of the most important aspects of patient selection (Boxes 61–2 and 61–3). It allows the physician to differentiate between VCFs and other common spinal pain syndromes such as nerve root compression, spinal stenosis, disk herniation, symptomatic degenerative changes, and others. Additionally, it is important to determine the degree of back pain, level of mobility, and therapeutic maneuvers attempted to alleviate the pain.

A detailed physical examination is the cornerstone of diagnosis and management for VCFs. Close attention should be placed on sensory and motor neurologic examinations. The presence of hyperreflexia in the lower extremities suggests myelopathy resulting from significant spinal cord impingement. Patients also tend to have focused pain in the region of the fracture. The presence of radicular pain should alert the physician to look for other causes of pain. Traditionally, pain from vertebral compression fractures is not radicular in nature, and further workup (e.g.,

BOX 61–1. INDICATIONS FOR PERCUTANEOUS VERTEBRAL AUGMENTATION

Painful vertebral fractures
Progressive osteolytic compression fractures
Osteoporotic fracture refractory to medical therapy
Hemangioma, multiple myeloma, metastatic lesions
Benign bone lesions
Osteonecrosis
Possible structural reinforcement prior to surgical stabilization
Unstable fractures
Prevention of sequelae of immobilization (decubitus ulcers, deep vein thrombosis, urinary tract infections)
Multiple thoracic compression deformities

BOX 61–2. CONTRAINDICATIONS FOR PERCUTANEOUS VERTEBRAL AUGMENTATION

Absolute Contraindications
- Asymptomatic stable fracture
- Active infection (epidural abscess, sepsis, osteomyelitis, diskitis)
- Local or systemic infection
- Osteomyelitis of target vertebra
- Fractured pedicles
- Clinically effective medical therapy
- Allergy to any required component or contrast
- Pain unrelated to the vertebral collapse
- Osteomyelitis of target vertebra
- Uncorrected coagulopathy
- Acute traumatic fracture of nonosteoporotic vertebra
- Burst fracture

Relative Contraindications
- Radicular pain (radiculopathy caused by a compressive syndrome unrelated to vertebral body collapse
- Pain older than 1 year with a stable fracture
- Tumor extension into epidural space
- Vertebra plana
- Younger age

BOX 61–3. PATIENT SELECTION CHARACTERISTICS

- Fracture unresponsive to conservative medical therapy (analgesics, bed rest, immobilization)
- Fracture with activity on bone scan or edema on magnetic resonance imaging, if in combination with other selection criteria
- Subacute or acute fractures less than 1 year old are ideal to restore vertebral height; however older symptomatic fractures should also be treated
- Pain focused in the region of the fracture
- Fracture site tender to palpation
- Absence of radicular pain
- Pain from fracture negatively affecting mobility, activities of daily living (ADLs), and patient function

select a candidate for either vertebroplasty or kyphoplasty. MRI is currently recommended as the imaging modality of choice because it has been found to be more conclusive in assessing the acuteness of the fracture, assessing canal compromise, and ruling out tumor. In acute fractures, MRI shows an increased T2 signal secondary to bone marrow edema.[11] For a complete picture, MRI examinations should include both transverse and sagittal T1- and T2-weighted images. Sometimes MRI images are used in conjunction with computed tomography (CT) scans to show accurate visualization of the target level and to see if the fracture line extends past the posterior portion of the vertebral body. In order to target the most recent fractures in patients with multiple fractures, bone scan has been used.[12] Plain spinal radiographs also have a role in VCF management. They allow the physician to visualize pedicle anatomy. If the patient has smaller pedicles, it may be easier to undergo percutaneous vertebroplasty because smaller needles are used, or to use the extrapedicular kyphoplasty approach.[11]

TECHNIQUES

Vertebroplasty

Contraindications for any patient undergoing any type of percutaneous approach to repair VCFs include active infection, coagulopathy, burst fractures, osteoblastic or soft tissue tumors, patient refusal, young age, fractured pedicles, contrast allergy, and pregnancy.

Patients undergoing percutaneous vertebroplasty typically can be anesthetized with just local anesthesia, local with conscious sedation, or general anesthesia. The procedure usually takes about 30 minutes, with time increasing to between 15 and 30 minutes per level. A patient imaging device must be used during the procedure and is typically accomplished with fluoroscopy alone. Often physicians use two C-arm machines to visualize anteroposterior and mediolateral view, which allows one to assess trocar

MRI) can be helpful in diagnosis. Percussion of the spine is sometimes carried out to help delineate the symptomatic level of vertebral compression because often pain is elicited within one or two levels of the offending compression fracture. Percussion of the spine is not a sensitive measure of VCF level as noted in Gaughen and colleagues, who analyzed a series of 90 patients undergoing percutaneous vertebroplasty and found that 10 patients had no tenderness to percussion preoperatively.[10]

Radiologic techniques coupled with a detailed history and physical examination can provide the physician with all the necessary tools to properly depth as well as location. If an upper thoracic level is to be done, the scapulae often prevent sufficient view. A combination of fluoroscopy and CT guidance is also used because CT can provide an axial view for needle placement.[13] The axial view is helpful because it allows visualization of the entire length of the pedicle. Because the scapulae will not be superimposed on the images as is the case with fluoroscopy, the images on CT may provide the physician with a clearer view. Additionally, epidural leakage can be identified on CT. Leakage has been implicated in nerve root, ganglion, or spinal cord damage. Fluoroscopy also can detect bone cement leakage but is unable to detect a hematoma.

Prophylactic IV antibiotics are typically administered. Cefazolin 1 g intravenously is the most common primary antibiotic used. In patients who are allergic to penicillin or cephalosporin, Clindamycin 600 mg or vancomycin 1 g can be used.

Vertebral body access should be obtained via unipedicular or bipedicular approach. Controversy exists regarding venography prior to injection of PMMA. In theory, venography can give the physician a picture of the anatomy. Venography can show venous drainage and confirm needle placement into the bony trabeculae.[14] Venography is not essential for safety because contrast material and PMMA have different viscosity and flow patterns. Thus venography may not adequately predict flow patterns of PMMA.[15] Additional evidence was provided by Wong and Mathis, who studied more than 1500 percutaneous vertebroplasties without venography. They showed no significant complications secondary to cement leakage or extravasations.[16]

In the thoracic and lumbar regions, 2 to 6 mL of cement is usually enough for the procedure. The entire vertebral body does not have to be filled with cement to achieve pain relief.[17] In fact, as little as 2 mL of cement can be used to restore vertebral body strength.[18] Studies have shown that there is no correlation between volumes of cement injected and pain reduction.[19,20]

After completion of the procedure, the patient is to remain prone until the cement has hardened. Then the patient can be transferred to recovery. A CT scan is usually done postoperatively to evaluate for possible complications and assess cement distribution. This procedure can be done on an outpatient basis, although it is important to have the patient remain in a recumbent position for 3 to 5 hours, with assessment of neurologic status and evaluation for bleeding and hematomas.

Kyphoplasty

A variation of percutaneous vertebroplasty is kyphoplasty. Preoperative and postoperative evaluation of kyphoplasty is similar to percutaneous vertebroplasty. Kyphoplasty involves the percutaneous introduction of a balloon into the vertebral body. After insertion, the balloon is inflated in order to create a cavity for the placement of cement. Once the balloon is inflated, a void is created that can then be filled with PMMA that is more viscous than that used for percutaneous vertebroplasty.

Central Cavity Creation

One of the newer procedures described to treat vertebral compression fractures is known as central cavity creation (Figs. 61–1 to 61–3). Central cavity creation is a modified technique of percutaneous vertebroplasty that involves manually creating a cavity to inject more viscous cement (Figs. 61–4 to 61–6) with low resistance into fractured vertebral bodies under fluoroscopic guidance.[21] The procedure is performed under monitored anesthesia care with local anesthesia, and requires no hospital admission.

After a preoperative antibiotic, and standard prepping and draping, an oblique fluoroscopic view to image the "Scottie dog" is obtained. After injecting local anesthetic in the appropriate area, an awl-tipped probe is inserted and advanced through the pedicle and into the vertebral body. Continuous anteroposterior and lateral views are used to ensure correct placement at the junction of the posterior third and middle third of the vertebral body. Next, a 0.5-mm stainless steel cannula is advanced into the cancellous bone just past the cortical wall. The probe is removed and the cannula left in place. This is repeated on the other side. Then hinge-tipped curets are inserted to create and shape the cavity. Rotation of the curet is halted and repositioned if any resistance is felt. The cavity is enlarged using progressively larger-tipped curets. The cavity is then injected with cement under fluoroscopic guidance, one side at a time.

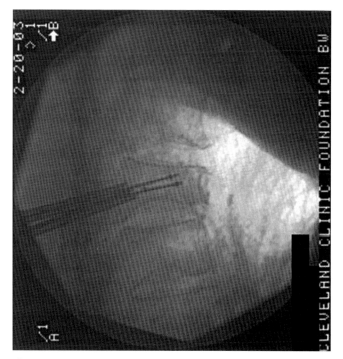

Figure 61–1. Lateral fluoroscopic view shows two trocars placed into the vertebral body just before balloon inflation.

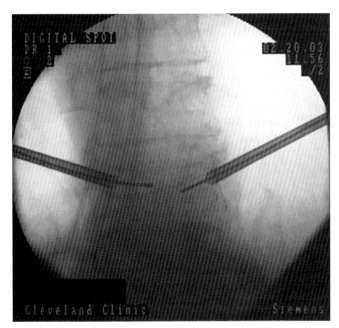

Figure 61–2. Anteroposterior fluoroscopic view demonstrates two trocars placed into the vertebral body just before balloon inflation.

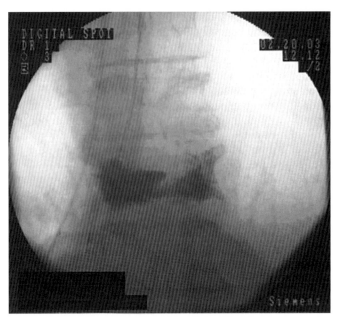

Figure 61–4. Anteroposterior fluoroscopic view of a kyphoplasty at the conclusion of the procedure.

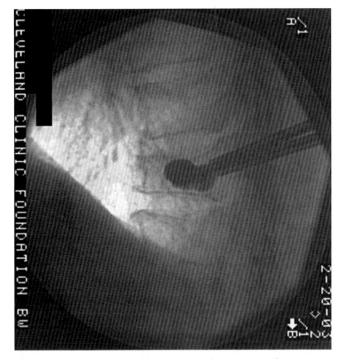

Figure 61–3. Lateral fluoroscopic image demonstrates the injection of cement into the vertebral body.

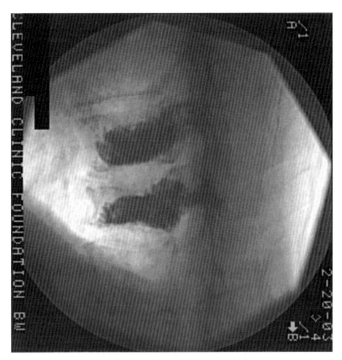

Figure 61–5. Lateral fluoroscopic image after a completed kyphoplasty done at two levels.

This procedure is associated with a decrease in VAS pain scores, use of postoperative narcotics, and significant improvement in function and general activity. Advantages include a low rate of cement extravasation, most likely a result of a more viscous cement. It also offers advantages over kyphoplasty in the sense that it is much less costly, with kits costing approximately $1175 compared with some kyphoplasty kits that cost $3400. Central cavity creation also has a shorter postoperative recovery time because this procedure can be done under local anesthesia with monitored anesthesia care. Some disadvantages of this procedure include the inability to have any substantial effect on restoring lost vertebral height or treating kyphosis. Cavity creation is also more labor intensive than traditional vertebroplasty, but less so than kyphoplasty. Central cavity creation is a relatively new procedure that has not undergone as extensive clinical study and review as traditional vertebroplasty and kyphoplasty.[21]

Complications

The complications surrounding percutaneous vertebral augmentation traditionally are categorized into two areas: procedural complications and leakage of cement. Leakage of cement is by far the most common complication associated with percutaneous vertebral augmentation. Many variables contribute to the degree and significance of leakage of cement including the level of injection, severity of fracture, and the amount of cement injected. The distribution of leakage of cement for vertebroplasty and kyphoplasty, respectively (Fig. 61–7) were 32% and 11% epidural, 32.5% and 48% paraspinal, 30.5% and 38%

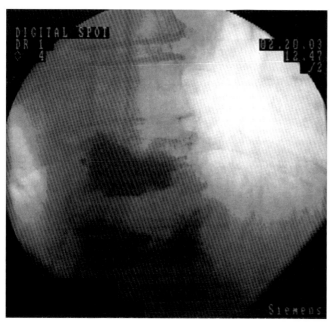

Figure 61–6. Anteroposterior fluoroscopic image of a two-level kyphoplasty at the conclusion of the procedure.

intradiskal, 1.7% and 1.5% pulmonary, and 3.3% and 1.5% foraminal.[22]

Although leakage of cement is noted as a common complication, severe clinical sequelae were noted in only a small percentage of patients. Severe clinical sequelae included pulmonary emboli, which occurred in 0.6% and 0.01% for vertebroplasty and kyphoplasty, respectively, and neurologic complications occurred in 0.6% and 0.03% of vertebrae.[23] Pulmonary embolism is usually caused by cement leakage into the paravertebral veins and cement extravasation into bone marrow or fat particles that enter circulation. Neurologic complications are categorized as radiculopathy, spinal claudication, and paraplegia (Fig. 61–8). Radiculopathy can occur secondary to cement leakage into the neural foramen. In regard to cement leakage, the vast majority is asymptomatic, with approximately 96% from vertebroplasty and 89% from kyphoplasty.

Other complications that can occur from percutaneous vertebral augmentation are procedural complications. These include infection, bleeding, and allergic reactions from the PMMA or venography dye, which has been associated with systemic hypotension and fever.

Outcomes and Efficacy

Both kyphoplasty and vertebroplasty have been used successfully to treat pain related to osteoporotic vertebral fractures. In addition to successfully treating pain conditions, restoration of vertebral height is another important outcome measure. As people age and vertebral bodies undergo osteoporotic degeneration, height loss as well as pathologic vertebral fractures often result. Kyphoplasty has been associated with a greater restoration of height at 97%, compared with only 30% with vertebroplasty. The magnitude of lost height restoration varies depending on the severity of the compression fracture, with average

Figure 61–7. Percentage of occurrence and distribution of cement leakage by location in vertebroplasty and kyphoplasty. (Data from Hulme P, Kebs J, Ferguson S, Berlemann U: Vertebroplasty and kyphoplasty: A systematic review of 69 clinical studies. Spine 2006;31:1983-2001.)

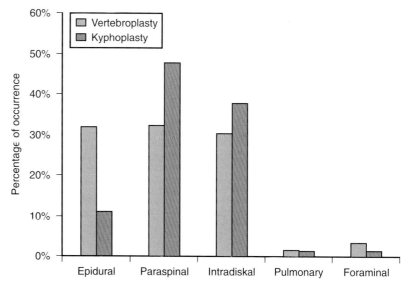

DISTRIBUTION OF CEMENT LEAKAGE

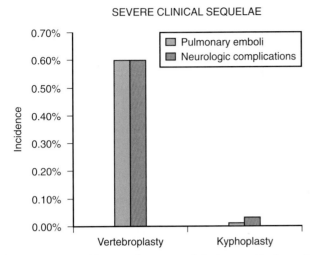

Figure 61–8. Incidence of severe clinical complications for vertebroplasty and kyphoplasty. (Data from Moreland DB, Landi MK, Grand W: Vertebroplasty: Techniques to avoid complications. Spine J 2001;1:66-71.)

estimates of 35% lost height restoration.[24] The restoration of vertebral body height can reverse the decrease in FEV_1 that can be found in kyphotic patients.

Pain reduction is often used as a measure of successful vertebral augmentation. Additionally, one must realize that the advantage of pain reduction is associated with an increase in physical activity as well as an improved mood. Cortet and associates showed that pain was reduced by 56% by day 3 in a prospective study of 16 patients undergoing 20 levels of percutaneous vertebroplasty.[25] This study found that patients also demonstrated an increase in physical activity and energy and a decrease in social isolation.

In terms of efficacy, the duration and onset of pain reduction in percutaneous vertebral body techniques are important outcomes. Numerous studies have shown that percutaneous vertebroplasty is safe and effective in providing both short- and long-term pain relief. Partial or complete relief was observed in 70% to 95% of patients in the first 3 days after the procedure.[25-27] Most patients notice a significant reduction in pain in the first 24 hours.[28]

In a prospective analysis of percutaneous vertebral augmentation, improvements in pain and physical and mental function were seen by 2 weeks and persisted in an 18-month follow-up.[29] This study was a prospective analysis of percutaneous vertebroplasty at 54 levels in patients with osteoporotic VCFs.

Debate surrounds the outcomes of percutaneous vertebral augmentation in comparison to conservative treatment. Often the patient population that is most susceptible to vertebral compression fractures is older adults and as such may be deemed poor surgical candidates. Often lost in translation is the fact that these techniques do not result in significant blood loss or fluid shifts, which thereby lead to fewer complications particularly in the frail older adult patient.

The procedures are often short and depending on technique may be done without general anesthesia. In regard to pain reduction, comparisons between invasive percutaneous vertebral augmentation versus noninvasive conservative treatment have been carried out. Diamond and colleagues provided valuable insight regarding percutaneous vertebroplasty in comparison with conservative treatment.[30] In a nonrandomized prospective study, Diamond followed patients who underwent vertebroplasty (70% of studied group) compared with those who underwent nonoperative, conservative therapy. Those treated with vertebroplasty noted a 53% reduction in pain and a 29% improvement in physical function 24 hours after the procedure. This patient group also was able to stop all analgesic medications in 24% of the patients studied. In the conservative group there was no noted change in pain scores in the first 24 hours and the patients were not able to stop analgesic medications. This supports the observation that most pain related to VCFs can improve in 2 to 12 weeks following the insulting event.[31] Another study analyzing the outcomes of percutaneous vertebroplasty was done by Perez-Higueras and associates, which assessed clinical and radiologic outcomes in 12 patients over a 5-year period.[31] The initial pain scores were found to be 9.1/10 and fell to 2.1/10 on postoperative day 3, and remained stable at 2.2/10 on the 5 year follow-up. At the 5-year follow up, all patients were "very" or "somewhat" satisfied with the procedure. Radiologic analysis with CT scan revealed cement leakage in 48% of cases, but only 1 patient was found to have transient neuritis.

One of the potential serious complications of a percutaneous vertebral augmentation technique is cement leakage. Often physicians and patients hear case reports of cement leakage causing an unwanted neuritis, paralysis, or embolism. Several radiologic analyses have demonstrated that cement leakages are relatively rare. Clinically significant sequelae of percutaneous vertebral augmentation from leakage of cement are rare.

In comparison with vertebroplasty, kyphoplasty was associated with a lower rate of cement extravasation secondary to the high viscosity of the PMMA and the lower injection pressure used.[32,33] Additionally, it is thought that another reason of less cement extravasation in kyphoplasty may be due to the inflatable bone tamp, which compacts trabecular bone and seals pathways for cement leakage.[34]

Pain scores and vertebral height augmentation, particularly in the first year following percutaneous vertebral augmentation, have been extensively studied. A retrospective study by Ledlie and Renfro[35] showed significant reductions in pain scores postprocedure. A reduction from a mean preprocedure level of 8.6/10 was reduced to 2.7/10 postprocedure. Patients were followed up for 1 year and were found to have a further reduced pain score of 1.4/10. Patients also demonstrated an increase in physical activity level and energy. Vertebral height showed dramatic improvement as well, from 65% preprocedure to 90%

Table 61–1. Vertebroplasty versus Kyphoplasty

PROCEDURE	ADVANTAGES	DISADVANTAGES
Vertebroplasty	Minimally invasive Short procedure time Increases vertebral body strength and stability Avoidance of general anesthesia Less expensive Improved pain score, patient satisfaction, and increased immobilization	Potential increased risk of cement leakage Does not correct lost vertebral body height or sagittal deformity
Kyphoplasty	Pain relief Restoration of lost vertebral body height Correction of sagittal imbalance Increased vertebral body strength and stability Allows for more viscous cement	General anesthesia is often used Increased cost Longer procedure time than vertebroplasty Requires bipedicular instrumentation

postprocedure. Various other studies have demonstrated an increase in vertebral body height after kyphoplasty.[36-38] Lieberman and coworkers showed a lost height restoration percentage of 35% after kyphoplasty.[39]

Extensive longer-term studies demonstrating the efficacy of pain reduction following percutaneous vertebral augmentation also have been carried out. The evidence demonstrates that even when followed for 5 years after intervention, patients demonstrate reduction in pain scores, not improved physical and mental function. In a study performed at the Cleveland Clinic Foundation, 900 consecutive kyphoplasties done in 300 patients over an approximately 5-year period were observed for changes in pain score, physical function postprocedure, and height restoration.[40-42] The mean age was 69 years, duration of symptoms was 7 months, and levels treated were between T3 and L5. Results demonstrated an increase in physical function, social function, and emotional and mental status. Visual Analogue Scale (VAS) pain scores showed improvement, and general health was unchanged. There were no significant neurologic symptomatic cement leakages in the 300 patients studied over a 5-year period.

CONCLUSION

Percutaneous vertebral augmentation is a safe minimally invasive technique that decreases pain from vertebral compression fractures. Improvements in pain scores, functional scores, and prevention of sequelae of immobility have been shown in many clinical studies. Kyphoplasty, vertebroplasty, and central cavity creation all are done percutaneously. Kyphoplasty can restore vertebral body height and improve kyphosis in 50% of patients. Vertebroplasty is associated with an immediate decrease in acute pain, and less narcotic usage. Serious complications associated with percutaneous techniques include cement leakage, causing neuritis or paraplegia, and emboli (Table 61–1).

Osteoporotic VCFs comprise a significant cause of disability in older adult patients. Patients often complain of severe pain with acute fractures, isolate themselves socially, and decrease their overall physical function. Patients who become sedentary following a VCF are at increased risk for developing other complicated medical disorders such as pneumonia, deep venous thrombosis, pulmonary embolus, decreased lung function, decubitus ulcers, and increased urinary tract infections.

Percutaneous vertebroplasty or kyphoplasty can provide patients with relief following an acute VCF. Vertebroplasty has the advantages of lower cost and shorter procedure time. Disadvantages include an increased risk of cement extravasation, although multiple studies have shown that this is an infrequent clinical sequela. It cannot correct lost vertebral body height or correct sagittal imbalance. In comparison, kyphoplasty can restore vertebral body height and correct sagittal imbalance, allows increased usage of viscous cement, has a lower extravasation of cement, and is found to have a lower complication rate. Disadvantages include higher cost and increased procedure time.

Although some authors believe that kyphoplasty should be standard of care in patients who have failed conservative therapy, both procedures provide excellent pain relief, decrease sequelae of immobility, increase vertebral body strength, and increase physical as well as emotional status.

References

1. Murphy KJ, Lin DD: Vertebroplasty: A simple solution to a difficult problem. J Clin Densitom 2001;4:189-197.
2. Aslan S, Karcioglu O, Katirci Y, et al: Speed bump induced spinal cord injury. Am J Emerg Med 2005;23:563.
3. Cooper C, Atkinson EJ, O'Fallon WM, Melton LJ 3rd: Incidence of clinically diagnosed vertebral fractures; a population based stuffy in Rochester, Minnesota, 1985-1989. J Bone Miner Res 1992;7:221.
4. Riggs BL, Melton LJ: The worldwide problem of osteoporosis: Insights afforded by epidemiology. Bone 1995;17:505-511.
5. Truumees E: Osteoporosis. Spine 2001;26:930-932.
6. Silverman SL: The clinical consequences of vertebral compression fractures. Bone 1992;13(suppl 2):27-31.
7. Lane JM, Johnson CE, Khan SN, et al: Minimally invasive options for the treatment of osetoporotic vertebral compression fractures. Orthop Clin North Am 2002;33:431-438.
8. Melton LJ, Kan SH, Frye MA, et al: Epidemiology of vertebral compression fractures in women. AM J Epidemiol 1989; 129:1000-1011.

9. Mendel E, Burton: Vertebroplasty and kyphoplasty. Pain Physician 2003;6:335-341.
10. Gaughen JR, Jensen ME, Schweickert PA, et al: Lack of pre-operative spinous process tenderness does not affect clinical success of percutaneous vertebroplasty. J Vasc Interv Radiol 2002;13:1135-1138.
11. Barr JD, Barr MS, Lemly TJ: Combined CT and fluoroscopic guidance for percutaneous vertebroplasty. Presented at the 34th annual meeting of the American Society of Neuroradiology, Seattle, 21-27 June 1996.
12. Maynard AS, Jensen ME, Schweickert PA, et al: Value of bone scan imaging in predicting pain relief from percutaneous vertebroplasty in osteoporotic vertebral fractures. Am J Neuroradiol 2000;21:1807-1809.
13. Gangi A, Kastler BA, Dietemann C, et al: Percutaneous verte-broplasty guided by CT and fluoroscopy. AJNR 1994;15:83-86.
14. Jensen ME, Evans AJ, Mathis JM, et al: Percutaneous PMMA vertebroplasty in the treatment of osteoporotic compression fractures: Technical aspects. Am J Neuroradiol 1997;18:1897-1904.
15. Gaughen JR Jr, Jensen ME, Schweickert PP, et al: Relevance of antecedent venography in percutaneous vertebroplasty for the treatment of osteoporotic compression fractures. AJNR 2002;23:594-596.
16. Wong W, Mathis J: Is intraosseous venography a significant safety measure in performance of vertebroplasty? J Vasc Interv Radiol 2002;13(2):137-138.
17. Belkoff SM, Mathis JM, Jasper LE, et al: The biomechanics of vertebroplasty: The effect of cement volume on mechanical behavior. Spine 2001;26:1537-1541.
18. Murphy KJ, Lin DD: Vertebroplasty: A simple solution to a difficult problem. J Clin Densitom 2001;4:189-197.
19. Cotton A, Dewatre F, Cortet B, et al: Percutaneous verte-broplasty for osteolytic metastases and myeloma: Effects of the percentage of lesion filing and the leakage of methylmethac-rylate at clinical followup. Radiology 1996;200:525-530.
20. Komemushi A, Tanigawa N, Kariya S, et al: Percutaneous verte-broplasty for compression fracture; analysis of vertebral body volume by CT volumetry. Acta Radiol 2005;46:276-279.
21. Vallejo R, Benyamin R, Floyd B, et al: Percutaneous cement injection into a created cavity for the treatment of vertebral body fracture: Preliminary results of a new vertebroplasty technique. Clin J Pain 2006;22:182-189.
22. Hulme Paul, Kebs J, Ferguson S, Berlemann U: Vertebroplasty and kyphoplasty: A systematic review of 69 clinical studies. Spine 2006;31:1983-2001.
23. Moreland DB, Landi MK, Grand W: Vertebroplasty: Tech-niques to avoid complications. Spine J 2001;1:66-71.
24. Weill A, Chiras J, Simon JM, et al: Spinal metastases: Indica-tions for and results of percutaneous injection of acrylic surgi-cal cement radiology 1996;199:241-247.
25. Cortet B, Cotton A, Boutry N, et al: Percutaneous vertebro-plasty in the treatment of osteoporotic compression fractures: An open prospective study. J Rheumatol 1999;26:2222-2228.
26. Do HM, Kim BS, Marcellus ML, et al: Prospective analysis of clinical outcomes after percutaneous vertebroplasty for painful osteoporotic vertebral body fractures. AJNR 2005;26:1623-1628.
27. Kobayashi K, Shimoyama K, Nakamura K, et al: Percutaneous vertebroplasty immediately relieves pain of osteoporotic vertebral compression fractures and prevents prolonged immobilization in patients. Eur Radiol 2005;15:360-367.
28. Martin JB, Jean B, Sugiu K, et al: Vertebroplasty: Clinical expe-rience and follow up results. Bone 1999;25:11-15.
29. Perez-Higueras A, Alvarez L, Rossi RE, et al: Percutaneous ver-tebroplasty: Long term clinical and radiological outcome. Neuroradiology 200;44:950-954.
30. Diamond TH, Champion B, Clark WA: Management of acute osteoporotic vertebral fractures: A nonrandomized trial com-paring percutaneous vertebroplasty with conservative therapy. Am J Med 2003;114:257-265.
31. Perez-Higueras A, Alvarez L, Rossi RE, et al: Percutaneous vertebroplasty: Long term clinical and radiological outcome. Neuroradiology 200;44:950-954.
32. Belkoff SM, Mathis JM, Fenton DC, et al: An ex vivo bio-mechanical evaluation of an inflatable bone tamp used in the treatment of compression fracture. Spine 2001;26:151-156.
33. Belkoff SM, Mathis JM, Deramond H, Jasper LE: An ex vivo biomechanical evaluation of a hydroxyapatite cement for use with kyphoplasty. Am J Neuroradiol 2001;22:1212-1216.
34. Philips FM, Wetzel FT, Leiberman I, Campbell-Hup PM: An in vivo comparison of the potential of the potential for extravertebral cement leak after vertebroplasty and kypho-plasty. Spine 2002;27:2173-2179.
35. Ledlie JT, Renfro MJ: Balloon kyphoplasty: One year outcomes in vertebral body height restoration, chronic pain, and activity levels. J Neurosurg 2003;98:21-30.
36. Garfin SR, Yuan HA, Reiley MA: Kyphoplasty and vertebro-plasty for the treatment of painful osteoporotic compression fractures. Spine 2001;26:1511-1515.
37. Fourney DR, Schomer DF, Nader R, et al: Percutaneous verte-broplasty and kyphoplasty for painful vertebral body fractures in cancer patients. J Neurosurg (Spine I) 2003;98:21-20.
38. Theodorou DJ, Theodorou SJ, Duncan TD, et al: Percutaneous balloon kyphoplasty for the correction of spinal deformity in painful vertebral body compression fractures. J Clin Imag 2002;26:1-5.
39. Lieberman IH, Dudeney S, Reinhardt MK, et al: Initial outcome and efficacy of kyphoplasty in the treatment of painful osteo-porotic vertebral compression fractures. Spine 2001;26:1631-1683.
40. Coumans JV, Reinhardt MK, Lieberman IH: Kyphoplasty for vertebral compression fractures: 1 year clinical outcomes from a prospective study. J Neurosurg 2003;99:44-50.
41. Dudeney S, Leiberman IH, Reihhardt MK, et al: Kyphoplasty in the treatment of osteolytic vertebral compression fractures as a result of multiple myeloma. J Clin Oncol 2002;20:2382-2387.
42. Wong X, Reiley MA, Garfin S: Vertebroplasty/kyphoplasty. J Womens Imag 2000;2:117-124.

CHAPTER
62 Lumbosacral Epiduroscopy

James E. Heavner, Hemmo Bosscher, and Mitchell Wachtel

Lumbosacral epiduroscopy is defined for purposes of this discussion as direct visualization of the lumbar and sacral epidural space with a percutaneously inserted flexible fiberoptic device that has a channel through which instruments can be inserted and fluids can be injected. Synonyms for this procedure include spinal canal endoscopy, spinal epiduroscopy, myeloscopy, spinal or lumbar epiduroscopy, and endoscopic adhesiolysis. The target population for epiduroscopy is patients with lumbar or sacral nerve radiculopathy or low back pain who are not clearly candidates for surgery, who have failed back surgery syndrome, or who have not received sustained benefit from more traditional therapy such as single epidural steroid injection. The objectives of epiduroscopy are (1) to gain information by direct visual inspection that contributes to the documentation of pathologic processes responsible for low back pain or radiculopathy and (2) to do therapeutic interventions under direct visual control to relieve pain.

HISTORY

Interest in viewing the contents of the bony vertebral canal using percutaneously placed devices has existed for a long time. As early as 1931 Burman[1] used arthroscopic equipment to examine the anatomy of vertebral column removed from cadavers. Pool[2] reported results of examination primarily of the subarachnoid space of almost 400 patients in 1942. Abnormalities recognized included varicose vessels; arachnoid adhesions of post-traumatic or postinflammatory origin, neoplasms, the presence of inflamed nerve roots associated with clinical neuritis, and the effects of a herniated nucleus pulposus or hypertrophied ligamentum flavum. Significant advancement toward clinical application of epiduroscopy in modern medical practice occurred only after introduction of flexible fiberscopes capable of delivering high-quality images, especially with computer enhancement, and development of suitable light sources. This equipment has been used to view the spinal epidural space as well as the spinal subarachnoid space.

Pursuit of the use of lumbosacral epiduroscopy for diagnostic and therapeutic purposes in pain management increased rapidly beginning in the mid 1980s. We and others began exploring the use of lumbosacral epiduroscopy as an aid to lysis of epidural adhesions.[3] The lysis procedure is based on evidence that adhesions in the epidural space are involved in the pathophysiology of low back pain or radiculopathy and prevent delivery of therapeutic agents to target sites.[4] The procedure involves (1) definition of a filling defect on epidurography that corresponds to the spinal segment innervating the painful area, (2) insertion of a catheter into the defect and injection of normal saline and hyaluronidase to remove tissue (fibrosis) barriers to fluid flow, and (3) injection of therapeutic agents through the catheter to the target site. It was reasoned that a flexible endoscopic device with a deflectable tip and a working channel would facilitate catheter placement, provide mechanical in addition to hydraulic forces to break tissue barriers, and provide visual information that would aid in diagnosis and prognosis.

CURRENT STATUS

Epiduroscopy is mostly focused on the L4, L5, and S1 areas because these are the most common dermatomal locations of painful neuropathies involving the lower extremities. Abundant clinical experience and published data demonstrate the safety and efficacy of epiduroscopy.[5,6] Literature reports claim that visualization of pathologic tissue and observation of targeted drug administration via epiduroscopy results in substantial and prolonged pain relief. The authors of one study stated that adhesions unreported by magnetic resonance imaging (MRI) can be identified.[7] Manchikanti and associates[8] concluded that endoscopic adhesiolysis with the administration of corticosteroids is also a safe and possibly cost-effective technique for relief of chronic intractable pain failing to respond to other treatment modalities. There are many reports showing that epiduroscopy is a safe procedure if precautions are taken such as to limit the rate and volume of fluid injected during the procedure.[6-15]

Epiduroscopy equipment continues to improve. Increased clarity of visualization and experience enhances the ability to recognize structures. Nevertheless, the objective of finding a bulging disk or a diseased nerve root, as is often the case, may be difficult to achieve. However, information may be obtained by evaluating more readily identifiable tissues such as dura, periosteum, fat and scar tissue, and blood vessels. By assessing these structures relative to other clinical findings and outcomes of prior treatment, we believe advancement has been made in the interpretation of epiduroscopy findings.

Like many pain therapies, high evidence-based standards demonstrating efficacy for epiduroscopy are limited, but the evidence published in peer-reviewed journals is increasing. In 2003, the Australian Royal College of Surgeons published a review of the literature about epiduroscopy based on a systematic search of MEDLINE, PREMEDLINE, EMBASE, Current Contents (until October 2002), PubMed, Cochrane Library, and Science Citation Index.[16]

List of Studies Found

Total number of studies	10
Systematic reviews	0
Randomized controlled trials	0
Nonrandomized comparative studies	1
Case series	6
Case reports	3

To date, visual information obtained during epiduroscopy in patients with low back pain or radiculopathy is presented as an important component of the data in only one study report.[9] In this study, two investigators evaluated without knowledge of medical history, epiduroscopy findings including amount of fatty tissue, amount of fibrous tissue, degree of adhesion, and degree of vascularity. There were two groups of study subjects, one with monosegmental radiculopathy and one with multisegmental radiculopathy. The amount of fatty tissue and degree of vascularity were less in the multisegmental group than in the monosegmental group.[9]

Fiberoptic Images of the Epidural Space

Examination with epiduroscopy is usually limited to the posterior, posterolateral, lateral, and anterolateral epidural spaces. Successful application of epiduroscopy requires unique knowledge of the anatomy of the contents of the bony vertebral canal. Interpreting images obtained through epiduroscopy is not easy without adequate training and experience. Most of the difficulties can be understood if one realizes that the visual field seen through the epiduroscope is only a small fraction of the epidural space. A larger spatial context depends on a sequence of images obtained by maneuvering the scope in the area of interest. Because anatomic landmarks are sparse, fluoroscopic orientation, using anteroposterior or lateral views, is needed to place these images in a larger anatomic context. However, as experience is acquired, reliance

---

BOX 62–1. GENERAL INDICATIONS FOR EPIDUROSCOPY

1. Observation of pathology and anatomy
2. Direct drug application
3. Direct lysis of scarring (with medication, blunt dissection, laser and other instruments)
4. Placement of catheter and electrode systems (epidural, subarachnoid)
5. An adjunct to minimally invasive surgery

---

on fluoroscopy decreases. Landmarks such as the filum terminale, dura, and pedicles of the vertebrae are useful for orientation. Another limiting factor is size of the epidural space. The spinal canal is occupied primarily by the dural sac and its contents, and epidural fat. Expected structures such as disks, disk herniations, and compressed nerve roots are difficult to see. Protruded or prolapsed disk material may not be recognized because there are no obvious features identifying the material as seen during epiduroscopy. In addition, an intervertebral disk is partially covered by the posterior longitudinal ligament, which in turn is covered by epidural fat obscuring the disk almost completely. A large disk herniation may be present, but shows itself as an irregular fibrotic mass that is difficult to penetrate, rather than a smooth disk bulge. Nerve roots are visible (just under the pedicle). However, they are easily missed if not actively looked for. Once a nerve root is identified, it may supply only limited information. The question arises: what does one look for? Pathologic processes in the epidural space are easily described by the absence of expected tissues and by the presence of abnormal tissues at these sites (Box 62–1).

ANATOMY AND PHYSIOLOGY

As an epiduroscope is advanced through the sacral and lumbar bony vertebral canal, it is directed through an anatomic area referred to as the epidural space. This space generally is considered to be a potential space. However, we know the area between the dura and the walls of the vertebral canal is a real space filled with fat, nerve roots, and fibrous tissue.

This canal varies in shape and size, and the contents differ depending on region. The spinal cord, which is surrounded by the pia mater, cerebrospinal fluid, arachnoid mater, and dura mater (from closest to the cord outward) ends in the adult at about L1 or L2. The spinal cord tapers at its end forming the conus medullaris and then the filum terminale. The filum terminale and lumbar, sacral, and coccygeal anterior and posterior nerve roots continue in the caudal sac. The caudal sac is filled with cerebrospinal fluid (CSF) and is bounded outwardly first by the arachnoid, then by the dura. Anterior and posterior nerve roots traverse through the caudal sac for varying distances, depending on where they exit the spinal cord proximally and where they exit the intervertebral foramen distally (Fig. 62–1). These nerve roots

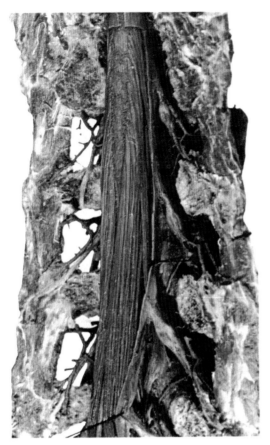

Figure 62–1. A photograph of the posterior surface of the conus medullaris and cauda equina from the spine of a female aged 18 years. (From Crock HV, Yoshizawa H: The Blood Supply of the Vertebral Column and Spinal Cord in Man. New York, Springer-Verlag, 1977.)

Gross Fiberscopic Anatomy of the Epidural Space

When the epiduroscope enters the normal sacral canal, the first view usually is of peridural fat with sparse small blood vessels running through it, and the filum terminale may be seen. More cephalad in the sacral and lumbar canal, the dura surrounding the caudal sac may be viewed as a bluish white structure. The epiduroscope advances most easily in the dorsal epidural space, which consists of lamina and fat. Nerve roots with an attached blood vessel may be observed through the dura and on the right and left sides of the canal. Occasional thin sheets of fibrous tissue may be seen in the fat or between fat deposits. Laterally, the vertebral pedicles are relatively easy to identify by their smooth, rounded shape. So is the medial aspect of the pars superior of the facet joint. The nerve roots are variable in size and are recognized by a characteristic blood vessel on their surface. The roots can be followed medial, then inferior to the pedicle. The epiduroscope can often be advanced through neuroforamen, into the paraspinous space. The nerve root is small relative to the large neuroforamen and abundant epidural fat in the neuroforamen, continuous with extra spinal fat, makes the nerve root sometimes difficult to find. The disk should be found superior to the pedicle but is hard to identify. The indentations of the dura and posterior longitudinal ligaments, between nerve root sleeves, are large and allow inspection of the anterior epidural space or at the least the lateral part of it. If no pathology obstructs the advancement of the scope and it is long enough, the lumbosacral epidural space from approximately S2 to L1 can be investigated in this fashion.

Fat Tissue

Fat tissue is derived from mesenchyme and may serve as a buffer between the hard spinal wall and the more delicate neural structures in the spine (Fig. 62–2). It differs from subcutaneous fat by the relative absence of connective tissue. The presence of fat may be a marker for adequate regional perfusion and lack of pathologic (inflammatory) processes. It is most easily recognized by its color. It is white with a globular appearance, and can be easily penetrated with the scope. It seems most abundantly present in the lateral recesses and the neural foramina and less so in the posterior epidural space except for the sacral epidural space, which is often completely filled with fat. Absence of fat may be the result of fat atrophy associated with the normal aging process or, more likely, as the result of an inflammatory process and local ischemia. Its absence may play an important role in the pathophysiology of back pain because epidural fat plays a role in the mechanical buffering of the thecal sac with flexion and extension. Whether fat tissue differentiates in an alternative direction (i.e., fibrous tissue) in response to noxious stimuli or is replaced by abnormal pathologic tissue is not known.

form the cauda equina. As the roots exit the caudal sac, they are covered by extensions of the meninges and travel between the lateral bounds of the bony vertebral canal and the dura for varying distances and at varying angles, depending on where they exit the canal. The distance becomes longer and the angle less steep from the lumbar to the sacral region. The diameter of the nerves varies from spinal segment to spinal segment. The dorsal root ganglion is very near or in the intervertebral foramen and the anterior and posterior nerve roots join to become the spinal nerve in the foramen. The caudal sac ends at approximately S2 and the filum terminale, fused with the filum of the dura, continues caudally from there to the coccyx, where it blends with the periosteum. Epidural fat normally is present in discrete pockets in the posterior and lateral epidural spaces.[17] Epidural veins are restricted to the anterior epidural space.[17,18] An open arterial plexus on the posterior surface of the dura has been described.[19] The plica mediana dorsalis, a connective tissue band in the dorsomedial epidural space attached at one end to the posterior dura and to the periosteum of the vertebral arch at the other, may or may not be seen.[20] Careful examination of lateral intervertebral spaces may reveal articular surfaces and vertebral pedicles.

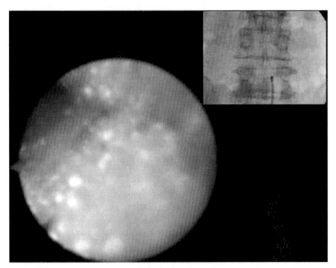

Figure 62–2. Normal peridural fat, right L5 normal fat.

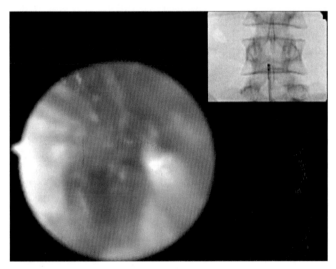

Figure 62–3. Neovascularization, just left of midline L4 neovascularization.

Vasculature

Arteries and veins traversing the posterior or postero-lateral epidural space normally are sparse or not present at all (Fig. 62–3). Arteries usually are small. Veins usually are transparent and may be difficult to differentiate from adhesions. Arteries are easy recognizable by their pulsating behavior. Obviously, in the absence of fat the number of visible vessels will increase. However, this may also be part of an inflammatory response. Abnormal vasculature is recognized by its increased density and chaotic orientation in areas of pathology. Because these arteries are dilated, they contain more blood and make a strikingly purple-red appearance. Obstruction to venous blood flow by pathologic processes leads to dilated, tortuous vessels, not only on an affected nerve root but at any site that is involved in the pathology. During epiduroscopy, some bleeding from ruptured vessels may occur; however, these vessels are often small, and bleeding seems relatively insignificant.

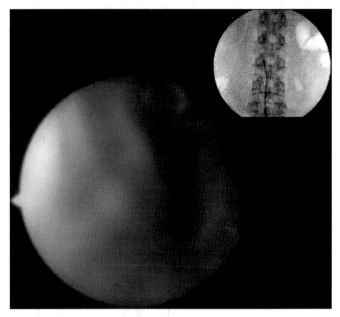

Figure 62–4. Active inflammation, left L3 active inflammation.

Inflammation

Inflammatory changes are common and to some extent may be part of the normal aging process (Fig. 62–4). They can be found diffusely throughout the epidural space and do not seem to lead to clinical symptoms. Inflamed tissue is recognized by a dark purple or inklike color. It is diffuse and heterogeneous. It is the result of hyperemia and is associated with increased vasculature, exudates, and fibrosis. If the area of inflammation is extensive or is located near the nerve root, touching the inflamed area with the tip of the epiduroscope is painful. Fragility of blood vessels in inflamed areas causes the tissues to bleed on the slightest touch with the scope. In some patients, inflammation is diffusely present in the entire lumbosacral epidural space. Total epidural fat is diminished or absent. The periosteum and dura are hyperemic, and maneuvering of the scope is painful and causes diffuse bleeding.

Fibrosis

One of the most striking images obtained through epiduroscopy is the one of white scar (Figs. 62–5 and 62–6). Fibrosis is most likely the result of direct trauma (i.e., surgery), chronic inflammation, or local ischemia. Independent of its cause, it is characterized by the *abnormal* presence of sheets or strings of white tissue. Because epidural fibrosis may play an important role in patients with chronic back pain and radicular pain, it is useful to grade the extensiveness of the epidural fibrosis.

Grade 1: The fibrosis consists of strings and sheets traversing the epidural space and attaching to bone or dura. It is often mixed with fat tissue and may be part of the normal aging process. It offers no resistance to advancement of the scope. Grade 1 fibrosis is unlikely to cause clinical symptoms.

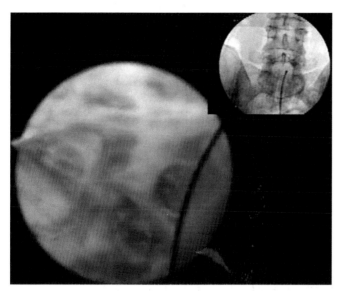

Figure 62–5. Grade 2 fibrosis with increased vascularity and inflammation, right L5 grade 2 fibrosis with increased vascularity and inflammation.

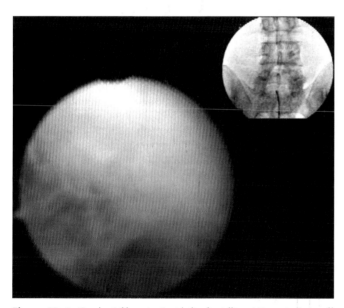

Figure 62–6. Grade 4 fibrosis, just left of midline L5 posterior wall of epidural space adhesions with inflammatory chains.

Grade 2: Strings and sheets of fibrosis increase in size and number and form a more continuous network. Inflammatory changes are often present as well. The fibrosis partially replaces epidural fat. There is some resistance to scope advancement. Maneuvering the scope may be painful. Grade 2 fibrosis clearly is abnormal and is likely part of a pathologic process that leads to clinical symptoms.

Grade 3: Fibrosis is continuous and occupies discrete areas of the epidural space. There is no epidural fat and inflammation may be less pronounced. The scope can be advanced with difficulty, if at all, in areas occupied by grade 3 fibrosis, and attempts to do so are painful.

Grade 4: Fibrosis is now one large dense mass that is continuous and occupies an anatomic region of the epidural space. The scope cannot be advanced at all.

It is important to recognize that epidural fibrosis is associated with multiple different pathologic processes and should be placed in the appropriate clinical context. For example, after back surgery, the dura may adhere to the walls of the spinal canal and be covered by strings and sheets of fibrosis or adhere to paraspinous tissue where a laminotomy was performed. In this case, the scope cannot be advanced because of dural adhesions. Large disk herniations may also appear as a white irregular fibrotic (grade 4) mass that is impossible to penetrate with the scope. This may be extruded disk material or a fibrotic response to chronic inflammation.

Nerve Roots

Nerve roots are surprisingly hard to find for structures that occupy 30% of the neuroforamen. The S3, S4, and S5 nerve roots are usually missed completely because the introducer accessing the epidural space for epiduroscopy is inserted to about S3. The S2 nerve root is usually easy to find. The S1 nerve root can be found in the lateral recess of the sacral epidural space on its way to the sacral neuroforamen. It passes medial and inferior to a bony structure equivalent to the pedicle of the lumbar vertebra. This is commonly the site of fibrosis and may explain persistent radicular pain in the S1 distribution after an L5-S1 fusion of the lumbar spine. The lumbar nerve roots can be found below and medial to the pedicle, the perpendicular space. A characteristic blood vessel accompanies the nerve root and can be seen through the root sleeve. Under normal conditions this vessel is straight; with pathology it becomes dilated and gives an effaced appearance. A tortuous vessel may be a sign of circulatory obstruction. The nerve root sleeve itself can make a large dilated appearance. Touching a healthy nerve root is not painful although a paresthesia may be felt. However, in pathology, touching the nerve with the tip of the epiduroscope is often very painful.

Disks, Dura, and Ligaments

As mentioned earlier, disk and disk material are difficult to identify. On gross examination, that is, during surgery, the disk is easily identified by its white, almost yellow, appearance in contrast with the darker brown vertebral bone. It is only partially covered by the longitudinal ligament. The disk can probably be seen during epiduroscopy by placing the scope in the neuroforamen just superior to the pedicle; however, color and texture of the disk seen through the scope and the presence of obscuring epidural fat make it difficult to obtain useful information with respect to disk pathology. A known disk herniation is characterized by the absence of epidural fat and the inability to place the scope in the neuroforamen. A dense white mass obstructs the advancement of the scope. Areas of inflammation and fibrosis may be seen as well. One does not see a nice smooth, possibly red disk protrusion (compressing a nerve root) as shown in textbook pictures. The dura is recognized by its white, smooth appearance. It may pulsate with changes in CSF pressure. Blood vessels can be seen on the dura, as may be fibrotic structures, possibly ligaments. In pathology, numerous areas of increased vasculature, hyperemia, and fibrosis cover the dura. These areas of inflammation may be continuous with inflammation that accompanies the nerve root.

TECHNICAL ASPECTS OF EPIDUROSCOPY

Epiduroscopy Equipment

- Epiduroscope with light source and video display. Epiduroscopes are available from Karl Storz, Myelotec and Equip. We prefer and use Karl Storz equipment (Fig. 62–7A, B) such as a video display system that allows simultaneous viewing of fluoroscopy and epiduroscopy images (Karl Storz Twin Video).
- Percutaneous introducer set and guidewire. (Supplied with Storz, Myelotec and Equip equipment. We prefer to use a 9- or 10-French Super Arrow-Flex vascular access set from Arrow International, Reading, PA.)
- 25-gauge, $^3/_4$-inch, and 18-gauge infiltration needles
- Two three-way stopcocks and IV set with extensions
- Number 10 blade scalpel
- Assorted syringes (5, 10, and 20 mL)
- 18-gauge Tuohy epidural needle
- 36-cm epidural (Tun-L) catheter with connector (optional)
- Two 2 × 2 split intravenous (IV) sponges
- Transparent surgical dressing
- Nerve stimulators (optional)

DRUGS

- 2% lidocaine for skin infiltration
- 0.25% bupivacaine or 0.2% ropivacaine
- Preservative-free normal saline
- 1500 units of hyaluronidase (Wydase)
- 10% hypertonic saline (optional)
- Steroid
- Iohexol (Omnipaque 240) radiographic contrast

PREPARATION OF THE PATIENT

Physical examination (including examination of the entry site for local infection and distorted anatomy), lumbosacral MRI, urology evaluation (if necessary), and laboratory studies including
- Complete blood count with platelets
- Prothrombin time, partial thromboplastin time
- Platelet function studies and bleeding time
- Urinalysis

For preoperative medication, we use the standard American Society of Anesthesiologists' recommendations for conscious sedation. Preprocedure sedatives, analgesics, and ancillary drugs are administered as

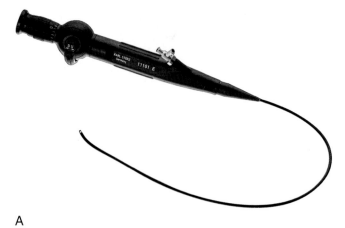

A

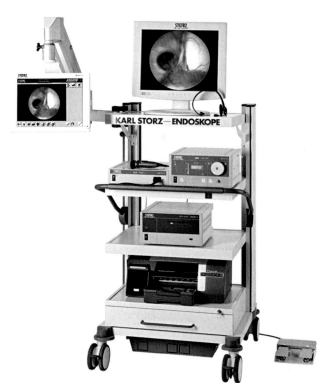

B

Figure 62–7. A, Karl Storz epiduroscope. **B,** Ancillary equipment for epiduroscopy.

needed in the surgical holding area. The patient is given 1 g of ceftriaxone (Rocephin) intravenously before the start of the case (ciprofloxacin [Cipro], 400 mg, given 1 hour before epiduroscopy, may be substituted if there is concern about allergy).

PROCEDURE

Location

At Texas Tech University Health Sciences Center/ University Medical Center, epiduroscopy is performed in the operating room.

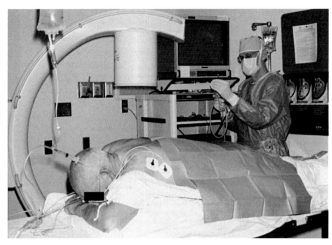

Figure 62–8. Patient in prone position prepared for epiduroscopy.

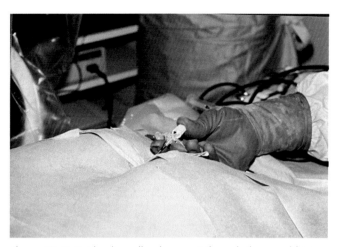

Figure 62–9. Epidural needle placement through the sacral hiatus.

Position of the Patient

The patient is placed in the prone position (Fig. 62–8). A pillow usually is placed under the abdomen to reduce lumbar lordosis. The epidural access site is prepared for sterile entry and a full-body sterile surgical drape is placed over the patient, leaving only the access site exposed.

Anesthetic Care

The goal for anesthetic care for epiduroscopy is to keep the patient comfortable and to provide amnesia. Local anesthetic is infiltrated at the epidural access site, hypnotic is administered to obtund consciousness, systemic opioid is administered for pain control, and an amnesic is administered (e.g., propofol with ketamine, fentanyl, midazolam).

We have begun injecting 5 mL of 0.2% ropivacaine into the epidural space before performing epiduroscopy to reduce pain provoked by scope manipulation in areas of pathology.

Patients do not describe feeling sensations during epiduroscopy when the scope is in normal areas, even in the absence of epidural local anesthetic injection.

Access to the Epidural Space

Access to the epidural space for epiduroscopy is via the sacral hiatus using the Seldinger technique. A skin wheal is raised over the sacral hiatus using 1 to 2 mL of 1% lidocaine and a 25-gauge needle. An 18-gauge needle is used to penetrate the skin. An 18-gauge Tuohy epidural needle is then inserted through the puncture site and into the sacral hiatus. The needle enters the gluteal fold parallel to the longitudinal axis of the patient's body (Fig. 62–9). It is directed cephalad through the hiatus parallel to the caudal portion of the sacral canal. This may be verified in both the posteroanterior and lateral fluoroscopic views. A guidewire is inserted through the needle and advanced to approximately the L5 or S1

level. A small stab wound is made through the skin and underlying tissue and sacrococcygeal ligament with a number 10 × 1-blade scalpel. The epidural needle is removed and a 10-French dilator is then inserted over the guidewire through the incision into the sacral canal. Then the dilator is removed and the dilator with a sheath is placed over the guidewire into the space. It is important to check the guidewire for freedom of movement to avoid kinking it. It also is important to advance the dilator and sheath together until the sheath passes through the sacrococcygeal ligament. This can be confirmed both by feeling a "pop" when the sheath passes through the ligament as well as by a lateral fluoroscopic view of the sacrum. The dilator and guidewire are removed, leaving the sheath in place. Before the sheath is inserted it is filled with saline and when in place, 5 mL of saline are injected through the injection port of the sheath to expand the epidural space.

Epiduroscopy

The epiduroscope allows for three-dimensional direct visual observation. As stated, we use equipment during epiduroscopy that displays on a monitor both the epiduroscopic image and the fluoroscopic image. Which is the primary image and which is the secondary image can be changed. We usually have the epiduroscopy image as the primary one except when we need more detail from the fluoroscopy image than can be obtained with it as a smaller secondary image. Our examination of the epidural space may extend from the sacrum to as far cephalad as the posterior border of L2, depending on the patient's area of symptoms and the extent of abnormalities encountered. Skill is required to manipulate the epiduroscope through the bony vertebral canal and to direct the scope tip to areas of interest.

The epiduroscope is inserted through the sheath (Fig. 62–10). Fluoroscopy is used to verify proper placement. During the epiduroscopy procedure, preservative-free 0.9% saline is injected through the working channel of the epiduroscope to expand the

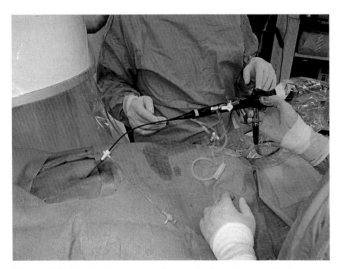

Figure 62–10. Epiduroscope inserted through sheath into the epidural space.

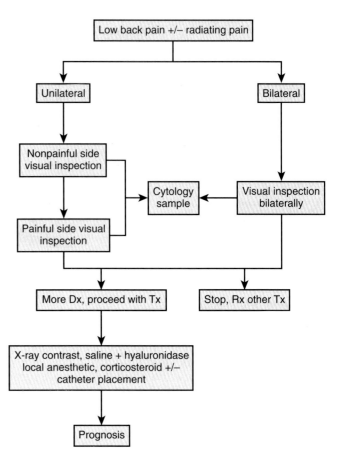

Figure 62–11. Epiduroscopy algorithm. Dx, diagnosis; Rx, medication; Tx, treatment.

epidural space and to flush away tissue debris and any extravasated blood to provide optimal viewing. How successful this is depends on many factors, including how fast fluid is infused, compliance of the contents of the space, presence of compartments, and how fast fluid exits through the intervertebral foramen into the paraspinal area. Care must be taken to use the minimal amount of saline. The total volume infused should generally not exceed 100 mL. In addition to monitoring the volume infused, epiduroscopy time should be monitored. At our institution, epiduroscopy time usually is less than 30 minutes.

If the patient has unilateral symptoms, we first examine the epidural space contralateral to the symptomatic side (Fig. 62–11). This provides the general appearance of the "normal" epidural space for the patient. Next, we examine the symptomatic side with emphasis on viewing the area where the nerve or nerves that innervate the symptomatic side transverse the epidural space and pass through the intervertebral foramen. The presence or absence and the character of fat, blood vessels, and fibrous tissue is noted as well as the presence of abnormal tissue and inflammation (Box 62–2). The scope tip readily exits a normal intervertebral foramen. The goal is to find an area or areas of pathology that when touched by the tip of the epiduroscope produce arousal or pain in the painful area identified during the preprocedure evaluation.

Abnormalities include discrete or diffuse inflammation and diffuse or discrete fibrosis that ranges from mild (through which the scope easily passes) to a dense, solid mass through which the scope cannot be passed. Increased vascularity (small or larger vessels) or engorged, distended blood vessels may be seen. Fibrous scars may be avascular or have varying degrees of vascularity (Box 62–3). We are in the process of obtaining specimens using a cytology inserted through the working channel of the epi-duroscope for examination. A variety of cell

---

BOX 62–2. ASSESSMENTS

- Evaluate normal or asymptomatic side areas
- Identify tissue and structure
  - Dura
  - Periosteum
  - Fat
  - Scar tissue
  - Blood vessels

BOX 62–3. FINDINGS

- Marked variability in "pathology"—objective documentation
- Possible subgroupings:
  - No abnormalities
  - Inflammation
  - Dural adhesions to perivertebral tissue
- Most common pathology noted
  - Increased vascularity
  - Decreased vascularity
  - Vascular distention
  - Fibrosis
  - Maturity, extent, intensity varies

types and tissue fragments have been obtained (Fig. 62–12A-D).

After the examination (diagnostic) phase of the procedure, we proceed with treatment, which includes breaking any existing fibrosis that was not lysed during the examination. The lysis is accomplished by using mechanical force delivered by moving the tip of the epiduroscope and by injecting hyaluronidase and normal saline through the working channel of the scope. Radiopaque contrast material is injected through the working channel to determine if there is a path for fluid to reach the area of pathology associated with the patient's symptoms. Then local anesthetic and corticosteroid are injected through the scope's working channel to the target site. More than one area may be treated depending on clinical presentation of symptoms and epiduroscopy findings. After the treatment is finished, the epiduroscope and the sheath are removed. The site is covered with antibiotic ointment and occlusive dressing. The patient is observed until criteria for discharge from the hospital are met.

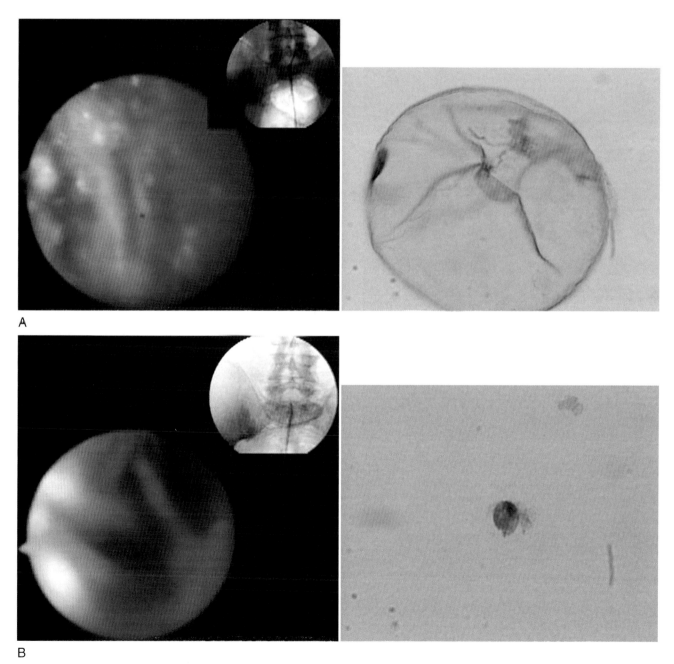

Figure 62–12. Epiduroscopy view of cytology sample site *(left frames)* and predominant cell type *(right frames)* obtained from the sample. **A,** 48-year-old male—FBS, Rt L4 radiculopathy. *Left frame,* right side, inflammation and scarring, fatty tissue. *Right frame,* cytology, fat cell. **B,** 68-year-old male—FBS, Lt L4-5 radiculopathy. *Left frame,* a little left of midline, scar tissue adhering to the dura. *Right frame,* cytology, durocyte.

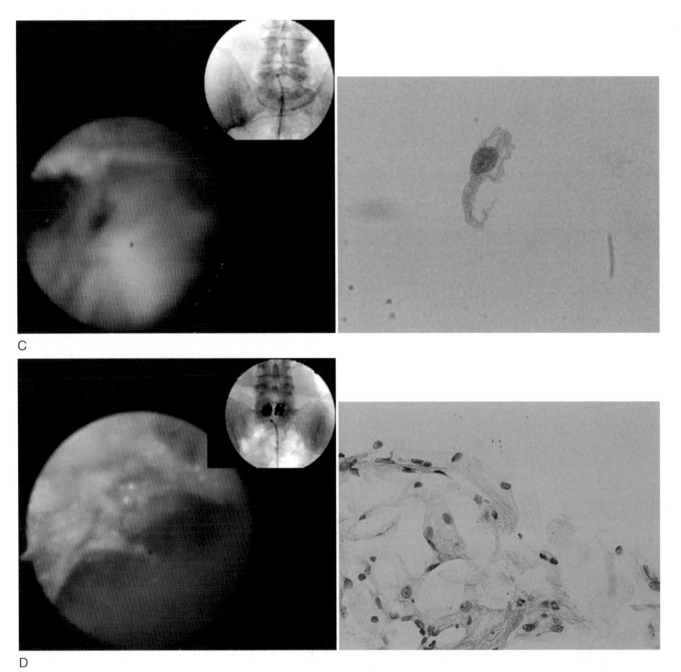

Figure 62–12, cont'd. C, 68-year-old male—FBS Lt L4-5 radiculopathy. *Left frame,* left side, fibrosis L5. *Right side,* cytology, big spindle cell. **D,** 44-year-old female—FBS (hardware), Lt L5 radiculopathy and low back pain. *Left frame,* left side, mostly hyperemia, an active inflammatory, bleeds easily. *Right frame,* cytology, tissue fragment with polymorphonuclear cells.

TREATMENT OF RADICULAR PAIN USING EPIDUROSCOPY

Targeted Drug Delivery

When an area of pathology is identified, the abnormality is treated by local drug injection through the working channel of the scope. The objectives of such an injection in the treatment of radiculopathy include the reduction or prevention of inflammatory lesions adjacent to the nerve root and reduction or prevention of epidural fibrosis through chemical adhesiolysis.

Placement of glucocorticosteroids at a site of inflammation may have an advantage over injection in the epidural space through other methods.

Mechanical Adhesiolysis

One of the most impressive images through epiduroscopy is of epidural fibrosis. Indeed, epidural scarring has been implicated in failed back surgery and chronic radicular pain.[21] The exact mechanism by which fibrosis may cause neuropathic pain is unclear, but local ischemia may play a role. Removal of perineural fibrosis may lead to improved local circulation and decrease of neuropathic symptoms. Multiple attempts to remove fibrosis or methods to prevent the buildup of epidural scar after surgery have been attempted with variable success. A mixture of 0.9% sodium chloride and hyaluronidase (1500 units; 10 mL) is part of the approach to remove fibrosis. Advancement of the scope in areas of fibrosis may have a mechanical lytic effect. Obviously, the effect will be more pronounced in areas of light fibrosis (grade 1 or 2) than in dense epidural scarring (grades 3 and 4). Significant amounts of normal saline are used to dilate the epidural space in order to obtain images. These normal saline injections in relatively closed compartments may lead to buildup of pressure and result in effective adhesiolysis. Forceful injections with saline, contrast material, hyaluronidase and other drugs have been studied. Outcomes of these injections have been variable. The effectiveness of these forceful injections on radicular pain is most likely highly dependent on the precise placement of the scope in the neuroforamen at the site of the pathology. Experience suggests that with precise placement of the scope, improvement of the epidurogram, that is, improved patency of the nerve root in the neuroforamen and lateral recess, is associated with clinical improvement. Several studies support this notion. Of course, these kind of observations need to be substantiated by more rigorously controlled studies. More involved techniques such as the use of fiberoptic laser in the ablation of fibrous material have been studied.[22]

Combined Adhesiolysis and Targeted Drug Delivery

There are an increasing number of studies that report on the effectiveness of epiduroscopy in the treatment of chronic radicular pain.[5,6] In general, these studies use a combination of drug delivery and mechanical adhesiolysis. Corticosteroids are injected with local anesthetics. A mixture of clonidine, hyaluronidase, and hypertonic saline may be injected in addition to variable amounts of saline to dilate the epidural space.[7] The emphasis is on fluoroscopic guidance of the scope to the area of the pathology. Very little description of epidural pathology as observed through the scope is provided in these studies—the scope is used mainly as a tool for targeted drug delivery and the exact target is not always clear.

INDICATIONS AND CONTRAINDICATIONS

Indications for lumbosacral epiduroscopy are shown in Box 62–1. In our opinion, the importance of epiduroscopy as a tool to help establish a diagnosis, guide therapy, and aid in prognosis following therapy is inadequately emphasized in patients with lower extremity radiculopathy with or without low back pain.

Contraindications for epiduroscopy include systemic infections, regional infection at the site of insertion, and in patients with bleeding disorders. The caudal area is prone to contamination and the

tract to the sacral hiatus may be a route of entry to the spinal canal. A prophylactic dose with antibiotics (e.g., ceftriaxone, ciprofloxacin) is recommended. Neurologic deficit is a relative contraindication because most of the patients will have neurologic abnormalities. Because decompression of the sacral nerve roots may lead to *improved* bladder and bowel function, neurogenic incontinence should not be an absolute contraindication to the procedure. Prior urodynamic evaluation in patients with symptoms of neurogenic bladder will provide a baseline status. Anatomic abnormalities of the sacrum may preclude placement of the scope. Resistance to scope placement may lead to scope damage and complications. Interestingly the distorted anatomy seen with Tarlov's cysts does not seem to interfere with epiduroscopy. Complications may arise from increased epidural and intracranial pressure with the infusion of dilating fluids in the epidural space. Therefore epiduroscopy in patients with increased intracranial pressure is contraindicated. Significant resistance to injection of fluids may indicate low compliance of the epidural space and forms a relative contraindication. Locally increased pressure may lead to circulatory abnormalities associated with compartment syndrome, with potentially devastating neurologic consequences. Because significant amounts of contrast material may be used during epiduroscopy, caution is advised in patients with impaired kidney function, particularly in older adults.

COMPLICATIONS

Complications of epiduroscopy are similar to other spinal procedures and include infection, bleeding with hematoma formation, and drug reactions (Box 62–4). Trauma to the sacral hiatus and canal may occur, but can be minimized with proper technique. Such trauma may result in persistent pain after the procedure. Infection may lead to a fistula or abscess. Any sign of infection at the puncture site should therefore be treated aggressively. Manipulation of the scope in the epidural spinal canal may lead to direct damage to neural structures or to circulatory compromise of these structures. In particular, this may occur in a region of pathology when injected drugs loccu-

---

BOX 62–4. COMPLICATIONS

1. Residual pain at insertion site
2. Residual numbness
3. Bowel, bladder, sexual
4. Somatomotor
5. Macular hemorrhage with visual impairment
6. Difficulty obtaining access to the epidural space
7. Subdural or subarachnoid space entry
8. Scope breakage

Note: There is no complication that is unique to epiduroscopy.

late and the extramural pressure increases sufficiently to jeopardize local blood flow. In addition, the dura may be punctured by the scope, especially in areas of pathology.[23] Gentle manipulation of the scope and use of direct vision may prevent this. The dura is surprisingly resilient to puncture by the scope. On occasion, the dural sac extends far into the sacral epidural space. Aspiration of CSF and the typical appearance of the subarachnoid space on first inspection will show that entry occurred and prevent the epiduroscopist from causing damage to neural structures. Persistent CSF leak has been reported; however, complications from this may be limited because the sacral epidural space is not a closed space.

One of the more feared complications of epiduroscopy is visual disturbance. Rapid epidural infusion generating a pressure gradient may explain disruption of retinal circulation and result in retinal hemorrhages. Avoiding infusion pressures and significant pressure *changes* may prevent these complications. Gill and Heavner[24] reviewed the mechanism whereby fluid injection into the epidural space may lead to retinal hemorrhage.

Advancement of a scope through a too narrow sacral epidural canal at the hiatus may damage the scope to the point of breakage requiring surgical removal. If significant resistance to the scope is encountered, the procedure should be aborted.

HELPFUL HINTS

In our experience, the most difficult technical aspects of epiduroscopy are placing the dilator and sheath and advancing the epiduroscope to the area(s) of interest. Anteroposterior (AP) and lateral fluoroscopic viewing should be used as needed to ensure that the dilator and sheath follow the guidewire and are directed as straight as possible toward the sacral hiatus. The dilator and sheath must be advanced as a unit and there must not be tissue between the stab wound and the path of the dilator and sheath. We usually use a 10-French dilator and sheath but if we encounter difficulty we will use a 9-French dilator then switch to a 10-French or continue with a 9-French sheath. Access usually is much easier in females than in males. We rarely fail with females but fail in about 1 of 15 males.

Before inserting the epiduroscope, be sure it is in focus and color balanced. Establish a neutral or reference position for the scope to aid orientation and to establish up/down, right/left for scope tip manipulation as well as for image interpretation. When advancing the scope, rotate it and deflect the tip so the scope follows the spinal canal. Identification of the correct spinal level is almost impossible without simultaneous fluoroscopy. We use fluoroscopy in the pulse mode. Total fluoroscopy time for a procedure is usually less than 1 minute.

Avoid introducing air into the injected fluid. This causes distortion of the epiduroscopic image and can be difficult to move out of the visual field.

Recognition of structures and pathology is challenging. It is absolutely essential to be familiar with the anatomy of the epidural space and other contents of the spinal canal, especially as viewed through an epiduroscope. Also essential is familiarity with the type and appearance of pathology that might be encountered.

EFFICACY

In a systematic review of spinal endoscopy, Chopra and colleagues[5] retrieved 112 articles using their search criteria, 8 of which were considered to be relevant reports of studies of spinal endoscopic adhesiolysis. Two randomized, double-blind evaluations, three prospective evaluations, and three retrospective evaluations and multiple case reports were available for review.

The randomized trials showed significant improvement in pain relief, as well as multiple other parameters including return to work at 3 months, 6 months, and 1 year. The prospective evaluations also showed improvement. Two retrospective evaluations included in the analysis showed positive short-term and long-term results.

Dashfield and colleagues[25] reported no difference among groups treated for chronic sciatica with targeted epidural drug delivery with or without epiduroscopy. In contrast, Manchikanti and coworkers[6] reported remarkably better outcomes in patients with low back and lower extremity pain when the epiduroscope was used for adhesiolysis compared with when it was not.

CONCLUSION

There is an abundance of evidence that epiduroscopy can be performed safely and provide benefit to patients with low back pain with or without radiculopathy. Visual information is obtained that aids in the diagnosis, treatment, and prognosis.

References

1. Burman MS: Myeloscopy or the direct visualization of the spinal cord. J Bone Joint Surg 1931;13:695-696.
2. Pool JL: Myeloscopy: Intraspinal endoscopy. Surgery 1942; 11:169-182.
3. Saberski LR: Spinal endoscopy: Current concepts. In Waldman (ed): Interventional Pain Management (2nd ed). WB Saunders, Philadelphia, pp 143-161, 2001.
4. Racz GB, Holubec JT: Lysis of adhesions in the epidural space. In Racz GB (ed): Techniques of Neurolysis. Boston, Kluwer Academic, 1989, pp 57-72.
5. Chopra P, Smith HS, Deer TR, Bowman RC: Role of adhesiolysis in the management of chronic spinal pain: A systematic review of effectiveness and complications. Pain Physician 2005;8:87-100.
6. Manchikanti L, Boswell MV, Rivera JJ, et al: A randomized, controlled trial of spinal endoscopic adhesiolysis in chronic refractory low back and lower extremity pain. BMC Anesthesiology 2005;5:10.
7. Geurts JW, Kallewaard JW, Richardson J, Groen GJ: Targeted methylprednisolone acetate/hyaluronidase/clonidine injec-

tion after diagnostic epiduroscopy for chronic sciatica: A prospective, 1-year follow-up study. Reg Anesth Pain Med 2002;27:343-352.

8. Manchikanti L, Pampati V, Bakhit C, Pakanati R: Non-endoscopic and endoscopic adhesiolysis in post lumbar laminectomy syndrome: A one-year outcome study and cost effectiveness analysis. Pain Physician 1999;2:52-58.

9. Igarashi T, Hirabayashi Y, Seo N, et al: Lysis of adhesions and epidural injection of steroid/local anaesthetic during epiduroscopy potentially alleviate low back and leg pain in elderly patients with lumbar spinal stenosis. Br J Anaesth 2004;93: 181-187.

10. Manchikanti L: The value and safety of epidural endoscopic adhesiolysis. Am J Anesthesiol 2000;275-278.

11. Richardson J, McGurgan P, Cheema S, Gupta S: Spinal endoscopy in chronic low back pain with radiculopathy: A prospective case series. Anaesthesia 2001;56:454-460.

12. Ruetten S, Meyer O, Godolias G: Endoscopic surgery of the lumbar epidural space (epiduroscopy): Results of therapeutic intervention in 93 patients. Min Invas Neurosurg 2003; 46:1-4.

13. Saberski L: A retrospective analysis of spinal canal endoscopy and laminectomy outcome data. Pain Physician 2000;3: 193-196.

14. Saberski LR, Kitahata LM: Direct visualization of the lumbosacral epidural space through the sacral hiatus. Anesth Analg 1995;80:839-840.

15. Schütze G, Kurtse G, Grol O, Enns E: Endoscopic method for the diagnosis and treatment of spinal pain syndromes. Anesteziol Reanimatol 1996;4:62-64.

16. Australian Safety and Efficacy Register of New Interventional Procedures—Surgical (ASERNIP-S). Epiduroscopy. Rapid Review. New and Emerging Techniques—Surgical, June 2003. www.surgeons.org/asernip-s/net-s.

17. Hogan QH: Lumbar epidural anatomy: A new look by cryomicrotome section. Anesthesiology 1991;75:767-775.

18. Gershater R, St Louis EL: Lumbar epidura venography: Review of 1200 cases. Radiology 1979;131:409-421.

19. Crock HV, Yoshizawa H: The blood supply of the vertebral column and spinal cord in man. New York, Springer-Verlag, 1977.

20. Blomberg RG: The dorsomedian connective tissue band in the lumbar epidural space of humans: An anatomical study using epiduroscopy in autopsy cases. Anesth Analg 1986;65: 747-752.

21. Ross JS, Obuchowski N, Zepp R: The postoperative lumbar spine: Evaluation of epidural scar over a 1-year period. Am J Neuroradiol 1998;19:138-186.

22. Epstein JM, Adler R: Laser-assisted percutaneous endoscopic neurolysis. Pain Physician 2000;3:43-45.

23. Shah RV, Heavner JE: Recognition of the subarachnoid and subdural compartments during epiduroscopy: Two cases. Pain Practice 2003;3:321-325.

24. Gill JB, Heavner JE: Visual impairment following fluid injection and epiduroscopy: A review. Pain Med 2005;6:367-374.

25. Dashfield AK, Taylor MB, Cleaver JS, Farrow D: Comparison of caudal steroid epidural with targeted steroid placement during spinal endoscopy for chronic sciatica: A prospective, randomized, double-blind trial. Br J Anaesth 2005;94: 514-519.

PART VIII

Pain Management in Special Situations and Special Topics

C. Argoff and C. Wu

CHAPTER

63 Pain Management in the Emergency Department

James R. Miner and Knox H. Todd

Emergency physicians provide acute care for an extraordinary broad range of illnesses and injuries, the majority of which involve some degree of pain. Emergency providers also cause pain in the course of therapeutic and diagnostic procedures. This chapter considers the prevalence of pain in the emergency department (ED), barriers to its adequate treatment, and a variety of treatment modalities. Space limitations prohibit a discussion of the wide variety of specific painful conditions that present to the ED. These can be found in other chapters of the text.

PREVALENCE AND ASSESSMENT OF PAIN IN THE EMERGENCY DEPARTMENT

Pain is the motivating factor for the majority of patients seeking emergency care, and as a presenting complaint accounts for up to 78% of visits to U.S. EDs.[1-3] Although arriving at a diagnosis and choosing the appropriate therapy to treat underlying conditions are principal goals for physicians, those who present to the ED with pain also desire recognition of their pain and rapid, effective pain treatment.

Patients face many barriers in their efforts to obtain superior medical care, especially in regard to pain. The ED serves as a fail-safe mechanism for our fragmented health care system, and pain is but one of the many conditions in which we not only face the problem of acute clinical presentations, but also care for those with chronic pain who have been failed by other parts of the health care system.

Notwithstanding the issue of providing compassionate care, pain that is not acknowledged and managed appropriately causes anxiety, depression, sleep disturbances, increased oxygen demands with the potential for end-organ ischemia, and decreased movement with an increased risk of venous thrombosis.[4,5] Failure to recognize and treat pain may also result in dissatisfaction with medical care, hostility toward the physician, unscheduled returns to the ED, delayed complete return to full function, and an increased risk of litigation.[6]

Pain is inherently subjective and inevitably complex. Our patients experience pain and suffering as individuals; we assess it only indirectly. The ED's task is to use a commonly understood vocabulary and classification system in assessing pain so that our findings can be communicated consistently. Only by quantifying the pain experience in meaningful ways can we move beyond myth and opinion toward a scientific approach to our many questions regarding the pain experience. This challenge is at the root of our difficulties in treating pain, thus issues surrounding pain assessment have primacy in our approach to understanding. Only when we use comparable methods in assessing pain can we begin to accumulate the scientific evidence that should drive our practice.

The most common response of physicians confronted by patient pain reports is skepticism. The validity of patient self-reports is often questioned, and attempts to "objectify" the pain experience are sought. This search is bound to disappoint the querulous clinician, as neither blood tests, tissue pathology, diagnostic imaging, physical assessments, nor patient behaviors reliably reflect the internal pain experience.

A number of practical pain assessment tools are available. The subjective nature of pain makes such instruments necessary, and revised standards of The Joint Commission (TJC) have fostered their widespread use. Pain intensity should be assessed for all patients presenting to the ED with either an 11-point numerical rating scale (NRS) or a graphic rating scale (GRS). The NRS is sensitive to the short-term changes in pain intensity associated with emergency care.[7,8] GRS or picture scales are particularly useful for populations with limited literacy, including children.[9,10] In one study of patients who have advanced cancer and pain, 81% were able to complete a picture scale, whereas only 75% could complete the Visual Analogue Scale (VAS).[11] In another study, the authors noted that male patients were uncomfortable with scales depicting severe pain using tears.[12] Picture scales with such depictions might profitably be avoided because they may be biased in the direction of less severe pain in male patients.

The VAS is another measure of pain intensity often used in research settings. It consists of a 100-mm line, oriented horizontally and bounded on each end by verbal descriptors of pain intensity, with "no pain" on the left side of the line and "worst pain possible" at the right. Patients are asked to place a mark on the line that best represents their pain intensity level. The distance from the left of the line to the mark is measured and pain intensity is reported in millimeters (0 to 100). There is no advantage in using a VAS over an NRS in clinical settings; both are reliable and valid measures of pain intensity.[13] In fact, certain patient populations find the NRS easier to complete; therefore, it is preferred over the VAS for routine use.[7,14]

No matter the specific pain scale used, assessments should be repeated after therapeutic interventions and at the time of ED discharge.

THE PROBLEM OF EMERGENCY DEPARTMENT OLIGOANALGESIA

Although adequate analgesia in the ED is an important goal of treatment, the underuse of analgesics, termed "oligoanalgesia" by Wilson and Pendleton in 1989, occurs in a large proportion of ED patients.[15-19] A variety of factors are felt to give provenance to pain undertreatment[20] (Box 63–1).

Recognized risk factors for ED oligoanalgesia include extremes of age[21-23] and minority ethnicity.[24,25] It has been suggested that patients' expectations for pain treatment and perceptions of pain intensity do not differ by ethnic groups when patients are matched for socioeconomic factors.[26-28] Differences have been noted, however, in the way that patients of different cultural backgrounds express their pain.[28] Differences in the interactions of physicians and patients of a different ethnic group have been described, and may affect physician assessment.[29,30] When affect, actual patient-physician interaction, and cultural expressions of ethnicity are removed from a case presentation, such as with written clinical vignettes, patients with similar pain are similarly treated by physicians.[31] Cultural discordance between the patient and the physician may hinder the ability of patients to confer an understanding of their pain to their physician.

Treatment of pain is dependent on the physician's accurate assessment of the patient's pain. In fact, the only predictor of treatment that Bartfield and colleagues found for patients with back pain was the physician's assessment, regardless of the patient's ethnicity, age, or insurance status.[32] Disparities in the treatment of pain likely come from variations in assessment rather than variations in treatment among patients assessed as having a similar degree of pain.

Although there is a general reluctance to accept patient report as the most reliable indicator of pain, and disparities between patients' and physician's pain intensity ratings may lead to inadequately treated pain, patients themselves may be reluctant to report pain presence and intensity. This may be a result of low expectations of obtaining pain relief, fear of analgesic side effects, and a notion that pain is to be expected as part of the underlying disease or from medical treatments. Some patients have an inappropriate fear of addiction when prescribed opioids or fear the stigma associated with opioid use.

Although federal regulators and state medical boards do not perceive emergency medicine as a specialty prone to inappropriate prescribing, and investigations of, or sanctions against, emergency physicians are rare, many emergency physicians express fears of such scrutiny or sanctions related to prescribing or administering opioids. In treating pain in patients receiving chronic opioid therapy, confusion over the concepts of physical dependence, tolerance, addiction, and pseudoaddiction may constitute a barrier to appropriate treatment. These phenomena are discrete, and standard definitions may be helpful in caring for patients managed with chronic opioids (Box 63–2).

ED personnel commonly identify patients who are thought to seek opioids for illegitimate purposes. Although drug addiction occurs in all patient populations, EDs are felt to be particularly rife with such patients. Unfortunately, the true prevalence of addiction and aberrant drug seeking behaviors is unknown. When the prevalence of such problems is overestimated, oligoanalgesia is the predictable result.

PAIN TREATMENT AND PROCEDURAL SEDATION

Effective pain management involves both pharmacologic and nonpharmacologic modalities. Simply asking about pain and validating the pain reports has a potent effect on patients' satisfaction with ED pain management. In one study, patient satisfaction with pain management was predicted more strongly by the perception that ED staff asked about pain than by the actual administration of an analgesic.[33] Other modalities, such as reassuring the patient that pain will be addressed, immobilizing and elevating injured extremities, and providing quiet, darkened rooms for patients with migraine headaches are essential aspects of quality pain management.

Pharmacologic therapies should begin as soon as is practical after presentation to the ED. Analgesic protocols allowing early pain treatment can decrease the

---

BOX 63–1. FACTORS UNDERLYING EMERGENCY DEPARTMENT OLIGOANALGESIA

1. Lack of educational emphasis on pain management
2. Inadequate emergency department (ED) quality improvement systems
3. Lack of ED pain research, particularly among older adult and pediatric populations
4. Emergency providers' concerns regarding opioid addiction and abuse
5. Fear of opioid adverse effects
6. Racial and ethnic bias

Table 63–1. Analgesics Administered in the Emergency Department (735 Doses Given to 506 Patients)

MEDICATION	N (%)
Morphine	148 (20.1)
Ibuprofen	127 (17.3)
Hydrocodone/acetaminophen	93 (12.7)
Oxycodone/acetaminophen	83 (11.3)
Ketorolac	60 (8.2)
Acetaminophen	53 (7.2)
Hydromorphone	36 (4.9)
Antacid	26 (3.5)
Meperidine	24 (3.3)
Fentanyl	23 (3.1)
Metoclopramide	13 (1.8)
Codeine/acetaminophen	12 (1.6)
Oxycodone	10 (1.4)
Naproxen	9 (1.2)
Other	18 (2.4)
Total	735 (100)

From Todd KH, Ducharme J, Choiniere M, et al: Pain in the emergency department: Results of the Pain and Emergency Medicine Initiative (PEMI) multicenter study. J Pain 2007;8:460-466.

time to effective treatment and improve patient outcomes.[34-36]

Analgesics may be administered by a variety of routes; however, the vast majority of medications are administered by the oral or parenteral routes. Oral therapies are most commonly used because they are convenient and inexpensive for patients who can tolerate oral intake. When pain is severe, analgesics must be given immediately and titrated to effect. The intravenous rather than intramuscular (IM) route is indicated in this context. IM injections are painful, they do not allow for titration, absorption is unpredictable, and they result in slow onset of drug action. Unless intravenous access is elusive, there is little to recommend the IM route.

In general, it is inappropriate to delay analgesic use until a diagnosis has been made. In the case of acute abdominal pain, a large number of studies find no deleterious effect of intravenous opioid therapy on our ability to make appropriate diagnoses.[37]

Specific Treatment Modalities

A wide variety of analgesics are used in emergency medicine practice. In a recent 20-site survey of ED analgesic practice, a total of 735 doses of 24 different analgesics were administered to 506 patients receiving analgesics while in the ED. The majority of analgesics administered were opioids (59%), morphine being the most commonly used analgesic (20%), followed by ibuprofen (17%). Analgesics recorded as being administered in the report are listed in Table 63–1.[38]

Non-Opioids

Commonly available analgesics include opioid and non-opioid agents. When opioids are required for pain treatment, non-opioids should be included in order to potentiate the opioid analgesic effect and decrease the severity of side effects. Non-opioids include salicylates, nonsteroidal anti-inflammatory drugs (NSAIDs), and acetaminophen. Unfortunately, non-opioid agents exhibit an analgesic ceiling effect and cannot be titrated to effect. This limits their usefulness in the setting of severe or fluctuating pain; however, they should be used as an adjunct to opioid therapies unless contraindicated, for the reasons noted earlier.

Acetaminophen is indicated for mild to moderate pain, and is often combined with opioid agents. Acetaminophen, unlike NSAIDs, has no antiplatelet activity or anti-inflammatory effect. Although a great deal of attention has been paid to acetaminophen hepatotoxicity, especially in the setting of chronic malnutrition, alcoholism, or liver disease, such effects are uncommon, particularly as compared to NSAID-related gastrointestinal toxicity.

NSAIDs, including salicylates, act to inhibit prostaglandin synthesis by interfering with cyclooxygenase (COX) enzymes. They cause platelet dysfunction and can precipitate renal failure in patients with renal insufficiency or volume depletion. They increase the risk of gastrointestinal bleeding when taken chronically.

Opioids

Opioid combination analgesics are commonly used for moderate to severe pain. Although the opioid component in these agents does not exhibit ceiling analgesic effects, the nonopioid component dose must be limited; thus one cannot titrate these analgesics. The convenience of combination therapy must be balanced against this limitation. Hydrocodone and oxycodone combination agents are associated with less nausea and vomiting and are preferable to codeine combinations agents. Also a significant proportion of the population are poor metabolizers of codeine, which must be metabolized to morphine in order to manifest analgesic effects, further limiting its effectiveness.

The tramadol-acetaminophen combination agent is indicated for acute pain; however, experience with this agent in the ED setting is limited. Its mechanism of action is unclear: the tramadol component binds only weakly to opioid receptors and inhibits the reuptake of both norephinephrine and serotonin.

Opioids are the mainstay of ED therapy for moderate to severe pain, and morphine is the standard of comparison for all agents of this class. If contraindicated because of allergy or other sensitivity, hydromorphone or fentanyl may be substituted. These opioids can be rapidly titrated intravenously to control severe pain, allowing institution of an oral regimen. Fentanyl has the advantage of being relatively short acting and is preferred in the setting of multiple trauma, head injury, and potential hemodynamic instability. Intravenous morphine is the standard of treatment for severe pain in the ED. Morphine 0.1 mg/kg bolus has been found to be safe but not usually adequate to effect pain relief.[39] Repeat boluses of 0.05 mg/kg every 5 minutes until pain relief represents a safe incremental strategy.[40,41]

Meperidine is a problematic opioid for a number of reasons. Many EDs have eliminated completely the use of meperidine because of its metabolism to normeperidine, a toxic metabolite causing central excitation and seizures, as well as its contraindication in patients taking monoamine oxidase inhibitors.[42] It is, however, frequently used. In a recent review of ED patients treated in the United States for isolated benign headache, meperidine was found to be the most common prescribed treatment, despite national recommendations for the use of nonopioid therapies supported by strong evidence.[43] This likely has more to do with the persistence of medical tradition than with pharmacology. Subtherapeutic doses of intramuscularly administered meperedine have been used to treat a wide variety of acute pain complaints by generations of physicians. The availability of other opioid agents of equal efficacy with fewer contraindications and fewer adverse effects argues against its continued use.

Agonist-antagonist opioids, such as nalbuphine and butorphanol, have mixed effects on opioid receptor subtypes, exhibiting ceiling effects on both analgesia and respiratory depression. Because clinically important respiratory depression is distinctly rare in the setting of acute pain treatment, it is difficult to justify their routine use. One possible exception is for patients with advanced pulmonary disease. In particular, one cannot titrate these drugs to maximal effect because of analgesic ceiling effects. Additionally, these drugs are contraindicated and will induce withdrawal symptoms in patients who are physically dependent on opioids, either because of opioid therapy for chronic pain, methadone maintenance therapy, or active opioid addiction.

Patient-Controlled Analgesia

The use of patient-controlled analgesia (PCA) has been described in emergency medicine in adults and children.[44,45] Although no specific advantage has been found over the titration of opioids, PCAs were found to be at least as effective. In the setting of high demands on nursing resources, PCAs could serve to ensure pain treatment.

Alternative Delivery Routes

Multiple alternative delivery routes for the administration of pain medications have been described. The use of nebulized fentanyl has been described and holds great promise as a route of opioid delivery that can be initiated before an intravenous (IV) needle has been placed.[46-48] The promise of nebulized pain medications, especially in children who have severe pain but have not had an IV needle placed yet could be very useful in the ED.

Procedural Sedation and Analgesia

Minimal, moderate, and deep sedation have all been described in the ED. Patients often present to the ED in need of painful or complex procedures that require compliance that must be done emergently, and procedural sedation and analgesia (PSA) has adopted a specialized format for procedures in the ED. Unlike most patients who are undergoing sedation in other settings, patients in the ED have unpredictable nothing per mouth (NPO) status, often have concurrent severe systemic disease, and usually are in severe pain before the procedure begins. In addition, unpredictable concurrent events and time or bed constraints in the ED complicate these procedures.

The indications for ED PSA range from pain control for short painful procedures to the need for patient compliance with a complex emergent procedure. Goals for level of sedation during ED PSA range from minimal through moderate and deep sedation, depending on the needs for the procedure. Although it is acknowledged that deep sedation can inadvertently result in patients achieving a level of sedation consistent with anesthesia, this is not typically the goal of ED PSA. Minimal sedation, a drug-induced state during which patients respond appropriately to their developmental age to verbal commands, is generally performed for procedures that require compliance but are not typically painful with the use of local anesthesia. Minimal sedation has been described for lumbar puncture, evidentiary examinations, simple fracture reductions (in combination with local anesthesia), and abscess incision and drainage.

During minimal sedation, cardiovascular and ventilatory function are usually maintained, although patients should be monitored for inadvertent oversedation to deeper levels with oxygen saturation monitors and close nursing supervision. Agents typical of minimal sedation include fentanyl, midazolam, combinations of the two, and low-dose ketamine.

Moderate sedation is performed on patients who would benefit from either a deeper level of sedation to augment the procedure or from amnesia of the event. Moderate sedation is a drug-induced depression of consciousness during which patients respond appropriately to their developmental age to verbal commands, either alone or with light tactile stimulation. Patients usually have an intact airway and maintain ventilatory function without support. As with minimal sedation, inadvertent oversedation to deeper levels can occur with moderate sedation, and appropriate monitoring including oxygen saturation, cardiac, and blood pressure should be done throughout the sedation, and direct observation of the patient's airway should be maintained throughout the procedure. Agents used for moderate sedation in the ED include propofol, etomidate, ketamine, and the combination of fentanyl and midazolam.

Deep sedation is performed on patients who would benefit from a deeper level of sedation in order to complete the procedure for which they were being sedated. Generally, amnesia of the procedure is similar between moderate and deep sedation, and it is not necessary to sedate patients to a deep level only to obtain amnesia of the procedure.[49] Deep sedation generally is achieved in the ED with the same agents as moderate sedation; the difference is in the intended level of sedation. Monitoring for deep sedation is the same as for moderate with oxygen saturation, cardiac and blood pressure monitoring, and direct observation of the airway. End-tidal carbon dioxide has also been described in ED PSA, but its use over direct observation of the patient's airway has not been established.[50] Deeply sedated patients can develop respiratory depression but generally maintain a patent airway and adequate ventilation. Patients sedated to this level can progress to a level of sedation consistent with anesthesia,[40,51-53] and there is some evidence that this may occur more frequently in patients intended to undergo deep sedation than in those who are to undergo moderate sedation.[54] For this reason, it is usually safer to use moderate than deep sedation in the ED unless the procedure for which the patient was being sedated requires a deeper level of sedation (such as hip reduction).

Patients who progress to an unintended level of sedation consistent with anesthesia are not arousable, even to pain. The ability to independently maintain ventilatory function is usually impaired, and patients often require assistance in maintaining a patent airway. Because patients can quickly progress to this level using the agents typical of moderate and deep sedation, physicians performing moderate and deep sedation must be prepared to provide ventilatory support until the patient has regained consciousness. In order to decrease the likelihood of aspiration, patients who are undergoing moderate or deep sedation in the ED should be kept NPO. It is difficult to find a consensus on the amount of time a patient should be kept NPO prior to PSA.[55,56] Many departments use 3 to 6 hours as a minimum.[57]

ED PSA has been described in patients who are medically stable (American Society of Anesthesiologists Physical classes 1 and 2) and in those who are not (classes 3 and 4). PSA for critically ill children has been described using ketamine[58] and in adults using propofol or etomidate.[41] The degree of respiratory depression noted in these patients was similar to patients with physical status scores of 1 or 2, but an increased rate of hypotension was seen in physical status 3 and 4 patients who received propofol. It may be that ketamine and etomidate are better suited for the emergent sedation of critically ill patients, but there is not yet sufficient data to make a definite recommendation.

Sedated patients are generally monitored by pulse oximetry, which is a sensitive measure of oxygenation. If a patient receives supplemental oxygen before starting PSA, this monitor may not be as sensitive to changes in the patient's ventilatory status.[50,59,60] Preoxygenation is generally recommended for ED PSA; however, there is no evidence that it decreases the incidence of transient hypoxia that has been noted as a complication of PSA. End-tidal carbon dioxide has been recommended as an additional modality for the monitoring of sedated patients.[57,61] Monitoring expired carbon dioxide during PSA allows for a graphic display of the patient's ventilatory status that can be a detector of respiratory depression before it becomes clinically apparent.[50] In the event of hypoventilation, the end-tidal CO_2 value increases as the respiratory rate decreases. In the event of increasing airway obstruction, the baseline end-tidal CO_2 value decreases along with a blunting of the waveform as a result of increased mixing of the nasal expiratory sample with ambient air caused by the turbulence from the obstruction.

Ketamine has been described in adults[62] but predominantly in children for use in ED PSA.[63] It is a dissociative anesthetic that provides 15 to 20 minutes of sedation when given intramuscularly, with a return to baseline mental status in 30 to 60 minutes. It can be given in doses of 1 to 4 mg/kg IM and should be combined with atropine 0.01 mg/kg to prevent hypersalivation. The addition of 0.1 mg/kg of midazolam to ketamine has been described to prevent emergence phenomena, but this has been shown to have unclear use.[64] The 1 mg/kg dose achieves light sedation sufficient for such procedures as lumbar puncture, dressing changes, and simple laceration repair. The doses ranging from 2 to 4 mg/kg result in increasingly deep levels of sedation but have all been shown to generally achieve moderate or deep sedation with a decreasing responsiveness to pain as the dose is increased. Patients sedated with ketamine usually maintain a patent airway and ventilate normally. Laryngospasm has been described with its administration at a fairly rare rate.[65] Patients undergoing PSA with ketamine should be monitored for respiratory depression and possible laryngospasm.[63] Emergence phenomena, described as an unpleasant perceptual experience by patients as they regain consciousness from sedation with ketamine, has been described in adults and children.[64,66,67] The use of ketamine IV has also been described for ED PSA.[62,68] It is generally given at 1 mg/kg IV and has an onset of 1 to 2 minutes, followed by moderate sedation lasting 8 to 12 minutes. The side effects have been described as similar to IM ketamine and similar precautions should be taken.

The combination of fentanyl and midazolam has been described for minimal, moderate, and deep sedation in the ED.[50,54,66,69,70] These medications result in the longest sedation of the agents described here and have been noted to have a high rate of respiratory depression that increases with the dose. Because of this, this combination of agents, whereas adequate for minimal sedation, is less useful for moderate and deep sedation, and its use for these levels of sedation is not recommended. Dosing for minimal sedation has been described as 0.1 mg/kg IV midazolam followed by 0.5 µg/kg IV fentanyl, with repeated fentanyl boluses every 3 minutes until the patient is adequately sedated. The sedation typically lasts 30 to 60 minutes, with a return to baseline mental status of 45 to 120 minutes. This method of PSA has increasing respiratory depression with increasing levels of sedation, and close respiratory monitoring is required. A sedation regimen similar in duration but without analgesic properties is pentobarbital. It is usually used for the sedation of children for radiologic procedures.[71,72] The medicine is usually started at 2.5 mg/kg IV, followed by 1.25 mg/kg IV every 5 minutes until sedation is achieved. This is usually used for minimal or moderate sedation, and pulse oximetry is required. The rate of respiratory depression is lower than for other protocols but the sedation is inadequate for painful procedures.[73]

Methohexital has also been described for moderate and deep PSA.[40,74,75] It is a very short-acting agent with dense amnestic capabilities. It can be given at 1 mg/kg IV with 0.5 mg/kg repeat boluses every 2 minutes as needed. It has an onset of 30 seconds. The sedation generally lasts 2 to 4 minutes with a return to baseline mental status of 10 to 15 minutes. It has been associated with respiratory depression and a quick progression to deeper levels of sedation than intended, and can result in oversedation even when carefully titrated. This agent therefore requires close respiratory monitoring throughout the sedation, as with other agents. When compared directly with propofol, it was found to be similarly effective and safe when only a single bolus was given, and less safe than propofol when multiple doses were required.[40]

It therefore should be used principally for very brief procedures that are expected to last less than 2 to 4 minutes, such as simple fracture and dislocation reductions.

Propofol is well described for ED PSA.[40,41,50-54,76-80] It is generally administered as a 1 mg/kg bolus with repeat boluses of 0.5 mg/kg every 3 minutes until the patient is adequately sedated for the procedure. The sedation persists 2 to 5 minutes after a single bolus, and longer for patients receiving multiple boluses, with a return to baseline mental status in 10 to 15 minutes. This medication has been associated with rates of clinically apparent respiratory depression from 4% to 7.7% in ED PSA, so close respiratory monitoring is required as with the other agents. It has also been associated with hypotension in critically ill patients and should be used with caution in this group.[41]

Another agent used in ED PSA is etomidate.[41,81-86] It is usually given as a single bolus of 0.1 to 0.3 mg/kg, with an onset of sedation in 30 to 60 seconds, and sedation lasting 7 to 10 minutes. It is not associated with hypotension and is therefore optimal in patients who are at risk for this. It is however, associated with myoclonic jerking in up to 25% of patients receiving the medication, which can sometimes complicate the procedure for which the patient has been sedated.[41] This makes it slightly suboptimal relative to propofol in healthy patients. Etomidate has been associated with adrenal suppression. This has been noted in studies of single boluses of 0.3 mg/kg, but no significant changes in cortisol levels were found, and the significance of this remains unclear.[87]

SUMMARY

- Failure to recognize and treat pain may cause unnecessary increases in anxiety and delayed return to function among emergency department patients.
- Barriers to superior emergency department pain management include knowledge deficits among providers and inadequate quality improvement efforts.
- The true prevalence of opioid addiction among emergency department patients is unknown and likely overestimated by emergency physicians and nurses.
- Few specialty-specific treatment guidelines exist to promote best practices for emergency department pain management.
- Emergency providers tend to disbelieve pain reports that do not conform to our expectations.

References

1. Cordell WH, Keene KK, Giles BK, et al: The high prevalence of pain in emergency medical care. Am J Emerg Med 2002; 20:165-169.
2. Johnston CC, Gagnon AJ, Fullerton L, et al: One-week survey of pain intensity on admission to and discharge from the emergency department: A pilot study. J Emerg Med 1998; 16:377-382.
3. Tanabe P, Buschmann M: A prospective study of ED pain management practices and the patient's perspective. J Emerg Nurs 1999;25:171-177.

4. Gureje O, Von Korff M, Simon GE, et al: Persistent pain and well-being: A World Health Organization Study in Primary Care. JAMA 1998;280:147-151.
5. Anderson FA Jr, Spencer FA: Risk factors for venous thromboembolism. Circulation 2003;107(23 suppl 1):I9-I16.
6. Furrow BR: Pain management and provider liability: No more excuses. J Law Med Ethics 2001;29:28-51.
7. Paice J, Cohen F: Validity of a verbally administered numeric rating scale to measure cancer pain intensity. Cancer Nurs 1997;20:88-93.
8. Sze FK, Chung TK, Wong E, et al: Pain in Chinese cancer patients under palliative care. Palliat Med 1998;12:271-277.
9. Breyer JE, Knott CB: Construct validity estimation for the African-American and Hispanic versions of the Oucher Scale. J Pediatr Nurs 1998;13:20-31.
10. Bellamy N, Campbell J, Syrotuik J: Comparative study of self-rating pain scale in osteoarthritis patients. Curr Med Res Opin 1999;15:113-119.
11. Shannon MM, Ryan MA, D'Agostino N, et al: Assessment of pain in advanced cancer patients. J Pain Symptom Manage 1995;10:274-278.
12. Ramer L, Richardson JL, Zichi Cohen M, et al: Multimeasure pain assessment in an ethnically diverse group of patients with cancer. J Trans Nurs 1999;10:94-101.
13. Bellamy N, Campbell J, Syrotuik J: Comparative study of self-rating pain scales in rheumatoid arthritis patients. Curr Med Res Opin 1999;15:121-127.
14. Fosnocht DE, Chapman CR, Swanson ER, et al: Correlation of change in visual analog scale with pain relief in the ED. Am J Emerg Med 2005;23:55-59.
15. Wilson JE, Pendleton JM: Oligoanalgesia in the emergency department. Am J Emerg Med 1989;7:620-623.
16. Stalnikowicz R, Mahamid R, Kaspi S, et al: Undertreatment of acute pain in the emergency department: A challenge. Int J Qual Health Care 2005;17:173-176.
17. Pines JM, Perron AD: Oligoanalgesia in ED patients with isolated extremity injury without documented fracture. Am J Emerg Med 2005;23:580.
18. Neighbor ML, Honner M, Kohn MD: Factors affecting emergency department opioid administration to severely injured patients. Acad Emerg Med 2004;11(12):1290-1296.
19. Fosnocht DE, Swanson ER, Barton ED: Changing attitudes about pain and pain control in emergency medicine. Emerg Med Clin North Am 2005;23(2):297-306.
20. Rupp T, Delaney KA: Inadequate analgesia in emergency medicine. Ann Emerg Med 2004;43:494-503.
21. Jones JS, Johnson K, McNinch M: Age as a risk factor for inadequate emergency department analgesia. Am J Emerg Med 1996;14:157-160.
22. Friedland LR, Kulick RM: Emergency department analgesic use in pediatric trauma victims with fractures. Ann Emerg Med 1994;23:203-207.
23. Selbst SM: Managing pain in the pediatric emergency department. Pediatr Emerg Care 1989;5(1):56-63.
24. Todd KH, Samaroo N, Hoffman JR: Ethnicity as a risk factor for inadequate emergency department analgesia. JAMA 1993;269:1537-1539.
25. Todd,KH, Deaton C, D'Adamo AP, et al: Ethnicity and analgesic practice. Ann Emerg Med 2000;35:11-16.
26. Miner J, Biros MH, Trainor A, et al: Patient and physician perceptions as risk factors for oligoanalgesia: A prospective observational study of the relief of pain in the emergency department. Acad Emerg Med 2006;13:140-146.
27. Pfefferbaum B, Adams J, Aceves J: The influence of culture on pain in Anglo and Hispanic children with cancer. J Am Acad Child Adolesc Psychiatry 1990;29:642-647.
28. Greenwald, HP: Interethnic differences in pain perception. Pain 1991;44:157-163.
29. Tait RC, Chibnall JT: Physician judgments of chronic pain patients. Soc Sci Med 1997;45:1199-1205.
30. Cooper-Patrick L, Gallo JJ, Gonzales JJ, et al: Race, gender, and partnership in the patient-physician relationship. Jama 1999;282:583-589.
31. Tamayo-Sarver JH, Dawson NV, Hinze SW, et al: The effect of race/ethnicity and desirable social characteristics on physicians' decisions to prescribe opioid analgesics. Acad Emerg Med 2003;10:1239-1248.
32. Bartfield JM, Salluzzo RF, Raccio-Robak N, et al: Physician and patient factors influencing the treatment of low back pain. Pain 1997;73:209-211.
33. Todd KH, Sloan EP, Chen C, et al: Survey of pain etiology, management, and satisfaction in two urban emergency departments. Can J Emerg Med 2002;4:252-256.
34. Zohar Z, Eitan A, Halperin P, et al: Pain relief in major trauma patients: An Israeli perspective. J Trauma 2001;51:767-772.
35. Kelly AM: A process approach to improving pain management in the emergency department: Development and evaluation. J Accid Emerg Med 2000;17:185-187.
36. Fry C, Aholt D: Local anesthesia prior to the insertion of peripherally inserted central catheters. J Infus Nurs 2001;24:404-408.
37. McHale PM, LoVecchio F: Narcotic analgesia in the acute abdomen—A review of prospective trials. Eur J Emerg Med 2001;8:131-136.
38. Todd KH, Ducharme J, Choiniere M, et al: Pain in the emergency department: Results of the Pain and Emergency Medicine Initiative (PEMI) multicenter study. J Pain 2007;8:460-466.
39. Bijur PE, Kenny MK, Gallagher EJ: Intravenous morphine at 0.1 mg/kg is not effective for controlling severe acute pain in the majority of patients. Ann Emerg Med 2005;46:362-367.
40. Miner JR, Biros M, Krieg S, et al: Randomized clinical trial of propofol versus methohexital for procedural sedation during fracture and dislocation reduction in the emergency department. Acad Emerg Med 2003;10:931-937.
41. Miner JR, Martel ML, Meyer M, et al: Procedural sedation of critically ill patients in the emergency department. Acad Emerg Med 2005;12:124-128.
42. Hershey LA: Meperidine and central neurotoxicity. Ann Intern Med 1983;98:548-549.
43. Vinson DR: Emergency department treatment of migraine headaches. Arch Intern Med 2002;162:845.
44. Melzer-Lange MD, Walk-Kelly MD, Lea CM, et al: Patient-controlled analgesia for sickle cell pain crisis in a pediatric emergency department. Pediatr Emerg Care 2004;20:2-4.
45. Evans E, Turley N, Robinson N, et al: Randomised controlled trial of patient controlled analgesia compared with nurse delivered analgesia in an emergency department. Emerg Med J 2005;22:25-29.
46. Fulda GJ, Giberson F, Fagraeus L: A prospective randomized trial of nebulized morphine compared with patient-controlled analgesia morphine in the management of acute thoracic pain. J Trauma 2005;59:383-388.
47. Ballas SK, Viscusi ER, Epstein KR: Management of acute chest wall sickle cell pain with nebulized morphine. Am J Hematol 2004;76:190-191.
48. Bartfield JM, Flint RD, McErlean M, et al: Nebulized fentanyl for relief of abdominal pain. Acad Emerg Med 2003;10:215-218.
49. Miner JR, Bachman A, Kosman L, et al: Assessment of the onset and persistence of amnesia during procedural sedation with propofol. Acad Emerg Med 2005;12:491-496.
50. Miner JR, Heegaard W, Plummer D: End-tidal carbon dioxide monitoring during procedural sedation. Acad Emerg Med 2002;9:275-280.
51. Bassett KE, Anderson JL, Pribble CG, et al: Propofol for procedural sedation in children in the emergency department. Ann Emerg Med 2003;42:773-782.
52. Frazee BW, Park RS, Lowery D, et al: Propofol for deep procedural sedation in the ED. Am J Emerg Med 2005;23:190-195.
53. Miner JR, Biros MH, Seigel T, et al: The utility of the bispectral index in procedural sedation with propofol in the emergency department. Acad Emerg Med 2005;12:190-196.
54. Miner JR, Biros MH, Heegaard W, et al: Bispectral electroencephalographic analysis of patients undergoing procedural sedation in the emergency department. Acad Emerg Med 2003;10:638-643.
55. Green SM: Fasting is a consideration—not a necessity—for emergency department procedural sedation and analgesia. Ann Emerg Med 2003;42:647-650.

56. Agrawal D, Manzi SF, Bupta R, et al: Preprocedural fasting state and adverse events in children undergoing procedural sedation and analgesia in a pediatric emergency department. Ann Emerg Med 2003;42:636-646.

57. American College of Emergency Physicians: Procedural sedation in the emergency department. Ann Emerg Med 2005;46:103-104.

58. Green SM, Denmark TK, Cline J, et al: Ketamine sedation for pediatric critical care procedures. Pediatr Emerg Care 2001;17:244-248.

59. Hart LS, Berns SD, Houck CS, et al: The value of end-tidal CO_2 monitoring when comparing three methods of conscious sedation for children undergoing painful procedures in the emergency department. Pediatr Emerg Care 1997;13:189-193.

60. Bennett J, Peterson T, Burleson V: Capnography and ventilatory assessment during ambulatory dentoalveolar surgery. J Oral Maxillofac Surg 1997;55:921-925;discussion 925-926.

61. Levine DA, Platt SL: Novel monitoring techniques for use with procedural sedation. Curr Opin Pediatr 2005;17:351-354.

62. Chudnofsky CR, Weber JE, Colone PD, et al: A combination of midazolam and ketamine for procedural sedation and analgesia in adult emergency department patients. Acad Emerg Med 2000;7:228-235.

63. Green SM, Krauss B: Clinical practice guideline for emergency department ketamine dissociative sedation in children. Ann Emerg Med 2004;44:460-471.

64. Wathen JE, Roback MG, Mackenzie T, et al: Does midazolam alter the clinical effects of intravenous ketamine sedation in children? A double-blind, randomized, controlled emergency department trial. Ann Emerg Med 2000;36:579-588.

65. Green SM, Nakamura R, Johnson NE: Ketamine sedation for pediatric procedures: Part 1, A prospective series. Ann Emerg Med 1990;19:1024-1032.

66. Kennedy RM, Porter FL, Miller JP, et al: Comparison of fentanyl/midazolam with ketamine/midazolam for pediatric orthopedic emergencies. Pediatrics 1998;102(4 Pt 1):956-963.

67. Green SM, Sherwin TS: Incidence and severity of recovery agitation after ketamine sedation in young adults. Am J Emerg Med 2005;23:142-144.

68. Green SM, Rothrock SG, Harris T, et al: Intravenous ketamine for pediatric sedation in the emergency department: Safety profile with 156 cases. Acad Emerg Med 1998;5:971-976.

69. Pena BM, Krauss B: Adverse events of procedural sedation and analgesia in a pediatric emergency department. Ann Emerg Med 1999;34(4 Pt 1):483-491.

70. Dionne RA, Moore PA, Gonty A, et al: Comparing efficacy and safety of four intravenous sedation regimens in dental outpatients. J Am Dent Assoc 2001;132:740-751.

71. Malviya S, Tait AR, Reynolds PI, et al: Pentobarbital vs chloral hydrate for sedation of children undergoing MRI: Efficacy and recovery characteristics. Paediatr Anaesth 2004;14:589-595.

72. Kienstra AJ, Ward MA, Sasan F, et al: Etomidate versus pentobarbital for sedation of children for head and neck CT imaging. Pediatr Emerg Care 2004;20:499-506.

73. Karian VE, Burrows PE, Zurakowski D, et al: Sedation for pediatric radiological procedures: Analysis of potential causes of sedation failure and paradoxical reactions. Pediatr Radiol 1999;29:869-873.

74. Zink BJ, Darfler K, Salluzzo RF, et al: The efficacy and safety of methohexital in the emergency department. Ann Emerg Med 1991;20:1293-1298.

75. Bono JV, Rella JG, Zink BJ, et al: Methohexital for orthopaedic procedures in the emergency department. Orthop Rev 1993;22:833-838.

76. Pershad J, Godambe SA: Propofol for procedural sedation in the pediatric emergency department. J Emerg Med 2004;27:11-14.

77. Burton JH, Miner JR, Shipley ER, et al: Propofol for emergency department procedural sedation and analgesia: A tale of three centers. Acad Emerg Med 2006;13:24-30.

78. Symington L, Thakore S: A review of the use of propofol for procedural sedation in the emergency department. Emerg Med J 2006;23:89-93.

79. Guenther E, Pribble CG, Junkins EP Jr, et al: Propofol sedation by emergency physicians for elective pediatric outpatient procedures. Ann Emerg Med 2003;42:783-791.

80. Havel CJ Jr, Strait RT, Hennes H: A clinical trial of propofol vs midazolam for procedural sedation in a pediatric emergency department. Acad Emerg Med 1999;6:989-997.

81. Falk J, Zed PJ: Etomidate for procedural sedation in the emergency department. Ann Pharmacother 2004;38:1272-1277.

82. Hunt GS, Spencer MT, Hays DP: Etomidate and midazolam for procedural sedation: Prospective, randomized trial. Am J Emerg Med 2005;23:299-303.

83. Burton JH, Bock AJ, Strout TD, et al: Etomidate and midazolam for reduction of anterior shoulder dislocation: A randomized, controlled trial. Ann Emerg Med 2002;40:496-504.

84. Vinson DR, Bradbury DR: Etomidate for procedural sedation in emergency medicine. Ann Emerg Med 2002;39:592-598.

85. Keim SM, Erstad BL, Sakles JC, et al: Etomidate for procedural sedation in the emergency department. Pharmacotherapy 2002;22:586-592.

86. Ruth WJ, Burton JH, Bock AJ: Intravenous etomidate for procedural sedation in emergency department patients. Acad Emerg Med 2001;8:13-18.

87. Schenarts CL, Burton JH, Riker RR: Adrenocortical dysfunction following etomidate induction in emergency department patients. Acad Emerg Med 2001;8:1-7.

CHAPTER

64 Pain in the Critically Ill Patient

Michael Erdek

Pain in the critically ill is a poorly studied entity. Only recently has attention and investigation turned toward the issues of pain assessment and treatment in this population, and the existing literature is scant. The prevalence of poorly treated pain in the critically ill is considerable, and greater than seemingly commonly believed among health care physicians. This chapter endeavors to examine some of the salient issues as well as the pertinent literature detailing the barriers to assessment and treatment of pain in the intensive care unit as well as some strategies to deal with this challenge.

PREVALENCE OF PAIN IN THE INTENSIVE CARE UNIT

Patients admitted to the intensive care unit (ICU), although often unable to communicate as a result of the severity of their disease process or the presence of impediments such as artificial airways or endotracheal tubes (ETTs), experience pain and discomfort that often goes unrecognized and untreated.

An observational study in 128 Italian ICUs of 661 postoperative patients found that 36.3% of patients did not receive any analgesia in the first 48 hours of their ICU stay.[1] In only 54.5% of instances in which opioid was given was "pain control" the reason for the administration. Fentanyl was the most commonly administered opioid (more than morphine). Although fentanyl's rapidity of onset makes it perhaps desirable in an ICU setting, its use by prolonged infusion may be counterproductive in that its lipophilicity contributes to a prolonged offset of action when weaning or discontinuing this medication.

One study attempted to characterize the experience of a group of critically ill patients at high risk for hospital death.[2] Between 55% and 75% of 100 cancer patient self-responders reported the experience of pain, discomfort, anxiety, sleep disturbance, or unsatisfied hunger or thirst.

One prospective cohort study of 400 medical ICU patients found that those patients for whom analgesics were prescribed had a higher concomitant incidence of hemodynamic monitoring, greater use of neuromuscular blocking agents, more mechanical ventilation days, and longer ICU and hospital lengths of stay.[3] Consistent with these findings, patients who received analgesics also had higher trauma injury severity scores (TISS) and predicted mortality.

BARRIERS TO PAIN ASSESSMENT IN THE INTENSIVE CARE UNIT

Given the potential compromise of patients' physiologic stability and communication skills secondary to underlying disease processes, the ICU presents a unique environment for the assessment and treatment of pain. There is, therefore, a unique challenge to clinicians that may not commonly be seen in other arenas of pain control. As mentioned, the presence of impediments to communication such as the presence of an ETT or the severity of underlying critical illness may prevent the typical ICU patient from communicating with the nursing or physician staff their level of discomfort (Box 64–1).

A critically ill patient may be obtunded secondary to the underlying disease process or physiologically compromised by a process such as sepsis or shock. The question has been raised as to how much real pain the patient is experiencing, and there is difficulty in answering this issue. Many patients may not remember these experiences, and even if these experiences are recalled, there are limitations of assessing pain retrospectively.[4] One of the chief challenges in the discussion of pain in the ICU is the assessment of pain in a population in which communication may be compromised. An increased vigilance by the physician and nursing staff as well as the development and use of alternative means of pain assessment are necessary when patients cannot verbalize pain.

A recent study examined the assessment and treatment of pain in two surgical ICUs in a university hospital setting.[5] After the investigators found poor results in both of these areas, the following action plans of improvement were sequentially implemented: (1) to educate the physician and nursing staff regarding the importance of pain and to measure pain with a modified Visual Analogue Scale (VAS) that is similar to a numeric rating scale (Fig. 64–1),

(2) to assure these modified VAS scales are readily available at patients' bedsides, (3) to have house physicians document and report patients' pain scores on daily ICU rounds, and (4) to create an expectation in these ICUs that a pain score greater than 3 is a cause for intervention. Although 42% of nursing interval assessments were not measured on a standard 10-point scale at baseline, after the 5-week period of implementation of these strategies, pain assessments according to this scale increased to more than 70%. The study also found that patients whose pain scores were less than 3/10 increased from 59% before these interventions were begun to greater than 90% after they were completed.

Additional methods of evaluating pain in patients unable to communicate verbally have been developed from similar techniques in the pediatric arena. This would include the various behavioral pain assessment scales, in which pain scores are recorded by assessing a variety of patients' nonverbal behaviors and sometimes including changes in vital signs. An investigation described above found that placing VAS cards at the patients' bedsides permits some patients to point at a spot on the scale that corresponds to their pain score.[5]

BOX 64–1. BARRIERS TO PAIN ASSESSMENT AND TREATMENT IN THE INTENSIVE CARE UNIT

Severe critical illness causing mental status compromise
Endotracheal intubation or positive pressure mask ventilation
Sleep deprivation
Failure to recognize pain issues in the face of hemodynamic/septic/other issues

---

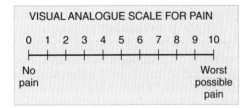

Figure 64–1. Modified Visual Analogue Scale for pain.

One group[6] recently attempted to validate a behavioral pain scale (Fig. 64–2)[7] for use in the ICU environment, noting that no pain scale for patients incapacitated by critical illness had yet been validated. Noting a significant difference between physiologic variables such as heart rate and mean arterial pressure, the observers were able to validate a behavioral pain scale at rest and during painful procedures. The behaviors evaluated in determining a score for pain were facial expression, upper limb movements, and compliance with mechanical ventilation. This scale was also felt to be feasible from a time standpoint, with an average assessment time of 4 minutes.

BARRIERS TO PAIN TREATMENT IN THE INTENSIVE CARE UNIT

The difficulty of treatment of pain in those hospitalized in the ICU has been clearly documented. The SUPPORT investigators examined more than 4000 ICU patients over 2 years. In the data-gathering, phase I portion, family members reported moderate to severe pain at least half the time for 50% of conscious patients who died in the hospital.[8] Similar results were found in another study, in which a sample of 24 surgical patients from two different hospitals was interviewed after transfer from the ICU. Sixty-three percent of the patients rated their pain as being moderate to severe in intensity while in the ICU.[9]

Another study analyzed the adequacy of pain control for 17 trauma patients during the initial aspect of their ICU admission.[10] In contrast to 47% of patients rating their pain as severe, 95% of house staff and 81% of nurses reported the patients had received adequate pain control. This is underscored by the fact that 53% of house staff did not ask patients if pain control was satisfactory. The impact of insufficient analgesia was evidenced by the fact that 68% of patients reported that pain affected their ability to cough and 55% had trouble deep breathing. Presumed barriers to adequate pain control were felt to include a disparity in the perception of pain between patients and caregivers, patients refusing to request pain medicine despite the presence of moderate to severe pain, and physician and nurse concerns about patients' adverse physiologic response to further or

Item	Description	Score
Facial expression	Relaxed	1
	Partially tightened (e.g., brow lowering)	2
	Fully tightened (e.g., eyelid closing)	3
	Grimacing	4
Upper limb movements	No movement	1
	Partially bent	2
	Fully bent with finger flexion	3
	Permanently retracted	4
Compliance with mechanical ventilation	Tolerating movement	1
	Coughing but tolerating ventilation for most of the time	2
	Fighting ventilator	3
	Unable to control ventilation	4

Figure 64–2. Behavioral pain scale.

increased doses of analgesics. It noted that 19% of patients reported a fear of addiction to opioids. Misconceptions regarding opioid pharmacology on the part of caregivers have been reported.[10] In one report, some members of a nursing staff felt that the use of anxiolytics negated the need for larger doses of opioids.

A critically ill patient's ability to communicate pain may be impaired by the severity of the injury or the presence of factors that impede communication, such as the presence of endotracheal or positive pressure ventilation. One study attempted to put forth guidelines regarding sedation and analgesia in the critically ill patient nearing death[11] (Box 64-2).

BOX 64-2. GUIDELINES FOR RELIEF OF PAIN AND SUFFERING IN THE INTENSIVE CARE UNIT

Relief of Pain and Suffering
In order to relieve pain and suffering at the end of life, both pharmacologic and nonpharmacologic means should be used. Nonpharmacologic interventions include ensuring the presence of family, friends, and pastoral care (if desired) and changing the technologic intensive care unit (ICU) environment to a more private and peaceful one.

Initial Dosage
Most ICU patients require narcotics and sedatives in order to ease the pain and suffering associated with their critical illness. The amount of drugs needed varies on an individual basis. As in active disease treatment, palliative care *must* be individualized.

Titration of Analgesics and Sedatives
Once analgesics and sedatives are initiated, they are increased in response to (1) patient's request; (2) signs of respiratory distress; (3) physiologic signs—unexplained tachycardia, hypertension, diaphoresis; (4) facial grimacing, tearing, vocalizations with movements, turns or other nursing care; and (5) restlessness.

Does a Maximal Dose Exist?
No maximum dose of narcotics or sedatives exists. The goal of palliative care is to provide relief of pain and suffering, and whatever the amount of drugs that accomplishes this goal is the amount needed for that individual patient.

Should Analgesics and Sedatives Be Administered in Response to Signs and Symptoms of Pain and Suffering or Before They Begin?
Support for both approaches exists among intensivists on this. The treatment of signs and symptoms of pain and suffering is good palliative care. When appropriate doses of narcotics and sedatives are used and the intent of the physician is clear and well documented, preemptive dosing in anticipation of pain and suffering is not euthanasia or assisted suicide but good palliative care.

In doing so, the panel recognized the difficulty of pain assessment in this setting as a result of several factors including communication problems particular to the ICU environment, the severity of critical illness and potential presence of multisystem organ failure, the possibility of decreased level of consciousness resulting from illness and drugs, and the difficulty in the interpretation and reporting of clinical signs. In the treatment of terminal disease, there are several possibilities for titrating sedation and analgesia: patient request, signs of respiratory distress, and physiologic signs such as tachycardia, hypotension, diaphoresis, facial grimacing, tearing, vocalization, or patient restlessness.

The use of a questionnaire to collect data on patients' stressful experiences associated with being in an ICU and with mechanical ventilation was used by one investigation.[12] Of those who remembered the ETT, 68% were significantly bothered by not being able to speak (68%), pain associated with the ETT (56%), and anxiety regarding the ETT (59%). It is not surprising that this study found that those who did not remember the ETT or ICU were on average more severely ill and subject to a longer duration of mechanical ventilation than the group who remembered these experiences. It is quite possible, given the severity of their disease process, that the former group may have been more likely to be chemically paralyzed or heavily sedated.

BENEFITS OF ASSESSING AND TREATING PAIN IN THE INTENSIVE CARE UNIT

ICU patients who are intubated may be at higher risk for pulmonary complications after surgery. Postoperative pain in these patients results in a pattern of shallow breathing with fewer sigh breaths. Complications of retention of secretion, atelectasis, hypoxemia, and pulmonary infections may be seen among this group.[13] Epidural analgesia, intrapleural analgesia, intravenous patient-controlled analgesia (PCA), and intercostal nerve blockade (the duration of which is based on the duration of the local anesthetic used) are options in this situation. Clinical situations in which placement of thoracic epidural analgesia may be of significant benefit to the patient in the ICU include patients with post-thoracotomy pain; these catheters may be left in place to provide coverage of chest tube site pain until the chest tubes are discontinued. The placement of epidural catheters for pain control may aid trauma patients with rib fractures, and also may provide benefit to facilitate weaning from mechanical ventilation.[14]

PCA in the ICU is useful in an awake and alert patient by allowing the patient to receive on-demand dosing of analgesic agents, either via the epidural or intravenous route. Ballantyne and colleagues published a meta-analysis of randomized, controlled trials to examine postoperative analgesic therapies and their effects on pulmonary outcomes.[15] Epidural opioids tended to decrease the incidence of atelectasis (respiratory rate [RR] = 0.53, 95% cardiac index

[CI] = 0.33-0.85) and showed a less impressive tendency to decrease the incidence of pulmonary infections (RR = 0.53, 95% CI = 0.18-1.53) and overall pulmonary complications (RR = 0.51, 95% CI = 0.20-1.33) when compared with systemically administered opioids. Epidural local anesthetics, compared to systemically administered opioids, were found to decrease the incidence of pulmonary infections (RR = 0.36, 95% CI = 0.21-0.65) and overall pulmonary complications (RR = 0.58, 95% CI = 0.42-0.80). There were no clinical or statistical significant differences found in other measures of pulmonary outcome, including forced expiratory volume in 1 second (FEV$_1$), forced vital capacity (FVC), and peak expiratory flow rate (PEFR). This meta-analysis sheds light on the value of postoperative epidural analgesia in reducing postoperative pulmonary morbidity, and questions the correlation of these spirometry values as predictors of postoperative pulmonary morbidity.

The benefit of controlling perioperative pain to attenuate the perioperative stress response has been debated. This response brings about an increase in sympathetic tone, increased secretion of catecholamines and catabolic hormones such as glucagon and cortisol, and decreased secretion of anabolic hormones such as insulin. It also increases antidiuretic hormone (ADH) and aldosterone secretion, electrolyte abnormalities, and protein catabolism. One theory suggests that opioids diminish the hyperglycemic and epinephrine responses because of efferent nerve blockade to the adrenal medulla yet have no effect on the cortisol response as a result of incomplete afferent nerve block.[16]

One group attempted to study the quality of the dying process in the ICU by retrospectively interviewing family members of 38 ICU decedents.[17] This investigation found that family members perceived that the patients experienced substantial physical symptoms during the last week of life, but felt that their loved ones' pain was under satisfactory control less than half the time. A review of the hospital records showed a near universal absence of data regarding pain assessment as well as records of how sedatives and analgesics were titrated to pain and symptom relief. Of the many items measured, the perception of how well the patient's pain was under control correlated strongly with the quality-of-dying ratings as measured in the study. The authors concluded that end-of-life care in the ICU include management of pain as well as support of dignity, respect, peace, and maximizing patient's pain control.

METHODS OF PAIN CONTROL IN THE INTENSIVE CARE UNIT

This topic is limited to discussion of methods of pain control (Box 64–3) as pertinent to the ICU setting, given that these issues are discussed in detail in other chapters in this text.

Analgesia may be administered by blocking afferent impulses carried along neural pathways, affecting

---

BOX 64–3. METHODS OF PAIN CONTROL IN THE INTENSIVE CARE UNIT

Opioids
Nonsteroidal anti-inflammatory drugs (NSAIDs)
Neuraxial (epidural and intrathecal) local anesthetics and opioids
Peripheral nerve blocks (including sympathetic nerve blocks)

---

integration in the central nervous system (which may display plasticity and central sensitization in response to pain), and blocking efferent impulses modulated by the neuroendocrine or sympathetic nervous system.[16]

Opioids mediate analgesia by binding with both central and peripheral opioid receptors, with the µ- and κ-receptors most important for analgesia. An "ideal" opioid would have rapid onset, ease of titration, and lack of accumulation of the drug or its metabolites, and low cost.[18] Morphine may precipitate histamine release and theoretically might cause hypotension in the ICU patient with diminished volume status. In addition, active metabolites such as morphine-3- and morphine-6-glucuronide may accumulate in the presence of renal insufficiency. Meperidine is a poor drug for use in the ICU. It is metabolized to normeperidine, the accumulation of which may lead to delirium and seizures in patients with renal compromise. Opioids are discussed in more detail in Chapter 31.

The Society of Critical Care Medicine put forth practice parameters with regard to the use of opioids in the intensive care unit.[19] The authors suggested that morphine is the initial agent of choice, and is best started at a loading dose of 0.05 mg/kg administered over 5 to 15 minutes. It was suggested that most adults require 4 to 6 mg/hr after an adequate loading dose. This report also suggested fentanyl (1 to 2 mcg/kg/hr after one or more loading doses of 1 to 2 mcg/kg) or hydromorphone (initiated at 0.5 mg and titrated by 0.5-mg increments to a general range of 1 to 2 mg every 1 to 2 hours) are acceptable alternatives to morphine. It is important to remember that opioid-tolerant patients often require higher doses of opioid analgesia than their opioid-naive counterparts.

The use of opioids may lead to hypotension in patients with intravascular volume compromise or those reliant on sympathetic tone for end-organ perfusion, which may be a significant issue in the ICU population. The route of administration is important. Subcutaneous and intramuscular injections, never optimal for pain relief in any setting, are not advisable given the uncertain perfusion and absorption seen in many ICU patients.[20] Transdermal fentanyl presents similar issues, and is suboptimal for acute pain management given the 12- to 24-hour delay in both onset and offset of analgesia.[21] Patients who are able to cooperate may benefit from the institution of intravenous patient-controlled analgesia (IVPCA). IVPCA possesses an inherent safety mechanism in that the patient stops using the demand feature when pain is controlled and when side effects such as sedation are more prominent. This property of IVPCA helps minimize the chance of opioid overdose and resultant respiratory depression while optimizing the timely delivery of analgesic agent to the patient.[22]

A group of authors examined the effect of thoracic epidural bupivacaine-morphine versus IVPCA morphine after thoracoabdominal esophagectomy.[23] Pain scores at rest and with mobilization were better in the epidural group on postoperative day one, as were the opioid-mediated side effects such as sedation. It was noted, however, that one third of those in the epidural group had their infusion discontinued earlier than planned because of technical failures such as insufficient analgesia or catheter displacement. Group assignment had no effect on ICU stay, duration of hospitalization, or mortality. Given the ability of epidural analgesia to decrease sympathetic tone, it is not surprising that this study found that the epidural group received larger amounts of colloid and crystalloid intravenously in the first 24 hours.

Intrathecal dosing of opioids may be done perioperatively, before a patient's transfer to the ICU. Questions have been raised regarding the need for monitoring these patients for delayed respiratory depression, as well as the subsequent timing of analgesics. This issue was examined by a prospective, randomized, double-blind study in postoperative lumbar spinal fusion patients.[24] Patients were randomized to receive intraoperative injection of either 0.2 mg (group 1), 0.3 mg (group 2), or 0.4 mg (group 3) of morphine into the dural sac under direct visualization. Pain levels were similar in groups 2 and 3 at zero hours and at 12 hours after surgery, but were significantly higher in group 1. The patients' respiratory rate was significantly lower in group 3 than in groups 1 and 2. The $PaCO_2$ was also higher in group 3. No difference, however, was found in pruritus or nausea among the three groups. Some intensivists have suggested that this would argue for 0.3 mg as an optimal perioperative intrathecal morphine dose. Some might extrapolate from these data that the use of a monitored bed for postoperative monitoring for delayed respiratory depression in patients receiving 0.3 mg or less of intrathecal morphine is unwarranted and may lead to an unnecessary use of resources.

Nonsteroidal anti-inflammatory agents (NSAIDs) should not be discounted as useful adjuncts in some ICU patients. Ketorolac, an intravenous NSAID, has been shown to have opioid-sparing effects and therefore may limit opioid-mediated side effects. This and other nonselective inhibitors of cyclooxygenase (COX) may have adverse effects on gastric mucosal perfusion, platelet aggregation, and renal perfusion in patients with suboptimal intravascular volume status. Therefore it is recommended that ketorolac be limited to only several days' use, and administered with caution in older adults.[25] Newer, highly selec-

tive COX-2 inhibitors are not in common use in the ICU setting and may be inappropriate in older adults given the recently documented increase in adverse cardiac events in this population.[26]

Interventional pain procedures also may have a role in the ICU. Thoracic epidural infusion of local anesthetic, with or without the addition of an opioid may be useful for patients with traumatic rib fractures, who often encounter difficulty weaning from mechanical ventilation secondary to significant chest wall pain.[14] The use of intercostal nerve blocks is debatable given that the relief only lasts as long as the duration of action of the local anesthetic used.

Another potential role for a pain procedure in the ICU is poor distal perfusion in an extremity. Sympathetic blocks may prove useful in such situations.[27] This may be achieved by either the direct performance of a sympathetic ganglion block, such as a stellate ganglion block or lumbar sympathetic block to improve perfusion in an affected upper or lower extremity, respectively. An indwelling axillary or femoral nerve sheath catheter might also be a means of providing local anesthetic on a continual basis, either with or without superimposed patient-demand dosing.[28]

EPIDURAL INFUSIONS IN THE INTENSIVE CARE UNIT

Epidural infusions may consist of a combination of a local anesthetic and an opioid. This allows the synergy of two mechanisms of action: local anesthetics work by blocking sodium channels on the nerve membrane, and opioids work through opioid receptors in the substantia gelatinosa of the dorsal horn of the spinal cord. This combination also minimizes the potential toxicity or side effects from each agent. The potential for seizures or cardiac toxicity from the local anesthetic or sedation or respiratory depression from the opioid may be attenuated because less of each agent is used when they are used in combination.[29]

Many local anesthetic-opioid combinations include fentanyl. Fentanyl is relatively lipophilic and tends to affect the neuraxis at or near the level of the spinal cord, where it is infused.[30] It will also achieve plasma levels relatively quickly because of its lipophilicity. Morphine, conversely, has relatively hydrophilic properties. It tends to ascend cephalad in the neuraxis, potentially contributing to delayed respiratory depression.

The clinical situation in the ICU may dictate the choice of opioid in the infusion. Thoracic epidural analgesia may be beneficial for pain control in postthoracotomy patients to cover incisional pain as well as pain from chest tube sites, which can be particularly problematic with regards to pain control.[31] Given the restricted use of intravenous fluids associated in many thoracic surgical cases, the patient may arrive in the ICU with a picture of uncontrolled pain in the face of relatively low blood pressure. A dose of local anesthetic given via the epidural catheter may precipitate hypotension as a result of interruption of sympathetic tone and may lead to compromise of end-organ perfusion. Given the desirability of maintaining the epidural catheter for ongoing pain control, one solution to this problem is to provide a continuous epidural infusion of morphine.[32] Excellent neuraxial anesthesia can be given without the hypotension that might ensue from a local anesthetic. There is a possibility of progressing to a local anesthetic-opioid combination as the patient progresses to euvolemia.

Attention has been given to the use of epidural analgesia in the ICU in the presence of posttraumatic rib fractures. Epidural analgesia has been compared with IVPCA and found to improve patients' pain scores.[14] This study reviewed the charts of 64 patients with three or more rib fractures after a motor vehicle accident and had initiation of intravenous (IV) PCA morphine or thoracic epidural analgesia with bupivacaine and fentanyl within 24 hours of admission. Despite the fact that the patients who received epidural analgesia were older and sustained more rib fractures, their pain scores on a five-point scale were significantly lower for up to 80 hours from baseline.

One recent study retrospectively reviewed more than 64,000 patients from the National Trauma Data Bank with one or more rib fractures.[33] The authors found that mortality and pulmonary morbidity increased with the number of rib fractures. It was found that only 2% of all patients with fractured ribs received epidural analgesia. This use was increased in those patients who suffered six or more rib fractures. The use of epidural analgesia was associated with a significant decrease in hospital mortality compared to alternative forms of analgesia, leading the authors to conclude that this modality of pain control appears to be underused.

SEDATION IN THE INTENSIVE CARE UNIT

Before treating anxiety in the critically ill patient, it is crucial to identify other underlying disorders that can contribute to this problem. These include hypoxemia, hypoglycemia, hypotension, metabolic disturbances, and drug and alcohol withdrawal. Agitation may lead to harmful sequelae such as breathing against the ventilator, increase in oxygen consumption, and removal of monitoring devices and catheters.[18] No one gold standard exists to quantify sedation, and the Ramsay, Riker, Motor Activity Assessment, and Vancouver scales all have been used for this process[34-37] (Tables 64-1 to 64-4).

Common sedatives used in the care of the critically ill patient include benzodiazepines such as midazolam and lorazepam, hypnotic agents such as propofol, and centrally acting α_2 agents such as dexmedetomidine. Titrating a given sedative to a defined end point has been recommended with subsequent systematic tapering of the dose or, alternatively, daily interruption of sedation with retitration to minimize prolonged sedation.[18]

The effect of the specific agent on weaning from mechanical ventilation was examined.[38] A remifentanil-based regimen (started at 0.1 to 0.15 mcg/kg/minute and titrated in 0.025-mcg/kg/minute increments every 5 to 10 minutes to optimum levels based on clinical judgment), when compared with a midazolam-based regimen (administered by infusion or by boluses and titrated to optimum levels based on clinical judgment), resulted in a decreased duration of mechanical ventilation by more than 2 days. It also reduced, by 1 day, the time from the start of the weaning process to the time of extubation. The authors did not comment on the relative cost of the two agents, and whether an overall cost savings was appreciated in the remifentanil-based group.

Table 64-1. Ramsay Scale

SCORE	ITEM
1	Anxious and agitated or restless or both
2	Cooperative, oriented, and tranquil
3	Responding to commands only
4	Brisk response to light glabelar tap
5	Sluggish response to light glabelar tap
6	No response to light glabelar tap

From Ramsay MA, Savege TM, Simpson BR, et al: Controlled sedation with alphaxalone-alphadolone. BMJ 1974;2:656-659.

Table 64-2. Riker Sedation-Agitation Scale

SCORE	CATEGORY	DESCRIPTION
7	Dangerous agitation	Pulling at endotracheal tube, trying to remove catheters, climbing over bedrail, striking at staff, thrashing side to side
6	Very agitated	Does not calm despite frequent verbal reminding of limits, requires physical restraints, biting endotracheal tube
5	Agitated	Anxious or mildly agitated, attempting to sit up, calms down on verbal instructions
4	Calm, cooperative	Calm, easily arousable, follows commands
3	Sedated	Difficult to arouse, awakens to verbal stimuli or gentle shaking but drifts off again, follows simple commands
2	Very sedated	Arouses to physical stimuli but does not communicate or follow commands, may move spontaneously
1	Unarousable	Minimal or no response to noxious stimuli, does not communicate or follow commands

From Riker RR, Picard JT, Fraser GL: Prospective evaluation of the Sedation-Agitation Scale for adult critically ill patients. Crit Care Med 1999;27:1325-1329.

Table 64–3. Motor Activity Assessment Scale

SCORE	DESCRIPTION	DEFINITION
0	Unresponsive	Does not move with noxious stimulus
1	Responsive only to noxious	Opens eyes *or* raises eyebrows *or* turns head toward stimulus *or* moves limbs with noxious stimulus
2	Responsive to touch or name	Opens eyes *or* raises eyebrows *or* turns head toward stimulus *or* moves limbs when touched or name is loudly spolen
3	Calm and cooperative	No external stimulus is required to elicit movement *and* patient is adjusting sheets or clothes purposefully and follows commands
4	Restless and cooperative	No external stimulus is required to elicit movement *and* patient is picking at sheets or tubes *or* uncovering self and follows commands
5	Agitated	No external stimulus is required to elicit movement *and* attempts to sit up *or* moves limbs out of bed *and* does not consistently follow commands (e.g., will lie down when asked but soon reverts back to attempts to sit up or move limbs of bed)
6	Dangerously agitated, uncooperative	No external stimulus is required to elicit movement *and* patient is pulling at tubes or catheters *or* thrashing side to side *or* striking at staff *or* trying to climb out of bed *and* does not calm down when asked

From Devlin JW, Boleski G, Mlynarek M, et al: Motor activity assessment scale: A valid and reliable sedation scale for use with mechanically ventilated patients in an adult surgical intensive care unit. Crit Care Med 1999;27:1271-1275.

Table 64–4. The Vancouver Interaction and Calmness Scale

INTERACTION SCORE /30	STRONGLY AGREE	AGREE	MILDLY AGREE	MILDLY DISAGREE	DISAGREE	STONGLY DISAGREE
Patient interacts	6	5	4	3	2	1
Patient communicates	6	5	4	3	2	1
Information communicated by patient is reliable	6	5	4	3	2	1
Patient cooperates	6	5	4	3	2	1
Patient needs encouragement to respond to questions	1	2	3	4	5	6

CALMNESS SCORE /30	STRONGLY AGREE	AGREE	MILDLY AGREE	MILDLY DISAGREE	DISAGREE	STONGLY DISAGREE
Patient appears calm	6	5	4	3	2	1
Patient appears restless	1	2	3	4	5	6
Patient appears distressed	1	2	3	4	5	6
Patient is moving around uneasily in bed	1	2	3	4	5	6
Patient is pulling at lines/tubes	1	2	3	4	5	6

From de Lemos J, Tweeddale M, Chittock D, et al: Measuring quality of sedation in adult mechanically ventilated critically ill patients: The Vancouver Interaction and Calmness Scale. J Clin Epidemiol 2000;53:908-919.

CONCLUSION

The assessment and treatment of pain in the critically ill population are challenging tasks given the frequent lability in patients' physiologic status and the compromise in their ability to communicate. Although undertreatment of pain in ICU patients has been well documented, data suggest that organizational changes and appropriate use of pharmacologic therapy may improve pain control in the critically ill patient. Intensivists have a variety of therapeutic options available including NSAIDs, opioids (both by infusion and by IVPCA), and central and peripheral nerve blockade such as sympathetic nerve blocks and continuous epidural analgesia.

References

1. Bertolini G, Minelli C, Latronico N, et al: The use of analgesic drugs in postoperative patients: The neglected problem of pain control in intensive care units. An observational, prospective, multicenter study in 128 Italian intensive care units. Eur J Clin Pharmacol 2002;58:73-77.
2. Nelson J, Meier D, Oei E: Self-reported symptom experience of critically ill cancer patients receiving intensive care. Crit Care Med 2001;29:277-282.
3. Freire A, Afessa B, Cawley P: Characteristics associated with analgesia ordering in the intensive care unit and relationships with outcome. Crit Care Med 2002;30:2468-2472.
4. van de Leur JP, van der Schans CP, Loef BG, et al: Discomfort and factual recollection in intensive care unit patients. Crit Care 2004;8:R467-473.
5. Erdek M, Pronovost P: Improving assessment and treatment of pain in the critically ill. Int J Qual Health Care 2004;16:59-64.

6. Aissaoui Y, Ali Zeggwagh A, Zekraoui A, et al: Validation of a behavioral pain scale in critically ill, sedated, and mechanically ventilated patients. Anesth Analg 2005;101:470-476.

7. Payen JF, Bru O, Bosson JL, et al: Assessing pain in critically ill sedated patients by using a behavioral pain scale. Crit Care Med 2001;29:2258-2263.

8. The SUPPORT Principal Investigators: A controlled trial to improve care for seriously ill hospitalized patients. JAMA 1995;274:1591-1598.

9. Puntillo K: Pain experiences of intensive care unit patients. Heart Lung 1990;19:526-533.

10. Whipple J, Lewis K, Quebbeman E: Analysis of pain management in critically ill patients. Pharmacotherapy 1995;15:592-599.

11. Hawryluck L, Harvey W, Lemieux-Charles L: Consensus guidelines on analgesia and sedation in dying intensive care unit patients. BMC Med Ethics 2002;3:3.

12. Rotondi A, Lakshmipathi C, Sirio C: Patients' recollections of stressful experiences while receiving prolonged mechanical ventilation in an intensive care unit. Crit Care Med 2002;30:746-752.

13. Goettler CE, Fugo JR, Bard MR, et al: Predicting the need for early tracheostomy: A multifactorial analysis of 992 intubated trauma patients. J Trauma 2006;60:991-996.

14. Wu CL, Jani ND, Perkins FM, et al: Thoracic epidural analgesia versus intravenous patient-controlled analgesia for the treatment of rib fracture pain after motor vehicle crash. J Trauma 1999;47:564-567.

15. Ballantyne J, Carr D, deFerranti S, et al: The comparative effects of postoperative analgesic therapies on pulmonary outcome: Cumulative meta-analyses of randomized, controlled trials. Anesth Analg 1988;86:598-612.

16. Lewis K, Whipple J, Michael K: Effect of analgesic treatment on the physiological consequences of acute pain. Am J Hosp Pharm 1994;51:539-554.

17. Mularski RA, Heine CE, Osborne ML, et al: Quality of dying in the ICU: Ratings by family members. Chest 2005;128:280-287.

18. Jacobi J, Fraser G, Coursin D: Clinical practice guidelines for the sustained use of sedatives and analgesics in the critically ill adult. Crit Care Med 2002;30:119-141.

19. Shapiro BA, Warren J, Egol AB, et al: Practice parameters for intravenous analgesia and sedation for adult patients in the intensive care unit: An executive summary. Society of Critical Care Medicine. Crit Care Med 1995;23:1596-1600.

20. Ariza-Andraca C, Altamirano-Bustamante E, Frati-Munari A, et al: Delayed insulin absorption due to subcutaneous edema. Arch Invest Med 1991;22:229-233.

21. Gourlay GK, Kowalski SR, Plummer JL, et al: The transdermal administration of fentanyl in the treatment of postoperative pain: Pharmacokinetics and phamacodynamic effects. Pain 1989;37:193-202.

22. Looi-Lyons LC, Chung FF, Chan VW, et al: Respiratory depression: An adverse outcome during patient controlled analgesia therapy. J Clin Anesth 1996;8:151-156.

23. Rudin A, Flisberg P, Johansson J, et al: Thoracic epidural analgesia or intravenous morphine analgesia after thoracoabdominal esophagectomy: A prospective follow-up of 201 patients. J Cardiothorac Vasc Anesth 2005;19:350-357.

24. Boezaart A, Eksteen J, Spuy G: Intrathecal morphine: Double-blind evaluation of optimal dosage for analgesia after major lumbar spinal surgery. Spine 1999;24:1131-1141.

25. Strom BL, Berlin JA, Kinman JL, et al: Parenteral ketorolac and risk of gastrointestinal and operative site bleeding. A postmarketing surveillance study. JAMA 1996;5:376-382.

26. Nussmeier NA, Whelton AA, Brown MT, et al: Complications of the COX-2 inhibitors parecoxib and valdecoxib after cardiac surgery. N Engl J Med 2005;352:1081-1091.

27. Baker RJ, Chunprapaph B, Nyhus LM: Severe ischemia of the hand following radial artery catheterization. Surgery 1976;80:449-457.

28. Horlocker TT, Hebl JR, Kinney MA, et al: Opioid-free analgesia following total knee arthroplasty—A multimodal approach using continuous lumbar plexus (psoas compartment) block, acetaminophen, and ketorolac. Reg Anesth Pain Med 2002;27:105-108.

29. Moizo E, Berti M, Marchetti C, et al: Acute pain service and multimodal therapy for postsurgical pain control: Evaluation of protocol efficacy. Minerva Anesthesiol 2004;70:779-787.

30. Sudarshan G, Browne BL, Matthews JN, et al: Intrathecal fentanyl for post-thoracotomy pain. Br J Anaesth 1995;75:19-22.

31. Milgrom LB, Brooks JA, Qi R, et al: Pain levels experienced with activities after cardiac surgery. Am J Crit Care 2004;13:116-125.

32. Suwanchinda V, Suksompong S, Prakanrattana U, et al: Epidural analgesia for pain relief in thoracic surgery. J Med Assoc Thai 2000;83:358-363.

33. Flagel BT, Luchette FA, Reed RL, et al: Half-a-dozen ribs: The breakpoint for mortality. Surgery 2005;138:717-725.

34. Ramsay MA, Savege TM, Simpson BR, et al: Controlled sedation with alphaxalone-alphadolone. BMJ 1974;2:656-659.

35. Riker RR, Picard JT, Fraser GL: Prospective evaluation of the Sedation-Agitation Scale for adult critically ill patients. Crit Care Med 1999;27:1325-1329.

36. Devlin JW, Boleski G, Mlynarek M, et al: Motor activity assessment scale: A valid and reliable sedation scale for use with mechanically ventilated patients in an adult surgical intensive care unit. Crit Care Med 1999;27:1271-1275.

37. de Lemos J, Tweeddale M, Chittock D, et al: Measuring quality of sedation in adult mechanically ventilated critically ill patients: The Vancouver Interaction and Calmness Scale. J Clin Epidemiol 2000;53:908-919.

38. Breen D, Karabinis A, Malbrain M, et al: Decreased duration of mechanical ventilation when comparing analgesia-based sedation using remifentanil with standard hypnotic-based sedation for up to 10 days in intensive care unit patients: A randomized trial. Crit Care 2005;9:R200-R210.

65 Pain Management at the End of Life

Perry G. Fine and David Casarett

The end stages of chronic, progressive, life-limiting diseases bring a host of difficult symptoms and causes of suffering. There are disease-mediated symptoms, such as pain, dyspnea, fatigue, and loss of mobility, and there are the accompanying emotional states, such as depression, anxiety, and a sense of uselessness.[1] These symptoms and states intertwine and interact in a complex manner, and each one deserves attention.

Of the many symptoms experienced by those at the end of life, pain is one of the most common and most feared.[2,3] Pain is often undertreated, even when prevalence rates and syndromes are well understood and the means of relief are within all physicians' capabilities to provide, directly or through consultation. With careful assessment and a comprehensive plan of care that addresses the various aspects of the patient's needs, pain can be controlled in the vast majority of cases. Awareness and provision of basic and specialized interventions can ensure comfort for all patients through the final stages of a terminal illness. This is equally important in order to prevent prolonged and pathologic grief in surviving loved ones.

All the members of a palliative care team play important roles in comprehensive pain management. Both physicians' and nurses' roles begin with assessment and continue throughout the development of a plan of care and its implementation. Rehabilitation specialists, clinical pharmacists, psychologists, social workers, and spiritual counselors also provide important elements in helping patients optimize their quality of life, stay comfortable, heal relationships, complete unfinished business, and find peace as they approach death. To provide optimal pain control, all health care professionals must understand the causes and prevalence of pain at the end of life, the treatments used to provide relief, and the barriers that prevent good management.

To illustrate some common scenarios, we present three different fictional, but typical, case studies.

CASE 1: Pain Assessment and Care Planning in a Cognitively Intact Patient

Judith is a frail 81-year-old who lives on her own with assistance from a home care nurse and from a daughter, who lives nearby. She was admitted to the hospital with acute respiratory failure resulting from bronchitis. She has advanced chronic obstructive pulmonary disease (COPD), with general fatigue and a poor appetite, and reports severe, debilitating pain in the mid-thoracic region from postherpetic neuralgia (PHN). She also struggles with coronary artery disease and attendant angina pectoris that is usually relieved with nitrates. Judith says that she has been feeling "pretty low" lately and finds herself becoming irritated at small events. She characterizes her pain as "bad as it can be" (Fig. 65–1). After a 2- to 3-day intensive care unit (ICU) stay, she will be ready for discharge. However, her pain from PHN is still not controlled, and her life expectancy is most likely limited because of her ongoing comorbidities. She does not have a written advance directive. The hospital staff discusses the next step.

PREVALENCE OF PAIN AT THE END OF LIFE

Assessing pain in patients approaching the end of life requires a multifactorial evaluation. It is important to acknowledge and address the prevalence, high incidence, and serious adverse consequences of pain in the end-stage conditions that affect patients with advanced medical illness, such as controlled and uncontrolled cancer, heart disease, human immunodeficiency virus (HIV) disease, neurodegenerative diseases (e.g., amyotrophic lateral sclerosis [ALS] and multiple sclerosis), and end-stage renal and respiratory diseases (Figs. 65–2 and 65–3).[4,5] These conditions may also be accompanied by other pain-producing disorders that may require separate treatments, as in the case mentioned.

The prevalence of pain in the terminally ill varies by diagnosis and demographics. Approximately one third of the people who are actively receiving treatment for cancer and two thirds of those with advanced malignant disease experience pain.[6-9] Almost 75% of patients with advanced cancer who are admitted to the hospital report pain on admission.[10] In a study of cancer patients who were very near the end of life, pain occurred in 54% and 34% at 4 weeks and 1 week prior to death, respectively.[11] In a recent study by Goudas and colleagues[12] that compiled the results of 28 epidemiologic surveys, the study authors found that in one study of more than 35,000 Japanese cancer patients, 68% to 72% of patients in the terminal stages reported pain. In another study of more than 13,000 cancer patients in U.S. nursing homes, an average of 30% of the patients reported daily pain. In those patients, pain varied according to age, sex, race, marital status, physical function, depression, and cognitive status.[13]

In other studies of patients admitted to palliative care units, pain often is the dominant symptom, along with fatigue and dyspnea.[2] Until recently it was widely believed that patients dying from nonmalignant disease did not have high levels of pain. However, it is now known that patients dying from cardiac failure, chronic obstructive pulmonary disease (COPD), end-stage renal disease, and other end-stage diseases suffer similar levels of pain to those found in patients with malignant disease.[14,15] People at particular risk for undertreatment include older adults, minorities, and women.[16,17]

More recently, an attempt has been made to characterize the pain experience of those with HIV disease, a disorder frequently seen in palliative care settings. More than 56% of patients with HIV disease report pain, with the most common manifestations being headache, abdominal pain, chest pain, and neuropathies.[4,5,18,19] Lower CD4+ cell counts and HIV-1 ribonucleic acid (RNA) levels are associated with higher rates of neuropathy.[19,20] There have been many reports of undertreatment of patients with HIV disease, including those patients with a history of addictive disease.[21]

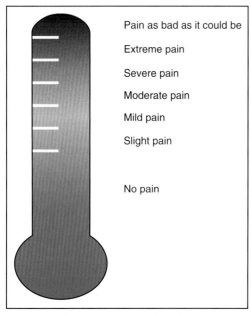

Figure 65–1. Pain thermometer. (Used with permission of Keela Herr, PhD, RN, College of Nursing, The University of Iowa, 2007.)

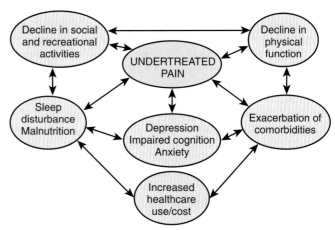

Figure 65–3. Consequences of undertreatment of pain. (Data from Davis MP, Srivastava M: Demographics, assessment, and management of pain in the elderly. Drugs Aging 2003;20:23-57.)

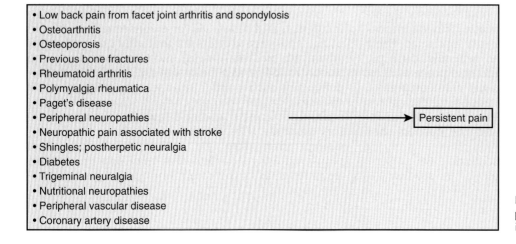

- Low back pain from facet joint arthritis and spondylosis
- Osteoarthritis
- Osteoporosis
- Previous bone fractures
- Rheumatoid arthritis
- Polymyalgia rheumatica
- Paget's disease
- Peripheral neuropathies
- Neuropathic pain associated with stroke
- Shingles; postherpetic neuralgia
- Diabetes
- Trigeminal neuralgia
- Nutritional neuropathies
- Peripheral vascular disease
- Coronary artery disease

Persistent pain

Figure 65–2. Common causes of persistent pain in advanced medical illness.

Table 65–1. Pain Scales Online

DESCRIPTION	WEB ADDRESS
Wong-Baker FACES Pain Rating Scale (Pediatrics)	www3.us.elsevierhealth.com/WOW/faces.html
Sample of Wong-Baker FACES Pain Rating Scale, with instructions for administration available in many languages	www3.us.elsevierhealth.com/WOW/facesTranslations.html
FACES Pain Scale—Revised (FPS-R), with instructions for administration available in many languages	http://painsourcebook.ca/docs/pps92.html
Verbal pain scale	www.intelihealth.com/IH/ihtIH/WSIHW000/29721/32087.html#verbal
Numerical pain scales	www.intelihealth.com/IH/ihtIH/WSIHW000/29721/32087.html#numerical
	www.medtronic.com/neuro/paintherapies/pain_treatment_ladder/drug_infusion/patient_management/drug_pat_mgmt_strat.html#maps
Pain map	www.medtronic.com/neuro/paintherapies/pain_treatment_ladder/pdf/prestim_pain_assess.pdf
McGill Pain Questionnaire	www.physiobase.com/Protocols/assessmentforms/pain_questionnaire_2.pdf
Short-Form McGill Pain Questionnaire	www.med.umich.edu/obgyn/repro-endo/Lebovicresearch/PainSurvey.pdf
Brief Pain Inventory	www.ohsu.edu/ahec/pain/paininventory.pdf
List of pain scales with evaluations	www.chcr.brown.edu/pcoc/Physical.htm
Pain scales in 17 languages	www.britishpainsociety.org/pain_scales.html

ASSESSING PAIN AT THE END OF LIFE

Assessment of pain, including a thorough history and comprehensive physical examination, guides the choice of diagnostic studies and the development of the pharmacologic and nonpharmacologic treatment plan. The primary source of information in a pain assessment should be a patient's self-report. There are many different pain rating scales available, ranging from complex multidimensional tools to very simple numeric and picture scales, which can help patients identify pain and then document the efficacy of treatment (see Table 65–1 for links to sample pain scales). When using pain scales, be sure to follow the directions for administration carefully.

A pain scale that suits a given patient's ability to self-report should be part of each patient's medical record. Health professionals should teach patients and their families to use these scales themselves to help in longitudinal pain assessment and continuity of care. Patients with terminal illnesses should be encouraged to describe their experiences of pain in their own words. However, many patients near the end of life are unable to provide detailed descriptions of their pain character, intensity, or location. Particularly for patients with cognitive impairment, self-assessments may be difficult to interpret. Nevertheless, even in these patients, self-assessments remain the cornerstone of pain management. For these patients, the use of the "pain thermometer" has been validated as a self-report instrument for pain intensity in patients with mild to moderate cognitive impairment.[22]

CASE 1: Pain Assessment and Care Planning in a Cognitively Intact Patient (Continued)

Judith describes her PHN as a "burning, needling pain" near her spine, spreading out across her back on the right, beneath her axilla, and around to her breast. Her pain subsides sometimes, but rarely goes away altogether. Knowing the character and location of her neuropathic pain allows her caregivers to pinpoint adjuvant pain relief. In contrast, Judith's angina pain is "a deep, heavy ache" in her chest. She notes that it is intermittent and that it is stressful, because she never knows quite when to expect it. By asking her to keep track of when her angina occurs, her caregivers are able to predict more precisely when it may be triggered, and advise her accordingly, perhaps reducing both severity and frequency.

A comprehensive evaluation of pain should include an assessment of the pain intensity, character, frequency, onset, duration, and location as well as a detailed history of pain, a physical and neurologic examination, and psychosocial assessment. Diagnostic evaluation that includes tests to determine the cause of pain are important to corroborate clinical impressions of the cause of pain and mechanisms, but diagnostic workup should neither delay empiric treatment nor add excessive burden to the patient, especially when death is imminent. It also is important to take into account common pain– and advanced illness–related comorbidities, such as sleep disturbances and depression, which can affect pain levels, suffering, and functioning.[23,24]

Terminally ill patients sometimes complain of pain as a way of expressing other forms of suffering, distress, grieving, anxiety, or depression. When this is the case, psychosocial or spiritual evaluation and intervention will be more effective than analgesics. It is well established that attention and emotion influence pain processing and perception, and conversely inadequately managed pain can lead to anxiety and depression.[7-9] Therefore comprehensive assessment is required to determine the optimal plan of care, as specific to pain etiology as possible. Particularly for health care providers unfamiliar with the care of patients near the end of life, involvement of other disciplines (e.g., nursing, social work, chaplaincy) can be very valuable in uncovering other sources of emotional or spiritual suffering that may be confusing the pain assessment.

DIFFERENTIATING PAIN MECHANISMS AT END OF LIFE

Patients in the terminal stage of an illness often experience multiple mechanisms of pain, for example, both nociceptive and neuropathic, operating simultaneously. Nevertheless, it is important to differentiate among different types of pain because the type of treatment and its success is largely dictated by the pain mechanism and its original source.[25,26] In some conditions, especially metastatic cancer, pain is often caused by a complex mix of nociceptive and neuropathic factors.

Effects of Unrelieved Pain

There is growing evidence that inadequate pain relief might hasten death, not only via the well-recognized morbid effects of increasing physiologic stress, reducing mobility, increasing proclivities toward pneumonia and thromboembolism, and increasing the work of breathing and myocardial oxygen requirements, but also through immune suppression.[27] Pain may lead to a spiritual despair and significant decrease in emotional well-being because the individual's quality of life is impaired.[4,5] It is the professional and ethical responsibility of clinicians to focus on and attend to adequate pain relief for their patients and to properly educate patients and their caregivers about analgesic therapies.[28]

CASE 1: Pain Assessment and Care Planning in a Cognitively Intact Patient (Continued)

Returning to Judith, who has COPD, coronary artery disease, and PHN, it is clear that discussions about care preferences (i.e., advance directives) are optimal before a medical crisis and while there is cognitive capacity for decision making. However, under the current circumstances, a care planning meeting with the attending clinician, consultant clinicians (e.g., palliative care/hospice team), and designated responsible family member is of paramount importance. The team must adequately control her pain before discharge with a follow-up plan in place, or they must transfer her to a skilled facility, such as an inpatient palliative care/hospice unit, where pain management expertise and focused attention are immediately available. Alternatively, with a prognosis of 6 months or less, if Judith prefers to go home immediately, a hospice program with the ability to manage her pain condition should be consulted. Regardless of setting, nonpharmacologic approaches to pain control along with titration of "first-line" agents for neuropathic pain (anticonvulsants, topical local anesthetic, and opioids) should proceed with close monitoring to balance therapeutic and adverse effects.

CASE 2: Pain Assessment and Care Planning in a Severely Cognitively Impaired Patient

Grace is a 74-year-old in the late stages of Alzheimer's disease with severe osteoarthritis in her knees and spine. She lives with her married daughter and two grandchildren. Her daughter and a son living nearby provide her essential care, and until recently she has remained active and ambulatory. She is beginning to experience severe pain from her arthritis, manifest by grimacing, crying, and moaning. The current caregivers are not always sure what she is expressing, but they understand that she is in some distress and are eager to help alleviate it. They meet with their family physician to talk about options. Because Grace is in the far-advanced stage of Alzheimer's disease, the physician refers her to hospice for comprehensive care and support of her family. During her initial evaluation, the family stresses that their primary goal is to make sure that Mom is comfortable. The hospice nurse evaluates Grace and determines that she responds well to a variety of nonpharmacologic interventions. Her family members express a willingness to use a variety of hands-on and nonpharmacologic techniques to help Grace live her last days relatively free of pain and suffering. Meanwhile, she is started on a regimen of around-the-clock acetaminophen (1000 mg four times daily) with the option for more potent pharmacologic therapies left open.

NONPHARMACOLOGIC APPROACHES TO PAIN MANAGEMENT IN PALLIATIVE CARE

An important aspect of any management strategy is the use of nonpharmacologic treatments.[23,29] Various nonpharmacologic approaches to pain are effective in alleviating pain for patients with advanced illness. These include physical interventions, such as positioning and active or passive mobilization (therapeutic exercise); techniques, such as transcutaneous electrical nerve stimulation (TENS), massage, and heat or cold; and complementary and alternative medicine techniques, music, and relaxation or imagery exercises. Table 65–2 offers a list of some of the most common nonpharmacologic interventions.

The type of intervention, or combination of interventions, depends on the source and severity of pain as well as the physical condition and receptivity of the patient. In an investigation of the prevalence of complementary and alternative medicine use in an end-of-life population, Tilden and colleagues,[30] through a series of phone interviews with family caregivers of recently deceased, found that 53.7% of the deceased used some kind of complementary therapy, were more likely to be younger with college degrees and higher household incomes, and to have used one or more life-sustaining treatments. Symptom relief was the most frequent reason given for complementary and alternative medicine use. A recent study by Weiner and Ernst[31] that reviewed common complementary and alternative treatment modalities for the treatment of persistent musculoskeletal

Table 65–2. Nonpharmacologic Approaches to Pain Management in Palliative Care

INTERVENTION	DETAILS
Rehabilitation/physical therapy	• Physical, occupational, and speech therapy can be beneficial in managing pain. • Mobility may be improved by strengthening, stretching, and using assistive devices. • Home settings vary in their use for a debilitated person, as does the degree of hands-on physical assistance that friends and family can provide. • The decision to use these modalities is made on a case-by-case basis.
Massage	• Family members can be taught simple, safe techniques of massage. • Hospice programs can often provide trained, certified massage therapists who are familiar with the clinical issues faced by cancer and noncancer patients with far-advanced disease.
Transcutaneous/percutaneous electrical nerve stimulation	• Evidence exists to support the use of percutaneous electrical nerve stimulation for persistent low back pain and knee pain.
Acupuncture	• Popular complementary therapy for patients with cancer and other end-stage pain • Many patients with cancer use acupuncture when symptoms persist with conventional treatments, or as a complement to their ongoing treatments. • Several researchers have found acupuncture to be an effective antidepressant. • Studies show that acupuncture has a significant positive effect on chronic obstructive pulmonary disease (COPD), dyspnea associated with end-stage cancer, and asthma.

Cognitive interventions	• Some common cognitive interventions:
	  • Psychological tools and strategies for the purposes of self-regulating emotions
	  • Distraction from noxious sensations and thoughts
	  • Methods for reducing negative attitudes
	• Involving patients in cognitive self-care may improve mood and increase coping behaviors.

Music therapy	• Music effectively reduces anxiety and improves mood for:
	  • Medical and surgical patients
	  • Patients in intensive care units
	  • Patients undergoing procedures
	  • Children as well as adults
	• Low-cost intervention
	• Often reduces chronic pain
	• Improves the quality of life, enhancing a sense of comfort and relaxation
	• Music to caregivers may be a cost-effective and enjoyable strategy for improving empathy, compassion, and relationship-centered care without interfering with technical aspects of care.

pain found that the use of these modalities is increasing in older adults. The study authors concluded that rigorous clinical trials examining efficacy are still needed before definitive recommendations regarding the application of these modalities can be made.

Aside from their objective efficacy, a medical sociologic study by Garnett[32] on the use of complementary therapies by palliative care nurses sees these therapies as an "emotional inoculation" that builds resiliency and an important bond between patient and caregiver. Nonpharmacologic interventions often comfort the patient while involving and empowering family and other caregivers. The necessity of feeling effective for caregivers should not be overlooked—it can have a direct effect on the experience of the patient as well as the emotional survival of the family caregiver in particular. A study by Keefe and colleagues[33] on the self-efficacy of family caregivers of cancer patients found that caregivers who rated their self-efficacy as high reported much lower levels of caregiver strain as well as lower negative mood and higher positive mood. Caregiver self-efficacy in managing the patient's pain was related to the patient's physical well-being. When the caregiver reported high self-efficacy, the patient reported having more energy, feeling less ill, and spending less time in bed.

REHABILITATION AND PHYSICAL THERAPY

Functional rehabilitation and physical therapy techniques in appropriately selected patients can add to quality of life even in the face of limited life expectancy. In the case presented, Grace typifies patients who respond well to nonpharmacologic pain interventions. A recent study by Montagnini and colleagues[34] assessing the use of physical therapy in a hospital-based palliative care setting found that a significant proportion demonstrated improvement in function after 2 weeks. The study authors found that patients with a diagnosis of dementia were most likely to show improvement in functional status and concluded that physical therapy assessment and use were uncommon in the studied group, but when implemented, 56% of the patients benefited.

Massage

Research suggests that patients with cancer, particularly in the palliative care setting, are increasingly using aromatherapy and massage. There is good evidence that these therapies may be helpful for anxiety reduction for short periods. A study by Soden and colleagues[35] was designed to compare the effects of 4-week courses of aromatherapy with massage and massage alone on physical and psychological symptoms in patients with advanced cancer. The study authors were unable to demonstrate any significant long-term benefits of aromatherapy or massage in terms of improving pain control, anxiety, or quality of life, but sleep scores improved significantly in both groups, and there were statistically significant reductions in depression scores in the massage group, suggesting that patients with high levels of psychological distress respond best to these therapies.

Acupuncture and Transcutaneous Nerve Stimulation

These modalities may be effective in selected patients based on meta-analyses of the literature and findings of National Institutes of Health (NIH) consensus panels.[36] For percutaneous procedures, appropriate cautions, skilled certified practitioners, and fastidious aseptic techniques are required to protect patients and staff from untoward adverse outcomes. Similarly, for therapies involving electrical stimulation, awareness of implanted devices (pumps, stimulators, implantable cardioverter defibrillators, or pacemakers) and precautions to prevent malfunction must be taken.

Cognitive Interventions

Simple psychological interventions can have a significant impact on pain. As an example, Paqueta and colleagues[37] explored the idea that everyday emotion regulation through a self-supporting maintenance or change in positive and negative emotions can help reduce pain intensity in the hospitalized older adult. Emotion regulation was found to be prospectively related to pain intensity for both overall emotion and anxiety-specific regulation. The study authors suggest that promoting emotion regulation as a self-management strategy could contribute to cost-effective pain management in general or targeted older adult populations.[37]

Music Therapy

There is growing interest in the therapeutic use of music. The difficulties inherent in the medical treatment of this population make the use of music, as a noninvasive therapeutic modality, attractive.[38] Music is often used to enhance well-being, reduce stress, and distract patients from unpleasant symptoms. Although there are wide variations in individual preferences, music appears to exert direct physiologic effects through the autonomic nervous system.[39]

Choosing the Best Approach

A combination of treatments is usually most effective when using nonpharmacologic approaches to pain management. Similar to pharmacotherapy, multimodal approaches offer the potential benefit of additive and synergistic effects. Because nonpharmacologic therapies need to be tailored to individual likes, dislikes, and effectiveness, knowledge of the various modalities, management of expectations, open-mindedness, and a "trial-and-error" approach should be embraced.

CASE 2: Pain Assessment and Care Planning in a Severely Cognitively Impaired Patient (Continued)

The hospice nurse was able to offer Grace's family a variety of hands-on and alternative modalities that could be used in addition to pharmacologic interventions to successfully comfort the patient. The nurse found that simple stretches and strengthening and mobilization exercises were effective for reducing the stiffness that was associated with Grace's musculoskeletal disease. This helped to relax the patient and prevent the usual anxiety that is associated with getting her out of bed in the morning and daily personal care, such as bathing and toileting. A simple TENS unit appeared to ease the patient's knee pain. The nurse was also able to guide the family in some interventions that reduced Grace's anxiety and increased the family's sense of involvement and effectiveness. They found that songs from her youth brought Grace a great deal of pleasure, and her son, a fan of the music, enjoyed spending listening time with her. Physical contact often calmed Grace, and the nurse trained Grace's granddaughter in simple massage techniques. These interventions seemed to be effective and helped the family to feel that they were contributing to Grace's care and well-being.

CASE 3: Complex Symptom Management in the Home Setting

Ben is a 79-year-old with metastatic colon cancer who has just returned to his home in an assisted living facility postoperatively after a bowel resection. He sees a geriatric nurse practitioner, in collaboration with a family physician, for ongoing primary care. It has become clear that there are widespread metastases, and his oncologist agrees that the current goal of care is comfort only. Ben is still ambulatory and in the early stages of his terminal illness. No further chemotherapy or radiation therapies are indicated, but the patient reports progressive abdominal pain, and symptoms suggestive of intermittent bowel obstruction develop. Ben refuses further hospitalization and surgery, and prefers noninterventional therapies, if at all possible. A consulting pharmacist and medical director from the local hospice are asked to come in and help the nurse practitioner choose the best pharmacotherapy for pain and bowel-related signs and symptoms, including types of drugs, route of drug administration, and the best way to minimize possible side effects. The explicit goals of care are a comfortable, dignified death, crisis prevention, and self-determined life closure (no prolongation of dying by medical intervention).

DRUGS FOR PAIN RELIEF IN PALLIATIVE CARE

Pharmacologic therapies for pain include nonopioids, opioids, adjuvant analgesics, disease-modifying therapies, and (in some cases) interventional techniques. Intractable pain and symptoms that are not responsive to basic therapeutic techniques, although not common, must be treated appropriately and aggressively.[1] In some highly selective cases, palliative sedation may be warranted.[40] A sound understanding of pharmacotherapy for pain treatment allows the palliative care/hospice team to create a comprehensive plan of care as well as recognize and assess medication-related adverse effects, understand drug-drug and drug-disease interactions, and educate patients and caregivers regarding appropriate medication usage. Recognition of the limits of usual therapies and the ability to muster expert assistance are important skills. This will ensure a comfortable process of dying for the well-being of the patient and for the sake of those in attendance.

Genetic factors, pathologic processes, concurrent medication, and aging all influence drug response and disposition. However, there are also a variety of nonmedical factors that influence responses to drug treatment in patients with far-advanced disease, including the social, environmental, and psychological milieu as well as the general vulnerability of this population. Understanding the clinical pharmacology of the drugs in question is essential for professional caregivers.[25] Commonly, there is a need to use drugs for non–U.S. Food and Drug Administration (FDA)-approved indications or routes of administration, simply because randomized controlled clinical trials have not been performed, because (usually) of financial constraints. Rational polypharmacy (combining drugs with different mechanisms of action to produce additive or synergistic effects and minimize adverse effects) is often necessary, but there is a high potential for drug interactions, so close monitoring is required.

The principles of effective symptom control are always paramount: diagnose the underlying cause of each symptom and tailor the treatment to individual circumstances and clinical context. Keep in mind that normal pharmacokinetics and pharmacodynamics may be considerably altered by end-stage disease states. For example, in patients with chronic liver disease or hepatic metastases, drugs may bypass hepatic metabolism altogether, increasing bioavailability. Similarly, renal clearance is almost always diminished during the dying process, leading to the accumulation of drug metabolites, some of which (e.g., those of morphine) may be toxic.[5,41]

COMMUNICATING WITH PATIENTS, FAMILIES, AND OTHER HEALTH CARE PROFESSIONALS

Communicating clearly about pharmacologic pain control with patients, families, and other members of the palliative care/hospice team is essential to providing effective pain management. It is important to be specific about the types of drugs that are available, how they are likely to affect the patient, how they are to be administered, and how they may interact with existing medications. Despite the importance of pain management at the end of life, there are often substantial roadblocks to overcome in getting patients the treatment that they need. Professional health care workers may have unsubstantiated but strong beliefs about analgesic use, especially opioid use, that lead to underprescribing.[13,42]

Several surveys show that physicians, nurses, and pharmacists express concerns about addiction, tolerance, and side effects of morphine and related compounds.[43] These fears are pervasive among patients and family members as well. Studies have suggested that these fears lead to undermedication and increased pain intensity.[44] Concerns about being a "good" patient or belief in the inevitability of cancer pain lead patients to hesitate in reporting pain. In these studies, less educated and older patients were most likely to express these beliefs.

Often a physician or other providers may be reluctant to offer the patient direct and objective information on his or her health, especially toward the end of life, seeking to "soften the blow" by keeping the details vague. Most patients, however, prefer complete information about their condition.[45,46] However, patients may wish to defer decision making to the physician or family members.[47,48] Physicians have a professional duty to determine patients' medical wishes. As a purely practical matter, by default or situational necessity, this responsibility may fall to the nurse or nurse practitioner. It is important to know that there are helpful tools, such as simple card sorting, that can be used to facilitate this exchange; for example, the five-card Control Preference Scale uses cards to portray different roles in treatment decision making with a statement and a picture.[49]

DISPELLING COMMON MYTHS ABOUT PAIN MANAGEMENT

Understanding the barriers that are faced when treating pain can lead professionals to better educate and counsel patients and their families.[33] Patients should be asked whether they are concerned about addiction and tolerance (often described as becoming "used to" or "immune" to the drug).[50] At the end of life, patients may need to rely on family members or other support persons to dispense medications. Studies suggest that patients' pain experiences and family members' perceptions about them don't correlate well, leading to inadequate provision of analgesia.[51,52] The interdisciplinary palliative care/hospice team is essential in the communication effort, with nurses, social workers, chaplains, physicians, volunteers, and others providing support in exploring the meaning of pain and barriers to pain relief. Education, counseling, reframing, and spiritual support are imperative.

OVERVIEW OF NON-OPIOID AND OPIOID THERAPY IN ADVANCED DISEASE

This section provides a brief overview of commonly used and newer pharmaceutical agents available in the United States for the treatment of persistent pain associated with advanced disease. Pain-relieving drugs can be categorized as non-opioid analgesics, opioid analgesics, and adjuvant analgesics. Detailed knowledge of these classes of agents is necessary to provide quality palliative care, and although a comprehensive review is beyond the scope of this chapter, links to more detailed lists of all drugs used for pain control throughout the world can be found in Table 65–3.

There are several possible methods of approaching pharmacologic pain management for patients with advanced diseases. Patients may require several different medications to deal with a variety of pain syndromes and disease- or treatment-related discomfort. For expedient and thorough treatment, it is often wise to adopt a stepwise approach to the use of pain medications. The World Health Organization (WHO) has developed a simple three-step model for managing cancer pain that can be applied to many different situations. It has been modified over time to adapt to the evolving fields of pain and palliative medicine (Fig. 65–4).[1] This revised approach recommends that mild pain (1 to 3 on a numeric analogue scale) should be treated with non-opioid pain relievers, such as aspirin, acetaminophen, and nonsteroidal anti-inflammatory drugs (NSAIDs), with or without adjuvant therapy. Higher pain intensities indicate the use of non-opioid analgesics along with opiate derivatives, such as hydrocodone, oxycodone, or tramadol. If pain is not relieved, then titration of opioids, such as morphine, hydromorphone, and fentanyl, in combination with non-opioid analgesics and adjuvants is indicated. Refractory pain syndromes will often require more invasive techniques, such as spinal opioids, nerve block, or neurostimulation.[1,26,53]

Table 65–3. Drugs for Pain Control at the End of Life

WEB ADDRESS	CONTENT
www.palliativedrugs.com	Palliative care formulary online
www.pallmed.net	Generic site, with drug-compatibility database
http://nccam.nih.gov	Information on complementary medicines
www.fda.gov/orphan	Information on orphan drugs

From Doyle D, Hanks G, Cherny NI, Calman K (eds): Oxford Textbook of Palliative Medicine (3rd ed). Oxford, UK, Oxford University Press, 2003.

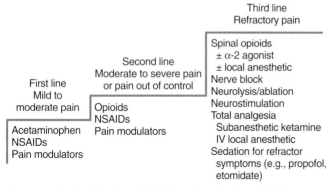

Figure 65–4. Modification of WHO 3-Step Ladder. NSAIDs, nonsteroidal anti-inflammatory drugs. (From Fine PG: The evolving and important role of anesthesiology in palliative care. Anesth Analg 2005;100:183-188.)

Non-Opioid Analgesics

Acetaminophen

Acetaminophen has been determined to be one of the safest analgesics for long-term use in the management of mild pain or as a supplement in the management of more intense pain syndromes. It is especially useful in the management of nonspecific musculoskeletal pain or pain associated with osteoarthritis, but should be considered an adjunct to any chronic pain regimen. It is often forgotten or overlooked when severe pain is being treated in terminally ill patients, but it can be quite effective as a "coanalgesic." It is important to take into account acetaminophen's limited anti-inflammatory effect and its hepatic effects. Reduced doses or avoidance of acetaminophen is recommended for patients with renal insufficiency or liver failure, particularly in individuals with significant alcohol use.[29,54]

NSAIDs

NSAIDs reduce the biosynthesis of prostaglandins by inhibiting cyclooxygenase (COX) and the cascade of inflammatory events that cause, amplify, or maintain nociception. NSAIDs also appear to directly affect the peripheral and central nervous systems. COX has been identified in spinal cord neurons, and may play a role in the development of neuropathic pain, but these agents do not appear to be useful in the treatment of neuropathic pain.[25] The "classic" NSAIDs (e.g., aspirin or ibuprofen) are relatively nonselective in their inhibitory effects on the enzymes that convert arachidonic acid to prostaglandins, so gastrointestinal ulceration, renal dysfunction, and impaired platelet aggregation are common.[4] The COX-2 selective NSAIDs rofecoxib and valdecoxib are off the market, and because of potential problems and concerns with gastrointestinal bleeding and thrombosis, celecoxib should be used with caution in high-risk palliative care patients for protracted periods.[55]

NSAIDs are useful in treating many pain conditions mediated by inflammation, including those caused by cancer.[56-58] These agents cause minimal nausea, constipation, sedation, or effects on mental function, although there is evidence that their use can impair short-term memory in older patients.[59] These agents may be very useful for moderate to severe pain control, either alone or as an adjunct to opioid analgesic therapy. Adding NSAIDs to an opioid regimen may allow a reduced opioid dose when sedation, obtundation, confusion, dizziness, or other central nervous system effects of opioid analgesic therapy alone become problematic.[57] Extended-release formulations are likely to increase compliance and adherence.[25] As with acetaminophen, decreased renal function and liver failure are relative contraindications for NSAID use. Platelet dysfunction or other potential bleeding disorders also contraindicate use of the nonselective NSAIDs because of their inhibitory effects on platelet aggregation, a clear advantage of the coxib class of NSAIDs. If NSAIDs are effective, but there is need for prolonged use or there is a history of gastrointestinal complications, proton pump inhibitors can be given to lower the risk of gastrointestinal bleeding.[60] For more information on NSAIDs, see Chapter 35.

Opioid Analgesics

Opioid analgesics are the most useful agents for the treatment of pain associated with advanced disease, including neuropathic pain.[61,62] There are few, if any, indications for the mixed agonist-antagonist agents, especially in older patients at end of life.[63,64] The pure antagonists are used to treat acute overdose and, in selected cases, prevent opioid-induced bowel dysfunction.[65,66] The opioids used most commonly in palliative care are morphine, hydromorphone, fentanyl, oxycodone, and methadone. A sustained-release form of oxymorphone is available and may add to this growing formulary.[67]

The only absolute contraindication to the use of an opioid is a history of a hypersensitivity reaction (e.g., rash, wheezing, and edema). Allergic reactions are almost exclusively limited to the morphine derivatives, and the prevalence of true allergic reactions to synthetic opioids is much lower. There is significant inter- and intraindividual variation in clinical responses to the various opioids, so dose titration is the best approach to initial management. Idiosyncratic responses may require trials of different agents in order to determine the most effective drug and route of delivery for any given patient. Table 65–4 lists more specific suggestions regarding optimal selection of opioids in end-of-life care, and Table 65–5 lists the commonly used opioids.

Opioid analgesics may accumulate toxic metabolites over time, especially when drug clearance and elimination decrease as disease progresses and organ function deteriorates.[68] Use of meperidine is specifically discouraged for repeated dosing over time because of its neurotoxic metabolite, normeperidine.[64] Use of propoxyphene is also discouraged because of the active metabolite norpropoxyphene, its weak analgesic efficacy, and the significant acetaminophen dose found in some formulations.[63] The mixed agonist-antagonist agents, typified by butorphanol, nalbuphine, and pentazocine, are not recommended for the treatment of pain in patients with advanced disease. They have limited efficacy, and their use may cause an acute abstinence syndrome in patients using pure agonist opioids.[69] For further information on opioids and chronic opioid therapy, see Chapter 31.

Morphine

Morphine, the prototype agonist, is considered the gold standard of opioid analgesics and is used as a measure for dose equivalence.[63] Although some patients cannot tolerate morphine because of pruritus, headache, dysphoria, or other adverse effects, common initial dosing effects, such as sedation and nausea, often resolve within a few days.[70] It is best to anticipate these adverse effects, especially constipation, nausea, and sedation, and prevent or treat appropriately (see following). Morphine-3-glucuronide, a metabolite of morphine, may contribute to myoclonus, seizures, and hyperalgesia, particularly

Table 65–4. Choosing an Opioid: A Matrix of Factors Leading to a "First Best Choice"

GENERAL PHARMACOMEDICAL CONSIDERATIONS	PHARMACOCLINICAL CONSIDERATIONS	PHARMACOGENETIC CONSIDERATIONS	PHARMACOECONOMIC CONSIDERATIONS
Allergies/sensitivities (e.g., morphine and its derivatives)	• Prior experience (subjective responses and preferences) • Adherence (compliance) issues • Social circumstances (cognitive capacity, reliable caregiver, etc.)	Cytochrome P-450 enzyme system genotypes (e.g., "slow metabolizers" at CYP2D6 ineffectively convert the prodrug codeine to the active drug morphine)	Insurance coverage and formulary restrictions
Drug-disease interactions (e.g., renal insufficiency; pulmonary disease)	Administration or absorption preferences and limitations (e.g., oral vs. transdermal formulation; once-a-day dosing vs. multiple dosings per day; G-tube "sprinkle" formulations)	Future possibilities of genotyping to match patient-specific opioid phenotypes to physiochemically different opioids	Indirect costs (e.g., caregiver time, use of clinical services, treatment of side effects such as constipation, etc.)
Drug-drug interactions (e.g., CNS depressants; MAOIs; SSRIs; shared metabolic pathways [i.e., inducers and inhibitors of at CYP2D6 and CYP3A4])	Monitor efficacy (e.g., activity, sleep, mood, pain intensity scores)		
Monitor changes in clinical condition (e.g., resolution or progression of disease; new disease; change in medications)	Monitor adverse effects (e.g., sedation, nausea, bowel function, ataxia, cognitive effects, "tolerance"/hyperalgesia)		

CNS, central nervous system; CYP, cytochrome P-450 isoenzyme; G-tube, gastrostomy tube; MAOIs, monoamine oxidase inhibitors; SSRIs, selective serotonin reuptake inhibitors.
Originally published in Fine PG: Opioid-induced hyperalgesia and opioid rotation. J Pain Palliat Care Pharmacother 2004;18:75-79. Reprinted with permission from Haworth Press, Inc.

Table 65-5. Pure μ-Agonists Used in End-of-Life Care for Pain Control in the United States

DRUG	EQUIANALGESIC (MG) DOSES*†	HALF-LIFE (HR)	PEAK EFFECT (HR)	DURATION (HR)	TOXICITY	COMMENTS
Morphine	10 IM/IV/subcutaneous; 20-30 PO‡	2-3; 2-3	0.5-1; 1-2	3-4; 3-6	Constipation, nausea, sedation most common; respiratory depression is rare when titrated to effect	Standard for comparison for opioids; multiple routes available
Controlled-release morphine	20-30 PO‡	2-3	NA	8-12	Typical opioid effects	Brand name and generics available
Sustained-release morphine	20-30 PO‡	2-3	4-6	12-24	Typical opioid effects	Once-a-day recently approved in the United States
Hydromorphone	1.5 IM/IV/subcutaneous; 7.5 PO	2-3; 2-3	0.5-1; 1-2	3-4; 3-6	Typical opioid effects	Potency and high solubility may be beneficial for patients requiring high opioid doses and for subcutaneous administration.
Oxycodone	20-30 PO	2-3	1-2	3-6	Typical opioid effects	Available as a single entity or combined with NSAIDs or acetaminophen
Controlled-release oxycodone	20-30 PO	NA	3-4	8-12	Typical opioid effects	Oral immediate releases and extended-release formulations available
Oxymorphone	1 IM/IV/subcutaneous; 10 PR; 10-15 PO	NA; NA	0.5-1; 1.5-3	3-6; 4-6	Typical opioid effects	
Levorphanol	2 IM/IV/subcutaneous; 4 PO	12-15; 12-15	0.5-1; 1-2	3-6; 3-6	Typical opioid effects	With long half-life, accumulation possible after beginning or increasing dose
Methadone	Variable	12-150	1-2	6-8	Typical opioid effects	Highly variable half-life and potential for accumulation require greater vigilance for development of opioid toxicity; can prolong the QTc interval
Hydrocodone	30 PO	2-4	1-2	3-6	Typical opioid effects	Only available combined with acetaminophen or NSAIDs
Fentanyl	50-100 mcg IV/subcutaneous	7-12	<10 min	1-2	Typical opioid effects	Can be administered as a continuous IV or subcutaneous infusion
Fentanyl transdermal system	NA	NA	12-24	48-72 per patch	Typical opioid effects	Refer to package for equianalgesic dosing guidelines for oral and parenteral medication. Not recommended for opioid-naïve patients; not recommended for acute pain.
Oral transmucosal fentanyl citrate	NA	7-12	15-30 min	1-2	Typical opioid effects	Not recommended for opioid-naïve patients. Recommended starting dose for breakthrough pain, 200-400 mcg, even with high "baseline" opioid doses

*Dose provides analgesia equivalent to 10 mg of morphine given by IM route. These ratios are useful guides when switching drugs or routes of administration. In clinical practice, the potency of the IM route is considered to be identical to the IV and subcutaneous routes.

†When switching from one opioid to another, incomplete cross-tolerance requires a reduction in the dose of the new drug by 25% to 50% to prevent excessive opioid effects. Provision of "rescue" medication during the conversion period (a few days) prevents breakthrough pain that may result from relative underdosing. When switching to methadone from another drug, the reduction in the equianalgesic dose should be greater, usually 75% to 90%.

‡Extensive survey data suggest that the relative potency ratio of IM to PO morphine, which has been shown to be 1:6 in an acute dosing study, is 1:2 to 1:3 with chronic dosing.

FDA, U.S. Food and Drug Administration; IM, intramuscular; IV, intravenous; NA, not applicable or no data available; NSAIDs, nonsteroidal anti-inflammatory drugs; PO, per mouth; PR, per rectum.

Originally published in Fine PG, Portenoy RK: A Clinical Guide to Opioid Analgesia. Minneapolis, McGraw-Hill Healthcare Information, 2004.

when patients cannot clear the metabolite as a result of renal impairment.[68,71] Side effects and metabolite effects can be differentiated over time. Side effects generally occur soon after the drug is absorbed, whereas metabolite effects are generally delayed by several days. Morphine's bitter taste may be prohibitive, especially if "immediate-release" tablets are left in the mouth to dissolve. In this case, several options are available. One available type of long-acting morphine comes in a capsule that can be opened, releasing small pellets that can be mixed in applesauce or other soft food.[72] Oral morphine solution can be swallowed, or small volumes (0.5 to 1 mL) of a concentrated solution (e.g., 20 mg/mL) can be placed in the mouth of patients whose voluntary swallowing capabilities are significantly limited.[73]

Fentanyl

Fentanyl is a lipophilic opioid that can be administered parenterally, spinally, transdermally, and transmucosally, and is nebulized for the management of dyspnea.[4] Because of its potency, dosing is usually conducted in micrograms. It should be noted that on July 15, 2005, the FDA issued a public health advisory to alert health care professionals, patients, and their caregivers of reports of death and other serious side effects from overdoses of fentanyl in patients using transdermal fentanyl for pain control.[74] Careful fentanyl dosing is particularly important in older patients; a recent study of transdermal fentanyl in postoperative patients found that absorption was significantly delayed in men 64 to 82 years of age compared with men 25 to 38 years of age.[75]

In consideration of the these cautions, transdermal fentanyl, often called the fentanyl patch, is particularly useful when patients cannot swallow, do not remember to take medications, or experience adverse effects from other opioids.[76] Opioid-naïve patients should begin with titrated immediate-release opioids to establish the needed 24-hour dose of opioid before determining that the lowest available dose, currently a 12-mcg/hour patch, can be tolerated. Patients should be monitored by a responsible caregiver for the first 24 to 48 hours of therapy until steady-state blood levels are reached. Transdermal fentanyl may not be appropriate for patients with fever, diaphoresis, cachexia, morbid obesity, and ascites, all of which may have a significant effect on the absorption, blood levels, and clinical effects of the drug.[77,78] Some patients experience reduced analgesic effects within 48 hours of applying a new patch. If so, determine whether a higher dose can be tolerated with increased duration of effect or whether a more frequent (every 48 hours) patch change is the better alternative. Under most circumstances, breakthrough pain medications should be available to patients using continuous-release opioids, such as the fentanyl patch. Several novel transdermal fentanyl delivery systems are under development, including ones that allow bolus dosing. There are insufficient data

or experience to make recommendations about their relative safety or efficacy at this time.

Oral transmucosal fentanyl citrate is composed of fentanyl on an oral applicator to provide rapid absorption of the drug. This formulation of fentanyl is particularly useful for breakthrough pain, as demonstrated in the first clinical report of its use for this indication in a terminally ill patient.[79]

Oxycodone

Oxycodone is a synthetic opioid available in a long-acting formulation (OxyContin), as well as immediate-release tablets (alone or with acetaminophen) and liquid. It is approximately as lipid-soluble as morphine, but has better oral absorption.[80] Side effects appear to be similar to those experienced with morphine, but one study comparing the two formulations in patients with advanced cancer found that oxycodone was less likely to cause nausea and vomiting.[81]

Methadone

Methadone has several characteristics that make it useful in the management of severe, chronic pain.[82-84] Methadone has a half-life of 24 to 36 hours with a much longer terminal half-life, allowing for prolonged dosing intervals. However, the analgesic half-life of methadone is often much shorter. Methadone is an N-methyl-D-aspartate (NMDA) receptor antagonist, which may be of particular benefit in neuropathic pain.[85] Methadone is much less costly than comparable doses of proprietary continuous-release formulations, making it potentially more available for patients without sufficient financial resources for more expensive drugs.

Despite these advantages, much is unknown about the appropriate dosing ratio between methadone and morphine, as well as the safest and most effective time course for conversion from another opioid to methadone.[86] Current data suggest that the dose ratio increases as the previous dose of oral opioid equivalents increases, and although the long half-life is an advantage, it also increases the potential for drug accumulation prior to achieving steady-state blood levels.[84] There may be a risk of oversedation and respiratory depression after 2 to 5 days of treatment with methadone. Close monitoring of these potentially adverse or even life-threatening effects is required.[25,41] Recent case reports suggest that high doses of methadone may lead to life-threatening QT interval prolongation, although it is not clear whether this is a result of the methadone or preservatives in the parenteral formulation.[86]

Patients currently receiving methadone as part of a maintenance program for addictive disease often develop cross-tolerance to opioids and require higher doses than opioid-naïve patients.[87] Prescribing methadone for addictive disease requires a special license in the United States, so prescriptions for methadone to manage pain in palliative care should specify "for pain."

Hydromorphone

Hydromorphone is a synthetic opioid that can be a useful alternative to morphine in patients at end of life. It is available in oral tablets, liquids, suppositories, and parenteral formulations, but the only long-acting formulation was recently recalled by the FDA because of interactions with alcohol that could lead to excessively rapid drug release.[88] As a synthetic opioid, hydromorphone can be useful if there is inadequate pain control or when patients experience true allergic responses to morphine or intolerable side effects occur. The metabolite hydromorphone-3-glucuronide may lead to the same opioid neurotoxicity seen with morphine metabolites: myoclonus, hyperalgesia, and seizures.[89] This is particularly likely in patients with renal dysfunction.[90,91]

Routes for Administering Opioids

The oral route is generally preferred when patients are capable and enteral absorption is not problematic. In the palliative care setting, alternative routes of administration must be available for patients who can no longer swallow or when other dynamics preclude the oral route.[4] These include transdermal, transmucosal, rectal, vaginal, topical, epidural, and intrathecal. In a study of cancer patients at 4 weeks, 1 week, and 24 hours before death, more than half of the patients required more than one route of opioid administration. As patients approached death and oral use diminished, the use of intermittent subcutaneous injections and intravenous or subcutaneous infusions increased.[11] Therefore in caring for patients near the end of life, it is essential to identify alternatives to oral administration that can be used if necessary.

Enteral feeding tubes can be used to access the gut when patients can no longer swallow. The rectum, stoma, or vagina can be used to deliver medication, although fecal contents, mucosal dryness, thrombocytopenia, or painful lesions may preclude the use of these routes. For morphine, commercially prepared suppositories, compounded suppositories, or microenemas can be used to deliver the drug directly to the rectum or stoma.[92] Sustained-release morphine tablets have been used rectally, with resultant delayed time to peak plasma level and approximately 90% of the bioavailability achieved by oral administration.[93]

Because the vagina has no sphincter, a tampon covered with a condom or an inflated urinary catheter balloon may be used to prevent early discharge of the drug.[92] Although useful, the rectal or vaginal routes may be unacceptable to many patients and their caregivers, especially when the patient is obtunded or unable to assist.[5]

Parenteral administration in palliative care is usually limited to subcutaneous and intravenous delivery because repeated intramuscular opioid delivery is excessively noxious. The intravenous route provides rapid drug delivery but requires vascular access that may not be easily obtained or maintained in a home or long-term care setting. In the absence of intravenous access, it must be remembered that subcutaneous boluses, although effective, have a slower onset and lower peak effect when compared with intravenous boluses.[4] Subcutaneous infusions as much as 10 mL/hour are usually absorbed, although most patients tolerate 2 to 3 mL/hour with least difficulty.[94,95]

Intraspinal routes, including epidural or intrathecal delivery, may allow administration of drugs, such as opioids, local anesthetics, and α-adrenergic agonists. A recent randomized controlled trial demonstrated benefit for cancer patients experiencing pain.[53] However, the equipment used to deliver these medications is complex, requiring specialized knowledge for health care professionals and potentially greater caregiver burden. Risk of infection and other complications along with up-front and maintenance costs are significant concerns when contemplating high-technology procedures. Selection should be based on greater than 6 months' life expectancy for implanted programmable pumps, and adequate organizational infrastructure to manage these devices should be in place.

ADJUVANT THERAPIES

The term *adjuvant analgesics* is often used synonymously with *coanalgesics, pain-modifying drugs,* and similar descriptives. A wide variety of non-opioid medications from several pharmacologic classes have been demonstrated to reduce pain caused by various pathologic conditions (e.g., tricyclic antidepressants) or to modify the ongoing disease process in a way that specifically reduces pain (e.g., bisphosphonates).[96] Under most circumstances these drugs are indicated for the treatment of severe neuropathic pain or bone pain, and opioid analgesics are used concurrently to provide adequate pain relief. Typical adjuvants include tricyclic antidepressants, serotonin-norepinephrine reuptake inhibitor (SNRI) antidepressants, anticonvulsants, corticosteroids, and other disease-modifying drugs, such as bisphosphonates for metastatic bone pain. See Table 65–6 for a listing of current adjuvant therapies for neuropathic pain. For more information on adjuvant analgesics, see Chapter 34.

Antidepressants

The analgesic effect of tricyclic antidepressants appears to be related to inhibition of norepinephrine and serotonin reuptake, making these neurotransmitters more available within central nervous system pain inhibitory pathways. There are many significant, controlled clinical trials for several pain conditions, and a recent consensus panel listed tricyclic antidepressants as one of five first-line therapies for neuropathic pain.[97,98] The significant side effects, especially in older patients, require careful titration and monitoring in palliative care populations, but their sleep-enhancing and mood-elevating effects

Table 65–6. Adjuvant Therapies for Neuropathic Pain

CATEGORY/AGENTS	COMMENTS
Corticosteroids Dexamethasone Prednisone Prednisolone	• Shown to reduce spontaneous discharge in injured nerves • Dexamethasone has the least mineralocorticoid effect (long duration of action for once-daily dosing) • May be dosed orally, intravenously, subcutaneously, or epidurally • May produce psychosis, proximal muscle wasting
Anticonvulsants Carbamazepine Gabapentin Valproate Phenytoin Clonazepam Tiagabine Levetiracetam Lamotrigine Topiramate Zonisamide Oxcarbazepine Pregabalin	• Older agents are used extensively, but potential for adverse events requires careful monitoring. Clinical experience is extensive for carbamazepine, but propensity for bone marrow suppression (i.e., leukopenia) limits its use in patients with cancer • Lamotrigine has demonstrated efficacy in HIV sensory neuropathy, painful diabetic neuropathy, and post-stroke pain, but requires slow titration. Also associated with Stevens-Johnson syndrome and severe rash • The role of newer agents (e.g., levetiracetam, oxcarbazepine, tiagabine, etc.) has not been established • Gabapentin approved for PHN • Pregabalin approved for painful diabetic neuropathy
Tricyclic Antidepressants Amitriptyline Nortriptyline Desipramine Imipramine Clomipramine	• Use is associated with significant tolerability issues • Nortriptyline has fewer anticholinergic/anti–α-adrenergic effects, and therefore has better tolerability, especially in older adults • Should be administered at night to reduce daytime sedation and support good sleep hygiene
Local Anesthetics Mexiletine Lidocaine IV	• Oral lidocaine analogues are effective in some patients, but long-term use may lead to clinically significant adverse events • Infusional lidocaine is gaining greater acceptance; may be particularly effective for visceral or central pain • A lidocaine challenge can assess whether a patient's pain is responsive, i.e., 1-3 mg/kg IV or subcutaneous over 30-60 min. If challenge is effective or partially effective, continuous infusion consists of 1-2 mg/kg/hr • Perioral numbness suggests toxicity. Infusion should be halted and restarted at a slower rate on resolution
Anticancer Therapies Radiation therapy Surgery	• Local, half-body, or whole-body radiation therapy can enhance efficacy of analgesia by directly affecting tumor and other causes of pain • Curative excision or palliative debulking of tumor may relieve pain directly, decrease symptoms of obstruction or compression, and improve prognosis

HIV, human immunodeficiency virus; PHN, postherpetic neuralgia.
Adapted and reprinted with permission from Fine PG, Miaskowski C, Paice JA: Meeting the challenges in cancer pain. J Support Oncol 2004;2(suppl 4):5-22.

may be beneficial enough to outweigh their disadvantages.[99] The newer mixed SNRIs—selective serotonin reuptake inhibitors (SSRIs), such as venlafaxine and duloxetine—may offer some of the advantages of tricyclic antidepressants without the anticholinergic side effects.[100] See Chapter 33 for a more complete discussion of antidepressants.

Anticonvulsants

The older anticonvulsants, such as carbamazepine and clonazepam, putatively relieve pain by blocking sodium channels.[99] These compounds are very useful in the treatment of certain types of neuropathic pain, especially pain with episodic, lancinating qualities such as trigeminal neuralgia. Gabapentin seems to have several different mechanisms of action, although calcium ion channel blockade is thought to be its main pain-inhibiting mechanism.[101]

The analgesic doses of gabapentin reported to be effective in a typical and common neuropathic pain condition, painful diabetic neuropathy, ranged from 900 mg/day to 3600 mg/day in divided doses.[102] Additional evidence supports the use of gabapentin in neuropathic pain syndromes seen in palliative care, such as thalamic pain, pain due to spinal cord injury, cancer pain, and restless legs syndrome and HIV-associated sensory neuropathies.[24,103] Withdrawal from gabapentin, if indicated due to ineffectiveness or adverse effects, should be gradual to prevent possible seizures.[104] In the authors' experience, other anticonvulsants that have been used effectively in treating neuropathies causing pain in patients at end of life include lamotrigine, pregabalin (newly approved for painful diabetic neuropathy), levetiracetam, tiagabine, and oxcarbazepine, but no clinical trials in this specific population are available.[23,25,105]

Corticosteroids

Corticosteroids are particularly useful for neuropathic, visceral, and bone pain syndromes in patients with far advanced disease, including plexopathies and pain associated with stretching of the liver capsule as a result of metastases.[106,107] Dexamethasone produces the least amount of mineralocorticoid effect, making it the least toxic choice. Dexamethasone is available in oral, intravenous, subcutaneous, and epidural formulations. The standard dose is 16 to 24 mg/day and can be administered once daily due to the long half-life of this drug, but divided doses are usually used to mitigate high-dose toxic effects, such as psychosis and severe blood sugar abnormalities in diabetic patients. Doses as high as 100 mg may be given with severe pain crises, similar to the doses used in acute neurologic emergencies. Intravenous bolus doses should be administered over several minutes to reduce untoward reactions, such as burning sensations.

Local Anesthetics

Local anesthetics are useful for relieving neuropathic pain. They can be given orally, topically, intravenously, subcutaneously, or spinally.[108] Mexiletine has been reported to be useful when anticonvulsants and other adjuvant therapies have failed. Doses start at 150 mg/day and increase to levels as high as 900 mg/day in divided doses.[109,110] Pretreatment electrocardiogram evaluation is recommended to evaluate for conduction blocks that can be exacerbated by oral local anesthetics. Local anesthetic gels and patches have been used to prevent the pain that is associated with needlestick and other minor procedures. Both gel and patch (lidocaine 5% patch) versions of lidocaine have been shown to reduce the pain of PHN.[111] Intravenous lidocaine at 1 to 5 mg/kg (maximum, 500 mg) administered over 1 hour, followed by a continuous infusion of 1 to 2 mg/kg/hour, has been reported to reduce patients' intractable neuropathic pain in inpatient palliative care and home hospice settings.[23] Epidural or intrathecal lidocaine or bupivacaine delivered with an opioid can reduce neuropathic pain.[112]

Bisphosphonates

Bisphosphonates inhibit osteoclast-mediated bone resorption and alleviate pain related to metastatic bone disease and multiple myeloma, reduce the incidence of pathologic fractures, and are used to treat tumor-related hypercalcemia.[113] In patients with breast cancer and multiple myeloma, zoledronic acid has demonstrated improved safety and efficacy compared with pamidronate.[114,115] Similarly, there appears to be more sustained pain relief with zoledronic acid compared with other bisphosphonates in patients with metastatic prostate cancer.[116] Clinical trials in patients with lung and renal cell carcinoma have also shown therapeutic benefit from regular infusions of zoledronic acid.[117]

Calcitonin

Subcutaneous calcitonin may be effective in the relief of neuropathic or bone pain, although studies are inconclusive.[118] The nasal form of this drug may be more acceptable in end-of-life care when other therapies are ineffective. Usual doses are 100 to 200 IU/day subcutaneously or nasally.

Chemotherapy and Radiation Therapy

Palliative chemotherapy is the use of antitumor therapy to relieve the symptoms that are associated with malignancy. Patient goals, performance status, sensitivity of the tumor, and potential toxicities must be considered.[4] Examples of symptoms that may improve with chemotherapy include relief of chest wall pain from reduced tumor ulceration through the use of hormonal therapy in breast cancer. Similarly, newer agents, such as docetaxel, reduce pain and improve quality of life in hormone-refractory prostate cancer, and topotecan and epidermal growth factor receptor inhibitors accomplish similar results for patients with lung cancers.[119-121]

Radiation therapy is also a highly useful adjunct to control pain from bone metastasis and pressure-inducing and ulcerative malignancies. Single-fraction and hypofractionated regimens are proving to be effective in very sick patients and those with limited life expectancy in whom the opportunity costs of multiple treatment sessions are untenable.[122,123] These therapies are often underused in hospice or palliative care, and they should be considered for any patient with a life expectancy of more than a few weeks.[124]

Other Adjunct Analgesics

Baclofen, a skeletal muscle relaxant, is also useful for the relief of spasm-associated pain, and it may be helpful in the treatment of intractable hiccups, which can be painful and cause sleep disturbance.[125] Doses begin at 10 mg/day, increasing every few days. Feelings of weakness and confusion or hallucinations often occur with doses greater than 60 mg/day. Slow downward titration is necessary to prevent withdrawal-related seizures.

Calcium channel blockers are believed to provide pain relief in certain pain syndromes as well. For instance, nifedipine 10 mg orally may be useful to relieve ischemic or neuropathic pain syndromes.[126,127] There are few randomized controlled clinical trials to support these mostly anecdotal findings.

BEGINNING THERAPY, ADDING OR CHANGING DRUGS, AND BREAKTHROUGH PAIN

Application of practical and mechanism-based approaches, coupled with context-appropriate follow-up, will optimize drug and other palliative therapies. The "best first choice" and subsequent timing of opioid rotation will depend on patient-specific medical, psychological, and social considerations and a sound knowledge of opioid pharmacotherapy. If adverse effects exceed the analgesic benefit of the drug, convert to an equianalgesic dose of a different opioid. Because cross-tolerance is incomplete, reduce the calculated dose by one third to one half and titrate upward based on the patient's pain intensity scores.[4]

Titration and combining drugs that may provide additive or synergistic effects should proceed along rational lines, based on the pharmacokinetics and monitored pharmacodynamics of the drugs. Frail patients and those with pain crises may require observation in a monitored setting in order to provide safe and effective relief within an acceptable time frame.

Transitory flares of pain, or breakthrough pain, can be expected both at rest and during movement. If breakthrough pain lasts longer than a few minutes, rescue doses of the patient's current analgesics may provide relief.[128] In patients without parenteral access, oral transmucosal fentanyl may be useful for rapid episodic pain relief or during a brief but painful dressing change. Frail, older adults, or severely debilitated patients should start with the 200-mcg dose and efficacy should be monitored, advancing to higher dose units as needed.[129] Clinicians must be aware that unlike other breakthrough pain drugs, the around-the-clock dose of opioid does not predict the effective dose of oral transmucosal fentanyl. Some pain relief can usually be expected in about 5 to 10 minutes after administration. Patients should use oral transmucosal fentanyl citrate over a period of 15 minutes because more active sucking will result in more swallowing and less transmucosal absorption.

Because misunderstandings lead to undertreatment, all clinicians involved in the care of patients with advanced illness and pain must be able to differentiate and clearly explain to patients and their families the clinical conditions of tolerance, physical dependence, and the rarity of addiction related to opioid use at end of life. It also is critically important to be aware that there is no established relationship between titration of opioid analgesics to affect pain relief and timing of death in palliative care or hospice settings.[130,131]

MINIMIZING AND MANAGING ADVERSE EFFECTS

There are a variety of adverse effects that drugs for pain can cause patients in palliative care. The normal side effects associated with pain-relief medications are often exacerbated by changes in metabolism caused by end-stage disease, polypharmacy associated with advanced age, and other factors. Following are some of the more common adverse effects and an overview of possible approaches to preventing or alleviating them.

Constipation

Patients in palliative care frequently experience constipation, in part because of opioid therapy.[44] Always begin a prophylactic bowel regimen when commencing opioid analgesic therapy. Avoid bulking agents, such as psyllium because these tend to increase desiccation time in the large bowel, and debilitated patients can rarely take in sufficient fluid to facilitate

the action of bulking agents. Instead starting with cost-effective and palatable products, such as senna tea and fruit or senna plus docusate sodium (Colace) for patients with a history of "sluggish" bowel function is advised. If this is ineffective at creating regular laxation, then prescription therapies are indicated (e.g., bisacodyl, senna derivatives, propylene glycol).[41] Tables listing recommended regimens are readily available in clinical guidelines and texts.

Sedation

Excessive sedation may occur with the initial doses of opioids. If sedation persists after 24 to 48 hours and other correctable causes have been identified and treated, psychostimulants may be beneficial. These include dextroamphetamine 2.5 to 5 mg by mouth every morning and midday or methylphenidate 5 to 10 mg by mouth every morning and 2.5 to 5 mg midday (although higher doses are frequently used, and use later in the day may be required for wakefulness throughout the evening hours, if desired).[4] Adjust both the dose and timing to prevent nocturnal insomnia, and monitor for undesirable psychotomimetic effects (such as agitation, hallucinations, and irritability). Once-daily dosing of modafinil, a newer agent approved to manage narcolepsy, has been reported to relieve opioid-induced sedation.[132]

Respiratory Depression

Respiratory depression is rarely a clinically significant problem for opioid-tolerant patients who are in pain.[41] When respiratory depression occurs in a patient with advanced disease, the cause is usually multifactorial.[133,134] When depressed consciousness occurs along with a respiratory rate less than 8/minute or hypoxemia (O_2 saturation less than 90%) associated with opioid use, slow, cautious titration of naloxone should be instituted (0.4 mg [one ampule, 400 mcg, diluted in 10 mL injectable saline = 0.4 mcg/mL]) every 3 to 5 minutes while providing respiratory support and supplemental oxygen). Excessive administration may cause abrupt opioid reversal with pain and autonomic crisis.

Nausea and Vomiting

Nausea is common and vomiting is an occasional adverse effect associated with opioids as a result of activation of the chemoreceptor trigger zone in the medulla, vestibular sensitivity, and delayed gastric emptying, but habituation occurs in most cases within several days.[4] Assess for other treatable causes. In severe cases or when nausea and vomiting are not self-limited, pharmacotherapy is indicated. Usually, low doses of an H_1 blocker (e.g., diphenhydramine) are all that is required while the patient habituates to this unpleasant side effect. If there is no relief within a few days, metoclopramide or a different opioid is recommended; also consider transdermal rather than enteral therapy.[25,41]

Myoclonus

Myoclonic jerking can occur with high-dose opioid therapy. If myoclonus develops, switch to an alternate opioid, especially if using morphine. Evidence suggests that this symptom is associated with metabolite accumulation, particularly in the face of renal dysfunction.[4] A lower relative dose of the substituted drug may be possible because of incomplete cross-tolerance. Clonazepam 0.5 to 1 mg by mouth every 6 to 8 hours, to be increased as needed and tolerated, may be useful in treating myoclonus in patients who are still alert, able to communicate, and take oral preparations.[135] Lorazepam can be given sublingually if the patient is unable to swallow. Otherwise, parenteral administration of diazepam is indicated if symptoms are distressing. Grand mal seizures associated with high-dose parenteral opioid infusions have been reported and may be caused by preservatives in the solution.[136] Preservative-free solutions should be used when administering high-dose infusions.

Pruritus

Pruritus can occur with most opioids, although it appears to be most common with morphine. Fentanyl and oxymorphone may be less likely to cause histamine release. Most antipruritus therapies cause sedation, so the patient must see this as an acceptable trade-off. Antihistamines (such as diphenhydramine) are the most common first-line approach to this opioid-induced symptom. Ondansetron and paroxetine have been reported to be effective in relieving opioid-induced pruritus, but no randomized controlled studies exist.[137,138]

CASE 3: **Complex Symptom Management in the Home Setting** (Continued)

After examination and consultation, it is determined that Ben can continue to reside in the assisted-living facility, attended to by home-based hospice staff. Treatment proceeded with subcutaneous administration of octreotide and hydromorphone to relieve bowel symptoms and provide analgesia on an as-needed basis. In this way the unpleasantness of nasogastric suctioning, nausea, and vomiting was avoided, and he was able to die in a manner consistent with his preferences.

CONCLUSION

Effective pain management in advanced medical illness and at the end of life is a critical component of quality medical care to ensure dignified, safe, and comfortable dying. To quote Sir William Osler, the "father of modern medicine," "The study of morbid anatomy combined with careful clinical observations has taught us to recognize our limitations and to accept the fact that a disease itself may be incurable and that the best we can do is to relieve symptoms and make the patient comfortable."[139]

Principles to help improve this important domain of clinical care can be summarized with the following key points regarding pharmacotherapy for the relief of pain in far-advanced illness.

SUMMARY

- Ensure that communications about goals of care and treatment plans among professional caregiving staff and the patient and family members are clear and understood in order to optimize outcomes and minimize potential conflicts.
- Determine the etiology of pain and the social and prognostic circumstances that will affect the pain experience and pain therapy.
- Focus on discernible clinical end points
  - Pain reduction
  - Functional capacities
  - Mood
  - Sleep
  - Relationships
  - Pleasure in living
- Match the mechanism of pain with the class of drug whenever possible; initiate therapy and adjust dose according to therapeutic response, side effects, and known pharmacokinetics of the drug.
- Anticipate and monitor for adverse effects
  - Prevent side effects
  - Actively treat side effects
- Acetaminophen should be the first consideration in the treatment of mild to moderate pain of musculoskeletal origin.
- Use adjunctive drug therapies, especially for neuropathic pain.
- Opioid analgesic drugs are often necessary to relieve moderate to severe pain, and long-acting or sustained-release analgesic preparations should be used for continuous pain.
- Breakthrough pain should be identified and treated by the use of fast-onset, short-acting preparations.
- Last, and perhaps most important, know your limits. When a patient is not responding to therapy, be prepared to consult with someone who has more training, expertise, and experience.

References

1. Fine PG: The evolving and important role of anesthesiology in palliative care. Anesth Analg 2005;100:183-188.
2. Ng K, von Gunten CF: Symptoms and attitudes of 100 consecutive patients admitted to an acute hospice/palliative care unit. J Pain Symptom Manage 1998;16:307-316.
3. Caraceni A, Weinstein SM: Classification of cancer pain syndromes. Oncology (Williston Park) 2001;15:1627-1640, 1642; discussion 1642-1623, 1646-1627.
4. Paice JA, Fine PG: Pain at the end of life. In Ferrell BR, Coyle N (eds): Oxford Textbook of Palliative Nursing (2nd ed). New York, Oxford University Press, 2005.
5. Doyle D, Hanks G, Cherny NI, Calman K, eds. Oxford Textbook of Palliative Medicine (3rd ed). Oxford, UK, Oxford University Press, 2003.
6. Chang VT, Hwang SS, Feuerman M, Kasimis BS: Symptom and quality of life survey of medical oncology patients at a veterans affairs medical center: A role for symptom assessment. Cancer 2000;88:1175-1183.
7. Meuser T, Pietruck C, Radbruch L, et al: Symptoms during cancer pain treatment following WHO-guidelines: A longitu-

dinal follow-up study of symptom prevalence, severity and etiology. Pain 2001;93:247-257.

8. Wells N: Pain intensity and pain interference in hospitalized patients with cancer. Oncol Nurs Forum 2000;27:985-991.

9. Rabow MW, Petersen J, Schanche K, et al: The comprehensive care team: A description of a controlled trial of care at the beginning of the end of life. J Palliat Med 2003;6: 489-499.

10. Brescia FJ, Portenoy RK, Ryan M, et al: Pain, opioid use, and survival in hospitalized patients with advanced cancer. J Clin Oncol 1992;10:149-155.

11. Coyle N, Adelhardt J, Foley KM, Portenoy RK: Character of terminal illness in the advanced cancer patient: Pain and other symptoms during the last four weeks of life. J Pain Symptom Manage 1990;5:83-93.

12. Goudas LC, Bloch R, Gialeli-Goudas M, et al: The epidemiology of cancer pain. Cancer Invest 2005;23:182-190.

13. Bernabei R, Gambassi G, Lapane K, et al: Management of pain in elderly patients with cancer. SAGE Study Group. Systematic assessment of geriatric drug use via epidemiology. JAMA 1998;279:1877-1882.

14. Hall EJ, Sykes NP: Analgesia for patients with advanced disease: Part 1. Postgrad Med J 2004;80:148-154.

15. Cohen LM, Germain M, Poppel DM, et al: Dialysis discontinuation and palliative care. Am J Kidney Dis 2000;36: 140-144.

16. Cleeland CS, Gonin R, Baez L, et al: Pain and treatment of pain in minority patients with cancer. The Eastern Cooperative Oncology Group Minority Outpatient Pain Study. Ann Intern Med 1997;127:813-816.

17. Cleeland CS, Gonin R, Hatfield AK, et al: Pain and its treatment in outpatients with metastatic cancer. N Engl J Med 1994;330:592-596.

18. Nurmikko TJ, Haanpaa M: Treatment of postherpetic neuralgia. Curr Pain Headache Rep 2005;9:161-167.

19. Larue F, Brasseur L, Musseault P, et al: Pain and symptoms during HIV disease. A French national study. J Palliat Care 1994;10;95.

20. Vogl D, Rosenfeld B, Breitbart W, et al: Symptom prevalence, characteristics, and distress in AIDS outpatients. J Pain Symptom Manage 1999;18:253-262.

21. Swica Y, Breitbart W: Treating pain in patients with AIDS and a history of substance use. West J Med 2002;176:33-39.

22. Herr KA: Pain assessment in the older adult with verbal communications skills. In Gibson SJ, Weiner DK (eds): Pain in Older Persons. Seattle, IASP Press, 2005, pp 111-133.

23. Chang H-M: Pain and its management in patients with cancer. Cancer Invest 2004;22;799-809.

24. Miller KE, Miller MM, Jolley MR: Challenges in pain management at the end of life. Am Fam Physician 2001;64: 1227-1234.

25. Fine PG, Miaskowski C, Paice JA: Meeting the challenges in cancer pain management. J Support Oncol 2004;2(suppl4): 5-22.

26. Deer TR: Current and future trends in spinal cord stimulation for chronic pain. Curr Pain Headache Rep 2001;5:503-509.

27. Page GG: The immune-suppressive effects of pain. Adv Exp Med Biol 2003;521:117-125.

28. Fine PG: The ethical imperative to relieve pain at life's end. J Pain Symptom Manage 2002;23:273-277.

29. AGS Panel on Persistent Pain in Older Persons: Clinical guideline for assessment and management of persistent pain in older persons. J Am Geriatr Soc 2000;50:S205-S224.

30. Tilden VP, Drach LL, Tolle SW: Complementary and alternative therapy use at end-of-life in community settings. J Altern Complement Med 2004;10:811-817.

31. Weiner DK, Ernst E: Complementary and alternative approaches to the treatment of persistent musculoskeletal pain. Clin J Pain 2004;20:244-255.

32. Garnett M: Sustaining the cocoon: The emotional inoculation produced by complementary therapies in palliative care. Eur J Cancer Care (Engl) 2003;12:129-136.

33. Keefe FJ, Ahles TA, Porter LS, et al: The self-efficacy of family caregivers for helping cancer patients manage pain at end-of-life. Pain 2003;103:157-162.

34. Montagnini M, Lodhi M, Born W: The utilization of physical therapy in a palliative care unit. J Palliat Med 2003;6:11-17.

35. Soden K, Vincent K, Craske S, et al: A randomized controlled trial of aromatherapy massage in a hospice setting. Palliat Med 2004;18:87-92.

36. National Institutes of Health Consensus Development Statement. Acupuncture. November 3-5, 1997. Revised draft 11/5/97. Available at: www.healthy.net/LIBRARY/Articles/NIH/Report.htm Accessed March 1, 2006.

37. Paqueta C, Kergoata M-J, Dube L: The role of everyday emotion regulation on pain in hospitalized elderly: Insights from a prospective within-day assessment. Pain 2005;115: 355-363.

38. Myskja A: Therapeutic use of music in nursing homes. Tidsskr Nor Laegeforen 2005;125:1497-1499.

39. Kemper KJ, Danhauer SC: Music as therapy. South Med J 2005;98:282-288.

40. Rousseau PC: Palliative sedation in the management of refractory symptoms. J Support Oncol 2004;2(2):181-186.

41. Fine PG, Portenoy R: A Clinical Guide to Opioid Analgesia. Minneapolis, McGraw-Hill Healthcare Information, 2004.

42. Teno JM, Weitzen S, Wetle T, Mor V: Persistent pain in nursing home residents. JAMA 2001;285:2081.

43. Lasch K, Greenhill A, Wilkes G, et al: Why study pain? A qualitative analysis of medical and nursing faculty and students' knowledge of and attitudes to cancer pain management. J Palliat Med 2002;5:57-71.

44. Potter VT, Wiseman CE, Dunn SM, Boyle FM: Patient barriers to optimal cancer pain control. Psychooncology 2003;12: 153-160.

45. Bruera E, Neumann CM, Mazzocato C, et al: Abstract attitudes and beliefs of palliative care physicians regarding communication with terminally ill cancer patients. Palliat Med 2000;14:287-298.

46. Jenkins V, Fallowfield L, Saul J: Abstract information needs of patients with cancer: Results from a large study in UK cancer centres. Br J Cancer 2001;84:48-51.

47. Degner LF, Kristjanson LJ, Bowman D, et al: Information needs and decisional preferences in women with breast cancer. JAMA 1997;277:1485-1492.

48. Degner LF, Sloan JA: Decision making during serious illness: What role do patients really want to play? J Clin Epidemiol 1992;45:941-950.

49. Degner LF, Sloan JA, Venkatesh P: The Control Preferences Scale. Can J Nurs Res 1997;29:21-43.

50. Paice JA, Toy C, Shott S: Barriers to cancer pain relief: Fear of tolerance and addiction. J Pain Symptom Manage 1998; 16:1-9.

51. Ward SE, Berry PE, Misiewicz H: Concerns about analgesics among patients and family caregivers in a hospice setting. Res Nurs Health 1996;19:205-211.

52. Berry PE, Ward SE: Barriers to pain management in hospice: A study of family caregivers. Hosp J 1995;10:19-33.

53. Smith TJ, Staats PS, Deer T, et al: Randomized clinical trial of an implantable drug delivery system compared with comprehensive medical management for refractory cancer pain: Impact on pain, drug-related toxicity, and survival. J Clin Oncol 2002;20:4040-4049.

54. Tanaka E, Yamazaki K, Misawa S: Update: The clinical importance of acetaminophen hepatotoxicity in non-alcoholic and alcoholic subjects. J Clin Pharm Ther 2000;25:325-332.

55. US Food and Drug Administration, Department of Health and Human Services: Center for Drug Evaluation and Research. Questions and answers: FDA regulatory actions for the COX-2 selective and non-selective non-steroidal anti-inflammatory drugs (NSAIDs). Created April 7, 2005. Available at: www.fda.gov/cder/drug/infopage/COX2/COX2qa. htm. Accessed March 1, 2006.

56. Mercadante S: The use of anti-inflammatory drugs in cancer pain. Cancer Treat Rev 2001;27:51-61.

57. Lucas LK, Lipman AG: Recent advances in pharmacotherapy for cancer pain management. Cancer Pract 2002;10(suppl1): S14-20.

58. Mercadante S, Fulfaro F, Casuccio A: A randomised controlled study on the use of anti-inflammatory drugs in

patients with cancer pain on morphine therapy: Effects on dose-escalation and a pharmacoeconomic analysis. Eur J Cancer 2002;38:1358-1363.

59. Hoppmann RA, Peden JG, Ober SK: Central nervous system side effects of nonsteroidal anti-inflammatory drugs. Aseptic meningitis, psychosis, and cognitive dysfunction. Arch Intern Med 1991;151:1309-1313.

60. Wolfe MM, Lichtenstein DR, Singh G: Gastrointestinal toxicity of nonsteroidal antiinflammatory drugs. [erratum appears in N Engl J Med. 1999;341:548]. N Engl J Med 1999;340:1888-1899.

61. Inturrisi CE. Pharmacology of analgesia: Basic principles. In Bruera E, Portenoy RK (eds): Cancer Pain: Assessment and Management. Cambridge, UK, Cambridge University Press, 2003.

62. Rowbotham MC, Twilling L, Davies PS, et al: Oral opioid therapy for chronic peripheral and central neuropathic pain. N Engl J Med 2003;348:1223-1232.

63. American Pain Society: Principles of Analgesic Use in the Treatment of Acute Pain and Cancer Pain (5th ed). Glenview, Ill, American Pain Society, 2003.

64. Miaskowski C, Cleary J, Burney R, et al: Guideline for the Management of Cancer Pain in Adults and Children, APS Clinical Practice Guidelines Series, No. 3. Glenview, Ill, American Pain Society, 2005.

65. Pappagallo M: Incidence, prevalence and management of opioid bowel dysfunction. Am J Surg 2001;182(5A suppl): 11S-18S.

66. Paulson DM, Kennedy DT, Donovick RA, et al: Alvimopan: An oral, peripherally acting, mu-opioid receptor antagonist for the treatment of opioid-induced bowel dysfunction: A 21 day treatment-randomized clinical trial. J Pain 2005;6: 184-192.

67. Gabrail N, Dvergsten C, Ahdieh H: Establishing the dosage equivalency of oxymorphone extended release and oxycodone controlled release in patients with cancer pain; a randomized controlled study. Curr Med Res Opin 2004;20: 911-918.

68. Andersen G, Jensen NH, Christrup L, et al: Pain, sedation and morphine metabolism in cancer patients during long-term treatment with sustained-release morphine. Palliat Med 2002;16:107-114.

69. Ripamonti C: Pharmacology of opioid analgesia: Clinical principles. In Bruera E, Portenoy RK (eds): Cancer Pain: Assessment and Management. Cambridge, UK, Cambridge University Press, 2003, pp 124-149.

70. Mercadante S, Villari P, Ferrera P, Casuccio A: Opioid-induced or pain relief-induced symptoms in advanced cancer patients. Eur J Pain 2006;10:153-159.

71. Smith MT: Neuroexcitatory effects of morphine and hydromorphone: Evidence implicating the 3-glucuronide metabolites. Clin Exp Pharmacol Physiol 2000;27:524-528.

72. O'Brien T, Mortimer PG, McDonald CJ, Miller AJ: A randomized crossover study comparing the efficacy and tolerability of a novel once-daily morphine preparation (MXL capsules) with MST continuous tablets in cancer patients with severe pain. Palliat Med 1997;11:475-482.

73. Coluzzi PH: Sublingual morphine: Efficacy reviewed. J Pain Symptom Manage 1998;16:184-192.

74. US Food and Drug Administration, Department of Health and Human Services: MedWatch, The FDA Safety Information and Adverse Event Reporting Program. 2005 safety alerts for drugs, biologics, medical devices, and dietary supplements. Posted July 15, 2005. Available at: www.fda.gov/MedWatch/SAFETY/2005/safety05.htm#Fentanyl. Accessed March 1, 2006.

75. Fine PG: Opioid analgesic drugs in older people. Clin Geriatr Med 2001;17:479-487.

76. Muijsers RB, Wagstaff AJ: Transdermal fentanyl: An updated review of its pharmacological properties and therapeutic efficacy in chronic cancer pain control. Drugs 2001;61: 2289-2307.

77. Menten J, Desmedt M, Lossignol D, Mullie A: Longitudinal follow-up of TTS-fentanyl use in patients with cancer-related

pain: Results of a compassionate-use study with special focus on elderly patients. Curr Med Res Opin 2002;18:488-498.

78. Radbruch L, Sabatowski R, Petzke F, et al: Transdermal fentanyl for the management of cancer pain: A survey of 1005 patients. Palliat Med 2001;15:309-321.

79. Ashburn MA, Fine PG, Stanley TH: Oral transmucosal fentanyl citrate for the treatment of breakthrough cancer pain. Anesthesiology 1989;71:615-617.

80. Davis MP, Varga J, Dickerson D, et al: Normal-release and controlled-release oxycodone: Pharmacokinetics, pharmacodynamics, and controversy. Support Care Cancer 2003; 11:84-92.

81. Lauretti GR, Oliveira GM, Pereira NL: Comparison of sustained-release morphine with sustained-release oxycodone in advanced cancer patients. Br J Cancer 2003;89:2027-2030.

82. Shaiova L, Sperber KT, Hord ED: Methadone for refractory cancer pain. J Pain Symptom Manage 2002;23:178-180.

83. Bruera E, Palmer JL, Bosnjak S, et al: Methadone versus morphine as a first-line strong opioid for cancer pain: A randomized, double-blind study. J Clin Oncol 2004;22:185-192.

84. Davis MP, Walsh D: Methadone for relief of cancer pain: A review of pharmacokinetics, pharmacodynamics, drug interactions and protocols of administration. Support Care Cancer 2001;9:73-83.

85. Morley JS, Bridson J, Nash TP, et al: Low-dose methadone has an analgesic effect in neuropathic pain: A double-blind randomized controlled crossover trial. Palliat Med 2003;17: 576-587.

86. Gazelle G, Fine PG: Methadone for the treatment of pain. J Palliat Med 2003;6:621-622.

87. Doverty M, Somogyi AA, White JM, et al: Methadone maintenance patients are cross-tolerant to the antinociceptive effects of morphine. Pain 2001;93:155-163.

88. Otis JA, Fudin J: Use of long-acting opioids for the management of chronic pain. US Pharmacist. Available at: www.uspharmacist.com/index.asp?show=search. Accessed March 1, 2006.

89. Wright AW, Mather LE, Smith MT: Hydromorphone-3-glucuronide: A more potent neuro-excitant than its structural analogue, morphine-3-glucuronide. Life Sci 2001;69: 409-420.

90. Fainsinger R, Schoeller T, Boiskin M, Bruera E: Palliative care rounds: Cognitive failure and coma after renal failure in a patient receiving captopril and hydromorphone. J Palliat Care 1993;9:53-55.

91. Lee MA, Leng ME, Tiernan EJ: Retrospective study of the use of hydromorphone in palliative care patients with normal and abnormal urea and creatinine. Palliat Med 2001; 15:26-34.

92. McCaffery M, Martin L, Ferrell BR: Analgesic administration via rectum or stoma. J ET Nurs 1992;19:114-121.

93. Du X, Skopp G, Aderjan R: The influence of the route of administration: A comparative study at steady state of oral sustained release morphine and morphine sulfate suppositories. Ther Drug Monit 1999;21:208-214.

94. Nelson KA, Glare PA, Walsh D, Groh ES: A prospective, within-patient, crossover study of continuous intravenous and subcutaneous morphine for chronic cancer pain. J Pain Symptom Manage 1997;13:262-267.

95. Watanabe S, Pereira J, Hanson J, Bruera E: Fentanyl by continuous subcutaneous infusion for the management of cancer pain: A retrospective study. J Pain Symptom Manage 1998; 16:323-326.

96. Fine PG, Bellamy C: Bisphosphonates for metastatic bone pain. J Pain Palliat Care Pharmacother 2005;19:61-63.

97. Hammack JE, Michalak JC, Loprinzi CL, et al: Phase III evaluation of nortriptyline for alleviation of symptoms of cisplatinum-induced peripheral neuropathy. Pain 2002;98: 195-203.

98. Dworkin RH, Backonja M, Rowbotham MC, et al: Advances in neuropathic pain: Diagnosis, mechanisms, and treatment recommendations. Arch Neurol 2003;60:1524-1534.

99. Farrar JT, Portenoy RK: Neuropathic cancer pain: The role of adjuvant analgesics. Oncology (Huntingt) 2001;15:1435-1442, 1445; discussion 1445, 1450-1433.

100. Goldstein DJ, Yu Y, Detke MJ, et al: Duloxetine vs. placebo in patients with painful diabetic neuropathy. Pain 2005; 116:109-118.
101. Maizels M, McCarberg B: Antidepressants and antiepileptic drugs for chronic non-cancer pain. Am Fam Physician 2005;71:483-490.
102. Backonja M, Beydoun A, Edwards KR, et al: Gabapentin for the symptomatic treatment of painful neuropathy in patients with diabetes mellitus: A randomized controlled trial. JAMA 1998;280:1831-1836.
103. Hahn K, Arendt G, Braun JS, et al: German Neuro-AIDS Working Group. A placebo-controlled trial of gabapentin for painful HIV-associated sensory neuropathies. J Neurol 2004; 251:1260-1266.
104. Barrueto F Jr, Green J, Howland MA, et al: Gabapentin withdrawal presenting as status epilepticus. J Toxicol Clin Toxicol 2002;40:925-928.
105. Rosenstock J, Tuchman M, LaMoreaux L, Sharma U: Pregabalin for the treatment of painful diabetic peripheral neuropathy: A double-blind placebo-controlled trial. Pain 2004;110: 628-638.
106. Mercadante S, Fulfaro F, Casuccio A: The use of corticosteroids in home palliative care. Support Care Cancer 2001; 9:386-389.
107. Wooldridge JE, Anderson CM, Perry MC: Corticosteroids in advanced cancer. Oncology (Huntingt) 2001;15:225-234; discussion 234-226.
108. Mao J, Chen LL: Systemic lidocaine for neuropathic pain relief. Pain 2000;87:7-17.
109. Sloan P, Basta M, Storey P, von Gunten C: Mexiletine as an adjuvant analgesic for the management of neuropathic cancer pain. Anesth Analg 1999;89:760-761.
110. Wallace MS, Magnuson S, Ridgeway B: Efficacy of oral mexiletine for neuropathic pain with allodynia: A double-blind, placebo-controlled, crossover study. Reg Anesth Pain Med 2000;25:459-467.
111. Barbano RL, Herrmann DN, Hart-Gouleau S, et al: Effectiveness, tolerability, and impact on quality of life of the 5% lidocaine patch in diabetic polyneuropathy. Arch Neurol 2004;61:914-918.
112. Deer TR, Caraway DL, Kim CK, et al: of chronic pain related to failed back surgery syndrome and metastatic cancer pain of the spine. Spine J 2002;2:274-278.
113. Coleman RE: Bisphosphonates: Clinical experience. Oncologist 2004;9(suppl 4):14-27.
114. Rosen LS, Gordon D, Kaminski M, et al: Long-term efficacy and safety of zoledronic acid compared with pamidronate disodium in the treatment of skeletal complications in patients with advanced multiple myeloma or breast cancer: A randomized, double-blind, multicenter, comparative trial. Cancer 2003;98:1735-1744.
115. Rosen LS, Gordon DH, Dugan W Jr, et al: Zoledronic acid is superior to pamidronate for the treatment of bone metastases in breast cancer patients with at least one osteolytic lesion. Cancer 2004;100:36-43.
116. Saad F, Gleason D, Murray R, et al: Zoledronic acid is well tolerated for up to 24 months and significantly reduces skeletal complications in patients with advanced prostate cancer metastatic to bone. J Urol 2003;169(suppl):394.
117. Rosen LS, Gordon D, Tchekmedyian NS, et al: Long-term efficacy and safety of zoledronic acid in the treatment of skeletal metastases in patients with non-small cell lung carcinoma and other solid tumors: A randomized, phase III, double-blind, placebo-controlled trial. Cancer 2004;100: 2613-2621.
118. Martinez MJ, Roque M, Alonso-Coello P, et al: Calcitonin for metastatic bone pain. Cochrane Database Syst Rev 2003: CD003223.
119. Van Poppel H: Recent docetaxel studies establish a new standard of care in hormone refractory prostate cancer. Can J Urol 2005;12(suppl):81-85.
120. Gralla RJ: Quality-of-life considerations in patients with advanced lung cancer. Effect of topotecan on symptom palliation and quality of life. Oncologist 2004;9(suppl 6): 14-24.
121. Langer CJ: Emerging role of epidermal growth factor receptor inhibition in therapy for advanced malignancy. Focus on NSCLC. Int J Radiat Oncol Biol Phys 2004;58:991-1002.
122. Hartsell WF, Scott CB, Bruner DW, et al: Randomized trial of short- versus long-course radiotherapy for palliation of painful bone metastases. J Natl Cancer Inst 2005;97: 798-804.
123. Konski A, Feigenberg S, Chow E: Palliative radiation therapy. Semin Oncol 2005;32:156-164.
124. Lutz S, Spence C, Chow E, et al: Survey on use of palliative radiotherapy in hospice care. J Clin Oncol 2004;22: 3581-3586.
125. Walker P, Watanabe S, Bruera E: Baclofen, a treatment for chronic hiccup. J Pain Symptom Manage 1998;16:125-132.
126. George S, Pulimood S, Jacob M, Chandi SM: Pain in multiple leiomyomas alleviated by nifedipine. Pain 1997;73:101-102.
127. Fine PG: Analgesia issues in palliative care: Bone pain, controlled release opioids, managing opioid-induced constipation and nifedipine as an analgesic. J Pain Palliat Care Pharmacother 2002;16:93-97.
128. Fine PG: Breakthrough pain. In Bruera E, Portenoy R (eds): Cancer Pain. Cambridge University Press, New York, 2003, pp 408-411.
129. Coluzzi PH, Schwartzberg L, Conroy JD, et al: Breakthrough cancer pain: A randomized trial comparing oral transmucosal fentanyl citrate (OTFC) and morphine sulfate immediate release (MSIR). Pain 2001;91:123-130.
130. Bercovitch M, Adunsky A: Patterns of high-dose morphine use in a home-care hospice service: Should we be afraid of it? Cancer 2004;101:1473-1477.
131. Morita T, Tsunoda J, Inoue S, Chihara S: Effects of high dose opioids and sedatives on survival in terminally ill cancer patients. J Pain Symptom Manage 2001;21:282-289.
132. Webster L, Andrews M, Stoddard G: Modafinil treatment of opioid-induced sedation. Pain Med 2003;4:135-140.
133. Sykes N, Thorns A: Sedative use in the last week of life and the implications for end-of-life decision making. Arch Intern Med 2003;163:341-344.
134. Sykes N, Thorns A: The use of opioids and sedatives at the end of life. Lancet Oncol 2003;4:312-318.
135. Eisele JH Jr, Grigsby EJ, Dea G: Clonazepam treatment of myoclonic contractions associated with high-dose opioids: Case report. Pain 1992;49:231-232.
136. Hagen N, Swanson R: Strychnine-like multifocal myoclonus and seizures in extremely high-dose opioid administration: Treatment strategies. J Pain Symptom Manage 1997;14: 51-58.
137. Larijani GE, Goldberg ME, Rogers KH: Treatment of opioid-induced pruritus with ondansetron: Report of four patients. Pharmacotherapy 1996;16:958-960.
138. Zylicz Z, Smits C, Krajnik M: Paroxetine for pruritus in advanced cancer. J Pain Symptom Manage 1998;16:121-124.
139. Osler W: Canada Lancet 1909;42:899-912.

The cost of a parenteral opioid home infusion may be high. It includes rental of the pump, involvement of a home infusion agency including pharmacy overheads, delivery of the premixed medication to the home, and availability of home infusion nurses on a 24-hour basis. However, the cost of poorly controlled pain is even higher in human terms as well as from the need to rehospitalize the patient for uncontrolled pain.[47,48,51,52] Medicare, Medicaid, and most private insurance cover the cost of home infusion pain management as long as there is a clearly documented indication for such an approach. For Medicare patients, if an opioid other than morphine or hydromorphone is being used, a letter is usually needed to explain why the alternate opioid has been chosen. The specific insurance requirements regarding drug specificity must be clarified before the patient's discharge.

Group 3. This group consists of patients who are imminently dying and want to go home. Patients in this group may require a parenteral route of drug administration to control their pain. Systems are in place, however, to manage even the most complex patients at home if the family is strongly committed to this end. There are a variety of models in place to facilitate good pain control. Regardless of which model is selected as the optimal mechanism for the delivery of home pain management at end of life, the common theme for all models is one of an interdisciplinary team approach to care, with the patient and family at the center of such care.[44]

Hospice care, the most widely available model of home care for the dying, focuses on optimizing quality of life in those not seeking, and unlikely to benefit from, life-sustaining treatment. Hospice programs are run by both profit and nonprofit organizations and have become part of the standard of care offered to patients nearing the end of life. Eligibility requirement for a hospice program is a life expectancy of 6 months or less. A major advantage for patients and families followed in a hospice home care program is regular home visits by the hospice nurse and a 24-hour emergency support from skilled hospice nurses with backup from the hospice medical staff. In addition, all medication related to the terminal illness are covered by the hospice benefit at no additional charge to the patient.[53] However, medications not associated with terminal illness, for example, those related to long-standing hypertension or diabetes, are still the financial responsibility of the patient.

Because of the variety of hospice models, levels of sophistication, and breadth of services offered, the needs of the patient and the services offered through the program should be evaluated before referral of a patient.[44] For example, although most hospice programs have changed their policy toward the use of technology in end-of-life care, in contrast with an earlier "no high-tech" approach, restrictions on the financial reimbursement for hospice programs may limit the ability of smaller programs to deliver care to patients requiring the parenteral route of opioid

infusion to manage their pain, especially if they already have one or two such patients on their program. The physician who refers the dying patient to hospice care can remain actively involved in the patient's ongoing pain management. In some instances the referring physician or associated nurse practitioner remains the patient's primary clinician and works with the hospice team in titrating the opioids to ensure comfort. In other instances the referring physician asks the hospice physician to assume that role.

Group 4. Group 4 consists of patients with chronic cancer-related pain, who are going home to an environment where it is suspected that drug diversion may occur. Patients themselves may have a history of illicit drug use. In general, patients with a history of drug abuse are at risk for having their pain undertreated.[54,55] Three subgroups of patients can be identified: (1) patients who are actively using street drugs, (2) those who are in methadone maintenance programs, and (3) patients who have not used illicit drugs for many years.[56]

Patients in the first subgroup strain the resources of the most sophisticated home management pain team and require tight control during opioid therapy. It is recognized that these patients, like any others, may experience severe pain associated with their cancer but will probably require larger doses of opioids to control it because of tolerance development. One physician or nurse practitioner should be identified as the person to adjust analgesics and write all prescriptions, and one nurse identified as the person to organize and coordinate the plan of care.[44] If the patient is on an oral drug regimen, it may be necessary to give only a 1-week supply of the opioid at a time. Giving a larger amount at one time invariably results in "running out of the drug" regardless of the amount given. Psychiatric symptoms and comorbidities such as anxiety, depression, and bipolar disorders are frequently seen in this population and need to be addressed.[54,55] A team approach is essential in the care of these patients. If the patient is in a methadone maintenance program, it is important that the program be contacted for assistance in planning the overall care.

For some patients being discharged home into a drug abuse or chaotic environment, the use of an oral route of opioid administration is not feasible because of constant drug loss. Occasionally these patients are placed on a parenteral route of opioid administration to ensure adequate pain control and safety, maintain tighter control on the amount of drug used, and to minimize the risk of drug diversion. In these situations, *no* extra opioid bags are left in the home and neither the patient nor family is taught how to change the infusion bags (infusion bag changes are done by the home infusion nurse). If available, cassettes can be used for the infusion because there is less risk of "siphoning off" the medication. Personal experience in using this approach with several patients has been successful. The patient's pain has been controlled, and unaccounted-for drug use kept to a minimum. Patients also appear to appreciate the considerable amount of attention they receive. It is however, time intensive and requires close coordination and communication between the prescribing physician or nurse practitioner, the home infusion pharmacist, and the home infusion nurse.[44]

Group 5. This group consists of patients with cancer and pain who are unable to be cared for in their own home, and are to be discharged to an extended care facility that de facto becomes their home. Such facilities are rarely able to accommodate a patient whose pain requires a parenteral route of opioid administration. These patients are frequently older adults, debilitated, and receiving polypharmacy for chronic medical conditions. They are at high risk for having their pain inadequately assessed and are consequently undermedicated for pain.[57,58] In addition, the older adult and debilitated patient's therapeutic margin may be narrow, and the individual is at increased risk for developing distressing side effects including sedation and confusion. Close monitoring is required, with careful dose titration and adjustment based on ongoing assessment. This implies training, skill, and an institutional system in place that regularly screens for the presence of pain and adequacy of relief. Until recently, the staff in long-term care facilities had little training in pain management and end-of-life care. Such training is still limited although The Joint Commission (TJC) standards have made such training mandatory.[59]

Prior to a patient's discharge to a long-term care facility it is important that verbal communication be established between the pain management physician or nurse from the discharging institution and the physician and nursing supervisor from the extended-care facility. The two teams can then work together to ensure adequate pain relief for the patient. In the past 5 to 10 years some long-term care facilities have established contracts with community hospice programs and have developed palliative care approaches for their residents. However, this is not the norm, and the selection of a long-term care facility for someone with cancer and pain must be done with care.[44]

ADDITIONAL ASPECTS OF TRANSITION FROM HOSPITAL TO HOME

In preparing the patient and family to go home, the focus is on security, clarification of the pain management plan, and communication.[44] A family meeting before discharge is useful for consolidating this information.

Focus on Family Security

The central role of the family is acknowledged in the management of pain in the home. It is emphasized that the family will be given ongoing support and backup for their day-to-day pain management deci-

sions, for example, the when and how of rescue dose use, and the management of opioid side effects should they occur. The needs of the family when the patient is initially discharged home and their needs later on are different. When the patient is first discharged home the family is still learning the basic principles and skills required for pain management. Once these skills have been learned and a routine established, the need is for continuing support and validation.[44]

Clarification and Written Instructions on Pain Management

Patients and families benefit from specific, detailed written instructions in layperson language of the pain management approach—pharmacologic and nonpharmacologic—to be used at home. That analgesics should be taken to prevent pain rather than having to be "earned" through experiencing severe pain is emphasized. Included in the discussion are addressing concerns about the prevalence of addiction when opioids are used to manage pain, and the clinical significance of tolerance (e.g., that the opioids may no longer be effective when the pain gets bad if they are used early on in a disease process). In addition, safety issues surrounding opioids in the home are reviewed. These include that the opioids be kept in a safe place out of reach of children; that unused opioids be flushed down the toilet or returned to the prescribing institution for disposal; that if parenteral opioids are used, a syringe and needle disposal kit be obtained; and that needles and syringes, however well wrapped, should not be disposed of in household garbage containers.[44]

Communication of Pain Severity, Pain Relief, and Treatment Side Effects

The patient and family are given written directions on whom to call on a 24-hour basis if pain is not well controlled or if adverse side effects from the prescribed analgesics are experienced. Tools of communication are reinforced including keeping a daily diary to record pain level (using a numerical estimate, e.g., 0-to-10 scale or categorical scale, e.g., none, slight, moderate, severe), medication taken, other pain-relieving strategies, extent and duration of pain relief, activity level, and overall mood. Keeping a pain diary can heighten the patient's and caregiver's awareness of the pattern of pain, guide pain management behaviors, enhance a sense of control, and facilitate communication.[41,60]

Communicating with the Community: A Necessary Precursor to Pain Management at Home

A series of steps is helpful to ensure that a pain management plan instituted in the hospital is maintained by the patient at home. First, if home care nursing has been instituted the home care nurse should be contacted to discuss the pain management plan. Second, the community pharmacy should be contacted to ensure that they have the prescribed opioids in stock or if not are willing to obtain them. In addition, it should be established specifically when the drugs will be available in the home pharmacy so that the patient is not left uncovered.[44]

In the event that the local pharmacy neither has nor can obtain the prescribed opioid, another source for the patient must be located before discharge from the hospital. Third, the physician or nurse practitioner who will be responsible for writing the opioid prescriptions and titrating the drug must be clearly identified. Fourth, the family should be instructed to establish a routine where the amount of medication they have left is checked on a scheduled basis so that the medication does not "run out" (the Friday night and holiday syndrome). Some families find it helpful to keep a 1-week's supply of the medication to the side, and when they need to go into that medication it reminds them to call their prescribing clinician for a new prescription. These simple steps can help ease the transition from hospital to home for the patient and the family.[44]

Providing Continuity of Care for the Patient with Cancer and Pain at Home

The hospice movement has addressed the need for continuity of care of the dying patient.[53] A similar need of the cancer patient with chronic pain who is not imminently dying and the importance of bridging the gap between hospital and community have been recognized.[44,61] A palliative care approach, using hospital-based continuity of care or supportive care programs, which bring the expertise of a cancer center to the community, is seen as a valuable component to patient care, and addresses the needs of the cancer patient with chronic pain earlier on in the disease process. Such a model of care is also important for dying patients who either do not have access to a hospice program or who, for a variety of reasons, choose not to be followed by the hospice system of care.

CONCLUSION

Successful pain management at home depends on an informed and confident patient and family with collaboration and effective communication among the physician or nurse practitioner, home care nurse, and patient and family. Most important, a system of ongoing monitoring and support for the patient and family must be in place to ensure effectiveness of pain relief measures and early identification of undue stress on the part of the family. Careful discharge planning will help facilitate appropriate pain management and support for the patient at home as well as for the family and continuity of care.

SUMMARY

- There is a major shift in responsibility for day-to-day pain management when a patient is to be cared for at home.
- What was primarily the responsibility of the nurse/physician team becomes the responsibility of the patient and family. Pain management in the home is a family experience.
- When the patient is seriously ill, frail, or an older adult, assessment and management of pain become more complex
- Multiple symptoms and polypharmacy become the norm.
- A family is expected to keep track of and administer multiple medications frequently with minimal training, which may lead to an overwhelmed family, nonadherence to a pain management plan, and poorly controlled pain.
- Comprehensive patient and family assessment will help identify factors that make the patient at risk for having pain poorly controlled in the home setting.
- Tailoring a pain management regimen that fits the patient and family caregiver's values, goals, and capabilities is important if pain control is to be maintained at home.
- Family and patient education in pain and symptom management as well as ongoing support from competent pain practitioners are essential. Clear, straightforward communication, both verbal and in writing, is a critical component of the education and support.
- Continuity of care can be fostered through 24-hour telephone availability of a pain management expert to the patients, their families, and community professionals.

References

1. Arras JD, Dubler NN: Bringing the hospital home. Hastings Cent Rep 1994;Sept/Oct:S19-S28.
2. Leonard KM, Enzle SS, McTavisj J, et al: Prolonged cancer death: A family affair. Cancer Nurs 1995;18:222-227.
3. Siegel KS, Ravei VH, Houts P, et al: Caregiver burden and unmet family needs. Cancer 1995;68:1131-1140.
4. Miaskowski C, Zimmer EF, Barrett KN, et al: Differences in patients' and family caregivers' perceptions of the pain experience influence patient and family caregiver outcomes. Pain 1997;72:217-226.
5. Ferrell BR, Ferrell BA, Rhiner M, et al: Family factors influencing cancer pain management. Post Grad Med J 1991;67(suppl 2):S64-S69.
6. Hileman JW, Lackley NR, Hassanein RS: Identifying the needs of home caregivers in patients with cancer. Oncol Nurs Forum 1992;19:771-777.
7. Ferrell BR, Grant M, Boreman T, et al: Family caregiving in cancer pain management. J Palliat Med 1999;2:185-195.
8. Levine C (ed): Always On Call: When Illness Turns Families into Caregivers. New York, United Hospital Fund of New York, 2000.
9. Ferrell BR, Hastie BA: Home care. In Berger AM, Portenoy RK, Weissman DE (eds.): Principles and Practice of Palliative Care and Supportive Oncology (2nd ed). Philadelphia, Lippincott Williams & Wilkins, 2002, pp 775-788.
10. Meuser T, Pietruck C, Radbruch L, et al: Symptoms during cancer treatment following WHO guidelines: A longitudinal follow-up study of symptom prevalence, severity and etiology. Pain 2001;93:247-257.

11. Cleeland CS, Gonin R, Hatfield AK, et al: Pain and its treatment in outpatients with metastatic cancer. N Eng J Med 1994;330:592-596.

12. Bruera E, Kim HN: Cancer pain. JAMA 2003;290:2476-2479.

13. Miaskowski C: The need to assess multiple symptoms. Pain Manage Nurs 2002;3:115.

14. National Institute of Health. NIH state-of-the-science statement on symptom management in cancer: Pain, depression and fatigue. Accessed July, 2002. Available at: http://consensus.nih.gov/ta/022/022_intro.htm.

15. Portenoy RK, Thaler HT, Kornblith AB, et al: Symptom prevalence, characteristics and distress in a cancer population. Qual Life Res 1994;3:183-189.

16. Ferrell BA, Whiteman JE: In Morrison RS, Meier DE (eds): Pain in Geriatric Palliative Care. Oxford, UK, Oxford University Press, 2003, pp 205-229.

17. Miaskowski C: The impact of age on a patient's perception of pain and ways it can be managed. Pain Manage Nurs 2000; 1(suppl.1):2-7.

18. Ferrell BA: Overview of aging and pain. In Ferrell BR, Ferrell BA (eds): Pain in the Elderly. Seattle, IASP Press, 1996, pp 1-10.

19. Helme RD, Gibson SJ: Pain in older people In IK Cronbie IK, Croft R, Linton SJ, et al (eds): Epidemiology of Pain. Seattle, IASP Press, 2000, pp 103-112.

20. Herr KA, Mobily PR: Pain assessment in the elderly. J Gerontol Nurs 1991;17:12-19.

21. Herr KA: State of the art review of tools for assessment of pain in non verbal adults. City of Hope pain resource website: www.cityofhope.org/prc/elderly.asp, 2005.

22. Polomano RC, Farrar JT: Pain and neuropathy in cancer survivors. Cancer Nurs 106(3) Supplement to Volume 29 Nos 2S. State of the science and nursing approaches to managing long-term sequelae of cancer and cancer treatment, 2006.

23. MacDonald L, Bruce J, Scott NW, et al: Long-term follow-up of breast cancer survivors with post-mastectomy pain syndrome. Br J Cancer 2005;92:225-230.

24. Visovsky C: Chemotherapy-induced peripheral neuropathy. Cancer Invest 2003;21:439-451.

25. Dropcho EJ: Neurotoxicity of cancer chemotherapy. Semin Neurol 2004;24:419-426.

26. Quashoff S, Hartung HP: Chemotherapy-induced peripheral neuropathy. J Neurol 2002;249:9-17.

27. Bosompra K, Ashikaga T, O'Brien PJ, et al: Swelling, numbness, pain and their relationship to arm function among breast survivors: A disablement process model perspective. Breast J 2002;8:338-348.

28. Senturk M, Ozcan PE, Talu GK, et al: The effects of three different analgesic techniques on long-term post-thoracotomy pain. Anesth Analg 2002;94:11-15.

29. Von Roenn JH, Cleeland CS, Gonin R, et al: Physicians' attitudes and practice in cancer pain management: A survey from the Eastern Cooperative Oncology Group. Ann Intern Med 1993;119:121-126.

30. Grossman SA, Sheidler VR, Sweeden K, et al: Correlations of patient and caregiver ratings of cancer pain. J Pain Symptom Manage 1991;6:53-57.

31. Taylor EJ, Ferrell BR, Grant M, et al: Managing cancer pain at home: The decisions and ethical conflicts of patients, family caregivers and home-care nurses. Oncol Nurs Forum 1993; 20:919-927.

32. Yaeger KA, Miaskowski C, Dibble SL, et al: Differences in pain knowledge and perception of the pain experience between outpatients with cancer and their family care-givers. Oncol Nurs Forum 1995;22:1235-1241.

33. Magrum LC, Bentzen C, Landmark S: Pain management in home care. Semin Oncol Nurs 1996;12:202-208.

34. Coyle N: Focus on the nurse: Ethical dilemmas with highly symptomatic patients dying at home. Hospice J 1997;12: 33-41.

35. Ward SE, Berry PE, Misiewicz H: Concerns about analgesics among patients and family caregivers. Res Nurs Health 1996;19:205-211.

36. Ferrell BR, Grant M, Chan J, et al: The impact of cancer pain education on family caregivers of elderly patients. Oncol Nurs Forum 1995;22:1211-1218.

37. West CM, Dodd MJ, Paul SM, et al: The PRO-SELF: Pain control program: An effective approach for cancer pain management. Oncol Nurs Forum 2004;30:65-73.

38. Coyle N: In their own words: Seven advanced cancer patients describe their experience with pain and the use of opioid drugs. J Pain Symptom Manage 2004;17:300-309.

39. Elliot BA, Elliot TE, Murray DM, et al: Patient and family members: The role of knowledge and attitudes in cancer pain. J Pain Symptom Manage 2002;23:369-382.

40. Lobchuk MM, Kristjanson L, Degner L, et al: Perceptions of symptom distress in lung cancer patients: Congruence between patients and primary family caregivers. J Pain Symptom Manage 1997;14:136-146.

41. Schumacher LL, Koresawa S, West C, et al: Putting pain management regimens into practice in the home. J Pain Symptom Manage 2002;23:369-382.

42. Rhiner M, Ferrell BR: A structured non-drug intervention program for cancer pain. Cancer Pract 1993;1:137-143.

43. Pan CX, Morrison RS, Ness J, et al: Complementary and alternative medicines in the management of pain, dyspnea and nausea and vomiting at end of life. J Pain Symptom Manage 2000;20:374-385.

44. Coyle N: Pain management in the home: Current Pain and Headaches Report. Cancer Pain 2005;9:231-238.

45. Kanner RM, Portenoy RK: Unavailability of narcotic analgesics for ambulatory patients in New York City. J Pain Symptom Manage 1983;1:87-89.

46. Morrison RS, Wallenstein S, Natale DK, et al: "We don't carry that"—Failure of pharmacies in predominantly non-white neighborhoods to stock opioid analgesics. N Eng J Med 2000; 342:1203-1206.

47. Ferrell BR, Schaffner M: Pharmacoeconomics and medical outcomes in pain management. Semin Anesth 1997;16:152-159.

48. Kornick CA, Santiago-Palma J, Moryl N, et al: Benefit-risk assessment of transdermal fentanyl for the treatment of cancer pain. Review Article. Drug Safety 2003;26:969.

49. Miaskowski C, Dodd MJ, West C, et al: Lack of adherence with the analgesic regimen: A significant barrier to effective cancer pain relief. J Clin Oncol 2001;19:4275-4279.

50. Coyle N, Cherny N, Portenoy RK: Subcutaneous infusions at home. Oncol 1994;8:21-27.

51. Jacox A, Carr DB, Mahrenholz DM, et al: Cost considerations in patient-controlled analgesia. Pharmacoeconomics 1997;12(2 pt 1):109-120.

52. Grant M, Ferrell BR, Rivera LM, et al: Unscheduled hospital readmissions for uncontrolled symptoms. Nurs Clin North Am 1995;30:673-682.

53. Egan KA, Labyak MJ: Hospice palliative care: A model for quality end-of-life care. In Ferrell BF, Coyle N (eds): Textbook of Palliative Nursing. Oxford, Oxford University Press, 2006, pp 13-46.

54. Passik SD, Kirsh KL: Opioid therapy in patients with a history of substance abuse. CNS Drugs 2004;18:13-25.

55. Passik SD, Kirsh KL: Assessing aberrant drug-taking behaviors in the patient with chronic pain. Curr Pain Headache Rep 2004;8:289-294, 2004.

56. Foley KM: Pain assessment and cancer pain syndromes. In Doyle D, Hanks GW, MacDonald N (eds): Oxford Textbook of Palliative Medicine. Oxford, Oxford University Press, 1993, pp 154-155.

57. Teno JM, Kabumoto G, Wetle T, et al: Daily pain that was excruciating at some time in the previous week: Prevalence, characteristics, and outcomes in nursing home residents. J Am Geriatr Soc 2004;52:840-841.

58. Allcock N, McGarry J, Elkan R: Management of pain in older people within the nursing home: A preliminary study. Health Soc Care Community 2002;10:464-471.

59. Joint Commission on Accreditation of Hospital Organizations (JCAHO), www.jcaho.org, 2005.

60. Schumacher KL, Koresawa S, West C, et al: The usefulness of a daily pain management diary for outpatients with cancer-related pain. Oncol Nurs Forum 2002;29:1304-1313.

61. Coyle N: Continuity of care for the cancer patient with chronic pain. Cancer Suppl 1989;63:2289-2293.

Table 67–3.   Minimum Target Organ Radiation Doses to Produce Organ Pathologic Effects

ORGAN	DOSE (RAD)	DOSE (GY)	RESULTS
Eye lens	200	2	Cataract formation
Skin	500	5	Erythema
Skin	700	7	Permanent alopecia
Whole body	200-700	2-7	Hematopoietic failure (4-6 weeks)
Whole body	700-5000	7-50	Gastrointestinal failure (3-4 days)
Whole body	5000-10,000	50-100	Cerebral edema (1-2 days)

organ radiation doses that lead to pathologic effects are shown in Table 67–3. Radiation dermatitis still occurs in fluoroscopists with unknown long-term consequences.

Minimizing Patient Radiation Exposure

Minimize Dose and Time

Physicians using ionizing radiation should adhere to the ALARA principle ("as low as reasonably achievable"), combining optimal technique and shielding to minimize patient and personnel exposure. Because no dose of ionizing radiation is without biologic effects and can be considered absolutely safe, x-ray should be used only when necessary and the dose and exposure time should be limited. Dose is a factor of both the number of x-rays (proportional to mA × seconds of exposure) and the energy of the x-rays (proportional to kVp). Modern fluoroscopy units use ABC, which automatically controls mA and kVp settings to optimize brightness and contrast while minimizing dose. However, if you choose to use fluoroscopy in manual mode (e.g., to increase penetration in an obese patient), the kVp should be increased while minimizing mA. For an equivalent increase in exposure, the mA must be doubled, whereas the kVp must be raised only 15%. When using the ABC mode, the only element under practitioner control is the exposure time, and this should be held to the minimum required to complete the procedure. Short pulses of exposure rather than continuous exposure should be employed whenever feasible. Continuous fluoroscopy in the form of movies (cineradiography) exposes patients to markedly higher doses than brief spot images. Many modern units include an option termed *pulse* mode for use in place of a continuous technique: this mode substitutes brief, periodic spot images separated by an interval without exposure (e.g., a new image is displayed 1 or 2 times/second). Use of this mode in place of continuous fluoroscopy can reduce overall exposure dramatically and is suitable for procedures in the pain clinic where continuous fluoroscopy is needed (e.g., while threading an epidural catheter or spinal cord stimulation lead).

Optimize the Position of the X-Ray Tube

Radiation exposure to the patient is best minimized by starting with ensuring optimal distance between the patient and the x-ray tube (Fig. 67–2). When the x-ray tube is positioned close to the patient, a small area of skin will be exposed to radiation, but because of the proximity of the x-rays, the dose that this smaller area will be exposed to is much higher. When the tube is positioned farther from the patient, a larger area is exposed to a smaller dose of radiation. The x-ray tube should be positioned as far from the patient as possible without including unnecessary structures in the field of view.

Use Shielding Whenever Possible

The use of lead shielding can prevent exposure of regions adjacent to the area that is to be imaged from being exposed to any ionizing radiation. Small lead shields can be placed on the table underneath the patient, directly in front of the x-ray beam *before* it penetrates the patient to protect the gonads or the fetus, in the rare instance in which fluoroscopy is necessary in a pregnant patient. Although lead shields should be readily available in the fluoroscopy suite, they are seldom practical for use during image-guided injection of the lumbosacral spine because the shield would lie directly in the path of the structures to be imaged.

Use Collimation

Fluoroscopy units have built-in mechanisms that allow the emitted x-ray beam to be reduced in size and changed in shape (or *collimated*) so that the area of the patient exposed is minimized. All units have both linear and circular collimation. Linear collimation employs shutters that can be moved in from either side of the exposure field and are very helpful in imaging long, thin structures like the spine (Fig. 67–3). Circular collimation can be helpful when a small, circular area is to be imaged (Fig. 67–4). Collimation is also very helpful in optimizing image quality because the ABC mode attempts to optimize the image quality by taking into account the exposure needed across the entire field of exposure; it is often difficult to visualize both very radiodense and radiolucent areas in the same image. Collimation can exclude areas of greatly varying radiodensity to improve image quality by reducing the range of densities included in the field. Two good examples are imaging of the thoracic spine in which the large

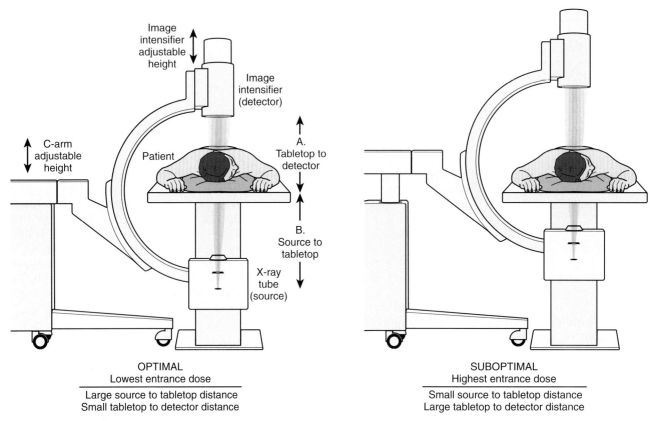

Figure 67–2. Optimal spacing between the x-ray source and the patient to minimize radiation exposure. (Reproduced with permission from Rathmell JP: Atlas of image-guided intervention in regional anesthesia and pain medicine. Philadelphia, Lippincott Williams & Wilkins, 2006, Figure 2–2, p. 12.)

density differences between the spine and the adjacent air-filled lungs can make it difficult to see the bony elements of the spine with any resolution. Linear collimation to limit the field to the spine itself will dramatically improve the image quality (see Fig. 67–3). Likewise, imaging in the cervical spine is fraught with the same difficulties when the air on either side of the neck is included in the x-ray field. Either linear collimation or circular collimation (see Fig. 67–4) can be used to limit the field to the area of interest, improving image quality and reducing radiation exposure. Modern fluoroscopy units also may allow for *magnification* of the image by electronically magnifying the area of interest. Magnification allows better visualization of a smaller area but leads to increased radiation exposure as the system increases output to compensate for losses in gain. To minimize the dose to the patient, the largest field of view, in conjunction with the tightest collimation, should be used.

Minimizing Personnel Exposure

Use Proper Shielding

Only the personnel needed to conduct the procedure should be in the fluoroscopy suite. Everyone should be shielded with lead aprons *before* fluoroscopy begins. The person using the fluoroscopy unit should

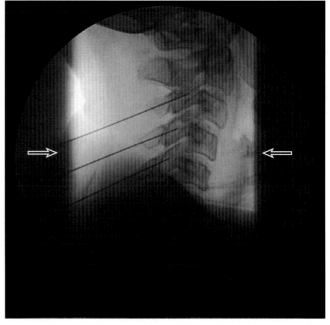

Figure 67–3. Use of adjustable (linear) collimator to decrease radiation exposure to the patient while improving image resolution by decreasing the range of tissue density included in the image field. Arrows point to the shutters of the linear collimator. (Reproduced with permission from Rathmell JP: Atlas of image-guided intervention in regional anesthesia and pain medicine. Philadelphia, Lippincott Williams & Wilkins, 2006, Figure 2–3, p. 13.)

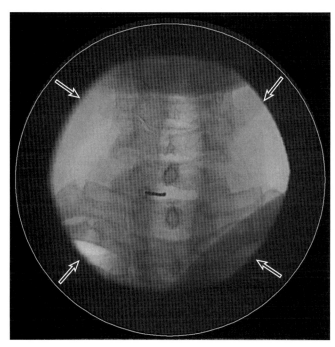

Figure 67–4. Use of adjustable (iris) collimator to limit the field to the area of interest reduces radiation exposure to the patient and improves image resolution by decreasing the range of tissue density included in the image field. Arrows point to the shutters of the iris collimator. (Reproduced with permission from Rathmell JP: Atlas of image-guided intervention in regional anesthesia and pain medicine. Philadelphia, Lippincott Williams & Wilkins, 2006, Figure 2–4, p. 13.)

alert everyone in the room that he or she is about to begin and ensure that all personnel are shielded. Routine use of thyroid shields can minimize the long-term risk of thyroid cancer. Although protective lead gloves can reduce the exposure of the hands to radiation, they can produce a false sense of security. When leaded gloves are used and the person's hands are in the field of exposure, units with ABC will increase their output to compensate for the radiodense leaded gloves, and negate their protective effects. Techniques that prevent the physician's hands from direct exposure within the x-ray field should be used at all times. Protective eyeglasses dramatically reduce eye exposure during fluoroscopy—leaded eyewear is recommended for personnel who accumulate monthly readings on collar badges greater than 400 mrem (4 Sv). Levels of exposure in this range are typically encountered only in areas where continuous cineangiography is conducted frequently (e.g., the cardiac catheterization laboratory).

Physician Position

Personnel must understand the geometry of the radiation path as it passes from the x-ray tube to the image intensifier, and adopt positions that minimize exposure during fluoroscopy (Fig. 67–5). The dose drops proportionally to the square of the distance from the x-ray source. Thus, standing as far from the

x-ray tube as practical is the first means to minimize exposure. Using an intravenous extension tube and taking a step back from the table when contrast is injected under continuous or live fluoroscopy will reduce exposure. When the x-ray tube is rotated to obtain a lateral image, the physician should step completely away from the table beneath the x-ray tube and out of the path of the x-ray beam or move to the side of the table of the image intensifier. Inverting the C-arm so that the x-ray tube is above the table and the image intensifier is below the table is used by some to increase the C-arm's range of lateral movement beyond the typical 45 to 55 degrees allowed by the unit. This practice dramatically increases exposure to both patient and physician by bringing them in proximity with the x-ray source.

Optimizing Image Quality

Modern fluoroscopy units use ABC, which automatically adjusts mA and kVp to optimize image brightness and contrast while minimizing radiation exposure. These controls can be adjusted separately. Increased kVp produces x-rays of higher energy that penetrate without attenuation, thus the resulting image is brighter with less contrast between different tissues, thereby reducing image detail. The clarity of small structures, or image detail, can be improved by lowering kVP, reducing the distance between the patient and the image intensifier, and by using collimation to limit the field of exposure to only those structures of interest. Fluoroscopic images also have less sharpness at the periphery of the image because of a falloff in brightness and spatial resolution, a phenomenon called *vignetting*. Placing the structure of interest in the center of the image yields maximum image detail. Finally, *pincushion distortion* occurs toward the periphery of the image because the x-rays emanate from a spherical surface and are detected on a flat surface. This results in an effect much like a fisheye camera lens, with a splaying outward of objects toward the periphery of the image. This can lead to particular difficulties when attempting to advance a needle using a coaxial technique if the needle is toward the periphery of the image.

Radiographic Contrast Agents

Iodine is the only element that has proven satisfactory as an intravascular radiographic contrast medium (RCM). Iodine produces the radiopacity, whereas the other portions of the molecule act as the carriers for the iodine while improving solubility and reducing the toxicity of the final compound. Organic carriers of iodine are likely to remain in widespread use for the foreseeable future. During image-guided injection, injection of RCM can prove invaluable in determining the final location and distribution of the injectate (Figs. 67–6 to 67–8). Use of RCM can improve the safety of many techniques by allowing for detection of intravascular (Figs. 67–9 and 67–10), subdural (see Fig. 67–7), or intrathecal (see Fig. 67–8) needle

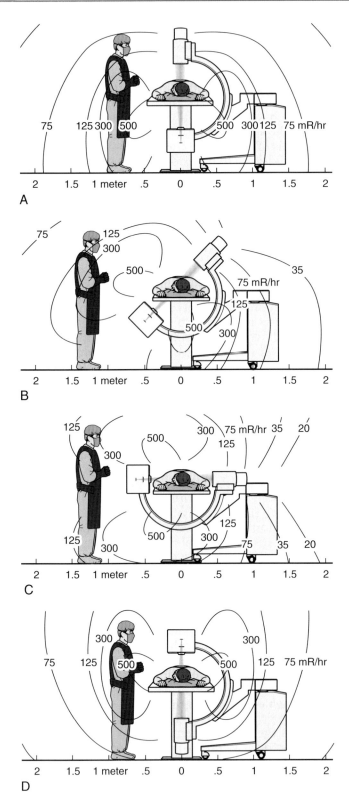

Figure 67–5. Radiation exposure dosage during fluoroscopy. **A,** During routine use in the anteroposterior (AP) plane, the x-ray tube (source) should be positioned below the patient and the director above the patient to minimize radiation exposure to both the patient and the physician. **B,** The oblique projection results in markedly increased exposure to the physician. **C,** During use in the lateral projection, the physician should step completely behind the x-ray tube (source) to minimize radiation exposure. When it is necessary to work close to the patient during lateral fluoroscopy, the physician should move to the side of the table opposite the x-ray tube to minimize exposure. **D,** Radiation exposure to both patient and physician is dramatically increased when the x-ray tube (source) is inverted above the patient. Some physicians invert the C-arm to allow for more extreme lateral angle (e.g., rotation beyond 35 to 45 degrees oblique to the side opposite the C-arm is not possible without *inverting* the C-arm on some units). Radiation exposure can be reduced by rotating the patient on the table and keeping the x-ray source below the table. (This figure was adapted with the assistance of Philips Medical Systems USA, Seattle, Washington, based on radiation exposure data for the Pulsera 9-inch mobile c-arm. Reproduced with permission from Rathmell JP: Atlas of image-guided intervention in regional anesthesia and pain medicine. Philadelphia, Lippincott Williams & Wilkins, 2006, Figure 2–5, p. 14.)

location *before* local anesthetic or steroid is placed. In cases in which iodine is not acceptable, such as with patients who have an iodine allergy, gadolinium may be an acceptable but less dense alternative (Fig. 67–11).

Pharmacology

There are four chemical varieties of iodinated RCM in widespread use: Ionic monomers, nonionic monomers, ionic dimers, and nonionic dimers. On intravascular injection, all four are redistributed rapidly via capillary permeability to the extravascular space, they do not enter the interior of blood or tissue cells, and they are rapidly excreted—more than 90% eliminated via glomerular filtration within 12 hours of administration. None of the four types of RCM have marked pharmacologic actions. All RCM agents come in a range of concentrations that vary according to the radiopacity; because iodine is the element that is responsible for the radiopacity, the iodine concentration in mg/mL represents the radiopacity. The nonionic monomers are now used almost exclusively in pain medicine—the nonionic dimers offer increased radiopacity at very low osmolar concentrations, but are not yet in widespread clinical use.

Several important chemical properties determine the characteristics of RCM in clinical use. *Osmolality* depends on the number of particles of solute in solution, and is highest for the ionic contrast agents. Adverse reactions, particularly discomfort on injection, have been reduced dramatically with the advent of a low-osmolar RCM. Contrast media with osmolality less than 500 mOsm/kg of water are virtually painless. *Radiopacity* is dependent on the iodine concentration of the solution and therefore depends on

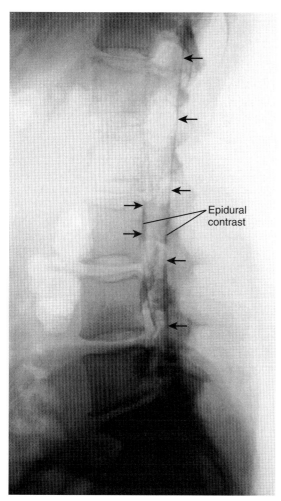

Figure 67–6. Epidural contrast injection. This typical lateral lumbar epidurogram demonstrates the "double-line" or "railroad track" appearance of radiographic contrast in the anterior and posterior epidural space *(arrows)*. (Reproduced with permission from Rathmell JP, Torian D, Song T: Lumbar epidurography. Reg Anesth Pain Med 2000;25:540-545.)

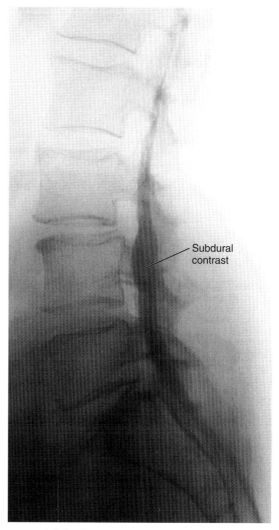

Figure 67–7. Subdural contrast injection. Injection of contrast in the subdural (epiarachnoid) space is recognized by the loculated appearance of the contrast collection on this lateral radiograph of the lumbar spine. The contrast does not extend to the anterior portion of the thecal sac, but is not limited to the epidural space. (Reproduced with permission from Ajar A, Rathmell JP, Mukerji S: The subdural compartment. Reg Anesth Pain Med 2002;27: 72-76.)

the number of iodine atoms per molecule and the concentration of the iodine-carrying molecule in solution. Digital subtraction electronically enhances the image, reducing the amount of needed contrast medium by a factor of two- to threefold; with use of digital subtraction, RCM with as little as 150 to 200 mg/mL of iodine can be used even for intra-arterial use. Ionic molecules dissociate into cation and anion in solution; nonionicity, or a molecule that does not dissociate in solution, is essential for myelography or use along the neuraxis, where placement within the cerebrospinal fluid (CSF) is possible during injection. The chemical properties of two of the most common contrast media used in clinical practice are compared in Table 67–4.

The most frequently used ionic monomers are dia-trizoate (Urografin), iothalamate (Conray), and metri-zoate (Isopaque). All ionic monomers are the salts of meglumine or sodium as the cation and a radio-opaque triiodinated fully substituted benzene ring as the anion. The ionic monomers are still used for

intravenous pyelography and similar applications, but have been completely replaced by the low-osmolar, nonionic RCM for many applications, including intrathecal adminiatration. The most common nonionic monomers in clinical use include iohexol (Omnipaque), iopamidol (Niopam), and ioversol (Optiray). The nonionic monomers appeared in the 1970s, and now represent the most common RCMs in clinical use. They are more stable in solution and less toxic than the ionic monomers.

Adverse Reactions to a Radiographic Contrast Medium

Modern contrast agents have reduced, but not elimi-nated, the risk of adverse reactions. To minimize the risk, the RCM should be used in the smallest

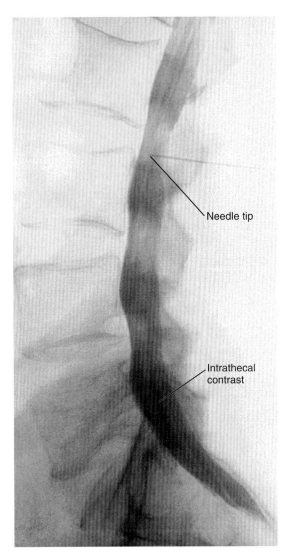

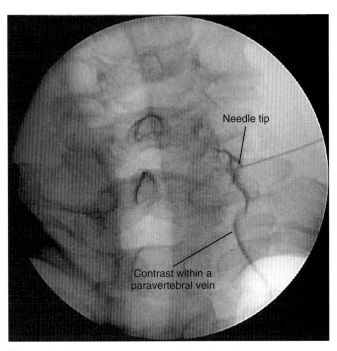

Figure 67–9. Intravenous contrast injection. Intravenous contrast injection is typically not seen on still images because the contrast material is rapidly diluted in the bloodstream. During real-time or live fluoroscopy, intravenous contrast injection *appears* as in this anteroposterior (AP) radiograph of the cervical spine taken during cervical transforaminal injection. The contrast can be seen flowing toward the heart with the venous blood.

Figure 67–8. Intrathecal contrast injection. This typical myelogram demonstrates contrast within the thecal sac on this lateral radiograph of the lumbar spine. The spinal cord and exiting nerve roots are visible as hypodense regions within the contrast collection. (Reproduced with permission from Rathmell JP, Torian D, Song T: Lumbar epidurography. Reg Anesth Pain Med 2000;25:540-545.)

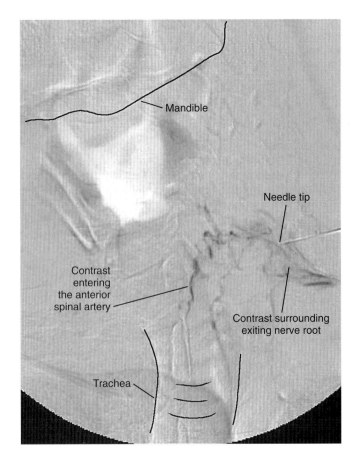

Figure 67–10. Intra-arterial contrast injection (digital subtraction). Intra-arterial contrast injection is typically not seen on still images because the contrast material is rapidly diluted in the bloodstream. During real-time or live fluoroscopy, intravenous contrast injection appears as in this anteroposterior (AP) digital subtraction radiograph of the cervical spine taken during cervical transforaminal injection. The contrast can be seen flowing away from the heart toward the end organ (in this image, toward the spinal cord) with the arterial blood. Use of *digital* subtraction cineradiography allows for detection of intravascular injection with small doses of radiographic contrast material. (Adapted with permission from Rathmell JP, Aprill C, Bogduk N: Cervical transforaminal injection of steroids. Anesthesiology 2004;100:1595-1600.)

concentrations and in the smallest total dose that will allow adequate visualization. Adverse reactions associated with RCM can be divided into idiosyncratic anaphylactoid reactions, nonidiosyncratic reactions, and combined reactions. The risk of adverse reactions is significantly greater with use of high-osmolar ionic agents when compared with low-osmolar nonionic agents. This discussion focuses on the risks associated with low-osmolar nonionic agents because they are used almost exclusively in pain medicine applications.

Idiosyncratic Anaphylactoid Reactions

Idiosyncratic reactions are the most feared, the most serious, and even fatal complications associated with RCM. They occur without warning, and at present we cannot predict or prevent them. These reactions usually begin within 5 minutes of injection and may be mild and self-limited or proceed rapidly to life-threatening cardiovascular collapse. The risk of anaphylactoid reaction is increased in those with previous reaction to RCM (sixfold), in asthmatic patients (eightfold), in allergic and atopic patients (fourfold), and in patients with advanced heart disease (threefold) (Table 67–5).

Nonidiosyncratic Anaphylactoid Reactions

Nonidiosyncratic reactions can be divided into chemotoxic reactions: those caused by chemical reactions to the iodine-carrying molecule, and osmotoxic reactions, or those caused by high osmolality of the contrast medium. These nonidiosyncratic reactions are dose dependent; this type of reaction should be exceedingly rare in those receiving the small volumes of RCM required to facilitate needle localization during image-guided pain treatment.

Chemotoxic reactions are rare and may result in direct organ toxicity and include cardiac (direct and prolonged decrease in cardiac contractility), neurologic (seizures), and renal toxicity (oliguria, impaired creatinine clearance, and reduced glomerular filtration rate that may progress to acute renal failure).

Osmotoxic reactions are much more common with high-osmolar contrast media, in which the osmolality of the RCM can reach several times that of physiologic osmolality of 300 mOsm/kg H_2O (see Table

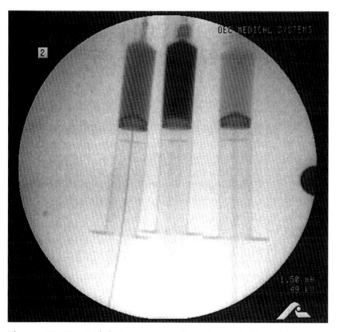

Figure 67–11. Gadolinium as an alternate to iodinated contrast. The appearance on fluoroscopy of a 10-mL syringe filled with 5 mL each of gadodiamide *(left)*, iohexol 180 mg/mL (Omnipaque 180) *(middle)*, and water *(right)*.

Table 67–5. Incidence of Severe Adverse Drug Reactions Following Intravenous Injection of Low-Osmolar Nonionic Radiographic Contrast Medium

CLINICAL HISTORY	SEVERE ADR (%)
No history of allergy or previous ADR to RCM	0.03
Renal disease	0.04
Diabetes mellitus	0.05
Heart disease	0.10
History of allergy	0.10
Atopy	0.11
History of previous ADR to RCM	0.18
Asthma	0.23

ADR, adverse drug reaction; RCM, radiographic contrast medium.
Adapted from Katayama H, Yamaguchi K, Kozuka T, et al: Adverse reactions to ionic and nonionic contrast media. A report from the Japanese Committee on the Safety of Contrast Media. Radiology 1990;175:621-628.

Table 67–4. Comparison of Two Common Radiographic Contrast Agents Used in Clinical Practice*

CHEMICAL COMPOSITION	TRADE NAME	IODINE (MG/ML)	OSMOLALITY (MOSM/KG H_2O)	VISCOSITY (CENTIPOISE AT 37° C)	RADIOGRAPHIC CONTRAST AGENT TYPE
Sodium/meglumine diatrizoate	Urografin 150	146	710	1.4	Ionic, high osmolar
Sodium/meglumine diatrizoate	Urografin 325	325	1650	3.3	Ionic, high osmolar
Iohexol	Omnipaque 180	180	360	2.0	Nonionic, low osmolar
Iohexol	Omnipaque 300	300	640	6.1	Nonionic, low osmolar

*The ionic, high-osmolar agent diatrizoate and the nonionic, low-osmolar agent iohexol. Iohexol (180 mg/mL) is the agent used almost exclusively in pain medicine applications. It provides a nonionic, low-osmolar RCM that balances a low risk of adverse reaction, safety for intrathecal administration, and sufficient radiopacity for identifying intravascular and intrathecal placement.

67–4). Osmotoxic reactions have been dramatically reduced with the advent of nonionic low-osmolar agents like iohexol, and should be exceedingly rare after administration of the small volumes used in pain medicine applications. Hyperosmolar reactions include erythrocyte damage (hemolysis), endothelial damage (capillary leak and edema), vasodilation (flushing, warmth, hypotension, cardiovascular collapse), hypervolemia, and direct cardiac depression (reduced cardiac contractility). The relative incidences of various adverse reactions to RCM are listed in Table 67–6.

Recognition and Treatment of Reactions to Radiographic Contrast Agents

Reactions can be generally grouped into mild, moderate, and severe. The incidence of these reactions following the small volumes of RCM used in pain medicine has not been detailed, but the incidence following intravenous administration of larger volumes of contrast is given later. Mild reactions occur in 5% to 15% of those receiving intravenous contrast and include flushing anxiety, nausea, arm pain, pruritus, vomiting, headache, and mild urticaria. These are generally mild and self-limiting and require no specific treatment. Occasionally an oral antihistamine (diphenhydramine 25 mg) can be useful in managing pruritus as well as anxiety. More serious reactions occur in 0.5% to 2% of those receiving intravenous contrast and include more pronounced severity of mild symptoms as well as moderate degrees of hypotension and bronchospasm. Suggested treatments for moderate reactions are given in Table 67–7.

Severe reactions are life threatening and occur in less than 0.04% of those receiving intravenous RCM and include convulsions, unconsciousness, laryngeal edema, severe bronchospasm, pulmonary edema, severe cardiac dysrhythmias, and cardiovascular collapse. Treatment of these life-threatening reactions is urgent and necessitates the immediate availability of full resuscitation equipment and trained personnel along with a practiced routine for responding to these rare events. The airway must be secured and oxygen, mechanical ventilation, external cardiac massage, and electrical cardiac defibrillation administered as required. Death may ensue following this type of severe adverse reaction; the incidence is not known with accuracy, but likely lies between 1/14,000 and 1/170,000 intravenous administrations of RCM.

Prevention of Reactions to Radiographic Contrast Media

Recognition of the factors that predispose patients to adverse reactions when receiving RCM is the first step in prevention (Box 67–1). The risk of reaction is increased in those with previous reaction to RCM (sixfold), in asthmatic patients eightfold), in allergic and atopic patients (fourfold), and in patients with advanced heart disease (threefold). If there is any chance that the injectate will end up in the subarachnoid space, then a low-osmolar, nonionic contrast agent must be used. Infrequent deaths have been reported following the inadvertent intrathecal administration of ionic RCM. Most pain medicine practitioners have adopted the universal use of a low-osmolar nonionic RCM in a moderate concentration (e.g., iohexol 180 mg/mL) for all applications.

There is no known premedication regimen that can reliably eliminate the risk of severe reactions to RCM. The most common suggested strategies combine pretreatment with corticosteroids (e.g., oral prednisone 50-mg doses 12 and 2 hours before RCM administration) and antihistamines (e.g., oral diphenhydramine 50 mg 1 to 2 hours before RCM administration). Some authors recommend addition of H_2 antagonists (e.g., oral ranitidine). This approach has been proven to reduce the incidence of subsequent adverse reactions in those with a history of previous reaction to high-osmolar contrast agents, but it is less clear if prophylactic treatment is needed before use of a low-osmolar nonionic contrast agent like iohexol. Patients thought to be at greater than usual risk are listed in Box 67–1. In many practices,

Table 67–6. Type and Relative Incidence of Adverse Drug Reactions Following Intravenous Injection of Low-Osmolar, Nonionic Radiographic Contrast Medium

PATIENT CHARACTERISTICS IN TRIAL	
Total number of patients	163,363
Total adverse reaction	3.13%
Total severe adverse drug reactions	0.04%
Death	1

SYMPTOMS	% OF ADR
Nausea	1.04
Heat	0.92
Vomiting	0.45
Urticaria	0.47
Flushing	0.16
Venous pain	0.05
Coughing	0.15
Dyspnea	0.04

ADR, adverse drug reaction.
Adapted from Katayama H, Yamaguchi K, Kozuka T, et al: Adverse reactions to ionic and nonionic contrast media. A report from the Japanese Committee on the Safety of Contrast Media. Radiology 1990;175:621-628.

Table 67–7. Suggested Treatment for Reactions to Radiographic Contrast Medium of Moderate Severity

ADVERSE REACTION	SUGGESTED TREATMENT
Urticaria	Diphenhydramine 25-50 mg PO, IM, or IV
Anxiety	Diazepam 5-10 mg PO or midazolam 1-2 mg IV
Bronchospasm	Mild: inhaled albuterol Severe: Hydrocortisone 100 mg IV Epinephrine 0.05-0.1 mg subcutaneous, IM, IV

BOX 67–1. PATIENTS CONSIDERED AT GREATER THAN USUAL RISK OF SEVERE ADVERSE REACTIONS TO RADIOGRAPHIC CONTRAST MEDIUM

Those with a history of previous adverse reactions to radiographic contrast medium (excluding mild flushing and nausea)

Asthmatics

Allergic and atopic patients

Cardiac patients with congestive heart failure, unstable dysrhythmia, or recent myocardial infarction

Patients with diabetic nephropathy or renal failure of any etiology

Frail, older adult patients

Those with severe, general debility or dehydration

Extremely anxious patients

Patients with specific hematologic or metabolic disorders (sickle cell anemia, polycythemia, multiple myeloma, pheochromocytoma)

Adapted from Grainger RG: Intravascular radiologic iodinated contrast media. In Grainger RG, Allison DJ, Adam A, Dixon AK (eds): Grainger & Allison's Diagnostic Radiology (4th ed). New York, Churchill Livingstone, 2001.

radiographic contrast is avoided altogether in those at elevated risk for adverse reaction. Most procedures in pain medicine can be carried out safely without use of radiographic contrast. In some instances (e.g., epidural placement), the location can be established using loss of resistance alone, and final needle position can be verified using anteroposterior (AP) and lateral radiography without contrast. However, some injections should not be attempted without radiographic contrast injection (e.g., transforaminal injection). In this case, injection of contrast under live or real-time fluoroscopy (with or without digital subtraction) is the only means to detect intra-arterial needle location (see Fig. 67–10) and prevent catastrophic injection of particulate material directly to critical vessels supplying the spinal cord. Performing interlaminar epidural steroid injection without contrast may well be a safe and effective alternative to transforaminal injection in the patient with greater than usual risk for adverse reaction to RCM.

Acknowledgments

The radiation exposure data shown in Figure 67–5 is based on isokerma data provided by Philips Medical Systems USA, Seattle, Washington, for their 9-inch Pulsera mobile C-arm.

Additional Reading

Radiation Safety

Berlin L: Malpractice issues in radiology: Radiation-induced skin injuries and fluoroscopy. AJR Am J Roentgenol 2001;178: 153-157.

Fishman SM, Smith H, Meleger A, Seibert JA: Radiation safety in pain medicine. Reg Anesth Pain Med 2002;27:296-305.

Norris TG: Radiation safety in fluoroscopy. Radiol Technol 2002; 73:511-533.

U.S. Food and Drug Administration: Public Health Advisory: Avoidance of serious x-ray induced skin injuries to patients during fluoroscopically guided procedures. Rockville, Md, Center for Devices and Radiological Health, U.S. Food and Drug Administration, September, 1994.

Radiographic Contrast Agents

Ajar A, Rathmell JP, Mukerji S: The subdural compartment. Reg Anesth Pain Med 2002;27:72-76.

American College of Radiology: Manual on Contrast Media (4th ed). Reston, Va, American College of Radiology, 1999.

Dawson P, Cosgrove DO, Grainger RG (eds): Textbook of Contrast Media. Oxford, UK, ISIS Medical Media, 1999.

Grainger RG: Intravascular radiologic iodinated contrast media. In Grainger RG, Allison DJ, Adam A, Dixon AK (eds): Grainger & Allison's Diagnostic Radiology (4th ed). New York, Churchill Livingstone, 2001.

Greenberger PA, Patterson R: The prevention of immediate generalized reactions to radiocontrast media in high-risk patients. Clin Immunol 1991;87:867-872.

Katayama H, Yamaguchi K, Kozuka T, et al: Adverse reactions to ionic and non-ionic contrast media. A report from the Japanese Committee on the Safety of Contrast Media. Radiology 1990;175:621-628.

Rathmell JP, Torian D, Song T: Lumbar epidurography. Reg Anesth Pain Med 2000;25:540-545.

Thomsen HS, Muller RN, Mattrey RF (eds): Trends in Contrast Media. Berlin, Springer-Verlag, 1999.

Spring DB, Bettman MA, Barkan HE: Deaths related to iodinated contrast media reported spontaneously to U.S. Food and Drug Administration 1978-1994: Effect of availability of low osmolality contrast media. Radiology 1997;204:333-337.

68 Chronic Pain Clinical Trials: IMMPACT Recommendations

Dennis C. Turk and Robert H. Dworkin

PREVALENCE OF PAIN AND COSTS OF TREATMENT

Pain is an extremely prevalent symptom. Chronic pain alone is estimated to affect 15% to 20% of the adult population of the United States,[1] upward of 50 million people.[2] Approximately 3.5 million people in the United States have cancer with moderate to severe pain reported by 35% to 45% at the intermediate stage of the disease and by 60% to 85% in advanced stages of cancer.[3]

An estimated 112 million adults reported monthly nonprescription analgesic use[4] and a national survey by the American Pharmaceutical Association revealed that 84% of respondents had used a nonprescription drug for pain the preceding year.[5] In 2002, more than 66 million prescriptions for opioids, nonsteroidal anti-inflammatory drugs (NSAIDs), and non-narcotic analgesics prescribed for pain were mentioned in emergency department reports alone.[6] Approximately 13 million Americans take prescription analgesics on a monthly basis.[4] Figures for surgery and other nonpharmacologic treatments are equally high. For example, in 2001 there were almost 600,000 surgeries (laminectomy, diskectomy, lumbar spinal fusions) performed for back pain alone,[7] with no indication that these figures are declining.

Pain is not only prevalent, it is also extremely costly. Annual estimates of direct costs for health care and indirect costs (e.g., disability compensation, lost tax revenue, lost productivity) exceed $150 billion annually.[7,8]

A large and growing number of treatments are available to manage acute and chronic pain. A critical question to ask about existing treatments as well as newly developed ones is how effective are they in ameliorating symptoms. It is impossible to provide a single answer to this deceptively simple question beyond "it depends." It depends on knowledge of the source or cause of pain, variations in patients treated, the criteria used to determine success, the methods used for assessing these criteria, the design of the studies that attempt to establish effectiveness, and the statistical analyses selected to evaluate the outcomes.

EVIDENCE-BASED MEDICINE

The prevalence of pain, the diversity of treatments available, the inconsistency in the outcomes of clinical trials, and the inability to directly compare results between studies has led to considerable consternation and call for more and better research. The inadequacy of the data and the practice of relying on clinical judgment have resulted in pleas for *evidence-based medicine* (EBM), a phrase that has progressed from a buzzword to a mantra. EBM refers to the use of evidence, specifically in the form of quantitative research data, concerning the effectiveness of medical interventions, to guide decisions about whether to use those interventions in medical practice. The primary goal of EBM is to improve health outcomes through the deployment of the most effective interventions.

The steps of EBM consist of (1) formulation of questions to answer information needs, (2) seeking answers supported by the best evidence, (3) examination of the quality of the evidence, (4) application of evidence to implement best health care practice, and (5) evaluation of health care practice. The sources of evidence are derived from published studies, available reviews, abstracts, and unpublished studies and data. The quality of the evidence is often ranked from low to high (Fig. 68–1). Although the methods described may sound good, there are a number of concerns that mitigate some of the enthusiasm for EBM (Box 68–1).

EBM has becomes almost synonymous with double-blind, randomized, controlled trials. The assumption by some is that such trials are the only way to determine the validity of the claim of treatment effectiveness. However, there is as much disagreement regarding what qualifies as acceptable evidence as there is regarding what qualifies as good clinical prac-

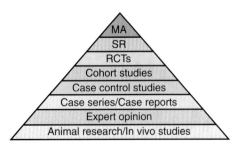

Figure 68–1. Hierarchy of evidence. MA, meta-analysis; SR, systematic reviews; RCTs, randomized controlled trials. (From http://cebm.jr2.ox.ac.uk/docs/levels.html, accessed 5/23/06.)

BOX 68–1. SOME CHALLENGES WITH THE EVIDENCE-BASED MEDICINE APPROACH

- Inconsistency among conclusions of different reviews even using similar quality ratings
- Variability of results among outcome criteria
- Inconsistency in use of inclusion criteria
- Variability in outcome criteria and measures (ease of measurement vs. relevance)
- Technical bias favors research that investigators know how to do
- Absence of published studies (*"Absence of evidence is not evidence of absence"*)
- Positive results more likely to be published: "file draw problem"
- Variability in entry criteria for inclusion
- Heterogeneity in quality of studies combined
- Combining marginally related studies
- Studies of interventions that likely to have commercial value most likely to be supported (e.g., drug trial vs. physical therapy trial)
- Data obtained in commercially supported studies more likely to be positive
- Generalization from clinical trials to clinical practice ("efficacy" vs. "effectiveness" trials)

BOX 68–2. SOME CHALLENGES WITH RANDOMIZED CONTROLLED TRIALS

- Sample included in clinical trials may not represent clinical practice (inclusion and exclusion criteria (e.g., exclude women of childbearing age, limits on age, presence of depression)
- Difficulties with blinding (participants and providers may be able to detect treatment received)
- Ethical concerns about use of placebo treatment
- Patient willingness to be in a placebo trial
- Method of recruitment will influence representativeness of the sample (e.g., referral bias, clinical vs. community sample)
- "Denominator problem": number of participants known but the number eligible unknown except in population based studies
- Characteristics of volunteers for randomized controlled trial (RCT) (not all eligible will volunteer)
- Studies of interventions likely to have commercial value more likely to be conducted (e.g., pharmacologic intervention vs. physical therapy)
- Precision of diagnoses
- Problem of dropouts
- Short trial duration (typically <3-6 mo)
- Determining appropriate comparators
- Appropriate statistical analyses (multiple end points)
- Provide information about groups, not individuals
- Publication bias (positive trials more likely to be published)
- Often report only statistical significance and not clinical meaningfulness or meaningful results to patients.
- Inconsistency in use of outcome criteria
- Bias toward studies that are easy (known methods) to conduct

tice. Some of the issues that needed to be considered when evaluating randomized trials are enumerated in Box 68–2.

ESTABLISHING THE EFFECTIVENESS OF TREATMENTS

Following the development of each new treatment come clinical trials designed to demonstrate its beneficial effects and safety. In order to determine the benefits of treatment, investigators must decide on the appropriate end points for establishing both the statistical significance and also the clinical importance of the effects of treatment. In a clinical trial of the efficacy or effectiveness of a treatment for chronic pain, pain reduction and safety are necessary outcome variables but they may not be sufficient for a comprehensive evaluation of the overall benefit or harm of a treatment. The complexity of pain, and particu-

larly chronic pain, and its negative effect on diverse aspects of function require the assessment of multiple outcome domains to evaluate treatments comprehensively. A number of considerations are important in deciding which outcome domains should be included in chronic pain clinical trials. The domains should match the purpose of the study, measure positive and negative outcomes of treatment, and be appropriate for the chronic pain syndrome studied and the specific characteristics of the sample (e.g., demographics, duration, and severity of symptoms). Central issues involve the identification of outcome domains that are clinically meaningful and for which there are measures that are responsive and provide a comprehensive yet efficient evaluation of treatment response.[9,10]

Once domains and measures have been selected, investigators must establish criteria not only for the statistical significance of the outcomes but also for their importance.[11-13] When evaluating importance, consideration must be given to the question of "importance to whom." The importance of different degrees of symptom reduction and of the presence and intensity of adverse effects associated with treatment can vary greatly between and among clinical investigators, patients, and disease conditions.[14,15]

When multiple outcome variables are included in a study, investigators must consider how inconsistencies among outcomes will be interpreted. Strategies for classifying participants as responders across multiple end points have been suggested,[16] and there are also statistical approaches available for analyzing outcomes when multiple measures have been used.

Variability among clinical trials in outcome assessments has impeded evaluations of the efficacy and effectiveness of treatments for chronic pain, and the use of different outcome domains and measures preclude meaningful comparisons among studies. One way to facilitate such evaluations would be through the use of a common set of outcome domains and measures, criteria for establishing importance of outcomes, preferred experimental designs, and data-analytic strategies. Although investigators may wish to augment a core set of measures with others that are specific to the situation or treatment being studied, and might have specific reasons for choices of end points, designs, and analytic strategies, development of guidelines would permit comparisons among different samples, treatments, and settings.

Development of a core set of procedures would have important advantages for clinicians and investigators. It would facilitate comparison and pooling of data while leaving investigators free to augment the core set with others of their choice. In addition, a consensus on measures and methods would encourage more complete investigation and reporting of relevant outcomes so that investigators do not simply present a single outcome while ignoring others. Another advantage is that it would encourage development of cooperative multicenter projects. Such standardization would simplify the process of designing and reviewing research proposals, manuscripts, and published articles. Finally, published results of clinical trials using common, agreed-upon procedures will allow clinicians to make more informed clinical decisions for each patient regarding the optimal treatment, especially with respect to its risks and benefits. With greater consensus about clinical trials should come improvements in studies conducted and the ability to combine information to make better decisions in a more timely fashion.

THE INITIATIVE ON METHODS, MEASUREMENT, AND PAIN ASSESSMENT IN CLINICAL TRIALS

To address the objective of improved clinical trials in pain, the Initiative on Methods, Measurement, and Pain Assessment in Clinical Trials (IMMPACT) was

established and has convened a number of consensus meetings. The objective of the first meeting was to develop consensus recommendations for core outcome domains for chronic pain clinical trials. Other initiatives provide precedents for this undertaking, including Outcome Measures in Rheumatoid Arthritis Clinical Trials (OMERACT)[17] and World Health Organization/International League of Associations for Rheumatology (WHO/ILARS)[18] in rheumatology, European Organization for Research and Treatment of Cancer (EORTC)[19] and the Research Network of the European Association of Palliative Care[20] in oncology, and an international consortium of back pain researchers.[21] Subsequent meetings focused on available measures for each of the core domains specified, appropriate methods for developing new and evaluating existing measures, methods for establishing clinically meaningful results as well as appropriate methods for analyzing data from clinical trials with multiple outcomes, and innovations in experimental designs. In the remainder of this chapter we will provide an overview of the IMMPACT process and consensus recommendations that have evolved to date.

IMMPACT is an international consortium of professionals from academia, regulatory agencies, the U.S. National Institutes of Health, U.S. Veterans Administration, industry, and consumers. The professional participants are engaged in research, clinical, or administrative activities relevant to the design and evaluation of pain treatment outcomes and they represent anesthesiology, biostatistics, clinical pharmacology, epidemiology, geriatrics, internal medicine, law, neurology, nursing, oncology, outcomes research, patient perspectives, pediatric pain, physical medicine and rehabilitation, psychology, and rheumatology. All participants have research, clinical, or administrative expertise relevant to evaluating pain treatment outcomes or represent people included in clinical trials. The authors of this chapter have served as the facilitators for each of the consensus meetings. Since its inception in November 2002, there have been six general IMMPACT meetings. The first two meetings focused on adults; four additional meetings have addressed issues of instrument development, methodology, and data analytic strategies that are applicable to all populations; and a seventh meeting was held that focused exclusively on issues specific to pediatric outcome domains and measures.

CORE OUTCOME DOMAINS AND MEASURES

The complexity of chronic pain suggests that multiple domains are relevant when evaluating the effects of treatment. A number of considerations are important in deciding what domains should be considered in any clinical trial. The domains should match the purpose of the study, measure positive and negative outcomes of treatment, and be appropriate for the chronic pain disorder and the population of interest. A central issue is identification of the set of domains that are clinically meaningful and that might be expected to change as a result of treatment.

IMMPACT[9] recommended that the core outcome domains and measures (Box 68–3) described below should be *considered* in the design of all clinical trials of the efficacy and effectiveness of treatments for any type of chronic pain. It is not the intention of these recommendations that use of these domains and measures should be considered a *requirement* for approval of applications by regulatory agencies or that treatments must demonstrate statistically significant or clinically important benefits with all of these outcomes to establish evidence of efficacy or effectiveness. There may be circumstances in which use of some or all of these core outcomes will not be appropriate, for example, in clinical trials in the cognitively impaired or in infants and children. As noted, a separate IMMPACT meeting (pedIMMPACT) was convened to examine the appropriateness of these domains for children and adolescents along with identifying measures that were appropriate for different ages for each domain.

Pain

Although a ubiquitous phenomenon, pain is inherently subjective. The only way to know about someone's pain is by what is said or shown by behavior. Because there is no "objective" method for assessing pain, self-report provides the gold standard in assessments of pain and its characteristics. Pain assessment therefore requires that patients and participants in clinical trials describe their own experiences. Although individuals interpret measures of pain in different and somewhat idiosyncratic ways, these interpretations can be expected to remain relatively constant within people over time, providing valid measures of change in pain as a result of treatment (or natural history).

Many different aspects of pain can be assessed in a clinical trial, for example, intensity; unpleasantness, onset, location, and durability of pain relief; whether pain is intermittent or constant; frequency of pain; qualities of pain (including the distinction between stimulus-evoked and stimulus-independent pain); radiation; use of rescue medications and other rescue treatments; and pain behaviors, including facial expression. Surrogate end points for pain also may be assessed (e.g., physiologic findings, including imaging measures); however, these cannot be considered primary end points because of the inherently subjective nature of pain. Most chronic pain clinical trials also will assess pain history, including measures such as age at onset, duration, and exacerbating and alleviating factors, but these variables are baseline characteristics. They may be used for inclusion criteria, as a basis for stratification, or as covariates in trials but not outcomes.

Pain Intensity

For most clinical trials of chronic pain treatments, a measure of pain intensity will provide the primary (but not sole) outcome measure. Each of the commonly used methods of rating pain intensity, including Visual Analogue Scale (VAS), numerical rating scales (NRS), and verbal rating scales (VRS), appears sufficiently reliable and valid, and no one method consistently demonstrates greater responsiveness in detecting improvements associated with pain treatment.[22] However, there are important differences among VAS, NRS, and VRS measures of pain intensity with respect to missing data from failure to complete the measure, patient preference, ease of data recording, and ability to administer the measure by telephone or with electronic diaries.

VRS and NRS measures tend to be preferred over VAS measures by patients, and VAS measures usually demonstrate more missing data than NRS measures. Greater difficulty completing VAS measures is associated with increased age and greater opioid intake, and cognitive impairment has been shown to be associated with inability to complete NRS ratings of pain intensity.[22] Patients who are unable to complete

NRS ratings may be able to complete VRS pain ratings (e.g., none, mild, moderate, severe). Other measures are available to assess pain in children and those who are unable to communicate (e.g., stroke patients, mentally impaired).[23]

On the basis of a review of the literature on pain measures prepared for the second IMMPACT meeting[24] and discussions among the participants, an 11-point (i.e., 0 to 10) NRS measure of pain intensity is recommended as a core outcome measure in clinical trials of chronic pain treatments. In order to facilitate consistency among studies, IMMPACT recommended that the specific format of this rating should be the numbers from 0 through 10 presented with the descriptor "No pain" centered below the "0" and "Pain as bad as you can imagine" centered below the "10," accompanied by the instructions, "Please rate your pain by indicating the number that best describes your pain on average in the last 24 hours." Pain "at its worst" or pain "at its least" could also be included in the assessment. Depending on the specific aims and design of the clinical trial, pain during the past week can also be assessed using the scale described.

There are circumstances in which reliable, valid, and responsive measures of pain intensity that do not use an NRS are routinely used; for example, the Western Ontario and McMaster Universities Osteoarthritis Index (WOMAC)[25] uses VAS ratings. These circumstances should be distinguished from those for which no such measures exist and NRS ratings of pain intensity are recommended. Of course, when other measures of pain intensity are used, it may be valuable to administer NRS ratings to compare with other diseases or treatments.

Investigators should also consider including a VRS measure of pain intensity (e.g., "none," "mild," "moderate," "severe") as a secondary outcome measure to limit the amount of missing data if study participants have difficulty with the primary NRS measure. Such measures describe the effects of pain treatment in terms of changes in categorical descriptors, which may be more readily interpreted than VAS and NRS ratings, but do not have the interval and ratio scale properties of VAS and NRS scales. In addition to analyzing and reporting absolute changes in pain intensity during the clinical trial, IMMPACT recommended that the percentages of patients obtaining various reductions in pain intensity from baseline be reported. Such responder curves can provide useful data by indicating the percentage of patients attaining the entire range of pain reduction from zero to 100%.[26]

Rescue Analgesics and Concomitant Pain Treatments

The use of all pain-related treatments during the course of a clinical trial should be assessed, including rescue analgesics and any other concomitant pain treatments. This is a straightforward task in single-dose analgesic trials that prohibit the concurrent use of other medications, but it is more difficult in chronic pain clinical trials that allow concurrent use of pain medications and other treatments for pain (e.g., physical therapy) for weeks or months. Some chronic pain trials have allowed pain medications being taken during the baseline period to be continued throughout the trial, and dosage stabilization is often required before patients are allowed to enroll in such trials. However, when changes in the use of concomitant pain treatments are permitted, they can be considered an outcome measure.[27]

Providing patients with access to rescue analgesics makes it easier to include a placebo group in treatment efficacy studies because patients not obtaining adequate pain relief are provided with an analgesic. This may reduce the number of participants who terminate from a trial prematurely. However, administration of rescue medication complicates the interpretation of differences in pain ratings between patients taking placebo and active treatments because of the reduction in pain expected in patients receiving rescue treatment. The use of rescue medications is affected by both patient and provider beliefs, and patients use rescue medications to achieve varying levels of pain relief as well as for a variety of other reasons, including to improve sleep or reduce anxiety, to prevent increased pain resulting from increased activity, and to treat an episode of pain (e.g., headache) unrelated to the clinical trial.

Rescue medication consumption has been used as an outcome measure in clinical trials, with assessments including amount used and time-to-use.[28,29] Scales have been developed that allow quantification of medication use in chronic pain patients based on dosage and medication class,[30] and composite measures have been proposed that combine rescue medication use and pain intensity ratings into a single score.[31,32] Although these may be used to compare different treatment groups in clinical trials, the psychometric properties of such composite measures are not well established.

Despite the complex issues involved in the interpretation of rescue medication use in a clinical trial, in many circumstances patients in a placebo group can be expected to take more of a rescue treatment than patients administered an efficacious investigational treatment. When considered together with pain intensity ratings, the amount of rescue treatment used by patients can provide an important supplemental measure of the efficacy of the treatment being evaluated. Assessments of rescue treatments are recommended as a secondary outcome in trials in which rescue treatment is provided.

Pain Quality

Pain is known to have different sensory and affective qualities in addition to its intensity, and measures of these components of pain may be used to more fully describe an individual's pain experience.[33,34] It is possible that the efficacy of pain treatments varies for different pain qualities, and measures of pain quality may therefore identify treatments that are efficacious for certain types of pain but not for overall pain intensity. Assessment of specific pain qualities at baseline also makes it possible to determine whether certain patterns of pain quality moderate the effects of treatment. The Short-Form McGill Pain Questionnaire[35] assesses 15 sensory and affective pain descriptors, and its sensory and affective subscales have demonstrated responsiveness in a number of clinical trials.[36,37] IMMPACT recommended this questionnaire for inclusion in clinical trials as a secondary outcome measure to evaluate the effects of pain treatment on specific pain qualities.

Temporal Aspects of Pain

Measures of the temporal aspects of pain—including variability in intensity; time to onset of meaningful pain relief; durability of pain relief; and frequency, duration, and intensity of pain episodes—have not received adequate attention in pain research. The available evidence indicates that measures of pain frequency have validity and represent a distinct dimension of pain.[22] Frequency of breakthrough pain (i.e., episodes of severe pain superimposed on ongoing pain) is an important temporal aspect of pain that has been used as an outcome measure in clinical trials.[38] When appropriate, investigators should consider administering measures of the temporal aspects of pain as secondary outcome measures in clinical trials. The temporal dimensions that should be considered include trial participants' reports of the time to onset of meaningful pain relief and its durability as well as the frequency and intensity of episodes of breakthrough pain.

Health-Related Quality of Life

It often has been assumed that chronic pain is highly associated with alterations in emotional and physical functioning and that reduction in pain will inevitably lead to improvement in function and satisfaction with treatment. This is not necessarily the case because pain and functioning are only modestly related in many published studies. Moreover, changes in pain severity may have only a limited relationship with participants' ratings of improvement and satisfaction.[16,39] Such data indicate that even though pain is typically considered the primary outcome in evaluating pain treatments, it is important to consider other outcomes in clinical trials.

Health-related quality of life (HRQOL) is a multidimensional construct that includes the physical, psychological, and social domains recognized by the World Health Organization, as well as the impact of disease-specific and treatment-related symptoms on self-perceptions of functioning.[40,41] HRQOL refers to those domains that are specifically related to health and that can be influenced by the health care system.[42,43] HRQOL outcomes are especially impor-

tant for evaluating the effect of treatment on chronic diseases for which cure is not possible and therapy may be prolonged. Moreover, when treatment extends over long periods, it is critical to examine whether the benefits of symptom reduction are compromised by reductions in HRQOL resulting from adverse effects of treatment.

There is a lack of agreement regarding the specific variables that should be included in assessments of HRQOL, which has important consequences for researchers, especially with respect to study design and instrument development.[44] Although the lack of a consensual definition of HRQOL is unfortunate, various measures have demonstrated reliability and validity and are widely used in clinical trials of diverse disorders. The consensus of IMMPACT is that two central components of existing HRQOL instruments, physical functioning and emotional functioning, are core domains that should be considered in all clinical trials of the efficacy and effectiveness of chronic pain treatments. This recommendation is supported by the results of studies in which exploratory and confirmatory factor analyses were used to identify the variables needed to comprehensively assess chronic pain patients, which suggested that three relatively independent domains—pain severity, physical functioning, and emotional functioning—are required to capture the multidimensionality of the pain experience.[45-47]

Physical Functioning

Functional status typically refers to the ability to perform particular defined tasks, such as walking a short distance; social role functioning and participation in social interactions also may also be assessed. A major decision to be made in assessing the impact of a treatment on physical functioning involves whether a generic or a disease-specific measure will be used. The tradeoffs between these two approaches have important implications for the interpretation of the results of a trial.

Disease-specific measures are designed to evaluate the effect of a specific condition (e.g., ability to wear clothing in patients with postherpetic neuralgia). Such specific effects of a disorder may not be assessed by a generic measure, and disease-specific measures may therefore be more likely to reveal clinically important improvement or deterioration in function that is a consequence of treatment. In addition, responses on disease-specific measures will generally not reflect the effects of comorbid conditions on physical functioning, which may confound the interpretation of change occurring over the course of a trial when generic measures are used. Generic measures, however, make it possible to compare the physical functioning associated with a given disorder and its treatment with those of different conditions.[48] Thus the use of disease-specific and generic measures in combination facilitates the achievement of both sets of objectives. Regardless of whether a generic or a specific measure of physical functioning is selected, physical functioning is a core outcome domain in clinical trials of chronic pain treatment efficacy and effectiveness.

Disease-specific measures may be more responsive to the effects of treatment on function, but generic measures provide information about physical functioning and treatment benefits that can be compared across different conditions and studies.[40,49] Each of these approaches has strengths. On the basis of reviews of the literature on generic and pain-related measures of physical functioning prepared for the second IMMPACT meeting,[50,51] IMMPACT recommended that a disease-specific measure of physical functioning in chronic pain clinical trials when a suitable and well-accepted one is available (e.g., WOMAC[25]; Roland and Morris Back Pain Disability Scale[52]) and a generic measure of physical functioning should be considered for chronic pain clinical trials.

Disease-specific measures of physical functioning have not been developed and validated for many chronic pain conditions. In clinical trials examining such disorders, use of either the Multidimensional Pain Inventory (MPI)[45] Interference Scale or the Brief Pain Inventory (BPI)[53,54] pain interference items (i.e., general activity, mood, walking ability, normal work, relations with other people, sleep, enjoyment of life) is recommended. The MPI and BPI interference scales provide reliable and valid measures of pain interference that have been translated into many languages and studied in diverse chronic pain conditions in multiple countries.

These two pain-specific measures of physical functioning have distinct advantages and disadvantages, and use of both may be considered when doing so would not impose an undue burden on participants. The MPI Interference Scale does not assess sleep, and if this measure of physical functioning is administered, then use of a measure of sleep is recommended; there are single-item[36] and multiple-item[55,56] measures of the impact of pain on sleep that can be used for this purpose. The BPI does include an item assessing pain interference with sleep, but also includes ratings of mood, social relations, and enjoyment of life, which may constitute a separate factor measuring affective state that is relatively independent of the remaining items.[54] Few clinical trials, however, have examined BPI factors separately and so administration and analysis of only the three BPI activity items (general activity, walking ability, normal work) as a measure of physical functioning cannot be recommended until such analyses become available.

Regardless of whether a disease-specific measure of physical functioning or the MPI Interference Scale or the BPI interference items are used in a clinical trial, administration of a generic measure of physical functioning should be considered to obtain data that will allow comparisons with other disorders and that could be used in cost-effectiveness analyses.[57,58] The SF-36 Health Survey[59] is the most commonly used generic measure of HRQOL, and it has been used in numerous clinical trials of diverse medical and psychiatric disorders. IMMPACT recommended that the SF-36 be considered as a generic measure for use in chronic pain clinical trails.

Emotional Functioning

The results of numerous studies suggest that chronic pain is often associated with emotional distress, particularly depression, anxiety, anger, and irritability. The presence of emotional distress in people with chronic pain presents a challenge when assessing symptoms such as fatigue, reduced activity level, decreased libido, appetite change, sleep disturbance, weight gain or loss, and memory and concentration deficits. These symptoms are often associated with pain and have been considered "vegetative" symptoms of depressive disorders. Improvements or deterioration in such symptoms therefore can be a result of changes in either pain or emotional distress. Although it is difficult to interpret changes in emotional functioning because of the many factors that contribute, this domain is central in people's assessments of their well-being and satisfaction with life, and the authors recommend that it should be considered a core outcome domain in clinical trials of the efficacy or effectiveness of treatments for chronic pain.

On the basis of a review of the literature of measures of emotional functioning prepared for IMMPACT,[60] the Beck Depression Inventory (BDI),[61] and the Profile of Mood States (POMS)[62] were recommended as core outcome measures of emotional functioning in chronic pain clinical trials. Both the BDI and POMS have well-established reliability and validity in the assessment of symptoms of depression and emotional distress, and they have been used in numerous clinical trials in psychiatry and an increasing number of chronic pain clinical trials.[60] In research in psychiatry and chronic pain, the BDI provides a well-accepted criterion of the level of psychological distress in a sample and its response to treatment.

The POMS[62] assesses six mood states—tension-anxiety, depression-dejection, anger-hostility, vigor-activity, fatigue-inertia, and confusion-bewilderment —and provides a summary measure of total mood disturbance. Although the discriminate validity of the POMS scales in patients with chronic pain has not been adequately documented, it has scales for the three most important dimensions of emotional functioning in chronic pain patients (depression, anxiety, anger) and assesses three other dimensions that are very relevant to chronic pain and its treatment, including a positive mood scale of vigor-activity. Moreover, the POMS has demonstrated beneficial effects of treatment in some (but not all) recent chronic pain trials.[36,37] For these reasons, administration of both the BDI and the POMS is recommended in chronic pain clinical trials to assess the major aspects of the emotional functioning outcome domain.

As noted, various symptoms of depression—such as decreased libido, appetite or weight changes, fatigue, and memory and concentration deficits—are also commonly believed to be consequences of chronic pain and the medications used for its treatment.[63] It is unclear whether the presence of such symptoms in patients with chronic pain (and other medical disorders) should nevertheless be considered evidence of depressed mood, or whether the assessment of mood in these patients should emphasize symptoms that are less likely to be secondary to physical disorders.[64] Because of the evidence that measures of emotional functioning are adequately reliable, valid, and responsive when used in the medically ill,[60] IMMPACT recommended that the principal analyses of the BDI and POMS in chronic pain clinical trials use the original versions without adjustment for presumed confounding by somatic symptoms. Depending on the specific objective of the clinical trial, supplemental analyses could be conducted to separately examine nonsomatic and somatic aspects of emotional functioning.

Patient Global Ratings of Improvement and Satisfaction

Assessments of individual outcome domains such as pain and physical and emotional functioning may not adequately characterize the clinical trial participant's overall assessment of treatment and the subjective meaningfulness of any improvement (or worsening). Global evaluations by participants in clinical trials of the benefits of treatment presumably reflect not only the magnitude of the changes in these outcomes but also the personal importance that these outcomes have for participants. Such perceptions of the importance of treatment-associated changes often differ considerably from those of health care professionals, and the value and significance of therapeutic changes differ greatly among individuals and are important determinants of their treatment satisfaction.

By soliciting patients' preferences, investigators acknowledge the unique values of different outcomes and their aggregate for individual patients. Patients' values and preferences are what distinguish global ratings from other measures, and such ratings are thought to provide sufficient unique information to warrant inclusion in all clinical trials of treatments for chronic pain.

Many different approaches have been used to assess clinical trial participants' overall evaluation of their benefit from and satisfaction with treatment provided. One of the most common involves assessments of improvement or worsening with treatment, for example, the Patient Global Impression of Change (PGIC) scale,[65] which requires participants to rate changes they have experienced since the beginning of a clinical trial. This measure is a single-item rating by participants of their improvement with treatment during a clinical trial on a seven-point scale that ranges from "very much improved" to "very much worse" with "no change" as the midpoint.

There has been widespread use of the PGIC in recent chronic pain clinical trials,[13,66] and the data provide a responsive and readily interpretable measure of participants' assessments of the clinical importance of their improvement or worsening over the course of a clinical trial. Impressions of change scores using different verbal outcome categories also have been used to determine the minimally important difference in quality-of-life measures.[67] Although these measures appear to have validity, additional research is necessary to determine the relative extent to which ratings on the PGIC and similar measures reflect reduced pain, improvement in functioning, side effect burden, or other variables and whether this varies for different people.

Other approaches to the global assessment of treatment response include ratings of participant satisfaction with treatment and global ratings of disease state from which changes from baseline can be calculated. These ratings may differ in the degree of emphasis given to rating the treatment's performance (e.g., degree of response to treatment, helpfulness or usefulness of treatment) versus the participant's feelings about the treatment (e.g., satisfaction, preference).

The use of assessments of participants' overall evaluation of treatment in clinical trials is not without controversy. First, many such assessments are based on rating a single item, and it is not possible to establish the internal consistency of one rating. In addition, global impressions of improvement may fail to detect important changes.[68] Moreover, the judgment of change requires that participants in clinical trials assess both their present and initial state and then perform what may be an unreliable mental subtraction; because participants may be unable to recall their initial state, their ratings may be based on an "implicit theory" of change beginning with their present state and working backward.[69] However, if a treatment is associated with severe adverse effects, the participant may not need to remember baseline pain to rate satisfaction with treatment. The role of memory may therefore be greater in rating global impression of change than overall satisfaction with treatment.

Despite the necessity for care in the use of participant global assessments, the results of recent research provide support for their validity. For example, Collins and colleagues[70] found that a global rating (How effective do you think the treatment was?) provided similar evidence of analgesic efficacy as an aggregate measure of relief of acute pain, and Fischer and associates[14] reported that retrospective measures were not only more responsive to change than serial pain assessments but also were more strongly associated with clinical trial participant satisfaction. These data illustrate that concerns about the influence of memory in evaluating improvement may not always be an impediment to the processes by which participants actually evaluate their satisfaction with treatment and assess its benefits.

Ultimately, patients decide whether the positive attributes of a treatment outweigh its negative aspects including costs, and this is an important determinant of whether they adhere to and continue with treatment. Participant ratings of improvement and satisfaction with treatment provide unique information in outcomes assessment in clinical trials because they may allow an integration of the benefits of treatment and adverse events and other costs from within the participant's personal perspective. On the basis of a review of the literature of measures of global outcome prepared for the IMMPACT-II consensus meeting,[71] IMMPACT recommended the use of the PGIC[10] in chronic pain clinical trials as a core outcome measure of global improvement with treatment.

Symptoms and Adverse Events

Most patients will experience some degree of side effect burden with any pharmacologic treatment, and the importance of monitoring adverse events in the evaluation of new drugs has long been recognized as a component of all clinical trials. Two treatments may be equally effective and their adverse events not significantly different on a statistical basis but patients may view the side effects of a treatment as sufficiently noxious to discontinue or not fully adhere to the treatment.[72]

Therapies, such as the medications that relieve pain, have a variety of other effects that may not only cause discomfort but also impair physical and emotional function and exacerbate comorbid symptoms, which thereby may offset the therapeutic benefit. Max and Laska[73] noted that common analgesic adverse events (e.g., gastrointestinal distress, sedation, depression) can limit the dosage that can be realistically prescribed. The challenge is finding the dosage that maximizes pain relief and functional improvements and minimizes side effects. The onset of new diseases and initiation of new treatments during a clinical trial complicates assessments of symptoms and adverse events. When initiated during a trial, concomitant treatments are often protocol violations. Characteristics of the disease are baseline features or covariates when present at the beginning of a trial but are an adverse event when it emerges or worsens.

The usual strategy for identifying side effects is to ask patients and clinicians to record the occurrence of any adverse events that might be attributed to the treatment. Several studies,[74] however, suggest that patients may not acknowledge the presence of many potentially important side effects spontaneously during open-ended inquiry. Although there may be many reasons for the differences (e.g., memory, embarrassment), the fact is that important side effects may be missed by the use of open-ended questions. Negative health consequences of treatment using standard lists of symptoms that patients can rate with respect to presence, severity, and importance are an important domain that should be systematically assessed and reported in all clinical trials of treatments for chronic pain. Investigators should consider broad-based measures rather than ones

more limited in scope because the latter may underestimate the symptom distress experienced by the patient.[72] Moreover, investigators should determine not only the presence of side effects but their severity and importance to the patient.

Assessment of the percentages of clinical trial participants experiencing adverse events based on passive capture is standard in clinical trials; however, assessments of their severity and importance to patients are much less common, although this may provide valuable information. IMMPACT recommends that the prospective assessment of symptoms and adverse events relevant to the specific trial is a core outcome domain that should be included in all pain clinical trials, and that the strategy used to assess these events should include trial participants' ratings of their presence, severity, and importance.

On the basis of a review of the literature on the assessment of symptoms and adverse events prepared for the IMMPACT meeting[75] and discussions among the participants, IMMPACT recommend that "passive capture" of spontaneously reported events and the use of open-ended prompts should be used in all chronic pain clinical trials to assess adverse events, ideally supplemented by periodic review of systems beginning at baseline. In describing the results of clinical trials, the incidence of individual adverse events and serious adverse events should be reported by the treatment group, including the percentages of participants who experienced at least one treatment emergent adverse event.

Active capture using structured interviews or questionnaires to assess specific symptoms and adverse events that are relevant to the disorder or treatment being studied will often be more sensitive and more informative than passive capture or general inquiries.[76,77] Depending on the objectives of a clinical trial, prospective capture of symptoms and adverse events can be conducted at periodic intervals throughout the trial, including baseline and the conclusion of the trial, ideally by the same investigator. The frequency, duration, intensity, distress, importance to the patient, impact on daily function, and causal attribution by investigator and patient of symptoms and adverse events can be assessed,[72,78] which will provide information about the clinical importance of safety and tolerability outcomes.

Patient Disposition

IMMPACT recommended that the Consolidated Standards of Reporting Trials (CONSORT) guidelines[79-81] should be adhered to when publishing the results of clinical trials, and these guidelines provide a valuable overview of the types of participant disposition data that should be obtained when conducting trials. All potential study participants screened for a clinical trial should be carefully described with respect to the proportion who are ultimately enrolled, and why those who were not enrolled were excluded. Detailed information should be provided regarding the extent and reasons for treatment nonadherence, prohibited concomitant medications, and all other protocol deviations that may affect the interpretation of the trial results, including treatment modification, premature participant withdrawal from the trial, and loss to follow-up. Investigators should report the number of withdrawals related to each of the symptoms and adverse events identified in each of the treatment groups. This detailed characterization of participant disposition is the sixth core domain that should be assessed in all clinical trials of pain treatment efficacy and effectiveness.

To be effective, a treatment must have a beneficial effect on the symptom or disease being treated and the clinical trial participant must adhere to the treatment regimen. The most potent analgesic may demonstrate less than its potential benefit if participants in a clinical trial fail to use the medication in the manner prescribed, are unable to tolerate a fully effective dose, or drop out of the trial because of unacceptable adverse events or inadequate pain relief. Furthermore, the benefit of the treatment being studied may be obscured if participants receive any treatments that are not allowed in the protocol.[82]

The dosage and duration of all treatments received by participants during the clinical trial must be recorded, not only the treatment being investigated but also all concomitant treatments. Treatments initiated during the trial often reflect inadequate pain relief or the presence of distressing or uncontrolled adverse events (the use of rescue medications and changes in concomitant medication use may be justifiable as pain outcome measures when specified in the protocol; see previous discussion). Assessments of the use of rescue and prohibited medications and alterations in prescribed treatment as a result of adverse events and symptoms must be considered in evaluating the results of chronic pain clinical trials.

Significant percentages of patients enrolled in clinical trials prematurely terminate participation in the study. The IMMPACT recommendations are in agreement with the CONSORT statement[82] as to the importance of reporting data on patient attrition and loss to follow-up, and emphasize that the reasons for nonadherence be provided and not just the percentage who fail to comply. Patient disposition, premature exit from a trial, nonadherence to treatment, and loss to follow-up form a core domain that should be reported as an outcome in all clinical trails.

Although the CONSORT guidelines provide a valuable enumeration of the core elements of information on participant disposition that should be recorded when conducting trials, consideration should be given to collecting and reporting the following additional information in chronic pain clinical trials: (1) the recruitment process and the percentages of participants enrolled from each recruitment method used; (2) the number of candidate participants who were excluded from participation and the reasons why; (3) the number of candidates who chose not to enter the trial and the reasons why; (4) the use of prohibited concomitant medications and all other protocol deviations that may affect the interpretation of the trial results; (5) the number and reasons for withdrawal from each treatment group, including deaths and patients lost to follow-up; and (6) the types, rates, and reasons for nonadherence with treatment in each treatment group. If there were reasons that this set of information was not collected, the investigator should note why this was the case.

Detailed information describing the extent to which each participant adhered to the protocol will make it possible for data analyses to be conducted that examine efficacy in patients who adhered to the protocol. Such *efficacy evaluable* or *per protocol* analyses can sometimes be valuable in interpreting the results of intention-to-treat analyses, although the benefits of comparing randomized groups are lost. Although an important component of patient disposition, withdrawal from a clinical trial because of a lack of treatment effectiveness also can be considered an end point.[83,84]

Although reasons for withdrawal are usually provided in reports of clinical trials, this information is often inadequate. For example, "drop out because of adverse events" may be given as a reason for withdrawal, but this is not informative without tabulation of the specific adverse events associated with the withdrawals. Similarly, "withdrawal of consent" is commonly given as a reason for withdrawals, but this is impossible to interpret without description of the reasons why patients withdrew.

Several factors may compromise the integrity of the double-blind used in a clinical trial.[85] Participants' and investigators' guesses regarding which treatment was administered should therefore be assessed, and the reasons for the specific guesses (e.g., medication side effects or pain relief) should be collected to assist in interpreting any unblinding that may have occurred.[86,87]

Comments on the Core Domains and Measures

IMMPACT recommends that investigators designing and conducting clinical trials of chronic pain treatment efficacy and effectiveness should consider each of the six core domains discussed. It is important to emphasize, however, it is not necessary for positive results to be obtained for all of the core domains for the treatment to be deemed efficacious. Also we want to emphasize the word *considered*. These core domains and measures should be considered and are not mandatory because it is possible that there are specific trials for which one or more of these domains might not be relevant. In such instances, the recommendation is that investigators should acknowledge that they have considered each outcome domain and provide the rationale when they decide not to include assessment of a particular domain. Of course there are many supplemental outcome domains that can be included in a chronic pain clinical trial (described later), and we expect that the core outcome domains will be supplemented by assessment of additional domains that are required to evaluate a specific treatment (or that the investigator wishes to include for exploratory purposes).

8. United States Bureau of the Census. Statistical abstract of the United States: 1996 (116th ed). Washington, DC, 1996.

9. Turk DC, Dworkin RH, Allen RR, et al: Core outcome domains for chronic pain clinical trials: IMMPACT recommendations. Pain 2003;106:337-345.

10. Dworkin R, Turk D, Farrar J, et al: Core outcome measures for chronic pain clinical trials: IMMPACT recommendations. Pain 2005;113:9-19.

11. Jaeschke R, Singer J, Guyatt GH: Measurement of health status: Ascertaining the minimal clinically important difference. Control Clin Trials 1989;10:407-415.

12. Juniper EF, Guyatt GH, Willan A, et al: Determining a minimal important change in a disease-specific quality of life questionnaire. J Clin Epidemiol 1994;47:81-87.

13. Farrar JT, Young JP, LaMoreaux L, et al: Clinical importance of changes in chronic pain intensity measured on an 11-point numerical pain rating scale. Pain 2001;94:149-158.

14. Fischer D, Stewart AL, Blich DA, et al: Capturing the patient's view of change as a clinical outcome measure. JAMA 1999;282:1157-1162.

15. Ganz PA: What outcomes matter to patients: A physician-researcher point of view. Med Care 2002;40(suppl):III-11-III-19.

16. Dougados M, LeClaire P, van der Heijde D, et al: A report of the Osteoarthritis Research Society International Standing Committee for Clinical Trials Response Criteria Initiative. Osteoarthritis Cartilage 2002;8:395-403.

17. Bellamy N, Kirwan J, Boers M, et al: Recommendations for a core set of outcome measures for future phase III clinical trials in knee, hip, and hand osteoarthritis. Consensus development at OMERACT III. J Rheumatol 1997;24:799-802.

18. Brooks P, Hochberg M for ILAR and OMERACT: Outcome measures and classification criteria for the rheumatic diseases. A compilation of data from OMERACT (Outcome Measures for Arthritis Clinical Trials), ILAR (International League of Associations for Rheumatology), regional leagues and other groups. Rheumatology 2001;40:896-906.

19. Aaronson NK, Ahmedzai S, Bergman B, et al: The European Organization for Research and Treatment of Cancer QLQ-C30: A quality-of-life instrument for use in international clinical trials in oncology. J Natl Cancer Inst 1993;85:365-376.

20. Caraceni A, Cherny N, Fainsinger R, et al: Pain measurement tools and methods in clinical research in palliative care: Recommendations of an expert working group of the European Association of Palliative Care. J Pain Symptom Manage 2002;23:239-255.

21. Deyo RA, Battie M, Beurskens AHHM, et al: Outcome measures for low back pain research: A proposal for standardized use. Spine 1998;23:2003-2013.

22. Jensen MP, Karoly P: Self-report scales and procedures for assessing pain in adults. In Turk DC, Melzack R (eds): Handbook of Pain Assessment (2nd ed). New York, Guilford Press, 2001, pp 15-34.

23. Hadjistavropoulos T, von Baeyer C, Craig KD: Pain assessment in persons with limited ability to communicate. In Turk DC, Melzack R (eds): Handbook of Pain Assessment (2nd ed). New York, Guilford Press, 2001, pp 134-152.

24. Jensen MP: The validity and reliability of pain measures for use in clinical trials in adults. Presented at the second meeting of the Initiative on Methods, Measurement, and Pain Assessment in Clinical Trials (IMMPACT-II), April 2003, Washington, DC (www.immpact.org/meetings.html).

25. Bellamy N, Buchanan WW, Goldsmith CH, et al: Validation study of WOMAC: A health status instrument for measuring clinically important patient relevant outcomes to antirheumatic drug therapy in patients with osteoarthritis of the hip or knee. J Rheumatol 1988;15:1833-1840.

26. Farrar JT, Dworkin RH, Max MB: Use of the cumulative proportion of responders analysis graph to present pain data over a range of cut-off points: Making clinical trial data more understandable. J Pain Symptom Manage 2006;31:369-377.

27. Kieburtz K, Simpson D, Yiannoutsos C, et al: AIDS Clinical Trial Group 242 Protocol Team. A randomized trial of amitriptyline and mexiletine for painful neuropathy in HIV infection. Neurology 1998;51:1682-1688.

28. Morrison BW, Daniels SE, Kotey P, et al: Rofecoxib, a specific cyclooxygenase-2 inhibitor, in primary dysmenorrhea: A randomized controlled trial. Obstet Gynecol 1999;94:504-508.

29. Eisenberg E, Lurie Y, Daoud D, Ishay A: Lamotrigine reduces painful diabetic neuropathy: A randomized controlled study. Neurology 2001;57:505-509.

30. Steedman SM, Middaugh SJ, Kee WG, et al: Chronic-pain medications: Equivalence levels and method of quantifying usage. Clin J Pain 1992;8:204-214.

31. Lehmann KA: Patient-controlled analgesia for postoperative pain. In Benedetti C, Chapman CR, Giron G (eds): Opioid Analgesia: Recent Advances in Systemic Administration. New York, Raven Press, 1990, pp 297-334.

32. Silverman DG, O'Connor TZ, Brull SJ: Integrated assessment of pain scores and rescue morphine doses during studies of analgesic efficacy. Anesth Analg 1993;77:168-170.

33. Melzack R, Torgerson WS: On the language of pain. Anesthesiology 1991;34:50-59.

34. Price DD, Harkins SW, Baker C: Sensory-affective relationships among different types of clinical and experimental pain. Pain 1987;28:297-307.

35. Melzack R: The short-form McGill Pain Questionnaire. Pain 1987;30:191-197.

36. Rowbotham MC, Harden N, Stacey B, et al: Gabapentin Postherpetic Neuralgia Study Group: Gabapentin for the treatment postherpetic neuralgia: A randomized controlled trial. JAMA 1998;280:1837-1842.

37. Dworkin RH, Corbin AE, Young JP, et al: Pregabalin for the treatment of postherpetic neuralgia: A randomized, placebo-controlled trial. Neurology 2003;60:1274-1283.

38. Farrar JT, Cleary J, Rauck R, et al: Oral transmucosal fentanyl citrate: Randomized, double-blinded, placebo-controlled trial for treatment of breakthrough pain in cancer patients. J Natl Cancer Inst 1998;90:611-616.

39. Dawson R, Spross JA, Jablonski ES, et al: Probing the paradox of patients' satisfaction with inadequate pain management. J Pain Symptom Manage 2002;23:211-220.

40. Guyatt GH, Feeney DH, Patrick DL: Measuring health-related quality of life. Ann Intern Med 1993;118:622-629.

41. Testa MA, Simonson DC: Assessment of quality-of-life outcomes. Curr Concepts 1996;334:835-840.

42. Varni JW, Seid M, Kurtin P: Pediatric health-related quality of life measurement technology: A guide for healthcare decision makers. JCOM 1999;6:33-40.

43. Seid M, Varni J, Jacobs J: Pediatric health-related quality-of-life measurement technology: Intersections between science, managed care, and clinical care. J Clin Psychol Med Settings 2000;7:17-27.

44. Gladis M, Gosch E, Dishuk N, Crits-Cristoph P: Quality of life: Expanding the scope of clinical significance. J Consult Clin Psychol 1999;67:320-331.

45. Kerns RD, Turk DC, Rudy TE: The West Haven-Yale Multidimensional Pain Inventory (WHYMPI). Pain 1985;23:345-356.

46. De Gagné TA, Mikail SF, D'Eon JL: Confirmatory factor analysis of a 4-factor model of chronic pain evaluation. Pain 1995;60:195-202.

47. Holroyd KA, Malinoski P, Davis MK, Lipchik GL: The three dimensions of headache impact: Pain, disability and affective distress. Pain 1999;83:571-578.

48. Dworkin RH, Nagasako EM, Hetzel RD, Farrar JT: Assessment of pain and pain-related quality of life in clinical trials. In Turk DC, Melzack R (eds): Handbook of Pain Assessment (2nd ed). New York, Guilford Press, 2001, pp 659-692.

49. Fowler FJ, Cleary PD, Magaziner J, et al: Methodological issues in measuring patient-reported outcomes: The agenda of the work group on outcomes assessment. Med Care 1994;32:JS65-JS76.

50. Haythornthwaite JA: The assessment of pain-related physical function for clinical trials in chronic pain. Presented at the second meeting of the Initiative on Methods, Measurement, and Pain Assessment in Clinical Trials (IMMPACT-II), April 2003, Washington, DC (www.immpact.org/meetings.html).

51. Stucki G, Cieza A: HRQL measures in chronic pain trials. Presented at the second meeting of the Initiative on

Methods, Measurement, and Pain Assessment in Clinical Trials (IMMPACT-II), April 2003, Washington, DC (www.immpact.org/meetings.html).

52. Roland M, Morris R: A study of the natural history of back pain, part I: Development of a reliable and sensitive measure of disability in low back pain. Spine 1983;8:141-144.

53. Cleeland CS, Nakamura Y, Mendoza TR, et al: Dimensions of the impact of cancer pain in a four country sample: New information from multidimensional scaling. Pain 1996;67:267-273.

54. Cleeland CS, Ryan KM: Pain assessment: Global use of the Brief Pain Inventory. Ann Acad Med 1994;23:129-138.

55. Peloso PM, Bellamy N, Bensen W, et al: Double blind randomized placebo control trial of controlled release codeine in the treatment of osteoarthritis of the hip or knee. J Rheumatol 2000;27:764-771.

56. Watson CPN, Moulin D, Watt-Watson J, et al: Controlled-release oxycodone relieves neuropathic pain: A randomized controlled trial in diabetic neuropathy. Pain 2003;105:71-78.

57. Thompson D: Toward a pharmacoeconomic model of neuropathic pain. Clin J Pain 2002;18:366-372.

58. Turk DC: Clinical effectiveness and cost-effectiveness of treatments for patients with chronic pain. Clin J Pain 2002;18:355-365.

59. Ware JE, Sherbourne CD: The MOS 36-item short-form health survey (SF-36). Med Care 1992;30:473-483.

60. Kerns RD: Assessment of emotional functioning in pain treatment outcome research. Presented at the second meeting of the Initiative on Methods, Measurement, and Pain Assessment in Clinical Trials (IMMPACT-II), April 2003, Washington, DC (www.immpact.org/meetings.html).

61. Beck AT, Ward CH, Mendelson M, et al: An inventory for measuring depression. Arch Gen Psychiatry 1961;4:561-571.

62. McNair DM, Lorr M, Droppleman L: Profile of Mood States. San Diego, Educational and Industrial Testing Service, 1971.

63. Gallagher RM, Verma S: Mood and anxiety disorders in chronic pain. In Dworkin RH, Breitbart WS (eds): Psychosocial Aspects of Pain: A Handbook for Health Care Providers. Seattle, IASP Press, 2004, pp 589-606.

64. Wilson KG, Mikail SF, D'Eon JL, Minns JE: Alternative diagnostic criteria for major depressive disorder in patients with chronic pain. Pain 2001;91:227-234.

65. Guy W: ECDEU assessment manual for psychopharmacology (DHEW publication no. ADM 76-338). Washington, DC, US Government Printing Office, 1976.

66. Just N, Ciccone DS, Bandilla EB, Wu W-H: Global impressions versus validated measures of treatment effectiveness in patients with chronic nonmalignant pain. Rehabil Psychol 1999;44:194-207.

67. Dunkl PR, Taylor AF, McConnell G et al: Responsiveness of fibromyalgia clinical trial outcome measures. J Rheumatol 2000;27:2683-2691.

68. Guyatt GH, Osoba D, Wu AW, et al: Clinical Significance Consensus Meeting Group: Methods to explain the clinical significance of health status measures. Mayo Clin Proc 2002;77:371-383.

69. Ross M: Relation of implicit theories to the construction of personal histories. Psychol Rev 1989;96:341-347.

70. Collins SL, Edwards J, Moore RA, et al: Seeking a simple measure of analgesia for mega-trials: Is a single global assessment good enough? Pain 2001;91:189-194.

71. Farrar JT: The global assessment of pain and related symptoms. Presented at the second meeting of the Initiative on Methods, Measurement, and Pain Assessment in Clinical Trials (IMMPACT-II), April 2003, Washington, DC (www.immpact.org/meetings.html).

72. Anderson RB, Hollenberg NK, Williams GH: Physical Symptoms Distress Index. A sensitive tool to evaluate the impact of pharmacological agents. Arch Intern Med 1999;159:693-700.

73. Max MB, Laska EM: Single-dose analgesic comparisons. In Max M, Portenoy R, Laska E (eds): Advances in Pain Research and Therapy, vol 18. New York, Raven Press, 1991, pp 55-95.

74. Anderson RB, Testa MA: Symptom distress checklists as a component of quality of life measurement: Comparing prompted reports by patient and physician with concurrent adverse event reports via the physician. Drug Inform J 1994;28:89-114.

75. Katz N: The measurement of symptoms and side effects in clinical trials of chronic pain. Presented at the second meeting of the Initiative on Methods, Measurement, and Pain Assessment in Clinical Trials (IMMPACT-II), April 2003, Washington, DC (www.immpact.org/meetings.html).

76. Rabkin JG, Markowitz JS, Ocepek-Welikson K, Wager SS: General versus systematic inquiry about emergent clinical events with SAFTEE: Implications for clinical research. J Clin Psychopharm 1992;12:3-10.

77. Testa MA, Anderson RB, Nackley JF, Hollenberg NK: Quality of Life Hypertension Study Group. Quality of life and antihypertensive therapy in men: A comparison of captopril with enalapril. N Engl J Med 1993;328:907-913.

78. Lingjaerde O, Ahlfors UG, Bech P, et al: The UKU side effect rating scale: A new comprehensive rating scale for psychotropic drugs and a cross-sectional study of side effects in neuroleptic-treated patients. Acta Psychiatr Scand Suppl 1987:334:1-100.

79. Begg C, Cho M, Eastwood S, et al: Improving the quality of reporting of randomized controlled trials: The CONSORT statement. JAMA 1996;276:637-639.

80. Altman DG, Schulz KF, Mohcr D, et al: CONSORT Group. The revised CONSORT statement for reporting randomized trials: Explanation and elaboration. Ann Intern Med 2001;134:663-694.

81. Moher D, Schulz K, Altman DG for the CONSORT Group: The CONSORT statement: Revised recommendations for improving the quality of reports of parallel-group randomized trials. Ann Intern Med 2001;134:657-662.

82. Turk DC: Reporting on participant disposition in clinical trials. Presented at the second meeting of the Initiative on Methods, Measurement, and Pain Assessment in Clinical Trials (IMMPACT-II), April 2003, Washington, DC (www.immpact.org/meetings.html).

83. International Conference on Harmonisation. Guidance for industry, E10: choice of control group and related issues in clinical trials, 2001, Washington, DC (www.fda.gov/cder/guidance/index.htm).

84. European Agency for the Evaluation of Medicinal Products. Note for guidance on clinical investigation of medicinal products for treatment of nociceptive pain, 2002 (www.emea.eu.int/pdfs/human/ewp/061200en.pdf).

85. Even C, Siobud-Dorocant E, Dardennes RM: Critical approach to antidepressant trials: Blindness protection is necesary, feasible and measurable. Br J Psychiatry 2000;177:47-51.

86. Moscucci M, Byrne L, Weintraub M, Cox C: Blinding, unblinding, and the placebo effect: An analysis of patients' guesses of treatment assignment in a double-blind clinical trial. Clin Pharmacol Ther 1987;41:259-265.

87. Turner JA, Jensen MP, Warms CA, Cardenas DD: Blinding effectiveness and association of pretreatment expectations with pain improvement in a double-blind randomized controlled trial. Pain 2002;99:91-99.

88. Acquadro C, Benson R, Dubois D, et al for the PRO Harmonization Group: Incorporating the patient's perspective into drug development and communication: An ad hoc task force report of the patient-reported outcomes (PRO) harmonization group meeting at the Food and Drug Administration, February 16, 2001, Washington, DC. Values in Health 2003;6:522-531.

89. Willke RJ, Burke LB, Erickson P: Measuring treatment impact: A review of patient-reported outcomes and other efficacy endpoints in approved product labels. Contr Clin Trials 4004;25:535-552.

90. Rothwell PM, McDowell Z, Wong CK, Dorman PJ: Doctors and patients don't agree: Cross sectional study of patients' and doctors' perceptions and assessments of disability in multiple sclerosis. BMJ 1997;124:1580.

91. Clinch J, Tugwell P, Wells G, Shea B: Individualized functional priority approach to the assessment of health related quality of life in rheumatology. J Rheumatol 2001;28:445-451.

92. Hewlett S, Smith AP, Kirwan JR: Values for function in rheumatoid arthritis: Patients, professional, and public. Ann Rheum Dis 2001;60:928-933.

93. Kvien TK, Heiberg T: Patient perspective in outcome assessments—Perceptions or something more? J Rheumatol 2003;30:873-876.

94. Kirwan J, Heiberg T, Hewlett S, et al: Outcomes from the patient perspective workshop at OMERACT 6. J Rheumatol 2003;30:868-872.

95. Casarett D, Karlawish J, Sankar P, et al: Designing pain research from the patient's perspective: What trial endpoints are important to patients with chronic pain? Pain Med 2001;2:309-316.

96. Stone AA, Shiffman S: Ecological momentary assessment (EMA) in behavioral medicine. Ann Behav Med 1994;16:199-202.

97. Joint Committee on Standards for Educational and Psychological Testing of the American Educational Research Association, the American Psychological Association, and the National Council on Measurement in Education. Standards for educational and psychological testing. Washington, DC, American Educational Research Association, 1999.

98. Nunnally J, Bernstein I: Psychometric Theory (3rd ed). New York, McGraw-Hill, 1994.

99. Gershon R, Cella D, Dineen K, et al: Item response theory and health-related quality of life in cancer. Exp Rev Pharmacoeconomics Outcomes Res 2003;3:783-791.

100. Roorda K, Molenaar IW, Lankhorst GJ, Bouter LM: Improvements of a questionnaire measuring activity limitation in rising and sitting down in patients with lower-extremity disorders living in home Arch Phys Med Rehabil 2005;86:2204-2210.

69 Outcomes, Efficacy, and Complications from Acute Postoperative Pain Management

Christopher L. Wu and Spencer S. Liu

Proper management of acute postoperative pain is vital because inadequate control of postoperative pain may lead to short- and long-term adverse outcomes. Postoperative pain continues to be undermanaged despite the introduction of national guidelines. The pathophysiology of postoperative pain provides a variety of theoretic avenues by which postoperative analgesia might beneficially affect postoperative outcomes. Attenuation of these detrimental pathophysiologic responses might improve patient outcomes for a variety of systems and end points, although use of different analgesic options (e.g., regional analgesia vs. systemic opioids) might result in different outcomes. In addition, each analgesic option is associated with a different side effect and adverse event profile. These complications may influence the over-all analgesic efficacy and acceptance of a particular analgesic option.

PATHOPHYSIOLOGY OF ACUTE POSTOPERATIVE PAIN

Acute postoperative pain may adversely affect a wide range of organ systems. These adverse pathophysiologies generally may not manifest themselves in healthy surgical patients but may contribute to perioperative morbidity in patients with a decreased physiologic reserve.

Cardiovascular

There is a high prevalence of cardiovascular disease in the general surgical population. Of the approximately 27 million patients in the United States who have surgery every year, 8 million have coronary artery disease or risk factors for cardiovascular disease. One million of these patients have perioperative cardiac complications at an estimated cost of $20 billion for in-hospital and outpatient care.[1] Thus it is not surprising that perioperative cardiac morbidity is the most common cause of death following anesthesia and surgery.[2]

Postoperative pain may contribute to cardiac morbidity by activation of the sympathetic nervous system and the coagulation cascade. Increased activity of the sympathetic nervous system may lead to angina, dysrhythmias, and increased areas of myocardial infarction.[3] Conversely, attenuation of perioperative sympathetic activity may decrease postoperative mortality from cardiovascular events (myocardial infarction, dysrhythmia, congestive heart failure) after noncardiac surgery.[3] Mechanisms by which increased sympathetic activity may result in cardiac morbidity may involve increased myocardial oxygen demand or a decrease in myocardial oxygen supply (Fig. 69–1). Increased heart rate, blood pressure, and contractility resulting from sympathetic efflux and catecholamines can increase myocardial oxygen demand. However, most perioperative episodes of myocardial ischemia are silent[1] and occur without major hemodynamic changes.[4] These observations suggest that decreases in myocardial oxygen supply may be more important than increases in oxygen demand as a cause for perioperative myocardial ischemia. Finally, sympathetic activation enhances postoperative hypercoagulability, thereby increasing the likelihood of coronary thrombosis and reduced myocardial oxygen supply.[5,6] Thus, reducing pain and the accompanying sympathetic activity from high-quality postoperative pain management may decrease postoperative cardiac morbidity.

Pulmonary

Postoperative pulmonary complications may occur more frequently than cardiac complications and are

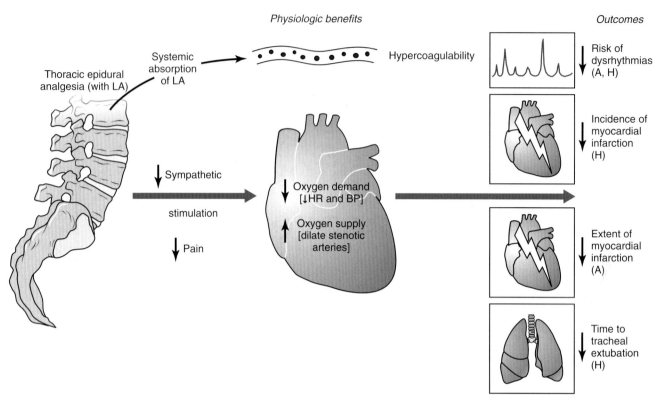

Physiologic benefits

Outcomes

Figure 69–1. The figure depicts the potential beneficial effects of epidural anesthesia and analgesia on attenuating adverse cardiac physiologic effects associated with surgery. Epidural anesthesia and analgesia may decrease sympathetic stimulation and pain. By attenuating adverse cardiac physiologic effects through decreasing hypercoagulability, decreasing oxygen demand, and improving oxygen supply, perioperative use of epidural anesthesia and analgesia may improve cardiac outcomes including decreasing the risk of dysrhythmias, incidence and extent of myocardial infarction, and time to tracheal extubation. A, animal studies; H, human studies; LA, local anesthetics.

associated with significantly longer durations of hospital stay.[7] A recent prospective study observed that incidence of pulmonary morbidity was 1.8% after minor surgery, 10.6% after major surgery, and as high as 33% after major upper abdominal surgery.[8] Postoperative pulmonary dysfunction occurs due to pain, surgical trespass, and residual effects of general anesthesia (Fig. 69–2). Postoperative pulmonary dysfunction is most severe after upper abdominal and thoracic surgery and relatively preserved after laparoscopic and peripheral surgery.[7] Vital capacity and the forced expiratory volume in 1 second (FEV_1) decrease by approximately 60% from preoperative values after upper abdominal surgery and by 40% after lower abdominal and thoracic surgery.[9] The most important postoperative change is probably the decrease in functional residual capacity (FRC), which starts at about 16 hours postoperatively, reaches a nadir at 24 to 48 hours, and returns to normal within a week.[9] The ventilation-perfusion imbalance and atelectasis accompanying postoperative loss of FRC can contribute to hypoxemia, pneumonia, and other pulmonary complications.[7,9] Other detrimental postoperative pulmonary changes associated with pain and surgical injury include a rapid, shallow breathing pattern and increased work of breathing.

In addition to pain, upper abdominal and thoracic incisions cause postoperative diaphragmatic dysfunc-

tion and decreased intercostal muscle tone.[7] Postoperative diaphragmatic dysfunction appears to be the result of a neural reflex inhibiting the phrenic nerve. Neither the vagus nerve nor intensity of postoperative pain appears to be involved.[10] Postoperative pulmonary complications are related to the disruption of normal coordination of respiratory muscles that occur postoperatively, and maneuvers that promote deep breathing appear to be most efficacious in reducing the incidence of postoperative pulmonary complications.[7] Thus postoperative analgesic techniques that provide good pain control and that can minimize surgical effects on diaphragmatic and intercostal muscle tone may improve postoperative pulmonary outcome.

Coagulation

Overall, an estimated 200,000 new cases of deep vein thrombosis and pulmonary embolism occur in the United States each year.[11] Surgical patients are especially vulnerable to developing coagulation-related complications. A hypercoagulable state develops during the perioperative period[5,12] that is associated with an increase in vaso-occlusive and thromboembolic morbidity (Fig. 69–3).[12,13] Activation of the stress response and sympathetic nervous system by pain and surgery appears to be a major contributor

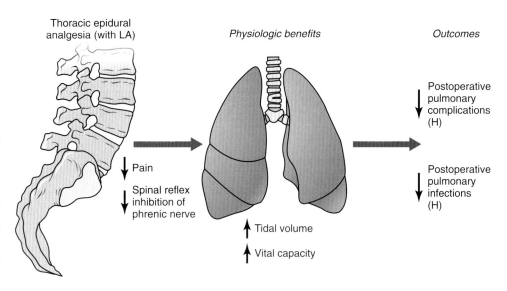

Figure 69–2. The figure depicts the potential beneficial effects of epidural anesthesia and analgesia on attenuating adverse pulmonary physiologic effects associated with surgery. Epidural anesthesia and analgesia may decrease pain and the spinal reflex inhibition of the phrenic nerve. By attenuating adverse pulmonary physiologic effects through increasing tidal volume and vital capacity, perioperative use of epidural anesthesia and analgesia may improve pulmonary outcomes including decreasing the incidence of postoperative pulmonary complications and infections. H, human studies; LA, local anesthetics.

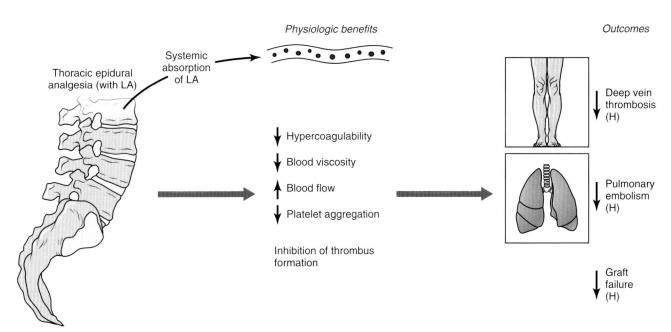

Figure 69–3. The figure depicts the potential beneficial effects of epidural anesthesia and analgesia on attenuating adverse coagulation-related physiologic effects associated with surgery. Epidural anesthesia and analgesia may provide many physiologic benefits including decreasing overall hypercoagulability, blood viscosity, and platelet aggregation. In addition, epidural anesthesia and analgesia may increase blood flow and inhibit thrombus formation. By attenuating adverse coagulation-related physiologic effects, perioperative use of epidural anesthesia and analgesia may improve coagulation-related outcomes including a decrease in risk of deep vein thrombosis, pulmonary embolism, and graft related failures. A, animal studies; H, human studies; LA, local anesthetics.

to the hypercoagulable state that can accompany the postoperative period.[5] Postoperative changes in coagulation include an increase in coagulation factors, enhanced platelet activity, decrease in coagulation inhibitor concentrations, and inhibition of fibrinolysis.[3]

Postoperative hypercoagulability affects the venous as well as the arterial circulation system. Venous thrombotic morbidity includes deep vein thrombosis with potential pulmonary embolization. Arterial thrombotic morbidity includes coronary artery thrombosis, leading to myocardial ischemia, and vas-cular graft occlusion, which leads to lower extremity ischemia. Methods of acute pain management that reduce pain and the accompanying stress response and activation of the sympathetic nervous system may therefore decrease vaso-occlusive and thromboembolic morbidity.

Gastrointestinal

Postoperative ileus is a virtually universal complication after abdominal surgery that prolongs duration of hospitalization and is estimated to have an annual

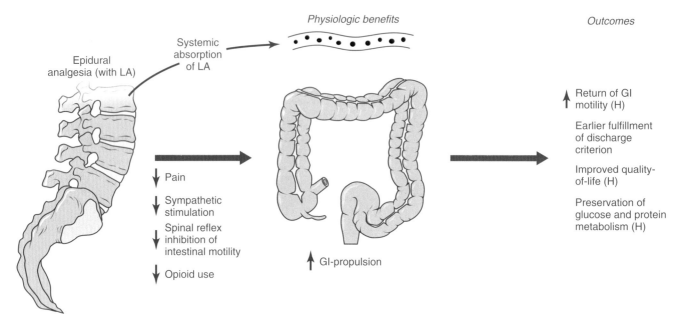

Figure 69–4. The figure depicts the potential beneficial effects of epidural anesthesia and analgesia on attenuating adverse gastrointestinal (GI) physiologic effects associated with surgery. Epidural anesthesia and analgesia may decrease pain, sympathetic stimulation, spinal reflex inhibition of intestinal motility, and opioid use. By attenuating adverse gastrointestinal physiologic effects, perioperative use of epidural anesthesia and analgesia may improve overall GI propulsion and outcomes including earlier return of GI motility, earlier fulfillment of discharge criteria, improved quality of life, and preservation of glucose and protein metabolism. H, human studies; LA, local anesthetics.

cost of $750 million the U.S. health care system.[14] Development of ileus also may increase postoperative morbidity by delaying resumption of enteral feeding. Early resumption of postoperative enteral feeding decreases stress response, promotes wound healing, and decreases septic complications.[15,16] Postoperative pain is thought to initiate a spinal reflex arc that inhibits intestinal motility. In addition, pain and surgical insult will activate the sympathetic nervous system and stress response, leading to further inhibition of intestinal motility (Fig. 69–4).[14,17] Reduction of pain, stress response, and sympathetic nervous system activity by postoperative pain management may decrease the duration and severity of postoperative ileus.

Stress Response

Surgical insult and pain elicit a metabolic response via local trauma, somatic neural pathways, and sympathetic neural pathways (Fig. 69–5). The stress response involves both neuroendocrine hormones and local tissue release of cytokines and prostaglandins. Physiologic effects of stress response mediators are varied and include tachycardia, hypotension, fever, hypercoagulability, ileus, and suppression of immune function.[3,17] Quantity of stress mediators released is dependent on the degree of surgical insult. More extensive surgery results in greater release of stress response mediators.[18] Physiologic effects of stress response are dose related[19] and are correlated with postoperative infection, vaso-occlusion, and mortality.[6,20] Thus, reduction in perioperative stress response by postoperative pain management may

decrease postoperative cardiovascular morbidity, infectious complications, ileus, and mortality.

EFFECTS OF ACUTE PAIN MANAGEMENT ON POSTOPERATIVE OUTCOME

The previous section has outlined potential mechanisms whereby postoperative pain management might decrease perioperative morbidity. This section reviews clinical trials, particularly focusing on data that are available in an evidence-based or systematic fashion (e.g., meta-analysis), examining effects of postoperative pain management on various outcomes. Although there are many analgesic options for postoperative pain management, this chapter focuses on the more commonly used agents, namely systemic opioids, nonsteroidal anti-inflammatory drugs (NSAIDs), and regional (epidural and peripheral) analgesia because the vast majority of the available systematic evidence is available when examining these agents. Throughout this section, the type of outcome used by each discussed study and the exact analgesic techniques being compared are specified.

INFLUENCE OF ANALGESIC OPTIONS

Systemic Opioids

Systemic opioids are a cornerstone for the treatment of acute postoperative pain. This class of analgesic agents is quite versatile. Opioids may be administered through a variety of routes (e.g., oral, intravenous, intramuscular, subcutaneous, intra-articular,

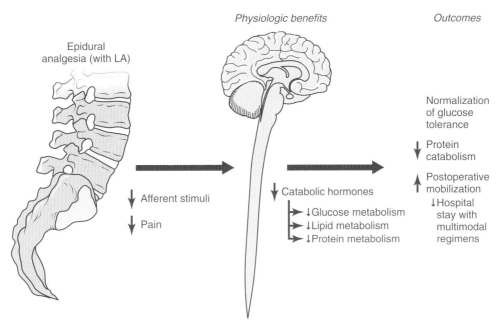

Figure 69–5. The figure depicts the potential beneficial effects of epidural anesthesia and analgesia on attenuating adverse neuroendocrine stress–related physiologic effects associated with surgery. Epidural anesthesia and analgesia may attenuate the overall neuroendocrine stress response in part by decreasing pain and afferent input. By attenuating adverse neuroendocrine stress–related physiologic effects including attenuating an increase in catabolic hormones with preservation of glucose, lipid, and protein metabolism, perioperative use of epidural anesthesia and analgesia may improve neuroendocrine stress–related outcomes including preservation of protein catabolism, normalization of glucose tolerance, and possibility decrease in hospital stay with a multimodal approach to patient convalescence. LA, local anesthetics.

neuraxial) and have a relatively quick onset of analgesia. Administration of opioids via an intravenous patient-controlled analgesia (IV PCA) device (compared with as needed intramuscular injection) may result in superior analgesia and greater patient satisfaction.[21,22] Although opioids are effective in providing analgesia, for the most part they do not provide any physiologic benefits per se in attenuating the adverse pathophysiology that occurs postoperatively. In fact, opioids may have some paradoxical detrimental antianalgesic properties, such as hyperalgesia and tolerance, although the specific clinical relevance and applicability need to be examined.

Nonsteroidal Anti-inflammatory Agents

NSAIDs are a valuable adjuvant for the treatment of acute postoperative pain. They exhibit both a peripheral and central mechanism of analgesic action. NSAIDs are presumed to exert their analgesic properties via inhibition of cyclooxygenase (COX) with traditional NSAIDs inhibiting both isoforms (COX-1 and COX-2), whereas newer agents (COX-2 inhibitors) inhibit the COX-2 isoform (which is upregulated during inflammation) to a greater extent. Although NSAIDs are traditionally though to be "weak" analgesics, single-dose data for postoperative pain suggest a surprising analgesic efficacy of these agents compared with opioids (Fig. 69–6).[23] As an adjuvant agent, NSAIDs (including COX-2 inhibitors) and acetaminophen are commonly used in the perioperative setting. Recent systematic reviews and

meta-analysis of randomized controlled trials indicate that when combined with IV PCA with morphine, NSAIDs (multiple dose or infusion only of nonspecific agents and COX-2 inhibitors), but not acetaminophen, do significantly decrease postoperative pain scores.[24-28] Although NSAIDs, COX-2 inhibitors, and acetaminophen in combination with IV PCA do provide an opioid-sparing effect, this decrease in opioid consumption does not consistently translate into a decrease in opioid-related adverse events or side effects.[24-26] The use of acetaminophen and COX-2 inhibitors does not appear to decrease the relative risk of opioid-related side effects and use of nonspecific NSAIDs appears to only decrease the relative risk of some opioid-related side effects (i.e., postoperative nausea and vomiting [PONV], sedation) but not others (i.e., pruritus, urinary retention, respiratory depression).[24-26]

Continuous Regional (Epidural and Peripheral) Analgesia

The use of continuous regional analgesia holds the greater possibilities in attenuating adverse perioperative pathophysiology and improving patient outcomes. Meta-analyses suggest that both epidural and continuous peripheral regional analgesia provide superior postoperative analgesia when compared with systemic opioids, including those delivered via IV PCA.[29-31] Compared with that for peripheral regional analgesia, there is enough information to examine the efficacy of epidural analgesia on many

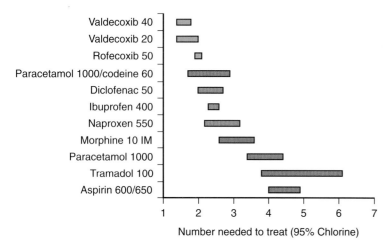

Figure 69–6. League table of number needed to treat (NNT) for at least 50% pain relief over 4 to 6 hours in patients with moderate to severe pain, for all oral analgesics except intramuscular morphine. (From Oxford League table of analgesics in acute pain. www.jr2.ox.ac.uk/bandolier/booth/painpag/Acutrev/Analgesics/Leagtab.html. Accessed December 18, 2005.)

types of patient outcomes although whether epidural anesthesia and analgesia improves all outcomes is uncertain because of the presence of methodologic issues in many of the available studies. For instance, the effect of epidural anesthesia and analgesia on patient outcomes is dependent on many factors including the congruency of epidural catheter location and surgical incision, type of analgesic regimen (local anesthetic vs. opioid [opioids may provide adequate analgesia but may not provide the physiologic benefit of local anesthetics]), duration of epidural analgesia (premature removal of epidural analgesia may negate any physiologic benefits), and use as part of a multimodal approach to patient convalescence.

Mortality

The use of opioids and NSAIDs per se does not appear to provide a beneficial effect in reducing perioperative mortality. Possibly because of the favorable effects in attenuating perioperative pathophysiology, use of perioperative epidural anesthesia and analgesia (particularly a local anesthetic-based solution) may be associated with a decrease in postoperative mortality. The largest set of randomized data to examine this issue is the CORTRA meta-analysis, which incorporated data from 142 randomized controlled trials (RCTs) up to January 1, 1997 (9553 patients analyzed).[32] The results of this meta-analysis suggested that intraoperative neuraxial (spinal and epidural) anesthesia was associated with a 30% decreased odds of death at 30 days after surgery although the decrease in mortality was attributed primarily to orthopedic subjects, which constituted approximately 60% of the subjects in the meta-analysis. There was no difference in odds of death between spinal and epidural anesthesia.

Another study examined the association of the presence of postoperative epidural analgesia and mortality using the Medicare claims dataset. A 5% nationally random sample of Medicare beneficiaries from 1997 to 2001 was analyzed to identify patients undergoing a variety of surgical procedures (e.g., lobectomy of the lung, colectomy, total abdominal

hysterectomy, pancreaticoduodenectomy, nephrectomy, gastrectomy, and radical retropubic prostatectomy) and patients were divided into two groups, depending on the presence or absence of a bill for postoperative epidural analgesia. Multivariate regression analyses noted that the presence of epidural analgesia was associated with a significantly lower odds of death at 7 days (odds ratio [OR] = 0.52) and 30 days (OR = 0.74) after surgery despite the fact that there was no difference between the groups with regard to overall major morbidity.[33] However, another analysis on a lower-risk surgical group (i.e., total hip replacement) using similar methodology revealed no benefit for postoperative epidural analgesia in decreasing postoperative mortality.[34] Thus some data suggest an association between perioperative epidural analgesia and decreased postoperative mortality but significant methodologic issues are present in these data that may preclude a definitive answer to whether epidural analgesia actually decreases postoperative mortality. Use of continuous peripheral analgesia would provide the same theoretic benefit in attenuating perioperative pathophysiology as epidural analgesia; however, there are few data examining the association of this technique and postoperative mortality.

Cardiovascular Morbidity

Postoperative pain management techniques that optimize analgesia, reduce sympathetic activity, and reduce perioperative hypercoagulability would be expected to decrease cardiac morbidity. The importance of excellent postoperative analgesia for improved cardiac outcomes has been demonstrated in pediatric cardiac,[20] adult cardiac,[35] and adult noncardiac surgery.[36] Some data suggest that administration of certain types of opioids may be associated with a reduction in cardiovascular morbidity in some cases. A randomized trial in neonates undergoing cardiac surgery observed that mortality was markedly reduced (0% vs. 27%) in the group receiving more effective postoperative analgesia.[20] Similar differences in intermediate outcome were observed in adults undergoing cardiac surgery randomized to postoperative analgesia with intravenous infusions of sufentanil versus morphine.[35] However, there is not enough consistent evidence to suggest that perioperative use of systemic opioids per se will decrease cardiovascular morbidity.

Conversely, there is evidence that use of epidural analgesia may be associated with a decrease in cardiovascular morbidity, which may be related to its ability to suppress the sympathetic nervous system during the perioperative period. Systemic opioids do not appear to block the sympathetic nervous system; in contrast, epidural opioids,[37] alpha agonists,[38] and especially thoracic epidural administration (TEA) of local anesthetics[39] appear to be effective suppressants of the sympathetic nervous system and may produce beneficial reductions in myocardial oxygen demand by lowering heart rate and blood pressure[40] and dilating stenotic epicardial coronary arteries,[41] which is critical in patients with severe refractory coronary artery disease. In contrast, lumbar epidural administration of local anesthetics may reduce myocardial oxygen supply by lowering coronary artery perfusion pressure (hypotension) without decreasing heart rate or dilating coronary vessels. Support for this concern has been demonstrated in studies of patients, with risk factors for coronary artery disease receiving thoracic or lumbar epidural analgesia. The thoracic group experienced improved segmental wall function,[42] whereas the lumbar group developed segmental wall motion abnormalities suggestive of myocardial ischemia.[43]

Two meta-analyses have examined the efficacy of epidural analgesia and postoperative cardiovascular events. The first meta-analysis examined all types of surgical procedures and included 11 randomized controlled trials (1173 patients).[44] Not unexpectedly, postoperative epidural analgesia provided better analgesia for the first 24 hours after surgery. Although there was no difference in the frequency of in-hospital death, the rate of myocardial infarction was significantly lower in those who received epidural analgesia (rate difference = −3.8%). This difference was pronounced in the subgroup analysis in which postoperative thoracic (but not lumbar) epidural analgesia showed a significant reduction in the rate of myocardial infarction (rate difference = −5.3),[44] corroborating experimental data showing a physiologic benefit for thoracic but not lumbar epidural analgesia with local anesthetics in improving various aspects of perioperative cardiac function.

A second meta-analysis examining the efficacy of TEA and cardiovascular events was performed in patients undergoing coronary artery bypass surgery.[45] Fifteen trials enrolling 1178 patients were included for analysis. Although there were no differences in the incidences of mortality or myocardial infarction between TEA and systemic opioids, the presence of TEA was associated with a significant reduction in the risk of dysrhythmias, time to tracheal extubation, and reduced analogue pain scores. Thus clinical and experimental studies suggest that TEA contain-

ing local anesthetic may beneficially attenuate the sympathetic nervous system and decrease cardiac morbidity.

Effects of analgesic technique on postoperative coagulability may affect coronary artery thrombosis and myocardial oxygen supply. Epidural administration of local anesthetics may reduce perioperative hypercoagulability via a number of mechanisms. In addition, use of nonspecific (traditional) NSAIDs (i.e., not COX-2 inhibitors) which exhibit antiplatelet effects would theoretically have a beneficial effect in attenuating perioperative hypercoagulability and improving cardiovascular outcomes. Although there is no systematic review on this specific topic, the addition of ketorolac to IV PCA morphine has been shown to decrease the number of episodes of myocardial ischemia in noncardiac surgery patients.[36] Thus both epidural analgesia with local anesthetics and systemic use of NSAIDs may decrease perioperative hyper-coagulability and improve cardiac outcome in high-risk patients.

Pulmonary Morbidity

Pain, surgical trespass, and decreased diaphragmatic and intercostal muscle activity all contribute to postoperative pulmonary dysfunction. Certain surgical populations (older patients, patients with preexisting pulmonary disease, type of surgical procedure) may be at higher risk for developing postoperative pulmonary morbidity. Postoperative pulmonary morbidity may be as high as 60% in some of these surgical patients with an associated increase in postoperative mortality rates (4.5%).[8] Through the provision of superior analgesia or attenuation of adverse perioperative pathophysiology, certain modalities of postoperative pain management might theoretically improve postoperative pulmonary outcome. IV PCA administration of opioids provides better analgesia than intramuscular as-needed administration[21] and a meta-analysis comparing IV PCA to as-needed administration of opioids suggested that PCA with opioids is associated with a decreased risk of pulmonary complications.[22]

It is recognized that epidural analgesia with a local anesthetic-based regimen provides better analgesia than IV PCA opioids,[30] which might theoretically provide greater benefit in decreasing the frequency of postoperative pulmonary complications. A meta-analysis of randomized controlled trials assessing the effects of seven analgesic therapies (including systemic opioids and epidural analgesia with local anesthetics) on postoperative pulmonary function after a variety of procedures demonstrated that patients who received epidural local anesthetics had a decreased incidence of pulmonary infections (relative risk [RR] = 0.36) and pulmonary complications overall (RR = 0.58) compared with systemic opioids.[21] Thus TEA offers the most attractive means to provide superior analgesia and lessened diaphragmatic dysfunction in high-risk patients after upper abdominal and thoracic surgery, and the available systematic analyses support the usefulness of epidural analgesia for reducing postoperative pulmonary morbidity.

Thromboembolic Morbidity

The hypercoagulable state that follows surgery is thought to be a primary determinant of postoperative thromboembolic morbidity. Use of acute pain management to reduce postoperative pain and the accompanying stress response and activation of the sympathetic nervous system may decrease vaso-occlusive and thromboembolic morbidity. Systemic administration of opioids[12] and NSAIDs[46] does not appear to significantly affect the perioperative increase in hemostasis. In contrast, epidural analgesia with local anesthetic regimens has been shown to attenuate perioperative increases in hemostatic function. Epidural analgesia attenuates perioperative increases in coagulation proteins[47] and platelet activity,[12] preserves fibrinolytic activity,[5] and increases arterial and venous blood flow. Systemic absorption of epidural local anesthetics may also be important because local anesthetics also have directly attenuated platelet aggregation and reduced blood viscosity.[3]

Current accumulation of data would suggest that regional anesthetic techniques followed by epidural analgesia containing local anesthetics would provide optimal benefit against thromboembolic morbidity. Randomized controlled trials and meta-analyses generally suggest that intraoperative epidural and spinal anesthesia will decrease postoperative hypercoagulable-related adverse events such as vascular graft thrombosis, deep vein thrombosis, and pulmonary embolism. A meta-analysis of 13 randomized controlled trials in patients undergoing femoral neck fracture repair suggests that those who received neuraxial anesthesia had a lower risk of deep vein thrombosis.[48] These findings are similar to the CORTRA subgroup analysis, which showed that use of neuraxial anesthesia was also associated with decreased odds of developing deep vein thrombosis by 44% and pulmonary embolism by 55%.[32] Use of epidural anesthesia followed by epidural analgesia has been shown to reduce the risk of deep vein thromboses (up to a fivefold reduction) and pulmonary emboli (threefold reduction) after orthopedic[49] and urologic surgery.[50]

Clinical trials suggest that use of epidural anesthesia followed by epidural analgesia also improves survival of lower extremity vascular grafts. Tuman and associates randomized patients undergoing vascular surgery to receive either general anesthesia followed by systemic opioids or a combined general-epidural anesthesia followed by epidural analgesia. Use of epidural analgesia was associated with a ninefold reduction in incidence of vascular graft occlusion.[12] Christopherson and colleagues reported similar results in patients undergoing lower extremity revascularization.[13] Patients were randomized to either general anesthesia followed by systemic opioids or epidural anesthesia followed by epidural analgesia.

Use of epidural analgesia was associated with a five-fold decrease in incidence of reoperation.[13]

Thus the modality of postoperative pain management may influence thromboembolic morbidity in selected patient populations. Use of epidural anesthesia followed by epidural analgesia appears to be associated with a reduced risk of lower extremity vascular graft failure and formation of deep vein thromboses after orthopedic and urologic surgery. One of the difficulties in interpreting these studies, however, is the fact that many early studies did not concurrently use systemic anticoagulant prophylaxis. As such, the true benefit of perioperative regional analgesia in decreasing deep vein thrombosis and pulmonary embolism remains uncertain.

Gastrointestinal Morbidity

Postoperative pain and resultant activation of the stress response and sympathetic nervous system are thought to be major determinants of the severity and duration of postoperative ileus. Analgesic modalities that have been suggested to favorably affect postoperative gastrointestinal (GI) function are epidural local anesthetics and NSAIDs. In addition to providing superior analgesia, epidural local anesthetics can block both the afferent and efferent limbs of the spinal reflex contributing to ileus.[17] Systemic absorption of epidural local anesthetics may also contribute to improved postoperative GI function. Both intraperitoneal and intravenous administration of local anesthetics speeds return of propulsive motility in the colon and shortens duration of postoperative ileus.[51,52] Proposed mechanisms for systemic effects of local anesthetics on the GI tract are a direct excitatory effect on intestinal smooth muscle, reduction of opioid analgesic requirement, and block of the inhibitory spinal reflex arc.[52] Furthermore, segmental neural block of thoracic and lumbar dermatomes with epidural local anesthetic would theoretically block inhibitory sympathetic outflow to the GI tract.[53] The parasympathetic nervous system promotes motility in the GI tract and is mediated via the vagus nerve and pelvic nerves originating from the sacral spinal cord. Thus segmental block of only the thoracic and lumbar dermatomes via a thoracic epidural catheter should preserve the beneficial activity of the parasympathetic system while providing pain relief and attenuation of the sympathetic system.

Systemic administration of NSAIDs, such as ketorolac, may reduce the severity and duration of postoperative ileus.[54-56] NSAIDs may favorably affect postoperative GI function by directly inhibiting production of prostaglandins contributing to ileus and decreasing the need for opioid analgesia.[55,57] Although some randomized trials have demonstrated faster recovery of GI function with ketorolac when added to systemic or epidural opioid, a recent meta-analysis suggested no benefit for NSAIDs (including COX-2 inhibitors) in preventing bowel dysfunction.[26] In addition, NSAIDs such as ketorolac have not been shown to be an effective sole analgesic agent for postoperative analgesia,[58,59] and are best used as adjunctive analgesics to epidural or systemic analgesia.

Numerous well-designed clinical trials examine effects of different epidural analgesic regimens on postoperative ileus. A systematic review of available randomized trials indicates a consistently faster recovery of GI function with epidural administration of local anesthetics (with and without opioid) when compared with systemic or epidural opioids.[60] TEA with local anesthetics may also provide earlier fulfillment of discharge criteria.[14] In contrast to the theoretic benefits of epidural local anesthetics and systemic NSAIDs, both epidural and systemic opioids have been shown to directly inhibit GI motility. Spinal cord activity of epidural opioids directly inhibits colonic motility and contributes to postoperative ileus.[3,14] Systemic administration of opioids has been clearly demonstrated to delay gastric emptying, delay colonic transit, and contribute to postoperative ileus.[54] Administration of systemic opioids with IV PCA does not lessen the severity or duration of postoperative ileus when compared to intramuscular administration on an as-needed basis.[54]

Patient-Oriented Outcomes

The vast majority of the available literature has focused on the effect of different analgesic regimens on "traditional" clinically oriented patient outcomes such as morbidity and mortality; however, far fewer studies have examined the effect of postoperative pain on patient-oriented ("nontraditional") outcomes such as patient satisfaction, quality of life, and quality of recovery. The emphasis on patient-oriented assessments reflects the increasing interest in these end points in other areas of medicine, mirrors the rise of consumerism of health care (e.g., "customer service"), and comes at a time when the incidence of anesthetic-related mortality and major morbidity has dramatically declined as more difficult to assess in clinical trials.[61] By affecting many physical and mental aspects of a patient's recovery, acute postoperative pain may have an adverse effect on a variety of patient-oriented outcomes.

Although we are just beginning to fully evaluate the effect of postoperative pain on patient-oriented outcomes, it is not difficult to appreciate that different analgesic options (systemic opioids vs. NSAIDs, vs. regional analgesia) provide different levels of analgesia, are associated with different side effects, and consequently may result in different levels of patient satisfaction or quality of recovery.[61] Postoperative epidural analgesia provides significantly superior analgesia when compared with that of systemic opioids,[29] and as such, epidural analgesia may have a beneficial effect on patient satisfaction, quality of life, or quality of recovery compared to systemic opioids. Two prospective, nonrandomized observational trials suggested that an increase in the level of postoperative pain is associated with a decrease in a patient's quality of life and quality of recovery in the immediate postoperative period.[62,63] In a randomized controlled trial, epidural analgesia compared to IV PCA with opioids provided superior postoperative pain control and was associated with preservation of health-related quality of life after abdominal surgery.[64] Although there is no valid study assessing patient satisfaction as a primary end point, a systematic review indicates that use of regional analgesic techniques, compared to systemic opioids, results in higher patient satisfaction.[65] Thus assessment of patient-oriented end points is a widely accepted outcome measurement and may be adversely affected by an increase in postoperative pain. Postoperative epidural analgesia may improve patient-oriented outcomes, although there are many methodologic issues in available trials.

Economic Outcomes

Although alleviation of acute pain by itself is a worthwhile endeavor, concerns over soaring costs of medical care have led to interest and debate over the best means to contain these costs. Currently, there are no studies that properly evaluate the economic effects of a specific analgesic technique or option. The cost savings of postoperative analgesia (reduction in morbidity, decreases in hospital stay) need to be weighed against the potential cost increases (personnel, drugs, complications) and evaluated in a comprehensive fashion.

Although an inclusive discussion of cost and cost analysis is beyond the scope of this chapter, the four most commonly used methods for economic analysis in health care are cost minimization, cost-benefit analysis, cost-effectiveness analysis, and cost-usefulness analysis.[66-68] Cost minimization is determination of the least amount of money required to provide a service regardless of patient outcome. Although cost minimization studies often focus on drug costs alone, it is also important to examine modality costs. For example, drug costs of inpatient opioid analgesia with morphine are highest with controlled-release morphine when compared with costs of conventional oral and parenteral morphine; however, the total direct costs of providing analgesia with controlled-release morphine are lower because of a lower pharmacy staff, nursing, and ancillary supply costs.[69] Thus a cheaper drug or more expensive modality may not portray the entire economic picture.

Cost-benefit analysis increases the scope of economic analysis by taking into account the monetary benefit acquired for the total cost spent for an intervention. The major difficulty in this analysis is the attachment of monetary numbers to a benefit. Cost-effectiveness analysis is similar to cost-benefit but sidesteps the issue of monetary value of a benefit. This approach defines a measure of effectiveness (e.g., Visual Analogue Scale pain score) and determines a cost per unit of effectiveness (e.g., $10 [U.S. dollars] per 5-mm reduction in pain score with the use of drug X). Thus by definition the most cost-effective treatment may not be the cheapest.[70] Difficulties with this type of analysis include agreement on the desired effect and ability to gather reliable data on incidence of complications and costs of complication management. It is also important to realize that cost-effectiveness analysis may be specific for the intervention, patient population, and for the work patterns and experiences of the sponsoring institution.[71] Finally, cost-usefulness analysis carries cost-effectiveness analysis one step further by assigning a value to the outcome of an intervention. In this analysis the outcome of an intervention is the number of additional years of life gained after adjustment for quality. This outcome is commonly expressed as quality-adjusted life years (QALY).[72] In this type of outcome, a year of good health has more value than a year of bad health and death may be better than a poor quality survival.

COMPLICATIONS FROM ACUTE POSTOPERATIVE PAIN MANAGEMENT

Potential benefits from postoperative pain management must be balanced against potential complications. Although a comprehensive risk-benefit analysis for each analgesic option discussed has not been published, it should be recognized that the presence of complications or side effects will reduce the overall analgesic efficacy of the particular analgesic option. The following section briefly reviews complications from systemic and epidural analgesia.

SYSTEMIC ANALGESIA

Systemic Opioids

All opioid agonists are capable of producing similar complications in equianalgesic doses. Common complications from use of systemic opioids are nausea, pruritus, urinary retention, sedation, constipation, and respiratory depression. Although most complications are dose dependent, individual responses to systemic opioids are highly variable.[73] Probably the most feared complication of opioid use is life-threatening respiratory depression. Fortunately, premonitory signs of central nervous system depression usually precede respiratory depression. Very few large-scale surveillance studies have been performed to determine the incidences of respiratory depression after systemic administration of opioids for postoperative pain management. Commonly quoted incidences are approximately 0.9% with an as-needed administration[74] and approximately 0.8% with IV PCA administration.[75] With such a low incidence, no real risk factors have been identified. Systemic opioids for postoperative analgesia have a long history of relatively safe use on hospital wards, with few serious side effects.

Nonsteroidal Anti-inflammatory Drugs

The three most serious perioperative complications from NSAID use are renal impairment, impaired hemostasis, and GI disturbance. In general, complications from NSAIDs can be minimized by avoiding high doses, avoiding long duration of therapy, and using caution with older adult patients. Renal impairment from NSAIDs may occur as acute renal failure or as nephrotic syndrome. Acute renal failure associated with NSAID use is rare, with an approximate incidence of 1.1%.[76] There appears to be an association between duration of NSAID therapy and development of acute renal failure. In a retrospective analysis of patients receiving 10,219 courses of ketorolac, use of ketorolac for greater than 5 days was associated with twice the risk of developing renal failure (OR = 1.08 to 4).[76] In contrast, incidence of acute renal failure after use of ketorolac for less than 5 days was no greater than the incidence observed after opioids (1.1%). Nephrotic syndrome is an idiosyncratic drug reaction to many NSAIDs and usually resolves after cessation of NSAID therapy.[77]

NSAIDs have depressant effects on platelet function. Potential hemostatic complications from NSAIDs are operative site and GI bleeding. A study comparing 10,272 courses of ketorolac to 10,247 courses of opioids determined no significant association between use of ketorolac and operative site bleeding.[78] Patients receiving ketorolac had a slightly greater chance of GI bleeding (OR = 1.3). Further risk factors for GI bleeding were use of ketorolac for greater than 5 days, increased dose of ketorolac, and age of patient of more than 75 years.

One of the more recent developments in the use of NSAIDs has been the association of the COX-2 inhibitors, with an increased incidence of cardiovascular events such as myocardial function. It is now recognized that the COX-2 enzyme may play an important cardioprotective role via prostacyclin I_2 (PGI_2).[79] By inhibiting PGI_2, COX-2 inhibitors may actually promote thrombosis via the unopposed action of thromboxane A_2. A meta-analysis of rofecoxib trials indicated that administration of rofecoxib is associated with an increased risk when compared to control.[80] Although rofecoxib was withdrawn because of cardiovascular adverse effects, celecoxib remained on the market because the data linking celecoxib to cardiovascular events did not seem as clear-cut as that for rofecoxib (possibly because of the greater selectivity for COX-2 by rofecoxib), although more recent data also suggested that celecoxib was associated with a higher incidence of cardiovascular events.[81-83]

Epidural Analgesia

Analgesic Agents

Commonly used agents for epidural analgesia include local anesthetics and opioids. Common complications from the use of local anesthetics for epidural analgesia include motor block, hypotension, urinary retention, and pressure necrosis.[17] Use of larger doses (e.g., higher concentrations) of local anesthetics appears to increase the risk of motor block and hypotension.[84,85] The site of epidural placement also affects incidence of motor and autonomic block. Placement of thoracic epidural catheters diminishes the risk of motor block[86] and results in incidence of hypotension comparable to systemic morphine.[87,88] Although there is a wide range reported for the incidence of motor block with epidural analgesia, partly because of the differences in definitions used, a meta-analysis of randomized controlled trials indicates that the incidence of motor block with postoperative epidural analgesia ranges from 1% to 7%.[29,89] Complications from epidural local anesthetics can be minimized by using small doses and placing thoracic catheters where appropriate.

Epidural administration of opioids results in pruritus (0% to 100% incidence), nausea (~30%), urinary retention (0% to 80%), and respiratory depression (0.2% to 1.9%).[90] None of these complications are clearly dose related, and all can occur with any commonly used opioid (morphine, fentanyl, sufentanil, hydromorphone, meperidine).[90] Respiratory depression is probably the most serious complication from epidural opioids. All commonly used opioids for epidural analgesia have been reported to result in clinically important respiratory depression.[90] Both early (less than 2 hours after administration) and late respiratory depression can occur with epidural opioids. Virtually all reports of clinically important respiratory depression with epidural opioids have involved morphine.[90] The hydrophilic nature of morphine with resultant cephalad cerebrospinal fluid migration well explains this observation.[91] Nonetheless, large-scale surveillance studies report similar incidences of clinical respiratory depression with the use of bolus morphine (0.2%),[74] infusions of morphine/bupivacaine (0.07%),[92] fentanyl/bupivacaine (0.4%),[93] sufentanil/bupivacaine (0.4%),[94] and patient-controlled epidural analgesia with fentanyl/bupivacaine (0.2%).[86] These low incidences have precluded the determination of important risk factors for respiratory depression and indicate that epidural analgesia can be safely used on hospital wards.

Catheter-Related Complications

Despite the fact that epidural analgesia provides superior pain control compared with systemic opioids in the postoperative period, a certain percentage of epidural catheters will become dislodged prematurely, which decreases the overall analgesic efficacy of this technique. A systematic review of 165 trials noted that actual premature epidural catheter dislodgement was 5.7%,[95] a rate similar (approximately 5% to 7%) to those reported for labor epidurals.[96] Epidural catheters also may migrate to other locations such as the intrathecal or intravascular space. Several large-scale observational trials indicate that the incidence ranges from 0% to 0.2%.[97-100] Migration of the epidural catheter from the epidural space into a blood vessel is also uncommon and large-scale observational trials indicate that the incidence ranges

from 0% to 0.7%.[98-101] This is similar to the intravascular migration rate (0.25%) reported in a large-scale cohort study of 19,259 neuraxial blocks for labor analgesia.[96]

Symptomatic epidural hematoma is probably one of the most serious complications from epidural analgesia. Puncture of epidural vessels during placement of epidural catheters occurs in approximately 3% to 12% of cases.[102] Although formation of asymptomatic hematomas is common (up to 60%),[103] development of symptomatic epidural hematomas is rare. Examination of large, mostly retrospective, series of patients suggests an incidence of approximately 1:150,000 for epidural hematoma after epidural anesthesia/analgesia.[104] Although epidural catheters have been safely used in patients receiving anticoagulants such as heparin,[105] warfarin,[106] and antiplatelet agents,[107] there appears to be an association between development of epidural hematoma and impaired coagulation. In a review of 61 cases of epidural hematoma, a hemostatic abnormality was present in 69% of the cases.[104] Recently, low-molecular-weight heparin (LMWH) has been introduced for deep vein thrombosis prophylaxis and the differences between LMWH and traditional heparin (higher and more predictable bioavailability, longer-half, and minimal affect on traditional tests of coagulation)[108] may have contributed to the higher incidence of epidural hematomas associated with LMWH use in North America[109] despite the fairly extensive European experience with LMWHs previously (approximately 100,000 patients with spinal or epidural anesthesia in combination with LMWH with 6 reported cases of epidural hematoma).[110] A set of consensus statements for the administration of regional anesthesia and analgesia in the anticoagulated patient has been developed by the American Society of Regional Anesthesia (www.asra.com).

Neurologic injury is another uncommon complication of epidural analgesia. Prospective studies suggest that incidence of neurologic injury is approximately 0.002% to 0.16% and is usually self-limited.[92,111-113] There is often a concern of increased risk of neurologic injury with placement of thoracic as opposed to lumbar epidural catheters. Clearly the epidural space is smaller and the spinal cord is present when thoracic epidural catheters are placed.[114] However, a prospective series examining 4185 patients undergoing placement of thoracic epidural catheters reported a 0.7% incidence of neurologic injury. None of these injuries clinically involved the spinal cord (paraplegia).[113] Thus risk of neurologic injury does not appear to be greater with placement of thoracic versus lumbar epidural catheters in experienced hands.

A final rare and serious complication of epidural analgesia is formation of an epidural abscess. An approximate incidence of occurrence with epidural analgesia is 0.02% to 0.05%.[92,115] Epidural abscesses may occur in the absence of epidural catheters as a result of hematogenous rather than direct spread,[116] and do not appear to be associated with duration of epidural catheterization.[117] A large-scale survey indicates that the patients with epidural abscess had a longer mean catheterization time, the majority of patients with epidural abscess were immunocompromised by one or more complicating diseases, and that the level of catheter insertion was not critical to the likelihood of abscess formation.[117] Nonetheless, an epidural catheter offers an obvious route of infectious entry into the epidural space. Daily assessment of benefits of analgesia versus risk of complications should be made for every patient.

CONCLUSION

The adverse pathophysiology that occurs postoperatively may contribute to increased perioperative morbidity and mortality. Pathophysiology of postoperative pain offers several avenues for acute pain management to beneficially influence outcome. Certain analgesic options, such as regional analgesia, may be possibly more efficacious in attenuating perioperative pathophysiology and providing superior analgesia. Although there are methodologic issues in the interpretation of available data, there is a suggestion that use of epidural analgesia in high-risk populations may improve cardiac, pulmonary, gastrointestinal, and coagulation-related outcomes. The benefits of these analgesic techniques must be weighed against the possible risks or complications associated with the techniques and assessed on an individual basis. Further well-designed studies are needed to determine effects of acute pain management on postoperative outcome, patient-oriented outcomes, and costs of medical care.

SUMMARY

- Perioperative pathophysiology affects many systems and may contribute to postoperative morbidity and mortality. Attenuation of perioperative pathophysiology might improve patient outcomes.
- Different classes of analgesic agents have different effects in their capability in attenuating perioperative pathophysiology. For instance, epidural analgesia with a local anesthetic-based analgesic regimen may attenuate perioperative pathophysiology to a greater extent than systemic opioids. This differential effect on perioperative pathophysiology may result in a difference in patient outcomes with different analgesic regimens.
- Use of postoperative epidural analgesia may be associated with an improvement in some patient outcomes such as a decrease in cardiovascular, pulmonary, gastrointestinal, and patient-oriented outcomes in high-risk patients. However, there are methodology issues in interpreting available data.
- Many factors (e.g., catheter incision congruency, duration of analgesia, analgesic agents used) in the use of epidural analgesia may influence patient outcomes.
- Any potential benefits from a particular postoperative analgesic regimen must be balanced against any potential complications, and the choice of a particular postoperative analgesic regimen should be made on an individual basis including consideration of patient preferences.

References

1. Mangano DT, Goldman L: Preoperative assessment of patients with known or suspected coronary disease. N Engl J Med 1995;333:1750-1756.
2. Mangano DT: Perioperative cardiac morbidity. Anesthesiology 1990;72:153-184.
3. Wu CL, Fleisher LA: Outcomes research in regional anesthesia and analgesia. Anesth Analg 2000;91:1232-1242.
4. Jain U, Laflamme CJ, Aggarwal A, et al: Electrocardiographic and hemodynamic changes and their association with myocardial infarction during coronary artery bypass surgery. Anesthesiology 1997;86:576-591.
5. Rosenfeld BA, Beattie C, Christopherson R, et al: The effects of different anesthetic regimens on fibrinolysis and the development of postoperative arterial thrombosis. Anesthesiology 1993;79:435-443.
6. Parker SD, Breslow MJ, Frank SM, et al: Catecholamine and cortisol responses to lower extremity revascularization: Correlation with outcome variables. Crit Care Med 1995;23:1954-1961.
7. Warner DO: Preventing postoperative pulmonary complications: The role of the anesthesiologist. Anesthesiology 2000;92:1467-1472.
8. Pedersen T, Eliasen K, Henriksen E, et al: A prospective study of mortality associated with anesthesia and surgery: Risk indicators of cardiopulmonary morbidity. Acta Anaesthesiol Scand 1990;34:144-155.
9. Craig DB: Postoperative recovery of pulmonary function. Anesth Analg 1981;60:46-52.
10. Mankikian B, Cantineau JP, Bertrand M, et al: Improvement of diaphragmatic function by a thoracic epidural block after upper abdominal surgery. Anesthesiology 1988;68:379-386.
11. Kroegel C, Reissig A: Principle mechanisms underlying venous thromboembolism: Epidemiology, risk factors, pathophysiology and pathogenesis. Respiration 2003;70:7-30.
12. Tuman KJ, McCarthy RJ, March RJ, et al: Effects of epidural anesthesia and analgesia on coagulation and outcome after major vascular surgery. Anesth Analg 1991;73:696-704.
13. Christopherson R, Beattie C, Frank SM, et al: Perioperative morbidity in patients randomized to epidural or general anesthesia for lower extremity vascular surgery. Anesthesiology 1993;79:422-434.
14. Liu SS, Carpenter RL, Mackey DC, et al: Effects of perioperative analgesic technique on rate of recovery after colon surgery. Anesthesiology 1995;83:757-765.
15. Moore FA, Feliciano DV, Andrassy RJ, et al: Early enteral feeding, compared with parenteral, reduces postoperative septic complications: The results of a meta-analysis. Ann Surg 1992;216:172-183.
16. Shou J, Lappin J, Minnard EA, et al: Total parenteral nutrition, bacterial translocation, and host immune function. Am J Surg 1994;167:145-150.
17. Liu SS, Carpenter RL, Neal JM: Epidural anesthesia and analgesia: Their role in postoperative outcome. Anesthesiology 1995;82:1474-1506.
18. Naito Y, Tamai S, Shingu K, et al: Response of plasma adrenocorticotropic hormone, cortisol, and cytokines during and after upper abdominal surgery. Anesthesiology 1992;77:426-431.
19. Douglas RG, Shaw JH: Metabolic response to sepsis and trauma. Br J Surg 1989;76:115-122.
20. Anand KJ, Hickey PR: Halothane-morphine compared with high dose sufentanil for anesthesia and postoperative analgesia in neonatal cardiac surgery. New Engl J Med 1992;326:1-9.
21. Ballantyne JC, Carr DB, deFerranti S, et al: The comparative effects of postoperative analgesic therapies on pulmonary outcome: Cumulative meta-analyses of randomized, controlled trials. Anesth Analg 1998;86:598-612.
22. Walder B, Schafer M, Henzi I, et al: Efficacy and safety of patient-controlled opioid analgesia for acute postoperative pain: A quantitative systematic review. Acta Anaesthesiol Scand 2001;45:795-804.

23. Oxford League: Table of analgesics in acute pain, 2005. Available at www.jr2.ox.ac.uk/bandolier/booth/painpag/Acutrev/Analgesics/Leagtab.html.
24. Marret E, Kurdi O, Zufferey P, et al: Effects of nonsteroidal antiinflammatory drugs on patient-controlled analgesia morphine side effects. Anesthesiology 2005;102:1249-1260.
25. Remy C, Marret E, Bonnet F: Effects of acetaminophen on morphine side-effects and consumption after major surgery: Meta-analysis of randomized controlled trials. Br J Anaesth 2005;94:505-513.
26. Elia N, Lysakowski C, Tramer MR: Does multimodal analgesia with acetaminophen, nonsteroidal antiinflammatory drugs, or selective cyclooxygenase-2 inhibitors and patient-controlled analgesia morphine offer advantages over morphine alone? Anesthesiology 2005;103:1296-1304.
27. Straube S, Derry S, McQuay HJ, et al: Effect of preoperative COX-II-selective NSAIDs (coxibs) on postoperative outcomes: A systematic review of randomized trials. Acta Anaesthesiol Scand 2005;49:601-613.
28. Kranke P, Morin AM, Roewer N, et al: Patients' global evaluation of analgesia and safety of injected parecoxib for postoperative pain: A quantitative systematic review. Anesth Analg 2004;99:797-806.
29. Block BM, Liu SS, Rowlingson AJ, et al: Efficacy of postoperative epidural analgesia: A meta-analysis. JAMA 2003;290:2455-2463.
30. Wu CL, Cohen SR, Richman JM, et al: Efficacy of postoperative patient-controlled and continuous infusion epidural analgesia versus intravenous patient-controlled analgesia with opioids: A meta-analysis. Anesthesiology 2005;103:1079-1088.
31. Richman JM, Liu SS, Courpas G, et al: Does continuous peripheral nerve block provide superior pain control to opioids? A meta-analysis. Anesth Analg 2006;102:248-257.
32. Rodgers A, Walker N, Schug S, et al: Reduction of postoperative mortality and morbidity with epidural or spinal anaesthesia: Results from overview of randomised trials. BMJ 2000;321:1493.
33. Wu CL, Hurley RW, Anderson GF, et al: Effect of postoperative epidural analgesia on morbidity and mortality following surgery in Medicare patients. Reg Anesth Pain Med 2004;29:525-533.
34. Wu CL, Anderson GF, Herbert R, et al: Effect of postoperative epidural analgesia on morbidity and mortality after total hip replacement surgery in Medicare patients. Reg Anesth Pain Med 2003;28:271-278.
35. Mangano DT, Siliciano D, Hollenberg M, et al: Postoperative myocardial ischemia. Therapeutic trials using intensive analgesia following surgery. Anesthesiology 1992;76:342-353.
36. Beattie WS, Warriner CB, Etches R, et al: The addition of continuous intravenous infusion of ketorolac to a patient-controlled analgetic morphine regimen reduced postoperative myocardial ischemia in patients undergoing elective total hip or knee arthroplasty. Anesth Analg 1997;84:715-722.
37. Breslow MJ, Jordan DA, Christopherson R, et al: Epidural morphine decreases postoperative hypertension by attenuating sympathetic nervous system hyperactivity. JAMA 1989;261:3577-3581.
38. Guyenet PG, Cabot JB: Inhibition of sympathetic preganglionic neurons by catecholamines and clonidine: Mediation by an alpha adrenergic receptor. J Neurosci 1981;1:908-917.
39. Stevens RA, Artuso J, Kao T, et al: Changes in human plasma catecholamines concentrations during epidural anesthesia depend on level of the block. Anesthesiology 1991;74:1029-1034.
40. Blomberg S, Emanuelsson H, Ricksten SE: Thoracic epidural anesthesia and central hemodynamics in patients with unstable angina pectoris. Anesth Analg 1989;69:558-562.
41. Blomberg S, Emanuelsson H, Kvist H, et al: Effects of thoracic epidural anesthesia on coronary arteries and arterioles in patients with coronary artery disease. Anesthesiology 1990;73:840-847.
42. Saada M, Catoire P, Bonnet F, et al: Effect of thoracic epidural anesthesia combined with general anesthesia on segmental wall motion assessed by transesophageal echocardiography. Anesth Analg 1992;75:329-335.
43. Saada M, Duval A-M, Bonnet F, et al: Abnormalities in myocardial segmental wall motion during lumbar epidural anesthesia. Anesthesiology 1989;71:26-32.
44. Beattie WS, Badner NH, Choi P: Epidural analgesia reduces postoperative myocardial infarction: A meta-analysis. Anesth Analg 2001;93:853-858.
45. Liu SS, Block BM, Wu CL: Effects of perioperative central neuraxial analgesia on outcome after coronary artery bypass surgery: A meta-analysis. Anesthesiology 2004;101:153-161.
46. Varrassi G, Panella L, Piroli A, et al: The effects of perioperative ketorolac infusion on postoperative pain and endocrine-metabolic response. Anesth Analg 1994;78:514-519.
47. Donadoni R, Baele G, Devulder J, et al: Coagulation and fibrinolytic parameters in patients undergoing total hip replacement: Influence of anaesthesia technique. Acta Anaesthesiol Scand 1989;33:588-592.
48. Sorenson RM, Pace NL: Anesthetic techniques during surgical repair of femoral neck fractures: A meta-analysis. Anesthesiology 1992;77:1095-1104.
49. Sharrock NE, Haas SB, Hargett MJ, et al: Effects of epidural anesthesia on the incidence of deep-vein thrombosis after total knee arthroplasty. J Bone Joint Surg Am 1991;73:502-506.
50. Hendolin H, Mattila MA, Poikolainen E: The effect of lumbar epidural analgesia on the development of deep vein thrombosis of the legs after open prostatectomy. Acta Chir Scand 1981;147:425-429.
51. Rimback G, Cassuto JH, Wallin G, et al: Effect of intra-abdominal bupivacaine instillation on postoperative colonic motility. Gut 1986;27:170-175.
52. Rimback G, Cassuto J, Tollesson P: Treatment of postoperative paralytic ileus by intravenous lidocaine infusion. Anesth Analg 1990;70:414-419.
53. Hogan QH, Stadnicka A, Stekiel TA, et al: Region of epidural blockade determines sympathetic and mesenteric capacitance effects in rabbits. Anesthesiology 1995;83:604-610.
54. Nitschke LF, Schlosser CT, Berg RL, et al: Does patient-controlled analgesia achieve better control of pain and fewer adverse effects than intramuscular analgesia? A prospective randomized trial. Arch Surg 1996;31:417-423.
55. Parker RK, Holtmann B, Smith I, et al: Use of ketorolac after lower abdominal surgery: Effect on analgesic requirement and surgical outcome. Anesthesiology 1994;80:6-12.
56. Grass JA, Sakima NT, Valley M, et al: Assessment of ketorolac as an adjuvant to fentanyl patient-controlled epidural analgesia after radical retropubic prostatectomy. Anesthesiology 1993;78:642-648.
57. Ready LB, Brown CR, Stahlgren LH, et al: Evaluation of intravenous ketorolac administered by bolus or infusion for treatment of postoperative pain: A double-blind, placebo-controlled, multicenter study. Anesthesiology 1994;80:1277-1286.
58. Cepeda MS, Vargas L, Ortegon G, et al: Comparative analgesic efficacy of patient-controlled analgesia with ketorolac versus morphine after elective intraabdominal operations. Anesth Analg 1995;80:1150-1153.
59. Bosek V, Miguel R: Comparison of morphine and ketorolac for intravenous patient-controlled analgesia in postoperative cancer patients. Clin J Pain 1994;10:314-318.
60. Jorgensen H, Wetterslev J, Moiniche S, et al: Epidural local anaesthetics versus opioid-based analgesic regimens on postoperative gastrointestinal paralysis, PONV and pain after abdominal surgery. Cochrane Database Syst Rev 2000;CD001893.
61. Wu CL, Richman JM: Postoperative pain and quality of recovery. Curr Opin Anesthesiol 2004;17:455-460.
62. Wu CL, Rowlingson AJ, Partin AW, et al: Correlation of postoperative pain to quality of recovery in the immediate postoperative period. Reg Anesth Pain Med 2005;30:516-522.
63. Wu CL, Naqibuddin M, Rowlingson AJ, et al: The effect of pain on health-related quality of life in the immediate postoperative period. Anesth Analg 2003;97:1078-1085.

64. Carli F, Mayo N, Klubien K, et al: Epidural analgesia enhances functional exercise capacity and health-related quality of life after colonic surgery: Results of a randomized trial. Anesthesiology 2002;97:540-549.

65. Wu CL, Naqibuddin M, Fleisher LA: Measurement of patient satisfaction as an outcome of regional anesthesia and analgesia: A systematic review. Reg Anesth Pain Med 2001;26: 196-208.

66. Joicoeur LM, Jones-Grizzle AJ, Boyer JG: Guidelines for performing a pharmaco-economic analysis. Am J Hosp Pharm 1992;49:1741-1747.

67. Detsky A, Naglie I: A clinician's guide to cost effectiveness analysis. Ann Intern Med 1990;13:147-154.

68. Wachta MF, White PF: Economics of anesthetic practice. Anesthesiology 1997;86:1170-1196.

69. Goughnour BR: Cost considerations of analgesic therapy: An analysis of dosing frequency and route of administration. Postgrad Med J 1991;67:S87-S91.

70. Neumann PJ, Rosen AB, Weinstein MC: Medicare and cost-effectiveness analysis. N Engl J Med 2005;353:1516-1522.

71. Trotter JP, Renhart SP, Katz RM, et al: Economic assessment of ketorolac versus narcotic analgesia in postoperative pain management. Clin Ther 1993;15:938-948.

72. Robinson R: Cost-utility analysis. BMJ 1993;307:793-795.

73. Gourley GK, Kowalski SR, Plummer JL, et al: Fentanyl blood concentration-analgesic response relationship in the treatment of postoperative pain. Anesth Analg 1988;67: 329-337.

74. Ready LB, Loper KA, Nessly M, et al: Postoperative epidural morphine is safe on surgical wards. Anesthesiology 1991;75: 452-456.

75. Wheatley RG, Madej TH, Jackson IJ, et al: The first year's experience of an acute pain service. Br J Anaesth 1991;67: 353-359.

76. Feldman HI, Kinman JL, Berlin JA, et al: Parenteral ketorolac: The risk for acute renal failure. Ann Intern Med 1997;126: 193-199.

77. Radford MG, Jr., Holley KE, Grande JP, et al: Reversible membranous nephropathy associated with the use of nonsteroidal anti-inflammatory drugs. JAMA 1996;276:466-469.

78. Strom BL, Berlin JA, Kinman JL, et al: Parenteral ketorolac and risk of gastrointestinal and operative site bleeding: A postmarketing surveillance study. JAMA 1996;275:376-382.

79. Howard PA, Delafontaine P: Nonsteroidal anti-inflammatory drugs and cardiovascular risk. J Am Coll Cardiol 2004;43: 519-525.

80. Juni P, Nartey L, Reichenbach S, et al: Risk of cardiovascular events and rofecoxib: Cumulative meta-analysis. Lancet 2004;364:2021-2029.

81. Solomon SD, McMurray JJ, Pfeffer MA, et al: Cardiovascular risk associated with celecoxib in a clinical trial for colorectal adenoma prevention. N Engl J Med 2005;352: 1071-1080.

82. Okie S: Raising the safety bar—The FDA's coxib meeting. N Engl J Med 2005;352:1283-1285.

83. Wright JM: The double-edged sword of COX-2 selective NSAIDs. CMAJ 2002;167:1131-1137.

84. Scott DA, Chamley DM, Mooney PH, et al: Epidural ropivacaine infusion for postoperative analgesia after major lower abdominal surgery—A dose finding study. Anesth Analg 1995;81:982-986.

85. Liu S, Angel JM, Owens BD, et al: Effects of epidural bupivacaine after thoracotomy. Reg Anesth 1995;20:303-310.

86. Liu SS, Allen HW, Olsson GL: Efficacy and incidence of side effects of patient controlled epidural analgesia with bupivacaine/fentanyl on hospital wards. Anesthesiology 1998;88: 688-695.

87. Moinche S, Hjortso N-C, Blemmer T, et al: Blood pressure and heart rate during orthostatic stress and walking with continuous postoperative thoracic epidural bupivacaine/morphine. Acta Anaesthesiol Scand 1993;37:65-69.

88. Crawford ME, Moiniche S, Orbaek J, et al: Orthostatic hypotension during postoperative continuous thoracic epidural bupivacaine-morphine in patients undergoing abdominal surgery. Anesth Analg 1996;83:1028-1032.

89. Wigfull J, Welchew E: Survey of 1057 patients receiving postoperative patient-controlled epidural analgesia. Anaesthesia 2001;56:70-75.

90. Chaney MA: Side effects of intrathecal and epidural opioids. Can J Anaesth 1995;42:891-903.

91. Shook JE, Watkins WD, Camporesi EM: Differential role of opioid receptors in respiration, respiratory disease, and opiate-induced respiratory depression. Am Rev Respir Dis 1990;142:895-909.

92. de Leon-Casasola OA, Parker B, Lema MJ: Postoperative epidural bupivacaine-morphine therapy: Experience with 4,227 surgical cancer patients. Anesthesiology 1994;81:368-375.

93. Scott DA, Beilby DSN, McClymont C: Postoperative analgesia using epidural infusions of fentanyl with bupivacaine: A prospective analysis of 1,014 patients. Anesthesiolology 1995;83:727-737.

94. Broekema AA, Gielen MJM, Hennis PJ: Postoperative analgesia with continuous epidural sufentanil and bupivacaine: A prospective study in 614 patients. Anesth Analg 1996;82: 754-759.

95. Dolin SJ, Cashman JN, Bland JM: Effectiveness of acute postoperative pain management: I. Evidence from published data. Br J Anaesth 2002;89:409-423.

96. Paech MJ, Godkin R, Webster S: Complications of obstetric epidural analgesia and anaesthesia: A prospective analysis of 10,995 cases. Int J Obstet Anesth 1998;7:5-11.

97. de Leon-Casasola OA, Parker B, Lema MJ: Postoperative epidural bupivacaine-morphine therapy: Experience with 4,227 surgical cancer patients. Anesthesiology 1994;81: 368-375.

98. Wheatley RG, Schug SA, Watson D: Safety and efficacy of postoperative epidural analgesia. Br J Anaesth 2001;87: 47-61.

99. Ready LB: Acute pain: Lessons learned from 25,000 patients. Reg Anesth Pain Med 1999;24:499-505.

100. Tanaka K, Watanabe R, Harada T, et al: Extensive application of epidural anesthesia and analgesia in a university hospital: Incidence of complications related to technique. Reg Anesth 1993;18:34-38.

101. Burstal R, Wegener F, Hayes C, et al: Epidural analgesia: Prospective audit of 1062 patients. Anaesth Intensive Care 1998;26:165-172.

102. Mulroy MF, Norris MC, Liu SS: Safety steps in epidural injection of local anesthetics: Review of the literature and safety recommendations. Anesth Analg 1997;85:1346-1356.

103. Wulf H, Striepling E: Postmortem findings after epidural anaesthesia. Anaesthesia 1990;45:357-361.

104. Vandermeulen EP, Aken V, Vermylen J: Anticoagulants and spinal-epidural anesthesia. Anesth Analg 1994;79:1165-1169.

105. Rao TLK, El-Etr AA: Anticoagulation following placement of epidural and subarachnoid catheters: An evaluation of neurologic sequelae. Anesthesiology 1981;55:618-620.

106. Horlocker TT, Wedel DJ, Schlichting JL: Postoperative epidural analgesia and oral anticoagulant therapy. Anesth Analg 1994;79:89-93.

107. Horlocker TT, Wedel DJ, Schroeder DR, et al: Preoperative antiplatelet therapy does not increase the risk of spinal hematoma associated with regional anesthesia. Anesth Analg 1995;80:303-309.

108. Horlocker TT, Heit JA: Low molecular weight heparin: Biochemistry, pharmacology, perioperative prophylaxis regimens, and guidelines for regional anesthetic management. Anesth Analg 1997;85:874-885.

109. Horlocker TT, Wedel DJ, Benzon H, et al: Regional anesthesia in the anticoagulated patient: Defining the risks. Reg Anesth Pain Med 2003;28:172-197.

110. Rauck RL: The anticoagulated patient. Reg Anesth 1996; 21(6S):51-56.

111. Moen V, Dahlgren N, Irestedt L: Severe neurological complications after central neuraxial blockades in Sweden 1990-1999. Anesthesiology 2004;101:950-959.

112. Auroy Y, Narchi P, Messiah A, et al: Serious complications related to regional anesthesia. Anesthesiology 1997;87:479-486.
113. Giebler RM, Scherer RU, Peters J: Incidence of neurologic complications related to thoracic epidural catheterization. Anesthesiology 1997;86:55-63.
114. Hogan QH: Epidural anatomy examined by cryomicrotome section: Influence of age, vertebral level, and disease. Reg Anesth 1996;21:395-406.
115. Wang LP, Hauerberg J, Schmidt JF: Incidence of spinal epidural abscess after epidural analgesia: A national 1-year survey. Anesthesiology 1999;91:1928-1936.
116. Baker AS, Ojemann RG: Spinal epidural abscess. N Engl J Med 1975;293:463-468.
117. Darchy B, Forceville X, Bavoux E, et al: Clinical and bacteriologic survey of epidural analgesia in patients in the intensive care unit. Anesthesiology 1996;85:988-998.

70 Outcomes, Efficacy, and Complications of the Treatment of Back Pain

Honorio T. Benzon

The lifetime prevalence of low back pain (LBP) is approximately 80%.[1] This condition is second only to the common cold as the reason patients seek medical care. The estimated cost of medical care for patients with LBP exceeds $8 billion annually.[2] In view of the high prevalence and high cost of back pain, the pain medicine physician should be aware of the outcomes, efficacy, and complications of the treatments of LBP. To present an overview of this subject, I discuss the following topics: (1) the presence of abnormal findings such as herniated disk and spinal stenosis in asymptomatic patients; (2) follow-up of asymptomatic patients including the resolution of herniated disks; (3) outcome measures and measurement tools used in the studies on LBP; (4) long-term results of surgery in patients with LBP; (5) results of interventional procedures in patients with LBP; (6) psychological management of back pain; and, (7) pharmacologic management of back pain. It is hoped that the reader will gain a better idea of the role of these treatments.

ABNORMAL DIAGNOSTIC FINDINGS IN ASYMPTOMATIC PATIENTS

The presence of abnormal findings in individuals who never had back pain or radiculopathy has been known for some time. Herniated disks were seen in 24% of patients who had myelograms for reasons other than back pain[3] and abnormal diskograms were noted in 37% of asymptomatic subjects.[4] Computed tomography (CT) also showed that 36% of individuals have disk herniations in the absence of symptoms.[5]

More recent studies using magnetic resonance imaging (MRI) confirmed the earlier findings on myelography and CT (Table 70–1). Boden and associates[6] performed lumbar MRI in 67 individuals who never had LBP, sciatica, or neurogenic claudication. Nineteen (28%) of the individuals had a major abnormality; herniated nucleus pulposus was noted in 16 subjects (24%) and spinal canal stenosis in 3 subjects (4%). The prevalence of abnormal findings was the same among the men and women but varied according to the ages of the subjects. Twenty percent of individuals less than 60 years sold had herniated nucleus pulposus (HNP) compared with 36% in the subjects 60 years old or older. One patient younger than 60 years old had spinal stenosis compared with 3 of 14 patients (21%) older than 60 years of age. Degeneration or bulging of the disk was present in 35% of the younger subjects compared with all but one in the 60- to 80-year-old subjects.

Jensen and colleagues[7] confirmed the findings of Boden and associates. MRI was performed in 98 asymptomatic people; 36% of the asymptomatic subjects had normal disks at all levels. Twenty seven percent had a protrusion, 52% had a bulgeiu in at least one level, and 1% had an extrusion.[7] The common nonintervertebral disk abnormalities were Schmorl's nodes in 19% of the subjects, annular defects in 14%, and facet arthropathy in 8%. Seven percent had spondylolysis, 7% had spondylolisthesis, 7% had spinal canal stenosis, and 7% had neural foraminal stenosis. Like the results of Boden and associates, the findings were similar in men and women.

MRI studies of the cervical spine also showed the presence of abnormal findings in volunteers who had no history of cervical disease. Nineteen percent of 63 volunteers had an abnormality: 14% of those who were less than 40 years old and 28% of those who were older than 40. Ten percent of the subjects less than 40 had an HNP, 4% had foraminal stenosis, and 25% had degenerated or narrowed disk. Five percent of the subjects older than 40 had an HNP, 3% had bulging disk, 20% had foraminal stenosis, and 60% had degenerated disk.[8]

The presence of abnormal findings in asymptomatic individuals (see Table 70–1) calls for caution in performing interventional procedures or surgery in patients with low back and neck pain. The results on the MRI should therefore be strictly matched with

Table 70–1. Abnormal Findings in Asymptomatic Patients with Low Back and Neck Pain

STUDY (REFERENCE NUMBER)	DIAGNOSTIC TOOL	FINDINGS
Lumbar Spine Abnormalities		
Hitselberger and Witten[3]	Myelography	HNP (24%)
Wiesel[5]	Computed tomography	HNP (36%)
Boden[6]	MRI	Abnormality in 28%: HNP (24%), spinal stenosis (4%)
Jensen[7]	MRI	Disk protrusion (27%), bulge (52%), extrusion (1%), annular defects (14%), facet arthropathy (8%), spondylolysis (7%), spondylolisthesis (7%), spinal stenosis (7%), foraminal stenosis (7%)
Holt[4]	Discograms	Abnormal findings (37%)
Cervical Abnormalities		
Boden[6]	MRI	Abnormality in 19%: HNP (15%), bulging disk (3%), foraminal stenosis (24%), degenerated disk (85%)

HNP, herniated nucleus pulposus; MRI, magnetic resonance imaging.

the patients' clinical signs and symptoms before therapy is started.[6-8]

Follow-up of Patients with Abnormal Findings

A 7-year follow-up study of the asymptomatic patients who had abnormal findings on the MRI[6] resulted in 50 patients being followed: 21 of the 50 patients developed back pain; their 1989 scans showed normal findings in 12, a herniated disk in 5, stenosis in 3, and moderate disk degeneration in 1.[9] Repeat MRI of the patients showed a greater frequency of disk herniation, bulging, degeneration, and spinal stenosis than the original scans. It should be noted that 29 of the 50 patients did not develop back pain in spite of abnormal findings on their MRI.

The spontaneous regression of HNP has been reported.[10] Eleven patients with herniated lumbar disk showed unequivocal regression or disappearance of their HNP. The repeat CT was prompted by persisting symptoms or new symptoms.[10] None of the 11 patients had interventional treatment(s); therapy included bed rest, physiotherapy, and exercises. The possible reasons for the disappearance of the HNP include regression of the HNP through the annulus via a tear in the annulus, fragmentation and sequestration at a distance from the annulus, and dehydration and shrinkage of the HNP. Teplick[10] considered the first reason as the most plausible. It should be noted that in the same study, 39 patients had similar or additional findings on repeat CT, that is, there was no regression of the HNP.[10]

The spontaneous regression of herniated disks has been demonstrated in other studies.[11-15] It appears that larger initial disk herniations have a greater tendency to regress.[16] Initial studies showed that sequestered disk herniations have a greater tendency to regress than subligamentous (the extruded or protruded disk materials are located beneath the posterior longitudinal ligament [PLL]) or transligamentous (the extruded material is partially exposed to the epidural space through a tear in the PLL) disk herniations.[10,11,13,14] To shed light on this issue further, Ahn and coworkers[16] compared the rates of regres-

sion among transligamentous, subligamentous, and sequestered herniations. Thirty-six patients with HNP on their MRI were treated conservatively: bed rest, oral steroids and nonsteroidal anti-inflammatory drugs (NSAIDs), massage, and physical therapy were prescribed during the acute phase. During the subacute and chronic stages, the treatments included NSAIDs and antidepressants, pelvic dynamic stabilization exercises, back school, and pelvic traction. None received epidural or selective nerve root injection. Two MRIs were performed, the first one at 1 to 28 months after the onset of the first symptoms (mean interval, 6.8 months) and the second MRI was obtained 3 to 27 months later (average interval, 8.5 months). The second MRI was performed when the radicular pain was markedly relieved or when the symptoms maintained a plateau for longer than 1 month. Of the 36 herniated disks, 25 decreased in size. Ten (58%) of 18 subligamentous herniations, 11 (79%) of 14 transligamentous herniations, and all 4 (100%) sequestered herniations were reduced in size.[16] Successful clinical outcome correlated with a decrease in herniation of more than 20%[16] and occurred in 13 of 18 patients (72%) in the subligamentous group, 11 of 14 patients (79%) in the transligamentous group, and 4 of 4 patients (100%) in the sequestered group. The decrease in herniation ratio was related to the presence of transligamentous extension and not related to the initial size of herniation. The better results in transligamentous extensions may be secondary to exposure of the herniated disk material to the rich vascular supply in the posterior epidural space, resulting in its resorption.[13,14]

OUTCOME MEASURES AND MEASUREMENT TOOLS IN LOW BACK PAIN RESEARCH

Outcome measures and measurement tools are necessary in quantifying the results of treatment.[17] The outcome domains for studies on LBP include pain, functional impairment related to the back, generic well-being, disability, and patients' satisfaction with their care (Table 70–2). The measurement tools for back-related function include the Roland-Morris and

Table 70–2. Selected Outcome Measures for Studies on Low Back Pain

OUTCOME DOMAIN	MEASUREMENT TOOL
Generic health status	Medical Outcomes Study SF-36 SF-36 PF$_{18}$
Back-related function*	Oswestry Disability Questionnaire Roland-Morris Disability Scale
Pain	Visual Analogue Scale for back and leg pain SF-36 Bodily Pain Scale
Pain symptom	Sciatica Bothersomeness Index Low Back Pain Bothersomeness Index Stenosis Bothersomeness Index
Satisfaction with care	Likert Self-rating Scale of global perceived recovery Patient Satisfaction Scale
Work disability	Work status

*Other proposed back-specific functional instruments include the North American Spine Society Lumbar Spine Questionnaire (NASS LSQ), Quebec Back Pain Disability Scale (QBPDS), Low Back Outcome Score (LBOS), and Waddell Disability Index (WDI).

From Benzon HT: Studies on diagnostic injections and surgery for low back pain: Problems, advances, and opportunities. Anesth Analg 2007;105:1523–1525 (with permission).

the Oswestry scales. The Roland-Morris questionnaire is simpler; it contains 18 questions that deal with the patient's activity, pain, dependence on others, and emotional status.[18] The Oswestry Disability Index contains 10 questions that deal with the pain, ability of the patient to perform personal care, activity level, social life, and travel activities.[19] The Roland-Morris Disability Scale is suited for telephone administration and is more useful in primary care settings. In contrast, the Oswestry scale is more useful in specialty care settings or in situations in which the disability level is likely to remain relatively high throughout the study period.[20] A change of at least 2 to 3 points in the Roland-Morris score and 7 to 10 points in the SF-36 physical function subscale is considered clinically significant.[21] The Roland-Morris and Oswestry scales have been modified to improve their measurement properties.[22,23] Other outcome measures include the sickness impact profile,[24,25] Quebec Back Pain Disability Scale,[26] Short Form (SF)-36 or its modification,[27] and the Sciatica Bothersomeness Index.[21,28] In the SF-36, changes in the bodily pain and physical functioning are considered relevant to back pain. These outcome measures have been assessed, and their strengths and weaknesses discussed.[21,29-31] Clinical investigators on back pain should know these outcome domains and measurement tools and include relevant measures in their studies to better confirm the effects of their treatment or intervention.

SURGICAL TREATMENT FOR HERNIATED DISK

Surgery for back pain involves treatment for primary radicular pain or primary back pain.[32] The primary cause of radicular pain is herniated lumbar disk; previous studies on the long-term results after surgery were limited by their retrospective nature, small number of patients studied, questionable follow-up results because the follow-ups were done by the surgeon, lack of confirmatory diagnostic tests such as MRI, and lack of adequate outcome measures. Three studies compared surgery versus conservative management for radicular pain secondary to herniated disk.[33-36]

The original randomized clinical trial on surgery for herniated disk was performed by Weber.[33] Two hundred eighty patients with sciatica were assigned to three groups: (1) group 1—126 patients in whom the recommended treatment was in doubt were randomized to either surgery (60 patients) or conservative management (66 patients); (2) group 2—67 patients who had surgery for definite indications (severe scoliosis, intolerable pain, sudden or progressive muscle weakness or bowel/bladder paralysis; and, (3) group 3—87 patients who continued their conservative treatment. The conservative treatments of the patients in group 1 included exercises, analgesics, and back school. At 1 year the patients who were randomized to surgery did significantly better—a greater percentage of the patients rated their results as "good" or "better." At the 4-year follow-up, there was a tendency to a more favorable effect in the patients who had surgery but the difference was not statistically significant. At the 10-year follow-up, only age correlated with unsatisfactory results—older patients had poor or bad results.[33]

The Spine Outcomes Research Trial (SPORT) group compared surgery with conservative management in the treatment of radicular pain from herniated disk: one was a randomized study[34] and another was an observational cohort study.[35] In the randomized study, 501 patients were randomized to either surgery such as open diskectomy (245 patients) or nonoperative management (256 patients) that consisted of education and counseling, medications with opioids or NSAIDs, epidural steroid injections, and activity restriction. The main outcome measures included the SF-36 bodily pain and physical function scales and the American Academy of Orthopedic Surgeons version of the Oswestry Disability Index, whereas secondary measures included patient self-reported improvement, work status, and satisfaction. The severity of symptoms was measured by the Sciatica Bothersomeness Index. Follow-up of the patients occurred at 6 weeks, 3 months, 6 months, and 1 and 2 years after enrollment. The investigators noted substantial improvements for all primary and secondary outcomes in both groups. For each measure and at each point, the treatment favored surgery. However, the differences for the primary outcomes were small and not statistically significant (the secondary measures showed significant advantages for surgery). In their cohort study, the SPORT investigators noted clinically important and statistically significant differences in the self-reported outcomes in the patients who had surgery.[35]

The improvement with surgery at the earlier stages of follow-up were noted in the SPORT trial, the study by Weber, the study by Carragee and colleagues,[36] and other studies.[37-39] The lack of long-term difference between surgery and conservative management supports the patient's involvement in the decision-making process.[32] Surgery may be the best option in patients in whom a more rapid resolution of disabling pain is important and may include patients who have experienced financial hardship with prolonged and recurrent absence from work. Delay of surgery does not seem to lead to neurologic deterioration, cauda equina syndrome, or progression of spinal instability.

The results of the studies showing lack of long-term benefit from surgery should not cloud the definite indications for surgery. These include major trauma with gross instability, unstable spondylolisthesis, persistent or complicated spinal infections, and spinal tumors with progressive neurologic loss.[32]

SURGICAL TREATMENT FOR SPINAL STENOSIS

Similar to the studies on surgery for herniated disk, the studies on surgery for spinal stenosis have been hampered by lack of randomization, small number of patients, inadequate outcome measures, and inadequate period of follow-up. Several studies fulfilled some of the noted criteria. Jonsson and associates[40] prospectively followed 105 patients with lumbar spinal stenosis who underwent surgical decompression (laminectomy without fusion); follow-up intervals were at 4 months and 1, 2, and 5 years after surgery. Excellent results (almost or totally pain-free) were reported by 63% to 67% of the patients at the 4-month and 2-year follow-ups and by 52% of the patients at the 5-year follow-up. Significantly better results were noted in the patients with an anteroposterior diameter of 6 mm or less at the narrowest site. They identified the ideal patient as someone who has pronounced constriction of the spinal canal, insignificant lower back pain, no concomitant disease affecting walking ability, and a symptom duration of less than 4 years.[40]

Amundsen and coworkers[41] assigned their patients into the following groups: (1) surgery group (19 patients), whose symptoms were quite severe and underwent surgery; (2) conservative group (50 patients), whose pain was mild to moderate to justify surgery; (3) randomized group, whose severity of pain left the treatment in doubt and patients were randomized to either the randomized surgery (RS) group (13 patients) or the randomized conservative (RC) group (18 patients). Surgery consisted of nerve decompression by partial or total laminectomy, facetectomy, diskectomy, and removal of osteophytes. The conservative management consisted of orthosis, back school, and physical therapy (ambulation and stabilizing exercises). Good results were reported by the surgery and conservative groups after 1 year and 4 years (84% of the surgery group and 57% of the conservative groups at 4 years). Of the randomized patients, results were good in 47% of the patients in the conservative group and in 92% of the patients in

the surgery group. After 10 years, results were reported good in the following: 71% of the patients who had surgery, 73% for the conservative group, and 79% for the randomized group (91% of the RS group and 44% in the RC group). The study by Amundsen and coworkers showed better results in the patients randomized to surgery.[41] It should be noted that the patients who had unsatisfactory results from their conservative treatment had surgery 3 to 27 months later. The final result in these patients was not inferior to that of the initial treatment. Their conclusion was that the outcome was most favorable for surgery (in the patients with severe symptoms). However, an initial conservative treatment is advisable for many patients because an unsatisfactory result can be treated with surgery later without reduction in the outcome.

The Maine Lumbar Spine Study is a nonrandomized observational study wherein patients with spinal stenosis were followed for 1, 4, and 10 years.[42-44] The treatment, whether surgery or conservative management, was determined in a routine clinical manner by the patient and physician. The surgically treated patients had decompressive laminectomy, and fusion was uncommon. Conservative management consisted of back exercises, bed rest, physical therapy, spinal manipulation, narcotic analgesics, and epidural steroids. Outcome measures included improvement in patient symptoms (improved, same, or worse), patient satisfaction, frequency and bothersomeness of the back and leg pain, functional status with a modified Roland-Morris disability scale, and health perception with the SF-36 questionnaire. Preliminary results at 1 year favored surgery with the relative benefit persisting, but narrowed at 4 years.[42,43] Long-term follow-up at 10 years showed a similar percentage of the surgical and nonsurgical patients improved (53% vs. 50%); their predominant symptom, either back or leg pain improved (54% vs. 42%), and they were satisfied with their treatment (55% vs. 49%).[44] The patients who had surgery reported less severe leg pain symptoms and greater improvement in back-specific functional status after 8 to 10 years. Some patients underwent subsequent surgical procedures (23% of the surgical patients underwent an additional lumbar spine surgery and 39% of the nonsurgical patients underwent surgery) and had worse outcomes than those who continued their initial treatment. The authors concluded that surgery may offer better outcomes compared with nonsurgical treatment over several years. However, long-term outcomes are similar.

The complications of surgery included cauda equina syndrome from an epidural hematoma, infection, chronic pain, nerve injuries, dural tear, deep vein thrombosis, pulmonary embolism, and blindness secondary to ischemic injury from position of the patient during the surgery.[40,45,46]

The role of spinal fusion surgery has been outlined by Deyo and Mirza.[46] Initially used for severe scoliosis, spinal tuberculosis, and fractures, its indication has been expanded to other conditions. These included spondylosis, spinal stenosis, and spinal stenosis with spondylolisthesis. There is little evidence to support the efficacy of spinal fusion in association with diskectomy for patients with herniated disks and radiculopathy. Discogenic pain is a controversial indication of spinal fusion. One randomized study showed some effectiveness of spinal fusion[47] but limitations of the study included lack of blinding, a small percentage of improvement in pain and function, and diminished improvement over time.[47] Another study showed no difference between spinal fusion and a standard rehabilitation treatment in terms of pain relief or improvement in function.[48]

Overall the studies showed better results with surgery in patients with spinal stenosis, but the favorable results were not maintained over time. Conservative management can therefore be initiated and surgery be delayed with no difference in the effect of surgery. The conservative management of spinal stenosis has been outlined by Yuan and Albert.[49] These include activity modification, avoidance of heavy lifting and excessive trunk extension, elastic lumbar binder, oral medications such as anti-inflammatory drugs, muscle relaxants, antidepressants, cryotherapy, hot packs, manual therapy, ultrasound, transcutaneous nerve stimulation, traction, chiropractic manipulation, and epidural steroid injections.[49] The active phase of nonsurgical treatment consists of flexion-based exercises, aquatic therapy, stretching of hip flexors, hamstrings, and paraspinal muscles, and strengthening of the back and abdominal muscles.[49]

INTERLAMINAR EPIDURAL STEROID INJECTIONS FOR RADICULAR PAIN SYNDROMES

Epidural steroid injections (ESIs) are the most commonly performed procedures in a pain clinic. The history, rationale for their use, results of studies, and complications of epidural steroid injections have been described in Chapter 55. Several reviews on the subject concluded the efficacy of ESIs in radicular pain syndromes and noted the lack of randomized controlled trials.[50-53]

There are now adequate randomized and controlled studies on lumbar interlaminar ESIs (Table 70–3). Dilke and associates[54] showed significantly better pain relief and better rates of return to work with ESI than with interspinous ligament saline injections at 3 months' follow-up. Snoek and colleagues[55] reported greater subjective and objective improvements after ESI compared with placebo injection, but this difference did not reach statistical significance. Their study used undiluted steroid in a 2-mL volume and evaluated patients after 24 to 48 hours (compared with 6 days in the study by Dilke and associates). Carette and coworkers[56] administered ESI up to three times and found that the differences in improvement between groups were not significant, except for improvements in the finger-to-floor distance ($P = 0.03$) and in sensory deficits at 3 weeks, and in leg pain at 6 weeks. These improvements were observed in the methylprednisolone group at 3 weeks and 6 weeks, but there were no significant differences after 3 months. ESI did not offer significant functional benefit or reduce the need for surgery in about 25% of these patients within 12 months. Cuckler and colleagues[57] compared epidural methylprednisolone-procaine with epidural saline and noted no difference in the results. There was no difference in the results between the patients who had herniated disk and the patients who had spinal stenosis.

In their Wessex Epidural Steroids Trial (WEST), Arden and coworkers[58] compared three lumbar ESIs with triamcinolone acetonide (80 mg in 10 mL 0.25% bupivacaine) with 2 mL interligamentous saline. There was a transient benefit of the ESI group over the placebo group at 3 weeks. However, there was no difference in results between the steroid and the control groups at 6 to 52 weeks. Wilson-MacDonald and colleagues[59] compared epidural and intramuscular steroid injections (80 mg methylprednisolone and 8 mL 0.5% bupivacaine). They noted superiority of the epidural steroid at 3 months but no difference in results at 24 months. There was no difference in the results between the patients who had herniated disk from those with spinal stenosis.

Table 70–3. Results of Prospective, Randomized, and Controlled Studies on Interlaminar Epidural Steroid Injections

AUTHOR	STUDY	ABNORMALITY	TREATMENTS	RESULTS
Dilke[54]	P, R, DB	HNP,	MP, 80 mg in 10 mL NS vs. 1 mL NS, lumbar	60% vs. 31% initial pain relief; better results of the steroid at 3 mo
Snoek[55]	P, R, DB	HNP	MP, 80 mg in 2 mL NS vs. 2 mL NS, lumbar	No difference between the two groups
Carette[56]	P, R, DB	HNP, 158 patients	MP, 80 mg in 8 mL NS vs. 1 mL NS, lumbar	Less sensory deficit and leg pain with steroid, functional disability and incidence of surgery the same
Cuckler[57]	P, R, DB	HNP, SS, 73 patients	MP, 80 mg in procaine vs. procaine (8 mL volume)	No difference in results (42% for steroid vs. 44% for control)
Arden[58]	P, R, DB	Sciatica 228 patients	TA, 80 mg in 10 mL 0.25% B vs. 2 mL NS	Superiority of the steroid at 3 wk No benefit from 6 to 52 wk
Wilson-MacDonald[59]	P, R, B	HNP, SS, 93 patients	MP, 80 mg in 8 mL 0.5% B; E vs. IM	Better relief with ESI at 3 mo, no difference at 24 mo

B, bupivacaine; DB, double-blind; E, epidural; ESI, epidural steroid injection; HNP, herniated nucleus pulposus; IM, intramuscular; MP, methylprednisolone; NS, normal saline; P, prospective; R, randomized; SS, spinal stenosis; TA, triamcinolone.

The randomized and blinded studies on lumbar interlaminar ESIs showed better results with the steroid injection.[54-59] However, such superiority was transient, on the average not lasting more than 3 months. These findings were noted by Wilson-MacDonald[59] and the Therapeutics and Technology Assessment Subcommittee of the American Academy of Neurology[60]; the subcommittee report recommended against the routine use of ESIs. This recommendation has to be viewed against the natural history of patients with herniated disk and spinal stenosis—these patients seem to do well over time with conservative management.[61-63] The transient relief provided by ESIs may prevent the use of addicting opioids; ESIs should be used as part, and not the sole modality, of the conservative management of sciatica.

There has been a paucity of well-controlled studies on cervical ESIs for cervical radicular pain. The few studies that have been done were mostly descriptive, and their results were the same as in lumbar ESIs, that is, transient relief from the injections.[64-66] To date, there has been no prospective, randomized, controlled, double-blind study on cervical ESIs.

Transforaminal Epidural Steroid Injections

To improve the efficacy of ESIs, the transforaminal (TF) approach was recommended. In this approach, the drug is deposited in the anterior epidural space and around the nerve root at the area of the intervertebral foramina. In relation to the interlaminar approach, in which the earlier studies were mostly observational and case series, a fair number of the studies on TF ESIs were randomized and controlled (Table 70–4). Riew and associates[67] compared TF ESI with betamethasone (6 mg) and bupivacaine (1 mL 0.25%) versus bupivacaine alone. The patients had radicular pain secondary to HNP or spinal stenosis and were considered candidates for surgery. A greater number of the patients in the steroid group (20 of 28 versus 9 of 27 patients) decided not to proceed with surgery. Karppinen and coworkers[68] compared TF ESI with methylprednisolone (40 to 80 mg) and 1 mL bupivacaine 0.5% versus normal saline in patients with sciatica secondary to a disk abnormality. At 3 months the steroid group had better results in terms of leg pain, straight-leg raise, and satisfaction.

However, the saline group had significantly lower back pain at 3 and 6 months and lower leg pain at 6 months. By 1 year, 18 patients in the steroid group and 15 in the saline group underwent surgery. The authors concluded that TF ESI has a short-term effect.[68] Ng and colleagues[69] compared TF ESI with methylprednisolone (40 mg) and bupivacaine (2 mL 0.25%) versus bupivacaine (2 mL 0.25%) only in patients with unilateral leg pain secondary to herniated disk or spinal stenosis. There was no significant difference in the outcome measures (Oswestry, pain, change in walking distance) between the two groups at 3 months. Their conclusion was that TF ESI with steroid did not provide additional benefit. In summary, two of the three controlled studies on TF ESI showed better results with TF ESI.

Interlaminar Epidural Steroid Injections versus Paramedian (Lateral Epidural Space) and Transforaminal Epidural Steroid Injections

Three studies compared interlaminar ESI with the paramedian and TF approaches (Table 70–5). Kraemer and associates performed two prospective studies[70]: the first one was a prospective randomized study that compared the interlaminar approach (40 patients), paramedian approach 47 patients), and paravertebral local anesthetic injections (46 patients). In their paramedian approach, which they called perineural approach, the authors inserted their needle at an oblique angle, and the tip of the needle ended up at the "lateral part of the anterior epidural space" (p. 358); triamcinolone 10 mg in 1 mL local anesthetic was injected. The authors noted better results in the perineural group compared with the interlaminar group (68% excellent or good results versus 54%). Both steroid groups had better results than the paravertebral approach (65% were unchanged). In their second prospective (double-blind) study, the epidural perineural triamcinolone (24 patients) was compared with epidural perineural saline (25 patients). The saline group had intramuscular triamcinolone to rule out any systemic effect of the perineural steroid. Patients who had the perineural steroid had better results (54% good versus 40%).[70]

Thomas and coworkers[71] performed a randomized double-blind study comparing interlaminar ESI with TF ESI. Their TF ESI was performed under fluoro-

Table 70–4. Results of Selected Prospective, Randomized, Controlled Studies on Transforaminal Epidural Steroid Injections

AUTHOR	STUDY	ABNORMALITY	TREATMENT	RESULTS
Riew[67]	P, R, DB	HNP, SS 55 patients	TF ESI (B vs. B/Bu	Greater number of patients in the steroid group did not have surgery (20 of 28 vs. 9 of 27)
Karppinen[68]	P, R, DB	Sciatica, disk abnormality, 160 patients	TF ESI (M/Bu vs. NS)	Steroid group better at 2 wk; back pain lower in NS group at 3 and 6 mo
Ng, et al[69]	P, R, DB	HNP, SS 86 patients	TF ESI (M/Bu vs. Bu)	No difference in outcome measures at 3 mo

B, betamethasone; Bu, bupivacaine; DB, double-blind; ESI, epidural steroid injection; HNP, herniated nucleus pulposus; M, methylprednisolone; NS, normal saline; P, prospective; R, randomized; SS, spinal stenosis; TF, transforaminal.

Table 70–5. Studies Comparing Interlaminar and Transforaminal Epidural Steroid Injections

AUTHOR	STUDY	ABNORMALITY	TREATMENT	RESULTS
Kraemer[70]	P, R	Sciatica, 133 patients	Perineural* TA/LA vs. interlaminar TA/LA vs. paravertebral LA	Better results with perineural TA; epidural steroid group better than paravertebral group
	P, R, DB	Sciatica, 45 patients	Perineural TA/NS vs. IM NS	Better results with perineural TA/NS
Thomas[71]	P, R, DB	HNP, 31 patients	TF ESI Dex vs. interlaminar Dex	Better results with TF ESI at 6 and 30 days and at 6 mo
Schaufele and Hatch[72]	R, CC	HNP, 40 patients	TF ESI vs. interlaminar ESI (M/lidocaine)	Better short term results with TF ESI

*Perineural approach: needle was inserted obliquely through the ligamentum flavum with the tip of the needle ending at the "lateral part of the anterior epidural space" (p. 358).
CC, case control; DB, double-blind; Dex, dexamethasone; ESI, epidural steroid injection; HNP, herniated nucleus pulposus; IM, intramuscular; LA, local anesthetic; M, methylprednisolone; NS, normal saline; P, prospective; R, randomized; T, triamcinolone; TF, transforaminal.

scopic control throughout the procedure and a neurogram was demonstrated. In contrast, they used fluoroscopy briefly in their interlaminar approach and no epidurogram was performed. Dexamethasone 5 mg in 2 mL solution was injected in both techniques. The authors showed significantly better results with the TF approach at 6 and 30 days and at 6 months. Schaufele and Hatch[72] performed a retrospective, case control study. The records of 40 patients who underwent TF ESI (20 patients) and interlaminar ESI (20 patients) were compared (the patients had low back or radicular pain secondary to herniated disks). Methylprednisolone 80 mg in lidocaine (1 to 2 mL for the TF approach and 2 to 3 mL for the interlaminar approach) was injected. The authors noted better results with the TF approach.

The retrospective case control nature of the study by Schaufele and Hatch[72] makes it hard for one to make definitive conclusions. In contrast, the prospective, randomized, double-blind study by Thomas and coworkers[71] showed significantly better results with the TF ESI. The favorable results were still noted at the 6-month follow-up, a finding that needs to be confirmed.

Complications of Epidural Steroid Injections

The complications from ESIs have been described in chapter 55. In addition, Abram,[73] Fitzgibbon and associates,[74] and Bogduk[75] discussed the complications from interlaminar and transforaminal epidural steroid injections. As Huntoon stated in Chapter 55, the complications are secondary to the technique (interlaminar or transforaminal), needle trauma, vasospastic or ischemic, infectious, drug injected, as well as the drug diluent or additives. The complications related to epidural steroid injections are summarized in Box 70–1. Complications related to transforaminal technique include central nervous system (CNS) injuries affecting the brain (cerebral embolism, infarct) or the spinal cord (paraplegia). This topic is partly related to the sizes of the particles in the steroid preparation and has been discussed in Chapter 38. Methylprednisolone has the largest particle size followed by triamcinolone and betamethasone; dexamethasone is pure liquid but its definite

---

BOX 70–1. COMPLICATIONS FROM EPIDURAL INJECTIONS

Interlaminar Epidural Steroid Injections (ESIs)
Nerve injury
Infection
Headache (dural puncture)
Death or brain damage
Arachnoiditis (unintentional intrathecal injection)
Spinal cord trauma (mostly related to cervical and thoracic approaches)
Corticosteroid effects
　Hypercorticism
　Adrenal suppression
　Increase in blood sugar
　Sodium retention (increased blood pressure, congestive heart failure [CHF])

Transforaminal ESIs (Includes Complications from Interlaminar Approach)
Central nervous system injuries
　Brain infarct or embolism
　Spinal cord injury (paraplegia)

---

role in ESIs has not been established by prospective controlled studies. The role of diluents and preservatives in the steroid preparation, including polyethylene glycol[76,77] and benzyl alcohol are also discussed in Chapter 38.

FACET JOINT INJECTIONS AND MEDIAL BRANCH BLOCKS FOR FACET SYNDROME

Pain emanating from the facet joints is discussed in Chapter 56. Briefly, patients with low back pain secondary to facet problems have pain in the low back that radiates to the ipsilateral posterior thigh that usually ends at the knee. Cohen and Raja[78] showed the referral patterns of facet pain, in the following descending order: the pain is usually felt across the low back, lower buttocks, posterior and lateral thigh, groin, lateral leg, and medial leg. Physical examination usually shows paraspinal tenderness and reproduction of pain with extension-rotation maneuvers of the back. It should be noted that there are no historic or physical examination findings that are characteristic of facet pain or reliably predict response to diagnostic facet injections.

Diagnosis of facet syndrome is made by a combination of the patient's history, physical examination findings, and response to diagnostic medial branch blocks or facet joint injections. A positive response to these injections or blocks usually confirms the diagnosis. For medial branch blocks, some investigators recommend the use of local anesthetics with different durations of effect, for example, lidocaine and bupivacaine, and correlate the duration of relief with the known duration of effect of the drug.[79] This is not routinely followed in clinical practice because the use of lidocaine may result in prolonged relief because the "cycle of pain" has been broken.

Some patients may have prolonged response to facet joint injections (up to 3 to 6; see Chapter 56).[80-83] If the patient has this prolonged response, then it is best to wait for recurrence of the pain. If the relief is short lived, especially after medial branch blocks, then thermal rhizotomy (RF) of the medial branches should be performed. There are few randomized, controlled studies on thermal rhizotomy of the lumbar medial branch blocks[84-88] (Table 70–6). The study by King and Lagger[84] was done in 1976 when equipment was not as advanced as today. The authors showed 27% response rate at 6 months in the patients who had the RF of the posterior ramus compared with 53% after RF of the area of maximum tenderness. Gallagher and coworkers[85] studied patients who had good or equivocal response to facet joint injections and randomized them to either RF denervation or a sham intervention. In the patients who had good response to the diagnostic blocks, better responses were noted in the RF group at the 1- and 6-month follow-up periods. Sanders and Zuurmond[86] studied patients who had more than 50% relief after intra-articular lidocaine and randomized them into either medial branch RF or intra-articular

RF. At 3 months' follow-up, both groups showed improvements, with better improvements in the intra-articular RF group. Van Kleef and colleagues[87] also studied patients who had favorable response to a medial branch block and randomized them into either a true RF or a sham procedure. At 3 months, 60% (9 of 15 patients) had more than 50% relief compared with 25% in the sham group. The significant difference was again noted at the 12-month follow-up: 47% (7 of 15) versus 12.5% (2 of 16). Leclaire and colleagues[88] included patients who had pain relief after an intra-articular injection and randomized them into either an RF or a sham procedure. At 1 month improvements were noted in the Roland-Morris scores in the RF group compared with the sham group. Van Wijk and associates[89] included patients who responded to intra-articular local anesthetic facet injections and randomized them into either an RF or a sham procedure. More patients in the RF group (62% vs. 39%) reported a *greater* reduction of their pain. Two controlled studies on thermal RF of the cervical medial branches showed different results. Lord and associates[90] showed better results after RF (return to work and relief of pain), whereas Stovner and coworkers[91] showed no difference between the RF and sham procedures. Overall, the randomized controlled studies showed improvements after thermal RF of the medial branches that may last 3 to 12 months.

PULSED RADIOFREQUENCY ABLATION (PULSED RADIOFREQUENCY) FOR BACK PAIN AND PERIPHERAL NEURALGIAS

The history of the development of pulsed RF has been chronicled[92] (Doctors Eric Cosman, Menno Sluijter, and William Ritman developed the technique). It is interesting to note that Slappendel and coworkers[93] studied RF ablation between 67° and 40° C in 1997; they did not use pulsed RF but decreased the temperature of the tip of their electrode to 40° C. They lesioned the cervical spinal

Table 70–6. Randomized, Controlled Studies on Radiofrequency Denervation of the Medial Branches (Facet Nerves)

STUDY	STUDY POPULATION	RESULTS
King and Lagger[84]	RF of the posterior primary ramus vs. RF of the area of maximum tenderness vs. control group (stimulation but no RF)	At 6 mo: 27% response rate for RF of primary ramus, 50% for RF of area of maximal tenderness, 0% in control group
Gallagher et al[85]	Patients previously who had good or equivocal response to facet joint injections randomized to RF or sham	Significantly better results noted in RF group at 1 and 6 mo
Sanders and Zuurmond[86]	Patients had ≧50% relief after intra-articular lidocaine, randomized to RF of medial branch vs. intra-articular RF	At 3 mo: improvements in both groups
Van Kleef, et al[87]	Patients had favorable response to MBB, randomized to RF or sham	Better results noted in the RF group at 3 mo (60% vs. 25%) and at 1 yr (47% vs. 12.5%)
Leclaire, et al[88]	Patients had relief after intra-articular injection, randomized to RF or sham	At 1 mo: improvements in Roland-Morris scores in the RF group
van Wijk, et al[89]	Patients responded to intra-articular injection, randomized to RF or sham	At 3 mo: ≧50% relief in 62% (RF group) vs. 39% (sham)

MBB, medial branch block; RF, radiofrequency.

dorsal root ganglion and noted no difference between the two temperatures.[93] Slappendel and coworkers gave credence to the theory that mechanism(s), other than heat, alters the transmission of pain impulses.

Thermal RF involves heating the needle tip to 80° C for 90 seconds, and in pulsed RF, the needle tip is heated to 42° C for 120 seconds. Pulsed RF is achieved by applying 500,000 Hz current for 20-millisecond pulses delivered every 0.5 second for a total duration of 120 seconds—the temperature does not exceed 42° C.[94] The exact mechanism of pulsed RF has not been established. The RF lesion was initially thought to be secondary to selective blockade of the small myelinated and unmyelinated fibers[95] but a subsequent morphologic study found destruction of both the small and large fibers.[96] Clinically, the EMG and SEP potentials remain after an RF of the DRG in the cervical region,[97] indicating that a majority of the large fibers remain intact. Pulsed RF may reversibly disrupt the transmission of impulses across small myelinated fibers without destroying them while the larger myelinated fibers are unaffected.[98] Pulsed RF, but not continuous RF, was associated with increased cFOS-immunoreactive neurons in laminas I and II in the dorsal horn of the rat spinal cord.[99] However, it should be noted that this increase does not necessarily mean antinociception.

Intuitively, the lower temperature in the pulsed RF results in less tissue destruction. This attractive feature of the procedure led to numerous publications, most of which were case series or retrospective in nature. Most of the publications involved use of pulsed RF of the dorsal root ganglion and peripheral neuralgias. Only few reports are cited in this chapter because of the deficiencies inherent in these kinds of studies.[100-106]

There are very few controlled studies on pulsed RF. The publication by Slujter and colleagues[107] contained two studies, one of which was a prospective study that compared the efficacy of PRF to continuous radiofrequency ablation (CRFA); the other study in their publication was a case series. The maximum temperature in their RF was 42° C. In the controlled trial, the patients underwent pulsed RF of the DRG (the vertebral levels were not stated). Better success rate was noted in the pulsed RF group: 56% of the patients had more than 75% global perceived relief at the 6-week follow-up compared with 4% in the continuous RF group (Table 70–7).

Erdine and associates[108] studied 40 patients with trigeminal neuralgia and compared pulsed RF (42° C for 120 seconds) with continuous RF (70° C for 60 seconds) of the trigeminal ganglion. Only 2 of the 20 patients who had the pulsed RF had decreases in their Visual Analogue Scale (VAS) score, and their pain recurred 3 months later. In contrast, the patients who had continuous RF had significant decreases in their VAS scores and improvement in their satisfaction scores. The patients who had pulsed RF were treated with continuous RF 3 months later, and their VAS and satisfaction scores improved significantly.

A recent study by Van Zundert and colleagues[109] compared pulsed RF with a sham intervention, wherein a needle was placed, sensory stimulation was performed, and the generator was "manipulated."[109] Twenty-three patients with cervical radicular pain were studied: 11 had the PRF treatment and 12 had the sham intervention. At 3 months' follow-up, the patients in the pulsed RF group had significantly better outcomes with regards to VAS (20-point reduction) and perceived global effect (greater than 50% improvement). The quality-of-life scales also showed a trend in favor of the pulsed RF group.

Pulsed RF is a new and exciting therapeutic modality. However, the results of the very few randomized controlled studies were conflicting: two studies showed it to be effective,[107,109] whereas one study did not.[108] A position statement paper commissioned by the International Spine Interventional Society concluded that pulsed RF has unproven efficacy.[110] It is too soon to be endorsing this technique because more randomized controlled studies are needed to definitely identify the role of this intervention. It may have a role in patients with radicular pain and patients with peripheral neuralgias.[103,104,106] Complications of pulsed RF are minimal,[111] a safety feature that makes it an attractive therapeutic modality.

OTHER INTERVENTIONAL PROCEDURES: INTRADISKAL ELECTROTHERMAL THERAPY AND PERCUTANEOUS DISK DECOMPRESSION

There are not enough randomized and controlled studies to merit discussion of these techniques in this

---

Table 70–7. Controlled Studies on Pulsed Radiofrequency

STUDY	STUDY POPULATION, TREATMENTS	RESULTS
Sluijter, et al[107]: P, C	Radicular pain, 60 patients, pulsed RF of DRG vs. continuous RF	Success rates: 56% (20 of 36 patients) with pulsed RF vs. 4% (1 of 24 patients) with continuous RF
Erdine, et al[108]: P, R, DB	Trigeminal neuralgia, 40 patients, pulsed RF of trigeminal ganglion vs. continuous RF	2 of 20 patients with pulsed RF had decreases in VAS compared with all patients in the continuous RF group
Van Zundert, et al[109]: P, R, DB, SC	Cervical radicular pain, 23 patients, pulsed RF of DRG vs. sham intervention	At 3 mo follow-up: significantly better outcomes in the pulsed RF group (VAS scores and global perceived effect)

C, controlled; DB, double-blind; DRG, dorsal root ganglion; P, prospective; R, randomized; RF, radiofrequency; SC, sham controlled; VAS, Visual Analogue Scale.

chapter. The few studies that have been performed on these interventions are discussed in Chapter 60, which deals with back pain and intradiskal procedures.

PSYCHOLOGICAL INTERVENTIONS FOR CHRONIC LOW BACK PAIN

Psychological treatments for low back pain usually consist of cognitive-behavioral treatment, behavioral treatment, and biofeedback and relaxation training. The efficacy of these treatments in low back pain has been the subject of several reviews[112-116] and meta-analysis[117] articles. In a recent meta-analysis, Kerns's group[117] looked at the efficacy of outpatient psychological interventions for adults with noncancer chronic low back pain. Out of 952 articles identified in their initial search, 22 studies published across 25 articles were included in their final analyses. Outcome measures in their meta-analysis included pain intensity, emotional functioning, physical functioning (pain interference or pain-specific disability, health-related quality of life), participant ratings of global improvement, health care use, health care provider visits, pain medications, and employment or disability compensation status. Their meta-analysis showed positive effects of psychological interventions, contrasted with various control groups, in terms of pain intensity, pain-related interference, health-related quality of life, and depression. The treatment modalities, when grouped together, were superior to control on pain intensity, pain interference, and health-related quality of life but were not superior for depression.[117] Cognitive behavioral treatment was superior to control group at reducing post-treatment pain intensity, whereas relaxation training was superior to control group at reducing post-treatment intensity and depression; relaxation training was more efficacious than cognitive behavioral therapy in relieving depressive symptom severity (Table 70–8). Multidisciplinary treatments that included a psychological component had positive short-term effects on pain interference and positive long-term effects on return to work. The conclusions of the review articles and the meta-analysis support the clinical impression that psychological treatments are necessary components of the multidisciplinary management of chronic low back pain.

PHARMACOLOGIC MANAGEMENT FOR CHRONIC BACK PAIN, SPECIFICALLY THE USE OF OPIOIDS

The pharmacologic management of low back pain includes opioids, nonsteroidal anti-inflammatory medications or cyclooxygenase-2 (COX-2) inhibitors, antidepressants, and anticonvulsants. With opioids, there are now adequate rigorous randomized controlled studies to permit a meta-analysis of the published results.[118] The results of six studies[119-124] that compared an opioid with a non-opioid or a placebo are shown in Table 70–9. The results of four studies[119-122] were included in the meta-analysis of Martell and colleagues.[118] Although the individual studies showed better results with opioids, the pooled results showed an insignificant reduction in pain in patients receiving opioid treatment compared with those receiving non-opioids or placebo.[118] Nine studies compared two or more opioids (see Table 70–9): five[125-129] of these nine[125-133] studies were included in the meta-analysis. The individual studies showed improvements with opioid therapy but the pooled results of Martell and colleagues[118] showed an insignificant reduction in pain with opioid treatment compared with baseline. They concluded that opioids may be efficacious only for short-term treatment (<16 weeks) of chronic low back pain.

The prevalence of opioid treatment for chronic low back pain ranged from 3% to 66%.[118] The patients who are more likely to be prescribed opioids include those who reported greater disability, poorer functioning, greater distress and suffering, and higher functional disability scores.[134,135] In patients seen in spine specialty clinics, those who received opioids were more likely to have neurologic signs, pain radiation, and dermatomal distribution of their pain.[136]

A review article on the efficacy and safety of opioids for chronic noncancer pain noted that no randomized trial on the subject was rated good quality and that the observational studies were generally of poor quality.[137] The studies that looked at low back pain

Table 70–8. Effects of Psychological Interventions for Chronic Low Back Pain

OUTCOME MEASURE	Psychological Intervention: Effect*		
	COGNITIVE BEHAVIORAL TREATMENT	BEHAVIORAL TREATMENT	RELAXATION TRAINING
Pain intensity	Positive	Positive	Positive
Pain interference	Positive	Positive	Positive
Health-related quality of life	Negative	+/−	+/−
Depression	Negative	+/−	Positive

*All treatment modalities combined together were superior to control with regards to pain intensity, pain interference, and health-related quality of life but not for depression.

Data derived from Hoffman Papas RK, Chatkoff DK, Kerns RD: Meta-analysis of psychological interventions for chronic low back pain. Health Psychol 2007;26:1-9.

Table 70–9. Studies on the Efficacy of Opioids for Chronic Low Back Pain

STUDY	TYPE OF STUDY	STUDY DRUGS	RESULTS*
Opioid Versus Non-Opioid Medication or Placebo			
Kuntz and Brossel[120]	R, DB	Acetaminophen/caffeine (AC) vs. acetaminophen/dextropropoxyphene (AD)	>50% relief: 51% in AC vs. 47% in AD
Hale, et al[121]	R, PC, DB	Oxymorphone ER vs. oxycodone CR vs. placebo	Both opioids superior to placebo
Jamison, et al[122]	R, OL	Oxycodone or oxycodone plus morphine vs. naproxen	Less pain and improved mood in opioid groups
Muller, et al[123]	R, DB, C	Acetaminophen/codeine (AC) vs. tramadol	AC as effective as tramadol
Opioid Versus Another Opioid			
Thurel[125]	R, DB	Acetaminophen/codeine (AC) vs. acetaminophen/dextropropoxyphene (AD)	Similar in efficacy
Gammaitoni[126]	NR, OL	Oxycodone/acetaminophen: 7.5/325 mg vs. 10/325 mg	Reduction of baseline pain
Schofferman[127]	OL, observational	Long-acting opioids (exact medication[s] not stated)	Improvements in NRS and Oswestry scale
Ringe[128]	OL, observational	Transdermal fentanyl	Significant reduction of baseline pain
Simpson[129]	OL, C	Transdermal fentanyl for 1 mo, then SA oral opioid	Significantly better results with transdermal fentanyl in terms of pain and disability

*Above results are from the individual studies. Meta-analysis of the pooled results did not show reduced pain with opioids when compared with a non-opioid or placebo. Pooled results of the efficacy of the different opioids showed an insignificant reduction in pain from baseline.[118]

C, crossover; CR, controlled release; DB, double-blind; ER, extended release; NR, nonrandomized; NRS, numerical rating scale; OL, open label; PC, placebo controlled; R, randomized; SA, short acting.

showed equal efficacy of the short- and long-acting opioids.[137] The lack of long-term effectiveness of opioids in chronic low back pain[118] should be considered when prescribing opioids. This is especially important in view of the high prevalence of lifetime substance abuse disorders (36% to 56%), prevalence of current substance use disorders (as high as 43%), and aberrant medication-taking behaviors (5% to 24%) in this population. Opioids should be prescribed on a short-term basis.[118]

The available evidence supports the effectiveness of nonselective nonsteroidal anti-inflammatory drugs in acute and chronic LBP, and of antidepressants in chronic LBP.[138] Low back pain from muscular, inflammatory, and neuropathic causes demands specific pharmacologic treatments. The physician should be able to recognize these causes and prescribe medications accordingly.

CONCLUSION

Low back pain is a result of several causes, some of which are characterized by appropriate historic and physical examination findings, whereas findings in the other back pain syndromes are nonspecific. Commonly the patient presents with multiple causes of back pain. Physicians should use their best judgment on which cause or syndrome is the predominant one and treat it accordingly. The treatments for chronic low back pain include surgery, interventional procedures, physical medicine, rehabilitation, chiropractic, psychological, and pharmacologic. In this chapter, the results of randomized and controlled studies and meta-analyses on these treatments were presented. The clinician should use the treatments that are backed by evidence.

SUMMARY

- Abnormal MRI and CT findings are not uncommon in patients who have no back pain. These abnormalities, including herniated disks, have been shown to spontaneously regress with time.
- Surgery appears to have a short-term beneficial effect on back pain secondary to herniated effect. It appears to be more efficacious in spinal stenosis.
- Interlaminar epidural steroid injections results in a short-term (3 to 6 months) relief.
- There is rationale for use of the transforaminal approach, which also appears to have a short-term effect. The cervical TF approach may result in central nervous system adverse events including cerebral embolism and paraplegia and may be related to spasm of the arteries supplying the spinal cord or embolization of the particles of the depot steroids.
- Thermal rhizotomy of the medial branches supplying the facet joint in the appropriate patient results in 6 to 12 months of pain relief.
- Pulsed RF is a new and attractive modality. There are very few randomized studies supporting its efficacy. Pulsed RF of the segmental dorsal root ganglion may be useful in patients with radicular pain. Case reports support its role in peripheral neuralgias.
- Psychological interventions, especially when grouped together, are effective in reducing pain intensity, pain-related interference, and health-related quality of life. Of the psychological interventions, relaxation training is superior to control in the management of depression.
- Opioids, which may be used short term, are not effective in the long-term treatment of chronic low back pain.

References

1. Robertson JT: The rape of the spine. Surg Neurol 1993;39:5-12.
2. Deyo RA, Tsui-Wu YJ: Descriptive epidemiology of low-back pain and its related medical care in the United States. Spine 1987;12:264-268.
3. Hitselberger WE, Witten RM: Abnormal myelograms in asymptomatic patients. J Neurosurg 1968;28:204-206.
4. Holt EP: The question of lumbar discography. J Bone Joint Surg (Am) 1968;50:720-726.
5. Wiesel SW, Tsourmas N, Feffer HL, et al: A study of computerized-assisted tomography. I. The incidence of positive CAT scans in asymptomatic group of patients. Spine 1984;9:549-551.
6. Boden SD, Davis DO, Dina TS, et al: Abnormal magnetic-resonance scans of the lumbar spine in asymptomatic subjects: A prospective investigation. J Bone Joint Surg (Am) 1990;72:403-408.
7. Jensen MC, Brant-Zawadzki MN, Obuchowski N, et al: Magnetic resonance imaging of the lumbar spine in people without back pain. N Engl J Med 1994;331:69-73.
8. Boden SD, McCowin PR, Davis DO: Abnormal magnetic-resonance scans of the cervical spine in asymptomatic subjects: A prospective investigation. J Bone Joint Surg (Am) 1990;72:1178-1184.
9. Borenstein DG, O'Mara JW, Boden SD: The value of magnetic resonance imaging of the lumbar spine to predict low-back pain in asymptomatic subjects: A seven year follow-up study. J Bone Joint Surg (Am) 2001:83-A:1306-1311.
10. Teplick JG: Spontaneous regression of herniated nucleus pulposus. AJR 1985;145:371-375.
11. Bush K, Cowan N, Katsz DE, Gishen P: The natural history of sciatica associated with disc pathology. Spine 1992;17:1205-1212.
12. Fraser RD, Sandhu A, Gogan WJ: Magnetic resonance imaging findings 10 years after treatment for lumbar disc herniation. Spine 1995;20:710-714.
13. Komori H, Shinomiya K, Nakai O, et al: The natural history of herniated nucleus pulposus with radiculopathy. Spine 1996;21:225-229.
14. Matsubara Y, Kato F, Mimatsu K, et al: Serial changes on MRI in lumbar disc herniations treated conservatively. Neuroradiology 1995;37:378-383.
15. Benoist M: The natural history of lumbar disc herniation and radiculopathy. Joint Bone Spine 2002;69:155-160.
16. Ahn SH, Ahn MW, Byun WM: Effect of the transligamentous extension of lumbar disc herniation on their regression and the clinical outcome of sciatica. Spine 2000;25:475-480.
17. Turk DC, Dworkin RH, Allen RR, et al: Core outcome domains for chronic pain clinical trials: IMMPACT recommendations. Pain 2003;106:337-345.
18. Roland M, Morris R: A study of the natural history of back pain: Part I: Development of a reliable and sensitive measure of disability in low back pain. Spine 1983;8:141-144.
19. Fairbank JC, Couper J, Davies JB, et al: The Oswestry low back pain disability. Physiotherapy 1980;66:271-273.
20. Deyo RA, Battie M, Beurskens AHHM, et al: Outcome measures for low back pain research: A proposal for standardized use. Spine 1998;23:2003-2013.
21. Patrick DL, Deyo RA, Atlas SJ, et al: Assessing health related quality of life in patients with sciatica. Spine 1995;20:1899-1909.
22. Stratford PW, Brinkley JM: Measurement properties of the RM 18: A modified version of the Roland-Morris disability scale. Spine 1997;22:2416-2421.
23. Daltroy LH, Cats-Baril WL, Katz JN, et al: The North American Spine Society lumbar spine outcome assessment instrument: Reliability and validity tests. Spine 1996;21:741-749.
24. Deyo RA: Comparative validity of the sickness impact profile and shorter scales for functional assessment in low back pain. Spine 1986;11:951-954.
25. Jensen MP, Strom RE, Turner JSA, Romano JM: Validity of the sickness impact profile Roland scale as a measure of dysfunction in chronic pain patients. Pain 1992;50:157-162.
26. Kopec JA, Esdaile JM, Abrahamowicz M, et al: The Quebec Back Pain Disability Scale: Measurement properties. Spine 1995;20:341-352.
27. Davidson M, Keating JL, Eyres S: A low back-specific version of the SF-36 physical functioning scale. Spine 2004;29:586-594.
28. Atlas SJ, Deyo RA, Patrick DL, et al: The Quebec Task Force classification for spinal disorders and the severity, treatment, and outcomes of sciatica and spinal stenosis. Spine 1996;21:2885-2892.
29. Kopec JA: Measuring functional outcomes in persons with back pain: Review of back-specific questionnaires. Spine 2000;25:3110-3114.
30. Bombardier C: Outcome assessments in the evaluation of treatment of spinal disorders: Summary and general recommendations. Spine 2000;25:3100-3103.
31. Davidson M, Keating J: A comparison of five low back disability questionnaires: Reliability and responsiveness. Phys Ther 2002;82:8-24.
32. Carragee E: Surgical treatment of lumbar disk disorders. JAMA 2006;296:2485-2487.
33. Weber H: Lumbar disc herniation: A controlled, prospective study with ten years of observation. Spine 1983;8:131-140.
34. Weinstein JN, Tosteson TD, Lurie JD, et al: Surgical versus nonoperative treatment for lumbar disc herniation. The Spine Outcomes Research Trial (SPORT): A randomized trial. JAMA 2006;296:2441-2450.
35. Weinstein JN, Tosteson TD, Lurie JD, et al: Surgical vs nonoperative treatment for lumbar disk herniation. The Spine Outcomes Research Trial (SPORT) observational cohort. JAMA 2006;296:2441-2450.
36. Carragee EJ, Han MY, Suen PW, Kim D: Clinical outcomes after lumbar discectomy for sciatica: The effects of fragment type and annular competence. J Bone Joint Surg (Am) 2003;85:102-108.
37. Buttermann GR: Treatment of lumbar disc herniation: Epidural steroid injection compared with discectomy: A prospective, randomized study. J Bone Joint Surg (Am) 2004;86:670-679.
38. Atlas SJ, Keller RB, Wu YA, et al: Long term outcomes of surgical and nonsurgical management of sciatica secondary to a lumbar disc herniation: 10 year results from the Maine Lumbar Spine Study. Spine 2005;30:927-935.
39. Osterman H, Seitsalo S, Karppinen J, Malmivaara A: Effectiveness of microdiscectomy for lumbar disc herniation: A randomized controlled trial with 2 years of follow-up. Spine 2006;31:2409-2414.
40. Jonsson B, Annertz M, Sjoberg C, Stromqvist B: A prospective and conservative study of surgically treated lumbar spinal stenosis. Part II: Five-year follow-up by an independent observer. Spine 1997;22:2938-2944.
41. Amundsen T, Weber H, Nordal HJ, et al: Lumbar spinal stenosis: Conservative or surgical management? A prospective 10-year study. Spine 2000;25:1424-1436.
42. Atlas SJ, Deyo RA, Keller RB, et al: The Maine Lumbar Spine Study: III: 1-year outcomes of surgical and nonsurgical management of lumbar spinal stenosis. Spine 1996;21:1787-1795.
43. Atlas SJ, Keller RB, Robson D, et al: Surgical and nonsurgical management of lumbar spinal stenosis: Four-year outcomes from the Maine Lumbar Spine Study. Spine 2000;25:556-562.
44. Atlas SJ, Keller RB, Wu YA, et al: Long-term outcomes of surgical and nonsurgical management of lumbar spinal stenosis: 8 to 10 year results from the Maine Lumbar Spine Study. Spine 2005;30:936-943.
45. Turner JA, Ersek M, Herron L, Deyo R: Surgery for lumbar spinal stenosis. Attempted meta-analysis of the literature. Spine 1992;17:1-8.
46. Deyo RA, Mirza SK: Spinal fusion surgery—The case for restraint. New Engl J Med 2004;350:722-725.
47. Fritzell P, Hagg O, Wessberg P, Nordwall A: Lumbar fusion versus nonsurgical treatment for chronic low back pain: A multicenter randomized controlled trail from the Swedish Lumbar Spine Study Group. Spine 2001;26:2521-2532.
48. Ivar Brox J, Sorenson R, Friis A, et al: Randomized clinical trial of lumbar instrumented fusion and cognitive interven-

tion and exercises in patients with chronic low back pain and disc degeneration. Spine 2003;28:1913-1921.

49. Yuan PS, Albert TJ: Nonsurgical and surgical management of lumbar spinal stenosis. J Bone Joint Surg (Am) 2004; 2320-2330.

50. Benzon HT: Epidural steroid injections for low back pain and lumbosacral radiculopathy. Pain 1986;24:277-295.

51. Koes BW, Scholten RJPM, Mens JMA, et al: Efficacy of epidural steroid injections for low back pain and sciatica: A systematic review of randomized clinical trials. Pain 1995;63: 279-288.

52. Watts RW, Silagy CA: A meta-analysis on the efficacy of epidural corticosteroids in the treatment of sciatica. Anaesth Intensive Care 1995;23:564-569.

53. Boswell MV, Shah RV, Everett CR, et al: Interventional techniques in the management of chronic spinal pain: Evidence-based practice guidelines. Pain Physician 2005;8: 1-47.

54. Dilke TFW, Burry HC, Grahame R: Extradural corticosteroid injection in management of lumbar nerve root compression. Br Med J 1973;2:635-637.

55. Snoek W, Weber H, Jorgensen B: Double blind evaluation of extradural methylprednisolone for herniated lumbar discs. Acta Orthop Scand 1977;48:635-641.

56. Carette S, Leclaire R, Marcoux S, et al: Epidural corticosteroid injections for sciatica due to herniated nucleus pulposus. N Engl J Med 1997;336:1634-1640.

57. Cuckler JM, Bernini PA, Wiesel SW, et al: The use of epidural steroids in the treatment of lumbar radicular pain. J Bone Joint Surg (Am) 1985;67:63-66.

58. Arden NK, Price C, Reading I, et al: A multicentre randomized controlled trial of epidural corticosteroid injections for sciatica: The WEST study. Rheumatology 2005;44:1399-1406.

59. Wilson-MacDonald J, Burt G, Griffen D, Glynn C: Epidural steroid injection for nerve root compression: A randomized, controlled trial. J Bone Joint Surg (Br) 2005;87:352-355.

60. Armon C, Argoff CA, Samuels J, Backonja MM: Assessment: Use of epidural steroid injections to treat radicular lumbosacral pain. Neurology 2007;68:723-729.

61. Vroomen PC, de Krom MC, Slofstra PD, et al: Conservative treatment of sciatica: A systematic review. J Spinal Disord 2000;13:463-469.

62. Benoist M: The natural history of lumbar disc herniation and radiculopathy. Joint Bone Spine 2002;69:155-160.

63. Benoist M: The natural history of lumbar degenerative spinal stenosis. Joint Bone Spine 2002;69:450-457.

64. Stav A, Ovadia L, Sternberg A, et al: Cervical epidural steroid injection for cervicobrachialgia. Acta Anaesthesiol Scand 1993;37:562-566.

65. Castagnera L, Maurette P, Pointillart, et al: Long term results of cervical epidural steroid injection with and without morphine in chronic cervical radicular pain. Pain 1994;58:239.

66. Bush K, Hillier S: Outcome of cervical radiculopathy treated with periradicular/epidural corticosteroid injections: A prospective study with independent clinical review. Eur Spine J 1996;5:319.

67. Riew KD, Yin Y, Gilula L, et al: The effect of nerve-root injections on the need for operative treatment of lumbar radicular pain: A prospective, randomized, controlled, double-blind study. J Bone Joint Surg (Am) 2000;82:1589-1593.

68. Karppinen J, Malmivaara A, Kurunlahti M, et al: Periradicular infiltration for sciatica: A randomized controlled trial. Spine 2001;26:1059-1067.

69. Ng L, Chaudhary N, Sell P: The efficacy of corticosteroids in periradicular infiltration for chronic radicular pain: A randomized, double-blind, controlled trial. Spine 2005;30: 857-862.

70. Kraemer J, Ludwig J, Bickert U, et al: Lumbar epidural perineural injection: A new technique Eur Spine J 1997;6: 357-361.

71. Thomas E, Cyteval C, Abiad L, et al: Effect of transforaminal versus interspinous corticosteroid injection in discal radicul-algia—A prospective, randomized, double-blind study. Clin Rheumatol 2003;22:299-304.

72. Schaufele M, Hatch L: Interlaminar versus transforaminal epidural injections in the treatment of symptomatic lumbar

73. Abram SE: Complications associated with epidural, facet joint, and sacroiliac joint injections. In Neal JM, Rathmell JP (eds): Complications in Regional Anesthesia and Pain Medicine. Philadelphi, Saunders, 2007, pp 247-257.

74. Fitzgibbon DR, Posner KL, Caplan RA, et al: Chronic pain management: American Society of Anesthesiologists Closed Claims Project. Anesthesiology 2004;100:98-105.

75. Bogduk N: Complications associated with transforaminal injections. In Neal JM, Rathmell JP (eds): Complications in Regional Anesthesia and Pain Medicine. Philadelphia, Saunders, 2007, pp 259-265.

76. Benzon HT, Gissen AJ, Strichartz GR, et al: The effect of polyethylene glycol on mammalian nerve impulses. Anesth Analg 1987;66:553-559.

77. Benzon HT, Chew TL, McCarthy R, et al: Comparison of the particle sizes of the different steroids and the effect of dilution: A review of the relative neurotoxicities of the steroids. Anesthesiology 2007;106:331-338.

78. Cohen SP, Raja SN: Pathogenesis, diagnosis, and treatment of lumbar zygapophyseal (facet) joint pain. Anesthesiology 2007;106:591-614.

79. Schwarzer AC, Aprill CN, Derby R, et al: The false-positive rate of uncontrolled diagnostic blocks of the lumbar zygapophyseal joints. Pain 1994;58:195-200.

80. Lynch MC, Taylor JF: Facet joint pain for low back pain: A clinical study. J Bone Joint Surg (Br) 1986;68:138-141.

81. Lilius G, Laasonen EM, Myllynen P, et al: Lumbar facet joint syndrome: A randomised clinical trial. J Bone Joint Surg (Br) 1989;71:681-684.

82. Carette S, Marcoux S, Trouchon R, et al: A controlled trial of corticosteroid injections into facet joints for chronic low back pain. N Engl J Med 1991;325:1002-1007.

83. Marks RC, Houston T, Thulbourne T: Facet joint injection and facet nerve block: A randomized comparison in 86 patients with chronic low back pain. Pain 1992;49:325-328.

84. King JS, Lagger R: Sciatica viewed as referred pain syndrome. Surg Neurol 1976;5:46-50.

85. Gallagher G, Petriccione di Vadi PL, Vedley JR, et al: Radiofrequency facet joint denervation in the treatment of low back pain: A prospective, controlled double-blind study to assess its efficacy. Pain Clin 1994;7:193-198.

86. Sanders M, Zuurmond WW: Percutaneous intra-articular lumbar facet joint denervation in the treatment of low back pain: A comparison with percutaneous extra-articular lumbar facet denervation. Pain Clin 1999;11:329-335.

87. van Kleef M, Barendse GA, Kessels A, et al: Randomized trial of radiofrequency lumbar facet denervation for chronic low back pain. Spine 1999;24:1937-1942.

88. Leclaire R, Fortin L, Lambert R, et al: Radiofrequency facet joint denervation in the treatment of low back pain: A placebo-controlled clinical trial to assess efficacy. Spine 2001;26:1411-1416.

89. van Wijk RM, Geurtz JW, Wynne HJ, et al: Radiofrequency denervation of lumbar facet joints in the treatment of chronic low back pain: A randomized, double-blind, sham lesion-controlled trial. Clin J Pain 2005;21:335-344.

90. Lord SM, Barnsley L, Wallis BJ, et al: Percutaneous radiofrequency neurotomy for chronic cervical zygapophyseal-joint pain. N Engl J Med 1996;335:1721-1726.

91. Stovner LJ, Kolstad F, Helde G: Radiofrequency denervation of facet joints C2-C6 in cervicogenic headache: A randomized, double-blind-sham-controlled study. Cephalalgia 2004; 24:821-830.

92. Richebe P, Rathmell JP, Brennan TJ: Immediate early genes after pulsed radiofrequency treatment: Neurobiology in need of clinical trials. Anesthesiology 2005;102:1-3.

93. Slappendel R, Crul BJ, Braak GJ, et al: The efficacy of radiofrequency lesioning of the cervical spinal dorsal root ganglion in a double-blinded, randomized study: No difference between 40 degrees C and 67 degrees C treatments. Pain 1997;73:159-163.

94. Mikeladze G, Espinal R, Finnegan R, et al: Pulsed radiofrequency application in treatment of chronic zygapophyseal joint pain. Spine J 2003;3:360-362.

95. Letcher FS, Goldring S: The effect of radiofrequency current and heat on peripheral nerve action potential in the cat. J Neurosurg 1968;29:42-47.

96. Smith HP, McWorther JM, Challa VR: Radiofrequency neurolysis in a clinical model. J Neurosurg 1981;55:243-253.

97. van Kleef M, Spaans F, Dingemans W, et al: Effects and side effects of a percutaneous thermal lesion of the dorsal root ganglia in patients with cervical pain syndrome. Pain 1993;52:49-53.

98. Slujter ME, Cosman ER, Rittman WB, van Kleef M: The effects of pulsed radiofrequency fields applied to dorsal root ganglion—A preliminary report. Pain Clin 1998;11:109-117.

99. Higuchi Y, Nashold BS, Sluijter M, et al: Exposure of the dorsal root ganglion in rats to pulse radiofrequency activates dorsal horn lamina I and II neurons. Neurosurgery 2002;50:850-855.

100. Munglani R: The long term effects of pulsed radiofrequency for neuropathic pain. Pain 1999;80:437-439.

101. Mikeladze G, Espinal R, Finnegan R, et al: Pulsed radiofrequency applications in treatment of chronic zygapophyseal joint pain. Spine J 2003;3:360-362.

102. Bayer E, Racz G, Day M, Heavner J: Sphenopalatine ganglion pulsed radiofrequency treatment in 30 patients suffering from chronic face and head pain. Pain Practice 2005;5:223-227.

103. Cohen SP, Foster A: Pulsed radiofrequency as a treatment for groin pain and orchialgia. Urology 2003;61:645.

104. Shah RV, Racz GB: Pulsed mode radiofrequency lesioning of the suprascapular nerve for the treatment of chronic shoulder pain. Pain Physician 2003;6:503-506.

105. Van Zundert J, Brabant S, Van de Kelft E, et al: Pulsed radiofrequency treatment of the Gasserian ganglion in patients with idiopathic trigeminal neuralgia. Pain 2003;104:449-452.

106. Cohen SP, Sireci A, Wu CL, et al: Pulsed radiofrequency of the dorsal root ganglia is superior to pharmacotherapy or pulsed radiofrequency of the intercostal nerves in the treatment of chronic postsurgical thoracic pain. Pain Physician 2006;9:227-236.

107. Sluijter ME, Cosman ER, Rittman WB, Van Kleef M: The effects of pulsed radiofrequency fields applied to the dorsal root ganglion—A preliminary report. Pain Clin 1998;11:109-117.

108. Erdine S, Ozyalcin NS, Cimen A, Celik M, et al: Comparison of pulsed radiofrequency with conventional radiofrequency in the treatment of idiopathic trigeminal neuralgia. Eur J Pain 2006 (ahead of print).

109. Van Zundert J, Patijn J, Kessels A, et al: Pulsed radiofrequency adjacent to the cervical dorsal root ganglion in chronic cervical radicular pain: A double-blind sham controlled clinical trial. Pain 2007;127(1-2):173-182.

110. Bogduk N: Pulsed radiofrequency. Pain Med 2006;7:396-407.

111. Cahana A, Van Zundert JV, Macrea L, et al: Pulsed radiofrequency: Current clinical and biological literature available. Pain Med 2006;7:411-423.

112. van Tulder MW, Koes BW, Bouter LM: Conservative treatment of acute and chronic nonspecific low back pain: A systematic review of randomized clinical trials of the most common interventions. Spine 1997;22:2128-2156.

113. Morley S, Eccleston C, Williams A: Systematic review and meta-analysis of randomized controlled trials of cognitive behavior therapy and behavior therapy for chronic pain in adults, excluding headache. Pain 1999;80:1-13.

114. Guzman J, Esmail R, Karjalainen K, et al: Multidisciplinary rehabilitation for chronic low back pain: A systematic review. Br Med J 2001;322:1511-5116.

115. van Tulder MW, Ostelo R, Vlaeyen JWS, et al: Behavioral treatment for low back pain: A systematic review within the framework of the Cochrane Back Review Group. Spine 2001;26:270-281.

116. Nielson WR, Weir R: Biopsychosocial approaches to the treatment of chronic pain. Clin J Pain 2001;17S:S114-S127.

117. Hoffman BM, Papas RK, Chatkoff DK, Kerns RD: Meta-analysis of psychological interventions for chronic low back pain. Health Psychol 2007;26:1-9.

118. Martell BA, O'Connor PG, Kerns RD, et al: Systematic review: Opioid treatment for chronic back pain: Prevalence, efficacy, and association with addiction. Ann Intern Med 2007;146:116-127.

119. Richards R, Zhang P, Friedman M, Dhanda R: Controlled-release oxycodone relieves moderate to severe pain in a 3-month study of persistent moderate to severe back pain (Abstract). Pain Med 2002;31:176.

120. Kuntz D, Brossel R: Analgesic effect and clinical tolerability of the combination of paracetamol 500 mg and caffeine 50 mg versus paracetamol 400 mg and dextropropoxyphene 30 mg in back pain. Presse Med 1996;25:1171-1174.

121. Hale ME, Dvergsten C, Gimbel J: Efficacy and safety of oxymorphone extended release in chronic low back pain: Results of randomized, double-blind, placebo- and active-controlled phase III study. J Pain 2005;6:21-28.

122. Jamison RN, Raymond SA, Slawsby ES, et al: Opioid therapy for chronic noncancer back pain: A randomized prospective study. Spine 1998;23:2591-2600.

123. Muller PO, Odendaal CL, Muller FR, et al: Comparison of the efficacy and tolerability of a parcetamol/codeine fixed-dose combination with tramadol in patients with refractory chronic back pain. Arzneimittelforschung 1998;48:675-679.

124. Tennant F, Moll D, DePaulo V: Topical morphine for peripheral pain (Letter). Lancet 1993;342:1047-1048.

125. Thurel C, Bardin T, Boccard E: Analgesic efficacy of an association of 500-mg paracetamol plus 30-mg codeine versus 400-mg paracetamol plus 30-mg dextropropoxyphene in repeated doses for chronic low back pain. Curr Ther Res 1991;50:463-473.

126. Gammaitoni AR, Galer BS, Lacouture P, et al: Effectiveness and safety of new oxycodone/acetaminophen formulations with reduced acetaminophen for the treatment of low back pain. Pain Med 2003;4:21-30.

127. Schofferman J: Long-term opioid analgesic therapy for severe refractory lumbar spine pain. Clin J Pain 1999;15:136-140.

128. Ringe JD, Faber H, Bock O, et al: Transdermal fentanyl for the treatment of back pain caused by vertebral osteoporosis. Rheumatol Int 2002;22:199-203.

129. Simpson RK, Edmondson EA, Constant CF, Collier C: Transdermal fentanyl as treatment for chronic low back pain. J Pain Symptom Manage 1997;14:218-224.

130. Salzman RT, Roberts MS, Wild J, et al: Can a controlled-release oral dose form of oxycodone be used as readily as an immediate-release form for the purpose of titrating to stable pain control? J Pain Symptom Manage 1999;18:271-279.

131. Hale ME, Speight KL, Harsanyi Z, et al: Efficacy of 12 hourly controlled-release codeine compared with as required dosing of acetaminophen plus codeine in patients with chronic low back pain. Pain Res Manag 1997;2:33-38.

132. Hale ME, Fleischmann R, Salzman R, et al: Efficacy and safety of controlled-release versus immediate-release oxycodone: Randomized double-blind evaluation in patients with chronic back pain. Clin J Pain 1999;15:179-183.

133. Zenz M, Strumpf M, Tryba M: Long-term oral opioid therapy in patients with chronic nonmalignant pain. J Pain Symptom Manage 1992;7:69-77.

134. Fillingham RB, Doleys DM, Edwards RR, Lowery D: Clinical characteristics of chronic back pain as a function of gender and oral opioid use. Spine 2003;28:143-150.

135. Turk DC, Okifuji A: What factors affect physicians' decisions to prescribe opioids for chronic noncancer pain patients? Clin J Pain 1997;13:330-336.

136. Fanciullo GJ, Ball PSA, Girault G, et al: An observational study on the prevalence and pattern on opioid use in 25,479 patients with spine and radicular pain. Spine 2002;27:201-205.

137. Chou R, Clark E, Helfand M: Comparative efficacy and safety of long-acting oral opioids for chronic non-cancer pain: A systematic review. J Pain Symptom Manage 2003;26:1026-1048.

138. Schnitzer TJ, Ferraro A, Hunsche E, Kong SX: A comprehensive review of clinical trials on the efficacy and safety of drugs for the treatment of low back pain. J Pain Symptom Manage 2004;28:72-95.

71 Outcomes, Efficacy, and Complications of Neuropathic Pain

Christopher L. Wu, Elaina E. Lin, and David N. Maine

Clinicians are confronted with a wide variety of options for the treatment of neuropathic pain. Traditionally, certain interventions have been used, although others deemed ineffective (e.g., opioids) for the treatment of neuropathic pain; however, with our increasing knowledge of the pathophysiology of neuropathic pain and development of newer analgesic agents and interventions, there has been a renewed effort in critically evaluating all available treatment options. In addition, the increased general interest in evidence-based medicine and critical examination of the literature, both individually and systematically, have led to increased interest in examining the analgesic efficacy of current options for the treatment of neuropathic pain.

OVERVIEW OF STUDIES

Over the past few years there has been an increase in the number and quality of randomized controlled trials evaluating various options for the treatment of neuropathic pain. In many cases, particularly for systemic analgesics, there have been enough high-quality trials to undertake meaningful systematic reviews and meta-analyses of specific treatment options for neuropathic pain. These systematic reviews are useful for clinicians not only because they summarize the available literature in a systematic fashion but also because in some cases, they provide clinicians the relative analgesic efficacy of a particular option compared with other choices. The most common, easiest method for a practitioner to use is the number-needed-to-treat (NNT) or number-needed-to-harm (NNH), which allows a comparison of analgesic efficacy and harm across drug classes. The NNT represents the number of patients a clinician must treat to expect to achieve that outcome (e.g., >50% pain reduction). For instance, an NNT of three is interpreted that we would need to treat three patients before we would expect that 1 patient would

achieve the outcome of interest. The lower the NNT, the greater the efficacy of that particular intervention. Likewise, the higher the NNH, the fewer adverse events are associated with that particular intervention (or the lower the NNH, the more adverse events). Although the majority of available trials have focused primarily on pain relief and side effects profile of a particular intervention, more recent studies are beginning to incorporate valid, psychometrically developed instruments (both generic and disease specific) to comprehensively assess the efficacy of an analgesic in the treatment of neuropathic pain.[1]

OUTCOMES AND EFFICACY

There are a wide variety of systemic analgesic and interventional options for the treatment of neuropathic pain. Because of the large variation in study quality, the presence of many types of neuropathic pain states, and the numerous agents and options studied, it may be difficult for a clinician to truly determine which systematic analgesic and interventional options are truly efficacious for the treatment of neuropathic pain. We focus on the more commonly available and used systematic analgesic and interventional options for the treatment of neuropathic pain, focusing on the results of systematic reviews and meta-analyses when available.

SYSTEMIC ANALGESICS

Opioids

Outcomes and Efficacy

Although opioid analgesics are commonly used for the treatment of nociceptive pain, the analgesic efficacy of opioids for the treatment of neuropathic pain is unclear. Available trials examining the analgesic efficacy of opioids for the treatment of neuropathic pain yield conflicting results and there are many methodologic issues regarding trial design, including inadequate sample sizes, type of opioids administered, and duration of opioid treatment.[2] Other considerations that may contribute to the controversial nature of the use of opioids for the treatment of neuropathic pain include the use of multiple definitions and pain assessments of neuropathic pain and the presence of interindividual differences in opioid responsiveness.[3] Other factors, including the fear of opioid-related side effects, development of tolerance, and overstated fear of addiction, also may contribute to the underuse of opioids for treating neuropathic pain.

There have been several systematic reviews and meta-analyses on the analgesic efficacy of opioids for the treatment of neuropathic pain, with both intravenous and oral routes of opioid administration shown to be effective. One meta-analysis examined analyzed randomized, double-blind, controlled trials through December 2004 and separated trials into short- (<24 hours) and intermediate-term (median, 47 days) groups depending on the duration of outcomes assessment.[2] A total of four short-term and eight intermediate-term trials were ultimately accepted for analysis. Although the evidence of short-term studies in significantly decreasing neuropathic pain intensity was equivocal, analysis of intermediate-term studies (which may be more clinically meaningful) revealed a statistically significant decrease in pain scores (a weighted mean of 14 on a 0 to 100 scale) with similar opioid responsiveness for pain of central and peripheral etiologies (Fig. 71–1).[2] A quantitative systematic review of randomized controlled trials for analgesic therapy in postherpetic neuralgia noted that opioids demonstrated analgesic efficacy for the treatment of this type of neuropathic pain such as that pooled analysis yielded an NNT of only 2.7 (95% confidence interval [CI] = 2.1 to 3.8).[4]

The relative underdosing of opioids may have contributed to the controversy of whether opioids are effective for the treatment of neuropathic pain. Possible mechanisms by which nerve injury may decrease the analgesic actions of opioids include disturbances in presynaptic opioid receptor sites, increased central sensitization due to activation of N-methyl-D-aspartate (NMDA) receptors, antagonism of the inhibitory action of opioids by the cholecystokinin (CCK) system, and alteration of the descending-facilitatory controls on spinal sensory processing.[5] As a result, there may be a difference in opioid responsiveness between neuropathic and nociceptive pain such that higher doses of opioids may be necessary to decrease neuropathic pain compared with that for nociceptive pain.[6] A double-blind, randomized controlled trial evaluated the analgesic efficacy of a low and high dose of oral opioid for the treatment of a variety of neuropathic pains refractory to conventional therapy.[7] Over the 8-week study period, the authors found that patients who received the high-dose opioid regimen had a significant lower reduction of pain, improved sleep, a decrease in affective

distress, and reduction in interference with functioning compared with that in the low-dose group.[7] Finally, the concurrent use of other analgesic agents such as gabapentin during opioid therapy for the treatment of neuropathic pain may provide better analgesia at lower doses of each drug than either given alone for the treatment of neuropathic pain.[8] Thus the available data seem to indicate that opioids are effective in the treatment of neuropathic pain; however, higher doses may be necessary in some patients to achieve pain relief.

Complications

Although opioids are widely recognized to result in nausea, vomiting, pruritus, urinary retention, sedation, and less commonly, endocrine dysfunction, loss of libido, and immunosuppression,[9] long-term administration, and use of sustained-release agents generally may result in a lower incidence of these side effects because they provide more stable and steady serum opioid level. Although potential cognitive and neuropsychological side effects from opioid administration are somewhat controversial, some available data suggest that chronic use of opioids does not have an adverse effect on cognitive function because patients on chronic opioids did not demonstrate any decrease in neuropsychological testing or experimental driving ability.[10-13] All patients on chronic opioid therapy will develop tolerance and physical dependence, but the risk of addiction appears extremely low in patients without a history of addiction and who are prescribed opioids for legitimate medical purposes.[14,15] Although the presence of active addiction may have an adverse effect on the treatment of chronic neuropathic pain, the incidence of opioid addiction is thought to be less than 1%[16,17] (compared with addictive disorders present in approximately 10% of the general population[18]), and there are several methods to screen for patients who are suspected to have active opioid addiction.[18]

Anticonvulsants

Outcomes and Efficacy

Anticonvulsant drugs have been one of the more common and traditional options for the treatment of neuropathic pain of both peripheral and central origin. The similarities in cellular and molecular changes between certain forms of epilepsy and neuropathic pain resulted in the use of anticonvulsant agents for the treatment of neuropathic pain.[19] Because the molecular changes in neuropathic pain generally are marked by a peripheral accumulation of a novel sodium channel (peripheral nerve 3 [PN3]), increased NMDA receptor activity, reduction in gamma-aminobutyric acid inhibition, and changes in the penetration of calcium into neurons, use of anticonvulsant drugs may reduce overall neuronal excitability in part by blocking sodium channel

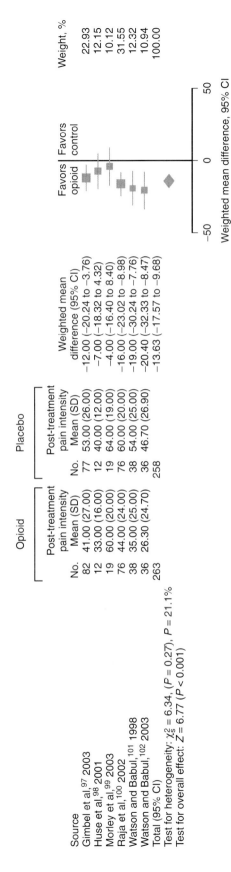

Figure 71–1. Results of the meta-analysis of intermediate-term trial efficacy. Data are presented as mean (95% confidence interval [CI]) differences in post-treatment pain intensity (on a Visual Analogue Scale from 0 to 100) between active treatment and placebo (fixed-effects model). Size of the data markers corresponds to the weight of the study in the meta-analysis. (From Eisenberg E, McNicol ED, Carr DB: Efficacy and safety of opioid agonists in the treatment of neuropathic pain of nonmalignant origin: Systematic review and meta-analysis of randomized controlled trials. JAMA 2005;293:3043-3052.)

activity.[19] Although carbamazepine and phenytoin were among the first anticonvulsants to be used for the treatment of neuropathic pain, newer agents such as gabapentin, lamotrigine, and pregabalin are more commonly used clinically.

Several systematic reviews of the efficacy of anticonvulsants for the treatment of neuropathic pain are available and the evidence is in favor of the use of anticonvulsants in decreasing neuropathic pain. Two systematic reviews indicate that gabapentin is effective for the treatment of neuropathic pain.[20,21] A systematic review of 14 trials (1398 subjects) examining the use of gabapentin for a variety of chronic neuropathic pain states revealed that the NNT for gabapentin is 4.3 (95% CI = 3.5 to 5.7) with 42% of subjects who received gabapentin showing an improvement compared with 19% on placebo.[20] The NNT for effective pain relief was lower for specific neuropathic pain states: 3.9 for postherpetic neuralgia and 2.9 for diabetic neuropathy.[20] A systematic review of both the controlled and uncontrolled literature also indicates that gabapentin seems to be effective in multiple neuropathic pain states.[21] A systematic review of the use of carbamazepine for the treatment of chronic neuropathic pain (including trigeminal neuralgia) examined 12 studies; however, only 2 of the studies provided evaluable data, which yielded an NNT of 1.8 (95% CI = 1.4 to 2.8), suggesting that carbamazepine is effective for the treatment of neuropathic pain although the size of the trials was relatively small.[20]

Other anticonvulsants have been examined for the treatment of neuropathic pain, although no systematic review or meta-analysis of trials is available at this time. Pregabalin, which interacts with the voltage-gated calcium channels that may be important in modulating neuropathic pain, has been shown to be effective in decreasing pain in a variety of neuropathic pain conditions including diabetic peripheral neuropathy and postherpetic neuralgia.[22-24] Higher doses (300 to 600 mg/day) produced more consistent results in reducing pain and improving quality of sleep and quality of life than lower doses (75 to 150 mg/day).[22-24] Both fixed and flexible regimens of pregabalin administration were effective in decreasing neuropathic pain over a 12-week period.[25] Oxcarbazepine, another newer anticonvulsant agent, was shown to be effective in reducing diabetic neuropathic pain when titrated to a maximum dose of 1800 mg/day.[26] However, it is not clear whether topiramate, a novel anticonvulsant with multiple neurostabilizing activities, is effective for the treatment of neuropathic pain because three randomized trials did not show efficacy in reducing diabetic neuropathic pain in doses up to 400 mg/day,[27] although other data suggest that topiramate may have some efficacy in reducing neuropathic pain of diabetic origin.[28,29] The available data examining the analgesic efficacy of lamotrigine in relieving neuropathic pain of different origins suggest that this agent may be useful in treating neuropathic pain, although not all randomized trials have demonstrated analgesic efficacy.[30-33]

Complications

Although individual anticonvulsant agents are associated with different side effect profiles, common side effects with anticonvulsants in general include sedation and cerebellar symptoms such as tremor, nystagmus, and incoordination.[19] Older anticonvulsants such as phenytoin and carbamazepine are associated with potential hematologic and cardiac side effects, whereas the newer agents may have a more favorable side effect profile. Common side effects from gabapentin include sedation-somnolence, fatigue, dizziness, dry mouth and occasionally ataxia, edema, blurry vision, headache, and nausea; however, the incidence of some of these side effects may be similar to those receiving placebo in some randomized trials.[8,21] The NNH for gabapentin for minor adverse events is 3.7 (95%CI = 2.4 to 5.4) and was not significant for adverse events leading to withdrawal from a controlled clinical trial (14% withdrew with gabapentin versus 10% for placebo).[20]

Antidepressants

Outcomes and Efficacy

Like the anticonvulsants, antidepressant agents have been traditionally used to treat neuropathic and chronic pain. Although antidepressant drugs, particularly the tricyclic antidepressants agents (TCAs), presumably exert the majority of their analgesic actions through the inhibition of presynaptic reuptake of monoaminergic transmitters, especially norepinephrine and to a lesser extent serotonin; other possible mechanisms of analgesic action include interference with the opioid system, interaction with NMDA receptors, and inhibition of ion channel activity.[34] Although the analgesic effects of antidepressants for the treatment of chronic pain occur independently from their antidepressant effects by blocking the reuptake of monoaminergic transmitters, antidepressant agents potentiate the inhibitory descending pathways on dorsal horn nociceptive transmission.[34]

TCAs may be the most effective classes of drugs for the treatment of neuropathic pain. A meta-analysis of 25 randomized controlled trials revealed that TCAs are a very effective treatment for a variety of neuropathic pains, with amitriptyline having an NNT of 2 (95% CI = 1.7 to 2.5) and desipramine having an NNT of 2.1 (95% CI = 1.5 to 3.2).[35] The analgesic efficacy of TCAs is not the same for all types of neuropathic pain; TCAs are most effective for diabetic neuropathy (NNT = 1.3; 95% CI = 1.2 to 1.5) and postherpetic neuralgia (NNT = 2.2; 95% CI = 1.7 to 3.1) but not effective in HIV-related neuropathies.[35] The findings in this systematic review are similar to those in other systematic reviews and meta-analysis.[4,36] Selective serotonin reuptake inhibitors (SSRIs) are less effective than TCAs in treating neuropathic pain. Compared with that for TCAs, the NNT for SSRIs for the treatment of neuropathic pain is much higher (NNT = 6.7; 95% CI = 3.4 to 43.5).[34,36] It appears that inhibition of norepinephrine rather than serotonin reuptake is more important for the analgesic effects of antidepressants.[34]

Newer antidepressants, such as venlafaxine and mirtazapine, also have been examined for their analgesic efficacy although there are not enough trials presently for a large-scale systematic review of these agents and their analgesic effects on neuropathic pain. Venlafaxine inhibits the reuptake of both norepinephrine, serotonin, and to a much lesser extent, dopamine. This agent also may interact with cholinergic, muscarinic, and α-adrenergic receptors and primarily inhibits serotonin reuptake at lower doses but preferentially inhibits norepinephrine at higher doses.[34] Several randomized controlled trials suggest that venlafaxine may be effective for the treatment of neuropathic pain including diabetic neuropathy and postmastectomy syndrome.[34,37] Classified as a noradrenergic and specific serotonergic antidepressant (NaSSA), mirtazapine facilitates noradrenergic transmission by blocking central presynaptic α_2-adrenegic receptors (thus preventing further norarenergic release) and facilitates serotonergic transmission by several possible mechanisms.[34] No large-scale randomized trials are available at this time, but animal studies suggest that mirtazapine and other similar newer antidepressants may be effective for the treatment of neuropathic pain.[38]

Complications

Although individual antidepressant drugs vary in their side effect profiles, SSRIs appear to be better tolerated than TCAs; however, TCAs demonstrate superior analgesic efficacy when compared with that of SSRIs.[34,36] TCAs typically exhibit stronger anticholinergic effects and patients have noted dry mouth, somnolence, palpitation-tachycardia, nausea, dizziness, constipation, and light-headedness. Nausea occurs more frequently with SSRIs.[39] The long-term dropout rate from side effects may be approximately 5%, but clinicians must remember that many TCAs are highly toxic in overdose, whereas the SSRIs appear much safer in this situation.[39] Overall, the NNH for minor adverse events was 4.6 (95% CI = 3.3 to 6.7) and 16 (95% CI = 10 to 45) for a major adverse event leading to withdrawal from a study.[35]

Local Anesthetics

Outcomes and Efficacy

Following peripheral nerve injury, a subtype of sodium channel (tetrodotoxin-resistant) known as the PN3 or sensory nerve specific (SNS), which exists only on sensory nerves accumulates at the end of the damaged nerve.[40] These sensory neuron-specific sodium channels may trigger neuropathic pain through spontaneous activation or nerve injury hyperexcitability.[40] Although anticonvulsants and antidepressants may potentially bock these sodium channels, the prototypical sodium channel blockers are local anesthetics, such as lidocaine. Lidocaine has the ability to attenuate ectopic discharges from neurons at concentrations below that for conduction blockade.[41]

Several systematic reviews examine the use of local anesthetics, particularly lidocaine (administered intravenously or topically) and mexiletine (administered orally), for the treatment of neuropathic pain. One recent systematic review of local anesthetic agents in the treatment of neuropathic pain examined 32 randomized, double-blind, crossover, controlled trials evaluating intravenous lidocaine (16 trials), mexiletine (12 trials), lidocaine followed by mexiletine (1 trial), and tocainide (1 trial).[42] Administration of intravenous lidocaine or mexiletine, the oral analogue of lidocaine, provided superior analgesia versus placebo and analgesic efficacy compared with carbamazepine, gabapentin, amantadine, or morphine.[42] A meta-analysis of 19 randomized controlled trials (10 lidocaine, 9 mexiletine) also demonstrated that both lidocaine and mexiletine provided superior analgesia (weighted mean difference of −10.6 on a Visual Analogue Scale of 0 to 100; 95% CI = −14.5 to −6.7) and were equivalent to morphine, gabapentin, amitriptyline, and amantadine for neuropathic pain.[41]

In examining individual types of neuropathic pain, intravenous lidocaine has been successfully used for the treatment of pain from amputation (phantom), spinal cord injury, peripheral nerve injury, diabetic neuropathy, lumbosacral radiculopathy, postherpetic neuralgia, and complex regional pain syndromes I and II.[41] The dose of intravenous lidocaine infusions in these studies were administered typically over 3 to 45 minutes and up to a total dose of 5 mg/kg.[41] Oral mexiletine has been successfully used for the treatment of neuropathic pain from spinal cord injury, diabetic neuropathy, and peripheral nerve injury.[41] Although the analgesic efficacy of mexiletine appears to be dose dependent and mexiletine doses of up to 675 mg administered three times per day have been reported,[40,43] typical doses are lower (100 to 200 mg three times per day) and higher dosages may be difficult to achieve clinically because of adverse side effects.[44]

Lidocaine may also be administered transdermally and is typically available as a 5% transdermal patch. Similar to that seen with intravenous or oral administration, transdermal lidocaine appears to attenuate ectopic neural discharges and the analgesia provided occurs in the absence of an anesthetic effect.[45] Randomized controlled trials indicate that lidocaine patch 5% is effective in relieving a variety of neuropathic pain states including postherpetic neuralgia and focal peripheral neuropathies.[46,47] The NNT for lidocaine pain to provide more than 50% pain relief is approximately 4.4, and the patch is very well tolerated with minimal side effects.[45,46]

Complications

Common side effects associated with administration of intravenous lidocaine and oral mexiletine include drowsiness, fatigue, nausea, and dizziness.[41] Other reported side effects with intravenous lidocaine include blurred vision, dysarthria, tremor, and light-headedness.[48] The most common side effects associated with mexiletine are nausea and sedation, although insomnia, trismus, headache, agitation, nightmares, and tremors have been reported.[49] No major adverse events were reported in controlled clinical trials with local anesthetics for treatment of neuropathic pain and the adverse event rate for systemically administered local anesthetics was equivalent to that of morphine, amitriptyline, or gabapentin.[41] When administered as a lidocaine patch 5%, lidocaine results in primarily local side effects (irritation) with minimal systemic adverse reactions and minimal systemic absorption of lidocaine.[47]

α_2-Adrenergic Blockers

Outcomes and Efficacy

Receptors for the α_2-adrenergic receptor are located in both the peripheral and central nervous systems. Activation of these receptors is mediated through G proteins, which leads to hyperpolarization of the cell membrane.[50] Although there are many receptor subtypes and physiologic functions mediated by these receptors, presynaptic α_2-adrenergic receptors may be especially important for analgesia because they regulate the release of norepinephrine and adenosine triphosphate.[50] Another proposed mechanism of analgesic action of α_2-adrenergic receptor agonists is related to the reduction of calcium entry through N-type voltage-gated calcium channels.[50]

Experimental data indicates that α_2-adrenergic receptor agonists may attenuate mechanical hypersensitivity in established nerve injury and may play a role in peripheral nerve injury.[51,52] Commonly available α_2-adrenergic receptor agonists are clonidine (transdermal, neuraxial) and dexmedetomidine (intravenous). There currently are no large-scale systematic reviews that examine the analgesic efficacy of α_2-adrenergic receptor agonists in the treatment of neuropathic pain; however, clonidine, which is only effective when administered near its site of analgesic action in the spinal cord, is the second most commonly administered neuraxial agent for chronic pain.[53] Even though there appears to be an analgesic benefit of clonidine for the treatment of acute postoperative pain,[54] the role for α_2-adrenergic receptor agonists in the treatment of chronic neuropathic pain is unclear, although clonidine may be useful for a subset of patients with diabetic neuropathy and may be especially useful for continuous intrathecal therapy.[55,56]

Complications

The most common side effects of the α_2-adrenergic receptor agonists include sedation, hypotension, and bradycardia (due to postsynaptic inhibition of the α_2-adrenergic receptor).

NMDA Receptor Antagonists

Outcomes and Efficacy

NMDA antagonists have been used to treat not only many types of chronic pain because of their central role in the long-term processing of nociception, but also other long-term neuronal processes such as memory and learning and possibly in the development of drug tolerance and dependence.[57] NMDA receptors are inotropic receptors for the excitatory neurotransmitter glutamate, with the glutamate binding site located in the NR2 subunit.[57] Compared with other glutamate receptors, the NMDA receptor is different in the sense that there is enhanced calcium ion permeability that is consistent with its role in long-term physiologic processes such as chronic pain (central sensitization) and memory.[57]

Administration of NMDA antagonists may decrease neuropathic pain because of their central role in neuroplasticity. There are few clinically available NMDA antagonists including ketamine, memantine, amantadine, and three clinically used opioids (methadone, dextromethorphan, and ketobemidone).[58] The studies examining the analgesic efficacy of NMDA antagonists for the treatment of neuropathic pain are equivocal. A systematic review of NMDA antagonists for the treatment of postherpetic neuralgia suggested that NMDA antagonists were not effective for the treatment of this type of neuropathic pain because the NNT was relatively high at 23.9.[4] Use of dextromethorphan and memantine did not appear to be effective for the treatment of neuropathic pain of traumatic origin, trigeminal neuralgia, and other types of chronic neuropathic pain.[59-62] However, higher doses of dextromethorphan may be effective to relieve diabetic neuropathic pain but not pain from postherpetic neuralgia.[63,64] Infusions of ketamine may provide a temporary decrease in the intensity of neuropathic pain including postherpetic neuralgia, central neuropathic pain, postamputation pain, and trigeminal neuralgia.[57,65]

Complications

The analgesic efficacy of NMDA antagonists is generally limited by the presence of side effects. Because of the varying affinities for the NMDA receptor and the lack of separation between therapeutic and side effects, the use of NMDA antagonists is restricted clinically. Side effects associated with analgesic doses of ketamine include auditory-visual disturbances, hallucinations, dizziness, and sedation, although different dosages, presence of coanalgesics or sedatives, and different routes of administration may result in a different incidence of side effects.[66] Dextromethorphan is associated with light-headedness, drowsiness, sedation, ataxia, visual disturbances, nausea, and euphoria.[62,63] Newer NMDA antagonists that exhibit greater receptor selectively are being developed and may ultimately result in fewer side effects.[57]

Tramadol

Outcomes and Efficacy

Tramadol is a centrally acting analgesic that exerts its analgesic action primarily through inhibition of serotonin and norepinephrine reuptake, although it may also exhibit weak opioid and a monoaminergic mechanism of action.[67] Tramadol is a versatile analgesic agent because it may be administered in a wide variety of routes (intravenous, intramuscular, subcutaneous, oral [including sustained-release and drops], and rectal) and is frequently used for postoperative pain in some areas. Because of its versatility and unique mechanism of action, tramadol has also been used to treat neuropathic pain.

A systematic review on the use of tramadol for the treatment of neuropathic pain examined five randomized controlled trials, with three of these trials comparing tramadol to placebo.[68] Tramadol appeared to be efficacious for the treatment of neuropathic pain with an NNT to reduce pain by at least 50% of 3.5 (95% CI = 2.4 to 5.9).[68] There were no sufficient data to determine if tramadol was superior to other agents such as morphine or clomipramine for the treatment of neuropathic pain.[68] Another systematic review noted that tramadol appeared to demonstrate analgesic efficacy for the treatment of postherpetic neuralgia with an NNT of 4.8 (95% CI = 2.6 to 27) although the number of patients studied was low.[4]

Complications

Side effects of tramadol commonly include nausea and dizziness. Caution should be used or tramadol should be avoided in patients with a history of seizures or who may be at higher risk for development of seizures.[69] Pooled analyses from randomized trials indicate that the NNH for tramadol was 7.7 (95% CI = 4.6 to 20).[68] Compared with opioids, tramadol exhibits a relative lack of respiratory depression, major organ toxicity and histamine release, and dependence and abuse potential.[70]

Capsaicin

Outcomes and Efficacy

Capsaicin, the active agent in hot peppers, interacts with the VR1 receptor, which not only is localized to sensory neurons but also releases peptides on activation. Although the primary mechanism of analgesia presumably is the result of desensitization of sensory (C-fiber) neurons containing VR1 receptors following release of substance P, other mechanisms may involve epidermal nerve fiber loss and desensitization of VR1 receptors on A-fibers.[45] The effect of capsaicin exposure on nociceptive processing is in part dependent on the dose and route administered; however, in humans, capsaicin is administered topically in concentrations of 0.025% and 0.075% although higher concentrations (5% to 10%) have been administered in conjunction with regional anesthesia.[45,71] Typically following topical capsaicin administration, there is a period of burning at the application site (activation of sensory neurons), followed by decreased sensitivity and with repeated applications, persistent desensitization.[45,72]

A systematic review of six double-blind, randomized, placebo-controlled trials (656 patients) examining the use of topical capsaicin for the treatment of neuropathic pain revealed that capsaicin overall has moderate to poor efficacy in the relief of neuropathic pain, but topical capsaicin may be useful for a subgroup of patients who are unresponsive or intolerant to other analgesic treatments for neuropathic pain.[72] Although topical capsaicin is superior to placebo, the NNT for topical capsaicin (6.4 [85% CI = 3.8 to 21] after 4 weeks and 5.7 [95% CI = 4 to 10] after 8 weeks of treatment) for the treatment of neuropathic pain is generally higher than that for other analgesic treatment options.[72] However, a pooled estimate of topical capsaicin for postherpetic neuralgia yielded a lower NNT (greater efficacy) of 3.3 (95% CI = 2.3 to 5.9).[4] Because of the typically modest pain relief obtained, topical capsaicin is considered as an adjunct therapy and not a first-line treatment option for neuropathic pain.[45]

Complications

Approximately 54% (compared to 15% with placebo) of patients will note local adverse events such as burning pain following initial application.[72] Coughing was noted in approximately 8% of patients using the higher concentration of capsaicin (0.075%).[72] Overall, the NNH is reported at 2.5 (95% CI = 2.1 to 3.1) for local reactions and 9.8 (95% CI = 7.3 to 15) for adverse events related to patient withdrawal.[72] The drop-out rate for capsaicin treatment may be high, with as much as 46% withdrawing from capsaicin treatment within 4 weeks.[73]

INTERVENTIONAL OPTIONS

The quality and quantity of controlled clinical trials examining outcomes, efficacy, and complications for interventional options for neuropathic pain are inferior to that for analgesic treatment options. Only a minority of available trials are randomized controlled trials and even fewer are double-blind and placebo-controlled partly because of the difficulty in conducting these types of trials for interventional options. Complications from these techniques are described in greater detail in previous chapters; however, general complications from these techniques are discussed here. Complications from interventional techniques typically result from either the technique itself or the drugs used in these techniques.

Neuraxial and Peripheral Nerve Blocks

Outcomes and Efficacy

Few randomized trials examine the analgesic efficacy of neuraxial and peripheral nerve blocks for the treatment of neuropathic pain, and there are no large-scale systematic reviews on this topic. The majority of trials have evaluated the efficacy of neuraxial nerve blocks for postherpetic neuralgia and low back pain. One randomized controlled trial enrolled 270 subjects who were randomly assigned to receive intrathecal methylprednisolone and lidocaine (3 mL of 3% lidocaine with 60 mg of methylprednisolone acetate), lidocaine alone (3 mL of 3% lidocaine), or no treatment once per week for up to 4 weeks.[74] Patients who were randomized to receive methylprednisolone had a significant decrease in pain relief that correlated with decreases in interleukin-8 concentrations, and no complications related to intrathecal methylprednisolone were noted.[74] A systematic review of epidural and intrathecal blocks used for the treatment of pain from herpes zoster and postherpetic neuralgia (PHN) found a beneficial effect of epidural local anesthetic and steroid for treatment of PHN[75]; however, the epidural injection of steroids and local anesthetics in the acute phase of herpes zoster does not appear to be effective for prevention of PHN.[76] A systematic review of clinical trials examining the usefulness of transforaminal epidural steroid injections or selective nerve root blocks for the treatment of lumbosacral radiculopathy found that transforaminal epidural steroid injections appeared to be a safe and minimally invasive adjunct treatment for lumbar radicular symptoms, but further prospective, randomized, placebo-controlled studies using sham procedures are needed.[77]

Complications

General complications associated with the neuraxial nerve block itself include failure of the technique, localized pain at the site of injection, infection or abscess, hematoma, and neurologic injury, which in rare cases may be permanent. Individual classes of medications are associated with different side effect profiles. Common side effects from neuraxial administration of local anesthetics (depending on dose and location of administration) include hypotension, motor blockade, and less commonly respiratory compromise from excessive blockade (e.g., "total spinal") and systemic central nervous and cardiac local anesthetic toxicity. Administration of neuraxial opioids may result in nausea, emesis, pruritus, sedation, or even respiratory depression. Neuraxial clonidine administration may result in hypotension, sedation, and bradycardia. Many analgesic agents have been reported (e.g., case reports of agents not commonly injected neuraxially) to be administered into the neuraxial, particularly intrathecally, but have not received federal regulatory approval for such purposes and there may be concern for the potential neurotoxicity of some agents, such as ketamine, adenosine, and neostigmine, because many of these agents have not been tested for safety in large-scale studies. Rare neurologic complications associated with neuraxial anesthesia include arachnoiditis, pneumocephalus, direct nerve injury that may manifest as severe burning pain in the lower back or lower extremities, dysesthesia, numbness, or bowel-bladder dysfunction.[78]

Similar to that seen with neuraxial techniques, general complications associated with the peripheral nerve block itself include failure of the technique, localized pain or bruising at the site of injection, infection or abscess, hematoma, and neurologic injury, which in rare cases may be permanent. The analgesic agents administered are similar to those administered neuraxially and carry the same potential risks, although the risk of a total spinal is not likely. However, one concern is the potential for intraneuronal (intrafascicular) injection of drug that may be associated with peripheral nerve injury (transient or permanent). The factors that contribute to the development of these injuries is controversial, but clinicians may consider readjusting the needle location if a patient notes severe pain on injection or if injection pressures seem excessively high on injection.

Sympathetic Nerve Blocks

Outcomes and Efficacy

Although sympathetic nerve blocks are used for the treatment of neuropathic pain, the overall efficacy of this technique is uncertain partly because of the relatively poor quality of studies available. A systematic review of sympathectomy (including surgical and chemical sympathectomies) for neuropathic pain called for more clinical trials because many of the currently available trials have significant methodologic flaws.[79] Other systematic reviews also noted that although chemical sympathectomy may provide temporary relief, long-term analgesic benefits have not been substantiated in well-designed large-scale studies.[80-83] Despite the lack of high-quality evidence supporting the use of sympathetic nerve blocks in the treatment of neuropathic pain, selective sympathetic nerve blocks may still play an important role in diagnosis and may become more important as a treatment option as we expand our understanding of the role of the efferent sympathetic system in neuropathic pain.[84]

Complications

The actual technique of sympathetic nerve block may be associated with different potential side effects in part because of the widely different locations of different sympathetic blocks. Any sympathetic nerve block may be associated with failure of the block to relieve pain, worsening of the pain, pain or bruising at the site of injection, or neurologic injury, which may be permanent. Injection of local anesthetics associated with sympathetic blocks may result in motor block if injected near a somatic nerve, accidental neuraxial injection, and systemic toxicity including central nervous system and cardiac toxicity. For stellate ganglion blocks, patients might experience Horner's syndrome, phrenic nerve inhibition (which may result in a sensation of shortness of breath), and rarely pneumothorax, or seizures from injection of small amounts of local anesthetics into the vertebral artery. For sympathetic blocks in the abdominal and pelvic region, potential complications include hematuria, hypotension, and rarely paraplegia.

Spinal Cord Stimulation and Intrathecal Pumps

Outcomes and Efficacy

Spinal cord stimulation (SCS) is a recognized interventional treatment option for neuropathic pain including that of sympathetic origin. A systematic review evaluated the effectiveness of spinal cord stimulation in relieving pain and improving functioning for patients with failed back surgery syndrome and complex regional pain syndrome and examined a total of 22 trials, most of which were not of high methodologic quality.[85] Although some of the trials indicated that SCS would be somewhat clinically effective in relieving pain at 12 months, the benefits of SCS on improving patient functioning were not consistently present.[85] In a randomized trial of patients who had had reflex sympathetic dystrophy for at least 6 months, patients who were randomized to receive electrical stimulation had reduced pain and improvement in health-related quality of life.[86] These results were similar to that found in a prospective nonrandomized trial in patients with complex regional pain syndrome (CRPS) I.[87] However, the use of SCS may not be as efficacious for other indications such as prevention of amputation in patients with critical limb pain and ischemia.[88] The cost-effectiveness of SCS has not been examined properly for each indication but some data indicate that SCS may be cost-effective for certain situations such as intractable angina, which is unsuitable for coronary revascularization.[89]

Implantable devices may allow for long-term infusions of analgesic medications (e.g., opioids, local anesthetics, adjuvants) in treating neuropathic and other types of chronic pain. A study of 18 noncancer patients (including some with neuropathic pain) who underwent implantation of programmable infusion pumps and received long-term intrathecal opioid infusion found that 11 of these patients (61%) had good or fair relief of pain with an average decrease of approximately 39%.[90] Two randomized controlled trials in cancer patients demonstrated that implantable drug delivery systems, when compared with comprehensive medical management, were associated with reduced pain scores, decreased analgesic-related drug toxicity, and increased survival for the duration of the trials.[91,92] A double-blind, placebo-controlled, randomized trial evaluating the analgesic efficacy of ziconotide, a selective N-type voltage-sensitive calcium channel blocker, found that intrathecal ziconotide provided clinically and statistically significant analgesia in patients with pain from cancer or AIDS, although there was some concern as to methodologic issues in this study.[93,94] Again, proper formalized cost-effectiveness studies have not been conducted for intrathecal drug therapy; however, some available data suggest that this interventional technique may be "cost-effective" in the long term despite the high initial costs associated with these devices.[95]

Complications

Like other surgical procedures, SCS and implantable intrathecal devices are associated with complications including device failure, infection, wound dehiscence, and neurologic injury. A systematic review of available literature found that although life-threatening complications with SCS were rare, minor adverse events were frequent, with approximately 34% of patients who received a stimulator experiencing an adverse event.[85] In one of the randomized controlled trials, 6 of the 24 patients (25%) enrolled experienced complications that required additional procedures, including removal of the device in 1 patient.[86] In a study evaluating the effect of SCS on critical limb ischemia, the total complication rate was approximately 27%, with loss of stimulation as a result of lead displacement occurring in 13 patients (22%) and local infection at the site of implantation occurring in 3 patients (5%).[96] Technical problems also may develop in implantable devices, and complications occurred in 6 of 18 patients (33%) in one trial.[90]

CONCLUSION

With our increasing knowledge of the pathophysiology of different types of neuropathic pain states, development of newer pharmacologic agents, and improvement in interventional technologies and procedures, clinicians have a wide range of options to decrease the severity of neuropathic pain in their patients. Although we have made significant strides in our attempts to optimize analgesia in a traditionally difficult type of pain to manage, further studies and analgesic drug development will be needed to not only improve analgesia but also minimize adverse events. Additional high-quality trials are needed (especially for interventional therapies) to allow for additional comprehensive (systematic) assessments of all available therapeutic options for the treatment of neuropathic pain.

SUMMARY

- Understanding the underlying pathophysiology of specific types of neuropathic pain states may facilitate proper treatment options for individual patients.
- Previously thought of as ineffective for the treatment of neuropathic pain, opioids have been shown to be effective for the treatment of different types of neuropathic pain states, although an increase in dosage may be needed.
- A number of systemic analgesics (e.g., antidepressants, anticonvulsants, opioids, local anesthetics, tramadol) have been shown to be relatively effective for the treatment of neuropathic pain in general. Other systemic analgesics (e.g., NMDA antagonists, capsaicin) overall may not be as effective but may be effective in some patients.
- The quality of studies examining the analgesic efficacy of interventional therapies for the treatment of neuropathic pain is inferior compared with that for systemic analgesics; however, certain interventional options may be more effective than others.
- Each analgesic or interventional option for the treatment of neuropathic pain is associated with a unique risk profile and clinicians should assess the analgesic benefits and associated risks when contemplating a specific therapy option.

References

1. Dworkin RH, Turk DC, Farrar JT, et al: Core outcome measures for chronic pain clinical trials: IMMPACT recommendations. Pain 2005;113:9-19.
2. Eisenberg E, McNicol ED, Carr DB: Efficacy and safety of opioid agonists in the treatment of neuropathic pain of non-malignant origin: Systematic review and meta-analysis of randomized controlled trials. JAMA 2005;293:3043-3052.
3. Dellemijn P: Are opioids effective in relieving neuropathic pain? Pain 1999;80:453-462.
4. Hempenstall K, Nurmikko TJ, Johnson RW, et al: Analgesic therapy in postherpetic neuralgia: A quantitative systematic review. PLoS Med 2005;2:e164.
5. Dickenson AH, Suzuki R: Opioids in neuropathic pain: Clues from animal studies. Eur J Pain 2005;9:113-116.
6. Benedetti F, Vighetti S, Amanzio M, et al: Dose-response relationship of opioids in nociceptive and neuropathic postoperative pain. Pain 1998;74:205-211.
7. Rowbotham MC, Twilling L, Davies PS, et al: Oral opioid therapy for chronic peripheral and central neuropathic pain. N Engl J Med 2003;348:1223-1232.
8. Gilron I, Bailey JM, Tu D, et al: Morphine, gabapentin, or their combination for neuropathic pain. N Engl J Med 2005;352:1324-1334.
9. Ballantyne JC, Mao J: Opioid therapy for chronic pain. New Engl J Med 2003;349:1943-1953.
10. Jamison RN, Schein JR, Vallow S, et al: Neuropsychological effects of long-term opioid use in chronic pain patients. J Pain Symptom Manage 2003;26:913-921.
11. Tassain V, Attal N, Fletcher D, et al: Long term effects of oral sustained release morphine on neuropsychological performance in patients with chronic non-cancer pain. Pain 2003;104:389-400.
12. Sabatowski R, Schwalen S, Rettig K, et al: Driving ability under long-term treatment with transdermal fentanyl. J Pain Symptom Manage 2003;25:38-47.
13. Galski T, Williams JB, Ehle HT: Effects of opioids on driving ability. J Pain Symptom Manage 2000;19:200-208.
14. Savage SR: Long-term opioid therapy: Assessment of consequences and risks. J Pain Symptom Manage 1996;11:274-286.
15. Portenoy RK: Opioid therapy for chronic nonmalignant pain: A review of the critical issues. J Pain Symptom Manage 1996;11:203-217.
16. Bannwarth B: Risk-benefit assessment of opioids in chronic non-cancer pain. Drug Saf 1999;21:283-296.
17. Porter J, Jick H: Addiction rare in patients treated with narcotics. N Engl J Med 1980;302:123.
18. Savage SR: Assessment for addiction in pain-treatment settings. Clin J Pain 2002;18:S28-38.
19. Jensen TS: Anticonvulsants in neuropathic pain: Rationale and clinical evidence. Eur J Pain 2002;6 Suppl A:61-68.
20. Wiffen PJ, McQuay HJ, Edwards JE, et al: Gabapentin for acute and chronic pain. Cochrane Database Syst Rev 2005;3:CD005452.
21. Mellegers MA, Furlan AD, Mailis A: Gabapentin for neuropathic pain: Systematic review of controlled and uncontrolled literature. Clin J Pain 2001;17:284-295.
22. Wiffen PJ, McQuay HJ, Moore RA: Carbamazepine for acute and chronic pain. Cochrane Database Syst Rev 2005;3:CD005451.
23. Lesser H, Sharma U, LaMoreaux L, et al: Pregabalin relieves symptoms of painful diabetic neuropathy: A randomized controlled trial. Neurology 2004;63:2104-2110.
24. Sabatowski R, Galvez R, Cherry DA, et al: Pregabalin reduces pain and improves sleep and mood disturbances in patients with post-herpetic neuralgia: Results of a randomised, placebo-controlled clinical trial. Pain 2004;109:26-35.
25. Freynhagen R, Strojek K, Griesing T, et al: Efficacy of pregabalin in neuropathic pain evaluated in a 12-week, randomised, double-blind, multicentre, placebo-controlled trial of flexible- and fixed-dose regimens. Pain 2005;115:254-263.
26. Dogra S, Beydoun S, Mazzola J, et al: Oxcarbazepine in painful diabetic neuropathy: A randomized, placebo-controlled study. Eur J Pain 2005;9:543-554.
27. Thienel U, Neto W, Schwabe SK, et al: Topiramate in painful diabetic polyneuropathy: Findings from three double-blind placebo-controlled trials. Acta Neurol Scand 2004;110:221-231.
28. Donofrio PD, Raskin P, Rosenthal NR, et al: Safety and effectiveness of topiramate for the management of painful diabetic peripheral neuropathy in an open-label extension study. Clin Ther 2005;27:1420-1431.
29. Raskin P, Donofrio PD, Rosenthal NR, et al: Topiramate vs placebo in painful diabetic neuropathy: Analgesic and metabolic effects. Neurology 2004;63:865-873.
30. McCleane G: 200 mg daily of lamotrigine has no analgesic effect in neuropathic pain: A randomised, double-blind, placebo controlled trial. Pain 1999;83:105-107.
31. Finnerup NB, Sindrup SH, Bach FW, et al: Lamotrigine in spinal cord injury pain: A randomized controlled trial. Pain 2002;96:375-383.
32. Simpson DM, McArthur JC, Olney R, et al: Lamotrigine for HIV-associated painful sensory neuropathies: A placebo-controlled trial. Neurology 2003;60:1508-1514.
33. Eisenberg E, Shifrin A, Krivoy N: Lamotrigine for neuropathic pain. Expert Rev Neurother 2005;5:729-735.
34. Coluzzi F, Mattia C: Mechanism-based treatment in chronic neuropathic pain: The role of antidepressants. Curr Pharm Des 2005;11:2945-2960.
35. Saarto T, Wiffen PJ: Antidepressants for neuropathic pain. Cochrane Database Syst Rev 2005;3:CD005454.
36. Sindrup SH, Jensen TS: Efficacy of pharmacological treatments of neuropathic pain: An update and effect related to mechanism of drug action. Pain 1999;83:389-400.
37. Reuben SS, Makari-Judson G, Lurie SD: Evaluation of efficacy of the perioperative administration of venlafaxine XR in

the prevention of postmastectomy pain syndrome. J Pain Symptom Manage 2004;27:133-139.

38. Bomholt SF, Mikkelsen JD, Blackburn-Munro G: Antinociceptive effects of the antidepressants amitriptyline, duloxetine, mirtazapine and citalopram in animal models of acute, persistent and neuropathic pain. Neuropharmacology 2005; 48:252-263.

39. Lader MH: Tolerability and safety: Essentials in antidepressant pharmacotherapy. J Clin Psychiatry 1996;57(suppl 2):39-44.

40. Kalso E, Tramer MR, McQuay HJ, et al: Systematic local anaesthetic-type drugs in chronic pain: A systematic review. Eur J Pain 1998;2:3-14.

41. Tremont-Lukats IW, Challapalli V, McNicol ED, et al: Systemic administration of local anesthetics to relieve neuropathic pain: A systematic review and meta-analysis. Anesth Analg 2005;101:1738-1749.

42. Challapalli V, Tremont-Lukats IW, McNicol ED, et al: Systemic administration of local anesthetic agents to relieve neuropathic pain. Cochrane Database Syst Rev 2005;4: CD003345.

43. Oskarsson P, Ljunggren JG, Lins PE: Efficacy and safety of mexiletine in the treatment of painful diabetic neuropathy. The Mexiletine Study Group. Diabetes Care 1997;20:1594-1597.

44. Kalso E: Sodium channel blockers in neuropathic pain. Curr Pharm Des 2005;11:3005-3011.

45. Sawynok J: Topical analgesics in neuropathic pain. Curr Pharm Des 2005;11:2995-3004.

46. Meier T, Wasner G, Faust M, et al: Efficacy of lidocaine patch 5% in the treatment of focal peripheral neuropathic pain syndromes: A randomized, double-blind, placebo-controlled study. Pain 2003;106:151-158.

47. Rowbotham MC, Davies PS, Verkempinck C, et al: Lidocaine patch: Double-blind controlled study of a new treatment method for post-herpetic neuralgia. Pain 1996;65:39-44.

48. Finnerup NB, Biering-Sorensen F, Johannesen IL, et al: Intravenous lidocaine relieves spinal cord injury pain: A randomized controlled trial. Anesthesiology 2005;102:1023-1030.

49. Wallace MS, Magnuson S, Ridgeway B: Efficacy of oral mexiletine for neuropathic pain with allodynia: A double-blind, placebo-controlled, crossover study. Reg Anesth Pain Med 2000;25:459-467.

50. Gertler R, Brown HC, Mitchell DH, et al: Dexmedetomidine: A novel sedative-analgesic agent. Proc (Bayl Univ Med Cent) 2001;14:13-21.

51. Romero-Sandoval A, Eisenach JC: Perineural clonidine reduces mechanical hypersensitivity and cytokine production in established nerve injury. Anesthesiology 2006;104:351-355.

52. Poree LR, Guo TZ, Kingery WS, et al: The analgesic potency of dexmedetomidine is enhanced after nerve injury: A possible role for peripheral alpha$_2$-adrenoceptors. Anesth Analg 1998;87:941-948.

53. Martin TJ, Eisenach JC: Pharmacology of opioid and nonopioid analgesics in chronic pain states. J Pharmacol Exp Ther 2001;299:811-817.

54. Brill S, Sedgwick PM, Hamann W, et al: Efficacy of intravenous magnesium in neuropathic pain. Br J Anaesth 2002;89:711-714.

55. Uhle EI, Becker R, Gatscher S, et al: Continuous intrathecal clonidine administration for the treatment of neuropathic pain. Stereotact Funct Neurosurg 2000;75:167-175.

56. Byas-Smith MG, Max MB, Muir J, et al: Transdermal clonidine compared to placebo in painful diabetic neuropathy using a two-stage "enriched enrollment" design. Pain 1995; 60:267-274.

57. Chizh BA, Headley PM: NMDA antagonists and neuropathic pain—Multiple drug targets and multiple uses. Curr Pharm Des 2005;11:2977-2994.

58. Sang CN: NMDA-receptor antagonists in neuropathic pain: Experimental methods to clinical trials. J Pain Symptom Manage 2000;19(1 Suppl):S21-25.

59. McQuay HJ, Carroll D, Jadad AR, et al: Dextromethorphan for the treatment of neuropathic pain: A double-blind randomised controlled crossover trial with integral n-of-1 design. Pain 1994;59:127-133.

60. Nikolajsen L, Gottrup H, Kristensen AG, et al: Memantine (a N-methyl-D-aspartate receptor antagonist) in the treatment of neuropathic pain after amputation or surgery: A randomized, double-blinded, cross-over study. Anesth Analg 2000; 91:960-966.

61. Gilron I, Booher SL, Rowan MS, et al: A randomized, controlled trial of high-dose dextromethorphan in facial neuralgias. Neurology 2000;55:964-971.

62. Carlsson KC, Hoem NO, Moberg ER, et al: Analgesic effect of dextromethorphan in neuropathic pain. Acta Anaesthesiol Scand 2004;48:328-336.

63. Nelson KA, Park KM, Robinovitz E, et al: High-dose oral dextromethorphan versus placebo in painful diabetic neuropathy and postherpetic neuralgia. Neurology 1997;48:1212-1218.

64. Sang CN, Booher S, Gilron I, et al: Dextromethorphan and memantine in painful diabetic neuropathy and postherpetic neuralgia: Efficacy and dose-response trials. Anesthesiology 2002;96:1053-1061.

65. Max MB, Byas-Smith MG, Gracely RH, et al: Intravenous infusion of the NMDA antagonist, ketamine, in chronic posttraumatic pain with allodynia: A double-blind comparison to alfentanil and placebo. Clin Neuropharmacol 1995;18:360-368.

66. Himmelseher S, Durieux ME: Ketamine for perioperative pain management. Anesthesiology 2005;102:211-220.

67. Grond S, Sablotzki A: Clinical pharmacology of tramadol. Clin Pharmacokinet 2004;43:879-923.

68. Duhmke RM, Cornblath DD, Hollingshead JR: Tramadol for neuropathic pain. Cochrane Database Syst Rev 2004;2: CD003726.

69. Desmeules JA: The tramadol option. Eur J Pain 2000;4(suppl A):15-21.

70. Shipton EA: Tramadol—Present and future. Anaesth Intensive Care 2000;28:363-374.

71. Robbins WR, Staats PS, Levine J, et al: Treatment of intractable pain with topical large-dose capsaicin: Preliminary report. Anesth Analg 1998;86:579-583.

72. Mason L, Moore RA, Derry S, et al: Systematic review of topical capsaicin for the treatment of chronic pain. BMJ 2004;328:991.

73. Paice JA, Ferrans CE, Lashley FR, et al: Topical capsaicin in the management of HIV-associated peripheral neuropathy. J Pain Symptom Manage 2000;19:45-52.

74. Kotani N, Kushikata T, Hashimoto H, et al: Intrathecal methylprednisolone for intractable postherpetic neuralgia. N Engl J Med 2000;343:1514-1519.

75. Kumar V, Krone K, Mathieu A: Neuraxial and sympathetic blocks in herpes zoster and postherpetic neuralgia: An appraisal of current evidence. Reg Anesth Pain Med 2004; 29:454-461.

76. van Wijck AJ, Opstelten W, Moons KG, et al: The PINE study of epidural steroids and local anaesthetics to prevent postherpetic neuralgia: A randomised controlled trial. Lancet 2006; 367:219-224.

77. DePalma MJ, Bhargava A, Slipman CW: A critical appraisal of the evidence for selective nerve root injection in the treatment of lumbosacral radiculopathy. Arch Phys Med Rehabil 2005;86:1477-1483.

78. Aldrete JA: Neurologic deficits and arachnoiditis following neuroaxial anesthesia. Acta Anaesthesiol Scand 2003;47:3-12.

79. Mailis A, Furlan A: Sympathectomy for neuropathic pain. Cochrane Database Syst Rev 2003;2:CD002918.

80. Furlan AD, Lui PW, Mailis A: Chemical sympathectomy for neuropathic pain: Does it work? Case report and systematic literature review. Clin J Pain 2001;17:327-336.

81. Wu CL, Marsh A, Dworkin RH: The role of sympathetic nerve blocks in herpes zoster and postherpetic neuralgia. Pain 2000;87:121-129.

82. Kingery WS: A critical review of controlled clinical trials for peripheral neuropathic pain and complex regional pain syndromes. Pain 1997;73:123-139.

83. Boas RA: Sympathetic nerve blocks: In search of a role. Reg Anesth Pain Med 1998;23:292-305.

84. Stanton-Hicks M: Nerve blocks in chronic pain therapy—Are there any indications left? Acta Anaesthesiol Scand 2001; 45:1100-1107.

85. Turner JA, Loeser JD, Deyo RA, et al: Spinal cord stimulation for patients with failed back surgery syndrome or complex regional pain syndrome: A systematic review of effectiveness and complications. Pain 2004;108:137-147.

86. Kemler MA, Barendse GA, van Kleef M, et al: Spinal cord stimulation in patients with chronic reflex sympathetic dystrophy. N Engl J Med 2000;343:618-624.

87. Harke H, Gretenkort P, Ladleif HU, et al: Spinal cord stimulation in sympathetically maintained complex regional pain syndrome type I with severe disability. A prospective clinical study. Eur J Pain 2005;9:363-373.

88. Klomp HM, Spincemaille GH, Steyerberg EW, et al: Spinal-cord stimulation in critical limb ischaemia: A randomised trial. ESES Study Group. Lancet 1999;353:1040-1044.

89. Merry AF, Smith WM, Anderson DJ, et al: Cost-effectiveness of spinal cord stimulation in patients with intractable angina. N Z Med J 2001;114:179-181.

90. Hassenbusch SJ, Stanton-Hicks M, Covington EC, et al: Long-term intraspinal infusions of opioids in the treatment of neuropathic pain. J Pain Symptom Manage 1995;10: 527-543.

91. Smith TJ, Coyne PJ, Staats PS, et al: An implantable drug delivery system (IDDS) for refractory cancer pain provides sustained pain control, less drug-related toxicity, and possibly better survival compared with comprehensive medical management (CMM). Ann Oncol 2005;16:825-833.

92. Smith TJ, Staats PS, Deer T, et al: Randomized clinical trial of an implantable drug delivery system compared with comprehensive medical management for refractory cancer pain: Impact on pain, drug-related toxicity, and survival. J Clin Oncol 2002;20:4040-4049.

93. Staats PS, Yearwood T, Charapata SG, et al: Intrathecal ziconotide in the treatment of refractory pain in patients with cancer or AIDS: A randomized controlled trial. JAMA 2004;291:63-70.

94. Staats PS: Notice of duplicate publication. JAMA 2004; 292:1681.

95. Kumar K, Hunter G, Demeria DD: Treatment of chronic pain by using intrathecal drug therapy compared with conventional pain therapies: A cost-effectiveness analysis. J Neurosurg 2002;97:803-810.

96. Spincemaille GH, Klomp HM, Steyerberg EW, et al: Technical data and complications of spinal cord stimulation: Data from a randomized trial on critical limb ischemia. Stereotact Funct Neurosurg 2000;74:63-72.

97. Gimbel JS, Richards P, Portenoy RK: Controlled-release oxycodone for pain in diabetic neuropathy: A randomized controlled trial. Neurology 2003;60:927-934.

98. Huse E, Larbig W, Flor H, Birbaumer N: The effect of opioids on phantom limb pain and cortical reorganization. Pain 2001;90:47-55.

99. Morley JS, Bridson J, Nash TP, et al: Low-dose methadone has an analgesic effect in neuropathic pain: A double-blind randomized controlled crossover trial. Palliat Med 2003;17: 576-587.

100. Raja SN, Haythornwaite JA, Pappagallo M, et al: Opioids versus antidepressants in postherpetic neuralgia. Neurology 2002;59:1015-1021.

101. Watson CP, Babul N: Efficacy of oxycodone in neuropathic pain: A randomized trial in postherpetic neuralgia. Neurology 1998;50:1837-1841.

102. Watson CP, Moulin D, Watt-Watson J, et al: Controlled-release oxycodone relieves neuropathic pain: A randomized controlled trial in painful diabetic neuropathy. Pain 2003; 105:71-78.

72 Outcomes, Efficacy, and Complications of Headache Management

Stephen D. Silberstein

Headache is a problem that has plagued humans since the beginning of recorded time. It is one of the most common medical complaints, accounting for more than 18 million outpatient visits per year in the United States. More than 1% of physicians' office and emergency department visits are primarily for headache.[1,2] In 1988, the International Headache Society (IHS) published a formal classification system for the diagnosis of headache disorders.[3] This system has been updated and improved (International Classification of Headache Disorders [ICHD]-2).[4] The IHS classification system (Box 72–1) continues to divide headache into primary and secondary disorders. In a primary headache disorder, headache itself is the illness and no other etiology is diagnosed. In a secondary headache disorder, headache is attributed to an identifiable structural or metabolic abnormality.

INSTRUMENTS AND SCALES IN HEADACHE

Headaches can severely interfere with daily functioning and productivity.[5,6] Research has demonstrated that improvement in symptoms and quality of life (QOL) are not perfectly correlated; symptoms may improve but function may not.[7] Consequently, it is important to include instruments that measure QOL. Instruments that assess migraine disability can improve headache care by facilitating physician-patient communication and guiding treatment decisions. Various headache scales are in use. They can be divided into two main groups: scales that measure the impact of a single migraine attack (with or without therapy) over 24 hours and those that measure the impact of migraine over weeks or months. The first group of scales has been used in randomized, placebo-controlled trials; these are highly sensitive to acute treatment effects.[8] The second group of scales has been chosen to compare results in randomized trials.[9]

The scales that measure the impact of an acute attack include (1) quality of life (Migraine-Specific Quality of Life Questionnaire [MSQOL] and Quality of Life Questionnaire [MSQ Version 2.1]); and (2) headache impact and disability (Headache Needs Assessment [HANA] Survey). The scales that measure long-term impact are (1) quality of life (Migraine-Specific Quality of Life [MSQoL]); (2) headache impact (Headache Impact Test [HIT], Headache Impact Questionnaire [HImQ], Headache Disability Inventory, or the Henry Ford Disability Inventory [HDI]); and (3) migraine disability (Migraine Disability Assessment [MIDAS]).

SCALES THAT ASSESS QUALITY OF LIFE

Quality of life (QOL) is influenced by environmental, economic, social, health-related, spiritual, and political factors. The fundamental domains of instruments that measure QOL include physical, psychological, and social areas. Generic as well as disease-specific measures have been used to measure QOL. The most commonly used generic measures are the Medical Outcomes Study (MOS) instrument, which include the Short Form 20 (SF-20),[10] the Short Form 36 (SF-36), and the Short Form 12 (SF-12).[11] Other generic QOL scales include the Sickness Impact Profile (SIP),[12] the Nottingham Health Profile (NHP),[13] and the Psychological General Well Being (PGWB) index.[14] The specific QOL scales for migraine fall into two broadly defined categories: those that measure QOL in a single migraine attack (MSQOL and MSQ Version 2.1) and those that measure the QOL over a period of weeks or months (MSQOL).

Migraine-Specific Quality of Life Questionnaire

The MSQOL is a questionnaire that assesses the short-term quality of life decrements associated with acute migraine headache attacks.[15] This questionnaire evaluates the impairment of QOL in the 24-hour period following the onset of a migraine headache. The questionnaire is self-administered and completed

**BOX 72–1. INTERNATIONAL HEADACHE
SOCIETY CRITERIA (INTERNATIONAL
CLASSIFICATION OF HEADACHE DISORDERS-2)**

Migraine
Migraine without aura
Migraine with aura
Childhood periodic syndromes that are commonly
   precursors of migraine
Retinal migraine
Complications of migraine
   • Chronic migraine
   • Status migrainosus

Tension-Type Headache
Infrequent episodic tension-type headache
Frequent episodic tension-type headache
Chronic tension-type headache

**Cluster Headache and other Trigeminal Autonomic
Cephalalgias (TACs)**
Cluster headache
Paroxysmal hemicrania
Short-lasting unilateral neuralgiform headache
   attacks with conjunctival injection and tearing

Other Primary Headaches
Primary stabbing headache
Primary cough headache
Primary exertional headache
Primary headache associated with sexual activity
Hypnic headache
Primary thunderclap headache
Hemicrania continua
New daily-persistent headache
Headache attributed to head and/or neck trauma
Headache attributed to cranial or cervical vascular
   disorders
Headache attributed to nonvascular intracranial
   disorders
Headache attributed to a substance or its
   withdrawal
Headache attributed to infection
Headache attributed to disorder of homeostasis
Headache or facial pain attributed to disorder of
   cranium, neck, eyes, ears, nose, sinuses, teeth,
   mouth, or other facial or cranial structures
Headache attributed to psychiatric disorder
Cranial neuralgias and central causes of facial
   pain

quickly and easily. MSQOL consists of 15 items with five domains: (1) work functioning, (2) social functioning, (3) energy/vitality, (4) migraine headache symptoms, and (5) feelings and concerns. There are three items within each domain. The response option for each of the items is on a 7-point scale in which 1 indicates maximum impairment of QOL and 7 indicates no impairment. Each domain has a maximum score of 21 and a minimum score of 3. The scores were compared between migraine-free and

migraine periods. The construct validity of the questionnaire was established by showing that there are significant relationships between a subject's 24-hour MSQOL scores and other indices of clinical migraine headache, such as headache severity, activity limitation, number of associated migraine symptoms, global change in migraine symptoms, and migraine duration.[15] The ability of the MSQOL to capture within-subject change in QOL was evaluated by comparing QOL scores during a "migraine-free" period with MSQOL scores 24 hours after migraine onset.[8] The MSQOL should be applicable to all adults suffering from episodic migraine headache. It was designed primarily for use in clinical trials to assess migraine management and to be responsive to subject changes in QOL in the 24 hours following the onset of a migraine headache. The MSQOL assesses subjective well-being and daily ability to function, in addition to measuring the typical associated symptoms of migraine such as nausea, photophobia or phonophobia, and head pain. The 24-hour MSQOL should not be used to measure global QOL between headache episodes.

Quality of Life Questionnaire

MSQ Version 2.1 is a disease-specific QOL instrument with three hypothesized scales; it has been developed, tested, and revised.[16] Version 2.1 was structured secondary to older versions of the MSQ (versions 1 and 2). The revised 14-item Version 2.1 consists of seven items in the role restrictive dimension that measure the degree to which performance of normal activities is limited by migraines; four items in the role preventive dimensions that measure the degree to which performance of normal activities is interrupted by migraines; and three items in the emotional function dimension that measure the emotional effects of migraine.[16] The MSQ dimensions had low to modest correlations with the two component scores of the SF-36 and were modestly to moderately correlated with migraine symptoms. The validation was structured in three separate analyses applied in 267 subjects.[17] The MSQ provides clinicians, researchers, and those who fund health care with a measurement tool to assess health-related QOL. The questionnaire was designed to be completed quickly and easily in a self-administered form (Box 72–2). These studies suggested the mean MSQ (version 2.1) scores 6 to 12 points higher (indicating better QOL).

Migraine-Specific Quality of Life

The MSQOL is used to assess a migraine patient's QOL over a long period (average 3 weeks). The MSQOL is a valid and reliable self-administered measure and a useful tool in clinical migraine research[18] (Box 72–3). It can add important information about a migraine's effect on QOL and the potential benefits of therapeutic interventions. This questionnaire has 25 items, each question having four answers. The general format and scoring is as follows: 1, very much; 2,

BOX 72-2. MIGRAINE DISABILITY ASSESSMENT (MIDAS) QUESTIONNAIRE

Please answer the following questions about *all* your headaches you have had over the past 3 months. Write your answer in the box next to each question. Write zero if you did not perform the activity in the past 3 months.

1. How many days in the past 3 months did □□ you miss work or school because of your headaches?
2. How many days in the past 3 months was □□ your productivity at work or school reduced by half or more because of your headaches? (Do not include days you counted in question 1 when you missed work or school.)
3. How many days in the past 3 months did □□ you not do household work because of your headaches?
4. How many days in the past 3 months was □□ your productivity in household work reduced by half or more because of your headaches? (Do not include days you counted in question 3 when you did not do household work.)
5. How many days in the past 3 months did □□ you miss family, social, or leisure activities because of your headaches?

TOTAL days □□

A. How many days in the past 3 months did □□ you have a headache (if a headache lasted more than 1 day, count each day)?
B. On a scale of 0 to 10, on average how □□ painful were these headaches (in which 0 = no pain at all, and 10 = pain as bad as it can be)?

Once you have filled in the questionnaire, add up the total number of days from questions 1 through 5 (ignore A and B).

Grading system for the MIDAS Questionnaire:

GRADE	DEFINITION	SCORE
I	Little or no disability	0-5
II	Mild disability	6-10
III	Moderate disability	11-20
IV	Severe disability	21+

From Stewart WF, Lipton RB, Dowson, AJ, Sawyer J: Development and testing of the Migraine Disability Assessment (MIDAS) Questionnaire to assess headache-related disability. Neurology 2001;56:S20-S28.

quite a lot; 3, a little; 4, not at all. The total score is then transferred to a scale of 0 to 100, a higher number representing a better QOL. For the MSQOL, Cronbach's alpha was 0.92, suggesting that the items are tapping into a single concept. The MSQOL has the potential to provide valuable information on a migraineur's QOL and be a useful adjuvant measure when assessing long-term treatment outcomes.

BOX 72-3. MIGRAINE WITHOUT AURA

Diagnostic Criteria
A. At least five attacks fulfilling B through D
B. Headache attacks lasting 4 to 72 hours and occur <15 days/month (untreated or unsuccessfully treated)
C. Headache has at least two of the following characteristics:
1. Unilateral location
2. Pulsating quality
3. Moderate or severe intensity
4. Aggravation by or causing avoidance from routine physical activity (e.g., walking or climbing stairs)
D. During headache at least one of the following:
1. Nausea and/or vomiting
2. Photophobia and phonophobia
E. Not attributed to another disorder

SCALES THAT ASSESS HEADACHE IMPACT AND DISABILITY

Headache impairs physical, social, and emotional functioning, but a diagnosis is not always made despite the availability of helpful tools. One reason for this is poor patient-physician communication. If the effect that headaches are having on a person's life can be communicated adequately to the physician, the likelihood of appropriate management will increase.[19] Impact and disability instruments are scored differently and have different interpretations. Generally the impact is scaled in a positive direction, with higher scores reflecting better QOL (i.e., lower impact). For disability measures, higher scores reflect greater activity limitation (i.e., higher impact). Measuring headache-related disability, together with assessments of pain intensity, headache frequency, tiredness, mood alterations, and cognition, can help assess the effect of migraine on sufferers' lives and on society.[20] The tools currently used for assessing headache impact are the HIT and HIT-6; Headache Impact Questionnaire (HImQ); Headache Needs Assessment (HANA) Survey; and HDI (or Henry Ford questionnaire). These scales, when properly used, can improve communication between patients and physicians, assess migraine severity, and act as outcome measures to monitor treatment efficacy. Impact tools also are used, along with other clinical assessments, to produce an individualized treatment plan.[20] Disability measures assess impairment in role functioning, that is, reduced ability to function in defined roles, such as paid work.[21] The disability instruments used are the HDI and MIDAS.

Headache Impact Test

The HIT is a tool that measures a headache's impact on a person's ability to function on the job, at home, and in social situations. The HIT was developed by the psychometricians who developed the SF-36 health assessment. HIT was designed for greater accessibility (on the Internet at www.headachetest.com and www. amlhealthy.com, and as a paper-based form known as HIT-6). The HIT-6 is a practical test consisting of six questions. A patient can complete the test in less than 2 minutes. The HIT-6 assesses disability over a 4-week period. The score range is 36 to 78: higher scores indicate greater disability impact. A score of 60 or more indicates a severe impact (headache stops family, work, school, or social activities), a score between 56 and 59 a substantial impact, a score between 50 and 55 some impact, and a score less than 49 indicates no impact.[22] The availability of this test on the Internet, with feedback provided, makes this a useful tool to help headache sufferers understand the burden of their migraines and seek appropriate management.

Headache Impact Questionnaire

The HImQ measures pain and activity limitations over a 3-month period. This instrument was the precursor to the MIDAS instrument. The HImQ score is derived from four frequency-based questions (number of headaches, missed days of work, missed days of chores, or missed days of non-work activity) and four summary measures of average experience across headaches (average pain intensity and average reduced effectiveness when having a headache at work, during household chores, and in non-work activity).[23,24] This scale was validated after assessing the pain and activity limitations in a population-based sample of 132 migraine-headache sufferers enrolled in a 90-day daily-diary study who completed the HImQ at the end of the study. Previous studies of the validity of retrospective pain and disability reporting were mixed.[23,25-32] Study participants completed the HImQ in person and then completed daily diaries for 90 days. The HImQ was developed to identify headache sufferers who have the greatest need for medical care. Self-administered questionnaires can adequately capture information to rate pain severity.

Headache Needs Assessment Survey

The HANA questionnaire was designed to assess two dimensions (frequency and bothersomeness) of a migraine's impact.[33] Seven issues related to living with migraine were used as ratings of frequency and bothersomeness. Validation studies were performed in a Web-based survey, a clinical trial-responsiveness population, and a retest reliability population. Headache characteristics (e.g., frequency, severity, and treatment), demographic information, and the HDI were used for external validation. The HANA can be used in medical practice groups (e.g., headache centers, managed care groups) as a screening tool to detect potential problems. The scores from the scale are compared before and after treatment to determine the headache's effect. Primary care physicians could use the HANA to screen patients with migraine for further evaluation. Once identified, those with severe migraine may be candidates for additional evaluation and immediate treatment. The HANA has several advantages: (1) it can select who should be treated; (2) it can increase productivity by adequately treating headaches; and (3) it can identify the need for aggressive treatment without the usual slow advancement through stepped-care algorithms. This brief self-applied questionnaire may be a useful screening tool to evaluate a migraine's impact. The two-dimensional approach to patient-reported QOL allows individuals to weight the impact of both frequency and bothersomeness of chronic migraines on multiple aspects of daily life.

Henry Ford Hospital Disability Inventory

The HDI is useful in assessing the impact of headache and its treatment on daily living.[34-37] It is a paper-and-pencil instrument that probes the functional and emotional effects of headache on everyday life. The HDI is a 25-item headache disability inventory, each item requiring a "yes" (four points), "sometimes" (two points), or "no" (zero points) response. Thus a maximum score of 100 points reflects severe self-perceived headache disability. The scale is easy to complete and simple to score and interpret. The HDI has high internal consistency reliability and good content validity; the long-term (2 months) test-retest stability of the HDI was robust.[34,35] The test-retest reliability for the beta-HDI was acceptable for the total score and functional and emotional subscale scores.[34] The HDI can be used to (1) assess the impact of headache on a patient's daily living; (2) monitor the effect of therapeutic intervention; and (3) plan for a global approach to coping with headache, involving the patient.

Migraine Disability Assessment Scale

The MIDAS was developed to measure headache-related disability and improve physician-patient communication about the functional consequences of migraine. The MIDAS questionnaire is based on five disability questions that focus on lost time in three domains: school work or work for pay; household work or chores; and family, social, and leisure activities.[38] This scale can be used by physicians, nurses, pharmacists, and alternative practitioners. The questionnaire is easy to complete and takes only a few minutes. The MIDAS questionnaire has demonstrated reliability,[39] as reported in two separate population-based studies in the United States and the United Kingdom, and validity, using a 3-month daily-diary study as the gold standard.[40] Scores on the MIDAS are highly correlated with physician judgments about the severity of illness and need for treatment.[41] The score of this instrument is as follows: little or no disability, 5 to 10; moderate disability, 1 to 20; and severe disability, more than 20. The MIDAS questionnaire is an important part of a package of educational, investigative, and therapeutic measures, and could play a major role in improving the care of patients with migraine and other types of headache.[20,42-49] A randomized, placebo-controlled trial showed that the MIDAS grade provides a basis for selecting initial treatment in stratified care.[50]

MIGRAINE

Migraine is a chronic neurologic disease characterized by episodic attacks of headache and associated symptoms. "Migraine" is derived from the Greek word *hemicrania* (Galen circa AD 200).[51] The diagnosis is based on the retrospective reporting of headache characteristics and associated symptoms.[52] The revised IHS diagnostic criteria for headache disorders[3] (ICHD-2, 2004) provide criteria for seven subtypes of migraine.[4]

Epidemiology

Migraine prevalence is similar and stable in Western countries including the United States.[53] A study performed in the United States in 1992 revealed that 17.6% of women and 6% of men had had one migraine attack in the previous year.[54] A second study 10 years later had similar prevalence estimates.[55] Migraine prevalence varies by age, gender, race, and income. Before puberty, migraine prevalence is approximately 4%[21]; after puberty it increases more rapidly in girls than in boys. It increases until approximately age 40, and then declines. Prevalence is lowest in Asian Americans, intermediate in blacks, and highest in whites.[21] In the United States, migraine prevalence decreases as household income increases.[21,54,56]

Migraine decreases sufferers' QOL. The World Health Organization ranks migraine among the world's most disabling medical illnesses.[57] Approximately 28 million Americans have severe, disabling migraine headaches.[55] Migraine's cost to employers is approximately $13 billion a year, and annual medical costs exceed $1 billion.[21] Instruments to quantify migraine disability include the MIDAS[40] and the HIT.[22]

Description of the Migraine Attack

The migraine attack can consist of premonitory, aura, headache, and resolution phases. Premonitory symptoms occur in 20% to 60% of migraineurs, hours to days before headache onset. They may include psychological, neurologic, constitutional, or autonomic features, such as depression, cognitive dysfunction, and bouts of food cravings.[58]

Aura

The migraine aura consists of focal neurologic symptoms that precede, accompany, or (rarely) follow an attack. Aura usually develops over 5 to 20 minutes; lasts less than 60 minutes; can be visual, sensory, or motor; and may involve language or brainstem disturbances.[3] Headache usually follows within 60 minutes of the end of the aura. Patients can have multiple aura types: most patients with a sensory aura also have a visual aura.[59] Simple auras include scotomata (loss of vision), simple flashes (phosphenes), specks, geometric forms, and shimmering in the visual field. More complicated visual auras include teichopsia or fortification spectra (the characteristic aura of migraine), metamorphopsia, micropsia, macropsia, zoom vision, and mosaic vision. Paresthesias are often cheiro-aural: numbness starts in the hand, migrates up the arm, and jumps to involve the face, lips, and tongue.[52,60] Weakness is rare, occurs in association with sensory symptoms, and is unilateral.[61] Apraxia, aphasia, agnosia, states of altered consciousness associated with déjà vu or jamais vu, and elaborate dreamy, nightmarish, trancelike, or delirious states can occur.[58]

Headache Phase

The median migraine attack frequency is 1.5 per month.[54] The typical headache is unilateral, of gradual onset, throbbing (85%),[62] moderate to marked in severity, and aggravated by movement.[3] Pain may be bilateral (40%) or start on one side and become generalized. It lasts 4 to72 hours in adults and 2 to 48 hours in children.[3]

Anorexia is common. Nausea occurs in almost 90% of patients, and vomiting occurs in about 33%.[63] Sensory hypersensitivity results in patients seeking a dark, quiet room.[52,63] Blurry vision, nasal stuffiness, anorexia, hunger, tenesmus, diarrhea, abdominal cramps, polyuria, facial pallor, sensations of heat or cold, and sweating may occur. Depression, fatigue, anxiety, nervousness, irritability, and impairment of concentration are common. Symptom complexes may be generated by linked neuronal modules.[64]

Formal Diagnostic Criteria

The IHS subdivides migraine into migraine with aura (Box 72-4) and migraine without aura (see Box 72-3).[4] To diagnose migraine without aura (see Box 72-3), five attacks are needed. No single feature is mandatory, but recurrent episodic attacks must be documented.[3] Migraine persisting for more than 3 days defines "status migrainosus."[3,4] Migraine occurring 15 or more days per month is called chronic migraine (CM) by the ICHD-2 (see Box 72-4).[65]

Migraine with aura is subdivided into typical aura, prolonged aura, hemiplegic migraine, basilar-type migraine, and migraine with acute-onset aura (see Box 72-4). The IHS classification now allows the association of aura with other headache types. Prolonged aura lasts from 1 hour to 1 week; persistent aura lasts for more than 1 week (but resolves); if neuroimaging demonstrates a stroke, a migrainous infarction has occurred.

BOX 72–4. MIGRAINE WITH AURA

1.2.1 Typical Aura with Migraine Headache: Diagnostic Criteria

A. At least two attacks fulfilling B through E
B. Fully reversible visual and/or sensory and/or speech symptoms but no motor weakness
C. Homonymous or bilateral visual symptoms including positive features (e.g., flickering lights, spots, lines) or negative features (i.e., loss of vision) and/or unilateral sensory symptoms including positive features (i.e., visual loss, pins and needles) and/or negative features (i.e., numbness)
D. At least one of two:
  1. At least one symptom develops gradually over ≥5 minutes and/or different symptoms occur in succession
  2. Each symptom lasts ≥5 minutes and ≤60 minutes
E. Headache that meets criteria B through D for migraine without aura begins during the aura or follows aura within 60 minutes
F. Not attributed to another disorder

Migraine Variants

Basilar-type migraine aura has brainstem symptoms: ataxia, vertigo, tinnitus, diplopia, nausea and vomiting, nystagmus, dysarthria, bilateral paresthesia, or a change in level of consciousness and cognition.[3] It should be considered when patients have paroxysmal brainstem disturbances. Some have suggested that hemiplegic migraine should be diagnosed if weakness is present.[61]

Ophthalmoplegic migraine is caused by an idiopathic inflammatory neuritis.[66] There is enhancement of the cisternal segment of the oculomotor nerve, followed by resolution over several weeks as symptoms resolve.

Hemiplegic migraine can be sporadic or familial.[52] Attacks are frequently precipitated by minor head injury.[61] Familial hemiplegic migraine (FHM) is an autosomal dominant, genetically heterogeneous disorder with variable penetration. FHM includes attacks of migraine without aura, migraine with typical aura, and episodes of prolonged aura, fever, meningismus, and impaired consciousness.[67] Headache may precede hemiparesis or be absent; hemiparesis onset may be abrupt and simulate a stroke. In 20% of unselected FHM families, patients have cerebellar symptoms and signs (nystagmus, progressive ataxia). All have mutations within CACNA1A.[68]

Treatment

Migraine varies widely in its frequency, severity, and impact on patients' QOL. Migraine treatment begins with making a diagnosis,[52] explaining it to the patient, and developing a treatment plan.[69] A treatment plan should consider not only a patient's diagnosis, symptoms, and any coexistent or comorbid conditions, but also the patient's expectations, needs, and goals.[70] Comorbidity indicates an association between two disorders that is more than coincidental.

Conditions that occur in migraineurs with a higher prevalence than would be expected include stroke, epilepsy, Raynaud's syndrome, and affective disorders, which include depression, mania, anxiety, and panic disorder. Possible associations include essential tremor, mitral valve prolapse, and irritable bowel syndrome.

The pharmacologic treatment of migraine may be acute (abortive) or preventive (prophylactic), and patients with frequent, severe headaches often require both approaches. Acute treatment attempts to relieve or stop the progression of an attack or the pain and impairment once an attack has begun. It is appropriate for most attacks and should be used a maximum of 2 to 3 days a week. Preventive therapy is given, even in the absence of a headache, in an attempt to reduce the frequency, duration, or severity of attacks. Additional benefits include improving responsiveness to acute attack treatment, improving function, and reducing disability.

Pharmacotherapy of the Acute Migraine Headache

Acute treatment can be specific (ergots and triptans), or nonspecific (analgesics and opioids). Nonspecific medications control the pain of migraine or other pain disorders, whereas specific medications are effective in migraine (and certain other) headache attacks but are not useful for nonheadache pain disorders. Triptans are effective in the range of mild, moderate, and severe migraine attacks.[71]

Treatment choice depends on attack severity, frequency, associated symptoms, coexistent disorders, prior treatment response, and the medication's efficacy, potential for overuse, and adverse events (AEs). A nonoral route of administration and an antiemetic should be considered when severe nausea or vomiting is present. Injections provide rapid relief. Headaches can be stratified by severity and disability (using MIDAS or HIT). Analgesics are used for mild to moderate headaches. Triptans or dihydroergotamine are first-line drugs for severe attacks and for less severe attacks that do not adequately respond to analgesics.[72] Patients with moderate or severe headaches with moderate or severe disability (based on the MIDAS) who were stratified to a triptan did better than patients given aspirin and metoclopramide.[73]

Early intervention prevents escalation and may increase efficacy.[74] Triptans can prevent the development of cutaneous allodynia, and cutaneous allodynia predicts the triptans' effectiveness.[75] Before deciding that a drug is ineffective, at least two attacks should be treated. It may be necessary to add an adjuvant or change the dose, formulation, or route of administration. If the response is inadequate, the headache recurs, or AEs are bothersome, a medication change may be needed. Limiting acute treatment to 2 to 3 days a week can prevent medication-overuse headache. When headaches are frequent, early intervention may not be appropriate.

All treatment occasionally fails; therefore rescue medications (opioids, neuroleptics, and corticosteroids) are needed. They provide relief, but often limit function because of sedation or other AEs.

Preventive Treatment

Preventive therapy is given in an attempt to reduce the frequency, duration, or severity of attacks. Additional benefits include improving responsiveness to acute attack treatment, improving function, and reducing disability. Preventive treatment may prevent episodic migraine's progression to chronic migraine and result in health care cost reductions. Silberstein and colleagues retrospectively analyzed resource information in a large claims database. The addition of migraine preventive drug therapy to therapy that consisted of only an acute medication was effective in reducing resource consumption. During the second 6 months after the initial preventive medication, as compared with the 6 months preceding preventive therapy, office and other outpatient visits with a migraine diagnosis decreased by 51.1%, emergency department (ED) visits with a migraine diagnosis decreased 81.8%, computed tomography (CT) scans with a migraine diagnosis decreased 75.0%, magnetic resonance imaging (MRI) scans with a migraine diagnosis decreased 88.2%, and other migraine medication dispensements decreased 14.1%.[76]

Preventive medications reduce attack frequency, duration, or severity.[52,77] According to the U.S. Headache Consortium Guidelines[78] as recently revised, indications for preventive treatment include the following:

- Migraine that significantly interferes with the patient's daily routine despite acute treatment
- Failure of, contraindication to, or troublesome AEs from acute medications
- Acute medication overuse
- Frequent headaches (more than 1/week; risk of chronic migraine or medication overuse)
- Patient preference
- Special circumstances, such as hemiplegic migraine or attacks with a risk of permanent neurologic injury

Prevention is not being used to nearly the extent it should be. Results from the American Migraine Study I and II and the Philadelphia phone survey 2 demonstrated that migraine preventive therapy is underused. In the American Migraine Study II, 25% of all people with migraine, or more than 7 million people, experienced more than 3 attacks per month, and 53% of those surveyed reported either having severe impairment because of their attacks or needing bed rest.[56] However, only 5% of all migraineurs currently use preventive therapy to control their attacks.[79]

BOX 72–5. HEADACHE ATTRIBUTED TO MEDICATION OVERUSE

A. Headache present on >15 days/month
B. Regular overuse for >3 months of one or more acute/symptomatic treatment drugs as defined under subforms of 8.2
  1. Ergotamine, triptans, opioids, or combination analgesic medications on ≥10 days/month on a regular basis for >3 months
  2. Simple analgesics or any combination of ergotamine, triptans, analgesic opioids on ≥15 days/month on a regular basis for >3 months without overuse of any single class alone
C. Headache has developed or markedly worsened during medication overuse

---

Preventive medication groups include β-adrenergic blockers, antidepressants, calcium channel antagonists, serotonin antagonists, anticonvulsants, and nonsteroidal anti-inflammatory agents (NSAIDs). Choice is based on efficacy, AEs, and coexistent and comorbid conditions (Box 72–5). The drug chosen is started at a low dose and increased slowly until therapeutic effects develop or the ceiling dose is reached. A full therapeutic trial may take 2 to 6 months. Acute headache medications should not be overused. If headaches are well controlled, medication can be tapered and discontinued. Dose reduction may provide a better risk-to-benefit ratio. Women of childbearing potential should be on adequate contraception.

Behavioral and psychological interventions used for prevention include relaxation training, thermal biofeedback combined with relaxation training, electromyography biofeedback, and cognitive-behavioral therapy.[80]

Coexistent diseases have important implications for treatment. In some instances, two or more conditions may be treated with a single drug. If individuals have more than one disease, certain categories of treatment may be relatively contraindicated.

The preventive medications with the best documented efficacy are the beta blockers, divalproex, and topiramate. Choice is based on a drug's proven efficacy, the physician's informed belief about medications not yet evaluated in controlled trials, the drug's AEs, the patient's preferences and headache profile, and the presence or absence of coexisting disorders.[52] The chosen drug should have the best risk-to-benefit ratio for the individual patient and take advantage of the drug's side effect profile.[81,82] An underweight patient would be a candidate for one of the medications that commonly produce weight gain, such as a tricyclic antidepressant (TCA); in contrast, one would try to avoid these drugs and consider topiramate when the patient is overweight. Tertiary TCAs that have a sedating effect would be useful at bedtime for patients with insomnia. Older patients with cardiac disease or patients with significant hypotension may not be able to use TCAs or calcium channel or beta blockers, but could use divalproex or topiramate. The athletic patient should use beta blockers with caution. Medication that can impair cognitive functioning should be avoided when patients are dependent on their wits.[81,82]

Comorbid and coexistent diseases have important implications for treatment. The presence of a second illness provides therapeutic opportunities but also imposes certain therapeutic limitations. In some instances, two or more conditions may be treated with a single drug. When migraine and hypertension or angina occur together, beta blockers or calcium channel blockers may be effective for all conditions.[83] For the patient with migraine and depression, TCAs or selective serotonin reuptake inhibitors (SSRIs) may be especially useful.[84] Divalproex and topiramate are the drugs of choice for the patient with migraine and epilepsy[85] or migraine and bipolar illness.[86,87] The pregnant migraineur who has a comorbid condition that needs treatment should be given a medication that is effective for both conditions and has the lowest potential for fetal AEs. When individuals have more than one disease, certain categories of treatment may be relatively contraindicated. For example, beta blockers should be used with caution in the depressed migraineur, whereas TCAs, neuroleptics, or sumatriptan may lower the seizure threshold and should be used with caution in the epileptic migraineur.

Although monotherapy is preferred, it is sometimes necessary to combine preventive medications. Antidepressants are often used with beta blockers or calcium channel blockers and topiramate or divalproex sodium may be used in combination with any of these medications. Pascual and associates[88] found that combining a beta blocker and sodium valproate could lead to an increased benefit for patients with migraine previously resistant to either alone. Fifty-two patients (43 women) with a history of episodic migraine with or without aura, and previously unresponsive to beta blockers or sodium valproate monotherapy, were treated with a combination of propranolol (or nadolol) and sodium valproate in an open-label fashion: 56% had a greater than 50% reduction in migraine days. This open trial supports the practice of combination therapy. Controlled trials are needed to determine the true advantage of this combination treatment in episodic and chronic migraine.

Conclusion

Migraine is an extremely common neurobiologic headache disorder that is caused by increased central nervous system excitability. It ranks among the world's most disabling medical illnesses. Diagnosis is based on the headache's characteristics and associated symptoms. The economic and societal impact of migraine is substantial. It affects sufferers' QOL such as work, social activities, and family life. There are many acute and preventive migraine treatments on the market. Acute treatment is either specific (triptans and ergots) or nonspecific (analgesics). Disabling migraine should be treated with triptans. Increased headache frequency is an indication for preventive treatment, which decreases migraine frequency and improves QOL. More treatments are being developed, which provides hope to the many sufferers who are still uncontrolled.

CHRONIC DAILY HEADACHE

Chronic daily headache (CDH) refers to headache disorders experienced frequently (15 or more days a month), including headaches associated with medication overuse. CDH can be divided into primary and secondary varieties.[89] Primary CDH is not related to a structural or systemic illness. Population-based studies in the United States, Europe, and Asia suggest that 4% to 5% of the general population have primary CDH,[90-92] and that 0.5% has severe headaches on a daily basis.[93-95] In population samples, chronic tension-type headache is the leading cause of primary CDH.[96] CDH patients account for the greatest number of consultations in headache subspecialty practices.[97] They often overuse medication, which may play a role in initiating or sustaining the pattern of pain. Anxiety, depression, and other psychological disturbances may accompany the headaches.[97]

Once secondary headache (including medication overuse headache [MOH]) has been excluded, frequent headache sufferers are subdivided into two groups, based on headache duration. When the headache duration is less than 4 hours, the differential diagnosis includes cluster headache, paroxysmal hemicrania, idiopathic stabbing headache, hypnic headache, and SUNCT. When the headache duration is greater than 4 hours, the major primary disorders to consider are chronic migraine (CM) (Box 72–6), hemicrania continua (HC), chronic tension-type headache (CTTH) (Box 72–7), and new daily persistent headache (NDPH).[97] CM, NDPH, and HC are primary CDH disorders that are now included in the second IHS classification.[4] Transformed migraine is similar, but not identical, to CM.[4]

Chronic migraine (see Box 72–6) has been called transformed migraine.[98] Most patients with this disorder are women, 90% of whom have a history of migraine without aura. Patients often report a process of transformation characterized by headaches that become more frequent over months to years, with the associated symptoms of photophobia, phonophobia, and nausea becoming less severe and less frequent. Patients often develop (or transform into) a pattern of daily or nearly daily headaches that phenomenologically resembles a mixture of tension-type headache and migraine, that is, the pain is often mild to moderate and is not always associated with photophobia, phonophobia, or gastrointestinal features. Other features of migraine, including aggravation by menstruation and other triggers, as well as unilateral-

BOX 72–6. REVISED INTERNATIONAL HEADACHE SOCIETY CRITERIA FOR CHRONIC MIGRAINE

A. Headache on 15 or more days per month for at least 3 months
B. Patient has had at least five attacks fulfilling criteria B through D for *Migraine without aura*
C. On 8 or more days per month for at least 3 months headache has fulfilled C.1 and/or C.2 below, that is, has fulfilled criteria for pain and associated symptoms of migraine without aura
   1. Has at least two of a through d
      a. Unilateral location
      b. Pulsating quality
      c. Moderate or severe pain intensity
      d. Aggravation by or causing avoidance of routine physical activity (e.g., walking or climbing stairs)
         and at least one of e or f
      e. Nausea and/or vomiting
      f. Photophobia and phonophobia
   2. Treated and relieved by triptan(s) or ergot before the expected development of C.1 above
D. No medication overuse and not attributed to another disorder

BOX 72–7. RISK FACTORS FOR CHRONIC DAILY HEADACHE

1. High headache frequency
2. Female gender
3. Obesity (body mass index >30)
4. Snoring
5. Stressful life events
6. High caffeine consumption
7. Acute medication overuse
8. Depression
9. Head trauma
10. History of migraine
11. Less than a high school education

ity and gastrointestinal symptoms, may persist. Attacks of full-blown migraine superimposed on a background of less severe headaches occur in many patients. The term *transformed migraine* (TM) has been used to refer to this process. The term *chronic migraine* (CM) is now being used by the IHS, in part because a history of transformation is often missing.

Drug Overuse and Medication Overuse (Rebound) Headache

MOH was previously called rebound headache, drug-induced headache, and medication-misuse headache

(see Box 72–5). Patients with frequent headaches often overuse analgesics, opioids, ergotamine, and triptans.[99] Although stopping the acute medication may result in the patient's developing withdrawal symptoms and a period of increased headache, subsequent headache improvement usually occurs.[100-104] Many primary CDH patients who were withdrawn from ergotamine and analgesics and given no further therapy no longer had daily headaches, although about 40% still had episodic migraine attacks.[92,105]

Definition and Classification of Medication Overuse Headache

In 1988, the IHS used the term *drug-induced headache* for MOH.[3] Overuse is now defined in terms of treatment days per month (see Box 72–5).

The epidemiology of MOH is uncertain. In European headache centers, 5% to 10% of patients have drug-induced headaches. One series of 3000 consecutive headache patients reported that 4.3% had drug-induced headaches.[106] Experiences in the United Kingdom (P. Goadsby, personal communication, June 2000) suggest that drug-associated headache is more common than the literature suggests. In American specialty headache clinics, as many as 80% of patients who presented with primary CDH used analgesics on a daily or near-daily basis.[92] Other headache clinics report a smaller percentage but a majority nonetheless.[107] In India, in contrast, medication overuse is less common.[108]

Diener and Dahlöf[109] summarized 29 studies that included 2612 patients with chronic MOH. Migraine was the primary headache in 65% of patients, tension-type headache (TTH) in 27%, and mixed or other headaches (i.e., cluster headache) in 8%. Women had more drug-induced headache than men (3.5:1; 1533 women, 442 men). This ratio is slightly higher than one would expect because of the usual migraine frequency gender differences. The mean duration of primary headache was 20.4 years. The mean admitted time of frequent drug intake was 10.3 years in one study, and the mean duration of daily headache was 5.9 years. Results from headache diaries show that the number of tablets or suppositories taken daily averaged 4.9 (range 0.25 to 25). Patients averaged 2.5 to 5.8 different pharmacologic components simultaneously (range 1 to 14).[110]

A prospective study of 98 patients investigated the pharmacologic features, such as mean critical duration until onset of MOH, mean critical monthly intake frequencies, and mean critical monthly dosages, as well as specific clinical features of MOH after overuse of different acute headache drugs. In this study, triptan overuse far outnumbered ergot overuse. This reflects the fact that despite high costs, triptans have become widely used (and overused) and suggests that they are about to become the most important group to cause MOH. Unlike patients who suffer from MOH following ergot or analgesic overuse, migraine patients (but not TTH patients) with triptan-induced headache did not describe the typical tension-type daily headache but rather a migraine-like daily headache (a unilateral, pulsating headache with autonomic disturbances) or a significant (and pure) increase in migraine attack frequency. Furthermore, the delay between the frequent medication intake and the development of daily headache was shortest for triptans (1.7 years), longer for ergots (2.7 years), and longest for analgesics (4.8 years). The intake frequency (single dosages per month) was lowest for triptans (18 single dosages per month), higher for ergots (37 single dosages per month), and highest for analgesics (114 single dosages per month). Hence, triptans not only cause a different spectrum of clinical features but also can cause MOH faster and with lower dosages than other substance groups.[111]

In addition to exacerbating the headache disorder, drug overuse has other serious effects. The overuse of acute drugs may interfere with the effectiveness of preventive headache medications. Prolonged use of large amounts of medication may cause renal or hepatic toxicity in addition to tolerance, habituation, or dependence. (Tolerance refers to the decreased effectiveness of the same dose of an analgesic, often leading to the use of higher doses to achieve the same degree of effectiveness. Habituation and dependence are, respectively, the psychological and physical needs to repeatedly use drugs.)

Epidemiology of Chronic Daily Headache

In population-based surveys using the Silberstein-Lipton criteria, primary CDH occurred in 4.1% of Americans, 4.35% of Greeks, 3.9% of older adult Chinese, and 4.7% of Spaniards. Population-based estimates for the 1-year period prevalence of CTTH are 1.7% in Ethiopia,[112] 3% in Denmark,[113] 2.2% in Spain,[94] 2.7% in China,[95] and 2.2% in the United States.[93]

Scher and colleagues,[93] using a validated computer-assisted telephone interview, ascertained the prevalence of CDH in 13,343 individuals ages 18 to 65 years in Baltimore County, Maryland. Those reporting 180 or more headaches a year were classified as having frequent headaches. Three mutually exclusive subtypes of frequent headache were identified: TM, CTTH, and unclassified frequent headache. The overall prevalence of CDH was 4.1% (5.0% women, 2.8% men; 1.8:1 women-to-men ratio). Prevalence was highest in the lowest educational category for both men and women. More than half (52% women, 56% men) met criteria for CTTH (2.2%), almost one third (33% women, 25% men) met criteria for TM (1.3%), and the remainder (15% women, 19% men) were unclassified (0.6%). Overall, 30% of women and 25% of men who were frequent headache sufferers met IHS criteria for migraine (with or without aura). On the basis of chance, migraine and CTTH would co-occur in 0.22% of the population; the fact that TM occurred in 1.3% of this population would suggest that their co-occurrence is more than random.

Castillo and associates[94] sampled 2252 subjects older than 14 years of age in Cantalucia, Spain. Overall 4.7% had CDH. Using the criteria of Silberstein and coworkers,[97] none had HC, 0.1% had NDPH, 2.2% had CTTH, and 2.4% had TM. Nineteen percent of CTTH patients and 31.1% of TM patients had a history of acute medication overuse. Eight patients had a previous history of migraine without aura and now had primary CDH with the characteristics of TTH only. These headaches met the criteria of CM but could have been migraine and coincidental CTTH.

In August 1993, Wang and associates[95] looked at the characteristics of primary CDH in a population of older adult Chinese (more than 65 years of age) in two townships on Kinmen Island; 77% of the eligible population (1533/2003) participated. Sixty patients (3.9%) had CDH. Significantly more women than men had primary CDH (5.6% and 1.8%, $p < 0.001$). Of the primary CDH patients, 42 (70%) had CTTH (2.7%), 15 (25%) had CM (1%), and 3 (5%) had other CDH. Only 23% of patients had consulted a physician for headache in the previous year.

Lu and coworkers[114] conducted a two-stage population-based headache survey among subjects older than 15 years of age in Taipei, Taiwan. Subjects who had had CDH in the past year were identified, interviewed, and followed up. CDH was defined as headache frequency of more than 15 days a month, with a duration of more than 4 hours a day. Of the 3377 participants, 108 (3.2%) fulfilled the criteria for CDH, with a higher prevalence in women (4.3%) than men (1.9%). TM was the most common subtype (55%), followed by CTTH (44%). Thirty-four per cent of the CDH subjects overused analgesics.

Risk Factors for Chronic Daily Headache

Wang and associates[95] ascertained that significant risk factors for CDH included analgesic overuse (odds ratio [OR] = 79), a history of migraine (OR = 6.6), and a Geriatric Depression Scale-Short Form score of 8 or more (OR = 2.6) (see Box 72-7). At follow-up, patients with persistent primary CDH had a significantly higher frequency of analgesic overuse (33% vs. 0%, $p = 0.03$) and major depression (38% vs. 0%, $p = 0.04$).

Granella and colleagues[115] found that risk factors that were associated with the evolution of migraine without aura into TM included head trauma (OR = 3.3), analgesic use with every attack (OR = 2.8), and long duration of oral contraceptive use.

Scher and associates[116] described factors that predict CDH onset and remission in an adult population. CDH was more common in women (OR = 0.65 [95% confidence interval [CI] 1.3 to 2]), those previously married (OR = 0.5 [95% CI 1.2 to 1.9]), with obesity (body mass index [BMI] > 30) (OR = 1.27 [95% CI 1 to 1.7]), and those with less education. Obesity, high baseline headache frequency, high caffeine consumption, habitual daily snoring, and stressful life events were significantly associated with new-onset CDH.[117] Having less than a high school education was associated with a threefold increased risk of CDH (OR = 3.56 [95% CI 2.3 to 5.6]).

Bigal and coworkers[118] in a clinic-based study, looked for risk factors associated with CDH and its subtypes. TM without MOH (in comparison with episodic migraine) was associated with allergies, asthma, hypothyroidism, hypertension, and daily caffeine consumption.

Zwart and colleagues[119] examined the relationship between analgesic use at baseline and the subsequent risk of chronic pain (>15 days/month) and the risk of analgesic overuse in a population-based study. In total, 32,067 adults reported the use of analgesics from 1984 to 1986 and at follow-up 11 years later (1995 to 1997). The risk ratios (RR) of chronic pain and of analgesic overuse in the different diagnostic groups (i.e., migraine, nonmigrainous headache, and neck pain) were estimated in relation to analgesic consumption at baseline. Individuals who reported using analgesics daily or weekly at baseline showed significant increased risk for having chronic pain at follow-up. The risk was most evident for chronic migraine (RR = 13.3, 95% CI 9.3 to 19.1), intermediate for chronic nonmigrainous headaches (RR = 6.2, 95% CI 5 to 7.7), and lowest for chronic neck pain (RR = 2.4, 95% CI 2 to 2.8). Among subjects with chronic pain associated with analgesic overuse, the RR was 37.6 (95% CI 21.3 to 66.4) for chronic migraine, 14.4 (95% CI 10.4 to 19.9) for chronic nonmigrainous headaches, and 7.1 for chronic neck pain (95% CI 5.5 to 9.2). The RR for chronic headache (migraine and nonmigrainous headache combined) associated with analgesic overuse was 19.6 (95% CI 14.8 to 25.9) compared with 3.1 (95% CI 2.4 to 4.2) for those without overuse. Analgesic overuse strongly predicts chronic pain and chronic pain associated with analgesic overuse 11 years later, especially among those with chronic migraine.

Treatment

Overview

Patients with CDH can be difficult to treat, especially when the disorder is complicated by medication overuse, comorbid psychiatric disease, low frustration tolerance, and physical and emotional dependency.[91,120] We recommend the following steps. First, exclude secondary headache disorders; second, diagnose the specific primary headache disorder (CM, CTTH, HC, or NDPH); and third, identify comorbid medical and psychiatric conditions and exacerbating factors, especially medication overuse. Limit acute medications (with the possible exception of the long-acting NSAIDs). Patients should be started on preventive medication (to decrease reliance on acute medication), with the explicit understanding that the drugs may not become fully effective until medication overuse has been eliminated.[121] Some patients

need to have their headache cycle terminated.[121] Patients need education and continuous support during this process. Outpatient detoxification options, including outpatient infusion in an ambulatory infusion unit, are available. If outpatient treatment proves difficult or is dangerous, hospitalization may be required.[89,122]

In some cases CDH reverts to episodic headache when preventive medication is initiated and acute medications are limited. In other cases, only moderate or no improvement may occur. Zeeberg and associates described the treatment outcomes in patients withdrawn from medication overuse. They studied 337 outpatients who were diagnosed with MOH and treated and dismissed from the Danish Headache Centre in 2002 and 2003. A 46% decrease in headache frequency from the first visit to dismissal occurred ($P < 0.0001$). Patients with no improvement 2 months after complete drug withdrawal ($N = 88$) subsequently responded to pharmacologic and/or nonpharmacologic prophylaxis, with a 26% decrease in headache frequency as measured from the end of withdrawal to dismissal. At dismissal, 47% of patients were on prophylaxis. In this population, about half of MOH patients benefit from drug withdrawal alone.[123]

Prognosis

The "natural history" of primary CDH, and rebound headache in particular, has never been studied and probably never will be for ethical and technical reasons. Recognition of the rebound process is probably therapeutic in and of itself and could affect the patient's behavior or the physician's approach. Retrospective analysis suggests that there may be periods of stable drug consumption and periods of accelerated medication use. Patients treated aggressively generally improve. There are no literature reports of spontaneous improvement of rebound headache, although this may happen. We[124] performed follow-up evaluations on 50 hospitalized primary CDH drug overuse patients who were treated with repetitive intravenous (IV) DHE and became headache-free. Once detoxified, treated, and discharged, most patients did not resume daily analgesic or ergotamine use. Seventy-two percent continued to show significant improvement at 3 months, and 87% continued to show significant improvement after 2 years. This would suggest at least a 70% improvement at 2 years in the initial group (35/50), allowing for patients lost to follow-up.

Our[124] 2-year success rate of 87% is consistent with the long-term success rates reported in the literature (Box 72-8). In a series of 22 papers[101-103,105,115,124-141] published between 1975 and 1999, the success rate of withdrawal therapy (often accompanied by pharmacologic or behavioral intervention) of patients overusing analgesics, ergotamine, or both was between 48% and 91%, with the rate being reported as 77% or higher in 10 papers (see Box 72-2).

BOX 72–8. DIAGNOSTIC CRITERIA FOR TENSION-TYPE HEADACHE

Infrequent Episodic Tension-Type Headache (International Headache Society [IHS] Diagnostic Criteria)

A. At least 10 previous headache episodes fulfilling criteria B through E listed below. Number of days with such headache <1 day per month (<12 days per year).

B. Headache lasting from 30 minutes to 7 days

C. At least two of the following pain characteristics:
   1. Pressing/tightening (nonpulsating) quality
   2. Mild or moderate intensity (may inhibit but does not prohibit activities)
   3. Bilateral location
   4. No aggravation by walking stairs or similar routine physical activity

D. Both of the following
   1. No nausea or vomiting (anorexia may occur)
   2. Photophobia and phonophobia are absent, or one but not the other is present

E. Not attributed to another disorder

Frequent Episodic Tension-Type Headache

A. At least 10 episodes fulfilling criteria B through E. Number of days with such headache is 1 day per month and <15 days per month for at least 3 months (≥12 days and <180 days per year)

B. Headache lasting from 30 minutes to 7 days

C. At least two of the following pain characteristics:
   1. Pressing/tightening (nonpulsating) quality
   2. Mild or moderate intensity (may inhibit, but does not prohibit activities)

   3. Bilateral location
   4. No aggravation by walking stairs or similar routine physical activity

D. Both of the following:
   1. No nausea or vomiting (anorexia may occur)
   2. Photophobia and phonophobia are absent, or one but not the other may be present.

E. Not attributed to another disorder

Chronic Tension-Type Headache (IHS Diagnostic Criteria)

A. At least 10 episodes fulfilling criteria B through F. Number of days with such headache >15 days per month for at least 3 months (>180 days per year)

B. Headache lasts hours or may be continuous

C. At least two of the following pain characteristics:
   1. Pressing or tightening quality
   2. Mild or moderate severity (may inhibit but does not prohibit activities)
   3. Bilateral location
   4. No aggravation by walking stairs or similar routine physical activity

D. Both of the following:
   1. No more than one of the following: photophobia, phonophobia, or mild nausea
   2. No moderate or severe nausea and no vomiting

E. No medication overuse

F. Not attributed to another disorder

TENSION-TYPE HEADACHE

Epidemiologic studies of the general population have shown that TTH is the most common type of headache, with a lifetime prevalence of 69% in men and 88% in women.[142] TTHs can begin at any age, but onset during adolescence or young adulthood is most common. The prognosis of frequent episodic tension-type headache (ETTH) and CTTH was favorable in a Danish follow-up to a cross-sectional headache study of 549 people. Among 146 subjects with frequent ETTH and 15 with CTTH at baseline, 45% experienced infrequent or no TTH (remission), 39% had frequent ETTH, and 16% experienced CTTH (poor outcome) at follow-up. Poor outcome was associated with baseline CTTH, coexisting migraine, sleeping problems, and not being married.[143]

Clinical Features and Associated Disorders

ETTHs are now classified as either infrequent (<1 day/month or 12 days/year) or frequent (>1 but <15 days/month or >12 but <180 days/year) (see Box 72–8). The IHS criteria for a TTH require that patients experience at least 10 previous headaches, each lasting 30 minutes to 7 days (median, 12 hours), with at least two of the following characteristics: a pressing/tightening (nonpulsating) quality, mild to moderate intensity, bilateral location, and no aggravation with physical activity. In addition, the patient should not have nausea or vomiting or a combination of photophobia and phonophobia. ETTH occurs less frequently than 15 days a month, whereas CTTH occurs 15 or more days a month.[144] The pain is a dull, achy, nonpulsatile feeling of tightness, pressure, or constriction (viselike or hatband-like), and it is usually mild to moderate, in contrast with the moderate to severe pain of migraine. The intensity increases with headache attack frequency.[145] Most patients have bilateral pain, but the location varies considerably within and between patients and can involve the frontal, temporal, occipital, or parietal regions, alone or in combination, and can change locations during an attack.[146] An occipital location is less common than a frontal or temporal location. Some patients have neck or jaw discomfort or frank problems with their temporomandibular joint.[147,148]

The onset of TTH is gradual, often occurring after or during stress, and the pain is typically worse late in the day. There is no prodrome. The pain is usually a nagging, tight, or viselike bilateral pressure that is located in the forehead, the temples, or the back of the head. It may radiate to the neck and shoulders. There are no associated autonomic or gastrointestinal symptoms except for occasional anorexia. The frequency of ETTH ranges from 2 to 12 days a month, with a median of 6 days a month. The headaches may be associated with menstruation.[144,149]

Twenty-five percent of TTH patients also have migraine.[150] What we call ETTH may be two distinct disorders. The first disorder may be mild migraine; the second may be a pure TTH that is not associated with other features of migraine (nausea, photophobia, or sensitivity to movement) or with attacks of severe migraine.[4] The fact that sumatriptan is effective for the TTH that migraineurs experience but not for the TTH that nonmigraineurs experience supports this concept.[151]

Patients with ETTH are no different from controls in terms of stress, depression, anxiety, emotional conflicts, sleeping problems, and fatigue. Patients with CTTH are often depressed.[149]

Differential Diagnosis

Migraine is the headache disorder that is most confused with TTH. Both can be bilateral, nonthrobbing, and associated with anorexia. Migraine is more severe, often unilateral, and frequently associated with nausea. Idiopathic intracranial hypertension, brain tumor headache, chronic sphenoid sinusitis, and cervical, ocular, and temporomandibular disorders need to be considered.[144,149]

Evaluation

Most patients with a long history of unchanged ETTHs do not require extensive evaluation if they have normal neurologic examinations and are otherwise healthy. Patients with CTTHs should be imaged with CT or MRI, even if their general and neurologic examinations are normal. A metabolic screen, complete blood count, electrolytes, and kidney and thyroid function studies also are appropriate.[149]

Management

TTH patients usually self-medicate with over-the-counter analgesics (aspirin, acetaminophen, other NSAIDs), with or without caffeine. If these medications are not effective, prescription NSAIDs or combination analgesic preparations can be used. Narcotics and combination analgesics that contain sedatives or caffeine should be limited because overuse may cause dependence. Symptomatic medication overuse can cause ETTHs to convert to CTTHs. Patients with both migraine and TTHs benefit from specific migraine medication, such as sumatriptan or DHE (see Boxes 72–7 and 72–8).[144,149]

Preventive therapy should be administered when a patient has frequent headaches that produce disability or may lead to symptomatic medication overuse. Medications used for TTH prevention include antidepressants, beta blockers, and anticonvulsants. Antidepressants, the medication of first choice, should be started at a low dose and increased slowly every 3 to 7 days. An adequate trial period of at least 1 to 2 months must be allowed. The addition of biofeedback therapy or beta-blocking agents may improve its therapeutic benefit.[144,149]

Prognosis and Future Perspectives

ETTH is a benign recurrent condition that usually improves with time. Some patients, however, progress to CTTH, especially when analgesic overuse is present. The prognosis of CTTH is controversial because many studies include patients with more severe headaches and coexisting conditions, such as migraine and psychiatric disorders.

CLUSTER HEADACHE AND OTHER TRIGEMINAL-AUTONOMIC CEPHALGIAS

The short-lasting primary headache syndrome may be conveniently divided into those that exhibit marked autonomic activation and those without autonomic activation. This group includes cluster headache (episodic or chronic) (see Box 72–8), paroxysmal hemicrania (episodic or chronic; Box 72–9), and short-lasting unilateral neuralgiform headache with conjunctival injection and tearing (SUNCT syndrome).

Pathogenesis and Pathophysiology

The pathogenesis of cluster headaches involves the trigeminovascular system, as demonstrated by a marked increase in the level of calcitonin gene-related peptide in the cranial venous circulation during attacks.[152] Parasympathetic system activation has been corroborated by the finding of dramatically elevated levels of vasoactive intestinal polypeptide during attacks[152] with robust ipsilateral autonomic features. Cluster events are probably related to alterations in the circadian pacemaker, which may be a result of hypothalamic dysfunction. Attacks increase following the beginning and end of daylight savings time, and there is a loss of circadian rhythm for blood pressure, temperature, and hormones, including prolactin, melatonin, cortisol, and β-endorphins. Evidence for the role of the hypothalamus in cluster headache pathogenesis has come from functional and morphometric neuroimaging. Using positron-emission tomography imaging, May and colleagues demonstrated marked activation in the ipsilateral ventral hypothalamic gray matter during nitroglycerin-induced acute cluster headache attacks.[153] Neurogenic inflammation, carotid body chemoreceptor dysfunction, central parasympathetic and sympa-

---

BOX 72–9. CLUSTER HEADACHE

A. At least five attacks fulfilling criteria B through E
B. Severe or very severe unilateral orbital, supraorbital and/or temporal pain lasting 15 to 180 minutes if untreated
C. Headache is accompanied by at least one of the following:
   1. Ipsilateral conjunctival injection and/or lacrimation
   2. Ipsilateral nasal congestion and/or rhinorrhea
   3. Ipsilateral eyelid edema
   4. Ipsilateral forehead and facial sweating
   5. Ipsilateral miosis and/or ptosis
   6. A sense of restlessness or agitation
D. Attacks have a frequency from one every other day to 8 per day
E. Not attributed to another disorder

Episodic Cluster Headache
A. Attacks fulfilling criteria A through E for *Cluster headache*
B. At least two cluster periods lasting 7 to 365 days and separated by pain-free remission periods of ≥1 month

Chronic Cluster Headache
A. Attacks fulfilling criteria A through E for *Cluster headache*
B. Attacks recur over >1 year without remission periods or with remission periods lasting <1 month

3.2 Paroxysmal Hemicrania
A. AT least 20 attacks fulfilling criteria B through D
B. Attacks of severe unilateral orbital, supraorbital, or temporal pain lasting 2 to 30 minutes
C. Headache is accompanied by at least one of the following:
   1. Ipsilateral conjunctival injection and/or lacrimation
   2. Ipsilateral nasal congestion and/or rhinorrhea
   3. Ipsilateral eyelid edema
   4. Ipsilateral forehead and facial sweating
   5. Ipsilateral miosis and/or ptosis
D. Attacks have a frequency of more than 5 per day for more than half of the time, although periods with lower frequency may occur
E. Attacks are prevented completely by therapeutic doses of indomethacin
F. Not attributed to another disorder

3.2.1 Episodic Paroxysmal Hemicrania
A. Attacks fulfilling criteria A through F for *Paroxysmal hemicrania*
B. At least two attack periods lasting 7 to 365 days and separated by pain-free remission periods of ≥1 month

3.2.2 Chronic Paroxysmal Hemicrania (CPH)
A. Attacks fulfilling criteria A through F for *Paroxysmal hemicrania*
B. Attacks recur over >1 year without remission periods or with remission periods lasting <1 month

---

thetic tone imbalance, and increased responsiveness to histamine have been proposed as the cause of cluster pain.[154]

Epidemiology and Risk Factors

With an incidence of 0.01% to 1.5 % in various populations, cluster headache prevalence is lower than that of migraine or TTH. Men have a higher prevalence than women, and black patients have a higher prevalence than white patients. Recent evidence suggests a progressively decreasing male preponderance: the male-to-female ratio based on the year of onset in Manzoni's study[155] decreased from 6.2:1 in the 1960s to 2.1:1 in the 1990s.[156] A family history of cluster headache is rare. The most common form of cluster headache is episodic cluster. The rarest form is chronic cluster headache without remissions, with only about 10% of patients suffering from this variety of cluster. Cluster headache can begin at any age, but it generally begins in the late 20s. Cluster headache rarely begins in childhood, and only about 10% of patients develop cluster when they are in their 60s.[154,157]

Clinical Features and Associated Disorders

Patients with cluster headache have multiple episodes of short-lived but severe, unilateral, orbital, supraorbital, or temporal pain. At least one of the following associated symptoms must occur: conjunctival injection, lacrimation, nasal congestion, rhinorrhea, facial sweating, miosis, ptosis, or eyelid edema. Episodic cluster consists of headache periods of 1 week to 1 year, with remission periods lasting at least 14 days, whereas chronic cluster headache has either no remission periods or remissions that last less than 14 days.[154,157]

The pain of a cluster attack increases to excruciating levels rapidly (within 15 minutes). The attacks often occur at the same time each day and frequently awaken patients from sleep. If the condition is left untreated, the attacks usually last from 30 to 90 minutes, but they may last as long as 180 minutes. The pain is deep, constant, boring, piercing, or burning in nature, located in, behind, or around the eye. It may radiate to the forehead, temples, jaws, nostrils, ears, neck, or shoulder. During an attack, patients often feel agitated or restless and feel the

139. Pringsheim T, Howse D: Inpatient treatment of chronic daily headache using dihydroergotamine: A long-term followup study. Can J Neurol Sci 1998;25:146-150.
140. Monzon MJ, Lainez MJ: Quality of life in migraine and chronic daily headache patients. Cephalalgia 1998;18:638-643.
141. Suhr B, Evers S, Bauer B, et al: Drug-induced headache: Long-term results of stationary versus ambulatory withdrawal therapy. Cephalalgia 1999;19:44-49.
142. Selby G, Lance JW: Observation on 500 cases of migraine and allied vascular headaches. J Neurol Neurosurg Psychiatry 1960;23:23-32.
143. Lyngberg AC, Rasmussen BK, Jorgensen T, Jensen R: Prognosis of migraine and tension-type headache: A population-based follow-up study. Neurology 2005;65:580-585.
144. Silberstein SD: Transformed and chronic migraine. In Goadsby PJ, Silberstein SD, Dodick DW (eds): Chronic Daily Headache for Clinicians. Hamilton, Ontario, BC Decker, 2005, pp 21-56.
145. Bakshi R, Mechtler LL, Kamran S, et al: MRI findings in lumbar puncture headache syndrome: Abnormal dural-meningeal and dural venous sinus enhancement. Clin Imag 1999;23:73-76.
146. Pakiam AS, Lee C, Lang AE: Intracranial hypotension with parkinsonism, ataxia, and bulbar weakness. Arch Neurol 1999;56:869-872.
147. Mokri B, Piepgras DG, Miller GM: Syndrome of orthostatic headaches and diffuse pachymeningeal gadolinium enhancement. Mayo Clin Proc 1997;72:400-413.
148. Rabin BM, Roychowdhury S, Meyer JR, et al: Spontaneous intracranial hypotension: Spinal MR findings. Am J Neuroradiol 1998;19:1034-1039.
149. Silberstein SD: Chronic daily headache and tension-type headache. Neurology 1993;43:1644-1649.
150. Fromm GH, Graff-Radford SB, Terrence CF, Sweet WH: Pretrigeminal neuralgia. Neurology 1990;40:1493-1495.
151. Lipton RB, Stewart WF, Cady R, et al: Sumatriptan for the range of headaches in migraine sufferers: Results of the spectrum study. Headache 2000;40:783-791.
152. Goadsby PJ, Edvinsson L: Human in vivo evidence for trigeminovascular activation in cluster headache. Brain 1994;117:427-434.
153. May A, Bahra A, Buchel C, et al: Hypothalamic activation in cluster headache attacks. Lancet 1998;352:275-278.
154. Silberstein SD: Pharmacological management of cluster headache. CNS Drugs 1994;2:199-207.
155. Manzoni GC: Male preponderance of cluster headache is progressively decreasing over the years. Headache 1997;37:588-589.
156. Manzoni GC: Cluster headache and lifestyle: Remarks on a population of 374 male patients. Cephalalgia 1999;19:88-94.
157. Manzoni GC, Prusinski A: Cluster headache: Introduction. In Olesen J, Tfelt-Hansen P, Welch KMA (eds): The Headaches (2nd ed). Philadelphia, Lippincott Williams & Wilkins, 2000, pp 675-678.
158. Silberstein SD, Niknam R, Rozen TD, Young WB: Cluster headache with aura. Neurology 2000;54:219-221.
159. Jarrar RG, Black DF, Dodick DW, Davis DH: Outcome of trigeminal nerve section in the treatment of chronic cluster headache. Neurology 2003;60:1360-1362.
160. Ford RG, Ford KT, Swaid S, et al: Gamma knife treatment of refractory cluster headache. Headache 1998;38:1-9.
161. Leone M, Franzini A: Stereotactic stimulation of the posterior hypothalamic gray matter in a patient with intractable cluster headache. N Engl J Med 2001;345:1428-1429.
162. Russell D, Vincent M: Chronic paroxysmal hemicrania. In Olesen J, Tfelt-Hansen P, Welch KMA (eds): The Headaches (2nd ed). Philadelphia, Lippincott Williams & Wilkins, 2000, pp 741-750.

Appendix of Useful CPT and ICD-9 Codes, Evaluation and Management Coding Template, and Useful Internet Resources

Douglas G. Merrill and David R. Walega

APPENDIX

A

CPT Codes Routinely Used in the Practice of Pain Medicine

CPT is a trademark of the American Medical Association.

SOFT TISSUE AND JOINT INJECTIONS

20550	injection of single tendon sheath, ligament or aponeurosis
20551	injection of single tendon origin/insertion
20552	injection of single or multiple trigger points, one or two muscles
20553	injection of single or multiple trigger points, three or more muscles
20600	arthrocentesis, aspiration or injection, small joint or bursa (e.g., fingers, toes)
20605	arthrocentesis, aspiration or injection, intermediate joint or bursa (temporomandibular, acromioclavicular, wrist, elbow, ankle, olecranon bursa)
20610	arthrocentesis, aspiration or injection, major joint or bursa (shoulder, hip, knee, subacromial)
27096	injection procedure for sacroiliac joint, arthrography and/or anesthetic/steroid

PERIPHERAL NERVE INJECTIONS AND CATHETERS

64400	injection, anesthetic agent; trigeminal nerve, any division or branch
64402	facial nerve
64405	greater occipital nerve
64412	spinal accessory nerve
64413	cervical plexus
	brachial plexus, single injection
64415	brachial plexus, continuous infusion by catheter (including catheter placement)
64416	including daily management for anesthetic agent administration
64417	axillary nerve
64418	suprascapular nerve
64420	intercostal nerve, single
64421	intercostal nerves, multiple, regional block
64425	ilioinguinal, iliohypogastric nerves
64430	pudendal nerve
64445	sciatic nerve, single
64446	sciatic nerve, continuous infusion by catheter (including catheter placement) including daily management for anesthetic agent administration
64447	femoral nerve, single
64448	femoral nerve, continuous infusion by catheter (including catheter placement) including daily management for anesthetic agent administration
64449	lumbar plexus, posterior approach, continuous infusion by catheter (including catheter placement) including daily management for anesthetic agent administration
64450	other peripheral nerve or branch

SYMPATHETIC INJECTIONS

64505	injection, anesthetic agent; sphenopalatine ganglion
64508	carotid sinus
64510	stellate ganglion (cervical sympathetic)
64517	superior hypogastric plexus
64520	lumbar or thoracic (paravertebral sympathetic)
64530	celiac plexus, with or without radiologic monitoring

SPINE INJECTIONS

64470	injection, anesthetic agent and/or steroid, paravertebral facet joint or nerve; cervical or thoracic, single level
64472	cervical or thoracic, each additional level list separately
64475	lumbar or sacral, single level
64476	lumbar or sacral, each additional level list separately
64479	injection, anesthetic agent and/or steroid, transforaminal epidural; cervical or thoracic, single level
64480	cervical or thoracic, each additional level list separately
64483	lumbar or sacral, single level
64484	lumbar or sacral, each additional level list separately

62310   injection, single (not via indwelling catheter), not including neurolytic substances, with or without contrast (for either localization or epidurography) of either diagnostic or therapeutic substance(s) (including local anesthetic, antispasmodic, opioid, steroid, other solution)

62311   epidural or subarachnoid; cervical or thoracic

62268   percutaneous aspiration of spinal cord cyst or syrinx

62270   spinal puncture, lumbar, diagnostic

62272   spinal puncture, lumbar, therapeutic, for drainage of cerebrospinal fluid by needle or catheter

62273   injection, epidural, of blood or clot patch

64999   unlisted procedure, nervous system

VERTEBRAL BODY INJECTIONS

22520   percutaneous vertebroplasty, one vertebral body, unilateral or bilateral injection, thoracic

22521   percutaneous vertebroplasty, one vertebral body, unilateral or bilateral injection, lumbar

22522   each additional thoracic or lumbar vertebral body, list in addition to primary level

22523   percutaneous vertebral augmentation, including cavity creation (fracture reduction and bone biopsy included when performed) using mechanical device, one vertebral body, unilateral or bilateral cannulation (e.g., kyphoplasty)

22524   lumbar

22525   each additional thoracic or lumbar vertebral body level
         See additional radiology codes to be used in conjunction with above codes

20225   percutaneous bone biopsy, with trocar or needle; deep (i.e., vertebral body)

INTRADISKAL INJECTIONS

62287   aspiration or decompression procedure, percutaneous, of nucleus pulposus of intervertebral disk, any method, single or multiple levels, lumbar *for fluoroscopic guidance use 76003*

62290   injection procedure for discography, each level; lumbar, *for radiologic supervision and interpretation see 72285, 72295*

62291   cervical or thoracic, *for radiologic supervision and interpretation see 72285, 72295*

62292   injection procedure for chemonucleolysis, including discography, intervertebral disk, single or multiple levels, lumbar

22526   Percutaneous intradiskal electrothermal annuloplasty, uni or bilateral, including fluoroscopic guidance, single level

22527   One or more additional levels

NEUROPLASTY/NEUROLYSIS/DENERVATION

62263   percutaneous lysis of epidural adhesions using solution injection (hypertonic saline, enzyme) or mechanical means (catheter) including radiologic localization, multiple adhesiolysis sessions; 2 or more days, includes codes 76005 and 72275

62264   1 day

62280   injection/infusion of neurolytic substance (alcohol, phenol, iced saline solutions) with or without other therapeutic substance; subarachnoid

62281   epidural, cervical, or thoracic

62282   epidural, lumbar, sacral (caudal)

64600   destruction by neurolytic agent, trigeminal nerve; supraorbital, infraorbital, mental, or inferior alveolar branch

64605   second and third branches at foramen ovale

64610   second and third branches at foramen ovale with radiologic monitoring

64612   chemodenervation of muscle(s); muscle(s) innervated by facial nerve (for blepharospasm, hemifacial spasm)

64613   cervical spinal muscle(s) (for spasmodic torticollis)

64614   extremity(s) and/or trunk muscle(s) (for dystonia, cerebral palsy, multiple sclerosis)

64650   chemodenervation of eccrine glands; both axillae

64653   other area(s) (e.g., scalp, face, neck), per day

64999   other area(s) of extremities (e.g., hands, feet)

95873   electrical stimulation for guidance in conjunction with chemodenervation

95874   needle electromyography for guidance in conjunction with chemodenervation

64620   destruction by neurolytic agent, intercostal nerve (for fluoroscopic guidance and localization for needle placement, use 76005)

64622   destruction by neurolytic agent, paravertebral facet joint nerve; lumbar or sacral, single level

64623   lumbar or sacral, each additional level (for bilateral procedure, use modifier 50 with 64622 or 64623)

64626   cervical or thoracic, single level

64627   cervical or thoracic, each additional level *list separately* (for bilateral procedure, use modifier 50 with 64626 or 64627)

64630	destruction by neurolytic agent; pudendal nerve
64640	other peripheral nerve or branch
64680	destruction by neurolytic agent, with or without radiologic monitoring; celiac plexus
64681	superior hypogastric plexus
64999	unlisted procedure, nervous system

SPINAL CATHETERS AND PUMPS

62318	injection, including catheter placement, continuous infusion or intermittent bolus, not including neurolytic substances, with or without contrast (for either localization or epidurography), of diagnostic or therapeutic substance(s) including anesthetic, antispasmodic, opioid, steroid, other solution, epidural or subarachnoid; cervical or thoracic
62319	lumbar, sacral (caudal)
62350	implantation, revision or repositioning of tunneled intrathecal or epidural catheter, for long-term medication administration via an external pump or implantable reservoir/infusion pump; without laminectomy
62355	removal of previously implanted intrathecal or epidural catheter
62360	implantation or replacement of device for intrathecal or epidural drug infusion; subcutaneous reservoir
62361	non-reprogrammable pump
62362	programmable pump, including preparation of pump, with or without programming
62365	removal of subcutaneous reservoir or pump, previously implanted for intrathecal or epidural infusion
62367	electronic analysis of programmable, implanted pump for intrathecal or epidural drug infusion (includes evaluation of reservoir status, alarm status, drug prescription status; without reprogramming
62368	with reprogramming
95990	refilling and maintenance of implantable pump or reservoir for drug delivery, spinal (intrathecal epidural) or brain (intraventricular)
95991	administered by a physician

PERIPHERAL AND EPIDURAL NEUROSTIMULATORS

63650	percutaneous implantation of neurostimulator electrode array, epidural
63655	laminectomy for implantation of neurostimulator electrodes, plate/paddle, epidural

63660	revision or removal of spinal neurostimulator electrode percutaneous array(s) or plate/paddle(s)
63685	insertion or replacement of spinal neurostimulator pulse generator or receiver, direct or inductive coupling
63688	revision or removal of implanted spinal neurostimulator pulse generator or receiver
95970	electronic analysis of implanted neurostimulator pulse generator system (rate, pulse amplitude and duration, configuration of wave form, battery status, electrode selectability, output modulation, cycling, impedance, and patient compliance measurements); simplex or complex brain, spinal cord, or peripheral, without reprogramming
95971	simple spinal cord or peripheral neurostimulator with intraoperative or subsequent programming
95972	complex spinal cord or peripheral neurostimulator, first hour
95973	complex spinal cord or peripheral neurostimulator, additional 30 minutes after first hour
64550	application of surface (transcutaneous) neurostimulator
64555	percutaneous implantation of neurostimulator electrodes; peripheral nerve (excludes sacral nerve)
64560	autonomic nerve
64561	sacral nerve (transforaminal placement)
64565	neuromuscular
64573	incision for implantation of neurostimulator electrodes; peripheral nerve (excludes sacral nerve)
64577	autonomic nerve
64580	neuromuscular
64581	sacral nerve (transforaminal placement)
64585	revision or removal of peripheral neurostimulator electrodes
64590	insertion or replacement of peripheral neurostimulator pulse generator or receiver, direct or inductive coupling
64595	revision or removal of peripheral neurostimulator pulse generator or receiver

MISCELLANEOUS

22010	incision and drainage, open, of deep abscess (subfascial) posterior spine; cervical, thoracic, or cervicothoracic
22015	lumbar, sacral, or lumbosacral

CONSCIOUS SEDATION

99143	moderate sedation services, provided by the same physician performing the diagnostic or therapeutic service that the sedation supports, requiring independent trained observer to assist in the

monitoring of the patient's level of consciousness and physiologic status; under 5 years of age, first 30 minutes intraservice time

99144   age 5 years or older, first 30 minutes

99145   each additional 15-minute interval

99148   moderate sedation services, provided by a physician other than the physician performing the diagnostic or therapeutic service that the sedation supports, requiring independent trained observer to assist in the monitoring of the patient's level of consciousness and physiologic status; under 5 years of age, first 30 minutes intraservice time

99149   age 5 years or older, first 30 minutes

99150   each additional 15 minute interval

RADIOLOGY CODES

76496   unlisted fluoroscopic procedure (diagnostic or interventional)

76499   unlisted diagnostic radiographic procedure

76000   fluoroscopy (separate procedure) up to one hour physician time

76003   fluoroscopic guidance for needle placement

76005   fluoroscopic guidance and localization of needle or catheter tip for spine or paraspinous diagnostic or therapeutic injection procedures (epidural, transforaminal epidural, subarachnoid, paravertebral facet joint, paravertebral facet joint nerve or sacroiliac joint), including neurolytic agent destruction

Injection of contrast during fluoroscopic guidance and localization is an inclusive component of codes 62263, 62264, 62270-62273, 62280-62282, 62310-62319

For percutaneous or endoscopic lysis of epidural adhesions, codes 62263, 62264 include fluoroscopic guidance and localization

76012   radiologic supervision and interpretation, percutaneous vertebroplasty or kyphoplasty, per vertebral body; under fluoroscopic guidance

76013   under CT guidance

73542   radiologic examination, sacroiliac joint arthrography, radiologic supervision and interpretation

Used in conjunction with 27096. If formal arthrography is not performed, recorded, and a formal radiologic report is not issued, use 76005 for fluoroscopic guidance for sacroiliac joint injections.

72275   epidurography, radiologic supervision and interpretation

Use code only when an epidurogram is performed, images documented, and a formal radiologic report is issued.

72285   discography, cervical or thoracic, radiologic supervision and interpretation

72295   discography, lumbar, radiologic supervision and interpretation

COMMON MODIFIERS

25   significant, separately identifiable E/M service by the same physician on the same day of a coded procedure or other service

50   bilateral procedure

51   multiple procedures

53   discontinued or aborted procedure

59   distinct procedural service, independent from other services performed on the same day

62   two surgeons performing procedure

each surgeon performs dictation, both working as primary surgeons during procedure

78   return to the operating room for a related procedure during the postoperative period

80   assistant surgeon

99   multiple modifiers

COMMENTS

There are newer procedures in pain medicine that have not been assigned a CPT code and are coded as an unlisted procedure or service. For example, 64999, unlisted procedure, nervous system, is used commonly for pulsed radiofrequency procedures. Under these circumstances, a detailed description of the procedure or service should be provided.

A special report should accompany any procedure or service that is rarely performed or is variable, new, or unusual. The information in such reports is often used to determine the appropriateness of the procedure or service. This report should include the specifics of the problem being treated, previous pertinent diagnostic findings, the equipment used for the procedure, the details of the procedure, and follow-up care.

As a general rule, the results of epidurography, discography, sacroiliac joint arthrography, and diagnostic fluoroscopy should be recorded in a separate report or dictation in the medical record.

The -59 modifier should be used when a "separate procedure" is performed. A "separate procedure" is independent of, unrelated to, or distinct from other procedures or services performed at the same visit. This may represent a different organ, tissue, or area of the body being treated, or a separate injection/aspiration site from others performed on the same visit. For example, if a patient underwent a left L5 transforaminal injection with fluoroscopic guidance for lumbar radiculitis and a right occipital nerve block for occipital neuralgia, one would code 64483, 76005, and 64405-59. The occipital nerve block is a "separate procedure," distinct from the lumbar spine injection, and performed for a separate and distinctly different diagnosis.

When multiple procedures are performed on the same day, the -51 modifier is used. The most important CPT should be listed first; the remaining additional CPT codes should be added with the -51 modifier.

The -25 modifier is added to an E/M code when this service is performed on the same day as a separately identifiable procedure or other service. The diagnosis for the E/M code should be separate and distinct from the diagnosis for which the procedure is being performed. For example, a patient undergoes a planned L4-5 facet joint injection with fluoroscopic guidance, but at the time presentation for the facet injection reports a new complaint of left arm numbness, tingling, and weakness consistent with C6 radiculopathy, for which a separate evaluation, physical exam, and medical decision-making process is performed by the physician. One would code 64475, 76005 for the facet injection performed, and a -25 modifier would be added to the E/M code selected based on the evaluation of the cervical radiculopathy (see E/M coding guidelines).

Reference

Current Procedural Terminology, Chicago, AMA Press, 2007.

APPENDIX

B ICD-9 Codes Routinely Used in the Practice of Pain Medicine

ICD-9 DESCRIPTOR

53.10	Herpes zoster with unspecified nervous system complication
53.12	Post-herpetic trigeminal neuralgia
53.13	Post-herpetic polyneuropathy
53.19	Post-herpetic neuropathy (other)
53.20	Post-herpetic neuropathy with ophthalmic complications
53.90	Herpes zoster without mention of complication (NOS)
141.00	Malignant neoplasm tongue
150.00	Malignant neoplasm esophagus
153.00	Malignant neoplasm colon
154.00	Malignant neoplasm rectum
157.00	Malignant neoplasm pancreas
174.00	Malignant neoplasm female breast
188.00	Malignant neoplasm bladder
199.00	Malignant neoplasm, disseminated, without specification of site
250.60	Diabetes mellitus with neurologic manifestations
296.30	Major depressive disorder, recurrent
300.02	Generalized anxiety disorder
300.40	Depression with anxiety (dysthymic disorder)
300.82	Somatoform disorder—undifferentiated
307.80	Pain disorders with psychological factors/ psychogenic pain
307.81	Tension headache
334.90	Spinocerebellar disease, unspecified
335.24	Primary lateral sclerosis, motor neuron disease
337.20	Reflex sympathetic dystrophy, CRPS unspecified locale
337.21	Reflex sympathetic dystrophy/CRPS upper limb
337.22	Reflex sympathetic dystrophy/CRPS lower limb
337.29	Reflex sympathetic dystrophy/CRPS other location
337.9	Unspecified disorder autonomic system
340.00	Multiple sclerosis
343.9	Cerebral palsy, infantile, unspecified
344.00	Quadriplegia unspecified
346.00	Classic migraine
346.10	Common migraine
346.20	Variant of migraine (cluster, etc.)
346.90	Migraine unspecified
348.0	Cerebral cysts
349.0	Headache post lumbar puncture
349.2	Disorder meninges, not otherwise specified
350.10	Trigeminal neuralgia
350.2	Atypical facial pain
351.8	Facial nerve disorders, other
353.00	Brachial plexus lesion
353.2	Cervical root lesions NOS
353.30	Thoracic root lesions NOS
353.40	Lumbosacral root lesions NOS
353.60	Phantom limb syndrome
354.00	Mononeuritis upper limb
354.40	Causalgia upper limb
355.0	Sciatica or pyriformis syndrome
355.1	Meralgia paresthetica (lateral femoral cutaneous nerve compression)
355.71	Causalgia lower limb
355.80	Mononeuritis lower limb unspecified
355.9	Mononeuritis or causalgia NOS
356.90	Peripheral polyneuropathy unspecified
357.50	Alcoholic polyneuropathy
356.4	Idiopathic progressive polyneuropathy
438.90	Unspecified late effects of cerebrovascular disease
443.00	Raynaud's disease
443.10	Thromboangiitis obliterans (Buerger's disease)
577.1	Chronic pancreatitis
595.10	Chronic interstitial cystitis
595.2	Chronic cystitis NOS
617.9	Endometriosis, site unspecified
625.30	Dysmenorrhea
625.9	Unspecified symptoms associated with female genital organs
705.21	Hyperhidrosis, primary focal
714.00	Rheumatoid arthritis
714.90	Inflammatory polyarthropathy, unspecified
715.00	Osteoarthrosis, generalized
715.10	Osteoarthrosis, localized
715.80	Osteoarthrosis, multiple sites but not generalized
715.90	Osteoarthrosis, unspecified localized vs. generalized
719.40	Pain in joint NOS
720.00	Ankylosing spondylitis
720.2	Sacroiliitis
721.0	Cervical spondylosis without myelopathy

721.10	Cervical spondylosis with myelopathy
721.20	Thoracic spondylosis without myelopathy
721.3	Lumbosacral spondylosis without myelopathy
721.41	Thoracic spondylosis with myelopathy
721.42	Lumbar spondylosis with myelopathy
721.60	Ankylosing vertebral hyperostosis
722.0	Cervical disk displacement without myelopathy
722.10	Lumbar disk displacement without myelopathy
722.11	Thoracic disk displacement without myelopathy
722.4	Degeneration of cervical intervertebral disk
722.51	Degeneration of thoracic intervertebral disk
722.52	Degeneration of lumbar intervertebral disk
722.71	Cervical disk disorder with myelopathy
722.72	Thoracic disk disorder with myelopathy
722.23	Lumbar disk disorder with myelopathy
722.80	Postlaminectomy syndrome unspecified area
722.81	Postlaminectomy cervical
722.82	Postlaminectomy thoracic
722.83	Postlaminectomy lumbar
722.90	Diskitis
723.0	Spinal stenosis, cervical
723.1	Neck pain
723.4	Cervical radiculitis or brachial neuritis
723.8	Occipital neuralgia
724.01	Spinal stenosis, thoracic
724.02	Spinal stenosis, lumbar
724.1	Thoracic pain

724.2	Low back pain
724.30	Sciatica
724.4	Lumbar or thoracic radiculitis
724.5	Backache unspecified
724.60	Sacral disorders (ankylosing, instability) including SI joint
724.79	Coccygodynia
725.00	Polymyalgia rheumatica
728.85	Muscle spasm
729.0	Rheumatism (pain and stiffness of muscle, tendon, nerve, joint)
729.1	Fibromyalgia, myalgia, myositis
729.2	Neuralgia unspec
729.5	Limb pain
733.13	Vertebral pathologic/spontaneous/compression fracture
756.11	Lumbar spondylosis
756.12	Lumbar spondylolisthesis
781.0	Abnormal involuntary movements
784.0	Headache
786.50	Chest pain
789.00	Abdominal pain unspecified
789.01	Abdominal pain right upper quadrant
789.02	Abdominal pain left upper quadrant
789.03	Abdominal pain right lower quadrant
789.04	Abdominal pain left lower quadrant
789.05	Abdominal pain periumbilical
789.06	Abdominal pain epigastric
789.07	Abdominal pain generalized
789.09	Abdominal pain multiple sites
799.30	Debility, unspecified
799.40	Cachexia—wasting (exclude nutritional marasmus 261)

C Evaluation and Management Template

This template has served as a useful tool in considering which E and M code to use in the setting of pain medicine practice. Its terminology derives from CPT. The authors and the publisher make no warranty as to the value of this template to any practitioner. Use of this template is *not* a guarantee of correct coding compliance and all practitioners should maintain regular consultations with qualified coding experts to be sure that their coding methods are in compliance.

DEFINITIONS

There are three components required in the chart to support any coding that is chosen: history, examination, and decision making. CPT specifically defines these terms and the reader is directed to the manual for that information.* A short version is as follows:

A. History

1. *Problem-focused:* a chief complaint and a "brief" history of the present illness (HPI)
2. *Expanded problem-focused:* adds a pertinent review of systems (ROS)
3. *Detailed:* adds an extended HPI and ROS, as well as a pertinent past, family, and social history directly related to the current problem
4. *Comprehensive:* adds a full review of all body systems and a complete past, family, and social history

B. Examination

1. *Problem-focused:* a "limited" examination only of the affected organ system or body area
2. *Expanded problem-focused:* adds a "limited" examination of any other symptomatic or related organ systems
3. *Detailed:* the same as expanded problem-focused but the examination becomes "extended"
4. *Comprehensive:* either a general multisystem examination or a complete examination of a single organ system.

* American Medical Association. Evaluation and management (E/M) service guidelines. In *CPT 2006 Current Procedure Terminology Professional Edition.* Chicago, AMA, pp 1-34.

CPT defines "body areas" and "organ systems" very specifically and the reader is directed to the CPT text to review these.

C. Decision Making

1. *Straightforward:* minimal or no diagnoses or management options, complexity or amount of data for review, or risk of complications and/or morbidity and mortality
2. *Low:* limited rather than minimal diagnoses or management options, low complexity or amount of data for review, and low risks
3. *Moderate:* moderate diagnoses or management options, moderate complexity or amount of data for review, and moderate risks
4. *High:* extensive diagnoses or management options, high complexity or amount of data for review, and high risk

D. Time

Strictly speaking, time is not an element of determination of level of complexity, but on occasion there will be an inordinately long time spent in counseling the patient or family, so-called face-to-face time. In this case, such time spent may outweigh the complexity of the other three elements.

In general, CPT recognizes only face-to-face time in determining if time should be a primary determinant of outpatient complexity level. It is not accurate to include time spent before or after the patient encounter, because that is time that was factored into the original work assigned to the CPT code. Fifty percent of face-to-face time must have been spent counseling and/or coordinating care for time to play a role in determining the code.

For inpatient work, "time on the floor" may also be included, to the extent that this time was spent in the care of or arranging services for the patient.

E. A Note About Number of Components Necessary

For office-established patients, subsequent hospital care, and other subsequent or established patient care, only two of the three key components are necessary. All other codes require all three of the three key components and must meet or exceed the stated requirements.*

TEMPLATE FOR DETERMINING SELECTED E AND M CODING CHOICES

3 "Key components" plus time* ▶

ELEMENTS ▶ CHOICE OF CODE ▶	I. History: Chief Complaint	HPI	Expanded	ROS	II. Exam: Body Areas	Organs	III. Medical Decision Making: Complexity**	Time if applicable* (in minutes)
I. New outpatient visit (all 3—history, exam, decision making—required) ▶								
99201	Yes	Problem focused	Problem focused	Problem focused	Problem focused	Problem focused	Straightforward	10
99202	Yes	Expanded problem focused	Expanded problem focused	Expanded problem focused	Expanded problem focused	Expanded problem focused	Straightforward	20
99203	Yes	Detailed	Detailed	Detailed	Detailed	Detailed	Low	30
99204	Yes	Comprehensive	Comprehensive	Comprehensive	Comprehensive	Comprehensive	Moderate	45
99205	Yes	Comprehensive	Comprehensive	Comprehensive	Comprehensive	Comprehensive	High	60
II. Established outpatient visit (2 of 3 required) ▶								
99211	N/A	N/A	N/A	N/A	N/A	N/A	N/A	5
99212	Yes	Problem focused	Problem focused	Problem focused	Problem focused	Problem focused	Straight-forward	10
99213	Yes	Expanded	Expanded	Expanded	Expanded	Expanded	Low	15
99214	Yes	Detailed	Detailed	Detailed	Detailed	Detailed	Moderate	25
99215	Yes	Comprehensive	Comprehensive	Comprehensive	Comprehensive	Comprehensive	High	40
III. Consultation Outpatient ▶								
99241	Yes	Problem focused	Problem focused	Problem focused	Problem focused	Problem focused	Straightforward	15
99242	Yes	Expanded problem focused	Expanded problem focused	Expanded problem focused	Expanded problem focused	Expanded problem focused	Straightforward	30
99243	Yes	Detailed	Detailed	Detailed	Detailed	Detailed	Low	40
99244	Yes	Comprehensive	Comprehensive	Comprehensive	Comprehensive	Comprehensive	Moderate	60
99245	Yes	Comprehensive	Comprehensive	Comprehensive	Comprehensive	Comprehensive	High	80
IV. Consultation Inpatient ▶								
99251	Yes	Problem focused	Problem focused	Problem focused	Problem focused	Problem focused	Straightforward	20
99252	Yes	Expanded problem focused	Expanded problem focused	Expanded problem focused	Expanded problem focused	Expanded problem focused	Straightforward	40
99253	Yes	Detailed	Detailed	Detailed	Detailed	Detailed	Low	55
99254	Yes	Comprehensive	Comprehensive	Comprehensive	Comprehensive	Comprehensive	Moderate	80
99252	Yes	Comprehensive	Comprehensive	Comprehensive	Comprehensive	Comprehensive	High	110

NOTES:
*See CPT re: time import
*See CPT for definitions

APPENDIX

D   Useful Internet Sites (Links as of May 2006)

A. JOURNALS

The *Journal of Regional Anesthesia and Pain Medicine* is at www.rapm.org

The *Journal of Pain* is at www.jpain.org

Pain may be read online at www.sciencedirect.com/pain

Spine is at www.spinejournal.com

Anesthesiology is at www.anesthesiology.org

The *International Journal of Acute Pain Management* is at http://www.elsevier.com/wps/product/cws_home/622996

The *Journal of Pain and Symptom Management* is at http://www.elsevier.com/wps/product/cws_home/505775

The *European Journal of Pain* is at http://www.elsevier.com/wps/pr oduct/cws_home/623037

The *Year Book of Anesthesiology and Pain Management* is at http://www.elsevier.com/wps/product/cws_home/623204

Seminars in Pain Medicine is at http://www.elsevier.com/wps/product/cws_home/623186

The Spine Journal is at www.spine.org/tsj.cfm

B. PROFESSIONAL SOCIETIES

The American Society of Anesthesiologists (including access to the Relative Value Guide) is at www.asahq.org

The American Society of Regional Anesthesia and Pain Medicine is at www.asra.com

The International Association for the Study of Pain is at www.iasp-pain.org

The American Medical Society (with CPT resources) is at www.ama-assn.org

The American Pain Society is at www.ampainsoc.org

The American Academy of Pain Medicine is at http://www.painmed.org/

The International Spine Intervention Society is at www.spinalinjection.com

The North American Spine Society is at www.spine.org

The American Society of Interventional Pain Physicians is at http://www.asipp.org/

C. BILLING AND CODING INFORMATION

The *Pain Management Coding and Billing Answer Book* may be ordered at www.decisionhealth.com

The Anesthesia and Pain Management Coding Alert may be ordered at www.codinginstitute.com

D. CMS

A variety of CMS websites are of interest, such as

For monitoring Carrier Medical Decisions:
http://www.cms.hhs.gov/mcd/search.asp

For reference regarding correct coding of evaluation and management services:
http://www.cms.hhs.gov/MLNProducts/downloads/eval_mgmt_serv_guide.pdf

For reference regarding ICD-9 correct coding:
http://www.cms.hhs.gov/ICD9ProviderDiagnosticCodes/

For reference regarding edits for coding:
http://www.cms.hhs.gov/physicians/cciedits/default.asp

For reference specifically for anesthesiologists and pain physicians:
http://www.cms.hhs.gov/center/anesth.asp

Index

Note: Page numbers followed by the letter f refer to figures; those followed by the letter t refer to tables. The letter b refers to boxed material.

A

AAHPM (American Academy of Hospice and Palliative Medicine), 10
AAOP (American Academy of Orofacial Pain), 10
AAPM (American Academy of Pain Medicine), 8-9
AAPManage (American Academy of Pain Management), 10
Abdominal aortic dissection, after celiac plexus block, 919
Abdominal pain
  during pregnancy, 573-574, 574f
  recurrent, in children, 354
Abducens nerve (VI), examination of, 178
A-beta fibers
  activation of, 135-136
  first-order synapse of, 138
  sprouting of, 147
Ablative therapy
  in intractable pain management, 402t, 405
  in visceral pain management, 532
  efficacy of, 534
ABPM (American Board of Pain Medicine), 9
Abscess, epidural
  after epidural steroid injections, 999, 999f
  after spinal cord stimulation, 981
  catheter-related, 1229-1230
Abuse, substance. See also Addictive disorders.
  criteria for, 796
  prevalence of, 794
Accessory nerve (XI), examination of, 179
Accreditation
  of medical practice, for improved patient safety, 100
  of pain practice, 91
Accreditation Council for Graduate Medical Education (ACGME)
  pain medicine curriculum recommended by, 112b-113b
  programs recognized by, 112
Accredited fellowship training, in pain medicine, 111-112
Acetaminophen, 618-620
  clinical use of, 620
  delivery and side effects of, 300t
  dosing considerations for, 619, 619b
  for burn pain, 322
  for headache, 494t
  for lumbar spine stenosis, 374
  for mild-to-moderate head pain, 318
  for opioid-tolerant patients, 325
  for pain management
    at end of life, 1166

Acetaminophen (Continued)
  during pregnancy, 568, 569t
  in children, 544, 544t
  in elderly, 323t, 324
  in emergency department, 1145
  for postoperative pain, 302
  mechanism of action of, 618-619
  metabolism of, 619, 619f
  properties and dosages of, 676
  risks and precautions associated with, 619-620, 620t
Acetic acid derivatives, 676-678. See also specific agent.
N-Acetyl-aspartate, decreased levels of
  in chronic pain, 168
  in disease states, 167-168
Acetylsalicylic acid, neuraxial delivery of, 700t, 708
Action potential
  generation of, 812-813, 812f
  of neuronal cells, electrophysiologic basis of, 812-813, 812f, 814f-815f, 815-817, 816t
  propagation of, 815
  refractory period of, 817
Acupuncture, 785-789
  clinical use of, 786-789
  for carpal tunnel syndrome, 788
  for headache, 788
  for herniated lumbar disk, 371
  for low back pain, 787-788
  for myofascial pain syndrome, 788
  for nausea and vomiting, 787
  for neck pain, 788
  for neuropathic pain, 788-789
  for postoperative pain, 787
  for temporomandibular joint dysfunction, 788
  in palliative care setting, 1163t, 1164
  referral for, 789
  research into, 785-786
  side effects of, 786
Acupuncture points, 789
Acute pain
  burn injury–related, analgesia for, 321-323, 321t
    non-opioid, 321t, 322
    opioid, 321t, 322
    peripheral regional, 321t, 322
  in cancer patient. See also Cancer pain.
    classification of, 415
  in children, 541-548. See also Children, acute pain in.
  in elderly, 557. See also Elderly, pain in.
  management of
    in older adults, 323-324, 323t

Acute pain (Continued)
  in opioid-tolerant patients, 324-325
  inpatient. See Inpatient pain management service(s).
  perception of, role of cerebral cortex in, 162
  postoperative, 299-315
    outcome of, 1222
    pathophysiology of, 1219-1222, 1220f-1223f
    treatment option(s) for
      acupuncture as, 787
      complications of, 1228-1230
        analgesia-related, 1228-1229
        catheter-related, 1229-1230
      continuous epidural analgesia as, 304-305, 304t, 1223-1224
      continuous subcutaneous local anesthetic infusions as, 305-306
      economic outcomes of, 1227-1228
      extended-release morphine as, 304, 304t
      intra-articular analgesia as, 314-315
      lower extremity nerve blocks as, 309-313, 310t, 312t
      morbidity associated with
        cardiac, 1224-1225
        gastrointestinal, 1226-1227
        pulmonary, 1225-1226
        thromboembolic, 1226
      mortality associated with, 1224
      obesity and, 325
      obstructive sleep apnea and, 325
      patient-oriented outcomes of, 1227
      peripheral analgesia as, 305
      single-dose neuraxial spinal opioids as, 303-304, 304t
      single-injection peripheral nerve blocks as, analgesic additives for, 313-314
      systemic non-opioid analgesics as, 300t, 302-303, 1223, 1224f
      systemic opioid analgesics as, 299-302, 300t, 1222-1223
      upper extremity nerve blocks as, 306-309, 307t
  traumatic injury–related, 315-321, 316t
    analgesia for
      evaluation of need for, 316-317
      in alcohol-intoxicated patient, 318
      in blunt chest trauma patient, 319-321, 319t
      in head injury patient, 318-319
      neuraxial techniques of, 317-318
      peripheral regional, 318
    inpatient hospitalization for, 317
    systemic opioids for, 317